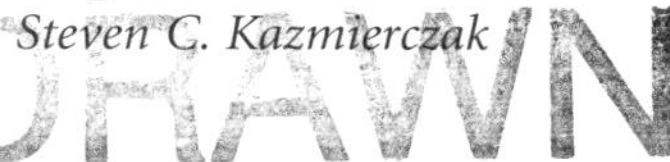

CLINICAL Chemistry

Theory
Analysis
Correlation

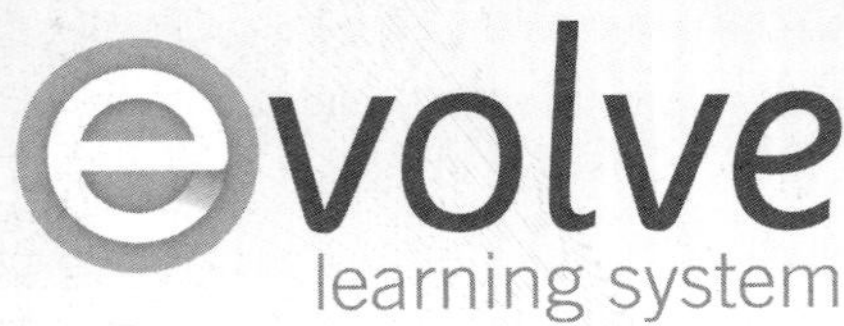

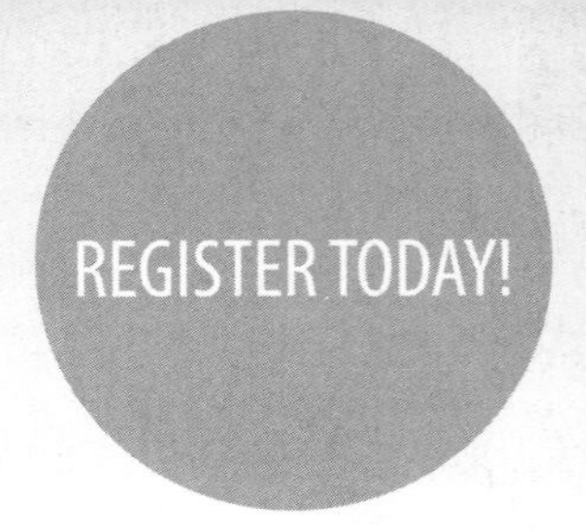

To access your Student Resources, visit:

http://evolve.elsevier.com/Kaplan/chemistry

Evolve Student Resources for Kaplan: Clinical Chemistry: Theory, Analysis, Correlation offers the following features

- **Methods of Analysis**
  A set of 144 Methods of Analysis describe current methodology in great detail.

- **Weblinks**
  Links to places of interest on the web specifically for clinical chemistry students.

- **Additional Resources**
  More content that complements the book's information

- **References**
  Linked electronically to the PubMed database of articles and abstracts

- **Content Updates**
  Find out the latest information on relevant issues in the field of clinical chemistry.

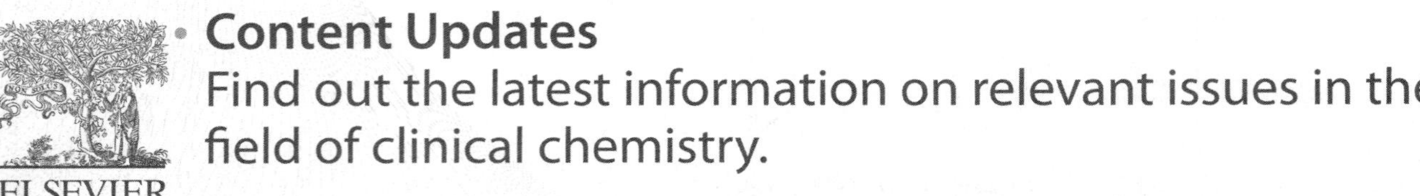

FIFTH EDITION

Theory
Analysis
Correlation

CLINICAL Chemistry

Lawrence A. Kaplan, PhD, DABCC
New York, New York

Amadeo J. Pesce, PhD, DABCC
Professor Emeritus
Department of Pathology and Laboratory Medicine
College of Medicine
University of Cincinnati
Cincinnati, Ohio;
Adjunct Professor
Department of Pathology and Laboratory Medicine
School of Medicine
University of California, San Diego,
Laboratory Director
Millenium Laboratories of California
San Diego, California

Methods of Analysis
Methods Section Editor
Peter E. Hickman, MB BS, PhD, FRCPA
Associate Professor
Australian National University Medical School;
Director of Chemical Pathology
The Canberra Hospital
Australian Capital Territory, Australia

Methods Associate Section Editor
Gus Koerbin, BAppSci, AFAIM
Principal Scientist ACT Pathology
Adjunct Professional Associate
University of Canberra
ACT Pathology
The Canberra Hospital,
Garran, Australian Capital Territory, Australia

Consulting Editor
Karol S. Sublett, BS, MT(ASCP)
Clinical Instructor, Chemistry
Clarian Health Partners
Clinical Laboratory Science Program
Medical Technologist, Laboratory (Generalist)
MidAmerica Clinical Labs
Indianapolis, Indiana

With 509 illustrations and 25 color plates

MOSBY

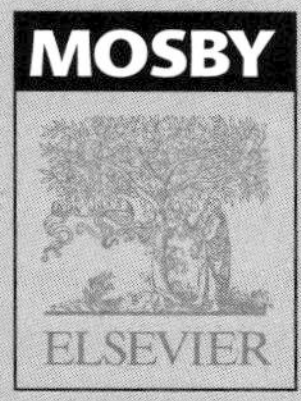

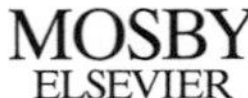

MOSBY
ELSEVIER

11830 Westline Industrial Drive
St. Louis, Missouri 63146

Clinical Chemistry: Theory, Analysis, Correlation ISBN: 978-0-323-03658-0

Library of Congress Cataloging-in-Publication Data

Clinical chemistry : theory, analysis, correlation / [edited by] Lawrence A. Kaplan, Amadeo J. Pesce.—5th ed.
p. ; cm.
Includes bibliographical references and index.
ISBN 978-0-323-03658-0 (hardcover : alk. paper) 1. Clinical chemistry. I. Kaplan, Lawrence A., 1944- II. Pesce, Amadeo J.
[DNLM: 1. Chemistry, Clinical. QY 90 C6415 2010]
RB40.C58 2010
616.07′56—dc22

2009009252

Publishing Director: Andrew Allen
Managing Editor: Ellen Wurm-Cutter
Publishing Services Manager: Catherine Jackson
Senior Project Manager: Rachel E. McMullen
Designer: Margaret Reid

Printed in the United States of America

Last digit is the print number: 9 8 7 6 5

To all those who worked with the editors over the past decades who are also in the process of moving on:

"Retirement requires the invention of a new hedonism, not a return to the hedonism of youth."
Mason Cooley (b. 1927), U.S. aphorist

To all those who will hopefully transfer this textbook safely to the next generation:

"Each age, it is found, must write its own books; or rather, each generation for the next succeeding."
Ralph Waldo Emerson (1803-1882)

" . . . *the way of man's contribution to ultimate fulfillment, is whenever one generation encounters the next, whenever the generation which has reached its full development transmits the teachings to the generation which is still in the process of developing, so that the teachings spontaneously waken to new life in the new generation.*"
Martin Buber, from *The Writings of Martin Buber*

We dedicate this textbook to the next generation of clinical chemists
and, with love, to our personal next generation—our grandchildren:

Clarice and Sonia Pesce
Shmuel and Tzippora Kaplan

Reviewers

Jeffrey M. Barksdale, PhD, MT(ASCP)
Director, Clinical Laboratory Science
Auburn University Montgomery
Montgomery, Alabama

Carol E. Becker, BS, MS, MT(ASCP), CLS(NCA)
Program Director
School of Clinical Laboratory Science/School of Histotechnology
OSF Saint Francis Medical Center
Peoria, Illinois

Donna Bedard, EdD, MT(ASCP)DLM
Professor and Chair
Clinical Laboratory Science Department
Winston-Salem State University
Winston-Salem, North Carolina

Karen S. Chandler, MA MT(ASCP), CLS(NCA)
Assistant Dean and CLS Program Coordinator
College of Health Sciences and Human Services
University of Texas-Pan American
Edinburg, Texas

Diane Davis, PhD, MT, SC, SLS(ASCP), CLS(NCA)
Associate Professor and Clinical Coordinator
Health Sciences Department
Salisbury University
Salisbury, Maryland

Karen Escolas, EdD, MT(ASCP)
Associate Professor
Department of Medical Laboratory Technology
Farmingdale State University of New York
Farmingdale, New York

Stephen M. Johnson, MS, MT(ASCP)
Program Director
School of Medical Technology
Erie, Pennsylvania

Linda M. Kasper, EdD
Retired Associate Professor
Department of Pathology and Laboratory Medicine
Indiana University School of Medicine
Indianapolis, Indiana

Richard Tulley, BS, MA, PhD, ABCC
Professor, BEST Coordinator
School of Human Ecology
Louisiana State University Agricultural Center
Baton Rouge, Louisiana

Contributors

Nancy W. Alcock, PhD, DABCC, FACB
(Contributor to a previous edition)

Rita R. Alloway, PharmD, BCPS, FCCP
Research Professor of Medicine
Director, Transplant Clinical Research
Director, Transplant Specialty Residency and Fellowship
University of Cincinnati
College of Medicine
Cincinnati, Ohio

Victor W. Armstrong, PhD
Professor
Department of Clinical Chemistry
George-August University
Goettingen, Germany

Hassan M. E. Azzazy, PhD, DABCC, FACB
Professor and Chairman
Department of Chemistry
The American University in Cairo
Cairo, Egypt

Kenneth E. Blick, PhD, ACS, DABCC, FACB
Professor
Department of Pathology
College of Medicine
University of Oklahoma Health Sciences Center
Oklahoma City, Oklahoma

John M. Brewer, PhD
Professor of Biochemistry and Molecular Biology
University of Georgia
Athens, Georgia

John R. Burnett, MB ChB, MD, PhD, FRCPA, FAHA
Head of Department
Department of Core Clinical Pathology & Biochemistry
PathWest Laboratory Medicine WA
Royal Perth Hospital
Perth, Western Australia, Australia;
Clinical Professor
School of Medicine & Pharmacology
University of Western Australia
Crawley, Western Australia, Australia

T. Andrew Burrow, MD
Clinical Fellow, Medical Biochemical Genetics
Department of Pediatrics
University of Cincinnati College of Medicine
Division of Human Genetics
Cincinnati Children's Hospital Medical Center
Cincinnati, Ohio

Elizabeth Ann Byrne, MS, CLS
(Contributor to a previous edition)

Demetra D. Callas, PhD, MBA
Director, Laboratory Administration
Northwest Community Hospital
Arlington Heights, Illinois

R. Neill Carey, PhD, FACB
Clinical Chemist
Peninsula Regional Medical Center
Salisbury, Maryland

John F. Chapman, Jr., DrPH, DABCC, NRCC, FACB
Professor
Department of Pathology and Laboratory Medicine
School of Medicine
University of North Carolina at Chapel Hill,
Director, Point-of-Care Testing
Associate Director, Core and Clinical Chemistry Laboratories
W.W. McLendon Clinical Laboratories
UNC Hospitals
Chapel Hill, North Carolina

Dan Chen, PhD, DABCC
Assistant Professor
Department of Pathology
New York University School of Medicine,
Associate Director
Clinical Chemistry Laboratory
Bellevue Hospital
New York, New York

David Chou, MD
Professor
Director, Laboratory Computer Services
Department of Laboratory Medicine
University of Washington Medical Center,
Chief Technology Officer
Information Technology Services
University of Washington Medicine
Seattle, Washington

Robert H. Christenson, PhD, DABCC, FACB
Professor of Pathology
Professor of Medical and Research Technology
University of Maryland School of Medicine,
Director, Core Laboratories
University of Maryland Medical Center
Baltimore, Maryland

Gregory A. Clines, MD, PhD
Assistant Professor of Medicine
Division of Endocrinology and Metabolism
School of Medicine
University of Virginia
Charlottesville, Virginia

Niel T. Constantine, PhD
Professor of Pathology
Director, Clinical Immunology
University of Maryland School of Medicine
Institute of Human Virology
Baltimore, Maryland

Lawrence Crolla, PhD, DABCC
Adjunct Assistant Professor
Department of Pathology
Stritch School of Medicine
Loyola University
Maywood, Illinois;
Consulting Clinical Chemist
Departments of Pathology and Respiratory Care
Alexian Brothers Medical Center
Elk Grove Village, Illinois;
Northwest Community Hospital
Arlington Heights, Illinois
West Suburban Hospital
Oak Park, Illinois;
Consulting Clinical Chemist
Department of Pathology
Ingalls Memorial Hospital
Harvey, Illinois

Laurence M. Demers, PhD, FACB, DABCC
Distinguished Professor of Pathology and Medicine
Director; Core Endocrine Laboratory and GCRC Core Laboratory
The Pennsylvania State University College of Medicine
The Milton S. Hershey Medical Center
Department of Pathology
Division of Clinical Pathology
Hershey, Pennsylvania

Richard F. Dods, PhD, DABCC, FACB
Illinois Mathematics and Science Academy
Aurora, Illinois

D. Robert Dufour, MD
Emeritus Professor of Pathology
George Washington University Medical Center,
Consultant Pathologist
Veterans Affairs Medical Center
Washington, DC

Barry N. Elkins, PhD
Chief of Chemistry
St. Vincent's Catholic Medical Center
New York, New York

Benjamin Eloff, PhD
U.S. Food and Drug Administration (FDA)
Rockville, Maryland

Jason J. Everly, PharmD, BCOP
Research Assistant Professor
University of Cincinnati
College of Medicine
Department of Surgery, Division of Transplantation
Cincinnati, Ohio

Matthew J. Everly, PharmD
University of Cincinnati
Cincinnati, Ohio

Carolyn S. Feldkamp, PhD, DABCC
Division Head, Clinical Chemistry
Department of Pathology
Henry Ford Hospital
Detroit, Michigan

M. Roy First, MD
Vice President, Research and Development
Global Immunology and Transplantation
Astellas Pharma US, Inc
Deerfield, Illinois

Kenneth J. Friedman, PhD, FACMG
Discipline Director—Molecular Genetics
Laboratory Corporation of America
Center for Molecular Biology and Pathology
Research Triangle Park, North Carolina

Carl C. Garber, PhD, FACB
Director, Statistical Applications
Quest Diagnostics Incorporated
Madison, New Jersey

Lewis Glasser, MD
(Contributor to a previous edition)

R. Jeffrey Goldsmith, MD
Professor of Clinical Psychiatry
Department of Veterans Affairs
Department of Psychiatry
College of Medicine
University of Cincinnati
Cincinnati, Ohio;
Posttraumatic Stress and Anxiety Disorders Program
Cincinnati VAMC
Ft. Thomas, Kentucky

Gregory A. Grabowski, MD
Professor
Department of Pediatrics
University of Cincinnati College of Medicine,
Director, Division of Human Genetics
Cincinnati Children's Hospital Medical Center
Cincinnati, Ohio

David G. Grenache, PhD, DABCC
Medical Director, Special Chemistry
ARUP Laboratories;
Assistant Professor of Pathology
University of Utah Health Sciences Center
Salt Lake City, Utah

Ann M. Gronowski, PhD
Associate Professor
Pathology & Immunology and Obstetrics & Gynecology
Washington University School of Medicine,
Assistant Medical Director
Special Chemistry, Serology and Immunology
Barnes-Jewish Hospital
St. Louis, Missouri

Anne Catherine Halstead, MD, FRCP(C)
Clinical Associate Professor
University of British Columbia,
Division Head, Central Laboratory Services
Department of Pathology
Children's and Women's Hospital of British Columbia
Vancouver, British Columbia, Canada

Catherine Hammett-Stabler, PhD, DABCC, FACB
Associate Professor
Department of Pathology and Laboratory Medicine
University of North Carolina,
Director, Toxicology
McLendon Clinical Laboratories, UNC Hospitals
Chapel Hill, North Carolina

William R. Heineman, PhD
Distinguished Research Professor
Department of Chemistry
University of Cincinnati
Cincinnati, Ohio

Peter E. Hickman, MB BS, PhD, FRCPA
Associate Professor
Australian National University Medical School;
Director of Chemical Pathology
The Canberra Hospital
Australian Capital Territory, Australia

W.E. Highsmith, Jr., PhD
Associate Professor of Laboratory Medicine and Pathology, and Medical Genetics
Mayo College of Medicine
Mayo Clinic
Rochester, Minnesota

David C. Hohnadel, PhD, FACB
(Contributor to a previous edition)

Paul S. Horn, PhD
Professor
Department of Mathematical Sciences
University of Cincinnati,
Visiting Professor
Department of Neurology
Cincinnati Children's Hospital Medical Center,
Statistician
Mental Health Care Line
Cincinnati Veteran's Affairs Medical Center
Cincinnati, Ohio

Oussama Itani, MD, FAAP, FACN
Clinical Associate Professor of Pediatrics and Human Development
Michigan State University
Kalamazoo Center for Medical Studies,
Medical Director of Neonatology
Borgess Medical Center
Kalamazoo, Michigan

Mark A. Jandreski, PhD, DABCC, FACB
Siemens Healthcare Diagnostics
Senior Manager, Manufacturing
Technical Operations
Walpole, Massachusetts

Sarah H. Jenkins, PhD
Director, Laboratory Services
Dayton Children's Medical Center
Dayton, Ohio

Stephen E. Kahn, PhD, DABCC, FACB
Professor, Pathology, Cell Biology, Neurobiology, and Anatomy
Vice Chair, Laboratory Medicine
Director of Laboratories
Loyola University Medical Center
Maywood, Illinois

Tiffany E. Kaiser, PharmD, BCPS
Research Assistant Professor
Department of Internal Medicine
Division of Digestive Disease
University of Cincinnati Medical Center
Cincinnati, Ohio

Joshua M. Kaplan, MD
Assistant Professor
Department of Medicine
University of Medicine and Dentistry for New Jersey
New Jersey Medical School
Newark, New Jersey

Lawrence A. Kaplan, PhD, DABCC
New York, New York

Rakesh Khatri, MD
University of Cincinnati Medical Center
Cincinnati, Ohio

Jon R. Kirchhoff, PhD
Professor of Chemistry
Department of Chemistry
University of Toledo
Toledo, Ohio

Ruth-Ann Lee, PharmD
University of Cincinnati
Cincinnati, Ohio

Michael Lehrer, PhD
Associate Professor of Pathology
Albert Einstein College of Medicine
Bronx, New York;
Chief Forensic Toxicologist
Medical Examiner's Laboratory of Suffolk County
Hauppauge, New York

Dailin Li, PhD, DABCC, FCACB
Clinical Chemist
Vancouver General Hospital,
Clinical Assistant Professor
Department of Pathology and Laboratory Medicine
University of British Columbia
Vancouver, British Columbia, Canada

Gillian Lockitch, MBChB, MD, FRCPC
Professor Emerita
Department of Pathology and Laboratory Medicine
Faculty of Medicine
University of British Columbia
Vancouver, Canada

John M. Lorenz, MD
Professor of Clinical Pediatrics
College of Physicians and Surgeons
Columbia University
Morgan Stanley Children's Hospital of New York-Presbyterian
New York, New York

Craig E. Lunte, PhD
Professor of Chemistry
Courtesy Professor of Pharmaceutical Chemistry
University of Kansas
Lawrence, Kansas

Andre Mattman, MD, FRCPC
Clinical Assistant Professor
Department of Pathology and Laboratory Medicine
University of British Columbia,
Medical Biochemist, Department of Pathology
Children's and Women's Health Center of British Columbia
Vancouver, British Columbia, Canada

Fermina M. Mazzella, MD
Associate Professor
Department of Pathology and Laboratory Medicine
University of Medicine and Dentistry for New Jersey
New Jersey Medical School
Newark, New Jersey

Gerald P. Morris, MD, PhD
Resident Physician
Department of Pathology and Immunology
Division of Laboratory and Genomic Medicine
Washington University School of Medicine,
Resident Physician
Barnes-Jewish Hospital
St. Louis, Missouri

Herbert K. Naito, PhD, MBA
(Contributor to previous edition)

Michael Nardi, MS
Associate Professor of Pediatrics and Pathology
Technical Director, Hematology and Special Hematology Laboratories
Bellevue Hospital Center, Department of Pathology
New York University School of Medicine
New York, New York

Marilyn Nelson, MBA, MT(ASCP)
Laboratory Director
Ingalls Memorial Hospital
Harvey, Illinois

Sally J. Newsome, BMedSc, BMBS, FRACP
Staff Specialist Endocrinologist
Bankstown-Lidcombe Hospital
Sydney, Australia

James H. Nichols, PhD, DABCC, FACB
Associate Professor of Pathology
Tufts University School of Medicine
Boston, Massachusetts;
Medical Director, Clinical Chemistry
Baystate Health
Springfield, Massachusetts

Elisabeth Nye, MBBS, FRACP, PhD
Endocrinologist
Greenslopes Private Hospital
Greenslopes, Queensland, Australia

Michael Oellerich, MD, FFPath (RCPI), FRCPath
Director, Department of Clinical Chemistry
George-August University
Goettingen, Germany

Richard B. Passey, PhD
(Contributor to a previous edition)

Amadeo J. Pesce, PhD, DABCC
Professor Emeritus
Department of Pathology and Laboratory Medicine
College of Medicine
University of Cincinnati
Cincinnati, Ohio;
Adjunct Professor
Department of Pathology and Laboratory Medicine
School of Medicine
University of California, San Diego,
Laboratory Director
Millenium Laboratories of California
San Diego, California

Michael A. Pesce, PhD
Clinical Professor of Pathology
College of Physicians and Surgeons
Columbia University,
Director of the Specialty Laboratory
New York Presbyterian Hospital
Columbia University Medical Center
New York, New York

Michael D. Privitera, MD
Professor of Neurology
Director, Cincinnati Epilepsy Center
University of Cincinnati Medical Center
Cincinnati, Ohio

Morris Pudek, PhD, FCACB
Regional Medical Discipline Leader
Clinical Chemistry
Vancouver Coastal Health
Department of Pathology and Laboratory Medicine
Vancouver General Hospital,
Clinical Professor
Department of Pathology and Laboratory Medicine
University of British Columbia
Vancouver, British Columbia, Canada

Lisa Reninger, MT(ASCP)
Laboratory Administrative Director
Alexian Brothers Medical Center
Elk Grove Village, Illinois

Adele Rike Shields, PharmD
Research Assistant Professor of Surgery
University of Cincinnati
College of Medicine,
Transplant Clinical Pharmacist
The Christ Hospital
Cincinnati, Ohio

Wolfgang A. Ritschel, MD, PhD
(Contributor to previous edition)

Wendy R. Sanhai, PhD, MBA
Senior Scientific Advisor
Office of the Commissioner
U.S. Food and Drug Administration (FDA)
Rockville, Maryland

Hans-Gerhard Schneider, MD, FRACP, FRCPA, FACB
Director of Pathology and Head of Clinical Biochemistry
Alfred Pathology Service
Alfred Health,
Clinical Associate Professor
Department of Medicine and Department of Immunology
Monash University
Melbourne, Victoria, Australia

William E. Schreiber, MD
Professor, Department of Pathology & Laboratory Medicine
The University of British Columbia,
Consultant Pathologist
Vancouver General Hospital
Vancouver, British Columbia, Canada

Harold R. Schumacher, MD, Capt., MC, USN (Retired)
Professor Emeritus
Department of Pathology and Laboratory Medicine
College of Medicine
University of Cincinnati
Cincinnati, Ohio

Bette Seamonds, PhD, DABCC
Department of Pathology
Mercy Health Laboratory
Clinical Chemist and Director of POCT Services
Darby, Pennsylvania

Shenaz Seedat, MBBS, FRACP
Advanced Trainee in Endocrinology
Greenslopes Private Hospital
The Princess Alexandra Hospital
Brisbane, Australia

John E. Sherwin, PhD
(Contributor to previous edition)

Anita Snodgrass
Manager of Microbiology
Microbiology Department
Michael Reese Hospital and Medical Center
Chicago, Illinois

Paul W. Stiffler, PhD (ABMM), F(AMM)
Executive Vice President and Director of Regulatory Affairs
Medtrol, Inc
Niles, Illinois

Stephan G. Thompson, PhD
Santa Barbara, California

Reginald C. Tsang, MD
Professor of Pediatrics
Department of Pediatrics
Cincinnati Children's Hospital Medical Center
Cincinnati, Ohio

Nicole A. Weimert, PharmD, MSCR, BCPS
Clinical Specialist, Solid Organ Transplantation
Clinical Assistant Professor, SC-COP
Medical University of South Carolina
Department of Pharmacy Services
Charleston, South Carolina

John F. Wheeler, PhD
(Contributor to a previous edition)

Tarek Zakaria, MD
University of Cincinnati Medical Center
Cincinnati, Ohio

Kejian Zhang, MD, MBA
Assistant Professor
Department of Pediatrics
University of Cincinnati
College of Medicine
Division of Human Genetics
Cincinnati Children's Hospital Medical Center
Cincinnati, Ohio

Contributors to Methods of Analysis

Zakaria Ahmed, PhD
Clinical Chemist
Department of Pathology and Laboratory Medicine
Rochester General Hospital
Rochester, New York

Hassan M. E. Azzazy, PhD, DABCC, FACB
Chairman and Associate Professor
Department of Chemistry
The American University in Cairo
Cairo, Egypt

Tony Badrick, BAppSc, BSc, BA, MLitSt (Math), MBA, PhD, FAIMS, FAACB, FQSA, FAIM, FACB, FRCPA (Hon)
Executive Manager—Laboratories
Sullivan Nicolades Pathology
Taringa, Queensland, Australia

John Beilby, BSc(Hons), PhD, FAACB, MHGSA, ARCPA
Principal Scientist
PathWest
Nedlands, Western Australia, Australia

Marion Black, BSc(Hons), Dip. Ed, MAACB
Senior Scientist
Clinical Biochemistry, Alfred Pathology Service
Victoria, Australia

John R. Burnett, MB ChB, MD, PhD, FRCPA, FAHA
Clinical Professor
PathWest Laboratory Medicine
Royal Perth Hospital
Perth, Western Australia, Australia

Kevin Carpenter, PhD, FHGSA
Principal Scientist and Head of Department
NSW Biochemical Genetics Service
The Children's Hospital at Westmead
Westmead, New South Wales, Australia

Kee Cheung, BSc(Hons), PhD, GradCert. Mgt.
Manager
Pathology Queensland—Princess Alexandra Hospital
Woolloongabba, Queensland, Australia

William Clarke, PhD, MBA, DABCC
Director, TDM and Toxicology, Director, CPOCT
Department of Pathology
Johns Hopkins School of Medicine
Baltimore, Maryland

Paul F. Coleman, PhD
Research Fellow
Infectious Disease Core R&D
Abbott Diagnostics
Abbott Park, Illinois

Joe D'Agostino, BSc, Grad Dip FMI, MAACB
Senior Scientist
Clinical Biochemistry Unit
Alfred Pathology Service
Alfred Hospital, Melbourne, Australia

Sheila Dawling, PhD, CChem, FRSC
Associate Professor of Pathology
Director, Toxicology
TDM Laboratory,
Associate Director
Clinical Chemistry
The Vanderbilt Clinic
Nashville, Tennessee

Joris R. Delanghe
Professor of Clinical Chemistry
Department of Clinical Chemistry
Ghent University Hospital
Gent, Belgium

Goce Dimeski, BSc
Supervising Scientist
Pathology QLD
Princess Alexandra Hospital
Woolloongabba, Brisbane, Australia

Angela Ferguson, PhD
Clinical Chemistry Fellow
Washington University School of Medicine
Department of Pathology and Immunology
St. Louis, Missouri

Michael J. Figursk, PhD
Research Associate
University of Pennsylvania
Hospital of University of Pennsylvania
Philadelphia, Pennsylvania

John Galligan
Supervising Scientist
Pathology Queensland Central Laboratory
Royal Brisbane Hospital
Herston, Queensland, Australia

Karen Golemboski, PhD, MT(ASCP)
Program Director and Chair
Clinical Laboratory Science
Bellarmine University
Louisville, Kentucky

Ronda F. Greaves, BSc, Grad Dip Ed, MAppSc, PhD, MAACB
Senior Scientist
Complex Biochemistry Department
The Royal Children's Hospital
RCH Laboratory Services
Parkville, Victoria, Australia

Kathryn Green, BSc(Hons), MSc(Med)
Senior Scientist
NSW Biochemical Genetics Service
The Children's Hospital at Westmead
Westmead, New South Wales, Australia

Elizabeth M. Hall, BSc, MSc, FRCPath
Principal Clinical Scientist
Department of Clinical Biochemistry
East Kent Hospitals University
NHS Trust
Kent and Canterbury Hospital
Canterbury, Kent, United Kingdom

Peter E. Hickman, MB BS, PhD, MPH, MAACB, FRCPA
Associate Professor
Australian National University Medical School;
Director of Chemical Pathology
The Canberra Hospital
Australian Capital Territory, Australia

Gregory A. Hobbs, PhD, DABCC
Clinical Laboratory Science
Bellarmine University
Louisville, Kentucky

David W. Holt, BSc, PhD, DSc(Med), CSci, EurClin Chem, FESC, FRCPath
Professor of Bioanalytics
ASI, Ltd
London, United Kingdom

David G. Hughes, BAppSci, Grad Dip Sci
Scientist
Clinical Chemistry, ACT Pathology
The Canberra Hospital
Garran, Australian Capital Territory, Australia

Mind Jin, PhD
Temple University
Philadelphia, Pennsylvania

Atholl Johnston, BSc, MSc, PhD, FBPharmacolS, FRCPath
Professor of Clinical Pharmacology
William Harvey Research Institute (School of Medicine and Dentistry)
Queen Mary
University of London
London, United Kingdom

Graham Jones, MBBS, DPhil, FRCPA, FAACB
Staff Specialist in Chemical Pathology
Department of Chemical Pathology
St. Vincent's Hospital
Darlinghurst, New South Wales, Australia

Saeed A. Jortani, PhD, DABCC, FACB
Associate Professor of Pathology and Laboratory Medicine
University of Louisville
School of Medicine
Louisville, Kentucky

Lawrence A. Kaplan, PhD, DABCC
New York, New York

Steven C. Kazmierczak, PhD, DABCC
Professor of Pathology
Director of Clinical Chemistry and Toxicology
Oregon Health and Science University
Department of Pathology
Portland, Oregon

Sandra Klingberg, B App Sci
Supervising Scientist, Protein Laboratory
Pathology Queensland, Central Laboratory
Royal Brisbane Hospital
Herston, Queensland, Australia

Gus Koerbin, BAppSci, AFAIM
Principal Scientist ACT Pathology
Adjunct Professional Associate
University of Canberra
ACT Pathology
The Canberra Hospital
Garran, Australian Capital Territory, Australia

Magdalena Korecka, PhD
Senior Research Investigator
School of Medicine
University of Pennsylvania
Philadelphia, Pennsylvania

William J. Korzun, PhD, DABCC, MT(ASCP)
Associate Professor
Department of Clinical Laboratory Sciences
Virginia Commonwealth University
Richmond, Virginia

Edmund Lamb, PhD, FRCPath
Clinical Scientist (Biochemistry) and Head of Department
Department of Clinical Biochemistry
East Kent Hospitals
NHS Trust
Kent and Canterbury Hospital
Canterbury, Kent, United Kingdom

Stanley S. Levinson, PhD, DABCC
Professor of Pathology and Laboratory Medicine
University of Louisville
Director of Clinical Chemistry and Immunochemistry
Department of Veteran Affairs Medical Center
Louisville, Kentucky

Barry Lewis, MD, FRCPA, FHGSA
Head, Department of Clinical Biochemistry
PathWest Laboratory Medicine WA
Princess Margaret Hospital
Perth, Western Australia, Australia

Jinong Li, PhD
Clinical Chemistry Fellow
Johns Hopkins Medical Institutions
Baltimore, Maryland

Greg Maine, PhD
Manager, Global Scientific Affairs
Associate Research Fellow
Abbott Laboratories
Abbott Park, Illinois

Christopher R. McCudden, PhD, DABCC, NRCC
Assistant Professor
Department of Pathology and Laboratory Medicine
School of Medicine
University of North Carolina
Chapel Hill, North Carolina

Denise A. McKeown, MSci, AMRSC
Senior Analyst
St George's, University of London
Analytical Unit
Department of Cardiac and Vascular Sciences
London, United Kingdom

Brett McWhinney, BSc, MSc, MBA, MPhil
Supervising Scientist
HPLC Section, Department of Chemical Pathology
Royal Brisbane Hospital
Herston, Queensland, Australia

Danni L. Meany, PhD
Clinical Chemistry Fellow
Johns Hopkins Medical Institutions
Baltimore, Maryland

James J. Miller, PhD, DABCC, FACB
Professor
University of Louisville
School of Medicine
Department of Pathology and Laboratory Medicine
Louisville, Kentucky

Michael Milone, MD, PhD
Assistant Professor of Pathology and Laboratory Medicine
Associate Director, Toxicology Laboratory
School of Medicine
University of Pennsylvania
Philadelphia, Pennsylvania

Gerald J. Mizejewski, BS, MS, PhD
Senior Research Scientist
Wadsworth Center
New York State Department of Health
Albany, New York

Scott A. Muerhoff, PhD
Volwiler Research Fellow
Infectious Diseases Research and Development
Abbott Diagnostics
Abbott Laboratories
Abbott Park, Illinois

Anthony O. Okorodudu, PhD, MBA
Professor
Director, Clinical Chemistry Division
UTMB/CMC Outreach Laboratory Services
Department of Pathology
University of Texas Medical Branch
Galveston, Texas

Peter O'Leary, BSc, MAACB, AFACHSE, ARCPA, PhD
Adjunct Professor, School of Public Health (Curtin)
Adjunct Associate Professor
School of Women's & Infants' Health (UWA),
Director, Office of Population Health Genomics
Public Health Division
Health Department of Western Australia
Perth, Western Australia, Australia

Matthew T. Olson, MD
House Officer, Department of Pathology
Johns Hopkins Medical Institutions
Baltimore, Maryland

Felix O. Omoruyi, PhD
Fellow
Department of Pathology
Clinical Chemistry
University of Texas Medical Branch
Galveston, Texas

Mauro Panteghini, MD
Professor of Clinical Biochemistry and Clinical Molecular Biology
University of Milan Medical School
Laboratorio Analisi
Milan, Italy

Gerardo Perotta, MPA
Interim-Coordinator, Pathology Education
Department of Pathology and Laboratory Medicine
University of Cincinnati College of Medicine
Cincinnati, Ohio

Michael A. Pesce, PhD
Professor Emeritus of Pathology and Cell Biology
Columbia University Medical Center
New York Presbyterian Hospital
New York, New York

Julia M. Potter, B Med Sc(Hons), MB BS, PhD, FRCPA
Professor of Pathology
Australian National University Medical School
Executive Director, ACT Pathology
The Canberra Hospital
Garran, Australian Capital Territory, Australia

Terry Pry, PhD
Retired-Manager Scientific Affairs, Asia-Pacific
Abbott Diagnostic Division
Abbott Laboratories
Auckland, New Zealand

Kishor Raja, BSc(Hons), MSc, PhD, CSci
Principal Clinical Scientist/Honorary Senior Lecturer
Clinical Biochemistry Department
King's College Hospital
London, United Kingdom

Jordan Reynolds, MD
Resident Physician
University of Cincinnati
Department of Pathology and Laboratory Medicine
Cincinnati, Ohio

Ken Robertson, BSc, AAIMS
Senior Scientist in Charge (Research)
PathWest Laboratory Medicine
Royal Perth Hospital
Wellington St. Perth, Western Australia, Australia

Andrea M. Rose, PhD, MBA
Senior Clinical Support Consultant
Roche Diagnostics
Indianapolis, Indiana

Enrico Rossi, PhD, MAACB
Research Biochemist
PathWest Laboratory Medicine
Nedlands, Western Australia, Australia

Randal J. Schneider, MS, PhD
Director of Clinical Chemistry and Toxicology
ProHealth Care Laboratories
Waukesha, Wisconsin

Les Shaw, BS, PhD
Professor
University of Pennsylvania
School of Medicine
Philadelphia, Pennsylvania

Run Zhang Shi, PhD
Instructor
Assistant Director of Clinical Chemistry and Immunology
Department of Pathology
School of Medicine
Stanford University
Stanford, California

Ravinder Jit Singh, PhD
Co-Director, Endocrine Laboratory Organization
Mayo Clinic
Rochester, Minnesota

Patricia Slev, PhD
Assistant Professor of Pathology (Clinical)
University of Utah,
Medical Director
Serologic Hepatitis and Retrovirus Laboratory
ARUP Laboratories
Salt Lake City, Utah

Ramasamyiyer Swaminathan, MBBS, MSc, PhD, FRCPath
Professor and Head of Department of Chemical Pathology
St. Thomas' Hospital
London, United Kingdom

Danyal B. Syed, BSc, MA, PhD, C(ASCP), CC(NRCC), DABCC, FACB
Laboratory Director
William F. Ryan Community Health Center
New York, New York

Danyel H. Tacker, PhD, FACB
Clinical Chemist
Ochsner Medical Center—New Orleans
New Orleans, Louisiana

Jillian R. Tate, BSc(Hons), MSc
Senior Scientist
Pathology Queensland
Chemical Pathology Department
Royal Brisbane and Women's Hospital
Brisbane, Queensland, Australia

John G. Toffaletti, PhD
Professor in Pathology
Clinical Laboratories and Department of Pathology
Duke University Medical Center
Durham, North Carolina

Susan Vickery, MSc, PhD
Senior Clinical Scientist
East Kent Hospitals University
NHS Trust
Kent and Canterbury Hospital
Canterbury, Kent, United Kingdom

Ping Wang, PhD, DABCC
Medical Director of Clinical Chemistry
The Methodist Hospital
Houston, Texas

Gregory Ward, BSc(Hons), MSc, MAACB, FAACB
Head, Biochemistry and Endocrinology
Sullivan Nicolades Pathology (Sonic Healthcare)
Brisbane, Queensland, Australia

Alan H. B. Wu, PhD
Professor, Laboratory Medicine
University of California, San Francisco
Clinical Chemistry and Toxicology Laboratories
San Francisco General Hospital
San Francisco, California

Odette Youdell, BAppSci(Hons), MAACB
Senior Scientist
Clinical Biochemistry
Alfred Pathology Service
Melbourne, Victoria
Australia

Preface

The first edition of this textbook was published in 1984. The field reviewed in this textbook, as well as its editors, have changed over the ensuing 25 years. It has always been our goal to have the text reflect the current, if not hint at the future, science of clinical chemistry. To this end we have had the special opportunity to work with some of the best clinical scientists practicing their craft in a large number of countries.

THE FIFTH EDITION TEXTBOOK: WRITTEN AND ELECTRONIC

The continuing multi-decade trend of laboratory consolidation is reflected in this current book. We have "encroached" on the traditional fields of Microbiology and Hematology to include new chapters that review tests from these specialty areas that are increasingly being performed in the more automated core clinical chemistry laboratory. These new chapters are on *Laboratory Analysis of Hemoglobin Variants*, *Laboratory Approaches to Serology Testing*, *Viral Hepatitis: Diagnosis and Monitoring*, and *The Newborn*.

All chapters from the Fourth Edition have been updated by the authors. Their material is supplemented with references (in electronic format on Evolve), bibliographies, and Internet sites.

As the science of clinical chemistry evolves, so does the technology used to bring expanded knowledge to our readers. And so we are using Elsevier's Evolve website to make available the huge amount of material that describes 144 methods used for routine and specialty analysis. Changes in the field and continuing space constraints in the textbook also necessitated removing some of the printed material to the Evolve site. So students who still need to review the excellent chapter by I-Wen Chen on Radioisotopes can find that chapter on this Internet site. A complete list of the contents of the Evolve website for the Fifth Edition is found on the inside front cover of this book.

STUDENT READERS

The editors were faced, more than ever, with the difficulty of balancing the needs of undergraduate students and the needs of professionals and more advanced students of clinical chemistry. While keeping the writing as straight-forward as possible, we hold all readers to a high hurdle of excellence. However, we commiserate with students of medical technology who will be assigned to read this textbook. You are facing the daunting task of having to understand this hugely expanded, complex science. We have thus added aids for the students; signposts that indicate the minimal material for which the student should have some basic understanding. So, at the beginning of every major section within the printed chapter the student will find a list of learning objectives for that section. At the completion of that section the student will find the most important concepts that we believe he or she should understand. Both the lists of ***Section Objectives*** and ***Key Concepts*** could not be exhaustive, and so, as usual, the editors as well as the students, must ultimately depend on the teachers for guidance. These aids and teachers will guide students as they navigate through this landscape.

At the beginning of each of the routine Methods of Analysis on Evolve, the student will find a boxed section, ***Students' Quick Hyperlink Review,*** which is hyperlinked to provide easy access to core information.

ANCILLARIES

For the Instructor

Evolve

We are offering several assets on Evolve to aid instructors:

- Test bank: a test bank of 1000 multiple-choice questions that feature rationales, cognitive levels, and page number references to the text. This can be used as review in class or for test development.
- Image Collection: all of the images from the book are available as JPGs and can be downloaded into PowerPoint presentations. These can be used during lectures to illustrate important concepts.
- Instructor's Manual: an instructor's manual is available that contains Chapter Focus, Teaching Strategies, Chapter Outline, Chapter Objectives, Key Words, Critical Thinking Questions, and Learning Activities.

For the Student

Evolve

The student resources on Evolve include:

- Methods of Analysis: a set of 133 routine methods describe current methodology in great detail
- Additional Resources: includes helpful information on radioisotopes, urinalysis, and other topics
- References: all of the references from the book are linked electronically to the PubMed database of articles and abstracts
- Weblinks, which link to places of interest on the web specifically for clinical chemistry students

Acknowledgments

As usual we thank the many people who have helped make this edition possible. We greatfully thank our many authors, who have borne the nagging of cranky old(er) clinical chemist editors, we once again acknowledge their patience and knowledge. They are listed, and they truly represent the best and brightest in clinical chemistry.

Special thanks must go to Peter Hickman and Gus Koerbin who have performed the impossible task of organizing and editing the Evolve Method's section, essentially another textbook.

We thank Karol Sublett, our consulting educator for helping us provide the Section Objectives and Key Concepts.

We greatly thank our editor, Ellen Wurm-Cutter, for her warm patience, advice, and encouragement, and Rachel McMullen, Senior Project Manager, for her steady and wise forbearance.

Contents

Color insert follows p. 600.

Basic Laboratory Principles and Techniques

Chapter 1

Bette Seamonds and Elizabeth Ann Byrne

Chapter Outline

Chapter Outline—cont'd

Key Terms

balances Instruments used to measure weight accurately; often electronic.

beakers Laboratory utensils used to contain liquids or solids.

bloodborne pathogens Potentially infectious agents in blood and body fluids.

buret (burette) Laboratory utensil used to deliver a wide range of volumes accurately.

centrifuge Instrument used to separate materials from solution through application of increased gravitational force produced by rotating or spinning samples rapidly.

Chemical Hygiene Plan A laboratory plan that follows Occupational and Safety Health Administration (OSHA)-mandated regulations, to protect employees against chemical hazards.

desiccant Material used in a desiccator to absorb water from the air.

desiccator Large container used to store material in a water-free environment.

dilution Process of preparing less concentrated solutions from a solution of greater concentration.

Erlenmeyer flask Laboratory utensil used to contain liquids.

funnel Laboratory utensil used to transfer liquids or solids into a container; also used for extraction of liquids.

graduated cylinder Laboratory utensil used to measure a volume of liquid.

heating block A temperature-controlled device used to warm and maintain materials at a specified temperature.

metric system A system of measurement of weights, distances, and volumes.

Occupational Safety and Health Administration (OSHA) Government agency responsible for mandating regulations to ensure safety in the workplace.

pipet (pipette) Laboratory utensil used to transfer a specific or varying volume of liquid.

sanitization The process used to maintain cleanliness in a water purification system.

syringe A device used for drawing up a specified quantity of liquid and then dispensing it volumetrically.

Système Internationale d'Unités (SI) An internationally accepted system of measurements.

thermometer A device, physical, electronic, or optical, that is used to measure temperature.

volumetric flask Laboratory utensil used to contain a specific volume of liquid.

water bath A temperature-controlled device filled with water, used to warm and maintain materials at a specified temperature.

water purification A treatment process (distillation, deionization, reverse osmosis, ultraviolet irradiation, ultrafiltration, or ozonolysis) used to remove water contaminants.

water purity Three levels of purity are defined, based on the amount of biological and dissolved organic and inorganic material present in the water.

PART 1: Basic Laboratory Principles and Techniques

Bette Seamonds

To provide accurate and precise clinical data, the clinical chemistry laboratory must be concerned with the analytical components used to provide this information. Familiarity with the purity of chemicals, solvents, and reagent water is essential. In addition, selection and use of appropriate analytical equipment and safe work practices are essential.

SECTION OBJECTIVES BOX 1-1

- Name all the grades of water used by a clinical laboratory.
- Describe the methods used for water purification and the specifications, uses, and storage and handling procedures associated with the different grades of reagent water.
- Describe the quality control and impurity testing procedures used for different grades of reagent water.

WATER AS A REAGENT

Water is one of the most important and commonly used reagents in the clinical laboratory. Because of its importance as a laboratory reagent, and because it often is "produced" within each laboratory, water is discussed more fully in the following section.

Reagent Grade Water

Organic and inorganic impurities in the reagent water can introduce significant error into an analysis. Some impurities are easy to detect, but others are far more difficult to observe. The need for high-purity reagent water in the clinical laboratory cannot be overemphasized.

Water systems that are improperly designed or inadequately maintained actually may add contaminants not originally found in the source water (feedwater). Thus the quality of reagent water produced by different purification systems can differ greatly. In general, systems that continually recirculate the water provide protection against stagnation and consequently minimize bacterial growth. However, the system must be decontaminated at regular intervals. The material used for the construction of pipes is important; plastics such as polyvinyl chloride (PVC) were commonly used but do not necessarily represent the best choice. PVC, in particular, leaches organic impurities into the purified water. In addition, it has a porous surface that tends to harbor bacteria and other biological impurities. For more detailed information, the reader is referred to the guideline, *Preparation and Testing of Reagent Water in the Clinical Laboratory: Approved Guideline,* 4th edition, published by the Clinical and Laboratory Standards Institute (CLSI).[1]

Water quality is not defined solely by the purification process used. Different types of purification processes may be employed, and in many laboratories, multiple processes are used. The quality of the feedwater is important, often dictating the purification processes to be used and ultimately the types of contaminants likely to remain. Many of the characteristics of feedwater are affected by geographical and seasonal variations. Seasonal variability depends on rainfall, ground drainage, sewage, and industrial waste, whereas geographical location determines the hardness (mineral content) of the feedwater. The laboratory should work closely with a reputable manufacturer to design a water purification system that meets its specific needs.

Purification Process

Distillation

Distillation of water in glass effectively removes bacteria, pyrogens, particulate matter, dissolved ionized solids, and, to a lesser extent, dissolved organic contaminants. It is not useful for elimination of dissolved ions derived from gases such as ammonia, carbon dioxide, and chlorine or low–boiling point organic compounds.

Deionization

In the deionization process, water is passed through a bed of mixed cation- and anion-exchange resins. Hydrogen and hydroxyl ions on the surface of the resins are displaced by cationic and anionic impurities. This process is excellent for removal of dissolved ions derived from gases and solids but is ineffective for all other contaminants. In addition, the resin must be frequently replaced or regenerated. Deionization is used in conjunction with carbon adsorption, which is very effective in removal of dissolved organic compounds. The characteristics of the carbon employed dictate the efficacy of removal of the different organic contaminants. Neither deionization nor carbon adsorption will remove particulate matter, bacteria, or pyrogens.

Reverse Osmosis

In reverse osmosis, water is forced under pressure through a semipermeable membrane, and remnants of dissolved organic, ionic, and suspended impurities, including microbial and viral contaminants, are left behind. Reverse osmosis, however, does not remove dissolved gases effectively. This method is used frequently to pretreat water before it undergoes purification by deionization.

Ultrafiltration

In ultrafiltration, water is passed through semipermeable membranes of pore size ≤0.2 mm, removing particulate matter, emulsified solids, most bacteria, and pyrogens. Increasingly, 0.1 μm postmembrane filters are being used to achieve an improved bacteria-free and pyrogen-free product. Ultrafiltration does not effectively remove dissolved ionized solids and gases and most organic contaminants.

Ultraviolet Oxidation and Sterilization

Ultraviolet (UV) oxidation and sterilization are used after other purification processes are performed to remove trace quantities of organic contaminants (oxidation) and bacteria (sterilization). Different wavelengths are used for these processes—185 nm for oxidation and 254 nm for sterilization. UV treatment is limited by intensity, contact time, and flow rate. Sterilization is the more commonly used procedure, but it frequently is referred to as UV oxidation.

Ozone

Ozone treatment, used primarily in industrial settings, effectively removes organic contaminants. However, smaller, less expensive ozone generators are becoming available and possibly will begin to find their way into clinical laboratory settings. After it is introduced into the pretreated water, the ozone kills bacteria by rupturing the cell membrane almost instantaneously (≈2 sec). Chlorine, on the other hand, simply diffuses into the cell and requires approximately a half hour to achieve its effect. The actual rate of lysis depends on the ozone level: higher ozone concentrations are used for highly contaminated systems, whereas lower concentrations are used for maintenance. After the microorganisms are lysed, the cytoplasmic constituents are oxidized by the ozone. The ozone then is removed by UV irradiation at 254 nm. Removal is crucial because ozone is incompatible with deionization resins. Ozone treatment can be used to effectively combat microbial contamination in pipes and purified water.

Grades of Water Purity

CLSI now defines Clinical Laboratory Reagent Water (**CLRW**) as "water that meets the specification for most routine clinical laboratory testing." Purified water with a resistivity of at least 10 mΩ•cm, referenced to 25° C, meets the specifications of CLRW. However, CO_2 readily dissolves in this water, causing its resistivity to drop; therefore, the water no longer meets the specifications. However, the water will still be adequate for many laboratory applications. Water that falls into the "Special" (SRW) category will likely require additional treatment to meet more specific requirements and applications.

Water that conforms to specifications published by other agencies such as the American Society for Testing and Materials (ASTM), the American Chemical Society (ACS), and the United States Pharmacopeia (USP) may or may not be equivalent to water that conforms to CLSI specifications. The reader is referred to the CLSI document, *Preparation and Testing of Reagent Water in the Clinical Laboratory: Approved Guideline,* 4th edition.[1]

Storage and Handling of Reagent Water

CLRW should be used immediately after it is produced, because its resistivity will rapidly decrease as carbon dioxide is absorbed. If storage is required, containers should be constructed of opaque materials with low gas permeability so that contamination will be held to a minimum. These materials should also be resistant to damage by the sanitizing agents and should be designed to minimize the growth of autotrophic bacteria. The containers should be as small as is possible their contents must be refilled at least every few days; drained between fillings to prevent stagnation, and sanitized regularly (e.g., quarterly).[2]

Storage tanks that are an integral part of a permanent system should be as small as is practical. The water in the reservoir may be recirculated continuously or intermittently through the purification process to maintain purity. Additional features and requirements are described in the CLSI document.[2]

Under some conditions, purchased stored water may be used. One example is water that is provided as a diluent by the manufacturer of a specific analytical system. In this case, the water has been validated by the manufacturer for use as stated in the product insert. Under no conditions can such a product be substituted for reagent water. Similarly, sterile water is not equivalent to reagent grade water and therefore is not an acceptable substitute. Other purchased products may include those used in high-performance liquid chromatographic (HPLC) procedures in facilities where the quality of in-house reagent water is not satisfactory for this purpose.

If water must be purchased, several important issues should be considered. The purchased product should define ion content, bacterial contamination, and resisistivity at the time of manufacture. The water should be purchased in quantities appropriate to usage. The packaged water should be protected from environmental contamination and from the leaching effects of the container. When the container is opened, the bacterial count and conductivity should be measured for assessment of quality degradation since manufacture. When required analytically, the water should be poured into an appropriate secondary container from which it will be sampled. Care must be taken to avoid touching the inside lid or dipping a pipet directly into the primary vessel. Unused portions of water must not be returned to the primary container. Water from the primary container should be discarded after a period of no longer than 1 week.

Suggested Uses

The scientific literature contains little documentation of the analytical difficulties caused by poor-quality water. However, many users of the document on reagent water have reported specific instances of analytical problems attributed to water quality. These include difficulty with coagulation and hematological analyses, interference with some immunoassay procedures, instrumentation problems (including background absorbance difficulties), leaching of contaminants from improperly regenerated deionization resins, and absorption of perfume into highly purified water causing difficulty with cell culture procedures. In addition, bacteria, silicate, and other ion contaminants have been suspected to interfere with enzyme and bilirubin analyses.[3] As techniques become more sensitive, more definitive information may become available.

CLRW should be used in all quantitative and most qualitative laboratory procedures, for electrophoretic analyses, for toxicology screening procedures, and in the preparation of buffers, standards, and controls. Further treatment of CLRW may be necessary for trace element and heavy metal analyses.

Special purpose reagent water may be necessary for specific procedures such as HPLC, chromosome analyses, human leukocyte antigen (HLA) testing, and in vitro fertilization (IVF) and gamete intrafallopian transfer (GIFT) procedures. Systems can be designed to produce water that meets specific requirements, or CLRW can be purified further.

Quality Control and Impurity Testing

Water must be monitored at regular intervals to evaluate the performance of a **water purification** system. Because of the variety of contaminants found in water, no single test can measure **water purity.** The schedule for regular evaluations may vary with the season and with the contaminants found. In addition to ensuring that the purification system is functioning acceptably under routine conditions, monitoring ensures the purity of the water after a component or components of the system have been changed. At a minimum, frequent bacterial surveillance and resistivity determinations are necessary (see below). The monitoring of other parameters such as pH, silicate content, pyrogens, organic contamination, and particulate matter depends on many factors. Each laboratory should determine frequency guidelines based on the history, system design, and use of its water purification system. In general, if the source water and the purification system produce a product that is consistently negative for a particular contaminant, the laboratory may test for that contaminant infrequently. Some tests must be performed by the laboratory, and other tests may be referred out.

Microbial Monitoring

Bacteria can inactivate reagents by metabolizing certain components. In addition, they contribute to the total organic contamination and can alter optical properties of test solutions. Although microbial monitoring is retrospective, it provides the laboratory with useful information and may be helpful in detecting impending problems.

Over the past several years, the importance of microbial biofilms and their contribution to the causes of contamination and infection has been confirmed. The characteristics of bacteria in biofilms are distinctly different from those of planktonic forms of the same species. Biofilms may consist of homogeneous or heterogeneous colonies. The structure of the colonies is such that water channels through the colonies enable provision of nutrients. The colonies adhere to surfaces such as those of medical devices, and it has been found that biofilm cells are at least 500 times more resistant to antibacterial agents as compared with their planktonic forms.[4] Because biofilm bacteria appear to predominate both numerically and metabolically, this poses a major challenge in terms of monitoring bacteria in the water supply. However, standard methods used for monitoring reagent water continue to apply until such time that the specialized equipment that is required becomes available.

Microbial contamination of water quality should be tested weekly. Several acceptable methods are available, although no single method can be assumed to quantitate all bacteria in a water sample. Therefore, the number of viable bacteria may be higher than the number of colony-forming units (cfu) as determined by any given method. Several criteria may be applied in choosing a method, but regardless of the method selected, the first step in obtaining a reliable result is to collect an appropriate sample.

Before collection, the spigot should be fully opened for at least 1 minute. This procedure flushes the system adequately and should be employed when water is drawn for use in reagent preparation. One of the most common causes of rapid bacterial contamination in water is inadequate flushing. The volume of water collected for analysis varies with the procedure used. An amount from 1 mL (for bacteriologic samplers) to 100 mL (standard plate count or filtration methods) may be collected. After collection, the sample should be processed as soon as possible. The sample should not be stored for longer than 1 hour at room temperature or for longer than 6 hours in the refrigerator. For certain procedures, the sample must be vortexed vigorously to ensure distribution of organisms within the sample. The most commonly found organisms are gram-negative rods. Previous editions of the CLSI water document defined 10 cfu/mL as the upper limit for bacterial contamination of reagent grade water.

Resistivity

Resistivity measurements are used to assess the ionic content of purified water. The higher the ion concentration, the lower is the resistivity. Ion-exchange tanks should be equipped with an in-line "resistivity" light that is calibrated to go off when the resistivity falls below 2 mΩ•cm, at which point the capacity of the tanks is exhausted. Systems that supply CLRW must have an in-line resistivity meter that is capable of reading to 18 mΩ•cm. Resistivity must be 10 mΩ•cm at a minimum (preferably 15 to 18 mΩ•cm) to meet CLRW specifications. Monitoring is performed daily.

pH

Monitoring of the pH of purified water generally is not necessary, but methods are available for use if a pH problem is suspected.[1] Anecdotal reports have suggested that in some facilities, source water pH problems have led to product water pH problems. Some systems now allow in-line pH measurements, but these are not yet used in clinical laboratories.

Pyrogens

Pyrogens are not monitored routinely in the clinical laboratory. However, anecdotal reports from manufacturers indicate that some immunoassay reagents are affected by interference from pyrogens. Therefore, testing for these contaminants may become more important with time. Procedures for pyrogen testing are readily available.[1,5,6]

Silica

Silica in the water supply can be a major problem in some geographical areas. Silica can interfere with trace metal and electrolyte analyses, enzyme determinations, and some spectrophotometric assays, and removal of this contaminant is essential. Colloidal silica is readily removed by distillation and certain reverse osmosis membranes. Other schemes for addressing contamination are cited.[1] Soluble silica may be measured by spectrophotometric analysis. Because the procedure requires the use of a narrow–band pass instrument, preferably capable of reading at ≈800 nm, and because the reagent blanks frequently generate absorbances higher than those of the water being tested, it is preferable to refer samples for analysis by inductively coupled plasma (ICP) spectrometry.

Organic Contaminants

Bacteria can multiply in the resin beds, significantly increasing the organic contamination of water. Methods routinely used to assess contamination, although plentiful, are not sufficiently specific (permanganate) or are impractical (e.g., requiring research grade spectrophotometers and HPLC). If the laboratory has access to HPLC, the measurement is easily accomplished.[7]

However, the best approach to dealing with organic contamination is to design and maintain the system optimally. Semiannual **sanitization** (or more frequently if quality control data dictate) helps control bacterial levels. Use of carbon adsorption and UV treatment also helps remove organic contaminants. Constant surveillance of the system ensures the production of reagent water of the desired quality. Current CLSI recommendations include the measurement of total organic carbon. This is most readily accomplished by the inclusion of an on-line instrument that is connected directly to the purified water stream. Such instruments are designed to detect CO_2 selectively. The detectors respond minimally, if at all, to other products of organic oxidation.[1]

System Documentation and Record Keeping

A procedure manual that includes the following should be developed for the water purification system[1,8]:

1. A quality assurance plan that defines the responsibilities of personnel
2. Procedures for preventive maintenance
3. Quality control checklists
4. Worksheets for documenting daily, weekly, monthly, and other testing
5. Documentation of corrective actions taken

KEY CONCEPTS BOX 1-1

- Types of water used by a clinical laboratory include feedwater (tap water) and Clinical Laboratory Reagent Water (CLRW).
- CLRW, which is used to prepare analytical reagents and sample dilutions, usually is prepared with a combination of filtration, ion exchange and carbon absorption chromatography, and ultraviolet (UV) light treatment.
- Quality control (QC) testing of CLRW includes microbial monitoring, resistivity measurements (dissolved solutes), silica measurements, and biannual decontamination.

SECTION OBJECTIVES BOX 1-2

- List and describe four grades of chemicals, and explain how they differ in their degree of purity.
- Describe the specifications associated with the quality of reagent chemicals and solvents.
- Differentiate between a primary standard and a Standard Reference Material (SRM).
- Define a desiccant and explain how it is used.

CHEMICAL LABORATORY SUPPLIES

Chemicals

Chemicals are available in varying degrees of purity, and in many instances, the types and concentrations of impurities are known. Less pure grades of chemicals include chemically pure, practical grade, technical grade, and commercial grade. Such chemicals are unsuitable for use in analytical work. Certain chemicals, especially pharmaceuticals, are produced to meet the specifications defined in the USP, The National Formulary, and The Food Chemical Index. These specifications define impurity tolerances that are not injurious to health.

Most qualitative and quantitative analyses performed in the clinical laboratory require the use of chemicals that meet the specifications of the ACS; such chemicals are described as analytical grade or reagent grade. ACS specifications establish the maximum quantities of impurities allowed in each chemical or provide impurity contents on a lot-to-lot basis. Some manufacturers sell certified or very pure materials when specifications have not been established by the ACS.

Additional standards of purity for certain chemicals have been specified by the International Union for Pure and Applied Chemistry (IUPAC). These include atomic weight standards (grade A); ultimate standards (grade B); primary standards (grade C), which are commercially available and have less than 0.002% impurities; working standards (grade D), which are commercially available and have less than 0.05% impurities; and secondary substances (grade E), which are defined or standardized by an acceptable reference method with a primary standard (grade C) used as the reference material.

Primary Standards

Primary standards are supplied with certificates of analysis for each lot. These preparations must be stable, nonhygroscopic substances of definite composition that can be dried without a change in composition.

Standard Reference Materials

Standard Reference Materials (SRMs) are available from the National Institute of Standards and Technology (NIST). Not all SRMs are as pure as primary standards; however, NIST defines their chemical and physical properties and provides a certificate documenting results of characterization. These standards may be used to characterize other materials. SRMs are available in solid, liquid, or gaseous form. The solids may be crystalline, powder, or lyophilized products.

Organic Solvents

Classification of organic solvents follows the same guidelines as those used for other chemicals. Thus for many analyses, in particular those involving spectroscopy and chromatography, reagents of even higher purity than reagent grade are required. These solvents frequently are referred to as spectrograde, nanograde, or HPLC grade, and information about the presence of contaminants is supplied with the solvent. The purity ensures minimal spectral interference and minimal residual contamination after sample extraction and evaporation of the solvent are performed as part of an analytical procedure. In general, these solvents are more than 99% pure (as determined by gas chromatography), and no single impurity exceeds 0.2%.

Gases

Gases, particularly those used in gas chromatography and atomic absorption analyses, must be extremely pure. Helium purity must be 99.9999% for gas chromatographic procedures. As with other reagents, information regarding contaminants and their concentrations is of utmost importance. (See Appendix D for more specific information.)

Chemical Safety

Many chemicals and solvents are flammable, teratogenic, and carcinogenic. Therefore, all chemicals should be handled with the utmost care, and inhalation of fumes or dust should be avoided. Similarly, the handling of gas cylinders requires adherence to specific regulations. Specifics of safe practices are discussed in the laboratory safety section.

Desiccants

A **desiccant** is a material that is used to absorb and remove water from the air or from another substance (Table 1-1). Some desiccants are deliquescent and therefore lose their efficiency

Table 1-1 Some Common Drying Agents (Desiccants)

Desiccant	Properties	Uses
Anhydrous $CaCl_2$	High-capacity, slow-acting, works well below 30° C	Most conditions, very inexpensive
Anhydrous $MgSO_4$	Neutral, rapid action	Most conditions, inexpensive
Anhydrous Na_2SO_4	Neutral, high capacity, works only below 32° C, slow action	Can remove large volume of water
Anhydrous $CaSO_4$	Extremely rapid action, chemically inert, limited capacity to absorb water (6% to 10% of its weight in water)	More expensive than $MgSO_4$ and Na_2SO_4; sold commercially as Drierite; can be easily regenerated for 3 hours
Al_2O_3 (activated alumina)	Can absorb 15% to 20% of its weight in water	Can be activated repeatedly by heating at 175° C for 7 hours

after liquefaction occurs. Others produce dust and therefore should be avoided. The most commonly used desiccants are manufactured with a moisture-sensitive indicator salt, such as cobalt chloride, to indicate exhaustion. Silica gel and anhydrous calcium sulfate (Drierite) are examples. These agents can be regenerated by heat, making them cost efficient.

KEY CONCEPTS BOX 1-2

- Laboratory chemicals are defined by grades of purity; analytical and reagent grades are purer than technical and commercial grades.
- Primary standards, prepared from the purest chemicals, are used to prepare working calibrators and standards.
- Standard Reference Materials (SRMs) are preparations of stated composition that may be used as primary standards.
- Desiccants are chemicals that usually are found in a solid form and can absorb water. It may be used to dry, or keep dry, another chemical.

SECTION OBJECTIVES BOX 1-3

- List examples of types of glass and plastics used in laboratory supplies and describe their most useful qualities.
- Compare and contrast the use and care of glass and plastic supplies.

LABORATORY PLASTIC AND GLASSWARE COMPOSITION AND CLEANING

Laboratory supplies that are used for the preparation, measurement, and storage of fluids and other products of reactions include tubing, glassware, and plasticware. Glass must be used for procedures involving HPLC and gas-liquid chromatography (GLC) because solvents readily attack plastics. On the other hand, many solutions with a pH above 6.0 can attack glassware, and alkaline solutions should be stored in plastic.[9] Glass also tends to adsorb metal ions, possibly altering significantly the concentrations of standard solutions.

Tubing

Natural latex rubber tubing is durable and can be used for glass connections. It is, however, affected by contact with oils, alkalis, corrosives, and hot water. Neoprene (synthetic) rubber tubing may be substituted for latex tubing in most situations. It should not be used with chlorinated or aromatic hydrocarbons.

More expensive than rubber tubing, synthetic plastic Tygon tubing (Saint-Gobain Performance Plastics, Beaverton, MI) is the most useful type. Tygon is resistant to chemicals and inert to chemicals. It can be used in many applications such as peristaltic pumps; it also can be joined to other tubing through a heat welding process. Over time, it tends to discolor and become slightly brittle. Polytetrafluoroethylene (Teflon) tubing (Zeus Industrial Products, Inc., Orangeburg, SC) is also available; it is more expensive than Tygon tubing but serves as a substitute in certain situations.

Types of Glass

Many types of glass are available. They differ in their tensile strength, resistivity to certain agents, and heat or light resistance. Most reusable glassware in the clinical laboratory is made from borosilicate glass, which is available under the brand names of Pyrex (Corning Glass Works, Corning, NY) and Kimax (Kimble Glass Company, Vineland, NJ). Borosilicate glass has a low alkaline earth content and is free of contaminants such as heavy metals. Therefore, liquids can be heated in borosilicate glass with minimal contamination. This type of glass can be heated safely to approximately 600° C for short periods. Table 1-2 lists additional types of glass and their uses.

Types of Plastic

Plastic laboratory utensils are made from polymerized organic monomers. The properties of the plastics depend on the nature of the monomer and the final polymer forms used to prepare the plastic materials. The most commonly used plastics include the polyolefins (i.e., polyethylene, polypropylene), polystyrene, polycarbonate, Teflon, and PVC.

Polyolefins, which are relatively chemically inert, are resistant to most acids, alkalis, and salt solutions. Organic acids and hydrocarbons cause swelling and penetration of the plastic. Concentrated sulfuric acid attacks polyethylene at room temperature. Polyethylene is used in most disposable plasticware and cannot be sterilized. Polypropylene may be sterilized.

Polycarbonate is stronger than polypropylene and has better temperature tolerances. Its chemical resistance is not as good as that of the polyolefins. Its primary characteristics include its clarity and resistance to shattering, which makes it the material of choice for items such as centrifuge tubes.

Table 1-2 Types of Commonly Used Glass and Their Properties

Glass	Properties	Purpose
Kimax/Pyrex	Relatively inert borosilicate glass, high resistance to heat and cold shock	All purpose
Vycor	Good resistance to drastic conditions of heat, shock, chemical treatment, and high temperature; acid and alkali resistant	Ashing, ignition techniques
Corex	Aluminosilicate glass, about sixfold stronger than borosilicate glass; scratch resistant; resistant to alkaline etching	Used under conditions of stress
High silica	>96% silicate; comparable to fused quartz; heat, chemical, and electrical tolerance; excellent optical properties	For high-precision analytical work, optical reflectors, and mirrors
Boron-free	Alkali resistant; poor heat resistance; soft; <0.2% boron	Highly alkaline solutions
Low actinic	Amber or red color reduces light exposure of contents	For use with light-sensitive materials in range of 300 to 500 nm (e.g., bilirubin, vitamin A, carotene)
Flint	Soda-lime glass containing oxides of sodium, silicon, and calcium; poor resistance to high temperature or temperature change, poor chemical resistance; also may leach organic contaminants	Used for disposable glassware items (e.g., pipets)
Coated	Thin, metallic oxide fire-bonded to glass surface	Conducts electricity, acts as electrostatic shield; protects against infrared
Optical	Made of soda lime, lead, and borosilicate	Prisms, lenses, and optical mirrors
Pyroceram*	High thermal resistance, chemically stable, corrosion resistant	Hot plates, heat exchangers

*Corning Incorporated Life Sciences, Lowell, MA.

Teflon is an extremely inert plastic with excellent temperature tolerance (−270° C to +255° C) and chemical resistivity. Because of its nonwettable surface and antiadhesive properties, it is an excellent material for stir bars, bottle-cap liners, stopcocks, and tubing. It is one of the most desirable materials for use in water distribution systems; however, it is considerably more costly than other plastics used for this purpose. Although it is easy to clean and dry, it scratches and warps readily.

PVC plastic is soft and flexible but porous. It is used frequently in the form of tubing, particularly in older reagent water systems, and its drawbacks are discussed in the section on reagent water. Vendors of water systems now, in general, refrain from using PVC piping.

In many instances, plastic utensils should be used instead of glass because plastic utensils do not release ions into solution, and they are unbreakable. However, some plastics such as polyethylene are porous, and evaporation may be a problem. Therefore, long-term storage in partially filled plastic containers is undesirable. In addition, polyethylene and other plastics can adsorb proteins and other compounds such as dyes, stains, and some salts, resulting in analytical problems. Nevertheless, plastic containers are preferable for use in trace metal analyses. One can remove small quantities of trace metals in the plastic by soaking the plastic in 1 M HCl and rinsing with water purified to eliminate trace metal contamination. Long-term soaking (>8 h) in acid should be avoided because it makes the plastic brittle. Plastic also can be cleaned with alcohol, alkalis, or alcoholic alkalis to remove trace organic contaminants that contribute to trace metal adsorption.

Cleaning of Glass and Plastic Utensils

Glassware must be cleaned thoroughly before it is used in any analytical procedure. Unclean glassware causes chemical contamination. In addition, if glassware is not clean, the surface of the glass does not wet uniformly, and volume errors result, caused by incomplete drainage of dispensing devices or distortion of the meniscus.

Dirty utensils should be rinsed immediately after use and soaked in a weak detergent solution or a tenfold dilution of household bleach. Any vessels in which hazardous materials were contained should be handled separately to prevent unintentional exposure to the hazardous agent. Numerous effective cleaning agents are available for washing laboratory glassware and plasticware. Some items, such as pipets, require additional soaking before washing. In many institutions, washing is done by an automatic glassware washer. The manufacturers of automatic washers usually recommend or require specific detergents. In general, metal-free, nonionic detergents that are not highly alkaline are used. The washer must be equipped with the appropriate purified water rinse cycles to prevent contamination. If utensils are washed manually, they must be thoroughly rinsed with tap water and then rinsed three to five times with purified, preferably CLRW, water. When glassware is clean, purified water drains as a continuous film, whereas unclean vessels will have small drops of water clinging to the surface. After drying, the appearance of spots indicates unclean glassware, possibly the result of inadequate rinsing. This procedure is not appropriate for nonwettable plastics. Incomplete detergent removal can be detected by rinsing a vessel with a dilute (20 mg/L) aqueous solution of sulfobromophthalein (bromsulphalein) dye or some other acid-base indicator, or by measuring the pH of purified water added to the glassware.

As was previously mentioned, acid washing may be necessary in some instances. Dilute HCl (1 M) or dilute HNO_3 (1 M) is preferred. Chromic acid is no longer used for this procedure because of residual contamination and the hazards of handling and preparing the solutions.

Ultrasonic cleaners may be used to supplement the action of detergents. These may be particularly helpful in cleaning protein-coated utensils.

Both glassware and plasticware should be dried at room temperature or at temperatures below 100° C. This prevents degradation of the plastic and changes in the volume designations of glassware. If solvents are used to assist in drying, they should be of high quality and water miscible. Any gases used should also be of high purity.

KEY CONCEPTS BOX 1-3

- Borosilicate glass is best for laboratory work because it is pure, hard, and chemically resistant. Flint glass is a lower-quality glass that is used for disposable glass products.
- Polyolefin plastics are the most chemically resistant, and they are inert to most chemicals except hydrocarbons and organic acids.
- Teflon may be needed in special cases because of its excellent temperature tolerance and high chemical resistivity.
- Laboratory glassware/plasticware should be soaked in nonionic, metal-free detergent or bleach after use, washed in detergents, and rinsed with Clinical Laboratory Reagent Water (CLRW).

SECTION OBJECTIVES BOX 1-4

- List commonly used laboratory supplies, and describe the specific functions of beakers, funnels, graduated cylinders, flasks, and pipets.
- Differentiate between the terms "to contain" and "to deliver."
- Explain the difference between volumetric pipets and graduated pipets.
- Describe the construction and use of micropipets.
- List a procedure for the preparation of a reagent.
- Describe the proper procedures for using pipets.

LABORATORY UTENSILS

Beakers

Beakers (Fig. 1-1, 4) are wide-mouthed, straight-sided, cylindrical vessels that are available in both glass and plastic. Beaker volumes range from 5 mL to several liters. They are used for general mixing and preparation of nonvolumetric liquid reagents.

Funnels

Funnels are used most commonly to transfer liquids or solids into containers. Filtering funnels (Fig. 1-1, *7*) are usually 58- or 60-degree angled funnels with short or long, thin stems. They are used with filter paper to remove particles from solution. Many funnels have ridges that increase the surface area available for filtering. Powder funnels for use in transferring solids (see Fig. 1-1, *8*) have wide-mouthed stems that allow easy passage of solids. The inner surface of these funnels is smooth. Both filtering and powder funnels are available in plastic and glass. Separatory funnels (see Fig. 1-1, *2*) are constructed with a ground-glass stoppered opening at one end and a stopcock opening at the other end. These devices are used for manual liquid-liquid extractions of relatively large volumes of samples. The lower phase is separated from the upper phase through the stopcock, allowing salvage of one or both phases.

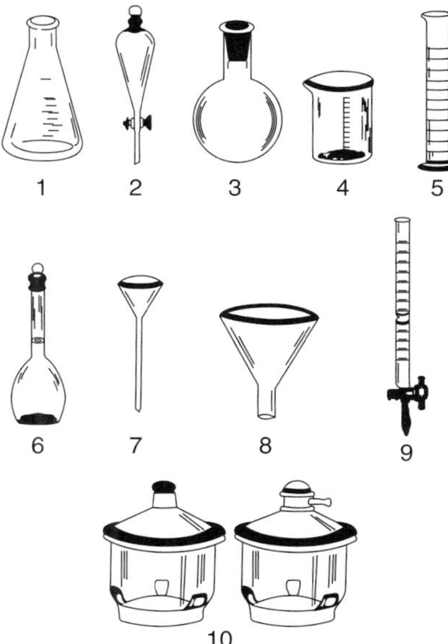

Fig. 1-1 Examples of commonly used laboratory utensils. *1,* Erlenmeyer flask. *2,* Separatory funnel. *3,* Round-bottom flask. *4,* Beaker. *5,* Graduated cylinder. *6,* Volumetric flask. *7,* Long-stem funnel (filtering). *8,* Powder funnel. *9,* Buret. *10,* Desiccators.

Desiccators

Desiccators (see Fig. 1-1, *10*) are used to dry, or keep dry, solid or liquid materials. The desiccant usually is placed in the bottom of the desiccator and a shelf is placed above the desiccant. The material then is stored on top of the shelf. The top of the desiccator has a wide, flat, ground-glass lip that fits snugly against an opposing lip on the bottom part of the desiccator. Stopcock grease usually is placed on the surface of the lips to provide an airtight seal. Many desiccators also have a stopcock outlet on the upper portion that allows the desiccator to be evacuated. Laboratories often have several desiccators to allow for storage at different temperatures, including ambient, refrigerator, and freezer temperatures. The types of desiccants available are described in Table 1-1.

Graduated Cylinders

Graduated cylinders are narrow, straight-sided vessels that are used to measure specific volumes (see Fig. 1-1, *5*). They are available in plastic and glass in sizes ranging from 5 mL to several liters. They may be calibrated to deliver (TD) or to contain (TC) the volume indicated at specific temperatures, and they are graduated into subdivisions of approximately 100 portions of the total volume of the cylinder. Sometimes they are equipped with stoppers and are used to prepare

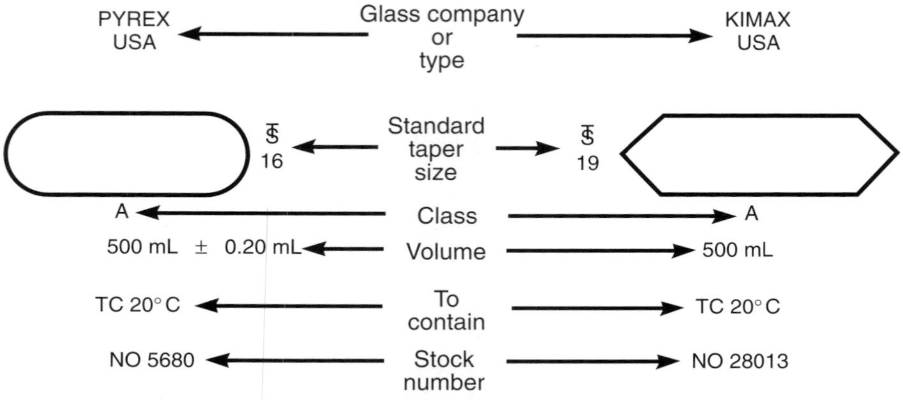

Fig. 1-2 Example of National Institute of Standards and Technology (NIST) specifications found imprinted on Class A volumetric flasks.

solutions that require less accuracy than those prepared volumetrically.

Burets

Traditional **burets** are long, graduated glass tubes with a stopcock at one end (see Fig. 1-1, *9*). These devices are used to deliver, accurately, known amounts of liquid into a container. Through measurement from graduated line to graduated line, fractional volumes of less than 1 mL may be dispensed with a high degree of accuracy. Microprocessor-controlled automatic burets now are available with accuracy as high as 0.1%. Dispensed volumes are monitored on a digital display capable of reading to 0.001 mL.

Flasks

Flasks of many types are used in the clinical laboratory; the most commonly used are the volumetric and **Erlenmeyer flasks** shown in Fig. 1-1, *1* and *6*. Round-bottom flasks often are used to evaporate a sample to dryness. The sizes of laboratory flasks range from 1 mL to several liters.

Volumetric Flasks

Volumetric flasks are essential for the accurate preparation of solutions of known concentration. Class A specifications for volumetric flasks are defined by the NIST and imprinted on the glass (Fig. 1-2). These specifications are accurate only at the temperature specified on the flask (Table 1-3). Volumetric flasks are used to contain (TC) an exact volume when the flask is appropriately filled to the indicator line. Such flasks therefore do not deliver an exact volume and cannot be used as transfer devices. The top of the volumetric flask is capped by a tight-fitting ground-glass or Teflon stopper. This allows the flask to be inverted without loss of liquid. Under no circumstances should a volumetric flask be heated because heating can distort the shape and volume of the flask. Volumetric flasks should not be used for reagent storage.

Table 1-3 Accuracies of Volumetric Flasks

Capacity, mL	Limit of Error, mL	Percent Error
25	0.03	0.1
50	0.05	0.1
100	0.08	0.08
250	0.11	0.04
500	0.15	0.03
1000	0.30	0.03

Syringes

Syringes may be used for accurate volumetric work such as injection of small volumes of a sample, liquid or gas, for chromatographic analysis. Syringes are available in a range of sizes from 1 to 500 μL. They are constructed of glass and have a precision-bore hole into which a tight-fitting plunger is placed. The dispensing tip of the syringe is a very fine diameter metal needle that is able to pierce the septum of the injection port. For syringes of greater than 5 μL volume, manufacturers claim that inaccuracy will not exceed 1% of the total syringe volume, and repeated measurements will not differ by more than 1% of the dispensed volume. For devices with less than 5 μL volume, 2% inaccuracy is the best that is achievable. In general, syringes are not calibrated because internal standards are employed in chromatographic procedures, allowing for correction of transfer errors. For gas chromatographic work with volatile samples, the syringes must be airtight.

Automatic syringes are used to deliver reagents and samples in automated laboratory instruments (see p. 370, Chapter 20).

Pipets

Most **pipets** are made of glass, although plastic serological pipets are available. Two general categories of manual pipets have been defined: transfer (volumetric) and measuring. Within these categories, three subclassifications exist to contain (TC), to deliver (TD), and to deliver/blow-out (TD/blow-out).

TC or rinse-out pipets must be refilled or rinsed with the appropriate solvent after the initial liquid has been drained from the pipet. These pipets contain or hold an exact amount of liquid that must be completely transferred for accurate measurement. Some examples of TC pipets are Sahli

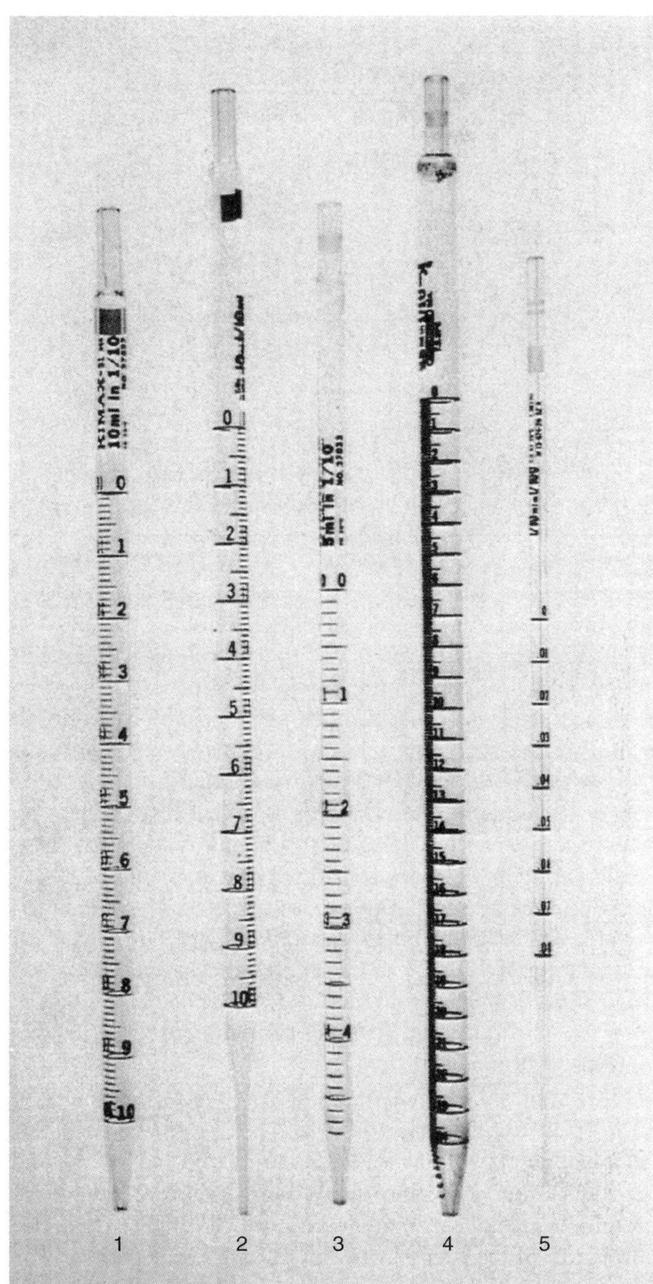

Fig. 1-3 Examples of transfer to deliver (TD) pipets. *1,* Mohr. *2,* Mohr long tip. *3,* Serological. *4,* Serological large opening. *5,* Serological long tip.

hemoglobin (Ward's Natural Science, Rochester, NY), transfer micro, and Lang-Levy pipets (Beilco Glass, Inc., Vineland, NJ). None of these devices meets Class A specifications. TD/blow-out pipets are filled and allowed to drain; afterward, the remaining fluid in the tip is blown out. These devices thus transfer or deliver an exact amount of liquid and are not rinsed out. Pipets belonging to this group include Ostwald-Folin (Thermo Fisher Scientific, Inc., Waltham, MA) and serological devices. These are easily identified by two frosted bands near the mouthpiece of the pipet (Fig. 1-3). Serological pipets are long, glass (or plastic) tubes of uniform diameter. They have volume graduations that extend to the delivery tip of the pipet. Thus the last drop of liquid blown out is included in the delivery volume. These pipets have long, tapered tips and variable tip openings that allow for controlled delivery. Pipets with large-tipped openings are used for delivery of viscous fluids.

Table 1-4 Accuracies (in mL) of Manual Pipets

Type of Pipet	1.0 mL	5.0 mL	10.0 mL	25.0 mL
NIST standard	—	0.01	0.02	0.025
Class A volumetric	0.006	0.01	0.02	0.03
Mohr	0.01	0.02	0.03	0.10
Mohr long tip	0.02	0.04	0.06	—
Serological	0.01	0.02	0.03	0.10
Serological large opening	0.05	0.10	0.10	0.20
Serological long tip	0.02	0.04	0.06	—

NIST, National Institute of Standards and Technology.

TD pipets are filled and allowed to drain by gravity. To ensure complete drainage, the flow rates are set to specifications defined by the NIST. The pipet must be held vertically and the tip placed against the side of the accepting vessel but not touching the liquid in it. Graduated TD pipets provide for accurate delivery of volumes smaller than the total pipet capacity by using the graduated lines to control the amount of liquid delivered. Pipets classified in this group include volumetric transfer, Mohr, and serological pipets (see Figs. 1-3 and 1-4). TD pipets meet Class A standards.

Volumetric (TD) pipets (see Fig. 1-4) consist of (1) an open-ended bulb, which holds the bulk of the liquid; (2) a long, glass tube at one end with a line (mark) indicating the extent to which the pipet is to be filled; and (3) a tapered delivery portion. After draining, these devices deliver the exact volume specified with a high degree of accuracy (Table 1-4). Ostwald-Folin (TD) pipets are similar in appearance to volumetric pipets, but their bulbs are closer to the delivery tip. They are used for accurate measurement of viscous liquids such as blood or serum and require that the contents be blown out. Thus they have etched bands near the top. To ensure complete delivery of the viscous fluid, the liquid is blown out after the pipet is allowed to drain freely to the last drop.

Mohr (TD) pipets are uniform in diameter with tapered delivery tips. Graduations are incised on the stem at uniform intervals so that calibration occurs above but not on the tip. The accuracy listed for these pipets is valid only when the pipet is filled. If smaller volumes are dispensed, the accuracy decreases proportionately. Mohr pipets with long tips are used for dispensing liquids into small vials. They are less accurate than the standard tapered-tip variety. Mohr pipets are never used as blow-out devices. The accuracy of Mohr and other pipets is summarized in Table 1-4.

Micropipets

Micropipets contain or deliver small volumes of liquid ranging from 1 to 1000 μL. Inexpensive disposable tubes with specific

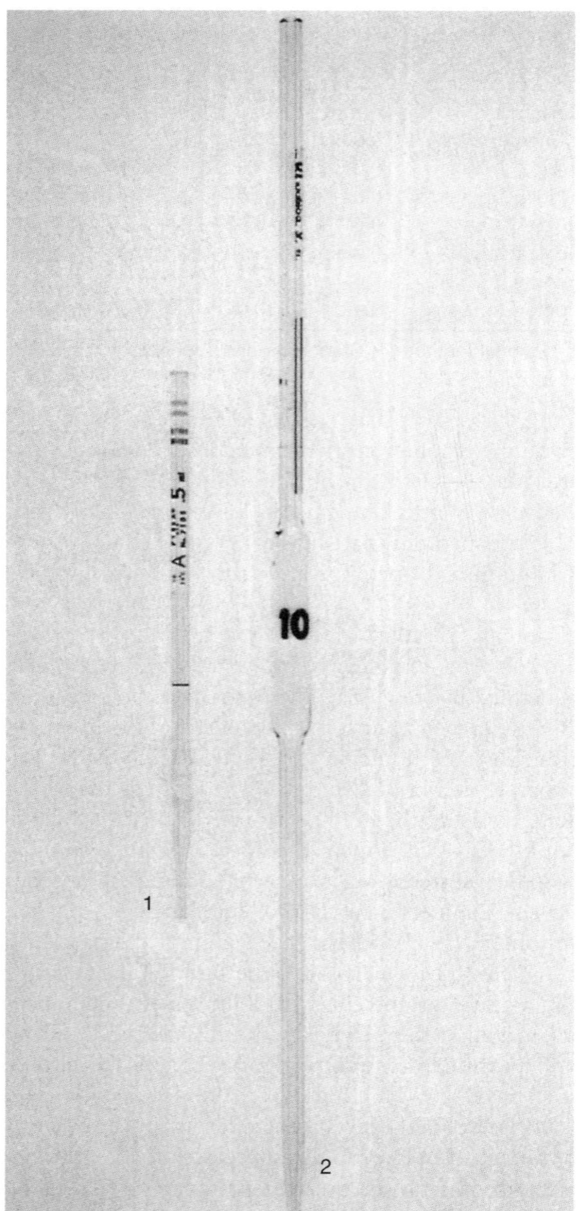

Fig. 1-4 Examples of to deliver (TD) pipets. *1,* Ostwald-Folin. *2,* Class A volumetric.

Fig. 1-5 Steps in using Eppendorf type of micropipet. **A,** Attaching proper tip size for range of pipet volume and twisting tip as it is pushed onto pipet to give an airtight, continuous seal. **B,** Holding pipet before use. **C,** Detailed instructions for filling and emptying of pipet tip. Follow manufacturer's complete instructions for care and use of micropipets.

volume demarcations are available. They are filled by capillary action, and the liquid is blown out of the tube by a device that is similar to a medicine dropper.

The most common type of micropipet is a semiautomated device that uses air displacement or positive displacement to dispense the contained liquid. Models with a digital volume adjustment are also available. Many brands of air displacement pipets are available, but all are piston-operated devices. A disposable and exchangeable polypropylene tip is attached to the pipet barrel, and liquid is drawn into and dispensed from this disposable tip (Fig. 1-5). Some instruments can automatically eject the used pipet tip and reload a new one, thereby minimizing analytical contamination. Several brands of positive displacement pipets are also available. The capillary tips, which may be made of siliconized glass, glass, or plastic, can be reused. These devices are particularly useful for handling reagents that react with plastics. Positive displacement pipettors deliver liquid by means of a Teflon-tipped plunger that fits snugly inside the capillary. Carryover of liquid is negligible in properly maintained instruments. In some instances, a washing step is used between samples.

The precision and accuracy of these devices are excellent if they are properly maintained. Sample recovery is at least 99%, with reproducibility errors of 0.6% to 0.3% for volumes between 10 and 500 μL. For volumes less than 10 μL, the errors are significantly larger. For this reason, manual procedures involving small volumes should be avoided.

Dilutors and Dispensers

Manual dispensers and pipettors frequently are used in the laboratory to add repeatedly a specified volume of reagent or diluent to a solution. Several types are commercially available, but all consist of a reagent bottle to which a plunger with a valve system is attached. The dispenser is fitted with a tube or a straw that reaches to the bottom of the bottle. The device must be primed with liquid to ensure removal of any air bubbles. Once primed, depression of the plunger delivers a selected amount of liquid. Return of the plunger to the original position refills the dispenser chamber. Manufacturers claim an error rate of 1% and a reproducibility rate of 0.1% for these devices at full deflection of the plunger. Manual dispensers require frequent cleaning to remove material that can hamper piston action.

Repetitively dispensing pipettors are useful for the serial dispensing of relatively small volumes of the same liquid. The volume dispensed is determined by the pipettor setting and by the size of the disposable syringe tip, which also acts as the liquid reservoir.

Automated dilutor-dispensers frequently are used to prepare many samples for analysis. Such devices can be an integral part of an automated chemistry analyzer. The dispensers pipet a preset volume of sample and diluent into a receiving vessel or instrument. The frequently used dual-piston dispenser allows adjustment of both sample and diluent volumes. One motor-driven syringe processes the sample, the other the diluent. The syringes are activated by a microprocessor, which allows each piston to fill the syringes simultaneously. A second signal repositions the valves to allow diluent to flow through the sample syringe. This displaces the sample, forcing it through the pipet tip and rinsing it in preparation for the next sample. Variable ratios of sample to diluent can be selected. However, a tenfold volume of diluent ensures adequate rinsing and negligible carryover. The inaccuracy is considered to be less than 0.5% of dispensed volume, and reproducibility is on the order of 0.05% of full-syringe volume, or 0.1% when at least 10% of the syringe volume is dispensed.

VOLUMETRIC TECHNIQUES

Class A Pipets

Clinical chemistry analytical procedures require exact volumetric measurements and transfers to ensure accurate results; Class A glassware therefore is required. In fact, the College of American Pathologists (CAP) specifies that volumetric pipets must be of certified accuracy (Class A), or the volumes of the devices must be verified (e.g., by a gravimetric or photometric procedure). In addition, automatic pipets and diluting devices must be checked periodically for accuracy and precision. Therefore, most laboratories routinely use Class A glassware.

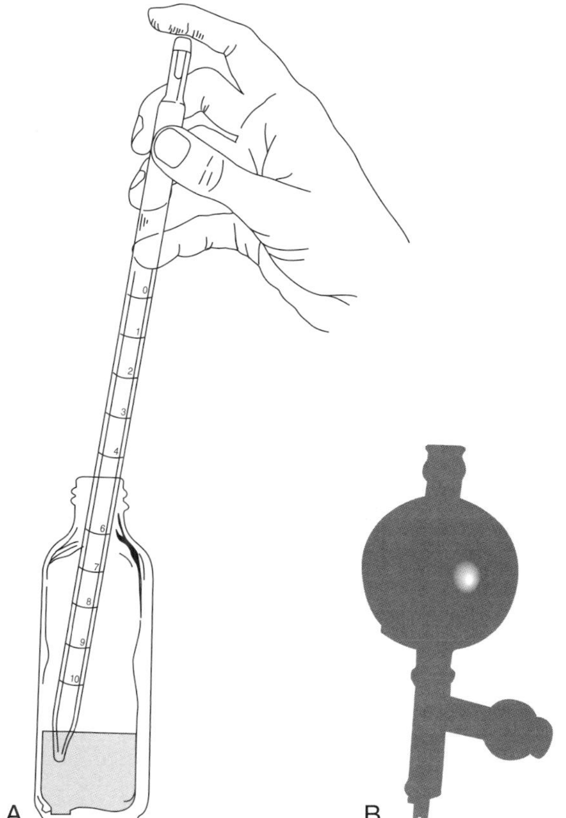

Fig. 1-6 A, Proper pipetting technique as described in text. **B,** Example of rubber pipetting bulb used to aspirate sample into pipet.

In addition, the glassware must be scrupulously clean; beads of liquid cling to the sides of dirty vessels and pipets, and volume measurements are inaccurate. Borosilicate glass pipets must be inspected frequently. Pipets with broken tips or etched glass should be discarded.

Class A pipets are filled with the aid of a rubber bulb or similar device. Under no circumstances is mouth pipetting permissible. The bulb is used to fill the pipet to above the calibration mark. The pipet is grasped by the thumb and the middle finger, with the index finger placed over the upper opening to control the flow of liquid (Fig. 1-6). After the pipet is filled above the mark, the tip is wiped with a lint-free tissue to remove excess fluid. The liquid then is allowed to drain so that the lowest part of the meniscus, sighted at eye level, is lined up with the mark; after this, the pipet is transferred to the receiving vessel. Next, the pipet is held in a vertical position with the tip against the side of the receiving vessel, and the liquid is drained as the index finger is removed from the pipet orifice. TD pipets must be held in position long enough (≈2 sec) to permit delivery of the specified volume. With TC or blow-out pipets, the rubber bulb is used to blow out the last remaining solution after drainage is complete.

Micropipets

Air displacement micropipets may be used in either of two modes, the forward mode or the reverse mode. The reverse mode is used with two-component stroke mechanism systems only. The precision of these devices in the forward mode depends on the precise draining caused by the air pressure, and they are relatively sensitive to the physical characteristics of the liquid being pipetted. Reverse mode operation, on the other hand, is considerably less sensitive to the type of liquid that is being dispensed. In the forward mode, the piston is depressed to the first stop position on a two-stroke device, the tip is placed in the liquid, and the piston is allowed to rise back slowly to the original position. This fills the tip with the designated volume of liquid. The pipet tip then is drawn up the sidewall of the vessel so that any adhering liquid is removed. If any extraneous droplets are visible, the tip is wiped carefully with a lint-free tissue, with care taken not to "wick" out any sample from the pipet tip. The tip then is placed on the wall of the receiving vessel, and the piston is depressed smoothly to the first stop position on a two-stroke device, allowing the liquid to drain. After 1 second, the piston is depressed to the second stop, blowing out the remaining liquid. When the reverse mode is used, the liquid is aspirated after depression to the second stop position. This overfills the pipet with sample. To dispense the liquid, the piston is depressed to the first stop, and, after 1 second, the pipet is removed.

Positive displacement micropipets are used in the same manner as forward mode air displacement devices. Again, careful wiping of the tip is crucial in order not to wick out a sample from the tip. The need for maintenance of the Teflon tip cannot be overemphasized. More detailed information on this technique is published elsewhere.[10]

General Procedures for Solution Preparation

Solution preparation requires accurate measurement of solute and solvent. The degree of accuracy required dictates the specific glassware to be used. The following procedure may be used for solution preparation:

1. Measure the solute by weighing, pipetting, or dispensing from a graduated cylinder or pipettor (as examples).
2. Prepare volumetric solutions by quantitatively transferring the solute to the receiving flask. If the solute exists as a stock solution, a volumetric pipet is used for transfer.
3. Add sufficient solvent to dissolve the solute where necessary.
4. If the receiving flask is a volumetric flask, add the solids or liquids to the flask, and then add diluent to approximately two-thirds the volume of the flask. Dissolution of the solid or liquid can be effected by swirling the liquid. Bring the solution to volume after the solute is completely dissolved. After dissolution, continue adding diluent until the meniscus, sighted at eye level, reaches the line etched into the neck of the flask. Completely mix the solution by placing a cover on the opening of the flask, holding the neck of the flask in your hand, and swirling the liquid while simultaneously inverting the flask. Alternatively, the **dilution** or dissolving of a solid in diluent can be achieved in an Erlenmeyer flask. The solution then is transferred to a volumetric flask; this is followed by several washes of the Erlenmeyer flask with diluent, transferring the liquid used for the washes to the volumetric flask.
5. If the use of a magnetic stir bar is necessary, remove the bar and rinse it with solvent before bringing the solution to volume.
6. Bring the solution to volume at room temperature only.
7. Mix the solution well to ensure homogeneity.
8. Transfer the solution to an appropriate reagent storage container (amber/clear, plastic/glass).

Quality Control of Micropipets, Dispensers, and Dilutors

General

The accuracy and precision of each manual micropipet should be verified on acquisition and monitored during the course of the year. The frequency of verification depends on the amount of use. Heavily used devices may need monthly verification, whereas rarely used devices may need to be checked only once or twice per year unless more frequent validation is mandated by an inspection agency. Manufacturers of newer micropipets are claiming 2-year calibration stability; however, more frequent calibrations will be required by inspection agencies.

Routine maintenance is crucial. Air displacement pipets have a fixed stroke length that must be maintained. In addition, such pipets have seals that prevent air from leaking into the pipet when the piston is moved, and these must be greased to maintain proper operation. The manufacturer will provide guidelines for performing this maintenance. Any worn parts must be replaced, and devices that do not meet specifications for precision or accuracy generally require servicing by the manufacturer.

Positive displacement pipets, in general, require similar maintenance with regard to spring checks and replacement of Teflon tips. Many of these devices also are supplied with a slide wire that is used to quickly check the plunger setting. This device cannot be used in place of routine performance checks. Again, the manufacturer provides guidelines for performing routine maintenance.

Quality Control Validation

The long established method for validating performance of micropipets is a gravimetric technique. Gravimetric methods are described in two different international standards.[11,12] Details vary slightly between the two standards, but these methods give equivalent results at larger volumes (for pipetting of hundreds of microliters or greater). At smaller volumes, gravimetric methods may produce different results because of details of how evaporation is measured and compensated for, and at very small volumes, below 20 μL, extreme care and strict environmental controls are necessary to achieve consistent results. Balance resolution requirements vary with test volume. A four-place analytical balance is suitable for volumes above 100 μL, and a six-place balance (single microgram resolution) is required for volumes of 10 μL and smaller.

Spectrophotometric procedures have been used for some time, and methods based on potassium dichromate, or single-dye commercial kits, are available. In 2005, the method was

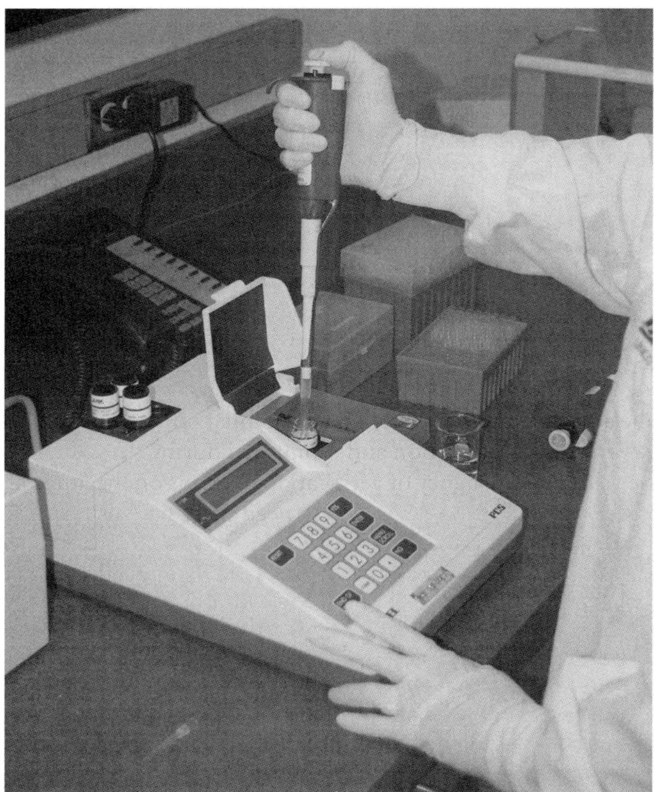

Fig. 1-7 Spectrophotometric apparatus for pipet calibration. (Courtesy of Artel, Westbrook, ME.)

made into an international standard,[13] which states that "uncertainty with this method tends to become lower as test volumes decrease." This makes the photometric method well suited for small volumetric micropipets, or for use in laboratories that lack high-resolution microgram balances.

The spectrophotometric method has gained in popularity because of the availability of commercial systems offered by Artel (Westbrook, ME). Systems include a dedicated spectrophotometer, Pipette Calibration System (PCS), and prepackaged and certified dye reagents (Fig. 1-7). The system uses a dual-dye ratiometric approach, which the company claims provides better precision and accuracy at low volumes when compared with the gravimetric method, which is prone to evaporation and other environmental factors. The PCS calculates and records calibration results automatically, thereby meeting the requirements of inspecting agencies. The results may be printed out to provide the hard copies needed for inspection. Artel also offers the Multichannel Verification System (MVS), which is used for assessment of multichannel and automated devices.

The following protocol, which describes the gravimetric method of verification, is based on the procedure described in the older National Committee on Clinical Laboratory Standards (NCCLS) guideline, *Determining Performance of Volumetric Equipment*[10]:

1. Make sure that all items used (water, weighing vials, and pipets) are at room temperature.
2. All measurements require the use of Type I water.
3. Measure and record the barometric pressure and the ambient temperature (t) of the water to 0.1°C.
4. To minimize evaporation errors, place a small amount of water in the weighing vessel (between 2 and 30 sample volumes, or a minimum of 0.5 mL). Cover with a square of Parafilm (Pechiney Plastic Packaging Company, Des Moines, IA) or a stopper. Ensure that all manipulations are performed without direct handling of the vial.
5. Weigh the vial (water and cover) and record the weight to the nearest 0.1 mg (W_v), or preferably, set to zero the weight of the vial, water, and cover.
6. Transfer the aliquot of water to be measured to the weighing vial using the pipet to be tested. Recover the vial.
7. Reweigh the vial to the nearest 0.1 mg and record the weight (W_t).
8. Repeat these measurements (W_v and W_t) to obtain 10 readings so as to evaluate both accuracy and precision. (A "quick check" method of four samplings allows rough assessment of precision.)
9. Calculate the mean weight ($\bar{W}_t$) as follows:

$$\bar{W}_t = \sum \frac{W_t}{n} - \sum \frac{W_v}{n}$$

   where *n* is the number of repetitive weighings.
10. Refer to *The Handbook of Chemistry and Physics* (*88th ed*, Taylor and Francis Group, 2008, LLC) to obtain the correction factor for the water temperature. Assess the conversion factor *z* (μL/mg), while incorporating the density of water at the test temperature and pressure.
11. Calculate the volume measured as follows:

$$\text{Mean volume, } \bar{V}_t = \text{Mean weight, } \bar{W}_t \times z$$

   where $\bar{W}_t$ is calculated from #9 above.
12. The accuracy is computed by evaluating the difference between the actual mean volume measured and the nominal volume as stated by the manufacturer, expressed as %:

$$\frac{\text{Mean volume}}{\text{Nominal volume}} \times 100\%$$

13. The precision is derived from the distribution of the individual weighings about their mean and is expressed as percent coefficient of variation (%CV).

In general, an error of 0.1% or less in accuracy may be ignored when the pipet is used. Larger errors may have to be evaluated more critically and the pipet adjusted, if necessary, to achieve a more accurate volume. Manufacturers may use mercury in place of water to assess performance. This practice is not acceptable in a routine laboratory setting.

The practice of using radioisotopes and enzymes is unacceptable because of large inherent errors and poor standardization. Other methods such as acid-base titration and coulometry have been suggested, but adequate documentation is not available to validate these methods.

Many laboratories today no longer have access to an appropriate analytical balance to perform micropipet accuracy and precision. This has led to the appearance of purchased micropipet services. The vendors of these services come to the laboratory with an analytical balance and perform the weighings required to verify pipet performance. In addition, they generally have the supplies needed to service any devices that require maintenance. If a laboratory uses such services, it is crucial that the vendor provide hard copies of each calibration, as well as documentation of certification of the balance used to perform the testing. Inspection agencies will require such documentation regardless of whether the testing is performed by the laboratory staff or by a vendor.

The accuracy of a dispenser can also be evaluated by a gravimetric procedure. The volume to be tested is set and the device is primed to ensure that no air bubbles are present. The water then is carefully dispensed into a preweighed test tube or other container, and the resulting volume is determined by the same equation used for pipet testing. A graduated cylinder can be used to make a rough assessment of the dispenser's performance. This procedure is helpful when one is making adjustments to the dispenser volume and provides a mechanism for daily verification. The gravimetric procedure should be performed at regular intervals (monthly, quarterly), depending on the use of the pipettor. Because this procedure involves larger volumes of liquid, a standard precision balance is adequate to assess the accuracy of the settings on the dispenser.

Automatic dilutors are best evaluated with the use of a potassium dichromate spectrophotometric method. A series of dilutions ($n = 20$) are prepared by the dilutor, measured spectrophotometrically, and then compared with a manual dilution made in the same volume ratios. The manual dilution must be prepared in volumetric flasks with sufficiently large volumes of sample (no less than 1 mL) to ensure accuracy. The absorbance of the samples prepared with the automatic dilutor then is compared with that of the sample diluted manually, and the accuracy of the automatic dilutor is computed as previously described. Agreement should be within 2%. Similarly, precision is computed with the distribution of individual absorbances about the mean, expressed as %CV. The %CV should be no more than 1%. This procedure can be used to evaluate some dilutor systems incorporated into automated instruments. Again, procedures involving the use of enzymes are unacceptable. The frequency of verification is determined by the amount of use. Monthly determinations are sufficient for most devices, including dilutors incorporated into automated equipment. As was mentioned previously, Artel has a device that is commercially available to perform automatic dilutor validation.

Pipets, dilutors, and dispensers must be reevaluated whenever the devices are serviced or repaired. All procedures must be documented and records maintained according to federal, state, and local inspection agency guidelines.

KEY CONCEPTS BOX 1-4

- "To contain" (TC) labware is designed to contain the volume specified on the container. "To deliver" (TD) labware is designed to deliver the volume specified on the container.
- Beakers are wide-mouthed, straight-sided vessels that are used to mix and prepare reagents.
- Funnels are designed to allow transfer of solids or liquids into a container.
- Cylinders, which are narrow-mouthed, straight-sided vessels, are designed TC or TD with a specified volume listed on the side of the cylinder.
- Flasks have narrower mouths and are used to mix and prepare reagents. Volumetric flasks are designed to prepare reagents with exact concentrations.
- TD pipets usually are designed to deliver the volume specified on the pipet, by passive drainage of liquid from the upright pipet. Type A pipets are required for the most exact volume transfers. Some TD pipets require blowing out the last remaining liquid in the pipet. TC pipets require rinsing the pipet out to deliver the specified volume. All pipets must be filled only with the use of rubber pipetting bulbs, with eyeing of the meniscus at eye level. Care must be taken when the tips of the pipets are wiped.
- Graduated pipets deliver a specified volume by draining liquid from graduated point to graduated point drawn on the pipet.
- Micropipets deliver volume through disposable glass or plastic tips. The accuracy and reproducibility of micropipets can be monitored through gravimetric or spectrophotometric procedures.

UNITS OF MEASUREMENT

SI Units

The **Système International d'Unités (SI)** system, which is based on the **metric system,** consists of seven basic units[14] (Table 1-5). Two or more basic units may be combined by multiplication or division to form SI-derived units (Table 1-6). Basic and derived units may be too large or too small for convenient use. Prefixes that form decimal multiples or submultiples of the units are permissible (Table 1-7). A few non-SI units have been retained because of difficulties encountered

Table 1-5 Basic Quantities and Units of the Système International d'Unités (SI)

Quantity	Basic Unit	Symbol
Length	Meter	m
Mass	Kilogram	kg
Time	Second	s
Electrical current	Ampere	A
Temperature	Kelvin	K
Luminous intensity	Candela	cd
Amount of substance	Mole	mol

Table 1-6 SI-Derived Units Used in Medicine

Derived Quantity	Derived Unit	Symbol
Area	Square meter	m^2
Volume	Cubic meter	m^3
Speed	Meter per second	m/s or $m \times s^{-1}$
Substance concentration	Mole per cubic meter	mol/m^3, or $mol \times m^{-3}$
Pressure	Pascal	Pa
Work energy or quantity of heat	Joule	J
Celsius temperature	Celsius degree	°C
Activity (radionuclide)	Becquerel	Bq
Power	Watt	W
Electrical charge or quantity	Coulomb	C
Electrical potential	Volt	V
Resistance		Ω
Conductance	Siemens	S

Table 1-7 SI Prefixes

Prefix*	Factor	Symbol
atto-	10^{-18}	a
femto-	10^{-15}	f
pico-	10^{-12}	p
nano-	10^{-9}	n
micro-	10^{-6}	μ
milli-	10^{-3}	m
centi-	10^{-2}	c
deci-	10^{-1}	d
deka-	10^{1}	da
hecto-	10^{2}	h
kilo-	10^{3}	k
mega-	10^{6}	M
giga-	10^{9}	G
tera-	10^{12}	T
peta-	10^{15}	P
exa-	10^{18}	E

*It is recommended that only one prefix be used.

in converting them to SI units or because of their widespread use. Non-SI units relevant to clinical chemistry and its symbols include time, expressed in minutes (min), hours (hr), or days (d); and volume, expressed as liters (L) or deciliters (dL). The General Conference of Weights and Measures (Conférence Générale des Poids et Mésures [CGPM]) has approved l, *l*, or L as the volume designation; however, L is the official abbreviation accepted in the United States.

SI Units in the Clinical Laboratory

The SI unit describes the concentration of body constituents in terms of the number of dissolved molecules, measured in moles (mol, mmol, and so on), rather than the amount of dissolved mass (mg, g, and so on).[14-18] A mole of a chemical contains the number of grams equivalent to its formula mass (see p. 33). The SI unit of enzyme activity is the katal, which is defined as the amount of enzyme that will catalyze the transformation of 1 mole of substrate per second in an assay system. This terminology has been approved by the Joint Commission on Biochemical Nomenclature of the International Union of Biochemistry (IUB) and the IUPAC but has not been approved by CGPM. Thus, the use of International Units (IU or U) to describe enzyme activity will undoubtedly continue (see Chapter 15). There is a constant relationship between the katal and the IU (1 katal = 16.67 IU) when measured under identical conditions of temperature, pH, substrate, and coenzyme concentration.

Often SI units are not used when the molecular weight of a protein is uncertain. However, even under these conditions, it is possible to express substance concentration rather than mass concentration, provided that the approximate molecular weight is included in the documentation. Such an approach also applies to hormones. IUs are used to express enzyme activity, whereas SI units are used for reporting osmolality. The SI unit for reporting pressure is the pascal. However, the numerical values expressed in pascals for blood pressure and blood gas partial pressures are too large; therefore, the kilopascal is the preferred unit. For further information regarding the SI system, the reader should refer to the NIST publication, *Guide for the Use of the International System of Units.*[16]

SECTION OBJECTIVES BOX 1-5

- Describe the proper operation, maintenance, and quality control of balances, centrifuges, water baths, and heating blocks in the clinical laboratory.
- Describe the use and calibration of thermometers.
- Define an immersion thermometer.
- List the liquids that can be used in liquid-in-glass thermometers.
- Describe the differences in operation of a swing-bucket and a fixed-angle centrifuge.
- Given a desired relative centrifugal force (RCF) and the known radius of a centrifuge, calculate the revolutions per minute (rpm) needed to achieve the desired RCF.

MEASUREMENT OF MASS

Mass may be defined as the quantity of matter. Weight is a function of mass under the influence of gravity as expressed by the equation:

$$\text{Weight} = \text{Mass} \times \text{Gravity}$$

Thus two objects of equal mass that are subject to the same gravitational force have equal weights. The gram (g) is a unit of mass. Measurement of mass or weight is achieved through use of a balance. The type of balance selected depends on the function that is being performed. Different **balances** are required for measuring kilogram (kg) weights (e.g., for fecal fat analysis) and microgram weights (e.g., for preparation of drug standards for toxicology analyses). Laboratories are equipped with different balances so that all necessary weight measurements can be performed.

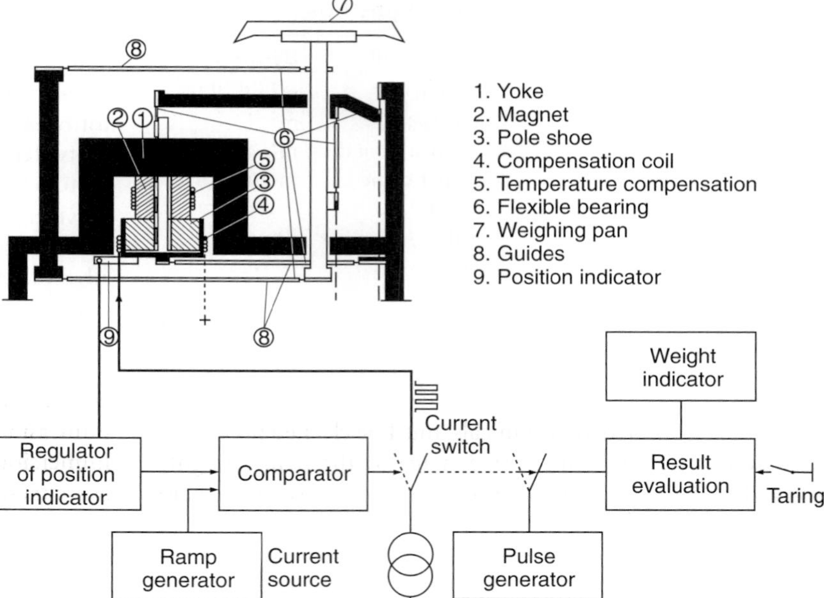

Fig. 1-8 Switching principle of an electronic force compensator balance. (Courtesy Mettler Toledo, Inc., Columbus, OH.)

Types of Balances

The electronic balance is a single pan balance that uses an electromagnetic force instead of weights to counterbalance the load placed on the pan (Fig. 1-8). The pan is attached directly to a coil suspended in the field of a permanent magnet. A current is passed through the coil, producing an electromagnetic force that keeps the pan in a constant position. When a load is placed on the pan, a photoelectric-cell scanning device attached to the lever arm changes position and transmits a current to an amplifier that increases the current flow through the coil and restores the pan to its original position. This current, which is proportional to the weight of the load on the pan, produces a measurable voltage that is converted by a microprocessor to a numerical display or data output that gives the mass of the load. The accuracy of an electronic balance depends on the linearity of both the torque motor and the digital voltmeter. Some electronic balances have a built-in electronic vibration damper. Excessive vibration can be detected when variation of the pointer or oscillation of numbers in the last decimal place of the digital display is observed. Most electronic balances have built-in taring ability that allows the weight of the weighing vessel to be "zeroed." This is a great convenience when performing multiple weighings, as for pipet calibrations. In addition, electronic balances can be interfaced with data processing equipment, thus providing calculations such as weight averaging and statistical analysis of multiple weighings. Electronic balances allow completion of weighings in 5 seconds or less. Table 1-8 summarizes the performance characteristics of balances.

Table 1-8 Characterization of Types of Balances in Relation to Their Operation

Type of Balance	Weighting Capacity, g	Readability	Reproducibility
Precision balances	32,000	0.1 g	±0.1 g
	16,000	0.1 g	±0.05 g
	6000	0.01 g	±0.01 g
	2000	0.01 g	±0.005 g
	1200	0.001 g	±0.001 g
	110	0.001 g	±0.0005 g
Analytical balances	210	0.1 mg	±0.1 mg
	205	0.01 mg	±0.03 mg
	50	0.1 mg	±0.1 mg
	20	2 μg	±3 μg
Microbalances	5.1	1 μg	±0.9 μg
	2.1	0.1 μg	±0.25 μg

Requirements for Operation

All balances should be located away from direct sunlight and drafts that can interfere with the weighing process. Analytical balances should be placed in a vibration-free location, preferably on an isolated heavy (such as marble) table. The more sensitive the balance, the more crucial these requirements are. Before a balance is used, it should be leveled by adjusting the foot screws and centering the bubble in the spirit level. The optical zero also should be verified. All weighings must be performed with the use of weighing paper, plastic boats, **beakers,** or some other container. Under no conditions should chemicals be placed directly on the pan. After the weighing process has been completed, all loose chemical crystals must be removed from the balance area. Similarly, any liquid spills,

Table 1-9 Individual NIST Tolerances for Class S Weights

Nominal Mass	Individual Tolerance, mg	Maintenance Tolerance, mg
1, 2, 3, 4, 10, 20, 30, 50 mg	±0.014	±0.014
100, 200, 300, 500 mg	±0.025	±0.05
1, 2, 3, 5 g	±0.054	±0.11
10, 20, 30 g	±0.074	±0.148
50 g	±0.12	±0.25
100 g	±0.25	±0.5

NIST, National Institute of Standards and Technology.

particularly of corrosive chemicals, must be cleaned up immediately to prevent permanent damage to the pans. Weights should be handled with the use of forceps, never with bare hands. Direct contact with skin causes oils, salts, and moisture to be deposited on the weights. The smaller the weight, the more significant is the effect.

Maintenance Procedures

In addition to the requirements already described, balances should be serviced at least annually, more frequently if they are heavily used. Service must be performed by the manufacturer or its representative. Periodic checks to verify weight accuracy are required, and records must be kept to document quality control and maintenance procedures. Verification procedures should be performed at least monthly and before any crucial analytical procedure is undertaken. Verification of performance requires the use of NIST Class S weights. The CAP also requires that approved laboratories validate balance performance with the use of Class S weights.[19] A 100 g weight should weigh 100 g ± 0.5 mg. Class S weights should be checked to verify that their apparent weights are within NIST specifications (Table 1-9). Unacceptable performance indicates the need for service. Some newer analytical balances have a single built-in weight for performing this function. Such balances still require verification of the entire measuring range.

THERMOMETRY

Types of Thermometers

Water baths and **heating blocks** must be maintained at constant temperature when temperature-sensitive assays are performed. Refrigerators and freezers must be maintained at constant temperature when used to store temperature-sensitive materials. Liquid-in-glass **thermometers,** thermistors, and electronic digital thermometers are used to monitor the temperature of these devices.

The temperature of every temperature-controlled device must be checked and recorded, along with any corrective action, every day as part of the quality control procedures performed in the laboratory. The accuracy of the thermometers used to monitor the heating baths should be verified regularly, usually every 6 to 12 months. It has been recommended[20] that the thermometer have an accuracy range of one-half that of the desired temperature range. For instance, if the desired accuracy for a heating bath is ±0.1° C, the thermometer should have a maximum uncertainty (error) of ±0.05° C.

Liquid-in-glass thermometers are available for partial or total immersion. Partial immersion thermometers are used to measure the temperature of water baths, heating blocks, and ovens. The immersion depth is engraved on the stem and usually is located about 76 mm from the bulb. Total immersion thermometers generally are used to check refrigerator and freezer temperatures but can be substituted for partial immersion thermometers if they are verified at the same immersion depth at which they will be used in the laboratory. Mercury-containing thermometers are no longer acceptable for use, and the mercury has been replaced by other liquids designed for general laboratory use.

Calibration of Liquid-in-Glass Thermometers

Calibration of thermometers requires the use of an NIST-certified or NIST-traceable thermometer. The NIST SRM program ensures that certified thermometers are available that can be used to calibrate thermometers at 0° C and in the range of 24° C to 38° C. NIST-traceable thermometers have wider operating ranges. The following procedure outlines the steps that must be followed to validate noncertified thermometers; it is based on the NCCLS (now CLSI) standard *Temperature Calibration of Water Baths, Instruments, and Temperature Sensors,* 2nd edition[20]:

1. Check the liquid column for separation or gas bubbles. (If any are present, refer to the NCCLS standard for procedures to correct the problem.)
2. Perform an ice point determination.[20] This will check for changes in bulb volume. After completion, set the thermometer aside for a few days to ensure recovery of the bulb.
3. Adjust the heating bath to the temperature required for analysis. It is important that the volume of the bath be at least 100 times greater than the volume of the fluid in which the thermometer being calibrated is placed. This ensures maintenance of a uniform temperature throughout the bath.
4. Place the reference and noncertified thermometers in test tubes filled with water to the appropriate depth. The thermometers should be placed close to one another but with sufficient space between to ensure adequate circulation in the bath.
5. If a total immersion thermometer is being calibrated for use as a partial immersion device, it must be immersed in the heating bath to the same depth used for test applications. Proper immersion of the thermometer is essential.
6. After thermal equilibrium is reached (this will require several minutes for liquid-in-glass thermometers), determine the temperature reading for both thermometers.

7. Electronic thermometers that use thermistor probes may be calibrated similarly. Thermal equilibrium of these devices occurs in a few milliseconds.

Thermometers that differ from the reference thermometer by more than 1° C should be discarded or returned to the supplier. Agreement within 0.1° C is required for critical laboratory purposes such as enzyme analyses. If discrepancies between 0.2° C and 1° C occur, the thermometer can be used for less critical functions such as monitoring ovens, refrigerators, and freezers. Each thermometer should be assigned a log number and the results of the calibration documented in a thermometer log book; this is useful for inspection purposes.

Also available from NIST is a gallium melting point cell, which can be used to calibrate electronic thermistor probes to a temperature of 29.772° C. These probes can be used to verify the accuracy of liquid-in-glass thermometers in the 20° C to 40° C range.[20]

WATER BATHS, HEATING BLOCKS, AND OVENS

Water baths may be either circulating or noncirculating in design. For clinical chemistry applications, noncirculating baths, in general, are unacceptable because temperature control is inadequate (±1° C). Circulating water baths, which have a tighter temperature control, are necessary. Such baths are equipped with an external or internal circulating pump that maintains adequate thermal equilibrium. In some instances, the pump may be coupled to a refrigeration unit to provide temperature control below room temperature. The bath liquid should consist of high-quality reagent water, to which is added a bactericidal agent such as alkyldimethylbenzyl ammonium chloride (Clear Bath; Spectrum Laboratories, Rancho Dominguez, CA). The bactericidal agent controls bacterial growth, reducing the frequency with which the bath water must be changed. The use of high-quality water is necessary to control salt deposits on the heat exchangers; such deposits interfere with maintenance of adequate temperature control.

Metal heating blocks are somewhat less efficient in maintaining a constant temperature and usually operate within ±0.5° C. Blocks that are incorporated into the cuvette compartment of a spectrophotometer operate with greater accuracy, usually within ±0.2° C or better.

The temperature of water baths and heating blocks should be measured daily with a thermometer calibrated against an NIST thermometer or NIST-certified thermometer. All measurements must be recorded and any corrective action documented.

Laboratory ovens may be used to dry chemicals, extracts, electrophoretic support media, thin-layer chromatography plates, and glassware. For most purposes, a temperature control of ±1° C is adequate. Thermometers used to monitor oven temperature should be checked for accuracy at least annually. The temperature of the oven should be measured daily to check for malfunction of the heating elements or thermistor controls. All gaskets also should be checked to verify integrity. Worn gaskets require replacement to ensure adequate temperature control. All measurements must be recorded and any corrective action documented.

CENTRIFUGES

Types

Three general types of **centrifuge** are available: swinging-bucket, or horizontal-head, centrifuges; fixed-angle, or angle-head, centrifuges; and ultracentrifuges. These are available as floor or table models, allowing the laboratory to purchase the instrument that best suits its needs.

Centrifuges are used in the clinical laboratory to separate substances of significantly different masses or densities. The two substances to be separated can be a solid (particles) and a liquid or two liquids of different densities. Centrifuges are used in the chemistry laboratory primarily to separate clotted blood or cells from serum or plasma and body fluids. Although the choice of a specific relative centrifugal force (RCF) to carry out these separations is not crucial, a force of 1000 to 1200 × g for 10 ± 5 min is recommended.[21] In some instances, more time may be necessary (see Chapter 18).

Swinging-bucket, or horizontal-head, rotors hold the tubes in a vertical position when the centrifuge is at rest; the tubes move to and remain in a horizontal position when the rotor is in motion. During centrifugation, particles constantly move along the tube while it is in the horizontal position, distributing the sediment uniformly against the bottom of the tube. After centrifugation is complete and the rotor has ceased turning, the surface of the sediment is flat with a column of liquid above it.

Fixed-angle rotors keep the tubes at a specified angle, 25 to 52 degrees to the vertical axis of rotation. During centrifugation, particles move along the sides of the tube to form a sediment that packs against the sides and bottom of the tube. The surface of the sediment in this case is parallel to the shaft of the centrifuge. As the rotor slows and then stops, gravity may cause the sediment to slide down the tube, forming a poorly packed pellet. Fixed-angle rotors are used when rapid sedimentation of small particles is required. The design of these rotors is more aerodynamic, allowing operation at speeds higher than those achievable with a swinging-bucket rotor. This capability allows microhematocrit centrifuges to operate at 11,000 to 15,000 revolutions per minute (rpm), with an RCF as high as 14,000 × g.

Ultracentrifuges are high-speed centrifuges that use fixed-angle or swinging-bucket rotors. They often are refrigerated to counter the heat generated as a result of friction. A small air-driven ultracentrifuge, the Airfuge (Beckman Coulter Inc., Spinco Division, Palo Alto, CA), is a miniature air turbine with a small rotor that operates at 90,000 to 100,000 rpm, generating a maximum RCF of 178,000 × g. This type of centrifuge has been used to separate chylomicrons from serum, allowing accurate analyses to be performed on the clear infranatant.

It also has been used to fractionate lipoproteins, perform drug-binding assays, and prepare tissue for hormone receptor assays. Analytical ultracentrifuges are used to determine sedimentation coefficients of proteins, allowing assessment of molecular weights.

Centrifuge Components

All centrifuges have a motor, a drive shaft, and a head or rotor, which may be in the form of a chamber with a cover. A power switch, timer, speed control, tachometer, and brake are the components that control the centrifuge. When necessary, refrigeration units are included. Some centrifuges are equipped with an alarm that sounds when a malfunction such as a tube imbalance occurs. Some centrifuges automatically shut down under these conditions, preventing tube breakage and the potential for exposure to biohazardous agents. All modern centrifuges have a required safety latch that prevents the operator from opening the instrument before the rotor has stopped.

Swinging-bucket rotors use pairs of buckets or carriers that swing freely. The carriers are designed to accept a variety of cushioned inserts, allowing centrifugation of small tubes or large bottles. Different fixed-angle rotors are required for containers of different sizes.

The motor in a large centrifuge is usually a direct-current, heavy-duty, high-torque, electrical motor. In smaller centrifuges, the current is usually alternating. Power is transmitted to the rotor by the commutator and brushes. The rotor shaft usually is driven by a gyro system, and the bearings usually are sealed, minimizing vibration and the need for lubrication. Centrifuge speed is controlled by a potentiometer that modulates the voltage supplied to the motor. Speed is also determined by the mass of the load in the rotor. The tachometer measures rotor speed in rpm. The brake decelerates the rotor by reversing the polarity of the current to the motor. The timer permits the rotor to reach a preprogrammed speed; the rotor then decelerates, with or without braking, after a set time has elapsed.

Refrigerated centrifuges are used when the heat generated during centrifugation could cause evaporation or denaturation of protein or leakage of cellular components in the sample. The temperature can be controlled at between −15° C and 25° C, allowing centrifugation at higher speeds and for prolonged periods.

The selection of centrifuge tubes and bottles is of importance. Plastic tubes (polystyrene, polypropylene) have a higher speed tolerance and can withstand RCFs as high as 5000 × g. Tubes with tapered bottoms, which form more compact pellets, may be required under certain conditions such as when sediment is prepared for microscopic urine analysis and some radioimmunoassay procedures. The tubes must fit snugly into the carriers; small tubes placed in too large a carrier result in improperly packed pellets. The top of the tube must not protrude so far above the carrier that the rotor is impeded. Balancing of tubes within the carriers is crucial. Newer centrifuges automatically decelerate and shut down when carriers are improperly balanced. Figure 1-9 demonstrates appropriate balancing. Improper balancing can cause the centrifuge to vibrate, disrupting the formed pellet. Whenever possible, tubes that contain biohazardous materials should be centrifuged with caps or stoppers in place to minimize aerosols.

Maintenance and Quality Assurance

Daily cleaning of the inside surfaces of the centrifuge with a tenfold dilution of household bleach or an equivalent disinfectant is crucial. When tube breakage occurs, the portions of the centrifuge in contact with the blood or other potentially infectious agent must be decontaminated immediately. The centrifuge bowl should be cleaned with a germicidal disinfectant, and the rotor heads and buckets should be autoclaved. All broken glass or plastic must be removed carefully and disposed of appropriately.

Centrifuge speeds that are used routinely should be checked periodically with a reliable photoelectrical or strobe tachometer in accordance with CAP inspection guidelines.[19] Measured and rated speeds should not differ by more than 5% under specified conditions. The accuracy of the centrifuge timer also should be checked and verified according to CAP inspection guidelines.[19] The temperature of refrigerated centrifuges should be checked at least monthly (daily is preferred) under standardized conditions. The agreement between measured and expected (or programmed) temperatures should be within 2° C.

Manufacturers' instructions for lubrication, maintenance, and replacement of brushes should be followed. (Centrifuges of recent manufacture do not have brushes.) Failure to replace worn brushes may cause the motor to fail and require replacement. All maintenance function checks must be recorded and all corrective actions documented.

Principles of Centrifugation

The speed of a centrifuge is expressed in rpm, whereas the RCF generated is expressed as a number times the gravitational force, g. The relationship between rpm and RCF is expressed by the following equation:

$$\text{RCF} = 1.12 \times 10^{-5} \times \text{r} \times (\text{rpm})^2$$

where *r* is the radius of the centrifuge expressed in centimeters and is equal to the horizontal distance from the center of the centrifuge bucket to the rotor shaft, and 1.12×10^{-5} is an empirical factor. Fig. 1-10 shows a nomogram used for determination of the RCF when the radius and the rpm are known. The RCF applied to a tube in a swinging-bucket rotor may be considerably greater than that applied to the same tube in a fixed-angle rotor because the tube never reaches a horizontal position under the latter condition. For this reason, it is preferable to process serum separator tubes with swinging-bucket horizontal rotors, which operate at higher RCFs.

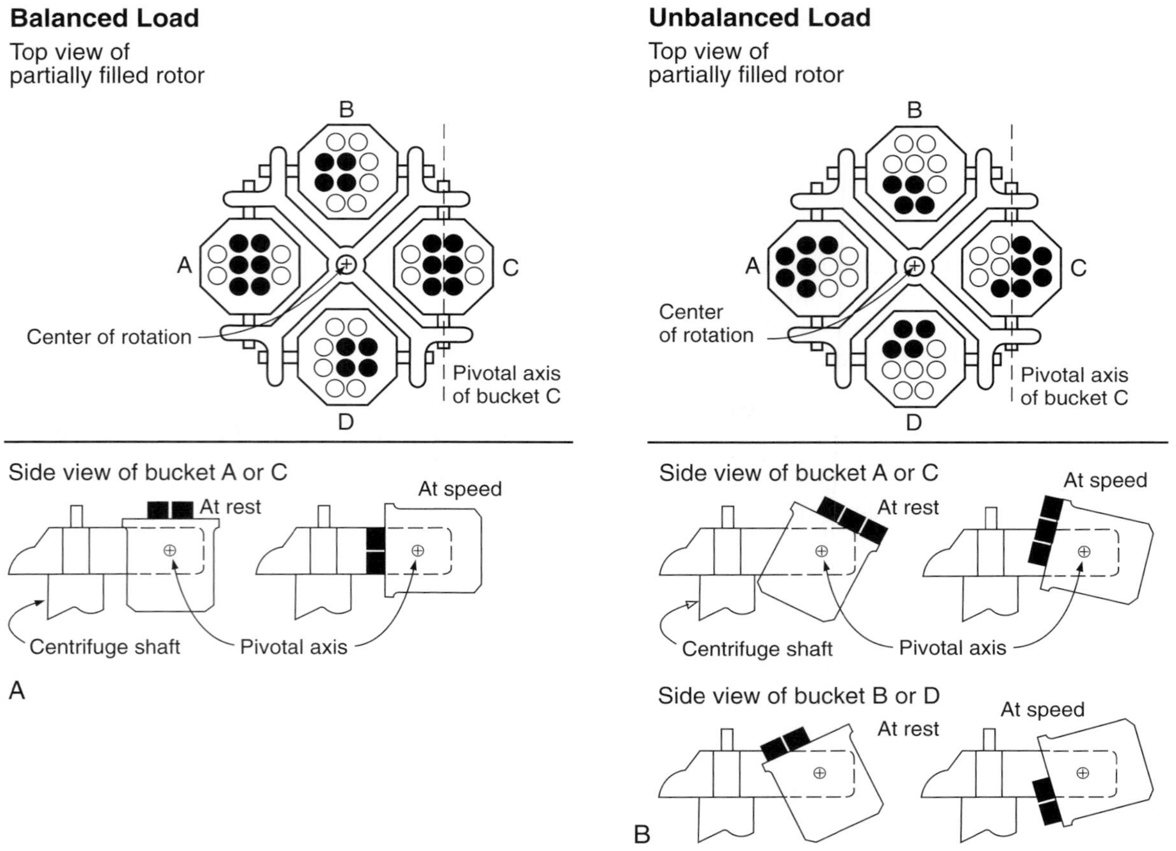

Fig. 1-9 Examples of balanced and unbalanced loads. **A,** If it is assumed that all tubes have been filled with an equal amount of liquid, this rotor load is balanced. The opposing bucket sets *A-C* and *B-D* are loaded with an equal number of tubes and are balanced across the center of rotation. Each bucket also is balanced with respect to its pivotal axis. **B,** Even if all the tubes are filled equally, this rotor is loaded improperly. None of the bucket loads is balanced with respect to its pivotal axis. At operating speed, buckets *A* and *C* will not reach the horizontal position. Buckets *B* and *D* will pivot past the horizontal. Also note that the tube arrangement in the opposing buckets *B* and *D* is not symmetrical across the center of rotation. (From *A Centrifuge Primer,* Palo Alto, CA, 1980, Spinco Division Beckman Instruments, Inc. [out of print].)

At times, it may be necessary to duplicate centrifugation conditions in two different instruments. This may be achieved by applying the following equations.

Calculation of adjusted speed[22]:

$$\text{rpm (new rotor)} = 1000 \times \frac{\text{RCF (original rotor)}}{1.12 \times \text{r (cm, original rotor)}}$$

Calculation of adjusted time[22]:

$$\text{Time (new rotor)} = \frac{\text{Time (old rotor)} \times \text{RCF (original rotor)}}{\text{RCF (new rotor)}}$$

These calculations do not take into account the differences between instruments in terms of the time necessary to reach full speed or to decelerate. Therefore, additional adjustments are necessary.

KEY CONCEPTS BOX 1-5

- The accuracy and reproducibility of electronic balances used by clinical laboratories must be validated 1 to 2 times a year with the use of Class S weights.
- Liquid-in-glass thermometers can no longer use Hg as the liquid. Certified thermometers must be checked annually for accuracy against a National Institute of Standards and Technology (NIST)-certified or traceable thermometer, or as specified, controlled temperatures (ice/water mix @ 4° C, boiling water @ 100° C; at sea level).
- The depth to which an emersion-type thermometer must be placed is determined by the line on the lower part of the thermometer.
- Water in a water bath should include an antimicrobial agent.

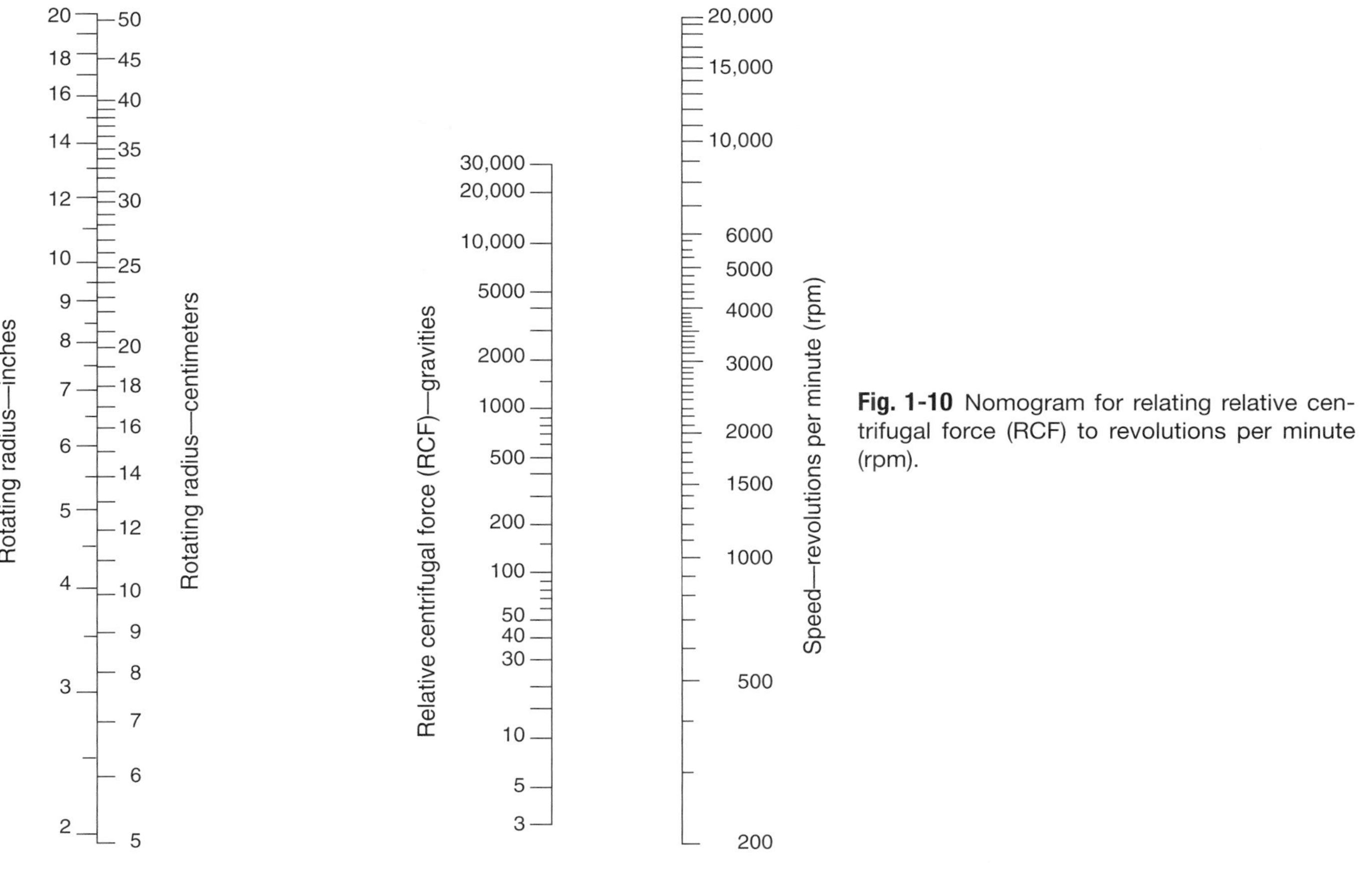

Fig. 1-10 Nomogram for relating relative centrifugal force (RCF) to revolutions per minute (rpm).

SECTION OBJECTIVES BOX 1-6

- List general laboratory safety regulations.
- List at least five components of the Occupational Safety and Health Administration (OSHA)-mandated Chemical Hygiene Plan.
- Define the term MDS, and explain its use.
- Describe the function of a chemical inventory and describe the elements of the National Fire Protection Association (NFPA) diamond.
- Describe the purpose of universal precautions, and explain how they are applied in the clinical laboratory.
- Describe the plan for protection against bloodborne pathogens.
- Define "latex allergies," and explain the precautions that should be taken to protect patients and hospital workers from an adverse latex exposure.

LABORATORY SAFETY

The **Occupational Safety and Health Administration (OSHA)** has mandated three programs to ensure the safety of laboratory and other health care personnel. The first, which deals with occupational exposure to chemical hazards,[23] became law in January 1991. The second deals with occupational exposure to **bloodborne pathogens**[24] and became law in March 1992. The third, which became law in April 2001, concerns the use of safer needle devices and is a revision of the earlier Bloodborne Pathogen Standard.[25] In addition to these mandated programs, the laboratory is responsible for the practice of general safety procedures.

Each clinical laboratory is responsible for designating a safety officer. This individual may also function as the chemical hygiene officer and program coordinator for the bloodborne pathogen program. Responsibilities of this employee include the preparation and updating of manuals that address safety policies and procedures, maintenance of records of training and continuing education, and maintenance of records of exposure to hazardous materials. The safety officer also may be responsible for ensuring that protective devices are available and are being properly and consistently used, and that the laboratory is functioning as a safe working environment. In a large facility, these functions are shared by several employees; however, the safety officer plays a key role in ensuring that all regulations are followed.

General Safety Practices

Fire safety is of utmost importance in the clinical laboratory. All equipment used for fire protection should meet the standards set by the National Fire Protection Association (NFPA). The equipment, which should be accessible to laboratory workers, may include fire extinguishers, fire blankets, cabinets for storage of flammable solvents and chemicals, fire alarms, smoke detectors, and sprinkler systems. Selection of the appropriate type of extinguisher is important, as is frequent inspection to ensure that it is in good working order. Tables 1-10 and 1-11 classify types of fires and compare types of fire extinguishers. Halotron extinguishers generally are used for areas in which computers are housed. Warning signs must be posted in these areas, and self-contained breathing equipment must be provided. Several extinguishers are necessary in a larger laboratory, and different types may be appropriate. All employees must be familiar with their use, and annual retraining is mandatory.

Electrical safety is also crucial because the potential for both electrical shock and fire exists. All equipment must be Underwriters Laboratories (UL) approved. This also includes extension cords, which should be used as temporary solutions only. All electrical outlets and equipment must be grounded, and wires should be checked for fraying or wear. Regular inspection decreases the likelihood of electrical accidents. Laboratory workers should document these inspections.

Any equipment used in an area where organic solvents are present must be equipped with explosion-free fittings such as plugs and outlets.

General safety equipment includes safety showers and eyewashes provided in each large work area. The safety program must include measures for routinely verifying that this equipment is operational, and maintenance records must be kept. Asbestos (heat-resistant) gloves are required for handling hot equipment, hot glassware, and dry ice. Other personal protective equipment is discussed in the sections involving chemical and biological hazards.

Table **1-10** Classes of Types of Fires

Class	Hazard
A	Cloth, wood, paper, ordinary combustibles
B	Flammable liquids (greases, solvents), flammable gases (natural or manufactured)
C	Operating electrical equipment (if electricity is turned off, fire is reclassified as A or B)

The Chemical Hygiene Plan

OSHA has mandated that as of January 31, 1991, laboratories must develop a **Chemical Hygiene Plan** for the protection and education of employees.[23] This plan should contain the elements indicated in Box 1-1.

Standard Operating Procedures

Standard operating procedures include protocols for handling accidents and chemical spills. In general, if chemicals have come into contact with eyes or skin, the contact areas require flushing with copious amounts of water followed by medical attention when necessary. Because the eye-washing procedure requires a 15-minute eyewash, portable eyewash stations are unacceptable. If a system that attaches to a spigot is selected, the water temperature must be adjusted to cut off the hot water supply or a controller installed to ensure that scalding

Table **1-11** Comparison of Fire Extinguisher Types

Type	Advantages	Disadvantages	Notes
Halotron (Class A, B, C, or BC)	• Quick fire knockdown • Will reach hidden fires • No damage to equipment • Good discharge range • Heat absorber • Rechargeable	• Requires rapid discharge • More expensive • Not for deep-seated fires	• Most common system for electrical/electronics • Maximum effectiveness requires rapid detection
Triclass dry chemical (Class A, B, C)	• Good on oil/grease • Good knockdown • Low cost • Rechargeable	• Limited personnel hazard • Equipment damage likely • Cleanup required • Not suitable for hidden fires	• Compatible with other agents • Subject to equipment interference
Carbon dioxide (Class B, C)	• Good fire suppression and cooling capability • Will reach hidden fires • No equipment damage • No messy cleanup/odor • Rechargeable	• May be toxic to personnel • May cause thermal/static (shock) damage • Heavy vapor settles out, limiting total discharge rate	• Secondary choice to Halotron for fighting Class B and C fires
Dry chemical regular (Class B, C)	• Won't bake on • Easy cleanup • Good knockdown • No odor • Nonconductive • Rechargeable	• Not suitable for hidden fires • Slight respiratory hazard	• Secondary choice to Halotron for fighting Class B and C fires

Box 1-1

Elements of a Chemical Hygiene Plan

1. Description of standard operating procedure
2. Material Safety Data Sheets (MSDSs)
3. List of chemicals in inventory
4. Information on appropriate chemical storage
5. Labeling requirements
6. Description of required engineering controls
7. List of required personal protective equipment
8. Information on waste removal and disposal
9. Information on mandated environmental monitoring where appropriate
10. Housekeeping requirements
11. Requirements for employee physicals and medical consultations
12. Training requirements
13. Record-keeping requirements
14. Designation of a chemical hygiene officer and committee
15. Other information deemed necessary for safety assurance

cannot occur. Cleanup procedures should be individually defined for specific chemicals when necessary and should specifically designate the protective clothing to be used during the cleanup procedure.

Rules for avoiding unnecessary chemical exposure must be defined. Smoking, eating, drinking, and applying cosmetics must be prohibited in all work areas. Long hair and loose clothing should be secured; sandals and canvas shoes should be prohibited. Contact lenses should not be worn in the laboratory because they prevent proper washing of the eyes in the event of a splash. In addition, plastic lenses may be damaged by organic vapors, leading to chronic eye infections. Hand washing after handling chemicals and before leaving the laboratory for the purposes of eating or drinking should be emphasized.

Cracked or chipped glassware should be discarded immediately because it can break during use. All glassware that has been in contact with a toxic or corrosive substance should be rinsed well with water or alcohol (depending on the solubility) before it is placed with other soiled glassware.

The laboratory is required to maintain an alphabetized, up-to-date file of material safety data sheets (MSDSs) to comply with local, state, and federal Right-to-Know laws. This may be achieved through the use of hard copy or electronic libraries. MSDSs are required for all chemicals, reagents, and kits used by the laboratory but not for any pharmaceutical agents such as aspirin.[26] The MSDS contains information about the physical and health hazards of each product. This file must be accessible to all employees and outside contractors who work in the laboratory.

Inventory

A chemical inventory that lists all hazardous agents used or stored in the laboratory is completed annually. A substance can be classified as hazardous by the Department of Transportation (DOT), by the Environmental Protection Agency (EPA), or by the NFPA diamond (see the following section on labeling). The inventory should be arranged alphabetically and should include the manufacturer and manufacturing address, physical state, quantity stored, Chemical Abstract Service (CAS) number if known, location of storage, and any hazard classification for health risks, fire, reactivity, or corrosiveness. A separate list must be maintained for carcinogens or suspected carcinogens.

Storage of Chemicals

Quantities of chemicals stored in the laboratory should be as small as practical. All refrigerators used for chemical storage must be marked clearly. Under no conditions may food or drink be stored, even temporarily, in a refrigerator used for chemical storage. Explosion-proof refrigerators, clearly labeled, are necessary for the storage of solvents with a low flash point.

Toxic chemicals, including carcinogens, must be stored in unbreakable, chemically resistant secondary containers in well-ventilated areas. These containers must be labeled to indicate that the compound is a CANCER SUSPECT AGENT or has HIGH CHRONIC TOXICITY.

Large amounts of volatile solvents must be stored in special safety cabinets approved by the NFPA. Where possible, these cabinets should be vented to the outside. Bench storage of volatile solvents is limited on the basis of OSHA classification of the solvent. This classification is determined by flash point and boiling point, with Class IA and IB solvents being the most combustible. Bench storage of such solvents may be limited to as little as 1 pint; however, some local fire departments may require compliance with more stringent regulations. Larger quantities must be transferred to safety cans with spring-loaded spouts. All cabinets where in-use solvents are kept should be labeled appropriately.

Large cylinders of compressed gas may be used in the laboratory. The most commonly used gases are oxygen, hydrogen, nitrogen, helium, carbon dioxide, and, to a lesser extent, acetylene and propane. Usually the tanks are color-coded and the contents are labeled by the NFPA diamond label system. OSHA regulations governing gas cylinders are based on publications of the Compressed Gas Association, Inc.[27] Cylinders should be stored away from the laboratory in a secure, upright position, preferably in a locked, ventilated, fire-resistant space with the empty cylinders well separated from the full ones. The cylinder must always be secured on a dolly or hand truck during transport. The protective cap must be left in place until the cylinder is connected. Gas cylinders (even when empty) must be securely fastened to a wall or bench or placed in a floor retainer because a fall can rupture the outlet valve, allowing the cylinder to be propelled like a torpedo. The laboratory worker should mark each cylinder with a tag that lists the date it was put into use. An exhausted cylinder should be replaced before it is completely empty to avoid contamination with foreign materials; it should be labeled with an EMPTY sign. In general, empty cylinders are recycled by suppliers. Small cylinders that contain propane, however, are not. These should be disposed of according to local fire codes.

Reduction valves for different types of gases are not interchangeable. Never substitute one regulator, with or without an adaptor, for another. Laboratory personnel should never attempt to force or free stuck or frozen regulator valves. All connections should be tested for leaks with soapy water. Very small leaks of oxygen or nitrogen are of little consequence, but leaks of hydrogen, acetylene, and other flammable gases are unacceptable. When a cylinder of flammable gas is shut down, it should be turned off at the main intake valve and the gas allowed to burn out. The reduction valves are then closed. A cylinder valve is not turned on unless the reduction valve is off. It is important to remember that propane is heavier than air, and therefore, a small quantity of leaking gas can flow along the top of the bench and be ignited by a flame elsewhere. For this reason, small, single-use cylinders of propane are more convenient and safer to use.

Labeling and Handling Requirements

OSHA regulation 29 CFR 1910.1450[23] defines specific labeling requirements. The labels of chemicals in the original containers must not be removed or defaced. For chemicals not in the original container, labeling information must include the following:

1. Identity of the hazardous chemical
2. Route of body entry (eyes, nose, mouth, skin)
3. Health hazard
4. Physical hazard
5. Target organ affected

Labeling requirements apply to all substances with a rating of 2 or greater according to the Hazards Identification System developed by the NFPA. This system consists of four small, diamond-shaped symbols grouped into a larger diamond shape (Fig. 1-11). The left diamond is blue and indicates a health hazard, the top is red and identifies a flammability hazard, the right diamond is yellow and indicates a reactivity-stability hazard (used for substances that are capable of explosion or violent chemical change), and the bottom white diamond is used for provision of special hazard information such as water reactivity. The degree of hazard is rated on a scale from 0 to 4, with 4 indicating the most severe risk. Such common items as isopropanol (isopropyl alcohol) or diluted bleach in squirt bottles therefore require regulatory labels. It may be desirable to use additional warning labels such as those used by the DOT and shown in Fig. 1-12. Labels also must indicate any available antidote or treatment modes.

The handling of hazardous chemicals requires great care. A discussion of the handling and disposal of radioactive chemicals is presented on Evolve. All flammable and toxic liquids must be used in an area with good ventilation, preferably in a fume hood. A properly operating fume hood should have a minimum air flow of 150 linear ft^3/min. Corrosive solutions such as acids, alkalis, and mercury salts also should be used in a fume hood. Stock bottles of concentrated acids should be transported in acid carriers to prevent and contain breakage. The use of personal protective equipment must be enforced. When reagents are prepared with concentrated acid, the acid must be added slowly to the water. Precautions for handling powdered carcinogens include the use of disposable equipment and a respirator, in addition to all other standard safety measures. After the compound has been handled, the area should be cleaned carefully and the glassware rinsed with strong acid or an organic solvent before regular washing.

Engineering controls are an important part of the daily operation of the laboratory. In addition to the provision, inspection, and documentation of functionality of fire

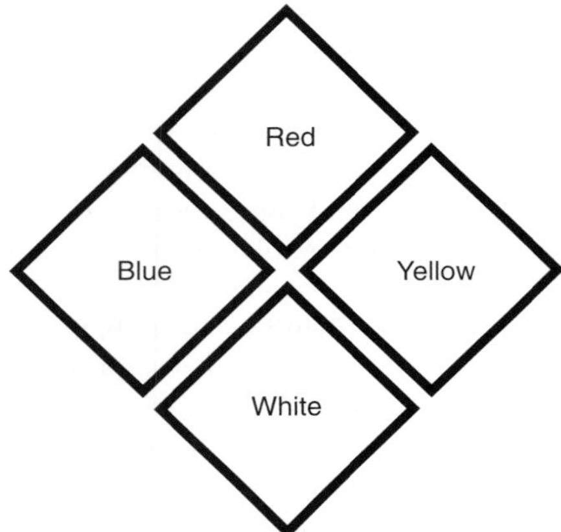

Fig. 1-11 Identification system of the National Fire Protection Association. (From Bauer JD: *Clinical Laboratory Methods*, ed 9, St. Louis, 1982, Mosby.)

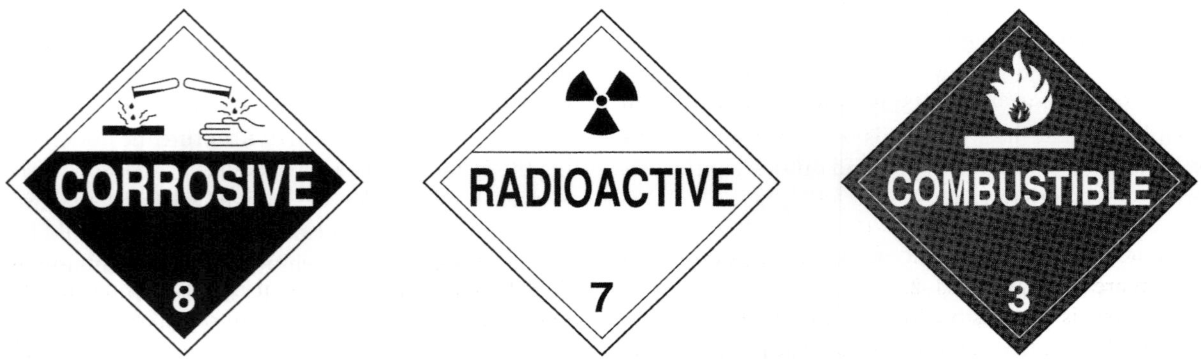

Fig. 1-12 Department of Transportation (DOT) labels.

extinguishers, eyewashes, and safety showers, other aspects of the laboratory environment must be monitored and validated. The quality and quantity of laboratory ventilation (4 to 12 air changes per hour) must be documented on a quarterly basis. All areas where hazardous substances are handled or stored such as storerooms, glove boxes, and cold rooms must have adequate ventilation and exhaust ducting. All fume hoods must be inspected after installation, and then annually by a reputable company. Inspection should include an evaluation of flow patterns and a flow-velocity profile. Any hood that fails inspection must be taken out of service immediately. A weekly safety checklist should be maintained that includes the following items: adequate air flow, no unnecessary items in the hood, correct baffle settings, and functioning guard window. Before a hood is used, acceptable hood performance should be confirmed by the technologist. This can be accomplished with the use of a permanent flowmeter or through observation of the disappearance of smoke or fumes produced after two applicator sticks whose cotton tips have been dipped in strong ammonia and hydrochloric acid, respectively, have been brought together carefully. (The tips are drenched with running water before disposal.) Alternatively, a paper wipe such as Kimwipe (Kimberly-Clark, Roswell, GA) may be held firmly under a baffle in the down position and the force of the exhaust evaluated. Care must be taken not to release the tissue into the exhaust system.

OSHA has defined the personal protective equipment required for laboratory operations involving chemical hazards. (Much of this equipment is identical to that required for protection against bloodborne pathogens, as will be described on p. 28 in the following section.) Handling of hazardous chemicals requires the use of gloves (the type to be used depends on the type of chemical hazard). Laboratory coats protect clothing; if chemical splashes are probable, an impervious full body apron offers additional protection. Masks, safety glasses with side shields, or full-face shields are necessary if the potential for eye, nose, or mouth contamination exists. Respirators must be provided and used according to the requirements listed in 29 CFR 1910.134. All personal protective equipment should be removed before a laboratory worker leaves a work area.

Waste and Chemical Control

Chemical waste and hazardous chemical disposal procedures must comply with all local and state regulations. Most laboratories are considered small-quantity generators by the EPA and are required to secure a generation number from the regional EPA office. Certain chemicals can be disposed of in the sanitary sewer system. Specific information must be obtained from local sources, but only those chemicals that are reasonably soluble (at least 3%) in water can be poured down the drain, and they must be flushed with at least 100 volumes of excess water. Compounds that should never be poured down a drain are listed in Box 1-2.

The laboratory is responsible for determining the disposition of chemical waste that is removed from the premises. The MSDS sheets and other sources may provide useful information for disposal of specific chemicals.[26,28] Incineration in an environmentally acceptable manner is common for combustible liquids. Placing volatile chemicals in a hood for the purpose of evaporation is unacceptable. The laboratory staff must familiarize itself with the rules and regulations that govern storage and disposition of toxic chemicals such as solvents and formaldehyde. Records of disposal must be maintained.

Box 1-2

Compounds That Cannot Be Disposed of in a Drain

Organic solvents with a boiling point of less than 50° C
Hydrocarbons
Halogenated hydrocarbons
Nitro compounds
Mercaptans
Most oxygenated compounds that contain more than five carbon atoms (such as Freon)
Organic compounds such as azides and peroxides
Concentrated acids and bases
Highly toxic, malodorous, or lacrimatory (tear-producing) compounds

Sodium azide, another troublesome chemical, still is used as a bacteriostatic agent. Azides form explosive salts with many metals, including copper and iron. These salts are readily detonated by mechanical shock. Although the amount of sodium azide used as a preservative is relatively small, continued use can result in a buildup of the metallic salts in sewer pipes. These salts are extremely explosive; even the use of a wrench on such a drain line can result in a violent explosion. The removal of azides from pipes is difficult. One method involves closing the lower end of a section of pipe and allowing a 10% solution of sodium hydroxide to remain in contact with the pipe for at least 16 hours. The pipe then is rinsed with copious amounts of water for at least 15 minutes. The use of azides should be avoided or minimized because in addition to their explosive potential they are carcinogenic.

Mercury, a neurotoxin (see p. 816, Chapter 42) and common environmental pollutant, was identified as a pollution problem in hospitals. An agreement between the EPA and the American Hospital Association in 1998 required hospitals to minimize the production of mercury-containing pollutants and reduce the number of products that contain mercury. This included replacing mercury-containing thermometers; as a consequence, mercury-containing thermometers are no longer acceptable in the hospital environment in the United States. Reagents and procedures using mercury-containing preservatives/bactericidal agents have been replaced by alternatives that no longer pose a threat to the environment.

Environmental monitoring may be necessary if the laboratory uses any chemical defined in the OSHA publication 29 CFR 1910 Subpart Z, three or more times per week. Included in this list is formaldehyde. Monitoring consists of semiannual room air monitoring over an 8-hour period, as well as individual badge monitoring of one or more employees exposed to the chemical. In the event that permissible exposure limits are exceeded, monitoring is required more frequently (quarterly) until acceptable exposure levels are achieved. Although xylene is not officially included on the list, a similar procedure should be followed for this chemical. Glutaraldehyde is also a potent sensory irritant that has the ability to precipitate proteins; excessive exposure may cause necrotic or inflammatory lesions of the upper respiratory tract.

Housekeeping such as floor cleaning and general laboratory cleaning should be done regularly according to a defined schedule; housekeeping personnel must be informed of the risks associated with working in the laboratory. The laboratory should be maintained as a clutter-free environment. Hallways and stairwells should be free from obstruction, waste must be handled carefully, laboratory supplies should be stored appropriately, and all spills should be cleaned thoroughly. Spill cleanup kits must be readily available for use. Multipurpose products such as sand and soda ash are useful, as are commercial products such as those marketed by chemical companies and safety product suppliers. The laboratory can assemble a kit that contains equivalent supplies (rubber gloves, towels, scoop, and various chemicals for neutralizing and absorbing organic solvents and corrosive chemicals). Kits must be labeled and highly accessible. Spills should be cleaned up immediately by laboratory workers with the use of appropriate personal protective equipment. Special cleanup kits are available for handling formaldehyde and mercury spills. The formaldehyde kits neutralize the spill and allow the contents to be disposed of in the regular trash under most conditions. Spilled mercury tends to break up into very small droplets, which are difficult to pick up. Even after collection, disposal tends to be a problem because metallic mercury must not be incinerated or burned. Many mercury kits are available that contain a material (sulfur and zinc compounds) that absorbs mercury droplets, producing a less toxic substance, which may be disposed of by burial. Some kits may include waste disposal through the kit manufacturer. The benches and floors in older laboratories may contain fine cracks in which mercury droplets can lodge. These droplets are difficult to remove, but the cracks should be cleaned, if possible, because mercury is somewhat volatile at room temperature. Rubbing powdered sulfur or sodium polysulfide into the cracks may help to change mercury into the less volatile sulfide salt. OSHA regulations mandate that personnel exposed to hazardous chemicals must be provided with medical consultations and examinations on a regular basis (such as annually). The extent of the physical examination is determined by the amount and type of exposure. In addition to regular examinations, personnel should be evaluated medically whenever a major spill occurs, when environmental monitoring indicates exposure above action levels, or when signs and symptoms of toxicity develop. Employees then should be continuously monitored and counseled until a medical clearance is given. Medical records must be maintained for 30 years after the employee leaves the workplace.

Training is a necessary and important part of the Chemical Hygiene Plan. Refresher training sessions or competency examinations must be given at least annually and attendance records documented. Training should ensure that the employee knows the extent of chemical exposure, understands the labeling system, knows the meaning of and location of the laboratory's MSDS book, is familiar with the required personal protective equipment, and knows how to react to and handle spills. Many training methods such as videotapes, handouts, and demonstrations may be used. In addition, the College of American Pathologists requires that the laboratory document the efficacy of the Chemical Hygiene Plan.[19]

Record keeping is a crucial component of the laboratory safety program. The laboratory must maintain records of (1) accident and incident reports, (2) inventory and usage for high-risk substances, (3) environmental monitoring where appropriate, (4) medical consultations, (5) training attendance, (6) housekeeping procedures, and (7) safety inspections.

Protection Against Biohazards and Medical Wastes

Universal Precautions

OSHA promulgated a final rule on December 6, 1991, which dealt with occupational exposure to blood and other potentially infectious materials. The program for protection against biohazards was to be instituted fully by July 6, 1992.[24] Many of the requirements of the program are similar to those contained in the Chemical Hygiene Plan, including development of a document that describes the following:

1. Extent of exposure for all employees
2. Engineering and work practice controls
3. Personal protective equipment
4. Task assessment
5. Housekeeping procedures
6. Spill cleanup procedures
7. Laundry requirements
8. Labeling requirements
9. Waste disposal
10. Provision of vaccinations
11. Medical consultations
12. Training
13. Record keeping

Some occupational exposure to bloodborne pathogens is probably inherent in every task in the chemistry laboratory. Therefore, all personnel are at risk. Even though this is the case, it is necessary to define the extent of exposure.

Universal precautions, as defined by the Centers for Disease Control and Prevention (CDC) and adopted by OSHA, are observed to prevent contact with blood and other potentially infectious materials.[24,25,29] General recommendations include the following:

1. All personnel must routinely use barrier precautions to prevent skin and mucous membrane exposure when contact with blood or body fluids from any patient is expected. Gloves must be worn during the performance of venipuncture and when one is handling blood, body fluids, or items soiled with blood or fluids. Protective eyewear or face shields must be worn during procedures that are likely

to cause splashing, to prevent exposure of the mucous membranes of the mouth, nose, and eyes to droplets of blood or body fluids. Gowns and aprons must be worn during procedures that are likely to generate splashing.
2. If the hands or the skin becomes contaminated with blood or other body fluids, it should be washed immediately and thoroughly. Hands should be washed immediately after gloves are removed.
3. Health care workers must avoid injuries from needles, scalpels, and other sharp devices. Needles must not be recapped, bent, broken, or removed from disposable syringes. After use, disposable syringes, needles, scalpel blades, and other sharp items must be placed in puncture-resistant containers.
4. Health care workers who have exudative skin lesions or weeping dermatitis must avoid direct patient care and contact with blood and other potentially infectious materials until the condition has been resolved.
5. Pregnant women are particularly cautioned to follow these rules.

Other work practice controls include the following:

1. Specimens of blood and other potentially infectious materials must be transported in leakproof containers. The laboratory worker should take care to avoid contaminating the outside of the container and any accompanying laboratory requisition.
2. Biological safety cabinets should be used for procedures such as blending, sonicating, and vigorous mixing, which can generate droplets.
3. Mouth pipetting is prohibited. Mechanical devices are used to pipet all liquids.
4. Eating, drinking, smoking, applying cosmetics or lip balm, and handling contact lenses are prohibited in biohazardous work areas, just as they are prohibited in areas where chemicals are used.
5. Only authorized personnel are permitted in the laboratory. Casual visitors are discouraged. Any visitor to the work area, including instrument service personnel, should be provided with personal protective equipment to the extent necessary.
6. Instruments that require service should be decontaminated before repair.
7. Chemistry analyzers that generate fine sprays of sample from the sample probe should be equipped with shields, if possible.
8. All employees must wash their hands and remove laboratory coats and other personal protective equipment before leaving the work area.

A revision of the Bloodborne Pathogen Standard 29 CFR 1910.1030 went into effect in April 2001. This revision includes the Needlestick Safety and Prevention Act,[25] which requires that needles used for withdrawing blood must have a "built-in safety feature or mechanism that effectively reduces the risk of an exposure incident." Such a device is shown in Fig. 1-13. The standard requires that the laboratory not only must provide the devices but also must monitor use of the devices as part of a quality improvement program. The Bloodborne Pathogen Manual must reflect these changes in technology; in addition, input should be documented from nonmanagerial employees, such as physicians and technologists, who are responsible for direct patient care. Such individuals are at high risk for injury caused by contaminated sharps.

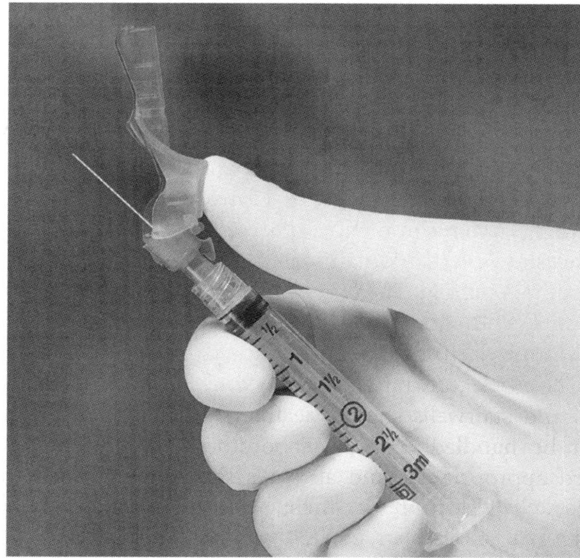

Fig. 1-13 Safety blood collection needle and adaptor.

As the result of continued efforts to reduce exposure to bloodborne pathogens, manufacturers of such devices have developed safer products. The costs associated with needlestick injuries are high; costs can exceed $5,000 per exposure as a result of medical management of the exposure and the development of new drugs to treat new and existing bloodborne infections.[29,30] In 2003, it was estimated that in the United States, the rate of injury from contaminated sharps was about 650,000 annually,[31] and that more than 200 health care workers die each year from acquired infections, primarily hepatitis.[32] However, at least 30 different pathogens have been shown to have been transmitted via a needlestick,[33] and even though an overt infection may not occur, the cost of follow-up to employees, employers, and insurance companies is extensive.[34]

Personal Protective Equipment

Safety equipment in the appropriate size must be provided by the employer at no cost to the employee. Laboratory coats must be impervious to fluids, offering optimal protection against biohazardous agents. Aprons may be used to provide additional protection. Safety glasses, masks, or full-face shields are used to protect the eyes, mouth, and nose.

Task Assessment

Safety policies should be established for each task performed by the laboratory. These policies should include engineering and work practice controls and requirements for personal protective equipment. For much of the work performed in the chemistry laboratory, coats, glasses, and gloves are necessary. For some tasks, additional protection is required.

Housekeeping Procedures

In accordance with a written schedule, laboratory workers must decontaminate all equipment and work surfaces with a chemical germicide such as a 1:10 dilution of household bleach (1) after completing specified procedures, (2) when surfaces are overtly contaminated, (3) immediately after any spill of a potentially infectious material, and (4) at the end of the work shift.

Routine cleaning procedures should be instituted for items such as waste cans and other receptacles. Broken glassware that may be contaminated is handled by mechanical means and is disposed of appropriately.

Spills of biological material are decontaminated as soon as possible by absorbing the spilled fluid with disposable absorbent material such as paper towels or gauze, flooding the contaminated area with bleach or wiping it with bleach-soaked towels, and then wiping the area with clean, dry towels or gauze. All contaminated items are placed in a biohazard bag and disposed of according to laboratory policy. Spill cleanup requires the use of personal protective equipment.

Contaminated laundry must be packed in red bags at the location where it is used or labeled with a biohazard sign if placed in another type of bag. All laundering and repair of laboratory coats are provided by the employer. Under no conditions may employees launder their own laboratory coats. When handling soiled laundry, personnel must wear gloves. Storage of clean and dirty coats must be well separated.

Warning labels (Fig. 1-14) must be used to identify (1) the entrances to work areas; (2) refrigerators and freezers that contain blood and other potentially infectious agents; (3) all containers used to store, transport, or ship potentially infectious materials; and (4) containers of regulated waste (other than red bags). Areas where food is stored should be labeled as nonbiohazard (clean) areas.

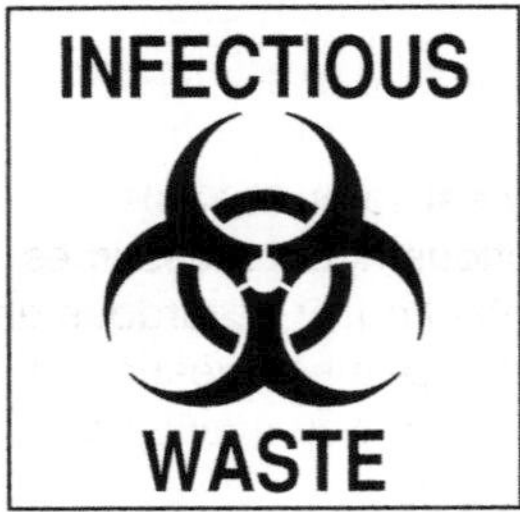

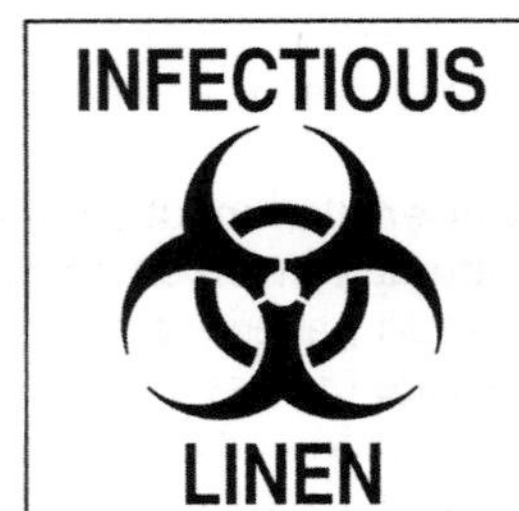

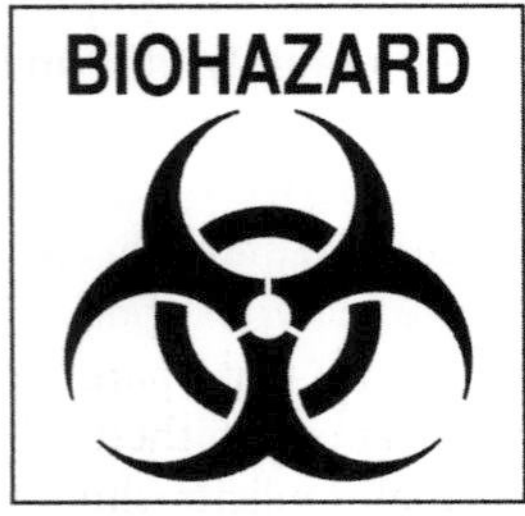

Fig. 1-14 Biohazard labels. (Courtesy Lab Safety Supply, Inc., Janesville, WI.)

Disposal

Regulated medical waste (infectious waste) must be disposed of in accordance with local and state regulations.[35] Contaminated materials should be segregated at the point of use into categories such as needles or sharps and other infectious waste. Containers must be leakproof and should be disposed of when three-fourths full. Any biohazardous waste that is decontaminated by a procedure such as autoclaving is exempt from these regulations and may be disposed of by standard processes. Several types of systems now available for waste treatment render the treated product unrecognizable; these include pulverizing and high heat processes. The legality of these devices is determined on a state-by-state basis.

Vaccination

Vaccinations against hepatitis B virus (HBV) must be offered to all employees without cost. Any employee who declines the vaccination must sign a form indicating that the continued risk of exposure to bloodborne pathogens is understood. These employees are at liberty to change their minds at any time. The vaccine is administered in a series of three doses over 6 months. Protective levels of antibodies are induced in 90% to 99% of adults; however, follow-up studies 3 to 5 years after vaccination have shown that in many individuals, titers are no longer measurable. These individuals should receive a single booster vaccination. No time frame for further follow up has been suggested.

Medical consultations and evaluations must be provided if an employee is exposed to a biohazardous agent through a needlestick, a cut, a mucous membrane exposure (eyes, nose, or mouth), or an exposure involving skin contact with large amounts of blood. The source patient is requested to consent to testing for both HBV and human immunodeficiency virus (HIV), if necessary by law. If consent is not required, testing is performed, and the employee is informed of the results. The employee's blood is collected and tested as soon as possible. If the employee does not consent to HIV testing, the sample must be preserved for at least 90 days to allow for a change of mind.

High-risk exposures from patients known to be HIV positive or patients at risk of being HIV positive are handled as emergencies. A medication such as azidothymidine (AZT) must be administered, preferably within 4 hours of the exposure.

Follow-up study of the exposed employee, including antibody or antigen testing, counseling, and postexposure prophylaxis, is conducted. The employee is retested at 6, 12, and 26 weeks after exposure if the patient is HIV positive or is a high-risk subject.

Training

All new employees require specific training sessions to ensure that they understand the epidemiology of bloodborne disease and the modes of transmission. Explanation of the types and the appropriate use of personal protective equipment is essential, as is explanation of emergency procedures to be followed in the event of exposure. All employees must be familiar with the laboratory's policies for protection against transmission of bloodborne pathogens. Adherence to all policies must be monitored regularly; counseling or retraining should be provided when failures are evident.

Records of the employee's HBV vaccination status are mandatory. In addition, results of physical examinations and consultations must be documented. All such records must be maintained for the duration of employment plus 30 years.

Documentation of all training sessions is kept for 3 years and includes dates of all programs, a summary of each program's content, names and qualifications of all instructors, and an attendance list, including names and job titles.

Quality control of all safety procedures as defined by OSHA is a major issue in today's laboratory. All records necessary to meet current government regulations covering chemical hygiene and biohazard protection should be readily available and carefully maintained.

Latex Allergy

Since 1991, when OSHA required employers to provide gloves and other protective measures for their employees,[36] laboratory workers have shown a marked increase in the development of latex allergy. An allergy may occur in response to proteins from the rubber tree itself or to chemicals used in the production of latex. Latex products can produce three types of responses:

1. Irritant contact dermatitis, which is the most common reaction but is not a true allergy
2. Allergic contact dermatitis (delayed hypersensitivity with a rash that usually appears 24 to 48 hours after contact), which results from the addition of chemicals to latex during harvesting, processing, and manufacturing
3. Latex allergy, which is more serious and can cause severe reactions such as respiratory symptoms (see Chapter 29)

The amount of latex exposure required to produce sensitization or an allergic response is unknown. However, the proteins responsible for latex allergies can be adsorbed onto the powder used on many latex gloves, resulting in increased skin exposure. In addition, the removal of powdered gloves can produce an aerosol of latex-contaminated powder, which can increase the risk for respiratory symptoms. Therefore, powder-free gloves should be used whenever possible to minimize the quantities of allergy-causing proteins.[36] Moreover, wearing latex gloves during episodes of dermatitis of the hands may increase skin exposure and the risk of developing latex allergy. The risk of progression from rash to a more serious reaction is unknown, but a rash could be the first sign of allergy.[37]

Recommendations from the National Institute of Occupational Safety and Health (NIOSH) include the provision that reduced-protein, powder-free gloves should be available to every employee. Employees also should be provided with continuing education programs and training materials about latex allergy, and high-risk workers should be periodically screened for allergy symptoms. Some hospitals have adopted a program to screen newly hired employees for a latex allergy or sensitization. Employees should be aware that "hypoallergenic" gloves do not decrease the risk of latex allergy. They may, however, reduce reactions to the chemical additives used in the production of latex (allergic contact dermatitis). Appropriate work practices also include the following:

- Do not use oil-based hand creams or lotions (they cause deterioration of the gloves) unless they have been shown to reduce latex-associated problems and maintain barrier protection.
- Wash hands with mild soap after glove removal and dry thoroughly.
- Keep work area clean to minimize latex dust.
- Be aware of procedures for preventing latex allergy.
- Learn to recognize the symptoms of latex allergy, including rashes, hives, flushing, itching, nasal and eye symptoms, asthma, and shock.
- Report these symptoms to your employee health service.
- Avoid direct contact with latex gloves and other latex-containing products until seen by a physician; if a latex allergy is demonstrated, use a medical alert bracelet.

KEY CONCEPTS BOX 1-6

- Clinical laboratories are under the safety regulations of the Occupational and Safety Health Administration (OSHA). OSHA requires that laboratories have a Chemical Hygiene Plan and a fire safety plan.
- The OSHA Chemical Hygiene Plan requires the use of material safety data sheets (MSDSs) that describe the safety rating of every chemical in the laboratory, a chemical inventory, chemicals appropriately stored, and a proper disposal plan for waste chemicals.
- Chemical storage practice will depend on the hazard associated with a chemical, as indicated by the National Fire Protection Association (NFPA) diamond. The NFPA diamond uses four colored subdiamonds to indicate health, fire, flammability, and chemical reactivity hazards, on a scale of 1 to 4, for each subdiamond.
- Universal precaution, a policy set to protect all laboratory workers from infectious agents, assumes that all patient samples are infectiously hazardous and require utmost care (no mouth pipetting, wearing of disposable gloves, and wearing of face masks) to ensure protection.

PART 2: Calculations in Clinical Chemistry[38-40]

Elizabeth Ann Byrne

DILUTION

In several areas of the medical laboratory, an employee must dilute blood or body fluids to prepare a measurable concentration. Accurate preparation of these dilutions is mandatory for reporting the actual concentrations of body fluid constituents. Diagnosis, prognosis, and therapy depend on these test results.

Dilution can be defined as expressions of concentrations. Dilutions express the amount, either volume or weight, of a substance in a specified total final volume. A 1:5 dilution contains 1 volume (weight) in a *total* of 5 volumes (weights)—that is, 1 volume and 4 volumes.

Expression of a 1:5 dilution can be stated as the common fraction $^1/_5$. This fraction enables a technician to calculate the actual concentration of a diluted solution.

Example

A 100 mg/mL nitrogen standard is diluted 1:10. The concentration of the resulting solution is $100 \times {}^1/_{10} = 10$ mg/mL.

The most commonly used equation for preparing dilutions is:

$$V_1 \times C_1 = V_2 \times C_2 \qquad \text{Eq. 1-1}$$

where V_1 is the volume, C_1 is the concentration of solution 1, and V_2 and C_2 are the volume and concentration of the diluted solution. These may be expressed as % (weight/volume, w/v), molarity, or normality concentration. V_2 and C_2 are similarly related. This basic equation can be expressed as follows:

$$\frac{V_1}{V_2} = \frac{C_1}{C_2} \qquad \text{Eq. 1-2}$$

The most common error in setting up any equation of this type is not placing the related volumes or concentrations in the proper place and having the units cancel out, leaving the final, uncanceled units.

One helpful practice for successfully solving laboratory calculations is to label all numbers in any equation with their respective units of measurement. This may take an extra minute but will save many minutes of reviewing calculations when the final result appears illogical or incorrect. A problem that does not properly cancel out units cannot be solved successfully. A second helpful practice is to reduce fractions to their least common denominators before calculating the results.

Example

Prepare 500 mL of 0.5MNaCl (molecular weight of NaCl = 58.5 g/mol):

$$500\text{ mL} \times \frac{1\text{ Liter}}{1000\text{ mL}} \times \frac{0.5\text{ mol}}{\text{Liter}} \times \frac{58.5\text{ g}}{\text{mol}} = \frac{0.5 \times 58.5\text{ g}}{2}$$

$$= \frac{29.25\text{ g}}{2} = 14.6\text{ g}$$

14.6 g of NaCl dissolved in 500 mL = 0.5 M NaCl

Example

Prepare 250 mL of 0.1 M HCl from stock 1 M HCl:

$$\text{Using } C_1 \times V_1 = C_2 \times V_2$$

where V_1 is the unknown

$$V_2 = 250\text{mL}$$

$$C_1 = 1.0\text{mol/L} \quad C_2 = 0.1\text{mol/L}$$

$$1.0\text{mol/L} \times V_1 = 250\text{mL} \times 0.1\text{mol/L}$$

$$V_1 = 25\text{mL}$$

Measure 25 mL of 1 M HCl; dilute to 250 mL with distilled water. This diluted solution has a 0.1 M HCl concentration. (Mathematical reasoning indicates that a 1:10 dilution of stock 1 M HCl results in a 0.1 M concentration, and 25 mL diluted to 250 mL equals a 1:10 dilution.)

Another Application of Dilutions

So that a 24-hour urine creatinine concentration could be assayed, the specimen had to be diluted 1:5 before measurement. Calculate the 24-hour excretion if the 24-hour urine volume is 1800 mL and the measured creatinine concentration is 260 mg/L:

$$\text{Total excretion} = \text{Total urine volume} \times \text{Concentration} \times \text{Dilution}$$

$$\text{Total excretion} = 1800\frac{\text{mL}}{24\text{hr}} \times 260\frac{\text{mg}}{\text{L}} \times 5 \times \frac{1\text{L}}{1000\text{mL}}$$

$$\text{Total excretion} = 2340\text{mg/24hr or } 2.34\text{g/24hr}$$

Exercises

Calculate the concentrations (answers are at the end of this chapter).

1. 10 M NaOH diluted 1:20 = ___ M.
2. 2 M HCl diluted 1:5 = ___ M.
3. 1000 mg/L glucose diluted 1:10 and then 1:2 = ___ mg/L.

Serial dilutions are those in which all the dilutions after the first one are the same. Exceptions to this general description of preparation of serial dilutions are included with certain techniques in serology, such as the antistreptolysin titer.

Serial Dilution Example

To determine the anti-Rh_0 (D) titer, serum is diluted 1:5 by the addition of 0.2 mL of serum to 0.8 mL of saline solution in tube 1. Tubes 2 through 8 contain 0.5 mL of saline as diluent. Dilution is performed by transferring 0.5 mL of tube 1 to tube 2, mixing, and then transferring 0.5 mL of tube 2 to tube 3, continuing through the tubes to tube 8 and mixing after each transfer. The concentration of serum in the tubes decreases by a factor of 2 with each dilution as follows: 1:5, 1:10, 1:20, 1:40, 1:80, 1:160, 1:320, and 1:640.

Exercises

4. For an ABO titer, tube 1 contains 0.9 mL of diluent, tubes 2 to 8 contain 0.5 mL of diluent, 0.1 mL of serum is added to tube 1, and serial dilutions using 0.5 mL are carried out in the remaining tubes. If the last tube showing agglutination with A cells is tube 6, what is the anti-A titer of the serum? (This is equal to the dilution in tube 6 = 1:___?)

5. All tubes for a serial dilution contain 0.5 mL of saline solution, 0.5 mL of serum is added to tube 1, and 0.5 mL is transferred through the row of tubes. Sheep cells are added to the tubes, and agglutination is demonstrated through tube 7. What is the titer of sheep cell agglutinations?

WEIGHTS AND CONCENTRATIONS

Definitions and Examples

Percent Concentrations

Percent concentrations generally are expressed as parts of solute per 100 parts of total solution; hence the expression percent, or per one hundred. The use of percent concentration is derived historically from the early pharmaceutical chemists. Although these terms still are commonly used in the United States, major organizations (American Association for Clinical Chemistry [AACC], CAP) are attempting to use unified SI units. Concentrations in SI units are described in moles per liter when the molecular weight of the substance is known. If the molecular weight is unknown, weight (mass) per milliliter or weight per liter is used.

The three basic forms of concentration are as follows.

Weight per Unit Weight (w/w)

Both solute and solvent are weighed, with the total equaling 100 g.

Example

5% w/w of NaCl contains 50 g of NaCl + 950 g of diluent.

Volume per Unit Volume (v/v)

The volume of liquid solute per total volume of solute and solvent is expressed.

Example

1% of HCl (v/v) contains 1 mL of HCl per 100 mL (or 1 dL) of solution.

Weight per Unit Volume (w/v)

The most frequently used expression, concentrations of w/v are reported as grams percent (g%) or g/dL, as well as mg/dL and μg/dL. When percent concentration is expressed without a specified form, it is assumed to be weight per unit volume. SI units express w/v in terms of weight per microliters (μL), milliliters (mL), or liters (L).

Example

To prepare 100 mL of 100 g/L of NaCl, weigh 10 g of NaCl and dilute to volume in a 100 mL volumetric flask.

Molarity

Molarity expresses concentration as the number of moles per liter of solution. One mole is the molecular weight of the substance in grams. A millimole is $^1/_{1000}$ of a mole. A molar solution contains 1 gram molecular weight of a substance per liter.

$$1 \text{ mol} = 1000 \text{ mmol}$$

$$1 \text{ mmol} = 1000 \text{ μmol}$$

$$1 \text{ μmol} = 1000 \text{ nmol}$$

Examples

1 M NaOH (molecular weight [MW] = 40.0 g/mol) contains 1 gram–equivalent molecular weight per liter, or 40 g diluted to 1000 mL with distilled water. A millimolar (1 mM) solution, or 0.001 molar (0.001 M), contains 1 mmol/L. 1 mM of NaOH is $^1/_{1000}$ of 40 g, that is, 0.040 g (or 40 mg). When diluted to 1000 mL, the concentration of the solution is 0.001 M.

Normality

Normality expresses concentration in terms of equivalent weights of substances. Equivalent weights are determined by the valence, which reflects the number of combining or replaceable units. A 1 normal (1 N) solution contains 1 equivalent weight per liter. The equivalent weight of an element or compound is equal to the molecular weight divided by the valence.

Normality and molarity relationships can be calculated readily if their definitions are understood.

Examples

1M HCl = 1N HCl, since 1 mole of H^+ or Cl^{-1} reacts for every mole of HCl.

1M H_2SO_4 = 2N H_2SO_4, since 2 moles of H^+ (i.e., equivalents) react for every mole of H_2SO_4.

1M H_3PO_4 = 3N H_3PO_4, since 3 moles of H^+ react for every mole of H_3PO_4.

1M $CaCl_2$ = 2N $CaCl_2$, since 2 Cl^- can react for every mole of $CaCl_2$.

1M $CaSO_4$ = 2N $CaSO_4$, since 2 mole volume electrons are available for reaction with either Ca^{++} or SO_4^-.

Equivalent weight is known as the number of grams of an element (or compound) that will react with another element (or compound). This so-called law of combining weights is operable for all chemical compounds.

To simplify chemistry procedures and reports, factors can be used to express a quantity of one compound as an equivalent quantity of another compound. This process can be termed equivalency.

Example

Calculate the amount of urea if a patient's urea nitrogen level is 800 mg/L. The formula for urea is NH_2-CO-NH_2, and its molecular weight is 60 g/mol. The molecular equivalent weight for nitrogen in the mole is 14 g/mol × 2 molecules = 28. The urea/nitrogen factor is determined by the following equation:

$$\frac{\text{MW of urea (60)}}{2 \times \text{MW of nitrogen (28)}} = \frac{x \text{ g of urea}}{1 \text{ g of urea nitrogen}}$$

$$28x = 60$$

$$x = 2.14 \text{ (factor)}$$

This factor states that 2.14 g of urea equivalently represents 1 g of urea nitrogen, so 800 mg/L urea nitrogen × 2.14 equals 1712 mg/L of urea. Laboratory results today are reported as urea nitrogen because historical methods for this particular test are based on measurement of urea nitrogen.

Competent laboratory personnel should be able to convert mg/dL to mEq/L. Electrolyte equivalents can be calculated from the following equation:

$$\text{mg/dL} \times 10 = 10\ \text{mg/L}$$

because mg/mEq weight is the millimolar weight in milligrams divided by the valence

$$\frac{\text{mg/L}}{\text{mg/mEq}} = \text{mEq/L}$$

or

$$\frac{\text{mg/dL}}{\text{mg/mEq}} \times 10\frac{\text{dL}}{\text{L}} = \text{mEq/L}$$

Example

What is the mEq/L concentration of serum chloride reported as 250 mg/dL? Since the millimolecular weight of chloride is 35.5 (i.e., 1 mmol = 35.5 mg), the milliequivalent weight of chloride is as follows:

$$\frac{\text{MW}}{\text{Valence}} = \frac{35.5\ \text{g/mol}}{1}$$

$$\frac{250\ \text{mg/dL}}{35.5\ \text{mg/mEq}} \times 10\frac{\text{dL}}{\text{L}} = 70\ \text{mEq/L}$$

Specific Gravity

Specific gravity can be used to determine the mass (weight) of solutions. It relates the weight of 1 mL of the solution to the weight of an equal volume of pure water at 4°C (1 g). One particular use of specific gravity is in preparation of dilutions from concentrated commercial acids, with the equation as follows:

$$\text{Specific gravity} \times \text{Percent assay} = \text{Grams of compound per milliliter}$$

Example

Concentrated HCl has a specific gravity of 1.25 g/mL and is assayed as being 38% HCl. What is the amount of HCl per milliliter?

$$1.25\,\text{g/mL} \times 0.38 = 0.475\,\text{g of HCl per mL}$$

One common error is neglecting to change the percent assay to its proper decimal; in the previous example, 38% = 0.38!

Exercise

6. How many milliliters of concentrated HCl is needed to prepare 1 L of a 0.1 N HCl solution if the molecular weight of HCl = 36.5?

Water of Hydration

Some salts are available in forms that are either anhydrous (no water) or hydrated (with water molecules). The form of the available salt, including the water of hydration, is listed on the manufacturer's label. To prepare accurate weight concentrations of these salts, calculations must include the molecules of water present in the compound. This is done most easily by calculating the percentage of the compound that is in the anhydrous form. With this percentage, the weight of the hydrated form can be corrected to that of the anhydrous form.

The advantage of using molar concentrations is that the water of hydration does not have to be accounted for in the calculations. For example, 1 mol of $CuSO_4$ = 160 g, and 1 mol of $CuSO_4 \cdot 5H_2O$ = 250 g. One gram–equivalent molecular weight of each compound contains 1 mol of $CuSO_4$, that is,

$$250\,\text{g}\ CuSO_4 \cdot 5H_2O = 1\,\text{mol of}\ CuSO_4 = 160\,\text{g of}\ CuSO_4$$

Example

How many grams of $MgCl_2$ are in 1 g of $MgCl_2 \cdot 3H_2O$?

Mg	24	Mg	24
Cl_2	71	Cl_2	71
	95 MW	$3H_2O$	54
			149 MW

$$\frac{95}{149} = \frac{x}{1}$$

$$149x = 95$$

$$x = 63.8\%$$

One gram of $MgCl_2 \cdot 3H_2O$ contains 0.638 g of $MgCl_2$.

Mole Fraction

Mole fraction refers to the ratio of the amount of a component to the total mixture of components. Mole fraction is a derived unit that is expressed as either a percent or a decimal.

Example

What percent Mg is contained in $MgCl_2 \cdot 3H_2O$?

$$\text{Mg} = 24$$

$$\text{Cl} = 35.5 \qquad \frac{24}{149} = 16.1\%$$

$$MgCl_2 \cdot 3H_2O = 149$$

Mg is 16.1% of the molecule $MgCl_2 \cdot 3H_2O$.

Example

To determine mole percent calcium in calcium carbonate (MW = 100). 1 mol of $CaCO_3$ weighs 100 g, comprising 40 g (Ca) + 12 g (C) + 48 g (3 × O). Since 40 g is calcium, the mole fraction of calcium in 1 L of 1 mol of calcium carbonate equals 40%.

Example

How much $CuSO_4 \cdot 5H_2O$ must be weighed to prepare 1 L of a solution containing 80 mg of $CuSO_4$?

$$\text{Total MW of } CuSO_4 \cdot 5H_2O = 250$$

$$\text{MW of } CuSO_4 = 160$$

The proportion of $CuSO_4 \cdot 5H_2O$ that is $CuSO_4$ is 160/250 = 0.64. Therefore, 1 g of $CuSO_4 \cdot 5H_2O$ contains 1 g × 0.64 = 0.64 g of $CuSO_4$. The rest, 0.36 g, is water. Thus:

$$\frac{80 \text{ mg}}{0.64} = 125 \text{ mg of } CuSO_4 \cdot 5H_2O$$

Examples of Calculations

a. What is the normality of concentrated HCl that has a specific gravity of 1.19 g/mL and a 38% assay?

$$\text{Specific gravity} \times \text{Percent} = \text{Grams/milliliter}$$

$$1.19 \times 0.38 = 0.452 \text{ g/mL} = 452 \text{ g/L}$$

$$1 \text{ equivalent weight of HCl} = 36.5 \text{ g}$$

$$\frac{452 \text{ g/L}}{36.5 \text{ g/Eq}} = 12.4 \text{ N}$$

b. If 24.5 g of H_2SO_4 (MW = 98 g/mol) is dissolved in a 1L solution,
   1. What is its molarity?
   2. What is its normality?

(Answer 1) 1 mol of H_2SO_4 = 98 g; therefore, 24.5 g equals

$$\frac{1 \text{ mol}}{98 \text{ g}} = \frac{x}{24.5}$$

$$x = 0.25 \text{ mol}$$

$$0.25 \text{ mol in } 1 \text{ L} = 0.25 \text{ mol/L} = 0.25 \text{ M}$$

(Answer 2) The valence of H_2SO_4 equals 2; therefore, the equivalent weight of H_2SO_4 is expressed as follows:

$$\text{Equivalent weight} = \frac{\text{Molecular weight}}{\text{Valence}} = \frac{98 \text{ g}}{2}$$

$$\text{Equivalent weight} = 49 \text{g}$$

To solve for the number of equivalents in 24.5 g,

$$\frac{1 \text{ equivalent}}{49 \text{ g}} = \frac{x}{24.5 \text{ g}}$$

$$x = 0.5 \text{ equivalent}$$

$$0.5 \text{ equivalent in } 1 \text{ L} = 0.5 \text{ Eq/L} = 0.5 \text{ N}$$

c. The molecular weight of $CaCO_3$ is 100 g/mol, and the atomic weight of calcium is 40 g/mol; how many grams or milligrams of $CaCO_3$ is needed to prepare the following?
   1. 1 L of 0.1 M $CaCO_3$?
   2. 10 mL of 100 mg/dL of Ca^{++} using $CaCO_3$?
   3. 50 mg/L of $CaCO_3$?
   4. 0.2 mEq/L of Ca^{++} using $CaCO_3$?

(Answer 1) 10 grams; 1 mol of $CaCO_3$ = 100 g; therefore, 0.1 mol = 10 g, since 0.1 molar = 0.1 mol/L = 10 g/L.

(Answer 2) The percentage weight Ca^{++} in $CaCO_3$ is

$$\frac{\text{Atomic weight } Ca^{++}}{\text{Molecular weight } CaCO_3} = \frac{40}{100} = 40\%$$

In 10 mL, 10 mg of Ca^{++} is needed or

$$\frac{10 \text{ mg}}{\% \text{ Ca in } CaCO_3} = \frac{10 \text{ mg}}{40\%} = \frac{10 \text{ mg}}{0.4} = 25 \text{ mg of } CaCO_3.$$

Therefore, 25 mg of $CaCO_3$ = 10 mg Ca^{++}.

(Answer 3) For 1 L, 50 mg of $CaCO_3$ is needed.

(Answer 4) 1 equivalent weight of $CaCO_3$ equals

$$\frac{\text{Molecular weight of } CaCO_3}{\text{Valence}} = \frac{100 \text{ g/mol}}{2 \text{ Eq/mol}} = 50 \text{ g/Eq}$$

To convert to milliequivalents,

$$1 \text{ mEq} = \frac{1 \text{ Eq}}{1000}$$

$$\therefore \frac{50 \text{ g}}{1 \text{ Eq}} \times \frac{1 \text{ Eq}}{1000 \text{ m/Eq}} = 50 \text{ mg/mEq}$$

To calculate the amount needed to prepare 1 L of 0.2 mEq

$$\frac{1 \text{ mEq wt}}{50 \text{mg}} = \frac{0.2 \text{ mEq wt}}{x}$$

$$x = 10 \text{ mg of } CaCO_3$$

Exercises

7. 3 M $CaCl_2$ (MW = 111.1) = ___ N $CaCl_2$
8. 2 N H_3PO_4 (MW = 98) = ___ M H_3PO_4
9. 2 M H_2SO_4 (MW = 98) = ___ N H_2SO_4
10. 250 mL of 5% NaCl contains ___ g of NaCl.
11. How much $CuSO_4 \cdot 5H_2O$ must be weighed to prepare 100 mL of 5% $CuSO_4$? (MW $CuSO_4$ = 159.61; MW H_2O = 18)
12. What percent of $CuSO_4 \cdot 5H_2O$ is water? ___%

CALCULATIONS BASED ON PHOTOMETRIC MEASUREMENTS (BEER'S LAW)

Refer to Chapter 2 for a description of the relationship between percent transmittance, absorbance, and concentration.

Colorimetry

Colorimetry is the measurement of the kind and amount of light absorbed or transmitted by a solution. These measurements of absorbance or transmittance are logarithmically related. Beer's law reflects the relationships between the absorbance and the concentration of a known standard solution, which states that the absorbance of a solution is directly related to its concentration. If Beer's law is true, then solutions of unknown concentration—the patients' samples—can be calculated as:

$$C_u = \frac{A_u}{A_s} \times C_s \qquad \text{Eq. 1-3}$$

C_u and A_u represent concentration and absorbance of the unknown samples, whereas C_s and A_s reflect those of the standard solution. When preparing a colorimetric method for clinical chemistry analysis, the technician must be sure that Beer's law is followed, or this formula cannot be used. In other words, this formula can be used only if the absorbance and the concentration are directly related, that is, if the absorbance doubles with doubling of concentration. A standard curve can be used to determine concentration values graphically. Standard curve preparations are described on p. 38.

Absorbance and Transmittance

Absorbance measures the amount of light that is blocked or absorbed by a solution. Absorbance is also termed optical density (OD), a term found in the older literature that is not in common use today.

Transmittance measures the amount of light that passes through a solution. Transmittance usually is expressed as a percentage, or %T. The %T scale is linear, as is noted on a colorimeter readout scale.

As is discussed in Chapter 2, absorbance and percent transmittance are logarithmically related because absorbance is a logarithmic function. Interconversion of absorbance and percent transmittance is commonly expressed by the following formula:

$$\mathrm{A} = -\log \frac{\%\mathrm{T}}{100} \qquad \text{Eq. 1-4}$$

This equation can be algebraically converted to the following form:

$$\mathrm{A} = -(\log \%\mathrm{T} - \log 100)$$

$$\mathrm{A} = -(\log \%\mathrm{T} - 2)$$

$$\mathrm{A} = -\log \%\mathrm{T} + 2$$

$$\mathrm{A} = 2 - \log \%\mathrm{T} \qquad \text{Eq. 1-5}$$

A laboratory worker can obtain absorbance from a hand calculator using this formula by punching in the numbers for %T, converting to the log form, placing a minus sign, and adding 2.

Examples

Determining Concentrations Using Absorbance (A) Readings

a. If absorbance of an unknown is 0.25 and the concentration of a standard is 4 mg/L with an absorbance of 0.40, the concentration of the unknown can be calculated using these equations:

$$C_u = \frac{A_u}{A_s} \times C_s$$

$$C_u = \frac{0.25}{0.40} \times 4 \text{ mg/L}$$

$$C_u = 2.5 \text{ mg/L}$$

b. To calculate the concentration of glucose if the following information is known,

$$C_s = 2000 \text{ mg/L}, A_s = 0.40, A_u = 0.25$$

Using the same formula above,

$$C_u = \frac{0.25}{0.40} \times 2000 \text{ mg/L}$$

$$C_u = 1250 \text{ mg/L}$$

c. To calculate the glucose concentration of unknown (C_u) if the %T is given. If the 1000 mg/L glucose standard (C_s) reads 49% T, and the unknown reads 55% T, the %T must be converted to absorbance because only absorbance is linearly proportional to concentration:

$$A_s = 2 - \log\%\mathrm{T} \qquad A_u = 2 - \log\%\mathrm{T}$$

$$A_s = 2 - 1.690 \qquad A_u = 2 - 1.740$$

$$A_s = 0.31 \qquad A_u = 0.26$$

$$49\%\ \mathrm{T} = 0.31\ \mathrm{A} = A_s$$

$$55\%\ \mathrm{T} = 0.26\ \mathrm{A} = A_u$$

$$C_s = 1000 \text{ mg/L}, A_u = 0.26, A_s = 0.31$$

Using the formula as in (a) and (b) previously,

$$C_u = \frac{0.26}{0.31} \times 1000 \text{ mg/L} = 839 \text{ mg/L}$$

Molar Extinction Coefficient

Molar extinction coefficients are used in the clinical laboratory to calculate concentrations and activities of enzymes in IU and to determine the purity of dissolved substances. Specific applications include checking standard solutions such as hemoglobin or bilirubin. The molar extinction coefficient, or the molar absorbance coefficient, or ε, is defined as the absorbance at a given wavelength of a 1 M solution of the substance in a 1 cm cuvette at 25° C. It is related to absorbance by the following formula:

$$A = \varepsilon c l \qquad \text{Eq. 1-6}$$

where A is absorbance at a specified wavelength, c is the concentration of the substance being measured in moles/L, and l is the path length in centimeters.

A suitable bilirubin standard, as a 1 M solution in chloroform, would have a theoretical absorbance of 60,700 (mean)

± 800 at 453 nm, when measured in a 1 cm cuvette at 25° C. Logical reasoning suggests that if this standard were diluted to 1:60,700, the absorbance would read 1.

Example

1 M bilirubin standard is diluted to 1:60,700 and then to 1:2, with the final dilution being 1:121,400. The absorbance of this dilution reads 0.495 in a 1 cm cuvette. What is the extinction coefficient of this bilirubin standard?

$$\varepsilon = \frac{0.495\,(121{,}400)}{1\text{ mol/L}\,(1\text{ cm})}$$

$$\varepsilon = 60{,}093\text{ liters} \times \text{mol}^{-1} \times \text{cm}^{-1}$$

A major application of ε is the measurement of concentrations of substances. If the ε of a substance is known and a 1 cm cuvette is used, Beer's law is simplified to the following:

$$c = \frac{A}{\varepsilon}$$

Example

The ε of NADH at 340 nm is 6.22×10^3 L × mol^{-1} × cm^{-1}. If the absorbance of NADH at 340 nm reads 0.350 in 1 cm curette, what is the concentration?

$$c = \frac{0.350}{6.22 \times 10^3\text{ L}\cdot\text{mol}^{-1}}$$

$$c = 5.6 \times 10^{-5}\text{ mol/L}$$

Exercises

13. NADH has a molar absorptivity of 3.3×10^3 at a wavelength of 366 nm. Calculate the concentration of a solution that has an A (absorbance) of 0.175 at 366 nm.
14. A chemistry technologist is checking a bilirubin standard. What is the molar absorptivity of a 1 M solution diluted to 1:60,700 and reading 0.70 in a 7 mm cuvette?
15. The chemistry technologist has a solution of NADH with a concentration of 0.05×10^{-3} mol/L. Calculate the molar absorptivity if it measures 0.300 at 334 nm.

BUFFERS

Buffers resist changes in acidity by forming a weakly ionized acid or base with the added H^+ or OH^- ions. For example, when HCl is added to a solution of Na^+Ac^- (sodium acetate) plus H^+Ac^- (acetic acid), the H^+ of HCl will react with the Ac^-, forming more HAc, which is only slightly ionized. The acetate–acetic acid effectively buffers by removing H^+ from the solution.

The Henderson-Hasselbalch equation is used to express acid-base relationships. Several forms of this equation can be used. They will not be delineated at this time but can be used for calculating acid-base problems. The simplest equation is as follows:

$$\text{pH} = \text{pK} + \log \frac{\text{Concentration of conjugate base}}{\text{Concentration of weak acid}} \quad \text{Eq. 1-7}$$

The pK value depends on a specific set of conditions, including degree of dissociation, temperature, and pH. The pK for the bicarbonate buffer system in serum or plasma is 6.10 at 37°C. Chemical reference books such as *The Handbook of Chemistry and Physics* contain pK values. Capable medical technologists should grasp the basic calculations of the Henderson-Hasselbalch equations even though laboratory instruments provide direct "read-out" values on patients' acid-base tests.

Examples

a. Calculate the pH of an acetate buffer composed of 0.20 M sodium acetate and 0.05 M acetic acid. (The pK for acetic acid is 4.76.)

$$\text{pH} = \text{pK} + \log \frac{[\text{Salt}]}{[\text{Acid}]}$$

$$= 4.76 + \log \frac{0.20}{0.05}$$

$$= 4.76 + \log 4$$

$$= 5.3621$$

$$\text{pH} = 5.36$$

b. Now for a complicated example. Prepare 1 L of an acetate buffer whose acetate concentration is 0.2 M with a pH of 5.0. (The pK of acetic acid is 4.76; the molecular weight of acetic acid is 60; the molecular weight of sodium acetate is 82.)

$$\text{pH} = 4.76 + \log \frac{[\text{Salt}]}{[\text{Acid}]}$$

$$\log \frac{[\text{Salt}]}{[\text{Acid}]} = 5.0 - 4.76$$

$$[\text{Salt}]/[\text{Acid}] = \text{antilog } 0.24$$

$$[\text{Salt}]/[\text{Acid}] = 1.7$$

The number 1.7 is the ratio of moles per liter of salt to moles per liter of acid. Any molar concentrations of salt to acid yielding a ratio of 1.7 will result in a 5.0 pH acetate buffer. *Note:* The problem specifies a concentration of 0.2 M solution, or HAc + Ac^- = 0.2 M.

If

$$Ac^-/HAc = 1.7$$

then

$$Ac^- = 1.7\text{ HAc}$$

or

$$HAc + 1.7\text{ HAc} = 0.2\text{ M}$$

and

$$2.7\ \text{HAc} = 0.2$$
$$\text{HAc} = 0.074\ \text{mol/L of acid}$$
$$\text{MW} \times \text{M} = \text{g/L}$$
$$60\ \text{g/mol} \times 0.074\ \text{mol/L} = 4.44\ \text{g/L of acid needed}$$

To calculate the weight of salt needed for 1 L use,

$$\text{Moles of salt} = \text{Total moles} - \text{Moles of acid}$$
$$= 0.2 - 0.074$$
$$= 0.126\ \text{moles of salt}$$

As done for the acid:

$$\text{MW of salt} \times \text{M} = \text{Grams of salt/liter}$$
$$82\ \text{g/mol} \times 0.126\ \text{mol/L} = 10.33\ \text{g of salt/L}$$

When 4.44 g of acid and 10.33 of salt are dissolved in a total volume of 1L, the resulting buffer concentration is 0.2M at a pH of 5.0.

ENZYME CALCULATIONS

Expressing enzyme activity in U has been generally accepted since its recommendation by the IUB in the early 1960s. One U of an enzyme is defined as the amount that will catalyze the transformation of 1 μmole of the substrate per minute under standard conditions. Activity is expressed in terms of enzyme units per liter of serum, or milliunits per milliliter, in the following relationship:

$$1\ \text{U/L} = \mu\text{mole/min/liter of serum}$$

Explanation of the basic equation for the conversion of absorbance data to U is not provided in this portion of laboratory calculation. Suffice it to state that any change in factors such as temperature or volume must be accounted for in the following basic equation (see Chapter 15):

$$\text{U/L} = \frac{\Delta A/\text{min} \times V_t \times 10^6\ (\mu\text{mol/mol})}{\varepsilon \times V_s \times l} \qquad \text{Eq. 1-8}$$

$\Delta A/\text{min}$ = Absorbance change per minute

V_t = Total reaction volume, including sample, reagent, and diluent

V_s = Serum volume

l = Cuvette path length

ε = Extinction coefficient

The factor of 10^6 μmol/mol is added to convert the answer to μmol/min/L (U/L).

Example

What is the lactate dehydrogenase (LD) activity of 0.1 mL of serum + 3 mL of substrate if the NADH being formed showed a 0.002 ΔA/min at 340 nm? ε for NADH = $6.22 \times 10^3 \times \text{L} \times \text{mol}^{-1} \times \text{cm}^{-1}$. Using the previously provided formula,

$$\text{U/L} = \frac{0.002\ (10^6\ \mu\text{mol/mol})(3.1\ \text{mL})}{1\ \text{min}\left(6.22 \times 10^3\ \dfrac{\text{L}}{\text{mol} \cdot \text{cm}}\right)(0.1\ \text{mL})(1\ \text{cm})}$$

$$\text{U/L} = 9.9$$

Example

Calculation of U units per liter of alkaline phosphatase activity using p-nitrophenol standard requires attention to all factors of the formula:

$$\text{U/L} = \frac{\Delta A/\text{min} \times V_t \times 10^6\ (\mu\text{mol/mol})}{\varepsilon \times V_s \times 1}$$

If ΔA of sample = 0.070, the ε for p-nitrophenol is 50,000 L/mol × cm; timing = 15 min; V_t = 5.5 mL; V_s = 0.005 mL.

$$\text{U/L} = \frac{0.070\left(10^6\ \dfrac{\mu\text{mol}}{\text{mol}}\right)(5.5\ \text{mL})}{15\ \text{min}\left(50{,}000\ \dfrac{\text{L}}{\text{mol} \cdot \text{cm}}\right)(0.005\ \text{mL})(1\ \text{cm})}$$

$$\text{U/L} = \frac{0.070 \times 5.5 \times 1000}{50 \times 0.75}$$

$$\text{Alkaline phosphatase activity} = 103\ \text{U/L}$$

STANDARD CURVES

Preparing standard curves on graph paper is an essential way of examining data for validity. Often calculations or computers do not reveal abnormalities of the system but calculate averages of results. Therefore, graphing of data is an important way to validate assays.

Previously in this chapter, Beer's law was defined as the direct relationship of the absorbance and concentration of a solution. This means that if a 2% solution reads 0.1 A, then a 4% concentration will read 0.2 A, and an 8% solution will read 0.4 A. Most solutions obey Beer's law; that is, concentration and absorbance are directly proportional only over specified ranges of concentrations.

Graphs

Figure 1-15 indicates that absorbances of glucose standard concentrations plotted on linear paper result in a straight line, confirming that Beer's law is followed for concentrations up to 3000 mg/L. The Fig. 1-16 graph, which plots the %T values of the same glucose concentrations used in Fig. 1-15 on linear paper, features a semicurved line; %T values are not linear versus concentrations. (Recall the logarithmic relationship of absorbance and %T.) Plotting %T values on semilog paper results in a straight line, which can be used to interpolate the concentrations of glucose from %T values (Fig. 1-17).

Exercises

Find glucose concentrations for the following readings, using Figs. 1-15 and 1-17.

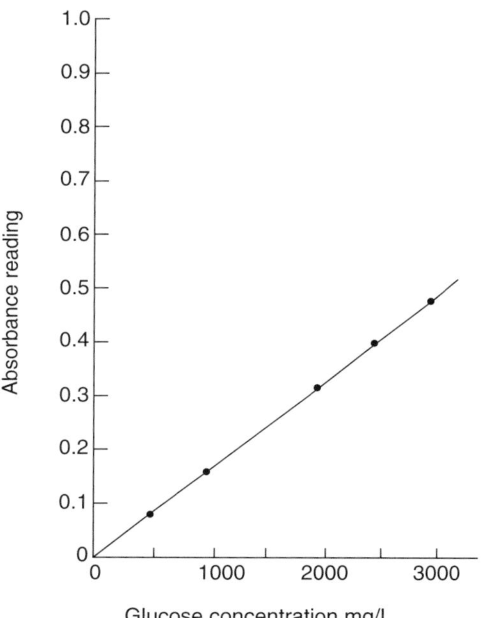

Fig. 1-15 Standard curve for glucose analysis: absorbance versus concentration on linear-linear graph paper.

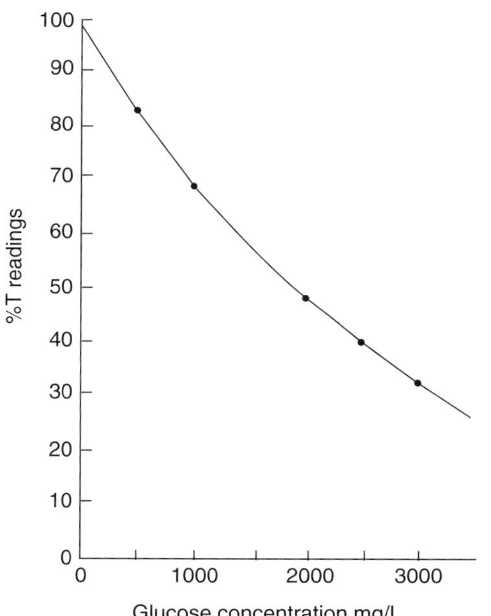

Fig. 1-16 Standard curve for glucose analysis: percent transmittance (%T) versus concentration on linear-linear graph paper.

16. 0.3 A = ___ mg/L
17. 0.39 A = ___ mg/L
18. 49% T = ___ mg/L
19. 52% T = ___ mg/L

Exercises Using One Known Standard Value to Determine Concentrations of Unknowns

What are the glucose concentrations of the following patients' samples if the 2000 mg/L standard reads 0.32 A?

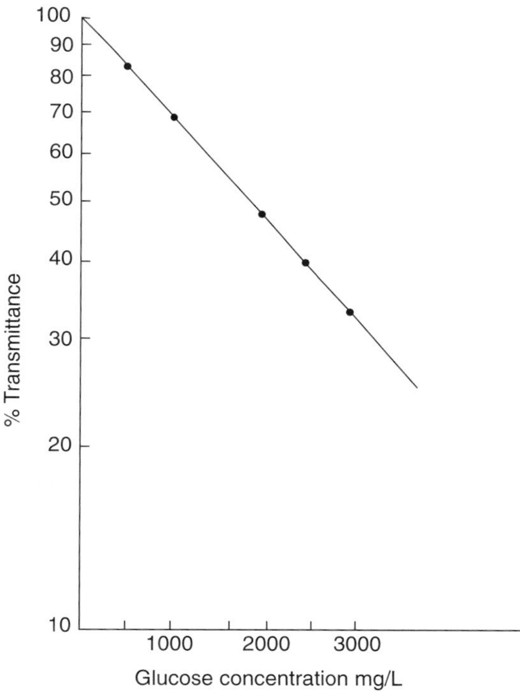

Fig. 1-17 Standard curve for glucose analysis: percent transmittance (%T) versus concentration on log-linear graph paper.

We can employ either of the following:

$$C_u = \frac{A_u}{A_s} \times C_s$$

or

$$\frac{C_u}{C_s} = \frac{A_u}{A_s}$$

20. 0.22 A = ___ mg/L
21. 0.14 A = ___ mg/L
22. 0.46 A = ___ mg/L

Renal Clearance Test Calculations

Renal clearance tests are used to assess kidney function. Renal clearance is a rate measurement that expresses the volume of blood cleared of the substance being studied (typically creatinine or urea) per unit of time. Therefore, the unit for the clearance test is milliliters per minute.

To calculate creatinine clearance, the following information is required:

Serum concentration (S)

Urine concentration (U) (Caution: The serum and urine concentrations must be in the same units, e.g., mg/L or mg/dL.)

Volume of urine excreted per minute (V) (volume of urine collected divided by time period in minutes)

$$\text{Clearance (uncorrected)} = \frac{\text{U} \times \text{V}}{\text{S}}$$

This calculation does not account for the patient's body surface area. If the physician requests a corrected value, the equation must be multiplied by 1.73/*A*, where 1.73 equals the average body surface area in square meters, and *A* equals the patient's body surface area:

$$\text{Clearance (corrected)} = \frac{\text{U} \times \text{V}}{\text{S}} \times \frac{1.73}{A}$$

The patient's body surface area is computed from a nomogram, using the patient's height and weight, or it is calculated with the following formula:

$$\log A = (0.425 \times \log W) + (0.725 \times \log H) - 2144$$

where *A* is the body surface area in square meters, *W* is the patient's weight in kilograms, and *H* is the patient's height in centimeters.

Examples

a. Determine the uncorrected creatinine clearance for a patient with a serum creatinine of 25 mg/L. The urine creatinine was 500 mg/L and the urine volume was 312 mL/4 h.

$$312 \text{ mL}/240 \text{ min} = 1.3 \text{ mL/min}$$

$$\text{C} = \frac{\text{U}}{\text{S}} \times \text{V} = \frac{500}{25} \times 1.3 = 26 \text{ mL/min}$$

b. Calculate the corrected creatinine clearance for a child who weighed 22.7 kg, was 95 cm long, and passed 500 mL of urine during a 24-hour period. Serum and urine creatinine values were 0.14 mmol/L and 4.75 mmol/L, respectively.

$$\log \text{A} = (0.425 \times \log 22.7) + (0.725 \times \log 95) - 2144$$

$$\log \text{A} = 0.576 + 1434 - 2144 = 0.134$$

$$\text{A} = 0.734$$

$$500 \text{ mL}/1400 \text{ min} = 0.35 \text{ mL/min}$$

$$\text{C} = \frac{\text{U}}{\text{S}} \times \text{V} \times \frac{1.73}{A}$$

$$= \frac{4.75}{0.14} \times 0.35 \times \frac{1.73}{0.734}$$

$$= 28.0 \text{ mL/min}$$

Timed Urine Tests

Results of urine tests may be reported in several ways. Values can be reported as concentration units, quantity per total volume, and quantity per unit of time. The clinical usefulness of urine tests is increased when quantitative results are expressed as amount per total volume or amount excreted in a given period. Good laboratory practice dictates that the urine total volume and the beginning and end time periods of collection be recorded.

When urine test results are reported as quantity per total volume, the concentration is measured and the results are corrected as follows:

$$\frac{\text{Amount}}{\text{Total volume}} = \text{Measured concentration} \times \text{Total volume}$$

This calculation requires that both the urine and the instrument concentration be reported using the same volume units.

Examples

a. Calculate the amount of protein in 2400 mL of urine with a concentration of 30 mg/dL.

$$\frac{\text{Amount}}{\text{Total volume}} = \frac{30 \text{ mg}}{100 \text{ mL}} \times 2400 \text{ mL} = 720 \text{ mg}$$

b. Determine the amount of sodium in 1800 mL of urine with a sodium concentration of 35 mEq/L.

$$\frac{\text{Amount}}{\text{Total volume}} = \frac{35 \text{ mEq}}{1000 \text{ mL}} \times 1800 \text{ mL} = 63 \text{ mEq}$$

When results are reported as quantity per time period of collection, the calculation of amount of substance per total volume must be performed first and the result reported for the length of time instead of for total volume.

ADDITIONAL EXERCISES

23. The hemoglobin standard solution contains 200 g/L. What amounts would be used to prepare 6 mL of the following concentrations?
    200 g/L?
    150 g/L?
    100 g/L?
    50 g/L?
24. a. What fraction of urea is nitrogen? Urea is $CO(NH_2)_2$.
    Atomic weights:
    C = 12
    O = 16
    N = 14
    H = 1

    b. What percent of urea is nitrogen?
25. There is available concentrated HCl with a 38% assay and a specific gravity of 1.170.
    a. What is the weight of HCl present in 1 mL?
    b. For the preparation of 100 mL of 10% wt/vol HCl, what mL of HCl would be diluted to a total volume of mL?
26. Normal saline solution is 0.85% concentration. What is its molarity? (NaCl molecular weight is 58.5.)
27. If a protein standard reads 0.48 A, and a patient's sample reads 0.36 A, what is the patient's protein concentration? Select one of the following answers:

a. Twice the standard concentration
b. Equal to the standard concentration
c. Three-fourths of the standard concentration
d. Not enough data for calculation

28. A patient in a diabetic coma has high blood glucose levels; serum from this patient is diluted 1:2 and again 1:2 before it is readable from the glucose chart as 1900 mg/L. What is the actual concentration in (a) mg/L, (b) mg/dL and (c) g/L?
29. How many mEq/L is in a solution that contains 27.7 mg/dL of potassium? (Atomic weight of K = 39.)
30. How many milliliters of 0.4 N NaOH can be made from 20 mL of 2 N solution?
31. What is the normality of a solution containing 40 mEq of NaOH per 50 mL?
32. What is the dilution of serum in a tube containing 200 mL of serum, 500 mL of saline, and 300 mL of reagent?
33. Calculate the alkaline phosphatase activity in U/L for the following:
    CE of standard (p-nitrophenol) = 5×10^4 L $\times$ mol^{-1} $\times$ cm^{-1}
    $\Delta A_{sample} = 0.150$
    $V_{sample} = 0.2$ mL
    $V_{total} = 2.2$ mL
    Timing = 15 minutes
34. What is the extinction coefficient for the following?
    Solution concentration = 1.2 molar
    Dilution of solution = 1/121,400
    Reading in a 1 cm cuvette = 0.6
35. A 0.01 M Na_2HPO_4 solution needs to be prepared (MW of Na_2HPO_4 = 141.98). Only the hydrated salt, $Na_2HPO_4 \cdot 7H_2O$ (MW = 267.98) is available. How many grams is needed to prepare 250 mL?
36. If a 50 mg/mL solution of Na_2HPO_4 needs to be prepared, how many grams of the hydrated salt described in question 35 must be weighed to make a 1L solution?
37. A medical technologist desires to prepare 50 mL of a 10 mg/mL solution of NADH (MW = 663.44). To do this accurately, the technologist first prepares a stock solution containing approximately 50 mg/mL. The absorbance of a 1:1000 dilution of the stock solution is measured at 340 nm and from the known molar absorbance of NADH at this wavelength (6.22×10^3), the actual concentration is calculated. A suitable dilution then is made to prepare 50 mL of the desired 10 mg/mL solution. Presume that the technologist, following these directions, has prepared a dilution of the stock solution with an absorbance of 0.562. Calculate the concentration of NADH in this stock solution as mmol/L and mg/L. What dilution should be made to prepare the 10 mg/mL of NADH solution?
38. A patient's serum calcium level is 3.5 mEq/L. The expected normal range is 90 to 110 mg/L. Is the patient's calcium level lower than, within, or higher than the expected normal range?
39. A sodium concentration is reported as 3500 mg/L. What is the concentration in mEq/L? (Atomic weight of sodium = Equivalent weight = 23 g/mol or 23 mg/mmol.)
40. If the cyanmethemoglobin standard, with a concentration of 200 g/L, reads 0.426 A, and a patient's blood sample reads 0.297 A, what is the concentration of hemoglobin in the sample?
41. A 200 mg/L urea nitrogen standard reads 0.30 A and a patient's sample reads 0.40 A. The concentration of the standard compared with the patient's level is
    a. Higher
    b. Twice as much
    c. $^3/_4$ as much
    d. $^4/_3$ as much
42. A glucose standard of 2000 mg/L reads 0.4 A and a patient's sample reads 1.0 A. The technologist should
    a. Report the result as 500 mg/dL
    b. Repeat the test before reporting
    c. Repeat the test on the diluted sample
    d. Prepare a fresh glucose standard

APPENDIX: ANSWERS TO PROBLEMS

1. 0.5 M
2. 0.4 M
3. 50 mg/L
4. 1:320
5. 1:128
6. 8.55 mL
7. 6
8. 0.667
9. 4
10. 12.5
11. 7.82
12. 36.05
13. $c = 53 \times 10^{-6}$ mol/L
14. CE = 60,700 L $\times$ mol^{-1} $\times$ cm^{-1}
15. 6.0×10^3 L $\times$ mol^{-1} $\times$ cm^{-1}
16. 1900 mg/L
17. 2400 mg/L
18. 1920 mg/L
19. 1740 mg/L
20. 1375 mg/L
21. 875 mg/L
22. 2875 mg/L
23. 200 g/L = 6 mL + 0 mL of diluent
    150 g/L = 4.5 mL + 1.5 mL of diluent
    100 g/L = 3.0 mL + 3 mL of diluent
    50 g/L = 1.5 mL + 4.5 mL of diluent
24. a. 28/60 = 7/15
    b. 46.6%
25. a. 0.445 g
    b. 22.5 mL will be diluted to 100 mL
26. 0.145 mol/L
27. c
28. a. 7600 mg/L
    b. 760 mg/dL
    c. 7.6 g/L
29. 7.1 mEq/L
30. 100 mL

31. 0.8 N
32. 1:5
33. 2.2 U/L
34. 6.07×10^4
35. 0.67 g
36. 94.4 g
37. The concentration of NADH in stock solution is 90.4 mmol/L, or 60 mg/mL. Take 8.3 mL of the stock and dilute to 50 mL to prepare the 10 mg/mL of solution.
38. 70 mg/L; lower than the expected range
39. 152 mEq/L
40. 139 g/L
41. c. $^3/_4$ as much
42. c

REFERENCES

1. *Preparation and Testing of Reagent Water in the Clinical Laboratory,* ed 4, Clinical and Laboratory Standards Institute (CLSI) Approved Guideline C3-A4, Villanova, PA, 2006, CLSI.
2. Gabler R, Hegde R, Hughes D: Degradation of high purity water on storage, J Liquid Chromatog 6:2565, 1983.
3. Winstead M: *Reagent Grade Water: How, When and Why?* Austin, TX, 1967, American Society of Medical Technologists.
4. Costerton JW, Lewandowski Z, Caldwell DE, et al: Microbial biofilms, Ann Rev Microbiol 49:711, 1995.
5. Jorgenson JH, Smith RF: Rapid detection of contaminated intravenous fluids using the Limulus in vitro endotoxin assay, Appl Microbiol 26:521, 1973.
6. Sullivan JD Jr, Valoes FW, Watson SW: Endotoxins: the Limulus amebocyte lysate system. In Bernheimer AW, editor: *Mechanisms in Bacterial Toxicology,* New York, 1976, John Wiley and Sons.
7. Bristol DW: Detection of trace organic impurities in binary solvent systems: a solvent purity test, J Chromatog 188:193, 1980.
8. *Laboratory Documents: Development and Control,* GP2-A5, Villanova, PA, 2006, CLSI.
9. Statement from the Quadrennial Symposium on Measurable Properties (Quantities) and Units in Clinical Chemistry, Gaithersburg, MD, August 5 and 6, 1976, Am J Clin Pathol 71:465, 1979.
10. *Determining Performance of Volumetric Equipment,* National Committee on Clinical Laboratory Standards (NCCLS) Proposed Standard I8-P, Villanova, PA, 1984, NCCLS.
11. ASTM E1154, 1989, Standard specification for piston or plunger operated volumetric apparatus. Available at www.astm.org.
12. ISO 8655-6, 2002, Piston-operated volumetric apparatus—gravimetric methods for the determination of measurement error. Available at www.iso.org.
13. ISO 8655-7, 2005 Piston-operated volumetric apparatus—non-gravimetric methods for the assessment of equipment performance. Available at www.iso.org.
14. Lide DR, editor: *Handbook of Chemistry and Physics,* ed 88, Boca Raton, FL, 2007-2008, CRC Press.
15. Lashor TW, Macurdy LB: *Precision Laboratory Standards of Mass and Laboratory Weights,* National Bureau of Standards, Circular 547, Washington, DC, 1954, U.S. Department of Commerce.
16. McCoubrey AO: *Guide for the Use of the International System of Units: The Modernized Metric System,* National Institute of Standards and Technology, Special Publication 811, Washington, DC, 1991, U.S. Department of Commerce.
17. The National Committee for Clinical Laboratory Standards Position Paper (PPC-11): Quantities and Units (SI), Clin Chem 25:657, 1979.
18. Committee on Hospital Care, American Academy of Pediatrics: Metrication and SI units, Pediatrics 65:659, 1980.
19. College of American Pathologists: General Checklist, 2008.
20. *Temperature Calibration of Water Baths, Instruments, and Temperature Sensors,* ed 2, NCCLS Approved Standard I2-A2, Villanova, PA, 1990, NCCLS.
21. *Procedures for the Handling and Processing of Blood Specimens,* ed 2, NCCLS Approved Guideline H18-A2, Villanova, PA, 1999, NCCLS.
22. *A Centrifuge Primer,* Palo Alto, CA, 1980, Spinco Division Beckman Instruments, Inc. (out of print).
23. Occupational exposures to hazardous chemicals in laboratories, Final rule, Federal Register, 29 CFR Part 1910.1450, Washington, DC, 1990, U.S. Department of Labor, Occupational Safety and Health Administration.
24. Occupational exposure to bloodborne pathogens, Final rule, Federal Register, 29 CFR Part 1910.1030, Washington, DC, 1991, U.S. Department of Labor, Occupational Safety and Health Administration.
25. Needlestick and other sharps injuries, Final rule, Federal Register, 29 CFR Part 1910, Washington, DC, 2001, U.S. Department of Labor, Occupational Safety and Health Administration.
26. *Sigma-Aldrich Library of Chemical Safety Data,* St. Louis, Sigma Chemical Co. (available in printed or CD-ROM format).
27. Compressed Gas Association, Inc.: *Handbook of Compressed Gases,* ed 2, New York, 1981, Reinhold Publishing.
28. Lunn G, Sansone EB: *Destruction of Hazardous Chemicals in the Laboratory,* ed 2, New York, 1994, Wiley Interscience.
29. U.S. Department of Health and Human Services: Recommendations for prevention of HIV transmission in health care setting, MMWR 56:1, 1987.
30. EPINet: Summary report for needle-stick and sharp object exposure: category nurse-device: 6 needle, winged steel, Jan 1, 2002–Dec 31, 2002.
31. Perry J, Jagger J: Healthcare worker blood exposure risks: correcting some outdated statistics. Adv Exposure Prev 6:28, 2003.
32. Jagger J, Hunt EH, Brand-Elnagger J, Pearson RD: Rates of needle-stick injury caused by various devices in a university hospital. N Engl J Med 3219:285, 1988.
33. Jagger J, De Carli G, Perry J, et al: Chapter 31. Occupational exposure to bloodborne pathogens: epidemiology and prevention. In Wenzel RP, editor: *Prevention and Control of Nosocomial Infections,* ed 4, Baltimore, MD, 2003, Lippincott, Williams & Wilkins.
34. Cohen ML: U.S. House Committee on Education and the Workforce Subcommittee on Workforce Protections: OSHA's Compliance Directive on Bloodborne Pathogens and the Prevention of Needlestick Injuries, Supplement to the Statement of Dr. Murray L. Cohen, June 22, 2000. Available at http://edworkforce.house.gov/heatrings/106th/wp/needlestick62200/cohen.htm.
35. Rutale WA, Weber DJ: Infectious waste—mismatch between science and policy: soundboard, N Engl J Med 325:578, 1991.
36. Tarlo SM, et al: Control of airborne latex by use of powder-free latex gloves, J Allergy Clin Immunol 93:985, 1994.
37. Kelly KJ, Sussman G, Fink JN: Stop the sensitization, J Allergy Clin Immunol 98:857, 1996.
38. Campbell JM, Campbell JB: *Laboratory Mathematics: Medical and Biological Applications,* ed 5, St. Louis, 1997, Mosby.
39. Greenwell RL: Calculus for the Life Sciences, Upper Saddle River, NJ, 2003, Pearson Education.
40. Johnson CW, Timmons DL, Hall PE: *Essential Laboratory Mathematics: Concepts and Applications for the Chemical and Clinical Laboratory Technician,* ed 2, Florence, KY, Delmar Cengage Learning, 2002.

INTERNET SITES

www.MSDS.chem.ox.ac.uk/—Oxford University safety
www.mhhe.com/biosci/genbio/dolphin5e/labprep.mhtml—A number of sections on practical lab technique, including calculations
www.practicingsafescience.org—Online safety course
http://www.osha.gov/pls/oshaweb/owadisp.show_document/p_table=STANDARDS&p_id=10106—Occupational Safety and Health Administration (OSHA) Regulations (Standards—29 CFR): Occupational exposure to hazardous chemicals in laboratories—1910.1450
www.clsi.org/—Clinical and Laboratory Standards Institute
http://www.epa.gov/—Environmental Protection Agency
http://www.epa.state.oh.us/ocapp/p2/hospital.html—Mercury pollution
www.medal.org—The Medical Algorithms Project; has a calculations program
http://www.phys.ksu.edu/area/jrm/safety/msds.html—Link for MSDS
http://www.intute.ac.uk/healthandlifesciences/medicine—BIOME, Greenfield Medical Library, Queens Medical Centre, Nottingham; target audience is the UK learning, teaching, and research community

Chapter 2

Spectral Techniques

Amadeo J. Pesce

Chapter Outline

Light and Matter
- *Properties of Light and Radiant Energy*
- *Interactions of Light With Matter*

Absorption Spectroscopy
- *Radiant Energy Absorption*
- *Beer-Lambert Law*
- *Instrumentation*
- *Detectors*
- *Charge-Coupled Devices*
- *Instrument Performance*
- *Selection of Optimum Conditions and Limitations*
- *Quality Control Checks of Spectrophotometers*
- *Reflectance Spectrophotometry*
- *Recording Spectrophotometry*
- *Multiwavelength Spectrophotometry*

Atomic Absorption
- *Principle*
- *Instrumentation*
- *Sources of Error*

Flame Photometry
- *Principle*

Fluorometry
- *Principle*
- *Instrumentation*
- *Limitations*
- *Time-Delayed Fluorescence*
- *Chemiluminescence*
- *Electrochemiluminescence*
- *Fluorescence Polarization*

Nephelometry and Turbidimetry
- *Principle*
- *Detection of Scattered Light*
- *Instrumentation*
- *Limitations: Turbidimetry versus Nephelometry*

Refractivity
- *Principle*
- *Applications*
- *Interference*
- *Instrumentation*

Key Terms

absorbance Defined as 2 – log %T, it is directly proportional to the concentration of the absorbing species if Beer's law is followed.

absorption spectrum The range of electromagnetic energy that is used for spectroanalysis, including both visible light and ultraviolet radiation; also graph of spectrum for a specific compound.

absorptivity Absorbance divided by the product of the concentration of a substance and the sample path length.

angle of detection The angle at which scattered light is measured in nephelometry.

atomic absorption spectrophotometry A quantitative spectroscopic measurement in which the emitted light from a source composed of one element is absorbed by the same element in a vapor phase. The amount of light absorbed is directly related to the concentration of the element in a sample.

band pass The range of wavelengths that reaches the exit slit of a monochromator; usually referred to as the range of wavelengths transmitted at a point equal to half the peak intensity transmitted.

Beer-Lambert law (most commonly referred to as **Beer's law**) The concentration of a substance is directly proportional to the amount of radiant energy absorbed.

bioluminescence An enzyme-catalyzed reaction that uses complex organic molecules and adenosine triphosphate (ATP) to yield light.

blank A solution that consists of all components including solvents and solutes, except the compound to be measured. This solution is used to set I_o, the original light intensity.

chemiluminescence A chemical reaction that usually involves oxidation in which one of the products is light.

chromogen A colored compound.

cuvette The receptacle in a photometer in which the sample is placed.

electrochemiluminescence A chemical reaction in which an electrochemically activated molecule oxidizes a second molecule, which emits light.

electronic transition The change in the orbital position of an electron of an atom or molecule. In the case of absorption of a photon of light, the electron usually goes from the ground or the lowest energy level to some higher one with a consequent higher energy state (increased energy) of the molecule. Serves as the basis of fluorescence phenomena.

emission wavelength The wavelength of light (λ_{em}) that is used to monitor decay of excited molecules into fluorescence; usually refers to the wavelength of output photons measured by a fluorometer.

excitation wavelength The wavelength of radiant energy (λ_{ex}) that is absorbed by a molecule and causes it to be raised to a higher energy state; usually refers to the wavelength of incident energy of a fluorometer.

filter An optical device (usually glass) that allows only a portion of polychromatic, incident light to pass through. The amount of transmitted light is related to the band pass of the filter.

flameless atomic absorption An atomic absorption technique in which the element is converted to a vapor phase without the use of a flame.

fluorescence The light emitted by an atom or molecule after absorption of a photon. This light is at longer wavelengths (less energy) than the absorbed light and usually is emitted in less than 10^{-8} sec. However, some compounds emit the photon at a slower rate.

grating An optical device consisting of a reflecting, ruled surface that disperses polychromatic light into a uniform, continuous spectrum. Dispersion of light is attributable to interference phenomena at the ruled surface.

hollow-cathode lamp A lamp that consists of a metal cathode and an inert gas. When an electrical current is passed through the cathode; the metal is sputtered free and, after colliding with the gas in the lamp, emits a line spectrum of specific wavelengths related to the metal of the cathode.

infrared radiation The region of the electromagnetic spectrum that extends from about 780 to 300,000 nm.

internal standard An element or compound added in a known amount to yield a signal against which an instrument or an analyte to be measured can be calibrated.

light scattering The interaction of light with particles that cause the light to be bent away from its original path (cause of turbidity).

line spectrum Discontinuous emission spectrum of elements in which emitted light bands cover a very narrow (0.1 nm) range of wavelengths.

molar absorptivity (ε) The absorbance of light, at a specific wavelength, divided by the product of concentration in moles per liter and the sample path length in centimeters. Molar absorptivity is expressed as L/mol·cm.

monochromatic Light of one color (wavelength). In practice, this refers to radiant energy composed of a very narrow range of wavelengths.

monochromator Device used to isolate a certain wavelength or range of wavelengths. Usually refers to prisms or grating.

nephelometry A technique that measures the amount of light scattered by particles suspended in a solution.

phosphorescence Similar to fluorescence, the light emitted by an atom or molecule after absorption of a photon. The light usually is emitted at a time greater than 10^{-3} seconds after absorption of the photon.

photodetector A device that responds to light (photons), usually in a manner proportional to the number of photons striking its light-sensitive surface. Commonly, a current that is proportional to the incident light intensity is generated.

photometer An instrument that measures light intensity; composed of a source of radiant energy, filter for wavelength selection, cuvette holder, detector, and readout device.

photon A particle that consists of a discrete packet of radiant energy.

polarized fluorescence The orientation of emitted fluorescent light, which can be calculated from the polarization formula.

polychromatic Light of many colors (wavelengths), usually referring to white light or that encompassing a defined portion of the spectrum.

Rayleigh-Debye scatter The reflection of light at different angles by particles suspended in a solution. This scattering occurs when the wavelength of incident light is greater than the size of the particles.

reflectance spectrophotometry A quantitative spectrophotometric technique in which the light reflected from the surface of a colorimetric reaction is used to measure the amount of the reaction product.

refraction A process by which the path of incident light is bent after the light passes obliquely from one medium to another of different density.

refractive index The ratio of the speed of light in two different media; usually, the reference medium is air.

refractometer An instrument used to measure the refractive index (refractivity) of various substances, especially of solutions.

spectrophotometer An instrument that measures light intensity. It is composed of a source of radiant energy, entrance slit, monochromator, exit slit, cuvette holder, detector, and readout device. Measurements in these instruments can be made over a continuous range of the available spectrum.

stray light Radiant energy reaching the detector that consists of wavelengths other than those defined by the filter or monochromator.

time-delayed fluorescence A technique in which the fluorescence of slowly emitting compounds such as metal chelates is measured. Usually, the time between 400 and 1000 msec is monitored.

transmitted light The portion of radiant energy that passes through an object.

ultraviolet radiation The region of the electromagnetic spectrum from about 180 to 390 nm.

visible light The radiant energy in the electromagnetic spectrum visible to the human eye (approximately 390 to 780 nm).

wavelength The linear distance traversed by one complete wave cycle of electromagnetic energy.

SECTION OBJECTIVES BOX 2-1

- Describe the relationship between percent transmittance (%T) and absorbance (A), and explain how this relationship affects the color of a solution.
- Describe the Beer-Lambert law and its limitations.
- Illustrate the construction and operation of photometric monochromators and detectors, and explain the advantages or disadvantages associated with the use of each in spectral instruments. Further describe the principles of spectral isolation and band pass.
- Draw a block diagram of the essential components of the atomic absorption spectrophotometer and the fluorometer, and state the principle of the operation of each, highlighting similarities and differences. Explain the interferences associated with each.
- Describe how the instrumentation and basic principles of photometry are modified by the application of turbidimetry, nephelometry, or fluorometry, and identify any unique interferences or sources of error associated with each.

LIGHT AND MATTER[1,2]

Properties of Light and Radiant Energy

Electromagnetic radiant energy is a form of energy that can be described in terms of its wavelike properties. Electromagnetic waves travel at high velocities and do not require the existence of a supporting medium for propagation.

The **wavelength,** λ, of a beam of electromagnetic radiant energy is the linear distance traversed by one complete wave cycle; it usually is given in nanometers (nm, 10^{-9} m). The frequency, ν, is the number of cycles that occur per second and is obtained by the following relationship:

$$\nu = \frac{c}{\lambda} \qquad \text{Eq. 2-1}$$

The velocity, c, varies with the medium through which the radiant energy is passing ($c = 3 \times 10^{10}$ cm/sec when measured in a vacuum).

Radiant energy can be shown to behave as if it were composed of discrete packets of energy called **photons.** The energy of a photon depends on the frequency or wavelength of the radiant energy. The relationship between the energy, E, of a photon and frequency is given by the following formula:

$$E = h\nu \qquad \text{Eq. 2-2}$$

in which h is Planck's constant and has a numerical value of 6.62×10^{-27} erg•sec. The equivalent expression involving wavelength is as follows:

$$E = \frac{hc}{\lambda} \qquad \text{Eq. 2-3}$$

This equation shows that shorter wavelengths have higher energy than longer wavelengths have.

The electromagnetic spectrum covers a very large range of wavelengths, as is shown in Table 2-1. The areas of the electromagnetic spectrum that are used commonly in the clinical laboratory include the **UV radiation** and **visible light** regions; the **infrared radiation (IR,** >780 nm) is also used. The visible region generally is specified as the region between 390 and 780 nm, whereas the UV spectrum usually referred to in the clinical chemistry laboratory falls between 180 and 390 nm. Sunlight or light emitted from a tungsten filament is **polychromatic light,** which is a mixture of radiant energy of different wavelengths that the eye recognizes as "white." The breakdown of the visible region into color absorbed and color reflected is shown in Table 2-2. If a solution absorbs radiant energy (light) of between 400 and 480 nm (blue), it will transmit all other colors and appear yellow to the eye. Therefore, yellow is the complementary color of blue. If white light is focused on a solution that absorbs energy of between 505 and 555 nm (green), the **transmitted light** and thus the solution will appear red. If a red light is focused on a red solution, red light will be transmitted because this solution cannot absorb red light. On the other hand, if green light is focused on the red solution, no light is transmitted because the solution absorbs all light but red. The human eye responds to radiant energy of between 390 and 780 nm, but laboratory instrumentation permits measurements at both shorter wavelengths, such as UV, and longer wavelengths, such as IR, of the spectrum.

KEY CONCEPT BOX 2-1

- Light and energy can be described by equations.
- Light interacts with matter in several ways. One is by moving an electron to a higher energy.

Table 2-1 Electromagnetic Spectrum

	Gamma Rays	X-Rays	Ultraviolet (UV)	Visible	Infrared (IR)	Microwave
Wavelength (nm)*	0.1	1	180	390	780	400×10^3

*This is the wavelength interval at which the lowest type of respective radiant energy occurs.

Table 2-2 Colors and Complementary Colors of Visible Spectrum

Wavelength*, nm	Color Absorbed†	Complementary of Solution Color Transmitted
350 to 430	violet	yellow
430 to 475	blue	orange
475 to 495	blue-green	red-orange
495 to 505	blue-green	orange-red
505 to 555	green	red
555 to 575	yellow-green	violet-red
575 to 600	yellow	violet
600 to 650	orange	blue
670 to 700	red	green

From Brown TL, Lemay HE: *Chemistry: The Central Science,* Englewood Cliffs, NJ, 1977, Prentice-Hall.
*Because of the subjective nature of color, the wavelength ranges are only approximations.
†If a solution absorbs the light of the color listed in the second column, the observed color of the solution (i.e., the transmitted complementary light) is given in the third column.

Interactions of Light With Matter

Photons and Matter Interactions

Some materials are light sensitive, that is, when they are struck by a photon, an electron is moved to a higher energy state. The energy imparted to the electron is dependent upon the energy of the incident photon. When photons strike the surface of certain materials (such as silicon), the energized electron may be released as a free electron. The free electrons can be quantitated by a number of recording devices (see below) used in analytical instruments. In contrast, matter may emit light if an electron falls from a higher energy level to a lower one.

Absorption Process

When an atom, ion, or molecule absorbs a photon, the added energy results in an alteration of state, and the species is said to be excited. Excitation may involve any of the following processes:

1. Transition of an electron to a higher energy level
2. A change in the mode of vibration of the molecule's covalent bonds
3. Alteration of its mode of rotation about the covalent bonds

Each of these transitions requires a definite quantity of energy, a specific **excitation wavelength;** the probability of occurrence for a particular transition is greatest when the absorbed photon supplies this exact quantity of energy.

The energy requirements for these transitions vary widely. Usually, elevation of electrons to higher energy levels requires greater energy absorption than is needed to cause vibrational changes. Rotational alterations usually have the lowest energy requirements. Therefore, absorption of energy in the microwave and in far-infrared regions results in shifts in rotational energy levels because the energy of the radiant energy is insufficient to cause other types of transitions. Changes in vibrational levels are caused by absorption in the near-infrared and visible regions. Promotion of an electron to a higher energy level occurs after energy is absorbed in the visible, ultraviolet, and x-ray regions of the spectrum. The energy content of the electrons of covalent bonds varies with the nature of the bonds. The energy of a photon of light needed to excite an electron therefore varies with the bond, and each type of bond has its own characteristic pattern of optimum wavelengths of light that can be absorbed by that bond. Table 2-3 gives the electronic absorption bands for many organic groups.[4]

The absorption pattern of a complex organic molecule that contains tens of thousands of bonds therefore must describe the cumulative sum of the absorption of all the individual covalent bonds.

The absorption of radiant energy by a solution can be described by means of a plot of the **absorbance** as a function of wavelength. This graph is called an **absorption spectrum** (Fig. 2-1). The absorption spectrum reflects the sum of the energy transitions characteristic of a molecule at each wavelength of light. Absorption spectra are often helpful for qualitative identification purposes. This is particularly true for low-energy absorptions such as those found in the IR region. Irrespective of the amount of energy absorbed, an excited electron tends to return spontaneously to its unexcited, or ground, state; in this process, it releases energy as kinetic (movement), vibrational, or light (see the later discussion of **fluorescence**) energy.

Emission Process

Some elements and compounds can be excited in such a fashion that when the electrons return from the excited state to the ground state, the energy is dissipated as radiant energy. Radiant energy may consist of one or several energy levels and therefore may include different **emission wavelengths.** This principle is used in flame photometry and fluorometric methods and is discussed further with these topics.

SECTION OBJECTIVES BOX 2-2

- Describe the relationship between percent transmittance (%T) and absorbance (A), and explain how this relationship affects the color of a solution.
- Describe the Beer-Lambert law and its limitations.

ABSORPTION SPECTROSCOPY[4-11]

Radiant Energy Absorption

Consider a beam of radiant energy with an original intensity, I_o, impinging on and passing through a square cell (whose sides are perpendicular to the beam) that contains a solution of a compound that absorbs radiant energy of a certain wavelength (Fig. 2-2). The intensity of the transmitted radiant

Table 2-3 Electron Absorption Bands for Representative Chromophores

Chromophore	System	λ_{max}	ε_{max}	λ_{max}	ε_{max}	λ_{max}	ε_{max}
Ether	—O—	185	1000				
Thioether	—S—	194	4600	215	1600		
Amine	$—NH_2$	195	2800				
Thiol	—SH	195	1400				
Disulfide	—S—S—	194	5500	255	400		
Sulfone	$—SO_2—$	180	—				
Ethylene	—C=C—	190	8000				
Ketone	>C=O	195	1000	270 to 285	18 to 30		
Ester	—COOR	205	50				
Aldehyde	—CHO	210	Strong	280 to 300	11 to 18		
Carboxyl	—COOH	200 to 210	3 to 25				
Nitro	$—NO_2$	210	Strong				
Azo	—N=N—	285 to 400	3 to 25				
Nitrate	$—ONO_2$	270 (shoulder)	12				
	$—(C=C)_2—$ (acyclic)	210 to 230	21,000				
	$—(C=C)_3—$	260	35,000				
	$—(C=C)_5—$	330	118,000				
	C=C—C≡C	219	6500				
Benzene		184	46,700	202	6900	255	170
Anthracene		252	199,000	375	7900		
Quinoline		227	37,000	270	3600	314	2750
Isoquinoline		218	80,000	266	4000	317	3500

From Willard HH, Merritt LL, Dean JA: *Instrumental Methods of Analysis,* ed 4, Princeton, NJ, 1965, Van Nostrand. See also Spectral Database for Organic Compounds, SDBS, organized by National Institute of Advanced Industrial Science and Technology (AIST), Japan. Available at http://riodb01.ibase.aist.go.jp/sdbs/cgi-bin/cre_index.cgi?lang=eng.

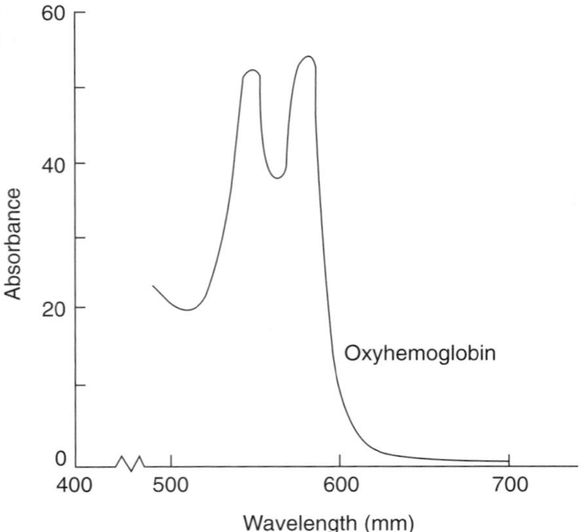

Fig. 2-1 Absorption spectrum of oxyhemoglobin.

energy, I_s, will be less than that of the I_o. Some of the incident radiant energy may be reflected by the surface of the cell or absorbed by the cell wall or the solvent. Therefore, these factors must be eliminated if only the absorption of the compound of interest is to be considered. This is done with the use of a **blank** or reference solution that contains everything but the compound to be measured. The amount of light passing through the blank solution is set as the new I_o (relative to the reference cell and solution). The transmittance for the compound in solution is defined as the proportion of incident light that is transmitted:

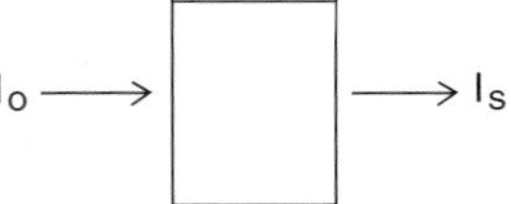

Fig. 2-2 Transmittance of radiant energy through a cuvette. I_O is the incident radiation; I_s is the transmitted radiation.

$$\text{Transmittance} = T = I_s/I_o \qquad \text{Eq. 2-4}$$

Usually, this ratio is described as a percentage:

$$\text{Percentage Transmission} = \%T = I_s/I_o \times 100\% \qquad \text{Eq. 2-5}$$

The concept of transmittance is important because only transmitted light can be measured.

As the concentration of the compound in solution increases, more light is absorbed by the solution and less light is transmitted. Percent T varies inversely and logarithmically with concentration. However, it is more convenient to use absorbance, A, which is directly proportional to the concentration. Therefore,

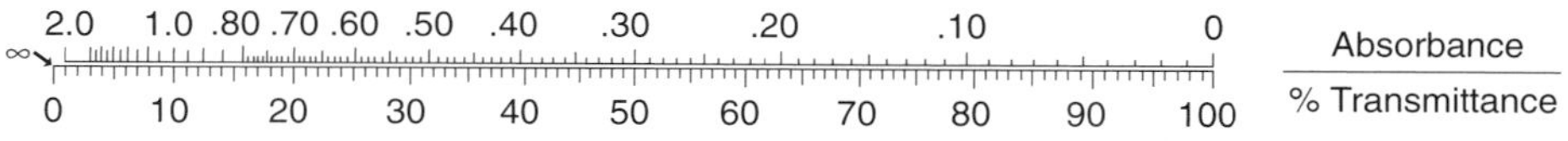

2.0 1.0 .80 .70 .60 .50 .40 .30 .20 .10 0 — Absorbance

0 10 20 30 40 50 60 70 80 90 100 — % Transmittance

Fig. 2-3 Scale showing relationship between absorbance and percent transmittance.

$$A = -\log I_s / I_o = -\log T = \log \frac{1}{T} \qquad \text{Eq. 2-6}$$

To convert T to %T, the denominator and the numerator are multiplied by 100%:

$$A = \log \frac{1}{T} \times \frac{100\%}{100\%} = \log \frac{100\%}{\%T} \qquad \text{Eq. 2-7}$$

This can be rearranged to

$$A = \log 100\% - \log \%\text{T} \qquad \text{Eq. 2-8}$$

or

$$A = 2 - \log \%\text{T} \qquad \text{Eq. 2-9}$$

It is important to remember that absorbance is not a directly measurable quantity, but that it can be obtained only by mathematical calculation from transmittance data.

The relationship between absorbance and %T is shown in Fig. 2-3, in which the linear %T scale runs from 0% to 100%, whereas the logarithmic absorbance scale runs from infinity to 0.

Beer-Lambert Law

The **Beer-Lambert law** (most commonly referred to simply as **Beer's law**) states that the concentration of a substance is directly proportional to the amount of radiant energy absorbed or is inversely proportional to the logarithm of transmitted radiant energy. If the concentration of a solution is constant and the path length through the solution that the light must traverse is doubled, the effect on the absorbance is the same as that caused by doubling the concentration because twice as many absorbing molecules are now present in the radiant energy path. Thus, the absorbance is also directly proportional to the path length of the radiant energy through the cell.

Beer's law states the mathematical relationship that connects absorbance of radiant energy, concentration of a solution, and path length:

$$A = abc \qquad \text{Eq. 2-10}$$

A is absorbance; *a,* **absorptivity;** *b,* light path of the solution in centimeters; and *c,* concentration of the substance of interest.

This equation forms the basis of quantitative analysis by absorption photometry or absorption spectroscopy. Absorbance values have no units. Absorptivity is a proportionality constant that is related to the chemical nature of the solute; it includes units that are reciprocal of those for *b* and *c*.

When *c* is expressed in moles per liter and *b* is expressed in centimeters, the symbol ε called the **molar absorptivity,** is used in place of *a* and is a constant for a given compound at

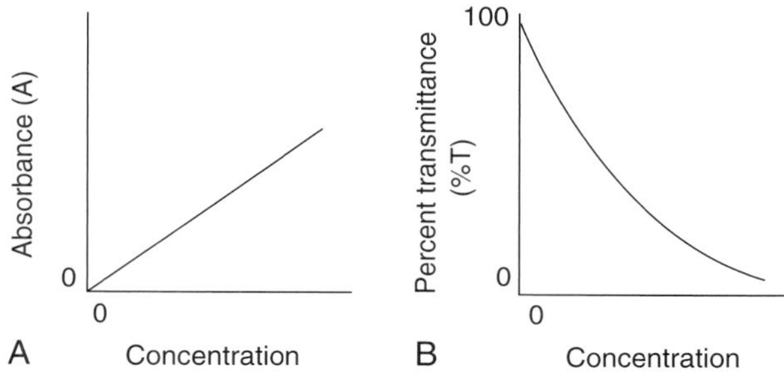

Fig. 2-4 Relationships of absorbance **(A)** and percent transmittance **(B)** to concentration.

a given wavelength under specified conditions of solvent, pH, temperature, and so on. It has units of L/mol•cm. A compound with higher molar absorptivity has a higher absorbance for the same molar concentration than a compound with lower molar absorptivity. Therefore, when selecting a colored product (**chromogen**) for spectrophotometric methods, the chromogen with higher molar absorptivity is used, to impart a greater sensitivity to the measurement.

Once a chromogen has been proved to follow Beer's law at a specific wavelength (i.e., a linear plot of *A* versus *c* with a zero intercept; Fig. 2-4, *A*), the concentration of an unknown solution can be determined by measurement of its absorbance and interpolation of its concentration from the graph of the standards. In contrast, when %T is plotted versus concentration (on linear graph paper), a curvilinear relationship is obtained (see Fig. 2-4, *B*). Because of the linear relationship between absorbance and concentration, it is possible to relate unknown concentrations to a single standard by a simple proportional equation. Therefore,

$$\frac{A_s}{A_u} = \frac{C_s}{C_u} \qquad \text{Eq. 2-11}$$

and

$$C_u = \frac{A_u}{A_s} \times C_s \qquad \text{Eq. 2-12}$$

in which C_u and C_s are the concentration of the unknown and the standard, respectively, and A_u and A_s are the absorbance of the unknown and the standard.

These equations are valid only if the chromogen obeys Beer's law and both standard and unknown are measured in the same cell. The concentration range over which a chromogen obeys Beer's law must be determined for each set of analytical conditions.

Beer's law is an ideal mathematical relationship that contains several limitations. Deviations from Beer's law, that is,

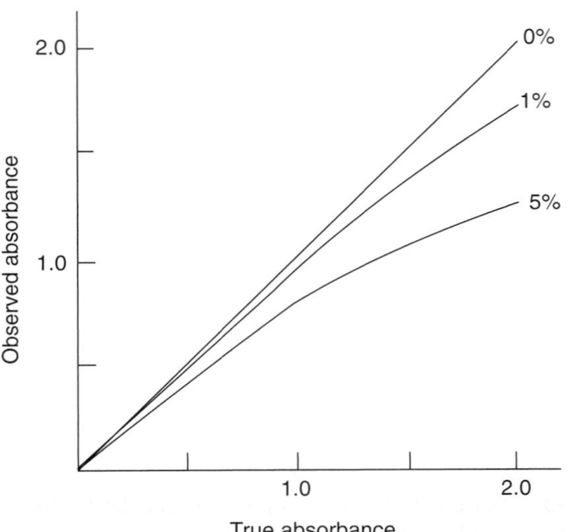

Fig. 2-5 Effect of stray radiation on true absorbance. (From Frings CS, Broussard LA: Calibration and monitoring of spectrometers and spectrophotometers, Clin Chem 25:1013, 1979.)

variations from the linearity of the absorbance versus the concentration curve (Fig. 2-5), occur when (1) very elevated concentrations are measured, (2) incident radiant energy is not monochromatic, (3) the solvent absorption is significant compared with the solute absorbance, (4) radiant energy is transmitted by other mechanisms (stray light), and (5) the sides of the cell are not parallel. If two or more chemical species are absorbing the wavelength of incident radiant energy, each with a different absorptivity, Beer's law will not be followed. If the absorbance of a fluorescent solution is being measured, Beer's law may not be followed.

Stray radiation (**stray light**) is radiant energy that reaches the detector at wavelengths other than those indicated by the **monochromator** setting. All radiant energy that reaches the detector, with or without having passed through the sample, will be recorded. Fig. 2-5 shows the effects of stray light on Beer's law. As the amount of stray light increases (or monochromicity decreases), deviation from Beer's law also increases (i.e., linearity decreases).

KEY CONCEPT BOX 2-2

- Absorption of light and concentration of a chemical in solution is quantified by Beer's law.

SECTION OBJECTIVE BOX 2-3

- Illustrate the construction and operation of photometric monochromators and detectors, and explain the advantages or disadvantages associated with the use of each in spectral instruments. Further describe the principles of spectral isolation and band pass.

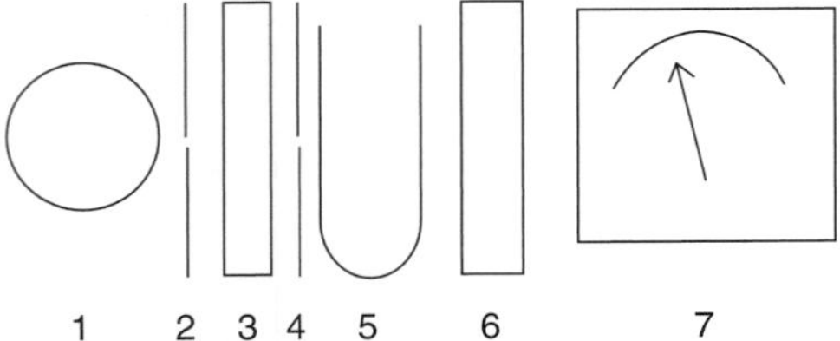

Fig. 2-6 Components of a spectrophotometer. *1,* Source of radiant energy; *2,* entrance slit; *3,* wavelength selector; *4,* exit slit; *5,* cuvette and cuvette holder; *6,* detector; *7,* readout device.

Instrumentation

Single-Beam Spectrophotometer

The major components of a single-beam **spectrophotometer** are shown in Fig. 2-6. The apparatus can be divided into seven basic components: (1) a stable source of radiant energy; (2) an entrance slit to focus the light; (3) a wavelength selector; (4) an exit slit to focus the light; (5) a device to hold the transparent container (**cuvette**), which contains the solution to be measured; (6) a radiant energy detector; and (7) a device to read out the electrical signal generated by the detector. If a **filter** is used as the wavelength selector, **monochromatic** light at only discrete wavelengths is available, and the instrument is called a **photometer.** If a monochromator is used (i.e., a prism or grating, see later discussion) as the wavelength selector, the instrument can provide monochromatic light over a continuous range of wavelengths and is called a spectrometer or spectrophotometer. Spectrophotometers can be double-beam instruments with two cuvette holders, one for the sample and the other for the blank, or reference sample. Advantages of the double-beam instrument include the capability of making simultaneous corrections for changes in light intensity, grating efficiency, slit width variation, and so on. It is particularly useful for obtaining spectral curves.

Sources of Radiant Energy

A variety of light sources are used. A tungsten filament lamp is useful as the source of a continuous spectrum of radiant energy from 360 to 950 nm (Fig. 2-7). Tungsten iodide lamps often are used as sources of visible and near-UV radiant energy. The tungsten halide filaments are longer lasting, produce more light at shorter wavelengths, and emit a higher intensity radiant energy than tungsten filaments do.

Hydrogen and deuterium discharge lamps emit a continuous spectrum and are used for the UV region of the spectrum (220 to 360 nm). Mercury vapor lamps emit a discontinuous or line spectrum (313, 365, 405, 436, and 546 nm) (see Fig. 2-7) and are used in photometers or spectrophotometers employed for high-performance liquid chromatography (HPLC).

Light-emitting diodes (LEDs) are also used as light sources. The solid material that makes up the diode is a semiconductor, a substance between a metal, which conducts an electrical

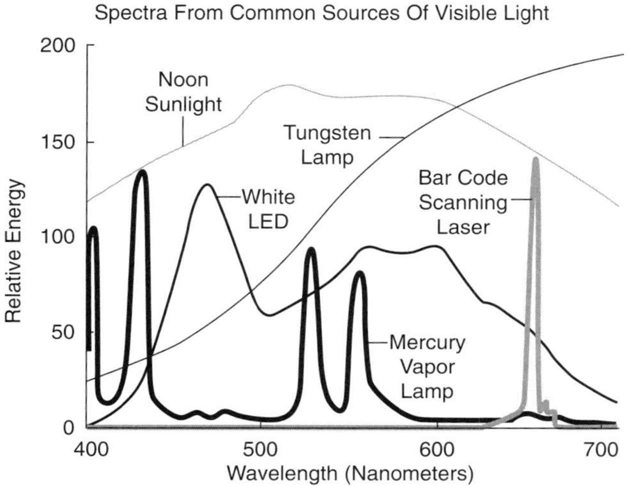

Fig. 2-7 Intensity of radiant energy versus wavelength for a variety of light sources. (Courtesy Microscopy Resource Center, Olympus America, Inc., Center Valley, PA.)

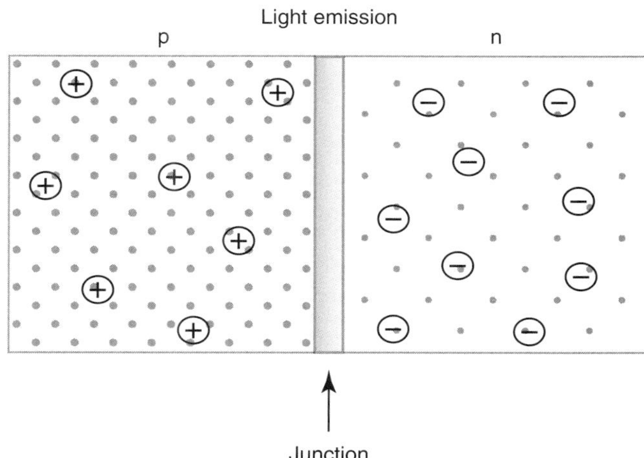

Fig. 2-8 Diagram of a simple light-emitting diode (LED). The electrons flow from the *n* to the *p* side and cross the junction underneath when voltage is applied. When they move, the electrons fall into "holes" in the *p* side. The energy of the "fall" is converted into light. The composition of the *p* and *n* semiconducting materials and the applied voltage define the wavelength of the emitted light.

current, and an insulator, which does not. LEDs use two types of semiconductors. N-type semiconductors usually consist of aluminum-gallium-arsenide with small amounts ("doped") of other elements so that the material has loose electrons. P-type semiconductors are similar, but have small quantities of different elements, so that the material has places, often termed 'holes', where loose electrons will be collected. These two types of semiconductors are "joined" so that the electrons will flow from the n to the p materials.[12,13] In the presence of an electrical field electrons from the n-type semiconductor fall into the "holes" of a p-type semiconductor (Fig. 2-8). The energy of this "fall" is released as a photon. The wavelength of the released photon is dependent on energy change of the "fallen" electron. Thus the process of an LED emitting light may be considered the reverse of the process occurring when light strikes matter.

It is important to understand that the amount of light given off by a radiant energy source is not constant over a continuous range of wavelengths. Thus, a typical lamp has a complex spectrum with maxima and minima (see Fig. 2-7). Lamps of different types and even from different manufacturers can vary. Therefore, care must be taken in choosing a lamp for a particular analysis, because the amount of light emitted at the desired wavelength may be too little or too much. For example, hydrogen or deuterium lamps, used for UV analysis, have a maximum output of UV radiation in the 250 to 300 nm range. The output of radiant energy at longer wavelengths (greater than 340 nm) is considerably less and can be too weak for many analyses.

Wavelength Selectors

Isolation of the required wavelength or range of wavelengths can be accomplished with the use of a filter or a monochromator. Filters, the simplest devices, consist of only a material that selectively transmits the desired wavelengths and absorbs all other wavelengths. In a monochromator, a **grating** or prism disperses radiant energy from the source lamp into a spectrum from which the desired wavelength is isolated by mechanical slits.

Filters

There are two types of filters: (1) those with selective transmission characteristics, including glass and Wratten filters; and (2) those based on the principle of interference (interference filters). The Wratten filter consists of colored gelatin between clear glass plates; glass filters are composed of one or more layers of colored glass. Both types of filters transmit more radiant energy in some parts of the spectrum than in others.

Interference filters work on a different principle, which is the same as that underlying the play of colors from a soap film, namely, interference. When radiant energy strikes the thin film, some is reflected from the front surface, but some of the radiant energy that penetrates the film is reflected by the surface on the other side. The latter rays of radiant energy now have traveled farther than the first by a distance two times the film thickness. If the two reflected rays are in **phase,** their resultant intensity is doubled, whereas if they are out of phase, they destroy each other. Therefore, when white light strikes the film, some reflected wavelengths will be augmented and some destroyed, resulting in colors.

Monochromators

Monochromators can give a much narrower range of wavelengths than filters can and are easily adjustable over a wide

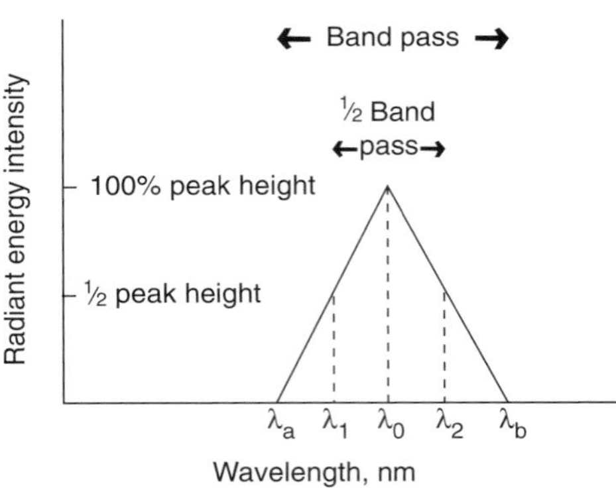

Fig. 2-9 Idealized distribution of radiant energy emerging from exit slit of wavelength selector. For a filter or a monochromator with entrance and exit slits of equal width, a symmetrical distribution of transmitted energy occurs, as shown.

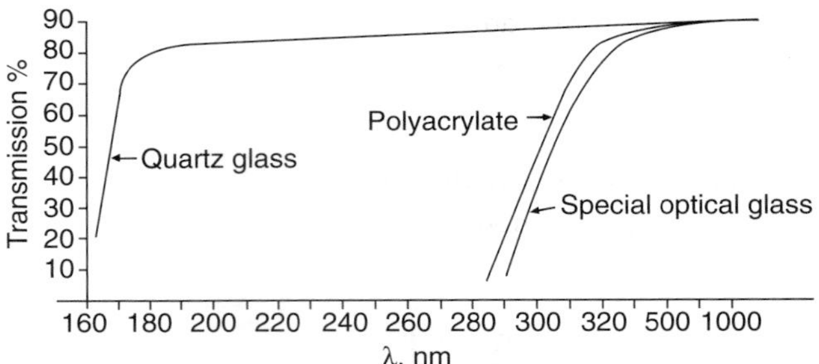

Fig. 2-10 Transmission characteristics of several types of optical materials used for cuvettes. (From Keller H: Optical methods of measurement. In Richterich R, Colombo JP, editors: *Clinical Chemistry,* New York, 1981, Wiley & Sons.)

spectral range. The dispersing element may be a prism or a grating.

Dispersion by a prism is nonlinear, becoming less linear at longer wavelengths (over 550 nm). Therefore, in certifying wavelength calibration, three different wavelengths must be checked. Prisms give only one order of emerging spectrum and thus provide higher optical efficiency because the entire incident energy is distributed over the single emerging spectrum.

A grating consists of a large number of parallel, equally spaced lines ruled on a surface. Dispersion by a grating is linear; therefore, only two different wavelengths must be checked to certify wavelength accuracy.

Band Pass

Except for laser optical devices, the light obtained by a wavelength selector is not truly monochromatic (i.e., of a single wavelength) but consists of a range of wavelengths. The degree of monochromicity is defined by the following terms. **Band pass** is that range of wavelengths that passes through the exit slit of the wavelength-selecting device. The nominal wavelength of this light beam is the wavelength at which the peak intensity of light occurs. For a wavelength selector such as a filter or a monochromator whose entrance and exit slits are of equal width, the nominal wavelength is the middle wavelength of the emerging spectrum.

The range of wavelengths obtained by a filter that produces a symmetrical spectrum usually is noted by its half-band width (or half-band pass). This describes the wavelengths obtained between the two sides of the transmittance spectrum at a transmittance equal to one-half the peak transmittance (Fig. 2-9). For monochromators, the degree of monochromicity is described by the nominal band width, which corresponds to those wavelengths that are centered about the peak wavelengths and transmit 75% of the total radiant energy present in the emerging beam of light. For monochromators with variable exit slits, the band pass also will vary.

Slits

Two types of slits are present in monochromators. The first, at the entrance, focuses the light on the grating or the prism, where it can be dispersed with a minimum of stray light. The second slit, at the exit, determines the band width of light that will be selected from the dispersed spectrum. When the width of the exit slit is increased, the band width of the emerging light is broadened, with a resultant increase in energy intensity but a decrease in spectral purity. In diffraction-grating monochromators, the exit slit may be of fixed width, resulting in a constant band pass. In contrast, prism monochromators have variable exit slits. The purposes of the two slits in filter photometers are to make the light parallel and to reduce stray radiation.

Cuvettes

In Fig. 2-6, the receptacle in which a sample is placed for spectrophotometric or photometric measurement is called a cuvette, or cell. These can have many shapes. The optical properties depend on their composition. Glass is used in the range of 320 to 950 nm. Below 320 nm, it is necessary to use quartz (silica) cells. Such cells can be used at higher wavelengths also. Fig. 2-10 shows the transmission patterns of several types of cuvettes. Although different shapes and path lengths are used, instruments usually are calibrated to a path length of 1 cm.

Detectors

Photomultiplier Tubes

A photomultiplier tube is an electron tube that is capable of significantly amplifying a current. The cathode is made of a light-sensitive metal that can absorb radiant energy and emit electrons in proportion to the radiant energy that strikes the surface of the light-sensitive metal. These surfaces vary in their response to light of different energies (wavelengths) and so also in the sensitivity of the photomultiplier tube (Fig. 2-11). Electrons produced by the first stage go to a secondary surface, where each electron produces between four and six additional electrons. Each of the electrons from the second stage goes on to another stage, again producing four to six electrons. As many as 15 stages (or dynodes) can be present in today's photomultiplier tubes (Fig. 2-12). Photomultiplier tubes have rapid response times, do not show as much fatigue as other detectors, and are very sensitive.

Photodiodes

Photodiodes are semiconductors that change their charged voltage (usually 5 V) upon being struck by light. The change is converted to current and is measured. A photodiode array is a two-dimensional matrix composed of hundreds of thin semiconductors spaced very closely together. Light from the instrument is dispersed by a grating or a prism onto the photodiode array. Each position or diode on the array is calibrated to correspond to a specific wavelength. Each diode is scanned, and the resultant electronic change is calculated to be proportional to absorption. This allows the entire spectrum to be recorded within milliseconds.

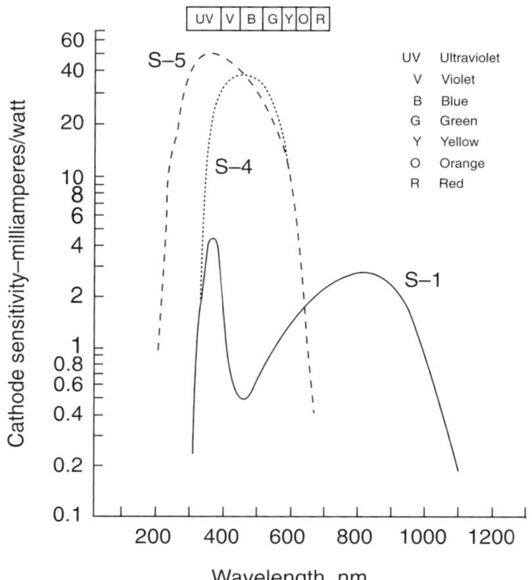

Fig. 2-11 Response of cathodes of several photomultiplier tubes to energy of different wavelengths. Sensitivity is expressed as milliamperes of current generated per watt of incident radiation.

Charge-Coupled Devices

These are solid-phase devices that are made of small silicon cells. When light impinges on the silicon surface, electrons are released. The electrons of each silicon cell are captured and quantified. The quantity of captured electrons are related to the amount of light originally hitting the cell.[14,15]

Instrument Performance

The sensitivity of response of a spectrophotometer results from combined effects of lamp output, efficiency of the filter or monochromator in the transmission of light, and response of the photomultiplier. Because these factors are all functions of wavelength, it is clear that the instrument must be reset when the wavelength is changed. This resetting most often takes the form of adjustment of the blank solution to read 100% T (zero absorbance) by changing the photomultiplier gain.

A series of recommendations on instrument specifications that cover many aspects of instrumentation used for photometric analysis have been proposed.[16,17] These specifications are listed in Table 2-4.

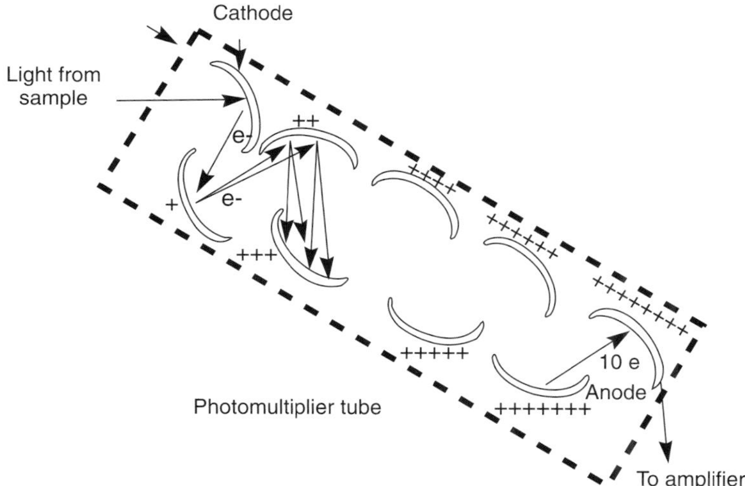

Fig. 2-12 Schema of photomultiplier tube. Each dynode (electrode used to generate secondary emissions of electrons) is represented by a crescent. Light impinges on each cathode and frees an electron. Electron is drawn toward first dynode (stage) by applied voltage. Secondary electrons are released and are passed on to successive dynodes, which are at increasingly higher voltages, as depicted by the + symbols. Increasing numbers of secondary electrons are generated at each stage. In this diagram, a tenfold amplification of the initial signal is produced at the anode. A photomultiplier tube may increase the signal several thousand–fold. (From Simonson MG: The application of a photon-counting fluorometer for the immunofluorescent measurement of therapeutic drugs. In Kaplan LA, Pesce AJ, editors: *Nonisotopic Alternatives to Radioimmunoassay,* New York, 1981, Marcel Dekker. Reprinted by courtesy of Marcel Dekker, Inc.[27])

Table 2-4 Guidelines for Photometric Enzyme Instruments

Parameter	Error or Range (95% Confidence, ±2 SD)
Carryover	
Sample to sample	<0.3%
Temperature accuracy	±0.1° C
Equilibration time	20 sec
Sample handling	
Accuracy	1%
Precision	0.5%
Size	50 μL or less
Reagent handling	
Mixing time	≤10 sec
Photometric performance (at a rate of 0.1 A/min)	
Initial absorbance 0 to 1 A	<3%
Initial absorbance 1 to 2 A	<5%
Wavelength accuracy	±2 nm
Band width	<8 nm
Wavelength range	Variable
Absorbance range	0 to 2 A
Linearity	<2%
Cell path/placement	<0.6%
Absorbance drift (10 to 60 min)	<2%
Absorbance accuracy	<2%
Absorbance reproducibility	
Low 0 to 1 A	±2%
High 1 to 2 A	±4%

From Instrumentation Guidelines Study Group, Subcommittee on Enzymes: Clin Chem 23:2160, 1977.

Selection of Optimum Conditions and Limitations

When a new spectrophotometric procedure is established, it is important to record the absorption spectrum of the material that is being measured. This absorption spectrum should be recorded in relation to either water or a reagent blank, depending on the actual method of analysis chosen. Examples of such spectra are presented throughout sections of this text. This spectrum will help to determine the best wavelength for the spectrophotometric analysis.

The optimum wavelength for a specific analysis depends on several factors, including the absorption maxima of the chromogen, the slope of the absorption peak, and the absorption spectra of possible interfering chromogens. An example of an absorption spectrum is shown in Fig. 2-13. According to Beer's law, the higher the molar absorptivity, the greater is the absorption at a given concentration and wavelength, and the higher is the sensitivity of the analysis. This spectrum includes three peaks of absorption (highest absorption coefficient): λ_1, λ_2, and λ_3 nm. The absorptivity at λ_2 is too low, and so the use of λ_2 can be ruled out immediately.

If an absorption peak is narrow, as it is for λ_1, any small error in the setting of the spectrophotometer at this wavelength results in a large change in absorbance. Because spectrophotometers use manually set wavelengths, this can cause large run-to-run imprecision and analytical error. A filter photometer requires a high-quality, accurate filter to ensure accuracy when monitoring is provided at a narrow absorption peak.

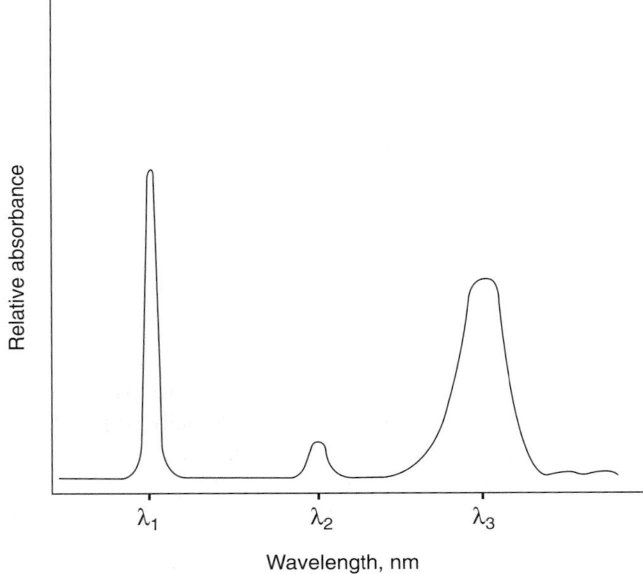

Fig. 2-13 Schema of idealized absorption spectrum. λ_1, λ_2, and λ_3 represent the absorption bands of a chromophore.

These problems can be avoided by using a wider absorption peak (λ_3). With this absorption peak, small changes in wavelength adjustment result in only small changes in absorptivity, and precision and accuracy are high.

The sensitivity of many methods may be improved by the use of absorption bands at shorter wavelengths (such as UV), because very often these have higher extinction coefficients. However, often there is additional nonspecific absorption from buffers or other chemical moieties in the solution at shorter wavelengths. Therefore, appropriate blanks must be used to obtain accurate measurements. In some techniques, the analyte is purified before analysis, and detection at short wavelengths (UV) is feasible and provides optimum sensitivity.

Knowledge of the wavelengths at which commonly interfering chromogens absorb light also helps in determination of the wavelength of choice. A general rule for selecting the optimum wavelength at which to monitor a spectrophotometric reaction includes three criteria: (1) choose an absorption peak with the greatest possible molar absorptivity, (2) choose a relatively broad peak, and (3) choose a peak that is as far as possible from the absorption peaks of commonly interfering chromogens.

Quality Control Checks of Spectrophotometers[17]

Several quality control checks should be performed to certify that spectrophotometers are functioning within specifications. These checks include wavelength accuracy, linearity of detector response, stray radiation (stray light), and photometric accuracy. Details of the spectrophotometer performance checks can be found in references 5 and 17.

Wavelength Accuracy

If the wavelength calibration of an instrument changes, the measured absorbance will change. The magnitude of the absorbance error attributable to inaccurate wavelength calibration depends on the relative location of the point on the absorption spectrum of the chromophore to be measured, that is, the absorbance error relative to the wavelength error is greater when the absorbance measurement is on the slope of the absorbance band than when the absorbance measurement is on or near the peak of the absorbance band. Maintenance of wavelength calibration is especially important for analyses such as spectrophotometric enzyme assays.

One method of checking wavelength accuracy involves replacement of the source lamp with a radiant energy source that has strong emission lines at well-defined wavelengths. Useful radiant energy sources are (1) the mercury vapor lamp, which has strong emission lines at 313, 365, 405, 436, and 546 nm (see Fig. 2-7); and (2) the deuterium or hydrogen lamp, which has useful emission lines at 486 and 656 nm.

A second method for checking wavelength calibration involves the use of rare earth glass filters such as holmium oxide and didymium. Holmium oxide has strong absorption lines at approximately 241, 279, 287, 333, 361, 418, 453, 536, and 636 nm. Didymium has much broader absorption bands at approximately 573, 586, 685, 741, and 803 nm. Because of the possibility of filter deterioration, this wavelength accuracy should be checked periodically.

A third method for checking wavelength calibration involves the use of a solution of a stable chromogen. In this case, it is used as a secondary wavelength calibration standard to determine whether the wavelength accuracy of an instrument has changed after a primary wavelength standard has previously verified the calibration. Disadvantages of using chemical solutions for wavelength calibration are that the absorption peaks are generally broad and spectral shifts may result from contamination, aging, or preparation errors.

Irrespective of the method used, calibration at two wavelengths is necessary for grating instruments, and calibration at three wavelengths is necessary for prism instruments.[18]

Linearity of Detector Response

A properly functioning spectrophotometer must exhibit a linear relationship between the radiant energy absorbed and the instrument readout. Instrument linearity is a prerequisite for spectrophotometric accuracy and analytical accuracy. Solid glass filters may be used to check instrument linearity. The most common method for certifying linearity of detector response involves the use of solutions of varying concentrations of a compound known to follow Beer's law. Some compounds used for this purpose are oxyhemoglobin at 415 nm; *p*-nitrophenol at 405 nm; cobalt ammonium sulfate at 512 nm; copper sulfate at 650 nm; and green food coloring at 257, 410, and 630 nm.

The absorbances of solutions that contain increasing concentrations of one such compound are plotted against the known concentrations. A nonlinear plot of absorbance versus concentration indicates either an error in dilution or an instrument problem. Besides a faulty detector, stray radiation or too wide a slit may cause a nonlinear response.

Stray Radiation

An increase in stray radiation often is observed at the extreme ends of the spectral range, where detector response or source energy is at its lowest. Stray radiation usually causes a negative deviation from Beer's law. Methods used to detect stray radiation employ filters or solutions that are highly transmitting over a portion of the spectrum but are essentially opaque below an abrupt "cutoff" wavelength. Several solutions have been used to check for stray radiation, including Li_2CO_3 below 250 nm, NaBr (0.1 mol/L) below 240 nm, and acetone below 320 nm. Many filters can detect stray radiation. If solutions or filters that transmit no radiant energy at the measurement wavelength are used, the measured transmittance is the amount of stray radiation present. Multiplication of this transmittance by 100 gives the percentage of stray radiation. An instrument malfunction is indicated whenever the amount of stray radiation exceeds 1%.

Actions taken to eliminate stray radiation include changing the light source, verifying wavelength calibration, sealing light leaks, realigning instrument components, and cleaning optical surfaces.

Photometric Accuracy

When analyses that do not use chemical standards are performed, absorbance accuracy is essential. An absorbance standard should have a constant, stable absorbance at a suitable wavelength that is insensitive to the spectral band width of the instrument and to variations in the configuration of the light beam. Such standards should be easy to use and readily available. The National Institute of Standards and Technology (NIST) provides a set of three neutral-density glass filters (SBM 930) that have known absorbances at four wavelengths for each filter. These filters are not completely stable and must be recalibrated periodically by the NIST.[19]

Potassium dichromate solution, cobalt ammonium sulfate solution, and potassium nitrate solution have been used as standards for checking photometric accuracy. Standard solutions are subject to absorbance changes with time, temperature, and pH; this makes them unsuitable as long-term calibration standards for photometric accuracy.

Reflectance Spectrophotometry

In **reflectance spectrophotometry**, a beam of light is directed at a flat surface, and the reflected light is quantified. The light reflected from the surface is focused onto a photomultiplier tube. The instrumentation can be similar to that of a single-beam filter spectrophotometer (Fig. 2-14). A lamp generates light that passes through a filter and a series of slits and is focused on the test surface. Some of the light incident to a test sample is absorbed by the chromophores on the surface, and

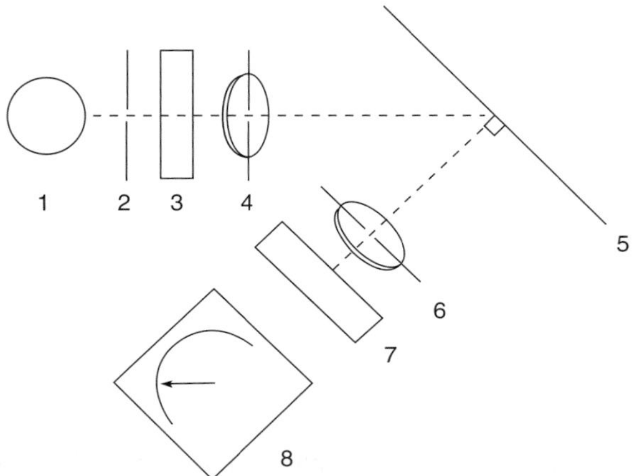

Fig. 2-14 Diagram of reflectance spectrophotometer. *1,* Light source; *2,* slit; *3,* filter or wavelength selector; *4,* collimating lens or slit; *5,* test surface; *6,* collimating lens or slit; *7,* detector; *8,* readout device.

the remainder is reflected. (This is analogous to light passing through a solution, for in this case also, some light is absorbed and the remainder passes through.)

The reflected light is passed through a series of slits and lenses and on to a photodetector. The signal then is converted to an appropriate readout. The term *reflection density* is used to describe the absorption of light by chromophores at the surface. Reflection density is related to the intensity of light reflected by the sample.[20] The reflection density, D_R, of the test sample is related to the ratio of the light reflected by the standard reflector (usually a barium sulfate–coated surface), R_0, to the light reflected by the test sample, R_{test}, as described by the equation

$$D_R = \log(R_0/R_{test}) \quad \text{Eq. 2-13}$$

This is analogous to the equation that relates %T (and thus absorbance) to incidental transmitted light (see equation 2-9, p. 49). In general, the optical properties of different surfaces vary considerably. The optical properties of test paper or plastic strips differ from those of dry film. Therefore, to calibrate an instrument for the measurement of reflection density, a standard with the specific surface employed by the test system must be used. The D_R value in the equation 2-13, may be corrected for stray reflectance. A black standard with the same surface characteristics as the test sample can be used to give a value for maximum absorbance. Any reflection read by the instrument under these conditions is stray reflection. This value can be subtracted from the test value to correct for this variable. The use of reflectance allows quantitative measurement of reactions on surfaces such as a dipstick or dry film.

The amount of light reflected and subsequently measured is instrument dependent. The angle at which the reflection is measured, the surface area monitored, and so on are variables. In addition, test surface variations (caused during the manufacturing or handling process) can alter surface reflectance properties.

Recording Spectrophotometry

The recording of entire absorption spectra is used either for the identification of compounds or to convert the spectra mathematically to their first or second derivatives. Recording of spectra can be done by spectrophotometers of the type described earlier or by diode array detection systems, in which there is a spatial relationship between the spectral lines spread by a prism or grating and the diode light detector. First- and second-derivative spectroscopy is the mathematical conversion of the absorption curve into the derivative function. These derivatives, which are used to eliminate interference with the observed absorption spectral lines, permit more accurate analyses.[21]

Multiwavelength Spectrophotometry[22]

The previous examples have described simple cases of light measurement under the assumption that the color or fluorescence of the analyte of interest was predominant at the chosen wavelength. Commonly, there is a spectral background in test solutions. One way to correct for this background is to subtract it out by measuring light at a second wavelength somewhat removed and at a longer wavelength from the first peak measurement. The difference between the two is considered to be the true absorption value. This is termed a bichromic measurement. Measurement at more than one wavelength is used to quantify several components that have spectral overlap. For this purpose, the extinction coefficient of each component at each measured wavelength must be known. In the case of blood hemoglobin, not all of the analyte is in one form, and the spectra of these forms (reduced hemoglobin, oxyhemoglobin, carboxyhemoglobin, methemoglobin, and sulfhemoglobin) overlap each other. The predominant forms of hemoglobin can be quantified by taking measurements at a series of wavelengths. Because the extinction coefficients of each form of hemoglobin are well established at each of these wavelengths, a matrix equation can be set up so that the measurements at six wavelengths (535, 560, 577, 622, 636, and 670 nm) can be used to calculate each component. This principle is used in most cooximeters.

Similar multiple wavelength measurements can be used for examination of fluorescence emission spectra to differentiate multiple fluorescent labels from each other.

KEY CONCEPT BOX 2-3

- Light measuring instruments usually have components to generate light of a desired wavelength, as well as a detector system to measure the amount of light passing through or emitted by the test system.
- Fluorescence is light emitted after a molecule is excited, usually by light or chemical means.

SECTION OBJECTIVES BOX 2-4

- Draw a block diagram of the essential components of the atomic absorption spectrophotometer and the fluorometer, and state the principle of the operation of each, highlighting similarities and differences. Explain the interferences associated with each.
- Describe how the instrumentation and basic principles of photometry are modified by the application of turbidimetry, nephelometry, or fluorometry, and identify any unique interferences or sources of error associated with each.
- Compare and contrast the principles of absorption and emission spectroscopy.
- Describe one of the chemical reactions that result in chemiluminescence.
- Compare and contrast the principles of absorption and emission spectroscopy.

ATOMIC ABSORPTION[23,24]

Atomic absorption (AA) **spectrophotometry** can be used in the clinical laboratory for determining calcium, magnesium, lithium, lead, copper, zinc, and other metals.

Principle

Vaporized atoms in the ground (unionized) state absorb light at very narrowly defined wavelengths. These absorption bands are on the order of 0.001 to 0.01 nm in width, and thus the entire absorption spectrum of atoms is called a **line spectrum.** If these atoms in the vapor state are excited, they can return to the ground state by emitting light of the same discrete wavelengths as the line spectrum. In AA spectrophotometry, the ionic form of the element is not excited in the flame but is dissociated from its chemical bonds and, by attracting free electrons produced by the combustion process, is placed in the atomic ground state. In this form, it is capable of absorbing light at the specific wavelengths of its line spectrum.

In AA, a beam of radiant energy containing the line spectrum of the element to be measured is passed through a flame that contains the vaporized test metal. The source emitting such radiant energy is called a **hollow-cathode lamp.** The wavelength of the absorbed radiant energy is the same as would be emitted if the element were excited. With the aid of a monochromator, the attenuation of one of the wavelengths of the incident light is measured. This attenuation is caused by interaction of the photons with ground state atoms in the flame. Beer's law is valid for relating the concentration of atoms in the flame to transmission or absorption of light. Only a small percentage of atoms in the flame are excited, and most atoms are in a form capable of absorbing radiant energy emitted by the hollow-cathode lamp.

Instrumentation

Fig. 2-15 shows the major components of an AA spectrophotometer.

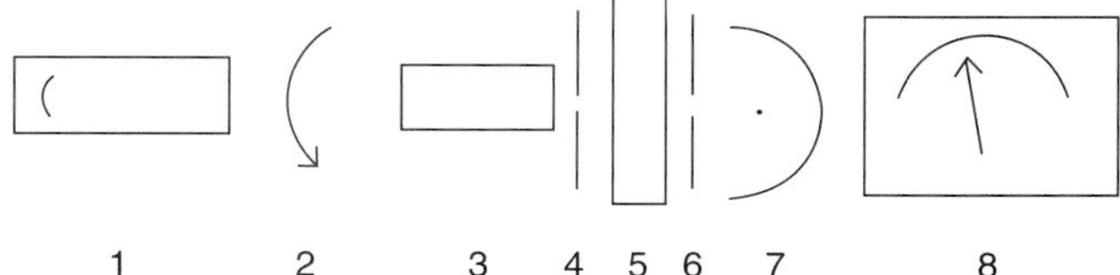

Fig. 2-15 Essential components of atomic absorption spectrophotometer. *1,* Hollow-cathode lamp; *2,* chopper; *3,* flame and burner assembly; *4,* entrance slit; *5,* wavelength selector; *6,* exit slit; *7,* detector; *8,* readout device.

Hollow-Cathode Lamp

The lamps have a hollow or cuplike cathode that is lined with the pure metal of the element to be determined or with an appropriate alloy. A separate lamp is used for each element, except in a few instances in which the cathode can be constructed in such a manner that a single lamp serves for two or three elements (such as calcium and magnesium). The lamp is filled with an inert monatomic gas, usually argon or neon, at low pressure, which varies with the analyte to be measured. For example, lead and iron can be better analyzed with neon-filled lamps, whereas lithium analysis is better performed with argon-filled lamps. Quartz or a special glass that allows transmission of the proper wavelength is used as the window. A current is supplied to the cathode, and metal atoms are released continually (sputtered) from the inner surface of the cathode, filling the lamp with an atomic vapor. Atoms in this vapor undergo electronic excitation by collision with the inert gas, and the resulting excited atoms emit their characteristic radiant energy when returning to the ground state electron level. This results in a beam of radiant energy with the correct wavelength for absorption by ground state atoms in the flame.

Burner

In AA spectrophotometry, the sample solution must be converted into the vapor phase. One technique converts the sample into a fine spray or aerosol while it is being introduced into the flame. This process is called nebulization. The nebulizer usually is considered part of the burner. Within the flame, solvent evaporates from the aerosol, leaving microscopic particles that disintegrate under the influence of heat to yield atoms. This phenomenon is termed atomization. Acetylene is the fuel that is commonly used in the burner. Temperatures of 2300° C usually are achieved in flame AA.

Flameless AA

The purpose of the flame is to convert the sample into an atomic vapor. Other atomization processes can replace the flame. In a more frequently employed atomization technique, the sample is dried on a carbon support platform or tube. The sample is vaporized in an inert atmosphere when an electrical current is passed through the support to create instantaneously a temperature sufficiently elevated to vaporize the analyte. These atomizers occupy the space normally occupied by the flame in flame AA instruments. The temperatures achieved by **flameless atomic absorption** (up to 2700° C) are necessary to vaporize heavier metals. Flameless AA instruments have a greater sensitivity than do flame AA instruments.

Monochromator and Detector

Monochromators (grating or prisms) and photomultiplier tubes can isolate a pure radiant energy signal and measure the intensity of that signal. Extraneous radiant energy, both from other wavelengths of the line spectrum and from light generated by the flame, is kept from reaching the photomultiplier tube by the monochromator. The photomultiplier tube converts the radiant energy that was not absorbed in the flame into a signal and amplifies this signal to drive a recorder or meter.

Sources of Error

Chemical, ionization, matrix, and burner interferences can occur in AA measurements. Additional factors that may cause variable behavior from sample to sample or between unknowns and standards include temperature, solvent composition, salt content, viscosity, and surface tension. A more complete description may be found in the third edition.

FLAME PHOTOMETRY[25]

Flame photometry was widely used in the clinical laboratory to determine sodium, potassium, and lithium concentrations in biological fluids. This technique is now rarely used.

Principle

Atoms of some metals, when given sufficient heat energy as supplied by a hot flame, become excited and reemit this energy at wavelengths characteristic of the element as described previously. The reactions undergone by ions in the flame are as follows:

$$A^+ + e^- \rightarrow A^0 \qquad \text{Eq. 2-14}$$

$$A^0 + \text{Heat} \rightarrow A^* \qquad \text{Eq. 2-15}$$

$$A^* \rightarrow A^0 + h\nu \qquad \text{Eq. 2-16}$$

A^* represents the excited atom in the flame, A^0 an atom with ground state electron energy, and $h\nu$ a photon. Alkali metals are relatively easy to excite in a flame. Lithium produces a red emission; sodium, a yellow emission; and potassium, a red-violet color in a flame. These colors are characteristic of the metal atoms that are present as cations in solution.

The intensity of the characteristic wavelength of radiant energy produced by the atoms in the flame is directly proportional to the number of atoms excited in the flame, which is directly proportional to the concentration of the substance of interest in the sample. The actual number of atoms present in the excited state is a small fraction of the total number of atoms present in the flame. For reproducible quantitation, an **internal standard** such as cesium is used.

Inductively Coupled Plasma Atomic Emission Spectroscopy (ICP-AES)[26]

The test samples are raised to about 10,000° F through the use of a radio-induced magnetic field and a neutral gas plasma. In this state, they emit photons as in flame photometry. The wavelengths of emission can be isolated and quantified. An alternative method sends some of the plasma output into a mass spectrometer, where the individual elements are separated and quantified.[26] The advantage of the ICP-AES technique is its ability to measure a number of metals simultaneously.

FLUOROMETRY[27-30]

Principle

Fluorescence may be considered one of the results of the interaction of light with matter. When light impinges on matter, it can simply pass through, as in a transparent solution; it can be scattered by the interaction; or it can be absorbed. When light is transmitted, there is no loss of energy. When light is scattered, there is no change in energy; the light is of the same wavelength before and after it interacts with matter. But when light is absorbed, the light energy is converted into any one of a number of forms, including radiationless **electronic transitions** (converting the energy into heat) and others, such as fluorescence and **phosphorescence,** in which photons are emitted (Fig. 2-16). Absorption of the light can be used, of course, to determine the concentration of compounds, as is done in absorption spectroscopy. If the absorbed light is reemitted, the emitted photons can be used to quantitate the amount of the light-emitting compound (fluor). Quantitation is also possible with the use of scattered light because the amount of scattered light is related to the number and size of the particles in solution. Methods that use light scattering are termed **nephelometry** and turbidity (see p. 62).

Fluorescent light is the result of the absorbance of a photon of radiant energy by a molecule. Once the molecule absorbs a photon, the molecule has an increased energy level, and because the molecular energy is greater than that of its environment, it seeks to eject the excess energy. When the energy is lost as an ejected photon, the result is fluorescence or phosphorescence emission.

For fluorescence to occur, there must be a high probability that the energy of the excited state can be converted to the ground state by the ejection of a photon. Not all compounds fluoresce; indeed, only a very few fluoresce. In those that do fluoresce, not every single photon absorbed is converted to fluorescent light. Some excited compounds lose energy by radiationless transitions, that is, by transfer of the energy to the solvent. For the same amount of light absorbed, molecules

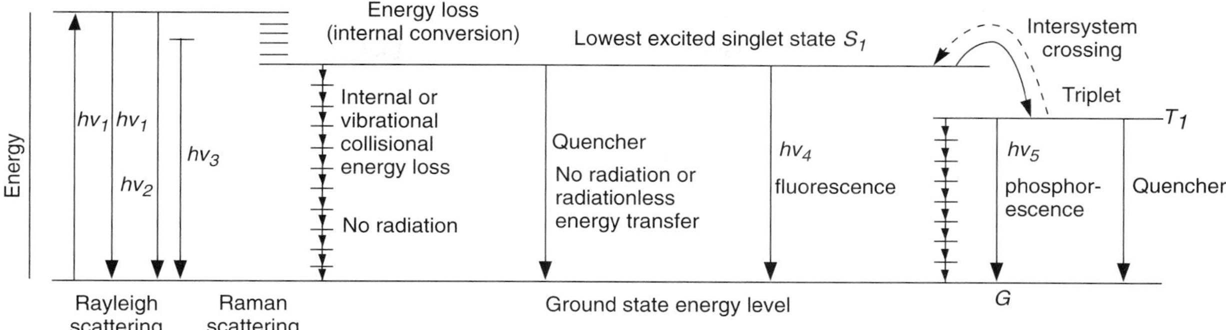

Fig. 2-16 Schema showing conversion of light energy into different forms of molecular and radiant energy. (From Pesce AJ, et al, editors: *Fluorescence Spectroscopy,* New York, 1971, Marcel Dekker. Reprinted by courtesy of Marcel Dekker, Inc.[28])

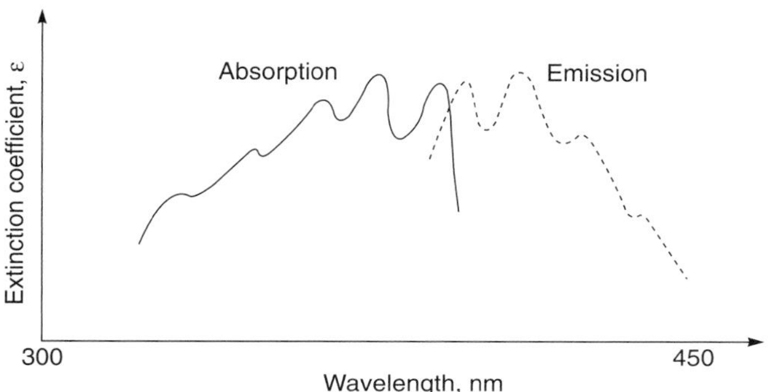

Fig. 2-17 Absorption (excitation) and emission (fluorescence) spectra of a fluorescent compound. (From Pesce AJ, et al, editors: *Fluorescence Spectroscopy,* New York, 1971, Marcel Dekker. Reprinted by courtesy of Michael Dekker, Inc.[28])

with higher fluorescence efficiency have brighter or more intense fluorescence. In solutions, when a molecule returns to the ground state by emitting a photon, there is less energy in the emitted photon than was present in the one initially absorbed. In other words, the emitted fluorescent light is at a longer wavelength than the exciting or absorbed radiation (Fig. 2-17).

Instrumentation

The basic components of a fluorometer are similar to those of an absorption spectrophotometer. The major difference is the introduction of a set of filters or a monochromator before the cell and after the cell to isolate the emitted light. A diagram of a fluorometer is presented in Fig. 2-18.

The principal components are the excitation light, filters or monochromators to separate the exciting light from the emitted light, and a sensitive detector. Most often, the measurement of fluorescent light is made at an angle of 90 degrees to the exciting light. This is done to maximize the sensitivity of the instrument by minimizing the amount of excitation light that can reach the photodetector. The detector is a photomultiplier or similar device that can quantitate the very small fluorescent light signal and thus achieve the desired level of sensitivity. Because the spectrum of absorption and emission varies from one compound to another, the instrument must be optimized for every analyte measured. This is done by adjusting the exciting wavelength to achieve the maximum absorption of photons, which usually means setting the instrument to the absorption maximum of the compound. By the same token, the wavelength of maximum emission of the fluorescent photons must also be ascertained, and this is the wavelength at which the fluorescence signal is recorded most often.

Limitations

The fluorescence signal of a compound is affected by many variables, including (1) solvent, (2) pH, (3) temperature, (4) absorbance of the solution, and (5) presence of interfering or specifically quenching compounds. Standardization is not usually done by an absolute procedure as in absorption spectroscopy because the fluorescence varies depending on (1) the intensity of the incident light on the sample, (2) the amount of light intercepted by the detector as controlled by the slits, (3) the band width of light analyzed, and (4) the efficiency of the detector. The quantum yield or efficiency of light emission of a photon is constant if solvent, pH, temperature, and so on are kept constant, but in general, the instrument will not be constant on a daily basis. Therefore, relative fluorescence yield is used for most measurements. For a reagent blank in a fluorometric assay, only the zero, or null, fluorescence can be set. There is no equivalent to the 100% scale of transmission. Therefore, the electronic signal varies from instrument to instrument for the same concentration of analyte.

To enable a series of fluorescent standards to form a curve that is linear with concentration, the absorbance of the solutions should not exceed 0.1. Above this absorbance, all portions of the solution are not uniformly illuminated, that is, the initially illuminated layer of the solution absorbs more light than the final layer, and thus the initial layer fluoresces more than the final layer. In dilute solutions, such as those with absorbance of less than 0.1, this does not occur. However, certain assays employ the inverse quantitative relationship between fluorescence intensity and the amount of light

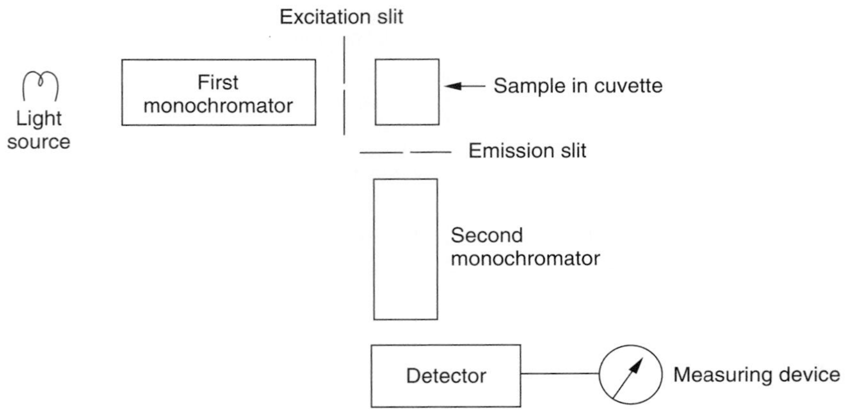

Excitation slit
Light source
First monochromator
Sample in cuvette
Emission slit
Second monochromator
Detector
Measuring device

Fig. 2-18 Essential components of a fluorometer. (From Brewer JM, et al, editors: *Experimental Techniques in Biochemistry,* Englewood Cliffs, NJ, 1974, Prentice-Hall.)

absorbed by a solution whose absorbance is greater than 0.1. Such assays are termed fluorescence attenuation assays. In these systems, a constant amount of fluorescent dye is placed in each test and control solution. In the test solution, the analyte causes a reaction in which a light-absorbing compound is produced. The greater the amount of colored reaction product formed by the analyte, the smaller is the amount of light absorbed by the fluorescent dye. Thus, the decrease in light passing through the solution results in a proportionate decrease in fluorescence intensity that can be related to the concentration of the analyte.

Time-Delayed Fluorescence[30]

One approach that can be used to improve the sensitivity of fluorescence techniques is the use of **time-delayed** or time-resolved **fluorescence.** The fluorescence emission time of most fluorescent molecules, such as fluorescein, is in the range of nanoseconds (nsec); that is, the fluorescence signal decays within 100 nsec. Some compounds such as the metal chelate diketone-europium have very long fluorescence lifetimes of 10 to 1000 microseconds (μsec). By measuring the fluorescence after 400 μsec, over a period of an additional 400 μsec, the fluorescence intensity of these compounds can be obtained without interference from light scattering or from any other molecules that may fluoresce. Aside from increasing the specificity of analysis, this technique provides greatly increased sensitivity.

Specialized instruments that use this technique illuminate the sample for a time, stop the illumination, and measure the emitted fluorescence over a specified time from 400 to 800 μsec after the illumination (Fig. 2-19). A limitation of this technique is the requirement for separation steps because the chelates cannot be measured directly in body fluids (see Chapter 9 for additional details).

Chemiluminescence[31,32]

A **chemiluminescence** reaction is any chemical reaction in which one of the products of the reaction is light. The enzyme peroxidase can react with molecules such as luminol

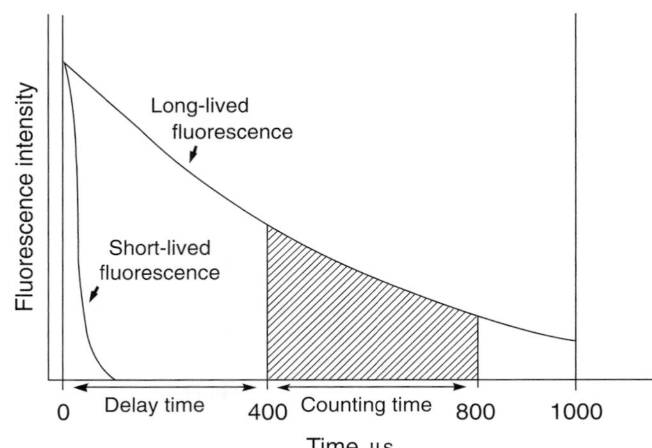

Fig. 2-19 Schema showing difference between short- and long-lived fluorescence.

(5-amino-2,3-dihydro-1,4-phthalazinedione) to yield light as part of the reaction product. The luminol reaction results in photon emission in the range of 400 to 450 nm. The low photon yield of this reaction has limited its sensitivity and its application. However, through the addition of enhancer molecules (luciferin, 6-hydroxybenzothiazole), the reaction can be followed for many minutes (30 or more) with a several thousand–fold increase in photon output. The products of these reactions are not known. A partial reaction may be written as follows:

$$2\,H_2O_2 + \text{Luminol and enhancer} \xrightarrow{\text{Peroxidase}} 2\,H_2O + h\nu + \text{Oxidized luminol} \qquad \text{Eq. 2-17}$$

The peroxidase is often part of an enzyme-labeled immunoassay system in which peroxidase is the label. The reaction can be measured by very sensitive photomultiplier tubes. The advantage of this technique is that it can be very sensitive. One molecule of peroxidase can turn over several million molecules of substrate per minute. Thus, detection can be more sensitive than that achievable with radioisotopes. A disadvantage of the system is that the reaction is performed in a heterogeneous system in which the peroxidase is attached to a solid phase. The H_2O_2 and luminol must be in a system that is free from common biological matrices, such as serum, and therefore a separation step is necessary.

Other dye systems that produce quantitative chemiluminescent reactions use the aromatic acridinium esters and the dioxetanes. The acridinium esters are oxidized most often by hydrogen peroxide to yield light, whereas the dioxetanes are made into stable phosphate ester derivatives that, when hydrolyzed, become spontaneously degraded, yielding light as one of the products. The LOCI analytical system discussed in the competitive binding chapter (see Chapter 9) uses a modification of these principles. A light beam at 680 nm is used to create singlet oxygen atoms $^1O_2{}^*$. These very reactive singlet oxygen atoms react with a dye to yield light, which in turn is transferred to a fluorophore dye that emits fluorescent light. These molecules must be located near each other for the reactions to take place. If they are not close together, the reaction does not occur.

Bioluminescence, the naturally occurring chemiluminescence phenomenon, has been extensively studied, and the reaction involving the molecule luciferin, adenosine triphosphate (ATP), and luciferase in the presence of oxygen is the best understood.

$$\text{Luciferin} + \text{ATP} + O_2 \xrightarrow{\text{Luciferase}} \text{Oxyluciferin} + \text{Light} \qquad \text{Eq. 2-18}$$

The reaction is quantitative because one photon of light is released for every ATP consumed. The sensitivity of the reaction is limited only by the photodetector's ability to count photons.

Electrochemiluminescence[33]

The **electrochemiluminescence** process is based on the formation of an excited state chemical intermediate that returns to the ground state by emitting a photon. This technique of excitation is different from those in which an excited state is achieved by absorption of a photon. In this case, the excited state is reached through a chemical reaction. One commercially successful system is based on the chemiluminescent properties of ruthenium complexes when they encounter free radicals. In this system, a ruthenium(II)-tris(bipyridyl) $[Ru(bpy)_3{}^{2+}]$ complex is oxidized from the 2^+ state to a 3^+ state by interaction with the cathode. This 3^+ complex reacts with a free radical, reducing the complex to a highly excited 2^+ state. The excited complex then emits a photon to return to the ground state where it may be recycled to undergo these same reactions. The free radicals in the Igen system are generated by the reaction of tripropylamine (TPA) with the anode, which yields a positively charged TPA free radical. This species gives up a hydrogen ion to form the TPA free radical. This free radical reacts with the 3^+ complex.

$$\text{Ru (complex)}^{2+} \xrightarrow{\text{electrode}} e^- + \text{Ru (complex)}^{3+} \qquad \text{Eq. 2-19}$$

$$\text{TPA} \xrightarrow{\text{electrode}} e^- + \text{TPA}^{\bullet+} \rightarrow \text{TPA}^{\bullet} + H^+ \qquad \text{Eq. 2-20}$$

$$\text{Ru (complex)}^{3+} + \text{TPA}^{\bullet+} + e^- \rightarrow \text{TPA degradation products} + \text{excited Ru (complex)}^{2+} \qquad \text{Eq. 2-21}$$

$$\text{excited Ru (complex)}^{2+} \rightarrow \text{Ru (complex)}^{2+} + h\nu \text{ (light at 620 nm)} \qquad \text{Eq. 2-22}$$

The light from the excited Ru $(\text{complex})^{2+}$ is released over about 0.6 second. Therefore, this is a luminescent process. The ruthenium complex can be attached to proteins, nucleic acids, and ligands. These labeled molecules are used in a variety of immunoassay formats.

Fluorescence Polarization[28,34,35]

Light is considered to be composed of an electronic vector and a magnetic vector. Normal light has these vectors in randomized orientations. If the light is polarized, all the electronic vectors have the same orientation.

When light is absorbed by a fluorescent molecule, it results in the transition of an electron to a higher energy level. The excited molecule emits light as the electron (fluorescent oscillator) returns to a lower energy level. Fluorescence polarization measurements require a dye with an electronic orientation such that the emitted light retains the initial orientation of the incident beam. An example of such a molecule is fluorescein. If polarized light is used to excite fluorescein molecules, the reemitted fluorescent light also can be polarized. However, molecules in solution rotate, and so this orientation and the fluorescence polarization can be lost. In fluorescence polarization, the dye must be selected so that its molecular rotation is so great between the times of light absorption and emission that the molecule becomes randomly oriented during this time and the fluorescence is minimally polarized. The quantity that is measured is the intensity of the oriented (polarized) light or the difference between the polarizer light is measured when the input is oriented vertically versus when the input light polarizer is oriented in the horizontal position.

For measuring polarized light, several options are available. One approach is to excite the test solution with light polarized in one dimension and to record the amount of the emitted fluorescence. The polarizer is placed immediately after the first monochromator as shown in the diagram of a fluorometer given in Fig. 2-18. The solution then is excited by light that is polarized at 90 degrees to the light used in the first excitation, and the emitted fluorescence is recorded. Polarization (P) can be determined from the following equation:

$$P = \frac{I_{vv} - I_{hv}}{I_{vv} + I_{hv}} \qquad \text{Eq. 2-23}$$

in which I_{vv} equals the signal recorded when the vertically polarized light is used to excite the sample, and I_{hv} is the response when the horizontally polarized light is used to excite the sample. Emitted light is measured from the vertical polarizer at a 90-degree orientation from the incident light by use of a second polarizer that is placed before the second monochromator.

Numerous processes affect the final polarization. For many fluorescent dyes, including the most popular one, fluorescein, polarization of light is retained if the molecule is held rigid. When the molecule randomly rotates by the process of brownian motion, polarization is lost. The ability of a molecule in solution to rotate partially depends on the viscosity of the solution and on the molecular volume of the molecule. When the viscosity of the solution or the molecular volume increases, the fluorescent molecules rotate more slowly and the polarization increases. In the case of the fluorescence polarization immunoassay, when the drug-fluorescein derivative is bound by antibody, the molecular volume increases. Therefore, the **polarized fluorescence** increases. When the derivative is unbound, the molecular volume is low and the fluorescence polarization is low (see Chapter 9).

Fluorescence polarization measurements can be made very accurately, and they are less affected by variations in fluorescence intensity than are standard fluorescence measurements (see Eq. 2-23). Thus, precision on the order of 1% or greater of measurement is readily achieved, which translates into more precise assay measurements. Another advantage of fluorescence polarization is that the technique can be used as a homogeneous assay. Disadvantages include the following: (1) the technique is limited to assays that can use fluorescent dyes, (2) the instrumentation required for performing fluorescence polarization measurement is often very specialized and may measure only fluorescence intensity or polarization, and (3) the system is less flexible than absorption spectroscopy. In addition, when fluorescence polarization measurements are performed, it is crucial to control temperature and viscosity.

KEY CONCEPT BOX 2-4

- Atomic absorption spectroscopy uses special lamps to generate line spectra and requires that the sample be in the vapor phase. Measurement is similar to that of other absorbance systems.
- Fluorescent light can be polarized. The amount of polarization can be related to bound and unbound forms of the fluorescent molecule.
- Light is scattered when it interacts with particles. This can diminish the light going through a solution and can be related quantitatively to the concentration of particles. Similarly, the scattered light can be examined at an angle and also can be related to particle concentration.

NEPHELOMETRY AND TURBIDIMETRY[36-38]

Principle

Interaction of Light With Particles

To understand the principle of nephelometric or turbidimetric assays, we must first examine the concept of light scattering. When a collimated (i.e., parallel, nondivergent) beam of light strikes a particle in suspension, some light is reflected, some is scattered, some is absorbed, and some is transmitted. Nephelometry is the measurement of the light scattered by a particulate solution. Turbidity measures **light scattering** as a decrease in the light transmitted through the solution.

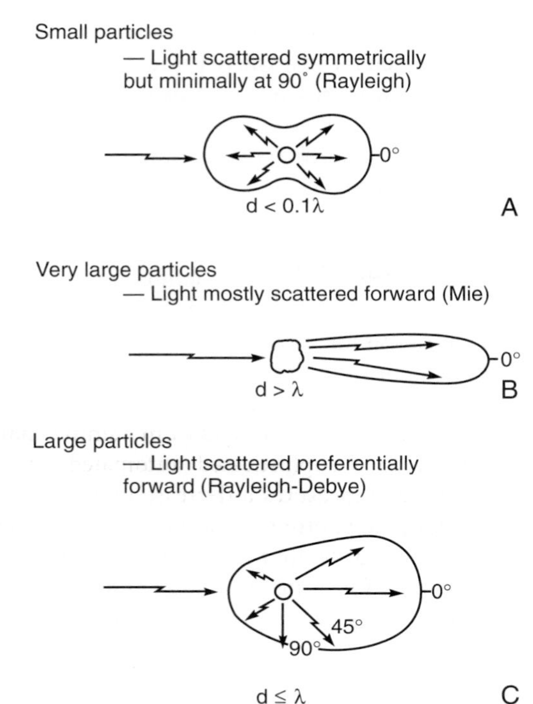

Fig. 2-20 Effect of particle size on scattering of incident light in a homogeneous solution. *d,* Particle diameter; *λ,* wavelength of incident light. (From Gauldie J: Principles and clinical applications of nephelometry. In Kaplan LA, Pesce AJ, editors: *Nonisotopic Alternatives to Radioimmunoassay,* New York, 1981, Marcel Dekker. Reprinted by courtesy of Marcel Dekker, Inc.[38])

In considering nephelometry, the question of how light is scattered by a homogeneous particle suspension must be examined. Three types of scatter can occur. If the wavelength, λ, of light is much larger than the size of the particle ($d < 0.1\lambda$), the light is symmetrically scattered around the particle, with a minimum in the intensity of the scatter occurring at 90 degrees to the incident beam, as described by Rayleigh (Fig. 2-20, *A*).

If the wavelength of the incident light is much smaller than the size of the particle ($d > 10\lambda$), then most of the light appears to be scattered forward because of destructive out-of-phase backscatter, as described by the Mie theory (see Fig. 2-20, *B*).

If, however, the wavelength of light is approximately equal to the size of the particles, more light appears scattered in a forward direction than in a backward direction (see Fig. 2-20, *C*), as described by **Rayleigh-Debye scatter.**[36]

One of the most common uses of light-scattering analyses is the measurement of antigen-antibody reactions. Because most antigen-antibody complex systems are heterogeneous with particle diameters of 250 to 1500 nm, and the wavelengths used in most light-scattering analyzers are 320 to 650 nm, the scatter seen is essentially Rayleigh-Debye, with the blank scatter being primarily described by Rayleigh scatter. Thus, the ability to detect light scatter in a forward direction (θ = 15 to 90 degrees) leads to greater sensitivity for nephelometric determinations. Such is the case in the newer rate and laser nephelometers.

Detection of Scattered Light

Turbidimetry

Turbidimetry measures the reduction in light transmission caused by particle formation, and it quantifies the residual light transmitted (Fig. 2-21). The instrumentation required for turbidimetric measurements ranges from a simple manual spectrophotometer to a sophisticated automated analyzer. Because this technique measures a decrease in a large signal of transmitted light, the photometric accuracy and sensitivity of the instrument primarily limit the sensitivity of turbidimetry. Instruments used for turbidimetry can be used for many other assays, such as enzyme assays and those assays based on color development.

Nephelometry

Nephelometry, on the other hand, detects a portion of the light that is scattered at a variety of angles (Fig. 2-22). The sensitivity of this method primarily depends on the absence of blank or background scatter because the instruments are detecting a small increment of signal at a scatter angle, θ, on a supposedly black, or null, background. Ideally, no light is detected in the absence of a scattering species, and so subsequent scatter in samples is measured against this black background. The signal is magnified by the use of a photomultiplier, and so the detection range is increased. However, such measurements require the committed use of a nephelometer, which has limited use in other assays.

Instrumentation

Schematic Layout of Instruments. A schematic layout of the basic components of a nephelometer is shown in Fig. 2-23. Typical systems consist of a light source, a collimating system, a wavelength selector such as a filter (the last two items are unnecessary with laser light sources), a sample cuvette, a stray light trap, and a photodetector.

Light Source. Fluoronephelometers use a medium-pressure mercury arc lamp as a light source, which serves for both nephelometry and fluorometry. The relatively high-intensity light and short-wavelength emission bands make this a good source. Other light sources range from simple low-voltage tungsten filament lamps and light-emitting diodes to sophisticated low-power lasers. Lasers produce stable, highly collimated, and intense beams of light (typically 1 milliradian divergence) that require no additional optical collimators as other light sources do. In optical systems that use laser light,

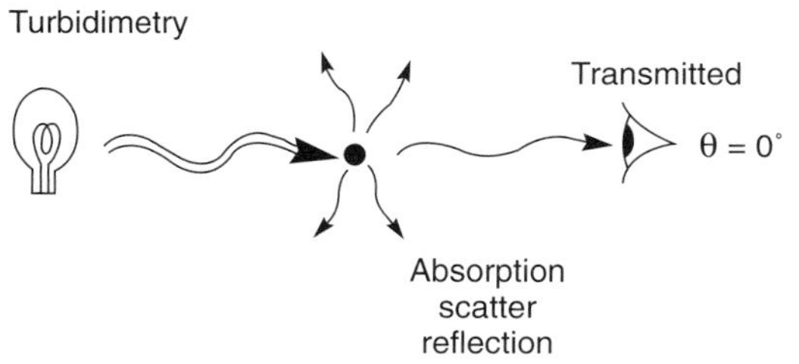

Fig. 2-21 Schema of turbidity measurement. *θ,* Angle of detection. (From Gauldie J: Principles and clinical applications of nephelometry. In Kaplan LA, Pesce AJ, editors: *Nonisotopic Alternatives to Radioimmunoassay,* New York, 1981, Marcel Dekker. Reprinted by courtesy of Marcel Dekker, Inc.[2])

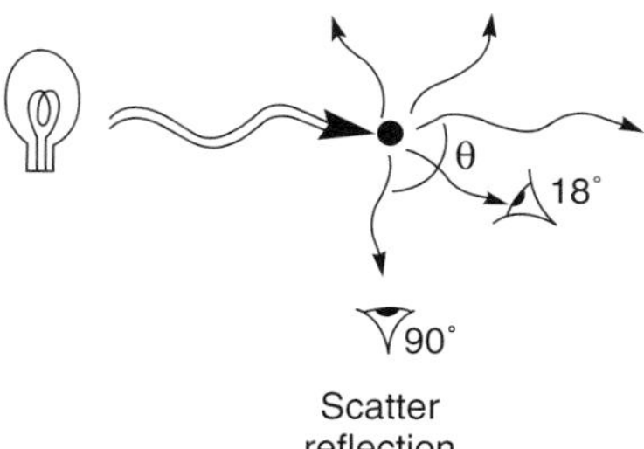

Fig. 2-22 Schema of nephelometric measurements. *θ,* Angle of detection. (From Gauldie J: Principles and clinical applications of nephelometry. In Kaplan LA, Pesce AJ, editors: *Nonisotopic Alternatives to Radioimmunoassay,* New York, 1981, Marcel Dekker. Reprinted by courtesy of Marcel Dekker, Inc.[2])

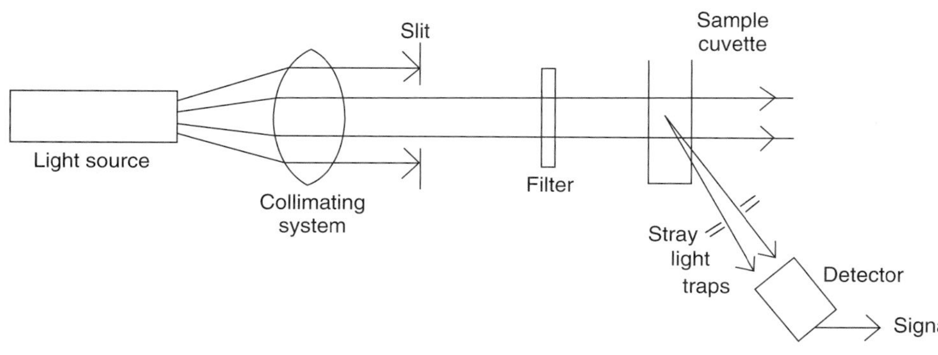

Fig. 2-23 Schema of basic components of a nephelometer.

it is easier to reduce stray light, which contributes to background scatter, and to mask the transmitted beam, thus allowing measurement of forward scatter. The increase in light intensity achievable with lasers also results in an improvement in signal-to-noise ratio, but this is limited somewhat by detector saturation. Disadvantages of laser sources include cost, safety problems, and the restricted availability of limited fixed wavelengths. Because particle size may continually change during the course of reaction analysis, as during immune precipitate formation, light scatter at a single wavelength may change while the average light scatter over many wavelengths remains relatively constant. The Beckman Array employs a broad-band filter for selection of a wavelength region from a normal tungsten lamp source to overcome this problem, which is obviously more acute in rate methods when the size of the particle is changing most rapidly.

In all cases, the photodetector system must be matched to the wavelength or wavelengths of scattered light, which, for nephelometry and turbidimetry, correspond to the incident light wavelength or wavelengths.

Angle of Detection[39]

Because particles the size of antigen-antibody complexes appear to scatter light more in the forward direction, the signal-to-noise ratio is increased as the detector is placed nearer the transmitted path (0 degrees).

The blank signal, described best by Rayleigh scatter (see Fig. 2-20, *A*), is not so affected by an altered **angle of detection.** Thus, although most early nephelometers detected light scattered at 90 degrees for reasons of manufacturing ease, which limited low-angle measurement capability, the detection of forward light scatter should provide theoretically greater sensitivity. The newer instruments tend to operate with lower detection angles, optimized in many cases to give the highest signal-to-noise ratio for the particular instrument's optics. Obviously, detection at 0 degrees is not possible because of the high intensity of the transmitted beam, but some laser-equipped fast analyzers that use a mask to block the transmitted beam are able to operate at very low angles. Instruments that employ low-angle detectors tend to have greater sensitivity than the 90-degree type of instruments.

Limitations: Turbidimetry versus Nephelometry

Although the principle of nephelometry—detection of a small signal (amplifiable) on a black background—should lend high sensitivity to this method, the sophistication and specifications of the available instruments do not achieve this promise. Turbidimetry—detection of a small decrease in a large signal—should be limited in sensitivity; however, current instruments have excellent discrimination and can quantify small changes in signal, thereby allowing turbidimetric measurements to achieve high sensitivity.

Turbidimetry and nephelometry have similarities to absorption spectrophotometry, and many sources of interference and errors are common to all these systems. Many techniques (discussed in Chapter 17) that can be used to minimize absorption interferences are also applicable to turbidimetry and nephelometry. Nevertheless, sample turbidity can interfere with both techniques.

Endogenous Color and Choice of Wavelength

Basic light-scattering theory predicts that the intensity of scattered light increases as shorter wavelengths of incident light are used. Most immunological assay reactions employ serum protein reactions that require the choice of a wavelength at which neither the proteins nor the colored serum components absorb appreciably. Because proteins absorb strongly at wavelengths shorter than 300 nm and serum has an absorption peak at 400 to 425 nm because of porphyrins, instruments tend to operate in the 320 to 380 or 500 to 650 nm range. Reduction of the protein concentration by dilution decreases background absorption. Most immunochemical reactions measured by nephelometry use high-affinity antibodies that allow for large dilutions of protein and consequent improvement in sensitivity.

Comparison of Sensitivity

Sensitivity in nephelometers is largely controlled by the amount of background scatter from sample and reagents. Because background scatter can be high relative to specific scatter, instruments do not reach their full potential of sensitivity. This limitation, coupled with the higher wavelengths generated in laser instruments, accounts for the fact that laser instruments show no great increase in sensitivity over conventional nephelometers.

Sensitivity in turbidimetric measurements depends on the ability of the detector to resolve small changes in light intensity. With the use of low wavelengths and high-quality spectrophotometers with their highly precise detection systems, sensitivity in turbidimetry is usually adequate for many measurements and, in many cases, compares well with nephelometry.

End Point versus Kinetic Analysis

Examination of light scattered as a function of time, after there is mixture of an antibody and antigen, shows that after an initial delay, there is an almost linear increase in scatter followed by a slower attainment of plateau scatter. The secondary reaction occurs much more slowly than the first because larger particles form and begin to flocculate, and they distort the scatter intensity seen at forward angles. Both turbidity and nephelometry measurements behave in this manner.

There are two basic ways of measuring light scatter caused by this reaction: end point analysis and rate analysis. End point analysis requires blank (reagent) determinations and a reasonable amount of elapsed time before final measurement. Fig. 2-24 shows the forward scatter developed at 70 degrees of a rate nephelometric analyzer.[38] When the two graphs are compared, the differences between an end point analysis (blank value and reading vs. reading at $t = x$, see Fig. 2-24, *A*) and a rate or kinetic analysis (increase in scattered intensity over a set time interval, see Fig. 2-24, *B*) can be seen. The kinetic approach, which electronically subtracts any blank signal, does not require a separate reagent blank to be run.

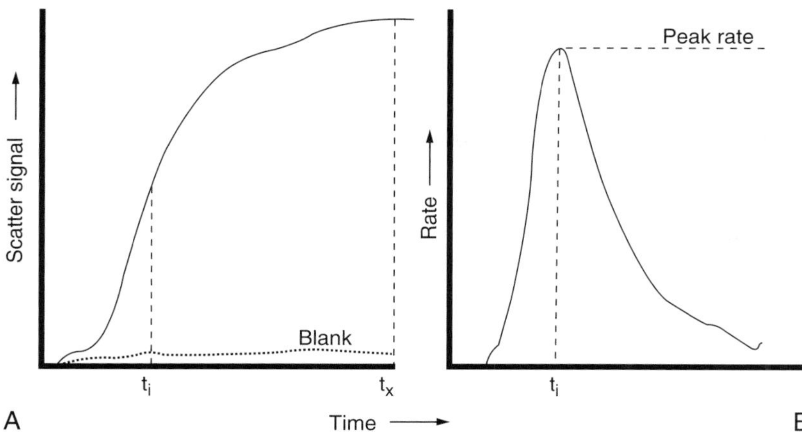

Fig. 2-24 Kinetic analysis of light scattering. **A,** Intensity of scattered light signal versus time. **B,** Rate of change of scattered light signal versus time.

Both kinetic and end point analysis can be applied equally to turbidimetry and nephelometry.

REFRACTIVITY

Principle

When a beam of light impinges on a boundary surface, it can be reflected or absorbed, or, if the material is transparent, it can pass into the boundary and emerge on the other side. When light passes from one medium into another, the path of the light beam changes direction at the boundary surface if its speed in the second medium is different from that in the first (Fig. 2-25). This bending of light is called **refraction.**[40]

Because the degree of refraction of a light beam depends on the difference in the speed of light between two different media, the ratio of the two speeds has been expressed as the index of refraction, or the **refractive index.** The relative ability of a substance to bend light is called refractivity. The expression of a refractive index, n, is always relative to air with the convention that n of air = 1. The measurement of the refractive index requires the measurement of angles because the light is bent at an angle proportional to the relationship of n in the medium through which the light is passing:

$$\frac{n}{n_1} = \frac{\sin\theta}{\sin\theta_1} \qquad \text{Eq. 2-24}$$

The refractivity of a liquid depends on (1) the wavelength of the incident light, (2) the temperature, (3) the nature of the liquid, and (4) the total mass of solid dissolved in the liquid. If the first three factors are held constant, the refractive index of a solution is a direct measure of the total mass of dissolved solids.

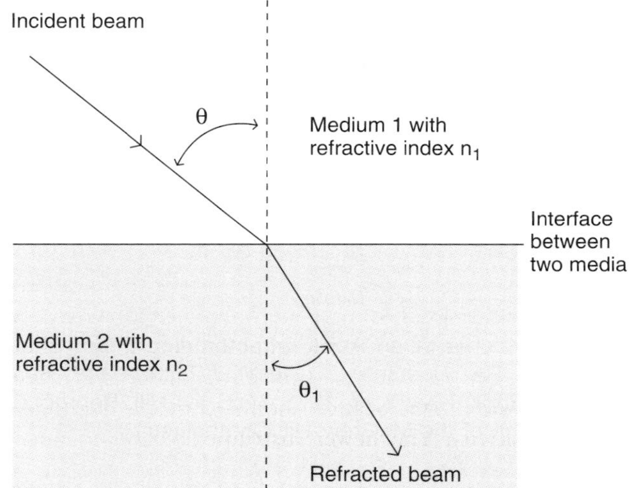

Fig. 2-25 Schema illustrating bending of light when it passes from a medium of one density into a medium of a different density, with an angle of deflection, θ_1.

Applications

Refractometry has been applied to the measurement of total serum protein concentration.[41] The assumption of this analysis is that the serum matrix (i.e., the concentration of electrolytes and small organic molecules) remains essentially the same from patient to patient. Because the mass of protein is normally so much greater than the mass of other serum constituents, small variations in these other substances have no significant effect on the refractive index of serum. **Refractometers** are calibrated against "normal" serum, and total protein concentrations are read directly from a scale.

Refractometry is also used to estimate the specific gravity of urine samples. The refractive index is linearly related to the total mass of dissolved solids and thus to specific gravity. This remains valid over most of the range normally encountered for urine (i.e., up to 1.035 g/mL).

Interference

When the concentration of small molecular weight compounds or particulate matter greatly increases, positive interference results. This interference occurs in the presence

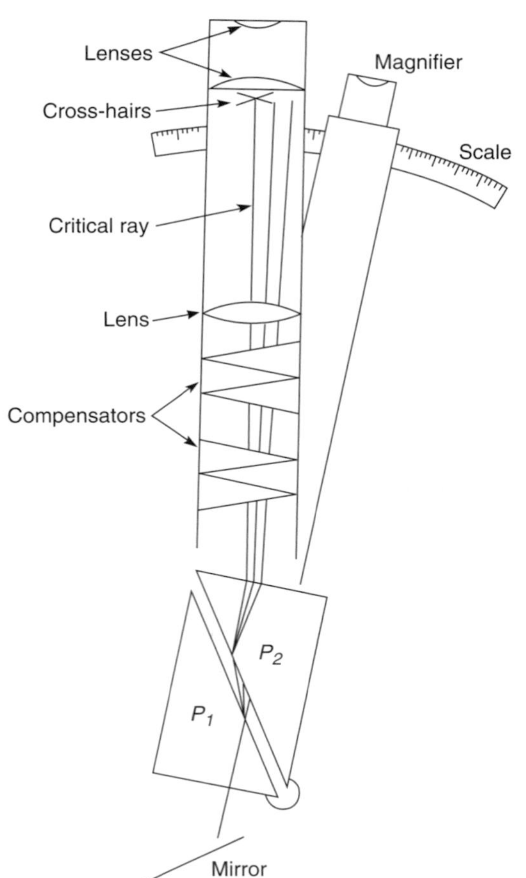

Fig. 2-26 Schema of an Abbé refractometer. (From Shugar GJ, Shugar RA, Bauman L: *Chemical Technicians' Ready Reference Book,* New York, 1973, McGraw-Hill. Reproduced by permission of the McGraw-Hill Companies.)

of hyperglycemia, hyperbilirubinemia, azotemia (increased serum urea), lyophilized samples, and hyperlipidemia. Hemolysis also results in false-positive values for total serum protein.

Instrumentation

Most clinical refractometers are based on the Abbé refractometer (Fig. 2-26), marketed by American Optical Corporation (Southbridge, MA). This refractometer consists of two prisms and a series of lenses. Light passes through the first prism, where the light beam is dispersed. The dispersed light passes into and through the thin layer of the liquid sample, where it is refracted. The light beam passes through a second prism, where the light again is dispersed and on leaving is refracted again. The boundary at the edge of the refracted light beam is aligned perpendicularly to the scale on which serum protein concentrations or specific gravity can be read. The scale for reading serum protein (g/dL or g/L) is established by calibration of the instrument against a "normal" serum solution. This type of refractometer is extraordinarily simple, having no moving or electrical parts. Thus, it is easily reproducible, measuring protein with a precision of ±1% and an accuracy of ±1 g/L. The sample size is on the order of 50 μL.

More complex refractometers are used to monitor column effluents for high-performance liquid chromatography analysis (see Chapter 6).

KEY CONCEPT BOX 2-5

- Light "bends" when going from a solution of one density to another. The amount of bending can be used to calculate the quantities of dissolved solids in a solution.

REFERENCES

1. Yehuda B: *Light and Matter,* New York, 2006, Wiley & Sons.
2. Richards WG, Scott RR: *Structure and Spectra of Molecules,* New York, 1985, Wiley & Sons.
3. http://www.its.caltech.edu/~ch24/lecture2324_2004.pdf
4. Willard HH, Merritt LL, Dean JA, Settle FA Jr: Instrumental Methods of Analysis, ed 7, Boston, MA, 1988, Wadsworth Publishing Company.
5. Frings CS, Broussard LA: Calibration and monitoring of spectrometers and spectrophotometers, Clin Chem 25:1013, 1979.
6. Brewer JM, Pesce AJ, Ashworth RB, editors: *Experimental Techniques in Biochemistry,* Englewood Cliffs, NJ, 1974, Prentice-Hall.
7. Haven MC, Tetrault GA, Schenken JR: *Laboratory Instrumentation,* ed 4, New York, 1994, Wiley & Sons.
8. Ward KM, Harris E: Spectrophotometry. In Ward KM, Lehmann CA, Leiken AM, editors: *Clinical Laboratory Instrumentation and Automation: Principles, Application, and Selection,* Philadelphia, 1994, WB Saunders.
9. Narayanan S: *Principles and Applications of Laboratory Instrumentation,* Chicago, 1989, ASCP Press.
10. Khazanie P: Spectrophotometry. In Anderson SC, Cockagne S, editors: *Clinical Chemistry: Concepts and Applications,* Philadelphia, 2002, WB Saunders.
11. CFRS 493.1215 Standard equipment maintenance and function checks. Federal Register 57(4):7164-7165, 1992.
12. http://www.howstuffworks.com/led2.htm
13. http://micro.magnet.fsu.edu/primer/java/leds/basicoperation/index.html
14. http://www.reference.com/browse/wiki/Charge-coupled_device
15. http://en.wikipedia.org/wiki/Electron-multiplying_CCD
16. Instrumentation Guidelines Study Group, Subcommittee on Enzymes: Guidelines for photometric instruments for measuring enzyme reaction rates, Clin Chem 23:2160, 1977.
17. Alexander LR, Barnhart ER: *Photometric Quality Assurance Instrument Check Procedures,* Atlanta, GA, 1980, U.S. Department of Health and Human Services, Centers for Disease Control, Bureau of Laboratories.
18. ASTM E275-01: *Standard Practice for Describing and Measuring Performance of Ultraviolet, Visible, and Near-Infrared Spectrophotometers,* West Conshohocken, PA, ASTM International.
19. Molecular Spectrometry and Microfluidic Methods Group, Analytical Chemistry Division, National Institute of Standards and Technology: Frequently Asked Questions Regarding UV/Visible Reference Materials, Gaithersburg, MD, NIST. Available at http://www.cstl.nist.gov/nist839/839.04/faqs.htm; NIST standards and calibrators for Optical Radiation Measurements. Available at http://ts.nist.gov/MeasurementServices/Calibrations/opticalproperties.cfm#38010C.
20. Curme HG, Columbus RL, Dappen GM, et al: Multilayer film elements for clinical analysis: general concepts, Clin Chem 24:1335, 1978.
21. Copeland BE, Dyer PJ, Pesce AJ: Plasma hemoglobin by first derivative spectro-photometry, Semin Diagn Hematol 1-8, 1988.

22. Zijlstr WG, Buursma A, Zwart A: Performance of an automated six-wavelength photometer (Radiometer OSM3) for routine measurement of hemoglobin derivatives, Clin Chem 34:149, 1988.
23. *Journal of Analytical Atomic Spectrometry* (JAAS), Cambridge, UK, Royal Society of Chemistry (United Kingdom).
24. Sperling MB, Welz B: *Atomic Absorption Spectrometry,* Weinheim, 1999, Wiley-VCH.
25. http://en.wikipedia.org/wiki/Spectrum_analysis
26. Evans E, Giglio J, Castillano T, et al: *Inductively Coupled and Microwave Induced Plasma Sources for Mass Spectrometry RSC, Analytical Spectroscopy Monographs,* Cambridge, UK, 1995, Royal Society of Chemistry.
27. Simonson MG: The application of a photon-counting fluorometer for the immunofluorescent measurement of therapeutic drugs. In Kaplan LA, Pesce AJ, editors: *Nonisotopic Alternatives to Radioimmunoassay,* New York, 1981, Marcel Dekker.
28. Pesce AJ, Rosen CG, Pasby TL, editors: *Fluorescence Spectroscopy,* New York, 1971, Marcel Dekker.
29. Lakowicz JR: *Principles of Fluorescence Spectroscopy,* Berlin, 2006, Springer.
30. Hemmilä I: Fluoroimmunoassays and immunofluorometric assays, Clin Chem 31:359, 1985.
31. *Enhanced Luminescence: A Practical Immunoassay System,* Medicine Publishing Foundation Symposium Series 18, Oxford, UK, 1986, Medicine Publishing Foundation.
32. Scholmerich J, et al, editors: *Bioluminescence and Chemiluminescence: New Perspectives,* New York, 1987, Wiley & Sons.
33. Wang J: *Analytical Electrochemistry,* Germany, 2006, Wiley-VCH.
34. Spencer RD: Fluorescence polarization. In Kaplan LA, Pesce AJ, editors: *Nonisotopic Alternatives to Radioimmunoassay,* New York, 1981, Marcel Dekker.
35. Jolley ME, Stroupe SD, Wang CH, et al: Fluorescence polarization immunoassay. I. Monitoring aminoglycoside antibiotics in serum and plasma, Clin Chem 27:1190, 1981.
36. Ritchie RF, editor: *Automated Immunoanalysis,* Parts 1 and 2, New York, 1978, Marcel Dekker.
37. Deverill I, Reeves WG: Light scattering and absorption developments in immunology, J Immunol Methods 38:191, 1980.
38. Gauldie J: Principles and clinical applications of nephelometry. In Kaplan LA, Pesce AJ, editors: *Nonisotopic Alternatives to Radioimmunoassay,* New York, 1981, Marcel Dekker.
39. Kusnetz J, Mansberg HP: Nephelometry. In Ritchie RF: *Automated Immunoanalysis,* Part 1, New York, 1978, Marcel Dekker.
40. Glover FA, Gaulden JDS: Relationship between refractive index and concentration of solutions, Nature 200:1165, 1963.
41. Rubini MD, Wolf AV: Refractometric determination of total solids and water of serum and urine, J Biol Chem 225:868, 1957.

BIBLIOGRAPHY

http://www.bertholf.net/rlb/Lectures/Lectures/Review%20of%20Analytical%20Methods%20I.pps —PowerPoint lecture by Robert L. Bertholf PhD, Associate Professor of Pathology, Chief of Clinical Chemistry and Toxicology University of Florida Health Sciences Center.

Light and color. http://www.sylvania.com/LearnLighting/LightAndColor/

Rouessac F, Rouessac A: *Chemical Analysis: Modern Instrumentation Methods and Techniques,* New York, 2007, Wiley & Sons.

Chromatography: Theory, Practice, and Instrumentation

3

Chapter

Michael Lehrer

Chapter Outline

Key Terms

adsorption Process whereby one substance adheres to another because of attractive forces between surface atoms of the two substances.

analyte The substance or component in a sample that is being measured.

band A chromatographic zone, that is, a region where the separated substance is concentrated.

capacity factor The ratio of the elution volume of a substance to the void volume in the column.

chromatography A method of analysis in which the flow of a mobile phase (gas or liquid) that contains the sample promotes the separation of sample components.

dipole The attractive force of compounds with centers of both positive and negative charges that are the result of an unequal sharing of bonding electrons between the two.

dispersive force The attractive force (also termed *van der Waals forces*) of compounds that results from the induction of a temporary dipole.

efficiency A measure of chromatographic performance that usually is related to the sharpness of peaks in the chromatogram.

electrostatic interaction The attractive force between compounds with formal positive or negative charges.

equilibrium concentration distribution coefficient (K_D) The ratio of the concentration of a sample component in one phase to its concentration in a second phase at equilibrium.

hydrogen bonding Attractive force of compounds formed when a hydrogen atom covalently linked to an electronegative element, like oxygen, nitrogen, or sulfur, has a large degree of positive character relative to the electronegative atom.

N Number of theoretical separating plates in a chromatographic column.

nonpolar A term that describes molecules that have a hydrophobic affinity, that is, those that are "water hating." Nonpolar substances tend to dissolve in nonpolar solvents.

normal phase A chromatographic mode in which the mobile phase is less polar than the stationary phase.

partition Process by which a solute is distributed between two immiscible phases.

peak A band or zone of a component that is being separated in the chromatographic instrument.

pK_a The pK of a weak acid is the pH at which it is half-dissociated.

polar A term that describes molecules that have a hydrophilic affinity, that is, those that are "water loving." Polar substances tend to dissolve in polar solvents.

polarity The attractive forces that encompass the total interaction of solvent molecules with sample molecules and of solvent or sample molecules with the stationary phase.

resolution (R or R_s) The degree of separation between two eluting components by chromatography.

retention time (t_R) The time that has elapsed from injection of an analyte into the chromatograph until it elutes into the detector.

selectivity (α) The ratios of the capacity factors for two substances measured under identical chromatographic conditions; sometimes termed *separation factor*.

theoretical plate number (N) A theoretical number that defines the efficiency of the chromatographic column.

void volume (V_0) Volume of solvent required to elute an unretained compound. Also, the volume of mobile phase imbibed in the pores and around the stationary phase in a column (related to total volume of column).

SECTION OBJECTIVES BOX 3-1

- Discuss the purposes of the mobile and stationary phases in chromatography.
- Explain the meaning of both small and large values for the capacity factor.
- Define "selectivity factor" (α) and explain how the selectivity factor may be changed in both gas and liquid chromatography to improve separation.
- List four attractive forces that form the physicochemical basis for polarity.

OVERVIEW OF CHROMATOGRAPHY

Chromatography is a physical technique that separates mixtures into individual components. It is a collective term that refers to a group of separation processes whereby a mixture of solutes, dissolved in a common solvent, are separated from one another by a differential distribution of the solutes between two phases. One phase, the solvent, is mobile and carries the mixture of solutes through the other phase, the fixed or stationary phase. Chromatographic methods encompass a great number of variations in technique in which the mobile phase ranges from liquids to gases and the stationary phase ranges from sheets of cellulose paper to capillary glass tubes as fine as a human hair that are internally coated with a covalently bonded complex or complex organic polymers.[1-4]

Branches of Chromatography

Chromatographic methods are classified according to the physical state of the solute carrier phase, that is, the mobile phase. These branches are represented in Figs. 3-1 and 3-2 as solution and gas chromatography, referring to the respective liquid and gaseous states of the mobile phase. In Fig. 3-1, these branches are classified further according to how the stationary-phase matrix is contained for a particular chromatographic method. For example, solution chromatography is divided into methods in which the stationary phase is a thin layer mechanically supported on a sheet (flat) or packed into a column. The flat method of support may involve the use of a sheet of paper, such as cellulose, or a thin layer on a mechanical backing, such as glass or plastic.

Column method is a term that is generally used to subdivide solution chromatography, wherein the stationary phase is packed into a glass or metal tube. However, it is noted that gas chromatography is strictly a column method because a column must be used for containment of the stationary phase.

The main divisions of chromatography, based on the mobile phase, may be subdivided according to the mechanism of solute interaction with the stationary phase (see Fig. 3-2). Two mechanisms, **adsorption** and **partition,** are the most commonly encountered for both solution and gas mobile-phase separations. Adsorption chromatography (liquid-solid [L/S] or gas-solid [G/S]) is a process whereby solutes of a sample are separated by their differences in *attraction* to the stationary versus the mobile phase. Partition chromatography (liquid-liquid [L/L] or gas-liquid [G/L]) is a process whereby the solutes of a sample are separated by differences in their *distribution* between two liquid phases (L/L) or between a gas and a liquid phase (G/L). In both cases of partition chromatography, the stationary phase is a liquid, and the mobile phase is a liquid or a gas.

These and other mechanistic divisions of solution chromatography are discussed below after chromatographic theory and principles are briefly discussed.

General Principles

Only a few general concepts of the theoretical principles of chromatography are discussed in this section. For more extensive discussions and additional reference leads, refer to a representative review, books,[1,5,6] and other specialized chromatographic techniques.[7,8]

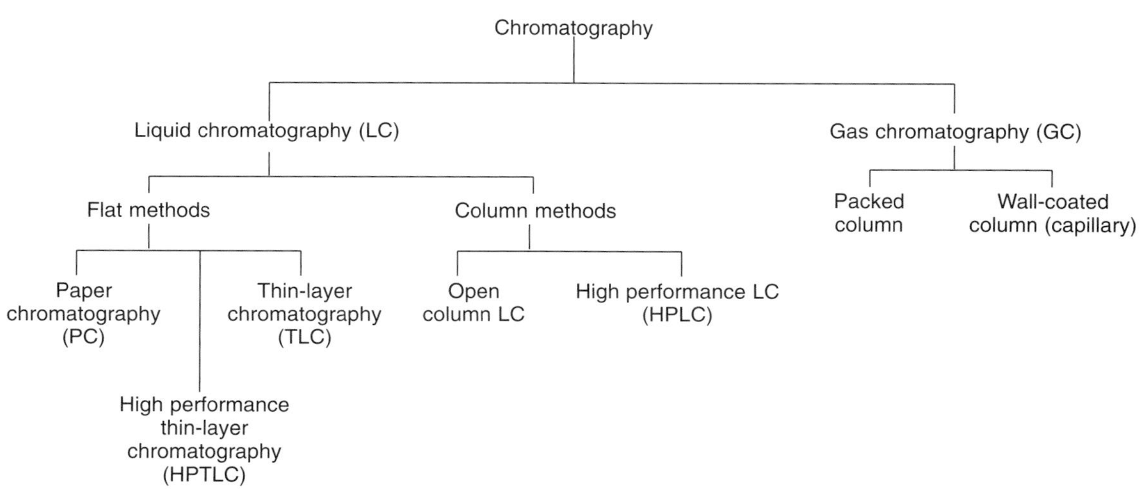

Fig. 3-1 Branches of chromatography according to mobile phase and physical apparatus.

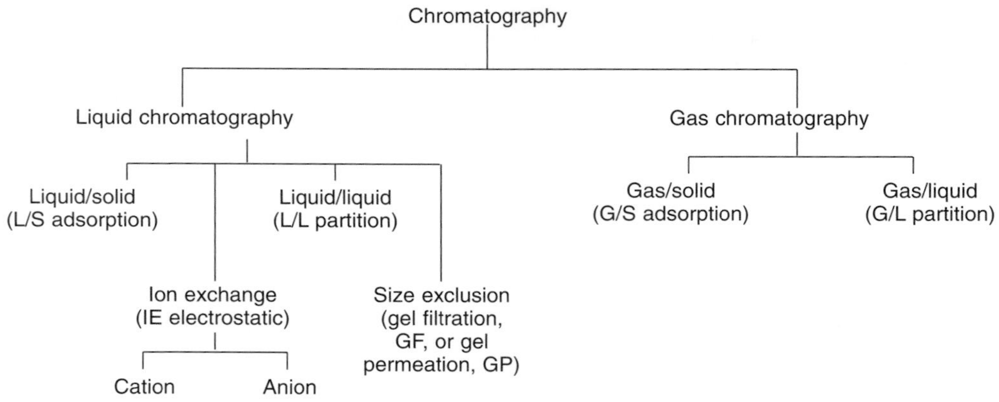

- Chromatography
  - Liquid chromatography
    - Liquid/solid (L/S adsorption)
    - Liquid/liquid (L/L partition)
    - Ion exchange (IE electrostatic)
      - Cation
      - Anion
    - Size exclusion (gel filtration, GF, or gel permeation, GP)
  - Gas chromatography
    - Gas/solid (G/S adsorption)
    - Gas/liquid (G/L partition)

Fig. 3-2 Branches of chromatography according to mechanism of separation on stationary phase.

The separation of a mixture that contains two or more components is performed with the goal of producing fractions, with each fraction having an increased concentration of one component relative to the other components contained in the original mixture. The physicochemical basis of chromatographic separation techniques is principally distribution equilibrium, which refers to the differences in solubility and adsorption of a component in two immiscible phases.[6]

Distribution equilibrium can be visualized as the distribution of a solute, *S*, between two immiscible phases, upper phase (u) and lower phase (l), at constant temperature and pressure. The ratio of the solute concentrations in the two phases determines the separation, which can be defined by an **equilibrium concentration distribution coefficient (K_D)** for the molar concentration (moles/L), C_u and C_l, of solute in the upper and lower phases, respectively:

$$K_D = \frac{C_u}{C_l} \qquad \text{Eq. 3-1}$$

The distribution coefficient is sometimes referred to as a *partition ratio.* A K_D of 1.0 means that 50% of the solute is distributed in the upper phase and 50% is distributed in the lower phase (Fig. 3-3, *A*); however, a K_D of 9.0 means that 90% of the solute is distributed in the upper phase and 10% in the lower phase (see Fig. 3-3, *B*).

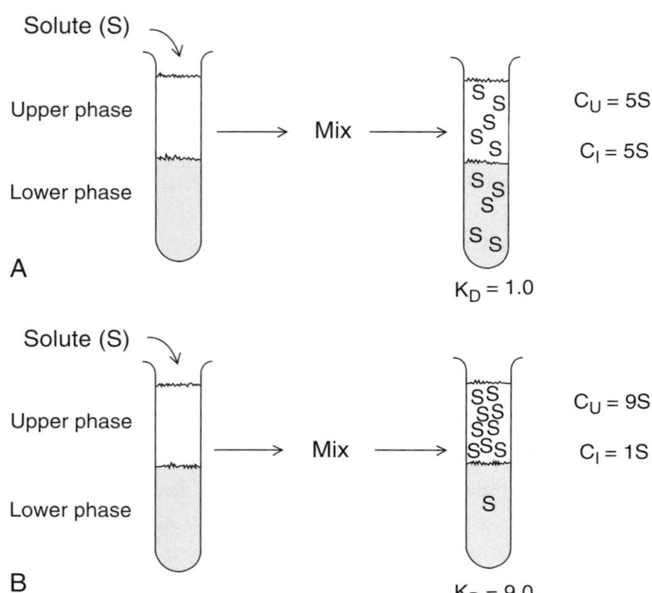

Fig. 3-3 Separation of a solute, *S,* by partition into two different solvent systems. In the first system, **A,** solute has a distribution coefficient, K_D, of 1.0, indicating an equal partitioning between upper and lower phases after mixing. In the second system, **B,** solute has a K_D of 9.0, indicating a partitioning of nine parts of the solute in the upper phase and one part of the solute in the lower phase after mixing. C_u, Upper-phase concentration; C_l, lower-phase concentration.

Resolution, Efficiency, and Speed of Analysis

Resolution

The ultimate goal of any given chromatographic technique is to separate the components of a given sample within a reasonable time in order to detect or quantitate in pure form a particular component or group of components. The degree to which components are separated from one another is a measure of the adequacy of the chromatographic separation. The question of what is adequate **resolution** can be answered by defining the objectives of the chromatographic separation. Generally, objectives for the analyst in a chemical laboratory depend on the following questions: (1) Is a particular substance present in a sample, that is, should a qualitative analysis be followed? (2) How much of a particular substance is present in a sample, that is, should a quantitative analysis be followed? In the following discussion of the theory of resolution, the principal emphasis (and corresponding illustrations) will be on column techniques, gas or liquid, rather than on flat methods.

Note that, by convention, the concentrations of solutes separated in a chromatographic system are plotted out versus time, units of elution volume, or distance. The **bands** (or zones) of **analytes** separated usually are referred to as a **peak.** Resolution is dependent on the positions of the centers of the

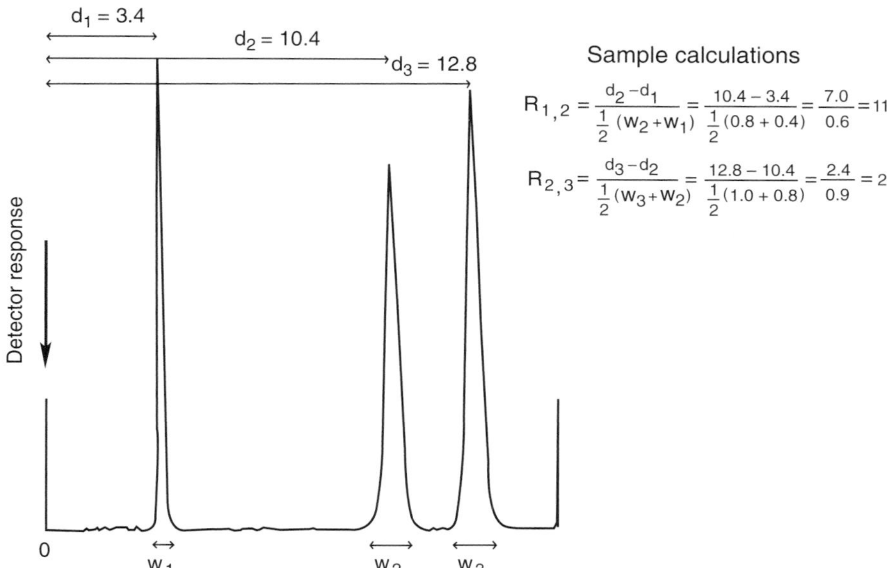

Fig. 3-4 Calculation of resolution of sample components actually separated by HPLC. The distances d_1 to d_3 are the actual amounts of time from injection (↓) to apex of eluting peak for each component, 1 to 3, respectively. Peak widths w_1 to w_3 are measured by triangulation at the base of each peak for components 1 to 3, respectively. Both d and w must be measured the same way from the time of injection, that is, in units of time (minutes or seconds), length (inches or centimeters), or elution volume (milliliters). Resolution, R, is unitless.

peaks that correspond to each compound and on the width of the peak between the points at which it is indistinguishable from the background signal. If the peak tracing reaches the background level before rising for the second peak, baseline resolution has been achieved.

An actual chromatographic separation of a three-component mixture by high-performance liquid chromatography is shown in Fig. 3-4, indicating important parameters for assessment of resolution, R. The quantity R for any two components is defined as the distance, d, between the peak centers of two peaks divided by the average base width, W, of the peaks:

$$R = \frac{d_2 - d_1}{\frac{1}{2}(w_1 + w_2)} \qquad \text{Eq. 3-2}$$

For this calculation, both the distance, d, and the peak width, w, are measured in the same units.

A resolution value of 1.25 or greater is required for good quantitative or qualitative chromatographic analyses. If the resolution is 0.4 or less, the peak shape does not clearly show the presence of two or more components. The actual value of the resolution depends on two factors: width of the peak and distance between peak maxima for column separations or diameter of the circular spots and distance between these spots for flat method separations. The high-efficiency separation shown in Fig. 3-5 demonstrates excellent resolution, while the low-efficiency separation demonstrates unacceptable resolution. It is considered unacceptable because of the significant co-elution of the 2 peaks. Optimal resolution requires baseline separation of two peaks that are being separated.

Because resolution depends on peak widths, stationary phases designed for the chemical nature of the components being separated should be selected to optimize efficiency of separation. These are readily available and featured in column supplier's catalogues. **Theoretical plates (N, Efficiency)** is a mathematical approach used in the early days of chromatography to estimate how to optimize a column's separation capabilities. Historically, such calculations were often more theoretical than practical and have been rendered obsolete by suppliers who customize stationary phases for specific applications. For an in-depth discussion of this aspect, the reader is referred to several books detailing theoretical aspects of efficiency.[9-12] Resolution of peaks also affects quantitation, as is discussed later in this chapter,

Chromatographic Efficiency

These determinant factors of resolution also are indicative of the efficiency of the chromatographic process. Efficiency is decreased by the broadening of a solute band as it migrates through the stationary phase. If broadening occurs to any significant extent during the chromatographic process, resulting peaks will be wide or resulting spots will be diffuse. The separation of components then is poor, and the sensitivity with which they can be detected is reduced. An example of high- versus low-efficiency separation is illustrated in Fig. 3-5 for both column and flat method separations.

Solute band broadening occurs during the actual chromatographic process and may be described as follows for a column separation. The sample, in a small volume of solvent, is introduced into the mobile phase at a point near the inlet end of the column. Once it has entered the column, the sample begins to disperse through thermal diffusion processes, which continue as it passes through the column. The longer the time

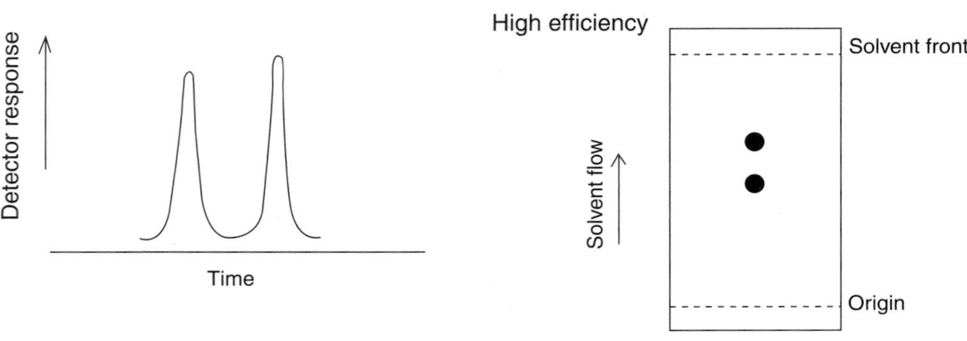

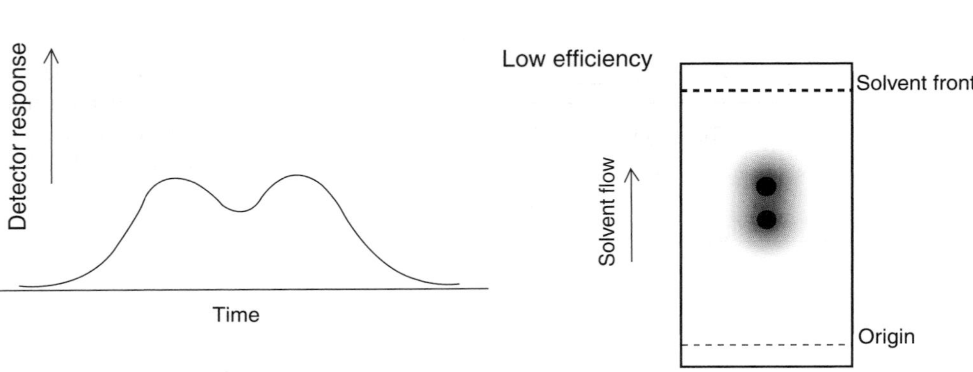

Fig. 3-5 Model chromatograms exemplifying high-efficiency separations and low-efficiency separations.

a solute band spends in a column (i.e., the longer the **retention time**), the greater is the opportunity for thermal diffusion and the greater is the band dispersion. The result is broader but Gaussian (symmetrical) elution peaks for the more retained solutes. Several additional factors contribute to solute band broadening. These include nonuniform regions of the stationary phase, nonuniform particle size distribution, and nonuniform column packing, which may result in nonuniform passage of solute molecules. In this case, some molecules in a solute band spend more time in the separation system than others do, that is, they have a longer path. These processes result in broader, nongaussian dispersion of solute bands, such as asymmetrical eluting peaks or trailing spots.

Retention

Optimal resolution depends on many factors. One of these is the ratio of the volumes of mobile and stationary phases in the column, that is, the **capacity factor,** k, which can be calculated from the chromatogram (Fig. 3-6, *A*) by Equation 3-3.

$$k = \frac{V_e - V_0}{V_0} = \frac{t_R - t_0}{t_0} \qquad \text{Eq. 3-3}$$

Void volume (V_0) is the volume of the mobile phase in the column, and V_e is the elution volume of solute retained by the stationary phase and undergoing chromatography. The HPLC chromatogram for Fig. 3-6, *B,* was obtained by injection of a sample that contained the two solutes retained by the stationary phase. The volumes V_1 and V_2 were measured from the injection point to the apex of the peak of each component. As was indicated previously, the capacity factor can be calculated also through the measurement of time from sample injection to the apex of the peaks of the components (t_R).

Small values of k indicate that the sample components are little retained by the stationary phase and elute close to a substance unretained by the column. Large values of k indicate that the sample components are well retained by the stationary phase, and that long analysis times are required.

The k value for a particular solute is constant for any given chromatography system at constant mobile-phase compositions and stationary-phase size and composition. Within these limits, the capacity factor varies neither with flow rate of the mobile phase nor with column dimensions, that is, length and diameter.

Selectivity

Another parameter on which resolution depends is the **selectivity** factor, α (alpha), a term that describes the ability of a chromatographic system to separate two solutes on the basis of how well they are retained. The selectivity factor is the ratio of the capacity factors for two solutes:

$$\alpha = \frac{k_2}{k_1} \qquad \text{Eq. 3-4}$$

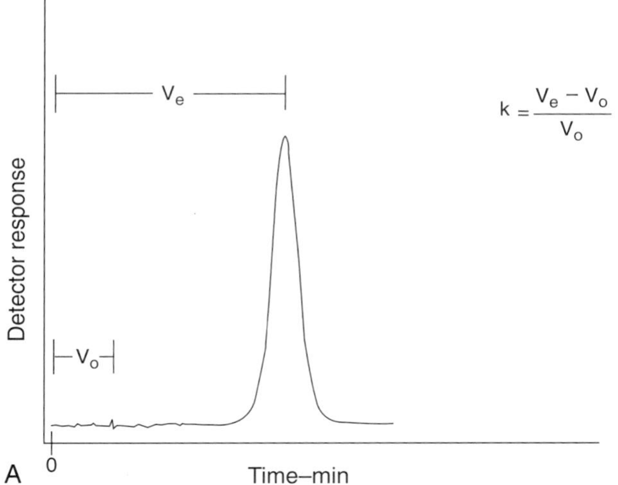

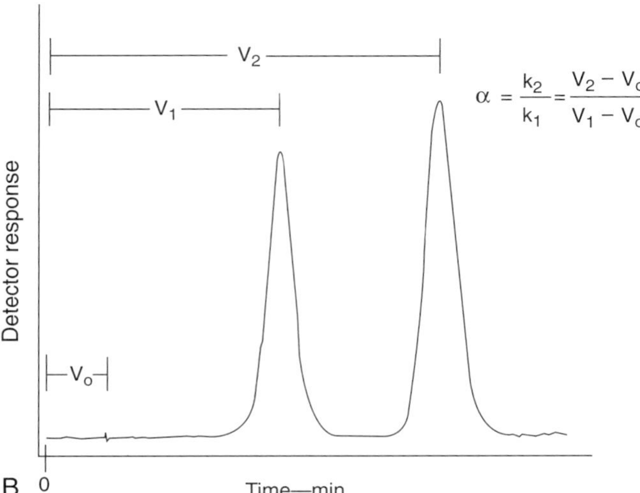

Fig. 3-6 A, Calculation of capacity factor, *k,* from a high-performance liquid chromatogram (HPLC). Sample was retained by stationary phase and underwent chromatography. **B,** Calculation of selectivity factor, α, from HPLC chromatogram. Solutes *A* and *B* were retained by stationary phase and underwent a chromatographic separation as indicated.

The capacity factor for a solute is determined as shown in Fig. 3-6; from this, the resultant selectivity of the system can be calculated, as is shown in Fig. 3-6, *B*. The selectivity of a given chromatographic system is a function of the process of solute exchange between the mobile phase and the stationary phase.[5] Therefore, to affect selectivity, one can change the chemical composition of the mobile phase or the stationary phase to increase the preference of the test solute for one phase or the other. In gas chromatography (GC), changes in stationary-phase chemistry are used for selectivity improvement; for liquid chromatography (LC), changes usually are made in either the stationary or the mobile phase.

Polarity

The concept of **polarity** is central to an understanding of the interaction of molecules in the liquid or gaseous state, as well as the overall chromatographic process. Polarity[13] encompasses both the interaction of solvent molecules with sample molecules and of solvent and sample molecules with the stationary phase. The physicochemical basis for polarity is the interaction of attractive forces that exist between molecules. These four attractive forces are more specifically referred to as ***dispersive***, *dipolar*, *hydrogen-bonding*, and *dielectric interactions*. As is illustrated in Fig. 3-7 and discussed below, all four of these interactions involve the attraction of induced, partial, or formal positive and negative charges.

Dispersion interactions of molecules, sometimes termed *van der Waals forces*, refer to the induced attraction between two molecules. This temporary separation of opposite charges (**dipole**) in one molecule induces the polarization of electrons in an adjacent molecule, thereby causing the two molecules to be attracted to each other by **electrostatic interactions** (see Fig. 3-7, *A*). The formation of temporary dipoles in molecules is the physical basis for existence in the liquid state of many compounds composed of elements with small differences in electronegativity, for example, the elements carbon and hydrogen. Generally, dispersive **polar** interactions are important only when the other forces are not present, or when some elemental constituents of molecules are electron-rich species such as halogens in halohydrocarbons.

Some molecules possess permanent rather than temporary dipoles (see Fig. 3-7, *B*). These compounds have centers of partial positive and negative charge that are the result of an unequal sharing of bonding electrons between two elements with large differences in electronegativity. This overall molecular dipole is enhanced by the presence of elemental nonbonding electron pairs within a compound. Elements such as oxygen, sulfur, halogens, and nitrogen possess nonbonding electrons when covalently linked to other atoms in the same compound. The resulting permanent dipole is directional, with one end of the molecule being partially positive and the other being partially negative.

One special category of dipolar molecules is composed of those with hydrogen covalently linked to an electronegative element such as oxygen, nitrogen, or sulfur. In these molecules, the hydrogen has a large degree of positive character relative to the electronegative atom to which it is bonded. Because of the small size of the hydrogen atom compared with other atoms, this positive end of the dipole can approach close to the negative end of a neighboring dipole. The force of attraction between the two is quite large, about 10 times that of normal dipolar interactions. This special case of dipole-dipole interactions is termed **hydrogen bonding** and is one of the most important types of weak attractive forces. This bonding is illustrated in Fig. 3-7, *C*, for the alcohol methanol.

The fourth type of attractive force is the electrostatic or dielectric interaction. In this case, the solute molecule of the stationary phase is a charged ionic species having either a formal positive or a formal negative charge. A small counter ion, such as H^+ or Cl^-, is present but is generally separated from the charged solute or stationary phase because of solvation by the mobile phase (see Fig. 3-7, *D*), that is, it is

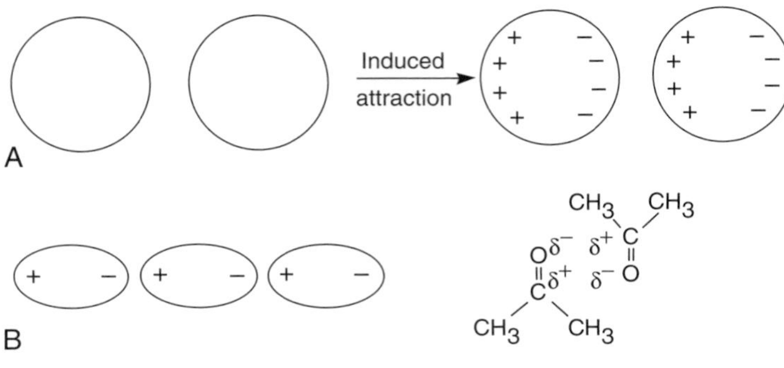

Fig. 3-7 Physicochemical interactions between molecules that constitute concept of polarity. **A,** Dispersive or van der Waals interactions. **B,** Dipole interactions. **C,** Hydrogen bonding. **D,** Electrostatic interactions.

surrounded by solvent molecules. These ionic species increase the dipolar character of the solvent. Dielectric interactions are quite strong and favor the dissolution of ionic or ionizable sample molecules in strongly dipolar solvents such as water or methanol.

The polarity of a solute molecule is the result of the four attractive forces described above and affects its interactions with the mobile and stationary phases. The more polar molecules have this property primarily because of strong dipoles, an ionic character, an ability to form strong hydrogen bonds, or a combination of the three forces. The less polar (**nonpolar**) molecules have dispersive forces as a primary basis of interaction with a very weak ability to interact through dipolar, hydrogen-bonding, or dielectric forces. The practical aspects of these interactive forces and the degree of polarity or nonpolarity form the basis for the mechanisms of chromatography.

Stationary-Phase Polarity

The stationary phase is the fundamental component of the chromatographic separation. The role of the stationary phase depends on its selectivity, which, in turn, is determined by the polarity of the phase. The forces constituting stationary-phase polarity are the same interactions responsible for mobile-phase (solvent) polarity: dispersion, dipole, hydrogen bonding, and dielectric.

The relative strength of polarity of stationary phases is more difficult to ascertain than the relative strength of polarity of liquid mobile phases. In GC, the two major variables determining the separation are the stationary phase itself and the temperature of the column, and study of the affinity of solute molecules of varying polarities has led to a classification system for stationary-phase polarity.

KEY CONCEPTS BOX 3-1

- Differential attraction of compounds to the stationary phase allows chromatographic separation of sample components. The mobile phase serves to conduct the samples past the stationary phase; in liquid chromatography (LC) the mobile phase also serves to affect the attraction of analytes to the stationary phase.
- The capacity factor (k) describes the relative retention of analyte in a chromatographic system, the higher the k, the greater the attraction to the stationary phase and the longer the retention time.
- The degree of chromatographic separation of 2 compounds is described by the "selectivity factor" (α). By changing the chemistry of the mobile and stationary phases in LC and the stationary phase in gas chromatography (GC), one can change the α and improve separation.
- The four attractive forces that explain the interaction of a compound with the stationary and mobile phases are dispersive, dipolar, hydrogen-bonding, and ionic.

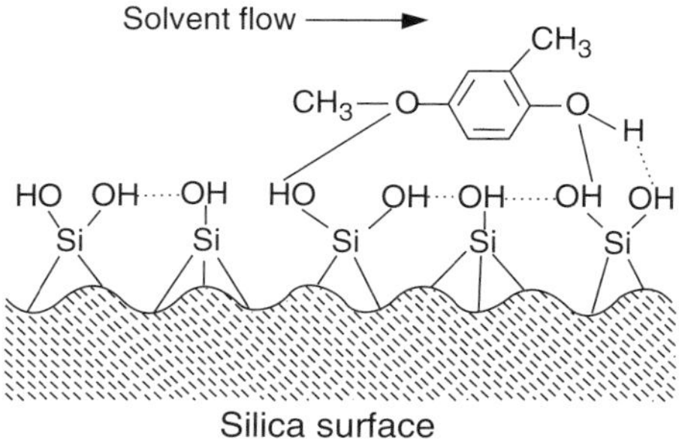

Fig. 3-8 Mechanism of separation of a metabolite of methylanisole by silica gel chromatography. Hydrogen bonds, · · · · · ·; covalent bonds, —.

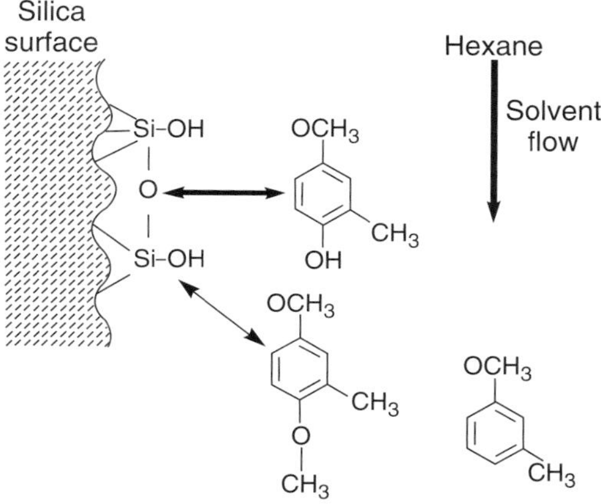

Fig. 3-9 Mechanism of adsorption chromatography by separation of 3-methylanisole and two of its biochemical metabolites. The most polar sample components, such as 3-methyl-4-hydroxyanisole, are retained the most by polar silica gel stationary phase *(heavy arrow)*. Sample components of intermediate polarity, such as 2,5-dimethoxytoluene, are retained to a much lesser degree *(light arrow)*, whereas relatively nonpolar components, such as 3-methylanisole, are not retained and prefer the nonpolar mobile phase, hexane.

SECTION OBJECTIVES BOX 3-2

- Differentiate the principles of adsorption and partition chromatography, including the relative retention times of polar and non-polar compounds.
- State the relative retention times for polar and non-polar compounds in reversed-phase vs. normal phase LLC.
- Explain the principle of ion-exchange chromatography, including interactions of the sample with the stationary phase and the importance of the pH of the mobile phase.
- Explain the principle of gel-permeation chromatography.

MECHANISMS OF CHROMATOGRAPHY

The mechanisms by which a chromatographic method can separate sample components generally are founded on polar interactions and physical interactions based on the size and shape of the solute molecules. The latter interaction is the mechanism for gel-permeation chromatography. The other broad mechanistic classes of chromatography are adsorption, partition, and ion exchange. Each is briefly discussed in the following sections.

Adsorption

The interactions of solute or mobile-phase molecules at the surface of a solid particle form the basis of the adsorption mechanism. There are fundamentally two types of adsorbents: nonpolar and polar. The latter category includes those that are acidic (i.e., with electron-accepting surfaces) and those that are basic (i.e., with electron-donating surfaces).

The principal polar adsorbents used in LC are silica and alumina.[14] Both hydrogen-bonding and dipole interactions between the solute and the surface hydroxyl (silica and acid-washed alumina) or the oxygen anionic (base-washed alumina) groups of the stationary phases constitute the mechanisms of separation (Fig. 3-8). The number and topographic arrangement of these groups, along with the total surface area, determine the activity and strength of the adsorption. Retention of solutes on these phases increases with increasing polarity of the compound class (Fig. 3-9). Retention of a solute molecule requires displacement of adsorbed solvent molecules. Adjustments in mobile phase polarity determine the strength of adsorption of the solute to the stationary phase and the retention characteristics of the system.

Adsorption chromatography offers many advantages for use in LC separations because (1) an extensive separation literature is available based on thin layer chromatography (TLC) methods that are readily transferable to adsorption HPLC; (2) the flexibility, speed, and low cost of TLC allow its use in experimental development; (3) TLC has great value for use in the preliminary investigation of samples of unknown constituents; and (4) adsorption chromatography, particularly with silica gel, has been widely used for the separation of drugs in both the HPLC and TLC modes.

Partition

Partition chromatography is based on the separation of solutes by the use of differences in their distribution between two immiscible phases. In liquid-liquid chromatography (LLC), the phase support is usually coated with a polar substance (**normal phase**), with separations accomplished through the use of an immiscible mobile phase. A normal-phase partition system would consist of silica coated with a monolayer of water or some other polar liquid and a relatively nonpolar mobile phase system. Separations in this system are based on solute polarity, with the least polar compounds eluting first and the most polar substances retained the longest in the polar stationary phase (Fig. 3-10 and Table 3-1). A similar separation system operates in paper chromatography, in which the cellulose is coated with an aqueous monolayer, and immiscible apolar solvents are used as the mobile phase.

A variation in the stationary phase for LLC has the silica support chemically modified to produce a monolayer of a nonpolar organic substituent. These chemically bonded

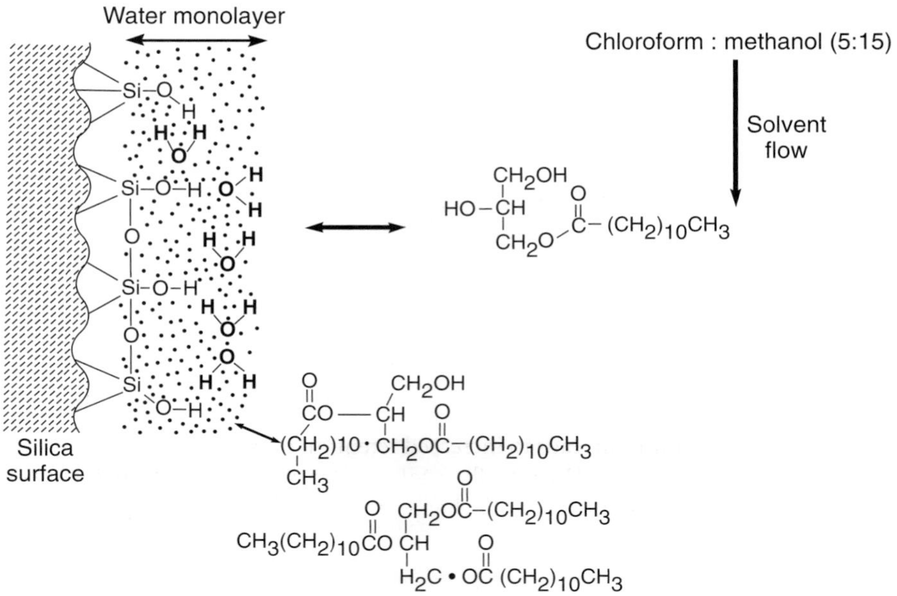

Fig. 3-10 Mechanism of liquid-liquid chromatography as exemplified by separation of the monoglycerides, diglycerides, and triglycerides of lauric acid. Silica gel stationary phase has a monolayer of water strongly held by hydrogen bonding. Solute molecules are partitioned between the liquid mobile phase (chloroform : methanol) and the liquid stationary phase, or water monolayer. The most polar sample components, the monoglycerides, are retained most by the polar stationary phase *(heavy arrow)*. Sample components of intermediate polarity, such as the diglycerides, are retained to a much lesser degree *(light arrow)*, whereas relatively nonpolar components, such as the triglycerides, are not retained and prefer the relatively nonpolar stationary phase.

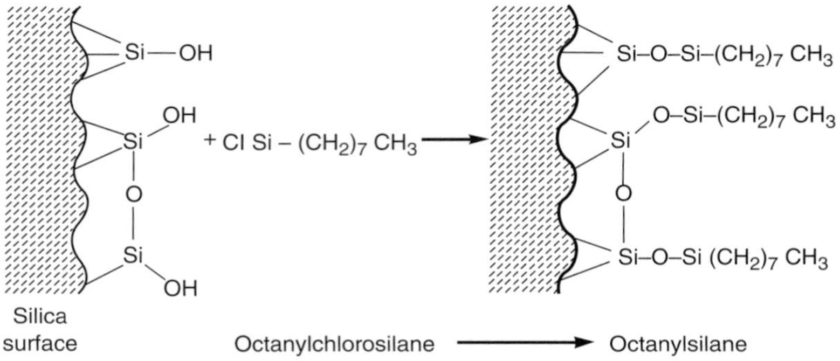

Fig. 3-11 Chemical preparation of bonded, stationary phase (reversed phase). Organochlorosilane reacts with nucleophilic hydroxyl (OH) groups of silica gel, forming siloxane covalent bond (Si—O—Si).

Table 3-1 Selected Groups of Solutes in Order of Increased Retention in Normal-Phase and Reversed-Phase Chromatography

Reversed Phase	Solute Type	Normal Phase
Most retained	Fluorocarbons	Least retained
↓	Saturated hydrocarbons	↓
	Unsaturated hydrocarbons	
	Halides and esters	
	Aldehydes and ketones	
	Alcohol and thiols	
Least retained	Acids and bases	Most retained

stationary-phase supports are available with a variety of functional groups. The most commonly used bonded phases are hydrocarbon phases such as octadecyl or octyl groups bonded to silica (Fig. 3-11). The organic nature of the bonded phases imparts a nonpolar character to the stationary phase. Therefore, the mobile phases commonly used, such as water, methanol, or acetonitrile, are highly polar. Solutes are separated by their relatively nonpolar character (i.e., the most polar eluting first), whereas nonpolar solutes are retained longer. From this type of separation characteristic, the use of bonded phases in LLC is termed *reversed-phase chromatography*. A further discussion and examples of normal-phase and reversed-phase LC are given later in this chapter.

Another example of chromatography in which a partition mechanism operates is gas-liquid chromatography (GLC). The forces of interaction between solute molecules and the liquid-coated stationary phase are the same as in LLC. However, for GC, the mobile phase serves as an inert carrier for the sample constituents, whereas in LLC, the mobile phase is an active, interacting component in the partition mechanism.

Ion Exchange

Ion-exchange chromatography uses stationary phases that possess formal positive or negative charges. The most common retention mechanism is the exchange of sample ions, *A*, and mobile-phase ions, *B*, with the charged groups, *R*, of the stationary phase:

$$A^- + R^+B^- \rightarrow B^- + R^+A^- \quad \textit{Anion exchange} \qquad \text{Eq. 3-5A}$$

$$A^+ + B^+R^- \rightarrow B^+ + A^+R^- \quad \textit{Cation exchange} \qquad \text{Eq. 3-5B}$$

In the first case, anion exchange is occurring, whereas cation exchange is shown for the second; sample ions compete with mobile-phase ions for ionic sites on the stationary phase. The sample ions with the weakest charge that interact less well with the stationary phase will be retained least, whereas those that interact strongly will be retained the most and will be eluted later. The principal force of these interactions is electrostatic, or the attraction of opposite charges.

To effect a separation of sample constituents, the extent of ionization of sample molecules is controlled by variations in pH of the mobile phase. Because the solutes are predominantly weak acids (HA) or weak bases (B), a change in pH will shift the following ionization equilibriums either to the right or to the left:

$$\text{pH}\downarrow \quad \text{pH}\uparrow$$

$$HA \rightleftharpoons H^+ + A^- \qquad \text{Eq. 3-6A}$$

$$BH^+ \rightleftharpoons H^+ + B \qquad \text{Eq. 3-6B}$$

An increase in ionization leads to increased retention of the sample. Factors other than pH controlling solute retention in ion-exchange chromatography are (1) charge strength of the solute ion, (2) ionic strength of the mobile phase, and (3) charge strength of the counterion on the stationary phase. One can decrease the retardation of solutes by increasing the ionic strength of the mobile phase and decreasing the strength of the counterion, such as through the use of Na^+ instead of H^+ for cation-exchange phases, or by adjusting the pH of the mobile phase in a manner that decreases dissociation of either solute, the counterion on the packing, or both.

Gel-Permeation (Molecular or Size Exclusion) Chromatography[15]

Gel-permeation chromatography (GPC) differs from the others because its separation is based on molecular size. The stationary phase for GPC contains pores of a specific average size, and if the sample molecules are too large to enter the pores, they are not retained (excluded) by the stationary phase and are eluted from the column first. Small sample molecules permeate deeply into the pores and are retained the longest. They ultimately diffuse from the pores and are swept away by the flow of the mobile phase. Intermediate-sized sample molecules enter the pores but do not penetrate as deeply into the pores and thus are not retained as well as the small sample molecules. They are eluted from the column in volumes between those used to elute the largest solute (small V_e) and smallest solutes (large V_e). This mechanism is illustrated in Fig. 3-12.

The major advantage of this mode of chromatography is that the GPC method can be used to separate any sample soluble in a mobile phase. Additionally, it is applicable to soluble species that range from 50 to more than 10 million daltons. Stationary-phase choice for GPC is based on the expected molecular weight range of the solute molecules and compatibility with the mobile phase. Lists of the available phases for GPC are tabulated in the manufacturers' literature, in reviews,[3,4] and in books.

The boundaries between different types of chromatography are not finite in that for some chromatographic separations, more than one mechanism may be operating. For example, in gel filtration chromatography, adsorptive interactions between the solute molecules and the stationary phase are common, in addition to the prevailing size exclusion mechanism.

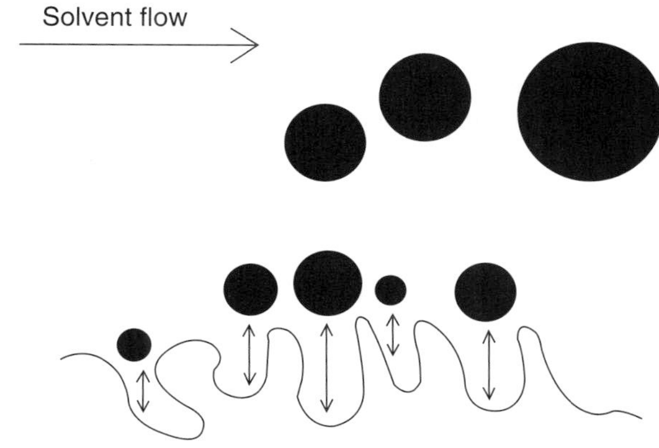

Fig. 3-12 Mechanism of size-exclusion chromatography. Stationary phase, in form of porous beads, contains pores of varying diameter. Mobile phase outside and inside pores is the same, except the liquid inside is immobilized. When a sample containing solutes varying from small to large molecules elutes through the column, small molecules penetrate all pores and are retained, thus being eluted later than large molecules, which move only in mobile phase. Molecules of intermediate size penetrate only some pores, thereby being retained to a lesser degree than small molecules.

KEY CONCEPTS BOX 3-2

- In adsorption chromatography compounds are separated by the tendency to be adsorbed onto the polar stationary phase. More polar compounds are adsorbed more strongly (large retention time) whereas less polar compounds have shorter retention times.
- In normal phase LC compounds are separated by the tendency to be adsorbed onto the polar stationary phase. More polar compounds are absorbed more strongly (large retention time) whereas less polar compounds have shorter retention times. In reversed-phase LC, less polar compounds are retained.
- Ion-exchange LC separates compounds based on their ability to be attracted (retained) by the ionized groups on the stationary phase. By changing the pH of the mobile phase, the ionic character of analytes changes and thus their retention on the stationary phase.
- Compound of differing molecular size can be separated by gel-permeation chromatography; larger compounds have short retention times whereas smaller ones spend more time in the stationary phase and have longer retention times.

SECTION OBJECTIVES BOX 3-3

- Explain four factors that are important in selecting a solvent for analyte isolation extraction methods.

SAMPLE PREPARATION FOR CHROMATOGRAPHY

Nature of Problem

In many cases, chromatographic analyses cannot be conducted on the sample as submitted to the clinical laboratory. The complexity of a biological sample matrix can render the chromatographic separation ineffectual by (1) interaction of sample impurities with the stationary phase, causing a reduction in the resolving power of the system; (2) saturation of most chromatographic detector systems, tending to raise the noise level and thereby decreasing sensitivity; (3) interaction of the component of interest with other matrix components, leading to irreproducibility of the separation from sample to sample; and (4) poorly resolved components that interfere with the analysis. To minimize these sample effects in the chromatographic separation, a strategy for initial separation of the analyte from many interfering components *(sample cleanup)* is required.

Any separation method employed in the laboratory must meet the criteria of yield, separation, capacity, and cost-effectiveness. The advantages of having high yield in any sample manipulation step are obvious, but if recovery is quantitative with little purification, the method is unsatisfactory. The corollary is also true: If the separation from impurities is excellent, but there is a low yield, the method is of little value. Many separation methods are readily applied on a large scale, where large amounts of sample are available, but others are applicable only to small-scale separations. The criterion of cost-effectiveness, which includes time, equipment, reagents, and labor, may render a separation method impractical.

The strategy of sample preparation for chromatographic analysis should include consideration of automation strategies[16,17] and of whether the objective of the analysis is to detect the substance under investigation qualitatively or quantitatively.[18]

Mechanical Methods for Initial Isolation of Analyte

The type of sample matrix received by the analyst in a clinical chemistry laboratory varies from a simple homogeneous-appearing liquid such as perspiration to a complex heterogeneous solid such as feces. The initial step in analyte preparation for chromatography will vary according to matrix. Solid samples, such as tissues or brain, are first disrupted or treated for preparation of a homogeneous solution or suspension from which the analyte can be isolated. Homogenization of tissues in a blender such as a Polytron (Brinkmann Instruments, Inc., Westbury, NY) with an appropriate solvent may solubilize the desired analyte. The use of a Potter-Elvehjem tissue grinder (VWR Supplies, Westchester, PA) is also effective. Tissue can also be extracted in a mortar with a pestle and a small amount of solvent. In addition to these grinding or shearing techniques, solid samples can be disrupted by sonication in solvent or hydrolyzed by acid, base, or enzymes.

Liquid samples may also require an initial treatment for removal of analytes sequestered by matrix components. Whole blood can be diluted with sterile water to disrupt blood cells osmotically before analyte isolation. Another initial treatment applied to blood or urine samples is to remove proteins and other macromolecules through precipitation. Two of the more commonly used protein-precipitating agents are trichloroacetic acid and barium sulfate.

In other mechanical methods of matrix disruption, such as homogenization in a solvent or buffer, centrifugation is commonly employed to remove cell debris, particulate matter, or other large contaminants. An alternative method for the removal of insolubles is filtration through an inert material, such as glass wool or nylon membrane.

Chromatographic Methods for Initial Isolation of Analyte

A common method for the initial isolation of components of interest from aqueous solutions, such as urine or blood, is the use of XAD-2 resin chromatography. This stationary phase of polydivinylbenzene has a large surface area and is of a nonionic character, making it capable of adsorbing many classes of organic compounds from aqueous solution, principally by dispersive and dipole interactions. The adsorbed organics are eluted from the XAD-2 by organic solvents such as methanol, acetone, diethyl ether, hexane, methylene chloride, or combinations of these solvents. The XAD-2 method has been applied most often to urine- or blood-screening methods for drugs of abuse and their metabolites, but it can also be applied to isolate trace amounts of many types of compounds.

Another very common chromatographic technique for initial analyte isolation is the use of small columns of silica, or the octadecylsilyl-bonded phase.[19] The analytes from a relatively large volume of sample are adsorbed from aqueous solution by forces similar to those operating in the XAD-2 procedure. Desorption is accomplished when a small volume of an appropriate solvent is passed through the silica or reversed-phase cartridge; the sample may then be processed for any mode of chromatography. Many additional resins of the type just described are currently available for the isolation of compounds of interest to the clinical chemist.[20]

Other types of chromatographic methods have been used in the preparation of samples for analysis. Ion-exchange chromatography has been widely used to isolate charged analytes. Anion exchange has been widely used for the isolation of acidic constituents from biological fluids. Ion-exchange stationary phases include diethylaminoethyl (DEAE)-Sephadex and the anion exchangers AGIX and Dowex 3.

Extraction Methods for Analyte Isolation

Liquid-liquid and liquid-solid partition methods have been widely used as extraction steps in a wide variety of clinical chemistry analyses before the chromatographic quantitation step. The reasons for the use of these extraction procedures are numerous, including isolation of the analyte from large quantities of contaminating materials and its concentration into a small volume of solvent, which makes detection easier. Liquid-liquid extraction procedures are easily accomplished, usually permitting the workup of multiple samples simultaneously.

The success of an extraction step depends on knowledge of the polarity of the analyte. This information is used to select an extracting solvent that will effectively remove the analyte from the sample. A general rule of solvent selection is that compounds tend to favor solvents that have the same polarity interaction forces. It is critical that the chosen solvent be immiscible with the sample matrix.

Other points must be considered in solvent selection. The solvent must be chemically compatible with the analyte, that is, no chemical reaction should be possible between the two. The solvent must be compatible with all subsequent operations after the extraction. For example, a solvent with a high boiling point would be difficult to remove, and so the analyte solution would be difficult to concentrate by evaporation. The solvent should not introduce any contaminants that would make the analysis difficult. Many laboratory supply companies offer common solvents of high purity grades, such as (1) *HPLC-grade solvents,* which are compatible with most detector systems and do not contain particulate matter that would foul the HPLC equipment; (2) *pesticide-grade solvents,* which are compatible with electron-capture GC detectors because they do not introduce any contaminating substances; and (3) *lipograde-grade solvents,* which do not contain any greases or other substances that would interfere with the analysis of lipids. The most common extraction contaminant is plasticizers, which usually come from cap liners and other plastic materials.[21] These contaminants, various alkyl phthalates, can interfere with some chromatographic analyses. Most such contamination problems can be eliminated by using screw-cap liners made of Teflon.

In general, a repeated series of extractions with smaller volumes of solvent will be more efficient than a single extraction with a large volume. For solid samples, the solvent may be introduced during the mechanical disruption step, as was previously mentioned. The cycle of grinding, sonication, and so on is repeated several times with several volumes of solvent. However, doing this sometimes does not effectively extract the desired analyte. In this case, the pulverized solid sample may have to be extracted with a Soxhlet extractor or a continuous infusion extractor. Both of these methods are more efficient than manual operations for extracting substances from a solid matrix. However, the requirements for these methods include a reasonably volatile extracting solvent and stability of the analyte at the boiling point of the solvent.

Samples undergoing chromatographic separations often need to be dissolved in a nonaqueous solution. The pH of the sample solution is then adjusted to below the **pK_a** of acidic components or above the pK_a of basic components with the addition of acid or base, respectively, to convert the analyte, 95% or greater, into its extractable (nonionized) form. A monograph relating pK_a values of acids to percent ionization at various pH values has been published by Hopgood.[22] If the pK_a of the analyte is not known, a lowering of the pH of the aqueous solution to a pH of 2.0 by the addition of acid is usually sufficient to permit the extraction of most acidic analytes. Likewise, raising the pH to 12 is usually sufficient to permit the extraction of most basic analytes of unknown pK_a.

For liquid-liquid extraction, an increase in the ionic strength of the aqueous layer will enhance the ease of extraction of the analyte, causing it to favor the extracting solvent. An ionic neutral salt, such as sodium chloride or potassium bromide, is commonly used for this purpose.

One of the problems frequently encountered in liquid-liquid extractions is the formation of emulsions, that is, one of the immiscible phases becomes dispersed as fine droplets in the other. To avoid emulsion formation, several precautions can be taken during the actual extraction process: (1) If the two liquid layers have a large contact surface, avoid vigorous mixing of the phases. The use of gentle agitation will accomplish the extraction. (2) Filter all finely divided particulate matter before extraction. (3) Use solvent pairs with large differences in density.

Processing of Sample Extracts

Many analyte extracts are too dilute for direct chromatographic analysis or for derivatization reactions before gas chromatography and usually are concentrated by evaporation of the extracting solvent.

Any solvent evaporation procedure must be conducted with care to avoid loss of the analyte. Such a loss of analyte can occur if traces of water are present in the extract. These can be removed by use of an anhydrous salt, such as sodium carbonate or sodium sulfate. Alternative desiccating salts, such as calcium oxide or magnesium sulfate, can also be used. Other purposes for drying an extract may be to subsequently conduct a derivatization procedure, such as acetylation or silylization, or to prevent interference with the chromatography step.

The analyte may also be lost by irreversible binding to the walls of the concentration vessel during concentration. This can be avoided by prior silylization of the glassware. Some substances are sufficiently volatile to form azeotrope mixtures with the solvent and be lost during evaporation. To avoid this, many gentle concentration methods or apparatuses are available. If the analyte is heat or oxygen sensitive, evaporation of the solvent under a stream of purified inert gas, such as nitrogen or argon, can be employed. In this case, warm the vessel to a range of 35° C to 50° C to expedite the evaporation process. The use of a rotary evaporator under reduced pressure is another gentle method for solvent evaporation. Such variations emphasize the importance of method validation and the key role that quality assurance samples, such as samples spiked with analyte, play in the use of a specific approach to cleanup.

Another method for concentrating the analyte is back-extraction of the compound of interest from the solvent. For example, Kossa and associates[23] have published a variety of methods whereby the analyte in the original extracting solvent is back-extracted into a small volume of analyte-derivatizing solvent before gas chromatography. Methods of this type expedite the analysis in that solvent evaporation steps are not required. Other examples of analyte cleanup procedures for preparing samples for chromatography are detailed in a review by Moldoveanu and David.[19]

These general principles of chromatography will be applied to both liquid and gas chromatographic systems in the next chapter.

KEY CONCEPTS BOX 3-3

- The ability to affect separation and detect the analytes may be adversely affected by other material in the sample.
- Thus most specimens must be extracted and partially purified prior to chromatography.

REFERENCES

1. Cazes J: *Encyclopedia of Chromatography,* 2nd ed, New York, Taylor & Francis, 2005.
2. Eiceman GA, Clement RE, Hill HH Jr: Gas chromatography, Anal Chem 64:170R, 1992.
3. Dorsey JG et al: Liquid chromatography: Theory and methodology, Anal Chem 64:353R, 1992.
4. Sherma J: Planar chromatography, Anal Chem 64:134R, 1992.
5. Miller JM: *Chromatography: Concepts and Contrast,* 2nd ed, New York, 2005, Wiley & Sons.
6. Wong HY: *Therapeutic Drug Monitoring and Toxicology,* Chromatographic Science Series, vol 32, New York, 1985, Marcel Dekker.
7. Rial-Otero R et al: Chromatographic-based methods for pesticide determination in honey: An overview, Talanta 71:503, 2007.
8. Baczek T: Improvement of peptides identification in proteomics with the use of new analytical and bioinformatic strategies, Current Pharmaceutical Analysis 1:31, 2005.
9. Meyer VR: *Practical High-Performance Liquid Chromatography,* 3rd ed, New York, 1998, Wiley & Sons.
10. Katz E et al, editors: *Handbook of HPLC,* New York, 1998, Marcel Dekker.
11. Wilson ID, editor: *Encyclopedia of Separation Science*, San Diego, 2000, Academic Press.
12. Scott RPW: *Liquid Chromatography Column Theory,* New York, 1992, Wiley & Sons.
13. Forgács E, Cserháti T: *Molecular Basis of Chromatographic Separation*, Boca Raton, FL, 1997, CRC Press.
14. Sadek PC: *Troubleshooting HPLC Systems*, New York, 2000, Wiley & Sons.
15. Hunt BJ, Holding SR, editors: *Size Exclusion Chromatography,* New York, 1989, Chapman & Hall.
16. Wells DA: *High Throughput Bioanalytical Sample Preparation—Methods and Automation Strategies, Progress in Pharmaceutical and Biomedical Analysis,* 5th ed, Amsterdam, 2003, Elsevier, pp 505-573.
17. Zhou S, Song Q, Tang Y, Naidong W: Critical review of development, validation, and transfer for high throughput bioanalytical LC/MS/MS methods, Current Pharmaceutical Analysis 1:3, 2005.
18. Scott RPW: *Chromatographic Detectors: Design, Function, and Operation*, New York, 1996, Marcel Dekker.
19. Moldoveanu SC, David K: *Sample Preparation in Chromatography*, 1st ed, Amsterdam, 2002, Elsevier Science.
20. Dietz C, Sanz J, Camara C.: Recent developments in solid-phase microextraction coatings and related techniques, J Chromatogr 1103:183-192, 2006.
21. DeZeeuw RA, Jonkman JHG, van Mansvelt FJW: Plasticizers as contaminants in high purity solvents: A potential source of interference in biological analysis, Anal Biochem 67:339, 1995.
22. Hopgood MF: Nomogram for calculating percentage ionization of acids and bases, J Chromatogr 47:45, 1970.
23. Kossa WC, MacGee J, Ramachandran S, Webber AJ: Pyrolytic methylation/gas chromatography: A short review, J Chromatog Sci 15:177, 1979.

BIBLIOGRAPHY

Books

American Society of Testing Materials: *ASTM Standards on Chromatography,* 2nd ed, ASTM Subcommittee E19.07 on Compilation of Chromatographic Methods, Philadelphia, 1989, ASTM.

Cazes J: *Encyclopedia of Chromatography* (Den New Dekker Encyclopedias), New York, 2001, Marcel Dekker.

Fried B, Sherma J: *Practical Thin-Layer Chromatography: A Multidisciplinary Approach*, New York, 1996, CRC Press.

Fritz JS, Gjerdec DT: *Ion Chromatography*, 3rd ed, New York, 2000, John Wiley & Sons.

Grob RL: *Modern Practice of Gas Chromatography,* 2nd ed, New York, 1985, Wiley & Sons.

Heftman E: *Chromatography: Fundamentals and Applications of Chromatography and Related Differential Migration Methods,* 5th ed, Journal of Chromatography Library, vol 51 A and B, New York, 1992, Elsevier Science.

Hermanson GT, Mallia AK, Smith PK: *Immobilized Affinity Ligand Techniques*, New York, 1997, Academic Press.

McNair HM, Miller JM: *Basic Gas Chromatography* (techniques in analytical chemistry), New York, 1991, John Wiley & Sons.

Papadoyannis IN: *HPLC in Clinical Chemistry,* Chromatographic Science Series, vol 54, New York, 1990, Marcel Dekker.

Sherma J, Fried B, editors: *Thin Layer Chromatography,* Chromatographic Science Series, vol 55, New York, 1990, Marcel Dekker.

Snyder LR, Glajch JL, Kirkland JJ: *Practical HPLC Method Development,* New York, 1988, Wiley & Sons.

Weston A, Brown PR: *HPLC and CE: Principles and Practice*, New York, 1997, Academic Press.

Comprehensive Abstracts, Journals, and Series in Chromatography

Advances in Chromatography, New York, Marcel Dekker, Inc.

Analytical Abstracts, London, Royal Society of Chemistry.

Chemical Abstracts, Columbus, Ohio, American Chemical Society.

Chromatographia, New York, Pergamon Press.

Chromatographic Reviews, Amsterdam, Elsevier Scientific Publishing Co.

Chromatographic Science Series, New York, Marcel Dekker, Inc.

Chromatography Symposium Series, New York, Elsevier Scientific Publishing Co.

Gas and Liquid Chromatography Abstracts, Barking, Essex, Applied Science Publishers.

Gas Chromatography Abstracts, London, Butterworth & Co.

Journal of Chromatography, New York, Elsevier Scientific Publishing Co.

Journal of Chromatography Library, New York, Elsevier Scientific Publishing Co.

Journal of Chromatographic Science, Niles, IL, Preston Publications.

Journal of High Resolution Chromatography and Chromatography Communications, Heidelberg, NY, Muthing Press.

Journal of Liquid Chromatography, New York, Marcel Dekker, Inc.

Progress in Thin-Layer Chromatography and Related Methods, Ann Arbor, MI, Lewis Publishers.

INTERNET SITES

www.chromatographyonline.com

www.spectroscopynow.com

www.fda.gov/cder/guidance/cmc3.pdf—Center for Drug Evaluation and Research (need Adobe Acrobat)

www.separationsnow.com

www.asms.org—American Society for Mass Spectrometry

www.sisweb.com/mslinks.htm

www.agilent.com/chem

www.bmss.org.uk/education.htm

www.ionsource.com

Chapter 4

Chromatographic Techniques

Michael Lehrer

Chapter Outline

Key Terms

active sites Sites on the stationary phase that reversibly bind the compound to be separated.

atmospheric pressure ionization (API) Ionization technique occurring near room atmospheric pressure that allows large molecules and other nonvolatile compounds to be analyzed by mass spectrometry.

base peak The most intense peak in the mass spectrum.

bonded phase A chromatographic packing material in which the stationary phase is covalently bound to the surface of the support.

capillary column An open tubular column with an inside diameter of 0.20 to 0.35 mm.

chemical ionization (CI) Low-energy ionization technique based on charge-transfer collision with an inert reagent gas.

daughter ions The ionic output of the second mass spectroscopy (MS) analyzer of an MS/MS system.

Deans switch A microfluidic valve that directs mobile-phase gas flow from one GC column to another.

derivative A molecule chemically altered from the original one.

effluent Mobile phase that has left the column.

electron ionization (EI) High-energy electron bombardment that transforms molecules into fragment ions.

electron-capture detector (ECD) A GC detector that uses beta particles to detect electronegative components such as halogens.

eluate A compound or mixture that has been separated in the column and has left it.

fingerprint The unique fragmentation pattern of organic compounds.

flame ionization detector (FID) A detector with a flame fueled by hydrogen that burns eluted components and converts them to ions that can be measured electrically.

Fourier-transform infrared spectrometer (FTIR) A specialized GC detector that measures infrared spectral lines of compounds as they elute from the GC column.

fragmentation pattern A display of the intensity of ion fragments formed versus mass-to-charge ratio.

full scan A mass spectrometric scanning sequence in which all ions in the entire mass range of interest are detected.

gas chromatography A physical technique that separates components based on their distribution between a gas and a stationary phase.

gas-liquid chromatography A separation technique that uses a liquid stationary phase.

gas-solid chromatography A separation technique that uses a solid stationary phase.

GC/MS Gas chromatograph interfaced with a mass spectrometer.

gradient elution An elution system where the mobile-phase composition is varied

ion trap detector (ITD) Mass spectrometer that operates on the principle of ion accumulation over time.

ionization potential The amount of energy required to displace an electron from the outer shell of a compound.

ionization source Area within the mass spectrometer where molecules are ionized by an electron beam.

IonSpray A variation of thermospray technique used to introduce liquid chromatograph eluent into the ion source of the mass spectrometer at ambient temperature.

isocratic elution Elution with a solvent mixture of constant composition.
isotope dilution Quantitation of chemicals different only in their isotope composition.
LC/MS Liquid chromatograph (LC) interfaced with a mass spectrometer (MS).
liquid phase Nonvolatile fluid that coats the support medium in the separation column.
magnetic sector Mass spectrometer that separates ion fragments based on their passage through a magnetic field.
mass filter The electronic or magnetic device that separates ions based on their mass-to-charge ratio.
mass fragmentation The breakdown of a large unstable molecular ion, usually in a defined pattern unique to the test molecule.
mass spectrometer A device to separate ions based on their mass-to-charge ratio.
mass spectrum (MS) The output of a mass spectrometer that displays mass-to-charge (m/z) ratios versus intensity of the ion fragment.
mass-to-charge (m/z) Ratio of the mass of an ion fragment divided by its ionic charge.
mobile phase Mixture of solvents that is percolated through the LC column.
molecular ion (M^+) The initial ion fragment that corresponds to the molecular weight of the compound.
negative-ion chemical ionization (NICI) Chemical ionization technique that focuses on the generation of negatively charged ions.
nitrogen-phosphorus detector (NPD) A GC detector especially sensitive to nitrogen- or phosphorus-containing compounds.
open tubular column A gas chromatographic column in which the stationary phase coats the inside walls of the column.
packed column A gas chromatographic column in which the stationary-phase support consists of particulate material that fills the column.
parent ion The ionic output of the first mass spectrometer analyzer of an MS/MS system.
quadrupole Mass spectrometer that separates ion fragments based on their passage through an electronic field.
retention time (t_R) Time that has elapsed from the injection of the sample into the chromatograph until it elutes into the detector.
reversed phase Chromatographic mode in which the mobile phase is more polar than the stationary phase
selected ion monitoring (SIM) Selective scanning of a few preselected ion fragments by the detector.
selected ion profile Selective scanning and area integration in the SIM mode of a significant ion fragment.
silanization The chemical process of converting the SiOH moiety of a stationary phase to the ester form.
soft ionization A low-energy ionization technique such as chemical ionization.
solids probe A probe used to introduce crystalline material directly into the mass spectrometer.
sorbent A material that has the property of interacting with the compound of interest, usually to make it bind.
stationary phase The portion of the separation system that is immobilized in the column.
SAMHSA (Substance Abuse and Mental Health Services Administration) The agency within the U.S. Department of Health and Human Services (DHHS) that works to improve substance abuse prevention and addiction treatment programs and associated mental health services and regulates NLCP laboratories
tandem mass spectrometry (MS/MS) The coupling of two or more mass analyzers.
thermal-conductivity detector A device that measures the difference between the heat conductivities of the carrier gas and those of the sample gas effluents.
thermospray A technique used to introduce liquid chromatography eluent into the ion source of the mass spectrometer.
time-of-flight (TOF) mass spectrometer A spectrometer that separates ion fragments based on their transit time through a given path.
total ion current (TIC) Chromatographic integration and display of ion currents in GC/MS applications.
triple-stage quadrupole (TSQ) Instrumental configuration of a quadrupole MS/MS.
two D-GC/MS An instrument that couples two GC columns to a MS detector (GC/GC/MS).
V_R (retention volume) The volume of the mobile phase required to elute a compound from a chromatographic column.
wide-bore column An open tubular column with an inside diameter of 0.50 to 0.75 mm.

SECTION OBJECTIVES BOX 4-1

- Discuss the role and utility of liquid chromatography (LC).
- Discuss quantitation and the role of internal standards.
- Discuss the selection of LC separation mode using various techniques, including size-exclusion, ion-exchange, absorption, partition, reverse-phase, ion-pair, and affinity and enantiomer chromatography.
- Discuss the utility of different types of LC support material.
- Discuss LC instrumental components, including solvent/sample introduction systems, columns/connectors, and detectors.

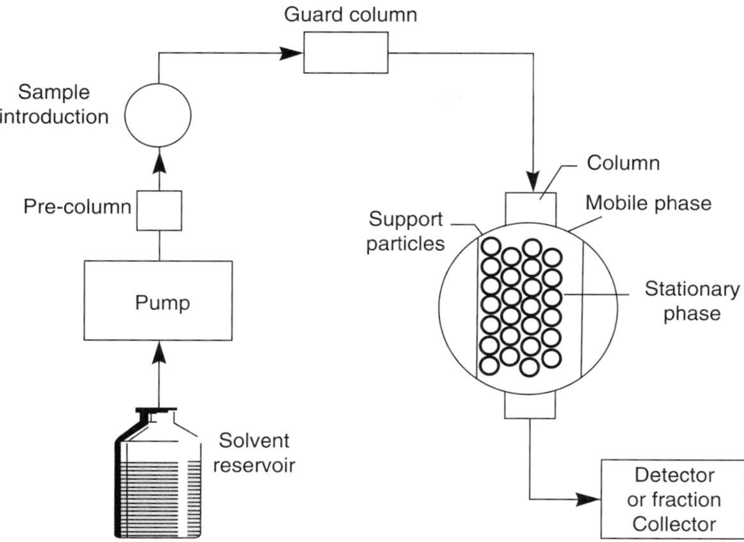

Fig. 4-1 Schematic diagram of a column liquid chromatographic system. (From Bowers LD, Carr PW: *Quantitative Aspects of HPLC Workshop,* Minneapolis, 1983.)

LIQUID CHROMATOGRAPHY

Fig. 4-1 shows a schematic diagram of a column chromatograph used in liquid chromatography (LC). The liquid **mobile phase** is taken from the reservoir and is moved through the column, usually by a pump. A method of introducing the sample into the chromatographic system is also required. The column is filled with packing material, which consists of small particles on which specific sites or a layer of solvent (both referred to as **stationary phase**) is held. Finally, the column **effluent** can be collected for further analysis or can be analyzed with an on-line detector, such as a photometer. The recording of any parameter that allows the analyte or analytes to be monitored as a function of elution volume or time is called a *chromatogram.*

Liquid chromatography is well suited for use in the clinical laboratory because most clinical samples contain relatively polar compounds that readily dissolve in commonly used mobile-phase solvents. This is in contrast to gas chromatography, which requires volatile analytes.

With the development of small (≤10 μm), totally porous particles in the early 1970s, liquid chromatography was able to achieve speed and resolution comparable with those of packed-column gas chromatography (GC). The introduction of covalently bonded stationary phases resulted in the further utilization of high-performance liquid chromatography (HPLC). Good books on HPLC at the beginning[1] and at more advanced[2] levels have been published. A comprehensive encyclopedia on the theory, techniques, and applications has also been published[3]; a glossary of 500 terms, abbreviations, and equations is available.[4]

Quantitation

Approaches

Quantitation in liquid chromatography is achieved when either the peak height or the peak area is related to the concentration of analyte in the sample. The chromatographic trace is a recording of the concentration of the analyte or analytes as sensed by the detector. (Fig. 3-6 is an example.) The greater the peak height for any given concentration, the more sensitive is the method. Thus minimizing the retention volume and maximizing the peak height results in the greatest assay sensitivity. Factors that decrease the retention volume include a small column void volume and a small retention factor. Low flow rates and small support-particle diameters lead to higher efficiencies and thus greater peak heights.

The second approach to quantitation of an analyte is measurement of the peak area. Most liquid chromatography detectors are concentration dependent; that is, they measure a concentration within the flow cell. This is in contrast to most GC detectors, which are mass flow dependent. The peak area obtained from a concentration-dependent detector is inversely proportional to flow rate, that is, the slower the flow rate, the greater is the integrated signal area. As a consequence, significant variation in peak area can occur if the flow rate changes during a chromatographic run. In addition, less resolution is required for an equal degree of accuracy when peak heights rather than peak areas are used because the overlap of peaks affects peak area but does not affect peak maximum.[5] A rough rule of thumb is as follows: Use peak *height* when there are interfering peaks or when maximum accuracy is required, but use peak area when precision is the main requirement. For peaks barely above the baseline noise, peak heights should always be used because it is difficult to accurately estimate the beginning and end points of the analyte.

Standardization

Standardization in liquid chromatography can be accomplished in any of three ways: external standardization, internal standardization, or standard addition. For external standardization, a calibration curve is constructed from the peak height (or peak area) values obtained with known concentrations of analyte and a constant injection volume. The slope of the curve is the sensitivity factor, *S*, in peak-height units per concentration unit (such as millimeters of chart height per millimole of analyte, mm/mM). The concentration of the unknown is then simply its peak height divided by the sensitivity factor. If the calibration curve is linear, the sensitivity factor can be obtained from a single standard. However, it is recommended in this case to check several control specimens to verify the validity of the sensitivity factor. The principal sources of error in external calibration are variable losses in the preparative steps before LC analysis and sample injection variability. It is thus important to treat the standards and samples in the same way. It should be possible to achieve 1% precision with external calibration, but up to 5% is commonly observed.

Internal standardization uses a compound that is usually structurally similar to the analyte to correct for losses during sample preparation, injection imprecision, and detector variation. The same amount of internal standard is added to each sample and standard before sample pretreatment and chromatography are performed. The calibration curve then is constructed from the ratio of the peak heights (or areas) of the standard and the internal standard at various standard concentrations (Fig. 4-2). It is assumed that any losses or variations that occur will affect the analyte and internal standard equivalently, allowing unknown concentrations to be measured by using the sensitivity factor or interpolating the value from the calibration curve. An internal standard can be used not only to improve accuracy and precision but also as a quality control check because peak height should be the same in all chromatograms. Several requirements must be met in the selection of an internal standard. These are summarized in Box 4-1. In some cases, internal standards do not improve precision and accuracy and may reduce precision because of the imprecision involved in measuring two peaks. When the detector is a mass spectrograph, the internal standard is usually the deuterated form of the test analyte.

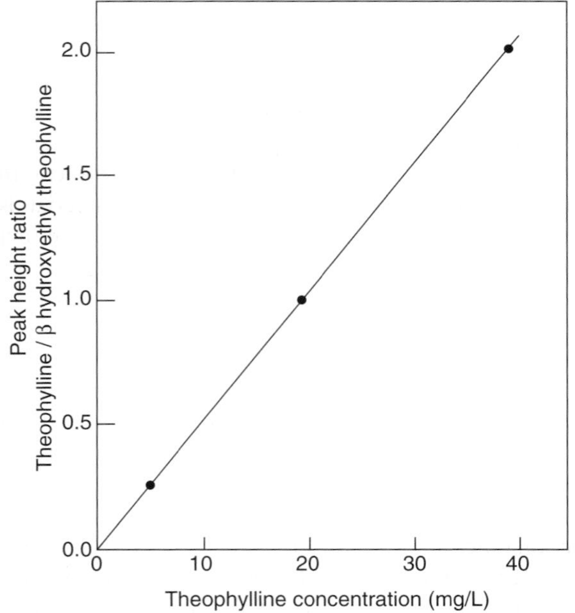

Fig. 4-2 Calibration curve for theophylline using internal standard technique.

Selection of a Chromatographic Mode

Use of a mobile phase with a constant composition is referred to as **isocratic elution.** The alternative to this is to change the mobile-phase composition during the chromatographic run. This can be done as a single change from one mobile phase to another (step gradient) or as a continuous change in any of a variety of shapes (such as linear, segmented linear, or exponential gradient), usually automated through the solvent delivery system. Complete treatment of **gradient elution** is described elsewhere.[6] In brief, the peak retention volume, width, and resolution are determined primarily by the rate of solvent composition change. Thus, many of the parameters such as selectivity and capacity are affected by gradient elution. Quantitative analyses developed with the use of gradient elution require pumps and controllers that can accurately reproduce the gradient. When gradient elution is used, the column requires equilibration with the original mobile-phase conditions before the next run. This adds to the total run time, particularly with **reversed-phase** analysis, which has made isocratic techniques preferred in the clinical laboratory.

The various mechanisms of chromatography, including ion exchange, gel permeation, size exclusion, absorption, and partition, were previously discussed (see pp. 74–77, Chapter 3). These modes are available in liquid chromatography; the selection of the best mode is a significant decision for the chromatographer. A brief description about selection of a chromatographic mode is presented.

Size-Exclusion Chromatography

One of the first considerations is the size of the molecules to be separated. If the molecules are relatively large (>100,000 daltons [D]), *size* (or *steric*) exclusion (SEC) is a logical first choice. If, on the other hand, the molecular weights are less than 1000 D, size exclusion is probably not the mode of choice.

Box 4-1

Requirements for Internal Standard (IS) Selection and Use

1. The internal standard must be completely resolved from all peaks in the sample.
2. It must be eluted near the analyte, with $k \pm 30\%$ being preferable.
3. It must behave similarly to the analyte in pretreatment if losses are to be corrected. This may require more than one internal standard.
4. It must have a peak height or area approximately equal to a standard in the concentration range desired.
5. It must not normally be present in the sample.
6. It should be commercially available in pure form.
7. It should be added as a liquid.

Ion-Exchange Chromatography

A second consideration is whether or not the analyte is an ion and whether an ionizable group is present on the molecule. In this case, ion exchange is a logical choice for molecules that can be charged. Ion exchange is based on the interaction of analyte charges with an oppositely charged group bound to the chromatographic support. Retention can be varied by varying pH or ionic strength. The greater the number of charges on the analyte, the greater is the retention. Increasing mobile phase ionic strength, combined with an increase in the number of charged groups (such as Na^+) competing with the analyte for exchange sites on the support, reduces retention. *Ion-pair* chromatography, which uses reversed-phase packing materials, can be used to separate ionic compounds. An updated review of biological compounds determined by ion-exchange chromatography has been published.[7]

Adsorption Chromatography

If the molecule has a molecular weight less than 1000 D and is not ionizable, the third consideration is whether the compound has the ability to form hydrogen bonds. Adsorption chromatography is based on the interaction of the analyte with a three-dimensional binding site on the support matrix, which may involve hydrogen bonding. Thus the structure and polarity of the solute are important in determining retention. For example, it is relatively easy to separate *p*-dinitrobenzene from *o*-dinitrobenzene using adsorption chromatography because of structural differences between the two compounds. On the other hand, separating caproic acid (with six carbon atoms) from caprylic acid (with eight carbon atoms) is very difficult because the parts of the molecules that interact with the stationary phase are identical.

In adsorption chromatography, compounds are eluted from the column because of competition between the analyte and the solvent for the binding site. A solvent that elutes compounds more rapidly and therefore competes better for the chromatographic sites is called a *strong solvent*. Water is a strong solvent for silica adsorbents because it interacts strongly with the silanol (SiOH) groups responsible for the adsorption mechanism. A solvent that does not compete well for sites is called a *weak solvent*. Hexane is a weak solvent for silica adsorbents. Solvent strength can be adjusted by using mixtures of solvents. A solvent strength scale called the *eluotropic series* has been developed to extended solvent strength theory to binary and ternary[8] mixtures. It is interesting to note that solvent mixtures of the same strength can show differences in selectivity because Snyder's theory considers only the adsorption process, whereas in reality the solute can also interact with the solvent.

Partition and Bonded-Phase Chromatography

A fourth consideration is partition chromatography. The interactions between solute and the stationary phase in partition chromatography are not nearly so well defined as those for adsorption systems. Any chemical forces that exist between molecules, including hydrogen bonding, van der Waals forces, ion-ion interactions, and so on, can be used in partition-based separations. The basis of partition systems is the distribution of a solute between two liquid solvent layers—one stationary and the other mobile. It is essentially analogous to thousands of liquid extractions taking place in a column. In classical partition chromatography, a polar liquid, such as β, β′-oxydipropionitrile (β, β′-ODPN), was coated onto the support particles, and an immiscible solvent such as hexane was used as the mobile phase. Because solvent-solute interactions involve the entire molecule, a typical partition system as given here would separate a homologous series (C6, C7, and C8 carboxylic acids) from some positional isomers. A partition system with a polar stationary phase and a nonpolar mobile phase is called *normal phase* because it was the first type of system developed. Later, a system with a nonpolar stationary phase, such as squalane, and a polar mobile phase, such as a water-acetonitrile mixture, was developed and called **reversed phase.** The development of chemically bonded stationary phases eliminated most of the instability problems of earlier systems. These materials are prepared by covalent bonding of an organic moiety onto the surface of the support particle, usually silica. The organic groups include nonpolar functions, such as octadecylsilane (ODS, or C18) or octylsilane (C8), and polar groups, such as cyanopropyl (CN), aminopropyl (NH_2), or glycidoxypropyl (diol) silanes. The advantages of **bonded phases** are that (1) polar and ionic compounds are readily separated, (2) the stationary phase does not strip off, (3) a gradient elution can be used, and (4) the columns are easy to use and take care of. The main disadvantage of bonded phases is that at pH values below 2, the bonded group is cleaved from the support, and at pH values above 8, the silica support particles dissolve, although packing materials with supports other than silica have been developed that can be used at up to pH 12 to 14 (see later discussion). Because most separations for clinical laboratory applications can be performed within this workable pH window, bonded phases are very popular. A separate section has been included to discuss the variety of separations feasible with reversed-phase systems.

Reversed-Phase Chromatography[9]

In a survey of HPLC users, approximately 70% of the HPLC separations were performed on reversed-phase columns.[10] The most popular reversed-phase packing material is the ODS, or C18, packing material. The mobile phase in reversed phase is most commonly water that contains an organic modifier such as methanol, acetonitrile, or tetrahydrofuran. In general, retention of an analyte on the reversed-phase column depends on the relative amounts of polar and nonpolar character of the analyte, as shown in Fig. 4-3 for the amino acid tyrosine. Retention on the reversed-phase packing material is favored by increased nonpolar content of the analyte, whereas residence in the mobile phase leading to early elution from the column is favored by increased content of polar functionalities present on the analyte. The organic modifier component of the mobile phase competes with the stationary phase for the nonpolar part of the analyte molecule; thus retention is decreased with an increased organic modifier in the mobile phase.

The actual description of the retention mechanism is more complex.[11] Although a partition mechanism has been proposed by some (in which solute is fully encompassed by the stationary phase), an adsorption mechanism (in which the solute is retained on the stationary phase through surface contact only), or a combination of both, has also been proposed.

It is normally necessary to remove proteins from plasma and serum samples before reversed-phase and normal-phase chromatography because the organic composition of the mobile phases used in these modes causes the denaturation and precipitation of proteins. These absorb onto the packing material, leading to pressure buildup, decreased column efficiency, and decreased column capacity.

Stationary-Phase Considerations

As was noted earlier, the separation obtained for any group of analytes is a function of both the stationary phase and the mobile phase. The analyst has the ability to vary mobile-phase conditions but is dependent on manufacturers for the stationary phase, particularly for bonded-phase packing. If chromatography is to be reproducible, the behavior of the stationary phase toward nonpolar, polar, and ionic compounds must be the same from column to column and from lot to lot. In addition, the durability of columns is important because of their expense.

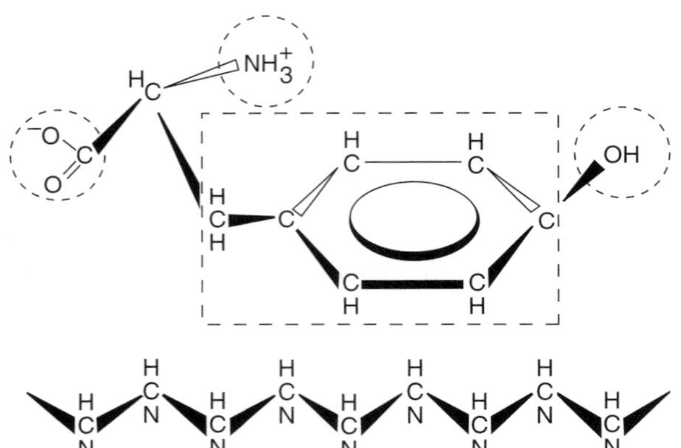

Fig. 4-3 Retention in reversed-phase chromatography is the result of the interaction of the nonpolar portion of the compound such as tyrosine *(enclosed in box)* with the nonpolar stationary phase. Hydrophilic groups *(circled)* tend to decrease retention.

The preparation of an ODS or C18 stationary phase is usually accomplished when the silanol (SiOH) groups on the silica gel are reacted with an ODS such as octadecyldimethylchlorosilane. The resulting surface contains octadecyl groups bound to the surface by siloxone (Si-O-Si) bonds, as shown in Fig. 4-4. Most manufacturers of columns use silanes with only one chloride group, and the resulting stationary phase is called *monomeric.* Because of the stereochemistry of the silica gel surface, only about one third of the silanol groups can react with the ODS groups. The remaining silanol groups are polar and can interact with polar analytes, changing the selectivity of the stationary phase. Trimethylchlorosilane can react with about an additional 20% of the surface silanol groups with a resultant increase in the nonpolar character of the support (see Fig. 4-4). This process is called *end capping* and is used in many commercially available packing materials. As might be expected, differences in the surface morphology of the silica gel, reaction conditions in the ODS-bonding step, and the presence or absence of end capping make columns purchased from different manufacturers perform differently. In fact, variations from lot to lot of packing material may be quite noticeable in the separations obtained for certain analyses. Thus it is not surprising that in adapting a method to a laboratory, significant changes in the mobile phase may be required if a C18 column from a manufacturer other than that named in the original report is used. Choice of a reversed-phase column still requires trial and error.

The most utilized reversed-phase functionalities are C18 and C8 (straight-chain hydrocarbons of 18 and 8 carbons, respectively). Functionalities from C1 to C30 are available. Other available functionalities include fluorinated alkyl phases, amide-alkyl phases, and polar embedded phases. Polar embedded phases consist of alkyl-bonded phases (usually C18, C8), and either contains a polar functionality within the alkyl chain or uses a hydrophilic end-capping reagent; they display stable retention in highly aqueous mobile phases that have little or no organic modifier present and are useful for basic compounds.

Fig. 4-4 Schematic diagram of a silica-based octadecyl reversed-phase support that has been end capped. Notice presence of residual silanol groups on surface.

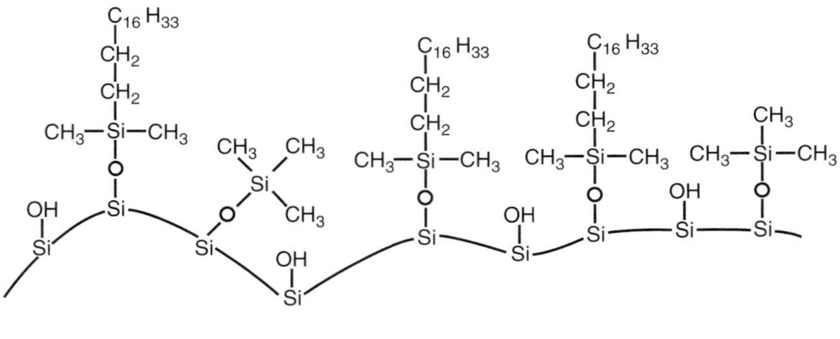

Mobile-Phase Considerations

The separation power in liquid chromatography arises from the fact that changes in mobile-phase composition can have major effects on selectivity and thus on resolution. In reversed-phase systems, two types of changes can be made: (1) changes in the type of organic solvent used and (2) additions to the mobile phase that affect its pH, ionic strength, or complexing ability.

Solvent Strength. The type of organic solvent used effects both retention and selectivity. In some cases, a change from methanol to acetonitrile actually alters the elution order of the compounds. The use of solvents to vary selectivity is largely empirical, and the exact role of each solvent in a separation is poorly defined. However, the relative strength of solvents is well defined with solvent strength; therefore, the ability to elute solutes increases in the following order: methanol < dimethyl sulfoxide (DMSO) < ethanol ≤ acetonitrile < tetrahydrofuran < dioxane < isopropanol. As a rule, when the retention of a solute is adjusted, a 10% increase in the fraction of organic solvent (such as methanol or acetonitrile) in water causes a twofold or threefold decrease in the *k* value.

Ion Suppression. Mobile-phase modifications that change retention by introducing a second chemical equilibrium process in the mobile phase have been used since the inception of reversed-phase chromatography. The first approach was control of pH to effect retention. If, for example, ascorbic acid was to be separated by HPLC, there would be a strong influence of pH on retention. At pH values above the pK_a of ascorbic acid, the acid would be deprotonated and charged and therefore would not partition itself strongly into the nonpolar stationary phase. Retention would be relatively low. On the other hand, at pH values below the pK_a, the acid would be protonated and uncharged and so would be much more strongly retained. In the area about one pH unit on either side of the pK_a, the retention changes rapidly as a function of pH, as is shown in Fig. 4-5. The use of pH control to increase retention for acids has been termed *ion suppression.* It is a very useful method of adjusting retention behavior. Buffers are normally used to control the pH. It is important to remember that an acid-base pair is a good buffer only within one pH unit of the pK_a. Table 4-1 lists some useful buffers for reversed-phase HPLC.

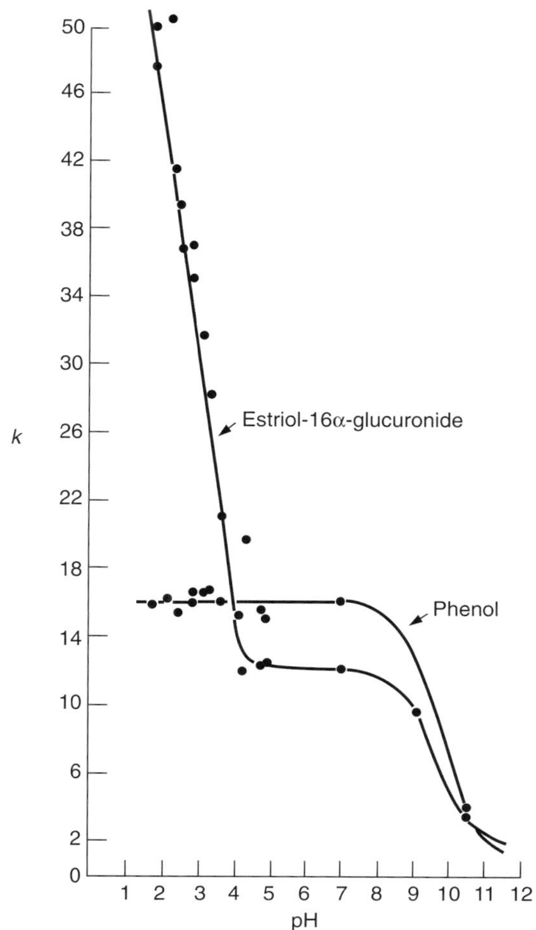

Fig. 4-5 Change in *k* as a function of pH for estriol-16α-glucuronide and phenol. Decrease in *k* at pH 2 is attributable to ionization of glucuronic acid; decrease at pH 10 is attributable to ionization of phenolic group. (From Oliphant C, Bowers LD, unpublished data.)

Table 4-1 Useful Buffers for Reversed-Phase HPLC

Buffer Pair	pK_a
Phosphoric acid/dihydrogen phosphate	2.12
Chloracetic acid/chloracetate	2.87
Succinic acid/monohydrogen succinate	4.23
Acetic acid/acetate	4.77
Piperazine phosphate	5.33
Monohydrogen succinate/succinate	5.65
Tetramethylethylenediamine phosphate	6.13
Dihydrogen phosphate/monohydrogen phosphate	7.20
Tris(hydroxymethyl)aminomethane	8.19

Chromatography of Basic Compounds on Conventional Reversed-Phase Packing Material

Basic compounds can be chromatographed on conventional reversed-phase packing materials by making modifications in the mobile phase. The biggest difficulty in chromatographing basic compounds on silica reversed-phase packing materials is the presence of silanol groups on the silica surface. As was mentioned previously, approximately 50% of the silanol groups remain on the silica support after synthesis of the reversed-phase packing material. A small percentage of these remaining silanol groups are strongly reactive, leading to adverse chromatographic effects, including severe tailing and irreversible adsorption of basic compounds and variable retention for different reversed-phase columns. At the mobile-phase pH values normally used in reversed-phase analysis (neutral pH), a basic analyte is positively charged. The highly reactive silanol groups on the silica surface, which are acidic and thus negatively charged, interact with the positively charged basic compound through an ion-exchange mechanism. Addition of amine modifiers (such as triethylamine) to the mobile phase prevents adverse chromatographic effects of silanol on basic analytes through a mechanism by which the positively charged amine modifier binds to the silanol ion-exchange sites on the reversed-phase packing material, thus blocking the silanol sites from interaction with the basic analyte. Low pH and high ionic strength mobile phases, which drive the equilibrium of the silanol groups to the protonated or counterion-associated form (which does not interact with positively charged basic compounds), are additional strategies used in conventional reversed-phase chromatography of basic compounds. In addition to the silanol ion-exchange mechanism mentioned above, silanol hydrogen bonding and metal impurities present within the silica have been implicated in the adverse chromatography effects seen for silica supports.

Ion-Pair Chromatography

The most popular method for chromatographing ionizable analytes (such as weak bases or weak acids) and ionic analytes on a reversed-phase column is ion-pair chromatography.[9] Use of ion suppression that employs silica-based, reversed-phase packing material is limited by the range of pH stability of the silica support (which is stable from pH 2 to 8). Thus the requirement of a low-pH mobile phase for the ion-suppression chromatography of weak acids limits the column lifetime, whereas ion suppression of weak bases is not possible on silica-based, reversed-phase materials because the pH requirement is too high. The advantage of ion-pair chromatography over ion-exchange chromatography is that it can separate both ionic and nonionic compounds simultaneously.

In ion-pair chromatography, a hydrophobic ionic species *(counterion)* that has the opposite charge to the analyte is added to the mobile phase, which is pumped through a reversed-phase column. The complex of the counterion and ionic analyte is called an *ion pair.* Several retention mechanisms have been proposed for ion-pair chromatography. One mechanism depicts the role of the counterion as a neutralizing agent that combines with the analyte ion in the mobile phase to form a neutral species that is retained on the reversed-phase column. The other model depicts the role of the counterion in terms of a modifier of the stationary phase, with the adsorption of the counterion on the reversed-phase packing material, thus changing the packing material into an ion exchanger that retains the ionic analyte.

Optimization of the separation in ion-pair chromatography is achieved through the manipulation of several mobile-phase variables, including type and concentration of ion-pair reagent, pH, type and concentration of organic modifier, ionic strength, and temperature.

Affinity Chromatography[12-14]

Affinity chromatography is a powerful tool in the analysis of biochemicals. In affinity chromatography, the principle of specifically interacting biochemical pairs is employed. Examples of biochemical pairs used in affinity chromatography are given in Table 4-2. In affinity chromatography, one of the components of the pair (termed the *affinity ligand*) is immobilized onto a support and packed into a column, making it a very specific chromatographic technique for the complementary component of the pair.

Table 4-2 Biochemical Pairs Used in Affinity Chromatography

Affinity Ligand	Complementary Component
Inhibitors, cofactors, substrate analogs	Enzymes
Immunoglobulins	Antigens, haptens
Receptors	Hormones
Nucleic acid components	Complementary nucleic acid components, polynucleotide-binding proteins
Lectins	Carbohydrates, glycoproteins
m-Aminophenylboronic acid	*cis*-diol–containing compounds (carbohydrates, nucleic acid components, catecholamines, glycoproteins)
Protein A, protein G	Immunoglobulin G
Heparin	Coagulation proteins
Dye molecules	Various proteins and enzymes
Metal chelators	Proteins, peptides, nucleic acid components

There are three stages to the affinity chromatographic separation process. The first stage is the injection of the sample into the aqueous *application buffer* (usually pH 7) pumped through the column, with all species passing through the column as nonretained, except for the complementary analyte, which is retained by the column. After all nonretained components pass through the column, the second stage of the chromatographic process is initiated, and the mobile phase is switched to an aqueous *elution buffer,* which causes disruption of the binding forces between the analyte and the affinity ligand, leading to elution of the analyte from the column. There are two categories of elution buffers, biospecific and general. Biospecific elution buffers contain a species that specifically interacts with the affinity ligand or analyte to affect elution. Biospecific elution thus adds a second step of specificity to the chromatographic process because there is specificity not only in retention, but also in elution of the analyte. Examples of biospecific elution include addition of sugars to the mobile phase in affinity chromatography using lectin supports and enzyme inhibitors to the mobile phase in the affinity chromatography of enzymes. General elution buffers affect elution by nonspecific means, through disruption of the electrostatic, hydrogen bonds, van der Waals, and hydrophobic forces that bind the analyte to the stationary phase. Strategies for general elution include changing mobile-phase pH or ionic strength, adding organic modifiers to the mobile phase, and using denaturing conditions in the mobile phase (5 to 8 M urea or 6 M guanidine). The disadvantage of general elution schemes is that species that nonspecifically adsorb to the support may elute with the analyte. The third stage of the affinity chromatographic process is re-equilibration of the column with application buffer before injection of the next sample.

The development of high-performance silica supports in which the surface was modified by the covalent attachment of a hydrophilic layer and of hydrophilic high-performance polymeric affinity chromatography have made these techniques applicable to the clinical laboratory. *High-performance affinity chromatography (HPAC)* is done by incorporation of high-performance packing material with covalently attached affinity ligands. A review on the determination of various clinically relevant analytes by HPAC has been published.[14]

An example is affinity chromatography in which *m*-aminophenylboronic acid columns are commonly used in the determination of glycated hemoglobins. The affinity ligand *m*-aminophenylboronic acid is a general ligand that binds compounds that contain a *cis*-diol functional group, which is present in the carbohydrate portion of many glycoproteins. In the determination of glycated hemoglobins, hemolysate of red blood cells is injected onto an *m*-aminophenylboronic acid column, which retains the glycated hemoglobin, allowing nonglycated hemoglobins to pass through the column. Changing the mobile phase to one containing the sugar alcohol sorbitol elutes the glycated hemoglobin, while the eluate is monitored at 415 nm. See Chapter 5 for additional discussion of this technique.

Affinity chromatography has limitless flexibility through the use of antibodies as affinity ligands; this subclassification of affinity chromatography is referred to as *immunoaffinity chromatography.*

Chromatography of Enantiomers[15]

Separation of enantiomers (chiral compounds) has its greatest application in the determination of pharmaceuticals because approximately 50% of the most frequently used drugs exist as enantiomer pairs. A compound that has one chiral center (which is most commonly a carbon atom that has four different groups bonded) exists in two isomeric forms that differ from one another in terms of spatial arrangement of the atoms around the chiral center. Each of the enantiomer pairs has identical physical properties (making separation difficult) but differs in reactivity toward chiral reagents and in reactivity in biological systems. The activity, metabolism, and sometimes the toxicity of a drug depend on the enantiomeric form; thus the separation of drug enantiomers is critical in pharmaceutical analysis. HPLC is the method of choice for the determination of enantiomers.

Enantiomers can be determined by HPLC in three general ways: chromatography on conventional columns after derivatization with a chiral reagent, chromatography on conventional columns with the use of mobile phases that contain chiral complexing reagents, and chromatography on columns that contain a *chiral stationary phase.*

Derivatization of the enantiomer analyte with a chiral reagent leads to the formation of a diastereomer. One diastereomer isomer is formed when a particular enantiomer reacts with the derivatizing agent, whereas a different diastereomer isomer is formed when the other enantiomer reacts. Diastereomer isomers have different physical properties, which facilitate their separation on conventional HPLC columns. In a similar manner, the presence of chiral reagents in the mobile phase leads to the formation of a different diastereomer isomer complex for each component of a particular enantiomer pair. Conventional HPLC columns can readily separate these diastereomer isomer complexes.

Specialized packing material containing a chiral compound as a stationary phase separates enantiomers as a result of differential spatial interaction of each enantiomer with chiral support. Determination of enantiomers with the use of chiral stationary-phase columns is advantageous compared with the derivatization or mobile-phase complexation methods because these previously described methods require reagents that have a high degree of optical purity. Chiral stationary phases include both biological and synthetic stationary phases. Biological stationary phases include covalent attachment to support of the following: (1) derivatized biological polymers such as polysaccharides, proteins, and peptides; (2) modified small biological molecules such as amino acids and alkaloids; and (3) macrocyclic antibiotics. In addition, there are native biological-like polymer supports such as cellulose triacetate and cellulose tribenzoate. Synthetic stationary phases include brush-type (Pirkle) phases, poly(meth)acrylates, polysiloxanes and polysiloxane copolymers, and imprinted polymers. In addition, chiral ligand exchange is used, which consists of a ligand with a bound transition metal immobilized onto a support. Many different types of chiral stationary phases are commercially available, the suitability of which for a particular enantiomer separation must largely be determined empirically. Thus no one universal chiral stationary phase is applicable to all enantiomer separations; the choice of column is dependent on the enantiomer compound determined.

Different Types of HPLC Packing Materials

Useful references that provide information on HPLC packing materials have been published.[16,17] Tables 4-3 through 4-5 provide general information and list commercially available packing material for the different HPLC modes. Advances in packing materials have occurred along three lines: (1) development of packing materials that are designed to alleviate the problems of silica supports; (2) development of packing materials, known as restricted access media, that allow direct chromatography of serum (or plasma); and (3) development of higher-efficiency supports for macromolecules. In Table 4-5, adsorption and polar-bonded packing materials are grouped together under normal-phase chromatography, which is consistent with a classification made by others, because both are polar packing materials.

Different Supports Addressing Problems of Silica Supports

Problems associated with the use of silica supports include a limited pH range ($2 < pH < 8$), poor performance in the reversed-phase chromatography of basic compounds, and problems with reproducibility. An ideal support material

Table 4-3 Reversed-Phase HPLC: General Information and Packing Materials

Mode	Reversed Phase
General Information	
Compounds determined	Low- and medium-polarity compounds
Comments	Most widely used chromatographic mode in clinical analysis
	Mobile-phase ion suppression or ion pairing is required for ionic or ionizable compounds
Commercially Available Packing Materials	
Bonded phase	*n*-Octadecyl (C18), *n*-octyl (C8) (Most widely used reversed-phase functionalities)
	n-Butyl (C4) (Preferred functionality for protein separations; however, less stable in acidic mobile phases [such as TFA] than C8, C18)
	Phenyl (Preferred functionality for compounds containing an aromatic group or groups)
	Cyano [—$(CH_2)_3CN$] (Used for retention of more polar compounds)
	C30 (See text)
	Fluorinated alkyl (See text)
	Polar embedded (See text)
	Others: Mixed phases such as C18/phenyl, amide/alkyl, and C18/ion exchange functionalities
	Other chain lengths (C1-C30)
	(These functional groups can be attached to the following supports: silica, polybutadiene modified/PM/alumina, PS-DVB, PVA, PM, hybrid organic-inorganic, octadecylphenyl modified carbon-coated zirconia)
Polymer covered	Silica modified with alkyl polysiloxanes, multifunctional alkyl silanes, alkyl PVA
	Alumina modified with polybutadiene (with or without attached alkyl groups)
	Polystyrene-coated zirconia or titanium dioxide
	Polybutadiene-coated or carbon-coated zirconia
Base support (native)	PS-DVB
	PAM
	Porous graphite
	Poly (divinylbenzene-methacrylate)
High speed	
Nonporous	PS-DVB (native), PM and silica (reversed-phase functionalities)
Perfusion	PS-DVB (native) (Applied Biosystems)
Monolithic	Silica (C18 functionality) (Merck Eurolab, Kyoto Jushi-Seiko)
Poroshell	Silica (solid core with porous outer shell, C18 functionality) (Agilent Technologies)
Styros	PS-DVB (native) (OraChrom)
Restricted access media	Internal surface reversed phase (ISRP) (Regis Technologies)
	(Glycine-L-phenylalanine-L-phenylalanine [GFF] on silica)
	Semipermeable surface (SPS) (Regis Technologies)
	(C8, C18, cyano and phenyl within polyoxyethylene bonded to silica)
	Shielded hydrophobic phase (SHP) (Supelco) (phenyl groups embedded in a hydrophilic network of poly[ethylene]oxide bonded to silica)
	Mixed functionalities
	• Capcell Pak MF (Phenomenex)
	• C1/C8/phenyl on polymer-coated silica
	• Diol-C8 silica (Merck KGaA)

PS-DVB, Poly(styrenemethyl-divinylbenzene); *PAM,* poly(alkylmethacrylate); *PM,* polymethacrylate; *PVA,* poly(vinyl alcohol); *TFA,* trifluoroacetic acid.

would have the high performance and pressure capabilities of silica supports but would be able to withstand a larger pH range, would be inert, and would have reproducible retention characteristics. Supports that are better than silica supports in some aspects but inferior to silica in other aspects have been developed.[18]

High-Performance Polymeric Supports[19]

Polymeric supports can be classified as either hydrophobic or hydrophilic. Poly(styrene-divinylbenzene) (PS-DVB), poly(alkyl methacrylate) (PAM), and polymethacrylate (PM), which includes poly(hydroxylalkyl methacrylate or acrylate), are the predominant hydrophobic polymeric supports used. The predominant hydrophilic polymeric supports that are commercially available are poly(vinyl alcohol) (PVA) and cross-linked agarose. The uses of these supports are given in Tables 4-3 through 4-5.

Ligands are covalently attached to these supports to produce reversed-phase, ion-exchange, and normal-phase packing materials. No modification of the polymer support is required for size-exclusion chromatography. It should be noted that PS-DVB reversed-phase packing materials are most often used without modification of the surface. These native PS-DVB

Table 4-4 Ion-Exchange HPLC: General Information and Packing Materials

Mode	ION EXCHANGE* Anion	Cation
General Information		
Compounds determined	Negatively charged compounds, acidic compounds, protein with pI <8	Positively charged compounds, basic compounds, proteins with pI >6
Comments	The charge of the stationary phase will vary with mobile phase pH (near pK_a of support functionality) for weak ion exchangers but not for strong ion exchangers	
Commercially Available Packing Material		
Bonded phase	*Weak* Primary, secondary, tertiary amines (—NH_2, —NHR, —NR_2) (Weak base functionalities with pK_a = 5-9; most utilized is DEAE [O—CH_2—CH_2—N—$(C_2H_5)_2$]) *Strong* Quaternary amine [—NR_3^+] (Strong base functionality with pK_a >13) (Note that various functional groups given above can be attached to silica, PS-DVB, PM, PVA, porous graphite)	*Weak* Carboxylic acid [—COO^-] (Weak acid functionalities with pK_a = 4-6; most utilized is carboxymethyl (CM) [CH_2—COO^-]) *Strong* Sulfonic acid [—SO_3^-] (Strong acid functionalities with pK_a <1) *Intermediate* Sulfoalkyl [—$(CH_2)_n$—SO_3^-] (Most utilized is SE and SP [pK_a for SP = 2.3]) (Note that functional groups given above can be attached to silica, PS-DVB, and PM)
Polymer covered	*Weak* Polyethyleneimine (PEI)-coated supports (silica, PS-DVB, and zirconia) *Strong* Latex with quaternary amine functionality coated onto poly(ethylvinyl-divinylbenzene) or PS-DVB supports	*Weak* Latex with carboxylic acid functionally coated onto poly(ethylvinyl-divinylbenzene) or PS-DVB supports Polybutadiene-maleic acid copolymer on silica *Strong* Polymer-coated silica with sufonic acid functionality
Base support (native)	None	None
High speed		
Nonporous	PM (PEI, DEAE, and NR_3^+ functionalities) Poly (dimethylaminopropylmethacrylamide) (dimethylaminopropyl functionality) Silica (various functionalities)	PM (carboxyl and SP functionalities) Silica (various functionalities)
Perfusion	PS-DVB with polyethyleneimine (weak), quaternized polyethyleneimine (strong) (Applied Biosystems)	PS-DVB with polyhydroxylated polymer [CM (weak) and SE and SP (strong) functionalities] (Applied Biosystems)
Monolithic	Polymer [such as poly(glycidylmethacrylate) co-ethyleneglycoldimethylacrylate (BIA Separations)] (DEAE, ethylenediamine, quaternary amine functionalities) (BIA Separations, Bio Rad)	Polymer [such as poly(glycidylmethacrylate)-co-ethyleneglycoldimethylacrylate (BIA Separations)] (sulfonyl and CM functionalities) (BIA Separations, Bio Rad)
Styros	PS-DVB (quaternary aminomethyl, polyamine, DEAE functionalities) (OraChrom)	PS-DVB (SP and SE functionalities) (OraChrom)
Others		Phosphonic acid and phosphonic acid derivative of EDTA adsorbed to zirconia

PS-DVB, Poly(styrene-divinylbenzene); *PM,* polymethacrylate; *PVA,* poly(vinyl alcohol); *PEI,* polyethyleneimine; *DEAE,* diethylaminoethyl; *SE,* sulfoethyl; *SP,* sulfopropyl.
*Mixed anion-cation packing exchange materials also exist, such as sulfonyl-quaternary amine on ethylvinyl benzene cross-linked with DVB.

packing materials, however, have selectivities different from those of conventional alkyl-bonded reversed-phase packing materials. PS-DVB supports require hydrophilic surface modification if they are to be used in modes other than reversed-phase modes. Polymeric supports have two advantages over silica supports. The first is an extended pH range. This allows reversed-phase determination of a basic compound without the need to add ion-pairing reagents. High-pH mobile phases can be used with polymeric supports, allowing basic compounds to be chromatographed as neutral species

Table 4-5 Normal-Phase and Size-Exclusion HPLC: General Information and Packing Materials

Mode	Normal Phase	Size Exclusion
General Information		
Compounds determined	Hydrophilic compounds (such as saccharides; complements reversed phase, which dose not retain hydrophilic compounds) Isomers (such as steroids) Class separation	Compounds >1000 daltons
Comments	(Low-performance normal-phase cleanup of sample is often done before HPLC or immunoassay procedure) Bonded normal phases compared to native silica and alumina: • Sharper peaks, no tailing • Less strength of retention • Faster mobile-phase equilibration, making gradient chromatography possible	Hydrophilic SEC (all packing materials listed below except PS-DVB) is used in clinical analysis
Commercially Available Packing Material		
Bonded phase	Diol [—$(CH_2)_3OCH_2CH(OH)CH_2(OH)$] Cyano [—$(CH_2)_3CN$] (also referred to as nitrile) Amino [—$(CH_2)_nNH_2$] (where $n = 3$ or 5) Fluorinated aromatic Dinitro-aromatic Polarity: amino > cyano > diol Almost all bonded phase supports are silica based, with a few exceptions such as aminopropyl on PS-DVB	Diol on silica [—$(CH_2)_3OCH_2CH(OH)CH_2(OH)$]
Polymer covered	Polyamine on PVA	Polyether and PVA on silica
Base support (native)	Silica Alumina Porous graphite Zirconia Titania (mixed adsorption/ion exchange properties)	PM, PVA, cross-linked agarose, PS-DVB
Monolithic	Silica (Kyoto Jushi-Seiko)	

PS-DVB, Poly(styrene-divinylbenzene); *PM,* polymethacrylate; *PVA,* poly(vinyl alcohol); *SEC,* size exclusion.

and thus retained on the reversed-phase column. The second advantage of polymeric supports is that they do not have reactive functional groups such as silanols on the surface and thus do not show adverse peak tailing and recovery effects when basic analytes are chromatographed.

The major disadvantage of polymeric supports is that they are less efficient than silica supports. PS-DVB supports also require at least 10% to 20% organic content in the mobile phase to prevent shrinkage of the support material. In comparison, hydrophilic polymeric supports are less susceptible to shrinkage and swelling effects when the concentration of the organic modifier is changed; these supports are thus compatible with completely aqueous mobile phases.

Other High-Performance Packing Materials

Other packing materials have been developed (in addition to polymeric packing materials) that address the problems associated with silica supports. Deactivated reversed-phase silica packing materials have been developed by various manufacturers and do not require the presence of amine modifiers in the mobile phase so that chromatography of basic compounds can be performed. One or more of the following strategies may be used to further deactivate the silica: excessive end capping, attaching a dense surface coverage of alkyl ligand, covering the silica surface with a polymer layer, employing proprietary treatments to modify the reactivity and distribution of the silanols on the surface, attaching novel ligands, and electrostatically shielding the silica surface.

High-Speed Analysis

Short columns design is one strategy used to speed up chromatographic analysis. Columns ≤5 cm have been used to decrease analysis time. Packing materials of decreased size (≤3 μm diameter) must be used for these short columns to achieve the same resolution as longer columns. Limitations of this strategy are that flow rates cannot be increased with porous packing materials because increased band spreading results from the longer distances that the molecules have to diffuse in the pores. In addition, there is a requirement for increased pressure in columns packed with smaller packing material (pressure increases by an exponential factor of a decrease in particle diameter). Finally, columns packed with small-diameter packing material have reduced application lives because of the high pressures and problems associated with plugging.

Instrumentation

As was mentioned previously, modern HPLC requires relatively sophisticated instrumentation to achieve difficult separations in less than 10 minutes. The separation system itself has four basic components: (1) a solvent delivery system to provide the driving force for the mobile phase, (2) a sample introduction system, (3) the column, and (4) the detector (see Fig. 4-1). In addition, a recorder or integrator, often used with computer data acquisition, is used to display or calculate the results. A useful and comprehensive discussion of proper operation, maintenance, and troubleshooting for all components of an HPLC system have been published.[20] Although the principles of instrumentation remain unchanged, new generations of LC and GC instruments in tandem with MS are introduced every 4 to 5 years, with higher sensitivities, better resolution, greater robustness, and more automation.[21,22]

Solvent Delivery Systems

The most common delivery system is based on the reciprocating piston pump. These systems minimize solvent delivery pulses, that is, stoppage of flow and compression of the solvent that occurred when the pump head refill. Pump pulsations are a source of detector noise.

Gradient elution can be attained when the solvents are mixed after they pass through the HPLC pumps. The gradient can be produced by continual adjustment of the flow rate of the multiple HPLC pumps, each pumping one solvent, to adjust the composition of the mobile phase (called *high-pressure mixing*). Alternatively, the solvents are mixed before they enter a single HPLC pump, with the gradient produced by a continual adjustment of the times that a proportioning valve allows a particular solvent to be pumped by the HPLC pump from one of several solvent reservoirs (called *low-pressure mixing*). High-pressure mixing gradient systems are considered the best according to current performance standards. Low-pressure mixing gradient systems are disadvantageous because of the high dead volume before the column; this is especially disadvantageous for microbore and capillary HPLC techniques because it leads to long delay times for the gradient to reach the column. In addition, low-pressure mixing has a greater susceptibility to outgassing of dissolved gases, which can occur with the mixing of different solvents (not thoroughly degassed) at low pressures before the column.

Sample Introduction Systems

The most widely used method of introducing a sample into the chromatographic system is the fixed-loop (fixed volume) injection valve. A sample aliquot is loaded into an external loop of stainless steel tubing. The valve is then rotated so that the sample loop is flushed onto the column by the mobile phase from the pump. Returning the valve to the original position allows loading of the next sample. Fixed-loop valves can be used in two ways: partial-fill method and full-loop method. In the latter, the entire loop (such as 20 μL) is filled with sample and injected. This is the most precise method. It should be recognized, however, that accurate results require flushing of the loop with 5 to 10 loop volumes of mobile phase before loading. In the partial-fill mode, the sample loop is not filled with sample. In this case, the loading syringe determines the precision of the injection volume.

In addition to the manual valve injector described above, many automatic sampling devices are available. These autosamplers allow unattended operation of the HPLC system, making 24 hr/day use possible. They are usually quite reliable and precise because of mechanical advances and computerization.

Columns and Connectors

The column is of course the most important part of the separation system. The packing material for columns has been discussed at length. In addition to the analytical (or preparative) column, which actually performs the separation, two types of protector columns might be used. A *guard column* (see Fig. 4-1) is located between the injector and the analytical column and is $^1/_{15}$ to $^1/_{25}$ the volume of the latter. It is packed with a material similar to that of the analytical column. Its function is to collect any particulate matter or any strongly retained components of the sample and therefore to protect the expensive analytical column. A *precolumn* is positioned between the pump and the injection valve for HPLC techniques employing silica-based packing materials. It is always packed with silica that can be used to saturate the mobile phase with silicate and thus prevent dissolution of the packing material in the analytical column. Capillary (0.1 to 0.5 mm), microbore (1 mm internal diameter [ID]), and small-bore (2 mm ID) columns are used because of the increase in sensitivity and the conservation of mobile phase, which is advantageous for cost, environmental, and detector compatibility reasons. Capillary/microbore columns with minimal amounts of mobile phase are required for mass spectrometric detection because these instruments require the removal of as much mobile phase as possible. In addition to the columns, the connections made between system components are critical because the fittings should introduce as little peak spreading as possible. They should be of zero dead volume or at least low dead volume type. An excellent article on the intricacies of HPLC plumbing is available.[23]

Detection Systems

The final component in the chromatographic system is responsible for detecting, identifying, and determining the concentration of compounds as they elute from the column. The position of the peak in the chromatogram (i.e., the **retention volume, V_R**) is helpful in qualitative identification. If a substance co-elutes with a known compound, it may be the same material; an identical retention, however, does not *prove* identity. Ideally, a detector would respond to any compound, would detect picograms or less of the analytes, would be immune to any solvent-related phenomena, and would respond linearly to a wide range of concentrations. Three types of HPLC detectors routinely used in the clinical laboratory are absorbance, fluorescence, and electrochemical detectors. These are not specific. Mass spectrometric detection, which meets all of the criteria, is important in clinical research, forensic toxicology, and specialized clinical testing. Selection of the appropriate detector depends on the required selectivity and sensitivity. Several books that provide a detailed description of various HPLC detection methods have been published.[24,25] Derivatization methods, although not covered in the following discussion, are an important means of enhancing sensitivity or specificity of detection in HPLC analysis.[26,27]

Absorbance Detection

(See Chapter 2.)

The most frequently used HPLC detection mode is absorbance spectrophotometry. The advantage of absorbance detectors over fluorescence or electrochemical detectors is that they can be used to detect a greater variety of compounds. However, absorbance detectors have poorer detection limit capabilities—a factor of 1000 lower compared with fluorescence and electrochemical detectors. The detection limit for absorbance detectors is approximately 5×10^{-10} g/mL. Wavelengths longer than 200 nm are required for absorbance detectors because mobile-phase solvents absorb appreciably at the low-ultraviolet wavelength region of the spectrum (<200 nm). In general, the number of compounds that can be detected increases as wavelength decreases. However, at shorter wavelengths, detection of interfering compounds is increased as are baseline shifts when gradient chromatography is used. It is thus desirable to use the longest wavelength at which a compound absorbs to increase the specificity of the technique.

Three types of LC absorbance detectors are available: fixed-wavelength, variable-wavelength, and multiple-wavelength. These detectors are described in the Spectroscopy, Chapter, 2.

Electrochemical Detection[28]

For a select group of compounds, electrochemical detection (LCEC) is the method of choice because of its superior sensitivity (femtomole to picomole). The types of compounds that can be measured undergo reversible electron transfer reactions. Characteristics of a small oxidation (or reduction) potential and fast kinetics are most desirable for sensitive and selective detection. The classes of organic compounds that have these characteristics are phenols (such as hydroquinones, catechols, and catecholamines), aromatic amines, thiols, nitro compounds, and quinones. Compounds such as aldehydes and ketones require too high a reduction potential, whereas alkyl amines and carboxylic acid functionalities require too high an oxidation potential for direct determination by LCEC detection. The most common LCEC analyses done in the clinical laboratory involve the determination of catecholamines, catecholamine metabolites, serotonin, and 5-hydroxyindoleacetic acid.

Amperometric and Coulometric Detection. In general, electrochemical detection of an analyte occurs through an electron transfer between the electrode surface and the analyte molecule, with subsequent measurement of the current. Please see Electrochemistry (Chapter 12) for more detail. Detectors are classified as either *amperometric,* in which 1% to 10% of the analyte reacts at the electrode, or *coulometric,* in which 100% of the analyte reacts. Increasing the electrode surface area or slowing the flow rates to increase the percentage of electroconversion does not increase detection limits because a concomitant increase in background electrolysis and hence noise occurs. Thus coulometric detectors have no detection limit advantage over amperometric detectors. Factors such as variations in temperature, flow rate, and mobile-phase impurities, which are important contributors to noise, must be controlled if the lowest detection limits are to be achieved. For this reason, gradients are not usually employed in LCEC detection.

Conductivity Detection. Similar to the LCEC techniques described previously, measurement of conductivity is considered an electrochemical detection method. The HPLC determination of inorganic anions uses anion-exchange chromatography with conductivity detection. See Electrochemistry (Chapter 12).

Mass Spectrometric Detection

Mass spectrometry (MS) has become a premier detection technique in HPLC because of its combined sensitivity/detection limit (down to femtomole amounts) and specificity (molecular mass determination) capabilities. The advent of two ionization technologies, electrospray ionization (ESI) (also called IonSpray) and atmospheric pressure chemical ionization (APCI), has revolutionized MS capabilities in bioanalysis by allowing the determination of ionic, polar, and nonvolatile compounds. This has paved the way for the direct interfacing of MS detectors with HPLC (see below).

Applications

Several books on HPLC of clinical and biochemical analytes have been published.[3,7,29] Table 4-6 contains a comprehensive list of the classes of clinically relevant compounds in which HPLC plays a significant role in analysis. The HPLC modes given in Table 4-6 for each compound class are the modes most prevalently used (as determined by a survey of recent literature).

KEY CONCEPTS BOX 4-1

- Resolution, efficiency, and speed of analysis in liquid chromatography (LC)
- Various LC chromatographic modes, including size-exclusion, ion-exchange, absorption, partition, reverse-phase, affinity, and enantiomeric separation.
- LC instrumentation components, including columns and type of packings and solvent/sample delivery components.

Table 4-6 Clinically Relevant Compounds Determined by HPLC

COMPOUND		
Class	**Subclass**	**Most Prevalent HPLC Mode or Modes Used**
Amino acids		Reversed phase, ion exchange
Anions	Oxalate, citrate, sulfate, phosphate, iodide, bromide, chloride, thiocyanate, nitrate, nitrite	Ion exchange
Bile acids		Reversed phase
Bilirubins		Reversed phase
Bioamines	Catecholamines and catecholamine metabolites	Reversed phase, ion pair
	Serotonin and serotonin metabolites	Reversed phase, ion pair
Carbohydrates	Monosaccharides and oligosaccharides	Reversed phase, ion exchange, ion-moderated partition, normal phase
Drug and drug metabolites		Reversed phase
Fatty acids and organic acids	Fatty acids	Reversed phase
	Organic acids	Ion exchange, ion-moderated partition, reversed phase
Hemoglobins		
	Glycated hemoglobins	Ion exchange, affinity
	Hemoglobin variants	Ion exchange
Isomers, positional		Normal phase
Lipoproteins		Size exclusion
Nucleic acid compounds		
	Nucleic acid bases, nucleosides, nucleotides	Reversed phase, ion pair
	Oligonucleotides	Reversed phase, ion exchange
	DNA restriction fragments	Reversed phase, ion exchange
Phospholipids		Normal phase
Porphyrins		Reversed phase
Prostaglandins		Reversed phase
Steroids		Reversed phase
Vitamins	Biotins, folates, nicotinamides, pantothenic acids, retinoids (vitamin A), riboflavins, thiamines, tocopherols (vitamin E), vitamin B_6, vitamin B_{12}, vitamin C, vitamin D, vitamin K	Reversed phase

SECTION OBJECTIVES BOX 4-2

- Discuss temperatures, type of columns, and molecules appropriate for gas chromatography (GC) separation.
- Discuss mobile/stationary-phase requirements and derivatization requirements.
- Discuss applications and selection of GC components, including carrier gas, sample injection port, column tubing, thermal compartment, and detectors.

GAS CHROMATOGRAPHY

Chromatography is a physical technique that separates two or more compounds based on their distribution between two phases, a stationary and a mobile one. In **gas chromatography** (GC), the stationary phase may be a solid or liquid, but the mobile phase is a gas that percolates over the stationary phase, moving the constituents through the column.

A gas chromatograph consists of six components (Fig. 4-6): (1) a pressurized carrier gas with ancillary pressure and flow regulators; (2) a sample injection port; (3) a column; (4) a detector; (5) an electrometer and signal recorder; and (6) thermostatted compartments encasing the column, detector, and injection port.

When separation of sample components is accomplished through the use of a mobile gas phase and a stationary phase consisting of a thin liquid layer held on a solid support, the technique is called **gas-liquid chromatography** (GLC). **Gas-solid chromatography** (GSC) employs a solid **sorbent** as the stationary phase. Both GLC and GSC may be further differentiated based on the stationary-phase support. When the **liquid phase** in GLC is coated over the surface of small particles, or the solid sorbent in GSC consists of small particles, the column acts as a container for the stationary phase. This technique is known as *packed-column GC.* When liquid-phase GLC or the solid sorbent coats the inner wall of the column, the column itself acts as a support for the stationary phase. This technique is known as *open-tubular GC,* or *capillary GC.* Regardless of the type of mobile or stationary phase, separation is achieved through the difference in partitioning of the various molecules of the sample between the two phases.

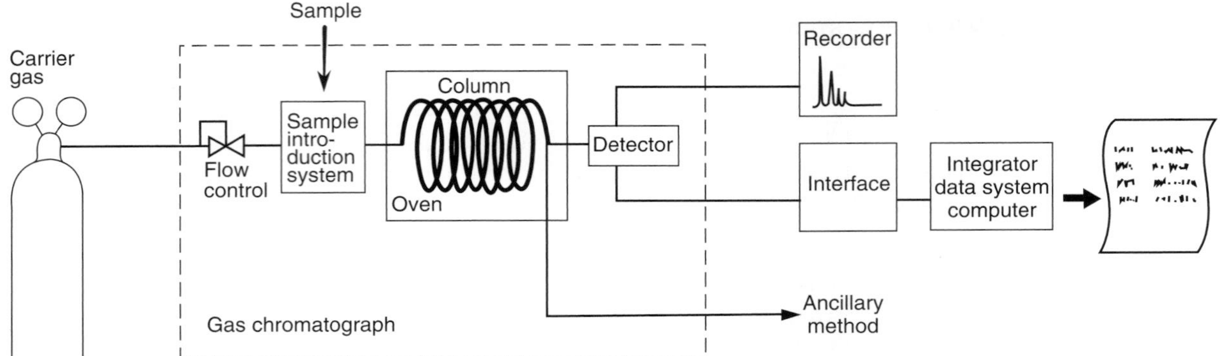

Fig. 4-6 Basic components of a gas chromatographic system. (From Ettre LS: *Practical Gas Chromatography,* Norwalk, CT, 1973, Perkin-Elmer Corp.)

Molecules That Can Be Separated by Gas Chromatography

Theoretically, any compound that can be vaporized or converted to a volatile **derivative** may be analyzed by gas chromatography. Compounds as small as carbon monoxide and methane and as large as 800 D have been successfully analyzed. Compounds larger than 800 D lack sufficient volatility. Generally, a compound must be stable as a vapor to produce a single identifiable chromatographic peak. Unstable compounds may be chemically converted (derivatized) to stable, volatile forms. However, if a compound degrades to known products or a consistent number of products, the resultant pattern of multiple compounds may be used as a means of tentative identification.

Inorganic compounds or the inorganic salts of organic acids and bases lack sufficient volatility for gas chromatographic analysis. Thus the technique is generally applied to analysis of organic molecules in their neutral nonionic forms. Before chromatographic analysis is performed, compounds are generally isolated and concentrated by means of solvent extraction and evaporation to dryness. The residues that contain the analytes are dissolved in small amounts of volatile organic solvents. The solvent-analyte solution is then chromatographed. The analyte vapor should not chemically interact with the solvent. The solvent should have greater volatility and much less affinity for the stationary phase than the analyte compounds do, thereby eluting far ahead of the analyte and not interfering with the chromatogram. The principles of chromatography discussed earlier in this chapter apply to instrumental GC. However, for complete treatment of the many complex variables that influence GC separations, consult Willett[30] and McNair.[31]

Temperature Dependence

Temperature is the most important single parameter in a gas chromatograph separation.

The time it takes the solute to travel through the GC column and reach the detector is called the **retention time (t_R)** and that time is directly dependent on the temperature. The retention times of solute molecules may be readily altered when one changes the column temperatures. Roughly, a 30° C decrease in column temperature will approximately double the retention time. Conversely, a 30° C increase in column temperature will approximately halve the retention time.

Table 4-7 Differences Between Packed and Capillary Columns

Parameter	Packed	Capillary
Length, meters	1.5 to 6.0	5 to 100
Inner diameter, millimeters	2 to 4	0.2 to 0.7
Specific permeability, (10^{-7}) cm^2	1 to 10	10 to 1000
Flow, mL/min	10 to 60	0.5 to 15.0
Pressure drop, psi	10 to 40	3 to 40
Total effective plates (2 meters, 50 meters)	5000	150,000
Effective plates per meter	2500 (ID 2 mm)	3000 (ID 0.25)
Capacity	10 μg/peak	<50 ng/peak
Liquid film thickness, μm	1 to 10	0.05 to 0.5

Column Performance

The ability of a column to produce optimum separations is measured by the quantities of *efficiency,* which is the ability to produce narrow peaks, and *resolution,* which is the ability to separate two adjacent peaks. **Open tubular columns** (i.e., when the packing material is on the sides of the column, leaving an open space for the gas flow) have greater efficiencies than **packed columns** (Table 4-7). The flow of gas in a GC propels the molecules that are being separated forward in the column. Typically, the optimum velocity chosen is ideal for only one compound; however, similar compounds have closely related optimum velocities, and a single flow rate is suitable for their separation. If the flow rate is too fast, the gas sweeps the diffusing molecules from the stationary phase before separation can occur, resulting in peak broadening. Because there is no support of sorbent particles that hinder movement in open tubular columns, the carrier-gas flow rate can be much lower than in packed columns (see Table 4-7).

Mobile-Phase Considerations

The most commonly used carrier gases are presented in Table 4-8. The carrier gas must be inert so as not to react with the

Table 4-8 Common Carrier Gases

Gas	Molecular Weight	Density (g/L)	Impurities (ppm)
Argon	39.944	1.784	
Helium	4.007	0.177	Hydrocarbons (1 to 100)
Hydrogen	2.018	0.089	
Nitrogen	28.014	1.251	Oxygen (20)

sample components. Large quantities of relatively pure gas must be commercially available because appreciable amounts of carrier gas are used for analysis. Common impurities in carrier gases are moisture, oxygen, and hydrocarbons. Each of these contaminants may adversely affect various detectors, producing unstable recorder baseline or extraneous peaks. In certain situations, carrier-gas impurities may interact with sample components and prevent their analysis. For example, pre-purified–grade nitrogen contains up to 20 ppm of oxygen. If high column temperatures are necessary to separate compounds that are readily oxidized, the oxygen impurity in nitrogen carrier gas may degrade the compounds on the column and prevent their detection or may produce multiple extraneous peaks of the degradation products. In such a situation, helium, which contains less oxygen contamination, should replace nitrogen as the carrier gas.

Stationary-Phase Considerations

Gas-Solid Stationary Phases

In gas-solid chromatography, the column is packed or the inner wall is coated with an adsorptive solid material on which the sample components are partitioned by adsorption on the surface of the solid. This material should possess a large surface area per unit volume to ensure rapid equilibrium between the stationary and gas phases. It should possess uniform particle size and pore structure and should be strong enough to resist breakdown during handling and column packing. Theoretically, the smaller the particle size of the support, the greater is the efficiency of the column. However, the smaller the particles, the greater is the resistance to flow, resulting in greater carrier-gas pressure.

The most common chromatographic solids for adsorption phases are made from diatomaceous earth (kieselguhr). Processed white kieselguhr is sold under many trade names: Chromosorb W, Celite, Gas Chrom, and Anakron. The diatomite may also be crushed, blended, pressed into brick, and processed so that mineral impurities form oxides and silicates, which give the material a pink color. It is marketed as crushed firebrick, or Chromosorb P. This material has greater density and is less fragile than the white material. The pore size of the pink material is only 2 mm compared with 9 mm for the white; therefore, greater efficiency is obtained with the pink material.

Each support possesses individual properties that may enhance or hinder its use for a particular application. The white material is slightly alkaline and will interact with acidic compounds. Its surface, however, is nonadsorptive, a property that favors its application for analysis of polar compounds. The pink material adsorbs polar compounds; thus it is best suited for the separation of nonpolar molecules like hydrocarbons.

Another type of solid stationary phase consists of porous polymer beads, which allow the analyte molecules to go into partition directly from the gas phase into the amorphous polymer. Porapak, a polymer of ethylvinylbenzene cross-linked with vinylbenzene, is the most popular polymer phase. The material may be modified by copolymerization with various polar monomers to produce beads of varying polarity. Porapak columns are thermally stable up to 250° C. At temperatures above 250° C, the column material will be degraded and eluted, a phenomenon called *column bleed.* These degradation products can be observed by the detector. Water and highly polar molecules are rapidly eluted from the polymer. Porapak is especially useful for baseline separation of aqueous samples containing low-molecular-weight alcohols, esters, halogens, hydrocarbons, ketones, and mercaptans (Table 4-9).

Gas-Liquid-Solid Supports for GLC

The stationary phase in gas-liquid chromatography is a thin film of liquid held on an inert support. In capillary chromatography, the liquid is coated on the walls of the tubing. In packed columns, the liquid is held in a thin-layer film across the surface of an inert support (Fig. 4-7). Many materials that act as stationary phases for GSC are also supports for the liquid phase in GLC. Both the pink and white solid phases described earlier are popular liquid supports. Although the support should be inert and should not influence separation, both pink and white materials have **active sites** because of metallic impurities and silanol (-SiOH) and siloxane (SiOSi-) groups, which form hydrogen bonds with polar compounds. This interaction gives rise to distorted (asymmetrical) peaks in the resultant GLC chromatogram. These active sites may be removed by acid washing of mineral impurities from the support and by conversion of the silanol groups to silyl esters (**silanization**) of dimethyldichlorosilane or hexamethyldisilazone. Silanization reduces surface activity but also reduces the surface area of the support so that no more than 10% (v/w) of the liquid stationary phase to total column weight may be applied. In certain instances, special additives are mixed with the liquid phase to block the active sites of untreated support material.

Liquid Phases

The universal popularity of GLC as a separation method is attributable to the large variety of liquid phases with differing solution properties and therefore different affinities for various classes of analytes. The range of liquids used as stationary phases is limited only by their volatility, thermal stability, and ability to coat the support. No single stationary phase will achieve all desired separations. Successful separation of 80% of a wide range of organic compounds may be achieved with the use of only four to seven phases: OV-101, OV-17, Carbowax 20M, OV-225, DEGS, OV-275, and OV-210.[34]

Table 4-9 Examples of Commonly Used Stationary Phases and Their Applications

Stationary Phase	Structures	Activity	Temperature (° C Min/Max)	Application	Specific Compounds
Silicone OV-1 (100% methyl)	$[-O-Si(CH_3)(R)-O-Si(CH_3)(R')-O-]_n$ R and R′ = CH_3 in above structure	Nonpolar	100/350	Bacteria, drugs	Fatty acid methyl esters, benzodiazepines
Silicone OV-17 (50%, phenyl)	R and R′ = Phenyl in above structure	Intermediate polarity	20/350	Drugs, steroids	Tricyclic antidepressants, barbiturates, cholesterol
Silicone OV-210 (50%, 3,3,3-trifluoropropyl)	R and R′ = $—CH_2—CH_2—CF_3$ in above structure	Polar	20/300	Drugs, pesticides	Basic drugs, lindane, aldrin, DDT
Silicone OV-225 (25% cyanopropyl, 25% phenyl)	R = Phenyl, R′ = $—CH_2—CH_2—CH_2—CN$ in above structure	Polar	20/275	Steroids	TMS derivatives of 17-ketosteroids
10% Apiezon L 2% KOH	Undefined mixture of high-boiling hydrocarbons	Nonpolar	50/225	Amines	Amphetamine
NPGS (neopentyl glycol succinate)	$[-CH_2-C(CH_3)_2-CH_2-O-C(=O)-CH_2-CH_2-C(=O)-O-]_n$		50/240	Volatile fatty acids	Acetic through caproic acids
Carbopack B/5%	$(-CH_2-CH_2-O-)_n$	Polar		Alcohols, aldehydes, ketones	Methanol, ethanol, acetaldehyde, acetone
DEGS (diethylene glycol succinate)	$(-CH_2-CH_2-O-CH_2-CH_2-O-C(=O)-CH_2-CH_2-C(=O)-O-)_n$	Polar	20/200	Bacteria	Fatty acid methyl esters
EGA (ethylene glycol adipate)	$(-CH_2-CH_2-O-C(=O)-CH_2-CH_2-CH_2-CH_2-C(=O)-O-)_n$		100/210	Amino acids	NBTFA derivatives of amino acids
Chromosorb 102 (styrene divinyl benzene polymer)	$(-CH=CH-CH=CH-C_6H_4-CH=CH-)_n$		<250° C	Alcohol, aldehydes	Methanol, ethanol, acetaldehyde
Porapak Q (ethylvinyl benzene + divinyl benzene polymer mixture)	$(-CH=CH-C_6H_4-CH=CH-)_n$		<250° C	Low molecular weight	Chlorinated hydrocarbons

TMS, Trimethylsilyl; *NBTFA*, nitroblue tetrazolium fatty acid.

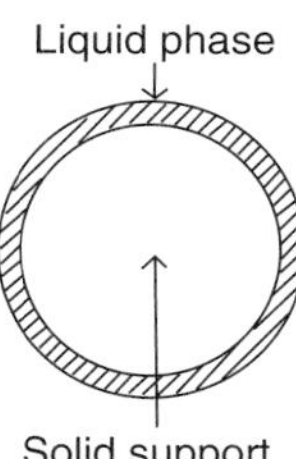

Fig. 4-7 Schema of solid support particle for gas chromatography with liquid stationary-phase coating.

Examples of liquid phases, characteristics, and applications are presented in Table 4-9.

Liquid phases may be generally classified into five categories: (1) nonpolar phases, which are hydrocarbon liquids such as squalane, silicone greases, Apiezon L, and silicone gum rubber. Generally, compounds are eluted from these phases in order of increasing boiling point; (2) intermediate-polarity phases that include polar or polarizable groups attached to a long nonpolar skeleton, such as esters of high molecular weight or alcohols such as diisodecylphthalate. Both polar and nonpolar compounds are separated by these phases, with the more polar ones eluted first; (3) polar phases, which contain a high concentration of polar groups, such as carbowaxes. These phases differentiate between polar and nonpolar compounds by interacting strongly only with polar compounds, separating these from the earlier eluting, less polar compounds; (4) hydrogen-bonding phases, which contain many hydrogen atoms readily available for hydrogen bonding, such as glycol phases. Polar compounds have greater affinity for the stationary phase and are eluted more slowly; and (5) special-purpose phases that can be prepared to use a specific chemical interaction between the sample and the stationary phase. An example of a special-purpose phase is silver nitrate dissolved in glycol to enhance separation of unsaturated hydrocarbons by charge-transfer interactions.

Each liquid phase has a specific temperature range for efficient use (see Table 4-9). The maximum temperature at which a phase may be used is determined by its volatility. Beyond this temperature, the phase is lost because of decomposition or volatilization and is carried into the detector, producing extensive background noise (column bleed). A column may be heated above the maximum temperature for brief periods of time as in temperature programming, but the maximum temperature must never be exceeded for isothermal (constant-temperature) analysis. Below the minimum temperature, the increased viscosity or solidification of the liquid does not allow reproducible analysis.

The amount of stationary phase in the column is expressed as percentage by weight of the liquid phase on the support. In general, packed columns contain 3% to 10% liquid phase. Deviations from these values may occur in specific applications: very low liquid loads for high-molecular-weight compounds and high loads for small, highly volatile compounds such as hydrocarbons that contain one to four carbon atoms. The amount of stationary phase directly affects the sample capacity and efficiency of the column. The greater the amount of liquid phase, the larger is the amount of sample that may be chromatographed.

The manufacturers of open tubular columns often use trade names for the liquid phases presented in Table 4-9. However, the name usually retains a numerical designation so that the chromatographer can recognize the composition of the liquid phase as given in the table. For example, a **capillary column** of HP-1 or DB-1 is a 100% dimethyl polysiloxane (simethicone) comparable with OV-1 (Table 4-9) produced by Agilent and J&W Scientific, respectively.

Variations in assay conditions and variations in stationary-phase packaging (lot to lot, company to company, and so on) affect the reproducibility of GC analysis. Relative retention times are converted to indices or constants to ensure reproducible identification of peaks of interest regardless of exact assay conditions. These values can then be used to compare data between analyses, within a laboratory, or between laboratories. The theory of stationary-phase efficiencies is complex and is well characterized by McReynolds and Rohrschneider as constant systems that classify stationary phases in terms of their separating power.[32]

Derivatization

Often it is desirable to modify a molecule chemically to form a new product with properties that are preferable to those of its precursors. Compounds are derivatized to make them volatile and stable as a gas and thus analyzable by GC. Derivatives are also prepared to achieve increased sensitivity, selectivity, or specificity for a given separation. Derivatives may be eluted from the column sooner, have less tailing, produce sharper peaks, provide stability to thermally labile compounds, and increase resolution. Derivatization involves a chemical reaction between some functional group on the sample molecule (usually a polar group, which reduces volatility or interacts with the stationary phase to increase retention time) and a smaller molecule (derivatizing agent), which forms a new product of increased volatility with a smaller partition coefficient (K_D). The derivatization may be carried out before sample injection or may occur in the injection port of the chromatograph ("on column" or "flash derivatization"). A few derivatization techniques are briefly presented, but for a more complete discussion, consult the literature.[27]

A popular GC derivatization technique is the replacement of an active hydrogen atom by a trimethylsilyl (TMS) group. The resultant *silyl* derivatives are usually less polar and more volatile and display greater thermal stability than their parent compounds. Silylizing reagents react vigorously with water or alcohol-containing solvents; therefore, the conversion reactions are carried out in anhydrous solvents such as acetonitrile or tetrahydrofuran. TMS reagents are flammable, and some are highly corrosive. They should be handled with care.

Esterification is often used for GC analysis of compounds that contain a carboxylic acid group. Methyl esters possess the greatest volatility and hence are most popular. Alkylation reactions with quaternary alkylammonium hydroxides or dimethylformamide-dialkyl acetals have become popular as

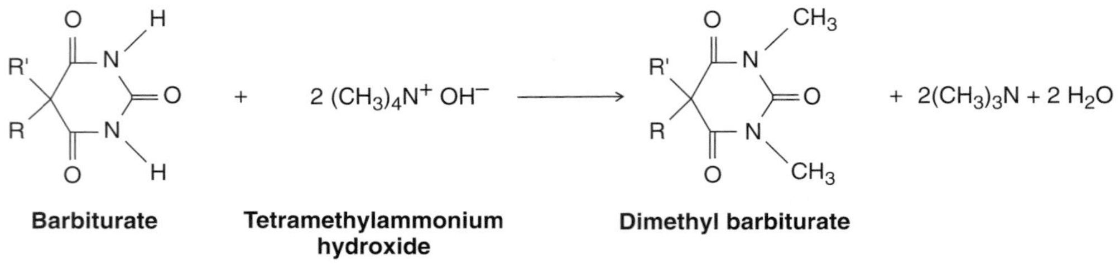

Fig. 4-8 Tetramethyl derivatization of barbiturate drugs.

"flash-derivatizing" reagents. Fig. 4-8 presents the flash derivatization reaction of tetramethylammonium hydroxide and barbiturate drugs.

Selection of a Mobile Phase

The mobile phase or carrier gas takes the vaporized sample through the column and into the detector. Selection of the proper carrier gas depends on three considerations: (1) the operating principles of the detector through which the gas will be continuously flowing, (2) the presence of impurities in the carrier gas, and (3) the desired speed of analysis and performance of the column. Compounds that are negligibly partitioned into a stationary phase cannot be separated from each other. Similarly, compounds with too great an affinity for the stationary phase will have unacceptably long, or irreversibly long, retention times.

Components of a Gas Chromatograph

See Fig. 4-6 for the components of a gas chromatograph.

Carrier Gas

The efficiency of a gas chromatograph depends on a constant flow of carrier gas. The carrier gas from a pressurized tank flows through a toggle valve, a flowmeter (range 1 to 1000 L/min), metal restrictors, and a pressure gauge (1 to 4 atmospheres). The flow is adjusted by a needle valve mounted at the base of the flowmeter. The gas moves more slowly at the head of the column than at the outlet because of a pressure drop in the column. Thus the flow rates are measured as the gas leaves the column. This is done with a soap-film flowmeter. A simple sidearm buret with a rubber bulb filled with soap solution is connected to the detector outlet. One determines the flow rate by noting the time required for a film (bubble) to pass between two calibrated volume marks on the buret.

Carrier gas should be inert, dry, and pure. The most common carrier gases are inert, but they may contain contaminants that affect column performance and the response of ionization detectors. Hydrocarbon gases and water are removed from the carrier gas by a molecular sieve trap between the gas cylinder and the chromatograph.

Sample Injection Port

Most GC analyses are performed on nonaqueous, liquid samples that are injected by a glass microsyringe. A needle is inserted through a septum into a heated block, where the sample is vaporized and swept by carrier gas into the column. The pressure inside the injection port is usually well above atmospheric pressure, and the stream of carrier gas sweeps away the sample and aids in vaporization. Thus a sample may be vaporized at temperatures below its atmospheric boiling point. However, the injection port temperature is usually set at 25° C to 50° C higher than the boiling point of the highest boiling components in the sample. This ensures that immediate vaporization will occur, and that the components will not be diluted by carrier gas and will enter the head of the column as a single band. The time required for vaporization is dependent on the amount and volatility of the sample. Dilute samples vaporize faster than concentrated samples. High-boiling or temperature-sensitive compounds may be diluted with volatile solvents, which lower injection temperatures significantly.

Because heated metal may catalyze the degradation of many biological compounds, many injection ports are equipped with a glass liner or a glass column that extends through the injectors flush to the septum. The latter approach is called *on-column injection*. For maximum efficiency, it is imperative that the sample be of the smallest possible volume (0.5 to 10 μL) consistent with detector sensitivity and that it be injected as a single, uniform band ("slug injection"). Gaseous samples are injected by a gas-tight syringe or a calibrated bypass loop. The loop consists of a glass system of three stopcocks, between two of which a standard volume of gas is trapped and introduced into the carrier gas stream when the stopcocks are switched.

Because of the low capacity of capillary columns, injection of undiluted samples will often overload the column. This problem is avoided with capillary systems by splitting the carrier gas flow after vaporization. In the split-injection technique, after vaporization of the sample, the carrier-gas flow is divided into two parts with a variable ratio of flows. The smaller part of the gas-sample mixture enters the column, while the larger flow bypasses the column inlet and leaves the system. The ratio of the flow to the column and the outlet is controlled by a needle value. Splitting ratios may be adjusted over a wide range (1:5 to 1:250).

A septum separates the chromatographic column from the laboratory environment. Septums are small disks of silicone rubber, or Teflon R–coated disks. Low-molecular-weight solvents used in the manufacture of septums may be released as the injection port is heated, producing unwarranted peaks (ghost peaks) in chromatograms and increasing the background level of the detector. Low-bleed septums from which the solvents have been extracted are available. Repeated injections through the septum will gradually destroy its mechanical strength, causing leakage that may affect retention time and sensitivity. This problem is easily avoided by regular insertion of new septums. Various specialized injection systems, including automatic sampling units, are commercially available.

Column Tubing

The column tubing contains the stationary phase (coating or packing material) and directs the carrier-gas flow. It should be inert and should not affect the separation by reaction with the stationary phase or the sample. The columns may be shaped as a U-tube, coiled in an open spiral or flat pancake shape. Stainless steel and copper columns are often used for analyses requiring temperatures greater than 250° C. However, for the analysis of drugs, steroids, or other biological compounds, metal columns may absorb these analytes or catalyze their degradation; thus glass is the tubing of choice for most clinical analyses. One disadvantage of glass is its fragility and inflexibility. Recently, nickel has been recommended as a substitute for glass. Nickel tubing has been effectively replacing glass in the analysis of specific drugs, pesticides, and cholesterol. However, the application of nickel tubing to the broad range of biological compounds has not yet been established.

The inside diameters of columns vary from capillary (0.2 mm) to packed columns (4 mm). Packed columns of 4 mm ID contain four times the stationary phase as 2 mm ID columns of the same length and therefore possess a greater sample capacity. However, the same separation will require higher temperatures and a longer analysis time on the wider column. In addition, columns should be only as long as necessary to effect the desired separation. A short column provides a short analysis time, low temperatures, a long column life, and less background in the detector. Packed columns of 0.7 to 2 m (2 to 6 feet) or **wide-bore columns** of 15 m (45 feet) are sufficient for most chemical separations.

Open tubular columns tend to contain small amounts of stationary phase that significantly reduce the capacity of the column, and the amount of sample injected must be consistent with the column's capacity. Internal diameter directly affects column capacity. Capillary columns with an ID of 0.2 mm have capacities of less than 100 ng of sample component, columns of 0.32 mm ID will accept up to 500 ng of sample component, and columns with 0.53 mm up to 2000 ng of sample component. "Wide-bore" columns with IDs of 0.75 mm approach the capacity of packed columns (15,000 ng).

Thermal Compartment (Oven)

Precise control of column temperature is imperative in gas chromatography. The column oven is controlled by a system that is sensitive to changes of 0.01 Celsius degree and maintains the column temperature at ±0.1 Celsius degree of the desired temperature. The column oven, injection block, and detectors should have separate heaters and controls. Analysis may be performed at a constant oven temperature (isothermal), or the temperature may be varied during the analysis

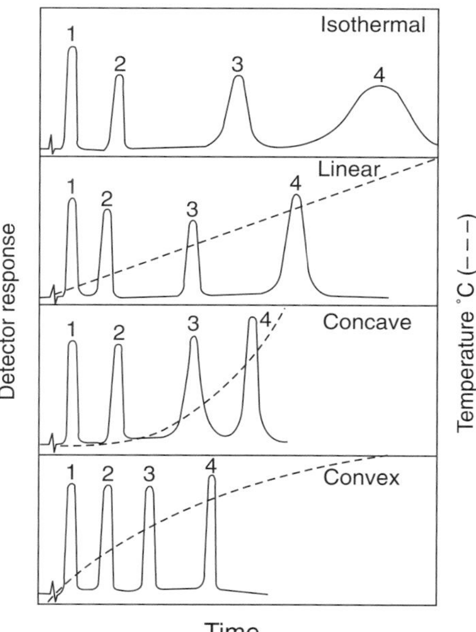

Fig. 4-9 Schema of theoretical separation of four compounds showing varying elution patterns with different temperature programming.

(temperature programming). The temperature change during analysis can be programmed to vary with time according to predetermined, reproducible patterns, giving linear, convex, or concave curves when column temperature is plotted against time (Fig. 4-9). Temperature programming is often used in separating a complex mixture, the components of which have widely varying affinity for the stationary phase. Initially, the column temperature is set low to permit separation and elution of the compounds with little affinity for the stationary phase. The temperature is then raised to elute compounds of higher stationary-phase affinity. Many chromatographs are equipped with specialized oven controls that uniformly raise the column temperature after each sample injection.

Detectors

As the carrier gas exits from the column, a detector senses the separated components of the sample and provides a corresponding electrical signal. Only a few devices are commonly used. For proper operation or optimum response, each type of detector requires a specific carrier gas (Table 4-10). The most widely used detectors are discussed in the following section.

Thermal-Conductivity Detector

A **thermal-conductivity detector** (TCD) measures the difference in ability to conduct heat (thermal conductivity) between pure carrier gas and the carrier with the sample mixture. A compound carried in the gas increases the thermal conductivity. Usually, four heat-sensing elements—thermistors or wires—are mounted in a brass or stainless steel heat sink and connected to form the arms of a Wheatstone bridge (Fig. 4-10). An electrical current is passed through the wires that make up the bridge. Two filaments in opposite arms

Table **4-10** Detectors and Appropriate Gases

Detector	Carrier Gas	Detector Gas
Thermal conductivity (TCD)	Helium, hydrogen	
Flame ionization (FID)	Helium, nitrogen	Air and hydrogen
Nitrogen-phosphorus (NPD)	Helium, nitrogen	Air and hydrogen
		Air and 8% hydrogen in helium
Electron capture	Nitrogen	5% methane in argon
	5% methane in argon	

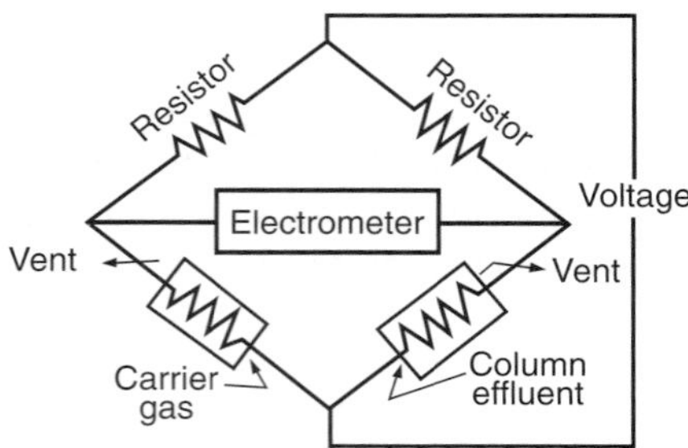

Fig. 4-10 Schema of thermal-conductivity detector. (From Werner M, Mohrbacher RJ, Riendeau CJ: In Baer DM, Dito WR, editors: *Interpretation of Therapeutic Drug Levels,* Chicago, 1981, American Society of Clinical Pathologists.)

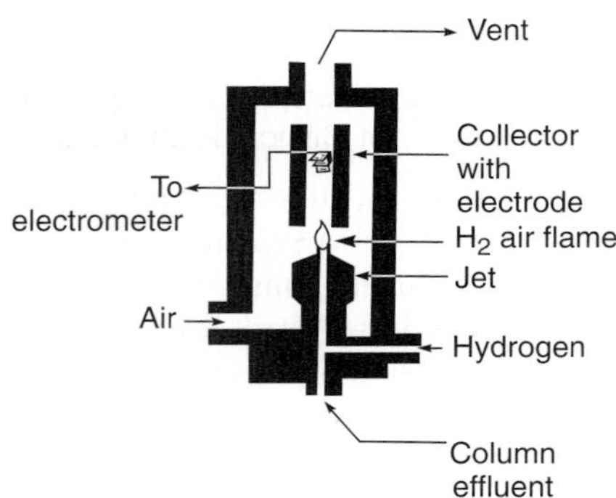

Fig. 4-11 Schema of flame ionization detector. (From Werner M, Mohrbacher RJ, Riendeau CJ: In Baer DM, Dito WR, editors: *Interpretation of Therapeutic Drug Levels,* Chicago, 1981, American Society of Clinical Pathologists.)

of the bridge are cooled by carrier gas (reference), and the other two by the column effluent (sample). The heat lost over both sets of wires is balanced by adjustment of the flow rate of the pure carrier gas. Emerging components from the column increase the rate of cooling of the sample wires because of the increased thermal conductivity of the gas mixture. This changes the electrical resistance of the sample wire pattern, causing the Wheatstone bridge to be out of balance. This imbalance causes a response on the recorder. Important variables in optimum TCD response are carrier gas, flow rate, filament current, and detector temperature. TCDs lack selectivity because any compound that cools the wire will cause a response. Also, they are not as sensitive as other detectors, with minimum detection ranging from 0.1 to 0.5 mg of analyte.

Flame Ionization Detector

In a **flame ionization detector (FID),** eluted components in the carrier gas are mixed with hydrogen and burned in air to produce a very hot flame to ionize organic compounds. A pair of electrodes, charged by a polarizing voltage, collect the ions and generate a current proportional to the number of ions collected. The resultant current is amplified by an electrometer, producing a response on the recorder. The response of an FID is directly proportional to the number of carbons in a molecule bound to hydrogen or other carbon atoms. It is insensitive to water, carbon monoxide, carbon dioxide, and most inorganic compounds. The FID is the most popular detector for the determination of organic compounds. Sensitivity depends on chemical structure; therefore, the detector response must be determined for each compound analyzed. At optimal conditions, the minimum detectable quantity of organic compound is 1 ng. A cross section of an FID detector is shown in Fig. 4-11.

Nitrogen-Phosphorus Detector

A **nitrogen-phosphorus detector (NPD)** is similar to an FID except that ions of an alkali metal (rubidium) are introduced into the hydrogen flame. When a compound that contains nitrogen or phosphorus is burned in the flame, the rate of release of alkali metal vapor is increased. The alkali metal vapor readily ionizes in the flame and increases the current flow, which results in enhanced sensitivity for nitrogen and phosphorus. The optimum response is greatly dependent on the flow of hydrogen. The selective interaction of alkali metal ions with these compounds is complex and poorly understood. However, the sensitivity to organonitrogen compounds and the lack of response to other organics make the NPD highly advantageous for the analysis of biological samples. At optimum conditions, the minimum detectable quantity of nitrogenous organic compounds is less than 1 ng. A cross section of an NPD detector is presented in Fig. 4-12.

Electron-Capture Detector

In an **electron-capture detector (ECD),** a radioactive isotope releases beta particles that collide with the carrier-gas molecules, producing many low-energy electrons. The electrons are collected on electrodes and produce a small, measurable, *standing current.* As sample components that contain chemical groups with high electron affinity (electrophilic species), particularly halogen atoms, are eluted from the column, they capture low-energy electrons generated by the isotope to form negatively charged ions. The detector

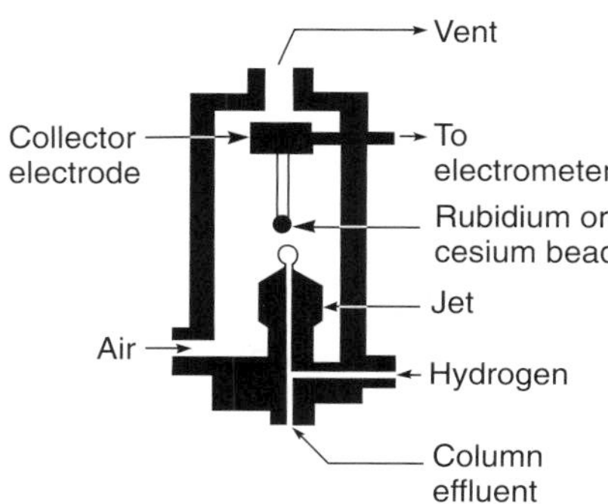

Fig. 4-12 Schema of alkali metal flame detector. (From Werner M, Mohrbacher RJ, Riendeau CJ: In Baer DM, Dito WR, editors: *Interpretation of Therapeutic Drug Levels,* Chicago, 1981, American Society of Clinical Pathologists.)

measures loss of cell current caused by the recombination of electrons. The sources of beta particles in an ECD are usually tritium and nickel-63. The ECD is the most sensitive detector available, since as little as 1 picogram of halogen-containing compound may be measured. Laboratories that use ECDs must be licensed by the Nuclear Regulatory Commission and are subject to all regulations concerning employee safety and possible environmental contamination set forth by the commission.

Mass Spectrometer as a Detector

The **mass spectrometer (MS)** is used as a specialized chromatographic detector to provide extremely sensitive detection (picogram quantities) and specific analyte identification. MS is the only analytical detector that yields a positive molecular identification of compounds. A detailed discussion of MS is found later in this chapter.

Fourier-Transform Infrared Spectrometer

The **Fourier-transform infrared spectrometer (FTIR)** obtains the infrared spectra of a compound as it elutes from the GC column. The report format of FTIR detectors is similar to that of MS detectors (see below, p. 111). A GC/FTIR produces chromatograms measured at specific IR bands similar to SIM mode GC/MS or records the entire IR spectrum of the compound just as an MS records the mass spectrum of a compound. Recent developments in narrow-range IR photon detectors and photo sample cells now give GC/FTIR sensitivity and specificity that rivals those of GC/MS.[35]

There are two types of interface for the GC to the FTIR detector: vapor phase and cryogenic deposition. In vapor phase, a heated fused silica line directs the GC effluent through a long narrow IR gas cell known as a *lightpipe.* An IR beam transmits through the lightpipe, which is sealed at each end with IR-transparent windows. In cryogenic deposition, the column effluent is directed into a vacuum chamber (10^{-5} torr) that ends with a fused silica restrictor positioned above a ZnSe IR-transparent plate. The effluent is deposited on the plate, which is held at liquid nitrogen temperatures. The plate with the frozen eluent is continuously exposed to the IR beam.

Both methods continuously collect the IR spectra of the eluted compounds. The detector does not destroy the compound, and the effluent for the FTIR may be directed into another detector system such as an MS (GC/FTIR/MS). GC/FTIR/MS is an extremely powerful identification technique. At present GC/FTIR is not routinely applied in the clinical chemistry laboratory; however, because of its low nanogram sensitivity, this technique is gaining popularity in forensic toxicology laboratories.

Chromatogram Readout

Strip-chart recorders have been commonly used readout devices in gas chromatography. Recorder sensitivity is usually 1 to 10 mV, with a full-scale response of 1 second or less. Quantitative determinations of separate compounds are performed in two ways: peak-height or peak-area measurements. In many cases, these have been replaced by a computerized data system that automatically records the response, identifies the sample components, integrates the signals, performs calculations, stores all data, and prints out the analytical results in final form.

GC Applications

GC is an extremely versatile and powerful analytical tool. Numerous sample components may be simultaneously separated, identified, and quantitated. By choosing the appropriate stationary phase, one can analyze any mixture of compounds that may be vaporized or converted to volatile derivatives. Selectivity and high sensitivity may be added by varying extractions,[36] as well as detectors. Yet, despite these advantages, application of GC in most clinical chemistry laboratories is limited to a few special areas of testing: therapeutic drug monitoring (TDM), toxicology, and testing for inborn errors of metabolism. The determination of drugs or toxicants has been the widest application for clinical laboratory use of GC because it provides a rapid, simple, reliable method for the simultaneous determination of volatile poisons such as methanol, ethanol, isopropanol, acetone, and acetaldehyde. Even in these areas, GC is applied to specific tests in only a relatively few laboratories because of the specialized training required for maintenance. Adoption of GC has also been limited by the need for manual sample preparation, its slow turnaround time, and the limited number of samples that each machine can process. GC is used to perform TDM analysis of psychoactive drugs, particularly those having active metabolites, which must be measured with the parent drug.

GC coupled to mass spectrometers has been the most successful adaptation of this technique. GC coupled with mass spectrometry is required when workplace confirmatory testing is performed for drugs of abuse in urine; these testing procedures are regulated by government agencies such as the Department of Defense, the Department of Transportation, and the Nuclear Regulatory Agency. Laboratories that perform such testing must be certified by the Department of Health and Human Services. As of this writing, about 45 laboratories, most associated with clinical laboratories, are so accredited.

GC is applied in highly specialized procedures of clinical chemistry, such as testing for inborn errors of metabolism. As a result of inherited defects in metabolism, unusual or inappropriate amounts of organic acids and other by-products of metabolism accumulate in serum and are excreted in urine. The determination of organic acids and their concentrations in urine or serum is a valuable tool for these rare defects.[37] Aciduria profiles are easily obtained with GC/FID, whereas serum profiles require more specific and sensitive GC/MS methods. At present, such testing is performed only in commercial reference laboratories or at university medical centers.

KEY CONCEPTS BOX 4-2

- Molecules being separated by gas chromatography (GC) must be in gaseous phase, requiring high temperature column performance.
- GC separation requires molecules to undergo repetitive partitioning between the mobile gas phase and the liquid or solid support phase.
- Derivatization of reactive moieties may improve GC separation significantly.
- The key components of a GC instrument include carrier gas, sample injection port, column in a heated oven compartment, and detector.

SECTION OBJECTIVES BOX 4-3

- Discuss the function of basic mass spectrometry (MS) components, including ion source, mass filter, and detector and formation of ions.
- Discuss creation of fragmentation patterns by electron and chemical ionization and comparative advantages.
- Discuss MS compound identification and quantitation using full-scan and selected ion monitoring.
- Discuss common combined separation techniques, including gas chromatography (GC)/MS, 2-D GC/MS, and liquid chromatography (LC)/MS, and describe their comparative advantages.
- Discuss the different types of mass spectrometers, including magnetic sector, quadrupole, ion trap, time-of-flight, and tandem MS/MS.
- Describe applications of MS, including forensic urine drug testing.

MASS SPECTROMETRY[33,38,39]

General Principles

Mass spectrometry uses the creation and analysis of ions to analyze a wide variety of molecules. Mass spectrometers are analytical devices that operate on the principle that charged particles moving through a magnetic or an electrical field can be separated from other charged particles according to their **mass-to-charge (m/z)** ratios. Because molecules do not have a net charge, mass spectrometers induce them through an ionization process. Charged molecules are not stable and can break down into fragments and lose their charge by interacting with other molecules or surfaces. Implicit in the use of a mass spectrometer is the assumption that the ionized (including fragmented) products are formed in a reproducible manner if the ionization, separation, and detection systems are kept constant.

Each of the resulting ions has a specific molecular mass and charge, which the mass spectrometer separates and detects. Because the mass of each ion is discrete to greater than a thousandth of an atomic weight unit, the resulting separation of the ion masses is displayed as spectral lines of intensity versus the mass-to-charge ratio. The intensity of each ion is proportionate to the numbers of that ion that reach the detector.

Most ions have a single unit charge; consequently, it is common practice to describe ions in terms of mass alone. However, doubly charged ions can occur, and such ion fragments have a mass value that is one-half of their true mass spectrometric value. The m/z value for each ion is plotted on the x-axis, and the intensity of the ion is plotted on the y-axis to yield a line graph output (Fig. 4-13). The most intense ion in the spectrum is termed the **base peak** and is arbitrarily assigned an abundance value of 100%. The intensity of other peaks is then normalized to the base peak intensity. The record of all ions formed and the relative abundance of each constitute the **mass spectrum** of that compound. This unique **fragmentation pattern** of the molecule is reproducible, and sample identification can be achieved when the ion values and intensities of an unknown compound are compared against reference spectra. A match constitutes the chemical identification of the unknown compound.

Mass Spectrometer

All mass spectrometers include a system by which a vacuum can be created and maintained; a device to introduce the samples (such as GLC, LC, and **solids probe**); an **ionization source,** which serves to ionize the sample; a **mass filter** or analyzer, with which charged particles are separated according to their m/z ratios; and ion collection, amplification, and detection devices (Fig. 4-14). Contemporary mass spectrometers also incorporate computer systems for control of the instrument and for acquisition, display, manipulation, and interpretation of data.

Ion Source

The ion source is maintained in a high-vacuum environment to enhance collision efficiency and ion formation. High-efficiency vacuum pumps maintain the ionization source pressure in the 10^{-5} to 10^{-7} torr range, which not only minimizes ion-molecule reactions (which complicate the analysis) but also optimizes the detection, resolution, and transmission of the ions generated.

Ions are generated in the ion chamber or ion source of the mass spectrometer (Fig. 4-15). The source may be viewed as a small closed box with several pinhole orifices that serve as inlets and outlets. Variable positive and negative electronic potentials are induced on specific metallic surfaces that define the ion source. An electron beam is directed into the source. Compounds that undergo analysis enter the ion source and are bombarded by the ionization beam operating at 70 eV (by convention). Some compounds are converted into positive

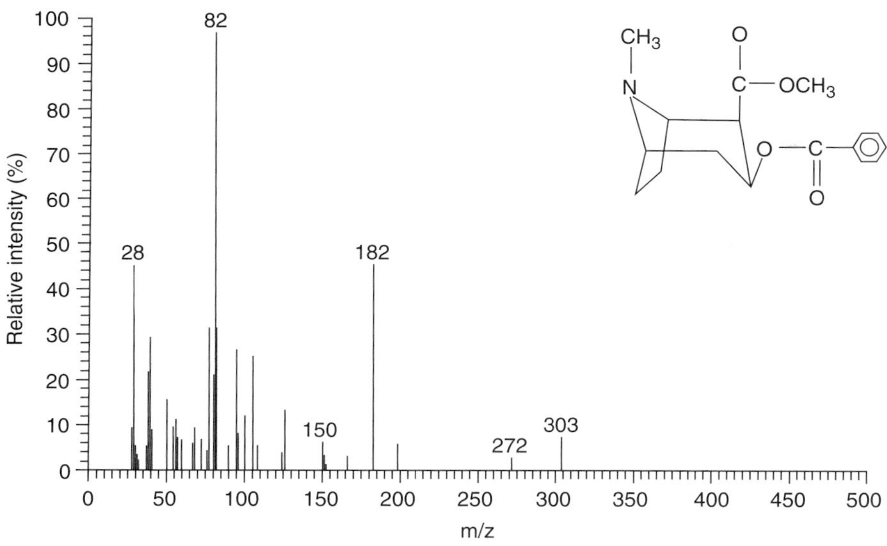

Fig. 4-13 Electron-impact mass spectrum of cocaine. (From Saferstein R: *Forensic Science Handbook,* Englewood Cliffs, NJ, 1982, Prentice Hall.)

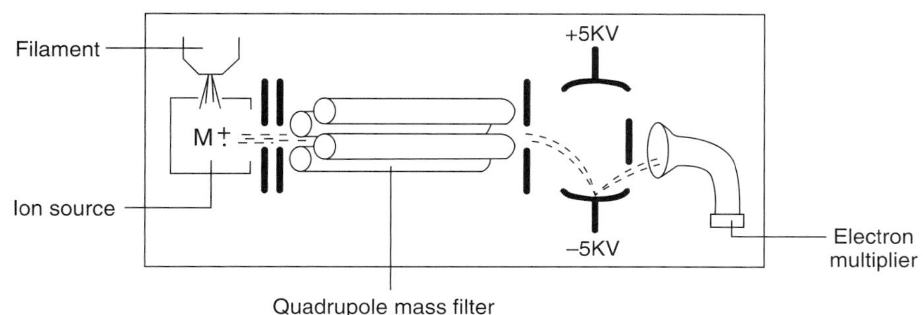

Fig. 4-14 A quadrupole mass spectrometer.

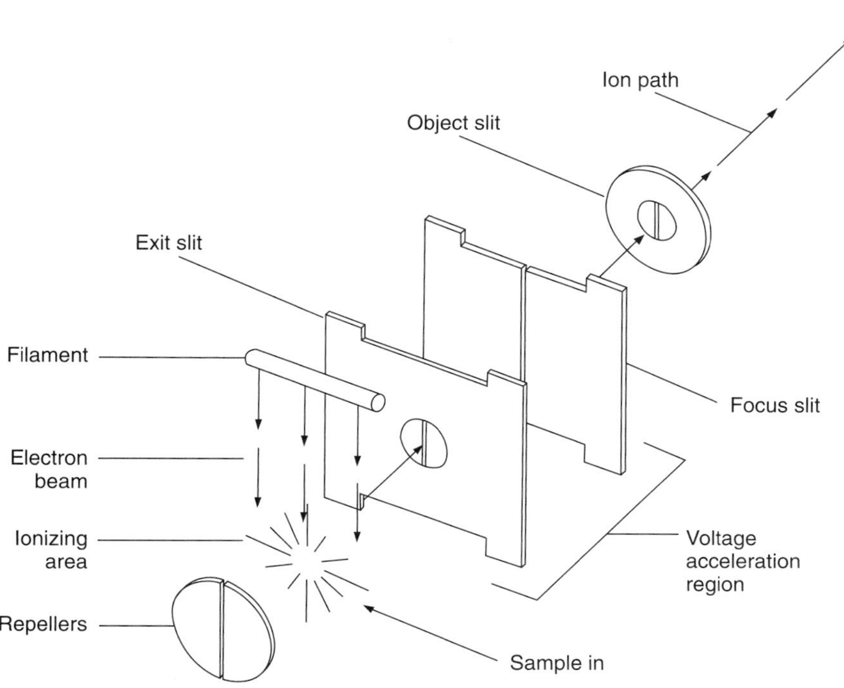

Fig. 4-15 Schema of an ion source. (From Saferstein R: *Forensic Science Handbook,* Englewood Cliffs, NJ, 1982, Prentice Hall.)

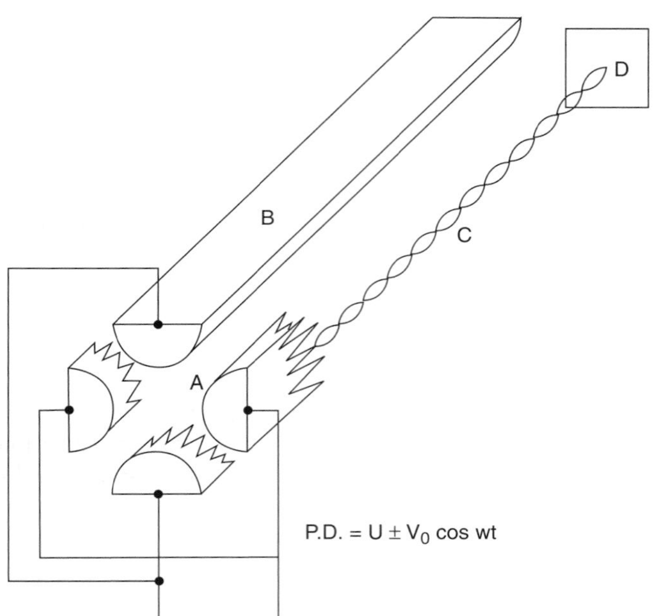

Fig. 4-16 Schema of quadrupole mass filter. *A,* Ion injection. *B,* Quadrupole rods. *C,* Oscillating ion beams. *D,* Collector. (From McFadden WH: *Techniques of Combined Gas Chromatography/Mass Spectrometry,* New York, 1973, Wiley & Sons. This material is used by permission of Wiley & Sons, Inc.)

and negative ions, and these ions are either attracted or repelled by the electronic potentials, that is, opposite charges attract, and like charges repel. Electronic voltage programming optimizes the preservation of ions of a given polarity (either positive or negative ions). For example, the negative potential maintains the positive ions in motion within the volume defined by the source. If an ion comes into physical contact with the metallic surface, it is instantly grounded and eliminated. By manipulating the magnitude and polarity of the electronic potentials, the ions within the source can be stored, accelerated, and directed in space to the outlets that lead to the mass filter.

Mass Filter

Electronic Separation

The mass filter separates the ions of interest according to their m/z ratios and allows these ions ultimately to reach the detector. Separation of ions by the mass filter can occur electronically with the use of a **quadrupole.** A quadrupole filter consists of a quadrant of four parallel hyperbolic or circular rods that provide a specific radio frequency field (Fig. 4-16). Opposite rods are electrically connected and their electrical charge (+ or −) is constantly altered, so that the negatively charged rods become positive and the positive rods become negative. The oscillating charge on the rods is what attracts (or repels) electrically charged ions that are being emitted from the ion source. The applied voltage consists of a constant direct current component U and a radio frequency component V_0 ($\cos wt$); and $w = 2\pi f$, in which f is the radio frequency.[38]

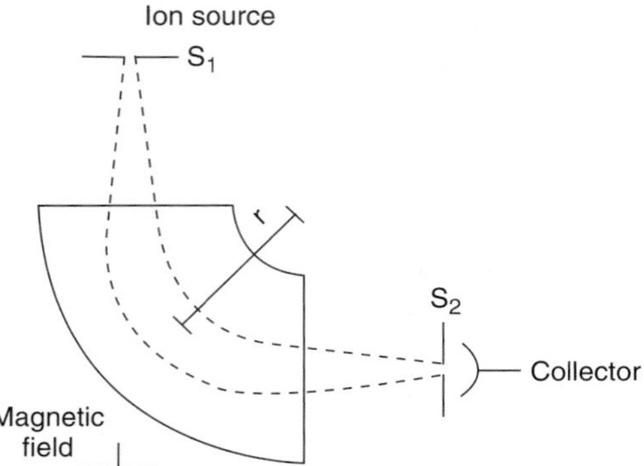

Fig. 4-17 Schema of 90-degree magnetic sector showing direction focusing of divergent ion beam. (From McFadden WH: *Techniques of Combined Gas Chromatography/Mass Spectrometry,* New York, 1973, Wiley & Sons. This material is used by permission of Wiley & Sons, Inc.)

The potential difference between the two sets of rods is thus $U \pm V_0 \cos wt$. This creates a unique oscillating field in which a positive ion injected into the quadrupole region will oscillate between the adjacent electrodes of opposite polarity. At a specified radio frequency, ions of a given mass undergo stable oscillation between electrodes. Ions of lower or higher mass undergo oscillation of increasing amplitude until they are grounded on the quadrupole electrodes. Within the quadrupole field, no force is exerted in the longitudinal direction, and so an ion with stable oscillation continues at its original velocity down the flight path to the detector. With 5 to 30 V of ion acceleration potential, the ions undergo a sufficient number of oscillations during the flight period to provide reasonable mass separation.

Magnetic Separation

Alternatively, the mass filter can separate the ions magnetically, as is the case in **magnetic sector** mass spectrometers. Ions formed in the source are accelerated toward a homogeneous magnetic field (Fig. 4-17). For ions with an electronic charge, *z,* and mass, *m,* the kinetic energy will be related to the accelerating voltage, *V,* by the following equation:

$$V = \frac{1}{2}mv^2 \qquad \text{Eq. 4-1}$$

in which v is the ion velocity. As the ions enter the magnetic field, *H,* they experience a force orthogonal to the field, which results in a curvature of the ion path. This accelerating force, *Hev,* is balanced by the centripetal force, so that

$$Hev = mv^2/r \qquad \text{Eq. 4-2}$$

in which r is the radius of the curvature. Elimination of the velocity term gives the equation

$$m/z = H^2r^2/2V \qquad \text{Eq. 4-3}$$

Thus, at a fixed radius, r, and for a singly charged ion, the mass focused at S_2 and collected by the detector is proportional to the square of the magnetic field and inversely proportional to the accelerating voltage. By varying either of these two parameters, ions of different mass-to-charge ratio can be deflected to the detector, and in this fashion, the mass spectrum is scanned.[38]

For most applications, it is preferable to vary the magnetic field and maintain constant accelerating voltage. When the voltage is varied over a course of a mass scan (with constant magnetic field), the efficiency of transmitting ions of low mass is much greater than that for ions of high mass. This mass discrimination is attributable to the fact that an ion of mass 400 will have one-tenth the accelerating voltage of an ion of mass 40. Because the higher mass region is the more important part of the spectrum, voltage scanning is used only for special cases in which magnetic scanning is impractical.

Magnetic Sector Mass Spectrometry

Magnetic sector instruments offer the highest resolution compared with all other types of mass spectrometers and are consequently more complex and expensive. Resolution specification is an important consideration when choosing among systems. Resolution is defined by the following equation:

$$\text{Resolution} = M/\Delta M \qquad \text{Eq. 4-4}$$

where M is the mass of the ion, and ΔM is the difference in mass between M and its adjacent ion. High-resolution systems have a resolution of 10,000 or greater. Such systems can separate an ion of mass 200.00 from an ion of mass 200.02. An instrument with a resolution of 800 will separate an ion of mass 800 from 801. Most clinical, environmental, and forensic applications have used the less expensive lower-resolution instruments.

Detectors

Almost all mass spectrometers detect ions by using electron multipliers. The impacting ion signal is amplified in the same manner as that described by Fig. 2-12 on p. 53. The detector is computer-interfaced to operate, record, and analyze the generated data.

Creation of Ion Fragments

Electron Ionization (EI)

Electron ionization (**EI,** electronic impact) is the most widely used method of ionization. For ionization to occur, the bombarding electrons must possess sufficient energy to displace an electron from the molecule's outer electron shell during the initial collision. The **ionization potential** of a molecule is the amount of energy required to displace that outer shell electron. Most organic compounds have ionization potentials in the 7 to 13 eV range. Thus the energy of the incoming ionization beam must exceed the ionization potential of the molecule that is being analyzed. Mass spectrometers are generally standardized on an ionization beam at 70 eV, which has sufficient energy to ionize incoming sample molecules efficiently. Additionally, bombardment at 70 eV imparts excess energy to the generated ions. This enhances their decomposition to secondary fragments that contain more structural information.

As gaseous sample molecules enter the ion source (see Fig. 4-15), the electron beam originating from a heated rhenium or tungsten filament bombards them. A small positive potential on the repeller plate focuses and repels the positive ions generated through the exit slit toward the mass analyzer. A much higher voltage potential is placed on one or more of the plates and is used to accelerate the velocity of the ions as they leave the exit slit. A focus slit is used to direct the ion's trajectory toward the mass analyzer.

Negative ions are also formed in the source. Such ions can be analyzed by reversing the voltage potentials of the repeller and accelerating plates. Compounds that can readily accommodate an extra electron such as halogen-containing drugs (or drugs derivatized with halogen-containing agents), polycyclic aromatics, and substituted phenols can generate significant negative ions, which allow sensitive detection by negative ion mass spectrometry. However, the resulting negative ion mass spectrum has fewer ion fragments, and these are usually at relatively low masses. Consequently, negative-ion EI provides less structural information than its positive-ion counterpart; therefore most applications center on positive-ion mass spectrometry.

Chemical Ionization

Chemical ionization (**CI**) is an indirect approach to sample molecule ion formation. A reagent gas is introduced into the source before the sample molecules enter. The 70 eV ionization beam ionizes the reagent gas molecules. When sample molecules enter the source, they collide with reagent gas ions, resulting in a charge transfer from the reagent gas ion to the sample.

The versatility of CI stems from its ability to select different reagent gases to influence the site and extent of sample ionization. Methane, isobutane, water, and ammonia are some of the more commonly encountered CI reagent gases; fragments generated can differ depending on both the reagent gas used and the chemical characteristics of the compound being analyzed. Choice of a particular reagent gas influences the ionization process. Several different mechanisms for charge transfer, such as proton transfer, charge exchange, or negative ionization, can occur. Proton transfer reactions and, to a lesser extent, negative ionization have received the most attention and widespread application.

Methane reagent gas exemplifies the proton transfer process. High-energy electron bombardment generates an abundance of CH_4^+ and CH_3^+ ions (Equation 4-5), which quickly react with excess methane gas to form stable CH_5^+ and $C_2H_5^+$ ions (Equations 4-6 and 4-7).

$$2CH_4 + 2e^- \rightarrow CH_4^+ + CH_3^+ + H^\bullet + 4e^- \qquad \text{Eq. 4-5}$$

$$CH_4^+ + CH_4 \rightarrow CH_5^+ + CH_3^\bullet \qquad \text{Eq. 4-6}$$

$$CH_3^+ + CH_4 \rightarrow C_2H_5^+ + H_2 \qquad \text{Eq. 4-7}$$

CH_5^+ and $C_2H_5^+$ are relatively stable adducts and constitute nearly 90% of the total methane ionization by the time the sample molecules enter the source. These ions react as Brönsted acids with most incoming sample molecules (M), protonating them to yield the quasimolecular ion $(MH)^+$ corresponding to their molecular weight plus one (Equations 4-8 and 4-9).

$$M + CH_5^+ \rightarrow MH^+ + CH_4 \quad \text{Eq. 4-8}$$

$$M + C_2H_5^+ \rightarrow MH^+ + C_2H_4 \quad \text{Eq. 4-9}$$

In a similar fashion, isobutane reagent gas yields a predominant number of *tert*-butyl reagent gas ions that protonate the sample molecules as follows:

$$M + C_4H_9^+ \rightarrow MH^+ + C_4H_8 \quad \text{Eq. 4-10}$$

CI is considered a **soft ionization** technique because of its low-energy transfer ionization process when compared with EI. Consequently, the quasimolecular ion produced is relatively stable and long lived when compared with the molecular ion produced in EI spectra. Because of this stability, the quasimolecular ion does not undergo as extensive fragmentation into secondary ion fragments as the molecular ion does in EI spectra. However, CI ionization does involve some energy transfer because the proton transfer reaction between the reagent gas ions and the sample molecule is an exothermic energy-producing process. The amount of energy transferred to the newly formed MH^+ ion is proportional to the exothermic reaction and determines the stability and hence survival of MH^+ in the source. The higher the exothermicity of the reaction, the more likely is MH^+ to decompose.

The formation of negative ions under CI conditions occurs through three primary pathways: electron capture, proton abstraction, and association. Of these three primary pathways, the electron capture (EC) process offers the most feasible approach for examining drugs and clinical samples. The EC ionization process takes place when the sample molecule captures a thermal or low-energy electron in the reagent gas plasma. For this to be the dominant process, the reagent gas must be one that generates low-energy electrons upon electron bombardment. Additionally, the gas itself must not form negative ions capable of reacting with the sample molecule. Methane fulfills these criteria. Upon ionization, methane forms CH_4^+ and CH_3^+ (see Equation 4-5) and low-energy electrons. Capture of these electrons by sample molecules and the subsequent decomposition of resultant negative ions produce the **negative-ion chemical ionization (NICI)** fragmentation pattern. An intense $(M{-}1)^-$ ion fragment is often generated. Very high sensitivity is characteristic of NICI. In many cases, the intensity of the base negative CI ion is 30 to 100 times greater than that of the base CI ion.[39] This can effectively extend routine detection levels to the femtogram level.

Mass Fragmentation

During the collision, energy is transferred from the ionization beam to the sample molecule. This resulting moiety can dissipate some of its excess energy by freeing its outer shell electron to give rise to a positively charged **molecular ion (M^+)** that corresponds to the molecular weight of the compound (Fig. 4-18). The molecular weight is an important piece of information obtained from a mass spectrum. The peak intensity of this molecular ion is directly proportional to the life span of the ion. A stable molecular ion lasts longer and hence generates an intense peak, whereas a short-lived ion generates a small peak. Most molecular ions are short lived and unstable because of their high energy level, and often they don't exist long enough to be detected. In such cases, the mass spectrum does not exhibit the molecular ion at all. In general, ions that can easily dissipate their excess energy internally, such as extensively conjugated fragments, are more stable and hence exist longer.

$$M + e^- \longrightarrow M^+ + 2e^-$$
$$M^+ \longrightarrow F_1 + F_2 + F_3^+ \ldots$$

Fig. 4-18 Electron ionization. *F,* Fragment; *M,* molecule; *M^+,* molecular ion.

In general, molecular ions are highly energized and thus inherently unstable. They dissipate their excess energy by breaking internal bonds and undergoing unimolecular decompositions that result in secondary ion fragments (F^+). Simultaneously, secondary fragments are formed by means of ion-molecule and ion-ion collisions that occur randomly in the ion source. Secondary fragments have lower masses; such fragments continue the process of dissipating their energy through further decomposition and by random collisions with other molecules and ions. The resulting effect is the formation of a large number of fragment ions with m/z values ranging from the molecular weight of the compound at the high end of the spectrum down to the lowest m/z values scanned. These fragments are detected and plotted according to their m/z ratios versus intensity to generate the mass spectrum of the compound. Fragmentation patterns provide a wealth of structural information about the molecule of interest. They provide the "**fingerprint**" specificity to make compound identification certain.

Spectral libraries are available to match these fingerprints and identify the test analyte. When there is no library match, the mass spectrum fragmentation pattern is examined for structural information. The initial investigation centers on matching the known molecular weight of the test molecule with the molecular ion that arises by the loss of the first electron. Subsequent fragmentation attributable to unimolecular decomposition and ion-molecule reactions yields other characteristic fragments that can help identify the chemical moieties present in the compound. In general, the higher m/z ion fragments are more helpful in compound identification than the lower ones. The reason is that higher m/z fragments represent fragmentation of the molecule of interest at the earlier stages of its breakdown in the ion source. Consequently, these fragments are closer to the molecule's original structure and are thus more "unique" than the lower m/z fragments. The lower m/z fragments are smaller parts of the molecule, and, although they can provide structural information, this information is less specific. Unfortunately, the most abundant ions in the EI mass spectra generally occur at low mass and may not necessarily be unique to the compound of interest. Low m/z ion data are still useful, provided that the compound being analyzed is pure. With either **GC/MS** or **LC/MS,** this requires good chromatographic separation and the avoidance of co-eluting interfering components.

Fig. 4-19 shows the postulated EI fragmentation decomposition of cocaine.[40] The molecular ion is m/z 303, and, although

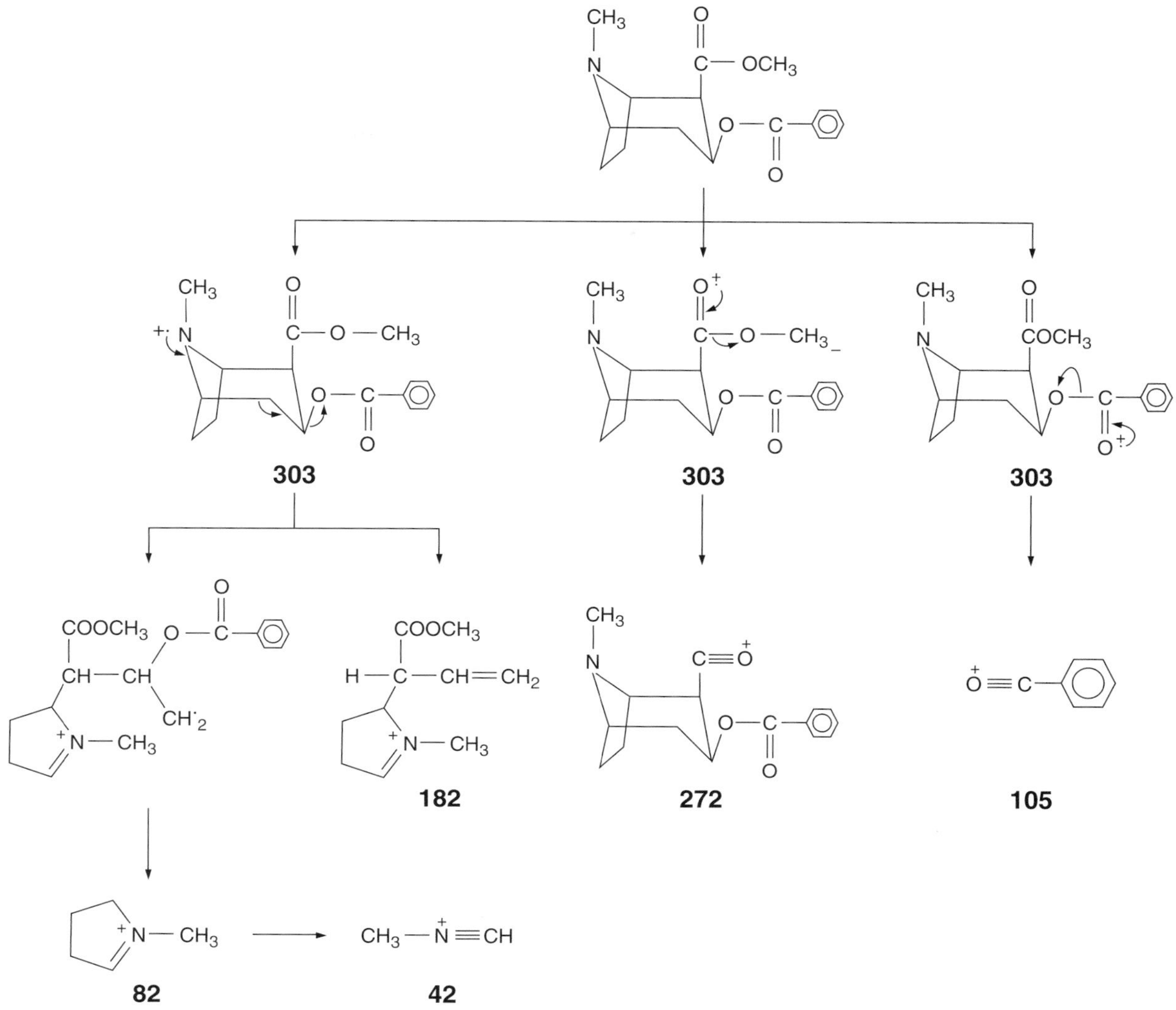

Fig. 4-19 Fragmentation pattern of cocaine.

weak, it is readily seen in the mass spectrum (see Fig. 4-13). The charge of the molecular ion is localized on the nitrogen atom and to a lesser extent on the two carbonyl oxygen atoms. Decomposition of the molecular ion occurs through several different pathways. Breakup of the molecular ion's six-membered ring with the loss of benzoic acid generates a relatively stable carbonium ion at m/z 182, which is seen as an intense fragment. The loss of the methoxyl moiety from the molecular ion generates the smaller fragment at m/z 272, and the aromatic carbonyl fragment at m/z 105 is also formed by cleavage from the molecular ion. The base peak is m/z 82 and represents the formation of a substituted pyrrole ring, which is very stable because of its highly resonant ring structure.

Certain elements that are often present in a wide variety of molecules, including drugs and their metabolites, have unique mass spectrometric behavior that imparts additional information. Nitrogen, for example, is the only commonly encountered element that has an even atomic mass and an odd valence. Thus, if the molecular ion has an even mass, it can be deduced that the compound of interest has no nitrogen atom or has an even number of nitrogen atoms. Additional structural information can be obtained from the mass spectrum when the compound of interest contains two or more abundant natural isotopes. Ion fragments containing halogen atoms have characteristic isotope clusters that arise from the two different isotopes present. For example, chlorine's natural isotopes are chlorine-35 and chlorine-37 with a relative abundance of 75.8% and 24.2%, respectively. Consequently, any fragments containing chlorine atoms always generate a characteristic pattern that consists of a doublet peak 2 atomic mass units (AMU) apart with a 3:1 ratio. Chlorine, bromine, and to a smaller degree, silicon and sulfur are the only elements with sufficiently abundant natural isotopes to generate useful information with low-resolution mass spectrometers. Another useful fact to remember is that carbon-13 to carbon-12 abundance is approximately 1.1%. Increasing the number of carbon atoms in an ion increases the probability that one of these atoms will be a ^{13}C isotope. The $(M + 1)^+/M^+$ ratio for a 10-carbon ion thus will exhibit 10 times the probability for ^{13}C, or $10 \times 1.1\% = 11\%$. Although an approximation, this

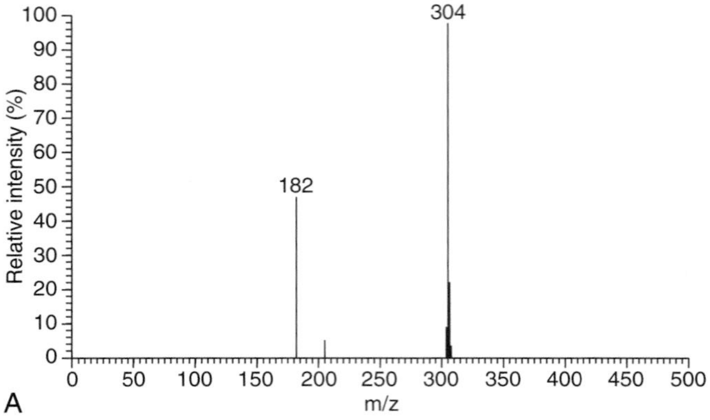

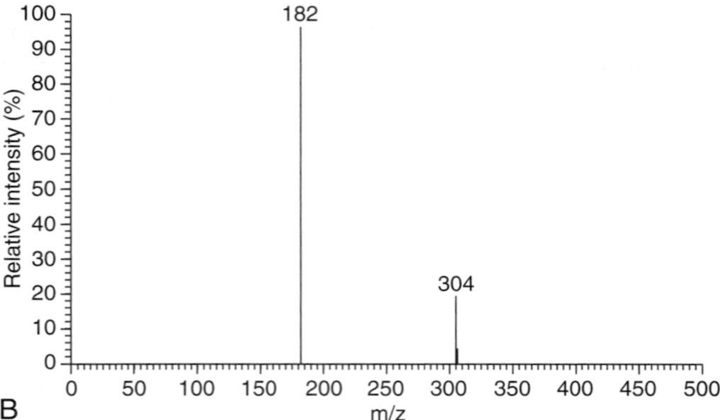

Fig. 4-20 A, Isobutane chemical ionization spectrum of cocaine. **B,** Methane chemical ionization spectrum of cocaine.

provides a means of determining the number of carbon atoms, which is paramount in interpreting the spectral lines of unknown organic compounds. To obtain more precise elemental composition, a high-resolution mass spectrometer is necessary.

Basic molecular structure and side chains of organic compounds can often be correlated to specific ion fragments in the mass spectrum. Metabolites frequently have similar structures and the same side chains as the parent compounds. Consequently, their mass spectra often contain similar or identical fragment ions. Chemically changing parent compounds by metabolism or by derivatization leads to anticipated fragment ions in the spectrum, making identification simpler. Such empirical pattern recognition observations are useful in the identification process, especially in the identification of drug metabolites and known poisons. Numerous molecular decomposition patterns of various chemical moieties have been systematically applied to interpretation of fragmentation patterns. A discussion of such interpretations is beyond the scope of this chapter; publications on this subject are available.[41]

A major advantage of CI spectra is their relative simplicity compared with the corresponding EI spectra. For example, the CI isobutane spectrum of cocaine (Fig. 4-20) is much simpler and contains few ions compared with the fragmentation patterns obtained by EI (see Fig. 4-13). The isobutane CI spectrum of cocaine is dominated by the quasimolecular ion that readily reveals the sample's molecular weight. As was discussed earlier, molecular weight is one of the most important pieces of information that may be obtained from the mass spectrum. Hence, CI is useful in obtaining molecular weight information that may not be always readily available by EI techniques. Other major CI fragmentations arise from the loss of protonated acid-labile groups from the quasimolecular ion. For example, benzoate esters (such as cocaine) may show the loss of benzoic acid, acetate esters the loss of acetic acid, and aliphatic alcohols the loss of water.

Comparison of Electron Ionization and Chemical Ionization

Sensitivity is another important factor that is affected by the ionization process. Typically, CI sensitivity can exceed that of EI by several orders of magnitude. This is attributable to CI's ability to concentrate **total ion current** into a small number of ions (because of the minimal fragmentation). Compare the cocaine CI fragmentation pattern with that obtained by EI. The CI spectrum (see Fig. 4-20) demonstrates that m/z 304 and 182 account for almost all the CI fragments generated. This is in stark contrast to the EI fragmentation (see Fig. 4-13) in which m/z 182 and 303 constitute only a small portion of the total number of fragments generated. As can be readily seen, the prominent CI ions typically have a higher response per unit weight of sample and hence greater sensitivity (compared with abundant EI ions). Additionally, such CI ions tend to have higher m/z values and hence are more unusual than the abundant EI ions, which tend to have a low m/z value. Notice that in the case of cocaine the base peak in EI is at a low mass (m/z 82), whereas the base peak with CI occurs at higher masses (m/z 182 with methane CI and m/z 304 with isobutane CI). This example also serves to demonstrate that the selection of CI reagent gas has a pronounced influence on the extent of fragmentation and the ultimate sensitivity of the analysis. Compounds that have different molecular weights generally give CI spectra with minimal overlap, enabling accurate identification of targeted compounds even when GLC fails to separate components of interest adequately.[42]

CI techniques should be viewed as complimentary to EI because they help minimize EI specificity gaps that may be encountered.[43] Incorporation of CI analyses in drug testing laboratories can be cost-effective because it can speed analytical analysis time by rapidly providing greater certainty of identification.

Negative ions produced under CI conditions are far more useful than those produced under EI conditions. Whereas negative ions in EI tend to have low mass fragments that impart little structural information, negative ions in CI tend to have more useful high-mass fragments. Information from NICI can also serve to complement information gained from positive-ion mass spectra generated under CI and EI conditions.

Analysis by Mass Spectrometry

Full-Scan Analysis

In the full-scan mode, the entire mass range of interest is repeatedly scanned. Scanning is programmed to start at the high m/z range and end at the low m/z value. In each scan, every ion fragment generated is monitored and displayed. The scan rate must be slow enough so that the detector can register a given fragment but fast enough so that multiple scans can occur during a given analysis. Multiple scans are necessary for the resulting ion statistics to be meaningful. The resulting mass spectrum, consisting of all ion fragments generated, offers a very high degree of specificity. In combination with mass spectrometry's high sensitivity, this full-scan fingerprint is extremely effective in providing positive identification of organic compounds such as drugs and their metabolites.[44]

Modern systems often rely on computer matching programs to identify unknown compounds. This is done by comparison of the acquired mass spectrum with an existing stored reference spectrum. A variety of different commercially available libraries exist. Many different library search algorithms are available to compare the unknown spectrum to existing stored reference spectra. Ten peak search, probability-based matching, forward or reverse search, purity search, and fit and reverse fit are commonly used search algorithms. Although a detailed description of search algorithms and libraries is beyond the scope of this chapter, a good discussion of the topic can be found elsewhere.[45,46]

Full-scan techniques are more demanding in terms of sample purity. Interfering or co-eluting compounds must be avoided. The presence of interfering compounds generates extraneous ions and complicates the resulting spectra. This can make identification difficult or even impossible. Consequently, most samples are purified before analysis is performed. Biological samples and those with particulate matter (such as organics in soil) need to be purified prior to mass spectrometric analysis. Common pre-analytical purification techniques utilized include: organic solvent extraction of components of interest from the aqueous matrix, recrystallization (if the sample is a solid), and purification by GC or LC separation prior to mass spectrometer analysis.

A total ion current (TIC) chromatogram is commonly generated when chromatographic separation is used. The total ion current is an integrated summary of all the mass ions produced. The resulting chromatographic output resembles the appearance of a conventional GLC chromatogram. The full-scan mass spectrum is typically generated at the top of the chromatographic peak to maximize sensitivity. However, multiple mass spectral lines can be generated from any part of the peak, which is helpful in assessing the purity and chromatographic resolution. Co-eluting components can be easily detected even in situations in which TIC peak shape is fully symmetrical. Although full-scan analysis offers the highest specificity, its sensitivity is limited. Scanning each fragment in the spectrum means that the detector spends significant time in regions where fragments give low-intensity adducts. Consequently, the same characteristics that make full-scan techniques highly specific are also responsible for limiting its sensitivity. Aspects that greatly influence sensitivity are discussed in greater detail later in this chapter.

Selected Ion Monitoring

Greater EI sensitivity can be obtained when the mass spectrometer is operated in the **selected ion monitoring (SIM)** mode, in which it monitors ion currents at only a few (generally three) preselected intense masses characteristic of the compound of interest. This increases the sensitivity of the response. Use of few ion fragments for compound identification is less specific than use of a **full scan** because all other ion fragments are discarded. This technique is frequently used for target compound identification applications such as forensic or clinical drugs of abuse analyses and is known by several names (such as SIM, selected, selective, or simultaneous ion monitoring; MID, multiple ion detection; and SMS, selective mass storage). Historically, the use of SIM techniques arose from sensitivity limitations of full-scan techniques in magnetic sector and quadrupole systems. For example, SIM analysis of cocaine can use ion fragments m/z 303, 182, and 82 (see Fig. 4-13). Selection of these three ions is preferred because of their relatively high intensity or uniqueness. The molecular ion at m/z 303 has a high m/z value and is considered unique, which helps increase the analytical specificity. The pyrrole ring with m/z 82 is a likely choice because of its high intensity (base peak). Although its relatively low m/z value makes it less specific, its intensity helps the SIM analysis achieve sensitivity at lower levels. It should be stressed that in SIM mode, all other ion fragments in the spectrum are lost, reducing the specificity of the analysis, particularly if other compounds generate ions with the same m/z value.

Often, SIM methods attempt to enhance specificity by comparing the relative ion intensities of major ions that are being monitored. This practice has been widely used in drugs of abuse testing and requires that the ratios of ion intensities in the unknown match, within ±20% of the standard. One limitation of this approach is that ion intensities and therefore ratios can vary depending on the amount of drug or metabolite present in the ion source. This can occur when the drug or metabolite concentrations are much higher or lower than those in the standard.[47]

Although identification in SIM techniques is less specific than in full-scan mode, it is adequate for many applications. However, care must be used because it is possible to incorrectly identify compounds when conditions are not optimized. For example, some drugs of abuse testing laboratories analyze amphetamine by means of GC/MS using m/z 44 as a quantification ion and m/z 58 as a qualifying ion.[48] These ions have low m/z values and are subject to potential interference from a variety of other compounds and background ion currents that may be present in the sample. For example, in addition to amphetamine, many other sympathomimetic amines exhibit a large peak at m/z 58, and carbon dioxide (a common background component) exhibits a peak at m/z 44. Significant identification errors can arise because commonly encountered legal drugs (such as ephedrine, phentermine, phenylpropanolamine, and other common over-the-counter [OTC] medications) have the same ion fragments as those selected to characterize illicit amphetamine. Such legal medications and OTC compounds are generally co-extracted in the sample preparation step, and their chromatographic retention times can be close to those of illicit drugs. If chromatography has shifted, the possibility of a false-positive or a false-negative result exists.

Quantitation

In MS, quantitative accuracy is best achieved by incorporating a known amount of an internal standard, which is added at the beginning of the analytical process (see p. 84). The internal standards should chemically resemble the test compounds as closely as possible so that their physical and chemical behavior matches those of the targeted analyte. This is the reason that, when available, deuterated analogues are used as internal standards. The technique of quantitation that uses chemicals different only in their isotope composition is termed **isotope dilution.**

In the case of drug analysis, the deuterated internal standard is the analyte with one or more hydrogen atoms substituted by deuterium atoms. This results in an internal standard that has very close characteristics in terms of polarity, extraction partition coefficient, derivatization, and chromatography compared with the drug itself (Fig. 4-21). In conventional GLC, a deuterated internal standard cannot be used because it must be chromatographically resolved from the compound of interest. In MS, this is not a problem because the atomic mass of a deuterium atom is 1 AMU greater than that of hydrogen. The deuterated internal standard has a different molecular weight and hence is differentiated from the drug by the difference in masses rather than in chromatographic retention time. Its fragmentation pattern will mimic that of the drug, but the fragments containing deuterium atoms will have a correspondingly higher m/z value.

The mass spectral SIM output displays only the ions that exhibit the m/z fragments that are being monitored. SIM quantitation simultaneously monitors the ion fragments of the compound and those of the internal standard. Fig. 4-21 shows **selected ion profiles** for two isotopes of silylated Δ^9-tetrahydrocannabinol analyzed by GC/MS. The internal standard contains the deuterated isotope (d_3), which is monitored at m/z 390. The ion profile of the compound of interest is the unlabeled analog, which is monitored at m/z 387. Chromatographic retention times of the two isotopes are essentially the same, and their identification is accomplished by taking advantage of the difference in molecular weights of the ion fragments. A quantitative value is obtained when the peak area or intensity of the compound of interest is compared with that of the internal standard. This ratio is then used to generate a quantitative value from a previously established calibration curve.

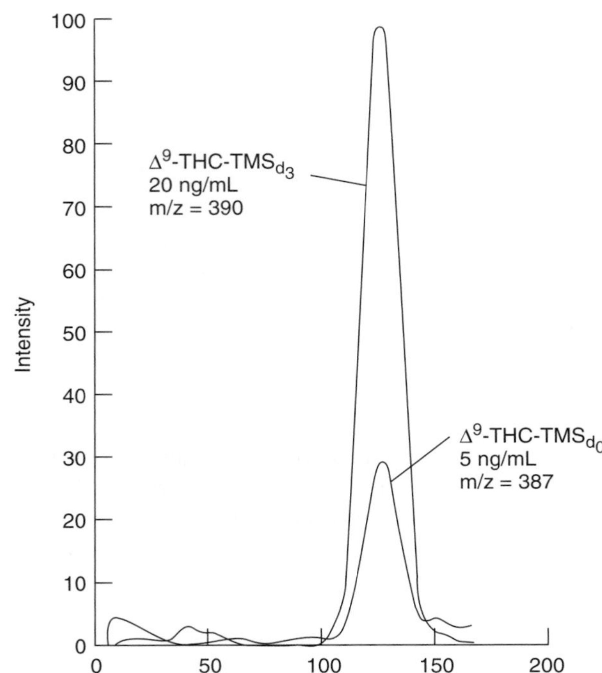

Fig. 4-21 Selected ion monitoring plot for quantitation of Δ^9-tetrahydrocannabinol in plasma. Undeuterated (d_0) and deuterated (d_3) drugs were monitored. (From Saferstein R: *Forensic Science Handbook,* Englewood Cliffs, NJ, 1982, Prentice Hall.)

Separation Techniques

Gas Chromatography/Mass Spectrometry (GC/MS)

The combination of GLC separation versatility coupled with specificity and sensitivity of MS makes GC/MS one of the most powerful techniques available for the identification of organic compounds.

The main technical issue in coupling these techniques arose from the incompatibility of pressure requirements. GLC requires a carrier-gas flow at approximately atmospheric pressure to move the sample through the column. Mass spectrometers, on the other hand, require high vacuum (10^{-5} to 10^{-7} torr) to operate effectively. Molecular jet separators combined with differential vacuum pumps have been used to evacuate the carrier gas selectively just before the GLC effluent entry into the ion source of the mass spectrometer.[38] Capillary columns have simpler interface requirements because capillary columns function effectively at much lower carrier-gas flow rates, which are within the pumping capacity of the mass spectrometer. Consequently, capillary column effluents can flow directly into the ion source.

Two different mass spectrometer data outputs are commonly obtained in GC/MS. The first, the TIC chromatogram, represents the integration of total ion current versus time of elution from the GLC column. The full-scan mass spectrum is the second output. This is used to validate the purity of a peak or the identity of a shoulder or minor peak component generating that ion current. The mass spectrum generated can be a full scan or an SIM. In either case, sensitivity is maximized when the mass spectrum is generated at the apex of the TIC peak. TIC can also be monitored exclusively in the SIM mode, which generates a selective ion chromatogram. This is a common practice in target compound identification applica-

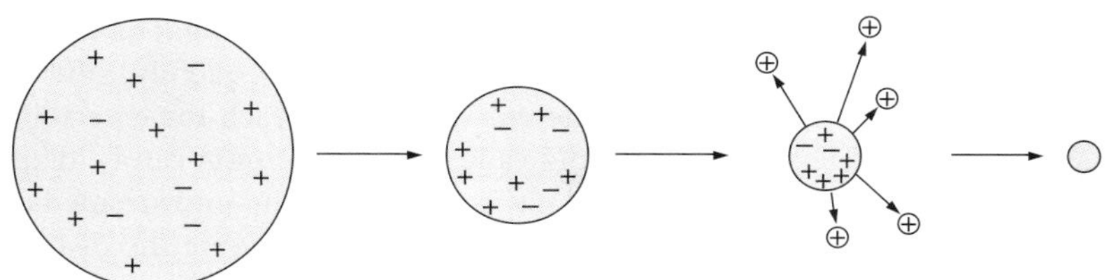
Original droplet contains ions of both polarities with one being predominant
As the solvent evaporates, the electric field increases and the ions move to the surface
At some critical field value ions are emitted from the droplet
Involatile residue remains as a dry particle

Fig. 4-22 Diagram of ion-evaporation process. (From *The API Book,* Eden Prairie, MN, 1992, Perkin-Elmer Sciex.)

tions. The output is then composed of only the ions with the m/z value being monitored. SIM quantitations rely on this technique by simultaneously monitoring the ion fragments of the compound of interest and those of the internal standard.

Two-Dimensional GC/MS (2-D GC/MS)

A relatively new technique that uses **two-dimensional gas chromatography** (GC/GC) was commercialized by Agilent in 2003. It is based on coupling two GC columns prior to MS detection to effect faster separation with greater resolution and enhanced sensitivity. A microfluidics **Deans switch** is used as a modulator to connect and control the mobile phase gas flow between the two GC columns.[49] The Deans switch modulator is equipped with a small storage volume that can be filled periodically with effluent from the first GC column, which is then swept at a high flow rate into a second GC column. The process of alternatively storing and then injecting portions of the first column effluent into a second column is termed GC/GC. The two-column system employed in GC/GC has a very high efficiency (large number of theoretical plates), which yields a dramatic increase in resolution with the added benefit of significant sensitivity enhancement.[50-52]

Liquid Chromatography/Mass Spectrometry (LC/MS)

Another useful combination consists of MS coupled to HPLC; which is suitable for the analysis of large, polar, ionic, thermally unstable, and nonvolatile compounds. It eliminates the need for the time-consuming chemical modifications often required for gas chromatographic separation. The interface of LC with MS requires removal of the less volatile mobile phase before mass spectrometric analysis is begun. This requires methods that can be used to volatilize the test samples into the gaseous state before they can be analyzed by MS.

Thermospray is one approach for connecting LC to an MS. The tip of the capillary tube from which the HPLC **eluate** emerges is heated by application of a high voltage. By optimizing the temperature, small charged droplets can be made to be ejected (sprayed) from the end of the tube into the MS ion source.

Thermospray relies on an ion-evaporation process in which ions are emitted from a liquid into the gas phase.[53] In theory, a charged droplet contains the solvent plus positive and negative ions, with ions of one polarity being dominant. The difference is the net charge; it has been postulated that the excess charge resides at the surface of the droplet. As the solvent evaporates, the electrical field at the surface of the droplet increases because of the decreasing radius. If the droplet evaporates far enough, a critical field is reached at which sample ions from the surface are emitted. Fig. 4-22 illustrates the ion-evaporation process.

IonSpray (also known as electrospray, ES) is a related technique suited to the introduction of thermally labile, complex, polar compounds into the mass spectrometer. It differs from thermospray in that it does not use heat to produce the spray, and it can readily occur at atmospheric pressure. Electospray generally operates in high vacuum, although it can be used at pressures up to atmospheric. It also generates a quasimolecular ion and is especially suitable for polar and thermally labile compounds. In addition to HPLC, IonSpray can be interfaced with other separation techniques such as capillary zone electrophoresis to allow the analysis of complex biological samples.

Atmospheric Pressure Ionization

Atmospheric pressure ionization (API) is a technique that allows the introduction of samples into the mass spectrometer at normal atmospheric pressure.[54] This facilitates MS analyses of large molecules such as proteins which cannot be vaporized effectively in the conventional high vacuum MS environment. API-MS ES has revolutionized proteomic analyses because such applications could previously not be analyzed by MS. Electrospray is the most versatile API-MS specimen introduction technique and is useful for analyzing samples that have multiple charges, such as proteins, peptides, and oligonucleotides, as well as for analyzing samples that are singly charged. It can be used to measure the molecular weights of most polymers, peptides, proteins, and oligonucleotides up to 150,000 D quickly and with high mass accuracy. API does not need high vacuum volatilization, which enables LC analyses of large relatively nonvolatile molecules. In biopharmaceutical and proteomic applications, chemists use API-ES to speed protein characterization, to accurately identify and characterize posttranslational modifications to proteins, and to quickly confirm the molecular weight of synthetic peptides.[55,56] Computerized MS with LC separation and flexible ionization techniques is the primary tool in the rapid progress of gene sequencing.[57,58]

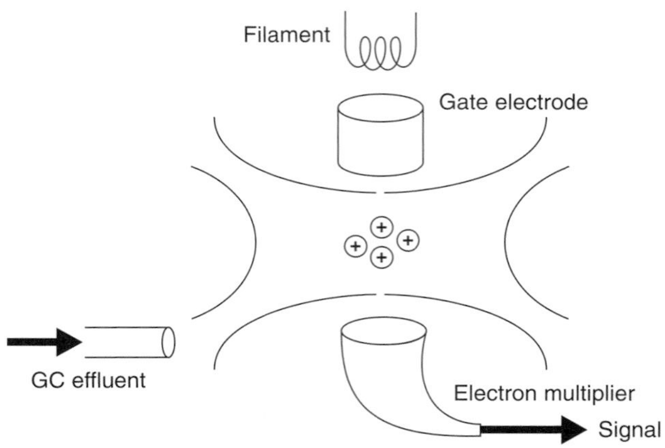

Fig. 4-23 The ion trap mass spectrometer.

Solids Probe

Direct MS with solids probe sample introduction has been used by toxicologists for many years to rapidly identify targeted compounds.[59] This technique is advantageous for compounds of low volatility, which can be introduced directly into the ion source. Another advantage of solids probe MS is that it eliminates the chromatographic separation step, allowing for very rapid analysis. MS analysis probing solids has been used extensively in the EI and CI modes with pure compounds. For biological specimens, CI is especially practical because compound identification can be done according to molecular weight.

Other Mass Spectrometers

Ion Trap Detector

Ion trap mass spectrometers combine the functions of an ion source with those of a mass analyzer. This is done in a simple three-electrode assembly that consists of a ring electrode and two end caps (Fig. 4-23). Electrons from a heated filament are pulsed by a gate electrode into the central cavity, where they ionize the sample molecules, resulting in conventional EI fragmentation patterns. The unique feature of ion trap mass spectrometers is that they "trap" and "store" ions generated over time within the ion source cavity. This is done through application of a radio frequency voltage to the central ring electrode, which causes ions of interest to be trapped and accumulated over time in the ion source. The trapped ions are then mass selectively ejected from the cavity according to their m/z ratio onto the electron multiplier, where they are detected. The effective trapping and accumulation of ions results in concentration of the ions of interest; consequently, very high sensitivities are obtained with an ion trap detector (ITD). The ion trap's superior sensitivity allows the user to obtain full-scan mass spectra with limits of detection comparable with those of SIM analyses in conventional quadrupole detectors.

Time-of-Flight MS

The **time-of-flight (TOF) mass spectrometer** is based on the principle that ions generated in the source must travel a fixed distance to reach the detector. The accelerating voltage propels the ions into a drift tube that is typically 1 m long. The velocity of ions is proportional to their mass. Consequently, different mass ions travel at different speeds and reach the detector at different times. The m/z value of any given ion can be determined mathematically when an accurate measurement is made of the time that the ion takes to traverse the distance and reach the detector. Currently, this type of mass spectrometer is used in research for the analysis of complex biopolymers at the picomole level. This type of instrument used with laser desorption ionization is suited for the measurement of high-mass molecules and can determine the molecular weights of peptides, intact proteins, and glycoproteins 300,000 D in size. TOF systems play a significant role in advancing the science of gene sequencing.

Tandem Mass Spectrometry

In general, improving the selectivity and detection limits of instrumental techniques can be achieved through extensive sample pretreatment (extraction, derivatization, chromatographic separation, and so on) before mass spectrometry is begun. An alternative approach to improve detection limits and enhance selectivity is the coupling of two or more analytical techniques in tandem.[60] GC/MS, GC/MS/IR, MS/MS, and GC/MS/MS are examples (as compared with MS alone).

Because of the minimum need for sample preparation, applications of **tandem mass spectrometry (MS/MS)** provide (1) increased speed of analysis; (2) decreased cost per sample; (3) improved limits of detection in complex mixtures; and (4) rapid, sensitive, and selective rapid analysis of complex mixtures.[61,62] Solids probe MS/MS can be performed on drugs that are difficult to chromatograph and hence cannot be run on conventional GC/MS. In tandem MS/MS, a mixture is introduced into the ion source of the first MS, where ionization of the mixture produces ions characteristic of the individual drug components, termed **parent ions.** A characteristic parent ion of the targeted drug of interest is then selected and isolated. This separates the analyte of interest from the other mixture components and can be thought of as analogous to the chromatographic separation step of GC/MS. The targeted parent ion is then subjected to second MS analysis, at which time it is further fragmented into secondary ion fragments termed **daughter ions.** This step is analogous to the fragmentation that occurs during the ionization step in GC/MS. Mass analysis of the daughter ions by the second mass analyzer provides a unique and highly specific identification of the targeted parent ion.

Fig. 4-24 demonstrates the schema of a tandem mass spectrometer. It consists of two mass analyzers connected sequentially. A collision chamber for fragmentation of selected ions is situated between the two mass analyzers. Although different types of mass spectrometers can be combined, the **triple-stage quadruple** configuration is one of the more popular. Many applications use CI techniques for the initial ionization to generate an intense quasimolecular ion fragment. The ion selected should be as specific and as intense as possible. This ion is then subjected to collisions with inert gas in the collision chamber. The second mass analyzer then separates the result-

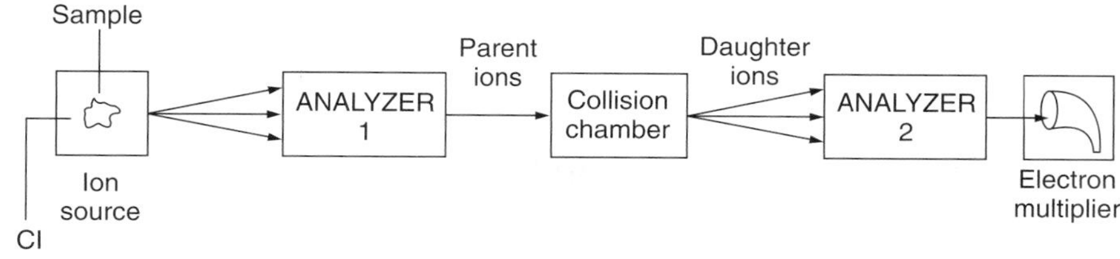

Fig. 4-24 Schema of a tandem mass spectrometer (MS/MS). *CI,* Chemical ionization. (From Yinon Y: *Forensic Mass Spectrometry,* Boca Raton, FL, 1987, CRC Press.)

ing daughter ions. Daughter ions' spectral lines resemble conventional EI spectral lines and are used for actual compound identification. MS/MS effectively generates highly characteristic fragmentation of a specific ion.

In summary, the first MS analysis is used to achieve separation of a mixture into components, a process performed by the GC in conventional GC/MS. With MS/MS, however, this separation process is instantaneous, whereas with GC/MS it can take 5 to 15 minutes. This time advantage is the feature that gives MS/MS the potential for very rapid analysis. Whereas the throughput of samples in conventional GC/MS may typically consist of four to six samples per hour, in MS/MS, 60 samples per hour can be analyzed. Additional time efficiency is gained because sample extraction and derivatization can be drastically minimized and in some cases totally avoided.

Forensic Drug Testing

In 1987, the Department of Health and Human Services (DHHS) charged the National Institute of Drug Abuse (NIDA) to develop and implement a laboratory accreditation program for laboratories that test government workers for drugs of abuse. The need for regulation arose from the fact that different laboratories were using different testing methods and performance standards to designate a result as positive for drugs of abuse. Thus, quality and reliability of results varied greatly.

Regulations[63] issued in 1988 covered all aspects of drugs of abuse testing. These included personnel requirements, security of facilities, chain-of-custody (COC), specimen handling, record keeping, confidentiality of results, proficiency testing, quality control (QC), independent inspection of facilities, and analytical testing requirements. The NIDA project, later called the **Substance Abuse and Mental Health Services Administration (SAMHSA)** program, has successfully implemented a rigorous accreditation program while propagating these standards; laboratories that fail to meet the standards have been decertified from the program. As of 2008, SAMHSA's National Laboratory Certification Program (NLCP) had certified approximately 40 laboratories. The goal of the program is to ensure that labs do not generate false-positive results, and that the results generated can stand up to legal challenges. Consequently, the term *forensic* drugs-of-abuse testing is used. The SAMHSA/NIDA analytical protocols for the detection of drugs of abuse in urine are based upon the use of two independent analytical techniques as follows:

1. A sensitive initial screening procedure to identify negative specimens and to select presumptive positive specimens for further testing. Screening had to be done using a U.S. Food and Drug Administration (FDA)-registered immunoassay technique.
2. A highly specific confirmatory technique that is at least as sensitive as the initial screen for confirmation of presumptive positive results. The confirmation method was limited to GC/MS.

Both screening and confirmation steps are incorporated into a forensic urine drug detection program in which the consequences of such an analysis will be the basis of actions taken against the individual who supplied the sample.[64] Because of the potential negative effect on the individual, only rigorous and conclusive procedures are used. GC/MS is generally accepted as a rigorous confirmation technique because it provides the best level of confidence in the result.[65]

It is worthwhile to remember that GC/MS is a technique that combines GLC separation with mass spectrometric detection. This means that good GC/MS results are highly dependent on good chromatographic separations. Although it may seem self-evident, many users encounter GC/MS problems that could be readily avoided by optimizing chromatographic and cleanup parameters. For several of the SAMHSA-regulated drugs, derivatization is necessary to increase the compound's volatility and optimize the chromatographic process.[47,66] Deuterated internal standards are used and are added to the biological samples before the extraction process is begun.

Misconceptions

Two widespread misconceptions about mass spectrometry are (1) that GC/MS is a specific method and (2) that GC/MS is 100% accurate. GC/MS is in fact an instrumental analytical technique with many variations and a diverse variety of instrumental configurational possibilities. Countless methods are based on GC/MS techniques, each with its own set of advantages and disadvantages. Some GC/MS methods may be appropriate for a given analyte, whereas others may not be. Although forensic testing laboratories are required to use GC/MS, they have great flexibility and freedom in selecting instrumentation, mode of operation, and actual analytical methods. When a correct method is performed correctly, it will result in the positive identification of a drug or metabolite. The result will be legally defensible if appropriate QC is part of the laboratory's analysis. The QC program should include the analysis of threshold-cutoff standards, drug-free samples, blind controls, and known controls that contain drugs below and above the threshold value with each batch of samples. In addition, forensic requirements call for strict chain of custody and laboratory security. Such requirements are part of the forensic package and are necessary because of the implications of laboratory results for job applicants, employees, and companies, and because of potential legal challenges to the laboratory's results. When all these aspects of testing are incorporated, the lab results are legally defensible.

REFERENCES

1. Meyer VR: *Practical High-Performance Liquid Chromatography*, ed 3, New York, 1998, Wiley & Sons.
2. Katz E et al, editors: *Handbook of HPLC*, New York, 1998, Marcel Dekker.
3. Wilson ID, editor: *Encyclopedia of Separation Science*, San Diego, 2000, Academic Press.
4. Majors RE, Carr PW: Glossary of liquid-phase separation terms, LCGC 19:124, 2001.
5. Snyder LR, Glajch JL, Kirkland JJ: *Practical HPLC Method Development*, New York, 1988, Wiley & Sons.
6. Ghrist BFD, Cooperman BS, Snyder LR: Design of optimized high-performance liquid chromatographic gradients for the separation of either small or large molecules. I. Minimizing errors in computer simulations, J Chromatogr 459:43, 1988.
7. Swadesh JK, editor: *HPLC Practical and Industrial Applications*, ed 2, Boca Raton, FL, 2001, CRC Press.
8. Snyder LR, Glajch JL, Kirkland JJ: Theoretical basis for a systematic optimization of mobile phase selectivity in liquid chromatography, J Chromatogr 218: 299, 1981.
9. Szepesi G: *How to Use Reverse-Phase HPLC*, New York, 1992, VCH.
10. Kazakevich Y: *HPLC for Pharmaceutical Scientists*, New York, 2007, Wiley & Sons.
11. Forgács E, Cserháti T: *Molecular Basis of Chromatographic Separation*, Boca Raton, FL, 1997, CRC Press.
12. Turkova J: *Bioaffinity Chromatography*, ed 2, Amsterdam, 1993, Elsevier.
13. Scouten WH: *Affinity Chromatography: Bioselective Adsorption on Inert Matrices*, St. Louis, 1992, Sigma-Aldrich.
14. Hage DS: Affinity chromatography: a review of clinical applications, Clin Chem 45:593, 1999.
15. Special review edition devoted to enantiomer separation, J Chromatogr A 906:1, 2001.
16. Unger KK, editor: *Packings and Stationary Phases in Chromatographic Analysis*, New York, 1990, Marcel Dekker.
17. Majors RE: Advances in the design of HPLC packings, LCGC 18:586, 2000.
18. Anderson DJ: High-performance liquid chromatography (advances in packing materials), Anal Chem 67:475R, 1995.
19. Mikes O, Coupek J: Organic supports. In Gooding KM, Regnier FE, editors: *HPLC of Biological Macromolecules*, New York, 1990, Marcel Dekker.
20. Sadek PC: *Troubleshooting HPLC Systems*, New York, 2000, Wiley & Sons.
21. de Villiers A et al: Evaluation of ultra performance liquid chromatography, J Chromatogr 1127:60, 2006.
22. Leandeo C et al: Ultra-performance liquid chromatography for the determination of pesticide residues in foods by tandem mass spectrometry, J Chromatogr 1144, 161, 2007.
23. Dolan J, Upchurch P: *Interchangeability of HPLC Fittings*, Oak Harbor, WA, 1983, Upchurch Scientific; also LC 2:20, 1984, and 3:92, 1985.
24. Scott RPW: *Chromatographic Detectors: Design, Function, and Operation*, New York, 1996, Marcel Dekker.
25. Parriott D, editor: *A Practical Guide to HPLC Detection*, San Diego, 1993, Academic Press.
26. Lingeman H, Underberg WJM, editors: *Detection-Oriented Derivatization Techniques in Liquid Chromatography*, New York, 1990, Marcel Dekker.
27. Lunn G, Hellwig LC: *Handbook of Derivatization Reactions for HPLC*, New York, 1998, Wiley & Sons.
28. Anderson DJ: High-performance liquid chromatography, Anal Chem 63:213R, 1991.
29. De Leenheer AP, Lambert WE, Van Bocxlaer JF, editors: *Modern Chromatographic Analysis of Vitamins*, ed 3, New York, 2000, Marcel Dekker.
30. Willett J, Kealy D: *Gas Chromatography*, New York, 1987, Wiley & Sons.
31. McNair HM, Miller JA: *Basic Gas Chromatography*, New York, 1998, Wiley & Sons.
32. McReynolds WO: Characterization of some liquid phases, J Chromatogr Sci 8:685, 1970.
33. Siuzdak G: *Mass Spectrometry in Biotechnology*, ed 2, San Diego, 2006, MCC Press.
34. Wong HY: *Therapeutic Drug Monitoring and Toxicology*, Chromatographic Science Series, vol 32, New York, 1985, Marcel Dekker.
35. Bourne S, et al: Performance characteristics of a real-time direct deposition gas chromatography/Fourier transform infrared spectrometry system, Anal Chem 62:2448, 1990.
36. Beceiro-Gonzalez E et al: Optimization and validation of a solid-phase microextraction method for the simultaneous determination of different types of pesticides in water by GC/MS, J Chromatogr 1141:165, 2007.
37. Forman DT: Role of the laboratory in diagnosis of organic acidurias, Ann Clin Lab Sci 21:85, 1991.
38. DeHoffman E, Stroobant V: *Mass Spectrometry: Principles and Applications*, ed 2, New York, 2001, Wiley & Sons.
39. Niessen WMA: *Liquid Chromatography–Mass Spectrometry*, ed 3, Boca Raton, FL, 2006, CRC Press.
40. Levine B: Principles of toxicology, AACC 227, 1999.
41. McLafferty FW: *Interpretation of Mass Spectra*, ed 3, Mill Valley, CA, 1980, University Science Book.
42. Lehrer M: Application of gas chromatography/mass spectrometry instrument techniques to forensic urine drug testing, Clin Lab Med 10:271, 1990.
43. deJong EG, Maes RA, van Rossum JM: Why do doping control labs need MS/MS? Presented at the International Symposium on Applied Mass Spectrometry in the Health Sciences, Barcelona, Spain, September 28, 1987.
44. Deutsch DG: *Analytical Aspects of Drug Testing, Chemical Analysis Series*, New York, 1989, Wiley & Sons.
45. Moffat AC et al: *Clarke's Analysis of Drugs and Poisons*, London, 2004, Pharmaceutical Press.
46. Aebi B, Werner B: Advances in the use of mass spectral libraries for forensic toxicology, J Anal Toxicol 26:149, 2002.
47. Peat MA: Analytical and technical aspects of testing for drug abuse: confirmatory procedures, Clin Chem 34:471, 1988.
48. Hewlett-Packard technical application: *GC/MS Confirmation of Amphetamines*, publication #23-5954-8146, Waltham, MA, 1987, Hewlett-Packard.
49. Mohler RE et al: Total-transfer, valve-based comprehensive two-dimensional GC, Analytica Chimica Acta 555:68, 2006.
50. Seeley JV et al: Microfluidic deans switch for comprehensive two-dimensional GC, Anal Chem 79:1840, 2007.
51. Apps P: Low cost, robust, in-house hardware for heart cutting two-dimensional GC, J Separation Sci 29:2338, 2006.
52. Quimby BD et al: Capillary flow technology for gas chromatography: reinvigorating a mature analytical discipline, LC/GC 25:4, 2007.
53. Pramanik BN, Ganguly AK: On the evaporation of small ions from charged droplets. In *Applied Electrospray Mass Spectrometry*, ed 1, New York, 2002, Marcel Dekker.
54. *The API Book*, Eden Prairie, MN, 1992, Perkin-Elmer Sciex.

55. Andregg RJ: Comprehensive on-line LC/LC/MS of proteins, Anal Chem 69:1518, 1997.
56. Premstaller A et al: High performance liquid chromatography–electrospray ionization mass spectrometry using monolithic capillary columns for proteomic studies, Anal Chem 73:2390, 2001.
57. Chong BE et al: Differential screening and mass mapping of proteins from premalignant and cancer cell lines using non-porous reversed-phase HPLC coupled with mass spectrometric analysis, Anal Chem 73:1219, 2001.
58. Udiavar S et al: The use of multidimensional liquid-phase separations and mass spectrometry for the detailed characterization of posttranslational modifications in glycoproteins, Anal Chem 70:3572, 1998.
59. Lehrer M, Karmen A: Chemical ionization mass spectrometry for rapid assay of drugs in serum, J Chromatogr 126:615, 1976.
60. Yost RA, Johnson JV: Tandem mass spectrometry for trace analysis, Anal Chem 57:758A, 1995.
61. Lee MS, Yost RA: Rapid identification of drug metabolites with tandem mass spectrometry, Biomed Environ Mass Spectrometry 15:193, 1988.
62. Weiss MD: Chemistry is winning the war against crime, Industrial Chemistry 15:28, 1988.
63. Federal Register: *Mandatory Guidelines for Federal Workplace Drug Testing: Final Guidelines,* April 11, 1988.
64. Lehrer M: Drug screening in the workplace, Clin Lab Med 7:389, 1987.
65. Hoyt DW et al: Drug testing in the workplace—are methods legally defensible? JAMA 258:504, 1987.
66. Hawks RL, Chiang CN: *Urine Testing for Drugs of Abuse,* National Institute of Drug Abuse Monogr no. 73, DHHS publ no (ADM) 87-1481, Washington, DC, 1987, DHHS.

BIBLIOGRAPHY

Books

American Society of Testing Materials: *ASTM Standards on Chromatography,* ed 2, ASTM Subcommittee E19.07 on Compilation of Chromatographic Methods, Philadelphia, 1989, ASTM.

Cazes J: *Encyclopedia of Chromatography* (Den New Dekker Encyclopedias), New York, 2001, Marcel Dekker.

Fried B, Sherma J: *Practical Thin-Layer Chromatography: A Multidisciplinary Approach*, New York, 1996, CRC Press.

Fritz JS, Gjerdec DT: *Ion Chromatography*, ed 3, New York, 2000, Wiley & Sons.

Grob RL: *Modern Practice of Gas Chromatography,* ed 2, New York, 1985, Wiley & Sons.

Heftman E: *Chromatography: Fundamentals and Applications of Chromatography and Related Differential Migration Methods,* ed 5, Journal of Chromatography Library, vols 51 A and B, New York, 1992, Elsevier Science Publishers.

Hermanson GT, Mallia AK, Smith PK: *Immobilized Affinity Ligand Techniques*, New York, 1997, Academic Press.

McNair HM, Miller JM: *Basic Gas Chromatography* (techniques in analytical chemistry), New York, 1991, Wiley & Sons.

Papadoyannis IN: *HPLC in Clinical Chemistry,* Chromatographic Science Series, vol 54, New York, 1990, Marcel Dekker.

Sherma J, Fried B, editors: *Thin Layer Chromatography,* Chromatographic Science Series, vol 55, New York, 1990, Marcel Dekker.

Snyder LR, Glajch JL, Kirkland JJ: *Practical HPLC Method Development,* New York, 1988, Wiley & Sons.

Weston A, Brown PR: *HPLC and CE: Principles and Practice*, New York, 1997, Academic Press.

Comprehensive Abstracts, Journals, and Series in Chromatography

Advances in Chromatography, New York, Marcel Dekker, Inc.

Analytical Abstracts, London, Royal Society of Chemistry.

Chemical Abstracts, Columbus, Ohio, American Chemical Society.

Chromatographia, New York, Pergamon Press.

Chromatographic Reviews, Amsterdam, Elsevier Scientific Publishing Co.

Chromatographic Science Series, New York, Marcel Dekker, Inc.

Chromatography Symposium Series, New York, Elsevier Scientific Publishing Co.

Gas and Liquid Chromatography Abstracts, Barking, Essex, Applied Science Publishers.

Gas Chromatography Abstracts, London, Butterworth & Co.

Journal of Chromatography, New York, Elsevier Scientific Publishing Co.

Journal of Chromatography Library, New York, Elsevier Scientific Publishing Co.

Journal of Chromatographic Science, Niles, IL, Preston Publications.

Journal of High Resolution Chromatography and Chromatography Communications, Heidelberg, NY, Muthing Press.

Journal of Liquid Chromatography, New York, Marcel Dekker, Inc.

Progress in Thin-Layer Chromatography and Related Methods, Ann Arbor, MI, Lewis Publishers.

INTERNET SITES

www.chromatographyonline.com

www.spectroscopynow.com

www.fda.gov/cder/guidance/cmc3.pdf—Center for Drug Evaluation and Research (need Adobe Acrobat)

www.chromatograhyonline.com/lcgc/

www.separationsnow.com

http://gc.discussing.info

www.asms.org—American Society for Mass Spectrometry

www.sisweb.com/mslinks.htm

www.agilent.com/chem

www.bmss.org.uk/education.htm

www.ionsource.com

Laboratory Analysis of Hemoglobin Variants

Michael Nardi

5

Chapter

Chapter Outline

Key Terms

See also Chapter 40.

α-like globin gene cluster A cluster of genes (ζ, α-2, and α-1) on chromosome 16, each of which codes for a positively charged globin chain, which forms a dimer with a β-like globin chain.

β-like globin gene cluster A cluster of genes (ε, γG, γA, δ, and β) on chromosome 11, each of which codes for a negatively charged globin chain, which forms a dimer with an α-like globin chain.

Hemoglobin (Hb) The major component of the red blood cell whose main function is to carry oxygen to human tissues; it is a heterotetramer that is composed of 2 α-like/2 β-like globin chain dimers.

Hemoglobin electrophoresis Hemoglobin preparation from washed and lysed red blood cells is applied to a membrane and exposed to an electrical field to allow the separation of normal and abnormal hemoglobin fractions on the basis of their charge.

Hemoglobin fraction In the normal adult, there are 3 major fractions: Hb A ($\alpha2\beta2$), Hb F ($\alpha2\gamma2$), and Hb A2 ($\alpha2\delta2$).

Hemoglobin variant A qualitative defect in the hemoglobin molecule that generally results from a single amino acid substitution caused by a mutation in the molecule.

Hemoglobinopathy A qualitative or quantitative abnormality in the production of the hemoglobin molecule.

Thalassemia A quantitative defect in the hemoglobin molecule that results from a deletion or a mutation in the molecule.

Methods on Evolve

Iron and TIBC
Ferritin

Hemoglobin (Hb), the most abundant protein found in erythrocytes (red blood cells [RBCs]), functions to carry oxygen to tissue. Hemoglobin is a heterotetramer composed of two α-like and two β-like globin chains, to each of which a heme group holding an iron molecule and a porphyrin ring is attached (see Chapter 40). Abnormalities of the hemoglobin molecule are called hemoglobinopathies.

Hemoglobinopathies are the most common monogeneic disease known to man. Sickle cell disease and **thalassemias** are seen most frequently, most likely the result of environmental pressure to provide a protective effect against malaria. Approximately 5% to 7% of the world's populations are carriers of some kind of inherited disorder of hemoglobin.[1] They can be divided into two groups. The first group is hemoglobin variants, of which presently more than 1000 variants are known.[2] More than 95% of these known variants have arisen from a single amino acid residue substitution in one of the chain types, with more than 60% involving the β-globin chain. Hemoglobin variants are generally qualitative defects that most often are detected by electrophoretic techniques. Accompanying clinical symptoms depend on the site of the mutation, with the vast majority not causing any clinical or hematological problems.

The second group is the thalassemias, which result from mutations or deletions of a specific globin gene that produce a quantitative abnormality (i.e., complete loss or significant reduction in production of the affected globin gene product). The α- and β-thalassemias are the most common and the most clinically and hematologically significant of the thalassemias. They generally are diagnosed by quantification of the minor **hemoglobin fractions,** Hb A2 and Hb F. Depending on the number of genes lost, the clinical and hematological consequences of the thalassemia that is present can range from benign to lethal.[1]

Certain variant hemoglobins, such as Hb E, Hb Constant Spring, and Hb Lepore, share features of structural hemoglobinopathies and thalassemias (i.e., production of structurally abnormal globin at a decreased rate or with reduced stability).

Many clinical indications suggest the need for testing for the presence of a **hemoglobinopathy** (Box 5-1). It is interesting to note that the vast majority of hemoglobinopathies have been detected serendipitously during investigation for clinically significant variants or thalassemias.[3,4] The laboratory diagnosis of hemoglobinopathies is of growing importance because of the requirement of many states for antenatal diagnosis of significant disorders of globin chain synthesis.[4]

Box 5-1

Clinical Indications for Testing for Hemoglobin Variants and Thalassemias

1. Antenatal screening to assess the risk for a fetus with a clinically significant hemoglobinopathy, permitting genetic counseling and adequate management of pregnant women
2. Newborn screening program to permit the early diagnosis of sickle cell disease, β-thalassemia major, and other clinically significant hemoglobinopathies to reduce their associated mortality and morbidity
3. Diagnosis of patients who present with clinical features suggestive of sickle cell disease or β-thalassemia major
4. Diagnosis of patients with an otherwise unexplained hemolytic anemia, polycythemia, anemia, or cyanosis
5. Determination of the presence of a hemoglobin variant that is responsible for abnormally elevated glycosylated hemoglobin (Hb A1c)

SECTION OBJECTIVES BOX 5-1

- Describe methods available for the quantification and identification of hemoglobin fractions.
- Describe the HPLC methods that are available for the quantification and identification of hemoglobin fractions, and compare currently available automated systems.
- Define the terms *retention time* and *window,* and explain how these are used to identify hemoglobin (Hb).

DETECTION, IDENTIFICATION, AND QUANTIFICATION OF HEMOGLOBIN FRACTIONS

In 1949, Linus Pauling used zone electrophoresis to demonstrate that electrophoretic mobility of hemoglobin from people with sickle cell anemia differed from that of normal people. Initially, **hemoglobin electrophoresis** in the clinical laboratory was undertaken with use of paper as the supporting medium and a borate discontinuous buffer system. For the past 35 years, hemoglobin electrophoresis has used cellulose acetate membranes at alkaline pH and citrate agar gels at acid pH as the support media, resulting in excellent separation and resolution of the variants. More recently, alkaline and acid gel supports have come into use. Other methods such as isoelectric focusing (IEF), globin chain electrophoresis, and immunoassay have been used. These latter techniques have limitations in the routine clinical laboratory, which are discussed later.[5]

The various electrophoretic techniques (see Chapter 6) are only qualitative assays that are capable of detecting hemoglobin fractions of varying mobility. Additional steps such as densitometry or elution must be taken for quantification of detected fractions. These additional steps have been shown to be subject to considerable imprecision and often are of limited use, especially for the minor hemoglobin fractions Hb A2 and Hb F, which are central to the diagnosis of α-thalassemia or β-thalassemia.[6] When the clinical laboratory uses such electrophoretic techniques, separate assays must be performed for the quantification of Hb A2 and Hb F (i.e., ion-exchange column chromatography [see Chapter 3] and alkali denaturation or radial immunodiffusion [see Chapter 7]), respectively. Besides being time consuming and technically complex, traditional manual methods of separating, identifying, and quantifying these hemoglobin fractions have other limitations and disadvantages.[7] The use in recent years of high-performance liquid chromatography (HPLC; see Chapter 4) technology, which allows the simultaneous quantification of Hb A2 and Hb F, as well as the detection, provisional identification, and quantification of variant hemoglobin fractions, has proved to be a powerful analytical tool in the clinical laboratory.[7-11]

DEVELOPMENT OF HPLC ANALYSIS OF HEMOGLOBIN FRACTIONS

Column chromatography has been used to separate both normal and abnormal hemoglobins and to quantitate Hb A2 for the diagnosis of β-thalassemia trait. Early automated cation-exchange HPLC instruments were developed as tools for hemoglobinopathy screening to meet the need created by expanded screening programs in larger medical centers, reference laboratories, and screening programs with large numbers of samples. HPLC instrumentation allows automated analysis in routine hospital laboratories for Hb A1c and for the normal and abnormal hemoglobin fractions used for the diagnosis and management of hemoglobinopathies.[5] Additional advancements have been made, in which the two different procedures (i.e., measurement of Hb A1c and of hemoglobin fractions) can be performed on the same equipment, thus allowing hemoglobinopathy screening to be brought into smaller laboratories because of its cost-effectiveness, in terms of both reagents and laboratory staffing.

Evaluations have been published for a number of automated HPLC systems that are now commercially available.[10,12-14] As the use of HPLC has dramatically expanded, result reporting for alkaline and acid electrophoresis, as well as isoelectric focusing, has been reduced by 50%.[15]

Overview of Technology for Detection of Hemoglobin Fractions by HPLC (see Chapter 4)

Alterations in amino acid composition of hemoglobin may result in changes not only in the net surface charge on the molecule but also in overall polarity (i.e., the introduction or loss of hydrophilic and hydrophobic groups), as well as alterations in the helical structure. These changes in the physical characteristics of hemoglobin may result in different electrophoretic migration rates for normal and abnormal hemoglobin fractions, as well as for different elution rates in different chromatography systems.

HPLC with anion-exchange stationary phases was used initially for analysis of undigested human hemoglobin to diagnose hemoglobin disorders such as Hb AS, Hb AC, Hb SS, Hb SC, Hb S/β-thalassemia, and Hb C/β-thalassemia. Anion exchange lacked the resolving capacity to classify other hemoglobin disorders and hemoglobin variants. These procedures were laborious, requiring days to achieve suitable separations in some cases. As a consequence, these methods were not applicable to routine clinical laboratories.[16]

To address these issues, cation-exchange materials that used cellulose and dextrans containing carboxymethyl groups were developed. Although they were successful because of their high capacity and hydrophilicity, these carbohydrate-based materials cannot withstand the high pressure used in HPLC. A simple cation-exchange material for HPLC was developed by reacting the polymer poly(succinimide) with the inorganic support aminopropyl-silica, thereby immobilizing the polymer on the surface through reactions with surface amino groups. Subsequent hydrolysis generated a cation-exchange group as an integral part of the polymer (see p. 91, Chapter 4). These coatings are reproducible and contain many carboxylic acid groups in a hydrophilic, polypeptide matrix. HPLC columns of this material feature excellent performance in terms of capacity, selectivity, recovery of enzyme activity, peak shape, and durability.[17]

Cation-exchange HPLC is a process by which a mixture of molecules (in this case, normal and variant hemoglobin fractions) with different net positive charges is separated into its components by absorption onto a negatively charged stationary phase. Components are eluted from the column by mobile phases containing different concentrations of cations that compete with proteins for the anionic binding sites on the stationary phase. The positively charged hemoglobin molecules are eluted from the column into the liquid phase in order of their decreasing affinity for the stationary phase. The eluted frations are detected spectrophotometrically in the eluate, provisionally identified by their retention time, and quantified by computing the area under the peak in the elution profile. Some correlation is noted between HPLC retention time and mobility on cellulose acetate electrophoresis at alkaline pH. The more positively charged hemoglobins (e.g., Hb S, Hb C) have a longer retention time, correlating with slower mobility on cellulose acetate at alkaline pH.[5]

COMPARISON OF DIFFERENT HPLC SYSTEMS FOR HEMOGLOBINOPATHY ANALYSIS

General Instrumentation (see Chapter 4)

Presently, three major manufacturers produce HPLC instruments for the detection, quantification, and identification of hemoglobinopathies in the clinical laboratory (Table 5-1).

All three systems positively identify samples with an internal barcode reader before patient samples are automatically mixed and diluted on the sampling station and injected to the analytical column. Pumps deliver a programmed buffer gradient of increasing ionic strength to the column to separate the hemoglobin fractions. The separated hemoglobin fractions pass through the flow cell of the filter photometer, where the absorbance is measured. Following elution of all the various hemoglobin fractions, initial buffer conditions are re-established prior to injection of the next sample. The computer software allows all critical events, including sample injection and reagent flow rates and composition, to be carefully controlled to provide maximum reproducibility of these processes. The software also reduces the raw data collected from each analysis (i.e., determination of the retention time and percent concentration of each peak). Retention time is the elapsed time in minutes from sample injection to the apex of the hemoglobin elution peak. The percent concentration of each peak is calculated as the integrated area for an individual peak divided by the total integration of area for all peaks present. Finally, a sample report and a chromatogram are generated for each sample (Fig. 5-1).[8]

To aid in the identification of results, intervals of retention time called "windows" have been assigned by the manufacturer (see Fig. 5-1). Within an assigned window, the most frequently occurring normal and abnormal hemoglobin fractions are expected to elute; a peak falling in the window associated with a specific hemoglobin is assumed to be that hemoglobin. Minor differences in the separation efficiency of individual analytical columns are compensated for by utilization of a calibrator with an assigned value for each hemoglobin to validate the time windows for each run and to aid in quantitation.

Table 5-1 Comparison of HPLC Systems for Analysis of Hemoglobin Variants

Specification		BioRad	Primus	Tosoh
Analysis time, min	Routine	6	4	7
	Enhanced	NA	10	NA
Wavelength, nm	Primary	415	412	415
	Secondary	690	NA	500
Temperature control		Yes	Ambient	Ambient
Number of buffers		2	2	3
Calibrators		A2/F	AFSC	A2/F

HPLC, High-performance liquid chromatography.
NA, Not applicable.

BioRad

BioRad Laboratories (Hercules, CA) provides several different hemoglobin testing systems for routine clinical laboratories, all of which use the same basic technology. BioRad employs a calibrator that contains Hb A2/F. Reference values for the Hb A2/F calibrator are based on correlation studies that compare the respective system with commercially available methods for Hb A2 and Hb F. Analysis of the calibrator yields separate calibration factors for both Hb A2 and Hb F, that is, the calculated ratio of the assigned value to the observed value. These calibration factors then are applied to the observed area percent for Hb A2 and Hb F in all subsequent analyses in the run, correcting for run-to-run differences in the allocation of area to these peaks. Because elution time is temperature dependent, the temperature at which the HPLC column is maintained is adjusted to allow the elution time of Hb A2 to occur at approximately 3.65 minutes. Although monitoring commences at the start of the elution process, the computer software does not integrate peaks that have elution times less than 0.73 minute. Thus, elution peaks for such hemoglobin fractions as Hb Barts, Hb H, and acetylated Hb F will not be integrated, quantified, and reported on the chromatograph report (Fig. 5-2, *A*).[8]

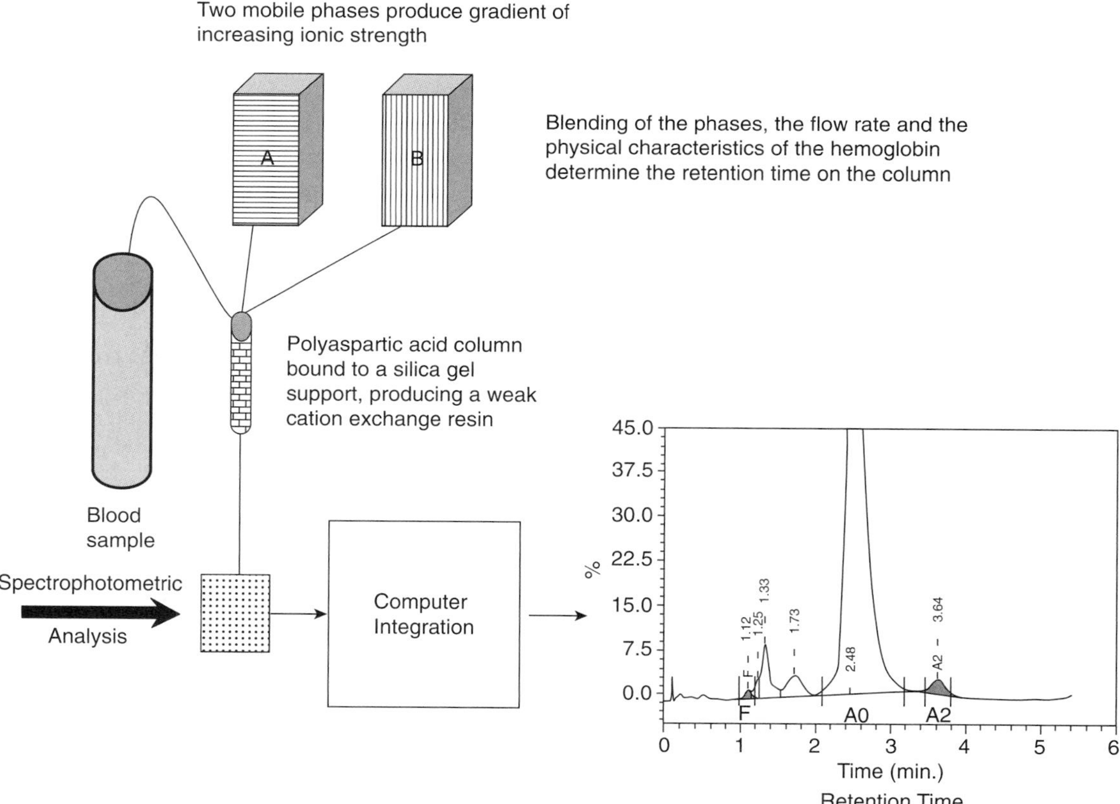

Fig. 5-1 Schematic representation of the performance of automated high-performance liquid chromatography (HPLC) analysis of hemoglobin fractions. Vertical lines on either side of the peaks indicate the manufacturer's assigned "windows" for Hb F, Hb Ao, and Hb A2, respectively.

Peak Name	Calibrated Area %	Area %	Retention Time (min)	Peak Area
F	0.8	---	1.12	12737
Unknown	---	1.1	1.25	20294
F2	---	4.9	1.33	89787
F3	---	3.6	1.73	66938
A0	---	87.2	2.48	1609996
A2	2.6	---	3.64	45938

Total Area: 1845691

F Concentration = 0.8 %
A2 Concentration = 2.6 %

Analysis connents:

Fig. 5-2 Examples of chromatograms from **(A)** BioRad on the Variant II, **(B)** Primus on the Ultra2, and **(C)** Tosoh on the G7.

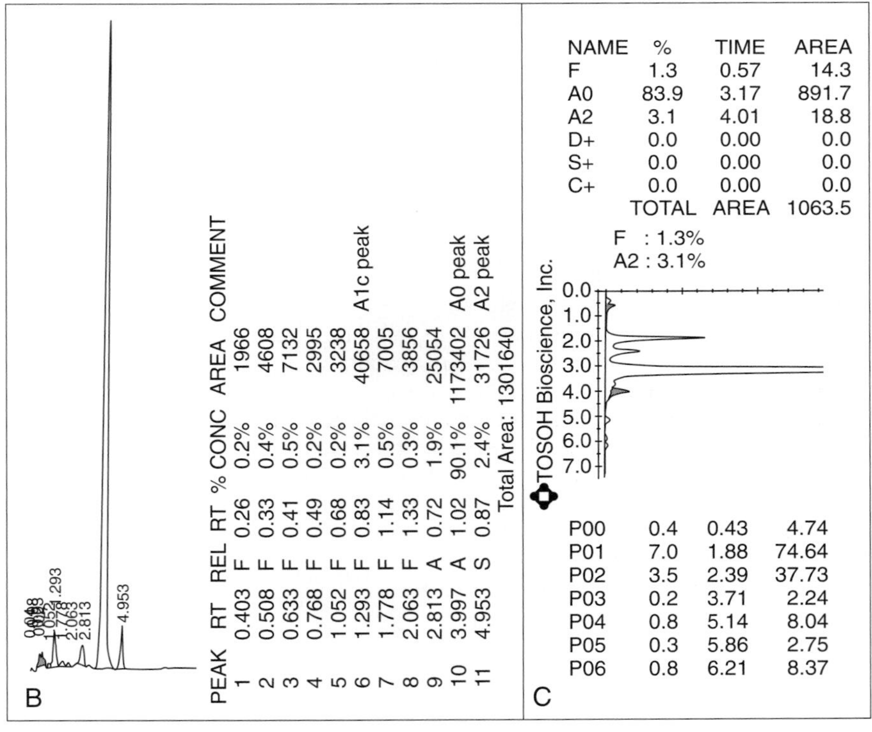

Primus

The HPLC equipment manufactured by Primus Corporation (Kansas City, MO) uses similar technology. In contrast to the BioRad systems, here the analytical column is maintained at ambient temperature. To adjust for any fluctuation in temperature, the Primus system automatically runs a calibrator containing hemoglobins F, A, S, and C prior to analysis of each set of 10 specimens. The detector in this system uses only a single wavelength at 413 nm, resulting in more background noise in the chromatographs. In addition, in lieu of the assignment of windows, a relative retention time is calculated and reported for each peak by dividing its retention time by that of one of the control peaks to aid in the identification of peaks. The Primus system begins to integrate the peaks from the beginning of the elution period, so Hb Barts, Hb H, acetylated Hb F, and other fast eluting hemoglobin fractions will be quantified. In addition, the Primus system has two analytical modes. All specimens are analyzed via the quick analysis program with a 4-minute elution period. With the use of computer set criteria, if abnormal peaks or higher than expected values of particular peaks are detected, the system will reflex to a high resolution program with a 10-minute chromatography period, allowing for more precise identification of the peak in question (Fig 5-2, *B*).[18]

Tosoh

A fully automated HPLC system from Tosoh (S. South Francisco, CA) employs technology that is very similar to both the BioRad and Primus systems. Although the BioRad and Primus systems use a two-buffer system, column elution in the Tosoh system is accomplished with use of a three-buffer system with a sample reading at 415 nm and a reference reading at 500 nm. The sequence is eluent 1 (lowest pH and salt concentration), followed by eluent 2 (same pH as eluent 1 but higher salt concentration), leading to a 1:1 ratio gradient between eluent 1 and eluent 3 (eluent 3 has the most alkaline pH and the highest salt concentration), and ending with a $^1/_4$ ratio gradient between eluent 1 and eluent 3. The column is maintained at ambient temperature. The elution program per sample lasts approximately 7 minutes. As with the BioRad system, windows are defined for the expected retention time for frequently found hemoglobin fractions. The Tosoh analyzer uses software that permits user-defined flag parameters to set alarms for different variables (Fig. 5-2, *C*).[19]

KEY CONCEPTS BOX 5-1

- Electrophoresis and cation-exchange HPLC are the primary tools for the detection of Hb variants. HPLC is superior to electrophoresis for quantification of individual Hb types.
- HPLC systems automatically dilute, hemolyze, and inject a sample and elute the Hb from the column. A chromatogram of the eluted Hb peaks is recorded, along with the retention times and tentative identification of peaks within critical windows.
- The expected retention time for a Hb is called the "window". All automated HPLC systems use the Hb retention time to identify that Hb.

QUANTIFICATION AND IDENTIFICATION OF HEMOGLOBIN FRACTIONS

Quantification of Hb A2

Quantification of Hb A2 is central to the differentiation and identification of α-thalassemia and β-thalassemia. It also is elevated or decreased in other hematological and medical conditions (Box 5-2). Quantification of Hb A2 involves the separation of Hb A2 from other hemoglobin fractions that are present, followed by determination of the relative proportion of Hb A2 that is present. This generally is undertaken through one of two procedures: micro-column chromatography or HPLC. Micro-column chromatography, although accurate for the measurement of this hemoglobin fraction, is labor intensive and imprecise. Quantification of Hb A2 via electrophoresis and densitometry is no longer recognized by the College of American Pathology (CAP) as an acceptable method for the quantitation of Hb A2 because CAP hemoglobinopathy

SECTION OBJECTIVES BOX 5-2

- Describe and compare methods available to quantitate Hb A2 and Hb F.
- Describe common normal and abnormal fractions seen in HPLC.
- List the advantages of HPLC over IEF and electrophoresis for the quantification and identification of Hb.
- Describe the use of retention time and peak quantity, and list hemoglobin characteristics that facilitate identification of a Hb variant.

Box 5-2

Causes for Alterations in Quantity of Hb A2

Congenital

Elevated

- β-Thalassemia trait
- Sickle cell trait
- Unstable hemoglobin variants

Reduced

- α-Thalassemia and hemoglobin (Hb) H disease
- δ-Thalassemia
- δβ-Thalassemia
- Hereditary persistence of fetal hemoglobin (HPFH) (deletional form)
- Hb Lepore
- Hb Kenya
- Presence of α- or δ-variant

Acquired

Elevated

- Hyperthyroidism
- Megaloblastic anemia due to vitamin B_{12} or folate deficiency
- Treatment of patients with human immunodeficiency virus (HIV) infection

Reduced

- Anemia of chronic disease
- Some cases of acute myeloid leukemia
- Hypothyroidism
- Iron deficiency
- Juvenile myelomonocytic anemia
- Lead poisoning
- Sideroblastic anemia

surveys have shown this technique to have intralaboratory coefficients of variation (%CVs) of greater than 30% for samples that contain Hb A2 in the reference interval.

Measurement of Hb A2 using cation-exchange HPLC is not, however, without problems. A number of hemoglobin variants, including Hb E, Hb G-Copenhagen, Hb Korle-Bu, Hb Lepore, and Hb Osu-Chritiansbourg, co-elute with a retention time identical or similar to that of Hb A2. The presence of any of these variants results in absurdly elevated levels of Hb A2. As a general rule, when the quantity of Hb A2 is greater than 8%, the presence of another hemoglobin fraction should be suspected.[1] Conversely, individuals with Hb D-Punjab trait have falsely decreased Hb A2 values because of an integration error that is caused by a rising baseline.[20]

Additionally, patients that are heterozygote for Hb S have physiologically elevated Hb A2 values.[1,4,7] It has been postulated that, in the presence of β-chain hemoglobin variants, the association of the α-globin chain with the β-globin chain variant is impaired, fostering the association of α-chains with δ-chains, thus increasing the Hb A2. Another factor that may play a role in the increase is the accumulation of Hb S adducts (post-translational modification products, such as glycated or acetylated Hb S).[21] Reporting of the elevated Hb A2 may lead to the incorrect diagnosis of a β-thalassemia, in addition to the heterozygote state for Hb S. To avoid this, many laboratories report different reference ranges for Hb A2 for patients with Hb AA and for patients with Hb AS, or they append the laboratory report with a statement that Hb A2 may be elevated in the presence of sickle trait and does not necessarily indicate the presence of β-thalassemia. Given these issues, automated HPLC provides a more accurate and precise quantitation of Hb A2 than does micro-column chromatography.[5]

Box 5-3

Conditions Associated With Elevated Quantity of Hb F

Congenital

- β-Thalassemia intermedia
- β-Thalassemia major
- β-Thalassemia trait
- Hemoglobin (Hb) Kenya
- Hb Lepore
- Hereditary persistence of fetal hemoglobin
- Sickle cell anemia
- Sickle cell trait, particularly Saudi/Indian haplotype
- Unstable hemoglobins

Acquired

- Aplastic anemia (Fanconi's anemia)
- Blackfan-Diamond syndrome
- Congenital dyserythropoietic anemia
- Diabetes mellitus
- Drug induced (treatment of sickle cell disease)
- Erythroleukemia
- Hydatidiform mole
- Juvenile myelomonocytic leukemia
- Kala-azar
- Metabolic disorders
- Paroxysmal nocturnal hemoglobinuria
- Pernicious anemia
- Pregnancy
- Schwachman-Diamond syndrome

Quantification of Hb F

Hb F is the major **hemoglobin variant** that is present in neonates (up to 90% in premature infants). Hb F is gradually replaced by Hb A, which reaches adult levels by the end of the first year of life. The accurate quantification of Hb F is important as an aid in the diagnosis of various hematological conditions (Box 5-3).

Historically, Hb F has been measured by utilizing its resistance to alkali solutions. The Singer 1-minute denaturation test gives reproducible results with accuracy suitable for clinical use when the Hb F level is above 5%, but it is less useful at lower levels. The Betke 2-minute alkali denaturation test is much better in the range usually found in clinical situations; better still is the modification published in 1974 by Pembrey, which can give precise and accurate results within the reference interval (0.2% to 0.8%) and up to Hb F levels as high as 50%. Above 50% Hb F, this method may underestimate the Hb F, but this is rarely of any clinical significance, and such specimens are rare after the neonatal period. Immunodiffusion techniques are labor intensive and relatively insensitive.[5] Densitometric scanning of Hb F bands can be performed on clarified cellulose acetate membranes or agarose gels after visualization by staining with amido black or acid violet. However, because Hb A and Hb F are not always clearly resolved, it is often difficult to accurately quantify Hb F with this technique, especially in healthy adults or in those with marginally increased Hb F.[5]

HPLC measures Hb F accurately and precisely from Hb F levels of ≈90% down into the reference interval.[7] However, the peak detectors are not always able to recognize Hb F. When greatly elevated, its elution peak frequently falls outside the generally assigned window and is not properly recognized and labeled as Hb F, resulting in labeling of the peak as "unknown." Similarly, in the lower half of the reference interval, no discernible peak may be detected by the system, resulting in no value for Hb F as reported from the chromatogram. If this happens, it is clinically satisfactory to report the result as <1%, although this can cause problems with the statistical analysis of some quality assessment schemes that cannot cope with a result that is "less than."[5]

Hb F is capable of being acetylated, and in the presence of large amounts of Hb F, as are seen in neonates, the acetylated form is approximately 15% of the total Hb F. The true Hb F value is the sum of the acetylated and non-acetylated forms of this hemoglobin. Because the acetylated form is a fast-eluting fraction, it elutes prior to initiation of the integration of peaks in the BioRad HPLC, resulting in artifactual underestimation of the amount of Hb F.[8] However, this underestimation is rarely, if ever, clinically significant.

Table 5-2 Examples of Retention Times for Common Variants

Variant	BioRad	Primus	Tosoh
Hb Barts	0.2	0.20-0.30 (RT/F)	0.28-0.35
Hb H	0.5	0.80-0.87 (RT/F)	0.29-0.39
Hb Fac	0.5	0.44-0.54 (RT/F)	NA
Hb F	1.10 ± 0.017	1.00-1.10 (RT/F)	0.58-1.02
Hb Hope	1.39 ± 0.007	1.00-1.03 (RT/F)	1.94-2.02
Hb N-Baltimore	1.70 ± 0.031	1.33-1.50 (RT/F)	NA
Hb J-Mexico	1.80 ± 0.015	0.76-0.78 (RT/A)	NA
Hb A	2.43 ± 0.041	0.97-1.05 (RT/A)	3.05-3.35
Hb Lepore	3.37 ± 0.019	1.11-1.15 (RT/A)	4.10-4.55
Hb D-Iran	3.49 ± 0.015	1.14-1.18 (RT/A)	4.61-4.65
Hb A2	3.63 ± 0.035	0.88-0.93 (RT/S)	3.65-4.75
Hb E	3.69 ± 0.069	0.82-0.86 (RT/S)	4.13-5.00
Hb Korle-Bu	3.92 ± 0.050	0.90-0.93 (RT/S)	NA
Hb D-Punjab	4.18 ± 0.007	0.94-0.96 (RT/S)	5.15-5.41
Hb G-Philadelphia	4.22 ± 0.037	0.90-0.92 (RT/S)	5.28-5.52
Hb S	4.51 ± 0.030	0.99-1.05 (RT/S)	5.50-6.50
Hb A2′	4.59 ± 0.030	1.00-1.03 (RT/S)	5.92-5.96
Hb Hasharon	4.83 ± 0.016	1.06-1.08 (RT/S)	6.29-6.33
Hb O-Arab	4.91 ± 0.008	0.91-1.03 (RT/C)	6.11-6.37
Hb C	5.18 ± 0.013	1.00-1.06 (RT/C)	6.50-7.50

Hb, Hemoglobin; *RT,* retention time; *RT/F, A, S, C,* relative retention time vs. HSF, A, S, and C; *NA,* not applicable.

At least seven hemoglobin variants have elution times similar to those of Hb F; therefore, when the Hb F value is greater than the age-specific expected value, confirmatory electrophoresis should be performed to verify the identity of the peak.[2]

The intra-assay and interassay imprecision of the HPLC measurement of Hb F is generally less than 5% for normal Hb F values and less than 2% for elevated Hb F values.[7,9,10]

Identification and Quantification of Other Hemoglobin Fractions

The application of HPLC to the identification of variant hemoglobins depends on the fact that, for each normal and hemoglobin variant fraction on a specified system, there is a characteristic retention time at which the hemoglobin appears to elute. The retention time for a particular hemoglobin fraction has been shown to have a low degree of imprecision, allowing tentative prediction of the variant that is present.[2,7-11] Retention time plus relative percentage of total hemoglobin and peak characteristics of variant hemoglobin fractions have been shown to provide important clues as to the identity of the unknown hemoglobin fraction. The relative retention times and elution sequences of normal and abnormal hemoglobin fractions have been published and are provided by specific manufacturers (see Table 5-2 for examples).

When the initial result suggests the presence of Hb S trait, the sickle solubility test should be performed for confirmation. Where the variant detected is clearly not sickle hemoglobin, hemoglobin electrophoresis at alkaline and acid pH or IEF is indicated. When an unusual variant cannot be reasonably identified by HPLC in tandem with hemoglobin electrophoresis or IEF, it is both analytically and clinically useful to determine whether it is an α- or β-variant in origin. Whereas the relative amount of the unknown fraction or the presence or absence of a variant Hb A2 fraction often suggests the type of globin chain variant that is present, additional studies may be warranted. Globin chain electrophoresis can be useful. This method, however, generally is restricted to reference laboratories.[5]

Because the quantification of Hb F or Hb S can be useful for monitoring the clinical care of patients with certain hemoglobinopathies, accurate and timely quantification of these hemoglobin fractions is becoming more widespread. For example, most often, hospital treatment of patients with Hb SS disease includes presurgical transfusion, the use of prophylactic hypertransfusion regimens, or the administration of hydroxyurea protocols. In cases of medical emergency, rapid and accurate identification of Hb S and quantification of Hb F, as well as other clinically significant hemoglobin variants associated with sickling syndromes and thalassemias, are frequently essential for establishing a diagnosis and beginning therapy. For patients with β-thalassemia major and Hb E/β-thalassemia, periodic quantification of transfused Hb A is required.

Imprecision and Linearity Studies

Proper laboratory utilization of HPLC technology includes verification of the minimal detectable concentration and establishment of the reportable range for the clinically important hemoglobin fractions that are to be quantitatively reported. This must occur at initial instrument installation and at regular intervals during operation and include hemoglobins A, A2, C, F, S, and other hemoglobin variants that are commonly encountered.[22]

The difficulty involved in obtaining appropriate standards for these studies makes these tasks quite difficult to perform. The basis for the integration of all Hb peaks and the calculation of the relative percentage for each peak is handled identically by the computer software (except for Hb F and Hb A2 on the BioRad systems). Thus, it is reasonable to assume that determination of imprecision at two different levels and linearity of a single abnormal hemoglobin variant should be sufficient for all the various fractions quantitatively reported by the laboratory.

Linearity studies can be accomplished by using a sample from a patient homozygote for a hemoglobin variant. Levels should range from approximately 90%, which corresponds to the amount generally found in the homozygote patient or a neonate, to at least 2%. This can be accomplished by making a series of admixtures of Hb AA blood and homozygote blood (such as Hb SS) for the variant of interest and plotting the linear regression of the expected percentage versus the actual percentage of the variant hemoglobin fraction. Precision studies should be performed at approximately 40% and 20%, corresponding to the amount of Hb S found in sickle trait patients and the target value for Hb S in those Hb SS patients on a hypertransfusion regimen, respectively.

Initial HPLC validation studies should be performed by comparing the identity and the relative percentage of the variant hemoglobin on HPLC versus the current method. If there is no method, it is acceptable to perform a correlation study with another established laboratory using HPLC. Correlation study versus densitometry has its limitations in that the lower level of sensitivity is approximately 5% for this technique. Accurate quantification of concentrations of hemoglobin fractions below 5%, except for Hb F and Hb A2, is not clinically relevant.

Advantages and Cautions for the Use of HPLC

The laboratory must understand the power and the limitations of the HPLC technique, which are common to all three current systems. In addition, because of the many normal and abnormal elution peaks displayed on the chromatogram, the performing laboratory must acquire considerable expertise and experience to understand which peaks, especially minor peaks, should be considered clinically relevant. A solid understanding of the complex subject of hemoglobin synthesis and assembly is central to accurate interpretation because the data produced can be complex at times (see Chapter 40 for details).

Similar to all laboratory technologies, a full understanding of not only the capabilities, but also the limitations, of HPLC is necessary. A larger range of variant hemoglobins can be provisionally identified by HPLC rather than by alkaline and acid electrophoresis. As a result of the quantification of Hb A2 and Hb F for each sample analyzed, various forms of thalassemia (α-, β-, δ-, and $\delta\beta$-thalassemia), as well as hereditary persistence of fetal hemoglobin (HPFH), can be diagnosed in a single procedure, thus eliminating the need for the more labor-intensive and less precise ion-exchange chromatography and alkali denaturation methods. Because of overlap in the worldwide distribution of hemoglobin variants and the thalassemias, it is to be expected that patients heterozygote for both molecular defects will be encountered frequently.[1]

Different hemoglobins often can co-elute in HPLC, demonstrating the limitation of using specific retention times for identification of a specific hemoglobin. For example, there are variants that do not separate from Hb A on HPLC, but do separate from Hb A on hemoglobin electrophoresis. On the other hand, there are hemoglobin variants that separate from Hb A on HPLC and that have identical migration as Hb A on alkaline and acid hemoglobin electrophoresis. At least seven variants elute in the Hb F window. Hb F may merge with the glycated Hb A peak and may not be detected when it is 0.6% or less. Elution of certain hemoglobin variants may overlap with Hb A2, resulting in absurdly elevated levels of Hb A2 (see above). Hb A2 often is elevated in the presence of Hb S and may be falsely reduced in the presence of Hb D-Punjab. Hemoglobins that can be distinguished from each other vary somewhat between different instruments and reagent systems.[8,18,19,22]

Despite this, HPLC has been shown to be the single most powerful tool for the differentiation of the more common hemoglobin variants available in the routine clinical laboratory. This includes differentiating Hb D-Punjab and Hb G-Philadelphia from Hb S, and Hb E and Hb O-Arab from Hb C, which are not conclusively identified by alkaline and acid hemoglobin electrophoresis. The presence of an Hb A2 variant often can be detected easily, allowing the ready diagnosis of β-thalassemia trait when a δ-chain variant is present, most commonly Hb A2′.[9] The presence of an Hb A2 variant also can facilitate the determination of whether an unknown hemoglobin fraction includes the presence of either an α-chain or a β-chain variant (even those with identical retention times).

Use of Retention Times and Peak Quantity and Characteristics for Hb Identification

The relative percentage of an uncommon variant many times will yield clues as to whether the variant in question is a mutant α- or β-globin chain variant. Commonly, α-chain variants are 15% to 25% of the total hemoglobin, whereas β-chain variants constitute 30% to 45%. There are many exceptions to this general rule, including the unstable hemoglobin variants and/or the presence of concomitant α- or β-thalassemias.[1] This is discussed in greater detail in a later section.

As with most column chromatography procedures, HPLC systems are highly sensitive to temperature, with different temperatures producing different retention times. Therefore, it is recognized that a hemoglobin variant can be only provisionally identified based on retention time alone since minor changes in retention time can result in incorrect identification of peaks.[3,6]

HPLC has the disadvantage that it separates hemoglobins that have undergone post-translational modification, such as acetylated Hb F and glycated forms of Hb A, Hb S, Hb C, and other variants, not only from each other but also from the unmodified forms, making interpretation on some systems more challenging. An increased amount of glycated Hb A or methemoglobin might be mistaken for a hemoglobin variant. An elevated percentage of glycated Hb A may lead to factitious elevation of Hb F. Glycated Hb S has a retention time the same as, or very similar to, that of Hb A, so that patients with sickle cell anemia may be thought to have a small amount of Hb A. The fact that glycated and other post-translationally modified variant hemoglobins often elute with the same retention time as the normal hemoglobin fractions can cause problems with automatic transfer of data.

Bilirubin is a common interferent, whose retention time leads to a sharp peak in the same general area of Hb Barts, thus mimicking an uncommon hemoglobinopathy. These specimens come primarily from treated patients with Hb SS, especially those undergoing hydroxyurea therapy.[23] It also would be expected to be seen in cases of hemolytic anemia and in neonates with hyperbilirubinemia associated with glucose-6-phosphate dehydrogenase (G6PD) deficiency.

It is imperative that all chromatograms be visually inspected by an experienced analyst prior to final verification to ensure that all peaks have been properly identified and quantified, especially prior to on-line transfer of results to a laboratory information system. This review will allow any necessary corrections to be made, such as elevated Hb A1c levels, questionable results for Hb A2, correction of Hb F values resulting from the presence of acetylated Hb F, or misidentification of a highly elevated peak as a variant. The laboratory may choose to have a set of standard comments added to the report, such as "Hb A2 cannot be quantified because of co-elution of an abnormal hemoglobin fraction," or "Hb A2 is elevated in the presence of sickle trait and does not necessarily indicate the presence of a β-thalassemia."

KEY CONCEPTS BOX 5-2

- Automated cation HPLC and electrophoresis can quantitate Hb fractions, but HPLC is the superior technique.
- Hb A, Hb A2, and Hb F are the normal Hb fractions seen in HPLC. Variant Hb is typically seen as Hb S and Hb C.
- Identification of Hb S should be confirmed with a solubility test.
- The proportion of Hb of the total Hb can help identify a variant Hb.

SECTION OBJECTIVES BOX 5-3

- Describe the differences between hemoglobin variants, hemoglobinopathies, and thalassemias.
- Describe possible interactions between hemoglobin variants and thalassemias.
- Discuss the advantages and disadvantages of different methods for the quantification and identification of hemoglobin fractions.

ABNORMAL VARIANT FRACTIONS

An understanding of the changes in globin subunit synthesis and of the biochemistry involved in the assembly of hemoglobin tetramers during human development from embryo through infancy to adulthood is needed to assist in the correct interpretation of the data produced by HPLC technology.

Human α-like and β-like globin genes are located on chromosome 16 and chromosome 11, respectively. The globin genes are ordered in the 5′ to 3′ direction of DNA according to the sequence of expression from embryogenesis to adult life (see Chapter 40, p. 773). As different globin gene products are produced throughout life, the positively charged α-like globins combine with negatively charged β-like globins, forming first an αβ dimer and then the complete hemoglobin heterotetramer.

During embryonic life, the α-like and β-like globin genes combine to produce Hb Portland (ζ2γ2), Hb Gower 1 (ζ2ε2), and Hemoglobin Gower 2 (α2ε2). Hb F (α2γ2) constitutes the vast majority of hemoglobin during fetal life, with a small amount of Hb A (α2β2) present. After birth, the amount of Hb F decreases and Hb A increases rapidly, reaching normal adult levels at 12 to 18 months of age.[1,5] Hb A2 (α2δ2) begins production at birth, reaching normal levels at approximately the same time as Hb F.

HPLC chromatograms for a normal adult and for a normal full-term neonate are shown in Figs. 5-3, *A* and *B*, respectively. The chromatogram for the neonate illustrates the very high percentage of Hb F seen at birth, along with the absence of Hb A2. The initial peak seen in the chromatogram represents the acetylated form of Hb F.

For interpretation of peaks seen on an HPLC chromatogram, it is best to view the peaks as representing dimers. When hemoglobin is placed in an electric field or an ionic solution, the hemoglobin heterotetramer disassembles into its two dimer components. For example, in the chromatogram of the normal adult, the peaks do not represent heterotetrameric Hb F, Hb A, and Hb A2, but the dimers αAγA, αAβA, and αAδA, respectively (see Fig. 5-3, *A*).

β-Variants

When a variant β-chain (βV) or α-chain (αV) is present, the hybrid hemoglobin tetramer is predominant inside the erythrocyte as αAβA/αAβV or αAβA/αVβA. Therefore, αAβA and αAβV are the predominant dimer forms found in the presence of a β-variant. Because an individual inherits only two β-globin genes (one on each chromosome), a heterozygous β-chain variant should constitute half of the total hemoglobin in the red cells. The formation of αβ dimers generally is considered to be facilitated, at least in part, by the electrostatic attraction between positively charged α-globin and negatively charged β-globin subunits. Many common β-globin variants acquire a positive charge, thereby reducing their ability to compete with βA-chains for αA-chains. In such cases, fewer variant hemoglobin dimers (αAβV) than normal Hb (αAβA) accumulate. The opposite situation is seen when

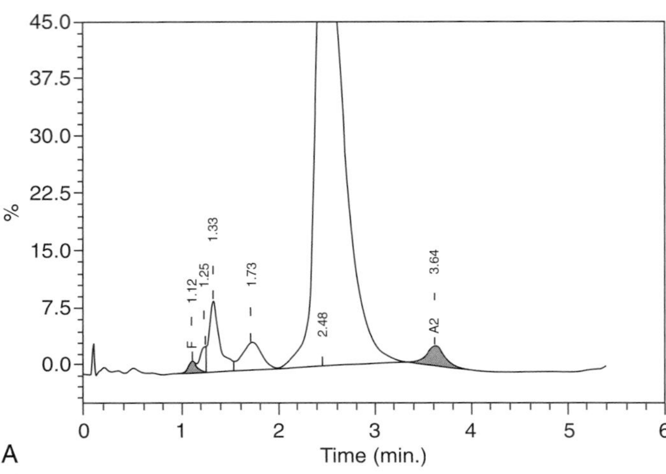

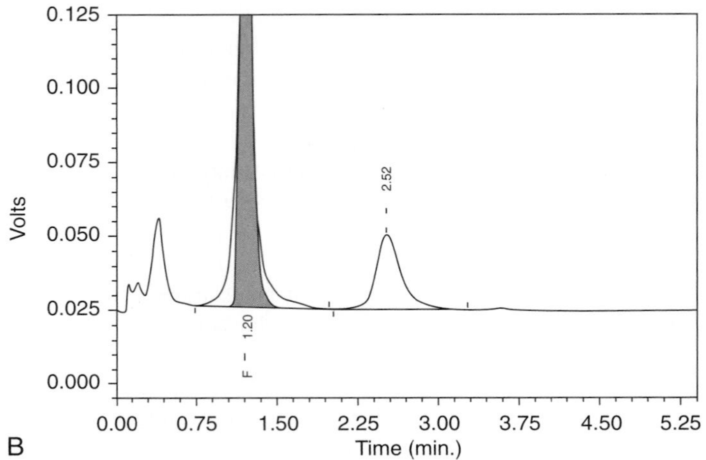

Fig. 5-3 Sample chromatograms for **(A)** a normal adult and **(B)** a normal neonate on the BioRad Variant II. Time (minutes) represents the retention time (RT) for each fraction to elute. The RT for each fraction is shown at the peak. For the normal adult, the RT for Hb F is 1.12, for Hb A is 2.48, and for Hb A2 is 3.64. For the normal neonate, the RT for Hb F is 1.20 and for Hb A is 2.52. The peak preceding Hb F is the acetylated Hb F (RT ≈0.4). In the absence of Hb A2 the variant system labels the vertical axis as Volts.

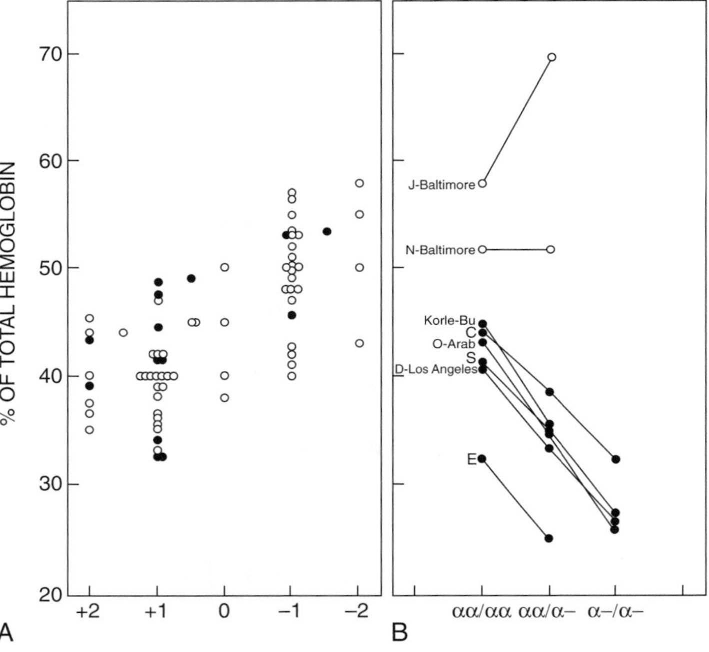

Fig. 5-4 A, Effect of charge on the proportion of abnormal hemoglobin in individuals heterozygous for 72 stable β-variants. Each data point represents a mean value for a given variant. The solid points (•) denote measurements of Huisman (Am J Hematol 14:393, 1983) with the use of high-resolution chromatography. Substitutions involving a histidine residue were scored as a change of $^1/_2$ charge. The "−1" group differs significantly from the "+1" group ($p < 0.001$) and from the "0" group ($p \leq 0.05$). **B,** Effect of α-thalassemia on a proportion of six positively charged β-variants (•) and of two negatively charged variants (o). (From Bunn HF, McDonald MJ: Nature 306:498, 1983.)

the mutation results in a β-chain variant with an additional negative charge, such as in Hb N-Baltimore. This phenomenon is in reality more complicated than this, since the overall surface charge of the subunits appears to play an important role in the rate of assembly. The final amount of abnormal hemoglobin tetramer produced is dependent not only on the rate of assembly of the α-like and β-like dimers, but also on the rate of synthesis and the stability of these dimers and tetramers. It is not surprising that heterozygotes for β-chain variants show a wide range of different levels of the abnormal hemoglobin (Fig. 5-4).

α-Variants

In the presence of an α-variant, αAβA and αVβA are the predominant dimers present. Similarly, since individuals normally have a total of four α-globin genes (two on each chromosome), an α-chain variant would be expected to constitute 25% of the total hemoglobin. However, in most cases, detected amounts of the α-chain variant are generally lower than expected for many of the same reasons as described above for β-chain variants.

Examples of the heterozygote state for the β-variant Hb S and the α-variant Hb G-Philadelphia are shown in Fig. 5-5,

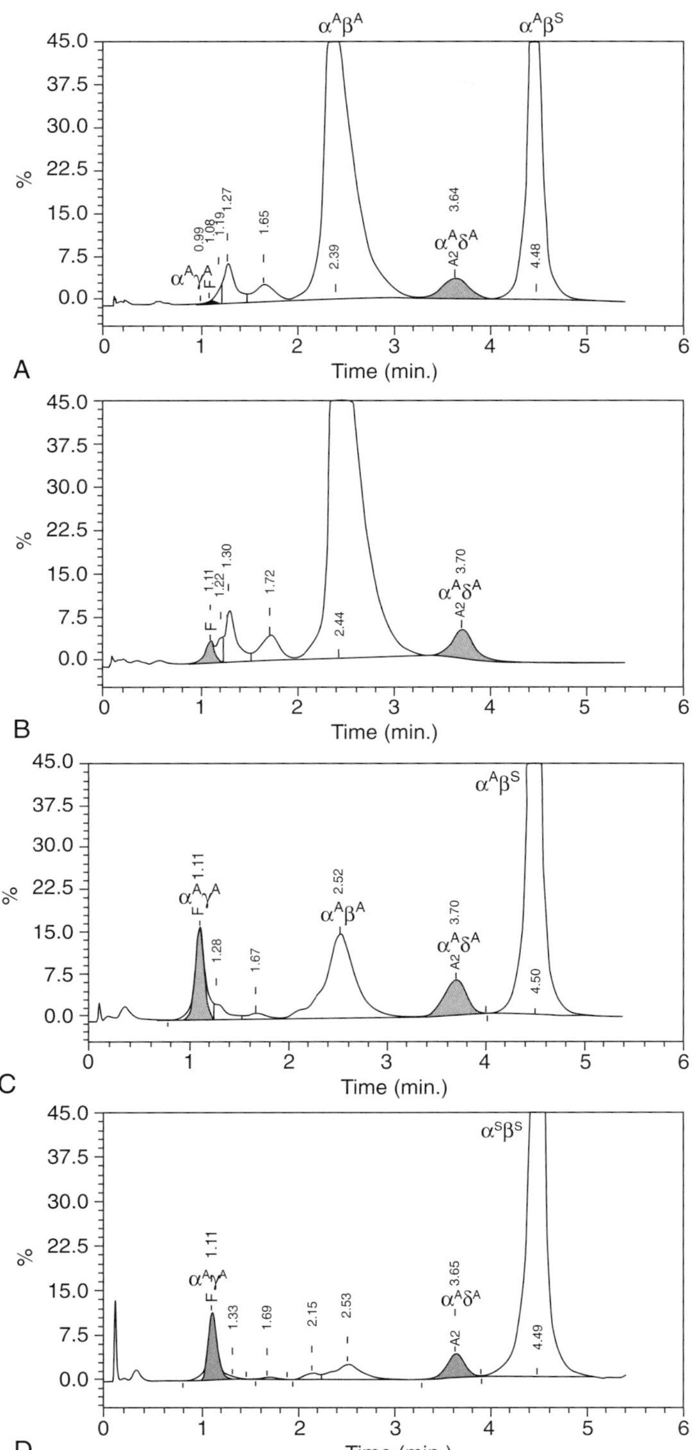

Fig. 5-5 Sample chromatograms on the BioRad Variant II of patients for **(A)** Hb S trait (αAγA = 0.2%, αAβA = 61.9%, αAδA = 3.8%, αAβS = 34.1%), **(B)** β-thalassemia trait (αAδA = 5.2%), **(C)** Hb S/β-thalassemia (αAγA = 7.0%, αAβA = 18.1%, αAδA = 6.4%, αAβS = 68.5%), and **(D)** homozygous Hb S (αAγA = 6.4%, αAδA = 4.1%, αAβS = 89.5%). Note the sharp peak at the beginning of the chromatograph in 6C. This peak represents contaminating bilirubin. Time (minutes) represents the retention time (RT) for each fraction to elute. The RT for each fraction is shown at the peak.

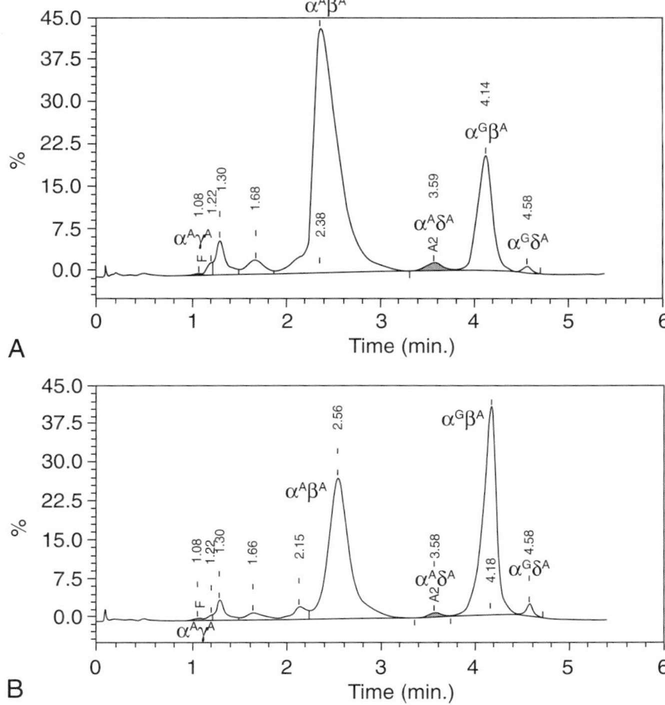

Fig. 5-6 Sample chromatograms on the BioRad Variant II of patients for **(A)** Hb G-Philadelphia trait (αAγA = 0.2%, αAβA = 79.3%, αAδA = 1.2%, αGβA = 18.8%, αGδA = 0.5%) and **(B)** heterozygous for Hb G-Philadelphia and α-thalassemia (αAγA = 0.3%, αAβA = 67.9%, αAδA = 0.8%, αGβA = 29.2%, αGδA = 1.1%). Time (minutes) represents the retention time (RT) for each fraction to elute. The RT for each fraction is shown at the peak.

A, and Fig. 5-6, *A*, respectively. In sickle trait (Hb AS, αAβA/αAβS), the relative percentage of "Hb S" (αAβS), generally ≈30% to 40%, is always less than "Hb A" (αAβA). The mutation that causes the Hb S variant (β6glu → val) involves substitution of the negatively charged glutamic acid by the neutrally charged valine, resulting in a more positively charged β-globin chain. Therefore, the assembly rate to the positively charged αA by the negatively charged βA will be greater than the positively charged βS, accounting for the difference in their relative amounts.

The relative amount of Hb G-Philadelphia (generally 16% to 20%) is significantly less than the expected 25%, again because of the difference in the rate of assembly of the variant αG-globin chain with the normal βA-globin chain. Therefore, the differentiation between an α-variant and a β-variant can often be aided by the relative percentage of the unknown fraction present. Hb D-Punjab (Fig. 5-7, *A*) has a retention time similar to Hb G-Philadelphia (see Fig. 5-6, *A*). In Fig. 5-6, *A*, the minor peak following the Hb G-Philadelphia peak (αGβA) represents αGδA, the variant Hb A2 peak indicative of the presence of an α-variant. Just as Hb A2 falls behind Hb A, the variant Hb A2 falls behind the variant hemoglobin peak. The true Hb A2 value is, therefore, the sum of the normal and variant Hb A2 peaks.

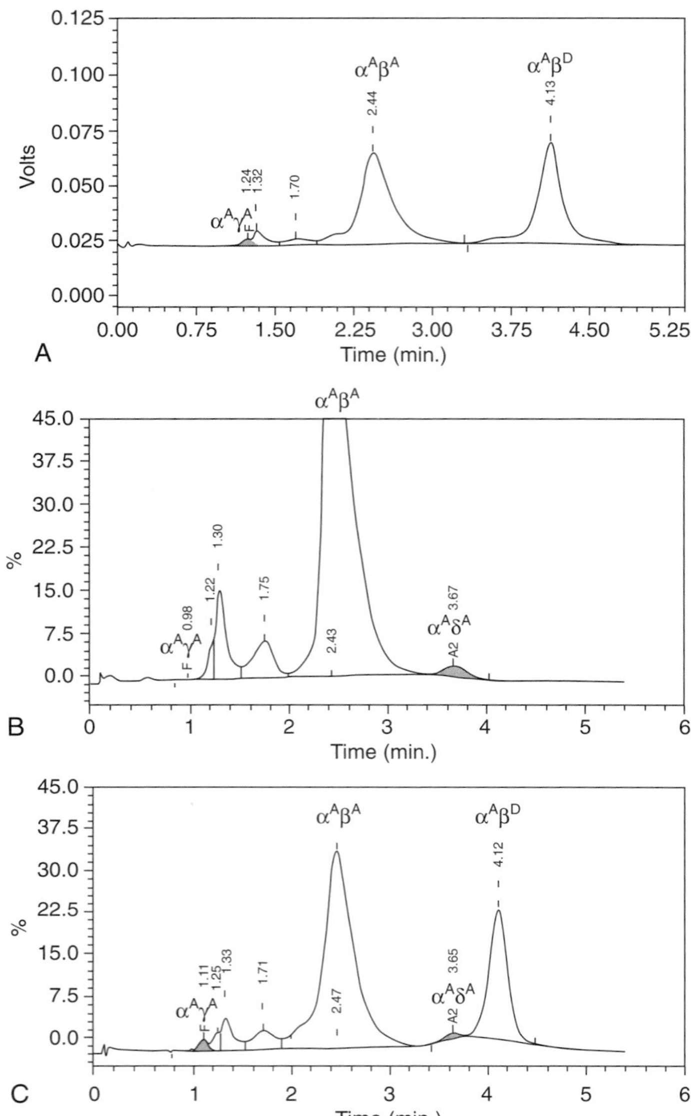

Fig. 5-7 Sample chromatograms on the BioRad Variant II of patients for **(A)** Hb D-Punjab trait (αAγA = 1.1%, αAβA = 56.3%, αAβD = 42.6%), **(B)** α-thalassemia trait (αAγA = 0.1%, αAβA = 98.0%, αAδA = 1.9%), and **(C)** heterozygous for Hb D-Punjab trait and α-thalassemia (αAγA = 1.2%, αAβA = 55.4%, αAδA = 0.9%, αAβD = 25.1%). Note the absence of Hb A2 in 7A caused by co-elution of the variant hemoglobin fraction. In the absence of Hb A2 the variant system labels the vertical axis as Volts. Time (minutes) represents the retention time (RT) for each fraction to elute. The RT for each fraction is shown at the peak. The peak seen at RT = 1.30 represents Hb A1c.

ABNORMAL QUANTITIES OF HEMOGLOBIN FRACTIONS: THE THALASSEMIAS

β-Thalassemia

Fig. 5-5, *B,* is an example of a β-thalassemia. The β-thalassemias are a diverse group of disorders of β-globin synthesis that result more commonly from mutations, but also from deletions, of the β-globin gene. A thalassemia is associated with complete blood count (CBC) indices that indicate the presence of a hypochromic, microcytic anemia, in the absence of iron deficiency anemia. Hb A2 generally is elevated in β-thalassemia trait, as in this example. Because the Hb S and β-thalassemia genes both are found in the African population, it is not surprising that cases of double heterozygosity (sickle β-thalassemia) are commonly found in this population. The form of β-thalassemia that is found among those of African origin results from mild mutations, commonly involving the β-globin gene promoters, that cause reduction (designated β+) rather than total loss (designated β0) of β-globin synthesis. Therefore, some βA-globin is being produced, resulting in low amounts (up to ≈40%) of Hb A. It is most important that in such cases (see Fig. 5-5, *C*), the relative amount of "Hb S" (αAβS) always exceeds that of "Hb A" (αAβA), whereas in sickle cell trait (see Fig. 5-5, *A*), the opposite is true. Fig. 5-5, *D,* is an illustration of a patient homozyogous for Hb S; the small amount of hemoglobin in the A window is glycated Hb S.

α-Thalassemia

Normally, four α-globin genes (αα/αα) are active. The α-thalassemias, generally resulting from deletions rather than mutations of the **α-globin gene cluster,** can be seen with several different genotypic forms (−α/αα, −α/−α, —/αα, −α/—) and are commonly found in many different ethnic populations. Complete loss of all four α-globin genes is incompatible with life. The Hb A2 level is generally normal or reduced in α-thalassemia trait. Fig. 5-7, *B,* is an example of a patient with α-thalassemia (−α/−α).

The chromatographic pattern of α-thalassemia should be expected to be affected by the presence of both β-variants and α-variant chains. Fig. 5-7, *A,* demonstrates the HPLC chromatogram for a patient heterozygote for the β-variant Hb D-Punjab (αAβA/αAβD). In α-thalassemia, in which reduced quantities of α-chains are synthesized, the number of negatively charged βA-chains that combine with the limited number of positively charged αA-globin chains increases. The number of positively charged βV-chains that can combine with positively charged αA-globin is decreased in proportion to the deficit in α-globin chains (see Fig. 5-4). This is demonstrated in Fig. 5-7, *C,* which shows a patient with a hypochromic, microcytic anemia in the absence of iron deficiency; this patient has both the β-variant Hb D-Punjab and α-thalassemia. The relative amount of variant hemoglobin is significantly lower than the expected amount. The presence of a β-thalassemia can be eliminated because the relative amount of Hb A is greater than the variant.

INTERACTION OF VARIANTS AND THALASSEMIAS: INTERPRETATION OF CHROMATOGRAMS

The presence of α-thalassemia in the presence of an α-variant, on the other hand, generally results in a higher than expected amount of the variant. Hb G-Philadelphia often is associated with an α-thalassemia in cis, that is, on the same chromosome

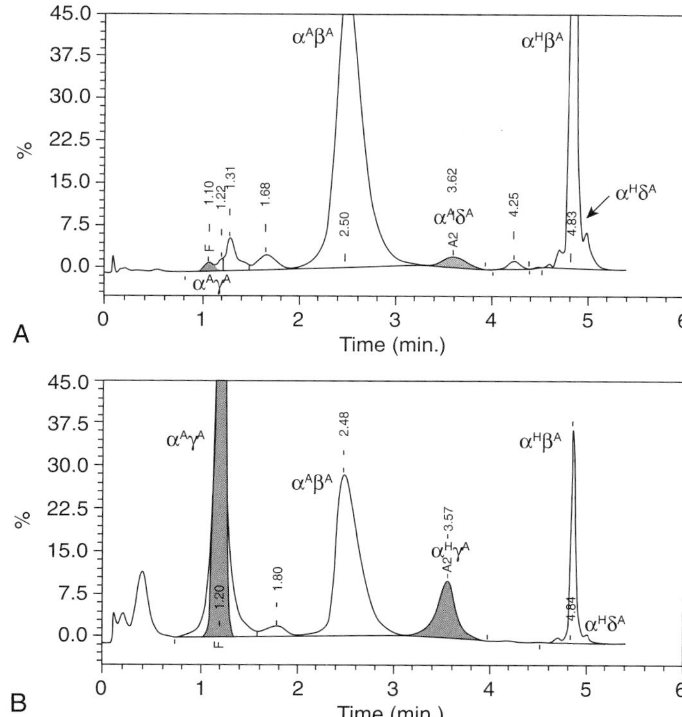

Fig. 5-8 Sample chromatograms on the BioRad Variant II of **(A)** an adult with Hb Hasharon trait (αAγA = 0.7%, αAβA = 63.6%, αAδA = 1.8%, αHβA = 21.9%) and **(B)** a newborn with Hb Hasharon trait (αAγA = 44.3%, αAβA = 34.9%, αHγA = 10.1%, αHβA = 10.7%). Time (minutes) represents the retention time (RT) for each fraction to elute. The RT for each fraction is shown at the peak. The two small, characteristic peaks preceding the Hb Hasharon peak are unknown but may represent the glycated Hb Hasharon. The small, unintegraged peak following Hb Hasharon is presumably the variant Hb A2 fraction, αHδA.

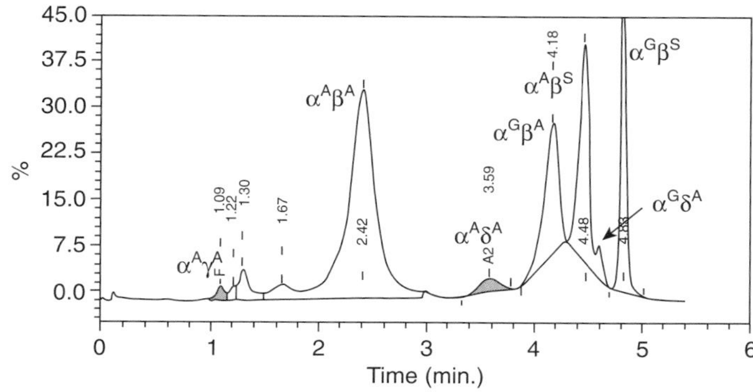

Fig. 5-9 Sample chromatogram on the BioRad Variant II of a patient double heterozygous for the α-variant Hb G-Philadelphia and the β-variant Hb S (αAγA = 0.9%, αAβA = 51.6%, αAδA = 2.4%, αGβA = 14.5%, αAβS = 17.6%, αGβS = 14.0%). Time (minutes) represents the retention time (RT) for each fraction to elute. The RT for each fraction is shown at the peak. Note the small, unintegrated peak following Hb G-Philadelphia, which is the variant A2 fraction, αGδA.

(αα/α^{G}–); therefore, the expected amount of αGβA produced would be 33%. The actual amount detected is generally ≈25%, consistent with the decreased rate of assembly of αGβA compared with αAβA (see Fig. 5-6, *B*). When a carrier for an α-chain variant has a β-thalassemia gene, the level of the α-chain variant is usually lower in the doubly affected individual than in the simple heterozygote.

The central tenet to the successful interpretation of HPLC chromatograms is an understanding of which globin chains, and in what relative amount, are expected to be produced in the patient's stage of life. Fig. 5-8, *A*, shows an HPLC chromatogram for a patient with the α-variant Hb Hasharon. This chromatogram demonstrates the classic characteristics of an α-variant, that is, relative amount of the variant (αHβA) less than 25%, reduced amount of Hb A2 (αAδA), and presence of the Hb A2 variant (αHδA). Fig. 5-8, *B*, shows the HPLC chromatogram of a 39-day-old infant who presented with an abnormal variant detected in a newborn screening program. The retention time and the peak characteristics of the late eluting hemoglobin fraction are suggestive of Hb Hasharon. At this stage of life, the baby, if indeed heterozygote for Hb Hasharon, would be expected to be producing relatively high numbers of normal αA-globin and variant αH-globin chains (ratio 3:1, respectively), reduced numbers of β-globin and δ-globin chains, and high numbers of γ-globin chains. Therefore, one would expect the following combinations to be present: αAγA, αHγA, αAβA, αHβA, αAδA, and αHδA. The relatively high amount of Hb A2, especially at this age, should make the observer very suspicious. Because Hb A2 normally is produced in significantly reduced amounts at this age, the peak essentially represents the dimer αHγA, which would be expected to decrease with increasing age of the infant.

Because the α-globin and **β-globin gene clusters** are found on separate chromosomes, it would be expected to find a patient double heterozygote for both types of variants. Fig. 5-9 shows the results of the offspring of parents, one with Hb S trait and the other with Hb G-Philadelphia trait. Again, knowledge of which combination of globin chains (αAγA, αAβA, αAδA, αGβA, αAβS, αGδA, and αGβS) and which relative amounts are expected quickly allows interpretation of this apparently complicated chromatogram.

Hb E and Hb Lepore (Figs. 5-10, *A* and *B*, respectively) elute at retention time similar to that of Hb A2. However, the relative percentage of each is statistically different for each other and from Hb A2. It generally is agreed that when the quantity of Hb A2 is greater than 8%, co-elution of another hemoglobin fraction should be considered.

It is important to remember that the interpretation and final diagnosis of a hemoglobinopathy cannot always be made solely from analysis of the hemoglobin fractions by HPLC and by other conventional laboratory methods. For clinicians to give definitive clinical or genetic advice about a variant or thalassemia found during hemoglobinopathy screening, further testing may be necessary to evaluate the variant Hb, including abnormality of solubility, production rate, stability, and the capacity to deliver or carry oxygen.[6]

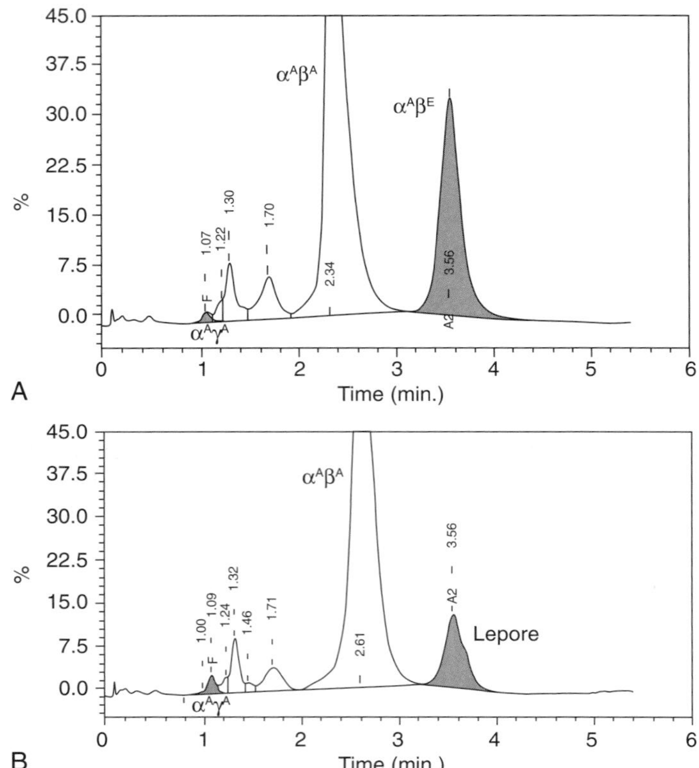

Fig. 5-10 Sample chromatograms on the BioRad Variant II of patients for **(A)** Hb E trait (αAγA = 0.7%, αAβA = 66.8%, αAβE = 32.5%) and **(B)** Hb Lepore trait (αAγA = 1.4%, αAβA = 85.5%, Lepore = 13.1%). Time (minutes) represents the retention time (RT) for each fraction to elute. The RT for each fraction is shown at the peak. Hb Lepore is a δβ-globin chain. Both Hb E and Hb Lepore co-elute with Hb A2.

Box 5-4

Factors* to Be Considered in Hemoglobin Variant Identification

High-performance liquid chromatography (HPLC)
- Retention times
- Relative peak heights of hemoglobin fractions
- Peak elution characteristics
- Other peaks associated with specific variants (i.e., A2′)

Personal and family clinical and hematological history (including ethnic origin)
Iron status (iron, ferritin, transferrin levels)
Hematologic evaluation (red blood cells [RBCs], hemoglobin [Hb], mean corpuscular volume [MCV], mean corpuscular hemoglobin [MCH], reticulocyte count, RBC morphology)
Hemoglobin electrophoresis (alkaline and acid pH, globin chain)
Isoelectric focusing electrophoresis
Hemoglobin functional studies (P_{50}, chemical and heat stability, Heinz bodies)
Kleihauer-Betke stain
Nucleic acid–based methods
- Polymerase chain reaction (PCR)
- Reverse-transcribed PCR
- DNA sequencing
- Sequencing of Fourier transform–based PCR (FT-PCR) amplified globin complementary DNA (cDNA) of the gene of interest

Family history and studies

*Factors are listed in order of consideration.

Clinical significance arising from the variant hemoglobin may be attributable to any of these factors. Collaboration of the laboratory and the clinician generally is required for the interpretation of all clinical and medical information. For this reason, the evaluation of the patient's complete hematological picture, a concise clinical history of the patient and family, and knowledge of the patient's ethnicity often are very important for an accurate final diagnosis (Box 5-4).[3,6]

HPLC VS ELECTROPHORESIS METHODS FOR VARIANT DETECTION

Alkaline (cellulose acetate membrane, pH 8.6) and acid hemoglobin electrophoreses (citrate agar, pH 6.2) presently remain the most widely used methods for investigating hemoglobinopathies. Alkalkine and acid agarose gels recently have become more popular because of their availability and cost-effectiveness. These gels are supplied ready-to-use, require minimal preparatory work, and can be used on semiautomated systems.

Alkaline electrophoresis is capable of separating normal and common hemoglobin variant fractions, such as Hb A, Hb F, Hb S, and Hb C. However, Hb S, Hb D-Punjab, Hb G-Philadelphia, and Hb Lepore are unresolved from each other, as are Hb C, Hb O-Arab, and Hb E. In addition, there are other variants with electrophoretic mobilities identical or similar to those of Hb S and Hb C. Consequently, acid electrophoresis is needed to aid in identification of the aforementioned variants. Nevertheless, the combination of these electrophroetic methods is still not able, in most cases, to separate Hb D-Punjab, Hb G-Philadelphia, and Hb Lepore from each other and, in some cases, Hb E from Hb O-Arab.[8] Therefore, none of these clinically important hemoglobin variants or combinations of variants can be conclusively identified by a single electrophoretic technique.

Except for Hb S, because of the availability of the solubility test, the identification of hemoglobin variants is often presumptive, based on characteristic electrophoretic mobility, quantity, and/or ethnic origin. A false-positive diagnosis of sickle cell anemia is unavoidable, and incorrect or unresolved diagnoses of hemoglobinopathies sometimes are encountered.

In addition, there are numerous hemoglobin variants, for example, Hb Twin Peaks and Hb Ty Gard, that are electrophoretically silent (i.e., identical migration rates to Hb A) but separate from Hb A on HPLC. Hb D-Punjab and Hb D-Iran both have identical migration with Hb S on alkaline and Hb A on acid hemoglobin electrophoresis but have distinct retention times on HPLC. Their differentiation by HPLC can have a significant impact on genetic counseling. Coinheritance of Hb S with Hb D-Punjab results in a clinically significant disease, but its interaction with Hb D-Iran is totally asymptomatic. This is also true for Hb E versus Hb E-Saskatoon. On the other hand, there are variants that do not separate from Hb A on HPLC, for example, Hb New York and Hb Knossos. The latter is an example of a clinically significant hemoglobin variant that does not separate from Hb A on electrophoresis or HPLC. Isoelectric focusing is required for its identification. Genetic analysis often is necessary for the identification of variants for which problems of co-migration are an issue and are suspected to have significant clinical and/or hematological implications.

QUANTIFICATION OF HB F AND HB A2

Quantification of hemoglobin fractions by densitometry is inaccurate for low concentrations of hemoglobin fractions such as Hb A2. Hb A and Hb F are not always clearly resolved, resulting in inaccurate quantification of Hb F by densitometry on alkaline electrophoresis. Carbonic anhydrase and its variants can cause confusion when electrophoretic preparations are stained with protein stains rather than with heme-specific stains, such as *o*-dianisidine.

Electrophoresis methods generally are reproducible and capable of separating common hemoglobin variants; they can be slow and labor intensive, although more rapid with certain systems. Variables such as hemoglobin concentration, amperage, running temperature, and length of electrophoresis run, separately or in combination, can limit the quality of separation and the relative positioning of bands, making identification of abnormal hemoglobin variants by electrophoresis tentative. The preparation of samples for hemoglobin electrophoresis is cumbersome, labor intensive, and time-consuming.

Isoelectric focusing uses thin agar gels to separate hemoglobin fractions based on their isoelectric points (see Chapter 6). This leads to the formation of discrete sharp bands and often separates hemoglobins that do not separate on conventional hemoglobin electrophoresis. It is used most often in reference laboratories and in large-scale screening programs, notably newborn screening programs, where it is convenient to batch and analyze samples in this manner. It has much better resolution than other electrophoretic methods but is comparatively more expensive and labor intensive and lacks accurate quantification capabilities. The hemoglobin migration allows resolution of Hb C from Hb E and Hb O-Arab and Hb S from Hb D-Punjab and Hb G-Philadelphia. Hb A and Hb F are clearly resolved. However, it separates post-translationally modified forms of the hemoglobins, such as glycated and oxidized hemoglobins, making interpretation difficult. As with alkaline and acid electrophoresis, many hemoglobin variants are silent on isoelectric focusing.[3,5] On the other hand, there are hemoglobin variants that are not separated on either alkaline or acid electrophoresis or HPLC that can detected by isoelectric focusing.

It is important to remember that electrophoresis techniques are qualitative by nature, and accurate quantification of the various hemoglobin fractions requires additional tests. HPLC can be used not only for the detection, provisional identification, and quantification of variant hemoglobins, but also for quantification of the normal hemoglobin fractions, Hb A, Hb F, and Hb A2. HPLC offers many other advantages over electrophoresis—automated and less labor intensive, minimal sample preparation, small sample volume requirement, routine quantification of Hb A2, providing diagnosis of β-thalassemia in a single procedure, and provisional identification of a large range of variant hemoglobins. The main disadvantages of HPLC—the higher capital and reagent costs and lack of HPLC knowledge by many laboratories—are balanced by the availability of highly automated HPLC platforms, which allow hemoglobinopathy analysis, as well as Hb A1c quantification on the same instrument. This makes HPLC technology more feasible in many more hospital clinical laboratories.

HEMOGLOBINOPATHY DETECTION PROTOCOL STRATEGIES

The number of hemoglobin variants discovered now exceeds 1000, and various analytical schemes involving electrophoretic and chromatographic methods have been developed for detecting many of these variants in a routine clinical laboratory.

A hemoglobinopathy detection protocol must be pragmatic, guided by the population studied, the type of service provided, and the technology employed. It is important to remember that in a diagnostic laboratory, the identification of a variant hemoglobin is most often presumptive rather than definitive. It may not be possible, let alone clinically relevant, to identify every hemoglobin variant encountered. The protocol chosen should ensure that a great majority of clinically relevant disorders are detected.

Except with newborn screening programs, in most cases, a stepwise approach guided by clinical features and hematological data has proved to be practical and useful in the decision of which patient should have a diagnostic workup of hemoglobinopathies.

The minimum requirements for the detection and identification of hemoglobinopathies should include a reliable screening test with a different and reliable test used for confirmation. Because reliable detection of hemoglobinopathies necessitates detection not only of abnormal hemoglobin fractions but of imbalanced ratios of those fractions, one of the methods used should be quantitative. Although each of the techniques reviewed above has limitations in its ability to unequivocally identify a variant hemoglobin, these minimum requirements can be achieved through a stepwise algorithmic approach, with the use of data from a number of laboratory techniques and integrated with clinical factors (see Box 5-4).

With use of a quantitative and specific method such as HPLC, the initial screen allows many of the pitfalls of detection programs to be avoided. There is relative certainty of the screening result and of the quantitative component for Hb A2 and Hb F, which can detect a potential thalassemia.

Examples of algorithms for antenatal screening with HPLC as the primary hemoglobinopathy screening tool have been discussed and recommended.[24]

KEY CONCEPTS BOX 5-3

- Knowledge of which hemoglobin (Hb) chains are produced and how they interact is critical for differentiating between an α- and a β-variant Hb and for identifying a thalassemia.
- Variant Hb chains also can interact with thalassemias to make HPLC identification difficult.
- HPLC is a superior method of identifying variant Hb, but electrophoretic techniques can be used in the identification process.
- HPLC is a far superior technique for quantification of Hb A2 and Hb F.
- Protocols are available that show the efficient use of all techniques for identification of Hb variants.

REFERENCES

1. Weatherall DJ, Clegg JB: *The Thalassaemia Syndromes,* Oxford, England, 2001, Blackwell Science Ltd.
2. Globin Gene Server website. Available at http://globin/cse.psu.edu. Accessed May 28, 2008.
3. Kutlar F: Diagnostic approach to hemoglobinopathies, Hemoglobin 31:243-250, 2007.
4. Wild B, Bain BJ: Detection and quantitation of normal and variant haemoglobins: an analytical review. Ann Clin Biochem 41:355-369, 2004.
5. Bain BJ: *Haemoglobinopathy Diagnosis,* Oxford, England, 2005, Blackwell Science Ltd.
6. Working Party of the General Haemotology Task Force of the British Committee for Standards in Haemotology: Guidelines: the laboratory diagnosis of haemoglobinopathies, Br J Haematol 101:783-792, 1998.
7. Papadea C, Cate JC IV: Identification and quantification of hemoglobins A, F, S, and C by automated chromatography. Clin Chem 42:57-63, 1996.
8. Jutovsky A, Nardi MA: Hemoglobin C and hemoglobin O-Arab variants can be diagnosed using the Bio-Rad Variant II High-Performance Liquid Chromatography System without further confirmatory tests, Arch Pathol Lab Med 128:435-439, 2004.
9. Joutovsky A, Hadzi-Nesic J, Nardi MA: HPLC retention time as a diagnostic tool for hemoglobin variants and hemoglobinopathies: a study of 60 000 samples in a clinical diagnostic laboratory, Clin Chem 50:1736-1747, 2004.
10. Riou J, Godart C, Hurtrel D, et al: Cation-exchange HPLC evaluated for presumptive identification of hemoglobin variants, Clin Chem 43:34-39, 1997.
11. Fucharoen S, Winichagoon P, Wiisepanichkij R, et al: Prenatal and postnatal diagnoses of thalassemias and hemoglobinopathies by HPLC, Clin Chem 44:740-748, 1998.
12. Waters HM, Howarth JE, Hyde K, et al: *Evaluation of the Bio-Rad Variant β Thalassemia Short Program: MDA Evaluation Report MDA/96/28,* London, 1996, Medical Devices Agency.
13. Bain BJ, Phelan L: *Evaluation of the Primus Corporation CLC330TM HPLC System for Haemoglobinopathy Screening: MDA Evaluation Report MDA/97/53,* London, 1997, Medical Devices Agency.
14. Bain BJ, Phelan L: *Evaluation of the Kontron Instruments Haemoglobin System PV for Haemoglobinopathy Screening: MDA Evaluation Report MD/97/53,* London, 1997, Medical Devices Agency.
15. Hematology and Clinical Microscopy Reference Committee: *Hemoglobinopathy Survey Proficiency Reports, 1994-2007,* Chicago, IL, 2007 College of American Pathologists.
16. Ou C-N, Buffone GJ, Reimer GL: High-performance liquid chromatography of human hemoglobins on a new cation exchanger, J Chromatogr 266:197-205, 1983.
17. Alpert AJ: Cation-exchange high-performance liquid chromatography of proteins on poly(aspartic acid)-silica. J Chromatogr 266:23-37, 1983.
18. *Primus Ultra2 Procedure Manual,* Primus Corporation, 2007, Kansas City, MO.
19. *Tosoh G7 Procedure Manual,* Tosoh Bioscience, Inc., 2006, South San Francisco, CA.
20. Dash S: Hb A2 in subjects with Hb D, Clin Chem 44:2381-2382, 1998.
21. Shokrani M, Terrell F, Turner EA, del Pilar Aguinaga M: Chromatographic measurements of hemoglobin A2 in blood samples that contain sickle hemoglobin, Ann Clin Lab Sci 30: 191-194, 2000.
22. Ou CN, Rognerud CL: Diagnosis of hemoglobinopathies: electrophoresis vs. HPLC, Clin Chim Acta 313:187-194, 2001.
23. Howanitz PJ, Kozarski TB, Howanitz JH, Chauhan YS: Spurious hemoglobin Barts caused by bilirubin, Am J Clin Pathol 125: 608-614, 2006.
24. Wacjman H, Prehu C, Bardakdjian-Michau J, et al: Abnormal hemoglobins: laboratory methods, Hemoglobin 25:169-181, 2001.

INTERNET SITES

http://globin.cse.psu.edu
http://www.labtestsonline.org
http://thalassemia.org
http://www.sicklecelldisease.org
http://www.hbpinfo.com/en/index.htm
http://www.bu.edu/sicklecell

Electrophoresis

John M. Brewer

Chapter 6

Chapter Outline

Key Terms

ampholyte A substance that has both acid and base properties; also a trade name for a mixture of substances with a range of isoelectric points that have high buffering capacities at their isoelectric points.

amphoteric A substance that can have a positive, zero, or negative charge, depending on conditions.

anion Negatively charged particle or ion.

boundary Edge of a zone, as of a macromolecule solution next to the solvent.

buffer A mixture of proton-donating and proton-accepting substances, the function of which is to keep the proton concentration (the pH) constant or nearly so. An example is a mixture of acetic acid and sodium acetate.

capillary electrophoresis Electrophoresis within a capillary tube or other small-diameter channel.

cation Positively charged particle or ion.

coion An ion of the same charge as the one under consideration; generally a much smaller ion.

conductivity The readiness of a substance to carry a current; in an ionic solution, the sum of the products of the charge concentrations and the charge mobilities.

convection Mass or bulk movement of one part of a solution relative to the rest, usually caused by density differences.

counterion An ion of charge opposite to the one under consideration; generally a smaller ion.

densitometry Measurement of the absorbance of analytes along the length of a support.

discontinuous solvent A solution consisting of at least two separate regions that have different ions in them.

disk electrophoresis A stacking or isotachophoretic step followed by zone electrophoresis, usually on a polyacrylamide gel.

effective mobility The actual mobility of a substance under certain conditions; generally less than the mobility because of a lower molecular charge or resistance by a supporting medium.

electrical field An influence measured in volts (or volts per centimeter) that is manifested by the behavior of a charged particle within it.

electrical neutrality A condition in which total positive charges equal total negative charges.

electroblot Substances separated on supporting medium by electrophoresis are transferred onto a facing sheet of material using an electrical field perpendicular to the original separating field. The material on the facing sheet adsorbs and immobilizes substances in the same pattern as the original separation.

electrochromatography Analyte movement through a chromatographic matrix produced by an electrical field rather than by hydrostatic pressure.

electrodes Substances in contact with a conductor. These substances are connected to the source of an electrical field.

electrolytes Ionic substances, usually of low molecular weight, added to provide as constant and uniform an ionic environment for electrophoresis as possible.

electro-osmosis Tendency of a solution to move relative to an adjacent stationary substance when an electrical field is applied.

electrophoresis Movement of charged particles caused by an external electrical field.

extinction coefficient The theoretical absorbance of a 1 M solution in a 1 cm path length cell at a specific wavelength.

frictional coefficient A measure of the resistance a particle offers to movement through a solvent.

gel A network of interacting fibers, or a polymer, that is solid but traps large amounts of solvent in pores or channels inside.

hydration Ions in water solution are surrounded by a cluster of water molecules, often a fixed number with a definite geometry.

ionic strength The sum of the concentrations of all ions in a solution, weighted by the squares of their charges.

isoelectric Condition of zero net charge on an amphoteric substance.

isoelectric focusing The ordering and concentration of substances according to their isoelectric points.

isoelectric point The pH at which a substance has a zero net charge.

isotachophoresis The ordering and concentration of substances of intermediate effective mobilities between an ion of high effective mobility and one of much lower effective mobility, followed by their migration at a uniform velocity.

Joule heating Heating of a conductor by the passage of an electrical current.

micellar electrokinetic chromatography A capillary electrophoresis technique in which separation of analytes, even uncharged ones, occurs after partitioning between the hydrophillic electrophoresis solvent and the hydrophobic interior of micelles that migrate in an electric field. The micelles are formed from ionic detergents. Separation will depend on the extent of the partitioning; see Chapter 3 for a review of partitioning theory.

mobility The velocity that a particle or ion attains for a given applied voltage. A relative measure of how quickly an ion moves in an electrical field.

molecular sieving Separation of molecules on the basis of their effective sizes.

polyacrylamide Polymer of acrylamide and usually some cross-linking derivative.

polyelectrolyte Substance with many charged or potentially charged groups.

resolving power Ability to separate closely migrating substances.

sodium dodecyl sulfate (SDS) A detergent and an especially effective protein denaturant.

solvation In water solutions, any polar substance is associated with some water molecules, although less strongly than in the case of ions (see "hydration").

Southern blot A kind of electroblot in which the substances separated and transferred are nucleic acids.

stacking Ordering or arranging and concentrating macromolecules according to their effective mobilities; compare with isotachophoresis.

Western blot A kind of electroblot in which the substances that are separated and transferred are proteins.

zeta potential The potential produced by the effective charge of a macromolecule, usually taken at the boundary between what is moving with the macromolecule and the rest of the solution.

zone A particular region or space within a larger one, which generally is distinguished by some property, such as its occupancy by a protein.

SECTION OBJECTIVES BOX 6-1

- Define the properties of the *cathode* and *anode* in electrophoresis.
- Describe the relationship between current, voltage, resistance, heat, conductivity, and power (wattage).
- State the molecular factors that affect the movement of a charged particle through an external electrical field.
- Describe the effect of pH on the movement of charged particles in electrophoresis.
- State the function of the buffer and the support media in electrophoresis.

Movement of charged particles caused by an *external* **electrical field** is called **electrophoresis.** Because charged molecules can be made to move, different molecules can be separated if they have different velocities in an electrical field. Therefore, electrophoresis is a separation technique, as is chromatography.

The electrical field is applied to a solution through oppositely charged **electrodes** placed in the solution (Fig. 6-1). An ion then travels through the solution toward the electrode of opposite charge: positively charged particles (**cations**) move to the negatively charged electrode (cathode), and negatively charged particles (**anions**) migrate to the positively charged electrode (anode).

APPLICATION OF ELECTRICAL FIELD TO A SOLUTION CONTAINING A CHARGED PARTICLE

Forces on a Particle

The force exerted on a charged particle depends on the electrical field, V (in volts or volts per centimeter), and the charge on the particle, Q. The force on the charged particle is the product:

$$F_{elec} = QV \quad \text{Eq. 6-1}$$

This electrical force, F_{elec}, when exerted on the particle, will cause it to move. However, a particle that is moving in a solvent will experience resistance because of the viscosity of

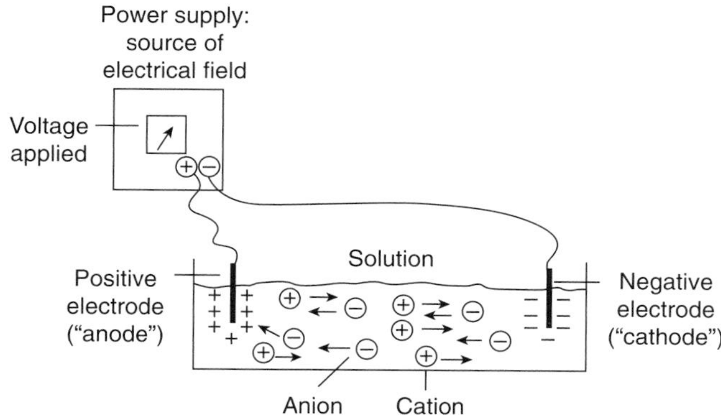

Fig. 6-1 Application of an electrical field to a solution of ions makes ions move.

the solvent. This resistance, which is itself a force, is proportional to the velocity:

$$F_{\text{resistance}} = fv \qquad \text{Eq. 6-2}$$

The proportionality constant, f, is called the ***frictional coefficient.***

The frictional coefficient depends on the viscosity of the solvent and the size and shape of the particle. The greater the viscosity, the slower is the movement. The bigger or more asymmetrical the particle, the slower is its movement through the solvent. The frictional coefficient of a large particle such as a protein is a characteristic property of the particle.

Mobility of a Particle

When an electrical field is applied to a charged particle, the particle begins to migrate. The electrophoretic and frictional forces oppose each other, and the particle's velocity increases until the forces are equal ($F_{\text{resistance}} = F_{\text{elec}}$). The velocity, v, that a particle attains for a given electrical field, V, is determined by two properties of the particle—its charge and its frictional coefficient. Consequently, the value of v/V is also a characteristic property of the particle and is called the ***mobility*** of the particle.

Effect of pH on Mobility

Each fully charged ion has a particular mobility. However, when a solution contains a substance whose pK is near the pH of the solution, that substance exists in both a charged and an uncharged form in the solution. The fraction of species with a charge depends on the pK of the substance and the pH of the solution. When the pH is equal to the pK_a of a weak acid, only 50% of the particles are charged. Because the effective (average) charge of a substance varies with the pH, its ***effective mobility*** also varies with the pH.

This is particularly true for substances such as proteins. Proteins are ***amphoteric*** substances, that is, they contain acidic and basic groups. Their overall (net) charge is positive at low pH values, zero (**isoelectric**) at a particular higher pH, and negative at still more alkaline pH values. Because mobility is directly proportional to the magnitude of the charge, the effective mobility of a protein is very much a function of the pH.

The most important practical consequence of this is that electrophoretic solutions usually are buffered so a constant pH is maintained. The ***buffer*** pH may be chosen to give an optimum net charge for maximum separation. For proteins, pH values in the 7 to 9 range generally are used. The buffer is used to maintain this pH and thus the net protein charge throughout the electrophoretic process. Buffers, which are ionic substances themselves, take part in any electrophoretic process—a fact that must also be considered.

Electrolytes

In electrophoresis, a substance such as a protein is put in one limited region, or ***zone,*** of the system and is made to move into another region, or zone. Therefore, much of the solution does not have protein in it at any particular time. If the protein and its associated counterions are not present to carry the current in a particular region, other ions must be present to carry the current. For this reason, it is a common practice to add an excess, usually about 0.1 M, of low-molecular-weight buffer to the solution through which the protein must travel. The buffer and salt ions (**electrolytes**) provide a constant electrical environment so that the overall movement of the protein is as constant as possible and will be minimally influenced by other protein molecules.

Ion Movement and Conductivity

In any electrical system, the current produced is proportional to the voltage applied:

$$V = \text{Resistance} \times \text{Current} \qquad \text{Eq. 6-3}$$

or

$$V = \text{Current/Conductivity} \qquad \text{Eq. 6-4}$$

In electrophoresis, the current is the flow of ions (in both directions). The **conductivity** is the sum of the concentrations times the effective mobilities of all ions present. An ion with a higher effective mobility carries a larger fraction of the current than one at the same concentration that has a lower effective mobility. The voltage, conductivity, and current thus all are related (Equation 6-4).

If the conductivity is increased by an increase in the salt concentration while the current is kept constant, the voltage must decrease. Such a decrease in voltage reduces the electrical force, F_{elec}, on charged particles, thus slowing the movement of macromolecules. This increases the time needed for a given separation, and the resolution decreases because of increased diffusion. If the conductivity is increased at a fixed voltage, the current must increase, thus increasing the electrical heat (**Joule heating**) generated by the system, because heating is proportional to the wattage, that is, to the square of the current. Excessive heating produces convective disturbances in the solutions, which distort the electrophoretic patterns and may denature macromolecules. The heat generated in any electrophoretic separation is the ultimate factor in how fast the separation can be done. Because increasing the conductivity at either a fixed voltage or current has deleterious effects, optimum results are achieved when the concentration of ions and therefore the conductivity are kept at moderate values.

FACTORS AFFECTING MOBILITIES OF MACROMOLECULES

Charge and Conformation

The clinical laboratory usually deals with **polyelectrolytes,** that is, substances with many charged or potentially charged groups on them. The net charge of a polyelectrolyte is determined by the total number of charged groups within the polyelectrolyte and its conformation. The folding, or *conformation,* of a protein produces binding sites for many small molecules. In some cases, electrolyte ions bind strongly and specifically to the macromolecule. For example, bovine serum albumin can bind several chloride ions. This changes the net charge of the macromolecule and therefore its mobility.

Ionic Atmosphere and Zeta Potential

Counterions, ions of opposite charge, naturally tend to hover in the vicinity of charged groups of macromolecules. In water, every polar substance interacts with the water (also polar) and ions interact with clusters of waters ("hydration"). Thus, counterions do not actually neutralize—bind directly to—charged groups on a macromolecule. Instead, they are located at a range of distances from the charged groups of the macromolecule, forming a double layer of charge about the macromolecule known as an *ionic atmosphere.*

The macromolecule moves with its entourage of hydration and hydrated counterions (Fig. 6-2). These reduce the effective charge of the macromolecule to a level given by the **zeta potential.** The zeta potential is the potential (voltage) produced by the effective charge of the macromolecule at the surface of shear. The surface of shear is the **boundary** between the entire macromolecular complex in solution (hydration layer and embedded counterions) and the material that is staying behind (the solvent).

Relaxation Effect

Because of random thermal motion, electrophoresing macromolecules move irregularly, in jumps, rather than in a continuous straight line. At each jump, the counterion atmosphere is left somewhat behind. The counterions (or their replacements from other parts of the solution) then move to catch up or reposition themselves, but this takes a little time. This is called a *relaxation effect.* It also tends to lower the mobility of the macromolecule because the retarded or misplaced counterions momentarily produce a field that acts in a direction opposite to that of the applied field.

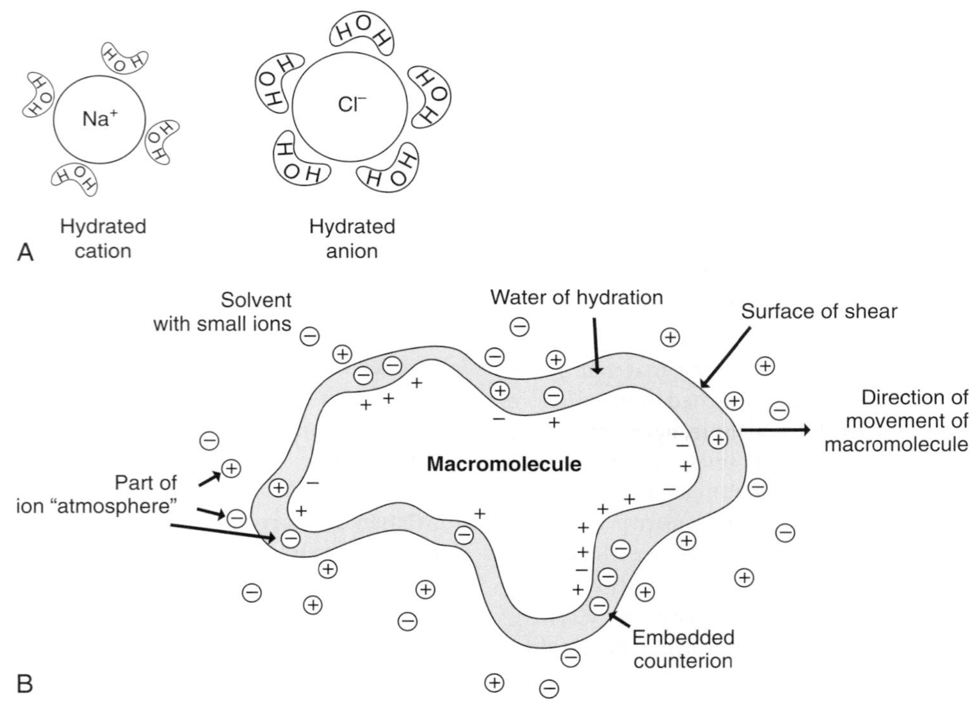

Fig. 6-2 State of charged substances in water solution. **A,** Small ions (Na^+ and Cl^-) with associated water molecules ("hydration"). **B,** Macromolecules in water move with water molecules associated with charged and polar groups on the surface of the macromolecule. Smaller ions of opposite charge also are associated with the charged groups, and these alter the effective charge of the macromolecule to an extent given by the "zeta potential." This is the effective electrical field strength (potential) of the macromolecule and of any smaller ions embedded in solvent carried along with the macromolecule ("water of hydration"). The zeta potential is measured at the "surface of shear": the boundary between what moves with the macromolecule and the rest of the solvent. Hydration of the small ions (Fig. 6-2, **B**) is not shown. *Gray area,* Water of hydration.

Electrophoretic Effect

Because ions in water solution are hydrated, the counterions of the electrolyte moving in the opposite direction carry solvent along with them. The macromolecule is thus moving against a *flow* of solvent, and its mobility is reduced by this factor also.

SUPPORT MEDIA

The goal of electrophoresis is to separate a mixture of substances, such as macromolecules, into completely separate zones. The narrower (thinner) the original zone of a mixture of macromolecules is, the smaller the migration distance necessary to achieve separation will be. Use of narrower zones means that complete separation can be effected in less time. Blurring or remixing of the separated zones as a result of diffusion is also reduced.

The major technical difficulty in using narrow (thin) zones of relatively concentrated macromolecules is a mechanical one. Such zones are considerably more dense than the solvent; thus the zones "fall" through the solvent faster than the macromolecules electrophorese. This is called *bulk flow*, or **convection.** One solution to this problem is to use a supporting medium.

Functional Basis

The supporting medium must allow as free a penetration of the material to be separated as possible and yet cut off bulk flow (convection). Most media do this by offering a restricted pore size for electrophoretic movement of the macromolecules. A capillary tube has the same effect. This is the basis of *capillary zone electrophoresis*. The capillary tubes are as little as 25 to 50 μm (0.025 to 0.05 mm) across.

Electro-Osmosis

Normally, the supporting medium should not interact with the molecules, because this might inhibit or stop migration (but see later discussion). The usual interaction problem encountered is not actual adsorption of the material. More common are effects of charged groups attached to the medium that result in **electro-osmosis.** For example, agar, often used as a supporting medium in electrophoresis, is a mixture of agarose and agaropectin. Agaropectin has a relatively large number of carboxyl groups in it, which at neutral pH have counterions. If a voltage is applied, the counterions move, but the carboxyl groups attached to the polysaccharide matrix cannot move. Counterions carry enough solvent with them to produce a net flow of solvent in *one* direction. This is electro-osmosis, sometimes called *endosmosis.* However, although electro-osmosis is more pronounced when charged groups are present in the supporting medium, it always occurs to some extent.

In capillary electrophoresis, the surface-to-volume ratio is high, so the surface characteristics of the capillary material become very important. Capillaries made of fused silica, which is transparent in the ultraviolet (UV), are almost always used. The surfaces of these consist of silanol groups that have a pK_a of 6.5, so capillary surfaces always bear some negative charge unless a low pH (2 or 3) is used, or unless they are derivatized or coated with an agent such as cellulose or a plastic. These may be done to reduce or eliminate electro-osmosis and such effects as actual adsorption of proteins to uncoated surfaces.

Types of Supporting Media

The supporting medium can be a solution such as a sucrose density gradient, but, in general, insoluble materials are used. Some are self-supporting, whereas the apparatus mechanically supports others. Paper or sheets of plastic such as cellulose acetate have enough mechanical strength to allow electrophoresis on sheets hung or stretched over rods.

Support media also can be classified as particulate or continuous. Particulate support media include glass beads, gel-permeation media (see p. 77, Chapter 3, and below) such as Sephadex, and cellulose fibers. Continuous support media include **polyacrylamide,** starch, and agarose gels.

Gels are jellylike solids in which considerable solvent is included. Starch gels, for example, are made from starch suspensions that are heated and cooled. The starch fibers interact, tangling with each other so that large gaps or pores filled with trapped solvent exist between the fibers. These gaps or pores are available for macromolecular movement. Similar gels can be made from agar, agarose, and some chemical polymers. Gels also can be made through polymerization of acrylamide with a small percentage of a bifunctional acrylamide derivative that cross-links the acrylamide polymers (Fig. 6-3).

Molecular Sieving

The porosity, or average pore size, of some media can be controlled, for example, by changing the gel concentrations of starch or agar. If the average pore size is near the average diameter of the macromolecules that are being electrophoresed, the supporting medium will produce **molecular sieving** effects.

Sequencing of deoxyribonucleic acid (DNA) is done by electrophoresis of a mixture of fluorescent labeled DNA

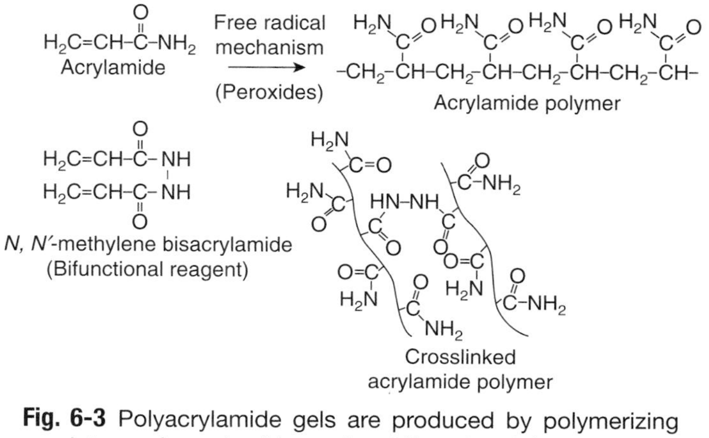

Fig. 6-3 Polyacrylamide gels are produced by polymerizing a mixture of acrylamide and a bifunctional (cross-linking) acrylamide derivative. The derivative shown is that in common use.

molecules that vary in length from a few nucleotides to many hundreds of nucleotides. These can be separated by electrophoresis in a capillary tube containing linear (un–cross-linked) polyacrylamide so efficiently that adjacent zones of separated polynucleotide differ in length by only one nucleotide. Several hundred base lengths can be separated (and "read") (Fig. 6-4). Note that oligonucleotides in general have one negative charge per nucleotide at neutral pH values, a constant "charge-to-mass ratio" in other words, and usually have the same shape and so are separated exclusively on the basis of their molecular weight.

The average pore size of polyacrylamide gels cast at 5% to 10% concentrations is also comparable to the effective diameters of many globular (relatively compact) proteins of 15,000 to 250,000 D. These gels will filter such solutions, separating proteins on the basis of *both* size and mobility. The molecular sieving effects can produce enhanced resolution, that is, narrower zones of macromolecules, as well.

KEY CONCEPTS BOX 6-1

- In an electric field, ions move to either the anode or cathode. Negatively charged cathodes are where cations (positively charged ions) move to; positively charged anodes are where anions (negatively charged ions) move to.
- The speed at which charged particles in solution move depends on (1) the voltage applied, (2) effective particle charge, (3) the viscosity of the solution, and (4) particle's effective size.
- Voltage is directly related to the sum of resistance and charge (Eq 6-3); conductivity is the inverse of resistance (Eq 6-4). Changing any one of these parameters will therefore affect the others. Increased power or wattage (volts × current or current squared ÷ conductivity) increases heat generation ("Joule heating"), which limits the speed of electrophoresis.
- The charge on a molecule's ionic groups can change with pH of the solution, which in turn can change the molecule's effective charge and movement in an electric field.
- Electrophoresis buffer functions to maintain a constant pH during electrophoretic separations and to carry the current. The support media restricts the sample to a defined 2-dimentional space.

SECTION OBJECTIVES BOX 6-2

- Discuss the uses of the following to affect electrophoretic separation.
  - Paper and cellulose acetate
  - Polyacrylamide gels
  - Starch and agar
- Discuss the advantages of capillary electrophoresis.
- Describe the electroblotting technique and its clinical utility.
- Describe the advantages and disadvantages of performing electrophoresis under conditions of constant current or voltage.

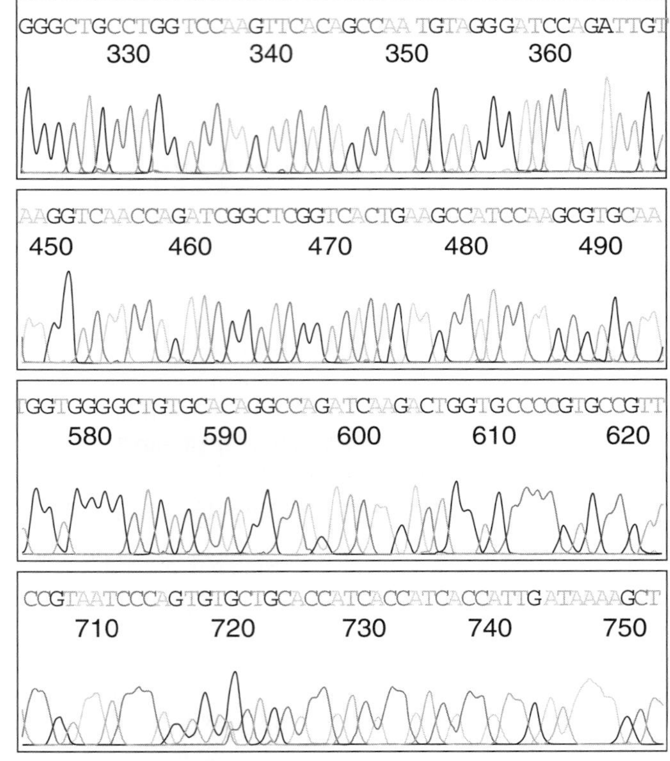

Fig. 6-4 Part of the data printout from a deoxyribonucleic acid (DNA) sequencing experiment. Each peak is from the fluorescence of a polynucleotide that is one residue (nucleotide) longer than the one that produced the peak to its left and one residue shorter than the polynucleotide that produced the signal to its right. The separation occurs by capillary electrophoresis (Applied Biosystems Prism apparatus) through linear (un–cross-linked) polyacrylamide. Each polynucleotide is terminated by an analog of adenine (A), cytosine (C), guanine (G), or thymine (T) that has a different fluorescence spectrum; these are recorded and identified as they migrate past the detector. The peaks get broader because of diffusion as polynucleotide length (numbers between the DNA sequence at the top and the profiles at the bottom) and electrophoresis time increase. (Data obtained at the Molecular Genetics Instrumentation Facility of the University of Georgia, courtesy of Dr. John Wunderlich.)

ENHANCED-RESOLUTION TECHNIQUES

Discontinuous Buffers

A solution with a lower conductivity is placed behind the protein zone, and a solution with a higher conductivity is placed in front. If the conductivities are suitable, the proteins become *stacked* between the two solutions: a series of proteins will arrange themselves according to their effective mobilities and will become concentrated, resulting in much greater (enhanced) resolution. Often solutions of ions at similar concentrations but with very different effective mobilities are used. However, simply diluting the analyte with water or an organic solvent like acetonitrile can produce **stacking** (Fig. 6-5).

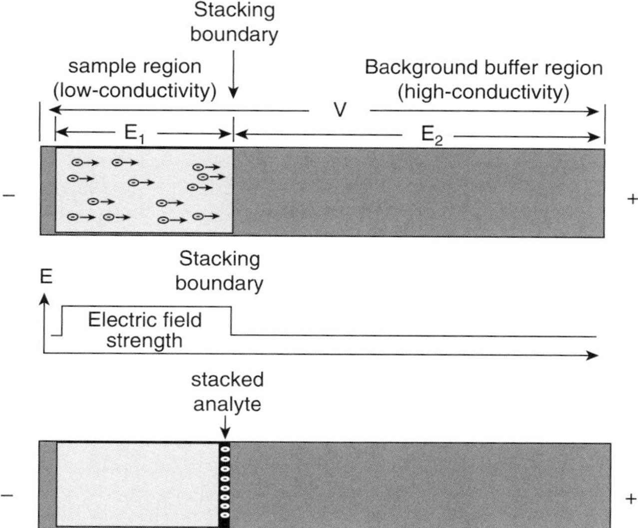

Fig. 6-5 "Stacking" of an analyte with a low charge-to-mass ratio, such as a protein in a discontinuous solvent system. The analyte is shown mixed in a solvent with a low(er) conductivity (lower concentration or effective mobility of ions or both) *(top).* With an electrical field applied, the current must be the same along the path, so the voltage is greater in the low-conductivity region *(middle).* The analyte has a greater effective mobility than the coion so moves to the boundary between the solutions and concentrates there, until its movement carries the same current as the low- and high-conductivity solutions *(bottom).* (From Peterson JR, Mohammad AA: *Clinical and Forensic Applications of Capillary Electrophoresis,* Totowa, NJ, 2001, Humana Press.)

There are three major applications of the use of **discontinuous solvent** systems to produce enhanced resolution: **isotachophoresis, disk electrophoresis,** and **isoelectric focusing.** These techniques, briefly described in Table 6-1, are used frequently to analyze proteins.

Separations Based on Molecular Size

By enabling separations on the basis of molecular size and molecular charge, the techniques briefly described in Table 6-2 also provide enhanced resolution. They usually employ polyacrylamide or agarose to prepare gels of known pore size. Molecules of smaller molecular size electrophorese faster than larger molecules that carry similar charges.

Electrophoresis of such substances sometimes is used analytically to estimate molecular weights from how far a given substance moves, compared with how far substances of known molecular weight ("standards") move under the same conditions.

SELECTION OF METHODS AND CONDITIONS

Knowledge of the **isoelectric point** and the molecular weight of the compound to be examined can help one to determine the optimum conditions for an electrophoretic separation. A buffer should be chosen with a pH that will provide the maximum separation without destroying the properties of the sample. Very acidic or basic conditions pose problems for any system, because an increasing fraction of the current is carried by protons or hydroxyl ions, resulting in poorer separation. A summary of the effects of the various variables on electrophoresis is provided in Table 6-3.

Support Media

Slabs or sheets are useful when different samples are compared, and routine clinical electrophoresis is done with the use of sheet supports. Gel cylinders sometimes are used in isoelectric focusing.

Paper and Cellulose Acetate

The main advantages of these materials are their thinness and their mechanical strength. A thinner support means greater sensitivity because less material is needed to produce a detectable spot or zone. In a thicker support, the same amount of sample in a zone is distributed in a greater volume and so is more dilute and hence more difficult to detect. Thicker supports are more likely to be used for preparative purposes.

Paper is especially favored for separation of low-molecular-weight substances in specialized biochemical laboratories. Cellulose acetate is prepared by treating cellulose with acetic anhydride. This puts acetyl groups on the sugar hydroxyl groups. The resulting material is pressed into sheets that are somewhat stronger than paper and a good deal more chemically uniform. Adsorption of material to any support leads to losses of material and to *tailing* of zones. Cellulose acetate is more inert in this respect, and because of its uniformity and ease of preparation (the strips are merely soaked in electrophoresis buffer so that no air is trapped), it is very widely used in routine clinical work.

Cellulose acetate sheets can be purchased in relatively uniform batches so that results of different electrophoresis experiments are more consistent. After electrophoresis, the strips can be sliced into bands containing stained or radioactive materials. These slices can be dissolved in a solvent such as acetone for easy quantitation.

On the other hand, resolution with cellulose acetate is not as good as with polyacrylamide (see later discussion). Eight or nine serum protein fractions can be resolved with the use of cellulose acetate, but up to 30 fractions can be detected with disk electrophoresis on polyacrylamide gels. So cellulose acetate is used because it lends itself to fast, easy, reproducible measurements, although of comparatively low resolution.

Gels

Gels can be cast with varying thicknesses to increase or decrease capacity (the amount of sample). Gels also offer the possibility of molecular sieving effects because their porosity can be controlled by changing their composition. On the other hand, their mechanical strength tends to be low.

Starch and Agar

Starch gels provide greater resolution than is obtained with agar or agarose. However, the inconvenience of preparing starch

Table 6-1 Enhanced-Resolution Techniques

Technique	Physical Basis	Mechanism	Effect	Limitations	Advantages and Uses
Isotachophoresis	Electrical neutrality; current in series circuit is constant. Lower conductivity solution after higher conductivity solution must move at same velocity and carry same current, and so the two solutions experience different voltages and adjust in concentration.	Solution of lower conductivity containing ion of lower mobility running behind solution of higher conductivity containing higher mobility ion (e.g., chloride); ion of intermediate mobility (e.g., protein) sandwiched between; concentration of protein increases to carry same current as lower and higher mobility ions.	Intermediate-mobility ions (e.g., proteins) stack in thin concentrated zones and move in discrete zones.	Ions not separated; resolution not as good as disk electrophoresis	No widespread clinical applications currently
Disk electrophoresis	Effective mobilities of some ions are pH dependent; it often is used with polyacrylamide gels.	As above, then stacked proteins overrun because of the pH change; change in pH produced using couterion	Proteins, now in thin zones, migrate independently.	Ion systems and pH values limited; technically more exacting than ordinary electrophoresis	High sensitivity and resolving power; used extensively to separate proteins, used most often as a research tool
Isolectric focusing	Migration of ions must occur in both directions; amphoteric ions (with both basic and acid groups) have zero effective mobility and zero net charge at their isoelectric point.	Ion movement stops because of zero counterion concentration, leaving all ions stacked in pH gradient; leading and trailing ions are an acid and a base.	Proteins in zones at isoelectric (isoionic) points; pH gradient is buffered by carrier ampholytes.	More complicated and exacting than ordinary electrophoresis	High capacity and resolution to 0.001 pH unit possible; primarily a research tool

gels has limited their use. The starch solution must be heated to 100° C, degassed—an awkward process—and then cast.

Agar and agarose (agar without the agaropectin) are easier to handle. Because agarose demonstrates a lower electroosmotic effect and exhibits fewer problems with adsorption, it is preferred over agar. The pore size of agarose is much greater than that of polyacrylamide. Therfore agar or agarose is used in most immunoelectrophoretic techniques because antigen and antibody must be able to migrate freely through the gel. Another advantage of agarose is that it may be poured after reheating to only about 50°C; thus some proteins, such as antibodies, can be mixed in without denaturing. Precast agarose gels with plastic backing are available commercially. These gels are used for separation of isoenzymes, hemoglobins, glycoproteins, and so on.

Polyacrylamide

Polyacrylamide gels are used less frequently in clinical laboratories but are a common research tool. They are clear, fairly easy to prepare, and exhibit reasonable mechanical strength over the acrylamide concentration range normally employed for proteins. In addition, they show a low endosmosis effect and have a pore size well suited for the separation of average proteins, ribonucleic acid (RNA) molecules, and smaller restriction fragments of DNA. A major clinical use of polyacrylamide gels is the separation of alkaline phosphatase isoenzymes. However, polyacrylamide gel preparation and casting are somewhat more exacting and time consuming, and complete reproducibility of gel preparation is not possible. Commercially prepared polyacrylamide sheets (some with plastic backing) are sold by several firms.

Table 6-2 Use of Supporting Media in Separation Based on Molecule Size

Method	Principle	Effect	Limitations	Advantages and Uses
Separation Based on Molecular Size				
Gradient gels	Gels cast with increasing gel concentrations going from origin to end of gel have gradient of pore sizes.	Larger macromolecules move more slowly as they encounter higher gel concentrations; can measure relative sizes and charges.	Difficult to reproduce gels	Research tool
Gels containing denaturants	Gels cast with denaturants (e.g., urea or SDS) so that macromolecules migrate in denatured forms; SDS binds uniformly and in large amounts to most proteins.	Proteins in SDS and oligonucleotides migrate inversely to subunit molecular weights or numbers of nucleotides.	Exacting technique: Disulfide bonds in proteins must be broken; not all proteins behave normally.	Research tool
Separations Based on Molecular Size and Charge				
Gel electrophoresis	Pore size is small enough to restrict diffusion.	Higher resolution	Reproducibility	Better resolution than cellulose acetate; agarose gels widely used; most often a research tool
Immunoelectrophoretic methods (see Chapter 8)	Antigen and antibody are brought together with the use of electrophoresis to form a precipitate.	Can identify and quantitate specific antigen and antibody	Sensitivity somewhat low	Better resolution than cellulose acetate; agarose gels widely used; most often a research tool
Two-dimensional electrophoresis	Separation occurs according to one parameter (e.g., isoelectric point) in one dimension (direction) and then according to a second parameter (e.g., size) at right angles.	Mixture of proteins spread over a surface; information proportional to square of length of side of surface	Exacting technique; difficult to reproduce patterns	High information content; widely used in clinical research

SDS, Sodium dodecyl sulfate.

Table 6-3 Common Effects of Electrophoretic Variables on Separation

Variable	Effect on Electrophoresis
pH	Changes charge of analyte and hence effective mobility; can affect structure of analyte, such as denaturing or dissociating a protein
Ionic strength	Changes voltage or current; increased ionic strength usually reduces migration velocity and increases heating
Ions present	Can change migration velocity if interaction is strong; can cause tailing of bands
Current	Too high a current causes overheating.
Voltage	Migration velocity is proportional to voltage.
Wattage	Heat generation depends on wattage (voltage × current). Limiting factor depends on cooling efficiency.
Temperature	Temperature gradients in support mediums cause bowed bands. Overheating can denature (precipate) proteins. Lower temperatures reduce diffusion but also reduce migration velocity; there is no effect on resolution.
Time	Separation of bands (resolution) increases linearly with time, but dilution of bands (diffusion) increases with the square root of time.
Medium	Major factors are endosmosis and pore size effects, which affect migration velocities.

Use of acrylamide substituted with ionizable groups that buffer at or near the isoelectric points of proteins to be separated greatly enhances the **resolving power** of isoelectric focusing. These substituted acrylamides produce what are called "immobilized pH gradient" gels.

Capillary Electrophoresis

The advantages of capillary electrophoresis techniques are the low volumes of buffers required, the very low amounts of analyte (nanoliters) used, the ease of changing conditions (buffer, pH, technique), and the low cost, because these techniques tend to be easy to set up and fast to perform. The greater speed of capillary electrophoresis separations derives from more efficient cooling of capillary tubes, which enables much greater voltages to be applied; some separations take less than 2 minutes. Even uncharged substances can be separated by electrophoresing micelles of charged detergents. Uncharged analytes partition into the interiors of moving micelles to varying extents. This technique is called ***micellar electrokinetic chromatography.***

Capillary electrophoresis must be done serially, one sample at a time. However, multicapillary instruments (currently up to 96 capillaries) are now available, so much higher sample throughput can be achieved. The major limitation is sensitivity, because of both the very low amounts of analyte electrophoresed and the very short (0.003 to 0.006 cm) optical path lengths across capillaries of 50 or 100 μm diameter. Direct observations of analytes as they migrate past an absorbance detector are possible if the analytes of interest have high "extinction coefficients"; otherwise, a variety of techniques for increasing sensitivity, such as fluorescence analysis or electrospray ionization mass spectrometry (MS), prior concentration of samples using stacking, ultrafiltration, or adsorbents, and so forth, are employed.

Currently, capillary electrophoresis in multicapillary devices is the method of choice for DNA sequencing because of severalfold increases in sample throughput resulting from shorter electrophoresis times (see Fig. 6-4). The U.S. Food and Drug Administration (FDA) has approved several capillary electrophoresis apparatuses for serum protein separations. One has seven capillaries and is also approved for analysis of proteins in urine and for analysis of serum proteins for monoclonal antibodies using an immunofixation method ("Western blot").

Considerable interest has developed in the use of short (ca. about 5 cm) capillaries or channels engraved or cast in silica or plastic blocks, called *microcapillary electrophoretic systems.* Even smaller volumes are used, and the very efficient cooling provided by the block of silica or plastic enables even higher voltages to be applied; consequently, shorter separation times, often of 1 to 2 minutes, result. Problems associated with detection are greater because the channels have even shorter optical path lengths, and currently, laser-induced fluorescence or electrochemical techniques are used most frequently for analyte detection. Very short analysis times make this technique possibly usable for emergency clinical situations.

Separation of proteins according to one property, usually isoelectric point, on a gel, followed by electrophoresis sideways onto a subsequently attached slab of polyacrylamide gel, usually in the presence of **sodium dodecyl sulfate (SDS),** is called "two-dimensional electrophoresis." About 1000 proteins can be resolved, and so comparisons performed between proteins from normal cells or tissues and cells or tissues from a diseased or drug-treated organism can be made to see what specific protein(s) increase or decrease as a result of the treatment or disease.

This can prove helpful in the development of treatment for disease, but sample preparation is exacting, and it is impossible to prepare polyacrylamide gels with exactly the same properties. Use is made of dyes with different fluorescent emission spectra, which form covalent bonds with lysyl residues in proteins. The dyes have the same molecular weights and one positive charge, so they do not change the charge (at alkaline pH values) of the proteins with which they react. In one application of this technique, one dye is reacted with proteins from normal cells and another with proteins from treated or diseased cells. The differently labeled proteins are *mixed* and electrophoresed *together,* so each protein zone resolved is from normal and treated/diseased cells, and *relative* amounts of the same protein from different cells or tissues are calculated much more reliably. This is "differential gel electrophoresis" (DIGE).

Electroblotting

An exception to the requirement that a supporting medium must not interact with the material being separated is the **Western blot** technique. In this technique, a gel slab that contains separated proteins is electrophoresed perpendicularly to the slab, with transferal of some or all of the separated proteins onto a facing sheet of material, often nitrocellulose, which adsorbs the proteins (see Fig. 8-2). The sheet is washed with some neutral protein, such as milk protein or bovine serum albumin, to block unoccupied adsorption sites. Then the locations of specific transferred adsorbed proteins are determined, usually by immunochemical assays. The resulting pattern may be compared with the original slab that is stained or examined by autoradiography for all proteins or all labeled proteins.

A major virtue of Western blots is their sensitivity. (The adsorption *concentrates* the proteins.) Adsorption of antigens or antibodies takes place at concentrations of antigen and antibody that are far too low for a precipitate to form. As little as 10^{-12} g/mm^2 of protein can be detected and hence identified. Consequently, antigens (and antibodies) in serum that are present at very low concentrations can be detected and even quantitated. This technique is used for detecting the antigens and antibodies in patients infected with the human immunodeficiency virus (HIV).

Electrochromatography

Originally, interactions between support media and analytes were minimized. However, because the aim is to produce separations of analytes, and because interactions with support media sometimes can facilitate separation, increasing attention has been directed to purposefully producing and using support media in which analyte-media interactions are important. This field is called **electrochromatography,** and it differs from conventional chromatography in that analyte movement through the chromatographic matrix is produced by an electrical field rather than by hydrostatic pressure.

Electrochromatography in tubes or capillaries that contain optically active substances affixed to their surface, such as cyclodextrins, is used to resolve racemic mixtures.

Conditions

Horizontal versus Vertical Position

Electrophoresis can be performed horizontally or vertically. Horizontal electrophoresis places less mechanical stress on the support, whereas vertical electrophoresis supporting media often are supported between glass plates.

If horizontal electrophoresis is used and the surface of the medium is open to air, evaporation of the solvent can cause salt concentrations to rise, usually unevenly along the support, leading to nonuniform current flow and heating. This can lead to uneven migration, especially at the sides of a horizontal, flat electrophoresis bed. "Submarine" electrophoresis is horizontal electrophoresis in which the support is covered with buffer solution, so that there is no evaporation from the support. The sample is inserted into slots or holes in the support and is electrophoresed through the support. If one buffer reservoir is higher than the other, convective flow of the buffer through the supporting medium may occur. Therefore, the electrophoresis apparatus should always be level.

Sample Application

Sometimes samples are simply applied to the surface of the supporting medium and are allowed to soak in. Commercial sample applicators can simultaneously apply to the support surfaces a desired number of 1 or 2 μL samples of, for example, blood or serum; such devices help to ensure greater uniformity of initial sample zone shapes and sizes, improving reproducibility of results in clinical laboratories. Sometimes special slots or holes ("wells") are cast or cut in a gel, and the sample, which is made denser than the solvent through the addition of sucrose or glycerol, is put into the well. The sample may be polymerized into the gel or cast with the gel. Injection of the sample is rarely used, except with isotachophoresis. In capillary zone electrophoresis, a very small quantity (a few microliters) of the sample may be electrophoresed into the capillary tube. If electrophoresis takes place in stages (as in two-dimensional electrophoresis), the gel that contains part or all of the sample may be cut out and reattached, sometimes with an agarose "glue," to another gel for the next stage in the separation.

Current and Voltage Considerations

Electrophoresis can be carried out at constant voltage, constant current, or constant power *(wattage)*. This often depends on the power supply available. Because diffusion increases with the square root of time, it is best to complete the electrophoresis as quickly as possible. This requires use of the maximum voltage. However, the maximum voltage is always limited by the efficiency of cooling of the apparatus. Some workers claim that temperature gradients of more than 0.1°C across a gel or other support lead to noticeable distortions of macromolecule zones. For some current clinical applications, temperature control does not appear to be necessary, and separations are carried out at ambient temperatures.

The conductivity of any electrophoretic system changes with time because of heating, and because the ionic composition changes as a result of movement (electrophoresis) of the sample along the system. Such changes are minimal in continuous systems, such as high-voltage paper electrophoresis, and application of constant voltage is satisfactory for these systems. For disk electrophoresis and isotachophoresis, a constant velocity of zone migration is desired, and a constant current is used. For isoelectric focusing, heating is usually the limiting factor (see earlier discussion), and so constant power (wattage) should be used.

Separation Time

In the case of isotachophoresis, electrophoresis is stopped when the trailing ion emerges. Isoelectric focusing is complete after the gradient has been formed and the current has dropped to a stable value. The time to stop a disk or ordinary zone electrophoretic separation usually is indicated by the position of the *tracking dye*—usually when the dye band reaches a predetermined position in the stationary support (typically at the end of the support). Dyes that have high mobilities, such as bromophenol blue, are employed. They usually are added to the sample. Because some proteins bind such dyes, their apparent mobilities may be changed.

KEY CONCEPTS BOX 6-2

- Solid sheets of paper and cellulose acetate are used for clinical electrophoresis applications to separate molecules.
- Gels made of agar, starch, and polyacrylamide can be prepared with varying sizes of the gel pores, allowing separation by molecular size as well as by charge.
- Analytes separated on a supporting medium can be electrophoresed onto another medium that strongly adsorbs and concentrates the separated analytes, increasing the detection sensitivity, for example in blotting techniques such as the "Western blot" and "Southern blot".
- Electrophoresis in extremely narrow capillary tubes uses very small sample sizes and affords very rapid separation times.
- Electrophoresis at constant, high voltage allows for the most rapid analysis, but produces large amounts of heat and cooling may be necessary. Uncooled apparatus may need lower voltage and longer separation times. Constant power (wattage) is needed for isoelectric focusing while constant current is best for disk electrophoresis.

SECTION OBJECTIVES BOX 6-3

- Classify commonly used electrophoresis stains according to the substance being visualized.
- Describe the physical or chemical reactions that allow the use of a stain to visualize a specific substance.
- Discuss some of the clinical applications of electrophoretic techniques.

LOCATING THE ANALYTE

Direct Observation

Direct spectrophotometric observation of analytes is often employed in capillary electrophoresis. Commercial capillary zone electrophoresis apparatuses use microfocused optics to enable direct measurement from absorbance or fluorescence of separated substances inside the capillary tube as they migrate past the light beam. Use of shorter wavelengths (such as 200 nm), at which most compounds absorb more strongly, improves the sensitivity of direct measurement at the cost of possible interference from other absorbing substances. With direct measurement, the patterns of separated substances must be obtained one at a time. Direct observation may be done when DNA molecules in gels are separated in the presence of a fluorescent intercalating agent such as ethidium bromide. Otherwise, the practice is to physically remove the support from the apparatus after the separation has been completed, to determine the distribution of analyte(s) on the support.

This can be accomplished by measurement of a physical property of a molecule, such as light absorption or refractive index, or through the use of a chemical reaction such as staining. Measurements of physical properties may lack specificity, sensitivity, or resolution. For example, not all proteins absorb strongly at 280 nm.

Staining

Staining of the support is routinely employed because it often achieves the desired goals of resolution, sensitivity, specificity, and speed (Table 6-4). Because the zones of material broaden by diffusion after electrophoresis has stopped, the first step in the analytical procedure is to eliminate diffusion. This can be done in paper electrophoresis by drying the paper or in autoradiography by drying or freezing the gels. In routine clinical electrophoresis, supports sometimes are dried in an oven before measurement is performed.

Proteins

Protein in gels often is denatured (i.e., precipitated in the gel matrix) by soaking the gels in dilute acetic acid or more effectively in trichloroacetic acid. Addition of sulfosalicylic acid further improves the denaturing ability of a staining solution. In the Western blot procedure, the proteins are immobilized by adsorption.

Sometimes heat must also be applied to make the proteins insoluble. However, some resist denaturation by all these conventional procedures and remain soluble in the stain. If detergents such as SDS or other soluble agents are present, they will interfere with precipitation. Inclusion of methanol in the acid solutions helps to remove such substances before staining.

Choice of Stain

Many types of stains are employed, depending on the need. Sometimes it is desirable to stain everything, such as all proteins. A dye called Stains-All is suitable. A silver stain, which reacts with both proteins and nucleic acids, is an alternative. Proteins, after electrophoresis on cellulose acetate, most often are stained with Ponceau S.

Stains and staining procedures are often specific for one chemical group. The ninhydrin (triketohydrindene hydrate) stain for amino groups, often used after paper electrophoresis of peptides or amino acids, is an example of this. Glycoproteins can be treated with periodic acid (for oxidation) and color developed with a dye (fuchsin) in the presence of a reducing agent (sulfite). This periodic acid-Schiff stain treatment oxidizes carbohydrate groups to aldehydes, which react with the dye to form a Schiff base. The sulfite reduces the Schiff base, making the stain permanent. There is also a spe-

Table 6-4 Commonly Used Stains and Support Media for Various Substances

Substance	Stain	Support Media	Comments
Amino acids	Ninhydrin	Cellulose acetate, Paper	Reacts with amino group
Proteins (general)	Ponceau S	Cellulose acetate, Polyacrylamide	About one-tenth as sensitive as Coomassie, but more specific for proteins; the most widely used stain; reversible
	Bromphenol blue Light green SF		About one-fifth the sensitivity of Coomassie, but can be used with ampholyte gels
	Coomassie blue R250		Can detect less than 0.2 μg of protein; usable with ampholyte gels
	Silver stain		50 to 100 times more sensitive than Coomassie; different proteins give different colors, for unknown reasons

Table 6-4 Commonly Used Stains and Support Media for Various Substances—cont'd

Substance	Stain	Support Media	Comments
	Stains-All		General sensitivity, including phosphoproteins
	Amido black 10B		About one-fifth as sensitive as Coomassie
	India ink		About 20-fold more sensitive than Coomassie; slow
	Colloidal gold		About 500-fold more sensitive than Coomassie; most sensitive stain currently available; used with Western blots; slow
	Colloidal Coomassie		About three times as sensitive as Coomassie; does not stain background
	Epicocconone		Fluorescent stain, usable with SDS gels; about 10 times as sensitive as silver stain; very linear with protein concentration
Serum proteins	Ponceau S		
	Coomassie blue R250		
Lipoproteins	Sudan black B	Agarose	
	Oil red O		
	Coomassie blue R250		Used with SDS gels
Glycoproteins	PAS	Agarose	Best for neutral glycoproteins; 40 ng of carbohydrate detectable with dansyl hydrazine (fluorescence)
	Stains-All		Best for sialic acid-rich glycoproteins and mucopolysaccharides
Immunoglobulins	Coomassie blue R250	Agarose	
Specific antigens by immunological electrophoretic techniques (e.g., Laurell rocket)	Amido black 10B		
Hemoglobins	Silver stain	Cellulose acetate, agar	
	o-Dianisidine		
	Ferricyanide		
	Peroxide		
Enzymes	NADH (fluorescence)	Agarose	
Dehydrogenases	Nitroblue tetrazolium chloride		
Esterases	β-Naphthyl esters and tetrazotized *o*-dianisidine		
Cholinesterases			
Phosphatases	1-Naphthyl phosphate and Fast blue B		
Isoenzymes			
Lactate dehydrogenase	Fluorescent NADH or tetrazolium	Agarose	
Creatine kinase	Fluorescent NADH or tetrazolium	Agarose	
Phosphatase (alkaline)	1-Naphthylphosphate, fast blue B or 5-Bromo-4-chloroindolyl phosphate	Polyacrylamide Cellulose acetate	
Nucleic acids	Stains-All	Agarose	Best for RNA, DNA
	Silver stain		2 to 5 times more sensitive than ethidium bromide
	Ethidium bromide		Fluorescent bands with DNA; less than 10 ng detectable
	TOTO-1		Fluorescence bands with DNA; 4 pg detectable; binds to ssDNA and RNA

Note: Sensitivity factors given are averages: Different proteins will stain with different intensities with any stain.
DNA, Deoxyribonucleic acid; *NADH,* reduced form of nicotinamide adenine dinucleotide; *PAS,* periodic acid-Schiff; *RNA*, ribonucleic acid; *SDS*, sodium dodecyl sulfate; *ssDNA*single-stranded DNA; *TOTO-1,* a brand name from Invitrogen; Carlsbad, CA.

cific stain for phosphoproteins. (See Table 6-4 for a list of commonly used stains.)

Once the stain has been introduced, usually by soaking the support in the stain solution, excess stain must be removed. This can be done electrophoretically or, most commonly, by diffusion. Electrophoretic removal is fast but can result in distortion of the stained zones. Diffusion involves repeatedly washing the support with a solvent or using a destainer to remove free stain.

The sensitivity provided by a stain depends on the molar absorptivity (extinction coefficient) of the stain. Stains in the form of colloidal particles, which adsorb to denatured proteins in gels like India ink or colloidal Coomassie, are more sensitive because of the higher absorbance provided by the very large number of molecules in each particle. Metal stains (silver, colloidal gold) are the most sensitive for the same reason. Fluorescent "stains" are potentially the most sensitive since fluorescence depends on the intensity of the exciting light, and SYPRO dyes are sensitive to the picogram range while epicocconone has a limit of detection down to 32 pg (32×10^{-12} g). The latter has a hydrophobic tail, so it binds well to SDS-protein complexes (the SDS does not have to be extracted first) and shows a linear response over a 10^4-fold concentration range.

Many enzymes are identified through the use of their colored or fluorescent substrates or products (zymograms), even in gels or other support media. For example, alkaline phosphatase hydrolyzes *p*-nitrophenylphosphate to *p*-nitrophenol, which has a yellow color at pH 8. Soaking a gel in such assay solutions produces colored bands where the enzymes are. If the product of enzymatic activity is of low molecular weight, rapid diffusion of the product may broaden the zone, making location of the enzyme or identification of the isozyme difficult. Products that form polymers or insoluble substances are better, but if this is not possible, a contact print method may be used. A sheet of paper or other material is impregnated with a chromophoric substrate and is pressed against the support that contains the separated enzyme or enzymes. Often the support is cut into slices, and the slices are incubated in an assay solution.

Other Localization Techniques

A common technique for localization of proteins and nucleic acids employs radioactive labels, such as iodine-125 or carbon-14, incorporated into the macromolecules. After electrophoresis, a piece of x-ray film is placed in contact with the stationary support in the dark for 12 to 24 hours. After the film has been developed, a dark area corresponding to the position of the radioactively labeled macromolecule will be present. This technique, autoradiography, is commonly employed in the Western blot technique for proteins and also is used in the **Southern blot** technique for nucleic acids (see Chapter 13).

Commonly encountered problems in electrophoresis, their most likely causes, and suggested corrective actions are listed in Table 6-5.

CLINICAL APPLICATIONS

For clinical research, high sensitivity of detection of analyte, high resolution of adjacent zones of analyte, and high reproducibility of separations are required. For routine clinical work, some resolution and sensitivity of detection are sacrificed for speed or throughput; reproducibility remains important but is ensured by frequent use of comparison samples from healthy individuals.

Table **6-5** Common Problems of Electrophoretic Separations

Problem	Likely Cause	Corrective Action
No migration	Instrument not connected	Check electrical circuits.
	Wrong pH; electrodes connected backward	Check isoelectric point of protein and pH of buffer; check electrode polarity.
Bowed electrophoretic pattern on edges of support	Overheating or drying out of support on edges of support	Humidify chamber; check buffer ionic strength; reduce wattage.
Tailing of bands	Chemical reaction: subunit dissociation or adsorption to support; precipitate in sample	Use different support; try different pH; centrifuge or filter sample first.
	Salt in sample	Check sample for salt; dialyze sample against electrophoresis buffer.
	Buffer coion effect	Use different buffer coion.
Holes in staining pattern	Analyte present in too high a concentration	Apply less concentrated sample.
Very thin, sharp bands	Molecular weight of sample very high for support pore size	Use support with larger pore size.
	Sulfhydryl oxidation and aggregation	Run sample with sulfhydryl reducing compound or at lower pH.
Very slow migration	High molecular weight	Use support with larger pore size.
	Low molecular charge	Change pH so that charge increases.
	Ionic strength too high	Check conductivity; dilute buffer.
	Voltage too low	Increase voltage.
Sample precipitates in support	pH too high or low	Run at different pH.
	Too much heating	Use lower wattage or external cooling.

From Westermeier R: *Electrophoresis in Practice,* ed 3, Weinheim, New York, 2001, Wiley-VCH.

The most common uses of electrophoretic techniques in the laboratory today include the following:

1. Specific protein electrophoresis
2. Quantitative analysis of specific serum protein classes, such as gamma globulins and albumin (see Chapters 53 and 31, respectively)
3. Identification and quantitation of hemoglobin and its subclasses (see Chapters 5 and 40)
4. Identification of monoclonal proteins in either serum or urine (see Chapter 53)
5. Separation and quantitation of major lipoprotein and lipid classes (see Chapter 37)
6. Isoenzyme analysis: separation and quantitation of enzymes such as creatine kinase, lactate dehydrogenase, and alkaline phosphatase into their respective molecular subtypes (see Chapters 16 and 36)
7. Immunoelectrophoresis: most often used to determine qualitatively the elevation or deficiency of specific classes of immunoglobulins; also can be used to semiquantitate serum proteins, such as transferrin and complement component C3 (see Chapter 8)
8. Western blot technique to identify a specific protein: used to confirm the presence of antibodies to viruses e.g., hepatitis, HIV (see Chapters 8 and 32)
9. Southern blot techniques to identify specific nucleic acid sequences (DNA or RNA) (see Chapter 13): used for prenatal diagnosis of inborn errors (see Chapter 45), diagnosis of viral infections (see Chapter 32), and identification of risk factors for cancer (see Chapter 53)

Two-dimensional techniques may replace some of the preceding procedures, but at this time, more attention is directed to capillary electrophoresis. All procedures involve measurement of alterations in an electrophoretic pattern compared with a normal control. These procedures often can be used to diagnose specific diseases (Fig. 6-6). Nephrotic syndrome, for example, may be accompanied by a decrease of more than 25% in α_2-globulin levels and a decrease of up to 25% in gamma globulin levels because of the loss of lower molecular weight proteins in the urine. The pattern of decrease or increase in several disease conditions is fairly characteristic, and hence quantitation of stained cellulose acetate strips is useful in diagnosis.

The stained support may be put through a strip scanner if the support is a strip or put through a modified spectrophotometer *(densitometer)* if it is not. Cellulose acetate supports sometimes must be "cleared," that is, made more transparent, before analysis by **densitometry.** This result is achieved by soaking the support in a solvent. With due care, the dye absorbance on the support is a good measure of the amount of protein. With cellulose acetate electrophoresis, normal serum is electrophoresed next to the serum to be tested. The plots of absorbance (color) versus distance obtained from a strip scanner allow immediate comparison of relative amounts of each class of separated proteins. Routine clinical electrophoresis of serum samples can be done with the use of highly automated instruments. Several companies such as Beckman-Coulter, Ciba-Corning, and Helena Laboratories sell such equipment.

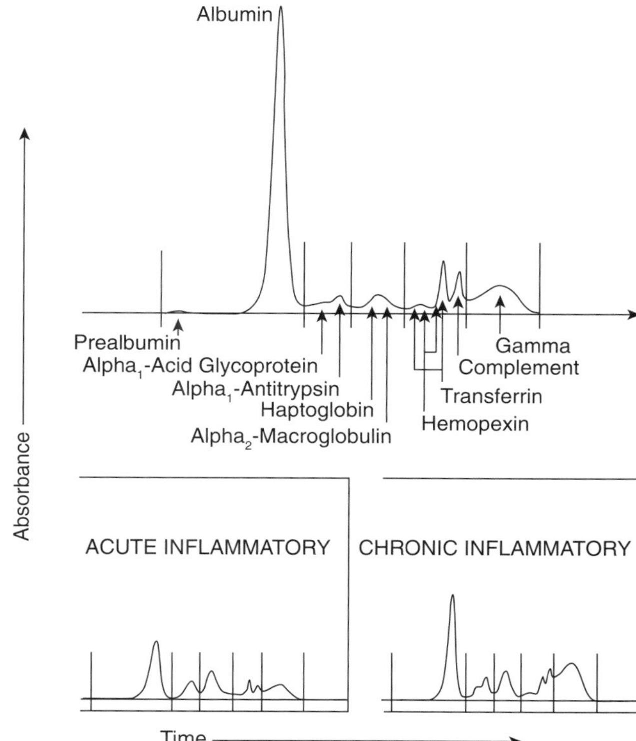

Fig. 6-6 Separations of serum proteins with the Beckman-Coulter Paragon CZE 2000. Separation times are 5 to 10 minutes; detection occurs by absorbance at 214 nm. *Upper trace,* Normal serum protein pattern, with categories of separated proteins identified. *Lower two traces,* Patterns produced with the use of serum from individuals with acute or chronic inflammatory conditions. (From Peterson JR, Mohammad AA: *Clinical and Forensic Applications of Capillary Electrophoresis,* Totowa, NJ, 2001, Humana Press.)

Use of electrophoretic techniques that provide higher resolution will increase diagnostic capabilities, but physicians will have to be trained to interpret the enhanced information.

Electrophoresis sometimes is used in assays of genetic defects. The two-dimensional techniques now being developed have tremendous potential in that area.

KEY CONCEPT BOX 6-3

- Analyte measurement usually requires removal of the supporting medium for staining, often with a dye, or sometimes with something that reacts specifically with an analyte of interest.
- Stains can be general, like a stain that visualizes all proteins, or more specific, such a stain that only visualizes lipoproteins. Compound that interact with nucleic acids are specific for DNA visualization.
- Analyte specificity can be achieved though the use of antibody-antigen interactions (Western blots) of the specific reactions of enzymes or isoenzymes.
- Clinical applications of blood, serum, and urine include measurements of hemoglobin variants, enzymes (alkaline phosphatase, CK isoenzymes), monoclonal antibody analysis, and serum protein and lipoprotein pattern identification.

BIBLIOGRAPHY

Baldo BA: Protein blotting: research, applications and its place in protein separation methodology. In: Chrambach A, Dunn MJ, Radola BJ, editors: *Advances in Electrophoresis,* New York, 1994, VCH.

Brewer JM, Ashworth RB: Disc electrophoresis, J Chem Educ 46:41, 1969.

Chrambach A, Jovin TM: Selected buffer system for moving boundary electrophoresis on gels at various pH values, presented in simplified manner, Electrophoresis 4:190, 1983.

Cutting JA: Gel protein stains: phosphoproteins, Methods Enzymol 104:451, 1984.

Gallagher SR, Winston SE, Fuller SA, Harrell JGR: Immunoblotting and immunodetection. In: Ausubel FM, Brent R. Kingston RE, Moore DD, Seidman JG, Smith JA, Struhl K, editors: *Current Protocols in Molecular Biology,* Unit 10.8, New York, 2000, Greene Publishing and Wiley Interscience.

Gander JE: Gel protein stains: glycoproteins, Methods Enzymol 104:447, 1984.

Haugland RP: *Handbook of Fluorescent Probes and Research Products,* ed 9, Eugene, OR, 2002, Molecular Probes.

Henry CS, editor: *Microchip Capillary Electrophoresis, Methods and Protocols, Methods in Molecular Biology,* vol 339, Totowa, NJ, 2006, Humana Press.

Kiriukin MY, Collins KD: Dynamic hydration numbers for biologically important ions, Biophys Chem 99:155-168, 2002.

Mackintosh JA, Choi HY, Bae SH, Veal DA, Bell PJ, Ferrari BC, Van Dyk DD, Verrills NM, Paik YK, Karuso P: A fluorescent natural product for ultra sensitive detection of proteins in one-dimensional and two-dimensional electrophoresis, Proteonomics 3:2273, 2003.

Marina ML, Rios A, Valcarcel M, editors: *Analysis and Detection by Capillary Electrophoresis,* vol XLV, *Wilson & Wilson's Comprehensive Analytical Chemistry,* New York, 2005, Elsevier.

Marouga R, David S, Hawkins E: The development of the DIGE system: 2D fluorescence difference gel analysis technology, Anal Bioanal Chem 382:669, 2005.

Merril CR: Gel-staining techniques, Methods Enzymol 182:477, 1990.

Mills GL, Lane PA, Weech PK: *A Guidebook to Lipoprotein Techniques,* Amsterdam, 1983, Elsevier.

Mosher RA, Saville DA, Thormann W: *The Dynamics of Electrophoresis,* Weinheim, Germany, 1992, VCH.

Peterson JR, Mohammad AA: *Clinical and Forensic Applications of Capillary Electrophoresis,* Totowa, NJ, 2001, Humana Press.

Righetti PG: *Immobilized pH Gradients, Theory and Methodology,* Amsterdam, 1990, Elsevier.

Rothe GM: *Electrophoresis of Enzymes: Laboratory Methods,* Berlin, 1994, Springer Verlag.

Rupley JA, Gratton E, Careri G: Water and globular proteins, Trends Biochem Sci 8:18-22, 1983.

Strege MA, Lagu AL, editors: *Capillary Electrophoresis of Proteins and Peptides, Methods in Molecular Biology,* vol 276, Totowa, NJ, 2004, Humana Press.

Van Holde KE: *Physical Biochemistry,* ed 2, Englewood Cliffs, NJ, 1985, Prentice-Hall.

Westermeier R: *Electrophoresis in Practice,* ed 3, Weinheim, NY, 2001, Wiley-VCH.

INTERNET SITES

www.aesociety.org—The Electrophoresis Society.

http://personal.cityu.edu.hk/~bhtan/Capillary%20electrophoresis.doc—Chemsoc website

www-lecb.ncifcrf.gov/EP/EPemail.html—Two-dimensional gel electrophoresis databases

www.life.uiuc.edu/molbio/geldigest/electro.html—Gel electrophoresis of DNA

www.uct.ac.za/microbiology/sdspage.html—SDS polyacrylamide gel electrophoresis (SDS-PAGE)

www.nal.usda.gov/pgdic/Probe/v2n3/puls.html—Pulsed field electrophoresis for separation of large DNA

http://ehs.berkeley.edu/pubs/factsheets/04electro.pdf—Guidelines for the Safe Use of Electrophoresis Equipment, The Office of Environment, Health & Safety (EH&S), University of California Berkeley

http://www.bertholf.net/rlb/Lectures/index.htm

http://www.bertholf.net/rlb/Lectures/index.htm lecture by Robert L. Bertholf, PhD, Associated Professor of Pathology, Chief of Clinical Chemistry and Toxicology

Immunological Reactions

Carolyn S. Feldkamp

Chapter 7

Chapter Outline

Key Terms

antibodies Proteins that combine specifically with antigens.

antibody affinity Measure of the binding strength of the antibody-antigen reaction.

antigenic determinant The portion of an antigen that reacts with antibody.

antigens Substances that induce an immune response.

avidity Measure of the binding strength of antibodies to multiple antigenic determinants on natural antigens.

B lymphocytes Lymphocytes that transform into plasma cells and produce antibodies.

chimeric antibodies Genetically engineered antibodies that contain murine variable regions and human constant regions.

conjugation Chemical attachment of a small molecule to a larger one, such as attachment of a cytotoxic agent to an antitumor antibody.

constant region C-terminus of light and heavy chains of antibodies, highly conserved. Not part of the antibody combining site.

cross-reactivity Binding of an antibody to an antigen other than the one initiating the immune response.

Fab fragment Portion of immunoglobulin molecule made by papain degradation and containing the antibody-combining site; composed of the light chain and a portion of the heavy chain.

Fc fragment Portion of immunoglobulin molecule produced by papain degradation and containing most of the heavy chain (including the complement-binding site).

flocculation A precipitation reaction that produces large, loose precipitates.

hapten Low-molecular-weight substance that can induce an immune response only when coupled to high-molecular-weight immunogenic molecules.

heavy (H) chain Portion of immunoglobulin molecule that consists of a polypeptide chain of about 50,000 daltons.

hypervariable regions Amino acid sequences in the variable regions of light and heavy chains that have an increased likelihood of variation.

idiotype Portion of immunoglobulin molecule that confers a unique character, most often including its antigen-binding site.

immunodiffusion Movement of antibody or antigen or both in a support medium from a region of high concentration to one of low concentration.

immunoelectrophoresis An immunoprecipitation technique in which antigens are separated from each other by migration in an electrical field, followed by reaction with antibody by immunodiffusion.

immunoglobulins (Ig) Proteins with antibody activity.

joining (J) chain Portion of immunoglobulin M (IgM) molecule that possibly holds the structure together.

lattice Cross-linked, three-dimensional structure formed by the reaction of multivalent antigens with antibody.

light (L) chain Portion of an immunoglobulin molecule that is composed of a polypeptide chain of about 22,000 daltons.

Ouchterlony technique A version of the original gel diffusion technique invented by Oudin, in which antigen and antibody in separate wells are allowed to diffuse toward each other.

plasma cells Immunoglobulin-producing cells that represent the end stage of B-cell differentiation.

precipitin reaction, or precipitin line Also called an immunoprecipitin, this refers to the precipitation of antigens and antibodies in gels. A precipitin line is an insoluble complex of antigens and antibodies that occurs when their relative concentrations are approximately equivalent or optimal for lattice formation.

radial immunodiffusion (Mancini technique) Measurement of antigen concentration by allowing antigen to diffuse into agarose containing the desired monospecific antibody. The area of the immunoprecipitin ring is proportional to the antigen concentration.

rocket (Laurell) immunoelectrophoresis Assay system in which the antigen, under the influence of an electrical field, migrates into agarose-containing antibody, with a resultant immunoprecipitation reaction. The precipitin lines appear rocket-shaped.

secretory piece Polypeptide chain attached to immunoglobulin A (IgA); may participate in secretion of IgA into mucosal spaces.

valency The effective number of antigenic determinants on an antigen molecule. Also sometimes used to describe the number of antibody-binding sites.

variable region N-terminal portion of immunoglobulin light and heavy chains whose amino acid sequence can change; this region includes the antigen-combining site.

zone of equivalence Region of antibody-antigen precipitin reaction in which concentrations of the two reactants are equal.

Immunological reactions can occur between two types of molecules—**antigens** and **antibodies.** This chapter examines these molecules and the interactions between them.

SECTION OBJECTIVES BOX 7-1

- Define the chemical nature of an antigen and antigen foreignness.
- Describe the physical nature and antigenicity of haptens.
- Define antigenicity, and list and explain eight factors that affect antigenicity.

ANTIGENS

Antigens, or immunogens, are defined as substances that induce an immune response. The immune response produced may be an antibody (humoral) response or may lead to the production of sensitized cells (cellular response). Usually, both humoral and cellular responses are stimulated.

Factors Affecting Antigenicity

Many factors determine the antigenicity of a molecule. The nature and dosage of an antigen, the route of administration, the organism immunized, and the sensitivity of the detection method are important factors in the evaluation of antigenicity. Many other conditions must be satisfied for a molecule to be immunogenic. These conditions are discussed below.

Chemical Nature

The first antigens investigated were bacteria and red blood cells that are complex macromolecular structures composed of many different proteins, carbohydrates, and lipids. Subsequent investigations have proved that immunogens are found in several chemical classes, including proteins, polysaccharides, glycolipids, nucleic acids, and polynucleotides.

Size

There is no absolute size requirement, but size is of considerable importance in determining the antigenicity of a molecule. The most potent immunogens are macromolecules with molecular weights greater than 100,000 daltons. The A and B polypeptide chains of insulin (2500 daltons) and of glucagon (3600 daltons) are immunogenic in guinea pigs. Nevertheless, most molecules with molecular weights less than 10,000 daltons are weakly immunogenic, if at all.

Haptens

Substances with low molecular weights can induce an immune response when coupled with higher-molecular-weight immunogenic carrier molecules. Such incomplete antigens, or **haptens,** do not elicit an immune response by themselves but do react with antibody produced against the hapten-carrier conjugate. Many low-molecular-weight compounds, including monosaccharides, lipids, peptides, hormones such as adrenocorticotropic hormone and prostaglandins, toxins such as arsphenamide, and drugs such as barbiturates and sulfonamides, have been shown to act as haptens.

Complexity

A molecule must exhibit a certain degree of chemical complexity to be antigenic. Synthetic amino acid homopolymers, composed of repeating units of a single amino acid, have been shown to be poor immunogens; copolymers of two or three amino acids are much better immunogens. Increasing immunogenicity follows increasing complexity. For example, the addition of aromatic amino acid residues such as tyrosine to synthetic amino acid copolymers increases their immunogenicity.

Antigenic Determinants

The portion of an antigen that is involved in the reaction with an antibody is called an **antigenic determinant,** or *epitope.* An antigen may contain more than one type of antigenic determinant; the number of antigenic determinants per antigen varies with the size and complexity of the molecule (Fig. 7-1). The effective number of antigenic determinants on an antigen is its **valency**. This is the number of antibody molecules that can be bound to an antigen at one time (see

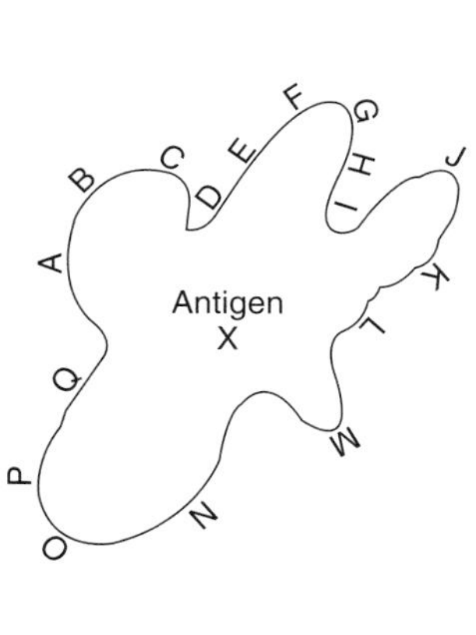

Antigenic determinants A to Q

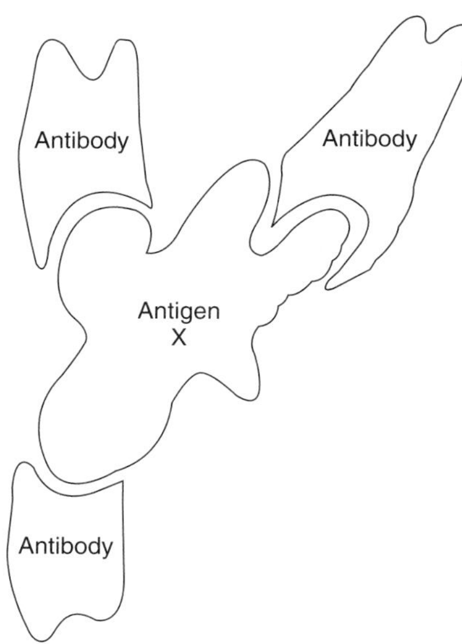

Valence = 3

Fig. 7-1 Antigen X contains many different antigenic determinants, designated *A* to *Q* in this schematic representation. Antibody molecules when combined with antigen X bind to different sites. The maximum number of molecules of antibodies bound in this figure is 3; therefore, the valence is 3.

Fig. 7-1). **Antibodies** recognize the three-dimensional shape of an antigenic determinant (conformational antigenic determinant), as well as its basic amino acid structure (sequential antigenic determinant). An antigenic determinant of a protein sometimes comprises as few as four amino acid residues. The combining site of an antibody molecule reacts with an antigenic determinant in the complementary lock-and-key manner of protein-enzyme interactions. The affinity of an antibody for an antigenic determinant is directly proportional to the closeness of fit.

Conformation and Accessibility

The tertiary structure or spatial folding of molecules is a significant factor in their immunogenicity. Antibodies to native proteins do not react with denatured molecules. They are directed primarily to conformational rather than sequential antigenic determinants.

In addition, accessibility or exposure to the environment is an important factor in determining immunogenicity. The terminal side chains of polysaccharides, the portions of a polysaccharide molecule that stick out from the main part of the molecule, are the most immunopotent regions of polysaccharide antigens. Accessibility of an antigen to the environment is related to the solubility of an antigen in aqueous medium. The more soluble an antigen is, the greater is the probability that it will interact with an antibody.

The influence of charge on immunogenicity may be a manifestation of accessibility. Charged or hydrophilic residues are more in contact with the environment than are hydrophobic residues, which tend to be sequestered in the interior of molecules.

Foreignness

The immune system is capable of distinguishing *self* from *nonself* in such a way that, under normal circumstances, a vigorous immune response is produced only to substances recognized as foreign. The more distant the evolutionary relationship between antigen and host is, the more immunogenic is the molecule. Thus guinea pig albumin will not evoke an immune response when injected into another guinea pig. This same guinea pig albumin will evoke a strong immune response, however, when injected into a different or more complex (higher) vertebrate, such as a rabbit or a monkey.

Genetics

It has recently been shown that the ability to recognize an antigen and the strength of the immune response produced may be under strict genetic control. Some strains of mice injected with synthetic polypeptides are capable of producing a vigorous immune response. Other mice, with closely related but nonidentical genetic backgrounds, may be poor responders or nonresponders.

In summary, many factors, including chemical nature, size, molecular complexity, conformation, accessibility, foreignness, and genetics, may influence the immunogenicity of an antigen.

KEY CONCEPTS BOX 7-1

- An antigen (Ag) is any chemical that is seen as foreign by an animal and induces antibody production in that animal.
- Most good Ags (i.e., proteins) have a high molecular weight (MW). A low-MW, poor Ag linked to a large compound can illicit an Ab response; these are called *haptens*.
- The three-dimensional (3D) structure determines a compound's antigenicity; a changed structure changes its antigenicity.
- The greater number of surface groups that have antigenicity, the greater is the valance, or antibody binding sites, of the compound.

SECTION OBJECTIVES BOX 7-2

- Describe the composition and structural differences of antibodies, and briefly describe how they are produced by animals.
- Describe light and heavy chains, their types, and how they combine to form antibody (Ab).
- Explain the functions of the V and C regions of antibodies.
- Name five human immunoglobulins, and describe the physiological role of each.

ANTIBODIES

Proteins that combine specifically with antigens are termed **antibodies.** Antibodies are produced by a subset of lymphocytes, called **B lymphocytes,** and by their progeny, **plasma cells.** B lymphocytes, through their production of antibodies, are responsible for the phenomenon of humoral immunity. Proteins with antibody activity are also called **immunoglobulins.** Immunoglobulins are an extremely heterogeneous group of molecules that account for approximately 20% of plasma proteins. Immunoglobulins are heterogeneous in their antigen specificity, amino acid sequence, migration within an electrical field, and functions. As many as 10,000 different molecules circulating in the human body may be classified as immunoglobulins.

Structure

An important advance in the study of immunoglobulin structure came with the discovery that electrophoretically homogeneous proteins found in the serum of patients with multiple myeloma were structurally homogeneous and were very closely related to normal immunoglobulin. Such myeloma proteins could be isolated in large quantities and chemically characterized. These studies produced an understanding of the precise structure of the antibody molecule.

H and L Chains

Antibodies are glycoproteins that are composed of 82% to 96% polypeptide and 4% to 18% carbohydrate. All immunoglobulin molecules have a common structure of four polypeptide chains. Two identical large chains, or **heavy (H) chains,** and two identical small chains, or **light (L) chains,** are held together by noncovalent forces and covalent interchain disulfide bonds (Fig. 7-2 and Color Plate 1).

The carbohydrate portion of the immunoglobulin molecule is bound covalently to amino acids in the polypeptide chains. The carbohydrates usually are found bound to the C-terminal half (Fc) of the molecule. Their function is poorly understood. They may be involved in transporting the molecule or protecting it from metabolic degradation.

Fab and Fc Fragments

Enzymatic digestion of immunoglobulin molecules has provided further evidence of their structure (see Fig. 7-2). Digestion with papain splits the molecule on the N-terminal side of the disulfide bonds, yielding three fragments of approximately equal size. Two of these fragments are identical and retain the antigen-binding capacity associated with an intact immunoglobulin molecule. Fragments with the antibody-combining site (**Fab fragments**) are each composed of an entire light chain and a portion of the heavy chain. The third fragment has no antigen-binding activity and is crystallizable (**Fc fragment).** The Fc fragment retains the other biological activities associated with immunoglobulin molecules—interaction with the complement system and binding to tissue. The Fc fragment is composed of the C-terminal half of the heavy chain.

Digestion with pepsin cleaves the antibody molecule on the C-terminal side of the disulfide bonds. This digestion results

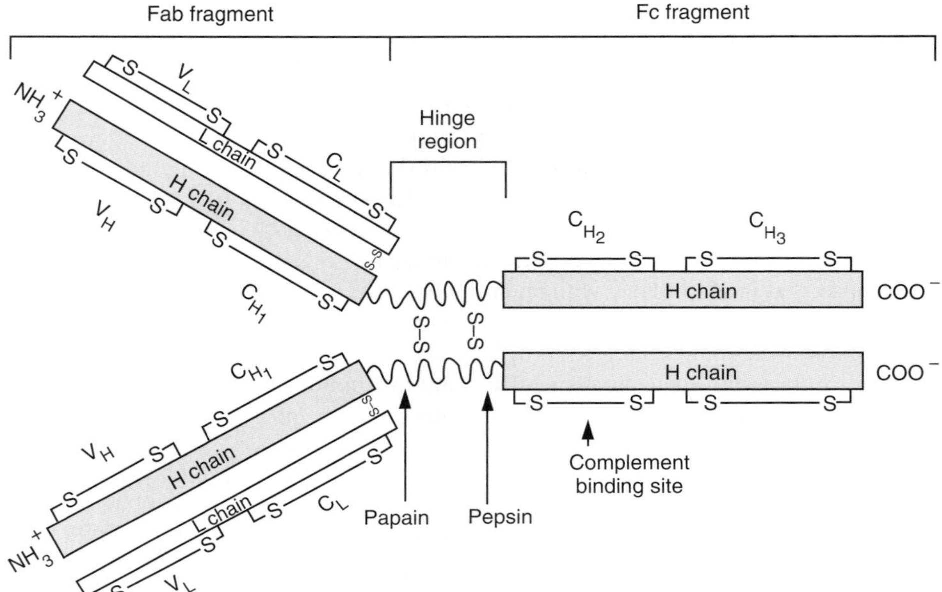

Fig. 7-2 Diagram of immunoglobulin G (IgG) molecule (immunoglobulin monomer). *C,* Constant region; *COO⁻,* C-terminus of immunoglobulin; *H,* heavy; *L,* light; NH_3^+, N-terminus; *S–S,* disulfide bonds; *V,* variable region. *Arrows* indicate papain and pepsin cleavage sites.

Table 7-1 Properties of Human Immunoglobulin Classes

Properties	IgC	IgA	IgM	IgD	IgE
Heavy chain	γ	α	μ	δ	ε
Subclasses	1 to 4	1 and 2	1 and 2	None	None
Light chain	κ and λ	κ and λ	κ and λ	κ and λ	κ and λ
Form	Monomer	Monomer and dimer	Pentamer (some monomer may circulate)	Monomer	Monomer
Formula	$\gamma_2\kappa_2$ or $\gamma_2\lambda_2$	$\alpha_2\kappa_2$ or $\alpha_2\lambda_2$	$\mu_{10}\kappa_{10}$ or $\mu_{10}\lambda_{10}$	$\delta_2\kappa_2$ or $\delta_2\lambda_2$	$\varepsilon_2\kappa_2$ or $\varepsilon_2\lambda_2$
J chain	No	On dimer	On pentamer	No	No
Molecular weight in daltons (approximate)	150,000	Monomer 160,000 Dimer 400,000	900,000	180,000	190,000
Complement fixation (classical pathway)	$G_3 > G_1 > G_2$	No	M_1 and M_2	No	No
Crosses placenta	Yes	No	No	No	No
Concentration in serum	8 to 16 mg/mL	1.4 to 3.5 mg/mL	0.5 to 2 mg/mL	Up to 0.14 mg/mL	≤300 ng/mL

Ig, Immunoglobulin.

in the $F(ab')_2$ fragment composed of two Fab fragments linked by disulfide bonds. The remainder of the molecule undergoes extensive degradation.

V and C Regions

Each polypeptide chain is composed of domains, or peptide sequences of uniform size (100 to 110 amino acid residues), that contain intrachain disulfide bonds. The domain of the N-terminal or antibody-combining site is more variable in its amino acid sequence than the rest of the polypeptide chain and is called the **variable region** (V region). The sequence and the spatial folding of the polypeptide chain are responsible for antibody specificity and affinity. The remainder of the polypeptide chain is composed of domains that are similar among immunoglobulin molecules of the same and other species. These domains are termed **constant regions** (C regions). Light chains are composed of one variable and one constant region (V_L and C_L). Heavy chains are composed of one variable and three or four constant regions (V_H and $C_{H1\text{-}4}$) (see Fig. 7-2).

The specific amino acid sequences of the variable regions of the light and heavy chains of an antibody molecule confer a unique three-dimensional structure to the antigen-binding potential antibody. These sequences are termed the **idiotype** of the molecule. The idiotype is determined by the antigenic determinant to which the antibody is directed. The structure of the idiotype permits the complementary fit of the antigenic determinant to the antibody-combining site.

Light-Chain Types

Two types of light chains are found in immunoglobulin molecules—kappa (κ) and lambda (λ). Kappa and lambda light chains differ in the amino acid sequence of their constant regions. A given antibody molecule always has two identical kappa light chains or two identical lambda light chains. An antibody molecule can never have both a kappa and a lambda light chain together. In human serum, the ratio of kappa to lambda antibody molecules is approximately 2:1.

Heavy-Chain Types

In humans, five types of heavy chains are distinguished on the basis of structural differences in the constant regions of the chains. These structural differences permit functional differences. The heavy-chain types, which are designated gamma (γ), alpha (α), mu (μ), delta (δ), and epsilon (ε), vary in molecular weight. The gamma, alpha, and delta heavy chains are composed of three constant regions. The mu and epsilon heavy chains have four constant regions. The heavy-chain type determines the class of immunoglobulin. In humans, five immunoglobulin classes correspond to the five heavy-chain types: immunoglobulin G (IgG), immunoglobulin A (IgA), immunoglobulin M (IgM), immunoglobulin D (IgD), and immunoglobulin E (IgE) (Table 7-1).

Some immunoglobulin classes consist of subclasses that are based on additional amino acid differences in their constant regions. IgG has four subclasses, and IgA and IgM each have two subclasses. The biological properties and concentrations of these subclasses may differ.

Immunoglobulin G

IgG molecules are monomers of the basic immunoglobulin subunit. They are composed of two kappa or two lambda light chains and two gamma heavy chains. IgG molecules therefore may be represented as $\gamma_2\lambda_2$ or $\gamma_2\kappa_2$. Approximately 75% of serum immunoglobulin is IgG. The frequency of IgG subclasses varies as follows: IgG_1, 60% to 70%; IgG_2, 14% to 20%; IgG_3, 4% to 8%; and IgG_4, 2% to 6%. Evidence indicates that antibodies to certain antigens may be restricted in their subclasses. Polysaccharide antigens tend to produce IgG_2 and IgG_4 antibodies. Antiviral and antinucleoprotein antibodies are found primarily in the IgG_1 and IgG_3 subclasses.

IgG molecules cross the placenta and are responsible for the immunological defense of the newborn. IgG molecules also fix to the surfaces of effector cells (T cells) and then are capable of antibody-mediated cytotoxic reactions, which are important in protecting the host. IgG molecules bind or "fix" complement, a complex of serum proteins that assists in the lysis or elimination of foreign particles. Complement proteins are bound to the IgG molecule at the midpoint of the heavy chain, near the disulfide bond in the C_{H_2} domain. This area of increased flexibility is called the *hinge region*. After reaction with large antigens, this region undergoes spatial changes to expose the complement-binding site (see Fig. 7-2). Molecules in the IgG subclasses differ in terms of their ability to fix complement proteins. IgG_3 is most active, followed by IgG_1, IgG_2, and IgG_4.

Immunoglobulin M

IgM accounts for approximately 10% of serum immunoglobulins and exists primarily as a pentamer of the basic immunoglobulin structure. The five immunoglobulin monomers are held in a circle by disulfide bonds between H chains of the subunits. In addition, the IgM molecule contains a polypeptide chain, called the **joining (J) chain,** which may help in maintaining its structure. The J chain is a small glycoprotein (15,000 daltons) that is covalently bound to the H chains of the molecule.

IgM is the predominant immunoglobulin in the initial immune response to an antigen. It is the most efficient immunoglobulin in fixing complement. This efficiency is a result of its pentameric structure. The presence of 10 Fab units conveys on the IgM pentamer molecule a theoretical valency of 10. This means that an IgM molecule should be able to bind 10 antigen molecules simultaneously. Although this value has been computed in some experimental systems, it is not normally observed. Steric hindrance may be responsible for this disparity.

Immunoglobulin A

IgA constitutes approximately 15% of serum immunoglobulins, but it is the predominant immunoglobulin in body secretions such as saliva, tears, sweat, human milk, and colostrum. In serum, IgA exists in both monomeric and polymeric forms. Polymeric serum IgA possesses the J chain. Secretory IgA exists as a dimer of the basic immunoglobulin unit combined with a J chain and an additional polypeptide chain called the **secretory piece.** The secretory piece is bound to dimeric secretory IgA by strong noncovalent linkages. It is important in secretory transport of the molecule and in its protection from proteolytic digestion in the gut. Secretory IgA provides the first line of defense against local infection and is important in the processing of food antigens in the gut.

Immunoglobulin D

IgD, a monomer of the basic immunoglobulin unit, is present in human serum in trace amounts. In addition, it is expressed on lymphocyte cell surface membranes. The main function of IgD is unknown, but it may be involved in lymphocyte differentiation.

Immunoglobulin E

IgE, which is also a monomeric immunoglobulin, is present in human serum in very low concentrations. IgE, which binds to cells by means of its Fc portion, is responsible for the physiological manifestations of allergy (see p. 562, Chapter 29).

Engineered Antibodies

Since 1975, monoclonal antibody technology has cloned natural antibodies to produce reagent quantities of antibodies for use in immunoassays, and as therapeutic and imaging agents (see Chapter 8). Subsequent advances in genetic engineering allowed the introduction of specific gene sequences into vectors so that proteins, including antibodies, with defined specificities could be designed. For example, antitumor antibodies have been created for use in cancer therapy. Modifications of antibody structure now are made for specific purposes. **Conjugation** techniques allow attachment of antitumor antibodies to imaging reagents like ^{90}Y (yttrium 90) or delivery of cytotoxic agents directly to tumor cells or to sites integral to the cancer process.

Other modifications to antibody structure are used to avoid some undesirable properties of antibodies synthesized in animals or clones of animal cells. For example, the therapeutic use of mouse monoclonal antibodies generates an immune response to the "foreign" protein. The presence of anti-mouse monoclonal antibodies (HAMA) makes multiple dosing of some agents ineffective for future therapies and causes significant and often unexpected interference in sandwich-type immunoassays. Toxic effects of therapeutic antibodies include cross-reaction with normal tissue and immune-mediated pulmonary, central nervous system (CNS), liver, and renal effects. Anti-HER-2/neu (Herceptin) used for breast cancer has been associated with cardiotoxic effects. Approaches to solutions for these problems include the use of Fab or Fab_2 antibody fragments that do not bind complement, that are dialyzable, and that reduce the exposure of the patient to many antigenic determinants.

Modifications to antibody structure for therapeutic antibodies include preparation of **chimeric antibodies,** a fusion of genes for the variable region from mouse antibody with human constant domains. "Humanized" antibodies are created from the gene combination of hypervariable regions of mouse antibody, with the rest of the molecule consisting of human antibody. Other antibodies have been "deimmunized," that is, amino acids not involved at the antigen binding site are removed and are replaced by amino acids that are relatively immunologically inactive.

KEY CONCEPTS BOX 7-2

- Antibodies (Abs) are proteins produced by B lymphocytes, which bind specific antigens.
- Monomeric abs are composed of four chains, 2 light and 2 heavy chains, connected by disulfide bonds.
- The three-dimensional (3D) structure of Abs brings together H and L chain amino acid sequences of variable composition to form the specific antigen (Ag)-binding portion of the Ab, or the Fab fragment formed by Ab digestion.
- G, M, A, D, and E are the five classes of Ab. G and M represent the primary humoral responses to Ag (late and early, respectively). The A class functions in body fluids, and the E class provides an allergic response.

SECTION OBJECTIVES BOX 7-3

- List and explain the forces involved in antigen-antibody reactions.
- List the factors that influence the specificity of immunochemical reactions.
- Explain the nature of cross-reactivity.

ANTIGEN-ANTIBODY REACTIONS
(see Color Plate 2)

Antigen-antibody reactions were first recognized by bacteriologists, who also surmised that such reactions exhibited specificity. These bacteriologists noted that the serum of patients recovering from infectious diseases could agglutinate the organism responsible for their disease but not unrelated organisms. Serum from persons not exposed to the disease or from patients before they contracted the disease could not agglutinate the same organisms. From such evidence, scientists have proposed the existence of antibody molecules, the specificity of their interactions with antigens, and the importance of such interactions in host defense.

The following sections consider the forces involved in antigen-antibody binding, the specificity of the reaction, and the mechanism of the reaction.

Binding Forces

The strength of the binding of an antigen to an antibody depends on the complementarity of fit of the antigenic determinant to the antibody idiotype and the resultant electrostatic attraction. It also depends on the sum of weak, noncovalent, intermolecular forces, such as hydrogen bonding, van der Waals forces, and hydrophobic interactions (see Table 27-2). Weak, short-range forces can operate between antigen and antibody if their closeness of fit brings them into proximity with one another.

In solution at physiological pH, charged polar groups on the amino acid residues of proteins can be strongly attracted to one another. These electrostatic forces are the strongest and most important contributors to the noncovalent attraction between antigen and antibody. Hydrogen bonding between the amino and carboxy groups of peptide bonds also contributes to the attractive forces. Hydrogen bonds are weaker than electrostatic forces, but their large numbers make them an important factor.

Van der Waals forces are the weakest forces involved and can function only within a very small radius because of their low strength. These van der Waals forces contribute to total binding strength.

The final component of the attractive forces involves hydrophobic bonding between apolar groups in solution. Hydrophobic bonding functions by the exclusion of polar water molecules to bring hydrophobic portions of molecules together. Such interactions also serve to attract polar water molecules to hydrophilic amino acid residues on protein molecules. Antibody molecules have large numbers of hydrophobic amino acid residues such as alanine, leucine, tyrosine, tryptophan, and methionine in their antibody-combining sites, where they enhance bonding to hydrophobic residues in antigenic determinants.

Antibody Affinity

The strength of the binding of a single antigenic determinant to an antibody is a function of the closeness of fit and is called **antibody affinity.** Antibody affinity is an expression of the attraction between molecules of antibody and antigen. It is a function of the sum of the short-range, noncovalent, intermolecular forces.

Binding of antigen to antibody is a reversible reaction. The equilibrium of the reaction favors antigen-antibody association if the fit between molecules is good and the forces that bind the molecules together are relatively strong and stable. The strength of the association between antigen and antibody is represented by the association constant, which may be derived as follows:

$$Ag + Ab \underset{k_2}{\overset{k_1}{\rightleftharpoons}} Ag \cdot Ab \qquad \text{Eq. 7-1}$$

$$\frac{[Ag \cdot Ab]}{[Ag][Ab]} = K_a \text{(Association constant)} \qquad \text{Eq. 7-2}$$

To study these reactions, one places solutions of a small antigen, or hapten, on either side of a semipermeable membrane. As the hapten diffuses across the membrane, the reaction proceeds to the right of Eq. 7-1, that is, hapten and antibody associate to form complexes. Eventually, equilibrium is reached. At equilibrium, the rate of the forward reaction and the rate of the reverse reaction are constant. One rate constant, k_1, expresses the tendency of the reaction to move toward the right, or the tendency for association. The other rate constant, k_2, expresses the tendency of the reaction to move to the left, or the tendency for dissociation. These reaction-rate constants differ for each antigen and antibody pair. The concentrations of antigen, antibody, and complex at equilibrium are described by Eq. 7-2. The equilibrium constant, K_a, expresses the tendency of the reaction to favor association between antigen and antibody.

Heterogeneity of Immune Response

Analysis of the binding of a simple hapten that contains a single antigenic determinant shows variation in the binding strength of antibody molecules. Immunization with a single antigenic determinant produces a variety of antibodies with different antibody-combining sites and with a range of antibody affinities. This is termed the heterogeneity of the immune response. Because haptens are three-dimensional, the immune system produces antibodies that have different areas of contact (Fig. 7-3). The antibody presents differing distributions of charged and hydrophobic residues, resulting in varying closeness of fit of hapten with each different antibody.

Antibody Avidity

In natural situations in vivo, a variety of antibody molecules are generated in response to a multivalent antigenic stimulus. Thus there are two areas of complexity: (1) multiple antibodies generated to different conformations on a single

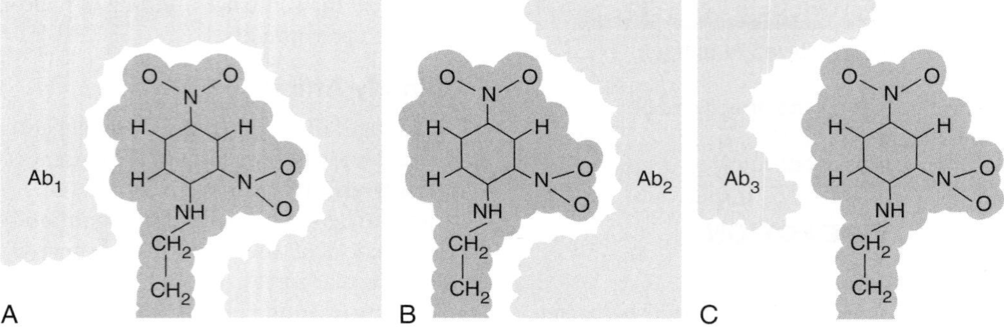

Fig. 7-3 Binding of antibodies (Ab) present in the same antiserum with different affinities to the same hapten (dinitrobenzene linked to amino group of lysine). **A,** Ab_1 fits with nearly whole hapten and is thus of high affinity. **B,** Ab_2 fits with less of molecule and not so closely and has a moderate binding affinity, whereas **(C)** the low-affinity Ab_3 is complementary in shape to such a small portion of hapten surface that its binding energy is very little above that occurring between completely unrelated proteins. Only a portion of the antibody-combining site is shown. (From Roitt IM: *Essential Immunology,* ed 4, Oxford, England, 1980, Blackwell Scientific Publications.)

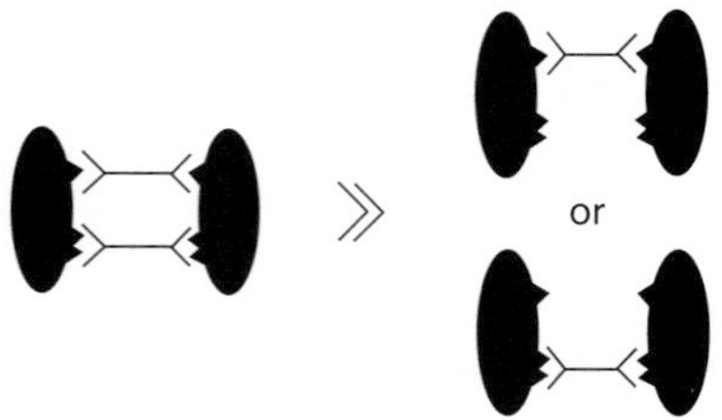

Fig. 7-4 Multivalent bonding of antigen-antibody increases bonding strength. A single bond created by divalent antibody molecules between a single antigenic determinant on two adjacent antigens is much weaker than a binding created by two divalent antibodies bound simultaneously to two unique antigenic determinants on two adjacent antigens. The strength and complexity of this multivalent bonding are described by the term *avidity.*

antigenic determinant and (2) multiple antigenic determinants on a single natural antigen. Both of these generate the *diversity* of the immune response. The measure of the binding strength of these heterogeneous antibodies to multiple antigenic determinants on natural antigens is termed **avidity.** Avidity is a measure of the cumulative binding strength of all the affinities of each antibody within the larger population for its complementary antigenic determinant(s). The sum of the bindings is greater than its individual parts because of the reversible nature of antigen-antibody bonds and because of the divalent nature of IgG molecules or the multivalent nature of IgM molecules (Fig. 7-4).

Cross-Reactivity

Cross-reactivity of antigen and antibody is a by-product of the heterogeneity of the immune response. As was stated previously, immunization with a simple hapten produces a variety of antibodies of differing affinities. Some of these antibodies will also combine with chemically related and structurally similar haptens. The reactivity of an antibody to a different antigen also may indicate that the two antigens in question share a previously unknown but common antigenic determinant. Thus cross-reactivity may result from similar or identical antigenic determinants in different antigens. Such cross-reactivity is often observed with antibodies produced to such drugs as penicillin. The reactivity of an antibody with penicillin may be very high, but metabolic derivatives that contain the basic drug structure also may react with an antibody produced to the original, parent drug.

In cases of prolonged antigenic challenge, such as that occurring in natural infection, the initial response occurs with low-affinity, low-specificity molecules, which may react with other closely related antigens. Over time, animals exhibit a natural selection for clones of plasma cells that produce high-affinity antibodies. As the heterogeneity of the antibody response narrows, the specificity of antigen-antibody reactions increases. This adaptation of the immune response promotes effective protection of the host against infection.

Genetic Basis of Antibody Diversity

The heterogeneity of the immune response or the variety of antibodies produced to a single antigen is known to be genetically determined. The variable (V) regions of light and heavy chains of the antibody molecule encode for antibody specificity. Some positions in the amino acid sequence of the V region have an even more increased likelihood of amino acid variation. These **hypervariable regions,** scattered throughout the amino acid sequence of the V region, are brought into proximity to one another by the natural folding (tertiary structure) of the antibody molecule. The amino acid sequence dictates possible attraction between polar amino acid residues, as well as the possibility of intrachain disulfide bonds. Folding of the protein so that the hypervariable regions are spatially close to each other forms the antibody-combining site.

KEY CONCEPTS BOX 7-3

- Weak (van der Waals, hydrophobic) and strong (hydrogen bonds), noncovalant bonds allow antibodies (Abs) to bind antigens (Ags).
- An Ab production to a large Ag will produce a heterogeneous population of Ab to different Ag determinants, with varying affinities to the determinants.
- The closeness of "fit" between an Ab and an antigenic determinant is the Ab affinity.
- The cumulative numbers and types of these bonds determine the strength of Ag-Ab binding, that is, the avidity of a heterogeneous population of Abs to an Ag determinant.
- The better the Ab affinity, the less frequently will the antibodies bind other Ags; thus they will have less cross-reactivity.

SECTION OBJECTIVES BOX 7-4

- Describe the lattice theory of antigen-antibody (Ag-Ab) precipitation and the various parts of a precipitation curve.
- Outline the mechanism of the following Ag-Ab gel-precipitation reactions, and state the principle of each: double immunodiffusion and radial immunodiffusion.

ANTIGEN-ANTIBODY PRECIPITATION REACTIONS

The primary reaction of antigen with antibody usually is detected by secondary manifestations of the reaction. The nature of the secondary manifestations depends on experimental conditions, the class of antibody involved in the reaction, the number of antigenic determinants on the antigen, and the size and solubility of the antigen. When an antibody reacts with soluble molecules that possess multiple antigenic determinants, cross-linking between antibody-antigen complexes can occur. This reaction can be detected by precipitation of the complex out of solution. The term **flocculation** may be used to describe a precipitation reaction that produces a large, loosely bound precipitate. The reaction of antibodies with large, particulate, multivalent antigens (such as red blood cells) is detected by agglutination of the antigen. These reactions are considered separately.

Precipitation Curve

When a known quantity of antibody is present in solution in a series of tubes to which increasing amounts of antigen are added, precipitation occurs in some of the test tubes. When the amount of precipitate is measured and correlated with the amount of antigen present, one obtains a curve similar to that shown in Fig. 7-5.

In the first phase of the reaction, called the *antibody-excess phase,* no free antigen (an antigen without bound antibody) can be detected in the fluid, and essentially no precipitate can be found. Free (unbound) antibody can be detected, however. As greater amounts of antigen are added, the amount of precipitate increases until a point of maximum precipitation is reached. At this point, no free antigen or free antibody can be detected in the fluid. This is called the **zone of equivalence.** As the amount of added antigen continues to increase, the amount of precipitate detected diminishes. Examination of the fluid phase of the reaction at this time shows no free antibody but increasing amounts of free antigen. This area of the curve is called the *antigen-excess phase.*

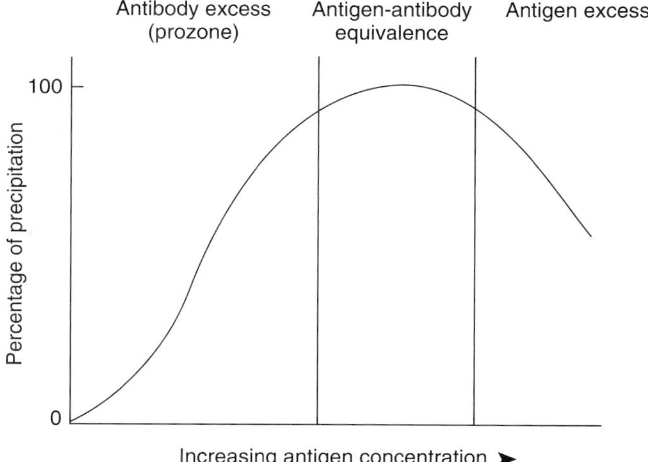
Antibody excess (prozone)
Antigen-antibody equivalence
Antigen excess
100
0
Percentage of precipitation
Increasing antigen concentration

Fig. 7-5 The quantitative precipitin curve in which the amount of antibody-antigen complex that precipitates is plotted as a function of antigen concentration.

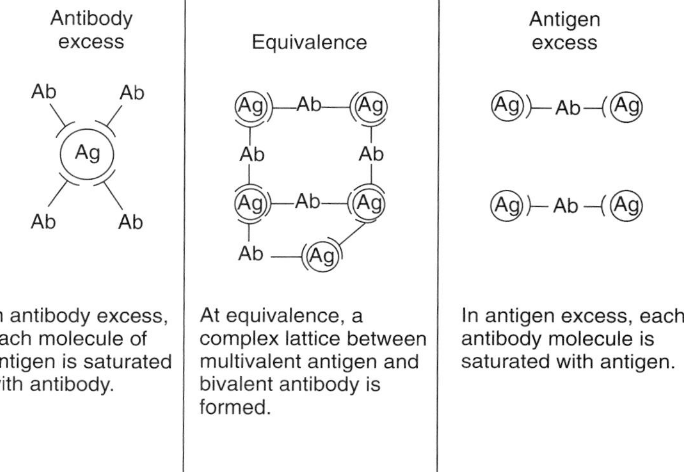
Antibody excess
Equivalence
Antigen excess
Ab
Ag
Ab-Ag
In antibody excess, each molecule of antigen is saturated with antibody.
At equivalence, a complex lattice between multivalent antigen and bivalent antibody is formed.
In antigen excess, each antibody molecule is saturated with antigen.

Fig. 7-6 Representation of sizes of molecular complexes formed at varying ratios of antigen and antibody.

Lattice Theory

Antigen-antibody complexes precipitate out of solution because of the multivalent nature of both molecules. The reaction of antigens that possess multiple antigenic determinants and antibodies with two (as in IgG) or more (as in IgM) antibody-combining sites produces a **lattice** of interlocking molecules. Antibody molecules can cross-link antigenic sites on the same or different molecules of antigen. As the size and complexity of the lattice increase, the lattice becomes insoluble and precipitates out of solution (Fig. 7-6).

In the antibody-excess zone, a single molecule of antigen binds to each antibody molecule. The excess of antibody ensures that each molecule of antigen can encounter a free antibody molecule. The absence of cross-linking produces small soluble complexes. As the antigen concentration increases and the zone of equivalence is reached, complexes of increasing size with increasing levels of cross-linking are formed. Such large, complex lattices precipitate out of solution.

As the antigen concentration continues to increase, the zone of antigen excess is reached. In this portion of the curve, smaller complexes are seen again. The size of the lattice decreases because there is sufficient antigen to permit binding of a free antigen molecule to each antibody-combining site. At high concentrations of antigen, lack of precipitation can result in false-negative results. Obviously, detection of antigen by antibody precipitation requires optimum concentration of both reactants. Formation of lattices best suited for precipitation occurs at an equal or equivalent concentration of antigen and antibody or at a slight antigen excess.

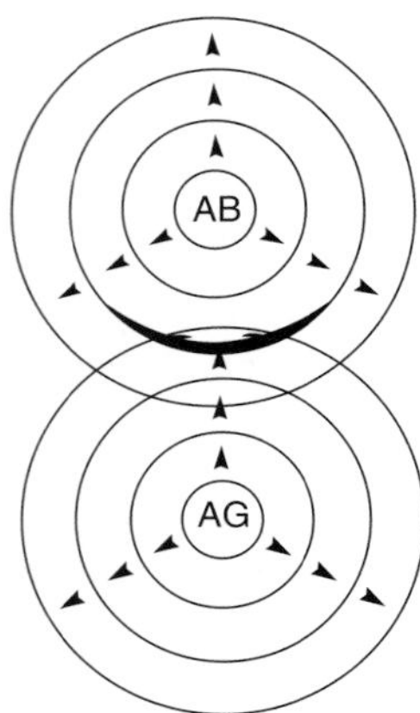

Fig. 7-7 Depiction of radial protein gradients in Ouchterlony immunodiffusion. Concentric circles represent decreasing protein concentrations. Both antigen (AG) and antibody (AB) diffuse radially from application wells. Precipitation *(heavy black arc)* occurs at the point of antigen-antibody equivalence. The precipitin line is closer to the well of lower concentration and is concave toward the reagent of higher molecular weight.

Other Factors Affecting Precipitation

The precipitation of antigen-antibody complexes out of solution can be affected by factors other than the ratio of antigen concentration to antibody concentration. Different antibody molecules can precipitate the same antigen to varying degrees. The efficiency of the antibody depends on its affinity and specificity. The charge and shape of the antigen-antibody complex are also important. Highly charged complexes are difficult to precipitate. The best precipitates are observed with protein antigens of molecular weights from 40,000 to 160,000 daltons. Proteins in this range are easily cross-linked by multivalent antibody molecules. Polysaccharide antigens, denatured proteins, and viruses produce broader precipitation curves. Their large size sterically hinders cross-linking. Precipitation also can be affected by temperature, pH, and ionic concentration. Such factors influence antigen-antibody interactions on a molecular level.

Precipitation Reactions in Gel

Precipitation reactions frequently are carried out in a gel-support matrix composed of agar or the more purified polysaccharide, agarose. The agar prevents convective mixing of antigen and antibody and thereby ensures establishment of concentration gradients of the two reactants. Precipitation in agar is only a moderately sensitive technique when compared with newer advances, such as chemiluminescent immunometric assays, but it is employed because of its ease and versatility. In addition, precipitation reactions in gels can be modified to permit the study of antigenic relationships among different compounds. The following section discusses two gel-precipitation reactions, double **immunodiffusion** and **radial immunodiffusion.**

Double Immunodiffusion

In double-immunodiffusion reactions, or **Ouchterlony technique,** agar or agarose is poured onto a solid support, such as a glass slide or a Petri dish. Wells are then cut into the agar, and antigen and antibody solutions are placed into separate wells. The solutions then diffuse toward one another in the gel in a radial fashion during room temperature incubation (Fig. 7-7). With diffusion into the agar, the solutions establish concentration gradients that diminish with distance from the well. At the point of antigen-antibody equivalence at the interface of the diffusing fronts, a **precipitin line** is formed (see Fig. 7-7). The positioning and shape of the line are dictated by the concentration of the reactants and the size of the molecules. The line will be closer to the well containing the reactant of lower concentration because the distance traveled is directly proportional to concentration. The rate of diffusion is also inversely proportional to molecular size. High-molecular-weight compounds, such as IgM, diffuse more slowly than lower-molecular-weight substances, such as IgG. The precipitation line that is formed at the interface of the two concentration gradients will be concave to the higher-molecular-weight compound, whose diffusion rate is slower. Because precipitation occurs at a range of antigen-antibody equivalence to slight antigen excess, an inappropriate ratio of antigen to antibody will result in failure to form a precipitate.

Radial Immunodiffusion

Because of its simplicity and accuracy, radial immunodiffusion can be easily used for the quantification of antigens. Radial immunodiffusion, the **Mancini technique,** is a precipitation reaction that is achieved by applying an antigen solution to a gel impregnated with a monospecific antibody solution. Wells are cut into the antibody-containing agar and dilutions of antigen are placed in the wells. Radial diffusion of antigen into the agar produces a concentration gradient that is inversely proportional to the distance from the well. At the point where antigen and antibody concentrations are equivalent, precipitation occurs. Because diffusion from the well is radial, the precipitation appears as a ring around the well. The precipitation reaction is dynamic rather than static;

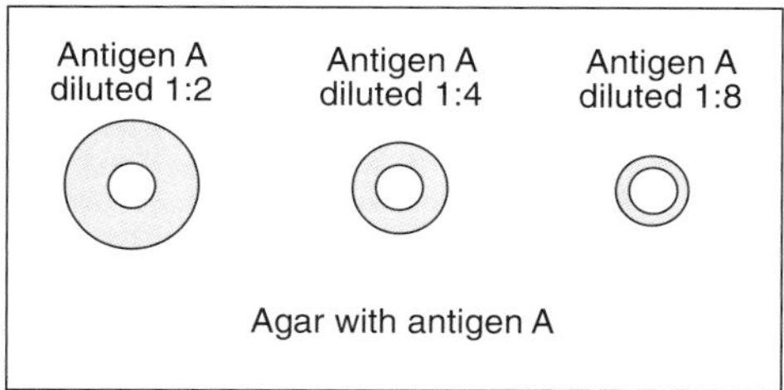

Fig. 7-8 Radial immunodiffusion patterns. The band of precipitation *(gray area)* extends as a disk from the center of each circular well. The area of precipitation is proportional to the concentration.

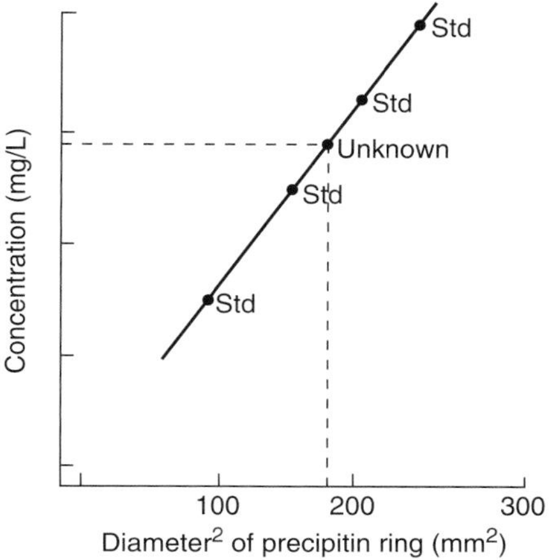

Fig. 7-9 Graph of the concentration of antigen expressed as milligrams per liter versus the square of the diameter of the precipitin ring. *Std,* Standard.

the ring first forms close to the well at the initial point of antigen-antibody equivalence. As antigen continues to diffuse from the well, antigen excess causes the precipitate to form soluble complexes that continue to diffuse outward. A new ring is formed at a new point of antigen-antibody equivalence. The square of the diameter of the ring (mm^2) is directly proportional to antigen concentration. The thickness of the ring is a function of the final concentration of antigen-antibody complexes at the equivalence point (Fig. 7-8).

When constant sample volume, temperature, pH, incubation time, and antibody concentration are maintained, an unknown antigen concentration can be determined. This is accomplished by comparing the area of the precipitation ring of the unknown antigen with those obtained for several dilutions of a standard antigen solution. When the concentrations of the diluted standard are plotted against ring area (or diameter squared, d^2), the concentration of the unknown can be easily determined (Fig. 7-9).

The assay is valid only over a rather narrow range of antigen concentrations. In part, this is dictated by the antibody concentration in the gel and by the ease of diffusion of the antigen into the gel. For some antigens, several dilutions are necessary to achieve the optimum concentration range. Urine and cerebrospinal fluid generally must be concentrated before they can be quantified by this technique. Excess salt must be removed from these specimens if they have been concentrated by lyophilization.

Monospecific antibody to the desired antigen is the only crucial reagent. If the antiserum binds more than one antigen, a double ring may be seen. Temperature should be kept constant. If the antigen is too large or aggregated, the resulting diffusion pattern will not be quantitative. This method is slow relative to other methods of antigen quantitation and has largely been replaced in the routine clinical laboratory.

Test sensitivity depends on antigen size; the greater the size, the poorer is the diffusion. For most serum proteins, the assay is sensitive to 50 μg/mL.

Other Quantitative Methods

Several methods are used for detecting or measuring antigens through adaptations and combinations of electrophoresis and precipitation reactions in gels. These include **immunoelectrophoresis** (immunoprecipitation after electrophoresis), counterelectrophoresis (movement of antigen and antibody into each other by electrophoresis), and **rocket (Laurell) immunoelectrophoresis** (electrophoresis of antigen into an antibody-containing gel). Although these methods have been replaced by faster and more sensitive techniques in contemporary clinical laboratories, they still may be used for research or for special applications. For details, please refer to earlier editions of this textbook.

KEY CONCEPTS BOX 7-4

- An antigen (Ag) with multiple determinants reacts with antibody (Ab) to form complex interlocking molecules, or lattices. As the lattice of Ag-Ab complexes grows large enough, they will precipitate.
- Early in the precipitation curve, with Ag excess, lattices are small, and there is no precipitation. With excess Ab, associated decreased precipitation occurs.
- Precipitation reactions serve as the basis for a number of qualitative and quantitative procedures.

BIBLIOGRAPHY

Abbas AK, Lichtman AH: *Cellular and Molecular Immunology,* ed 5, Philadelphia, 2005, Saunders.

Gosling JP, editor: *Immunoassays: A Practical Approach,* Oxford, 2000, Oxford University Press.

Gosling JP, Reen DJ: *Immunotechnology,* London, 1993, Portland Press.

Keren DF: *Protein Electrophoresis in Clinical Diagnosis,* ed 3, London, 2003, Oxford University Press.

Roitt IM, Brostoff J, Male DK: *Immunology,* ed 6, London, 2001, Mosby.

van Emon JM, editor: *Immunoassay and Other Bioanalytical Techniques,* Boca Raton, 2006, CRC Press.

Wild D: *The Immunoassay Handbook,* ed 3, Boston, 2005, Elsevier.

INTERNET SITES

http://learn.sdstate.edu/Deb_Pravecek/Chem383/immunology.htm

http://www.aaaai.org/—Professional medical organization of specialists in allergy, asthma, and immunology

http://www3.niaid.nih.gov/—The National Institute of Allergy and Infectious Diseases (NIAID)

Immunochemical Techniques

Carolyn S. Feldkamp

8
Chapter

Chapter Outline

Key Terms

agglutination Clumping or aggregating together by specific antibody of particles (e.g., red blood cells, latex beads) to which the specific antigenic determinant is attached.

agglutinin Specific antibody that causes agglutination.

antiantibody An antibody with specificity for immunoglobulins.

antigen reagent A stabilized solution containing a known amount of an antigen that is used as a standard.

antigenic determinant (epitope) Group of amino acids or other molecules exposed on the surface of a molecule, which can generate an antigenic response and bind antibody.

cold agglutinin An agglutinin that reacts better at temperatures less than body temperature; best reaction is usually at 4°C.

complement A group of serum proteins activated as a result of an antibody-antigen reaction. When the reaction occurs on the surface of a red blood cell, the activated complement can lyse the cell.

complement-fixation A term applied to a set of assays in which complement is activated or "fixed" by a test reaction system.

Coombs' test A type of agglutination reaction. A direct Coombs' test measures the presence of antibody on cells; an indirect test measures its presence in serum.

cross-reactant Molecule with a chemical or epitope structure similar to the antigen that binds the specific antibody, sometimes with a lower affinity.

cryoglobulin Protein that precipitates at temperatures less than body temperature; precipitates maximally at 4°C.

epitope See *antigenic determinant (epitope)*.

fluoroimmunoassay Any immunoprocedure that uses a fluorescent molecule as the indicator label.

functional sensitivity Lowest concentration of analyte that can be measured at a specified precision.

HAMA See *heterophilic antibodies (HAMA)*.

hemolysin Anti–sheep–red blood cell antibody.

hemolysis Damage to red blood cells that allows cellular contents to leak out. Detected by measuring released hemoglobin.

heterogeneous immunoassay Immunoassay format that uses two phases, usually liquid and solid, to separate reacted from unreacted components.

heterophilic antibodies (HAMA) Artifact seen in sandwich immunoassays in which patient's endogenous antibody to reagent antibodies links labeled antibody to capture antibody in the absence of antigen; results in false elevations of analyte.

high dose hook effect Artifact seen in sandwich immunoassays in which labeled antibody bound in the sandwich decreases in the presence of excess antigen; results in falsely low assay results.

homogenous immunoassay Labeled-analyte immunoassay format that does not require separation of bound and free antigen.

immunodiffusion Random, spreading movement of antibody or antigen or both in a support medium.

immunoelectrophoresis An immunoprecipitation technique in which antigens are separated from each other by migration in an electrical field, followed by reaction with antibody by immunodiffusion.

indicator The portion of an immunochemical reaction that can be measured; labeled antigen or antibody.

inhibition immunoassay A term for those types of immunoassays in which an excess of antigens prevents or inhibits the completion of either the initial or the indicator phase of the reaction.

matrix Sample type; everything in the sample that is not the analyte of interest.

monoclonal antibody A monospecific antibody that is produced by a single plasma cell or a single clone of plasma cells of a lymphocyte myeloma hybrid.

monospecific An antibody that will react with only one type of antigen molecule.

nephelometric assay Measurement of antigen or antibody by determination of the amount of light scattered as the result of the amount or rate of antibody-antigen aggregation.

nephelometric inhibition immunoassay (NINIA) Measurement of haptens by inhibition of formation of an antibody-antigen lattice.

nephelometry Measurement of light-scattering properties of large particles (such as antigen-antibody complexes) in solution.

polyclonal antiserum Serum from an immunized animal containing a heterogeneous mixture of antibodies with diverse affinities toward an antigen; produced by a large number of plasma cell clones.

prozone phenomenon Apparently lower reactivity or nonreactivity caused by a relative antigen excess.

RAST RadioAllergoSorbent Test assay; often used to indicate any assay of allergen-specific immunoglobulin (Ig)E.

reagent antibody A high-titer, high-affinity, immunoglobulin (Ig)G-class antibody prepared in animals for use in immunoassays.

sandwich assay Term applied to a solid-phase two-site immunometric assay in which the first layer is immobilized antibody, the second is antigen, and the third is labeled antibody.

sensitivity (analytical) Least detectable concentration of analyte. Usually defined as two or more standard deviations from the signal of a zero standard.

specificity (analytical) Property of an antibody molecule that restricts its reactivity to a defined molecule or group of molecules.

titer Maximum dilution of a specific antibody that gives a measurable reaction with a specific antigen; usually expressed as the reciprocal of that dilution.

Chapter 7 describes the molecular nature of antigens and antibodies and the general characteristics of the antigen-antibody reaction. This chapter deals with many techniques that use the antigen-antibody reaction as the basis for detecting, characterizing, or quantitating constituents in blood and other body fluids submitted to the laboratory for analysis. These constituents can range from low-molecular-weight drugs and their metabolites to high-molecular-weight proteins, such as immunoglobulin (Ig)M and α_2-macroglobulin. In most immunoassay formats, the patient's sample contains the antigen (analyte), and antibody is added as a reagent to detect or measure the antigen. On the other hand, in cases of infectious disease (see Chapter 32), serological determinations (see Chapter 10), allergy testing (see Chapters 1 and 29, p. 562), and autoimmune antibody testing, it is the antibody measurement in the patient's sample that is clinically important. For these antibody determinations, antigen of known composition is used. The antigen may be soluble or tissue based. This chapter concentrates on procedures that detect antigen in the patient's sample.

SECTION OBJECTIVES BOX 8-1

- Describe two ways of producing reagent antibody (Ab).
- List criteria for the selection of reagent Ab.
- Describe the types of molecules that can be measured as Ag.
- Explain the differences between immunological and biological activity.

REAGENTS

Antibody as Reagent

Reagent antibodies to protein antigens usually are prepared in animals, such as rabbits or goats, by repeated exposure of the animal to foreign substances. The foreign protein stimulates B lymphocytes to produce antibodies. Specific areas, **epitopes,** on the surface of the immunizing protein are major antigenic determinants of the antigen molecule that stimulate the production of the largest number of antibodies; minor determinants also stimulate antibody production. Because many different antibodies are attributable to the expansion of many clones of antibody-producing cells, the antiserum thus produced is termed a **polyclonal antiserum.** For example, an antiserum against the protein human serum albumin (anti-HSA) is a reagent that includes multiple antibodies to various antigenic determinants on HSA. This is also termed a **monospecific** antibody.

If this anti-HSA is to be used as a reagent in the clinical laboratory, its **specificity** (i.e., its reactivity only with HSA) must be verified by the same immunological test system that is used to generate patient results. For every reagent antibody, the specificity of its immunochemical reactivity is the single most important factor in the success or failure of any immunological technique used in the clinical laboratory.

Monoclonal Antibodies

Monoclonal antibodies are formed by a technology that hybridizes individual antibody-producing cells (plasma cells) with an immortal cell line (Fig. 8-1). Monoclonal antibodies have a single homogeneous primary structure and a unique antigen-binding site. These antibodies provide a reproducible reagent of known specificity and affinity. Monoclonal antibodies are used extensively in competitive and noncompetitive binding assays and in tissue assays to identify specific antigens.

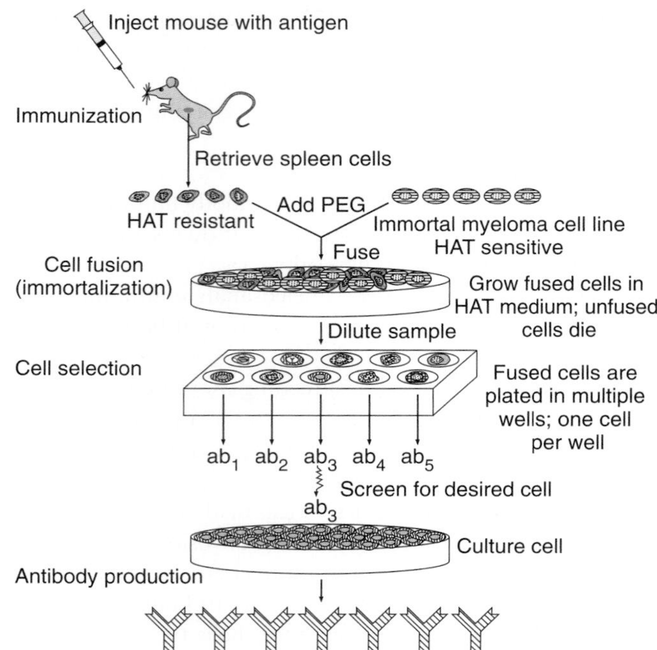

Fig. 8-1 Monoclonal antibody production. Antibody production is initiated by immunization of an animal with antigen. After the immune response, spleen cells are isolated, each of which produces a single, unique antibody. These cells are fused with an immortal myeloma cell line by exposure to polyethylene glycol (PEG). In the culture medium that contains HAT (a mixture of hypoxanthine, aminopterin, and thymidine), unfused myeloma cells, which cannot bypass the metabolic block caused by aminopterin, die. Unfused spleen cells also die naturally after 1 to 2 weeks. Fused cells survive, having the immortality of the myeloma cells and the HAT resistance of the spleen cells. Fused cells then are cultured at high dilution and are selected by screening for secretion of antibodies with the desired characteristics. Eventually, a culture of antibody-secreting cells derived from a single spleen cell produces reagent amounts of monoclonal antibody.

Selection

Selection of antibody as a reagent in an immunological procedure requires information about its characteristics such as the amount of specific antibody present (**titer**) and its affinity and specificity. Because not all of the immunoglobulin in an antiserum is reactive for a specific antigen, the amount of antibody that is available for reactivity in a specific immunological method is termed the *titer of the antibody.* The titer is the reciprocal of the maximum dilution of the antibody that gives a detectable reaction for a specific method. The titer of a reagent antibody may be different for each immunological procedure for which it is to be used. For example, anti-HSA may react in an immunoprecipitation technique at a maximum dilution of 1:32, but the same antiserum may react at a maximum dilution of 1:6400 in a competative binding immunoassay (IA) procedure.

Affinity

Reagent antibodies may be of high affinity or low affinity. Polyclonal antibodies in the reagent may be a mixture of both, but reagents in which high-affinity antibodies are predominant should be used. This results in a strong union with the antigen that is not readily reversible and that will not be influenced greatly by alteration of the reaction conditions. Low-affinity antibodies do not bind strongly with the antigen, and the union with antigen can be more strongly influenced by temperature, pH, and ionic strength with consequent changes in the reaction, resulting in dissociation of the antibody-antigen complex. Most commercial reagent antibodies are of the high-affinity type. If reagents are prepared in the laboratory, they should be tested to ensure that they are of the appropriate, preferably high, affinity.

Specificity

Specificity refers to the ability of an antibody to restrict its reaction to a defined group of molecules. Polyclonal antisera are a collection of antibodies directed at multiple antigenic determinants on a single antigen with multiple reactivities. Reagent antibodies also may react with antigenic determinants that are common to different molecules. For example, a reagent directed to the IgG molecule should recognize only the IgG molecule, but antibody in the reagent also may react with light chains of that IgG molecule. Because light chains are common to all immunoglobulin classes (i.e., IgA, IgM, and IgD), the reagent antibody then would react with all immunoglobulin molecules.

Specificity of the reagent antibody is particularly important in IAs that are used to measure the presence of small molecules such as drugs and hormones. Often there is a residual

Box 8-1

Examples of Molecules in Biological Fluids Frequently Measured by Immunological Techniques

Large Molecules
- Immunoglobulins (IgG, IgA, IgM, IgD, IgE)
- Complement components (C3, C4, factor B)
- Coagulation factors (factor VIII, fibrinogen)
- Lipoproteins
- Protein hormones
- Acute-phase proteins (α_1-antitrypsin, C-reactive protein)
- Albumin
- Selected urine and cerebrospinal fluid proteins
- Viral antigens and antibodies

Small Molecules
- Digoxin and digitonin
- Antibiotics
- Cytotoxic drugs
- Prostaglandins
- Hormones (steroids, thyroid hormones)
- Theophylline
- Anticonvulsant drugs
- Antiarrhythmic drugs
- Drugs of abuse

reaction between the reagent antibody and a closely related compound or metabolite. This reaction between antibody and the undesired antigen is termed *cross-reactivity.* When cross-reactivity with very similar antigenic determinants cannot be avoided, reagent manufacturers must state the degree of cross-reactivity with tested molecules, metabolites, and therapeutic drugs.

Because reagent antibody is protein, all precautions to prevent denaturation and degradation should be taken. The reagent should be kept free of bacterial contamination and should be stored in the refrigerator (4°C) if it is to be used within several days. Long-term storage at −20°C usually is adequate.

Antigen as Analyte

Range of Analytes

Numerous naturally occurring molecules or antigens that are proteins, glycoproteins, or lipoproteins can be detected and measured easily in biological fluids with specific reagent antibodies. In addition, many small molecules such as drugs and hormones can be measured (Box 8-1).

Sample Types and Stability

The biological fluids most commonly available to the laboratory for analysis are serum, urine, and cerebrospinal fluid. Antigens present in each of these fluids are subject to degradation depending on (1) the nature of the antigen, (2) its concentration, (3) its susceptibility to various enzymes in the body fluids, and (4) its relative stability at various storage temperatures (e.g., room temperature, 4°C, −20°C, −70°C). Each specimen must be stored and handled properly to ensure that the antigen molecule is unaltered and the reagent antibody can react with appropriate antigenic determinants on the molecule. **Cryoglobulins** are immunoglobulins that precipitate from serum or plasma as the temperature decreases from 37°C. Stability of antigens must be established for each biological fluid. For example, the C4 component of **complement** of serum is stable and can be measured accurately up to a week after receipt of the serum if the specimen is stored at 4°C before analysis. However, the C4 component in cerebrospinal fluid is very labile and usually is present at very low concentrations. If this kind of sample is stored longer than 8 hours at 4°C before analysis, the C4 will have been degraded and will be undetectable. Thus spinal fluid must be frozen and stored at −70°C.

Another example is that of antigen denaturation in urine specimens. Because most urine specimens are acidic, and proteins are degraded in an acid pH, many antigenic determinants on these proteins may be lost. β_2-Microglobulin is a protein that is found in both urine and plasma. In urine, it is used to estimate renal tubular dysfunction. It is rapidly destroyed if the pH of urine is less than 6.0. Quantitation of specific proteins in urine samples requires immediate neutralization of the acid pH at the time of collection. In contrast, the protein in serum is stable for a week when stored at 4°C. Antigen degradation may not be as significant when small molecules such as drugs are measured in urine. Nevertheless, it is always good laboratory practice to store biological fluids at 4°C if the analysis is not to be performed on the same day, and they should be stored in a frozen state if the analysis is to be performed much later.

Immunological versus Biological Quantitation

It should be emphasized that the immunological reactivity of a molecule may not be related to its biological activity. The importance of this distinction is illustrated by the examples of α_1-antitrypsin (α1AT) and parathyroid hormone (PTH).

α1AT is a potent inhibitor of the proteolytic enzyme trypsin. Certain genetic variations occur in which the variant is estimated to be present at normal levels when measured by immunochemical techniques, but the molecule's enzyme-inhibiting capability is greatly impaired. Immunochemically, the genetic variants react as well as the normally functioning molecule does; however, there is a great biological difference.

PTH degrades quickly in plasma, and the PTH molecule may not be present as the intact molecule released by the parathyroid gland. In patients with end-stage renal disease, these degradation products accumulate in plasma. When levels of PTH are obtained by some immunological methods, they can appear to be normal or increased when in fact there is a low level of the intact molecule. This discrepancy is attributable to the reaction of antibody with the breakdown products of PTH, which retain the appropriate antigenic determinants. Examples of immunological reactivity without biological activity occur frequently and demonstrate that normal levels of molecules assayed by immunological methods do not necessarily predict normal functional activity.

Reference Materials

Qualitative and quantitative measurements of antigen in biological fluids require the use of a highly specific reagent antibody and a known reference standard of **antigen reagent.** The reactivity of the antibody with the antigen in the patient's biological fluid is compared with the reactivity of the antibody with the standard antigen. For the most part, standards are supplied in comercially available immunological test kits. If the U.S. Food and Drug Administration (FDA) approves a test kit, the technologist is reasonably assured that the reagent antibody is detecting the antigen, as stated by the manufacturer. The World Health Organization (WHO) supplies reference antigen for many serum proteins as primary standards. Secondary standards have been developed by the College of American Pathologists (CAP) in collaboration with the Centers for Disease Control and Prevention (CDC) and are easily available. Federal regulations established by the Clinical Laboratories Improvement Act of 1988 (CLIA '88) define laboratory requirements to validate the accuracy and precision of clinical assays. Manufacturers' data may be used for kits used with no modification. Otherwise, thorough documentation of accuracy, precision, linearity, sensitivity, and normal ranges must be maintained.

KEY CONCEPTS BOX 8-1

- Assay-suitable antibody (Ab) can be produced as antiserum from animals exposed to a specific antigen (Ag) or as a monoclonal Ab.
- Important criteria for selection of reagent Ab include titer and affinity to and specificity for a specific Ag.
- For some molecules there is a difference between immunological quantitation and biological activity; immunoassays should be directed toward molecules of known biological activity.

SECTION OBJECTIVES BOX 8-2

- List assays that use the precipitation of antibody-antigen (Ab-Ag) complexes in gels.
- Explain the principle of the Western blot assay and its common applications.
- Explain the principle of immunonephelometry, and describe the common pitfalls of this technique.
- Explain the principle of the nephelometric inhibition immunoassay (NINIA) technique.
- Describe the compounds measured by immunonephelometry and NINIA.

QUANTITATION OF ANTIGENS AND ANTIBODIES BY IMMUNOLOGICAL REACTIONS IN GELS

Several techniques are available to measure antibodies and protein antigens by immunological reactions in gels laid onto a solid support. Antigen or antibody mixtures were separated in the gel by rate of diffusion, or electrophoresis. As antigen-antibody complexes were formed at concentrations of "equivalence" (see Chapter 7), the resulting precipitated complex could be visualized by eye. Quantitative relationships between the distance traveled in the gel and the concentration of reactants allowed quantitation. **Immunodiffusion, immunoelectrophoresis,** counterelectrophoresis, radial immunodiffusion, and Laurell ("rocket") immunoelectrophoresis have been replaced in clinical practice by nephelometric techniques and quantitative competitive binding and immunometric techniques that use labeled reactants. The latter techniques are quantitative, sensitive, and usually highly automated. Reactions of antigens and antibodies in gels still are used in laboratory specialties such as transfusion medicine or infectious diseases, as well as in research to test antisera and antigen mixtures for cross-reacting substances. Immunofixation still is used to qualitatively identify proteins and to establish light- and heavy-chain types of monoclonal proteins. **Agglutination** and techniques that use antigen migration and precipitation of immune complexes also are frequently used in point-of-care devices (POC). For details on the techniques that use immunological reactions in gels, please refer to earlier editions of this textbook.

IMMUNOFIXATION (WESTERN BLOT)

The immunoblotting technique known as the Western blot method is often used in clinical applications to confirm the presence of antibody (e.g., human immunodeficiency virus [HIV] antibody) to specific antigens. This technique also is used for the detection of specific proteins, such as apoE isoforms.

Principles

The method of immunoblotting is a three-stage procedure that uses electrophoresis to separate and transfer analytes. An antigen mixture first is electrophoresed in an appropriate support medium, such as polyacrylamide, neutral agarose, or paper strips, to separate the components by charge-to-weight differences. The support then is overlaid with a sheet of nitrocellulose-based filter paper. In a second electrophoretic step, the protein is transferred from the support to the nitrocellulose. The nitrocellulose has the property of effectively irreversibly binding the transferred protein. The nitrocellulose sheet then is treated with a protein solution, to block remaining binding sites and minimize nonspecific binding in the next step. Next, an antibody solution, usually serum from a patient, is allowed to react with the nitrocellulose sheet. Excess antibody then is removed by washing. The nitrocellulose sheet is incubated with a second labeled antibody that has specificity for the first antibody. The label allows detection of the original antigen-antibody reaction. If the label is an enzyme, such as peroxidase, the reaction is detected by substrate precipitation of, for example, a benzidine dye. A diagram is presented in Fig. 8-2.

Reagents

The reagent antibody's label must have a high specificity and specific activity so that it can detect only the desired antibody

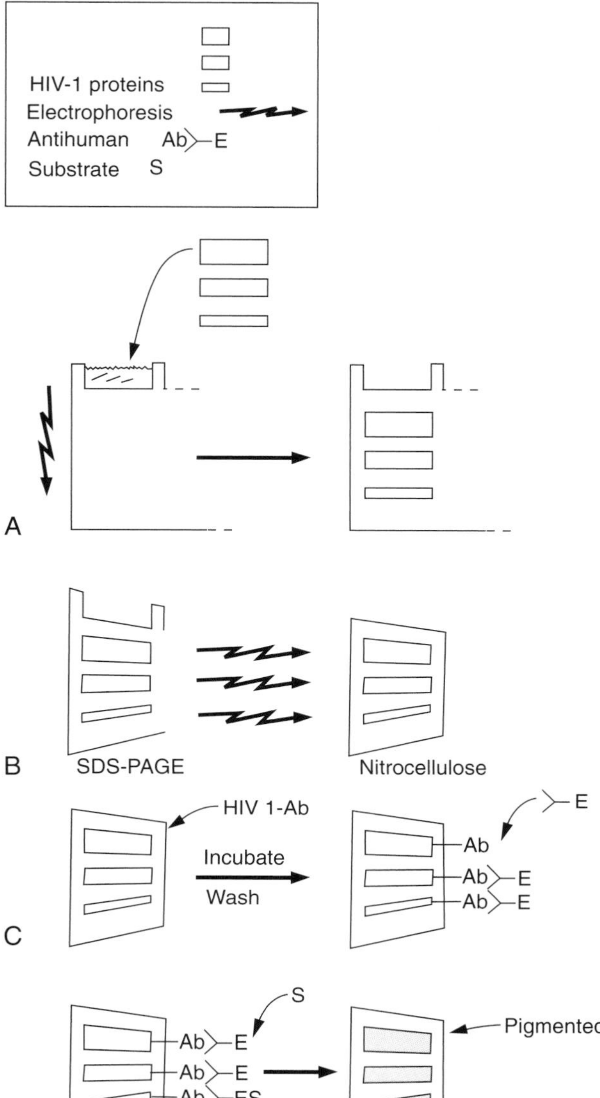

Fig. 8-2 Diagram of enzyme-linked immunoelectrotransfer blot technique (Western blot). **A,** Human immunodeficiency virus (HIV)-1 proteins are layered onto a sodium dodecyl sulfate–polyacrylamide gel electrophoresis (SDS-PAGE), subjected to electrophoresis, and separated according to their molecular weight. **B,** The discrete proteins then are electrophoresed (blotted) to a nitrocellulose matrix and are incubated, first with a specimen containing HIV-1 antibody (Ab), which binds to the discrete HIV-1 antigen (Ag) bands. **C,** Enzyme-labeled antihuman Ab then is added. The excess is washed away, and enzyme substrate is added. **D,** HIV-1 Ab directed toward discrete HIV-1 antigen bands is present; the discrete bands can be visualized as pigmented bands. (Reprinted from American Clinical Laboratory, vol 6, p 11, 1987. Copyright © 1987 by International Scientific Communications, Inc.)

or test protein, and so that the **sensitivity** of the assay will be great enough to detect the presence of the reaction.

Common Pitfalls

The assays commonly use peroxidase dye reactions to detect the presence of antibody or antigen. These assays often require skilled individuals to read the patterns.

Test Sensitivity and Interpretation of Results

This technique is nearly as sensitive as the enzyme immunoassay technique. However, whereas enzyme immunoassays are employed as quantitative assays, Western blots and other immunofixation methods are used primarily as qualitative techniques, that is, they are used to detect the presence or absence of a particular protein or antibody. A widely used application of the technique is for confirmation of the results of HIV screening. The sensitivity of the technique can be seen in the detection of less than 1 ng/mL of test protein.

IMMUNONEPHELOMETRY

Nephelometry

For a detailed discussion of **nephelometry,** see Chapter 2, pp. 62-65.

Principles

When an antibody and an antigen bind in solution, small complexes form quickly. Nephelometric, or light-scattering, assays measure this early second-order reaction, in which the antigen-antibody complex lattice is large enough to scatter light but is not large enough to precipitate (see pp. 62-64, Chapter 7). Clinically useful assays for specific plasma proteins are based on the direct relationship between the intensity of scattered light, the amount of precipitate formed, and the concentration of antigen, as long as the reaction was carried out in antibody excess conditions. Nephelometers used for these assays typically use a laser as a light source and measure either the end point of complex formation or the rate of complex formation. This aggregate formation can be greatly enhanced by the addition of the water-soluble polymer polyethylene glycol (MW 6000 D) at concentrations of 2% to 4%. The polymer causes a severalfold increase in light scatter while decreasing the reaction time tenfold. Fast (seconds to minutes) and precise methods for the specific measurement of plasma proteins such as albumin, immunoglobulins, complement components, and acute-phase reactants, are now available.

Antibody-antigen (Ab-Ag) lattice detection by turbidimetric analysis (see p. 159, Chapter 2) has been widely adapted to automated instruments. Both methods also have been adapted for application to small molecules such as hormones and therapeutic drugs (see pp. 62-64, Chapter 9).

Common Pitfalls

1. Antibody is not in excess. In these circumstances, the amount of precipitate formation will be recorded as a falsely low value.

2. Background scatter is too high. Rate nephelometric determinations are preferred to end-point determinations because they minimize the contribution of background. For example, it is possible to detect a 5% increase in scattering over background by using a rate measurement. In contrast, such a difference may not be measurable as an end-point change. Lipidemia causes high background scatter.
3. Interference is caused by colored solution. End-point methods are most often influenced by colored solutions. These absorb the scattered light, tending to yield lower values. However, even kinetic measurements are lower in highly colored solutions.
4. Mixing is insufficient. The rate method requires constant agitation to make uniform particles.
5. Pre-formed immune complexes in the patient serum may cause false-high or false-low values, depending on whether the rate of reaction is measured and how the background correction is done.

Limitations

For most assays, quantitation is valid only when the reagent antibody is in excess. Although each instrument manufacturer has devised ways of detecting antigen excess conditions, the measurement may have to be made at two different dilutions. This method is limited to measurements of antigens that form enough lattice to scatter light, such as proteins. Special test modifications are required for small molecules.

Monoclonal Antibody Reagents

The performance of light-scattering assays depends greatly on the quality of the antiserum used. With conventional polyclonal reagents, there is a continual need to monitor and adjust antiserum titer, specificity, and affinity. Such variability often is overcome by the use of a monoclonal antibody. However, unless the antigen has many identical antigenic sites, a single monoclonal antibody cannot form a lattice and will cause little or no light scatter. Some commercial reagent antibodies use a mixture of monoclonal antibodies, which will form large enough complex lattices to scatter light. This blending of monoclonal antibodies or the use of monoclonals in particle-enhanced light-scatter assays ensures constancy of reagent production and gives these assays greater stability and specificity. For a discussion of particle-enhanced light scatter assays, see Chapter 9.

Nephelometric Inhibition Immunoassay (NINIA)

Principles

If a small molecule such as a drug is covalently linked to a large carrier protein such as bovine serum albumin, the resulting conjugate acts as a large light-scattering antigen when reacted with antibody to the small molecule, or hapten. The complex formation can be inhibited by the addition of the specific hapten. The inhibition of binding is dose dependent, and a quantitative assay for the small molecule results. With appropriate manipulation of the variables, the number of haptenic groups on the carrier protein can be adjusted for adequate precipitation while allowing maximum sensitivity for inhibition by free hapten (Fig. 8-3). Nephelometric **inhibition assays** have been developed for rapid analysis of drugs occurring in mg/L amounts, such as phenytoin, phenobarbital, and theophylline.

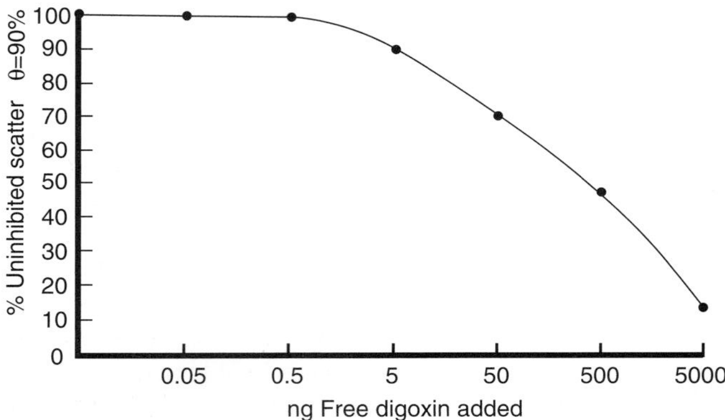

Fig. 8-3 Digoxin standard curve using nephelometric inhibition immunoassay.

KEY CONCEPTS BOX 8-2

- Immunodiffusion, immunoelectrophoresis, counterelectrophoresis, radial immunodiffusion, and Laurell ("rocket") immunoelectrophoresis all employ precipitation of antibody-antigen (Ab-Ag) in gel.
- The Western blot technique requires the separation of Ag by electrophoresis, transfer ("blotting") of the separated Ags onto nitrocellulose, and then the addition of sample to detect Ab against the Ags. This can be used to detect the presence of HIV Abs or specific proteins.
- Detection of small Ab-Ag complexes by scattering of incident light is called *immunonephelometry.* It is used to quantitate specific proteins in serum and cerebrospinal fluid (CSF).
- Nephelometric inhibition immunoassay (NINIA) requires the mixture of a molecule attached to a small particle, the small molecule from sample, and Ab to the molecule. The presence of small molecule in the sample inhibits Ab-Ag (particle) complexing. Used primarily for small molecules such as drugs.

SECTION OBJECTIVES BOX 8-3

- Define agglutination, and differentiate between direct agglutination, indirect agglutination, and agglutination-inhibition reactions.
- List important factors that must be controlled in agglutination assays.
- Describe the principles of direct and indirect Coombs' tests.
- Describe the principles of one- and two-stage complement-fixation tests.

AGGLUTINATION ASSAYS

Agglutination, the clumping and sedimentation of antigen after reaction with antibody, was first noted when the reaction of bacteria incubated with serum from an infected patient was observed. Observation of the agglutination of red blood cells after incubation with serum led to the discovery of ABO blood groups. Agglutination has been used extensively as a detection system because of its ease and versatility. However, it is only semiquantitative, showing reproducibility only within fourfold dilutions. Agglutinating antibodies (**agglutinins**) may be directed against naturally occurring antigens on the surfaces of cells (active or direct agglutination) or against substances that have been applied to the surfaces of cells or inert particles (passive or indirect agglutination).

Principles

Agglutination reactions depend on the formation of antibody bridges by bivalent (IgG) or multivalent (IgM) antibody between antigen particles with multiple **antigenic determinants.** Large particles, such as red blood cells or bacteria have many different antigens that appear hundreds of times on the cell or particle surface. Thus it is possible for antibody molecules to bind to more than one site on a single particle or to bind to equivalent sites on different particles. Such binding is called *cross-linking.* Antigens with a single antigenic determinant do not permit cross-linking and therefore do not agglutinate. Cross-linking may create a high-molecular-weight lattice that clumps together and precipitates. Because of its size and multivalency, IgM is said to be 750 times more efficient at agglutination than IgG. Agglutination reactions generally are used to detect antibody directed to particulate antigens; semi-quantitation is performed by serial dilution of serum. Reverse agglutination can be used to detect soluble antigen through the use of antibody adsorbed onto cell or particle surfaces. Agglutination reactions are read by the naked eye or with the aid of magnification. The extent of agglutination is scored 1+ to 4+ by estimation. The titer of the serum is the reciprocal of the highest dilution giving visible (1+) agglutination.

Factors Influencing Agglutination Reaction

Factors influencing agglutination include particle charge, antibody type, electrolyte concentration, viscosity of the medium, reactant concentrations, location and concentration of antigenic determinants, and time and temperature of incubation.

Particle Charge

Red blood cells, bacteria, and inert particles such as latex have a net negative surface charge called the *zeta potential.* These charges must be overcome to permit the cross-linking that results in agglutination.

Antibody Type

IgM antibodies are more efficient at agglutination because of their multivalency and because their size permits more effective bridging of the gap between cells caused by charge repulsion.

Electrolyte Concentration and Viscosity

The ionic strength of the medium used for the agglutination reaction can assist in reducing the negative surface charge of particles. This can be accomplished by addition of charged molecules, such as albumin, to the medium. The pH of the medium should be near that present under physiological conditions. At neutral pH, high electrolyte concentrations act to neutralize the net negative charge of particles. Increasing the viscosity of the medium with polymerized molecules, such as dextran, also assists in bringing the charged particles together.

Antigenic Determinants

As was stated earlier, antigens with multiple antigenic determinants are necessary for agglutination. A monovalent antigen does not permit cross-linking. Placement of the antigenic determinants onto the particle also can affect agglutinability. Antigenic determinants that are sparsely distributed are not as easily cross-linked as antigenic determinants that are densely distributed. Antigenic determinants also can be inaccessible to antibody binding because they are buried within cell membranes.

Concentration, Temperature, and Time of Incubation

The concentration of reactants can influence reaction time. At higher antigen concentrations, the reaction with antibody is more rapid. Agitation of the antigen suspension with antibody solution increases the reaction rate by increasing the surface area exposed to the antibody. At lower antigen concentrations, the reaction time can be shortened by centrifugation, which increases contact between the antigenic particles and the antibody. The temperature of incubation is also an important variable. Some antigens, including microbes, are bound most readily by antibody at 37°C. Some antigens react optimally with antibody at 4°C. These **cold agglutinins** include antibody to the i antigen on fetal and infant red blood cells. Optimum temperature for the agglutination reaction varies with different antigen-antibody systems. Temperature also affects the behavior of antibodies in vitro.

Direct Agglutination

Direct agglutination tests are frequently used in the immunological diagnosis of microbial infections. The titer of the serum reflects the concentration of the predominant antibody in the serum. Early detection of a high titer and documentation of a significant rise in titer are important tools in diagnosis. Antibodies to *Brucella* (brucellosis), *Salmonella* (typhoid fever), and *Proteus* (Rocky Mountain spotted fever) organisms are detected in this way. Direct agglutination tests also are used in the typing of human red blood cells in the blood bank.

Different bacterial antigens may give different patterns of agglutination. Antibodies to bacterial flagella cause cross-linking of the flagella themselves. These antibodies cause

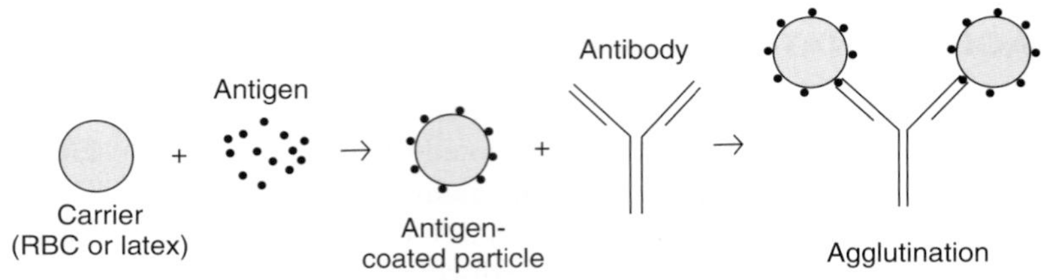

Fig. 8-4 Passive (indirect) agglutination reaction. Antigen is adsorbed onto the surface of the carrier particle, which then is agglutinated by antigen-specific antibody.

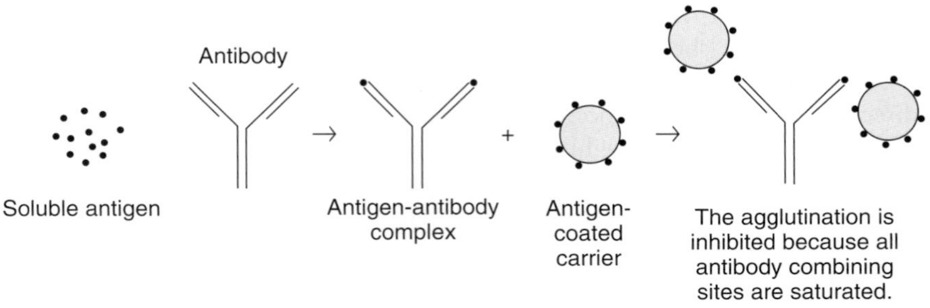

Fig. 8-5 Agglutination-inhibition reaction. Same reaction as that shown in Fig. 8-4, but inhibited by soluble antigen.

formation of a loose, rapidly formed agglutinate. Antibodies to antigens in the body of the bacterium cause cross-linking of the organisms themselves. This results in a granular, compact precipitate that develops more slowly.

Indirect Agglutination

Indirect agglutination involves the reaction of antibody with antigens that have been passively transferred onto the surfaces of particles (Fig. 8-4). Red blood cells, usually from humans, sheep, or turkeys, are employed. Inert particles such as latex (0.81 μm in diameter) and bentonite (clay) also are used. Polysaccharide and some protein antigens, such as albumin and purified protein derivatives, are easily adsorbed onto the particle surface. Other antigens require pretreatment of particles with tannic acid or chromium chloride, which modifies the cell surface. Antigen can be covalently bound to the cell surface by bifunctional molecules, such as bisdiazobenzidine or glutaraldehyde. Indirect agglutination is used in the diagnosis of syphilis. The Venereal Disease Research Laboratory (VDRL) test employs cholesterol crystals coated with cardiolipin antigen. Detection of rheumatoid factor, which is useful in the diagnosis of rheumatoid arthritis, uses agglutination of latex particles coated with human IgG. For the quantitation of rheumatoid factor, agglutination methods have been largely replaced by immunonephelometry.

Agglutination Inhibition

Agglutination inhibition is an adaptation of the agglutination reaction that permits detection and quantitation of soluble antigen. The concentrations of antibody and particles are carefully controlled to prevent antibody excess. Antibody is incubated with the test antigen solution, and antigen is bound to available antibody-combining sites. The antibody then is added to particulate antigen suspensions. The failure to agglutinate indicates that enough antibody-combining sites have been saturated with a soluble form of the same antigen that insufficient antibody-binding sites are available for binding and cross-linking of the particulate antigen. Quantitation of the soluble antigen can be accomplished by assessment of the degree of inhibition in serial dilutions of the antigen solution (Fig. 8-5).

ANTIGLOBULIN TESTING

Antiglobulin testing is a modification of the agglutination reaction that permits detection of certain immunoglobulins (incomplete antibody [IgG]) that may not produce agglutination even after binding to the particle surface. IgG is less effective at agglutination than IgM because its smaller size is less effective at bridging antigen particles. If an anti-immunoglobulin, or Coombs' reagent, is added to the unagglutinated IgG-coated particles, the Coombs' reagent will bridge the gap between particles through bivalent binding (Fig. 8-6). This enables cross-linking to achieve agglutination. The direct **Coombs' test** is used in blood banks to determine the presence of IgG antibodies to red blood cells.

The indirect Coombs' test is a variation of the antiglobulin test that is used to detect free antibody to red blood cells in patient serum (Fig. 8-7). Serum is screened against a panel of red blood cells of known and varied antigenicity. Agglutination of cells to which patient serum and antiglobulin reagent have been added indicates the presence of antibody in patient serum to an antigen present on the agglutinated cells.

Sample Requirements

Agglutination reactions can be used to measure components of plasma, serum, or cerebrospinal fluid. Urine must be buffered because of its usual acidity. Because serum complement may affect agglutination, complement inactivation or sample dilution to minimize complement activity may be necessary.

Reagents

Similarly to red blood cell agglutination techniques, factors that influence the reactions include particle charge, type of antibody, electrolyte concentration, and viscosity. Red blood

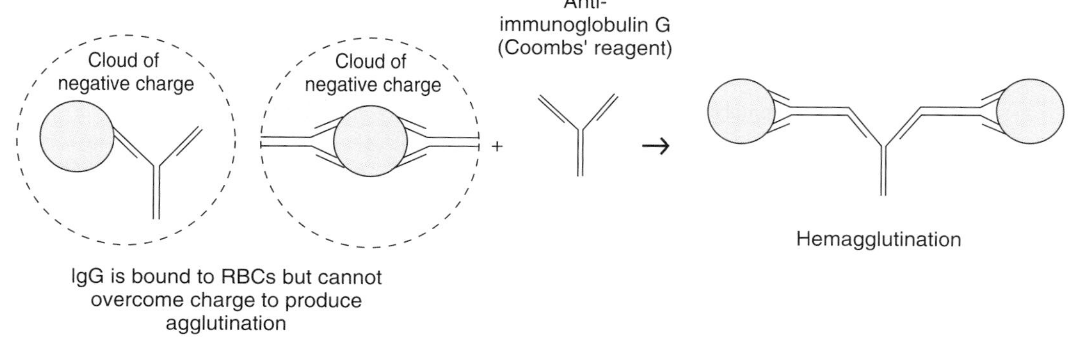

Fig. 8-6 Direct Coombs' test for antibody to red blood cells.

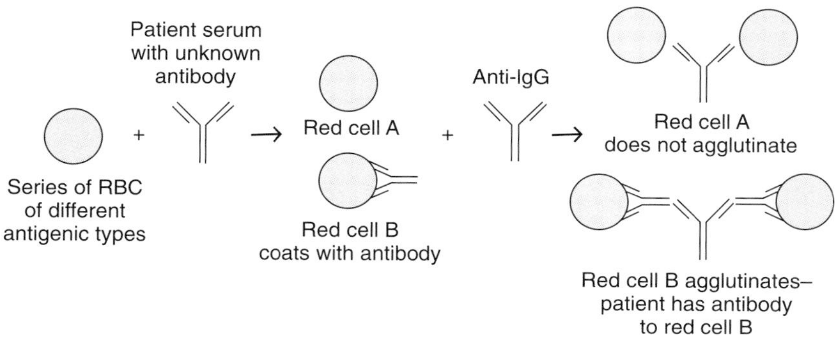

Fig. 8-7 Indirect Coombs' test for antibody.

cells, when used fresh, have a shelf life of about 2 weeks. Therefore, many manufacturers have developed fixed red blood cells (usually stabilized by tannic acid or glutaraldehyde) or latex beads to overcome the need to prepare the reagents every few weeks.

Instrumentation

The great advantage of this technique is the simplicity of instrumentation. Results can be detected by eye or with the aid of a mirror or magnifying glass.

Common Pitfalls

Antigen excess often results in a **prozone phenomenon** with false-negative results. Use of expired red blood cells or other reagents can result in lack of agglutination.

Limitations

This technique is only semiquantitative and thus allows estimates of the true value within a dilution factor of two.

COMPLEMENT-FIXATION ASSAYS

Complement-fixation tests are probably the most sensitive of the older immunological procedures. Although more sensitive, automated immunoassasys have largely replaced these older tests, complement-fixation tests are still important in the diagnosis of fungal, viral, and parasitic infections, and in the quantitation of functional complement levels (total hemolytic complement) and complement components.

Complement Proteins

The term *complement* is used to denote a series of plasma proteins that are activated in sequence after antigen-antibody reactions. Not all classes and subclasses of immunoglobulins are capable of activating complement or can activate it to the same degree (see Table 7-1, p. 155). The antigen-antibody complex used in **complement-fixation** tests therefore must involve an antibody that is capable of activating, or fixing, complement. As with agglutination reactions, pentameric IgM is 1000 times more efficient in fixing complement than is IgG.

The first protein in the complement sequence is bound to the second constant domain of the heavy chain (C_{H2}), which is inaccessible on an unreacted or unbound antibody. After interaction and binding with antigen, conformational changes in the immunoglobulin molecule cause the hinge region to open and the complement-binding site to become exposed. Subsequent complement proteins then are activated that can bind to the membrane of the cell to which the antigen-antibody complex is bound. Binding of the complete sequence of nine complement proteins results in small defects in the membranes of the cells. Cytoplasmic cell contents are lost through these holes, and extracellular fluid is admitted. This results in hypotonic swelling of the cell and ends in cell lysis. If cells used in the test are red blood cells, cell lysis results in release of hemoglobin into the medium. The amount of hemoglobin is directly proportional to the amount of complement fixed to the surfaces of the cells.

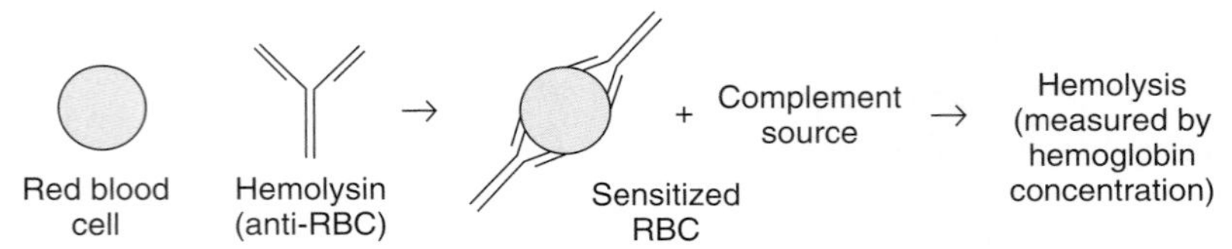

Red blood cell
Hemolysin (anti-RBC)
Sensitized RBC
Complement source
Hemolysis (measured by hemoglobin concentration)

Fig. 8-8 Complement fixation one-stage testing. For measurement of total hemolytic complement, test serum is added as source of complement. For measurement of complement components as complement source, test sera to which purified complement components are added are used; for example, to measure complement component 3, all components except C3 are added in excess to the test serum. Therefore, the reaction is limited only by the concentration of C3 in the test serum.

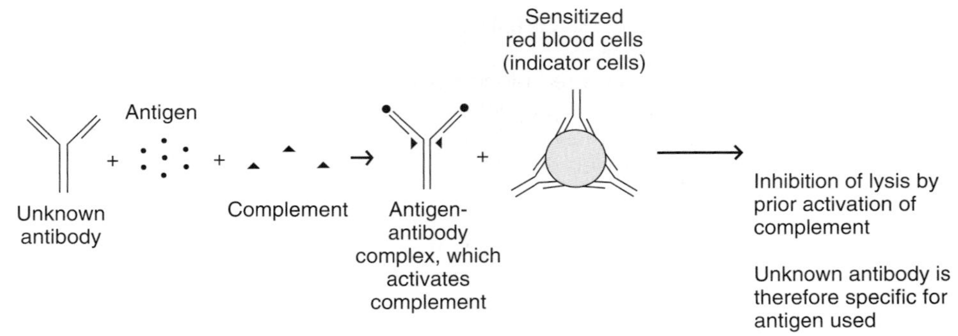

Unknown antibody
Antigen
Complement
Antigen-antibody complex, which activates complement
Sensitized red blood cells (indicator cells)
Inhibition of lysis by prior activation of complement
Unknown antibody is therefore specific for antigen used

Fig. 8-9 Complement-fixation two-stage testing. Antigen or antibody can be measured by holding constant all but the variable to be tested, in this case, unknown antibody.

One-Stage Testing

To assess total complement levels (complement activity that reflects all nine major complement proteins) or to assess individually the nine major complement proteins, a one-stage test system is used. A constant volume of red blood cells, usually sheep, is added to a constant amount of anti–sheep red blood cell, or **hemolysin.** A source of complement is added. For total complement measurements, dilutions of the unknown serum are used. For measurement of complement components, serum with an added excess of every complement component except the component to be measured is used. The degree of **hemolysis** is measured spectrophotometrically as hemoglobin and is directly proportional to the amount of complement available for fixation in the test serum (Fig. 8-8).

Some immunologically mediated diseases cause a decrease in total serum complement levels or in the levels of individual complement components. In addition, hereditary deficiencies of certain components of the complement system have been described.

Two-Stage Testing

Two-stage complement-fixation testing is used to measure antigen or antibody. In the first reaction, antigen and antibody are incubated with a known amount of complement. In the second stage, the residual complement activity in the solution is determined by an **indicator** system, such as sheep red blood cells that are coated with hemolysin. The degree of hemolysis of the indicator cells is inversely proportional to the amount of complement fixed in the first reaction and to the concentration of the test analyte (Fig. 8-9). To determine antigen levels, a constant volume of antibody is used. To determine antibody levels, a constant amount of antigen is used.

Sample Requirements and Preparation

Plasma collected in ethylenediaminetetraacetic acid (EDTA) preservative, serum, and cerebrospinal fluid may be analyzed. The samples cannot be hemolyzed. The endogenous complement of the sample is inactivated, usually by heating the specimen for 15 to 30 minutes at 56°C.

Reagents

Exogenous complement must be prepared daily and cannot be stored. The complement activity varies significantly from batch to batch and must be standardized daily.

Limitations

Complement-fixation tests are sensitive to many variables. They are inhibited by anticomplement activity (factors that inactivate or interfere with any of the complement proteins) in serum, including factors such as circulating immune (antigen-antibody) complexes, lipemic sera, aggregated immunoglobulins, and heparin.

It is critical to keep all components in the test constant except the one that is to be measured. Red blood cell number, concentration of complement, and concentration of antigen should be rigorously defined for antibody determinations. The instability of some complement proteins, variability in red blood cells, variation between lots of hemolysin, and the narrow range of optimum reactivity for many reagents can influence test results. The need for fresh reagents and the great variability make this assay one of the most difficult performed by a laboratory.

The CDC evaluates complement-fixation reagents and has developed standardized procedures for complement-fixation tests.

KEY CONCEPTS BOX 8-3

- Agglutination involves the coupling of large particles, such as red blood cells, by cross-linking antibodies (Abs).
- Agglutinating antibodies (agglutinins) can react against naturally occurring antigens (Ags) on the surfaces of cells (direct agglutination) or against Ags added to the surfaces of cells or inert particles (indirect agglutination).
- Agglutination inhibition, which is used to detect soluble Ags, requires mixing of sample and Ab. After the reaction, the mixture is added to Ag bound to particles; inhibition of agglutination indicates the presence of Ag in the sample.
- One-stage Coombs' test uses red blood cells (RBC), hemolysin, and the sample; the presence of complement in the sample causes RBC lysis.
- Two-stage complement fixation detects Ag or Ab. Ag and Ab are mixed with complement. Second stage measures residual complement by RBC coated with hemolysin.

SECTION OBJECTIVES BOX 8-4

- Describe the principles of solid-phase "sandwich" assays, while distinguishing between those that measure antigen and those that measure antibody.
- List the labels used for "sandwich" assays, while comparing their sensitivity and their ability to be used in heterogeneous and homogeneous assays.
- Define HAMAs, and explain how they can be detected and how their interference can be controlled.

INDICATOR-LABELED IMMUNOASSAYS

The immunoassays described earlier all use direct measurement of a physical property of the antigen-antibody complex or aggregates formed secondarily to the initial binding step (such as precipitation or light scatter). By introducing a labeled indicator antigen or antibody to trace the initial binding reaction, an enhanced analytical sensitivity can be achieved. These indicator-labeled immunoassays use as a detection system the sensitive measurement of some property of the indicator molecule. The indicators, or labels, most frequently used include enzymes and fluorescent or chemiluminescent molecules. The non-isotopic, indicator-labeled assays, suitable for both qualitative and quantitative measurements, are widely used because of their better sensitivity and reproduciblity; use of minimal, stable reagents; small sample size; and suitability for automation.

Quantitative immunoassays of this type usually use IgG as the reagent antibody. Although they are quite specific by virtue of the antibody specificity, the binding reactions are sensitive to the usual variations in temperature, pH, ionic strength, and sample or standard **matrix.** Analytical sensitivity to ng/mL range or even lower allows this type of assay to be used for analytes that are present in low concentrations, such as hormones, vitamins, and drugs.

Qualitative indicator-labeled immunoassays frequently are less sensitive but are convenient and very popular in the serology laboratory for the detection of antibodies to infectious organisms and for the characterization of autoimmune antibodies such as antinuclear antibody and antithyroid antibodies.

Indicator-labeled immunoassays generally may be classified as *competitive* or *noncompetitive* and as *heterogeneous* or *homogeneous.* Competitive reactions usually use labeled antigen and are carried out in the presence of excess antigen. The analyte and labeled analyte compete for binding sites on the antibody. Radioimmunoassay (RIA) is the older prototype of the heterogeneous type of competitive immunoassay, and the enzyme-multiplied immunoassay technique (EMIT) is an example of the **homogeneous immunoassay** type (see Chapter 9). Noncompetitive assays usually employ a labeled antibody and are carried out in the presence of excess antibody. Frequently, these assays are heterogeneous, using a capture antibody bound to a solid phase such as a plastic bead or test tube and a second phase consisting of the labeled antibody in solution. This latter type of assay is synonymous with the term *immunometric* or *sandwich assay.*

Labels

A label that is suitable for use as an immunochemical reagent must have certain qualities. The label must have high specific reactivity, that is, many detectable events per indicator molecule per unit of time. The specific activity must not be reduced, or quenched, by the conjugation of the indicator to the antigen or antibody. Enzyme labels should not be normally present in the sample in high enough concentrations to interfere with the measurement. This is crucial for homogeneous assays in which the sample matrix containing interfering substances remains in the reaction mixture during the measurement step. Several enzymes, metal chelates, radioisotopes, chemiluminescent dyes, and fluorophores fulfill most of these requirements and have been successfully used as labels in immunoassays. Examples of commonly used enzymes include horseradish peroxidase, alkaline phosphatase, glucose oxidase, and β-galactosidase. Selection of the enzyme for use as a label for the immunochemical reagents is often empirical, and each enzyme has distinct advantages and disadvantages. (For the properties of enzymes, see Chapter 15.) Radioisotopes can be used to label either antigens or antibodies. The most commonly used radioisotope is iodine-125, which has a high specific activity and a decay energy suitable for safe use in clinical laboratories (see Evolve).

In fluorometric immunoassays, either antigen or antibody can be conjugated, or covalently linked, with a fluorochrome molecule. The fluorochrome is a chemical that can absorb the electromagnetic energy of short-wavelength light (200 to 400 nm) and then emit light at a longer wavelength in the visible spectrum (400 to 700 nm) (see p. 59). The intensity of the emitted light is the measurable indicator in fluorometric immunoassays. Fluorescein isothiocyanate, often abbreviated FITC, has high molar absorptivity and can be easily conjugated to free amino groups in proteins. Some assays use

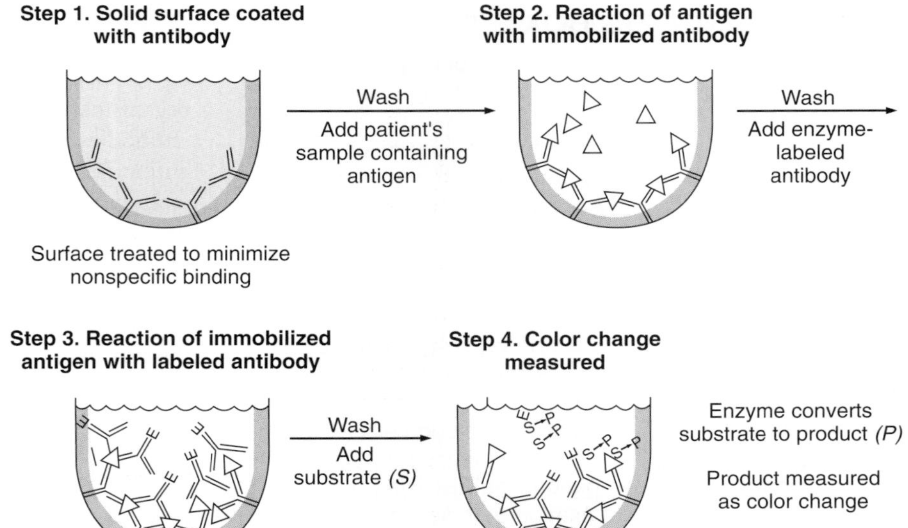

Fig. 8-10 Enzyme immunoassay. Sandwich technique with antibody label.

chelates of rare earth metals such as europium (Eu) or rubidium (Ru), which are naturally fluorescent and have half-lives up to 40 to 80 times that of fluorescein. New technologies use a variety of novel fluorescent molecules that have characteristics suitable for use in automated, multiplex, or point-of-care applications. Chemiluminescent dyes are used in a similar manner. In this case, the conjugate is activated by a chemical reaction and subsequently emits light that can be measured. The chemiluminescent molecule may be directly conjugated to the label, or a chemiluminescent substrate can be used with an enzyme label such as alkaline phosphatase.

IMMUNOMETRIC ASSAYS

Principles

Heterogeneous, Noncompetitive, Labeled Antibody (Immunometric Technique)

A popular format for this type of immunoassay is the **heterogeneous immunoassay,** which uses a solid phase coated with antibody for the first step of the assay. The first antibody reacts with the antigen that is being tested. The extent of this reaction is assessed by subsequent reaction with a second, labeled antibody. This forms the "sandwich" with the antigen between two different antibodies. The sandwich technique can be used to measure either antigens or antibodies (in which case, the solid phase is coated with antigen). Antibodies have been immobilized to polystyrene (microtiter plates), latex, or ferromagnetic particles.

For the antigen-measuring system, two different molecules of antibody must bind to the antigen. Thus, this type of immunoassay can measure only large antigens, such as proteins with multiple epitopes (Fig. 8-10). Antibody of the desired specificity is passively immobilized to a solid surface, such as the wells in a microtiter plate, a plastic test tube, or microparticles of metal or plastic. The solid surface is washed to remove all unreacted materials and then may be coated with a neutral protein to bind to other reactive sites on the solid support, to minimize nonspecific reactions and possible false-positive results ("blocking"). In the second step, the fluid that contains the antigen is reacted with the immobilized antibody. All nonreacting material then is washed away. In the third step, the labeled antibody reacts with the antigen that now has been immobilized by the antibody onto the solid phase. All unreacted labeled antibody then is washed away. If enzyme is used as the label, substrate with appropriate cofactors is added. Color, fluorescence, or light then is used to measure the amount of product. Either end-point or kinetic measurements may be used. The intensity of the measured product is directly proportional to the amount of antigen bound to the solid phase. If a radioisotope was used as the label, the radioactivity on the solid phase can be counted.

For an antibody-measuring system, the antigen of interest first must be immobilized on an insoluble matrix. A microtiter plate assay is depicted in Fig. 8-11. Immobilization with retention of antigenic reactivity is the first step of this procedure, with subsequent blocking of unreactive sites on the solid matrix. In the second step, the biological fluid containing presumptive antibody toward the immobilized antigen is allowed to react. Any antibody present is bound to the antigen immobilized on the solid phase. After separation of the unreacted components by washing of the support surface, the presence of antibody is detected and quantitated by addition of labeled **antiantibody** that is directed toward the class specificity of the antibody that is being measured. Finally, the label is quantitated.

An example of this format is the measurement of allergen-specific IgE, which generally is called the **RAST** test. The RadioAllergoSorbent Test was an early sandwich immunoassay in which individual allergens or mixtures of allergens were immobilized onto a solid capture matrix. After the addition of serum and the washing and labeling steps described above,

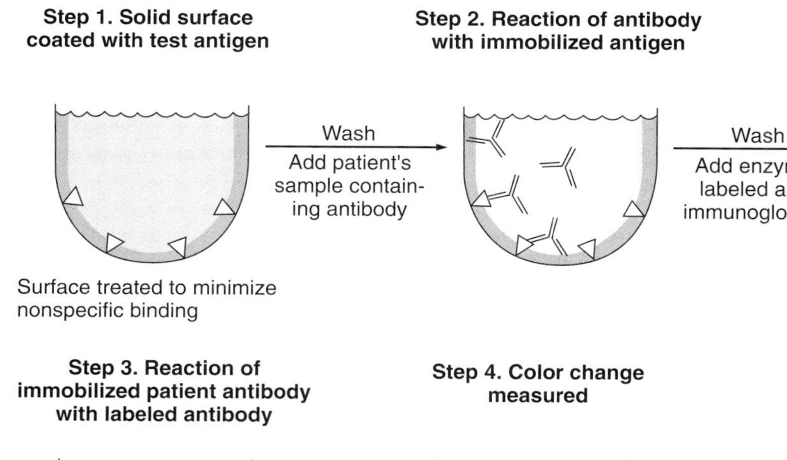

Fig. 8-11 Enzyme immunoassay. Detection of immunoglobulin (Ig)E specific for an allergen.

labeled anti-IgE is measured. This type of assay is standardized with IgE and is reported as KIU/L, or in arbitrary allergen-reactivity classes. Today, the original RAST has been replaced by several modifications. A popular example of commercially available assays is Phadia AB ImmunoCAP.

For both types of sandwich assays, the antibody or antigen that coats the solid phase must be in excess over the analyte that is being measured. If the amount of antigen present exceeds the binding capacity of the captured molecule immobilized on the solid phase, the assay will not be quantitative, possibly producing the so-called **high dose hook effect.** The labeled antibody also must be present in excess over the bound analyte to achieve a linear response and a quantitative assay.

Heterogeneous, Competitive-Binding Assays

The simplest competitive-binding assay uses labeled antigen (Fig. 8-12), and a thorough treatment is given in Chapter 9. For the case of enzyme immunoassay, the enzyme-labeled antigen is mixed with the test solution, which contains an unknown amount of the antigen. The solution that contains the labeled and unlabeled antigen is allowed to react with a limited amount of antibody that is bound to a solid matrix. Unbound antigen (both labeled and unlabeled) is removed by washing, and the amount of labeled antigen is measured by determination of the amount of enzyme bound to the solid surface. This assay is always performed in antigen excess. The test solution contains the enzyme substrate and cofactors, and the enzymatic reaction, which produces a colored product, proceeds continuously. The intensity of color is inversely proportional, but not linear, to the concentration of the antigen present in the test sample. This format of immunoassay can be used to detect small molecular antigens or hapten groups, including drugs and hormones such as steroids and thyroid hormones, in biological fluids.

Sample Requirements and Preparation

Many hormones, protein analytes, and antibodies in serum are stable for several days at refrigerator temperatures. For long-term storage, freezing is preferable.

Reagents

Solid Phase

The plastic, latex, or magnetic bead should be chosen such that the bound ("capture") reagent is not removed by the wash solution under the assay conditions. Several manufacturers have developed plastic microtiter plates and test tubes specifically for enzyme immunoassays.

Substrate

In the case of enzyme labels, the appropriate pure substrate specific for the enzyme is selected to maximize the catalytic activity of the enzyme. As in any enzyme assay, care should be taken to add sufficient substrate so that it will not be depleted during the standard reaction time even if a large amount of enzyme label is bound to the solid phase.

Instrumentation

A spectrophotometer usually is used to measure the color changes that result from enzyme activity. With contemporary instruments, this process can be automated and kinetic measurements are possible. When the reaction occurs in microtiter plates with reaction volumes of 100 to 200 μL, special spectrophotometers called *microtiter plate readers,* or *microELISA readers,* are used. A drawback to microtiter plate readers, however, is that they frequently are not as sensitive as a standard spectrophotometer. In addition, they usually are end-point readers. However, many have the ability to record the results of a standard 96-well microtiter plate in 1 to 2 minutes.

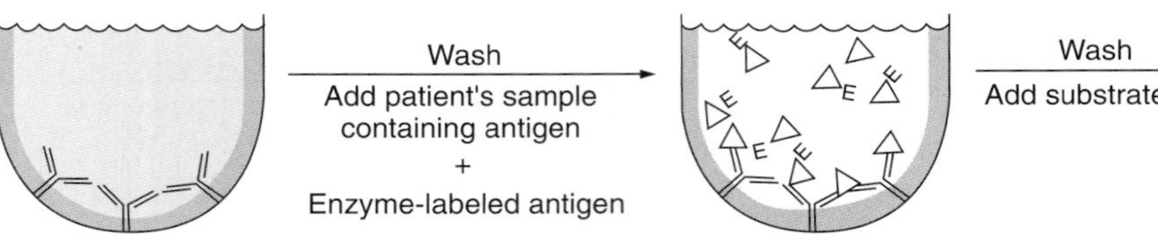

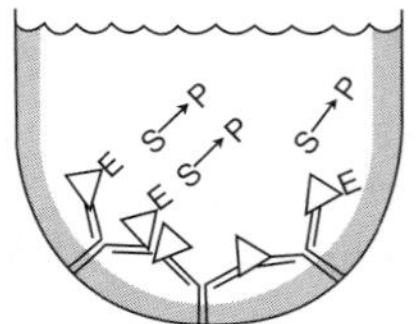

Fig. 8-12 Enzyme immunoassay. Competitive binding.

Instrumentation required for the measurement of radioisotopes is presented in Evolve. Iodine-125, the radioisotope that is used most commonly, requires a gamma counter. Specialized instrumentation also is required for the measurement of fluorescent labels. If metal chelates are employed, techniques such as time-resolved fluorescence may be used (see Chapter 2). Both indirect and direct **fluoroimmunoassays** require a fluorometer or spectrophotofluorometer to obtain an accurate reading of the fluorochrome-labeled antibody. Luminometers, or photon counters, measure light flashes or the "glow" emitted in chemiluminescent assays (see Chapter 2).

Interfering Substances

Substances in the sample matrix other than the analyte of interest may react with the reagent antibody **(cross-reactants),** may interfere with the antigen-antibody binding reaction or detection of the label, or may simulate specific binding by increasing nonspecific binding or by cross-linking the label with the solid phase. Analytical specificity depends on the ability of the antibody to bind unique epitopes.

Heterophilic Antibodies (HAMA)

Any component in the sample that can link the solid-phase antibody with the label will be measured as if it were analyte. Sandwich assays that use animal antibodies may show positive interference if a patient has *heterologous (antispecies)* antibodies in his serum (called *herophilic antibodies*). This type of interference has been reported with increased frequency with the introduction of analytical systems that use mouse monoclonal antibodies as reagents. One example of heterologous, antimouse antibodies is seen in patients who have been treated with mouse monoclonal antibodies for imaging or therapy and have subsequently developed human antimouse antibodies *(HAMA).*

Interfering heterophilic antibodies are not limited to those of mouse origin. Because there are genetically many homologous regions among animal species, heterophile antibodies often are detected even if the specific origin of the antigen cannot be identified. Heterophilic antibodies often are suspected clinically when a test result is unusually elevated and is inconsistent with the patient's condition. Important examples of such an interference have been seen in endocrinology or oncology studies, which use many protein hormones and tumor markers that are measured by sandwich immunoassays. For example, persistently elevated human chorionic gonadotropin (hCG) in a patient who is not pregnant and in whom there is no other evidence of trophoblastic disease might elicit some suspicion of a false elevation caused by some interfering substance. The false elevation need not be an exceedingly high value, just higher than the clinical situation warrants. A physician inquiry should be followed up immediately by appropriate investigation.

If HAMA or other heterophilic antibody interferences are suspected, they can be reduced or eliminated by preincubating the sample with, or including in the reaction mixture, sufficient nonimmune globulins from the same species to bind up the antimouse, or antispecies, antibodies without interfering with the specific analytical reaction. A significant drop in the result for the "treated" sample supports the hypothesis that the original, high result was caused by a heterophilic antibody. Blocking reagents, which contain a lyophilized mixture of different animal sera, are commercially available for this purpose. Also, the patient sample may be simply diluted to test for linearity. Frequently, an interference will disappear upon dilution. Nonlinear recovery in this experiment indicates that the original, high result was inaccurate, but it does not prove that the interference was caused by a heterophilic antibody. Reanalysis of the sample by an assay that employs antibodies of a totally different animal source may yield a more clinically reliable result. Manufacturers of commercial kits and instruments are aware of this type of interference and often include animal sera or other substances in their reaction mixtures to reduce the possibility of this interference.

Rheumatoid factor, which is anti-IgG, may interfere nonspecifically by linking solid-phase antibody with labeled antibody.

Nonspecific Binding

Nonspecific binding of labeled antigen or antibody to the solid support should be tested at the time of assay development by incubating the solid support or capture phase with tracer in the absence of reagent antibody.

Sample Interferences

The sample may contain substances that have enzyme activity or that fluoresce under assay conditions.

Interferences Affecting the Detection Reaction

Care must be taken to avoid contact with compounds that interfere with detection of the enzyme label, such as inhibitors or oxidizing reagents.

Common Pitfalls

Common problems with these assays include the following:

1. *Inappropriate plastic used for the microtiter plates or test tubes.* This is not a common problem when kits are used, but it is a consideration when new assays are developed. Lot changes, even from the same supplier, occasionally result in poor performance because of changes in the properties of the plastic support.
2. *Improper pH and ionic strength of buffer.*
3. *Nonspecific adsorption of reactants to plastic surface.* This nonspecific adsorption can be minimized by incubation of the solid phase with proteinaceous material, such as gelatin or bovine serum albumin, after initial adsorption of the capture reagent to the solid phase.
4. *Inadequate control of experimental conditions.* Precision in enzyme immunoassays depends on strict control of temperature, pH, ionic strength of buffers, and concentrations of the various cofactors necessary for the enzymatic conversion of substrate into product. Finally, because enzymes are proteins and are subject to rapid denaturation under improper incubation conditions, close attention must be paid to preserve the enzyme activity during analysis.
5. *Substrate depletion.* If a large quantity of enzyme-labeled reagent is captured on the solid matrix, substrate can be depleted very rapidly. Sufficient substrate must be included in the reaction mixture so that a suitable working range is available, and the upper limits of linearity should be carefully defined.

Test Sensitivity and Precision

Numerous formats have been described for the performance of indicator-labeled immunoassays. The sensitivity and precision of each of these immunoassays depend on the format selected and the instrumentation used to measure the label. Enzyme immunoassay (EIA) and immunometric techniques generally are considered to be sensitive in the ng/mL range, with a between-run coefficient of variation (CV) of less than 10% throughout the working range of the assay. Fluoroimmunoassays may have less sensitivity (about 100 to 200 μg/mL), but time-resolved fluoroimmunoassays and electrochemiluminescent assays are as sensitive as most EIA or immunometric assays. The CV observed within the same run typically range from 3% to 6%.

Immunoassay sensitivity depends on high specific activity labels, low nonspecific binding, and excellent precision. Immunoassay analytical sensitivity is conventionally defined as the concentration that has a measured response at 2 standard deviations from the response of the zero standard. **Functional sensitivity** is defined as the lowest concentration that has a precision of 20% CV or lower. This determination typically is made from a *precision profile,* a graph of CV versus analyte concentration.

KEY CONCEPTS BOX 8-4

- Immunometric ("sandwich") assays for antigen (Ag) detection have antibody (Ab) coated onto a solid phase. Sample is added and Ag binds to Ab on the solid phase. Following a wash, Ab with indicator is added. After a wash to remove excess indicator, indicator signal is measured.
- If Ag coats the solid phase, Ab in the sample can be detected after indicator anti-Ab Ab is added.
- Labels for indicator Ab include enzymes, chemiluminescent dyes, metal chelates, radioisotopes, and fluorophores.
- If Ag in the sample is added with a labeled Ag, a competitive-binding assay can be run, following wash to detect bound, labeled Ag. Used to measure small molecules.
- Human antimouse antibody (HAMA) is an Ab in sample that is directed againt the Ab used in an immunoassay. Often, the Ab is antimouse. Unusual results that do not correlate with the clinical condition are the best way to detect HAMAs. Rerunning the assay after dilution or with a totally different assay procedure can obviate the HAMA effect.

SUMMARY

The spectrum of immunological techniques is described and summarized in Table 8-1. Each of these procedures was developed to meet a specific need to identify or quantitate an antigen present in a patient's sample. Immunoprecipitation techniques are the least sensitive but have high specificity in detecting the presence of an antigen within the working range of the assay. Immunonephelometry is the most sensitive technique that uses precipitation as an end point and is a popular format for quantitating many specific proteins in serum and cerebrospinal fluid within an appropriate concentration range. Turbidimetric versions of these assays are commonly run on highly automated analyzers.

Immunofixation and Western blot techniques are qualitative tools. The former is commonly employed to identify an antigen present in a patient's sample, such as polyclonal IgG versus a monoclonal protein, or a C3 breakdown product

Table 8-1 Summary of Immunological Techniques

Technique	Assay End Point	Assay Sensitivity	Time Needed for Assay Results	Common Analytes	Comments
Immunodiffusion (Ouchterlony)	Precipitation (qualitative)	45 μg/mL	8 to 72 hours	Bacterial, viral, or fungal antigens	Most frequently used to screen for presence of antigen
Immunoelectrophoresis	Precipitation (qualitative)	500 μg/mL	12 to 24 hours	Serum, urine, and cerebrospinal fluid protein	Used to assay complex mixture of analytes in biological fluids
Counterimmunoelectrophoresis	Precipitation (qualitative)	3 μg/mL	2 to 3 hours	Bacterial, viral, or fungal antigens	Commonly used to screen for antigens associated with infectious agents; more rapid than immunodiffusion
Two-dimensional immunoelectrophoresis	Precipitation (qualitative)	500 μg/mL	8 to 10 hours	Serum proteins	Research, used to examine subtle differences in proteins
Radial immunodiffusion (Mancini)	Precipitation (quantitative), CV 10% to 15%	50 μg/mL	12 to 24 hours	Serum and CSF proteins	Most commonly used immunological technique to measure serum and CSF proteins
Laurell (rocket) immunoelectrophoresis	Precipitation (quantitative), CV 8% to 12%	50 μg/mL	4 to 8 hours	Serum and CSF proteins	More rapid than radial immunodiffusion
Turbidimetry	Light scattering of aggregates of antigen-antibody complexes (quantitative), CV ≈8%	50 μg/mL	15 minutes	Serum, urine, and CSF proteins	More rapid than radial immunodiffusion
Direct and indirect agglutination	Agglutination of bacteria or red blood cell–containing antigen (semiquantitative)	15 μg/mL	1 to 5 minutes	Antibodies to bacterial antigens (such as febrile agglutinins) and red blood cell antigens	Techniques commonly used by serology laboratory and blood bank; not often used in chemistry laboratory
Agglutination inhibition	Inhibition of agglutination (semiquantitative)	15 μg/mL	2 to 5 minutes	Detects antigens such as pregnancy hormones (hCG)	Rapid test procedure often used to screen the urine of pregnant women for hCG
Immunofixation	Reaction of enzyme-labeled Ab with antigens fixed after electrophoresis	10 μg/mL	1 to 4 hours	Serum proteins, including immunoglobulins	Used to study gammopathies and as Western blot to find antibodies to HIV
Complement fixation	Lysis of red blood cells or inhibition of red blood cell lysis (semiquantitative)	10 μg/mL	24 hours	Detect complement-fixing antibodies to bacterial, viral, or fungal antigens	Worldwide, commonly used serological procedure; sensitivity of assay approaches radioimmunoassay; assay difficult to perform
Immunonephelometry	Light scattering of aggregates of antigen-antibody complexes (quantitative), CV 3% to 8%	1 μg/mL	15 minutes	*Direct mode:* Serum, urine, and CSF proteins *Inhibition mode:* Drugs, such as theophylline and phenytoin	Popularly accepted technique to quantitate protein; in many laboratories, this technique has replaced radial immunodiffusion
Enzyme immunoassay (ELISA, sandwich)	Color reaction between enzyme and substrate (quantitative), CV 8% to 15%	<1 ng/mL	1 to 6 hours	Serum proteins (such as IgE); bacterial, viral, and fungal antigens; antibodies to infectious agents	Excellent assay for small amounts of antigen or antibody
RIA (competitive binding)	Measurement of radioactivity	<1 ng/mL	4 to 6 hours	Capable of measuring most molecules, large and small	Traditional assay, less popular because of radioisotope concerns
Enzyme immunoassay (competitive binding)	Color reaction between enzyme and substrate (quantitative), CV 8% to 15%	<1 ng/mL	1 to 2 hours	Small amounts of antigen (such as hormones, drugs, viral antigens)	Excellent assay for measuring ligands
Immunoradiometric	Radioisotope decay emission	<1 ng/mL	1 to 6 hours	Same as ELISA above	Excellent assay for quantitative measurement of low levels of antigens or antibodies; problem with radioactive wastes
Immunofluorometric	Fluorescence of dye	<1 ng/mL	1 to 2 hours	Same as ELISA and RIA above	Same as for immunoradiometric, but no waste problem
Chemiluminescent	Chemiluminescence of dye	<1 ng/mL	15 to 20 minutes	Same as ELISA and RIA above	Very sensitive for quantitative measurement of low levels of antigens

Ab, Antibody; *CSF,* cerebrospinal fluid; *CV,* coefficient of variation; *ELISA,* enzyme-linked immunosorbent assay; *hCG,* human chorionic gonadotropin hormone; *HIV,* human immunodeficiency virus; *IgE,* immunoglobulin E; *RIA,* radioimmunoassay.

versus C3 in native form. The Western blot is commonly used for verification of the presence of antibody to a specific antigen, such as HIV. The agglutination and complement-fixation techniques are procedures that are used primarily in serology and blood bank laboratories.

Indicator-labeled immunoassays predominate in the clinical laboratory because they extend the sensitivity and specificity of antigen detection. Non-isotopic immunoassays are the most frequently used immunoassays because of their sensitivity, specificity, and suitability for automation.

Selection of the appropriate immunological technique for detection of an antigen in the laboratory depends on many variables: sensitivity required (i.e., analyte concentration), available instrumentation, sample volume, desired turnaround time, availability of test in kit form, ease of the technique, and cost of performing the assay. Whatever assay format is selected, crucial factors that must be considered are the specificity of the reagent antibody, the antigen structure, and the sample stability.

BIBLIOGRAPHY

General

Gosling JP: *Immunoassays,* Oxford Univer Press, 2000.

van Emon JM: *Immunoassay and Other Bioanalytical Techniques,* CRC; 2006.

Wild D: *The immunoassay handbook,* ed 3. Elsevier Science, 2005.

Murphy KM, Travers P, Walport M. *Janeway's Immunobiology,* ed 7, Garland Science, 2007.

Diamandis EP, Christopoulos TK: *Immunoassay,* New York, 1996, Academic Press.

Wu, JT. Quantitative Immunoassay: A practical guide for assay establishment, troubleshooting, and clinical application. AACC Press; 2000.

Electrophoresis and Immunofixation

Keren DF: *Protein Electrophoresis in Clinical Diagnosis,* ed 3, London, 2003, Hodder Arnold.

Nephelometry

Marmer DJ, Hurtubise PE: Nephelometric and turbidimetric immunoassay (Chapter 17). In Diamandis EP, Christopoulos TK, editors: *Immunoassay,* New York, 1996, Academic Press.

Fluoroimmunoassays

Christopoulos TK, Diamandis EP: Fluorescence immunoassays (Chapter 14). In Diamandis EP, Christopoulos TK, editors: *Immunoassay,* New York, 1996, Academic Press.

Enzyme Immunoassays

Crother, J, The ELISA Guidebook, Humana Press; 2000.

Gosling JP: Enzyme immunoassay (Chapter 13). In Diamandis EP, Christopoulos TK, editors: *Immunoassay,* New York, 1996, Academic Press.

Chemiluminescent Immunoassays

Kricka LJ: Chemilluminescence immunoassay (Chapter 15). In Diamandis EP, Christopoulos TK, editors: *Immunoassay,* New York, 1996, Academic Press.

Precision Profile and Functional Sensitivity

Clinical Laboratory Standards Institute (CLSI): *Protocols for Determinantion of Limits of Detection and Limits of Quantitation (EP 17-A),* Wayne, PA, 2004, CLSI.

Spencer CA, Takeuchi M, Kazarosyan M, MacKenzie F, Beckett GJ, Silkinson E: Interlaboratory/intermethod differences in functional sensitivity of immunometric assays of thyrotropin (TSH) and impact on reliability of measurement of subnormal concentrations of TSH, Clin Chem 41:367, 1995.

Interferences

Clinical Laboratory Standards Institute (CLSI): *Immunoassay Interference by Endogenous Antibodies: Approved Guideline, I/LA 30-A,* Wayne, PA, 2008, CLSI.

Kricka LJ: Human anti-animal antibody interferences in immunological assays, Clin Chem 45:942, 1999.

Levinson SS, Miller JJ: Towards a better understanding of heterophile (and the like) antibody interference with modern immunoassays, Clin Chim Acta 325:1, 2002.

INTERNET SITES

General

www.uct.ac.za/microbiology/ababs.htm—Immunoassay techniques

http://www.waichung.demon.co.uk/webanim/Menu2.htm a list of animations of various types of immunoassays

http://www.bertholf.net/rlb/Lectures/index.htm the lecture for Immunochemical is listed on this page

Agglutination and Complement Fixation

http://www.itxm.org/TMU2000/tmu10-2000.htm

http://www.cehs.siu.edu/fix/medmicro/cfix.htm

Precision Profile and Functional Sensitivity

http://www.westgard.com/lesson29.htm

Principles for Competitive-Binding Assays

Stephan G. Thompson

9

Chapter

Chapter Outline

Key Terms

capture phase Ligand or specific binding protein attached to a solid surface or matrix to help separate bound from free label in a heterogeneous assay.

cloned-enzyme donor immunoassay (CEDIA) A homogeneous immunoassay in which a low-molecular-weight ligand is labeled with a genetically cloned fragment (enzyme donor) of β-galactosidase. The remaining portion of the molecule, complementary enzyme acceptor, is inactive unless the two components can combine to generate an active enzyme. In the assay, this combination is inhibited by antibody to the ligand-enzyme donor complex. Inhibition is relieved in a dose-response manner when the test ligand is present in the solution.

competitive-binding assay An analytical procedure that is based on the reversible binding of a ligand to a binding protein. The ligand competes in proportion to its concentration with a labeled derivative for binding to the limited number of binding sites.

conjugate Usually refers to the labeled reagent in which either the ligand (antigen) or the antibody is covalently attached to the label.

detection limit The smallest concentration of a ligand that can be statistically distinguished from a zero level in an assay. The detection limit also is referred to as the sensitivity or limit of a blank of an assay.

electrochemiluminescence Light emission resulting from the oxidation of a reactive label at the surface of an electrode upon application of an electric potential.

enzyme-linked immunosorbent assay (ELISA) A heterogeneous immunoassay that in one configuration employs an enzyme-labeled ligand and an antibody immobilized on a solid phase.

enzyme-multiplied immunoassay technique (EMIT) A homogeneous enzyme immunoassay in which a low-molecular-weight ligand is attached to an enzyme that is inhibited when the conjugate is bound by a specific antibody. Competitive binding of unlabeled ligand to the antibody relieves the inhibition in proportion to the ligand concentration.

fluorogen A nonfluorescent molecule that becomes fluorescent when modified by a chemical or enzymatic process.

heterogeneous assay A competitive-binding assay in which it is necessary to separate mechanically the protein-bound, labeled ligand from the unbound ligand before measurement of the signal generated by the label.

homogeneous assay Competitive-binding assay in which it is not necessary to separate protein-bound and free ligand fractions because the signal of the label is modulated by protein binding.

immunoassay Any binding assay in which the binding protein is an antibody.

immunogen A substance that stimulates an antibody response when administered to an appropriate animal. Immunogens include macromolecular antigens and otherwise nonantigenic haptens coupled to a macromolecular carrier.

label An atom or molecule attached to either the ligand or the binding protein, which is capable of generating a signal for monitoring the binding reaction.

ligand A molecule or part of a molecule that is reversibly bound by the binding protein in a competitive-binding assay. It usually is the analyte but it can be a cross-reactant.

luminescent oxygen channeling immunoassay (LOCI) Homogeneous luminescent immunoassay format based on a binding pair of microparticles in which the ligand-coated photosensitive member of the pair generates singlet oxygen upon illumination. The singlet oxygen reacts with its antibody-coated microparticle-binding partner, which luminesces in response. Only microparticles in close proximity to one another by binding to one another generate a signal that is inversely proportional to the concentration of ligand in the sample.

luminogenic substrates Enzyme substrates that emit light upon hydrolysis. Light emission is either a rapid (5- to 10-second) "flash" or a long-lived "glow," whereby the emission is measured up to 2 hours after the reaction is started.

paramagnetic particles Microparticles containing a ferrous core that are attracted to a magnetic field but do not contain any magnetic properties upon the field's removal.

rapid assays Semiquantitative immunoassays performed with a small hand-held device. The bound label most often is separated from the free label by "lateral flow" membrane chromatography.

sensitivity The degree of response to a change in the ligand concentration in an assay. Sensitivity often refers to the detection limit.

specificity The degree to which a binding protein binds its particular ligand while not binding structurally similar compounds.

time-resolved fluorescence Long-lasting fluorescence emitted from the chelates of lanthanide metals such as europium and terbium. Also characterized by its high quantum yield and an enormous Stokes shift.

Methods in Evolve

Radioisotopes in clinical chemistry

SECTION OBJECTIVES BOX 9-1

- Understand the principles of protein-ligand binding reactions.
- Understand the effects of endogenous binding proteins and their respective ligands.

PROTEIN BINDING AND THE LAW OF MASS ACTION

Competitive-binding assays are based on the noncovalent, reversible binding of a **ligand** to a specific binding protein. The binding assay most often is described by the following reaction:

$$\text{Ligand} + \text{Binding protein} \rightleftharpoons \text{Binding protein:ligand} \quad \text{Eq. 9-1}$$

where the binding protein has a measurable affinity for the ligand that interacts with it. In general, only one binding protein can bind a small molecule. This reaction can be considered simply as one molecule of ligand reacting with one protein binding site. The important molecular feature of binding proteins that enables them to be used in quantitative assays is their ability to bind compounds with a high **specificity** and affinity (see Chapters 7 and 8). Examples of specific binding proteins are listed in Table 9-1.

Nearly all competitive binding methods use antibodies as the binding protein for small molecules. These usually are gamma immunoglobulins (IgGs) that are directly produced in animals through a cellular response to immunization with the ligand, or that may be produced by monoclonal antibody hybridoma techniques with cells derived from an original antibody-secreting cell. These methods are discussed in great detail in Chapters 7 and 8, as well as in other sources listed in the bibliography at the end of this chapter.

Table 9-1 Specific Binding Proteins Present in Blood or Other Tissues

Binding Protein	Ligand
Antibodies	Varied antigens
Corticosteroid binding globulin (CBG)	Cortisol, corticosterone
Sex hormone–binding globulin (SHBG)	Estradiol, testosterone
Estrogen receptor	Estrogen
Intrinsic factor	Vitamin B_{12}
Thyroid-binding globulin (TBG)	Thyroxine (T_4) Triiodothyronine (T_3)
Vitamin D receptor	1-α,25-dihydroxyvitamin D_3

Small molecules by themselves normally do not provoke an immune response but do elicit antibodies when coupled with larger molecules; such small molecules are termed *haptens.* Because such small molecules participate in competitive-binding assays in which the binding protein is an antibody, the ligand may be referred to as a *hapten.*

The ligand in Equation 9-1 is the analyte to be quantified. Often ligands are drugs (digoxin, theophylline), hormones (cortisol, thyroxine [T_4]), or vitamins (B_{12}). For most competitive-binding reactions, the ligand refers to both the analyte and a **labeled** derivative of the analyte. Both must bind to the specific binding protein for the analyte to be measured. The final complex of binding protein and ligand is usually stable and dissociates only very slowly under favorable circumstances.

The binding reaction described in Equation 9-1 is more complex for larger ligands such as proteins because macromolecules have many different binding sites (antigenic determinants) on their surfaces. A protein therefore can have more than one antibody simultaneously attached to it. Such binding determinants can be structurally quite different from one another, and so the population of antibodies generated in an immune response to large molecules is heterogeneous (polyclonal antiserum). Antigenic determinants of high-molecular-weight **immunogens** and low-molecular-weight haptens are similar when one considers the behavior of antibody-binding reactions. Although macromolecules can be measured by competitive protein-binding assays, noncompetitive methods are employed more often. These are discussed in Chapter 8.

The law of mass action describes some aspects of the phenomenon that occurs when molecules bind to one another. This is best illustrated by examining the concentration of an antibody **(Ab)** and its ligand **(L)** or specific binding partner under equilibrium conditions. The bimolecular reaction

$$\mathrm{Ab} + \mathrm{L} \underset{k_{-1}}{\overset{k_1}{\rightleftharpoons}} \mathrm{Ab{:}L} \qquad \text{Eq. 9-2}$$

can be rearranged for calculation of the equilibrium association constant

$$K_a = \frac{k_1}{k_{-1}} = \frac{[\mathrm{Ab{:}L}]}{[\mathrm{Ab}][\mathrm{L}]} \qquad \text{Eq. 9-3}$$

where k_1 and k_{-1} are the respective rate constants for association and dissociation of the bound complex; [Ab] is the concentration of unbound or free antibody at equilibrium; [L] is the equilibrium concentration of unbound ligand (a term denoting the antigen, hapten, or other substance); and [Ab:L] is the equilibrium concentration of the ligand-antibody complex. K_a, also referred to as the *affinity constant,* is defined in reciprocal molar concentrations (M^{-1}) or liters per mole (L/mol). This is the volume into which a mole of the binding protein can be diluted to yield 50% binding of the ligand. The larger the K_a, the greater the affinity of the antibody for the ligand. It follows that for a constant amount of antibody in the reaction, less ligand is required for a high-affinity antibody to bind 50% of the ligand than is required for 50% binding by a low-affinity antibody. Antiserum produced by an animal that has been immunized with a high-molecular-weight immunogen usually contains a mixture of different populations of antibody (polyclonal antisera) to that antigen. These different populations of antibody vary in their ability to bind the ligand (affinity) and in their ability to recognize different sites on the protein's surface.

Only one uniform population of binding sites exists for a ligand when the binding protein or antibody is homogeneous, as in the case of monoclonal antibodies, which have a uniform binding affinity (K_a) and specificity for the antigen.

Low-affinity binding proteins and antibodies typically have association affinity constants on the order of 10^5 to 10^7 L/mol, whereas binders suitable for **immunoassays** and other competitive-binding assays have association constants between 10^8 and 10^{11} L/mol. A higher association constant makes it possible to design assays with sensitivities as low as 10^{-12} M, or lower, provided that the label itself is detectable at these low concentrations.

ENDOGENOUS BINDING PROTEINS

Many of the low molecular weight compounds measured in competitive binding assays, such as T_4, cortisol, estradiol, and testosterone, are bound by their respective endogenous serum binding proteins. To become available for measurement in "total ligand" assays, these compounds must be extracted or displaced from these proteins.

One means of accomplishing this is to change the sample pH to one that promotes conformational changes in the binding protein so that it releases its ligand. Another method is to add ligands similar in structure that have affinity for the binding protein and that by nature of an excess concentration, or greater affinity, competitively block and displace the ligand of interest from its binding protein. Some binding protein interactions are so strong that both methods, simultaneously altering the sample and displacing the analyte with another molecule, may be required. Examples include dihydroxytestosterone, which binds to sex hormone–binding globulin (SHBG) (see Table 9-1) with very high affinity to displace the female hormone estradiol for measurement in immunoassays, or anilino-naphthalene sulfonic acid, which can displace T_4 from one of its binding proteins, thyroxine-binding globulin (TBG).

In recent years, clinicians have found it important to not only measure the total concentration of hormone, such as thyroxine, but also the unbound or "free" fraction that is considered the biologically active fraction capable of eliciting a physiological response. Albumin also binds many hormones, but with such low affinity relative to the specific binding serum proteins and cellular receptors that the albumin-bound hormones also can be considered free or at least bioactive (see Chapter 48). Free hormone assays are constructed without the sample conditions or molecules required to liberate bound ligand from its binding proteins for measurement in total ligand assays.

KEY CONCEPTS BOX 9-1

- Law of mass action defines the binding reaction between a ligand and its binding protein.
- Ligand-specific proteins include antibodies and hormone-binding proteins.
- The affinity of a ligand-binding protein describes the degree to which the ligand will be bound.
- Some ligands require dissociation from their respective physiological binding proteins.

SECTION OBJECTIVES BOX 9-2

- Illustrate how the principles of protein binding form the basis for competitive-binding reactions.
- Identify the critical components of competitive-binding reactions.
- Distinguish the differences between heterogeneous and homogeneous assay formats.

BEHAVIOR OF COMPETITIVE-BINDING ASSAYS

The competitive-binding assay can be imagined as the addition of increasing amounts of unlabeled ligand to reaction mixtures that contain known, constant amounts of labeled ligand and a specific binding protein. In this case, labeled ligand, L*, and antibody, Ab, are added together in equimolar amounts. If one presumes that all the L* is bound, the reaction becomes

$$L^* + Ab \rightleftharpoons Ab{:}L^*$$

Two things happen with the addition of increasing amounts of unlabeled ligand (L): (1) unlabeled ligand competes with labeled ligand for antibody-binding sites, and (2) there is an excess of the total ligand (L and L*) in solution compared with the number of binding sites. The concentration of antibody-binding sites therefore is limiting with respect to total ligand, thus modifying the preceding reaction as follows:

$$L + AbL^* \rightleftharpoons AbL + AbL^* + L^* + L$$

Less L* is antibody bound (as Ab:L*); thus more L* is free as the amount of L increases. The amount or percentage of L* in bound form can be calculated from the amount of L and L* present.

When the percentage of labeled bound ligand is plotted as a function of the concentration of the unlabeled ligand, this yields the dose-response curve as shown in Fig. 9-1. The term *dose-response curve* applies to a plot of binding versus increasing amounts of ligand. The curvature of the dose-response plot in Fig. 9-1 is attributable to the logarithmic increase in the percentage of L that is bound when the concentration of L (dose) in the assay increases arithmetically. Thus the decrease in bound L* is also logarithmic. Conversion of the concentration of L to a logarithm makes the relationship become more linear.

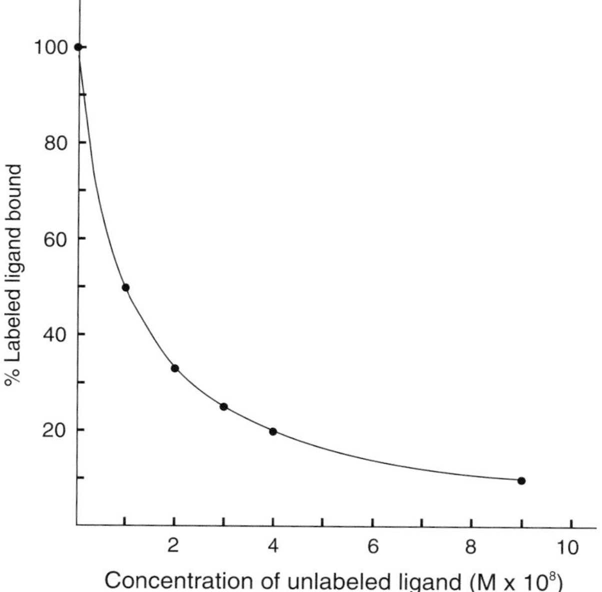

Fig. 9-1 Linear dose-response curve for a competitive protein-binding assay. Concentration (M) has been multiplied by 10^8.

COMPETITIVE-BINDING ASSAY FORMATS

Fig. 9-1 shows that to derive a dose-response curve, one must know the amount of labeled ligand that is antibody bound as a function of the amount of unlabeled ligand that is added. A variety of techniques have been developed to measure bound or free forms of the labeled ligand in a competitive-binding format.

Some of these techniques require that the antibody-bound labeled ligand be physically separated from the free labeled ligand. These assays are called **heterogeneous assays.** Immunoassay approaches that do not require physical separation of bound and free labeled ligand are called **homogeneous assays.** The activity of the label in a homogeneous assay is altered when the labeled ligand is bound to the specific binding protein; thus bound and free labeled ligands can be directly distinguished from one another.

Heterogeneous Assays

Table 9-2 lists some of the methods commonly used to separate protein-bound from free labeled ligand. In one example,

Table 9-2 Techniques to Separate Protein-Bound from Free Labeled Ligand

Technique	Principle
Specific adsorbents	Antibodies to the ligand or to the ligand-binding antibody are immobilized on the surface of a solid matrix such as glass fibers, latex microparticles, paramagnetic microparticles, membranes, or plastic. The immobilized antibody-ligand complex can be separated from the unbound ligand by decantation, washing, filtration, diffusion, or centrifugation.
Chromatography	The protein-bound ligand moves through the chromatographic medium at a rate that is different from that of the free ligand.
Precipitation by ammonium sulfate	The antibody-bound ligand is precipitated by ammonium sulfate (Farr technique); not commonly used anymore except for some manual assays.
Double antibody	The antibody-bound ligand is precipitated by the addition of a second antibody specific for the antibody in the antibody-ligand or antibody-antigen complex; not commonly used anymore except for some manual assays.

the ligand or antibody is covalently attached or adsorbed to the hydrophobic plastic surfaces of microtiter plate reaction wells or plastic beads, providing support for the capture phases of many different heterogeneous assays. The **capture phase** binds the labeled reactant in a competitive-binding heterogeneous assay, whether the latter is labeled ligand or is labeled antibody. Another system, the microparticle-based capture phase, is widely used for two reasons: (1) suspended microparticle capture phases approach solution-like kinetics in that diffusion distances are very short compared with the surface of a microtiter plate well or a coated polystyrene tube, and (2) microparticles in comparison provide a far greater surface area. For example, 1 mg of particles of 1 μm diameter consists of 60 cm^2 of surface area for immobilization of antibody or ligand compared with 1.0 to 1.5 cm^2 of surface area in a microtiter well. Both of these attributes shorten the assay time and potentially increase its **sensitivity.**

Latex and paramagnetic microparticles are used in similar heterogeneous assay formats; both can be used to readily separate the bound from the unbound label—one by filtration or radial diffusion through a porous filter and the other by magnetic attraction.

Other methods for separating bound from free labeled ligand are listed in Table 9-2. Both the ammonium sulfate technique and the double-antibody technique have been used with isotopic labels.

In some instances, competitive methods incorporate an indirect capture approach, in which an unrelated binding protein-ligand pair is used to bring the solid phase together with the capture antibody or ligand. In a classical example, immobilized streptavidin binds biotin that has been covalently attached to an antibody or to the ligand. Advantages of this approach are discussed below. Almost all of the methods described in Table 9-2 have been automated, resulting in improved precision (see Chapter 20, p. 374).

Homogeneous Immunoassays

By definition, the activity of the label in a homogeneous assay is modulated when it is bound to the specific binding protein. Modulation resulting from antibody binding can be direct, as when a ligand-specific antibody binds an enzyme-labeled ligand and inhibits the enzyme's activity, or indirect, as when the antibody-ligand interaction brings two reactants physically close enough to provide the coupled reaction needed to generate a measurable signal. An exception to this generalized definition for homogeneous immunoassays is based on the scattering of light by microparticles. Instead of an antibody modulating the signal per se, changes in light scattering are produced by the formation of antibody:ligand:particle complexes, in which either the antibody or the ligand or both are multivalently attached to latex particles; the corresponding binding partner is also multivalent, thus enabling the components to form larger, agglutinated complexes. An example is described later in this chapter.

KEY CONCEPTS BOX 9-2

- Ligand and labeled ligand compete for binding sites on proteins, usually antibodies (Abs).
- Binding sites on Abs are limiting relative to the total ligand (L + L*) concentration.
- Heterogeneous immunoassays require separation steps, and homogeneous immunoassays do not.
- The activity of the label is modulated by antibody binding in homogeneous assays.

SECTION OBJECTIVES BOX 9-3

- Distinguish between isotopic and non-isotopic labels.
- Provide examples of non-isotopic labels and order them in their relative sensitivities.
- Understand the relationship between each label and detection of its signal.

LABELED LIGANDS

Types of Labels

The types of markers commonly used to label ligands include radioisotopes, enzymes, fluorophores, and luminogens. These can be used in both homogeneous and heterogeneous competitive-binding assays. Types of labels, respective assays, and detection systems are presented in Table 9-3.

Factors Determining Choice of Label

Radioisotopes

Radioisotopic labels are used only with heterogeneous immunoassays because binding by antibody does not change the radioactive decay. In general, the desired sensitivity of the assay limits the choice of radioactive labels to certain specific isotopes that have high specific activity, high energy output, manageable half-lives, and ready availability. The radioisotope must be readily incorporated into or coupled to the ligand (or antibody) molecule, and its emission must be easily detected. Continued discussion of radioisotopes and of their application in a radioimmunoassay (RIA) can be found at the Evolve website.

Table 9-3 Some Labels for Competitive-Binding Assays

Label	Detector
Enzymes	
Chromogenic substrates	Photometer
Fluorogenic substrates	Fluorometer
Luminogenic substrates	Luminometer
Enzyme fragments	Photometer, fluorometer
Enzyme substrates	Photometer, fluorometer, luminometer
Fluorophores, fluorogens	Fluorometer
Luminogens	Luminometer
Electrochemiluminescence	Luminometer
Microparticles	Photometer, nephelometer
Radioactive isotopes*	Radioactivity counter

*Usable only in heterogeneous assays.

Table 9-4 Fluorophores Used as Labels in Competitive-Binding Assays

Fluorophore	Excitation Wavelength, nm	Emission Wavelength, nm	ε*	Fluorescence Quantum Yield†
Europium chelate‡	340	613	90,000	>0.95
Fluorescein	490	520	72,000	0.85
4-methyl umbelliferone	365	450	20,000	0.50

*ε is the absorbance of a 1 M solution through a 1 cm light path.
†The fluorescence quantum yield is relative to the quantum yield of acridine, which is 1.0.
‡Europium: β-diketone chelate.

Enzymes

Enzymes as labels differ from radioisotopes in that the antibody-ligand binding reaction can modify their activity. Again, enzymes must have high specific activity (i.e., conversion of many moles of substrate to product per minute per mole of enzyme) and must be easily attached to the ligand or antibody without losing significant activity. Commonly used enzymes include alkaline phosphatase, β-galactosidase, glucose-6-phosphate dehydrogenase, and peroxidase.

Some homogeneous enzyme immunoassays are based on the use of an inactive component of an enzyme molecule as the label. For example, in the **cloned-enzyme donor immunoassay (CEDIA),** the reactant label is a polypeptide fragment of β-galactosidase that complexes with the remainder of the enzyme. CEDIA is discussed in greater detail later.

Substrates

Substrates for enzyme labels also help to define the means for detection and, in some cases, the format by which the assay will be performed. Examples are shown in Table 9-3. The most commonly used substrates are either **fluorogenic** or luminogenic that become fluorescent or luminescent upon enzyme catalysis; these have been adopted for automated applications of the immunoassays of ligands that require greater sensitivity.

Although one usually can measure a thousandfold lower concentration of a fluorophore by fluorescence techniques rather than by colorimetric methods, the gain in assay sensitivity with fluorogenic substrates for enzyme labels is at best only tenfold to a few hundred–fold. Sensitivity greater than that seen with fluorescence or colorimetry generally is achieved with the use of **luminogenic substrates.** Because enzyme labels amplify the labeled ligand or antibody molecules that participate in the binding reaction, greater sensitivity can be achieved by longer incubation times for the conversion of substrate to product. This is an undesirable characteristic of some chromogenic substrates, particularly when more **rapid assays** are available that use either fluorogenic or luminogenic substrates. Two types of luminogenic substrates exist. When a "flash" reaction occurs, the emitted light is measured within 5 to 10 seconds after the reaction is initiated, whereas dioxetane substrates "glow" upon hydrolysis, so that the light measurement can be made from 2 minutes up to 2 hours after the reaction has started. The intensity of light and the duration of emitted light in some flash reactions catalyzed by peroxidase are increased several orders of magnitude by the addition of phenolic enhancer molecules. Also, the emission becomes a stable glow that can be measured any time between 2 and 30 minutes after the reaction is initiated.

Fluorophores

Fluorophores chosen as labels still fluoresce with a high degree of efficiency when attached to the ligand or antibody. Absorption (excitation) and emission wavelengths are well separated (Stokes shift) so that light scatter does not contribute to the fluorescence seen at the emission wavelength. Examples of fluorophores used as labels for competitive-binding assays and their properties are shown in Table 9-4. Of these, fluorescein and europium chelates are commonly used. Chelates of the rare earth lanthanide metals europium and terbium strongly absorb light and fluoresce with properties that depend on the chelating ligand. The quantum yield (photon output/photon input) is very high, and excitation and emission wavelengths are well separated. Europium and fluorescein have high extinction coefficients and quantum yields, but europium has the greatest separation between excitation and emission wavelengths (273 nm).

Luminogens

In addition to being enzyme substrates, luminogenic molecules are also used as direct labels for immunoassays. For example, both luminol and acridinium esters emit light upon chemical oxidation and hydrolysis by hydrogen peroxide under basic conditions. The light is emitted in a "flash" over a 2- to 4-second interval. The intensity of the total light emission is measured over 5 or more seconds.

Electrochemiluminescence (ECL)

Immunoassays based on ECL detection are composed of a label that emits light upon oxidation at the surface of an electrode when voltage is applied to it. The luminogenic label is a coordinated complex of ruthenium (Ru), ruthenium (II) tris(bipyridyl[bpy]), or $Ru(bpy)_3^{+2}$. Both $Ru(bpy)_3^{+2}$ and tripropylamine (TPA) are oxidized by the electrode to $Ru(bpy)_3^{+3}$ and the cationic radical, TPA^+. Both oxidized species then react to form the excited label $Ru(bpy)_3^{+2*}$, which emits light upon returning to its ground state, ready for another excitation/emission cycle. Labels not at the surface of the electrode are not oxidized and therefore do not emit light. A description of competitive binding formats in which ECL is used as the detection technology is presented later in this chapter.

Microparticles

When a microparticle multivalently coated with either antibody or ligand forms aggregated complexes upon binding to its specific binding partner, the increased particle size changes the amount and direction in which the light is scattered (see p. 62, Chapter 2). To minimize background signal, the measured particle should be smaller in diameter than the detection wavelength; thus optimal unaggregated particles are less than 1 μm in diameter. Both turbidimetry and nephelometry are commonly used to measure the binding reactions for microparticle-based competitive light-scattering reactions. Turbidimetry measures the decrease in incident light as a function of light scatter as the size of the aggregated particles increases. Thus these changes are detected as increases in absorbance at a particular wavelength. Nephelometry directly measures the scattered light reflected at a 70-degree forward angle (150 degrees from the source of the incident light; forward light scatter). Either kinetic or fixed time point measurements can be used, but use of the former is more efficient because it does not require a blank determination. The use of a near-infrared detection system, with its long wavelength, increases analytical sensitivity for turbidimetric measurements.

KEY CONCEPTS BOX 9-3

- Isotopic labels used for radioimmunoassay (RIA) are based on radioactive decay.
- Non-isotopic assay labels include enzymes, fluorophores, luminogens, and microparticles (in agglutination-based assays).

SECTION OBJECTIVES BOX 9-4

- Understand the quantitative relationship between sensitivity and antibody affinity.
- Describe the effects of label type, assay format, and interferences on sensitivity.
- Describe the relationship of antibody and ligand structure to assay specificity.
- Differentiate between classical and functional cross-reactivity measurements.

DETECTION LIMITS (SENSITIVITY)

The sensitivity of a binding-reaction assay is a function of the affinity of the binding protein for its ligand. Consequently, for 50% binding to occur, a ligand present at a concentration of 1×10^{-7} M would require an antibody with a K_a of 10^7 L/mol, whereas a ligand present at a concentration of 1×10^{-10} M would need an antibody with a K_a of 1×10^{10} L/mol.

Ideally, the binding protein in a competitive-binding assay would have the same affinity for both labeled and unlabeled ligands; however, this usually is not the case. In some instances, the label or the labeling procedure will alter the immunochemical properties of the ligand to the extent that antibody does not bind it as well as it does the unlabeled compound. In other instances, the converse is true: antibodies made against haptens can include affinity for the chemical bridge used to couple the ligand to the protein carrier. Such antibodies may have a higher affinity for the labeled ligand with the chemical bridge than they do for the unmodified ligand. In this case, the dose response for the unlabeled ligand would be low, and such an antibody would not be used to construct an assay.

The sensitivity of a competitive-binding assay often is improved if the ligand has sufficient time to bind to the antibody before the labeled ligand **conjugate** is added. This *sequentially* competitive-binding assay is particularly helpful when the antibody has greater affinity for the hapten conjugate than for the hapten alone compared with a *simultaneous* competitive format, in which the sample ligand and the ligand conjugate have equal access to the antibody. The response to the presence of sample ligand usually is greater in a sequential format, since the ligand has more opportunity to occupy the available antibody-binding sites than it would in a simultaneous format.

Besides the relationship to the affinity of the binding reaction, the **detection limit,** or the sensitivity of a competitive-binding assay, is dependent on the relative detectability of the labeled species. For example, a fluorophore should provide greater sensitivity than a chromophore; the fluorescent or luminescent product of enzyme-label catalysis will place the detection limit 1 to 2 orders of magnitude below that usually observed with chromogens as substrates; europium chelates can provide greater sensitivity than ^{125}I because of their greater label density compared with ^{125}I (which is limited to avoid damage to the radioactivity-labeled reagent).

Assay detection limit can be defined as the lowest concentration of a ligand that can be accurately and precisely distinguished from zero (ligand). Therefore, by definition, any nonspecific interaction that contributes to the signal in the absence of ligand compromises the detection limit by lowering the signal-to-noise ratio (S/N), thus making it more difficult to distinguish the signal derived from the specific binding reaction from that attributable to nonspecific binding (NSB) and other nonspecific interferences. Although other types of interference are prevalent in both homogeneous and heterogeneous assays, NSB is a common problem in the latter, where either a ligand-labeled conjugate or an antibody-labeled conjugate nonspecifically adheres to the solid phase. This phenomenon may be attributable to sites on the solid phase available for hydrophobic or ionic adsorption, because binding sites on the solid-phase surface are not covered, or because surface changes may occur after coating or chemical modification. Reduction of the NSB often is achieved by coating, "blocking," the solid phase with neutral proteins or synthetic high-molecular-weight polymers, or by including blocking proteins or detergents in the immunoassay reactions.

CROSS-REACTIVITY (SPECIFICITY)

The specificity of a binding protein for its ligand is measured by its ability to bind only the ligand in contrast to other substances. Cross-reacting molecules are structurally so similar to the ligand that they also are bound by the antibody. The greater the chemical difference between the ligand and a potential cross-reactant, the less likely it is that the cross-reactant will be bound. Examples of potential cross-reactants include drug analogs and metabolites for drug assays and low-molecular-weight hormones, such as estradiol and estriol, or their respective metabolites, which are similar in structure to each other. Differences in antibody binding of ligand and cross-reacting substances are a function of differences in affinity. These differences are reflected by responses to cross-reactants in competitive-binding assays. Table 9-5 gives two examples of the relationship between the K_a of the antibody for its ligand, two cross-reactants, and the concentration of each that is required in the assay to deliver the same binding response. The concentration of cross-reactant$_a$ required for 50% binding to antibody$_1$ is 10 times the concentration necessary to bind 50% of ligand$_1$. Similarly, 10,000-fold less ligand$_2$ is required to achieve 50% binding to antibody$_2$ than is necessary to bind 50% of cross-reactant$_d$. Table 9-5 shows that with a lower K_a, more antibody is required to bind 50% of the ligand or cross-reactant, further illustrating the relationship between sensitivity and K_a. The degree to which each cross-reactant in Table 9-5 interferes with the analysis of each ligand depends on the relative concentrations of ligand and cross-reactant in actual samples. For example, cross-reactants c and d probably would *not* interfere in the assay of ligand$_2$ unless they were present at concentrations 100 or 10,000 times higher, respectively, than that of ligand$_2$.

Table 9-5 Cross-Reactant Binding as a Function of Antibody Affinity

Antibody	Bound Species	K_a	Concentration (M) Required for 50% Binding*
1	Ligand$_1$	1×10^8	2×10^{-8}
	Cross-reactant$_a$	1×10^7	2×10^{-7}
	Cross-reactant$_b$	5×10^7	1×10^{-6}
2	Ligand$_2$	1×10^{10}	2×10^{-10}
	Cross-reactant$_c$	2×10^8	4×10^{-8}
	Cross-reactant$_d$	1×10^6	2×10^{-6}

*When 50% of the ligand or cross-reactant is bound, B/F = 1. Since $K_a = \frac{B}{F[Ab]}$; when B/F = 1, then $K_a = \frac{1}{[Ab]}$.

Ideally, antibodies or other binding proteins that participate in competitive-binding reactions are very specific for the ligand, with essentially no cross-reactivity with closely related molecules. In reality, the antibodies present in a heterogeneous antiserum bind the ligand with different affinities and orientations and therefore are likely to bind structurally similar molecules. One of the advantages of monoclonal antibodies (MAS) is the potential for selecting very specific antibodies that have essentially no cross-reactivity with other compounds. Examples of the cross-reactivity of antisera and a monoclonal antibody are shown in Figs. 9-2 and 9-3. The dose-response curves seen with antiserum (see Fig. 9-2) show that caffeine, which is structurally similar to the antiasthmatic drug theophylline, effectively competes only at much higher concentrations with the label for theophylline-binding sites. The degree of caffeine cross-reactivity, determined by the "classical" approach, is calculated by dividing the concentration of ligand (in this case, theophylline) at 50% of maximum binding (as indicated in Fig. 9-2) by the concentration of cross-reactant (caffeine), which also displaces 50% of the label according to the following equation:

$$\frac{[\text{Ligand}] \text{ at } 50\% \text{ binding}}{[\text{Cross-reactant}] \text{ at } 50\% \text{ binding}}(100) = \% \text{ cross-reactivity} \qquad \text{Eq. 9-4}$$

Caffeine cross-reactivity for the antiserum is 12.3% in Fig. 9-2, whereas only 1.2% cross-reactivity occurs with the theophylline monoclonal antibody, as shown in Fig. 9-3. Table 9-6 summarizes these results. A competitive-binding assay that uses the monoclonal antibody to theophylline is more specific than one that uses the antiserum; consequently, based on this analysis, the former assay would be less prone to caffeine interference.

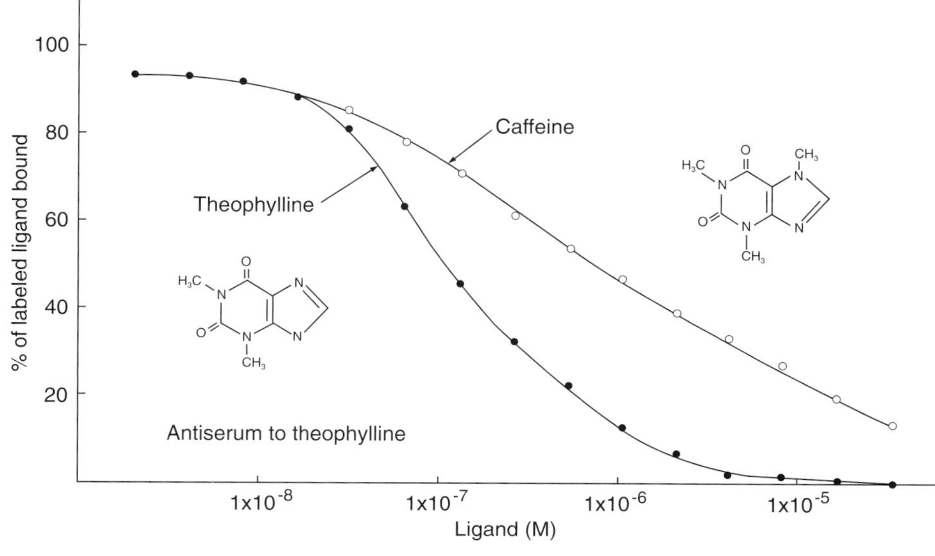

Fig. 9-2 Cross-reactivity of caffeine with a polyclonal antibody to theophylline in a homogeneous fluorescent immunoassay. Cross-reactivity is determined at concentrations of theophylline and caffeine required for 50% of the dose response. This is equivalent to 46.5% of the bound label. Refer to Table 9-6 for cross-reactivity data.

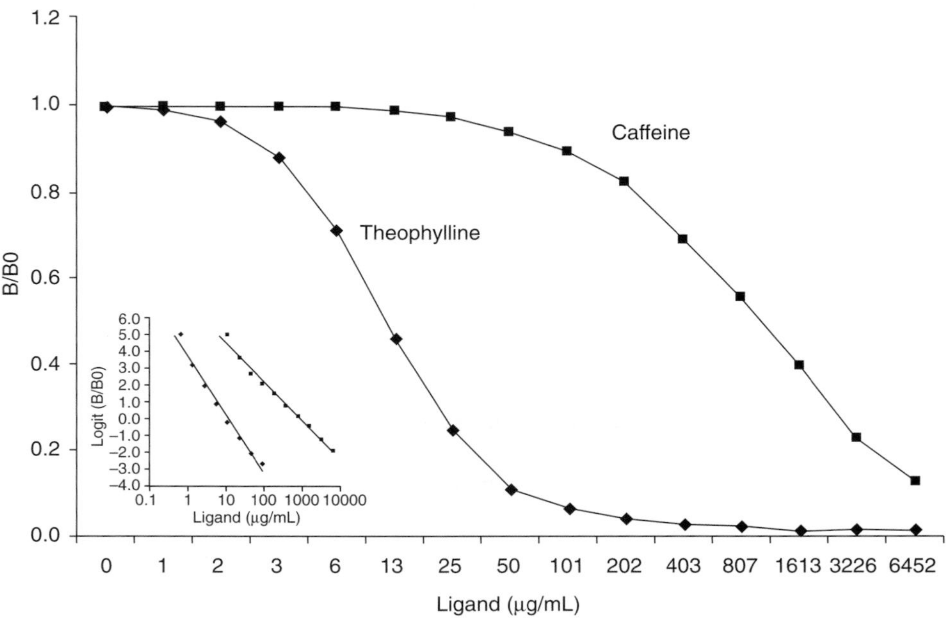

Fig. 9-3 Cross-reactivity of caffeine with a monoclonal antibody to theophylline in the same immunoassay indicated in Fig. 9-2. Cross-reactivity is determined at 43.2% of bound label, equivalent to 50% B/B_0. The figure insert shows dose-response curves after results are reduced and replotted, as described in the Data Reduction section (below).

Table 9-6 Caffeine Cross-Reactivity With Polyclonal or Monoclonal Antibodies to Theophylline

	CONCENTRATION (M) WHEN 50% OF LABEL IS BOUND		
	Theophylline	**Caffeine**	**% Cross-Reactivity**
Polyclonal	1.29×10^{-7}	1.05×10^{-6}	12.3
Monoclonal	6.15×10^{-8}	5.09×10^{-6}	1.2

Although the classical approach to determining cross-reactivity is useful for evaluating the comparative assay response of ligand and cross-reactant, the "functional" approach is more meaningful because it determines the contribution of a potential cross-reactant to the competitive-binding assay response in the presence of the ligand. For example, both the ligand and the cross-reactant are competing with each other and with the ligand-label conjugate for antibody-binding sites. Consequently, it is not surprising when a cross-reactant with cross-reactivity of 1% to 2% in the classical method increases the known concentration of a ligand by 10% to 20%. One approach that can be used to evaluate functional cross-reactivity is to determine the assay response to increasing concentrations of cross-reactant at different concentrations of ligand. Table 9-7 summarizes the cross-reactivity of caffeine, theobromine, and various theophylline metabolites at a midlevel theophylline concentration compared with that observed with the classical approach, whereas Fig. 9-4 illustrates the responses of various cross-reactants in a functional assay.

Now that the monoclonal antibodies produced from immortal cell lines can be readily screened for very high affinity ($K_a = 10^{11} - 10^{12}\ M^{-1}$) with almost absolute specificity, these binding proteins are preferred to polyclonal antibodies, which often are inconsistent in terms of quality and availability.

DATA REDUCTION

Earlier in this chapter, the displacement reaction was described by the equation

$$L + AbL^* \rightleftharpoons AbL + AbL^* + L^* + L$$

where Ab is the antibody or another binding protein that provides a limited number of ligand-binding sites. The concentration of the labeled ligand, L*, is constant and in excess of the binding-site concentration. The ligand, L, will compete with L* for available binding sites. As shown in Fig. 9-1, the amount of L* bound by the antibody is inversely proportional to the concentration of L in the assay. The dose response is a measure of either the bound L* or the free L* that has been displaced by L.

The dose response of a competitive displacement reaction usually is not linear, but S-shaped (see Figs. 9-1 and 9-2). It is difficult to interpolate a signal in the nonlinear portion of these curves to determine ligand concentration. To increase the linear, more readable, portions of the dose-response curve, the data are modified by a process called *data reduction.* Many different methods can be used to reduce the data. RIA data reduction is shown as an example on the Evolve website. For most automated immunoassay methods, computerized instruments offer various axis transformations, with polynomial and four-parameter curve-fitting equations that are well suited for generating curvilinear calibration lines and interpolating unknown results. Transformation of the y-axis can be plotted as B/B_0, the response at x dose divided by the response generated at zero dose (zero calibrator), more commonly as logit B/B_0. The logit transformation is the following:

$$\text{logit}(B/B_0) = \ln B/B_0/1 - B/B_0 \qquad \text{Eq. 9-5}$$

Either B/B_0 or logit B/B_0 can be plotted as a function of the arithmetic or logarithmic dose of the ligand concentration.

Table 9-7 Functional and Classical Cross-Reactivity Determinations for an Antitheophylline Monoclonal Antibody

	*CLASSICAL**		*FUNCTIONAL†*	
Cross-Reactant	**μg/mL**	**%**	**μg/mL**	**%**
1,3,7-trimethylxanthine (caffeine)	>10,000	<0.2	400	0.8
3,7-dimethylxanthine (theobromine)	760	2.8	390	0.8
1,3-dimethyluric acid	2900	1.0	580	0.5
3-methylxanthine	760	2.8	280	1.1

*Classical cross-reactivity determined as described by Eq. 9-4. Theophylline concentration at 50% binding was 21.3 μg/mL.
†Functional cross-reactivity is defined by the concentration of cross-reactant that increases the observed concentration of 15 μg of theophylline/mL control by 20%. Therefore functional cross-reactivity is calculated as follows:

$$\%\ \text{Cross-reactivity} = (100)\frac{3\,\mu\text{g theophylline/mL}}{\mu\text{g cross-reactant/mL at 20\% bias}}$$

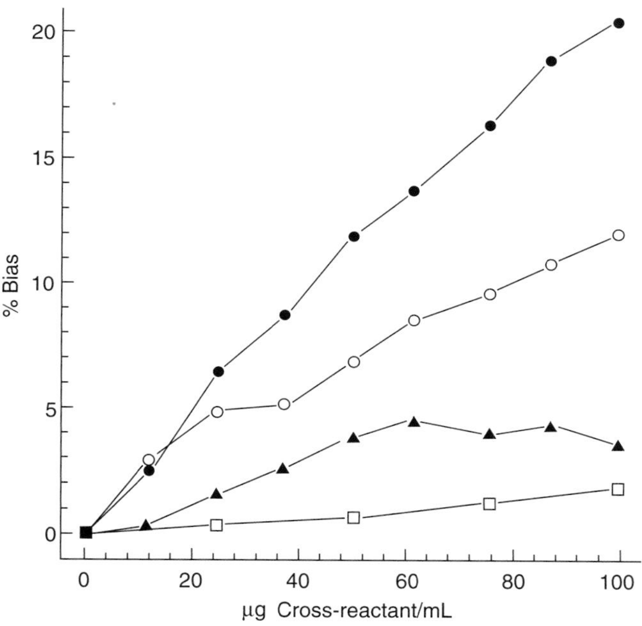

Fig. 9-4 Functional determination of cross-reactivity in a homogeneous turbidimetric inhibition assay. The observed increase in apparent concentration to a midrange control is measured in the presence of increasing concentrations of 1,3-dimethyluric acid, ●; 1-methylxanthine, ▲; 3-methylxanthine, ○; and caffeine, □.

The logit B/B_0 versus the logarithmic dose has been the most accepted empirical method for linearizing and reducing the data for competitive protein-binding dose-response curves (see insert Fig. 9-3).

Of the automated curve-fitting routines, two related equations are used most commonly. One is the four-parameter log-logistic (4PL) fit, an equation whereby the four parameters are estimated through a series of iterations of calibration responses that correspond to the respective calibrator concentrations. The other is a rearrangement of the 4PL, the logit-log equation, which is essentially equivalent to the 4PL. Both equations are described in detail in the Wild and Gosling references.

KEY CONCEPTS BOX 9-4

- Sensitivity of an immunoassay is primarily a function of the affinity of an anitbody for its ligand.
- The choice of label and assay format also help to define assay sensitivity.
- The antibody is the determinant for assay specificity.
- Cross-reactivity, a measure of assay specificity, is determined by classical and functional approaches.

SECTION OBJECTIVES BOX 9-5

- Understand the principles and limitations of heterogeneous and homogeneous assay techniques.
- Describe factors that are considered or evaluated for each immunoassay.
- Provide attributes for comparison for each immunoassay format.
- Understand potential limitations and interferences for each immunoassay format.

EXAMPLES OF NON-ISOTOPIC COMPETITIVE-BINDING ASSAYS

Heterogeneous Assay Techniques

Enzyme-Linked Immunosorbent Assay

The **enzyme-linked immunosorbent assays (ELISA)** are heterogeneous non-isotopic assays that usually have an antibody immobilized onto a solid support (see Table 9-2), whereas the ligand is labeled with an enzyme. Table 9-8 lists some enzymes used for ELISA (or other enzyme immunoassays). These enzymes are useful as labels because they satisfy the following criteria:

Table 9-8 Enzyme Labels for Immunoassays

Enzyme	Source	Molecular Weight	ACTIVITY Turnover Rate*	°C
Alkaline phosphatase	Calf intestine	140,000	420,000	37
β-Galactosidase	*Escherichia coli*	540,000	324,000	37
Glucose-6-phosphate dehydrogenase	*Leuconostoc mesenteroides*	130,000	93,600	30
Peroxidase	Horseradish	40,000	220,000	25

*The turnover rate is the number of moles of product released per minute per mole of enzyme at the designated temperature.

1. *High specific activity.* Signal amplification obtained with an enzyme label corresponds to the amount of substrate converted to product during the time of incubation. Enzymes with the highest specific activities yield the greatest amplification. Assays that use such enzymes have excellent sensitivity and are able to measure very low concentrations of ligand.
2. *Easily coupled to ligand.* Enzymes have sufficient acidic and basic amino acids, thiol groups, or carbohydrate to be coupled easily to the ligand without losing substantial enzymatic activity.
3. *Stability.* Enzyme labels are stable during the assay and under refrigerated storage conditions.
4. *Absent in fluid or tissue.* Enzymes usually are not present in the biological fluid or tissue sample that is to be analyzed.
5. *Retention of activity.* Enzymes retain most of their activity when attached to the ligand or antibody.

Alkaline phosphatase and horseradish peroxidase are inexpensively available in highly purified form. For this reason and those listed above, these two enzymes are used most often as labels for ELISA. Some of the enzymes listed in Table 9-8 can use chromogens, fluorogens, or luminogens as substrates. Fluorescent and luminescent products can be detected at concentrations that are 100 to 1000 times lower than those of chromophores, with an concomitant reduction of the incubation time.

Many configurations for ELISA have been devised. Some are based on competitive reactions, whereas others are direct immunometric "sandwich" assays. The sandwich ELISA is discussed in Chapter 8. The two basic formats for the competitive assays and the shapes of the respective typical dose-response curves that describe the signal remaining on the solid phase are shown in Figs. 9-5 and 9-6.

Of the two formats, the configuration in which the antibody has been immobilized onto the solid surface (Fig. 9-7) has been described more frequently. The ligand in the sample competes with the enzyme-labeled ligand for a limited number of antibody-binding sites fixed to the solid phase. After the binding reaction has taken place, the solid phase is washed with water or buffer to remove the unbound labeled ligand so that it does not contribute to the signal. The amount of enzyme bound to the solid phase is proportional to the absorbance, fluorescence, or luminescence of the product formed after the addition of substrate, and it is inversely proportional to the concentration of unlabeled ligand. This method is applicable to both low- and high-molecular-weight analytes.

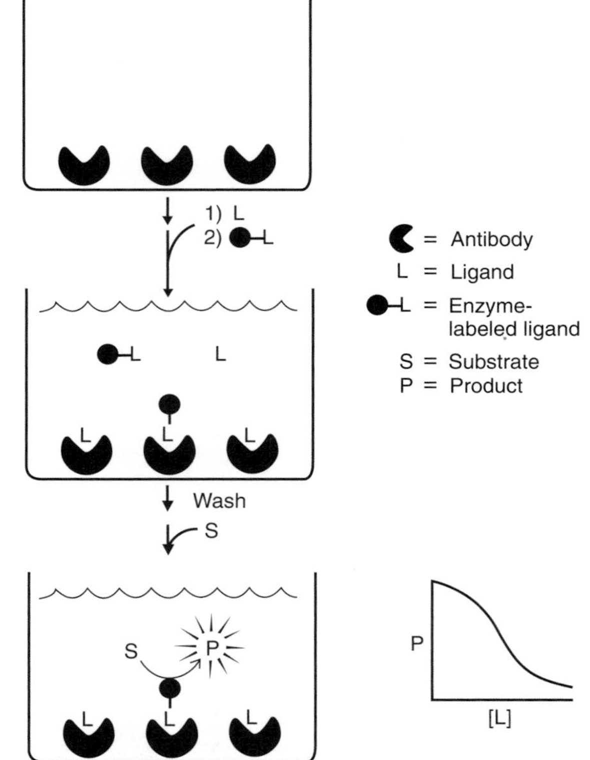

Fig. 9-5 Principle of the competitive enzyme-linked immunosorbent assay (ELISA) with the ligand labeled with an enzyme and a typical dose-response curve.

The ELISA dose response shown in Fig. 9-7 was generated on an automated analyzer, with alkaline phosphatase as the label and luminogen as its substrate.

Instead of antibody, the ligand can be attached to the solid phase, as shown in Fig. 9-6. Only those antibody-enzyme binding sites not occupied by the sample ligand will bind to the immobilized ligand. The solid-phase ligand:antibody-enzyme complex is washed before the substrate is added. Immunometric ELISAs have some of the same advantages as immunoradiometric assays (IRMAs) when compared with an enzyme-labeled ligand ELISA.

Although both ELISA formats illustrated in Figs. 9-5 and 9-6 measure the amount of labeled conjugate bound to the solid phase, the activity remaining in solution after the binding reaction has taken place also can be measured.

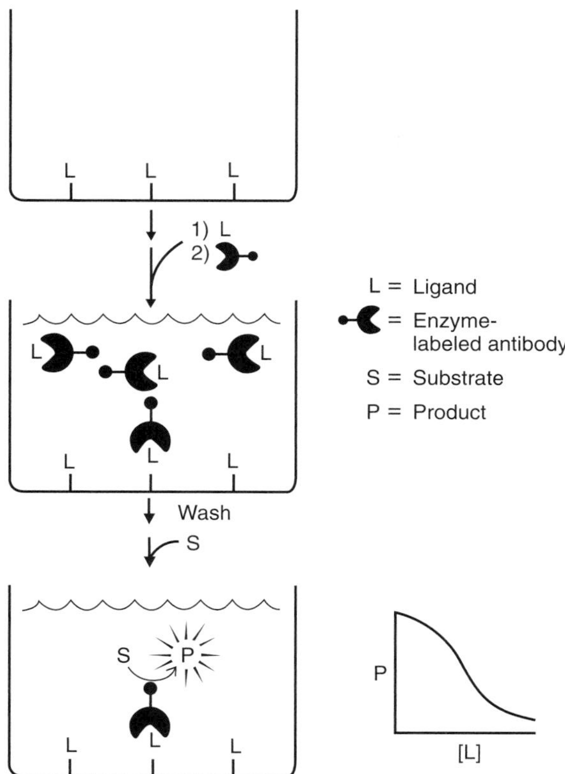

Fig. 9-6 Principle of the competitive enzyme-linked immunosorbent assay (ELISA) where the antibody is labeled with an enzyme. This is an immunometric assay.

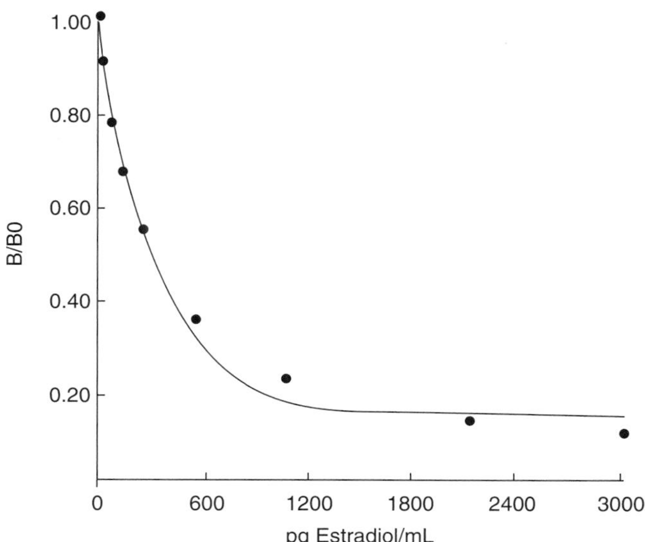

Fig. 9-7 Dose response for an automated chemiluminescent enzyme-linked immunosorbent assay (ELISA) for estradiol. The antiestradiol antibody is coupled to a plastic solid phase while the estradiol derivative is coupled to the alkaline phosphatase label.

In the earlier description of heterogeneous assays, some useful capture phases for separating antibody bound from unbound labeled ligand—namely, microtiter plates, latex, and various types of microparticles—were described. Paramagnetic microparticles are applicable to those systems that employ magnets, whereas latex microparticles are trapped by glass-fiber filters or membranes either before or after the binding reaction takes place but always before the washing steps and addition of the enzyme substrates. Similarly, antibody has been adsorbed to glass-fiber filters with the aid of a lattice formed with secondary antibodies, or it has been adsorbed to membranes. Both glass-fiber and membrane filter capture phase supports are components of flow-through or radial diffusion cassettes for automatic instruments, as are the capture support and reading areas for the rapid assay devices used so frequently as point-of-care assays for pregnancy, ovulation, and infectious disease testing (see p. 391, Chapter 21).

One of the drawbacks of adsorbing antibodies to solid surfaces such as the polystyrene of microtiter plates, beads, and microparticles or the membranes of rapid-assay devices is that both monoclonal and polyclonal antibodies can undergo substantial loss of antigen-binding capacity because of conformational changes that occur upon adsorption to such surfaces. Instances in which less than 5% of adsorbed monoclonals remained functional have been described. Major losses (≈50%) are also seen in cases where the antibodies have been covalently attached to the solid support. Indirect capture phases were developed to standardize assays and overcome losses in antigen-binding capacity. The avidin-biotin system is an example. Avidin (or streptavidin) binds biotin with very high affinity ($K_a = 10^{15}$ M^{-1}) and may retain two to three of its four binding sites upon attachment to a solid phase. The completed capture phase is formed when the immobilized avidin binds a biotinylated antibody or ligand so that immunobinding events occur with maximal antibody-ligand binding capacity. Fig. 9-8 illustrates increased capture capacity of a biotinylated antipeptide antibody bound to streptavidin immobilized to biotinylated latex particles. The figure demonstrates increased capacity as a function of antibody biotin density.

In addition to the biotin-avidin system, antifluorescein-fluorescein and antidigoxigenin-digoxigenin binding pairs have been used to form indirect capture phases. Aside from overcoming diminished antibody-capturing capacity, their use has a more practical advantage: the capture phase can be a universal reagent component for a family of different heterogeneous competitive-binding assays. For example, the same antifluorescein-coupled magnetic particles are used to capture fluoresceinated antiligand antibodies in competitive-binding assays for different steroid hormones.

Cascades or amplification schemes have also been devised for ELISAs, which theoretically enhance their sensitivity.

Time-Resolved Fluorescence
(see also Chapter 2, p. 60)

Lanthanide metal chelates have strong advantages as labels compared with other fluorophores used in competitive-binding assays. For example, the fluorescence lifetimes of europium chelates are extremely long—100 µsec and greater

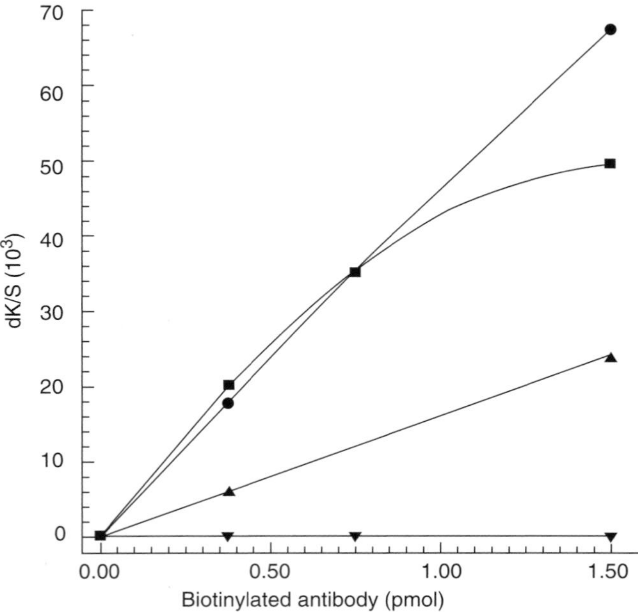

Fig. 9-8 Capture of biotinylated antipeptide antibody as a function of biotin density in an indirect capture assay, where dK/S is a measurement of reflected light. Streptavidin immobilized to biotinylated latex microparticles is incubated simultaneously with an increasing amount of biotinylated antibody containing 1.2, ▼; 4.3, ▲; 6.0, ■; or 10.7, ● biotins per molecule of antibody, respectively, and a constant concentration of peptide–alkaline phosphatase conjugate. The complex was retained on a glass-fiber filter and was washed before the addition of substrate.

than other fluorophores (5 nsec for fluorescein). With the appropriate instrumentation, one is able to measure such fluorescence 1 μsec or longer after a pulse of excitation light and to distinguish fluorescence from short-lived background fluorescent interferences. This is the basis for time-resolved fluoroimmunoassays, that is, heterogeneous assays with inherently low background capable of sensitivity as much as a thousandfold greater than that of other non–ELISA-based fluorescence methods.

Fluorescence of europium chelates is seen at wavelengths characteristic of the europium metal after light absorption by the chelator ligand with efficient energy transfer to the metal. The europium chelate complex is stable enough to withstand the washing conditions typical of heterogeneous assays. In the first **time-resolved fluorescence** immunoassays, highly fluorescent metal chelate complexes were insoluble in an aqueous environment, hence europium chelated by a poor energy-transferring ligand as the label was extracted and then recomplexed with a ligand appropriate for forming a highly fluorescent complex. Ligands have been synthesized to function as highly fluorescent labels when complexed with the metal, thereby eliminating the extraction step. Carrier proteins with a multiplicity (150) of europium chelate labels attached to antibodies by means of a biotin:streptavidin bridge have been shown to increase the signal up to 7000 times in some amplification configurations. Dose-response curves for time-resolved fluorescence assays are similar to those of other heterogeneous competitive immunoassays.

Rapid Assays

Immunoassays have been configured in small hand-held devices for qualitative and semiquantitative determinations. Similar to many home use pregnancy tests, these competitive assays have been made in flow-through and immunochromatographic (lateral flow) test formats. Labels for detection include enzymes, colored latex particles, and gold sols. Such devices do not require instrumentation because the results can be read visually. Consequently, they are ideal for screening. One example of such a device is used to screen for various combinations of drugs of abuse. A urine sample is first incubated with a high-affinity Mab and a ligand gold sol conjugate until the competitive binding reactions reach equilibrium. The antibody binds all of the conjugate and drug below a threshold concentration. The threshold drug concentrations are unique to different drugs, so it is necessary to manipulate the concentration of conjugate and antibody for each analyte to achieve the appropriate threshold. After incubation, the entire reaction mixture is applied to a solid phase in which a series of specific anticonjugate antibodies are immobilized in different zones on a nylon membrane. When a drug threshold has been exceeded, unbound gold sol-ligand conjugate is bound by solid-phase antibodies in proportion to the drug concentration in the sample, creating a colored band in a particular drug zone.

HOMOGENEOUS ASSAY TECHNIQUES

Homogeneous Enzyme Immunoassay

The first reported homogeneous immunoassay was an enzyme immunoassay for low-molecular-weight ligands, commonly known as the **enzyme-multiplied immunoassay technique (EMIT).** EMIT is used primarily for measuring analytes that are present in higher concentrations such as therapeutic drugs (theophylline, phenytoin) and drugs of abuse (opiates, cocaine). Binding of a specific antibody to the enzyme-labeled ligand changes the enzymatic activity of the label so that the antibody-bound enzyme can be distinguished from the unbound labeled ligand.

In most instances, binding of antibody to the enzyme-ligand conjugate sterically inhibits the enzyme by limiting access of the enzyme substrate to the catalytic site (Fig. 9-9). A typical enzyme-inhibition profile is shown in Fig. 9-10. Increasing the amount of gentamicin monoclonal antibody inhibits the activity of the enzyme label glucose-6-phosphate dehydrogenase (see Fig. 9-10). A dose-response curve for the competitive homogeneous enzyme immunoassay is shown in Fig. 9-11. The unlabeled ligand competes with enzyme-labeled gentamicin for limited numbers of antibody-binding sites, and as more unlabeled gentamicin is bound by the antibody, enzymatic activity increases. Usually, this response is reflected by a change in the rate of enzyme activity when two

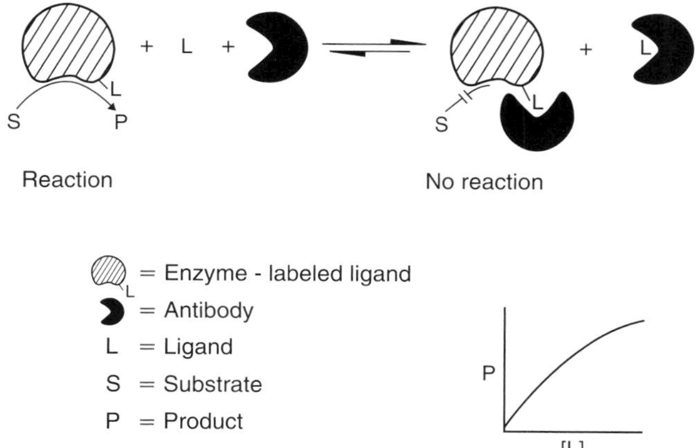

Fig. 9-9 Principle of the homogeneous enzyme immunoassay (enzyme-multiplied immunoassay technique, EMIT) and a typical dose-response curve.

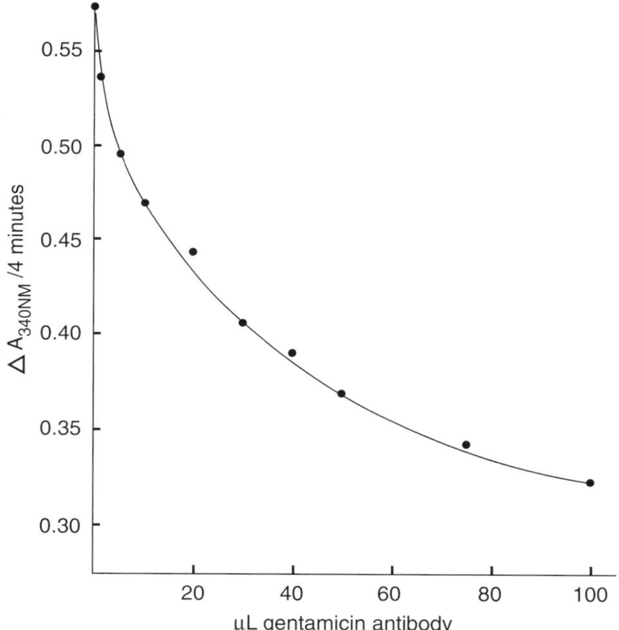

Fig. 9-10 Inhibition of activity of gentamicin–glucose-6-phosphate dehydrogenase conjugate by monoclonal antibody to gentamicin.

absorbance readings of the reaction are taken 30 seconds apart. Change in absorbance (ΔA) is used to calculate the dose response.

Another homogeneous enzyme immunoassay that, similar to EMIT, is particularly well suited for automated high-throughput immunoassay or chemistry systems is the CEDIA. The fundamental components of this method include an enzyme acceptor (EA), an inactive fragment of β-galactosidase that lacks the complementary enzyme donor (ED) fragment necessary for enzymic activity. The 10,000 dalton ED, when covalently conjugated to the haptenic ligand, is the labeled ligand for this competitive immunoassay for low-

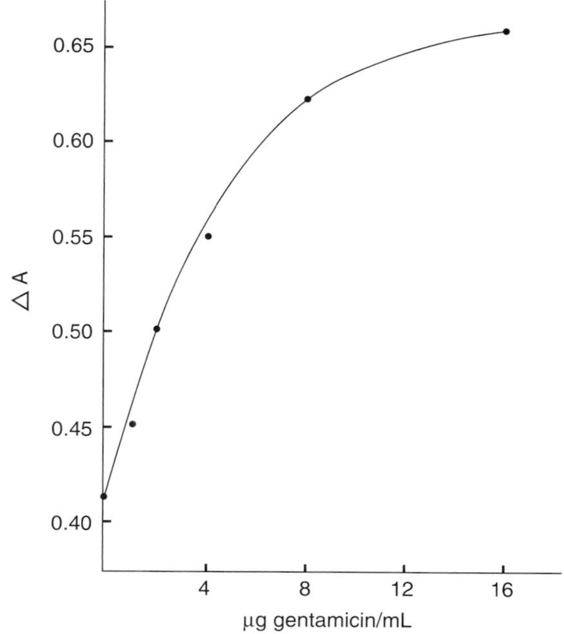

Fig. 9-11 Dose-response curve for the homogeneous gentamicin enzyme immunoassay.

molecular-weight analytes. Both β-galactosidase fragments are bioengineered by recombinant DNA techniques with the ligand attachment site to the ED so that it does interfere with the interaction of EA and ED. Reconstituted β-galactosidase activity approaches that seen with native enzyme.

When a ligand-specific antibody binds the ligand-ED, the re-combination of ED with EA is partially inhibited, thus making it possible to distinguish antibody-bound label from that which is free for interaction with EA. A time course for complementation-reconstituted β-galactosidase activity in the presence and absence of digoxin is shown in Fig. 9-12. The figure shows that although this technique is one of the more sensitive homogeneous methods, enzyme activity in the absence of analyte ligand is only partially blocked by the antiligand-antibody complex, even though the size of the antiligand antibody is increased by the addition of a second antispecies antibody to improve the steric hindrance of antibody-bound ligand-ED in generating an active enzyme. One can see in Fig. 9-12 that to improve the sensitivity of the assay, the reading would have to be taken beyond 5 minutes, preferably 10 or 15 minutes after the the reaction is initiated.

Fluorescence Polarization Immunoassay (see Chapter 2, pp. 61-62)

Fluorescence polarization immunoassay (FPIA) is based on the amount of polarized fluorescent light detected when the fluorophore label is excited with polarized light. The degree of polarization of the emitted fluorescent light depends on the rate of rotation of the fluorophore-ligand conjugate in solution. Small molecules rotate freely, and consequently, the fluorescent light emitted by the molecule is depolarized, whereas large molecules, such as proteins, rotate more slowly and emit

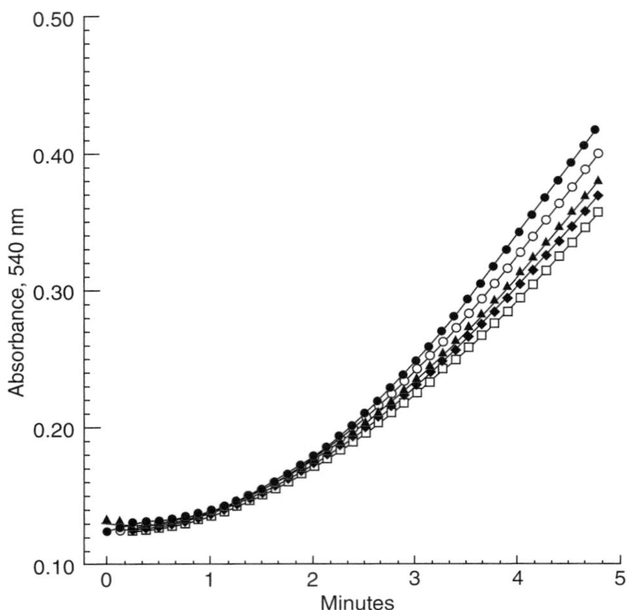

Fig. 9-12 Reaction time course for the cloned-enzyme donor immunoassay digoxin assay method. Response is in the absence, □, and the presence of 1.0, ◆; 2.0, ▲; 3.0, O; and 4.0 ng, ● of digoxin per milliliter of sample.

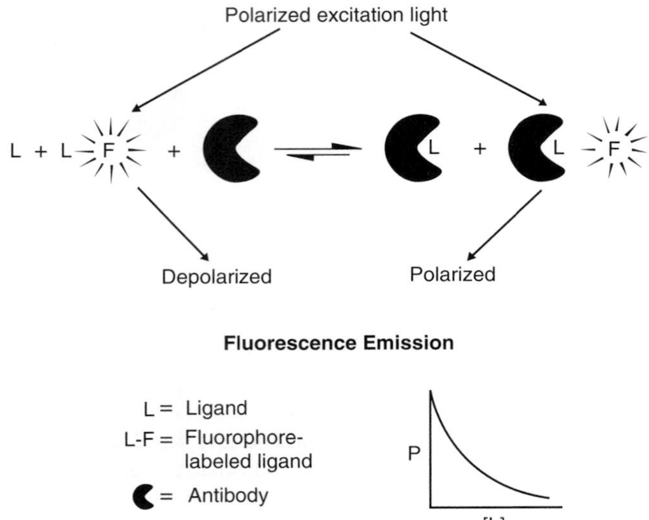

Fig. 9-13 Principle of the fluorescence polarization immunoassay (FPIA) and a typical dose-response curve.

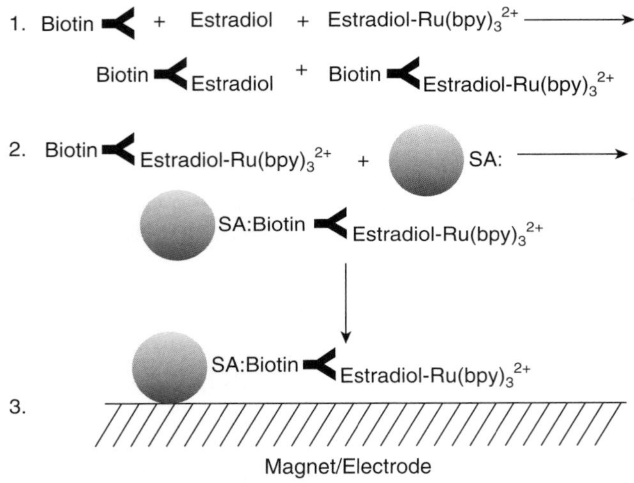

Fig. 9-14 Simultaneous electrochemiluminescence competitive binding reaction between estradiol and estradiol-labeled $Ru(bpy)_3^{2+}$ for antiestradiol binding sites (Step 1) followed by binding of labeled immune complexes to streptavidin-coated paramagnetic particles (Step 2), which then are bound and brought to the elctrode by the magnet (Step 3), where the label is oxidized, thus beginning the cascade of reactions that lead to light emission.

polarized fluorescent light. When an antibody binds a low-molecular-weight ligand labeled with a fluorophore, the fluorescence polarization of the labeled ligand is increased because rotation of the labeled ligand-antibody complex is much slower than that of labeled ligands alone. Unlabeled ligand will compete with labeled ligand for antibody-binding sites, and so the amount of polarized fluorescent light that results from a competitive-binding reaction is inversely proportional to the concentration of unlabeled ligand in the reaction. The principle of the FPIA and a typical dose-response curve are shown in Fig. 9-13. Similar to EMIT and micoparticle-based homogeneous assays, FPIAs are commercially available for all routinely monitored therapeutic drugs, as well as for drugs of abuse and other small molecules.

Electrochemiluminescence (see p. 61)

Electrochemiluminescent (ECL) competitive binding assays for haptens and higher-molecular-weight ligands are quasi-homogeneous assays in that they do not necessarily require a wash step to remove the unbound label. ECL assays incorporate a paramagnetic particle to capture and concentrate bound label on the surface of the electrode. In assays in which the hapten is labeled, a significant difference in ECL exists between the bound and free label as a result of decreased diffusion and steric hindrance of the antibody-bound label. Such assays are truly homogeneous in that antibody binding modulates the activity of the ruthenium complex label.

Both hapten-labeled and antibody-labeled approaches are used. For example, in a forward sequential competitive format for the hormone estradiol, shown in Figs. 9-14 and 9-15, the sample is incubated first with biotinylated antibody, then with $Ru(bpy)_3^{+2}$-labeled estradiol, and finally with streptavidin-coated **paramagnetic particles.** A magnet then concentrates the particle capture phase on the electrode prior to voltage application and subsequent ECL, shown in Fig. 9-15. Because the $Ru(bpy)_3^{+2}$ label is cycled while the TPA is consumed, the same label generates light as long as the voltage is applied to the electode and oxidizes both the label and the TPA.

4a. $Ru(bpy)_3^{2+} \xrightarrow[\text{Oxidation}]{\text{Electrode}} Ru(bpy)_3^{3+} + e^-$

4b. $TPA^* \xrightarrow[\text{Oxidation}]{\text{Electrode}} TPA^{+*} + e^- \longrightarrow TPA^*$

5. $Ru(bpy)_3^{3+} + TPA^* \longrightarrow Ru(bpy)_3^{2+*}$

6. $Ru(bpy)_3^{2+*} \longrightarrow Ru(bpy)_3^{2+} + 620\text{ nm Light}$

Fig. 9-15 Principle of the electrochemiluminescent reaction that follows the competitive binding reaction in Fig. 9-14. Both the label and tripropylamine (TPA) are oxidized simultaneously by the electrode, as shown in Steps 4a and 4b. Both oxidized species react, generating the excited unstable label (Step 5) that emits light when it returns to the ground state (Step 6).

Alternatively, in a simultaneous competitive immunoassay for the hormone thyroxine (T_4), sample T_4 competes with a T_4 ligand-biotin conjugate for $Ru(bpy)_3^{+2}$-labeled anti-T_4 antibody. Antibody-bound ligand-biotin conjugate then is captured by streptavidin-coated particles and is magnetically concentrated on the electrode. Both of these examples introduce a separation step by removing the bound label from solution so that only it participates in the electrochemiluminescent reaction. In this sense, ECL methods are a hybrid between homogeneous and heterogeneous formats in that there is a separation step without wash steps. Of course, wash steps can be introduced to lower the background and improve sensitivity.

Luminescent Oxygen Channeling Immunoassay

The **luminescent oxygen channeling immunoassay (LOCI)** is a homogeneous immunoassay format for both competitive and noncompetitive assays, which employs two sets of microparticles. In one competitive assay format, the first set of microparticles, ligand-coated sensitizer particles, is incubated with the sample and with the second set of microparticles, antibody-coated chemiluminescer particles. The sensitizer particles, impregnated with a photosensitive dye, generate singlet oxygen when illuminated with 680 nm light. The chemiluminescer particles, impregnated with a molecule that reacts with singlet oxygen, generates light energy that is transferred to an impregnated fluorophore and emits a fluoresecent signal. In the absence of ligand in the sample, ligand-coated sensitizer particles bind to the antibody-coated chemiluminescer particles, thus enabling the singlet oxygen to be "channeled" to the antibody-coated particles, as shown in Fig. 9-16. As sample ligand concentration increases, fewer sensitizer particles bind to the antibody-coated chemiluminescer particles with decreased signal. Chemiluminescer particles that are not part of a two-particle binding complex provide almost no signal. Very low background signal produces a very high S/N ratio and the most sensitive of homogeneous immunoassays.

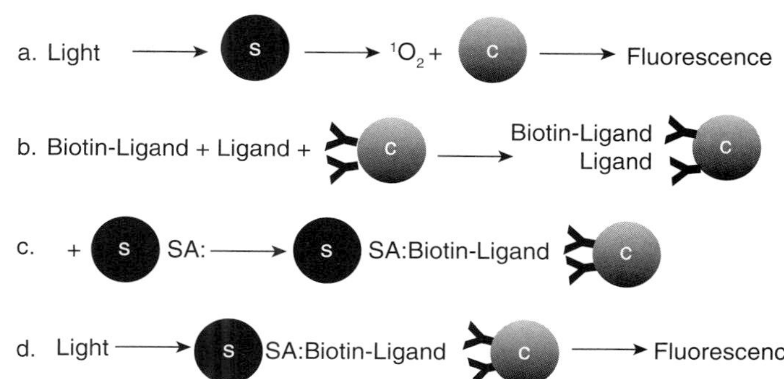

Fig. 9-16 Principle of the homogeneous luminescent oxygen channeling immunoassay (LOCI) method. Photosensitive dye in the sensitizer *(S)* particles generates singlet oxygen that reacts with dyes in the chemiluminescer *(C)* particles paired by antibody-ligand binding. The luminescent light energy produced upon reaction is transferred to a fluorescent dye, which then emits a fluorescent signal (Steps a and d). Steps b and c illustrate the competitive binding reactions and the indirect capture of the antibody-bound biotinylated ligand, thus creating complex aggregates of sensitizer-chemiluminescer particles. The dose reponse is indirectly proportional to the concentration of ligand in the sample. *SA,* Streptavidin.

Microparticle-Based Light-Scattering Inhibition Immunoassays

Competitive nephelometric and turbidimetric inhibition immunoassays differ only in how incident or scattered light is detected, as was discussed earlier. As with EMIT and FPIA, both turbidimetric and nephelometric inhibition assays are used for therapeutic drugs and drugs of abuse. The assay formats are similar: one of the the formats consists of an agglutinator, usually a water-soluble polymeric carrier substance, to which a number of haptenic ligands is coupled. Examples of carriers include dextran, polysucrose, and albumin. The antibody reagent is composed of antiligand antibodies adsorbed or covalently coupled to submicrometer-sized latex microparticles. The aggregated complex, formed when the agglutinator and the antibody reagent are combined, can be measured kinetically or at a single time point. The presence of the ligand in the assay inhibits the rate of aggregation by competing for the antibody-binding sites. The reaction time course for aggregation at different ligand concentrations in a turbidimetric inhibition assay is presented in Fig. 9-17. The density of both ligand on the agglutinator and antibody on the latex microparticles is optimized to obtain maximum kinetics in the absence of ligand with appropriate inhibition in its presence. Measuring the rate of agglutination early in the reaction provides for the greatest sensitivity, whereas the rate or fixed time point can be taken at any time during the reaction for those assays that do not require low detection limits.

For greater sensitivity, the ligands can be coupled to even smaller latex particles in a two-particle inhibition assay. In the absence of simple ligand, binding of the microparticles to antiligand creates aggregates whose increased forward light

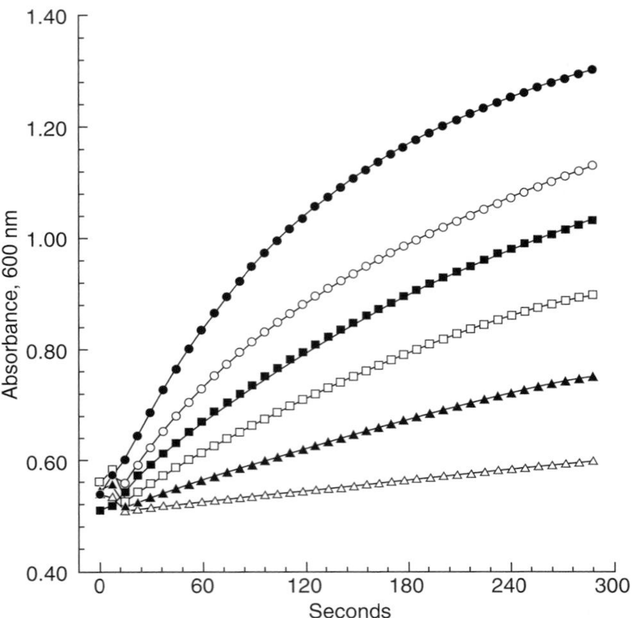

Fig. 9-17 Reaction time courses for a theophylline turbidimetric inhibition immunoassay in the absence, ●, and the presence of 2.5, ○; 5.0, ■; 10.0, □; 20.0, ▲; and 40.0, △ μg of theophylline per milliliter of sample.

scatter is measured nephelometrically. Ligand in the sample binds the antibody and inhibits particle aggregation in proportion to its concentration. More sensitive nephelometric measurements are made with rate near infrared particle immunoassay (rate NIPIA), which employs incident light in the near infrared at 940 nm. The level of endogenous spectral interferences such as lipemia, hemolysis, and icterus is reduced at this wavelength.

ATTRIBUTES AND LIMITATIONS OF DIFFERENT APPROACHES TO COMPETITIVE-BINDING ASSAYS

Before reviewing advantages and limitations of the competitive-binding assays described earlier, it is useful to discuss factors that should be considered when one designs or chooses a particular assay format. Convenience, cost-effectiveness, and performance for an assay must be addressed.

Convenience factors no longer are given as strong consideration as they once were because most if not all of the non-isotopic assays have been automated or are very amenable to automation. Still important, however, are sample volume, the time to first result, instrumental throughput (number of tests per hour), whether the assay requires manual sample pretreatment, costs of the assay and its analyzer, stability of reagents on and off the analyzer, frequency of calibration, and for RIA, radioactive waste disposal. The ideal assay should be performed quickly and cheaply, with very little operator hands-on time, with walk-away capability, and with a rapid data-reduction capability. The reagents would be stable for at least a year at room temperature or on board an automated system for at least 30 days. Finally, the calibration curve would be stable so that the assay would have to be recalibrated only when reagents had been changed or replaced.

Some of the most important performance factors are as follows:

1. Good assay response over the range of the standard curve.
2. A low background signal—that signal caused by nonspecific interactions of reagents in the assay or contributed by other substances in the samples. The background must be kept to a minimum to maximize S/N, detection limits, slope, and dynamic range.
3. High antibody affinity increases the slope of the dose-response curve and contributes to the sensitivity and detection limits of an assay. Sensitivity is related to the slope of the dose-response curve, to experimental error (accuracy and precision of the assay), and to the activity and detectability of the label.
4. Good precision and accuracy depend on the accuracy of the values used for the concentrations of standards or calibrators and on correct interpolation of the true shape of the dose-response curve between standards.
5. Specificity is determined by the ability of the antibody to discriminate between the ligand and similarly structured substances. In most cases, the screening and selection process for suitable antisera or monoclonal antibodies plays a very important part in determining antibody specificity. This is true for both native ligands (such as proteins) and the synthetic immunogens prepared to produce antibodies to low-molecular-weight substances.
6. Although some immunoassay interferences are related to antibody specificity, others that are contributed by the patient sample can affect either homogeneous or heterogeneous competitive-binding assays, or both.

For example, homogeneous assays may be influenced by endogenous binding proteins that could interfere with the immunoreaction or detection step. These may be removed by washing (heterogeneous method). Both types of immunoassay formats are subject to "heterophilic" antibody interferences from the patient sample. Heterophilic or endogenous antispecies antibodies can bind the assay antibody so that the signal is compromised. For example, human antimouse antibody (HAMA) will bind to the mouse immunoglobulin, coating the latex microparticle in a turbidimetric inhibition assay, with agglutination independent of the agglutinator, resulting in a falsely elevated signal. HAMA is commonly neutralized by the inclusion of excessive mouse immunoglobulin in the assay.

Table 9-9 compares some characteristics of previously described competitive-binding assays, and Table 9-10 lists some of the interferences. Heterogeneous assays have the greatest potential for sensitivity, with picomolar or lower detection limits. In addition to the high specific activities of radiolabels or enzyme labels, high-sensitivity fluorescent and luminescent labels are used routinely. Interferences that originate from substances in the sample or from impurities in the reagents are removed by the separation or wash step. Because it reduces the background signal, the heterogeneous proce-

Table 9-9 Characteristics of Some Competitive-Binding Assays

Immunoassay	Homogeneous or Heterogeneous	Detection Limit, M	Amplification	Low- or High-MW Ligands
CEDIA	Homogeneous	10^{-10}	Yes	Low
Chemiluminescence	Heterogeneous	10^{-13}	No	Both
ECL	Both	10^{-14}	Yes	Both
ELISA	Heterogeneous	10^{-11} to 10^{-15}	Yes	Both
EMIT	Homogeneous	5×10^{-10}	Yes	Low
FPIA	Homogeneous	5×10^{-9}	No	Low
Light scattering	Homogeneous	10^{-10}	No	Low
LOCI	Homogeneous	10^{-15}	No	Both
RIA	Heterogeneous	10^{-12} to 10^{-14}	No	Both
TRFI	Heterogeneous	10^{-12}	No	Both

CEDIA, Cloned-enzyme donor immunoassay; *ECL,* electrochemiluminescence; *ELISA,* enzyme-linked immunosorbent assay; *EMIT,* enzyme-multiplied immunoassay technique; *FPIA,* fluorescence polarization immunoassay; *MW,* molecular weight; *LOCI,* luminescent oxygen channeling assay; *RIA,* radioimmunoassay; *TRFI,* time-resolved fluorescence immunoassay.

dure also makes it possible to increase the volume of sample, which increases the sensitivity of the assay.

ELISA and the other non-isotopic immunoassays have many advantages, including the avoidance of radioisotope use. Because enzymes are biochemical amplifiers, systems that employ enzyme labels are capable of producing a greatly amplified signal, depending on the specific activity of the enzyme and the incubation time given for conversion of substrate to product. The use of fluorogenic or luminogenic substrates instead of chromogens can enhance the sensitivity of these assays 100 to 1000 times. Disadvantages of ELISA include the inconvenience of required washing steps compared with homogeneous assays, although available instruments automate these washing steps. Other factors are listed in Table 9-10.

The homogeneous enzyme immunoassay (enzyme-multiplied immunoassay technique, EMIT), although limited by absorbance of the product, is still sensitive to subnanomolar levels of ligand. EMIT and other methods that measure light absorbance are subject to possible interferences by hemolyzed, lipemic, and icteric samples. Because a rate measurement is used for EMIT, this method is difficult to perform manually but is quickly and easily accomplished with automated equipment. However, the assay is not suitable for high-molecular-weight ligands because antibody binding of the macromolecular enzyme conjugate does not provide sufficient enzyme inhibition for unlabeled ligand to elicit a response.

Fluorescence and luminescence assays are sensitive to subpicomolar concentrations of ligand, with chemiluminescent labels providing the greatest sensitivity. Homogeneous fluorescence assays avoid errors that can be introduced by the separation steps of heterogeneous systems. With the possible exception of the time-resolved fluoroimmunoassay, which is a heterogeneous assay, fluorescence assays are prone to interferences by hemolyzed, lipemic, and icteric samples. Possible sample interferences in homogeneous fluorescence immunoassays include light scattering from lipids and particulates, fluorescence quenching, and background fluorescence resulting from the presence of endogenous fluorophores. The fluorescence polarization immunoassay is sensitive to the depolarized scattered light of particulates in the assay and requires sophisticated instrumentation. Endogenous proteins may nonspecifically bind some fluorescein-labeled ligands, resulting in an increased polarization background.

CEDIA amplifies the signal because an active enzyme is generated in the assay. Unlike EMIT, antibody binds a ligand-label conjugate required to generate an active enzyme, rather than binding a ligand coupled to an enzyme that is already active. CEDIA, which has very high activity because of the generation of a high-turnover β-galactosidase label, would be more sensitive and would require a shorter incubation time if the antiligand antibody complex was a more effective inhibitor of the donor-acceptor complementation for generating active enzymes. In addition, both fluorogenic and luminogenic substrates are available for β-galactosidase, making this method readily adaptable to most automatic instrumentation.

Immunoassays based on electrochemiluminescence detection are versatile in that wash steps must be included in the format only if the assay sensitivity requires a separation step. ECL is capable of detecting subpicomolar levels of the label. In noncompetitive immunometric formats, the dynamic range can cover more than six orders of magnitude. The ruthenium complex labels are very stable, with shelf lives of over a year at room temperature. Finally, the assay can be rapidly performed on an automated system.

The luminescent oxygen channeling immunoassay is the most sensitive of the homogeneous immunoassays, similar in sensitivity to the most sensitive of the heterogeneous methods. Contributing to this high sensitivity is the very low background signal caused by the low diffusion of singlet oxygen to chemiluminescer particles not bound to sensitizer particles. The small particles, approximately 250 nm, provide for very fast kinetics and incubation times for some assays that can be as short as 3 minutes. Aside from human antispecies IgG antibodies (such as HAMA), the only endogenous interferent is ascorbic acid, which can react with singlet oxygen and lower the response. Normal plasma concentrations are much lower than those needed to cause significant inhibition.

Table 9-10 Some Potential Immunoassay Limitations and Interferences

Assay Type	Interferences/Limitations	Effect on Assay Response
Heterogeneous	Antibody or antigen deformation or steric hindrance at solid phase	Loss of binding affinity and capacity; reduces sensitivity
	Nonspecific binding of labeled conjugate to solid surfaces	Reduces S/N, sensitivity, detection limit
	Desorption of adsorbed binder	Loss of binding capacity over time; enhanced competitive response
	Conjugation of ligand or antibody to enzyme lowers its activity	Reduced signal that is compensated for by longer incubation times
	Increased enzyme labeling increases NSB	Lower S/N, sensitivity, detection limit
	Europium contamination with time-resolved fluorescence-labeled chelates	Increased background, lower S/N
Homogeneous	Increased sample background because of endogenous • Fluorescence • Spectral interferences • Label-like materials • Antibodies to label • Singlet oxygen scavengers	Lower S/N alleviated by dilution (which also lowers sensitivity) or by kinetic measurements (if appropriate)
General	Imprecision	Overall noise increases, thereby lowering S/N
	Exogenous substances	
	• Anticoagulants	Inhibit enzyme activity
	Endogenous substances	
	• Cross-reactants, metabolites	Increased signal response
	• Heterophilic antibodies, HAMA, rheumatoid factor	Bind antiligand antibody to simulate or interfere with normal response
	• Binding proteins—bind labeled ligand to decreased signal response	

From Nix B, Wild D: Calibration curve-fitting. In Wild D: *The Immunoassay Handbook*, Oxford, 2005, Elsevier.
HAMA, Human antimouse antibody; *NSB,* nonspecifically bound; *S/N,* signal-to-noise ratio.

Although the nephelometric inhibition immunoassay requires a special instrument, the turbidimetric inhibition method is applicable to most immunoassay and clinical automatic instrumentation. Although perhaps not so potentially sensitive as CEDIA and the homogeneous electrochemiluminescence immunoassay formats, in practice, this method is being used to quantitate lower-level analytes such as T_4 and digoxin.

KEY CONCEPTS BOX 9-4

- Enzyme-linked immunosorbent assay (ELISA), time-resolved fluorescence, and rapid assays are examples of heterogeneous formats.
- Enzyme-multiplied immnoassay technique (EMIT), fluorescence polarization immunoassay (FPIA), electrochemiluminescence (ECL), luminescent oxygen channeling immunoassay (LOCI), and rate nephelometric inhibition immunoassay (NINIA) are examples of homogeneous assays.
- Except for luminescent oxygen channeling immunoassay (LOCI), homogeneous assay detection limits generally are greater than those for heterogeneous assay methods.
- The heterogeneous assay wash steps remove many nonspecific sample interferences.
- Specific interferences such as those contributred by endogenous binding proteins can interfere with both heterogeneous and homogeneous assays.

BIBLIOGRAPHY

Immunoassays

Davies C: Introduction to immunoassays principles (Chapter 1) and Concepts (Chapter 6). In Wild D, editor: *The Immunoassay Handbook*, ed 3, Oxford UK, 2005, Elsevier Ltd.

Englebienne P: *Immune and Receptor Assays in Theory and Practice* (Chapters 4-6), Boca Raton, FL, 2000, CRC Press.

Gosling JP: *Immunoassays: A Practical Approach*, Oxford, UK, 2000, Oxford University Press.

Nix B, Wild D: Data processing. In Wild D: *The Immunoassay Handbook*, Oxford, 2005, Elsevier.

Price C, Newman D, editors: *Principles and Practices of Immunossays*, ed 2, New York, 1997, Stockton Press.

Price CP: The evolution of immunoassay as seen through the journal *Clinical Chemistry,* AACC 50th Anniversary Retrospective, Clin Chem 44:2071, 1998.

Enzyme Immunoassay

Hand C, Baldwin D: Immunoassays. In: Moffat A, Osselton MD, Widdop B, editors: *Clarke's Analysis of Drugs and Poisons,* ed 3, London, 2004, Pharmaceutical Press.

Porstmann T, Kiessig ST: Enzyme immunoassay techniques: an overview, J Immunol Methods 150:5, 1992.

Tijssen P: Practice and theory of enzyme immunoassays. In Burdon RH, van Knippenberg PH, editors: *Laboratory Techniques in Biochemistry and Molecular Biology,* vol 15, New York, 1985, Elsevier Science Publishing.

Enzyme-Linked Immunosorbent Assay (ELISA)

Avrameas S: Amplification systems in immunoenzymatic techniques, J Immunol Methods 150:23, 1992.

Lequin R: Enzyme immunoassay (EIA)/enzyme-linked immunosorbent assay (ELISA), Clin Chem 51:2415-2418, 2005.

Pesce AJ, Michael JG: Artifacts and limitations of enzyme immunoassay, J Immunol Methods 150:111, 1992.

Homogeneous Enzyme Immunoassay

Coty WA, Loor R: CEDIA, a homogeneous enzyme immunoassay system (Chapter 35). In Wild D, editor: *The Immunoassay Handbook*, ed 3, Oxford, UK, 2005, Elsevier Ltd.

Henderson DR, Friedman SB, Harris JD, et al: CEDIA, a new homogeneous immunoassay system, Clin Chem 32:1637, 1986.

Ullman EF: Homogeneous immunoassays (Chapter 12). In Wild D, editor: *The Immunoassay Handbook*, ed 3, Oxford, UK, 2005, Elsevier Ltd.

Immunoassay Interference

Kricka LJ: Interference in immunoassay—still a threat, Clin Chem 46:1037, 2000.

Levinson SS: The nature of heterophilic antibodies and their role in immunoassay interference, J Clin Immunoassay 15:108, 1992.

Pesce AJ, Michael JG: Artifacts and limitations of enzyme immunoassay, J Immunol Methods 150:111, 1992.

Valdes R Jr, Miller TI: Increasing the specificity of immunoassays, J Clin Immunoassay 15:87, 1992.

Time-Resolved Fluorescence Immunoassay

Diamandis EP: Multiple labeling and time-resolvable fluorophores, Clin Chem 37:1486, 1991.

Papanastasiou-Diamandis A, Christopoulos TK, Diamandis EP: Ultrasensitive thyrotropin immunoassay based on enzymatically amplified time-resolved fluorescence with a terbium chelate, Clin Chem 38:545, 1992.

Light-Scattering Assays

Newman DJ, Henneberry H, Price CP: Particle enhanced light scattering immunoassay, Ann Clin Biochem 29:22, 1992.

Luminescence Immunoassay

Blackburn GF, Shah HP, Kenten JH, et al: Electrochemiluminescence detection by development of immunoassays and DNA probe assays for clinical diagnostics, Clin Chem 37:1534, 1991.

Kricka LT: Chemiluminescent and bioluminescent techniques, Clin Chem 37:1472, 1991.

Ullman EF, Kirakossian H, Singh S, et al: Luminescent oxygen channeling immunoassay: measurement of particle binding kinetics by chemiluminescence, Proc Natl Acad Sci U S A 91:5426, 1994.

Ullman EF, Kirakossian H, Switchenko AC, et al: Luminescent oxygen channeling assay (LOCI): sensitive, broadly applicable homogeneous immunoassay method, Clin Chem 42:1518, 1996.

INTERNET SITES

www.curvefit.com/how_to_fit.htm—How to fit standard curves

Introduction to Immunoassays—http://www.abbottdiagnostics.com/Science/pdf/learning_immunoassay.pdf

http://www.elispot-analyzers.de/english/elisa-animation.html—active March 28, 2008

http://www.sumanasinc.com/webcontent/animations/content/ELISA.html—active March 28, 2008

http://www.waichung.demon.co.uk/webanim/Menu2.htm—active March 28, 2008

Laboratory Approaches to Serology Testing

Gerald P. Morris and Ann M. Gronowski

Chapter Outline

Key Terms

acute phase sample Serum sample taken at or near the time of onset of symptoms of infection.

affinity Measure of the binding strength of the antibody-antigen reaction.

agglutination Basic biochemical interaction that demonstrates the presence of antigen-specific antibody in classical serological reactions. Agglutination results from the formation of multimolecular lattice between antibodies and antigen molecules (or antigens complexed to larger carrier molecules or cells).

amnestic response Secondary antibody response when re-exposed to an antigen; has shorter lag phase, higher antibody titer, and more high-affinity IgG.

avidity Measure of the binding strength of antibodies to multiple antigenic determinants on natural antigens, which is a function of the affinity of the individual binding sites, as well as of the total number of binding sites in the molecule (e.g., two in IgG, IgA, IgE, and IgD; four in IgA dimers; and 10 in pentameric IgM).

complement fixation assay Assay designed to detect antibody to a specific pathogen through measurement of induction of complement-dependent lysis of red blood cells; antigen-specific Ab binds antigens and fixes complement, reducing the amount available to bind anti-RBC Abs.

convalescent phase sample Serum sample taken 3 to 4 weeks after initial presentation of illness. When compared with acute-phase samples, results can demonstrate a change in antibody response, indicative of infection.

cross-reactive antibodies Antibodies that recognize epitopes on multiple antigens (e.g., organisms).

ELISA The most common form of direct immunoassay; uses immobilized antigen in excess to capture antigen-specific antibodies from patient serum. Captured antibodies are measured by labeling with secondary enzyme-labeled anti-human immunoglobulin.

flocculation A type of agglutination reaction in which antigen-antibody complexes precipitate out of solution to form flakes.

IFA (indirect fluorescent antibody) Antibody detection technique whereby pathogen-specific antibodies are bound to killed and fixed pathogen, labeled with a secondary fluorophore-labeled anti-immunoglobulin antibody and visualized by fluorescent microscopy.

isotype Refers to the type of antibody as defined by the constant region of the antibody heavy chain. Antibodies have five isotypes—**IgM, IgD, IgG, IgE,** and **IgA**—which can be important to interpretation of serology results.

neutralization assay Demonstrates the presence of antibody by interference with a pathogenic mechanism. The most common neutralization assay currently in use is the **hemagglutinin inhibition (HAI)** assay, which inhibits agglutination of RBCs by viral hemagglutinins.

nontreponemal tests Serological assays sensitive for the diagnosis of syphilis, but not specific for *T. pallidum* antigens. The antigen recognized by nontreponemal tests is the phospholipid cardiolipin.

prozone phenomenon A rare, but important, source of false-negative reactions in serological testing that occur as the result of excess antibody and inhibition of lattice formation. This can be eliminated by dilution of suspected samples.

serology The study of noncellular immunological mediators in the serum. This term has become synonymous with measurement of antibody.

titer The lowest dilution of a serum sample that demonstrates immunological reactivity. Titer has limited utility in direct correlation with infection or protection but is useful primarily for comparing paired samples.

treponemal tests Serological assays sensitive for diagnosis of syphilis and specific for *T. pallidum* antigens.

Since the initial discovery of antibody response to infectious agents, measurement of this response, or serology, has played an important role in clinical medicine. The earliest serological assays of agglutination reactions and bactericidal activities were used to diagnose exposure to pathogens and still are used in the modern laboratory for the same purpose. The modern serology laboratory has added techniques such as nephelometry (see Chapter 2), immunofluorescence, and immunoblotting (see Chapter 8), which increase sensitivity, specificity, and throughput. Because many of the assays for serology can be performed with antigens bound to surfaces, similar to those of many other assays performed in the chemistry laboratory, and because these assays can be performed on similar if not the same instruments, many serology screening assays are currently performed in the chemistry, or core automated, laboratory. However, as we shall describe, confirmation is often performed with the use of specialized assays in a serology or immunology laboratory. Additionally, important performance and interpretive considerations in serology require a thorough understanding of the nature of antibodies, humoral immunity, and the performance of modern serological assays.

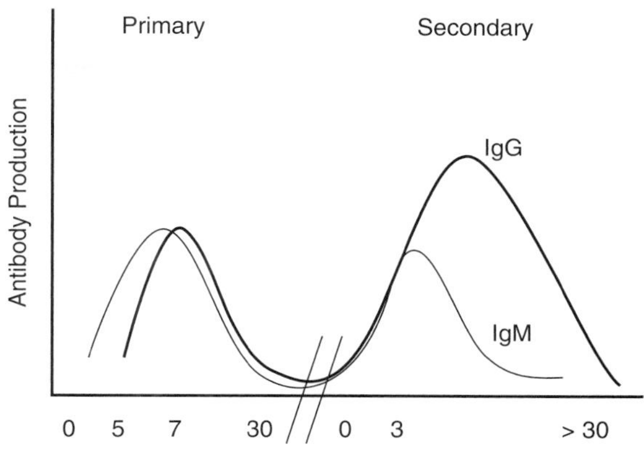

Fig. 10-1 Primary and secondary humoral immune responses. This figure illustrates the typical antibody response to exposure to antigen. Primary humoral immune responses are typified by the appearance of immunoglobulin (Ig)M within the first 3 to 5 days following exposure, followed by IgG production within the first week. Amnestic responses typically are mediated by IgG, which appears earlier (typically within 3 days) and in greater abundance than in a primary response.

SECTION OBJECTIVES BOX 10-1

- Define serology.
- List the classes of antibodies that constitute the humoral response.
- Describe the key concepts associated with clinical serological testing.
- Describe the principles of humoral immune responses, and explain how they relate to interpretation of serological testing.

HUMORAL IMMUNE RESPONSE

The term ***serology*** encompasses all noncellular immunological mediators in the serum; however, the term has become synonymous with measurement of antibody. The humoral immune system is capable of recognizing a vast array of diverse antigens, owing to the wide repertoire of antibodies, each with particular antigen specificity and **affinity.** The unique structure and function of antibodies[1] and their role in the humoral immune response are outlined in Chapter 7.

Although the antigen-binding properties of antibody molecules are defined entirely by the variable region, the constant regions can have important roles in mediating the effector functions of antibody and may be of interest in clinical evaluation. For light chains, there are two types of constant regions, κ and λ. The two types of light-chain constant regions are highly similar, differing by only a few amino acids, and no differences in their function are known. The constant regions of the heavy chains have greater diversity and more important correlations with the immunological function of the antibody. There are five main classes of heavy-chain constant regions—μ, δ, γ, ε, and α—which form the five classes, or **isotypes,** of antibodies—immunoglobulin (**Ig)M, IgD, IgG, IgE,** and **IgA,** respectively (IgG has four subclasses—IgG1, IgG2, IgG3, and IgG4).

The isotype identified is an important part of the interpretation of serology testing. For example, detection of IgM antibodies to a particular antigen implies recent exposure, as IgM antibodies are the first subclass produced during a primary humoral immune response. They typically have lower affinity for antigens but compensate through their pentameric structure, giving each IgM molecule 10 antigen binding sites, increasing the **avidity,** or stability, of the molecule for binding antigen. Over time, IgM is replaced by higher-affinity IgG antibodies, which dominate the latter portion of the primary immune response and subsequent **amnestic responses** (Fig. 10-1). IgG represents the majority of the humoral immune response; IgG antibodies are the largest portion of circulating antibodies by volume (≈80%), typically have the highest affinity for foreign antigens, and are the primary mediators of amnestic (remembered) humoral immune responses (see Fig. 10-1). IgA is the primary mediator of mucosal immunity but are detected at only low levels in serum. The physiological function of IgD is unclear, and detection of IgD is rarely clinically relevant, as it is present in only low concentrations in the circulation and has no known clinical significance. IgE is the primary mediator of allergic reactions, as the Fc region is recognized by mast cells and basophils, the primary mediators of allergic reactions. IgE production is stimulated greatly by some parasitic infections.

KEY CONCEPTS BOX 10-1

- Serology is the laboratory science of testing antibodies (immunoglobulin [Ig]) in serum. IgA, IgD, IgE, IgG, and IgM are the antibody classes produced by activated B lymphocytes. Each antibody has a tertiary structure that includes light and heavy chains.
- The humoral response to foreign antigen begins with the synthesis of IgM, which then is replaced with IgG. Both function in the blood. IgA functions in mucosa, and IgE works in blood against allergens.

SECTION OBJECTIVES BOX 10-2

- Define the term *titer,* and discuss its usefulness.
- Identify the basic types of serological methods, while describing the procedures of agglutination, complement fixation, enzyme-linked immunosorbent assay (ELISA), and direct antibody testing.
- List the advantages and potential interferences of each procedure listed above.
- List the "functional" assays that can be used to detect specific antibodies.
- Discuss the procedure performed to ensure a proper sample for serological testing.

APPLICATION OF SEROLOGY TO CLINICAL MEDICINE

Detection of Antibody

The basic function of serology is to define the presence or absence of antibodies to an antigen of interest, demonstrating exposure and subsequent immunological reaction. Serology can be done qualitatively or quantitatively, can be used for diagnosis or monitoring of disease, and can be performed by a variety of techniques that demonstrate binding of the antibody to a particular antigen.

As illustrated in Figure 10-1, antibody concentration and type change with time. Infectious agents comprise multiple antigens, and the host immune response to these antigens is time and antigen dependent. Serology techniques must be useful in detecting the host response to some of these antigens. It sometimes can be useful to determine the amount of antibody present. This is particularly useful when serum samples in a patient over time are compared; often, paired serum samples are required to differentiate between past exposure and vaccination (where antibody is persistent at low concentrations for a period of several years or longer) and recent infection that correlates with current disease. In these cases, an **acute phase sample** (taken at the time of patient presentation) is compared with a **convalescent-phase sample** (3 to 4 weeks following onset of symptoms).

Antibody quantity has been described historically by the term antibody **titer,** or the lowest dilution of a sample at which immunological reactivity is detectable by the method used. The term arose because historically it was not feasible to quantify the amount of reacting antibody; thus a comparable quantitative estimate was used. The question often arises as to whether a specific (typically high) titer can indicate an acute or ongoing infection, or whether a titer relates to immunological protection. The answer to both of these questions is no, as titer is not an independent indicator of humoral immunity. In some cases, there is a high basal titer for a specific antibody, which lessens the clinical significance of detection of a high titer antibody. Conversely, a low titer is often seen in acutely infected individuals who are not able to mount an appropriate immune response (i.e., immunosuppressed or immunodeficient). The only appropriate uses for titers are to establish a cutoff value for a serological test (many tests require a particular titer as a minimum for positivity because of performance issues of the assay or common low concentrations of antibody) and to compare consecutive serum samples from the same patient. In this last setting, at least a fourfold difference in titer between acute- and convalescent-phase sera is required to demonstrate active infection (the fourfold requirement represents the minimum accurately detectable analytical change). Comparison of titers in acute and convalescent sera is routinely used in the diagnosis of *Rickettsia* (Rocky Mountain spotted fever), *Mycoplasma*, leptospirosis, and brucellosis.

Thus the term titer is becoming antiquated, as modern assays typically are reported as positive/negative or describe the concentration of antibody present in terms of weight per volume. For enzyme-linked immunosorbent assays (ELISAs), individual manufacturers' package inserts should be consulted to determine whether acute and convalescent samples can be compared. Usually, a quantitative kit-specific formula is provided, and both samples should be analyzed at the same time to avoid differences between kits.

Agglutination Reactions

Among the most basic techniques used to demonstrate the presence of antibodies are **agglutination** reactions (see Chapter 8). Clinically, agglutination reactions are limited to a relatively narrow window of antigen concentration relative to antibody; if either the antibody or the antigen is in too great of excess, the lattice will not form optimally, and thus the agglutination reaction will not be visualized. This can lead to false-negative reactions when large amounts of antibody are present, a phenomenon known as the **hook effect** or the **prozone phenomenon.**[2] False negatives resulting from the prozone phenomenon can be corrected simply by diluting the serum sample and retesting. This type of false-negative reaction is uncommon but has been documented in rapid plasma reagin (RPR) tests for syphilis in patients with HIV.[3] As with all testing, the results of agglutination-based serology always should be evaluated in the context of the overall clinical setting.

Agglutination reactions are visualized by two principle methods—**flocculation** and **precipitation.** Flocculation reactions can be visualized by formation of antigen and antibody complexes in solution, resulting in microscopically or macroscopically visible clumps; the difference is that in agglutination reactions, the complexes sediment, and in flocculation reactions, they float in solution. The antigen can be attached to cells (as is the case when whole bacteria or antigens adsorbed onto red blood cells are used) or large microparticles (such as charcoal or fluorophores) for visualization, or they can be quantified by the use of nephelometric techniques. Attaching antigens to larger particles increases the sensitivity of agglutination reactions by 10- to 100-fold.[4] Agglutination reactions have been used widely because they are simple to perform, requiring only mixing of diluted patient serum and antigen preparation, and they are simple to interpret. However, they are manual procedures, so laboratories are changing toward higher-throughput automated assays.

In precipitation reactions, formation of the antigen-antibody lattice is visualized by the formation of aggregates in a gel or in solution.[5] Again, these assays are relatively simple to perform and interpret, although they are time- and labor-intensive, and laboratories continue to change toward higher-throughput assays.

Immunofluorescence

Antibodies to pathogen-specific antigens can be observed directly with the use of a fluorescently labeled secondary antibody (**indirect fluorescent antibody** [**IFA**]). The IFA technique uses a standard laboratory strain of pathogen (killed and heat- or formalin-fixed to a microscope slide) as the source of antigen to which patient serum is added. The sample then is washed from the slide, and a secondary fluorophore-labeled anti-immunoglobulin antibody is added to label any patient antibody that is bound to the pathogen. The fluorescent label is visualized under fluorescent microscopy, and the association of the fluorescent label with the pathogen demonstrates the presence of pathogen-specific antibody. IFA is relatively sensitive and has good specificity, although there are technical considerations, such as qualified personnel to interpret the staining and adequate washing to reduce nonspecific background staining, that require special technical training. Still, IFA is used widely because of its specificity and relative rapidity for diagnosis of infections with a variety of pathogens, including *Borrelia burgdorferi*[6] and *Treponema pallidum*,[7] and several viruses such as varicella, herpesviruses, and respiratory syncytial virus.[8]

Functional Assays

The presence of antibodies in serum also can be determined through observation of their immunological effector functions. One of the primary effector functions of immunoglobulin is to attract and activate the complement cascade on the surface of pathogens for lysis. **Complement fixation assays** have been in use in serology since the early 1900s (see Chapter 8). Complement fixation is used currently for a variety of pathogens, particularly fungal pathogens such as *Blastomyces, Coccidioides,* and *Histoplasma.*

The presence of pathogen-specific antibodies can be evaluated by examining their ability to inhibit pathogen functions. **Neutralization assays** demonstrate the presence of antibody by interfering with a pathogenic mechanism. The most common neutralization currently in use is the **hemagglutinin inhibition** (**HAI**) assay. Several viruses (notably influenza, adenoviruses, measles, mumps and rubella viruses, and arboviruses) possess adhesion molecules that enable adhesion and entry into cells, and that have the distinct property of agglutinating red blood cells (RBCs) in vitro. The reduction of RBC agglutination by exogenous viral antigen in the presence of sample serum demonstrates the presence of antigen-specific antibodies. Other measures of the neutralizing effects of pathogen-specific antibodies, such as plaque reduction assays (a measure of inhibiting viral infection of cultured cell lines) and toxin inhibition assays (such as *Clostridium tetani* or *Bacillus anthracis*), have been used previously but have fallen out of use in most laboratories because of the complicated nature of these assays, the difficulty associated with interpretation, and the fact that often paired sera are required to distinguish recent from previous exposures. However, an important exception is influenza, for which the HAI remains the gold standard, particularly in laboratories that use serotyping for epidemiological studies. Influenza strains are characterized by their use of one of sixteen hemagglutinin (HA) genes and one of nine neuraminidase genes; typically, only HA1 or HA3 has been observed to cause human disease, although recent human disease caused by avian influenza strains bearing HA5, HA7, or HA9 have led to increased interest in monitoring atypical HA gene usage by influenza.[9]

Direct Immunoassays

Classical serological techniques demonstrate the presence of antigen-specific antibodies by measuring the results of their binding to a target and forming an antigen-antibody complex, which can be measured by its physical properties (e.g., precipitation, increased molecular weight), or by demonstrating an effect of the antibody on the pathogen. However, these techniques have relatively limited sensitivity, often have poorly defined specificity, do not enable determination of the absolute amount of antibody present, are time-consuming and labor-intensive, and do not permit discrimination between immunoglobulin subclasses. All of these limitations are addressed through the use of direct immunoassay; direct immunoassays demonstrate the presence of specific antibodies by using an antigen-coated surface to bind, or capture, specific antibodies in patient sera, which then are labeled with the use of an enzyme-, fluorophore-, or radiolabeled secondary anti-immunoglobulin antibody.

The most common form of direct immunoassay is the **enzyme-linked immunosorbent assay** (**ELISA**). The ELISA method uses immobilized antigen (with the antigen in excess) to capture antigen-specific antibodies from patient serum. Following incubation with patient serum, there is a wash step, and a secondary enzyme-labeled antihuman immunoglobulin is added. The secondary antibody can be pan-immunoglobulin specific or can be specific for any of the immunoglobulin subclasses; as was discussed previously, examination for particular classes of antibodies also can provide specific information, particularly as related to the temporal relationship between exposure and immune response (recent primary infections elicit IgM as opposed to later primary or secondary responses, which are dominated by IgG). Following a wash step, bound antibody is detected by the addition of substrate that produces a colorimetric or fluorometric indicator. Use of ELISA has grown in the clinical serology laboratory because of its typically high sensitivity and specificity, high throughput, and increased precision, as well as the avoidance of radioactive substances.

The other type of direct immunoassay frequently used in clinical serology laboratories is the **immunoblot,** including the Western blot (see Chapter 8).

The primary utility of Western blots in modern serology laboratories is associated with their high specificity, which is a result of separation of multiple specific antigens by size on a single membrane. This allows detection of particular antigen-specific antibodies while permitting dismissal of cross-reactive or noninformative antibodies. Currently, Western blot testing is the gold standard technique for many clinically important infections, including human immunodeficiency virus (HIV) and Lyme disease. Most Western blots used in clinical serology laboratories are commercial kits that come with the antigens pre-adsorbed onto the nitrocellulose membrane, reducing variability and increasing assay standardization. However, Western blot assays are often difficult to interpret and require specialized training, specific to each assay.

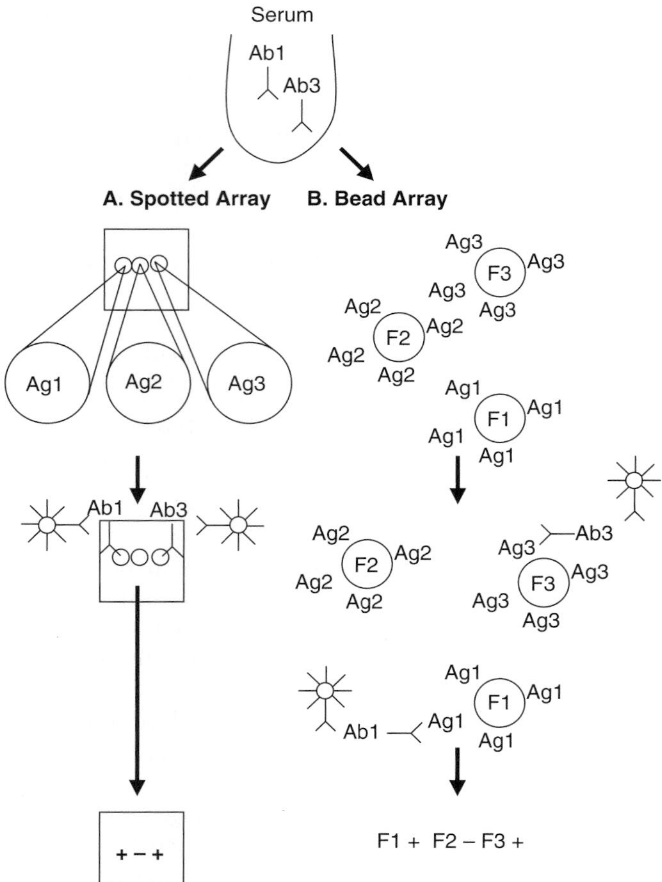

Fig. 10-2 Multiplexed serological testing. Multiplexed serological assays can be categorized into two broad categories. **A,** Microspotted arrays are sandwich immunoassays with individual antigens bound to small areas (<80 μm in diameter) on a polystyrene microchip. A single serum sample then is tested against the entire repertoire of antigens on the chip; antibodies that recognize antigens bind to specific areas of the chip and are labeled with a secondary fluorophore-labeled antibody. The pattern of fluorophore labeling on the chip is read by a laser scanner and is decoded to reveal the antibodies present in the serum sample. **B,** Bead-based arrays utilize multiple individual antigens bound to microspheres that can be differentiated on the basis of size or fluorophore labeling. Patient antibodies are labeled with a secondary fluorophore-labeled antibody, and the pattern of fluorophore labeling is analyzed by flow cytometry.

Multiplex and Array Assays

As in virtually all other areas of clinical laboratory analysis, there has been much interest in the development of new technologies to improve the throughput of serological assays. One way this has been addressed is by the development of multiplex serological tests (tests that measure multiple antibody specificities in a single assay). Multiplex serological assays can be categorized into two broad categories—microspotting or sectioning of antigens onto a microchip, and bead-based arrays (Fig. 10-2). Microspotted arrays are sandwich immunoassays with antigens bound to small areas (<80 μm in diameter) on a polystyrene microchip. Multiple antigens are combined on a single chip and bind multiple specific antibodies in specified areas of the microchip. Antibodies from patient serum are labeled with fluorophore-labeled anti-immunoglobulin antibodies, and the chip is scanned by an automated system to detect bound antibody.[10] Bead-based arrays are similar in concept, although they use multiple individual antigens bound to microspheres that can be differentiated on the basis of size or fluorophore labeling. Again, the basic concept is a sandwich immunoassay, with the amount of antibody binding to specific beads read by a flow cytometer.[11] Assays that use these techniques have been developed to examine several antibody specificities for a single pathogen such as EBV,[12] or to determine the presence of antibodies to multiple pathogens in a related diagnosis such as congenital infections[13] or common causes of infectious endocarditis. These multiplexed assays have demonstrated performance similar to ELISA, and they offer advantages in throughput that are useful to clinical laboratories.

Special Considerations

As with all laboratory testing, serological testing is dependent on proper sample collection, handling, and testing. Optimal specimens for serological testing are serum specimens collected by venipuncture into serum collection tubes. Following clot formation at room temperature, the serum should be separated within 2 hours. Serum samples can be stored at 4°C for several days until use, although storage for longer periods (often required in serology for paired samples) requires freezing of the sample at −20°C, thus avoiding repeated freeze/thaw cycles.[14] Serological testing should be performed at room temperature, unless otherwise indicated, as temperature affects the binding of antigen by antibody. Antigen binding also is affected by pH and ionic composition of the buffer, and these should be kept consistent.[15] Additionally, very high concentrations of an antibody can cause false-negative results (prozone effect), and these can be addressed by simple dilution of the serum sample (usually 1:100 or greater). False-positive results can arise from **cross-reactive antibodies,** or antibodies that recognize epitopes that are present on organisms other than the pathogen of interest. This type of interference can be addressed by adsorption of the test serum with nonspecific or potentially cross-reactive antigens prior to serological testing.

KEY CONCEPTS BOX 10-2

- *Antibody titer* is a term that is used to express the amount of antibody (Ab) in a sample. The higher the dilution needed to get a specific response, the greater is the Ab level, or titer. Titers provide little information regarding a patient's immune responsiveness to re-exposure to an antigen (Ag), and most assays report qualitative results. Titers have limited use today.
- Agglutination procedures (direct and indirect) employ the Ab-Ag reaction that causes agglutination, or precipitation, of the complexes. By attaching the reaction to cells or microparticles, the assays can become quantitative.
- Attaching Ag to red blood cells (RBCs) allows the reaction of Ab, in the presence of complement, with coated cells to be detected by lysis (direct) or absence of lysis (indirect) in the complement fixation assay.
- Specific Abs can be detected by various immunoassays, including enzyme-linked immunosorbent assay (ELISA) and immunometric (sandwich) assays. The latter are the most widely used assays because they have the advantages of being highly automated and very sensitive.
- Serum samples for serological testing should be centrifuged promptly and stored at 4°C and analysis performed at close to room temperature.

SECTION OBJECTIVES BOX 10-3

- State the methods, interpretation, and appropriateness of test utilization for serological tests commonly performed in clinical laboratories for the following:
  - Syphilis
  - Lyme disease
  - Peptic ulcer disease
  - HIV (human immunodeficiency virus)
  - Congenital (TORCH [TOxoplasma, Rubella, Cytomegalovirus, Herpes]) infections
  - Capsular polysaccharide antigen response

CURRENT CLINICAL APPLICATIONS

The clinical utility of serology, including important interpretive considerations, can best be illustrated by examination of a small number of current applications in the clinical laboratory.

Syphilis

Syphilis is a sexually transmitted disease caused by infection with *Treponema,* subspecies *pallidum* (referred to hereafter as *T. pallidum*). Syphilis initially manifests as a painless solitary lesion, or chancre, typically on the genital area, that forms at between 10 and 90 days after infection, and that usually resolves spontaneously in 1 to 6 weeks. This initial infection and resulting symptoms are referred to as *primary syphilis.* If untreated, the organism disseminates and, following an asymptomatic period of 1 to 5 weeks, causes a systemic infection that manifests as generalized rash, fever, and arthralgia. This systemic infection, secondary syphilis, lasts for 2 weeks to 1 year. Following secondary syphilis, the infection becomes latent for a number of years, during which the bacteria persist though a low-level infection. Approximately 35% of patients with latent syphilis will develop neurological symptoms, including headache, ataxia, focal deficits, and delirium known as *tertiary syphilis.*[16]

Microscopic detection of *T. pallidum* in fluid from lesions consistent with syphilis is diagnostic for primary and secondary syphilis. Direct detection of the pathogen is difficult as typical microscopic techniques do not allow direct visualization (special techniques of dark-field or fluorescent-labeled microscopy are required) and the organism cannot be cultured under standard laboratory conditions. However, there is a need to diagnose syphilis in patients without current chancres, whether prior to the development of primary disease or during latent infection. Serological testing remains the principal means of diagnosis of syphilis, and serological tests are broken into one of two categories—nontreponemal or treponemal—depending on the antigen specificity tested.

Nontreponemal tests refer to those serological assays that are sensitive for the diagnosis of syphilis but not specific for *T. pallidum* antigens. The antigen recognized by nontreponemal tests has been demonstrated to be the phospholipid cardiolipin,[17] a discovery that enabled standardization of nontreponemal assays. Currently, two standard nontreponemal tests primarily in use in the United States are the Venereal Disease Research Laboratory (VDRL) test[18] and the rapid plasma reagin (RPR) test.[19,20] Both tests are based on binding of phospholipid antigens by antibodies in the patient serum, with differences noted in the agent used to visualize the antigen and antibody binding; VDRL demonstrates binding by a flocculation reaction, resulting in formation of small particulate clumping; RPR uses charcoal particles to make the flocculation reaction easier to read. All of the standard nontreponemal tests have similar sensitivities and specificities for all stages of syphilis; sensitivities of 78% to 86% for primary, 100% for secondary, and 95% to 98% for latent syphilis, and specificities of 98% to 99%.[21] Serum is the specimen of choice for both nontreponemal and treponemal tests. RPR also can be performed with the use of plasma, but the VDRL test cannot, because the sample must be heated prior to use in VDRL testing. Nontreponemal tests will become positive 1 to 4 weeks following chancre formation during acute infection and will fade slowly with successful treatment, becoming negative

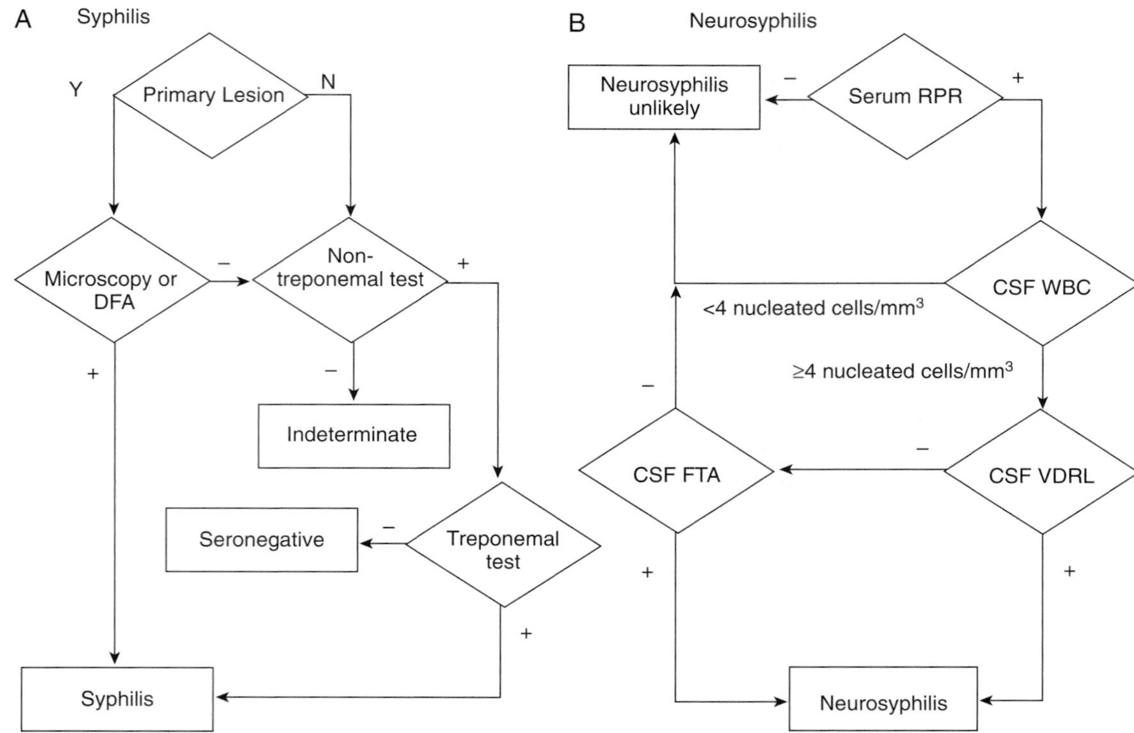

Fig. 10-3 Serological diagnosis of syphilis and neurosyphilis. **A,** Diagnosis of syphilis in the absence of a detectable organism in a primary lesion depends on serological diagnosis; serodiagnosis begins with a screening test, typically a nontreponemal antibody to demonstrate recent or active infection, and is followed by a treponemal test for specificity. **B,** Diagnosis of neurosyphilis should begin with a serum rapid nontreponemal test (such as plasma reagin [RPR] or a treponemal test to demonstrate prior exposure to *Treponema pallidum.* Evaluation of the cerebrospinal fluid (CSF) should begin with a count of nucleated cells in the white blood cells (WBCs) and should be followed by a fluorescent treponemal antibody test (FTA) for maximal specificity. Limited sensitivity of the FTA on CSF (30%) indicates that negative results should be followed by a Venereal Disease Research Laboratory test (VDRL) on CSF. *DFA,* Direct fluorescent antibody.

within 2 years of elimination of infection. All of the nontreponemal tests have the same sources of error; false-negative reactions occur in 1% to 2% of serum samples from patients with secondary syphilis[2] attributable to prozone reactions,[3] and false positives occur as the result of typical conditions that interfere with serological testing, including transient increases in immunoglobulins such as infectious mononucleosis, viral infections, or chronic conditions such as systemic lupus erythematosus or malignancy.[22]

The lack of specificity of nontreponemal tests necessitates confirmatory testing for all positive samples. **Treponemal tests,** serological tests specific for *T. pallidum* antigens, were developed for this purpose. Currently, three treponemal tests are in use—the fluorescent treponemal antibody test (FTA), the *T. pallidum* particle agglutination test (TP-TA), and the enzyme immunoassay (EIA). The FTA test demonstrates *T. pallidum*–specific antibodies by IFA of killed *T. pallidum;* however, non–*T. pallidum*–specific antibodies are first absorbed from the test serum with use of the sonicated Reiter treponeme (containing the cross-reactive antigens).[23,24] The TP-TA assay is an agglutination assay that uses *T. pallidum*–sensitized gelatin beads[25] and often is considered easier to perform, because there is no absorption step and no requirement for fluorescent microscopy. Newer ELISA treponemal tests have been developed with the use of *T. pallidum* sonicates or recombinant antigens; these offer the advantages of being automated and of demonstrating increased sensitivity and specificity.[26] The specificity of treponemal tests makes them useful for confirmation of exposure to *T. pallidum,* although they are limited in discerning current infection from past exposure. As in the case of many infectious agents, once a patient seroconverts, he or she remains positive for life.

Nontreponemal and treponemal tests are used in combination with clinical history in diagnosing syphilis at all stages. As was mentioned, microscopy is the gold standard for diagnosis of primary or secondary syphilis, although serology can be used in combination (Fig. 10-3, *A*); a reactive treponemal test in persons with no previous exposure or a fourfold increase in the titer of a reactive nontreponemal test as compared with the most recent previous result provides supporting evidence when microscopy does not reveal *T. pallidum.* Serology is the only method used for diagnosis of latent syphilis; seroconversion or a fourfold increase in the titer of a reactive nontreponemal test supports a diagnosis of latent syphilis.

Special consideration should be given to the diagnosis of **neurosyphilis** (Fig. 10-3, *B*) because the clinical symptoms are similar to those of many other diseases.[27] A nontreponemal or treponemal test should be the first test used for neurosyphilis to demonstrate exposure to *T. pallidum,* and an elevated count of nucleated cells in cerebrospinal fluid (CSF) (lymphocytosis of >4 cells/mm^3) should be used to demonstrate central nervous system (CNS) infection. If both of these are negative, the likelihood of neurosyphilis is extremely low, although there may be mitigating circumstances (poor antibody response in immunocompromised patients such as those with HIV[28] or a remote history of infection), and the entire clinical picture should be considered. If both are positive, then VDRL can be performed on CSF. Of particular note is that the VDRL test is the only test that can be used with CSF samples to investigate neurosyphilis, and the CSF sample is not heated as in the VDRL performed on serum.[22] The specificity of VDRL for neurosyphilis is near 100%, although its sensitivity is limited (50%). A positive result does not require confirmatory treponemal testing. Negative results should be followed by an FTA on CSF for increased sensitivity (near 100%). However, positive FTAs should be interpreted with caution as false positives can occur with as little as 5 μL of serum contamination.

Lyme Disease

Lyme borreliosis, or Lyme disease, is the syndrome that may follow infection with *Borrelia burgdorferi,* a spirochete transmitted by the bite of the *Ixodes* tick. Infection with *B. burgdorferi* typically begins with the appearance of erythema migrans, an annular rash at the site of the tick bite pathognomonic (indicative) for *B. burgdorferi* infection, and it may be accompanied by general signs of infection such as fever, headache, malaise, and arthralgia. The symptoms of primary infection typically resolve within 4 weeks, at which time, if left untreated, the organism disseminates to several organ systems, giving rise to a variety of symptoms that often include more severe symptoms from the primary infection, as well as meningitis, facial nerve palsy, and endocarditis. Late-stage Lyme disease occurs years after the initial infection and is typified by arthritis and neuropathy or encephalomyelitis.[29]

Diagnosis of Lyme disease is problematic, in that the symptoms (other than erythema migrans) are diffuse generalized symptoms that are similar to those of several other diseases, and they often occur well after the time of the initial tick bite and infection. Furthermore, *B. burgdorferi* is often present in very low numbers in lesions, making direct detection by microscopy or antigen assays poorly sensitive. Direct detection of *B. burgdorferi* in tissue samples from lesion sites has been enhanced by polymerase chain reaction (PCR) but has no benefit for diagnosis in patients with disseminated late Lyme disease.[6] *B. burgdorferi* cannot be cultured by routine clinical microbiological techniques; it has poor sensitivity (≈50%), takes as long as 6 weeks, and is performed only in Centers for Disease Control and Prevention (CDC) reference laboratories, limiting its use in clinical diagnosis. The difficulty associated with direct pathogen detection has made serology the primary method for diagnosis of Lyme disease.

Serodiagnosis of Lyme disease is complicated by the fact that *B. burgdorferi* has a large number of immunologically reactive antigens that are cross-reactive with other bacteria, as well as mammalian tissues. Furthermore, the pattern of antibody recognition changes during the course of infection.[6] Early infection is marked by antibody recognition of outer membrane protein OspC (p35) and flagellar proteins FlaA (p37) and FlaB (p41). These antibodies may be either IgM or IgG, as IgM responses can persist for months following infection and treatment, and the IgG response begins within the first weeks following disease onset. As infection progresses, *B. burgdorferi* modulates expression of antigens, which results in characteristic alterations in the antibody repertoire; IgG specific for BmpA (p39) and p58 are diagnostic in disseminated Lyme disease, and late-stage Lyme disease is characterized by a broad range of IgG recognizing OspA (p31), OspB (p35), OspC (p21), p28, p30, FlaA (p37), FlaB (p41), p45, p58, p66, and p93.[30,31] Of note are two antibody specificities that have been reported to correlate directly with specific symptoms—OspA in late-stage Lyme disease with arthritis,[32] and VlsE in late disease with neurological symptoms.[33]

Several methods are used for serodiagnosis of Lyme disease; serodiagnosis of Lyme disease is done through a two-tiered approach that combines the initial screening test of IFA or ELISA with a confirmatory Western blot.[34] IFA for IgM or IgG against fixed *B. burgdorferi* has demonstrated good sensitivity, and specificity is enhanced by adsorption of cross-reactive antibodies from patient sera by incubation with the Reiter treponeme prior to incubation with fixed *B. burgdorferi* (sera reactive at ≥1:64 are considered positive if adsorbed prior to IFA, and a titer of ≥1:256 is required if the serum is unadsorbed).[35,36] ELISA is the more common method used to screen for Lyme disease. Current ELISA kits suffer from lack of standardization of antigens, because most commonly, they are derived from sonicates of cultured *B. burgdorferi* (subject to antigenic variation, as well as containing several cross-reactive antigens), but newer commercial kits that use purified or recombinant antigens, which enhance specificity and reproducibility, are available.[37] Both IFA and ELISA have good sensitivity, and negative results are considered to exclude a diagnosis of Lyme disease. However, positive results with either should be followed by confirmatory testing by Western blot (Fig. 10-4). The use of Western blot enables examination of several *B. burgdorferi*–specific antigens, making it highly specific and enabling examination of antibodies to particular antigens, which differ at various stages of infection. Current criteria for a positive Western blot include IgM reactivity of at least two of OspC, BmpA, or Fla,[31] or IgG reactivity of five of p18, OspC, p28, p30, BmpA, Fla, p45, p58, p66, or p93.[30] The complex nature of the time variation in antigen specificity in the antibody repertoire and the appearance of cross-reactive bands require a high degree of training in interpretation of Western blot results. Both ELISA and Western blot can be used for diagnosis of neuroborreliosis from CSF. Comparison of CSF concentrations of IgG to serum IgG can be helpful in determining intrathecal production of antibody; a ratio of (CSF specific antibody × Serum total IgG)/(Serum specific antibody × CSF total IgG) ≥1.3 is indicative of intrathecal production.[38]

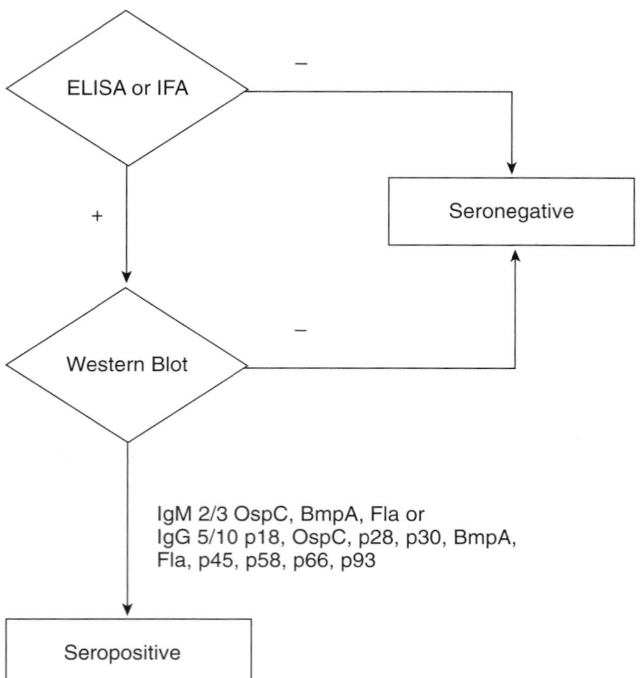

Fig. 10-4 Two-tiered serodiagnosis of Lyme disease. Serodiagnosis of Lyme disease is performed in a two-tiered manner to maximize sensitivity and specificity. Screening can be done by indirect fluorescent antibody (IFA) or enzyme-linked immunosorbent assay (ELISA), and negative results are considered to exclude a diagnosis of Lyme disease. Positive results should be followed by Western blot for specificity. Negative serodiagnosis in the setting of high clinical suspicion warrants repeat testing on a new serum sample.

Peptic Ulcer Disease

The identification of *Helicobacter pylori* as the causative agent of peptic ulcer disease in 1982 enabled a drastic change in the management of peptic ulcer disease; rather than symptomatic treatment, antibiotics could directly eliminate the causative agent.[39] Infection with *H. pylori* can be demonstrated in several ways, including direct pathogen detection on gastric epithelium biopsy (by culture or nucleic acid detection), measurement of urea production by organisms (urea breath test), and serology. Current recommendations are to use noninvasive tests such as the urea breath test or serology in all patients younger than 45 years of age, while older patients (with a higher prevalence of *H. pylori* infection) should have an upper endoscopy with biopsy for direct pathogen detection.[40] Serology traditionally has ranked as a third choice behind the urea breath test and the stool antigen test for noninvasive diagnosis of *H. pylori* infection. However, serology offers several special considerations that can make it a good choice for diagnosis. Serology is sensitive, in that 98% of infected patients seroconvert,[41] and it is particularly useful, in that patients treated with proton pump inhibitors (a common situation because of their over-the-counter availability) may have falsely negative urea breath tests. However, serology is not appropriate in all settings; high rates of seropositivity in older (>55 years of age) adults and in developing countries decrease the predictive value of the positive test, reducing the utility of serodiagnosis. Additionally, serology has limited benefit in monitoring the efficacy of treatment; several studies have suggested that a 25% decrease in titer may be significant, although antibodies to *H. pylori* may persist for months to years following successful treatment, and continued seropositivity may not reflect treatment failure.[42,43]

ELISA is the method of choice for the serological detection of *H. pylori* infection. Early ELISAs used whole cell sonicates, although this presented difficulty with high background and false-positive reactions, particularly caused by cross-reactivity with *Campylobacter.* To avoid these interferences, most commercially available ELISAs use a proprietary mixture of specific antigens and now routinely achieve sensitivities of >90% and specificities of >95%. Additionally, specificity for a particular antigen, CagA, has been correlated with peptic ulcer disease, gastric adenocarcinoma, and atrophy and often is included in commercial ELISA kits.

HIV

Human immunodeficiency virus (HIV), the causative agent of acquired immunodeficiency syndrome (AIDS), is a relatively newly emerged pathogen that quickly has become one of the leading causes of morbidity and mortality throughout the world. Since the description of the first patient with AIDS in 1981, HIV has spread to more than 37.8 million persons throughout the world, predominantly through sexual contact, but also through transfusion of contaminated blood products, sharing of contaminated needles by intravenous drug abusers, and maternal transmission to neonates. Although advances have been made in the treatment of HIV infection, there is no cure, and the focus of HIV has been on prevention and early diagnosis. Most new cases of HIV transmission occur through sexual contact, frequently when the infected person is unaware of his or her HIV status and is practicing high-risk behavior (such as having multiple sex partners). Furthermore, current treatments are much more efficacious during early infection, thus preventing progression to AIDS, than in later stages of disease. For these reasons, recent public health initiatives have suggested universal routine screening for HIV, replacing older recommendations for testing only high-risk populations.[44] Currently, the recommended testing strategy for diagnosing HIV infection consists of screening with either ELISA on serum or rapid point-of-care testing on buccal swab, followed by confirmatory IFA or Western blot (Fig. 10-5).[45]

Antibodies specific to HIV proteins typically can be detected within 1 to 8 weeks following exposure. The primary antigens targeted in the humoral immune response are the HIV envelope proteins gp120 and gp41, the envelope precursor protein gp160, the HIV polymerase proteins p10 (protease), p31 (endonuclease-integrase), and p66 (reverse transcriptase), the core proteins p7 (nucleocapsid), p18 (matrix), and p24 (internal capsid), and the core protein precursor p55. ELISA is the standard screening test because of its high sensitivity (>99.5%) and low false-negative rate (<1/40,000).[46] ELISA testing for HIV previously used viral lysates as target antigens, although

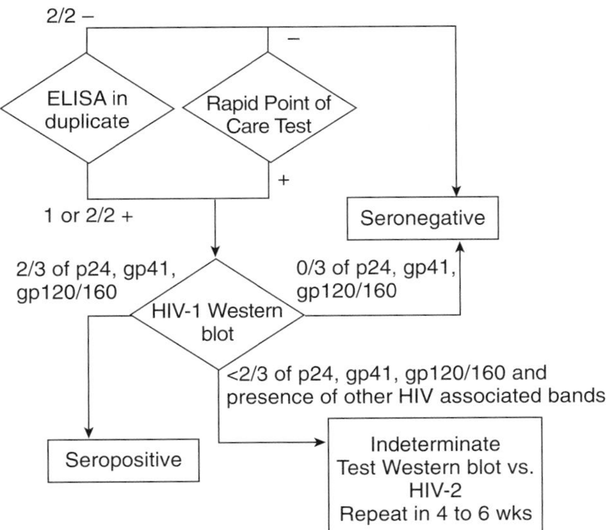

Fig. 10-5 Serological diagnosis of human immunodeficiency virus (HIV). Serodiagnosis of HIV begins with a screening assay of either an enzyme-linked immunosorbent assay (ELISA) or a rapid point-of-care device. A positive finding on either of these should be followed by confirmation by Western blot to HIV-1. Negative or indeterminate results should be tested by Western blot against HIV-2 and HIV-1 serotype O, and follow-up testing should be considered in 4 to 6 weeks.

most commercial kits now use recombinant proteins as target antigens, increasing reproducibility and interassay correlation. However, a drawback of the use of recombinant antigens is the more limited antigen repertoire, which has been implicated in false-negative results with HIV-1 subtype O infections. Most current HIV ELISAs use enzyme-labeled anti-IgG immunoglobulin as the label, although inclusion of anti-IgM has been reported to increase sensitivity in early infection. Newer, third-generation assays have been developed that use HIV antigens bound to the solid phase to capture HIV-specific antibodies, as well as enzyme-labeled antigens, to label the bound antibodies, primarily for detection of multiple HIV-specific antibody isotypes, and to reduce false-positive results from autoantibodies. ELISA also has a relatively high sensitivity (99.8%), but because of the number of samples tested, as well as the implications of a positive diagnosis, confirmatory testing is required.

Although ELISA is relatively simple in the context of a clinical serological laboratory, it remains too complex for use in developing countries, where HIV transmission is at its highest. For this reason, as well as to attempt to expand HIV testing availability to persons who may have limited health care access, and to provide rapid HIV results in acute care settings, rapid HIV immunoassays have been developed. These devices are lateral-flow devices that use recombinant HIV antigens to capture HIV-specific antibodies from serum or buccal swab, and colloidal gold-labeled detection antibodies capable of providing highly sensitive (>99.6%) and specific (>99.1%) results in minutes.[47] Confirmatory testing is recommended for all point-of-care HIV testing.[45]

Even though screening ELISAs and lateral-flow devices have relatively high specificities, confirmatory testing is required because of the low prevalence of HIV in low-risk populations, which results in a relatively high false-positive rate. Western blot is the most widely used HIV confirmatory test. HIV testing performed by Western blot is similar to other Western blot tests, although interpretation has important considerations. Western blot for HIV is subtype specific, and separate blots should be used for HIV-1 and HIV-2. Additionally, there is disagreement as to what degree of reactivity is required for a positive result; CDC guidelines suggest interpretation as positive for those sera that demonstrate reaction to two of p24, gp41, and gp120/gp160.[45] Furthermore, a negative result is assigned only to sera that demonstrate no reaction with known HIV proteins, while the appearance of any positive bands results in an indeterminate result, which requires retesting on a new serum sample in 4 to 6 weeks.

Epstein-Barr Virus

Epstein-Barr virus (EBV) is a human herpesvirus that is associated with a variety of diseases. Infection in infants and very young children is typically asymptomatic. In young adults, EBV infection often results in the most commonly associated disease, infectious mononucleosis, a self-limited lymphoproliferative disease characterized by fever, malaise, and marked lymphadenopathy lasting from a week to a year. In small numbers of patients, EBV infection can be chronic, resulting in prolonged symptoms of infectious mononucleosis, as well as complications in other organs, such as hepatitis, uveitis, and bone marrow suppression.[48] Additionally, EBV infection has been associated with several malignancies such as Burkitt's lymphoma, Hodgkin's disease, non-Hodgkin's lymphoma, and nasopharyngeal carcinoma, among others. These can be especially problematic in immunosuppressed persons, in whom EBV infection cannot be eliminated by the immune system. In X-linked lymphoproliferative disease, EBV infection results in fatal disease from a constellation of symptoms, including infectious mononucleosis, dysgammaglobulinemia, and lymphoproliferative disease.[49] Patients with concurrent HIV infection demonstrate markedly increased EBV viral load and an increased incidence of tumors, including non-Hodgkin's lymphoma, and CNS lymphomas, which demonstrate abnormal presence of EBV DNA.[48] EBV is also associated with lymphoproliferative disease in patients iatrogenically immunosuppressed following organ transplantation; post-transplant lymphoproliferative disorder (PTLD) affects approximately 1% of patients following hematopoietic stem cell transplants, but rates as high as 20% have been described in solid organ transplant recipients (see Chapter 54). The incidence of PTLD correlates with new infection during immunosuppression and with the degree of immunosuppression.[50]

Detection of EBV infection can be accomplished by nucleic acid detection or by serology, although each has particular limitations. Serology is used primarily to diagnose infectious mononucleosis following primary infection. The classical technique for serological diagnosis of EBV infection is the

Table 10-1 Antibody Reactivity to EBV Antigens

EBV Exposure	Heterophile	VCA IgM	VCA IgG	EA IgG	EBNA IgG
Seronegative	–	–	–	–	–
Current primary infection	+	+	+/–	+/–	–
Recovery/reactivation	+/–	+	+	+/–	+
Resolved past infection	–	–	+	+/–	+

EA, Early antigen; *EBNA,* Epstein-Barr nuclear antigen; *EBV,* Epstein-Barr virus; *Ig,* immunoglobulin; *VCA,* viral capsid antigen.

Paul-Bunnell assay, often referred to as the "heterophile antibody" test. This test involves agglutination of nonhuman RBCs by heterophile antibodies present in the serum of EBV-infected patients.[51] This original assay has been replaced in most clinical laboratories by agglutination or immunochromatographic assays with similar sensitivity.[52] Approximately 85% of patients with EBV will demonstrate heterophile antibodies. In the setting of classical symptoms in a patient with no prior history, a positive test for heterophile antibodies is sufficient for diagnosis. The relatively high false-negative rate, coupled with observations that the sensitivity of heterophile antibody detection drops to approximately 50% in very young children (<5 years old), indicates that negative results for heterophile antibodies should be followed by EBV-specific antibody testing.[53] Nucleic acid detection by PCR, although highly sensitive, is of limited use in the diagnosis of infectious mononucleosis, because there is no correlation between viral load and disease. However, PCR is useful in the detection of EBV DNA in associated lymphoproliferative diseases such as PTLD.

EBV-specific antibodies are directed against three main antigens—early antigen (EA), viral capsid antigen (VCA), and Epstein-Barr nuclear antigen (EBNA). The pattern of EBV-specific antibodies detected in patient serum correlates with the patient's exposure history (Table 10-1); following primary infection, IgM to VCA is typically the first antibody to be detected, developing concurrently with heterophile antibodies. These are followed closely by IgG to VCA and EA. Antibody response to EBNA typically is detected within 6 to 8 weeks following exposure. The initial IgM response declines after approximately 4 weeks, but IgG to VCA and, to a lesser extent, EBNA remain detectable for life; evaluation of VCA IgG is the most reliable method for demonstration of prior exposure to EBV. EBV-specific antibodies can be detected by IFA or ELISA, although ELISA is used more commonly because it is easier to perform and has higher sensitivity.[54]

Congenital (TORCH) Infections

Maternal infections during pregnancy can result in damage to the developing fetus; in particular, a set of pathogens that pose the greatest risk to the fetus have been defined. This group, identified by the acronym TORCH, includes *TOxoplasma gondii,* Rubella virus, Cytomegalovirus, and Herpes simplex (including varicella zoster virus, the causative agent of chicken pox) viruses. Perinatal infection with TORCH organisms in the mother can result in intrauterine growth restriction, chorioretinitis, epilepsy, and, in some cases, fetal death. Direct testing for TORCH organisms is problematic, as they are difficult to culture, and maternal infection is often asymptomatic. Serology is the best method used to evaluate maternal exposure to these pathogens, as it is able to differentiate between current primary exposure and past exposure to the pathogen, primarily by distinction of IgG and IgM antibody responses. Additionally, serology is attractive for diagnosis of perinatal infection because it does not require invasive procedures such as chorionic villus or umbilical cord blood sampling for direct pathogen detection by culture or PCR.

Toxoplasmosis refers to disease resulting from infection with *Toxoplasma gondii,* an obligate intracellular parasite that can be acquired by ingestion of undercooked meat or contaminated water, or by exposure to cat feces. Disease caused by *T. gondii* infection can be categorized into four main categories: self-limited flulike symptoms in immunocompetent patients, systemic toxoplasmosis seen in immunocompromised patients, chorioretinitis resulting from ocular infection, and congenital infection resulting in a spectrum of fetal malformations, which may include fetal demise.[55] Direct detection of the parasite by microscopy or culture has limited sensitivity, and detection by PCR, which is highly sensitive and specific, requires obtaining the appropriate specimen (chorionic villus or vitreous fluid), which often is problematic.[56] Therefore, diagnosis of *T. gondii* infection relies on serology.

Serological detection of antibodies to *T. gondii* is classically described by the Sabin-Feldman dye test, which is based on the observation that living *T. gondii* organisms bind methylene blue dye, but those that have been lysed in the presence of antibody and complement do not. Results are interpreted as the dilution of serum that results in 50% killing of organisms. However, serological testing for *T. gondii* is performed more typically with the use of ELISA or IFA.[55] Most ELISA or IFA assays test for the presence of IgM and IgG antibodies, although some kits also include IgA and IgE; the pattern of antibody production is reflective of the course of disease. IgM typically is produced within the first few days of exposure to *T. gondii* and is used to determine recent infection. However, several important considerations affect interpretation of the IgM result. In otherwise healthy patients, a negative IgM result excludes exposure to *T. gondii* over the previous 6 months. However, immunocompromised patients often do not produce detectable IgM, and a negative IgM should not preclude a diagnosis of recent infection. Additionally, commercial kits for detection of IgM to *T. gondii* have poor specificity, with high false-positive rates; according to the FDA, all positive *T. gondii* IgM results should be confirmed by a reference laboratory.[57-59]

Furthermore, the persistence of IgM from eradicated infection can give a false indicator of recent infection. IgA and IgE measurements have been described as adjunctive testing to IgM for distinguishing primary infection; IgA has demonstrated improved sensitivity over IgM in serological testing of newborns for congenital toxoplasmosis,[60] and IgE has demonstrated improved specificity as compared with IgM or IgA,[61] although typically, these are performed only in reference laboratories. Detection of *T. gondii* IgG is considered demonstrative of previous infection, as IgG appears within the first few weeks following infection and persists for life. Identification of *T. gondii* IgG does not differentiate recent infection from previous infection, although measurement of IgG is useful for ruling out exposure to *T. gondii*. Sensitivity for *T. gondii* IgG detection is comparable between commercially available kits.[55] Avidity testing of IgG has been reported to aid in the diagnosis of acute infection, with the idea that after primary antigen stimulation, antibody avidity is low, while remote infections demonstrate IgG with higher avidity[62]; avidity testing is complex and time-consuming because it involves dissociation of the antibody-antigen complex with the use of denaturing agents (such as urea). Interpretation of avidity results is also difficult with no standard cutoffs. It is agreed that low avidity results cannot be interpreted as diagnostic of recent infection, as low avidity antibodies can persist for several years. However, the presence of high-avidity antibodies rules out recent infection.

Current recommendations indicate screening of all women for rubella and of women with a negative or unknown history of varicella infection early in pregnancy,[63,64] although serological testing for other infections is recommended only for women who present with symptoms or an exposure history. Cytomegalovirus (CMV) testing is notable, in that >50% of the U.S. population is seropositive, and <10% of mothers positive for CMV IgM will pass the infection to the fetus.[65] Assessment of antibodies to TORCH-related infectious agents is typically performed by ELISA[28,55,57] Serological tests for each of the main organisms implicated in TORCH infections often are grouped for the convenience of the ordering physician into an orderable TORCH panel that can be used to detect and report IgM and IgG individually. False-negative results for all TORCH infections can occur very early in infection; IgM may be undetectable within the first 4 or 5 days following infection, and negative test results should result in retesting on a new sample after 10 to 14 days. Positive IgG results for TORCH organisms typically are taken as evidence of prior exposure, which presents little to no risk to the fetus. Additionally, a fourfold rise in IgG titers between acute and convalescent serum samples can be considered diagnostic for recent infection and may be required in circumstances where IgM results may be difficult to interpret (i.e., false positives in the setting of rheumatoid arthritis or juvenile arthritis). The presence of IgG in the absence of IgM is diagnostic of previous infection. This distinction is important in the setting of congenital infection in that most infectious agents pose minimal risk of transmission to the fetus during reexposure or reactivation. However, reactivation of latent infection and transmission resulting in congenital infection have been described without the reappearance of IgM, and the overall clinical presentation should be considered in the evaluation of serological results.[66]

Follow-up testing in the newborn should be performed by serological analysis and pathogen detection.[67] Serological testing of the newborn involves special considerations that dramatically affect the performance and interpretation of testing. First, detection of IgM in the newborn cannot be performed reliably until after the first month of life, as antibody production has not always begun. Additionally, maternal IgG passively transferred during gestation lasts for up to 3 months, which can make reliable detection of IgG production by the newborn difficult. These difficulties do not entirely preclude serological testing of newborns, although attempts at direct pathogen detection by culture and PCR should be included in follow-up testing for congenital infection.

CAPSULAR POLYSACCHARIDE ANTIGEN VACCINATION

In addition to demonstrating exposure to a particular pathogen, serological testing can provide information about the patient's immune system. Measurement of the production of antibody to vaccinated antigens enables qualitative assessment of the function of the humoral immune system; antibody production against protein antigens (e.g., tetanus toxoid) is demonstrative of antibody response to antigens that require T-cell help (T-dependent), while antibody response to polysaccharides provides evidence of response to antigens that elicit antibody without the help of T cells (T-independent).[1] Antibody responses to polysaccharides are particularly important, as they are the principal components of the bacterial capsule, an important virulence factor for several important pathogens such as *Haemophilus influenzae* type b, *Neisseria meningitidis,* and *Streptococcus pneumoniae.* Recent estimates suggest that as many as 10% of vaccinated persons have an inadequate antibody response and are susceptible to chronic and recurrent infection.[68,69] Serological testing for vaccine-specific polysaccharide antigens should be performed in patients who clinically demonstrate an inadequate immune response to capsulated bacterial infection, as evidenced by recurrent or chronic infection.

Quantitative measurement of antibodies directed against vaccine-specific polysaccharide antigens is performed by ELISA.[70,71] In the case of *Haemophilus influenzae,* serum is tested for antibodies against the b polysaccharide, and in *Neisseria meningitides* and *Streptococcus pneumoniae,* serum is tested for antibodies against multiple polysaccharide antigens that represent common infectious serotypes and multiple vaccine antigens. It is noteworthy that although these antigen preparations are pure (>98% purity), they still contain trace amounts of lipopolysaccharide and other cross-reactive polysaccharides, which can significantly alter the results of specific antibody testing, as the antibodies of interest are present in small amounts; care should be taken to use the minimal amount of antigen necessary for optimal detection to maximize specificity. Additionally, it has been recommended to absorb cross-reactive antibodies with heterologous polysaccharides prior to ELISA testing.[72]

Interpreting the results of polysaccharide-specific antibody testing is problematic, as there is significant variation in antibody concentrations between normal persons. Comparison of prevaccination antibody concentrations with a sample taken several weeks after vaccination is the most direct way to assess the adequacy of the humoral immune response. Well-characterized reference sera have been used to determine normal concentrations of antibody against *H. influenzae, N. meningitides,* and *S. pneumoniae* antigens following vaccination in children and adults.[73-77] However, because there is no definitive cutoff for antibody concentrations used to determine protection against subsequent infection, interpretation depends on comparison of the antibody response to antigens to which the patient has been exposed through vaccination versus established normal concentrations. Additionally, immunological protection against infection correlates better with the presence of bactericidal antibodies as measured by functional complement fixation assays.[75,76] All results must be correlated with the overall clinical presentation to determine the adequacy of the immune response.[78]

KEY CONCEPTS BOX 10-3

- Although the syphilis pathogen can be detected by microscopy, serological tests are used routinely. The nonspecific Venereal Disease Research Laboratory (VDRL) and reagin assays detect the phospholipid cardiolipin and are sensitive to prozone effects.
- Positive results by these assays should be confirmed by more specific assays that measure antibodies (Abs) to *Treponema pallidum* antigens, either by agglutination or by enzyme-linked immunosorbent assay (ELISA).
- Assays for Lyme disease are very nonspecific, and questionably positive results must be confirmed by nucleic acid testing. Both immunoglobulin (Ig)M and IgG Abs should be tested.
- Abs against *Helicobacter pylori* by ELISA or immunometric assay can be used to diagnose peptic ulcer disease caused by this agent. Molecular testing can be used to follow up on questionable results or to monitor treatment.
- Ab to HIV can be detected by ELISA testing and confirmed by the Western blot technique with the use of specific human immunodeficiency virus (HIV) antigen (Ag).
- Serological TORCH (TOxoplasma, Rubella, Cytomegalovirus, Herpes) testing detects Abs to a number of diseases that can cause congenital defects in a developing fetus. Both IgG and IgM Abs can be measured to differentiate between current infection and past exposure. Assay is typical by ELISA and immunometric techniques.
- Serological detection of Abs to polysaccharides of specific bacteria for which vaccinations are available can determine information about the immune status against re-exposure. ELISA is used most frequently.

REFERENCES

1. Abbas A, Lichtman AH, Pillaei S: Antibodies and antigens. In Abbas A, Lichtman AH, Pillai S, editors: *Cellular and Molecular Immunology,* ed 6, Philadelphia, 2007, Saunders Elsevier, pp 73-96.
2. Spangler AS, Jackson JH, Fiumara NJ, Warthin NJ: Syphilis with a negative blood test reaction, JAMA 189:113, 1964.
3. Jurado RL, Campbell J, Martin PD: Prozone phenomenon in secondary syphilis: has its time arrived? Arch Intern Med 153:2496, 1993.
4. Whicher JT, Price CP, Spencer K: Immunonephelometric and immunoturbidimetric assays for proteins, Crit Rev Clin Lab Sci 18:213, 1983.
5. Mancini G, Carbonara AO, Heremans JF: Immunochemical quantitation of antigens by single radial immunodiffusion, Immunochemistry 2:235, 1965.
6. Aguero-Rosenfeld ME, Wang G, Schwartz I, Wormser GP: Diagnosis of Lyme borreliosis, Clin Microbiol Rev 18:484, 2005.
7. Deacon WE, Falcone VH, Harris A: A fluorescent test for treponemal antibodies, Proc Soc Exp Biol Med 96:477, 1957.
8. Loeffelholz MJ: Rapid diagnosis of viral infections, Lab Med 33:639, 2002.
9. Beigel JH, Farrar J, Han AM, Hayden FG, Hyer R, de Jong MD, Lochindarat S, Nguyen TK, Tran TH, Nicoll A, Touch S, Yuen KY: Avian influenza A (H5N1) in humans, N Engl J Med 353:1374, 2005.
10. Ekins R: Ligand assays: from electrophoresis to miniaturized microarrays, Clin Chem 44:2015, 1998.
11. Fulton RJ, McDade RL, Smith PL, Keinker LJ, Kettman JR Jr: Advanced multiplex analysis with the FlowMetrix system, Clin Chem 43:1749, 1997.
12. Klutts JS, Liao RS, Dunne WM, Gronowski AM: Evaluation of a multiplexed bead assay for assessment of Epstein-Barr virus immunologic status, Clin Chem 42:4996, 2004.
13. Mezzazoma L, Bacarese-Hamilton T, DiCristina M, Rossi R, Bistoni F, Crisanti A: Antigen microarrays for serodiagnosis of infectious diseases, Clin Chem 48:121, 2002.
14. Pappin A, Grissom M, Mackay W, Huang Y, Yomtovian R: Stability of cytomegalovirus antibodies in plasma during prolonged storage of blood components, Clin Diagn Lab Immunol 2:25, 1995.
15. Kricka LJ: Principles of immunochemical techniques. In Burtis CA, Ashwood ER, Bruns DE, editors: *Tietz Textbook of Clinical Chemistry and Molecular Diagnostics,* ed 4, St. Louis, MO, 2006, Saunders, pp 219-243.
16. Tramont EC: Syphilis in adults: from Christopher Columbus to Sir Alexander Fleming to AIDS, Clin Infect Dis 21:1361, 1995.
17. Pangborn MC: A new serologically active phospholipid from beef heart, Proc Soc Exp Biol Med 48:484, 1941.
18. Harris AA, Rosenberg A, Riedel LM: A microflocculation test for syphilis using cardiolipin antigen: preliminary report, J Vener Dis Inform 27:159, 1946.
19. Escobar MR, Dalton HP, Allison MJ: Fluorescent antibody test for syphilis using cerebrospinal fluid: clinical correlation in 150 cases, Am J Clin Pathol 53:886, 1970.
20. Portnoy J, Carson W, Smith CA: Rapid plasma reagin test for syphilis, Public Health Rep 72:761, 1957.
21. Gregory N, Sanchez M, Buchness MR: The spectrum of syphilis in patients with human immunodeficiency virus infection, J Am Acad Dermatol 22:1061, 1990.
22. Larsen SA, Hambie EA, Wobig GH, Kennedy EJ: Cerebrospinal fluid serologic test for syphilis: treponemal and nontreponemal tests. In Morisset R, Kurstak E, editors: *Advances in Sexually Transmitted Diseases,* Utrecht, Netherlands, 1985, VNU Science Press, pp 157-162.

23. Deacon WE, Hunter EF: Treponemal antigens as related to identification and syphilis serology, Proc Soc Exp Biol Med 110:352, 1962.
24. Hunter EF, Deacon WE, Meyer PE: An improved FTA test for syphilis: the absorption procedure (FTA-ABS), Public Health Rep 79:410, 1964.
25. Pope V: Use of treponemal tests to screen for syphilis, Infect Med 21:399, 2004.
26. Schmidt BL, Edjlalipour M, Luger A: Comparative evaluation of nine different enzyme-linked immunosorbent assays for determination of antibodies against *Treponema pallidum* in patients with primary syphilis, J Clin Microbiol 38:1279, 2000.
27. Luger AF, Schmidt BL, Kaulich M: Significance of laboratory findings for the diagnosis of neurosyphilis, Int J Std AIDS 11:224, 2000.
28. Grangeot-Keros L, Enders G: Evaluation of a new enzyme immunoassay based on recombinant rubella virus–like particles for detection of immunoglobulin M antibodies to rubella virus, J Clin Microbiol 35:398, 1997.
29. Steere AC: Lyme disease, N Engl J Med 345:115, 2001.
30. Dressler F, Whalen JA, Reinhardt BN, Steere AC: Western blotting in the serodiagnosis of Lyme disease, J Infect Dis 167:392, 1993.
31. Engstrom SM, Shoop E, Johnson RC: Immunoblot interpretation criteria for serodiagnosis of early Lyme disease, J Clin Microbiol 33:419, 1995.
32. Askin E, McHugh GL, Flavell RA, Fikrig E, Steere AC: The immunoglobulin G (IgG) antibody response to OspA and OspB correlates with severe and prolonged Lyme arthritis and the IgG response to P35 correlates with mild and brief arthritis, Infect Immunol 67:173, 1999.
33. Zhang JR, Hardham JM, Barbour AG, Norris SJ: Antigenic variation in Lyme disease *Borreliae* by promiscuous recombination of VMP-like sequence cassettes, Cell 89:275, 1997.
34. Association of State and Territorial Public Health Laboratory Directors and the Center for Disease Control and Prevention: Recommendations. In *Proceedings of the Second National Conference on the Serologic Diagnosis of Lyme Disease,* Washington, DC, 1995, Association of State and Territorial Public Health Laboratory Directors, pp 1-5.
35. Magnarelli LA, Meegan JM, Anderson JF, Chapell WA: Comparison of an indirect fluorescent-antibody test with an enzyme-linked immunosorbent assay for serological studies of Lyme disease, J Clin Microbiol 20:181, 1984.
36. Russell H, Sampson JA, Schmid GP, Wilkinson HW, Plikaytis B: Enzyme-linked immunosorbent assay and indirect immunofluorescence assay for Lyme disease, J Infect Dis 149:465, 1984.
37. Kaiser R, Rauer S: Advantage of recombinant borrelial proteins for serodiagnosis of neuroborreliosis, J Med Microbiol 48:5, 1999.
38. Luft BJ, Steinman CR, Neimark HC, Muralidhar B, Rush T, Finkel M, Kunkel M, Dattwyler RJ: Invasion of the central nervous system by *Borrelia burgdorferi* in acute disseminated infection, JAMA 267:1364, 1992.
39. Warren JR, Marshall B: Unidentified curved bacilli on gastric epithelium in active chronic gastritis, Lancet 1:1273, 1983.
40. Malfertheiner P, Mergraud F, O'Morain C, Bazzoli F, El-Omar E, Graham D, Hunt R, Rokkas T, Vakil N, Kuipers EJ: Current concepts in the management of *Helicobacter pylori* infection: the Maastricht III consensus report, Gut 56:772, 2006.
41. Kuipers E, Pena A, Van Kamp G, Uyterlinde A, Pals G, Pels N, Kurz-Pohlmann E, Meuwissen S: Seroconversion for *Helicobacter pylori,* Lancet 342:328, 1993.
42. Hirschl AM, Brandstätter G, Dragosics G, Hentschel E, Kundi M, Rotter ML, Schütze K, Taufer M: Kinetics of specific IgG antibodies for monitoring the effect of anti-*Helicobacter pylori* chemotherapy, J Infect Dis 168:763, 1993.
43. Kosunen TU, Seppala K, Sarna S, Sipponen P: Diagnostic value of decreasing IgG, IgA, and IgM antibody titres after eradication of *Helicobacter pylori,* Lancet 339:893, 1992.
44. Centers for Disease Control and Prevention: Revised recommendations for HIV testing of adults, adolescents, and pregnant women in health-care settings, MMWR 55(RR14):1, 2006.
45. Centers for Disease Control and Prevention: Revised guidelines for HIV counseling, testing, and referral and revised recommendations for HIV screening of pregnant women, MMWR 50(RR19):1, 2001.
46. Ward JW, Holmberg SD, Allen JR, Cohn DL, Critchley SE, Kleinman SH, Lenes BA, Ravenholt O, Davis JR, Quinn MG, Jaffe HW: Transmission of human immunodeficiency virus (HIV) by blood transfusion screened as negative for HIV antibody, N Engl J Med 318:473, 1988.
47. Branson BM: Point-of-care rapid tests for HIV antibodies, J Lab Med 27:288, 2003.
48. Cohen JI: Epstein-Barr virus infection, N Engl J Med 343:481, 2000.
49. Gaspar HB, Sharifi R, Gilmour KC, Thrasher AJ: X-linked lymphoproliferative disease: clinical, diagnostic, and molecular perspective, Br J Haematol 119:585, 2002.
50. Cockfield SM: Identifying the patient at risk for post-transplant lymphoproliferative disorder, Transplant Infect Dis 3:70, 2001.
51. Paul JR, Bunnell WW: The presence of heterophile antibodies in infectious mononucleosis, Am J Med Sci 267:178, 1974.
52. Bruu AL, Hjetland R, Holter E, Mortensen L, Natas O, Petterson W, Skar AG, Skarpaas T, Tjade T, Asjo B: Evaluation of 12 commercial tests for detection of Epstein-Barr virus–specific and heterophile antibodies, Clin Diagn Lab Immunol 7:451, 2000.
53. Lennette ET: Epstein-Barr virus (EBV). In Lennette EH, Lennette DA, Lennette ET, editors: *Diagnostic Procedures for Viral, Rickettsial, and Chlamydial Infections,* ed 7, Washington, DC, 1995, American Public Health Association, pp 299-312.
54. Hess RD: Routine Epstein-Barr virus diagnostics from the laboratory perspective: still challenging after 35 years, J Clin Microbiol 37:3381, 2004.
55. Wilson M, Jones JL, McAuley JB: Toxoplasma. In Murray PR, Baron EJ, Jorgenson JH, Landry ML, Pfaller MA, editors: *Manual of Clinical Microbiology,* ed 9, Washington, DC, 2007, ASM Press, pp 2070-2081.
56. NCCLS: *Clinical Use and Interpretation of Serologic Tests for* Toxoplasma gondii: *Approved Guideline,* Wayne, PA, 2004, NCCLS.
57. U.S. Food and Drug Administration, 1997, FDA Public Health Advisory: Limitations of *Toxoplasma* IgM commercial test kits. Available at www.fda.gov/cdrh/toxopha.html.
58. Liesenfeld O, Montoya JG, Tathineni NJ, Davis M, Brown BW Jr, Cobb KL, Parsonnet J, Remington JS: Confirmatory serologic testing for acute toxoplasmosis and rate of induced abortions among women reported to have positive *Toxoplasma* immunoglobulin M antibody titers, Am J Obstet Gynecol 184:140, 2001.
59. Wilson M, Remington JS, Clavet C, Varney G, Press C, Ware D: Evaluation of six commercial kits for detection of human immunoglobulin M antibodies to *Toxoplasma gondii,* J Clin Microbiol 35:311, 1997.
60. Stepick-Biek P, Thulliez P, Araujo FG, Remington JS: IgA antibodies for diagnosis of acute congenital and acquired toxoplasmosis, J Infect Dis 162:270, 1990.
61. Montoya JG, Remington JS: Studies on the serodiagnosis of toxoplasmic lymphadenitis, Clin Infect Dis 20:781, 1995.
62. Liesenfeld O, Montoya JG, Kinney S, Press C, Remington JS: Effect of testing for IgG avidity in the diagnosis of *Toxoplasma gondii* infection in pregnant women: experience in a US reference laboratory, J Infect Dis 183:1248, 2001.
63. Centers for Disease Control and Prevention: Control and prevention of rubella: evaluation and management of suspected

outbreaks, rubella in pregnant women, and surveillance for congenital rubella syndrome, MMWR 50(RR12):1, 2001.

64. Grose C: Varicella infection during pregnancy, Herpes 6:33, 1999.
65. Lazzarotto T, Guerra B, Spezzacatena P, Varani S, Gabrielli L, Pradelli P, Rumpianesi E, Banzi C, Bovicelli L, Landini MP: Prenatal diagnosis of congenital cytomegalovirus infection, J Clin Microbiol 36:3540, 1998.
66. Centers for Disease Control and Prevention: *Manual for the Surveillance of Vaccine-Preventable Diseases,* Atlanta, GA, 1999, U.S. Department of Health and Human Services.
67. Centers for Disease Control and Prevention: Preventing congenital toxoplasmosis, MMWR 49(RR02):57, 2000.
68. Ambrosino DM, Siber GR, Chilmonczyk BA, Jernberg JB, Finberg RW: An immunodeficiency characterized by impaired antibody responses to polysaccharides, N Engl J Med 316:790, 1987.
69. Wasserman RL, Sorensen RU: Evaluating children with respiratory tract infections: the role of immunization with bacterial polysaccharide vaccine, Pediatr Infect Dis 18:157, 1999.
70. Madore DV, Anderson P, Baxter BD, Carlone GM, Edwards KM, Hamilton RG, Holder P, Kayhty H, Phipps DC, Peeters CC, Schneerson R, Siber GR, Ward JI, Frasch CE: Interlaboratory study evaluating quantitation of antibodies to *Haemophilus influenzae* type b polysaccharide by enzyme-linked immunosorbent assay, Clin Diagn Lab Immunol 3:84, 1996.
71. Phipps DC, West J, Eby R, Koster M, Madore DV, Quataert SA: An ELISA employing a *Haemophilus influenzae* type b oligosaccharide-human serum albumin conjugate correlates with the radioantigen binding assay, J Immunol Methods 135:121, 1990.
72. Frasch CE: Immune responses to polysaccharide and conjugate vaccines. In Detrick B, Hamilton RG, Folds JD, editors: *Manual of Molecular and Clinical Laboratory Immunology,* ed 7, Washington, DC, 2006, ASM Press, pp 434-443.
73. Elie CM, Holder PK, Romero-Steiner S, Carlone GM: Assignment of additional anticapsular antibody concentrations to the *Neisseria meningitidis* group A, C, Y, and W-135 meningococcal standard reference serum CDC1992, Clin Diagn Lab Immunol 9:725, 2002.
74. Jeurissen A, Moens L, Raes M, Wuyts G, Willebrords L, Sauer K, Proesmans M, Ceuppens JL, De Boeck K, Bossuyt X: Laboratory diagnosis of specific antibody deficiency to pneumococcal capsular polysaccharide antigens, Clin Chem 53:505, 2007.
75. Goldschneider I, Gotschlich EC, Artenstein MS: Human immunity to the meningococcus. II. Development of natural immunity, J Exp Med 129:1327, 1969.
76. Trotter C, Borrow R, Andrews N, Miller E: Seroprevalence of meningococcal serogroup C bactericidal antibody in England and Wales in the pre-vaccination era, Vaccine 21:1094, 2003.
77. Quataert SA, Kirch CS, Weidel LJ, Phipps DC, Strohmeyer S, Cimino CO, Skuse J, Madore DV: Assignment of weight-based antibody units to a human antipneumococcal standard reference serum, lot 89-S, Clin Diagn Lab Immunol 2:590, 1995.
78. Balmer P, Cant AJ, Borrow R: Anti-pneumococcal antibody titre measurement: what useful information does it yield? J Clin Pathol 60:345, 2006.

Measurement of Colligative Properties

Lawrence A. Kaplan

Chapter Outline

Key Terms

boiling-point elevation A phenomenon in which addition of solute molecules raises the temperature at which the solution will boil. For water, this is 1.86°C per mole of solute per kilogram of solvent.

colligative property A characteristic to which all the molecules of a solution contribute, regardless of their individual composition or nature.

colloid A large molecule, usually in aqueous solution. The term is commonly applied to protein solutions.

colloid osmotic pressure (COP) The osmotic pressure generated by that portion of a solution with high molecular weight (>30,000 daltons).

crystalloids The uncharged solute molecules of a solution.

dew point The temperature at which condensation of water from the vapor phase occurs.

diffusion The mixing or movement of molecules as a result of their random motion.

Donnan effect The distribution of ions caused by their having a high-molecular-weight ion on one side of a semipermeable membrane.

freezing-point depression A phenomenon in which the addition of solute molecules to a solution lowers the temperature at which the solution will freeze.

ketone bodies Acetone, acetoacetate, and other ketone-related molecules that are present in the serum of patients with diabetic ketoacidosis.

molality The number of moles of solute per kilogram of water or solvent.

oncotic pressure Another term for colloid osmotic pressure.

osmolal gap The difference between observed and calculated serum osmolarities; more frequently calculated as the osmolar gap. Calculated osmolar values include sodium concentration multiplied by 2, plus glucose and blood urea nitrogen.

osmolality The measurement of the number of moles of particles per kilogram of water.

osmolarity An alternative measure of colligative property that is clinically equivalent to osmolality; measurement of the number of moles of particles per liter of water.

osmometry The measurement of a colligative property of a solution in which the number of moles of a solute per unit volume (concentration) is determined.

osmosis Water flow across a semipermeable membrane.

osmotic pressure The hydrostatic pressure required to prevent a change in volume when two solutions of different concentrations are placed on opposite sides of a semipermeable membrane.

plasma expander Usually a high-molecular-weight dextran that is administered intravenously to increase the oncotic pressure of a patient.

Seebeck effect The voltage difference seen when two ends of a specially made wire are at two different temperatures.

semipermeable membrane A barrier that allows one type of molecule, such as water, to pass but does not allow another type of molecule, such as protein, to pass.

thermistor A temperature-measuring device in which the change of resistance is temperature dependent. The term is derived from the words *thermal resistor.*

thermocouple A device that generates a voltage (Seebeck effect) when the two ends of a wire are at different temperatures.

ultrafiltrate The solution that remains after passage through a semipermeable membrane. Usually, it contains only low-molecular-weight solutes.

vapor-pressure depression A phenomenon in which the addition of a solute molecule to a solvent decreases the amount of solvent in equilibrium between the vapor phase and the liquid phase.

SECTION OBJECTIVES BOX 11-1

- Identify the relationships among osmosis, osmotic pressure, osmolality, and osmometry.
- List four measurements that depend on colligative properties, and describe what happens to each property during sample concentration.

COLLIGATIVE PROPERTIES

All the molecules in a solution, regardless of their individual composition or nature, contribute to the **colligative properties** of that solution. The colligative properties affect the concentrations of biochemicals in physiological fluids and the movement of fluids across biological membranes.[1] We also use colligative properties to determine the composition of serum and urine.

Osmosis

Diffusion is the mixing of molecules that results from random motion caused by thermal kinetic energy (Brownian motion). For example, if an albumin solution is carefully overlaid with water, the albumin molecules will randomly move back and forth across the original interface boundary. Because there are more albumin molecules in the albumin solution, the odds are great that an albumin molecule will cross into the water side. Thus albumin will diffuse into the water layer until the solutions become homogeneous, that is, until the odds are equal that an albumin molecule will diffuse one way or the other across the original boundary because the concentration is equal on both sides.

The term **osmosis** specifically applies to water flow across a **semipermeable membrane** such as a cell membrane. A semipermeable membrane allows some particles in solution (molecules, ions, or aggregates of molecules) to diffuse through it but inhibits the passage of others; hence it is semipermeable. The simplest example of a semipermeable membrane is a dialysis membrane, which usually is made of cellophane. It has very small pores through which only water and some small molecules and ions pass (often termed an **ultrafiltrate**). However, large molecules, such as proteins, cannot pass through the membrane. To demonstrate, place an albumin solution in a section of dialysis tubing, and tie the ends of the tubing. If the tubing is placed in a beaker of water, the albumin molecules cannot move out of the membrane, but water molecules will diffuse in and affect dilution of the albumin. As a result, the tubing will swell as water flows into the albumin solution inside the tubing, increasing the pressure inside the membrane. If the tubing does not burst from this pressure, an equilibrium will be maintained between the water flowing in and the water being forced out by the internal pressure. The hydrostatic pressure built up and maintained by this process is called **osmotic pressure.**

Perhaps the most graphic example of osmosis is lysis of red blood cells when placed in water. So much water flows into the more concentrated intracellular fluid that the cell swells and bursts. Cells also can shrink if exposed to a fluid of high salt concentration. In this case, the water in the cell flows out of the cell into the concentrated solution outside. In the laboratory, this process affects the measurement of mean corpuscular volume (MCV). If the diluent is not isotonic, that is, of equal osmotic pressure with cellular fluid, the cells will swell or shrink, giving erroneous MCV and hematocrit values because the latter is calculated from the MCV.

Osmolality

The term **molarity** is used to characterize concentration, that is, the number of moles of solute per liter of water. **Molality** is the number of moles of solute per kilogram of water. Because a liter of water has a mass of 1 kg, the difference between these two expressions of concentration is usually small. Only for concentrated solutions is the difference appreciable. In practice, it is the difference between adding material to a liter of water (molality) and adding water to material to make a liter of solution (molarity).

Molality is the term best suited to **osmometry** because it gives a simpler theoretical formula for osmotic pressure than molarity does. The term *osmolality* is used to identify the number of moles of particles per kilogram of water. In practical clinical usage the two terms are used interchangeably.

Because the osmolality of a solution does not depend on the kind of particles but only on the number of particles, it is called a colligative property. A solution that is 1 millimolal in sodium chloride is 2 milliosmolal because in solution, sodium chloride separates into sodium and chloride ions, each ion representing a particle that contributes to the osmolality. Furthermore, a 1 millimolal calcium chloride solution is 3 milliosmolal because each molecule ionizes to give one calcium ion and two chloride ions.

Osmometry

Osmometry is the measurement of the concentration, not of a particular molecule, but of all molecules and ions in a solution. In this chapter, the principles and techniques for measuring osmolality are reviewed, examples of instrumentation are provided, and the clinical use of osmometry is discussed.

Osmolal Gap

There are just a few substances in plasma that contribute significantly to the osmolality, and they are mostly small molecules and ions. For example, plasma usually contains 40 g of albumin per liter, but the number of moles of albumin is very small (only about 0.62 mmol). In contrast, plasma contains about 150 mmol/L of sodium ion and 100 mmol/L of a corresponding anion such as chloride. This is about 5.8 g of sodium chloride per liter. Thus sodium chloride contributes 3000 times more to osmolality than does a similar mass of albumin.

Many formulas have been used to calculate the approximate osmolality of serum or plasma.[2] Most of these formulas sum up the major, measured contributors to the osmolality, and thus actually calculate the osmolarity. Calculated osmolarity, estimated osmolality, can be compared with measured osmolality; the difference is called the **osmolal gap.** An abnormal osmolal gap is an important indication of abnormal concentrations of unmeasured, low-molecular-weight substances in the blood. Because the formula predicts the plasma osmolality so well, there is little new information to be gained from routine measurements of the osmolality. However, in a few specific clinical situations described below, the measurement is informative and worthwhile.

The formulas shown below for calculation of serum osmolarity are approximations because they include only the most important *measured* contributors to osmolarity:

Historical units

$$\text{Calculated osmolality (mOsm/kg)} = 2 \times \text{Na}^+\text{(mEq/L)} + \frac{\text{Glucose (mg/gL)}}{18} + \frac{\text{BUN (mg/dL)}}{2.8} \qquad \text{Eq. 11-1}$$

SI units*

$$\text{Calculated osmolarity (mOsm/L)} = 2 \times \text{Na}^+\text{(mmol/L)} + \text{Glucose (mmol/L)} + \text{BUN (mmol/L)} \qquad \text{Eq. 11-2}$$

The SI units formula is very straightforward. The factor 2 in both equations counts the cation (sodium) once and the corresponding anions once. Glucose and blood urea nitrogen (BUN) are undissociated molecules that are counted once each. In the historical units formula, the dividing factors represent the respective molecular weights and the conversion from deciliters to liters. Note that these formulas use *molarity* rather than *molality.* This approximation compensates for some of the serum components and theoretical corrections that were ignored and produces a calculated osmolarity that is equivalent to the osmolality and agrees well with the measured osmolality.

The osmolal gap is defined as follows:

$$\text{Osmolal gap, Osm/kg} = \text{Measured Osm/kg} - \text{Calculated Osm/kg} \qquad \text{Eq. 11-3}$$

The average osmolal gap is near zero.

Colloid Osmotic Pressure

Osmotic pressure is a colligative property and hence reflects osmolality. This is strictly true for a semipermeable membrane that is permeable to water only. Measurement of the osmolal contribution of a group of molecules responsible for the **colloid osmotic pressure (COP)** is more practical and useful. COP is measured by the use of membranes that are permeable to small molecules. Small molecules—less than 30,000 D molecular weight—are called **crystalloids** if they are uncharged and ions if they are charged. Large molecules are called colloids. Hence COP measures only the contribution made to osmolality by large, essentially only protein, molecules. An alternative term is **oncotic pressure.**

KEY CONCEPTS BOX 11-1

- Osmolality is an important colligative property that is measured by osmometry.
- Plasma osmolarity can be calculated by summing the major, measured dissolved solutes.
- The calculated osmolar gap can be clinically important.

SECTION OBJECTIVES BOX 11-2

- State the relationship between freezing-point depression and moles of particles dissolved per kilogram of water, and calculate the osmolality from a given freezing point of a solution.
- Describe the techniques of freezing-point depression and vapor-pressure depression for osmolality determinations.

PRINCIPLES OF MEASUREMENT

Osmolality and osmotic pressure are colligative properties; thus any of four measurements that depend on colligative properties may be used to determine these properties. These measurements include (1) colloid osmotic pressure (COP), (2) **boiling-point elevation,** (3) **freezing-point depression,** and (4) **vapor-pressure depression.** Boiling-point elevation is not useful for clinical samples because proteins will coagulate, causing gross changes in the sample composition. Of the remaining three, freezing-point depression is the most frequently used technique for measuring osmolality.

Freezing-Point Depression

The use of salt to melt ice and snow is a well-known practice. This is an example of freezing-point depression, that is, dissolved salt increases the osmolality, thereby lowering the freezing point of the solution compared with that of the pure solvent (ice or snow). Ice forms when water molecules form a stable, crystalline structure (Fig. 11-1, *A*). The presence of dissolved molecules disrupts the formation of intermolecular water bonds, thus requiring a lower temperature to form the crystal structure (Fig. 11-1, *B*). The temperature at which ice and the water solution are in equilibrium is a function of the salt concentration. More precisely, the temperature at equilibrium is a function of the number of particles in solution. The freezing-point temperature is depressed 1.86°C for each mole of particles dissolved per kilogram of water. Because the osmolality of blood is about 0.285 Osm/kg (285 mOsm/kg), the freezing point is −0.53°C. Precise measurement of this temperature requires a sensitive thermometer. A **thermistor** (thermal resistor) is a semiconductor made from a mixture of oxides of transition metals such as manganese, cobalt, and nickel. Thermistors become better conductors of electricity as the temperature rises. The conductance or resistance of metals can be related to the temperature and hence to the osmolality.

Freezing-point depression is measured as follows:

1. The sample is cooled rapidly, usually by a cold block that is maintained at about −5°C by a solid electronic heat pump.

2. The sample is supercooled, that is, its temperature falls below the equilibrium freezing point. This occurs because pure ice crystals are slow to form.
3. Vigorous stirring induces the crystallization process. Once ice crystals begin to form, additional water molecules are added rapidly to the ice crystals. However, heat is released in the freezing process just as it is absorbed in the melting process. The heat that is released from the formation of ice crystals raises the temperature of the sample until the rapid freezing stops and an equilibrium temperature is established.
4. The temperature is measured at the plateau, that is, at the point at which the heat removed by the cooling bath is matched by the heat released by the freezing process. The temperature at this equilibrium is the freezing point of the solution and is inversely related to osmolality. The plateau temperature is measured electronically by the thermistor, and the temperature reading is converted to milliosmoles per kilogram and is displayed.

Because 1 osmol of solute lowers the freezing point by 1.86°C, osmolality can be calculated directly by the following formula:

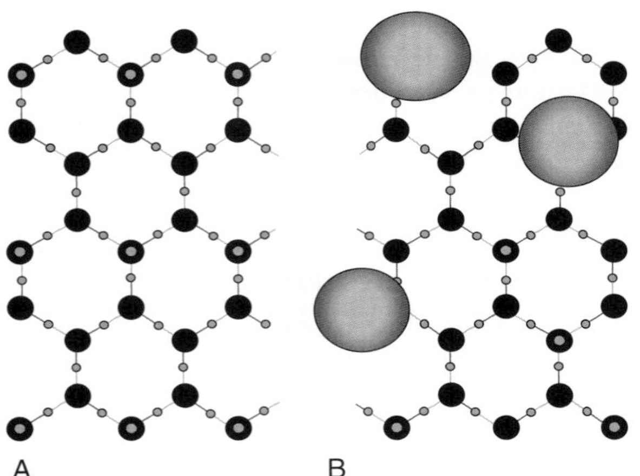

Fig. 11-1 Effect of solute on ice structure. **A,** Crystal structure of pure water. **B,** Crystal structure of water with added solute. ⚬, oxygen atom; ∘, hydrogen atom; ●, solute. (Courtesy Steven Dutch, Natural and Applied Sciences, University of Wisconsin, Green Bay, WI.)

$$\text{Osmolality (mOsmol/kg)} = \frac{\text{Freezing-point depression}}{1.86°\text{C}} \times \text{mOsmol/kg} \quad \text{Eq. 11-4}$$

However, it is more practical to calibrate the osmometer with the use of saline solutions. Calibration also corrects for systematic or procedural effects, such as the increase noted in concentration of the sample because pure water (as ice) is removed before the temperature is measured.

The sample entry port must be rinsed and wiped to minimize carryover from one sample to the next. This is especially important between samples of widely differing osmolality, such as standards and urine samples. The most common freezing-point osmometers are listed in Table 11-1, along with several key characteristics.

Vapor-Pressure Depression

Solvent molecules on the surface of a liquid are in constant thermal motion; some of these molecules escape from the surface into the atmosphere above the surface, forming a gaseous vapor phase in equilibrium with the liquid phase (Fig. 11-2, *A*). This process is called *evaporation.* If the liquid contains dissolved solute, some of these solute molecules will occupy the surface layer of the liquid. Generally, a solute molecule will not evaporate but will, by its presence, prevent a

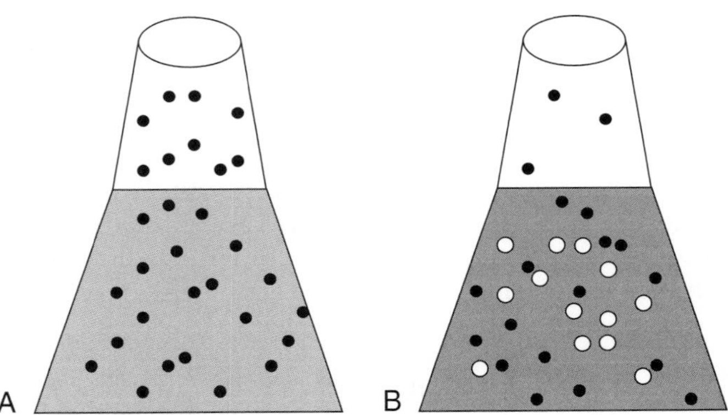

Fig. 11-2 Effect of solute on vapor pressure. **A,** Pure solvent. **B,** Solvent with added nonvolatile solute. ●, solvent molecule; ○, solute molecule.

Table 11-1 Characteristics of Clinical Osmometers

Manufacturer	Model*	Technique	Routine Sample Size, μL	Precision, %[†]	Measurement Time, Sec
Advanced Instrument, Inc. (Needham Heights, MA)	3320	FP	20	3.9	60
Fiske Associates, Inc. (Needham Heights, MA)	210	FP	20	4.1	90
Precision Systems, Inc. (Natick, MA)	Multi-Osmette	FP	30	4.2	60
Wescor, Inc. (Logan, Utah)	5520	VP	10	8.9	75
	4420	COP	350	10	180 to 300

COP, Colloid osmotic pressure; *FP,* freezing-point depression; *VP,* vapor pressure depression.
*All models are manually loaded with sample and have automated measurement and reporting. Variations in sample size, automated sampling, and printing are available.
[†]From 2005 College of American Pathologists' proficiency survey for osmolalities in normal range.

solvent molecule from evaporating. As the number of solute molecules increases, the chance that a solvent molecule will evaporate decreases, reducing the vapor phase in equilibrium above the liquid phase (see Fig. 11-2, *B*). Thus there is an inverse relationship between the concentration of dissolved solute particles (osmolality) and the vapor pressure above a solution. In vapor-pressure osmometry, the vapor-pressure depression of a solution is compared with that of a standard to determine the osmolality of a solution.

The temperature at which the atmosphere is saturated with solvent can be measured by a thermocouple. A **thermocouple** generates a voltage (**Seebeck effect**) between the ends of a wire. The voltage difference between the ends depends on the difference in temperature of the ends.

Thermocouples also exhibit the Peltier effect, which is the opposite of the Seebeck effect. An electrical current through the thermocouple transfers heat from one junction to the other. One junction cools while the other heats. The vapor-pressure osmometer passes an electrical current through the thermocouple in the measurement chamber, causing it to cool. When its temperature is low enough, water (solvent) begins to condense on it. The electrical current is discontinued, and the thermocouple comes to an equilibrium temperature at which the water condensing on it is matched by the water evaporating from it. This equilibrium temperature is measured by the Seebeck voltage, which is linearly related to the osmolality.

Vapor-pressure depression is measured as follows:

1. The sample is sealed in a chamber. The air quickly changes humidity until its humidity is in equilibrium with the sample.
2. The thermocouple cools until its temperature is below the **dew point.** The electrical current is turned off, and the junction temperature rises as vapor condenses on it.
3. The plateau temperature (the temperature at which an equilibrium exists between condensation and evaporation) is measured.
4. The vapor pressure of the sample is directly proportional to the thermocouple voltage. Again, it is more practical to calibrate this type of osmometer than to apply theoretical factors. Systematic or procedural effects that must be controlled include the sample volume, the size and composition of the sample absorbent disk, the time delay between sample application and sealing of the chamber, the cleanliness of the chamber, and changes in room temperature.

Table 11-1 provides information on the only available clinical vapor-pressure osmometer.

Colloid Osmotic Pressure

The COP is measured with a microporous filter or membrane that contains pores or channels whose diameters are carefully controlled to be impermeable to large molecules (proteins). Physiological saline is placed in a sealed chamber on one side of the membrane, and the sample is placed on the other. Saline solution flows into the sample until the back-pressure stops further flow. This back-pressure, or negative pressure, is sensed by a pressure gauge. Along with osmotic pressure, additional pressure is created by the **Donnan effect.** This effect arises because at physiological pH, most proteins are negatively charged. Because the sample is electrically neutral, positive charges are equal in number to negative charges on the proteins. These positive charges most often occur in the form of sodium ions. Charged sodium ions diffuse through the membrane, whereas the corresponding negatively charged proteins do not. This leads to a separation of electrical charges. Because of the charge separation, additional small, negatively charged molecules are attracted across the membrane. As a result, the number of particles that diffuse is larger than that resulting from simple osmosis, and the pressure across the membrane is greater. Because the net charge on proteins changes with pH, the measured COP also changes with pH.

Customarily, COP is reported in millimeters of mercury (mm Hg). In practice, maximum pressure occurs 30 to 90 seconds after the sample is placed into the instrument. This value is chosen because the pressure decays over time as a result of imperfections in the membrane that slowly allow large molecules to diffuse to the saline side, thus reducing the true pressure. Characteristics of a commercially available colloid osmometer are listed in Table 11-1.

KEY CONCEPTS BOX 11-2

- Dissolved molecules prevent ice from forming and decrease the temperature needed to freeze water.
- Osmolality usually is measured by the freezing-point depression osmometry technique.

SECTION OBJECTIVES BOX 11-3

- State the clinical utility of performing plasma osmolality and urine osmolality determinations.
- State the clinical situations in which measurement of the osmolal gap is useful.

CLINICAL USE OF OSMOMETRY AND COLLOID OSMOTIC PRESSURE

Plasma Osmolality

Osmolar Imbalance

Abnormally elevated plasma **osmolarity** can be caused by a number of disease states, such as diabetes, acidoses, and renal disease (see Chapter 30) and the measurement of plasma osmolarity can be an important diagnostic finding. A hypo-osmolar state caused by excess water intake can be life threatening and the measurement of a low plasma osmolarity a critical finding (see Chapter 28).

Screening for Toxin Ingestion

Only a few exogenous substances, usually alcohols, can be ingested in amounts sufficient to affect the plasma osmolality. Table 11-2 lists the osmolal gaps associated with potentially lethal concentrations of a number of toxins. If the measured concentration of ethanol (mmol/L) does not correspond within 10 mOsm to the calculated osmolal gap, an excess

Table 11-2 Toxic Substances Affecting Plasma Osmolality

Substances	TOXIC OR LETHAL CONCENTRATIONS Historical Units, mg/dL	SI Units, mmol/L	Corresponding Increase in Osmolality, mOsm/kg
Ethanol	350	80	80
Isopropanol	340	60	60
Methanol	80	24	24
Ethyl ether	180	24	24
Trichloroethane	100	9	9
Ethylene glycol	23	5	4
Acetone (including other ketones or ketone metabolites)	55	10	10

osmolal gap is present. An excess osmolal gap would suggest that another of the substances listed in Table 11-2 is also present.[3,4] Table 11-2 shows that trichloroethane and ethylene glycol can be at near-lethal levels in the blood without being readily detected by osmometry.

Although osmometry has long been recommended as a means to detect alcohol, it should be noted that vapor-pressure osmometers are not useful for the detection of alcohols because dissolved alcohol is also volatile and thus contributes to the solution's vapor pressure.

An increase in the osmolal gap may also reflect an increase in the anion gap in patients with metabolic imbalance. These changes can be caused by the presence of **ketone bodies** (see Chapter 38) or toxins (see Chapter 55).

Screening for Mannitol Toxicity

Mannitol is often used as an osmotic diuretic to treat patients with edema, especially cerebral edema, by reducing the amount of intracellular water. Although mannitol is a relatively nontoxic substance, it can cause renal damage at levels greater than 50 mmol/L. Measurement of the osmolality gap for patients undergoing mannitol therapy can be useful in estimating the serum levels of mannitol. If the osmolal gap is greater than 10 mOsm/L but less than 50 mOsm/L, it is likely that mannitol is present at a therapeutic, nontoxic level.

Urine Osmolality (see Chapter 30)

Renal concentrating ability is a sensitive measure of kidney function. The urine that is delivered to the bladder is typically one to three times more concentrated than the plasma. A random urine specimen whose osmolality is greater than 600 mOsm/kg is sufficient to demonstrate the kidney's ability to concentrate urine. However, if the random urine specimen is dilute, no conclusion about concentrating ability can be made. A definitive follow-up test involves overnight water restriction. After the morning void, at least one urine specimen should exceed 850 mOsm/kg. Patients who are compulsive water drinkers may require continuous observation to ensure that no water has been ingested.

The specific gravity as estimated by the refractive index or the dipstick dye technique can also be used to measure urine concentration. However, osmometry is less affected by the presence of protein or radiocontrast dyes.

Stool Osmolality

The measurement of the osmolality of watery (diarrheic) stools can be used to diagnose the cause of chronic diarrhea. Diarrheic stools can be caused by maldigestion of foods; the undigested nutrients cause an osmotic diuresis in the intestines, producing a stool with a high osmolality (see Chapter 35). Watery stools can also result from excessive intestinal excretion of fluids and electrolytes; this produces a stool with a low osmolality.

These two types of chronic diarrheic disorders often can be differentiated by calculating the stool osmolal gap. The stool osmolal gap is the difference between the measured stool osmolality and twice the sum of the measured stool sodium and potassium.

$$\text{Stool osmolal gap} = \text{Measured osmolality}_{\text{stool}} - 2([\text{Na}^+]+[\text{K}^+])_{\text{stool}} \quad \text{Eq. 11-5}$$

If the stool osmolal gap is less than 50 mOsm/L, the patient most likely has a secretional diarrhea.[5] A stool osmolal gap greater than 50 mOsm/L suggests the presence of unabsorbed, osmotic materials such as food. A large gap also may be seen in cases of excessive use of laxatives, some of which, such as the magnesium-containing laxatives, can be detected in stool water by the measurement of magnesium.

The osmolality of fresh liquid stool is approximately equal to that of serum. A hypo-osmolar watery stool (approximately <280 mOsm/L) might be suggestive of a factitious diarrhea, that is, one created by the patient, such as by adding water to the stool (Munchausen syndrome).[6]

Intestinal bacteria present in the stool can very rapidly convert stool carbohydrates into osmotically active fragments, raising the stool water osmolality. Thus stool osmolality measurements should be performed within 30 minutes of collection of the stool sample.

Serum or Plasma Osmolality

Sample collection technique is important in obtaining a valid specimen for measurement of osmolality. For example, stasis

Table 11-3 Estimated Effect of Anticoagulants on Osmolality (Compared with Serum)

Anticoagulant	Full Tube, mOsm/kg	Half-Full Tube, mOsm/kg
Heparin	+0	+0
EDTA (disodium salt)	+15	+30
Fluoride-oxalate (sodium fluoride–potassium oxalate)*	+150	+300
Iodoacetic acid (lithium salt)	+5	+10

*This hyperosmolal state accounts for the hemolysis that usually is observed in the plasma of these samples.

during phlebotomy should be avoided. In addition, the patient's position, supine or upright, affects the osmolality. Thus a sample from a fasting, hospitalized patient gives the most reproducible results.

Serum and heparinized plasma have similar osmolality values. The contribution to the osmolality by fibrinogen in plasma is small, and it is important only in the measurement of COP. Freezing-point depression techniques can use whole blood and are not affected by lipemia or hemolysis. Anticoagulants other than heparin increase the measured osmolality. Table 11-3 shows the estimated effect of four anticoagulants. On occasion, the type of anticoagulant used can be verified by measurement of plasma osmolality.

COLLOID OSMOTIC PRESSURE

The major use for the measurement of the COP is detection of conditions leading to pulmonary edema. In this condition, there is an accumulation of water in the lungs, which interferes with oxygen and carbon dioxide exchange. The actual diagnosis can be obtained from x-ray measurements. Two measurements are needed to predict pulmonary edema: left ventricular heart pressure and COP. As long as the COP is greater than the pulmonary blood pressure (as measured by the "pulmonary artery wedge pressure"), pulmonary edema is unlikely. If heart failure is not present, that is, if the pulmonary blood pressure is normal, COP measurements alone allow prediction of the probability of pulmonary edema.

Knowledge of the albumin or total protein content of the plasma permits estimation of the COP.[7]

$$COP_{plasma} = \alpha(2.8c + 0.18c^2 + 0.012c^3) + \beta(0.9c + 0.12c^2 + 0.004c^3)$$

(COP, mm Hg; c, protein content, g/dL, α, albumin content, g/dL; β, gamma content, g/dL) Eq. 11-6

However, the formula is inaccurate when used for acutely ill patients (especially patients with heart failure) and for patients who have received dextrans, or **plasma expanders.**

KEY CONCEPTS BOX 11-3

- Measurement of serum osmolality can be used to detect abnormal osmolar states resulting from disease.
- The osmolar gap can be used to screen for ingestion of toxins.
- Urine osmolarity can be used to access renal concentrating ability.
- Stool osmolarity can be used to determine the cause of diarrhea.

REFERENCES

1. Lord RCC: Review. Current concepts: osmosis, osmometry, and osmoregulation, Postgrad Med J 75:67, 1999.
2. Dorwart VW, Chalmers L: Comparison of methods for calculating serum osmolality from chemical concentrations and the prognostic value of such calculations, Clin Chem 21:190, 1975.
3. Glaser DS: Utility of the serum osmol gap in the diagnosis of methanol or ethylene glycol ingestion, Ann Emerg Med 27:343, 1996.
4. Darchy B, Abruzzese L, Pitiot O, et al: Delayed admission for ethylene glycol poisoning: lack of elevated serum osmol gap, Intensive Care Med 25:859, 1999.
5. Castro-Rodríguez JA, Salazar-Lindo E, León-Barúa R: Differentiation of osmotic and secretory diarrhoea by stool carbohydrate and osmolar gap measurements, Arch Dis Child 77:201, 1997.
6. Topazian M, Binder HJ: Brief report: factitious diarrhea detected by measurement of stool osmolality, N Engl J Med 330:1418, 1994.
7. Nitta S, Ohnuki T, Ohkuda K, Nakada T, Staub NC: The corrected protein equation to estimate plasma colloid osmotic pressure and its development on a nomogram, Tohoku J Exp Med 135:43, 1981.

INTERNET SITES

Giibs-Donnon—http://www.physioviva.com/movies/gibbs-donnan/index.html

Osmometry—1.1 http://www.aicompanies.com/PDFs/Articles/APP_Frz_2264_SP%20Rev1.pdf

Colligative properties—http://hyperphysics.phy-astr.gsu.edu/HBASE/chemical/meltpt.html#c1

http://hyperphysics.phy-astr.gsu.edu/HBASE/chemical/boilpt.html#c1

Colloid oncotic pressure—http://physioweb.med.uvm.edu/bodyfluids/

www.cvphysiology.com/Microcirculation/M012.htm

Electrochemistry: Principles and Measurements

12 Chapter

William R. Heineman, Jon R. Kirchhoff, John F. Wheeler, Craig E. Lunte, and Sarah H. Jenkins

Chapter Outline

Key Terms

activity (a) The effective concentration of a solution species that accounts for interactions with other solution species. The value used in a thermodynamically correct equilibrium expression.

activity coefficient (γ) Activity divided by molar concentration. A measure of the degree to which a species interacts with other solution species.

amperometry A controlled-potential technique in which current is measured at a fixed applied potential.

anode The electrode at which oxidation occurs.

auxiliary electrode The electrode in a three-electrode electrochemical cell that carries the current to maintain electrolysis at the working electrode.

cathode The electrode at which reduction occurs.

cell potential (E_{cell}) The quantitative measure of the energy of an electrochemical cell; the difference in electron energy between two electrodes.

charge (Q) A quantity of electricity that reflects the total current during a given time: $Q = \int_0^t i dt$ or $Q = it$ for constant i.

coulometry A technique that measures the charge required to electrolyze a sample completely.

current (i) The rate of charge flow (1 ampere = 1 coulomb/second).

electrolysis A nonspontaneous electrochemical reaction that results from the application of potential to an electrochemical cell.

electrolyte solution A solution of ions that provides a conducting medium for electrochemistry.

half-cell potential The quantitative measure of the energy of a half-cell reaction relative to a reference electrode.

half-cell reaction An electrochemical reaction that represents either an oxidation or a reduction at one of the electrodes in an electrochemical cell.

hydrodynamic voltammogram A graphical representation of current versus applied potential for a particular electrochemical reaction that occurs in a stirred or flowing solution.

indicator electrode An electrode whose half-cell or membrane potential varies as the concentrations of reactants and products change in solution. This potential is governed by the Nernst equation.

ionophore A neutral carrier molecule incorporated into an ion-selective electrode to detect a specific ion.

ion-selective electrode (ISE) An indicator electrode used in potentiometry to respond to specific ions in solution.

limiting current (i_l) The portion of a hydrodynamic voltammogram where electrolysis is occurring and the current remains constant as a function of increased applied potential.

liquid junction potential (E_{lj}) A potential that develops at the interface between two nonidentical solutions.

Nernst equation The expression that relates the cell potential to the standard cell potential and the activities of reactants and products within an electrochemical cell.

oxidation The process whereby a chemical species loses one or more electrons.

polarography Voltammetry performed at a dropping mercury working electrode.

potentiometry The technique in which the potential difference between two electrodes is measured under equilibrium conditions.

potentiostat An instrument that controls the potential of an electrochemical cell.

reduction The process whereby a chemical species gains one or more electrons.

reference electrode An electrode with a stable half-cell potential that is used to measure and control the relative potential of the working electrode.

salt bridge A device that allows ionic movement between compartments of an electrochemical cell to maintain electrical contact and at the same time prevent mixing of the separate solutions.

standard half-cell potential (E°) The electrochemical cell potential measured under standard state conditions.

stripping voltammetry A voltammetric technique that allows sample preconcentration at the electrode before voltammetric analysis.

voltammetry A technique whereby current is measured as a function of applied potential.

Electrochemistry involves the measurement of electrical signals associated with chemical systems that are incorporated into an electrochemical cell. The cell consists of two or more electrodes that interface a chemical system and an electrical system. The electrical system measures or controls the electrical parameters of voltage and **current *(i)*,** which are characteristic of a particular chemical system.

Electroanalytical chemistry makes use of electrochemistry for the purpose of analysis. In this application, the magnitude of a voltage or current signal originating from an electrochemical cell is related to the **activity** or concentration of a particular chemical species in the cell. Excellent detection limits coupled with a wide dynamic range are exhibited by many electroanalytical techniques, with an operating range of 10^{-8} to 10^{-1} M. Measurements generally can be made on very small volumes of sample, that is, in the microliter range and below. The combination of low detection limits and microliter volume samples allows picomole amounts of analyte to be measured routinely in some instances. Furthermore, electroanalysis lends itself to measurements made in vivo. For example, miniature electrochemical sensors are used to measure pH and partial pressure of oxygen (Po_2) in the bloodstream of patients with indwelling catheters.

In the clinical laboratory, electroanalysis is used routinely for the determination of many ions, drugs, hormones, metals, and gases. Methods are available for the rapid determination of analytes present at relatively high concentrations, such as blood electrolytes (Na^+, Cl^-, HCO_3^-), and analytes present at very low concentrations, such as lead and cardiac markers, in blood and urine samples.

The purpose of this chapter is to provide a fundamental background for understanding the electroanalytical techniques found in the clinical laboratory and to illustrate some of the practical applications of electroanalysis. These electrochemical techniques are divided into three basic categories: potentiometric, voltammetric, and coulometric. **Potentiometry,** the most widely used clinical application of electrochemistry, involves the measurement of a **cell potential (E_{cell})** under equilibrium conditions. **Voltammetry** and **coulometry** are considered dynamic techniques and are based on measurements made on a cell in which **electrolysis** is occurring. Many of the common definitions and symbols and much of the electrochemical nomenclature used in potentiometry, voltammetry, and coulometry are listed in Table 12-1.

Table 12-1 Electrochemical Terms, Units, Constants, Symbols, and Conversions

Term	Symbol	Unit of Constant	Symbol	Conversion or Value
Potential	E	Volt	V	V = J/C
Standard potential	(E^0)			E = i × R
Formal potential	($E^{0\prime}$)			
Current	i	Ampere	A	A = C/s
				1A = 1.05×10^{-5} mol of electrons per second
Charge	Q	Coulomb	C	C = A × s
				1C = 1.05×10^{-5} mol of electrons
Energy	H	Joule	J	
Resistance	R	Ohm	Ω	
Time	t	Second	s	
Temperature	T	Kelvin	K	
Activity	a	Moles per liter	mol/L	
Concentration	C	Moles per liter	mol/L	
		or moles per cubic centimeter	mol/cm^3	
Area	A	Square centimeters	cm^2	
Diffusion coefficient	D	Square centimeters per second	cm^2/s	
		Gas constant	R	8.31441 J/mol × K
		Faraday constant	F	9.64846×10^4 C/mol
		Number of electrons in electrode or redox reaction	n	

SECTION OBJECTIVES BOX 12-1

- Describe the scientific basis for potentiometric techniques.
- Describe the differences between a reference electrode and a detecting electrode.
- Explain the process by which ion-selective electrodes respond to the presence of an analyte and how they are used for clinical measurements.
- Describe how gas-sensing electrodes differ from other ion-selective electrodes (ISEs).
- Develop a knowledge of the methods and possible interferences associated with using electrochemistry in the clinical laboratory.

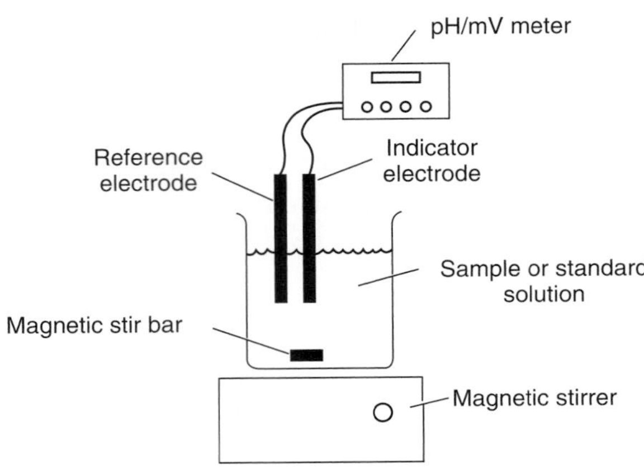

Fig. 12-1 Schema of apparatus for potentiometry.

POTENTIOMETRIC METHODS

Potentiometric methods are based on the measurement of a potential (voltage) difference between two electrodes immersed in solution under the condition of essentially zero current. The electrodes and the solution constitute an *electrochemical cell.* Each electrode in the electrochemical cell is characterized by a **half-cell reaction** with a corresponding **half-cell potential.** Potential, an important concept in electrochemistry, can be thought of as the power of the half-cell reaction. Potential is always measured against a fixed reference point or potential, which in electrochemistry terms is defined by a **reference electrode.** This allows direct comparison of the relative potential of two or more systems (i.e., half-cell reactions) to be easily made. The greater power (potential) of a half-cell reaction is indicated by a greater potential difference of the half-cell reaction relative to the reference point. By analogy, a baseball dropped from the top of a 10-story building will have greater potential (power) than a ball dropped from eye level with the ground used as the reference point.

Because essentially no current passes through the electrochemical cell during a potentiometric measurement, no net electrochemical reaction occurs. Thus, a potentiometric technique is an equilibrium method. Potentiometric techniques are important because they can provide accurate measurements of activities, concentrations, or activity coefficients of many solution species. In general, a solution of ions or molecules is characterized by its molar concentration. However, these species can interact with other ions, molecules, or solvent. Depending on the types of interactions that occur, the effective concentration of the species may be less than, equal to, or greater than the actual molar concentration of the species. The effective concentration is referred to as the **activity** of the species and is related to the molar concentration by an activity coefficient as shown in Eq. 12-1:

$$a_i = \gamma_i C_i \qquad \text{Eq. 12-1}$$

where a_i is the activity of an ionic species, γ_i is the **activity coefficient,** and C_i is the molar concentration of that species. Activity is the value used in a thermodynamically correct equilibrium expression, whereas concentration is the quantity of interest to clinical chemists.

A typical apparatus for potentiometry as shown in Fig. 12-1 includes two electrodes connected to a pH-millivolt meter to measure the potential difference between the two electrodes. One electrode, the **indicator electrode,** is chosen so that its half-cell potential (E_{ind}) responds to changes in the activity of a particular analyte species in solution. The other electrode is a reference electrode whose half-cell potential (E_{ref}) does not change.

Another important concept in potentiometry is that an individual half-cell potential is not measured. Only the potential difference between the indicator electrode half-cell and the reference electrode is measured. Furthermore, when the indicator electrode senses a change in analyte activity in solution, the potential difference changes, indicating a new analyte activity. The potential difference of the electrochemical cell, E_{cell}, is given by

$$E_{cell} = E_{ind} - E_{ref} + E_{lj} \qquad \text{Eq. 12-2}$$

where E_{lj} is the liquid junction potential. The liquid junction potential is the electrical potential that develops at the interface between two liquids as a result of differences in the rates with which ions move from one liquid to the other. For example, the liquid junction potential arises in Fig. 12-1 at the point where the tip of the reference electrode meets the solution because the ion types and concentrations inside the reference electrode usually differ from those of the sample into which it is immersed. Thus, E_{lj} is a potential that results from differences in **charge *(Q)*** rather than from an electrochemical reaction at an electrode, and typically it can be assumed to be constant for a given solution. The effect of the liquid junction potential can be minimized by adjusting the sample ionic strength. Because E_{ref} + E_{lj} are constant, it follows from Eq. 12-2 that E_{cell} changes only when E_{ind} changes with analyte activity. Therefore, the change in E_{cell} can be used for analysis.

Reference Electrodes

Since every electrochemical measurement is made with respect to a reference half-cell potential, a good understanding of the properties and types of reference electrodes is important.

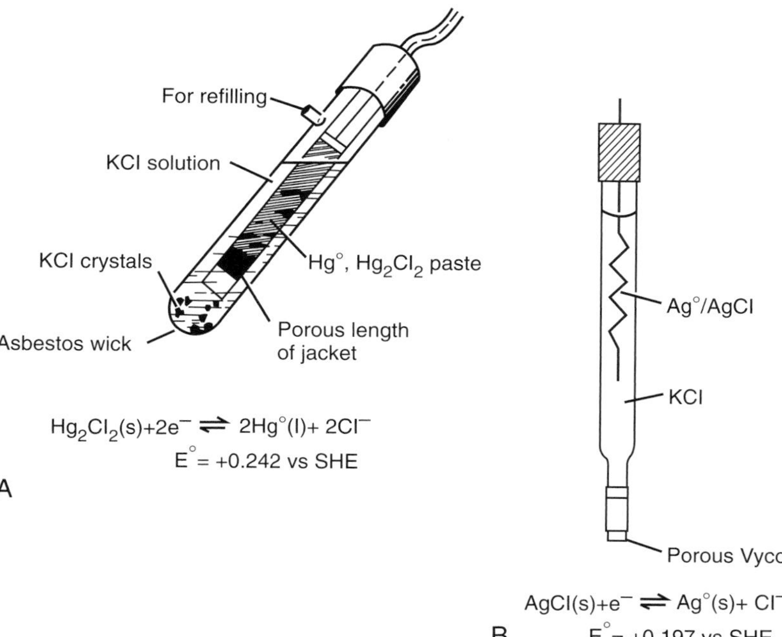

Fig. 12-2 Reference electrodes. **A,** Saturated calomel electrode *(SCE)* with asbestos wick for **salt bridge** function. **B,** Silver/silver chloride electrode (Ag/AgCl) with porous Vycor for salt bridge function.

A reference electrode is an electrochemical half-cell that is used as a fixed reference for the measurement of cell potentials. Ideally, a reference electrode should possess the following characteristics: a stable, easily reproducible half-cell potential; a reversible half-cell reaction; chemical stability of its components; and ease of fabrication and use. Three reference electrodes are discussed below; one is of fundamental significance, and two are of practical importance.

The *standard hydrogen electrode (SHE)* is the reference half-cell electrode on which tables of standard electrode potentials are based. In this half-cell, hydrogen gas at a pressure of 1 atmosphere is bubbled over a platinum electrode immersed in acid solution for which the activity of H^+ is unity. The potential of the SHE is defined as 0.0 V at all temperatures, and the potentials of other half-cell couples are referenced to this value. The potentials of other half-cells are either negative or positive of 0.0 V. Because other reference electrodes are easier to construct and use, the SHE is used rarely in practical applications of electrochemistry. However, it remains the reference electrode upon which tables of half-cell **reduction** potentials are based.

A commonly used reference electrode is the *saturated calomel electrode (SCE)*. A schema of a common type of SCE, its half-cell reaction, and its **standard half-cell potential** are shown in Fig. 12-2, *A*. The electrode consists of elemental mercury covered with a thin coating of calomel (Hg_2Cl_2) that is in contact with an aqueous solution saturated with KCl. The potential of the half-cell will be constant so long as the activity of Cl^- does not change. The easiest verifiable way to set the activity of Cl^- to a fixed value is to saturate the solution with a chloride salt such as KCl. So long as crystals of KCl are present, the experimenter knows that the solution is saturated, and that the activity of Cl^- is constant. Note that the other participants in the electrochemical reaction (Hg_2Cl_2 and Hg) are solid and liquid components and consequently exhibit unit activity, regardless of the amounts present in the cell. Thus the SCE offers the extraordinary convenience of being easily fabricated without the need for accurate preparation of the activities of any of the components.

Another commonly used reference electrode is the *silver/silver chloride electrode* (Ag/AgCl). A representative Ag/AgCl reference electrode is shown in Fig. 12-2, *B*. The electrode is prepared by coating a silver wire with a thin film of AgCl and immersing it in a solution of constant chloride concentration, which fixes the half-cell potential. The Ag/AgCl reference electrode is used routinely, especially as the inner reference electrode, in potentiometric membrane electrodes. The SCE and Ag/AgCl electrodes are commercially available or can be constructed conveniently.

Indicator Electrodes

The indicator electrode (or sensing electrode) is the essence of potentiometric analysis. This electrode should interact with the analyte of interest so that E_{ind} reflects the activity of this species in solution and not of other compounds in the sample that might interfere. The relative response of an electrode to one species and not to another species defines the selectivity of the electrode. The less an electrode responds to a non-analyte species, the better is its selectivity. The importance of having indicator electrodes that selectively respond to species of analytical significance has stimulated the development of many types of these electrodes.

Ion-Selective Electrodes

The most common indicator electrode used in clinical chemistry is the **ion-selective electrode (ISE).** The ISE is based on the measurement of a potential that develops across a selective membrane. The response of the electrochemical

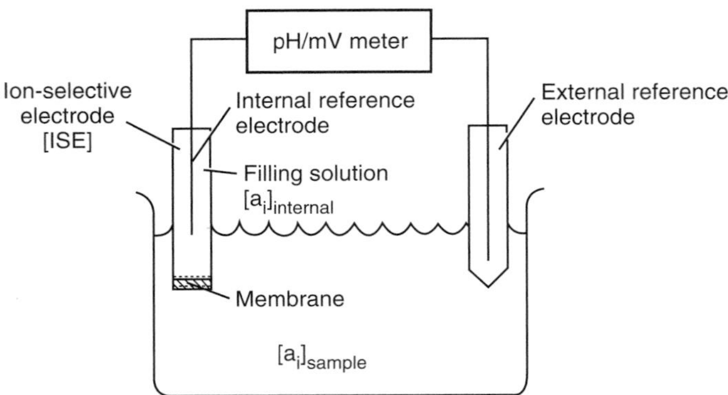

Fig. 12-3 Schema of an ion-selective electrode (ISE), external reference electrode, and pH/mV meter.

cell therefore is based on an interaction between the membrane and the analyte that alters the potential across the membrane. The selectivity of the potential response to an analyte depends on the specificity of the membrane interaction for the analyte.

A representative ISE is shown schematically in Fig. 12-3. The electrode consists of a membrane, an internal reference electrolyte of fixed activity, $(a_i)_{internal}$, and an internal reference electrode. The ISE is immersed in a sample solution that contains analyte of some activity, $(a_i)_{sample}$. An external reference electrode also is immersed in this solution. The internal and external reference electrodes constitute the two half-cells of the electrochemical cell. The potential measured by the pH/mV meter (E_{cell}) is equal to the difference in potential between the external ($E_{ref,ext}$) and internal ($E_{ref,int}$) reference electrodes, plus the membrane potential (E_{memb}), plus the **liquid junction potential (E_{lj})** that exists at the junction between the external reference electrode and the sample solution (Eq. 12-3). If the membrane is permeable to a particular ion [i], a potential develops across the membrane that depends on the ratio of activities of the ion on either side of the membrane. The half-cell potentials of the two reference electrodes are constant, sample solution conditions can be controlled so that E_{lj} is effectively constant, and the composition of the internal solution can be maintained so that $(a_i)_{internal}$ is fixed. Consequently, E_{cell} is described by the **Nernst equation** shown in Eq. 12-4, where K represents the constant terms and z is the charge on the analyte ion (cations: +1, +2, +3, and so on; anions: −1, −2, −3, and so on). This logarithmical relationship between cell potential and analyte activity serves as the basis of the ISE as an analytical device. A plot of E_{cell} versus log a_i for a series of standard solutions should be linear over the working range of the electrode and should have a slope of $2.3RT/zF$ or $0.0591/z$ for measurements made at 25°C. With the use of concentration instead of activity, calibration plots are readily constructed for analysis of the ion under consideration.

$$E_{cell} = E_{ref,ext} - E_{ref,int} + E_{memb} + E_{lj} \qquad \text{Eq. 12-3}$$

$$E_{cell} = K + 2.3\frac{RT}{zF}\log(a_i)_{sample} \qquad \text{Eq. 12-4}$$

$$E_{cell} = K + 2.3\frac{RT}{zF}\log[(a_i)_{sample} + k_{ij}a^{z/x}{}_j] \qquad \text{Eq. 12-5}$$

Many clinical samples are complex mixtures and potentially contain non-analyte ions that might interfere with analysis. As was noted above, ISEs have been developed to have the greatest selectivity possible. However, membranes may respond to a certain degree to ions other than the analyte (i.e., interferents). Thus, Eq. 12-5 provides a more general expression than Eq. 12-4 to account for membrane potential changes arising from the interferent(s). In Eq. 12-5, a_j is the activity of the interferent ion [j], x is the charge of the interferent ion, and k_{ij} is the selectivity constant. Small values of k_{ij} are characteristic of electrodes with good selectivity for the analyte, i.

The development of successful ISEs has hinged on the search for membranes that exhibit both sensitivity and selectivity for the analyte of interest. Of the two properties, selectivity is by far the more difficult to achieve. ISEs with selectivity for cations and anions have been developed with three basic types of membranes: liquid and polymer, solid state, and glass. All of these membranes function by selectively incorporating the analyte ion into the membrane, thereby establishing a membrane potential that depends on the activity of that ion in the sample. An ISE membrane must exhibit low solubility in the analyte medium to provide a durable electrode with a stable response. This requirement imposes a severe restriction on the material that can be used for membranes. Also, the membrane must exhibit some electrical conductivity to function in an electrochemical cell. The scope of ISEs has been expanded to include the measurement of gases and neutral organic compounds by combining ISEs with gas-permeable membranes and layers of enzymes, bacteria, and tissues. These general categories of electrodes and specific ISEs are considered in the following sections.

Liquid and Polymer Membrane Electrodes

A selective liquid membrane provides the basis for many excellent ISEs. The liquid consists of a water-insoluble, viscous solvent in which is dissolved an **ionophore,** a hydrophobic organic ion exchanger, or a neutral carrier molecule that has selective affinity for the ion of interest. The liquid typically is soaked into a thin, porous solid membrane such as cellulose acetate, which then is incorporated into the ISE. Alternatively, the ionophore can be incorporated in plasticized poly (vinyl chloride) as the membrane material.

Fig. 12-4 shows the schema of the membrane portion of a liquid membrane ISE and the mechanism whereby an electrode responds to the analyte ion (M^+) activity. The liquid membrane is in contact with internal and sample aqueous solutions of M^+. The neutral carrier ionophore (R) reacts with M^+ at each membrane-solution interface and extracts M^+ into the membrane as MR^+. The extraction of M^+ into the membrane generates a positive membrane potential at each interface as a result of the charge difference that occurs when M^+ is extracted into the membrane in the form of MR^+ and the counter anion X^- remains in the aqueous solution. As the

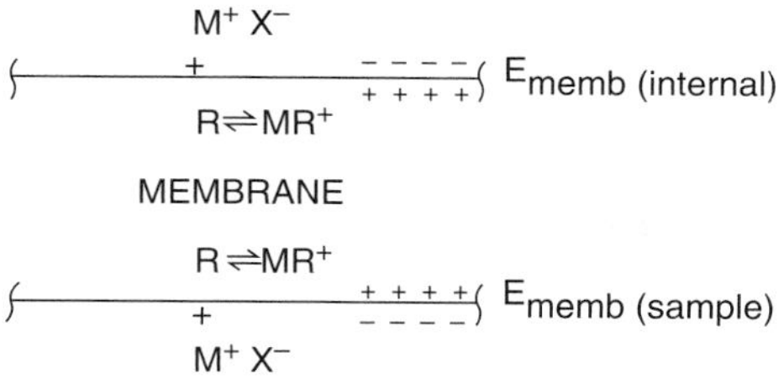

Fig. 12-4 Schema of liquid membrane ion-selective electrode (ISE), where M^+ represents analyte cation, and R represents neutral carrier ionophore.

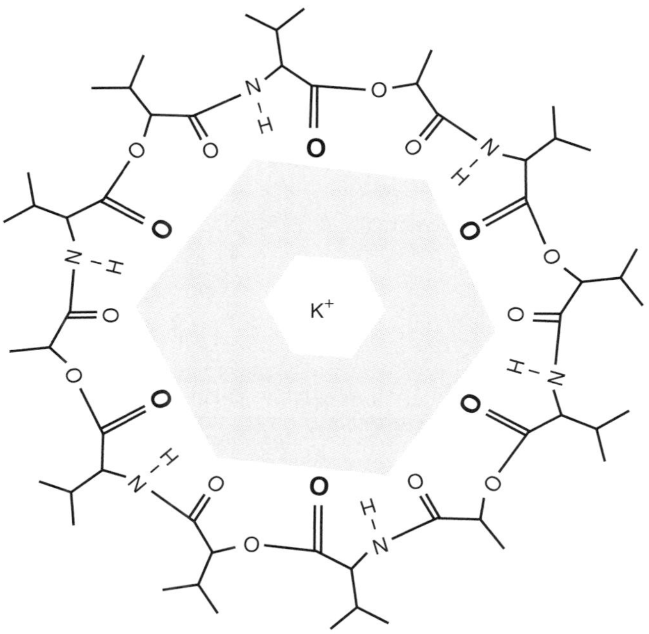

Fig. 12-5 Model of K^+ complex of valinomycin. Gray region represents K^+ ion. Bold oxygens are binding atoms.

activity of M^+ in solution is increased, the activity of MR^+ in the membrane increases and the membrane potential increases. This reaction exists at both the outer membrane surface, which is exposed to the sample, and the inner membrane surface, which contacts the inner filling solution of the ISE. The potential of the inner surface of the membrane, $E_{memb(internal)}$, is kept constant by maintenance of a constant activity of M^+ in the internal solution. Thus the only potential change measured in the circuit is the potential of the membrane surface contacting the sample, $E_{memb(sample)}$.

The availability of liquid and polymer membrane electrodes for a variety of ions is the result of the development of different neutral carrier ionophores and liquid ion exchangers that react selectively with particular ions. In the surface equilibria shown in Fig. 12-4, any ionic species other than M^+ that reacts to an appreciable degree with R will also generate a membrane potential and thereby cause an interference (Eq. 12-5). The selectivity of the electrode for M^+ therefore is determined by the relative affinity between R and M^+ and between R and the various interferent ions in the sample.

Several ionophores that selectively bind cations to nonaqueous membranes have been found. When a cation reacts with an ionophore, it is essentially inserted in a cavity within the ionophore that allows the cation to exist within a nonaqueous membrane medium. Selectivity for a particular cationic species is controlled by provision of an optimum environment in terms of number and position of binding atoms. An excellent example is the antibiotic valinomycin, which exhibits excellent selectivity for K^+. Fig. 12-5 illustrates the K^+ complex of valinomycin. The K^+ cation fits into a snug cavity surrounded by oxygen atoms. The electrode exhibits excellent selectivity for K^+ against Na^+ because the smaller Na^+ ion is bound less tightly in the valinomycin cavity. This feature is of considerable practical importance in the clinical determination of K^+ in serum, which contains higher concentrations of Na^+ than of K^+. Ionophores for the selective determination of NH_4^+, Ca^{2+}, Na^+, Li^+, and Mg^{2+} have also been incorporated into ISEs. The selective incorporation of these cations occurs by the same principle described for the K^+ electrode. The development of liquid and polymer membrane ISEs has allowed the measurement of ions in samples of diverse origin. The electrodes have been especially successful in clinical laboratories and now are used routinely for measuring Li^+, Ca^{2+}, K^+, Na^+, and Cl^- in biological fluids.

The response characteristics for liquid and polymer membrane ISE systems commonly used in biomedical investigations are shown in Table 12-2. Detection limits and linear ranges will vary among electrodes, especially for the liquid and polymer membrane type, depending on the ionophore and the filling solution used. Therefore, Table 12-2 summarizes typical linear ranges associated with current commercially available ISEs. Possible interferents are also given in Table 12-2. The impact of an interferent typically becomes greater as the concentration of the interferent increases or as the analyte concentration that is being measured decreases.

Recent advances in ISE technology for research applications have resulted in detection limits as low as 10^{-8} to 10^{-11} M, rivaling many trace analysis methods. New ion exchangers and neutral carriers are being evaluated continually in an effort to improve the selectivity of existing electrodes and to develop electrodes for other ions and molecules. Miniaturization also has allowed application of ISEs to determine analytes in low sample volumes. Continued research on ISE methods and materials will likely bring new innovations and applications in the future.

Solid-State Membrane Electrodes

Solid-state membranes consist of single crystals or pressed pellets of salts of the ions of interest. The crystal or pellet must have some degree of electrical conductivity and must exhibit very low solubility in the solvent in which the electrode is to be used—usually water. An excellent ISE for F^- uses LaF_3 crystals doped with Eu^{2+} to provide electrical conductivity. The membrane potential is generated by a selective surface reaction between LaF_3 and F^- in which solution F^- is incorporated into vacancies in the crystal lattice. The selectivity is very good

Table 12-2 Ion-Selective Electrodes (ISEs) Used in Clinical Chemistry

	Analyte	Linear Response Range, mol/L	Possible Interferences
Glass	H^+	10^{-12} to 10^{-2}	Na^+ (above pH 10)
	Na^+	10^{-6} to sat'd	K^+, Ag^+, Li^+
Solid state	F^-	10^{-6} to sat'd	OH^-
	Cl^-	5×10^{-5} to 1	Br^-, CN^-, S^{2-}, I^-
Liquid or polymer membrane	Na^+	10^{-5} to 1	Li^+, K^+, Ca^{2+}
	Cl^-	5×10^{-5} to 1	OH^-, Br^-, F^-
	K^+	10^{-6} to 1	NH_4^+, Cs^+, Tl^+
	Li^+	10^{-5} to 1	Ca^{2+}, Na^+, K^+
	Ca^{2+}	5×10^{-7} to 1	Pb^{2+}, Hg^{2+}, Cu^{2+}, Ni^{2+}, Fe^{2+}, Sr^{2+}
Gas sensors	CO_2	10^{-4} to 10^{-2}	Organic acids
	NH_3	5×10^{-7} to 1	Volatile amines

From http://www.thermo.com and https://www.fishersci.com.
Sat'd refers to saturated where the analyte has achieved itis maximum solubity under given solution conditions.

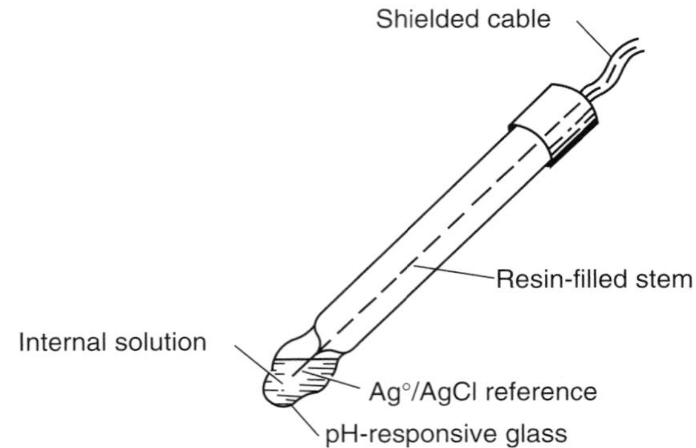

Fig. 12-6 Representative pH electrode.

because other anions do not fit well into the crystal structure. Another clinically important solid-state membrane electrode for determination of Cl^- is based on pressed-pellet membranes of the ionic conductor, Ag_2S, and AgCl. Similar electrodes have also been developed for the detection of Br^-, CN^-, I^-, SCN^-, S^{2-}, Ag^+, Cu^{2+}, Pb^{2+}, and Cd^{2+}.

Glass Membrane Electrodes

The first and most widely used ISE is the glass membrane electrode for pH measurements. Glasses of certain compositions respond to pH when a membrane potential develops as a result of an ion-exchange mechanism with H^+ that occurs in the thin, hydrated outer layer of the glass membrane that has been soaked in solution. The outstanding properties of the glass pH electrode are attributable to the remarkable selectivity of this surface reaction for H^+.

The basic design of the glass electrode for pH is shown in Fig. 12-6. The electrode consists of a glass or plastic tube with a thin, pH-sensitive glass membrane sealed within the tip. Ordinarily, the membrane is only about 50 μm thick and hence is very fragile. The bulb at the end contains an internal solution composed of 0.1 M HCl, into which is dipped a silver wire coated with AgCl, which provides an internal Ag/AgCl reference electrode. This solution also maintains a fixed activity of H^+, to which the internal surface of the membrane is exposed. A shielded cable provides electrical contact between the internal Ag wire and the external pH meter.

The pH response of the glass membrane is determined by the composition of the glass, which typically consists of Na_2O, CaO, and SiO_2. Pure SiO_2 is essentially an insulator that is unresponsive to pH. The addition of Na_2O to the glass formulation disrupts the neutral SiO_2 structure, so that negatively charged oxide sites (SiO^-) are paired with Na^+. The mobility of Na^+ in the glass renders the glass membrane slightly conductive to electrical charge. The negative oxide sites serve as ion-exchange sites in aqueous solution and provide the basis for pH response. The potential response to pH is extraordinarily accurate over a pH range of 0 to 14. At pH values above about 10, some pH electrodes exhibit significant response to other monovalent cations such as Na^+ and K^+. This response to alkali cations at high pH is termed the *alkaline error.* This error can be minimized to a certain extent by replacement of Na_2O and CaO within the glass with Li_2O and BaO.

On immersion of a dry glass membrane in an aqueous solution, the membrane surface becomes hydrated during the course of a few hours. The hydrated layer is only about 10 nm thick and is essential for establishing the cation exchange between Na^+ and H^+ ions at negatively charged oxide sites on the glass matrix. New electrodes will respond poorly until adequately soaked. Soaking the electrode in acid, for example, results in the replacement of Na^+ with H^+. The membrane response to H^+ can be understood in terms of a surface potential that results from the ion exchange of Na^+ with H^+ in the hydrated gel. Immersion of the electrode membrane in alkaline solution results in exchange of H^+ in the membrane with Na^+ as membrane H^+ moves into solution. The inner membrane potential is held constant by exposure to the fixed activity of H^+ in the internal solution. The hydration process also leads to a gradual dissolving of the glass layer, which generally

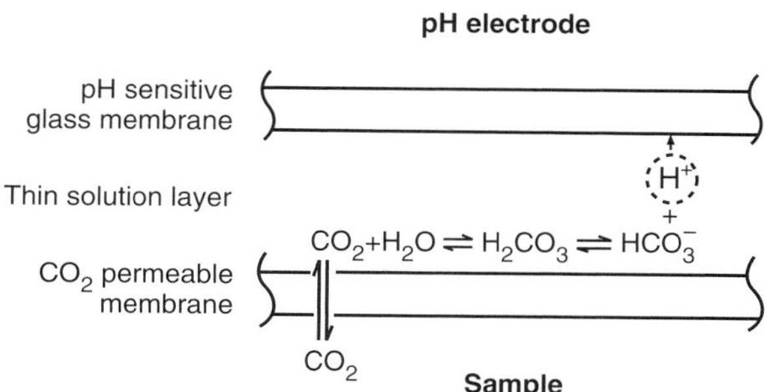

Fig. 12-7 Schema of gas-sensing electrode for carbon dioxide (CO_2).

determines the useful lifetime of an electrode. Glass electrodes for Na^+, Ag^+, and NH_4^+ have been developed by varying the composition of the glass.

Gas-Sensing Electrodes

Gas-sensing electrodes consist of an ISE in contact with a thin layer of aqueous electrolyte confined to the electrode surface by an outer membrane, as is shown schematically for a carbon dioxide (CO_2) electrode in Fig. 12-7. The outer membrane is very thin and is chosen so that it is permeable to the gas of interest; for CO_2, the membrane is made of silicone rubber. This membrane allows the passage of CO_2 gas in the sample. Dissolution of the CO_2 in the thin layer of electrolyte causes a change in pH that results from a shift in the equilibrium position of the chemical reaction shown in Fig. 12-7. The change in pH sensed by the internal ion-selective pH electrode is in proportion to the partial pressure of carbon dioxide (P_{CO_2}) of the sample. One of the most important applications of the CO_2 electrode is the measurement of blood P_{CO_2}.

The ammonia (NH_3) electrode in principle is identical to the CO_2 electrode; here the filling solution is aqueous ammonium chloride. The internal pH electrode senses the change in pH from the ammonium/ammonia (NH_4^+/NH_3) acid-base equilibrium. The pH change is thus proportional to the partial pressure of ammonia (P_{NH_3}) of the sample.

Gas electrodes have been used for other bioanalytical applications such as the measurement of CO_2 in general assays of decarboxylating enzyme activities and the measurement of NH_3 in tissue and serum. Characteristics of the CO_2 and NH_3 electrodes are shown in Table 12-2.

Care and Methodology

The care of ISEs is essentially similar for every ion type. Because the sensing tip of the electrode is made from fragile and sensitive materials, caution must be exercised to prevent breakage and to maintain the tip in a moist environment. Most commercially available electrodes are supplied with protective coverings to help prevent damage while they are not in use. Each ISE is also accompanied by the manufacturer's recommendations for specific cleaning and storage requirements. Storage and cleaning conditions depend on frequency of use, type of electrode, and application. For example, cleaning procedures are different for a pH electrode used in a protein solution versus an electrode used in a solution of inorganic ions. When exposed to proteins, electrodes are cleansed by rinsing with pepsin, bleach, or 0.1 M HCl, whereas an inorganic salt deposit might best be removed with a solution of ethylenediaminetetraacetic acid (EDTA). After each cleaning procedure, the electrode tip is rinsed thoroughly with distilled water, and the electrode is returned to the appropriate buffer or standard solution for storage.

Measurements of pH are easily made in the clinical laboratory with a two-point calibration procedure. Standard buffer solutions, which are commercially available, are chosen to bracket the pH of the sample solution. Electrode calibration is always initiated with a pH 7.00 buffer. The meter is adjusted to read 7.00 after the temperature control of the pH/mV/ion meter has been adjusted to the buffer temperature (alternatively, temperature is automatically compensated in many commercial meters with the use of a second probe). Depending on the sample to be measured, either an acidic (e.g., pH 4.00) or an alkaline standard buffer (pH 10.00) is used to complete the calibration, after which samples can be measured. Multiple calibrations may be necessary for large numbers of samples to compensate for electrode drift over time. In the case of pH measurements of physiological fluids, a two-point calibration with two buffers that tightly bracket the usual blood pH is used to ensure the greatest accuracy. Two such buffers are 0.08 M MOPSO, 0.08 M NaMOPSO, and 0.08 M NaCl (pH 6.865 at 25°C); and 0.08 M HEPES, 0.08 M NaHEPES, and 0.08 M NaCl (pH 7.516 at 25°C).

For other ISEs, an internal calibration procedure that relates the potential difference (in millivolts) to the log of the calibrant concentrations is used. Although ISEs measure an analyte's activity rather than concentration as strictly defined, the concentration can be logarithmically related to potential as long as the ionic strength is constant between standards and samples. This is accomplished by adding a small amount of a solution of high ionic strength to the calibrating standards and samples (e.g., 2 M $[NH_4]_2SO_4$, referred to as the ionic strength adjustment buffer), which must not contain any interfering ions. A recording of solution potential is made for each standard solution by the pH/mV/ion meter, beginning with the lowest concentration. A plot of log $(C_i)_{standard}$ versus potential is linear for a properly responding ISE until the limit of detection is approached, and the pH/mV/ion meter maintains a stored record of the calibration. Once calibrated, ion concentrations in samples are thus obtained by measurement of the potential response of the sample and use of the internal calibration curve to display sample concentration. Sample ion concentrations are valid as long as the matrix of the standard solutions is made to closely mimic the samples.

Most laboratory instruments routinely use a two-point standardization procedure to ensure similarity of response from analysis to analysis. Other standardization and analysis techniques have been developed for various electrodes and applications. For example, interference suppressor solutions are available from electrode manufacturers for use with some ISEs, to complex or precipitate ions that may interfere with the analyte of interest. Also, modern pH/mV/ion meters have alternative standardization procedures (e.g., method of linear segments) that can accomodate nonlinear curve fitting when one is operating close to the electrode's limit of detection.

In the clinical setting, the capacity to manage large numbers of samples and to make rapid measurements with the use of hand-held devices at the point of care (e.g., i-STAT™) is highly desirable. Thus, many ISEs are incorporated into automatic instruments that use a flow-through configuration, both for applications in the clinical laboratory and for portable analyzers (vide infra). This arrangement takes advantage of the rapid response of ISEs by placing them into multi-ion analyzers with large sample throughput capabilities and/or rapid analysis times. Calibrants, samples, and rinsing solutions are forced across the electrode surfaces of the ISEs by pumping or diffusion. A single reference electrode is used for all ISEs in a system with the exception of the CO_2 sensor in the clinical analyzer, which has its own reference electrode behind the gas-permeable membrane. Calibrants include a constant ionic strength buffer that closely matches the matrix of the physiological samples to minimize errors resulting from differences in liquid junction potentials between samples and standards. It must be emphasized that the proper care and use of ISEs either individually or as arrays in clinical analyzers are essential factors in ensuring accurate and reproducible analysis. This requires consistent monitoring of the performance of both the electrodes and the instruments as a whole. The following section presents a discussion of some of the common errors and interferences associated with ISE measurements.

Experimental Considerations and Interferences

Errors in ISE measurement can result for any ion determination if data are not collected for standards and samples at approximately the same temperature, since the Nernst equation that governs the calibration of potential versus concentration is temperature dependent. As noted above, some commercial instruments use independent temperature compensation to correct for this effect, but the analyst should be aware of the influence of temperature on response. Perhaps the most important source of error is the response of an ISE to a non-analyte or an interferent ion in the sample. It is thus critical to know the selectivity properties of the electrode that are being used, to ensure that non-analyte ions to which the electrode responds are not present in sufficiently high concentrations to constitute an interference, and/or to use suppressors as available to inhibit electrode response to interferents. Components in certain sample matrices also can change the sensitivity of an electrode by adsorbing to its surface, thereby blocking access of the analyte. Such electrode fouling is a particular problem in samples that contain surface-adsorbing species, such as proteins, which frequently are removed with pepsin/surfactant solutions. For single electrode determinations in whole blood or serum, techniques that isolate the ISE from direct contact with the sample are available, although the use of single electrode measurements is often impractical in the clinical setting. Modern multi-ion analyzers incorporate a small size-exclusion membrane that protects the ion-selective membrane from the high-molecular-weight components of biological fluids, while allowing analyte molecules access to the electrodes.

Although many ISEs are very selective, under certain conditions, some ions may interfere and contribute to erroneous results. Specific examples are listed in Table 12-2 and are discussed briefly below. Detailed descriptions of clinical analyses for many ions also can be found in the method reviews on Evolve associated with this text.

Measurements of *pH* have few specific interferences associated with them, and the linear response range is typically from pH 2 to 12. Sensitivity of the glass pH electrode may be reduced for some electrodes at pH values above 10 (i.e., "sodium error") because of the interference of monovalent cations in high concentrations, especially Na^+. Although monovalent cations can enter and move slowly through the hydrated layer, multivalent cations of 2+ or 3+ charge do not interfere. In solutions of pH less than 1, low water activities also may give rise to measurement error.

Na^+ ions are determined by either a glass electrode or a polymer type of liquid membrane electrode. Interferences are minimized because of the inherently high concentration of sodium in biological fluids, particularly blood. Interferences from K^+ and H^+ are seldom problematic in glass electrodes, although highly acidic urine samples can be a potential exception. In the case of the polymer-based ISE, Li^+ may be a potential interferent if the sample is derived from a patient who is being treated with a lithium pharmaceutical.

K^+ usually is measured by the valinomycin/polymer electrode described above. Good results are obtained for measurements in blood; however, in undiluted urine samples, a negative error may result because of the partitioning of a negatively charged lipophilic component of the urine that is permeable to the polymer. This component can be excluded by the use of an ISE that incorporates a silicone-rubber membrane instead of the polymer. Alternatively, accurate measurements can be obtained by sample dilution.

Determination of Na^+ and K^+ levels in undiluted blood and urine samples requires special mention. Measurements made by nondilutional ISE methods may yield different results from those obtained by dilutional-based ISE methods, which determine the concentration of ions in the total sample volume, which include dissolved solids as well as water. The dilution method brings all samples to a known ionic strength to compensate for any ionic composition differences. However, the clinically relevant value is the plasma water concentration and not the total plasma concentration. For the dilution method, plasma is considered to be 93.3% water and a constant. In the case of hyperlipidemia or increased plasma proteins, this is not true; the water content is lower than normal, and the calculated ion (i.e., Na^+) concentration therefore is low, sometimes strikingly so. The nondilution method does not suffer from this limitation as no assumption about the water content is required because the measurement is made directly in the plasma. However, nondilution methods may be affected by variations in sample ionic strength that can change the activity coefficient. Ionic strength is controlled in the dilution method. Also, changes to the electrode surface from plasma components are more likely with the nondilution method. Agreement between these methods usually is realized by calibration adjustment. Methodological differences may be greater in the case of Na^+ determinations, in particular because of the higher relative concentration of Na^+ in biological fluids. The influence of physiological effects on Na^+ and K^+ determinations in biological fluids is discussed in greater detail in the "Sodium and Potassium" method review on Evolve.

Special care must be taken in regard to the determination of Ca^{2+} and Mg^{2+}, which exist in both the bound form (with proteins or other biological molecules) and the unbound, ionized form. The Ca^{2+} and Mg^{2+} ISEs provide one of the best ways to measure the fully unbound, ionized forms of these metals, since the electrodes respond only to the ionized form, which is deemed physiologically relevant. It is important to note that since pH influences the fraction of free/bound, all measurements should be made at a standardized pH (e.g., 7.4).

The determination of Cl^- in biological fluids by an ISE can be compromised by fouling of the surface by proteins present in the sample. This problem can be minimized by using a semipermeable membrane to exclude these large molecules from the electrode surface. A liquid membrane electrode made of polymer that exhibits selectivity for chloride has been developed for use in electrolyte analyzers designed specifically for biomedical use. Chloride ISEs are subject to interference from Br^-, I^-, F^-, CN^-, OH^-, and S^{2-}, but, except for Br^-, these ions usually are not present in physiological samples at a level high enough to be problematic. Some chloride ISEs are also susceptible to interference from elevated levels of bicarbonate, leading to positive bias in the clinical measurement. The F^- ISE exhibits excellent selectivity and suffers only from interference of OH^- at high pH.

ISEs for the measurement of CO_2 are relatively straightforward and are interference-free. Undiluted blood can be used directly as the sample, and calibration typically is accomplished with 5% and 10% mixtures of CO_2 in an inert gas. Total CO_2 measurements require acidification to convert CO_3^{2-} and HCO_3^- to CO_2. In this case, calibration is performed with standard $NaHCO_3$ solutions. Response times for total CO_2 measurements are generally longer because of the necessity of establishing equilibrium conditions. Some CO_3^{2-}-selective membranes are currently available in certain instruments for total CO_2 measurements. Interferents are mainly organic acids to which the gas membrane is also permeable. The carbonate-selective membranes are subject to interferences from anions such as salicylate, but placement of the ISE behind a silicone-rubber membrane in the clinical analyzers alleviates this problem.

The NH_3 gas-sensing electrode responds selectively and rapidly (but indirectly) to P_{NH_3} in solution by measuring pH as described above; the major drawback is the questionable stability of the membrane and the electrode. Interference can result from nonpolar volatile amines present in the sample. With both the CO_2 and NH_3 electrodes, it is important to have a rapidly responding electrode. A decrease in response time signifies a loss in electrode performance and may require replacement of the membrane.

KEY CONCEPTS BOX 12-1

- Potentiometric techniques measure the potential of a chemical half-cell reaction versus a reference electrode.
- Commonly used reference electrodes are the Ag/AgCl and calomel electrodes. There must be a reference electrode against which the relative potential of the reaction (detecting) half-cell can be detected.
- Changes in the half-cell potential versus a reference electrode can indicate the concentration of an analyte that is causing the potential of the detecting electrode to change.
- Ion-selective electrodes (ISEs) work by having a surface that selectively interacts with a specific analyte; the interaction results in a change of the potential of that ISE versus the reference electrode.
- ISEs are used to measure Na^+, K^+, Cl^-, Ca^{2+}, and Li^+.
- Gas-sensing ISEs are covered with gas-permeable membranes that allow only the gases to interact with the ISE.

SECTION OBJECTIVES BOX 12-2

- Describe the scientific basis for voltammetric techniques.
- Describe in detail how glucose and oxygen electrodes work.
- Name several other clinical applications of the voltammetric technique.
- Describe the principles of anodic stripping voltammetry, and explain how the technique is clinically applied.

VOLTAMMETRIC METHODS

Electrochemical techniques in which a potential is applied to an electrochemical cell and the resulting current from an electrochemical reaction is measured generally are categorized as *voltammetric* methods. Electrochemical cells for voltammetry use a three-electrode configuration. The cell consists of a *working electrode, a reference electrode,* and an **auxiliary electrode.** The potential is applied between the working and the reference electrode by a **potentiostat;** this applied potential can force changes to occur to any electroactive species at the working electrode surface by electrolysis. Electrolysis can occur by a **reduction,** a gain of one or more electrons, or an **oxidation**—a loss of one or more electrons per molecule or ion. The current required to sustain the electrolysis at the

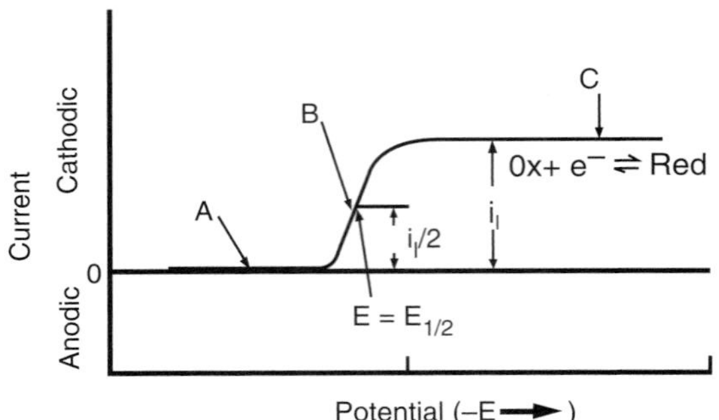

Fig. 12-8 Generalized hydrodynamic voltammogram for reduction of *Ox* to *Red.* Potential scanned negatively left to right. $E_{1/2}$ is half-wave potential; i_l, limiting current.

working electrode and to maintain electroneutrality in the cell is provided by the auxiliary electrode. This arrangement prevents the reference electrode from being subjected to large currents that could change its potential. Some voltammetry instrumentation is based on the two-electrode system. Here the auxiliary electrode is absent, and the reference electrode is subjected to the entire cell current.

The basic concept of applying a potential to an electrochemical cell and measuring the current that results from electrolysis can be implemented in numerous ways. Several different techniques have been developed by varying how the potential is applied or how the current is measured. Although the resultant output and the practical applications of these techniques are varied, they all share the common basis of applying a potential, *E,* and measuring a current, *i,* or a charge, *Q.* In addition, the solution may be moving or stationary with respect to the working electrode. Voltammetry in an unstirred solution is referred to as *stationary* solution voltammetry. *Hydrodynamic* voltammetry involves the forced movement of solution either by stirring the solution or flowing the solution over the electrode, as in liquid chromatography with *electrochemical detection* (LCEC; see Chapter 4).

The result of a voltammetric technique is called a *voltammogram* (i.e., a current-potential curve). Voltammograms give useful quantitative and qualitative information about the electrochemical reaction. A typical **hydrodynamic voltammogram** is shown in Fig. 12-8 for the reduction of species *Ox* by one electron to species *Red.* As the potential is scanned in the negative direction, the voltammogram can be described by three distinct regions. In region A, the potential applied at the working electrode is insufficient to cause electrolysis to occur; therefore, no current is observed. The onset of electrolysis is signaled by the rise in current in region B. The current continues to rise until a maximum value is reached. This takes place in region C, where electrolysis is occurring at the maximum rate possible. The maximum current in region C is defined as the **limiting current (i_l)** and is defined by Eq. 12-6:

$$i_l = \frac{nFAD_0C_0}{\delta} \qquad \text{Eq. 12-6}$$

where A is the electrode area, D_0 is the diffusion coefficient of Ox, C_0 is the concentration of Ox, and δ is the diffusion distance. As is illustrated by Eq. 12-6, the magnitude of i_l is directly proportional to the concentration of the electrochemically active analyte. Thus voltammetry can be used to quantitatively measure analyte concentration. The practical unit for current is the ampere (A), which represents the transfer of 1 coulomb of charge per second. This corresponds to the passage of 1.05×10^{-5} moles of electrons per second. Because the current involved in most electroanalytical techniques is very small, milliamperes (mA), microamperes (μA), and nanoamperes (nA) are commonly used units.

The *half-wave potential* ($E_{1/2}$) is defined as the potential at one-half the limiting current. $E_{1/2}$ is uniquely characteristic of the species undergoing electrolysis (just as the half-cell potential is for the reference electrode), and it can be used for qualitative identification. By convention, a reduction is described by a positive, or *cathodic,* current, whereas an oxidation is described by a negative, or *anodic,* current. The principles for an oxidation are similar and can be applied for a positive potential scan.

One specific type of voltammetry that is clinically useful is **amperometry.** Amperometric sensors are devices that measure the current generated at a fixed potential by an electroactive analyte in solution. The potential is set to a value of E where i_l occurs (Fig. 12-8, region *C*), and i_l then is measured for each sample. The current measured is directly proportional to the concentration of species present. Two clinically important amperometric sensors discussed below are the oxygen electrode and the glucose electrode.

Voltammetry Electrodes

Working Electrodes

Working electrodes have certain properties in common. Good electrical conductance is of foremost importance; consequently, working electrodes are generally metals or semiconductors. Chemical and electrochemical inertness is important in applications for which the electrode should function simply to transfer electrons to and from species dissolved in solution. This inertness allows a a wide range of applied potentials, minimum background contributions from the electrode, and solvent redox properties in which the electrochemistry of the analyte or analytes can be monitored easily.

Platinum, gold, mercury, and glassy carbon are commonly used materials for voltammetric electrodes. When used for voltammetry, mercury can be in the form of a *hanging mercury drop electrode.* To provide the working electrode surface, a reproducible mercury drop is extruded through a narrow glass capillary by means of a commercially available micrometer syringe. A new drop is formed by simply dislodging the old one and extruding more mercury. The *dropping mercury electrode* is the working electrode for **polarography.** With this technique, mercury is forced by gravity through a very fine capillary to provide a continuous stream of identical droplets. Each droplet expands, becomes too heavy to be suspended, and breaks loose from the capillary.

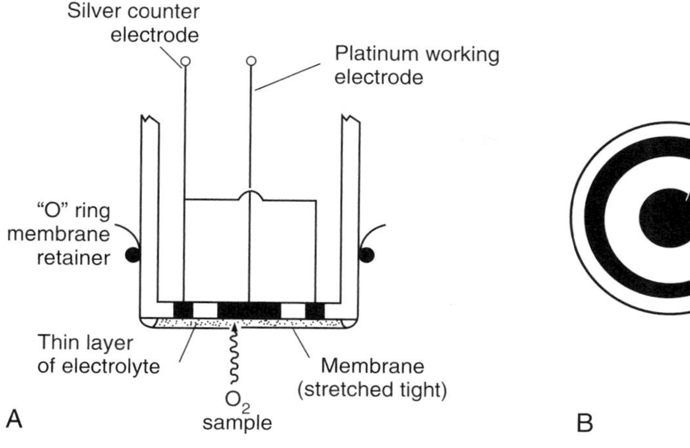

Fig. 12-9 Schema of oxygen electrode. **A,** Cross-sectional view showing diffusion of oxygen (O_2) sample through the membrane. **B,** View of electrode assembly from bottom.

Auxiliary Electrodes

Auxiliary electrodes are made from any conductive material, typically a piece of platinum wire.

Reference Electrodes

The commonly used reference electrodes for voltammetry are the SCE and Ag/AgCl electrodes, which have been described in detail previously.

Oxygen Electrode

The oxygen electrode is designed as a complete electrochemical cell. The basic design, which is shown in Fig. 12-9, incorporates a platinum disk as the **cathode** and an Ag/AgCl electrode as the **anode** in a buffered **electrolyte solution.** The electrochemical cell is isolated from the sample by an oxygen-permeable membrane. Oxygen diffuses through the membrane and is reduced electrochemically at the platinum electrode, which is held at a potential that quantitatively reduces oxygen (−0.5 to −0.6 V vs. Ag/AgCl).

$$O_2 + 2H^+ + 2e^- \rightarrow H_2O_2 \qquad \text{Eq. 12-7}$$

The current generated at the platinum electrode is directly proportional to the concentration (partial pressure) of oxygen dissolved in the sample. As with potentiometric indicator electrodes, the membrane inhibits electrode fouling from serum proteins in blood and also prevents other electroactive substances from being reduced at the electrode. Calibration of the electrode system is performed with standard solutions or gases that contain known concentrations of oxygen.

Few interferences are associated with the use of the oxygen electrode. Poor response times and variable results may indicate that degradation of the membrane or a change in pH of the buffer solution has occurred. Silver metal may deposit on the platinum cathode and also may affect the electrode response. Polishing the electrode with electrode polishing compound regenerates the platinum surface.

The oxygen electrode is incorporated into a blood gas analyzer, which measures oxygen, CO_2, and pH on samples of less than 250 μL of whole blood. Miniaturized O_2 electrodes have been developed for transcutaneous measurements, eliminating the need for drawing blood samples. However, the accuracy and response time of these electrodes depend on the physical characteristics of the patient's skin tissue. The oxygen electrode has been used to monitor enzyme-catalyzed reactions that involve consumption of O_2 to measure glucose (glucose oxidase), lactic acid (lactate oxidase), cholesterol (cholesterol oxidase), and uric acid (uricase).

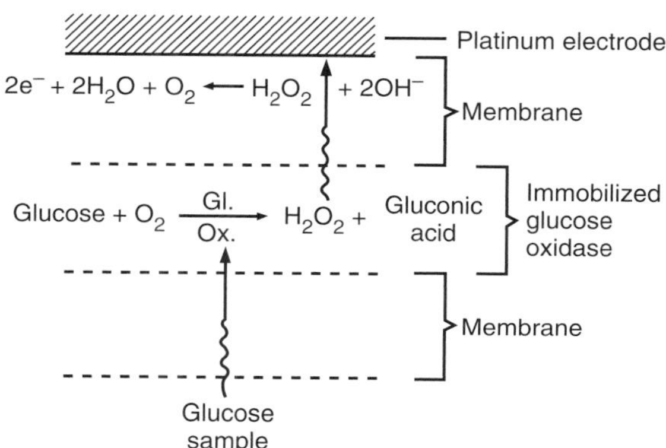

Fig. 12-10 Schema of glucose electrode.

Glucose Electrode

Glucose is another important constituent of serum and plasma that can be measured by an amperometric sensor. A diagram of a typical glucose electrode is shown in Fig. 12-10. The electrode uses the enzyme glucose oxidase immobilized between two membranes. Glucose oxidase (Gl. Ox.) catalyzes the oxidation of glucose in the sample by oxygen, also dissolved in the sample, generating hydrogen peroxide (H_2O_2) and gluconic acid. The inner membrane is permeable to H_2O_2, which is determined amperometrically by the underlying platinum electrode held at a positive potential sufficient to oxidize H_2O_2 to O_2 (the reverse of the reaction shown in Eq. 12-7). The current measured from the H_2O_2 oxidation is directly proportional to the glucose concentration; glucose concentrations have been reported to be quantified in the range of 10^{-7} to 10^{-3} M. Few interferences are noted for this electrode. The inner membrane is impermeable to ascorbic acid, uric acid, and acetaminophen, all of which are electroactive at the positive potential used to detect H_2O_2 and may be present in clinical samples. The design for this glucose electrode has been developed by the Yellow Springs Instrument Company (Yellow Springs, Ohio). The glucose electrode is often referred to as a **biosensor** because it incorporates a biological compound, glucose oxidase, as a key component in its operation. Analogous biosensors for other serum constituents can be made by simply using the appropriate enzyme to catalyze the oxidation. Glucose, lactic acid, and urea measuring electrodes are now common features of multi-analyte clinical analyzers.

Electrochemical test strips are commercially available for use in monitoring devices (glucometers) for patients with diabetes to measure whole blood glucose. These glucose meters are available for use in a physician office setting, for hospital use, or for personal use. Hospital glucose meters typically are used at the point of care, not only to manage diabetic patients but also in the treatment of trauma patients, premature babies, patients suffering from sepsis, and surgical patients. The glucose meters have disposable test strips that typically consist of thin electrodes deposited on a small strip of plastic. One electrode (carbon, gold, or palladium film) is converted to a glucose biosensor by addition of an enzyme; the other is made into a reference electrode. Glucose is rapidly determined electrochemically by adding a drop of blood to the test strip inserted into the small, hand-held, portable instrument. Most test strips use an electron transfer agent (mediator) to shuttle electrons to the electrode instead of detecting the enzyme-generated H_2O_2 as described above. For example, test strips that use glucose oxidase as the enzyme commonly use ferricyanide as the mediator. The reaction sequence is summarized below.

Solution reaction:

$$\text{glucose} + 2\ \text{ferricyanide} + H_2O \xrightarrow{Gl.\,Ox.} \text{gluconic acid} + 2\ \text{ferrocyanide} + 2H^+ \quad \text{Eq. 12-8}$$

Electrode reaction:

$$2\ \text{ferrocyanide} \xrightarrow{Gl.\,Ox.} 2\ \text{ferricyanide} + 2e^- \quad \text{Eq. 12-9}$$

Note that the mediator, ferricyanide, is regenerated by oxidation at the electrode. The current resulting from oxidation of the mediator is directly proportional to the glucose concentration. Using mediators instead of detecting H_2O_2 eliminates the reliance upon oxygen as a co-substrate, thereby reducing oxygen dependence. The oxygen-based reaction varies with the Po_2 of the sample, which could range from 40 mm Hg in venous samples to 400 mm Hg in arterial samples.

Anodic Stripping Voltammetry

Anodic **stripping voltammetry** is a voltammetric technique that is useful in clinical chemistry for the determination of heavy metals. An example of its use is the determination of Pb^{2+} in the biological fluids of patients suspected of having lead poisoning. Stripping voltammetry has the lowest detection limit of the commonly used electroanalytical techniques; analyte concentrations below 10^{-10} M have been determined. The technique consists of two steps. In the first step, analyte is deposited at a working electrode by the application of a potential sufficient to reduce the ionic species of interest to its metallic form. This step serves to preconcentrate the analyte by electrochemically depositing (plating) it on the electrode. If mercury is the working electrode, the deposited metal dissolves in the mercury (i.e., is extracted into the electrode). It is this preconcentration feature that enables such low concentrations to be reached by stripping voltammetry. In the second step, the deposited analyte is removed, or "stripped," from the electrode by application of increasingly positive potentials; the resulting current signal is a measure of the concentration of analyte in solution. Because the stripping step gives anodic current (i.e., the species is oxidized), the technique is termed *anodic stripping voltammetry.*

In anodic stripping voltammetry, only a fraction of the total analyte is deposited at the electrode by electrolysis during the preconcentration step. Complete deposition of all of the analyte at the electrode is time consuming and generally unnecessary, since adequate amounts usually can be deposited to give a satisfactory stripping signal in much shorter times. Because the deposition is not exhaustive, it is important to deposit the same fraction of analyte for each stripping voltammogram. The parameters of electrode surface area, deposition time, and stirring must be carefully duplicated for all standards and samples. Deposition times vary from 60 seconds to 30 minutes, depending on the analyte concentration, the type of working electrode, and the stripping technique used.

Anodic stripping voltammetry has become a useful method in the clinical laboratory for the determination of Pb^{2+} in blood and urine since the development of automated instrumentation by Environmental Science Associates (ESA). ESA also markets a digestion reagent, Metexchange, which frees bound Pb^{2+} from biological components of blood and urine. ESA has introduced a hand-held lead device (LeadCare) and a small CLIA (Clinical Laboratory Improvement Act)-waived analyzer (LeadCare II), appropriate for use in physician offices. The analyzer contains a unique gold particle electrode sensor that contains no mercury. Both devices require only 50 µL of blood that is pretreated with a reagent that releases bound Pb^{2+} from biological components. The solution is placed onto the electrode of the disposable sensor. The Pb^{2+} in the mixture is deposited onto the gold electrode for 140 seconds by reduction to Pb° at −530 mV versus a silver/silver chloride reference electrode. The plated Pb° then is removed (or "stripped") from the gold electrode through the application of a positive potential scan. The current generated is proportional to the lead concentration in the blood sample. Because most states require lead testing in children younger than 2 years old, these types of instruments, with analytical sensitivity of <3.5 µg/dL, will enhance compliance.

KEY CONCEPTS BOX 12-2

- Voltammetric electrodes used for amperometric measurements are kept at a constant voltage, which allows a specific analyte to react at the surface of the electrode. The amount of current formed from that reaction is proportional to the concentration of the analyte.
- The oxygen electrode allows oxygen (O_2) to react at the Pt surface to form hydrogen peroxide (H_2O_2) and a current.
- The oxygen electrode has been adapted to detect a number of analytes by incorporating onto the electrode surface an oxygen-reacting enzyme that changes the O_2 concentration, which is detected by the O_2 electrode.
- Examples of such applications include the glucose and lactate electrodes.
- Stripping voltammetry works by allowing a metal cation to be reduced at an electrode set at a specific voltage, which results in deposition of the metal on the electrode. The voltage is then changed to "strip" (reoxidize) the metal from the electrode with the production of a current. The amount of current needed to strip the metal is proportional to the initial concentration. This technique is used to measure blood lead.

SECTION OBJECTIVES BOX 12-3

- Describe how the coulometric method for the detection of chloride ions works.
- Describe the primary clinical application of this technique.

COULOMETRIC METHODS

Coulometry is a very useful electrochemical method for quantitative analysis. Clinical applications use one form of coulometry that involves the application of a constant current to generate a titrating agent. In principle, the time required to titrate a sample at constant current is measured and is related to the amount of analyte in a sample by Faraday's law (Eq. 12-10):

$$Q = it = nFN \qquad \text{Eq. 12-10}$$

where Q is the charge passed for a finite time, t, at constant current, i; n is the number of electrons involved in the electrochemical reaction; F is Faraday's constant; and N is the number of moles of analyte in the sample. Charge is a quantity of electricity. The unit for charge, the coulomb (C), corresponds to 1.05×10^{-5} moles of electrons. Because N is measured directly without the need for standards, coulometry is an absolute method that can be used for very precise determinations of analyte.

Titration of Chloride

Coulometry is still used in the clinical laboratory determination of chloride in sweat for the diagnosis of cystic fibrosis (CF). Patients with CF have a significantly higher concentration of chloride in their sweat when compared with normal individuals. Coulometric titration is the method for determination of chloride in sweat that is recommended by the Cystic Fibrosis Foundation. Most systems found in a clinical laboratory that use ISE technology have not been systematically validated for the determination of chloride in sweat. Typically, these ISEs also lack the sensitivity at lower concentrations to make ISEs a viable method. The determination of Cl^- takes advantage of the quantitative formation and low solubility of AgCl. Ag^+ ions (the titrating agent) are electrochemically generated at the Ag anode by application of a constant current. Cl^- ions in the sample are rapidly consumed as they react with Ag^+ to form insoluble AgCl. At any point in the titration, the Ag^+ concentration is very low.

$$\textit{Anode reaction: } Ag \rightarrow Ag^+ + e^- \qquad \text{Eq. 12-11}$$

$$\textit{Solution reaction: } Ag^+ + Cl^- \rightarrow AgCl(s) \qquad \text{Eq. 12-12}$$

However, the end point of the titration is signaled by a sudden increase in Ag^+ concentration that follows the consumption of all Cl^-. A second pair of Ag^+-specific electrodes detects the rise in concentration of Ag^+ in solution and immediately stops the titration. The amount of Cl^- in the sample is proportional to the number of Ag^+ ions generated at the anode.

Coulometric determination of chloride is very precise; however, other anions that form insoluble complexes with silver ion can result in Cl^- determinations that are falsely elevated. Also, poor reproducibility can be a problem at high chloride concentrations because of the large amount of precipitate.

KEY CONCEPTS BOX 12-3

- In the coulometric analysis of chloride (Cl^- ions), Ag^+ ions are generated from a Ag electrode. These ions react with Cl^- ions in the sample and precipitate as AgCl. When all of the Cl^- ions are reacted, the excess Ag^+ ions in solution are detected by an Ag^+-specific electrode. The time needed to generate the excess Ag^+ is proportional to the [chloride].
- The primary application of this technique is the sweat chloride test, which is used to diagnose cystic fibrosis.

MULTIANALYTE ELECTROCHEMICAL CLINICAL ANALYZERS

Instruments that measure a range of analytes simultaneously using potentiometric and voltammetric methods have been developed for use in clinical laboratories, physician offices, and point-of-care settings.

Benchtop Clinical Analyzers

Benchtop automated blood analyzers, incorporating several potentiometric and amperometric electrodes into a single flow-through instrument, can provide an array of measurements of blood gases and electrolytes using less than 250 μL and requiring less than 2 minutes for the complete analysis. Typical instruments incorporate a pH electrode, an amperometric oxygen electrode, and a range of ion-selective electrodes. Systems for the determination of blood gases, Na^+, K^+, Ca^{2+}, Mg^{2+}, Cl^-, and CO_2 are available. An amperometric glucose electrode, as described above, also is often incorporated into the clinical analyzer.

Point-of-Care Clinical Analyzers

Advances in the miniaturization of electrochemical sensors have allowed the development of small hand-held instruments, capable of determining a multitude of different analytes simultaneously and rapidly. This makes them very useful in the point-of-care setting, including emergency departments, intensive care units, operating rooms, and transport vehicles.

As with benchtop clinical analyzers, ion-selective electrode potentiometry is used to determine levels of sodium, potassium, chloride, and ionized calcium, in addition to pH and P_{CO_2}. Glucose, P_{O_2}, lactate, and creatinine are measured amperometrically in separate sensors. The oxygen and glucose electrodes operate according to the principles described earlier. One analyzer (i-STAT^{TM}) incorporates a hematocrit sensor that is based on the measurement of sample conductivity. Cardiac markers have been introduced as single cartridges for creatine kinase MB (CK-MB), cardiac troponin I (cTnI), and B-type natriuretic peptide (BNP), using a two-site enzyme-linked immunosorbent assay (ELISA sandwich) method with amperometric detection of the enzyme-generated product.

BIBLIOGRAPHY

General

Luppa PB, Sokoll LJ, Chan DW: Immunosensors—principles and applications to clinical chemistry, Clin Chim Acta 414:1, 2001.

Skoog DA, Holler FJ, Crouch SR: *Principles of Instrumental Analysis,* Belmont, CA, 2007, Thomson Brooks/Cole, Chapters 22-25.

Wang J: *Analytical Electrochemistry,* ed 3, New York, 2006, Wiley-VCH.

Wang J: *Electroanalytical Techniques in Clinical Chemistry and Laboratory Medicine,* New York, 1988, VCH Publishers.

Zoski CG, editor: *Handbook of Electrochemistry,* Amsterdam, 2007, Elsevier.

Potentiometric Methods

Bakker E, Meyerhoff ME: Ion-selective electrodes for measurements in biological fluids, Encyclopedia of Electrochemistry 9:277, 2002.

Bakker E, Pretsch E: Modern potentiometry, Angew Chem Int Ed 46:5660, 2007.

Bakker E, Pretsch E: Potentiometric sensors for trace-level analysis, Trends in Analytical Chemistry 24:199, 2005.

Bühlmann P, Pretsch E, Bakker E: Carrier-based ion selective electrodes and bulk optodes. 2. Ionophores for potentiometric and optical sensors, Chem Rev 98:1593, 1998.

Diamond D, Saez de Viteri FJ: Ion-selective electrodes and optodes. In Diamond D, editor: *Principles of Chemical and Biological Sensors,* New York, 1998, Wiley & Sons.

Dimeski G, Clague AE: Bicarbonate interference with chloride ion selective electrodes, Clin Chem 50:1106, 2004.

Meyerhoff ME, Opdyke WN: Ion-selective electrodes, Adv Clin Chem 25:1, 1986.

Voltammetric Methods

Bard AJ, Faulkner LR: *Electrochemical Methods,* ed 2, New York, 2001, Wiley & Sons.

Kissinger PT, Heineman WR, editors: *Laboratory Techniques in Electroanalytical Chemistry,* ed 2, New York, 1996, Marcel Dekker.

Lunte CE, Heineman WR: Electrochemical techniques in bioanalysis, Top Curr Chem 143:1, 1988.

Sawyer DT, Sobkowiak A, Roberts JL Jr: *Electrochemistry for Chemists,* ed 2, New York, 1995, Wiley-Interscience.

Coulometric Methods

LeGrys VA, et al: *Sweat Testing: Sample Collection and Quantitative Analysis: Approved Guideline,* ed 2, Pennsylvania, 2000, Clinical and Laboratory Standards Insitute.

i-STAT

Lauks IR: Microfabricated biosensors and microanalytical systems for blood analysis, Accounts of Chemical Research 31:317, 1998.

Biosensors

Blum LJ, Coulet PR, editors: *Biosensor Principles and Applications,* New York, 1991, Marcel Dekker.

Buerk DG: *Biosensors: Theory and Applications,* Boca Raton, FL, 1995, CRC Press.

Cunningham AJ: *Introduction to Bioanalytical Sensors,* New York, 1998, Wiley-Interscience.

Eggins B: *Biosensors: An Introduction,* New York, 1996, Wiley & Sons.

Ligler FS, Taitt CR: *Optical Biosensors: Today and Tomorrow,* ed 2, Philadelphia, 2008, Elsevier Science.

Newman JD, Turner APF: Home blood glucose biosensors: a commercial perspective, Biosens Bioelectron 20:2435, 2005.

Ramsey G, editor: *Commercial Biosensors,* New York, 1998, Wiley & Sons.

Wang J: Electrochemical glucose biosensors, Chem Rev 108:814, 2008.

Zhang X, Ju H, Wang J: *Electrochemical Sensors, Biosensors and their Biomedical Applications,* Boston, 2007, Academic Press.

INTERNET SITES

http://en.wikipedia.org/wiki/Ion-selective_electrode
Ion selective electrode

http://en.wikipedia.org/wiki/Glass_electrode
Glass electrode

Molecular Diagnostics

Hassan M. E. Azzazy, W. Edward Highsmith, Jr., Niel T. Constantine, and Kenneth J. Friedman

13 Chapter

Chapter Outline

Key Terms

allele A forms of a gene that occurs at a particular DNA location (locus); two alleles are usually present for each gene.

amplicon A DNA fragment that has been generated by using an amplification technique such as PCR.

base pairing The process by which purine and pyrimidine bases bind through hydrogen bonds. The bases pair in a specific complementary fashion: adenine with thymine (or uracil) and guanine with cytosine.

base sequence The exact order of purine bases (guanine and adenine) and pyrimidine bases (cytosine and thymine or uracil) found in nucleic acids. The order defines the primary sequence of the gene products, which are proteins.

complementary DNA (cDNA) DNA that contains an exact sequence of bases that will pair to a strand of DNA through base pairing. Complimentary DNA can be used as a probe for detecting specific sequences. When complimentary DNA is prepared from an mRNA transcript using reverse transcriptase it is termed cDNA and can be used as a probe for detecting specific sequences in Southern transfer analysis.

denaturation The process by which double-stranded nucleic acid separates to form single strands. Denaturation can be accomplished by heat, salts, or chemicals. Also termed *melting.*

double-stranded DNA Two complementary strands of DNA that are bound together through base pairing.

epigenetic code It is a system above the genetic code that consists of histone modifications (histone code) and DNA methylation. The epigenetic code is tissue and cell specific and can change gene expression without altering the underlying DNA sequence.

heteroduplex DNA A double-stranded DNA molecule in which the two DNA strands are perfectly base-paired except for a small number of bases (often one) which are mismatched or unpaired.

homoduplex DNA A double-stranded DNA molecule in which both strands are perfectly base-paired.

hybridization The process by which complementary single strands of nucleic acid form double-stranded complexes of nucleic acid through base pairing.

indels Point mutations that result form an insertion or deletion of a nucleotide base.

melting temperature The temperature at which one-half a population of identical DNA species exists in double-stranded form and one half exists in single-stranded (denatured) form. The melting temperature is dependent on the ionic strength of the solution.

Northern blot A process similar to the Southern blot, except that RNA is the molecule that is transferred and analyzed.

polymerase chain reaction (PCR) A process by which complementary DNA strands are enzymatically synthesized and amplified.

polymerases A class of enzymes that synthesize DNA from an existing template. Polymerases require a primer to begin synthesis, ribonucleotide or deoxynucleotide triphosphates as reactants, and magnesium as a cofactor.

proband The first member of a family that comes to medical attention for a genetic disorder.

probe A sequence of complementary DNA or RNA that is labeled with a radioisotope, enzyme, or other marker. Probes are used to detect specific sequences of nucleic acid by hybridization.

restriction endonucleases Class of nucleases (usually bacterial) that act within a strand of DNA at specific base sequences to cleave the DNA.

restriction fragment length polymorphism (RFLP) The pattern of DNA fragments observed in a test population when analyzed by restriction endonucleases and specific DNA probes.

restriction site The base sequence recognized and cleaved by a particular restriction endonuclease.

single-stranded DNA A length of DNA that is not paired with its complementary strand.

Southern transfer A process by which electrophoretically separated, denatured DNA is transferred from the electrophoretic gel (usually agarose) onto a nitrocellulose or nylon filter or membrane for subsequent hybridization analysis.

stringency The conditions under which a hybridization experiment is conducted. High stringency conditions (low ionic strength, temperature ≈ DNA melting temperature) allow the hybridization of only perfectly base-paired strands. Low stringency conditions (high ionic strength, temperature < DNA melting temperature) allow hybridization of homologous, but not perfectly base-paired, strands.

viral load The number of circulating viral particles, generally expressed as genome copies/mL or IU/mL.

The smallest unit of inheritance, the **gene,** codes for specific protein chains, each with a specific function in cell physiology. Chemically, genes are composed of deoxyribonucleic acid (DNA, see below). The **base sequences** are grouped into informational units of three bases (triplets), called codons. When transcribed into mRNA, each triplet sequence either codes for a specific amino acid or serves a regulatory function, such as stopping or starting protein chain synthesis. Structurally, the base sequence that composes a gene is linked to other genes, to regulatory sequences, and to (apparently) functionless DNA sequences. DNA is associated with a large number of proteins that serve regulatory functions and also package the genetic material into larger units called *chromosomes.*

As the complete human genome and its complement of genes have been sequenced, and as the relationship between these sequences and human diseases has grown, the clinical laboratory has begun to face new challenges. The laboratory now uses the techniques and technology of molecular biology to identify and characterize specific gene mutations associated with single gene disorders, such as cystic fibrosis (CF) or Duchenne's muscular dystrophy, as well as polygenic disorders, such as cancer and atherosclerosis. Molecular techniques are in standard use in the detection of infectious agents, including organisms that are difficult to culture or are present in low numbers. Additionally, these techniques are being used to determine appropriate drug therapy (pharmacogenetics) or even the likelihood of reading disorders (dyslexia).

SECTION OBJECTIVES BOX 13-1

- Review the structure of DNA, and describe how its properties of complementary base-pairing and digestion by specific nucleases can be used to identify specific sequences of DNA.
- Define and describe the basic types of mutations, and explain how they can cause cell dysfunction.

DNA STRUCTURE

Fig. 13-1 shows the unique arrangement of sugar, phosphate, and the purine and pyrimidine bases that form the double-helical structure known as DNA. Particular sequences of this structure form the *gene,* which codes for a specific protein (see Chapter 27, Part I).

DNA consists of two strands of base sequences that are bound to each other by hydrogen bonding between the bases of each single strand of DNA (see Fig. 13-1). The bases bind to each other in a specific, or *complementary,* fashion. This **base paring** results in adenine binding only to thymine, whereas guanine binds only to cytosine. Thus one chain of **double-stranded DNA** has a base sequence that is complementary to the other strand. A single strand of DNA will bind to another single DNA strand if the strands contain a high proportion of complementary sequences. For example, if a mixture consists of single strands of DNA-A and its complementary strand and an excess of other noncomplementary DNA strands, strand A will form *only* double-stranded complexes with its complementary strand and none other. In the laboratory, the process of allowing complementary single strands of DNA to form double-stranded DNA is called **hybridization.** Hybridization can also be performed between single strands of DNA and complementary strands of ribonucleic acid (RNA). For analysis of a specific DNA base sequence, a known copy of that base sequence is prepared. This copy of **complementary DNA (cDNA),** known as a DNA **probe,** is labeled in some fashion to allow monitoring of the hybridization reaction. The basis of the techniques described later in this chapter hinges on the hybridization properties of a specific sequence of bases that make up a single strand of the double-stranded helix of DNA.

Mutations and Gene Expression

A mutation is a change in the base sequence of the genetic material of an organism that occurs by insertion, deletion, or

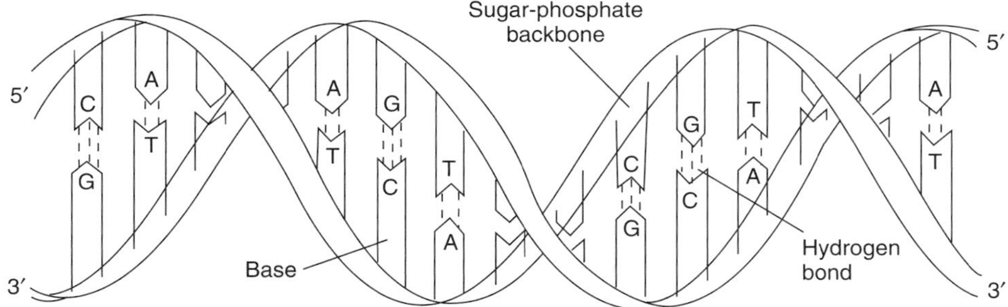

Fig. 13-1 Structure of DNA. DNA molecule is double helix that consists of two sugar-phosphate backbones with four bases—cytosine (C), guanine (G), adenine (A), and thymine (T)—attached. *C* and *G* residues and *A* and *T* residues on opposite strands pair through hydrogen bonding. (Reprinted with permission from LeGrys V, Leinbach SS, Silverman L: *CRC Crit Rev Clin Lab Sci* 25:255, 1987. Copyright CRC Press, Inc, Boca Raton, FL.)

substitution of a base. The base change may result in a change in the genetic code and the information residing in that code. A mutation that occurs in the portion of DNA that codes for a protein may result in a change in the amino acid sequence, and consequently the structure, of that protein. Changes in protein structure can result in no change in the function of the protein, a total loss of function, or a partial loss of function. It is the partial or total loss of function that usually results in a pathological state. The effect of a loss of function can be direct, such as the conformation dysfunction of hemoglobin that results in the disease sickle cell anemia (see Chapter 40), or indirect, such as the loss of function of regulators of gene expression that can result in cancers (see p. 253 and Chapter 53). A mutation that occurs in the nonstructural, regulatory regions of DNA can also result in a changed expression of a gene.

Mutations can occur by a wide variety of mechanisms. For the purposes of the discussion of cancer and inherited disease, mutations can be divided into germline and somatic events. A germline mutation is one that is present in all cells of the body and is passed from generation to generation by meiosis (creation of germ cells—sperm and egg) and sexual reproduction. Somatic mutations are those mutations that arise in tissue cells, generally as a result of some environmental insult or DNA replication error. For additional information on genetic inheritance, see Chapter 52.

Abnormal expression of genes can also result from inheritable changes to the chemical structure of genes that are not a result of a change of a base in a codon triplet. Methylation of the nucleotide bases, which classically occurs in the CpG dinucleotide, is a chemical modification that takes place after DNA synthesis. DNA methylation is a component of the **epigenetic code** that affects the expression of genes. Abnormal patterns of DNA methylation can cause abnormal gene expression (transcription) and disease states. Repeat base sequences that have no apparent informational content regarding protein structure exist throughout the DNA. The expansion of the number of repeats in a gene has been associated with specific diseases, and this change in the gene structure is inheritable.

KEY CONCEPTS BOX 13-1

- Purine and pyrimidine bases form the triplet codes in DNA that specify an amino acid in the protein that a gene codes for.
- When the bases correctly match, complementary DNA strands will bind to each other to form double-stranded DNA.
- Mutations represent a change—insertion, deletion, or replacement—in the base sequence in DNA that may affect the synthesis of the encoded protein. A normal protein may be produced, no protein may be synthesized, or none or part of its function may be preserved. The latter two cases may result in disease.
- Mutations can occur in a heritable manner in germline cells, or in a noninheritable form in somatic cells.

SECTION OBJECTIVES BOX 13-2

- Review how digestion of DNA by specific nucleases can be used to identify specific sequences of DNA.
- List the major clinical uses of techniques to identify specific DNA sequences.
- Describe the Southern blot technique.
- Describe the polymerase chain reaction.
- Compare and contrast specific and scanning mutation detection methods.

TECHNIQUES OF DNA ANALYSIS

Several core technologies are central to the modern practice of molecular biology. The first takes advantage of the ability of complementary strands of DNA to find each other in complex solutions and bind together to form the familiar DNA double helix. This specific binding, termed *hybridization,* forms the basis for almost all types of DNA detection methods. The second set of techniques that are crucial for manipulation and detection of specific nucleotide sequences involves a large number of enzymes that are commercially available. These enzymes in vivo are involved in DNA metabolism and repair or in bacterial host defense, and they provide the molecular tools with which nucleic acids can be manipulated with extraordinary specificity. One set of these enzymes are the **restriction endonucleases;** another set of enzymes that are broadly used are the **polymerases,** both DNA and RNA polymerases and reverse transcriptase. These enzymes are used in vivo to replicate DNA, to make RNA copies of DNA sequence; and, by retroviruses, to make DNA copies of RNA genomes. The third set of core techniques in modern molecular biology consists of the detection methods. These methods are required to possess extreme specificity, not for the chemical structure of DNA, which is identical for all genes in all species, but for the sequence of the bases, which determines the information that a particular piece of DNA is carrying. Further, as specific gene sequences form only a tiny fraction of the whole human genome, and because DNA is typically available only in microgram amounts, these methods must possess extreme sensitivity. The first of these methods to be described and widely adopted is the **Southern transfer.** The second is the **polymerase chain reaction (PCR).**

Restriction Digestion and Gel Electrophoresis

A specific property of DNA (and RNA) is its susceptibility to enzymes called *nucleases.* Nucleases hydrolyze the phosphodiester bonds that connect bases within a nucleic acid strand, resulting in cleavage of the strand. Certain nucleases have very high substrate specificity and will cleave a DNA strand only at specific base sequences, often as small as four to eight bases in length. Because these nucleases are employed by bacteria to restrict entry of foreign DNA into their cells, they are called *restriction endonucleases.* The sequences that the enzymes recognize and cleave are referred to as **restriction sites.** These enzymes require Mg^{++} ion for activity. More than 400 enzymes that recognize different restriction sites have been identified. Most of these are commercially available.

Restriction endonucleases are critical reagents in laboratories investigating DNA base sequences because they cleave the double-stranded nucleic acid only at specific points. After DNA is digested into a series of many smaller fragments, specific sequences can be more readily identified by the hybridization technique. To aid in the identification of a specific base sequence, the fragments can first be separated into molecules of differing molecular size. This is accomplished by either agarose or polyacrylamide (or their derivatives) gel electrophoresis.

The most common method for the visualization of DNA after electrophoretic size separation consists of staining with the intercalating agent, ethidium bromide, or the minor groove-binding agent, SYBR Green (Invitrogen, Carlsbad, CA). These compounds, when in solution, are free to lose energy acquired via incident radiation by increased rotation and collision with solvent molecules. However, when a molecule of ethidium bromide or SYBR Green is bound to the DNA double helix, these motions are lost, and the molecule rids itself of excess energy by fluorescence. The fragments of DNA generated by restriction enzyme digestion are equimolar with respect to each other, providing an easy method for determining the completeness of a given restriction digestion reaction. Hybridization of the separated fragments then is achieved by the Southern transfer technique.

Southern Transfer

Currently, Southern analysis is used in the clinical laboratory to detect large structural changes in DNA sequences that are not amenable to analysis by PCR. An example is the chromosome translocations involving the mixed lineage leukemia (MLL) gene at chromosome 11q23. Because this gene has been associated with translocation to more than 40 different chromosomes and genes, it is difficult to design PCR strategies that will detect all MLL rearrangements. Other uses for Southern analysis include genetic diseases in which an abnormal **allele** cannot be efficiently amplified or detected by PCR because of its large size or high G and C content. One such example is the fragile X syndrome.

For many gene targets of clinical interest, PCR has supplanted Southern analysis because it is much less costly and labor intensive, and it has a much quicker turnaround time. However, in some cases, the diagnostic sensitivity of PCR test strategies is not as great as for Southern transfer–based methods. An example is the detection of immunoglobulin gene rearrangements in leukemia and lymphoma. In this case, PCR will detect most (>95%), but not all, pathological events. Thus, Southern transfer analysis still retains a place in the clinical laboratory.

Blood samples for analysis are collected into acid-citrate-dextrose (ACD) or ethylenediaminetetraacetic acid (EDTA) anticoagulant tubes, and the white cells then are isolated from each sample. DNA is extracted from the white cells and is incubated with a restriction endonuclease to cleave the DNA into smaller fragments. The digested DNA sample is applied to an agarose gel and is electrophoresed to separate the fragments according to size. The fragments then are treated with alkali to separate the double-stranded DNA into single strands; this process is termed **denaturation.** The separated, denatured fragments are then transferred from the gel onto another support medium, such as a nitrocellulose or nylon membrane (the *Southern blot* procedure, different form the *northern blot* in which RNA is transferred) (Fig. 13-2). The fragment or fragments that contain the DNA sequence of interest are identified by incubating the membrane with a labeled DNA probe that contains sequences complementary to the sequence of interest. The label can be a radioisotope, an enzyme, or a chemiluminescent or a fluorescent dye. The complementary sequence of the probe permits it to hybridize to the sample DNA that contains linked probe sequences. In the case of radiolabeled cDNA, the membrane then is incubated with x-ray film to expose areas (bands) on the film where the probe has bound to the sample DNA, resulting in an autoradiogram.

Currently, non-isotopic detection methods that use colorimetric or luminescent detection are widely used because they reduce the time required for band visualization and exposure of technologists to ionizing radiation. These methods employ a second hybridization step that uses an enzyme-coupled antibody to a hapten that has been incorporated into the probe DNA instead of ^{32}P. The action of the enzyme then generates

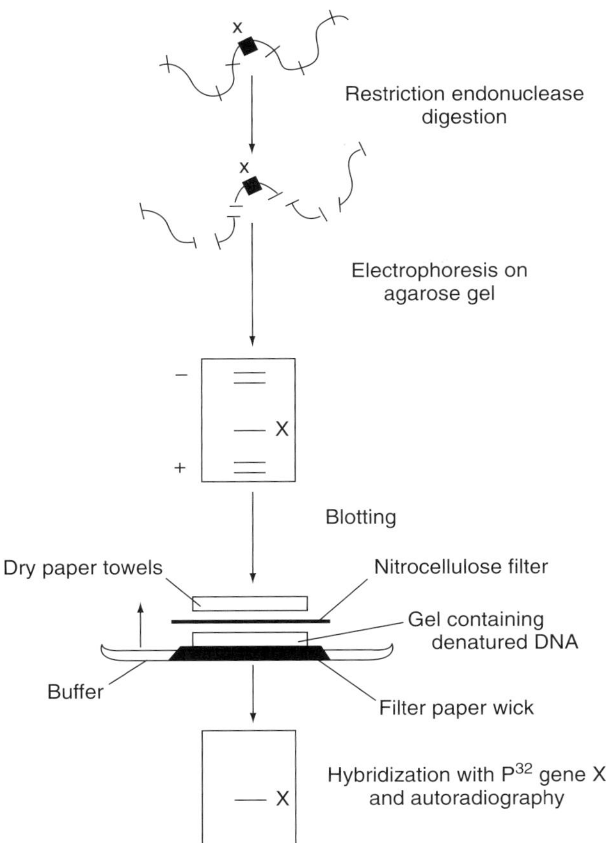

Fig. 13-2 Identification by Southern blot hybridization of DNA fragment containing gene X. DNA was digested with restriction endonuclease, and resulting fragments were fractionated according to size by electrophoresis in agarose gel. DNA fragments in gel were denatured and blotted to nitrocellulose filter as a result of flow of buffer through gel and nitrocellulose filter to dry paper towels. Subsequent hybridization of DNA on filter to ^{32}P-labeled gene X probe and autoradiography revealed single DNA fragment containing gene X. (Reprinted with permission from LeGrys V, Leinbach SS, Silverman L: *CRC Crit Rev Clin Lab Sci* 25:255, 1987. Copyright CRC Press, Boca Raton, FL.)

the colored or chemiluminescent product from a colorless or inactive substrate. Several non-isotopic detection systems are commercially available for use with Southern transfer; examples are the BrightStar kit from Ambion (Austin, TX) (chemiluminescent) and the AlkPhos Direct (colorimetric) and ECL (chemiluminescent) systems from GE Healthcare (Piscataway, NJ). The Southern blot procedure requires less than 24 hours from DNA extraction from whole blood to film development.

Polymerase Chain Reaction (PCR)

Although the Southern procedure combines reasonable sensitivity with excellent specificity, it is technically demanding, may require the use of hazardous, high-energy β-emitters such as ^{32}P, and has a long turnaround time. Several objections to the Southern procedure can be addressed by the use of the polymerase chain reaction (PCR). PCR is a technique for the rapid, in vitro amplification of specific DNA sequences. The introduction of PCR into clinical laboratories has revolutionized the practice of molecular diagnostics.

Knowledge of the sequence of the region of DNA flanking the DNA sequence of interest is required for PCR. Two synthetic oligodeoxynucleotides (primers), typically 20 to 30 bases in length, are synthesized (or purchased) such that one of the primers is complementary to an area on one strand of the target DNA 5′ to the sequences to be amplified, and the other primer is complementary to the opposite strand of the target DNA, again 5′ to the region to be amplified. A schematic is shown in Fig. 13-3.

To perform the amplification, the sample DNA is placed in a tube along with a large molar excess of the two primers, all four deoxynucleotide triphosphates (dNTPs), buffer, magnesium ion, and a thermostable DNA polymerase. The most commonly used polymerase is isolated from the thermophilic organism, *Thermus aquaticus.* This enzyme, termed *Taq polymerase,* has its optimal activity at 72°C but can survive for short periods at temperatures up to 95°C without being irreversibly denatured. The reaction is first heated to 95°C to melt the test DNA from a double-stranded to a single-stranded form. The temperature then is decreased, typically to 50°C to 60°C, to allow annealing, or hybridization, of the primers to their complementary sites on the **single-stranded DNA** of the sample. It should be noted that the vast molar excess of the primers, as well as their small size, ensures that the hybridization occurs between the sample DNA and the primers, and not between the two stands of the test DNA. The temperature then is increased to 72°C, the temperature optimum for Taq polymerase. The polymerase extends the primers in the 5′ to 3′ direction of each strand by incorporating the dNTPs into the growing complementary DNA strands. It is crucial that the polymerase extend far enough along each strand to create a new binding site for the opposite primer. After the temperature is held at 72°C for a period of time sufficient to synthesize a new DNA strand from one primer to the binding site of the other (typically 15 to 60 seconds), the process of temperature cycling is repeated. After heating is provided to denature the newly formed DNA, the temperature again is decreased to allow annealing of the primers, this time to the newly synthesized binding sites, as well as those on the original template DNA. The temperature again is increased to 72°C to extend the four bound primers (see Fig. 13-3). As the temperature changes are repeated, the DNA between the two primers is synthesized. The amount of DNA produced is exponential with respect to cycle number. After 30 cycles of annealing, extension, and denaturation, 2^{30}, or approximately 10^9, copies will have been generated.

In a typical experiment, starting with 20 to 100 ng of human DNA, 30 cycles of amplification will produce enough DNA from a single gene copy to be visualized on an ethidium bromide–stained gel. Because each cycle takes 2 to 5 minutes, amplification of a specific sequence can be accomplished easily in several hours. After amplification, the DNA can be analyzed by one of several techniques, depending on the specific problem.

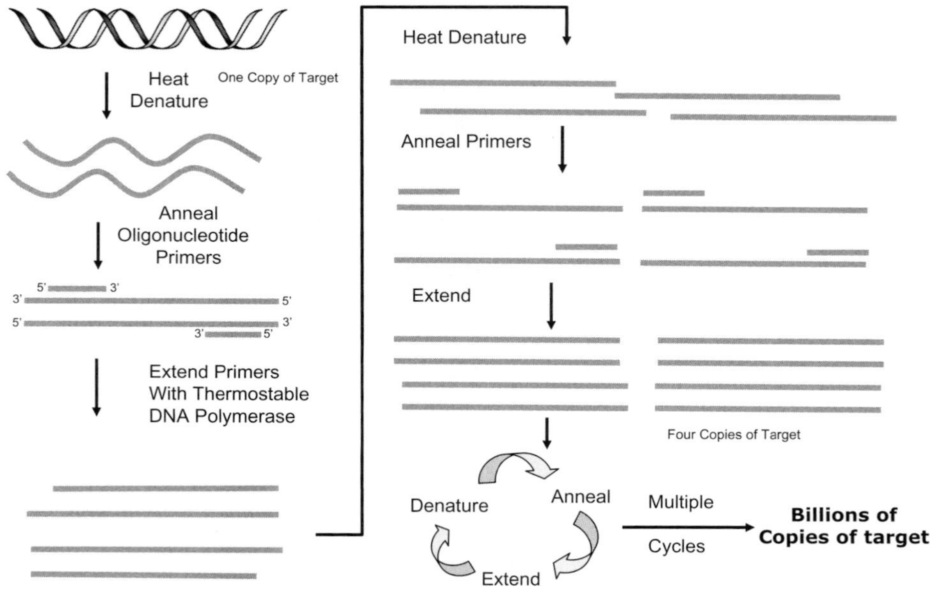

Fig. 13-3 Schematic representation of the first cycle of a PCR reaction.

PCR-Based Techniques and Applications

The application of PCR can be grouped into two broad categories: mutation detection techniques, which are used to investigate the actual base sequence at a particular locus, and quantitative methods, in which PCR-based techniques are used to quantify specific nucleic acid sequences. Mutation detection strategies can be grouped further into specific or scanning techniques.

Specific Mutation Detection Techniques

Specific mutation detection entails straightforward, and largely routine, procedures that can be used to analyze DNA samples for previously identified mutations using an assay designed for maximum specificity. This approach targets known mutations in potentially large cohorts of patients (such as factor V Lieden and sickle cell anemia) or panels of specific mutations in disorders characterized by one or a few common alleles (such as hereditary hemochromatosis [two mutations] and CF [typical panels range from 23 to 100 mutations]). Results from these types of analyses may confirm or establish clinical diagnoses. Furthermore, in families at risk for a particular genetic disease, specific or targeted mutation detection allows for rapid screening of an entire family for the mutation identified in the **proband,** thereby permitting accurate carrier determinations that aid reproductive decisions. Rapid testing of large numbers of patients permits an assessment of the mutation's frequency among disease-causing alleles, thereby determining which mutations are most prevalent in different patient populations and guiding the creation of effective clinical mutation testing panels.

The specific mutation detection methods themselves can be divided into those that use gel electrophoresis and those that use hybridization-based methods. Both types of approaches are robust and, in experienced hands, yield reproducible results. Both types of systems are in widespread use in clinical and research laboratories. One criterion for choice between these general platforms is the cost incurred per sample analyzed. In the authors' experience, when the number of samples to be analyzed at one time (samples per batch) is low, electrophoretic methods are often the most cost effective to develop, validate, and implement. However, when the number of samples per batch is larger (more than 8 to 12 samples), then hybridization-based techniques, many of which can be adapted to 96-well microplate formats, are often more cost effective.

Restriction Endonuclease Digestion

Mutations represent a change in the local DNA sequence and may involve single nucleotide substitutions, small deletions or insertions, or more complex rearrangements. Beyond their potential for clinical consequences, gene mutations may, by virtue of their changes in nucleotide sequence, create novel restriction endonuclease recognition sites or may destroy preexisting ones. For example, a DNA fragment that harbors a mutation might not be cleaved with a particular restriction enzyme that usually cleaves wild-type (normal) DNA. Conversely, a different mutation might create a novel restriction site not present in the wild-type DNA. In either case, mutated DNA produces a distinct restriction digestion pattern relative to that seen with nonmutated DNA when the digestion products of PCR-amplified DNA are compared after electrophoresis on either agarose or polyacrylamide gel. An example of this approach applied to mutation detection in CF is shown in Fig. 13-4.

The use of restriction enzymes to distinguish between alleles is one of the most common techniques used in clinical molecular laboratories. This method offers advantages over approaches associated with radioisotope usage and their collateral costs and concerns. The large variety of restriction endonucleases that are commercially available represents a

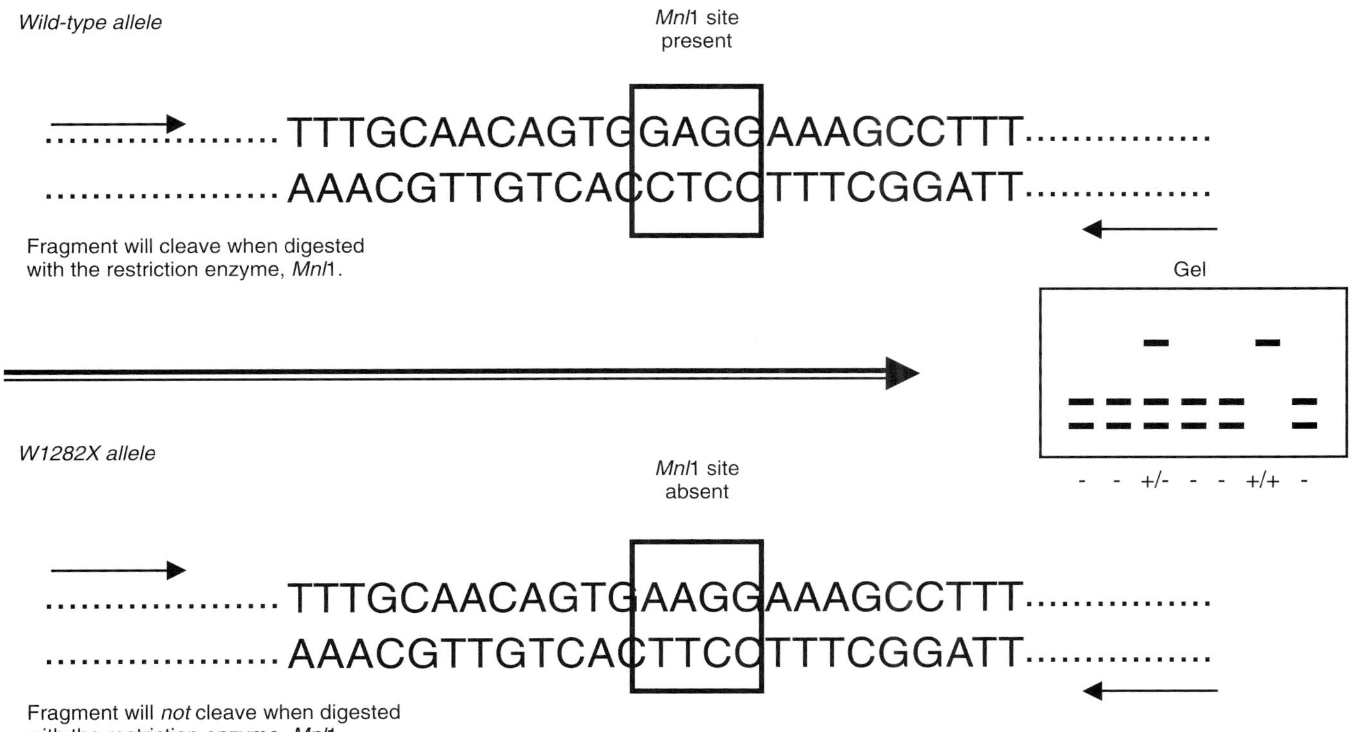

Fig. 13-4 Restriction endonuclease–mediated detection of the cystic fibrosis (CF) mutation, W1282X. The Mnl1 site is present in the wild-type allele and not in the mutant. –, normal; +/–, heterozygote (carrier); +/+, homozygous (affected).

substantial resource to molecular laboratories, and the wide variety of recognition sequences associated with these enzymes affords the investigator many choices for designing straightforward mutation detection strategies.

Despite this large supply of different restriction endonucleases, less than half of known DNA sequence variants independently alter restriction digestion patterns for a commercially available enzyme. Additionally, some enzymes are unreliable or are prohibitively expensive for use in routine, repetitive analyses. Other confounding factors include restriction enzymes with overly common recognition sites.

PCR-Mediated, Site-Directed Mutagenesis (PSM)

When confounding factors impede the design of simple restriction-based assays, laboratories may employ a modification of this approach. PSM is a technique by which a novel allele-specific restriction digestion pattern can be purposefully generated in association with virtually any mutation. This strategy is known by a variety of names other than PSM, including restriction site–generating PCR (RG-PCR) and amplification-created restriction site (ACRS). These techniques, identical in approach, involve the design of one PCR primer that abuts the mutation locus and includes typically one or two nucleotides mismatched relative to the template DNA. If properly designed, the mutagenic primer will retain sufficient complementarity to anneal specifically to its target DNA and support efficient amplification. All generated PCR products will include the mutation locus under study and will also incorporate the base change inherent to the mutagenic primer. The combination of the mutation and the novel base change of this primer engineers the creation of a novel restriction pattern where none was previously present. This method has been applied to a wide variety of clinically important mutations. An example of the application of PSM to detection of the α_1-antityrpsin Z allele is shown schematically in Fig. 13-5.

Amplification Refractory Mutation System (ARMS)

In this method, also known as *allele-specific PCR,* primers are designed that amplify only one of the alleles present at the locus of interest. This is accomplished with primers that are substantially mismatched relative to one allele but have sufficient complementarity to anneal to, and amplify, the other allele. Typically, ARMS is designed to amplify one allele, while a separate reaction is specific for the other allele at that locus. Although this assay avoids the need for a restriction enzyme, it is predicated on high allele specificity of amplification and requires two PCR reactions per patient sample, one each for the normal and mutant alleles. An example of the use of this technique for detection of the common connexin26 hereditary hearing loss allele, 35delG, is shown in Fig. 13-6.

Allele-Specific Oligonucleotide Hybridization (ASO, or Dot-Blot)

DNA is amplified by PCR and is spotted onto two nylon membranes. Each membrane then is hybridized with one of two synthetic, radiolabeled oligonucleotides that span the region of DNA that contains a specific mutation. One oligonucleotide has the sequence complementary to the wild-type, or normal, DNA sequence, whereas the other is perfectly complementary to the mutant allele. Under appropriate conditions of temperature and salt concentration (**stringency**),

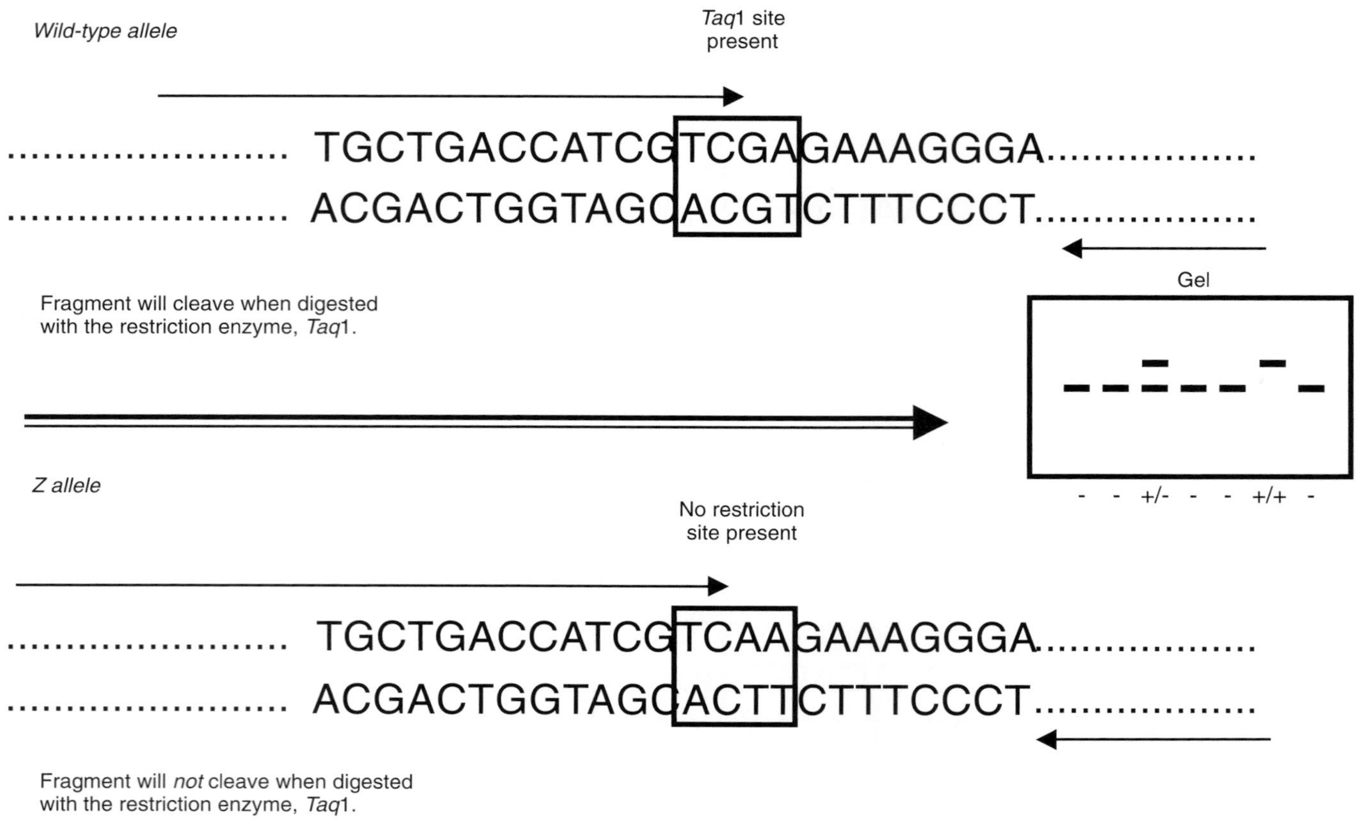

Wild-type allele

*Taq*1 site present

.... TGCTGACCATCGTCGAGAAAGGGA..................
.... ACGACTGGTAGCACGTCTTTCCCT..................

Fragment will cleave when digested with the restriction enzyme, *Taq*1.

Gel

- - +/- - - +/+ -

Z allele

No restriction site present

.... TGCTGACCATCGTCAAGAAAGGGA..................
.... ACGACTGGTAGCACTTCTTTCCCT..................

Fragment will *not* cleave when digested with the restriction enzyme, *Taq*1.

Fig. 13-5 PCR-mediated site-directed mutagenesis (PSM)-based detection of the α_1-antitrypsin Z mutation. After amplification containing a mismatched base, the Taq1 site is present in the wild-type allele and not in the mutant. –, normal; +/–, heterozygote (carrier); +/+, homozygous (affected).

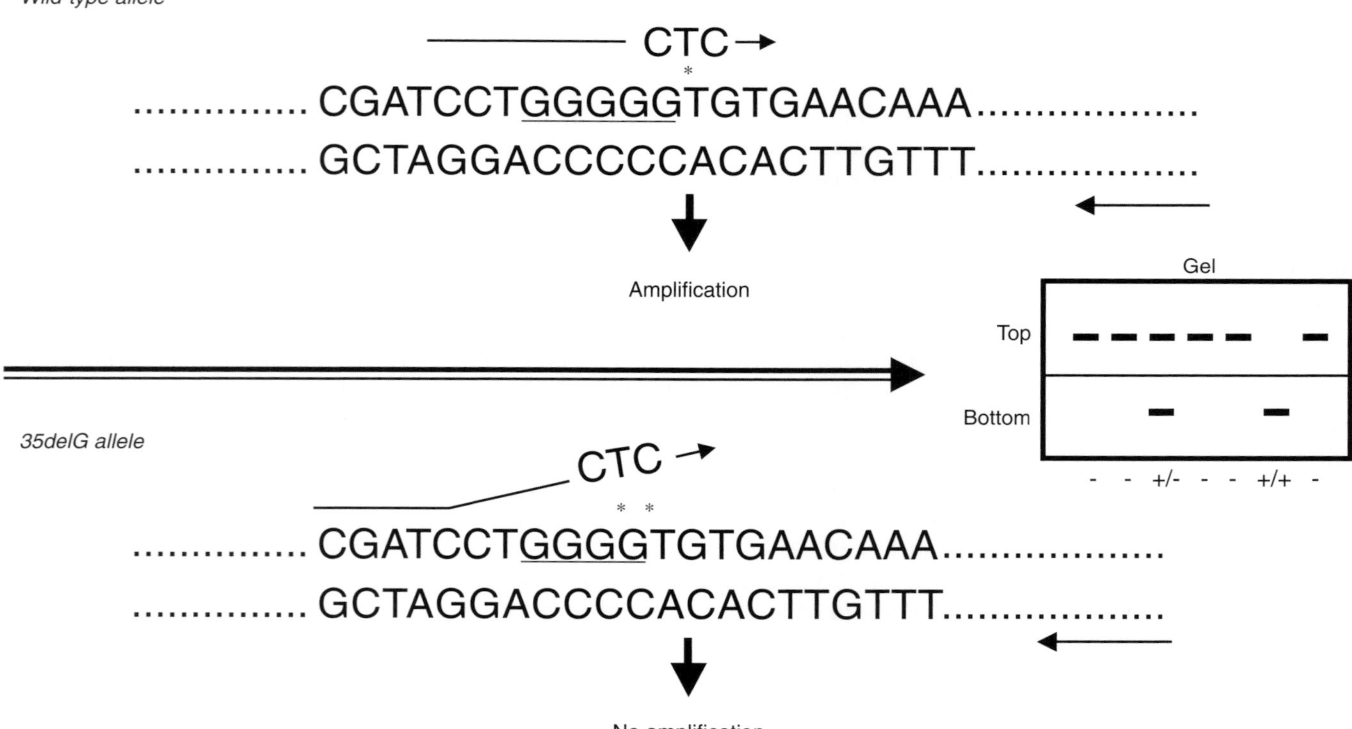

Fig. 13-6 Amplification refractory mutation system (ARMS)-based assay for the connexin26 hereditary deafness allele, 35delG. The primer complementary to the wild-type allele amplifies the wild type, but not the mutant. This result is shown in the top panel of the gel. A second polymerase chain reaction (PCR) is done with a primer complementary to the mutant allele, which amplifies the mutant but not the wild type. The result is shown in the bottom panel of the gel. –, normal; +/–, heterozygote (carrier); +/+, homozygous (affected).

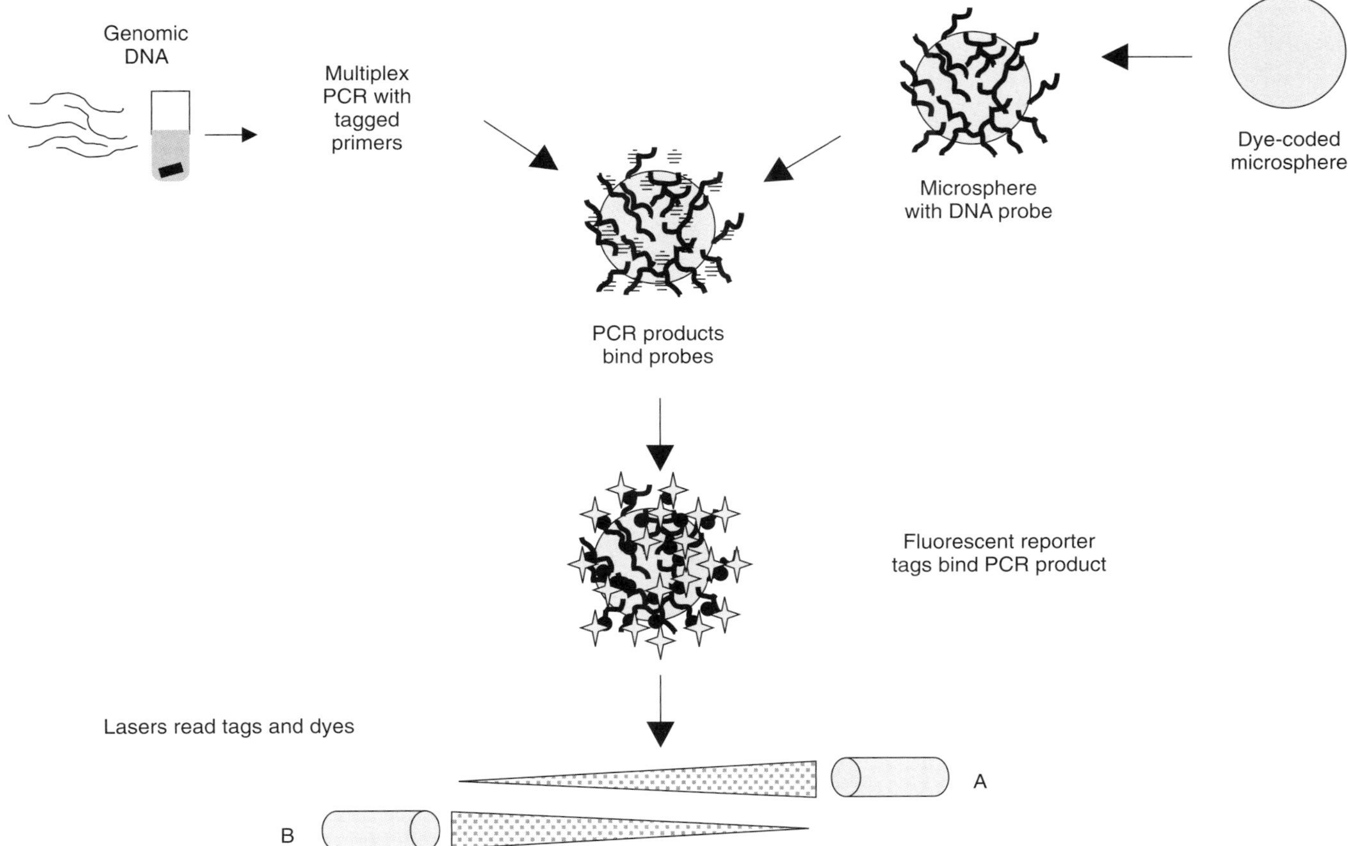

Fig. 13-7 Luminex-100 flow cytometry platform. Patient DNA is amplified with a sequence-tagged primer. The denatured polymerase chain reaction (PCR) product is hybridized to dye-labeled microspheres to which allele-specific oligonucleotide probes have been affixed. Fluorescent dye–labeled probes complementary to the sequence tags then are added. The presence of the fluorescent probes is detected by flow cytometry using a red *(A)* and a green *(B)* laser.

hybridization occurs only when the probe and the target DNA are perfectly base-paired. Thus the normal oligonucleotide binds only the normal amplified target, but the mutant oligonucleotide hybridizes only with the mutant allele. Detection is usually by autoradiography. Variants of this procedure include non-isotopic detection and hybridization in microtiter trays instead of on a membrane.

Reverse Dot-Blot

The reverse dot-blot is a variant of the ASO technique in which the allele-specific oligonucleotides (normal and mutant) are bound to a nylon membrane or are immobilized in microtiter tray wells. Amplification of the sample DNA is performed as usual but with one of the PCR primers labeled at the 5′ end with a biotin molecule. The amplified DNA is hybridized with the ASOs bound to the surface of a microtiter tray well under appropriately stringent conditions for allele-specific hybridization. After the hybridization and washing steps, avidin conjugated to alkaline phosphatase is bound to the biotin. Detection of the hybrids occurs by monitoring the action of the enzyme on a substrate to produce a colored, insoluble product. This system is the basis for the Roche Amplicor series of products (Roche Molecular Diagnostics, Pleasanton, CA).

Flow Cytometry

A powerful strategy is the Luminex X-Map System (Luminex Corp, Austin, TX). Luminex-100 is a microsphere-based flow cytometry assay that allows high-throughput sample processing for simultaneous detection of multiple sequence variants. Polystyrene microspheres are dyed internally with two spectrally distinct fluorochromes. An array is created that consists of 100 different microsphere sets, each set distinguishable by its internal dye ratios. Therefore, each set of microspheres can carry a different DNA probe, that is, for one allele at particular genetic locus and mixed with many other spectrally distinct microspheres in a multiplex reaction.

Oligonucleotide probes are bound to the surfaces of microspheres and are hybridized with biotin-tagged complementary PCR fragments derived from multiplex reactions amplifying several loci simultaneously. The spheres then are incubated with a fluorochrome that binds the biotin tag. Microspheres are interrogated individually in a rapidly flowing fluid stream as they pass by two separate lasers. High-speed digital signal processing classifies the microspheres on the basis of their spectral address and quantifies the fluorescence-labeled PCR fragment on the surface (Fig. 13-7). Thousands of microspheres are interrogated per second, resulting in an analysis

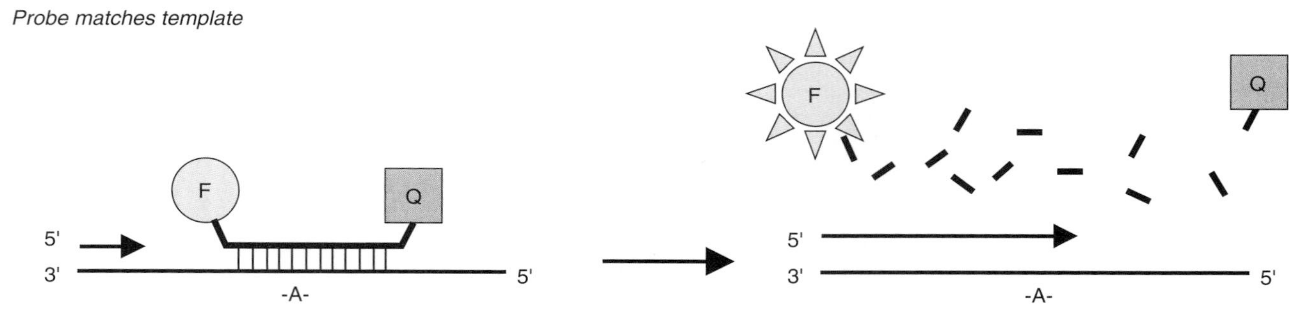

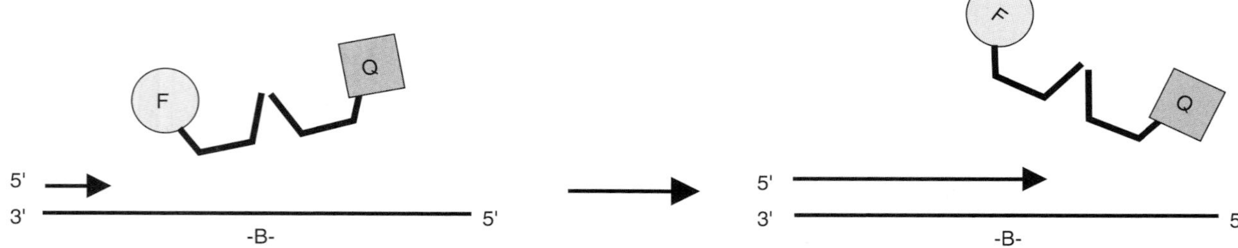

Fig. 13-8 TaqMan mutation detection. The TaqMan probe hybridizes to the wild-type allele and is degraded by the 5′ to 3′ exonuclease activity of Taq polymerase. The starburst figure depicts fluorescence of the fluorophore (*F*) after release from the effect of the Quencher *(Q)*. The probe does not bind to the mutant allele, the probe is not degraded, and fluorescence is not observed.

system capable of analyzing and reporting up to 100 different reactions in a single reaction tube in a few seconds. Approximately 1 hour is required for this system to analyze 96 samples arranged in a microtiter plate for multiple alleles.

Real-Time PCR

Instruments with both thermal cycling and fluorescence quantification capabilities have introduced automation to PCR analysis. These instruments allow for the quantification of a fluorescent signal from each PCR reaction vessel during the PCR reaction. The fluorescence signal changes as a function of cycle number and reflects the initial concentration of DNA template in the reaction mixture. Variations of real-time PCR techniques follow.

The 5′ Exonuclease Assay (TaqMan)

This strategy entails the use of a short DNA probe with a reporter dye attached to one end and a quenching agent linked to the other end. This probe is designed to perfectly match one allele at particular locus but to be mismatched relative to other alleles. As the polymerase advances during the extension phase of the PCR reaction, the 5′ to 3′ exonuclease activity of the polymerase digests any probe in its path, releasing the reporter dye from the quencher and generating a fluorescent signal (Fig. 13-8) that is proportional to the amount of allele that is present in the sample. This automated technique is useful for both nucleic acid quantification and specific mutation detection. For mutation detection, if the probe is mismatched relative to the template, its affinity for the template will be greatly reduced under appropriately stringent conditions, and probe not bound to the template will neither be digested nor generate a signal. A similar probe may be designed to detect the other alleles, and these assays may be pooled as long as each probe carries a different, separately detectable, reporter dye. For quantification of DNA templates, the cycle number at which a specified fluorescence intensity is attained is proportional to the initial DNA concentration. Thus, a sample with a relatively higher initial DNA concentration of any given DNA template, from, for example, a microorganism, will demonstrate detectable fluorescence at a lower cycle number than one with a lower concentration of template.

This chemistry is compatible with real-time PCR instrumentation from several vendors, including those manufactured by Cepheid, Roche, BioRad, Stratagene, and Applied Biosystems. Thus, the hybridization probe step, which prior to the development of "real-time PCR" instruments and chemistries required separate manipulations, now can be accomplished at the same time as the PCR reaction.

FRET Probe Analysis

Another specific mutation detection chemistry that uses the real-time PCR platform is FRET probe analysis. Similar to TaqMan chemistry, this technology uses fluorescence

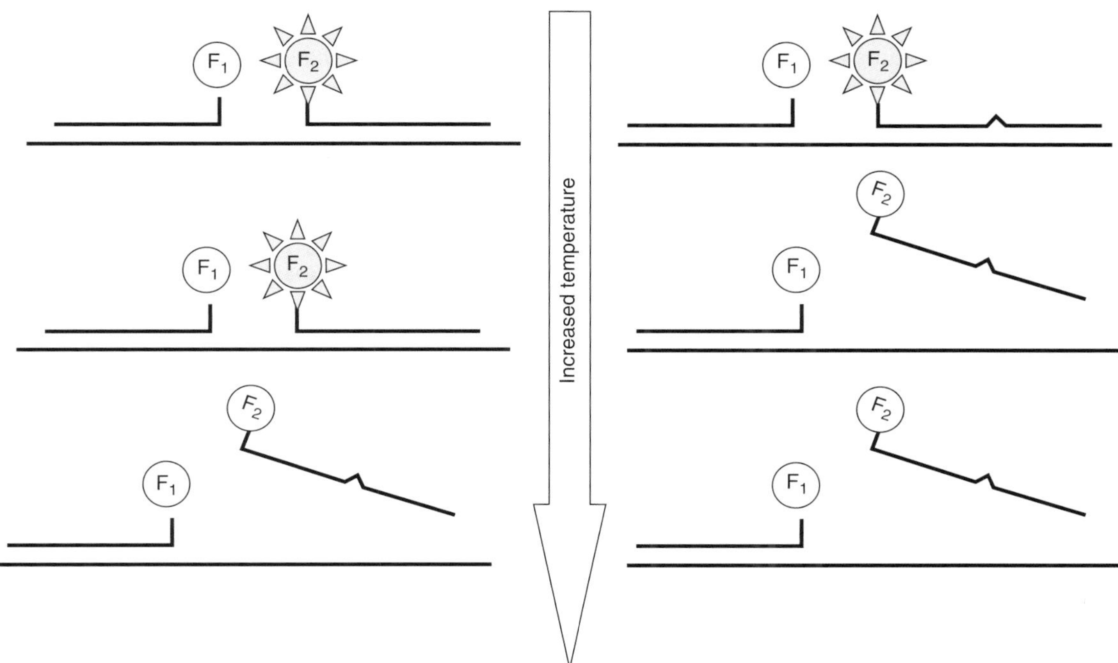

Fig. 13-9 Fluorescence resonance energy transfer (FRET) probe-specific mutation detection. *Left panel,* Both probes form perfectly base-paired double-stranded DNA. *Right panel,* One probe has a mismatch and melts earlier when the temperature is increased. The starburst figure depicts fluorescence of the second fluorophore (F_2) when it is in close physical proximity to the first fluorophore (F_1) and can be excited by FRET.

resonance energy transfer (FRET) between two fluorophores. FRET probe analysis employs two oligonucleotide probes, each labeled with a different fluorescent dye. The two fluorescent dyes are chosen so that the emission spectrum of one dye overlaps the excitation spectrum of the second dye. When the first dye is excited, it transfers its energy via a nonradiative mechanism (FRET) to the second dye, when the latter is in close physical proximity. This causes the second dye to emit a characteristic fluorescence. One probe, termed the *sensor* probe, overlays the site of the mutation to be detected and forms either a perfect DNA duplex or a **heteroduplex DNA.** The other probe, termed the *anchor* probe, is designed to hybridize to a nearby nonpolymorphic site and to have a **melting temperature** several degrees higher than the perfectly matched sensor probe. At low stringency, both sensor and anchor probes hybridize efficiently, and the close proximity of the two dyes causes illumination energy to be transferred efficiently from the first to the second dye. However, as the temperature is slowly increased, the mismatched sensor probe will melt before the perfectly matched anchor probe (Fig. 13-9). Thus, mutations are identified by differences in their melting curve profile compared with the wild-type allele. These differences can be seen in a plot of fluorescence intensity (of the anchor dye) versus temperature; however, the data are easier to interpret when displayed as the first derivative. Similar to Taq-Man chemistry, FRET probe analysis can be used for both mutation detection and template quantification. Although FRET probe analysis is compatible with most of the real-time PCR instruments that are currently available, it was developed for use with the Light Cycler (Roche Applied Sciences, Indianapolis, IN). With this instrument, which features very rapid cycle times, a batch of up to 32 samples can be analyzed for the presence of specific mutations in as little as 30 minutes. Other real-time PCR instruments, which use Pelletier heating and cooling systems, have slower cycle times but can analyze 96 or 384 samples per batch with the use of FRET probe technology.

MLPA (Multiplex Ligation Probe Amplification)

The real-time PCR techniques described above are notable for a very large dynamic range. The response of cycle number to DNA concentration is linear over up to six orders of magnitude. Thus, they have proved extraordinarily useful in clinical microbiology, where the numbers of pathogenic bacteria or viruses can be present over such a very large range. The detection of a twofold change, however, is more difficult.

Deletions (or duplications) of large regions of DNA (entire exons or entire genes) are an important class of pathogenic events that are not typically detectable with the use of specific or scanning mutation detection strategies described in this chapter. However, this type of mutation constitutes the majority of mutations that cause certain genetic disorders, such as Duchenne muscular dystrophy (DMD) or α-thalassemia. For example, two-thirds of all DMD is caused by insertions or deletions of one or more exons. There are point mutations in both DMD and α-thalassemia, but they constitute the minority. In other disorders (hereditary nonpolyposis colon cancer or CF), insertions or deletions constitute a small, but important, fraction of the mutational spectrum. For CF, >95% of mutant alleles result from point mutations (or small indels), but about 2% or so of CF mutant alleles have a large deletion or duplication in the CF gene. Because each PCR cycle doubles the amount of product DNA, the detection of insertion/deletion-type mutations in human genetics requires very precise assays, such as the MLPA method.

The MLPA assay uses oligonucleotide probes that are complementary to a region of interest, such that the 3′ end of one primer abuts the 5′ end of the other primer. In addition, the primers are designed to have "tails," or sequences, that are not complementary to the template DNA but are used as binding sites for PCR primers. If the two probes are hybridized perfectly to the template DNA, they can be ligated, or joined together, with DNA ligase, another DNA metabolic enzyme that can be used as a tool in the molecular laboratory. If the two probes are ligated together, they can be amplified by PCR using primers complementary to the tail sequences. Thus, this PCR-based method does not utilize amplification of the template, but of the probe.

The power of the MLPA technique (and the multiplex part of the name) is associated with the realization that multiple pairs of primers, targeting multiple loci (e.g., all the exons of a particular gene), can be designed with the same "tails," thus being amplifiable with a single pair of PCR primers. The use of the same primers for multiple loci greatly decreases the variability of amplification efficiency and allows comparison of the amount of amplified probe DNA from any locus versus what was amplified at a control locus. However, there must be a means for distinguishing the multiple probe amplicons from each other if a meaningful analysis is to be performed. This can be accomplished in several ways; in the commercial version, varying lengths of "stuffer" DNA (consisting of irrelevant sequences) are incorporated into various probe pairs. Thus, up to 40 amplified and fluorescently labeled probes can be separated and quantified by capillary electrophoresis.

The relative amount of DNA amplified at a locus heterozygous for a deletion (50% relative to a nondeleted control locus) or a duplication (150% relative to control) is readily determined and provides a robust assay for determining small values for gene dosage or copy number.

Mutation Scanning Techniques

Mutation scanning methods interrogate DNA fragments for all sequence variants present. By definition, these strategies are not predicated on specificity for specific alleles but rather are designed for highly sensitive detection for all possible variants. In principle, all sequence variants present will be detected without regard for advance knowledge of their pathogenic consequences. Once evidence for a sequence variant has been found, the sample must be sequenced to determine its molecular nature. The advantage of using a scanning method followed by sequencing of only positive PCR products is that the scanning methods typically are less costly to perform than DNA sequencing. Only when combined with appropriate genetic data and in vitro functional studies can investigators distinguish disease-causing mutations from polymorphisms without clinical consequences. In the research laboratory, mutation screening is a critical and obligatory final step toward identifying genes that underlie genetic disease. In the clinical laboratory, these methods are applied toward the detection of mutations in diseases marked by significant allelic heterogeneity.

Single-Stranded Conformational Polymorphism (SSCP) Analysis

This screening strategy takes advantage of the distinct secondary structures that single- and double-stranded DNA fragments will assume after they are denatured. The nature of these structures is highly dependent on the nucleotide sequence of the fragment. After amplification of a genomic fragment, the PCR product is denatured to single strands and is transferred immediately to ice. The sample then is electrophoresed on a nondenaturing polyacrylamide gel. Both double-stranded and single-stranded fragments will be apparent on the gel as distinctly migrating bands. The presence of a mutation or a polymorphism within the PCR product will be apparent through band shifts in the double- or single-stranded fragments or both, when compared with DNA fragments without sequence variants (Fig. 13-10). Multiple altered fragment conformations may arise from a single mutation.

Heteroduplex Analysis

Many mutation screening strategies are predicated on heteroduplex formation. Two single-stranded fragments of DNA such as recently synthesized PCR products will form fully matched, stable homoduplex structures if they have 100% sequence complementarity. DNA fragments with high, but incomplete, sequence complementarity will also form duplex structures, but these fragments may have subtly altered conformational properties and may become substrates for specific chemical and enzymatic reactions. When a DNA fragment from an individual heterozygous for a nucleotide substitution is amplified, the final PCR product will include homoduplex structures for each allele and heteroduplexes derived from the imperfect annealing of dissimilar fragments. Whenever heterozygosity is established, direct sequence analysis or other methods are used to identify the underlying mutation or polymorphism. When heteroduplexes are detected in large genes, DNA sequencing efforts may be targeted more effectively.

The conformational changes associated with heteroduplex structures often lead to fragments with altered electrophoretic mobility. Under appropriate conditions, these heteroduplex fragments will be separable from homoduplex forms, thereby establishing heterozygosity for a sequence variant in that sample. A method that exploits the differential migration of homoduplexes from heteroduplexes uses mutation detection enhancement (MDE) gels (BioWhittaker Molecular Applications, Rockland, ME). This proprietary gel matrix is formulated to enhance in a straightforward manner the electrophoretic separation between homoduplex and heteroduplex fragments. After PCR, DNA products are renatured slowly to enhance heteroduplex formation and are subsequently electrophoresed on MDE gels. The gel then is stained for DNA to resolve the fragments (Fig. 13-11). Differential migration of heteroduplex and homoduplex fragments is directly related to subtle structural differences between them.

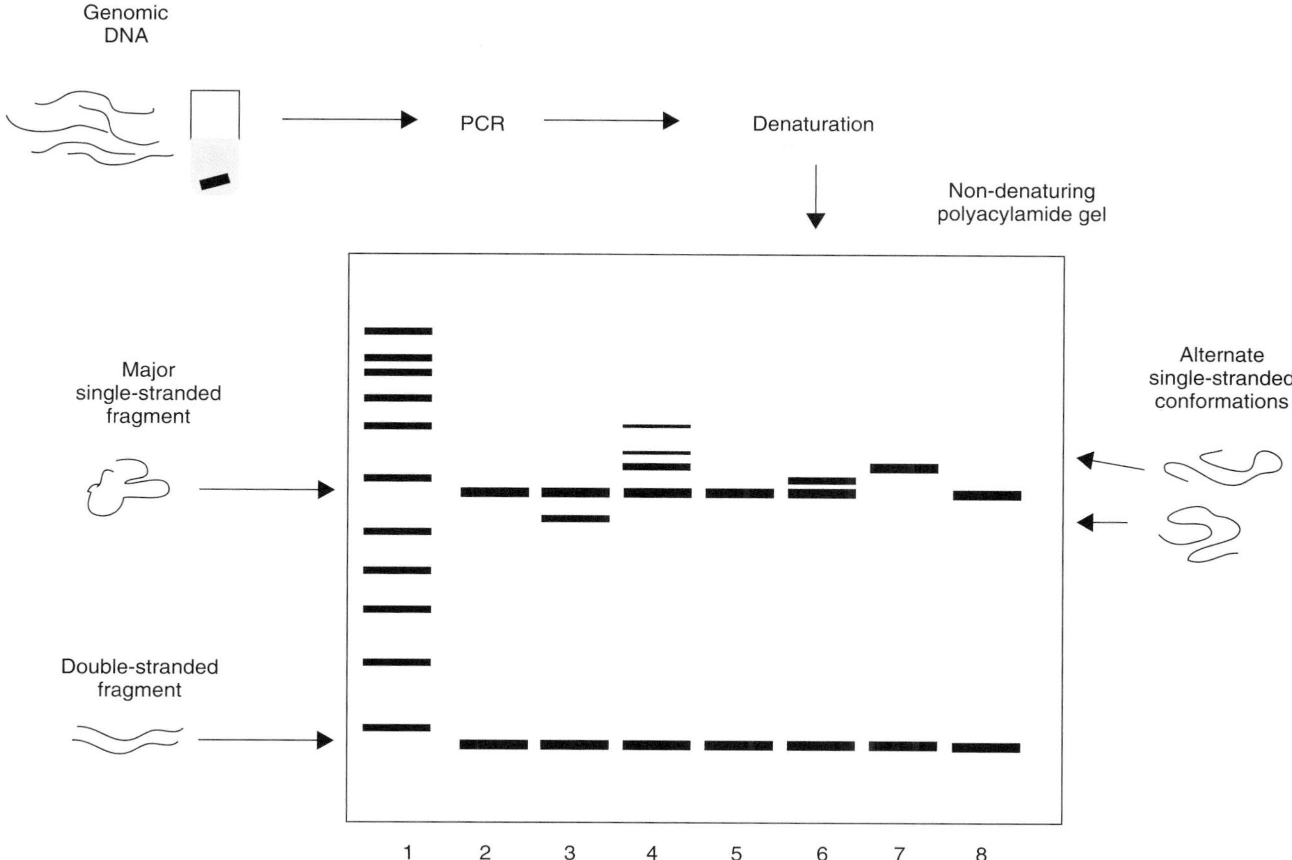

Fig. 13-10 Single-stranded conformational polymorphism analysis. Lane 1 depicts a size marker, Lane 2 shows a polymerase chain reaction (PCR) product from a normal control, Lanes 5 and 8 depict PCR products that have identical sequences. Lanes 3, 4, and 6 depict PCR products that have one allele with sequence identical to the control and another allele with a sequence variant, Lane 7 depicts a PCR product from an individual homozygous for a sequence variation.

Heteroduplex analysis on MDE gel electrophoresis is a simple, low-cost technique for mutation screening that is predicated on detecting mutations in the heterozygous state; some SSCP strategies use MDE gels that claim higher analytical sensitivity. It is important to note that no heteroduplex-based strategies have utility for detecting mutations present in the homozygous state. To overcome this limitation, DNA of a known genotype can be mixed with the patient sample prior to amplification, or a PCR product of known genotype can be mixed with the patient's PCR product to ensure the generation of heteroduplexes if the patient is homozygous for a mutation.

Denaturing Gradient Gel Electrophoresis (DGGE) and Temperature Gradient Gel Electrophoresis (TGGE)

The differential conformational properties of heteroduplex fragments may be exploited by other methods. As a result of their mismatched bases, heteroduplexes denature into single strands more readily than do the cognate homoduplexes (the original **homoduplex DNA** molecules from which they originate). DGGE uses a chemical gradient within the electrophoretic gel to take advantage of this difference. The chemicals involved, typically urea or formamide, serve to denature PCR fragments from double- to single-stranded fragments. TGGE uses a thermal gradient to achieve differential melting between homoduplexes and heteroduplexes. An advantage of the TGGE method is that it eliminates the need to prepare the gradient gels, a difficult and highly operator-dependent process. The availability of commercial apparatuses that can maintain a precise thermal gradient throughout a polyacrylamide gel has made TGGE a particularly popular mutation scanning method in recent years.

PCR of heterozygous samples with specially designed primers to optimize denaturation behavior and electrophoresis yields heteroduplex fragments with altered denaturation properties. Once denaturation of a fragment begins, its electrophoretic mobility through the gel slows dramatically. The appearance of these slowly migrating bands on denaturing gradient gels is indicative of heterozygosity for a DNA sequence variant in the underlying sample. The melting process is sensitive not only to the nature of the mismatch and the underlying mutation, but also to the sequence of the fragment as a whole. Particular advantages of gradient electrophoretic techniques include their high sensitivity to the detection of mutations—greater than 98% for most applications—and

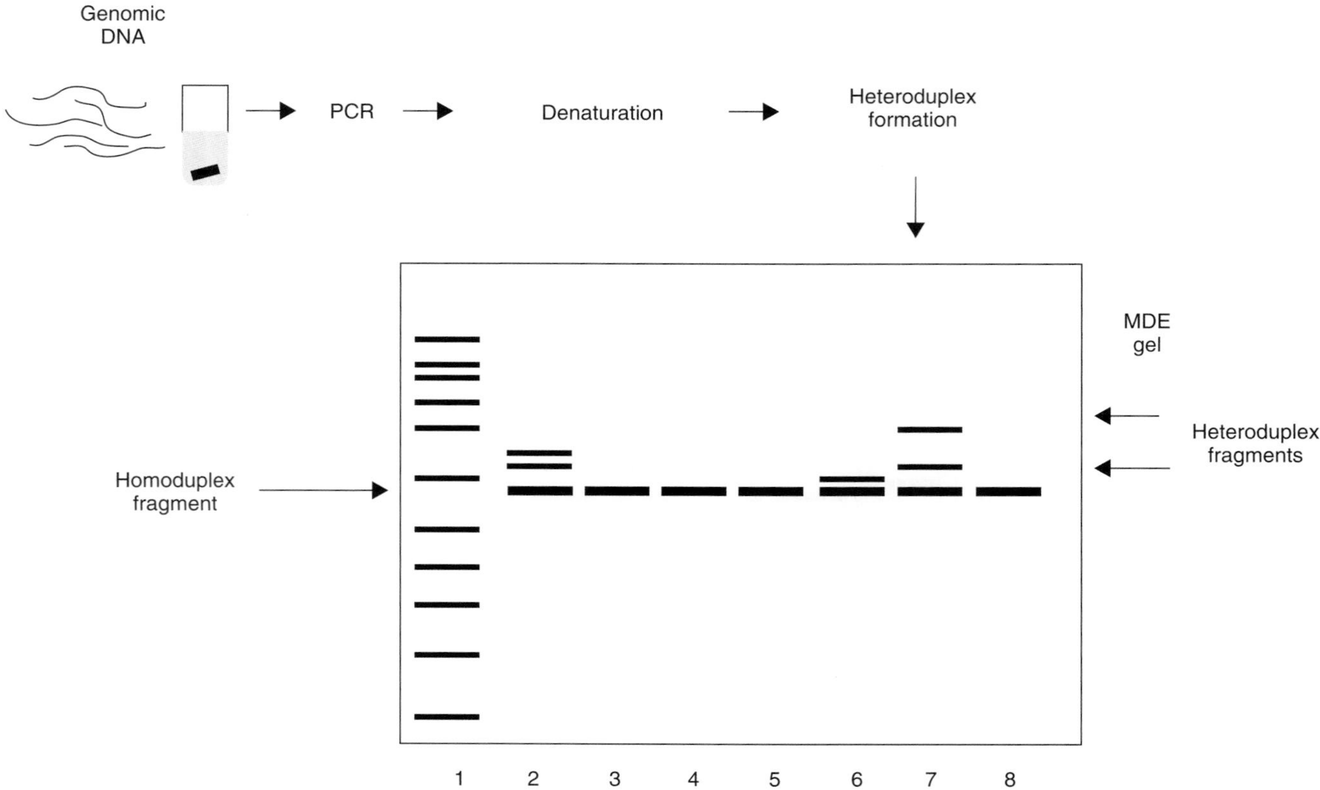

Fig. 13-11 Detection of mutations through heteroduplex analysis on MDE gels. Lanes 2, 6, and 7 depict polymerase chain reaction (PCR) products from individuals heterozygous for different sequence variants.

the existence of a theory that predicts melting behavior that can be used to design optimal PCR strategies for maximum sensitivity. An online tool for the prediction of melting behavior is available at the Physiological Biology Institute at the Heinrich-Heine University of Duesseldorf (www.Biophys.uni-duesseldorf.de/local/POLAND).

Denaturing High-Performance Liquid Chromatography (DHPLC)

DHPLC is a column-based technique used to detect heteroduplexes in a high-throughput manner with minimal operator involvement. This approach is well suited to evaluating large numbers of samples (≈150/day) for variants in a given DNA fragment. Unlike DGGE/TGGE, no special primers are required. For DHPLC, PCR products are eluted from a column with buffer that contains an ion-pairing reagent such as triethylammonium acetate (TEAA), which masks the DNA fragments' charge and binds them to the hydrophobic column packing. In this manner, size and conformation, not charge, influence elution from the column. The DNA fragments pass through the column with an increasing gradient of acetonitrile. Heteroduplexes that are partially melted elute from the column sooner than homoduplexes under appropriate denaturing conditions based on a temperature derived from readily available DNA melting software. Homoduplexes elute as single peaks. The presence of mutations or polymorphisms will elicit the formation of one or more heteroduplex conformations, which typically elute earlier than the homoduplexes (Fig. 13-12). Although the profile associated with a given mutation or polymorphism is typically reproducible between samples and repeat runs, direct sequencing is recommended to confirm the identity of the sequence variant.

Protein Truncation Test

With the human genome sequenced, interest now lies in the area of proteomics, the study of the entire set of proteins expressed by the genome of an organism under defined conditions. Cell-free expression systems can be used as a bridge between genomics and proteomics by converting nucleic acid sequence into protein sequence. An application of these in vitro expression systems for the detection of mutations is referred to as the protein truncation test (PrTT). This assay is useful for the detection of those mutations that alter the reading frame of the expressed protein, so called truncating mutations, which lead to a shortened protein product. This method is particularly useful in interrogating large genes that are frequently altered by nonsense and frameshift mutations (the result of small insertions or deletions), in addition to large deletions. Examples of underlying disorders include familial adenomatous polyposis, Duchenne and Becker muscular dystrophy, neurofibromatosis type 1, and hereditary breast and ovarian cancer defined by tumor suppressor genes such as *BRCA1* and *BRCA2*.

This method involves reverse transcription PCR (RT-PCR), in which total RNA is used to produce cDNA. PCR amplification, used with a forward primer that includes appropriate

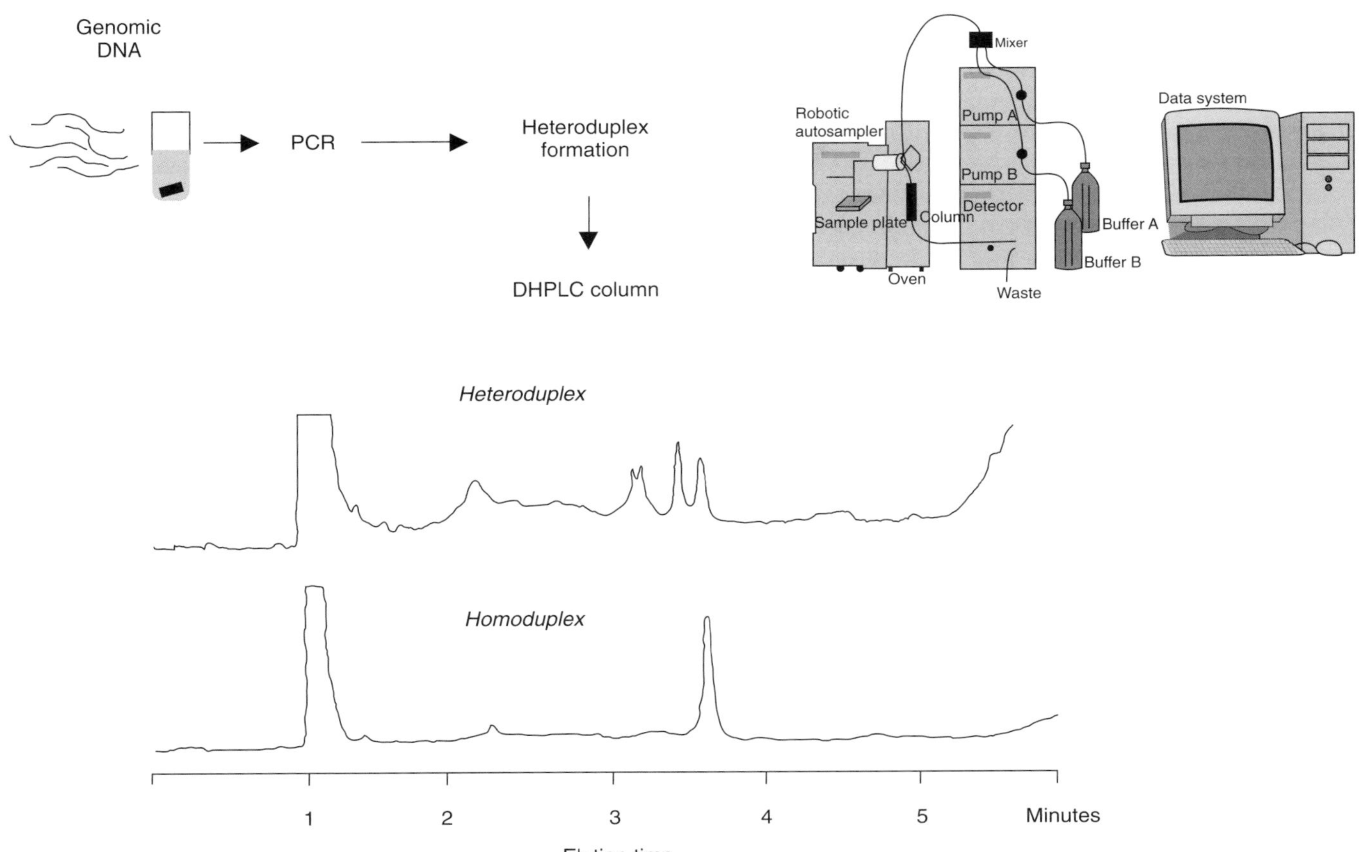

Fig. 13-12 Denaturing high-performance liquid chromatography (DHPLC). The homoduplex peak elutes at approximately 3.7 minutes. Heteroduplexes elute earlier.

signals for transcription and translation (Fig. 13-13), results in a functional protein-coding DNA segment coding for the *BRCA1* and *BRCA2* proteins. Protein synthesis is completed by coupling the product with an in vitro translation/transcription system that includes RNA polymerase, radiolabeled amino acids, ribosomes, transfer RNAs, and tRNA synthases. The processes of transcription and translation of the PCR product result in synthesis of a labeled protein product. The product can be sized by sodium dodecyl sulfate (SDS)–polyacrylamide gel electrophoresis. A novel, lower-molecular-weight band indicates the presence of a truncated polypeptide, representing a truncating mutation in that sample. The position of the band in the gel indicates the relative size of the product, from which the position of the mutation in the coding sequence can be extrapolated. Confirmation of the mutation is achieved by sequencing.

Missense mutations do not usually result in size alterations of proteins; therefore, other procedures must be used for missense detection. So for maximum analytical sensitivity, PrTT often is combined with other scanning techniques. Through this approach, sensitivity for *BRCA1* and *BRCA2* mutation detection can approach 90%.

DNA Sequencing

DNA sequencing is considered the "gold standard" for mutation detection. Although not perfect, when properly done, sequence analysis detects close to 100% of sequence variations present in analyte DNA. Two of the oldest techniques are the Maxim-Gilbert chemical sequencing and the Sanger enzymatic sequencing. Both involved the creation of pools of DNA fragments that are defined by their 3′ bases, that is, in the A reaction, the DNA must be broken into all of the possible oligonucleotides ending in an A. Similarly, the G reaction must produce all of the possible oligonucleotides that end in a G, and so on. Although Maxim-Gilbert sequencing still is used for some applications, such as sequencing of synthetic oligonucleotides, the great majority of DNA sequencing done in the years since 1977, including both public and private Human Genome Projects, utilized Sanger sequencing. Therefore, the rest of this discussion will focus exclusively on the enzymatic Sanger method. However, new methods, based primarily on pyrosequencing and "sequencing by synthesis," are emerging and will offer increased throughput and decreases in per-base cost of up to 100-fold versus automated Sanger sequencing.

The Sanger sequencing reaction is a multistep process. In the diagnostic laboratory, the first step is PCR amplification of the target of interest. Clearly, this is a critical step, and a poorly designed PCR strategy, with nonspecific amplification or poor yields, will result in an uninterpretable sequence. The next step involves the removal of excess dNTPs and PCR

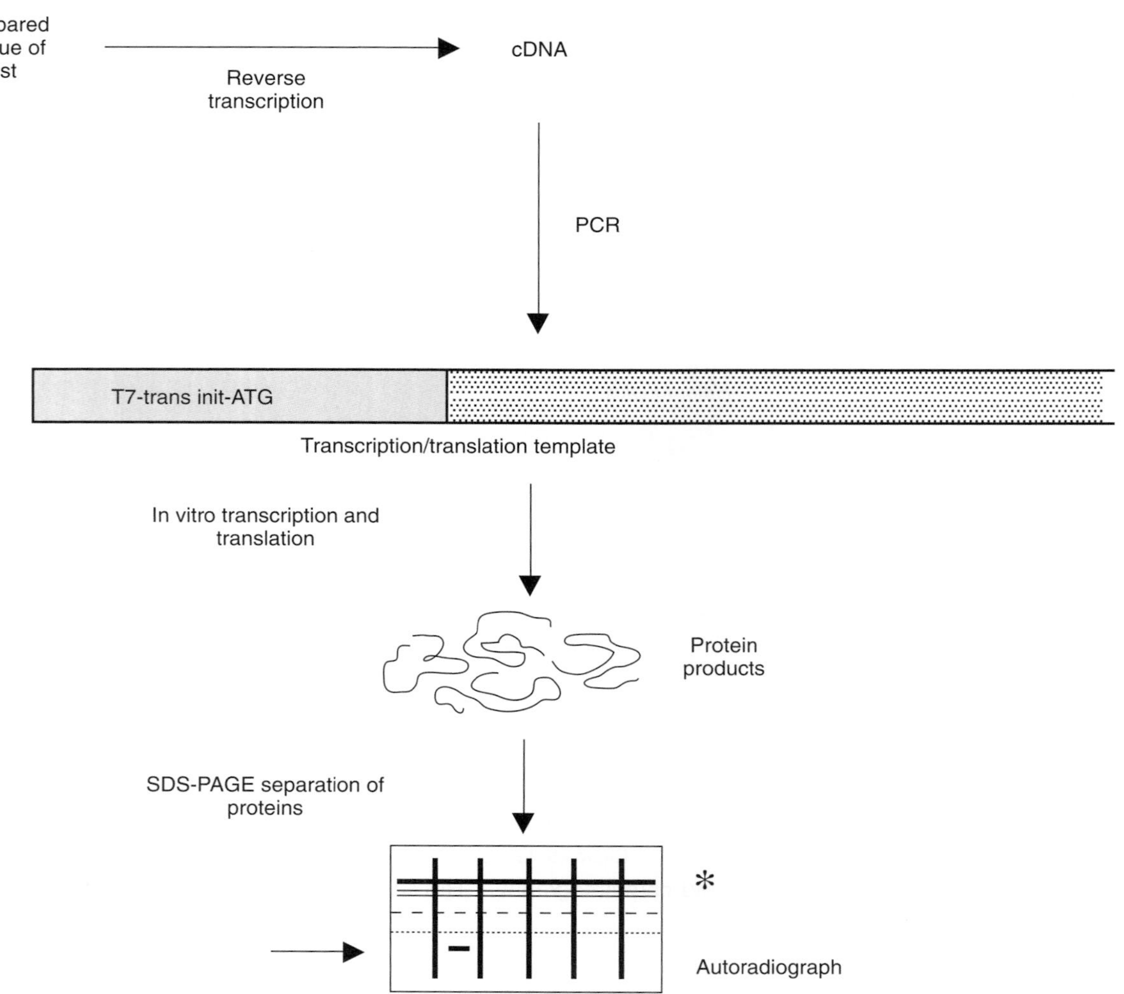

Fig. 13-13 Protein truncation test. After amplification with a primer containing T7 RNA polymerase promoter and transcription initiation sequences, the polymerase chain reaction (PCR) product is transcribed into RNA, and the RNA is translated into protein in vitro. The protein products are resolved by sodium dodecyl sulfate–polyacrylamide gel electrophoresis (SDS-PAGE). Lane 2 depicts a truncated protein caused by a mutation that results in an in-frame stop codon. The asterisk *(*)* identifies the full-length non-truncated protein.

primers. Next, the PCR product is denatured, and an oligonucleotide (the sequencing primer) is added and annealed 5′ to the region to be sequenced. A DNA polymerase (typically a recombinant thermostable enzyme) and a mixture of deoxynucleotide triphosphates (dNTPs) and dideoxynucleotide triphosphates (ddNTPs) then is added (and subjected to thermal cycling if a thermostable enzyme is used). The DNA polymerase will extend the annealed primer in the 5′ to 3′ direction, making a new strand of DNA that is complementary to the PCR product template. Because the ddNTPs retain a 3′ hydroxyl group, they can be incorporated into the growing complementary strand of DNA. However, because they lack the 5′ hydroxyl, they cannot be further extended by DNA polymerase. Thus, for example, when a dideoxyadenosine triphosphate is incorporated, the chain terminates at that A position, complementary to the corresponding T in the template. The rate at which ddNTPs are incorporated into the growing strand is dependent on both the ratio of dNTPs to ddNTPs in the reaction, and the efficiency with which the ddNTPs are recognized by the polymerase. Most applications in the clinical laboratory utilize dye-terminator chemistry. In this approach, the detectable label, in this case a fluorescent tag, is linked to the ddNTPs. Each of the four ddNTPs is labeled with one of four fluorescent molecules. Thus, the fragment terminated by incorporation of a ddATP will be labeled with one color, a fragment terminating in a G will be labeled with another color, and so on. The pool of DNA fragments then is subjected to high-resolution capillary electrophoresis, and the presence of each of the four fluorophores is scored as the DNA fragments migrate past a fixed, multiwavelength fluorescence detector. The output resembles a chromatogram and is read from the shortest fragment to the longer fragments, with a blue (for example) peak being read as an A, a red peak as a C, and so on. A schematic of the Sanger sequencing chemistry is shown in Fig. 13-14.

Enormous technical advances have been made in DNA sequencing technology since the first reports. In the early days of sequencing, the ability to read 100 bases after several days

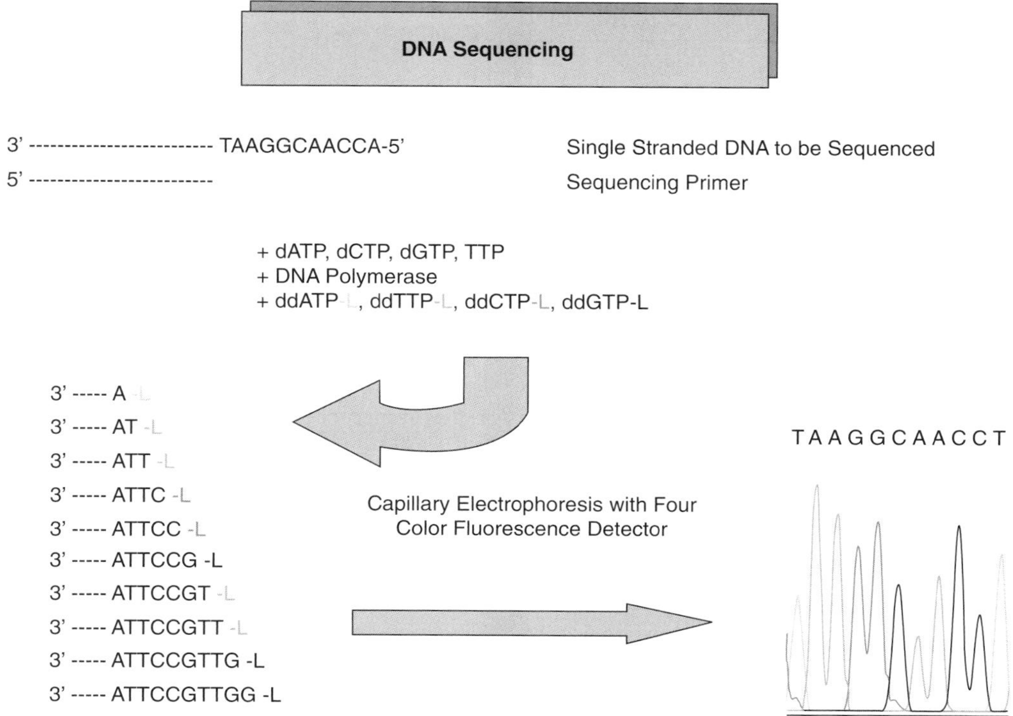

Fig. 13-14 A schematic of fluorescent Sanger sequencing using dye-terminator chemistry. A sequencing primer (5′-----) is annealed to the single-stranded template, or the DNA to be sequenced. DNA polymerase extends the primer in the 5′ to 3′ direction. The reaction is carried out in the presence of all four deoxynucleotide triphosphates and all four dideoxynucleotide triphosphates (ddNTPs). The ddATP is labeled *(L)* with dye 1, ddTTP is labeled with dye 2, etc. After the extension reaction is complete, a collection of fragments is obtained, each ending in a labeled dideoxynucleotide. These products are separated by electrophoresis in a single capillary and are detected with a multiwavelength fluorescence detector. The sequence of the original template is read from the resulting electropherogram.

of work was the state of the art. Automated capillary electrophoresis-based sequence analyzers capable of turning out sequences at the rate of up to 500,000 bases per day using Sanger sequencing chemistry are available. Increased demand for instrumentation as a result of the Human Genome Project has substantially decreased the cost of Sanger sequencing. Although still expensive, and still relatively labor intensive, DNA sequencing is standard practice in clinical microbiology laboratories and is rapidly replacing other mutation scanning methods in molecular genetics laboratories.

KEY CONCEPTS BOX 13-2

- The unique base specificity of restriction enzymes allows DNA to be cut at specific sites. Size-based separation of the DNA fragments after digestion allows mutated regions to be detected using different techniques. The Southern blot is one such technique that uses electrophoresis, transfer to nitrocellulose or nylon membranes, and hybridization with a detectable probe.
- Polymerase chain reaction (PCR) allows a specific DNA fragment to be amplified, or produced in large numbers, with specific oligonucleotide primers, which allows sensitive detection of the fragment.

SECTION OBJECTIVES BOX 13-3

- Define oncogenes and tumor suppressor genes, and describe how they can cause cancers.
- Differentiate between familial and sporadic cancers.
- Describe the molecular techniques that can be used to detect the mutations that cause these types of cancer.

CANCER (see also Chapter 53)

Genes and gene products serve to regulate cell growth and proliferation. When one or more of these gene products fail to fulfill their intracellular tasks, uncontrolled growth—a cancer—can result. The mechanism that brings about failure (inactivity or inappropriate activity) of these protein growth regulators is the occurrence of a mutation, or a change in the DNA coding for that particular protein. These mutations can occur as germline and somatic events. A germline mutation is one that is present in all cells of the body and is passed from generation to generation by meiosis (creation of sperm and egg) and sexual reproduction. Somatic mutations arise de novo in tissue cells, generally as a result of some environmental insult or DNA replication error. Although certain rare types of cancer are associated with germline transmission of mutant genes, the vast majority of cancers result from somatic mutations. Among the hundreds of thousands of genes in the human genome, mutation of only a few of them is necessary or sufficient to cause the deregulation of cell growth. According to our present understanding, there exist two broad classes of genes with these properties—oncogenes and tumor suppressor genes.

The molecular techniques described in this chapter are used to detect those mutations that are associated with cancer or a high risk of developing cancer.

Oncogenes

An oncogene is defined as a gene that, when activated inappropriately, results in uncontrolled growth of a cell population. Because only one copy of the gene needs to be mutated for the genotype to affect the phenotype (malignant vs. normal), oncogenes are said to act in a dominant fashion. The biochemical activities of oncogenes generally fall into one of three categories: (1) protein kinases and phosphorylases, (2) G-proteins and signal transduction proteins, and (3) transcription factors.

Several mechanisms for mutations activate protooncogenes to become oncogenes. Common mechanisms include (1) overproduction of the protooncogene by loss of the ability to regulate that gene, (2) increased concentration of the protooncogene by amplification of the number of genomic copies of that gene, and (3) activation of a protooncogene by chromosomal translocation in which the promoter region for a constitutively produced gene is brought into position to regulate an oncogene. Although several of these mechanisms have been studied, and some are common in particular types of cancer, the most common alteration of function or stability of a protooncogene occurs by a small mutation in the DNA coding for that gene.

Tumor Suppressor Genes

A class of genes that act as tumor suppressors (TSs) exist. TS genes act as recessive alleles, that is, a mutation in each tumor TS allele is required to release suppression of growth and allow a cancer to form. One mutation is germline and the second is a somatic one. TS genes were first observed in familial cases of bilateral retinoblastoma (RB). Other recessively acting tumor suppressor genes have been identified, including the Wilms' tumor gene *(WT)*, *p53,* the neurofibromatosis type 1 and 2 genes (*NF1* and *NF2*), the adenomatous polyposis coli gene *(APC)*, and the mismatch repair genes (*MSH2, MLH1,* and *MSH6*).

Because tumor suppressor genes are activated only by mutations that destroy the function of the gene, it seems reasonable that mutations that give rise to premature stop codons appearing in the reading frame of the gene would be overrepresented. This has been observed and will influence the choice of method used for the analysis of these genes.

Familial Cancer Syndromes

Extensive epidemiological evidence demonstrates that a number of cancers have a greater incidence in relatives of patients than in the general population. Most of these cancers follow straightforward Mendelian inheritance patterns (generally autosomal dominant with reduced penetrance, or, rarely, autosomal recessive) involving germline defects in single genes. Cancers in families in which Mendelian inheritance patterns cannot be demonstrated (i.e., relatives have risk levels that are elevated relative to the general population but are far lower than the risk predicted for single-gene disorders) are most likely the result of multiple factors, including genetic and environmental factors.

In more than 50 recognized Mendelian disorders, the risk of cancer approaches 100%. A particularly striking aspect of the inherited cancer syndromes is that multiple primary tumors often occur, whereas more than one tumor in a sporadic case is rare. The genes responsible for some of the cancer syndromes have been identified (Table 13-1). Most of these genes belong to the class of tumor suppressor genes. However, germline mutations of oncogenes, such as activating mutations in the RET oncogene in multiple endocrine neoplasia, also have been described.

Although the numbers of individuals affected by specific Mendelian familial cancers are small, in aggregate the numbers are significant, totaling approximately 5% of all cancers. The ability to detect germline tumor suppressor gene mutations is of extreme importance to families whose history shows them to be at risk for a cancer of this type. For these families, it is crucial to identify the causative mutation in the relevant gene and then trace that mutation through the family.

Sporadic Cancers

The great majority (95%) of cancers appear to arise without the inheritance of a mutant tumor suppressor gene. Rather, they arise de novo as a result of mutations in somatic (nongermline) cells.

An example is p53, a protein with multiple roles in the normal cell. It is associated with both the transcriptional activation of cellular growth factors and the downregulation of growth suppressor genes. Further, p53 has been shown to mediate the apoptotic (programmed cell death) pathway that is activated in response to severe cellular damage. Mutant *p53* can function as an oncogene in some tumors or as a mutated tumor suppressor gene in others. More than 1700 mutations in the *p53* gene have been described, a majority (approximately 80%) of which are missense mutations.

The identity of specific *p53* mutations may have implications for therapy. In the case of a long-lived *p53,* the apoptotic pathway is still viable; therefore, therapeutic maneuvers (e.g., radiation therapy) aimed at causing enough cellular damage for cells to undergo programmed death are effective. In the complete absence of *p53,* the apoptotic pathway cannot be engaged, resulting in a radiation-resistant phenotype. It has been shown that *p53* plays a central role in the spread (metastases) of tumors. Knowledge of *p53* mutations

Table 13-1 Genetic Alterations in Selected Cancers

Cancer	Population Affected	Gene(s) Affected	Mutations Detected	Technique(s)
Familial breast cancer	Ashkenazi Jewish heritage	*BRCA1* *BRCA2*	*BRCA1*: 185delAG *BRCA1*: 5385insC *BRCA2*: 6174delT	Targeted mutation analysis
	General population	*BRCA1* *BRCA2*	Sequence variants (mainly leading to protein truncation) *BRCA1* genomic rearrangements	Mutation scanning Sequence analysis Protein Truncation Test MLPA
Hereditary nonpolyposis colon cancer (HNPCC, Lynch Syndrome)	2% to 3% of all colon cancers	*MLH1* *MSH2* *MSH6*	Sequence variants Deletions and rearrangements	Mutation scanning Sequence analysis Southern blot MLPA
Non-Hodgkin's lymphoma (NHL)	—	*BCL-2* *BCL-6* *MYC*	Chromosomal translocations: → Fusing *BCL2* with IgH (80% of follicular lymphomas) → Fusing *BCL2, BCL6,* or *MYC* with *IgH* (50% of diffuse large B-cell lymphomas)	Southern blot Breakpoint specific PCR

will allow application of emerging targeted therapies in these cases. Several online databases are dedicated to the compilation and analysis of *p53* mutations. Representative examples include the IARC (International Agency for Research on Cancer) *p53* database (www.p53.iarc.fr) and the *p53* database at the P.M. Curie University in Paris (http://p53.free.fr).

Translocations in Leukemia and Lymphoma

The detection of specific chromosomal translocations often is required for the diagnosis of a specific leukemia or lymphoma. For example, many hematopathologists require cytogenetic or molecular evidence of the t(9:22) translocation to make a diagnosis of chronic myelogeneous leukemia. The presence of other translocations may not have 100% sensitivity but can indicate the diagnosis when identified. For example, the presence of the t(14:18) translocation, present in approximately 80% of follicular lymphomas, will identify most but not all cases of this malignancy.

The Cancer Genome Anatomy Project (CGAP) at the National Cancer institute maintains a database of cancer-related chromosomal abnormalities at http://cgap.nci.nih.gov/Chromosomes.

Detection of Minimal Disease

In addition to their diagnostic utility, the presence of unique molecular identifiers for a malignant clone can be used to monitor the efficiency of therapy, termed *detection of minimal residual disease.* The advent of quantitative PCR and RT-PCR with real-time analytical instrumentation has made these assays part of the standard of care. One issue to be addressed, however, is the level of analytical sensitivity required for monitoring of anticancer therapy. The analytical sensitivity of very sensitive PCR platforms may be too great, with many patients who display clinical remission still being PCR positive for the molecular marker. Additional studies should prove very helpful in defining appropriate cutoff values.

KEY CONCEPTS BOX 13-3

- Oncogenes are cell regulatory genes that when mutated can cause unrestricted cell growth.
- Tumor suppressor genes regulate cell growth; when they have mutated and lost function, cells have unrestricted growth. Both alleles of tumor suppressor genes must be mutated to cause cancer.
- Familial cancers are genetically inherited (germline mutations) and occur at much higher frequencies in families than in the general population. Sporadic cancers result from random gene mutation in somatic cells and are not inherited.
- Specific molecular techniques are applied for detection of oncogenes, tumor suppressor genes, and familial and sporadic cancers.

SECTION OBJECTIVES BOX 13-4

- Name at least two molecular methods that are used to monitor human immunodeficiency virus (HIV) infection.
- Describe the role of viral load testing in guiding retroviral therapy.
- Describe the differences between genotyping and phenotyping for HIV, list their purposes, and state one advantage and disadvantage of each.
- Describe the molecular assays used to monitor microbial resistance to therapy.

INFECTIOUS DISEASE

The application of molecular methods for the diagnosis and management of infectious diseases has revolutionized the way infections agents are identified and the way infections are monitored and managed (Table 13-2). Molecular methods have evolved to routinely offer a rapid (same day or overnight), sensitive, and specific diagnosis, and to monitor disease activity. Molecular methods have had a major impact on the

Table 13-2 Applications of Molecular Diagnosis for Management of Infectious Diseases

Application	Molecular Technique	Example Organism
Detection	PCR, LCR, TMA	HIV, Chlamydia, HCV
Screening	Hybrid capture	HPV
Quantification of viral load	PCR, Branched DNA	HIV, HCV, HBV
Detection of antimicrobial resistance	PCR, RFLP, Sequencing	*Mycobacterium tuberculosis,* staphylococci, etc.
Genotyping	PCR, Sequencing	HCV, HBV

HBV, Hepatitis B virus; *HCV,* hepatitis C virus; *HIV,* human immunodeficiency virus; *HPV,* human papillomavirus; *LCR,* ligase chain reaction; *PCR,* polymerase chain reaction; *RFLP,* restriction fragment length polymorphism; *TMA,* transcription-mediated amplification.

Table 13-3 Molecular Assays for HIV Detection and Quantification

Name	Company	Method	Limit of Detection, Copies/mL	Full Automation	Features
AMPLICOR HIV-1 MONITOR Test, v1.5	Roche	PCR	50	Yes, with COBAS AMPLICOR HIV-1 MONITOR	Approved for donor and cadaveric samples
NucliSens HIV-1 QT	bioMérieux	NASBA	40	No	Can be used with many sample types
VERSANT HIV-1 RNA 3.0	Bayer HealthCare	bDNA	50	No	
Abbott RealTime HIV-1 Viral Load Test	Abbott	Real-time PCR	40	Yes, with m2000 instrument system	Claim of better detection of variants
Cobas AmpliPrep/Cobas TaqMan HIV-1 Test	Roche	Real-time PCR	50	Yes with TaqMan analyzer	
APTIMA HIV-1 RNA Qualitative Assay	Gen-Probe	TMA	100		Only FDA-approved test for diagnosis
Procleix HIV-1/HCV assay	Gene-Probe	TMA	50		Used in a pooling strategy for donors

detection of organisms that are difficult or impossible to culture (e.g., viruses, *Mycobacterium* species, fungi), and they have increased sensitivity (level of detection) to as low as several organisms for agents for which culture and other methods have proved insensitive. Two of the most powerful applications of molecular techniques for infectious agents have been the quantification of HIV **viral load** and the analysis of HIV drug resistance; these are discussed below.

Human Immunodeficiency Virus (HIV) Viral Load and Drug Resistance Testing

HIV Viral Load

In addition to the qualitative identification of HIV infection by molecular methods, *quantitative* assessment of the number of circulating viral particles, or viral load, is now accepted as a standard practice in the management of HIV infection. Viral load is used to monitor the efficacy of combination antiretroviral pharmacotherapy and is a predictor of the progression time to acquired immunodeficiency syndrome (AIDS) and death.

HIV viral load is measured by assessing viral RNA, of which there are two copies per virion. Viral RNA is detectable in plasma about 2 weeks after infection is established, making it the earliest marker for identifying HIV infection. During early infection, RNA levels generally peak at about 1 million or more copies/mL, decrease by 2 to 3 logs with some fluctuation, and subsequently reach a "set point" by 6 months; once established, the set points remain fairly constant for months to years or increase slightly. Patients whose HIV RNA viral load levels exceed 100,000 copies/mL within 6 months of seroconversion (i.e., a high set point) are tenfold more likely to progress to AIDS within 5 years than are those with fewer than 100,000 copies/mL. Medical consensus suggests that physicians maintain their patients' plasma RNA levels at fewer than 10,000 copies/mL, and optimally below the analytical limits of detection (40 to 50 RNA copies/mL). Guidelines for the use of antiretroviral agents are posted on the U.S. Department of Health and Human Services HIV/AIDS Treatment Information Services website at http://www.hivatis.org/.

Several viral load assay systems are available to clinical laboratories throughout the world; however, only tests approved by the U.S. Food and Drug Administration (FDA) can be used in the United States. Table 13-3 lists the molecular assays used to detect and quantify HIV RNA. Each of these viral load tests has similar detection limits (40 to 50 copies/mL). Only one molecular test, the APTIMA HIV-1 RNA Qualitative Assay (Gen-Probe, San Diego, CA), can be used for the *diagnosis* of HIV infection, in contrast to others that are used to monitor infection. Therefore, this test can be used to assist in resolution of the status of patients who have an indeterminate serological result (as a confirmatory test) and to facilitate the early diagnosis of HIV infection before the appearance of antibody. Although all assays show good correlation with each other, they also show substantial inherent variation in intra-assay, interassay, interlaboratory, and intermethod testing, with coefficients of variations ranging from 10% to 40%, depending on the viral load. Further, because the quantitative results of any one test are not necessarily the same as those of other tests, it is recommended that laboratories that perform viral load testing consistently use the same type of assay to monitor patients' viral load over time (except for the Abbott Real-Time HIV-1 Test [Abbott Molecular, Des Plaines, IL], which can be used in conjunction with results from other assays). The Procleix HIV-1/hepatitis C virus (HCV) assay (Gen-Probe, San Diego, CA), which is used for the screening of donated blood, incorporates a *pooling* strategy wherein 16 or more samples are combined and screened as one to save on cost. Although the analytical sensitivity of this strategy is slightly less than that of single-donor testing, it is sufficient to detect nearly all cases of HIV infection.

These techniques are all similar, sharing the necessity for centrifugation for ultrasensitive analysis. All employ three common steps: (1) a preamplification step that usually includes sample preparation (e.g., cell lysis) and/or viral nucleic acid extraction; (2) an amplification step that consists of target nucleic acid sequence amplification or amplification of the signal; and (3) a back-end step that allows detection and/or quantification of the amplified products. Several instruments address the preamplification purification steps (e.g., use of silica technology for nucleic acid extraction). Several strategies may be used to detect viral RNA or DNA after preparation of samples. In the target (e.g., HIV RNA) amplification strategies, amplification methods are designed to "boost" by PCR the ability to detect the very low levels of nucleic acids that occur in blood. Alternatively, a signal amplification strategy can be used that increases the "marker" that shows that the target is present (e.g., by probe amplification).

Target amplification techniques for HIV include the reverse transcriptase polymerase chain reaction (RT-PCR) (AMPLICOR Monitor; Roche Molecular Diagnostics, Pleasanton, CA), transcription-mediated amplification (TMA) (Procleix; Gen-Probe, San Diego, CA), and nucleic acid sequence based amplification (NASBA) (NucliSENS; BioMerieux, Durham, NC). Probe amplification techniques include the branched chain DNA (bDNA) (Versant; Bayer Diagnostics, Tarrytown, NY) method and hybrid capture systems (Diagene, Gaithersburg, MD). The postamplification step (for detection) can be completed by using colorimetric, radioactive, or chemiluminescence- or fluorescence-generating reagents. Laboratories that use in-house RT-PCR methods may visualize the amplicons with ultraviolet light after electrophoresis in agarose gels that are stained with ethidium bromide (which binds to nucleic acids); however, most commercial kits for performing amplifications use probes to attach to the amplification products or to the viral target sequences. These probes are short nucleic acid sequences that are complementary to a portion of the viral target sequence and may be used to capture amplicons for subsequent detection, or they can be used to bind to the target sequence, in which case a coupled signal-generating unit is present (e.g., enzyme). Real-time measurement through fluorescence-generating probes is gaining in popularity and is allowing the attainment of rapid and sensitive results.

Other molecular methods have been introduced that may offer an increase in sensitivity over HIV RNA testing. The Immuno-PCR method couples a typical antigen detection enzyme-linked immunosorbent assay (ELISA) method for HIV p24 antigen with signal amplification, that is, rather than using a colorimetric indicator (as in ELISA), a double-stranded DNA molecule is coupled to the detector antibody of the ELISA through direct conjugation or a biotin-avidin bridge. Subsequently, PCR of the DNA molecule results in generation of a signal that is proportional to the quantity of target antigen. The increase in sensitivity is reflected by the fact that each virion has 3000 molecules of p24 antigen, as compared with only two copies of RNA, that is, there is more target. Immuno-PCR for HIV has been shown to have a sensitivity down into the attogram/mL (10^{-18} g/mL) level, an order of magnitude better than RNA tests (Constantine et al., unpublished observation). Immuno-PCR has been applied to a variety of infectious agents, including prions, bacteria, and parasites, and has been used for cancer markers (e.g., prostate-specific antigen [PSA]).

Viral Resistance

Although the use of highly active antiretroviral therapy (HAART) has transformed HIV infection to a manageable, chronic disease, it has been observed that any given combination of antiretroviral drugs may not decrease viral load levels to undetectable limits (<40 or 50 copies/ mL), or it may not maintain the viral load at undetectable levels for long periods of time. The principal reasons for drug failure include lack of compliance by patients and development of drug resistance by the virus.

Selective pressure from antiretroviral therapy and immunological responses of the host will promote the replication and propagation of certain variants, regardless of its original proportion in the HIV population. Under a specific selective pressure, those strains possessing mutations that provide a survival advantage will proliferate and emerge as the predominant viral species. The detection of specific mutations in the viral genome can indicate or predict resistance of the strain of HIV to the drug associated with the mutation. Evaluation of the genetic composition of HIV has become a clinically useful laboratory test that health care professionals use to select and tailor the appropriate antiretroviral agents in their efforts to manage HIV disease progression.

Viral Phenotyping

Phenotypical resistance assays evaluate the genetic "phenotype" of the virus related to drug resistance by directly determining the amount of drug necessary to inhibit HIV replication in cultured T lymphocytes. This is a measure, under controlled laboratory conditions, of the level of resistance of the HIV population derived from an individual patient to each of the anti-HIV drugs currently available. As a direct and quantitative measure of resistance, phenotyping is considered the reference method for determination of resistance of HIV to drugs.

These assays involve the insertion of PCR amplified reverse transcriptase and protease genes from the clinical isolate of the infected individual into a laboratory-derived molecular clone containing standardized envelope and accessory genes. The recombinant virus then is grown in viral culture in the presence of varying concentrations of the drug under evaluation, thereby enabling assessment of the phenotypical characteristics of the virus expressed by the inserted genes. In addition, a wild-type virus is grown alongside the recombinant test clone as a control for comparison. Resistance is measured in terms of the IC_{50} (the concentration of drug that inhibits replication of the virus by 50%). A fourfold or greater shift between the IC_{50} of the clone and that of the wild-type virus indicates drug resistance. These assays may be preferred in the management of individuals with extensive drug experience because they directly measure susceptibility, and results are easier to interpret because these assays measure how an individual strain of HIV will replicate in the presence of a particular drug or treatment regimen. Interpretation of drug susceptibilities is analogous to antibiotic sensitivity testing of bacteria.

Phenotypical analysis assesses the total effects of any mutations and mutational interactions that confer resistance to currently available antiretroviral agents by the subspecies of HIV within an individual. The disadvantages of phenotypical assays include their insensitivity for detecting minor species and the restricted availability of such assays. In addition, these tests have a lengthy turnaround time (2 to 3 weeks) and are labor intensive, cumbersome, and technically demanding. Lastly, clinically significant cutoff values are not always known because thresholds to define susceptibility are arbitrary and nonstandardized and do not vary on the basis of achievable drug concentrations; however, newer decision points are currently being evaluated. Table 13-4 presents the main commercially available HIV phenotypical assays.

For interpretation, the RT and protease gene sequences of the virus are established with the use of a DNA sequencing–based genotyping assay (see below). The sequence is analyzed by computer software that identifies mutations that confer resistance to any of the drugs and then scans the database for similar genotypes from previous samples that may match the patterns of mutations. Once any matches are identified, the phenotypes of these samples are retrieved from the database, and for each drug, an interpretive evaluation is provided. VIRCO Lab, Inc. (Bridgewater, NJ) offers an interpretive service, the *VirtualPhenotype,* which is based on a correlative database of more than 100,000 HIV phenotypes and genotypes.

Although the database was developed with use of the Virco genotyping system, the *VirtualPhenotype* is available via secure Internet to laboratories that use other genotyping products, including procedures developed in-house by individual laboratories.

Table 13-4 Commercially Available Phenotypical Assays for HIV

Name	Company	Features
Antivirogram	Virco, Mechelen	Interpretative Service (Virtual Phenotype)
PhenoSense	Monogram Biosciences	Interpretative Service (Therapy Guidance System)
Phenoscript	VIRalliance	Test is based on a single cycle of viral replication

Viral Genotyping

Genotypical antiretroviral resistance testing (GART) by DNA sequence analysis of reverse transcriptase and protease genes (some laboratories also provide the option of sequencing the region of the *env* that encodes gp41) and identification of specific mutations serve as the most common methods of evaluating HIV drug resistance. Those mutations that decrease the efficacy of drug binding to its active site are referred to as primary mutations. As a result of primary mutations, higher concentrations of drug generally are required to inhibit the activity of the enzyme. Secondary mutations are defined as those mutations that supplement the actions of the primary mutations by increasing the level of resistance through expansion of the viability of the virus encoding the primary mutation. In the absence of primary mutations, secondary mutations generally lack any effect on the level of resistance demonstrated by the virus.

GART results are often difficult to interpret. The virtual phenotype approach (see *VirtualPhenotype,* VIRCO Lab, Inc., above) uses an extensive database of genotype-phenotype correlations. In a rules-based approach, the information provided by genotyping is presented as a categorically resistant or sensitive prediction based on a rules algorithm. The rules-based interpretation, also known as the data analysis plan (DAP analysis), of genetic information relies on currently defined mutations or sets of mutations (stored in a computer database) that confer resistance. One version of an online rules-based interpretation software is currently available at Stanford University (http://hivdb.stanford.edu/hiv/). Sequence data are analyzed on the basis of rules created by panels of experts, such as HIV-1frenchreistance.org, the Stanford database, and others that interpret available data regarding mutations and their associated clinical significance.

Sanger sequencing on automated DNA sequence analyzers is the principle analytical platform currently in use for GART testing. Several vendors have developed total HIV genotyping systems, which include PCR amplification reagents, DNA sequencing reagents, and software that provides a rules-based interpretation of the sequence and generates a user-friendly, easily interpreted report. Two FDA-approved systems include the TruGene HIV-1 Genotyping Assay (Visible Genetics/Bayer Healthcare, Inc., Suwanee, GA) and the ViroSeq HIV-1 Genotyping System (Celera/Abbott, Rockville, GA), both of which use sequencing to determine the genotype; at least three other commercial systems are also available.

Another technique for viral genotyping is the Line Probe assay available from Innogenetics (INNO-LiPA; Innogenetics, Inc., Atlanta, GA), which is used for infectious agents such as hepatitis C virus and genetic disorders such as cystic fibrosis. This line probe assay or line immuno probe assay (LiPA) system uses a large set of oligonucleotide probes complementary to known sequence variants associated with drug resistance; these probes are immobilized on a nylon membrane in a reverse dot-blot format. Once targets are bound, they are detected through a biotin-avidin colorimetric signal. The advantages of this system are a higher sensitivity to minor species, a much shorter turnaround time, and significantly less technical expertise than is required for DNA sequencing. A disadvantage is that as new mutations are identified, new strips that incorporate new probes must be devised, validated, and manufactured.

KEY CONCEPTS BOX 13-4

Molecular nucleic acid testing can be used to
- Identify specific infectious agents with very high analytical sensitivity
- Monitor the numbers of organisms (e.g., viral load)
- Identify mutations within organisms
- Identify the resistance of organisms to drugs
- Provide prognostic information

Molecular methods used for these purposes include
- Preamplification (nucleic acid extraction)
- Amplification (of target or signal)
- Postamplification (detection on gels or in real time)

SECTION OBJECTIVES BOX 13-5

- Differentiate between autosomal recessive, autosomal dominant, and X-linked genetic disorders.
- Describe the limitations of molecular testing for genetic disorders.
- List several genetic diseases that are commonly tested for by molecular testing.

GENETIC DISORDERS

Abnormal variants of normal DNA sequences are associated with diseases of genetic origin (see Chapter 52). Whereas many genetic disorders can be diagnosed through classical clinical observational and nongenetic laboratory approaches, others are not so easily identified, especially for prenatal testing. The identification of a causal mutation can be integral to making a definitive diagnosis and, at a minimum, has confirmatory value. It may be used to make early diagnoses of these diseases and to give prospective parents the opportunity to assess their reproductive futures.

In general, genetic disorders can be grouped into the following categories: chromosomal abnormalities, multifactorial disorders, and single-gene disorders. Table 13-5 presents common mutations specific for a number of genetic diseases and molecular techniques used for their detection. The discussion in this chapter centers on single-gene disorders.

Single-gene disorders are inherited in one of the following patterns: autosomal dominant, autosomal recessive, or X-linked (see Chapter 52). The terms *autosomal* and *X-linked* refer to the chromosomal location of the disease-causing gene, or mutant gene. Generally, in X-linked disorders, males with the mutant gene express the disorder, whereas females with the same gene are *carriers.* Examples of X-linked disorders include Duchenne's muscular dystrophy and hemophilia. *Dominant* disorders are expressed whether an individual is heterozygous or homozygous, and the detection of a single causative mutation is diagnostic of the disease. Examples of these include achondroplasia and Huntington's disease. Autosomal *recessive* disorders include cystic fibrosis, sickle cell anemia, and phenylketonuria. For recessive disorders, detection of two causative mutations is needed to confirm the diagnosis. In the presence of clinical findings, the detection of a single mutation in the suspect gene is consistent with, but not sufficient for, a diagnosis; this presumes that a second mutation is present but is not detected. Individuals without clinical signs who are heterozygous for a recessive disorder are regarded simply as carriers; they have no personal risks regarding the gene-associated disorder in question but may find this information valuable when planning a family.

The number of disease-associated genes that have been identified has grown immensely (see www.ncbi.nlm.nih.gov). Theoretically, direct tests could be developed for all of these disorders. Although tests are available for many of them, *genetic heterogeneity* results in practical limitations to such testing. Genetic heterogeneity can take two primary forms—locus and allelic heterogeneity. *Locus heterogeneity* occurs when more than one gene can give rise to genetic diseases that are identical, or nearly so, in clinical presentation. Examples include the familial breast cancers (*BRCA1* and *BRCA2*), tuberous sclerosis (*TSC1* and *TSC2*), the many different spinocerebellar ataxias, polycystic kidney disease, and hereditary nonpolyposis colon cancer (*MLH1, MSH2, MSH6, PMS1,* and *PMS2*).

Allelic heterogeneity describes the presence of multiple mutations within a particular gene that result in a specific disorder. When the number of different mutations seen in a particular gene is very large, detecting all known mutations is not usually feasible, preventing the use of a few simple tests for diagnosis or carrier detection in all patients or families. An exception to this rule is sickle cell anemia. Every case of sickle cell anemia is caused by the same mutation, an A to T mutation in codon 6 of the β-globin gene (see Chapters 5 and 40). More typical are the mutational spectra of CF and Duchenne's muscular dystrophy (DMD), for which numerous different allelic mutations within these genes give rise to their respective diseases. There is one mutation (a three base-pair deletion termed ΔF508) in the CF transmembrane conductance

Table 13-5 Molecular Diagnosis of Selected Inherited Diseases

Inherited Disease	Description	Most Common Mutation(s)	Detection Technique
Duchenne muscular dystrophy	• Loss of muscle mass and function in male children • X-linked recessive	• Deletion of one or more exons of the dystrophin gene (79 exons; 2.2 Mb)	Multiplex PCR MLPA
Cystic fibrosis (CF)	• Most common autosomal recessive disease in Caucasians • Characterized by viscous mucus in the lungs with involvement of sweat glands, digestive and reproductive systems	• Multiple mutations in the *CFTR* gene that is located on chromosome 7 and codes for a chloride ion channel. 23 mutations account for 90% of CF alleles in Northern Europeans	PCR-OLA PCR-ASPE
Huntington's disease	• Neurodegenerative disease • Autosomal dominant	• Expansion of a CAG trinucleotide repeat in *IT15* gene	PCR + CE
Sickle cell anemia	• Autosomal recessive disease • Caused by S hemoglobin • Crescent-shaped RBCs • May become life threatening where blocked blood vessels may cause hemolytic or aplastic crisis	• Single mutation, *E6V,* in the β-hemoglobin gene on chromosome 11p15.5	PCR + RE digest PCR + Melt Curve analysis PCR-ASPE PCR-OLA
Charcot Marie Tooth 1A neuropathy	• A demyelinating disease of peripheral nerves • Characterized by distal muscle weakness and atrophy, sensory loss, and slow nerve conduction • Autosomal dominant	• 1.5 Mb duplication in chromosome 17p11.2-p12	MLPA PFGE FISH
Fragile X syndrome	• Most common form of inherited mental retardation • Atypical X-linked dominant • Carriers at risk for premature ovarian failure (females) or a tremor/ataxia syndrome late in life (males)	• Expansion of a *CGG* trinucleotide repeat in the 5′ untranslated region of *FMR1* gene	PCR + CE Southern blot
Hereditary hemochromatosis	• Autosomal recessive disease of iron metabolism • Excessive iron deposition in multiple organs	• 2 point mutations in the *HFE* gene on chromosome 6p	PCR + RE digest PCR + Melt Curve analysis PCR-ASPE PCR-OLA

ASPE-PCR, Allele-specific primer extension (ASPE) PCR; *CE,* capillary electrophoresis; *Mb,* megabase, one million base pairs; *MLPA,* multiplex ligation-dependent probe amplification; *PCR-OLA,* PCR-oligonucleotide ligation amplification; *PFGE,* pusled field gel electrophoresis; *RE,* restriction endonuclease.

regulator (CFTR) gene that accounts for approximately 70% of disease alleles in populations derived from Northern Europe. However, more than 1600 different mutations have been described on the CF gene, not including the most common mutation. A database of CFTR mutations is maintained at the Department of Genetics, Hospital for Sick Children, Toronto, Ontario, Canada (http://www.genet.sickkids.on.ca/cftr/). Large deletions in the dystrophin gene account for approximately 60% of cases of DMD. These deletions, although clustered in two hot spots, are heterogeneous, with few affected boys sharing the same deletion. The nondeletion cases are heterogeneous as well, with very few apparently unrelated boys sharing the same point mutation.

Thus even after a disease gene has been identified, it may not be possible to provide a direct test that provides complete information in a given family. For the many genetic disorders that are complicated by high allelic heterogeneity, one option is full gene sequencing, whereby each nucleotide of the gene's coding region and selected control regions is identified and compared with the sequence of the wild-type, or normal, gene sequence. In many instances, rare alleles associated with disease can be detected. Full gene sequencing, however, is not without its own set of pitfalls. These include the difficulty and expense of sequencing very large genes, as well as interpretive dilemmas associated with finding novel DNA sequence variations. Some of these variations are "real," in the sense of disrupting the expression or function of the gene's product; others are entirely benign. For some variants, the negative impact of gene function is obvious, such as for mutations that create premature translational stop codons, or gene deletions that derail the reading frame of the gene. In many cases, however, there are no such structural or contextual clues. These variants of unknown significance (VUS) are typically missense mutations that replace one amino acid with another. Even some silent mutations, DNA changes that do not influence the amino acid sequence, have been known to interfere with mRNA splicing, or to have even more subtle effects. In such cases, one is left to conjecture whether the change in DNA sequence is sufficiently disruptive to cause disease—a decidedly challenging task in the absence of exhaustive in vitro studies in model organisms designed to measure relevant loss of function. Interpretation of the clinical impact of the VUS is a relatively recent endeavor, and caution is recommended when gene sequencing or other mutation screening approaches are introduced into clinical practice.

One intriguing aspect about genetic testing is the potential for stratification of mutations according to the disease severity they invoke. A reliable correlation of genotype to phenotype, that is, disease expression, can be a valuable tool for the physician when answering questions from patients and families about the implications of genetic testing results. For example, Duchenne's and Becker's muscular dystrophies both arise predominantly from large deletions of the X-linked dystrophin gene. One might have postulated that larger deletions would cause the more severe, Duchenne's phenotype, or that specific regions in the gene are more sensitive to disruption and that severe mutations would cluster there. Neither theory is true. For the most part, it was found that deletions that disrupted the gene's reading frame led to more severe outcomes. In fact, these deletions entirely prevented synthesis of the dystrophin protein. Deletions that preserve the gene's reading frame enable an intact, if shortened, dystrophin protein molecular to be synthesized and are associated with the milder, later-onset Becker's phenotype.

The relationship between genetic mutations and disease severity is less clear for CF. Certainly translational stop mutations correlate with severe presentations of the disease, but different missense mutations can have widely divergent clinical consequences. No particular genotype defines a discrete clinical picture (e.g., age of onset, frequency of lung infection, pancreatic dysfunction, expected life span). Although detectable trends are evident when groups of CF patients are sorted according to genotype, CF genotyping is not currently a highly reliable prognostic tool.

In spite of these practical limitations, the number of single gene disorders for which molecular diagnostic tests are now available has expanded greatly in the past 15 years. A list of genetic tests and of the laboratories that offer them is maintained at http://www.genetests.org/. Online Mendelian Inheritance in Man (OMIM) is an Internet-accessible, comprehensive catalogue of human genes and genetic disorders maintained by the National Library of Medicine (http://www.ncbi.nlm.nih.gov:80/entrez/query.fcgi?db=OMIM). A very large database of human gene mutations, including links to more than 100 gene-specific databases, is maintained at the Institute of Medical Genetics in Cardiff, Wales (http://archive.uwcm.ac.uk/uwcm/mg/hgmd0.html and http://archive.uwcm.ac.uk/uwcm/mg/hgmd0.html).

Molecular genetics testing for at-risk families can be used for prenatal testing (see Chapter 52). Testing for known familial mutations can be performed on prospective parents (see below) or on cells derived from chorionic villus biopsy specimens or amniotic fluid. Preimplantation genetic diagnosis (PGD), whereby single cells derived by young embryos fertilized in vitro can be tested as well, permits the selection of embryos without the couple's mutations.

The utility of genetic testing is not limited to individual families with known risks for specific diseases. Population-based testing also may be considered for many diseases that have elevated prevalence in specific ethnic populations. Examples include sickle cell anemia in persons of African ancestry, and α- and β-thalassemia in individuals of Mediterranean, Indian, Chinese, or Southeast Asian backgrounds.

The prevalence of a number of genetic diseases, including CF, Tay-Sachs disease, Gaucher disease, Bloom syndrome, Fanconi anemia C, familial dysautonomia, Niemann-Pick disease, Canavan disease, and mucolipidosis type IV, is elevated in the Ashkenazi Jewish population. Carrier testing for each of these diseases is widely available, and testing recommendations for Tay-Sachs disease, CF, familial dysautonomia, and Canavan disease have been made by the American College of Medical Genetics (ACMG). For CF, which is common among Caucasians in general (about 4% of Caucasians are CF carriers), a joint statement was issued by the ACMG and the American College of Obstetricians and Gynecologists (ACOG) in 2001 (and amended in 2004) that recommended CF carrier screening for Caucasian couples contemplating a pregnancy or currently expecting. This testing, which may be offered to other ethnic groups as well, encompasses the 23 most common CF mutations, specifically, those with a frequency of 0.1% among patients with CF. This mutation panel will detect approximately 90% of carriers among Caucasians, and 97% of carriers among Ashkenazi Jews.

KEY CONCEPTS BOX 13-5

- Although specific gene defects associated with disease can be identified, allelic heterogeneity and rarity of the defect may make interpretation of results challenging.
- Interpretation of analysis is also made difficult because the exact relationship between a gene defect and disease, or penetrance, may not be known, or more than one mutation may cause the disease.
- For those diseases for which the gene defects have been well studied, molecular testing can be done as part of the carrier testing for preconception family planning, for newborn screening, or testing in high-risk populations.
- Diagnostic testing for a gene mutation in symptomatic patients for point mutations, deletions, and other mutations are performed for cystic fibrosis (CF), factor V Leiden–associated hypercoagulability, hemochromatosis, and the muscular dystrophies.

FUTURE APPLICATIONS

With completion of the Human Genome project and the identification of more disease-related genes, the demand for the application of this new knowledge to clinical practice will continue to increase. The clinical laboratory stands at the junction between the research laboratory and clinical practice. Through collaborative efforts by research laboratories, industry, governmental and private funding sources, and regulatory agencies, expanded genetic testing will become routine for a larger portion of the world's population.

BIBLIOGRAPHY

General

Bruns DE, Ashwood ER, Burtis CA, editors: *Fundamentals of Molecular Diagnostics,* Philadelphia, 2007, Saunders.

Buckingham L, Flaws ML, editors: *Molecular Diagnostics: Fundamentals, Methods and Clinical Applications,* Philadelphia, 2007, FA Davis Company.

Coleman WB, Tsongalis GJ, editors: *Molecular Diagnostics for the Clinical Laboratorian,* ed 2, Totowa, NJ, 2006, Humana Press.

Killeen A, editor: *Molecular Pathology Protocols,* Totowa, NJ, 2000, Humana Press.

Silverman LM, Hine R, editors: *Molecular Pathology,* Durham, NC, 1994, Carolina Academic Press.

Cancer Genetics

Coleman WB, Tsongalis GJ, editors: *The Molecular Basis of Human Cancer,* Totowa, NJ, 2001, Humana Press.

Diehl F, Li M, Dressman D, et al: Detection and quantification of mutations in the plasma of patients with colorectal tumors, Proc Natl Acad Sci U S A 102:16368, 2005.

Hodgson SV, Maher ER: *A Practical Guide to Human Cancer Genetics,* New York, 1993, Cambridge University Press.

Knudson AG: Chasing the cancer demon, Ann Rev Genet 34:1, 2000.

Roulston JE, Bartlett JMS, editors: *Molecular Diagnosis of Cancer: Methods and Protocols,* ed 2, Totowa, NJ, 2004, Humana Press.

Soussi T, Wiman KG: Shaping genetic alterations in human cancer: the *p53* mutation paradigm, Cancer Cell 12:303, 2007.

Vogelstein B, Kinzler KW, editors: *The Genetic Basis of Human Cancer,* ed 2, New York, 2002, McGraw-Hill.

Wood LD, Parsons DW, Jones S, et al: The genomic landscapes of human breast and colorectal cancers, Science 318:1108, 2007.

Infectious Disease and HIV

Barletta JM, Edelman DC, Constantine NT: Lowering the detection limits of HIV-1 viral load using real-time immuno-PCR for HIV-1 p24 antigen, Am J Clin Pathol 122:20, 2004.

Blum RA, Wylie N, England T, French C: HIV resistance testing in the USA—a model for the application of pharmacogenomics in the clinical setting, Pharmacogenomics 6:169, 2005.

Constantine NT, Saville R, Dax E: *Retroviral Testing and Quality Assurance: Essentials for Laboratory Diagnosis,* Ann Arbor, MI, 2005, Malloy Printers.

Hirsch MS, Brun-Vezinet F, D'Aquila RT, et al: Antiretroviral drug resistance testing in adult HIV-1 infection: recommendations of an International AIDS Society–USA panel, JAMA 283:2417, 2000.

International Perspectives of Antiretroviral Resistance: Special Issue. Journal of Acquired Immune Deficiency Syndromes, Supplement 1, 2001.

MacArthur RD: Drug resistance: an updated, user-friendly guide to genotype interpretation, AIDS Reader 10:652, 2000.

Scott JD, Gretch DR: Molecular diagnostics of hepatitis C virus infection: a systematic review, JAMA 297:724, 2007.

Vandamme AM, Sönnerborg A, Ait-Khaled M, et al: Updated European recommendations for the clinical use of HIV drug resistance testing, Antiviral Ther 9:829, 2004.

Vercauteren J, Vandamme AM: Algorithms for the interpretation of HIV-1 genotypic drug resistance information, Antiviral Res 71:335, 2006.

Vlahov D, Graham N, Hoover D, et al: Prognostic indicators for AIDS and infectious disease death in HIV-infected injection drug users, JAMA 279:35, 1998.

Weber B: Screening of HIV infection: role of molecular and immunological assays, Expert Rev Mol Diagn 6:399, 2006.

Genetics

Kanagawa M, Toda T: The genetic and molecular basis of muscular dystrophy: roles of cell-matrix linkage in the pathogenesis, J Hum Genet 51:915, 2006.

Rodriguez-Revenga L, Mila M, Rosenberg C, Lamb A, Lee C: Structural variation in the human genome: the impact of copy number variants on clinical diagnosis, Genet Med 9:600, 2007.

Shrimpton AE: Molecular diagnosis of cystic fibrosis, Expert Rev Mol Diagn 2:240, 2002.

The Human Genome: Special Issue. Nature 409:745, 2001.

The Human Genome: Special Issue. Science 291:1145, 2001.

Wang L, Freedman SD: Laboratory tests for the diagnosis of cystic fibrosis, Am J Clin Pathol 117(suppl):S109, 2002.

Chapter 14

Therapeutic Drug Monitoring

Michael Oellerich, Wolfgang A. Ritschel, and Victor W. Armstrong

Chapter Outline

Key Terms

absorption Uptake of unchanged drug into the circulation.

absorption rate constant Value describing how much drug is absorbed per unit of time.

active transport Movement of drug across a membrane by binding to a carrier molecule and delivery to the opposite side with expenditure of energy.

bioavailability The amount of drug in the formulation that the system of the patient can absorb.

biophase The site of interaction between the drug molecule and its receptor.

bound drug A pharmacological agent that exists in blood complexed with another molecule (usually protein or lipid).

C_{max} Maximum plasma level of drug.

C^{ss}_{av} Average steady-state concentration.

C^{ss}_{max} Maximum steady-state concentration (peak concentration).

C^{ss}_{min} Minimum steady-state concentration (trough concentration).

compartment A pharmacokinetic term for the drug concentration, *C*, and the volume of distribution of that drug.

distribution Proportional division of drug into different compartments of the body, such as blood and extracellular fluid.

elimination Final excretion of an agent.

first-order kinetics The rate of change of plasma drug concentration that is dependent on the concentration itself; that is, a constant proportion of drug is removed with time, or $dC/dt = -k \times C$.

free drug Pharmacological agent that exists in biological fluids unbound by other molecules.

half-life ($t_{1/2}$) The amount of time required to reduce a plasma drug level to one-half of its initial value. This term is also applied to the disappearance of the total amount of drug from the body.

LADME An acronym for the time course of drug distribution: *l*iberation, *a*bsorption, *d*istribution, *m*etabolism, and *e*limination.

liberation The process of drug release from the dosage form.

limited fluctuation method of dosing A method of dosing in which the drug given is not to exceed or go below specified limits.

maintenance dose The amount of drug required to keep a desired mean steady-state concentration.

MEC, MIC The minimum effective concentration, or the minimum inhibitory concentration, for a drug to be active. A drug is effective at any level above this value.

metabolism The biotransformation of the parent drug into metabolites.

Michaelis-Menten kinetics A method of transforming drug plasma levels into a linear relationship using the parameters of drug concentration and a constant, K_m.

passive diffusion The transport of drug by a concentration gradient across the membrane.

peak concentration The highest concentration reached after a dosage (usually soon after the dose is given).

peak method of dosing A method whereby the drug must reach a specified maximum level to be effective.

pharmacogenomics The science concerned with the identification and characterization of polymorphic genes encoding drug-metabolizing enzymes, transporters, receptors, and other drug targets.

pharmacokinetics The quantitative study of drug disposition in the body.

pharmacological effect The influence of a drug on a patient's biochemical or physiological state (such as lowering of blood pressure and bacteriostasis).

prodrug A parent compound that usually is not active and must be metabolized to the active form.

receptor The structure in the body with which the drug interacts, yielding its pharmacological effects. Most often, it is located on a cell membrane or on another cellular component.

slow release A dosage form of drug that allows the drug to be slowly placed into solution.

steady state A condition in which drug input and drug output are equal. This is obtained when, after multiple dosing, the peak concentration and the trough concentration after each dose oscillate within a specified range.

t Dosing interval.

t_{max} The time after dosing of maximum drug concentration.

terminal disposition rate constant The overall elimination of drug from the body per unit time.

therapeutic index The ratio between the plasma concentrations yielding the desired and undesired effects of a drug.

therapeutic range The relationship between the desired clinical effect of a drug and the concentration of drug in the plasma or blood. It is a range of drug concentrations within which the probability of the desired clinical response is relatively high and the probability of unacceptable toxicity is relatively low.

therapeutic window A term that describes a bell-shaped response curve of drug level versus pharmacological response.

total clearance (Cl_{tot}) A term that describes how much of the volume of distribution of a drug is cleared per unit of time.

toxic Implies poisonous or deleterious, sometimes fatal, side effects resulting from use of a therapeutic agent that is present at a level that is too high.

trough concentration The lowest drug concentration reached, usually before the next dose is given.

zero-order kinetics The rate of change of plasma concentration, independent of the plasma concentration. A constant amount is eliminated per unit of time, or $dC/dt = -k_0$.

zero-time blood level A hypothetical blood concentration obtained by extrapolation back to the initial, or zero, time of administration. Usually, this yields a maximal value.

Methods on CD-ROM

Anticonvulsant drugs
Carbamazepine
Cyclosporine A
Digoxin
Gentamicin and other aminoglycosides
Lithium
Methotrexate
Procainamide
Theophylline

FATE OF DRUG AND NEED FOR THERAPEUTIC DRUG MONITORING (TDM)

SECTION OBJECTIVES BOX 14-1

- Explain the difference between the concepts of reference intervals and therapeutic ranges.
- Apply the concepts of therapeutic range and therapeutic index to understand why frequent monitoring of certain drugs is necessary.
- Define the terms trough concentration, dosing interval, bioavailability, drug half-life, and steady state in the context of therapeutic drug monitoring.
- Discuss factors that affect the therapeutic range for a particular patient.
- Describe the components of the LADME system to describe drug disposition.
- Explain why patients with cardiac, hepatic, or renal disease may have a different clinical response to a drug, according to the effect these pathological factors have on the LADME system.

Table 14-1 Commonly Monitored Drugs, Recommended Sampling Times, Half-Lives, Therapeutic Ranges, and Critical Values

Drug	Recommended Sampling Time	[h]$t_{1/2}$, Hours	Therapeutic Range, μg/mL	Critical Range, μg/mL
Amikacin	0.5 to 1 hour after dose (peak) and end of dosing interval (trough)	0.5 to 3.0	Max 20 to 30, min < 5	Max > 35, min > 10
Amitriptyline	End of dosing interval	17 to 40	0.120 to 0.250	>0.500
Carbamazepine	End of dosing interval	10 to 60	4 to 12	>15
Clozapine	End of dosing interval	5 to 60[a]	0.35 to 0.6	>0.75
Cyclosporine	End of dosing interval[b]	4.7 to 12.7	0.1 to 0.3	>0.4
Digitoxin	8 to 24 hours after dose	72 to 384	0.01 to 0.025	>0.035
Digoxin	8 to 24 hours after dose	20 to 50	0.0008 to 0.002[c]	>0.0024
Ethosuximide	End of dosing interval		40 to 100	>150
Gentamicin	0.5 to 1 hour after dose and end of dosing interval	0.5 to 3.0	Max 5 to 10, min < 2	Max > 12, min > 2
Lidocaine	During infusion	1.2 to 2.3	1.5 to 5.0	>7
Lithium	End of dosing interval	14 to 33	0.6 to 1.2 (mmol/L)	>1.5 (mmol/L)
Phenobarbital	End of dosing interval	50 to 150	10 to 40	>50
Phenytoin	End of dosing interval	20 to 100	10 to 20	>20
Primidone	End of dosing interval	4 to 22	5 to 12	>15
Procainamide	End of dosing interval	3 to 5	4 to 10	>16[d]
Salicylate	1 to 3 hours after dose	3 to 20	150 to 300[e]	>400
Sirolimus	End of dosing interval	35 to 95[f]	0.004 to 0.012[g]	>0.015
Tacrolimus	End of dosing interval	5.5 to 16	0.005 to 0.015	>0.02
Theophylline	Intravenous infusion: 4 to 8, 12 to 24 hours, and 24-hour intervals after start of infusion; oral or intravenous injection: 2 hours after dose; oral sustained release: 4 to 6 hours after dose	3 to 12, nonsmokers; 2 to 6, smokers	8 to 20	>20
Tobramycin	0.5 to 1 hour after dose and end of dosing interval	0.5 to 3.0	Max 5 to 10, min < 2	Max > 12, min > 2
Vancomycin	1 hour after dose and end of dosing interval	4 to 10	Max 20 to 40, min 5 to 10	Max > 80, min > 20

[h]$T_{1/2}$, From healthy volunteers.
[a]Multiple dosing in schizophrenic patients.
[b]For absorption profiling, a 2-hour sampling time with respective therapeutic ranges has been proposed.[5]
[c]Heart failure, 0.0005 to 0.0009.
[d]Measure both parent and metabolite therapeutic range of combined; critical range >35 for both.
[e]Anti-inflammatory.
[f]$t_{1/2}$ from stable renal transplant recipients.
[g]Triple therapy with cyclosporine and corticosteroids, determination by liquid chromatography/mass spectrometry (LC-MS/MS).

Concept of Therapeutic Range

For many drugs, a relationship has been established between the clinical effects and the drug concentration in plasma or blood. In general, to achieve the desired **pharmacological effect** (such as lowering of blood pressure, pain relief, or bacteriostasis), a certain concentration must be reached at the site of interaction between the drug molecule and its **receptor** (cell membrane, cell component) to elicit the clinical effect.

Although **therapeutic ranges** have been empirically established in numerous clinical studies to assist in interpretation of drug measurements, drug concentrations must always be interpreted in the context of all clinical data. In contrast to the concept of reference intervals in clinical chemistry, there is no generally accepted concept or protocol on how to establish the therapeutic range of a drug. These therapeutic ranges, therefore, vary somewhat throughout the literature and should be used only as a general guide. They represent the range of drug concentrations within which the probability of the desired clinical response is relatively high and the probability of unacceptable toxicity is relatively low. Thus, it is important for the physician to know whether the drug is present in a concentration within the therapeutic range.

Clinicians should never assume, however, that a drug concentration within the therapeutic range is safe and effective for every patient. Recommended therapeutic ranges for some commonly monitored drugs are presented in Table 14-1. For most of the drugs listed in this table, concentrations are determined in serum or plasma. The exceptions are cyclosporine, tacrolimus, and sirolimus, for which whole blood measurements are recommended. Concentrations within the therapeutic range of a drug will produce a pharmacological response in most patients. At concentrations above the upper limit of the therapeutic range, an increased incidence of **toxic** side effects can be expected without, as a rule, any substantial improvement in the therapeutic effect. Absolute toxicity is less important than the ratio between the average toxic dose and the average therapeutic dose or concentration. The range between the concentration of drug required to produce the therapeutic response and that which produces a toxic effect determines how carefully the dosage of the drug must be monitored. The ratio of these concentrations is called the **therapeutic index** and is expressed as the minimum concentration (or dose) that produces toxicity divided by the minimum concentration (or dose) that causes the therapeutic response in a patient population. This ratio is narrow for some drugs (e.g., digoxin, lithium compounds, cyclosporine, tacrolimus) and wide for others. Hence the therapeutic range also may be narrow or wide. It is particularly desirable to monitor drug concentrations for drugs that have a narrow therapeutic range and a low therapeutic index (e.g., digoxin, lithium, gentamicin), that have dose-dependent elimination kinetics (phenytoin), or that show great individual variability in **metabolism** (tricyclic antidepressants). When this ratio is 2.0 or less, the compound can be difficult to use without significant toxicity being encountered. Toxic drug concentration values above which there is an enhanced or high probability of adverse effects are listed in Table 14-1.

Therapeutic ranges may require adjustment if other drugs with synergistic or antagonistic actions are also administered to the patient. A serum concentration of phenytoin considered within the therapeutic range may produce toxic symptoms when other central nervous depressants are present. The existence of pharmacologically active metabolites and alterations in protein binding also must be taken into consideration when one is interpreting serum concentrations. When certain drugs, such as phenobarbital, are administered over a long period, patients may develop a tolerance to the drug, and the upper limit of the therapeutic range may then be raised.

Target concentrations for cyclosporine or tacrolimus depend on the indication for treatment, the time after initiation of therapy, and concurrent immunosuppressive therapy (see Chapter 54).[1,2] Thus the therapeutic ranges for cyclosporine and tacrolimus can be taken only as a general guide. Most transplant centers recommend higher target concentrations during the early postoperative period followed by tapering of cyclosporine and tacrolimus doses to achieve a lower maintenance concentration range, usually 3 to 6 months after transplantation. Typically, **trough concentrations** of drug, measured at the end of a **dosing interval,** are used for immunosuppressive drug monitoring. Alternatively, abbreviated area under the concentration-time curve (AUC) strategies have been proposed to better assess drug exposure.[3,4] A disadvantage of these approaches in clinical practice is the necessity of exact timing of multiple blood samples. In the case of cyclosporine, the use of a single sampling point 2 hours post dose has been suggested as a surrogate for the abbreviated AUC.[5]

For correct interpretation of drug levels, knowledge of the time interval between administration of the last dose and blood sampling is imperative. With long-term therapy, blood samples should be taken in the **steady state.** In practice, samples usually are taken after four to five half-lives have elapsed, when more than 90% of the steady-state concentration has normally been reached (Fig. 14-1). Depending on the clinical question, either the peak concentration or the trough concentration taken directly before administration of the next dose is measured. When a drug is given by intravenous infusion, blood samples should be taken after the initial distribution phase has been completed, usually after around 1 to 2 hours. However, for digoxin and digitoxin, the time to equilibrium after oral or intravenous administration is usually 8 to 12 hours. For serum concentrations to best reflect the effects on cardiac activity, samples should be taken when drug equilibrium between serum and tissue has been achieved.[6]

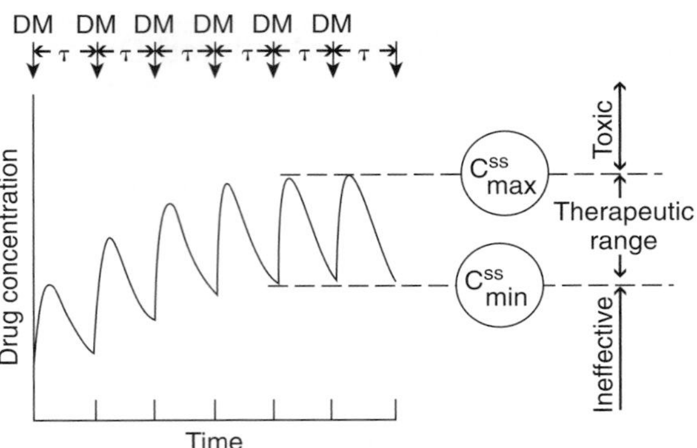

Fig. 14-1 Graph of blood-drug concentrations as function of dose and time. *DM,* Dose; τ, interval between doses; C^{ss}_{max}, concentration maximum at steady state; C^{ss}_{min}, concentration minimum at steady state. In this sample, τ is chosen to be equivalent to the half-life of elimination.

Monitoring of predose (trough) plasma/serum concentrations is an established procedure for lithium and some antidepressants and antipsychotics. Consensus guidelines and appropriate therapeutic ranges have been recommended for a large number of drugs used in psychopharmacotherapy.[7]

In the case of some drugs such as phenytoin or phenobarbital, the timing of the blood sampling is not important because fluctuations between peak and trough concentrations in the steady state are relatively small. With other drugs such as theophylline, which have a narrow therapeutic range and a short **half-life,** it may be necessary to obtain blood samples at both peak and trough levels to determine whether the correct dosage has been used. In the case of multiple daily dosings of the aminoglycosides, both peak and trough values should be monitored to prevent the administration of inappropriately high doses, which might predispose the patient to nephrotoxicity and ototoxicity.[8] Instead of multiple-dose regimens, once-daily dosing of aminoglycosides has been advocated to provide better antibacterial efficacy and less nephrotoxicity than conventional multiple-dose strategies with the same total daily dose. Although variation in the methods and conclusions has been noted, several meta-analyses and reviews have concluded that once-daily dosing is at least as efficacious as, and no more nephrotoxic than, multiple-daily dosing.[8] Some investigators suggest that only measurement of the trough concentration is required, and that the dose should be reduced if the concentration is above 1 to 2 mg/L. Others have recommended that dosage be guided by measurement of one or two

Box 14-1

Major Causes of Unexpected Serum Drug Concentrations Outside of the Therapeutic Range

- Noncompliance of patient
- Inappropriate dosage
- Malabsorption
- Poor bioavailability of the administered preparation
- Drug interactions
- Kidney and liver disease
- Altered protein binding
- Fever
- Genetically determined fast or slow metabolism

aminoglycoside concentrations at fixed time points after the infusion. Dosage is then adjusted according to a nomogram, by computer-assisted calculation of the daily AUC, or with the aid of a dose prediction software program.[8]

Some of the common causes of unexpected serum drug concentrations observed in patients are listed in Box 14-1. If these factors cannot be eliminated, and if adequate patient compliance can be ascertained, it will be necessary to adjust the dosage of the drug.

Therapeutic drug monitoring (TDM) is of particular importance in pediatric patients because drug metabolism changes with age,[9,10] and many of the factors listed in Box 14-1 can have a disproportionate effect on newborns.[11] In the first 6 months of life, hepatic and renal function is immature, and a much smaller dose per kilogram must be given to attain the same therapeutic concentration of a drug. As an example, the half-life of theophylline in the premature newborn is about 30 hours, decreasing in children to 2 to 6 hours before increasing again during puberty to values of 6 to 13 hours in nonsmoking adults. Children who are going through puberty and receiving drug therapy need to be monitored closely because the activity of the enzyme system metabolizing theophylline is changing substantially over this period.

LADME System to Describe Drug Disposition

It is generally accepted that changes in drug concentrations in the body that occur over time are related to the course of the pharmacological effects. The change in drug concentration over time is described by the **LADME** system, in which the **l**iberation, **a**bsorption, **d**istribution, **m**etabolism, and **e**limination of a drug are considered in sequence.

Liberation, or Drug Release, from a Dosage Form

To be absorbed, a drug must be present in the form of a true solution at the site of **absorption.** Hence the active ingredient of any dosage form except those that are already true solutions (such as intravenous injection, peroral elixir, peroral syrup, rectal enema, eye drops, and nose drops) has to be released from the dosage form before the drug can be absorbed. This release or liberation is the process of the drug passing into solution. When given orally by tablets, capsules, or suspensions, the drug dissolves in gastric fluid. After intramuscular or subcutaneous injection of suspensions, the drug dissolves in tissue fluid. After rectal administration, suppositories melt in the rectum, and the drug dissolves in rectal fluid. After application of ointments, the drug dissolves in the water of perspiration at the interface between the skin and the ointment. These are a few cases in which liberation is necessary for the drug to be absorbed.

Sustained or controlled-release dosage forms are preparations with **slow release** rates. These rates are designed for those drugs that do not remain in the body for a long time. Because the drug cannot be absorbed more quickly than it is released, the apparent absorption rate becomes a function of the release rate, and the entire absorption process takes longer, resulting in a prolonged duration of clinical effect.

Absorption

Absorption is the process by which the drug molecule is taken up into systemic circulation. Systemic circulation is usually defined as the bloodstream. The process of absorption must occur whenever a drug is administered *extravascularly,* that is, perorally, orally, intramuscularly, subcutaneously, rectally, or topically. Whenever a drug is given *intravascularly,* no absorption takes place because the drug is introduced directly into the bloodstream.

Absorption occurs through various mechanisms, including passive diffusion, active transport, facilitated transport, convective transport, and pinocytosis. **Passive diffusion,** which is applicable for about 95% of all drugs, depends on the concentration of nonionized drug being higher on one side of the membrane than on the other. As long as there is a concentration gradient across the membrane, the drug will be absorbed into the region of lower concentration. For weakly ionized drugs, the drug's pK_a and pH at the absorption site (such as stomach pH 1.5 to 3, intestines pH 5 to 7, rectum pH 7.8, or skin pH 5) influence the degree of ionization. The pH of blood is 7.4 and rather constant. As a general rule, ionized drug species are passively absorbed much less readily than nonionized species. At 2 pH units below an acid drug's pK_a and 2 pH units above a basic drug's pK_a, the drugs will be 99% nonionized and will exhibit maximal rates of absorption.

The next important absorption mechanism, **active transport,** requires binding of the drug molecule to a carrier (protein) in the membrane. The carrier delivers the drug to the opposite side of the membrane through an expenditure of energy. This process moves the drug (such as cardiac glycosides, hexoses, monosaccharides, amino acids, riboflavin) against a concentration gradient. *Facilitated transport* is a similar mechanism, but facilitated transport of a substance (such as vitamin B_{12}) follows the concentration gradient. *Convective transport* is the mechanism of absorption by which small molecules (such as urea) enter the systemic circulation through water-filled pores in the membrane. For all these mechanisms, the drug must be in true aqueous solution at the absorption site.

A unique absorption mechanism is that of pinocytosis of fats and solid particles. Engulfing vesicles form within the cellular membrane and open at the intracellular side, releasing the fat droplets or particles (such as vitamins A, K, D, and E; parasite eggs; fats; and starch).

Distribution

Once drug molecules have been absorbed, they are distributed within the bloodstream and can (1) be confined to the blood space, (2) leave the bloodstream and enter other extravascular fluids (such as interstitial fluid), or (3) migrate into various tissues and organs. The entire process of transfer of drug from the bloodstream to other body compartments is called **distribution.** This process usually takes between 30 minutes and 2 hours but may be completed within a few minutes or may take much longer than 2 hours (distribution time for methotrexate is 15 hours).

Metabolism

Metabolism is the process of biotransformation of the parent drug molecule to one or more metabolites. The metabolites are usually more polar, that is, more water soluble, and thus can be more easily excreted by the kidney or liver. Metabolism occurs primarily in the liver and the kidney but also takes place in plasma and muscle tissue. Usually, but not always, metabolites are less active and less toxic than their parent compounds. However, at this point, a group of drugs known as **prodrugs** should be mentioned. The prodrug as parent compound usually is not active and must be metabolized to the active form (e.g., mycophenolate mofetil is biotransformed to the active compound mycophenolic acid).[12] The active form of prodrug is unstable, is not readily soluble, or is poorly absorbed.

Some drugs form metabolites that are also active. For example, the active drug procainamide is biotransformed to the equipotent metabolite acetylprocainamide. The knowledge of active metabolites is particularly important for TDM to correlate the total concentration of all active forms with pharmacological effects.

Elimination

The final excretion of the drug from the body as unchanged parent compound or in the form of metabolites is called **elimination.** The major routes of excretion are through the kidney into urine and through the liver into bile and consequently into feces. Other pathways of elimination are through skin (sweat), lungs (expired air), mammary glands (milk), and salivary glands (saliva).

The elimination half-life is the time required to reduce the blood level concentration to one-half after equilibrium is obtained. After the drug is absorbed and distributed, it takes one half-life to eliminate 50% of the drug, seven half-lives to eliminate 99% of the drug, and ten half-lives to eliminate 99.9% of the drug.

Effects of Biological Variation on LADME

If a drug is given in identical amounts by the same route of administration at the same time of day to identical twins, the pharmacokinetic parameters will differ only very slightly. In fraternal twins, there will be larger differences. Greater differences will occur within a population group, even if this group is homogeneous with regard to sex, age, body weight, and health. These differences include genetically based variations in drug handling, which may influence absorption, distribution, metabolism, elimination, and drug-receptor interactions. Hence pharmacokinetic parameters for healthy subjects reported in the literature are means with ranges. They are actually valid only for the group studied.

Physiological and Pathological Factors Influencing Drug Disposition

Apart from biological variations caused by genetic differences, many physiological and pathological factors may alter considerably a drug's disposition.[13]

The most prominent physiological factors are body weight and composition, age, temperature (hyperthermia and hypothermia), gastric emptying time and gastrointestinal motility, blood flow rates (during rest and exercise), environment (high altitude, mountain sickness), nutrition, pregnancy, and circadian rhythm.

Among the most important pathological factors are renal impairment, liver impairment, acute congestive heart failure, burns, shock, trauma, and gastrointestinal disease.

Blood Levels as Indicators of Clinical Response

The rationale for the use of blood levels as indicators of clinical response is based on the concept that, for those drugs that interact at a receptor site without being changed, the drug concentration at the site of action determines the intensity and duration of the pharmacological effect. Because it is usually not possible to sample at the site of action or **biophase** (such as the cell membrane), the next alternative is to sample whole blood, plasma, or serum, which is the biological fluid in closest equilibrium with the receptor site that can be easily sampled. After the distribution phase is complete, the drug concentration in the central and peripheral **compartments** (i.e., blood) will decline in parallel. At this point, a pseudoequilibrium of distribution is obtained, regardless of whether the site of action is located in the central compartment or in any peripheral compartment. Although the total drug concentration may differ considerably between central and peripheral compartments, the concentration of **free (unbound) drug** will be the same. Hence, once the pseudoequilibrium of distribution is reached, a correlation should exist between pharmacological effect and drug concentration in blood. Usually, only the total drug concentration is measured, that is, both free and **bound drug,** in plasma. This is acceptable under normal conditions because individual differences in plasma-protein binding seem to be small; in some cases, however, this is not true.[14]

Blood Levels After Single Dose of Drug

Most graphical descriptions of a pharmacokinetic response are given as a plot of blood concentration versus time (Fig. 14-2). The shape and course of a blood level–time curve depend on the route of administration and the LADME system.

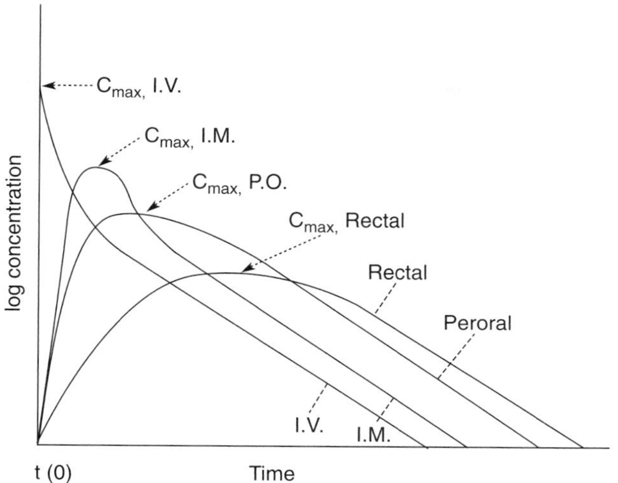

Fig. 14-2 Blood level–time curves of a hypothetical drug upon different routes of administration.

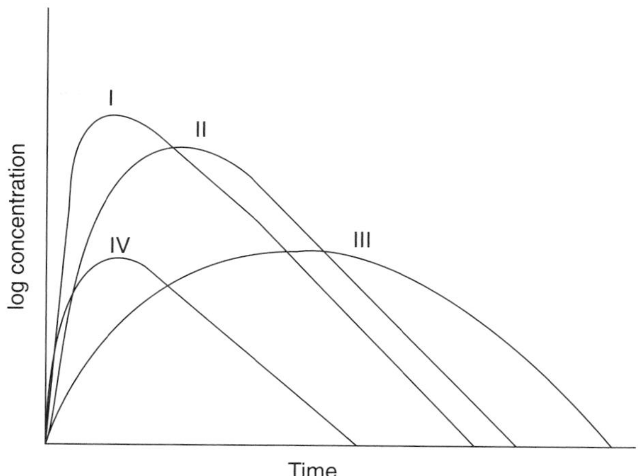

Fig. 14-3 Influence of liberation process on course of blood level–time curves. *I,* Fast-dissolving tablet; *II,* tablet with slower dissolution rate; *III,* sustained-release tablet; *IV,* tablet with poor bioavailability.

With rapid intravenous administration, each facet of the drug is instantly in the systemic circulation. If the drug is given by extravascular administration, none will be in systemic circulation at the moment of administration, that is, at time zero. After the drug is released from the dosage form, the blood level–time curve rises with continuous absorption. Once absorbed, a molecule is exposed to distribution, metabolism, and elimination. Because initially a greater proportion is absorbed than is distributed, metabolized, and eliminated, the blood level–time curve rises until input and output are equal. At this time (**t_{max}**), the **peak concentration** (**C_{max}**) is reached, and the blood level–time curve declines as elimination exceeds absorption (see Fig. 14-2).

Two liberation factors may change the shape of the curve: rate and extent of liberation. Drug products from different manufacturers may release the drug at various rates. A slow release may be intentional, as in the case of slow-release (sustained-release) dosage forms. However, if all the drug is released, the areas under the blood level–time curves of different formulations will be the same. If the drug is not fully released, a so-called **bioavailability** problem might be present, and the area under the curve will be reduced (Fig. 14-3). *Bioavailability* refers to the amount of drug that is systemically absorbed.

The absorption process can be influenced by many factors. Food (when the drug is given orally before, during, or after meals) may have no effect on the absorption, may accelerate or prolong the absorption, or may influence the extent of absorption. For example, the blood level of griseofulvin is greatly enhanced when the drug is given with fat, whereas a tetracycline blood level decreases when the drug is ingested with milk.

The volume of distribution may change in various pathological conditions. If the volume of distribution increases, the blood level decreases and vice versa. In congestive heart failure, (CHF) the volume of distribution usually increases, decreasing plasma levels of many drugs. But this effect also varies by drug. In CHF, the volume of distribution for certain drugs (digoxin, quinidine) is actually reduced. The same dose will therefore result in a higher concentration (Fig. 14-4).

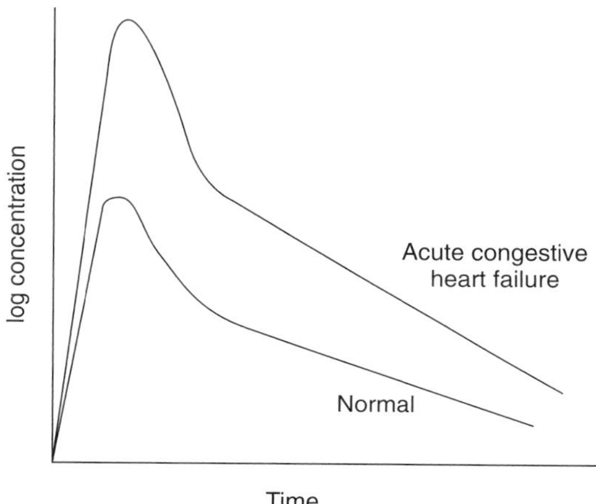

Fig. 14-4 Influence of distribution process on course of blood level–time curves of digoxin. In acute congestive heart failure, a higher blood level is observed because of decreased volume of distribution.

For drugs that are extensively metabolized, changes in blood levels may result from impaired metabolism (liver damage) or from other drugs given concomitantly that either compete for metabolic pathways (enzyme inhibition) or accelerate metabolism (enzyme induction) (Fig. 14-5).

Elimination of drugs, particularly of those predominantly eliminated through the kidney, may be tremendously prolonged in cases of renal failure and in aged persons with reduced renal function. The reduced elimination can result in a manyfold prolonged elimination half-life. Classic examples are the aminoglycosides. The normal half-life of gentamicin of 2 hours may be prolonged easily to 20 hours or longer (Fig. 14-6).

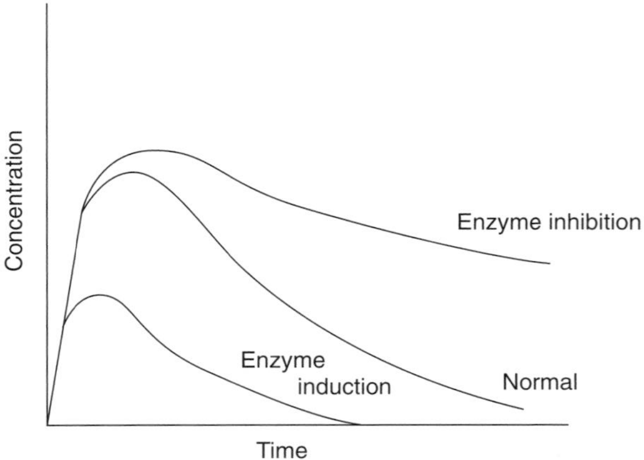

Fig. 14-5 Influence of metabolism processes on course of blood level–time curves. Enzyme inhibition and liver damage may greatly increase blood level, whereas enzyme induction may decrease it.

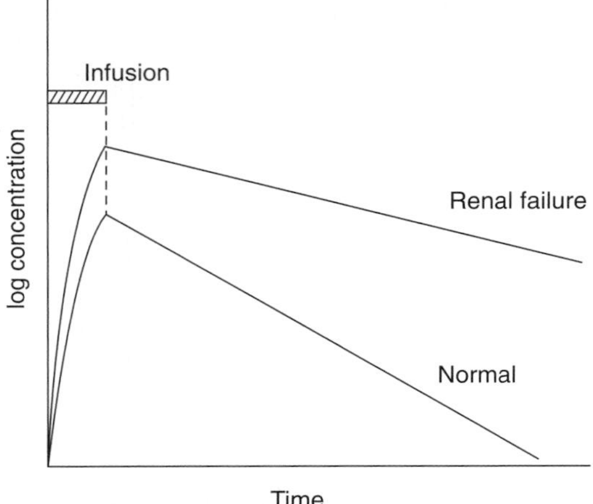

Fig. 14-6 Influence of elimination processes on course of blood level–time curve of gentamicin. In the presence of renal failure, peak concentration after short-term infusion is higher, and blood level remains elevated with a longer elimination half-life.

KEY CONCEPTS BOX 14-1

- The therapeutic range for a particular drug must be interpreted according to the level at which the probability of a desired clinical response exceeds the probability of unacceptable toxicity.
- Drugs with a narrow therapeutic range and a low therapeutic index, dose-dependent elimination kinetics, or high individual variability in metabolism are frequently monitored in the clinical laboratory.
- There are many factors, such as class of administered drug, clinical condition of the patient, means of drug administration, sampling time, etc. that affect therapeutic ranges.
- The trough concentration of a drug occurs right before the next dose. The Dosing interval is the time between dosing. The bioavailability of a drug describes how much of a drug dosage can be taken up. The half-life of a drug is the time needed to clear one-half of drug from the body.
- Knowledge of factors that affect each phase of the LADME system, such as route of administration and biochemistry of the drug, plus biological, physiological, and pathological features of the patient is necessary for proper interpretation of both clinical response and drugs levels obtained in the clinical laboratory.

SECTION OBJECTIVES BOX 14-2

- Differentiate five methods for dosing regimens and explain why knowledge of the dosing regimen for a particular patient is important in establishing proper sampling protocols for laboratory specimens.
- Differentiate the three types of kinetic processes used to characterize the disposition of drugs in the body: first-order, zero-order, and Michaelis-Menten.
- List drugs commonly measured in the clinical laboratory that follow first-order, zero-order, and Michaelis-Menten kinetics.

DOSAGE REGIMENS USED IN ACHIEVING THERAPEUTIC TARGET CONCENTRATION

Steady-State Therapeutic Drug Concentrations

Most drugs are not administered as a single dose. Instead they are administered in a series of doses given at specified intervals throughout the entire course of drug therapy. If the drug is administered repeatedly using dosing intervals shorter than the time required to eliminate the drug remaining in the body from the preceding dose, the drug will accumulate until a steady state is achieved, that is, one in which drug input and output are equal. Steady state is obtained when, with a specific regimen or dosage, the peak concentration (C^{ss}_{max}, or maximum steady-state concentration) and the trough concentration (C^{ss}_{min}, or minimum steady-state concentration) after each dose oscillate within a certain range; the goal is to achieve the therapeutic range. When a blood level–time curve is obtained after a single dose, the necessary parameters can be derived to predict the steady state and in turn the dose required to achieve a desired steady state.

The **maintenance dose** required to maintain a desired mean steady-state concentration, C^{ss}_{av}, at a given dosage interval, **t**, depends on the magnitude of C^{ss}_{av} (the drug concentration in blood required to elicit the pharmacological response), the pharmacokinetic parameters of drug disposition, and the patient's body weight. The generalized equation for determining the correct maintenance dose is given in Box 14-2.[15]

The dosing interval, *t*, is freely chosen within a wide range, most often at times less than $t_{1/2}$ (half-life). It may have to be increased in renal or hepatic diseases because $t_{1/2}$ often is greatly extended in these cases. In general, at the end of four half-lives (if a dosing interval less than the half-life is chosen), a steady-state level is reached with multiple dosing (see Fig. 14-1).

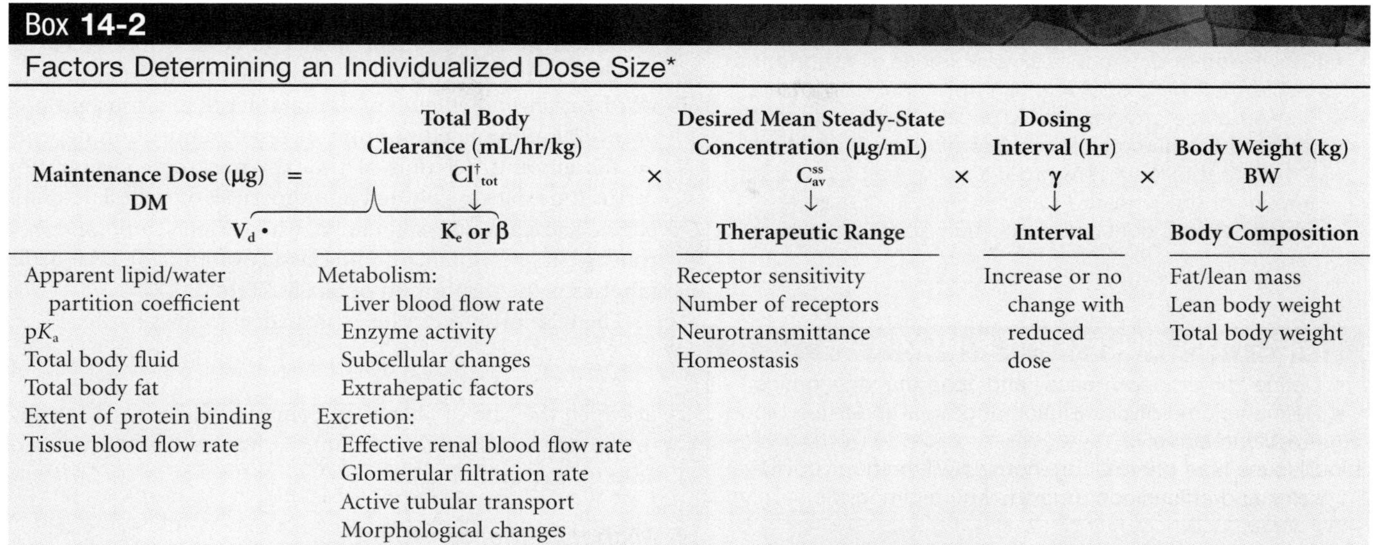

Box 14-2

Factors Determining an Individualized Dose Size*

$$\underset{\text{DM}}{\text{Maintenance Dose } (\mu g)} = \underset{Cl^{\dagger}_{tot}}{\text{Total Body Clearance (mL/hr/kg)}} \times \underset{C^{ss}_{av}}{\text{Desired Mean Steady-State Concentration } (\mu g/mL)} \times \underset{\gamma}{\text{Dosing Interval (hr)}} \times \underset{BW}{\text{Body Weight (kg)}}$$

$Cl^{\dagger}_{tot}$ → $V_d \bullet$ K_e or β; C^{ss}_{av} → Therapeutic Range; γ → Interval; BW → Body Composition

$V_d \bullet$	K_e or β	Therapeutic Range	Interval	Body Composition
Apparent lipid/water partition coefficient	Metabolism:	Receptor sensitivity	Increase or no change with reduced dose	Fat/lean mass
pK_a	Liver blood flow rate	Number of receptors		Lean body weight
Total body fluid	Enzyme activity	Neurotransmittance		Total body weight
Total body fat	Subcellular changes	Homeostasis		
Extent of protein binding	Extrahepatic factors			
Tissue blood flow rate	Excretion:			
	Effective renal blood flow rate			
	Glomerular filtration rate			
	Active tubular transport			
	Morphological changes			

List beneath each factor includes chemical and physiological determinants that influence each factor.
V_d, Apparent volume of distribution (mL/kg); K_e or β, overall terminal disposition rate constant (hr^{-1}).
*For further information see Ritschel WA: *Contemp Pharmacy Pract* 5:209, Washington, DC, 1982, American Pharmaceutical Association.
†$Cl_{tot} = V_d \bullet \beta$.

Dosing Regimens

The dosage regimen for multiple-dosing maintenance therapy can be designed according to five different methods, depending on the desired target concentration to be achieved or maintained throughout each dosing interval. For monitoring purposes, it is necessary to know which method will be used because the optimum blood sampling protocol for laboratory analysis depends on the method in question. Five methods for dosage regimen design follow:

- Minimum effective concentration **(MEC)** or minimum inhibitory concentration **(MIC)** method
- C^{ss}_{max}, or peak, method
- C^{ss}_{max}-C^{ss}_{min}, or limited fluctuation, method
- C^{ss}_{av}, or log dose-response, method
- TW, or **therapeutic window,** method

All methods refer to steady-state concentrations.

MEC or MIC Method

For some drugs to be effective, it is necessary to reach and maintain a minimum inhibitory concentration (MIC), or a minimum effective concentration (MEC), at steady state. Above the MIC or MEC, the drug will be effective, regardless of how high a peak level is reached, as long as the entire steady-state blood level–time curve is above the required MIC or MEC. If the blood level–time curve falls below the MIC or MEC level, the drug will be ineffective as long as the concentration stays below this level. Drugs such as bacteriostatic antibiotics and other antimicrobial agents (sulfonamides) that have a relatively large therapeutic index often are prescribed at dosages calculated by this method.

C^{ss}_{max}, or Peak, Method

For some drugs, it is desirable to reach a certain steady-state peak concentration during each dosing interval. However, for the remainder of the dosing interval, it is not required that the drug concentration remain above a minimum level. This is particularly the case with bactericidal drugs, which act only on proliferating microorganisms. In these cases, it is not desirable to inhibit growth of those microorganisms that have not been killed by the previous dose. Drugs that are often given in dosage regimens based on the C^{ss}_{max}, or **peak method of dosing,** include penicillins, cephalosporins, gentamicin, and kanamycin.

C^{ss}_{max}-C^{ss}_{min}, or Limited Fluctuation, Method

For some drugs, it might be desirable to maintain an MIC or MEC at steady state throughout the dosing interval but to never exceed a certain peak value. This is particularly the case if the drug has a narrow therapeutic range. Drugs that might be administered according to this **limited fluctuation method of dosing** to compute dosage include gentamicin, kanamycin, streptomycin, isoniazid, and theophylline.

C^{ss}_{av}, or Log Dose-Response, Method

For drugs whose clinical effect follows a log dose-response curve, drug doses are selected to achieve the desired steady-state concentration usually in the lower third of the log dose-response curve. For drugs following a log dose response, the intensity of effect (and of toxicity) increases with increasing peak size. Drugs whose dosages are often based on this pattern include digoxin, lidocaine, procainamide, theophylline, quinidine, bactericidal antibiotics, analgesics, antipyretics, and hypoglycemic agents.

TW, or Therapeutic Window, Method

With some drugs, such as antidepressants and antipsychotics, the clinical effect increases with dose size only up to a certain point and then actually diminishes as the dose size is further increased. Instead of a therapeutic range, there exists a therapeutic window that shows a more or less bell-shaped log dose-response curve.

KEY CONCEPTS BOX 14-2

- Knowledge of different dosing regimens is important to assure that the proper sampling protocol is followed.
- First-order, zero-order, and Michaelis-Menten kinetics are used to characterize the fate of drugs in the body. A drug that follows zero order kinetics has a constant amount of drug cleared per unit time; in first order drug kinetics a constant proportion of drug is cleared per unit time.

SECTION OBJECTIVES BOX 14-3

- Define "pharmacokinetics" and "pharmacogenomics."
- Define volume of distribution and area-under-the blood level time curve.
- Discuss how pharmacogenomics will help to provide safer and efficacious drug therapy regimens.

PHARMACOKINETICS

Pharmacokinetics is the quantitative study of drug disposition in the body. Pharmacokinetics permits (1) describing mathematically the fate of a drug after administration in a given dosage form by a given route of administration, (2) comparing one drug with others or one dosage form with other dosage forms, and (3) predicting blood levels of a drug with different dosage regimens or disease states.

Basically, in pharmacokinetics, three types of kinetic processes are used to characterize the fate of drugs in the body: first-order, or linear, kinetics; zero-order, or nonlinear, kinetics; and Michaelis-Menten, or saturation, kinetics.

First-Order Kinetics

Most processes of drug uptake (absorption), diffusion and permeation in the body (distribution), and excretion (urinary elimination) can be described by first-order, or linear, kinetics. This means that the rate of change of concentration of drug is dependent on the drug concentration. When the concentration versus time data are plotted on numerical, or cartesian, graph paper, a concave curve is obtained; when plotted on semilog paper, a straight line is obtained. The relationship is expressed as follows by Equation 14-1:

$$dC/dt = -k \times C \qquad \text{Eq. 14-1}$$

in which C is the concentration of the drug, k is the first-order rate constant, and t is time. The minus sign indicates that the drug concentration decreases with time. Drugs are eliminated in a manner that can be described by **first-order kinetics** when a *constant percentage* of drug is eliminated per unit of time. Drugs exhibiting first-order elimination kinetics are antibiotics, digoxin, lidocaine, procainamide, and theophylline. First-order kinetics describes the elimination of most drugs.

Zero-Order Kinetics

If the rate of elimination of a compound from the body is not proportional to the concentration of the drug taken, the elimination usually follows zero-order, or nonlinear, kinetics. This means that the rate of change of concentration is independent of the concentration of the particular drug. In other words, a *constant amount* of drug, rather than a constant proportion, is eliminated per unit of time (elimination depends on the amount per unit of time). When the concentration versus time data are plotted on numerical, or cartesian, graph paper, a straight line is obtained, whereas on semilog paper, a convex curve is obtained. The classic example for **zero-order kinetics** is the disposition of alcohol (ethanol).

The relationship can be expressed as follows by Eq. 14-2:

$$dC/dt = -k_0 \qquad \text{Eq. 14-2}$$

in which the rate of change of concentration, dC/dt, is equal to the zero-order rate constant, k_0, which has the units of amount per unit of time.

Michaelis-Menten Kinetics

In metabolism, nearly all biotransformation processes are catalyzed by specific enzyme systems with a limited capacity for the drug. Also, in active transport of drugs across membranes, the carriers have a limited capacity. Whenever the drug concentration present in a given system exceeds the capacity of that system, the rate of change of concentration is most precisely described by the Michaelis-Menten equation:

$$dC/dt = -(V_{max} \times C)/(K_m + C) \qquad \text{Eq. 14-3}$$

in which C is the drug concentration, t is the time, V_{max} is a constant representing the maximum rate of the process, and K_m is the Michaelis-Menten constant, the drug concentration at which the process proceeds at exactly one-half its maximal rate. Examples of drugs that show saturation-elimination or **Michaelis-Menten kinetics** are phenytoin, high doses of barbiturates, and glutethimide.

Compartment Models

To describe the quantitative processes of a drug in the organism, pharmacokinetics uses the concept of compartments. A compartment is a unit characterized by two parameters: the drug concentration, C, and the volume, V_d. By multiplying the drug concentration by the apparent volume of distribution, the amount, A, of the drug in that compartment is obtained:

$$A = C \times V_d \qquad \text{Eq. 14-4}$$

A given compartment model is not necessarily specific for a given drug. For example, a drug given intravenously is often described by a two-compartment open model, whereas the same drug given orally or by any other extravascular route may be described by a one-compartment open model. *Open* means that there is input to and output from the compartment.

In reality, the human body is a multimillion-compartment system. However, usually there exists in the intact organism easy access to only two kinds of biological fluids: blood (serum, plasma) and urine. Being restricted to blood or urine specimens, the drug has a fate in the body that usually is described by a one-compartment or a two-compartment open model.

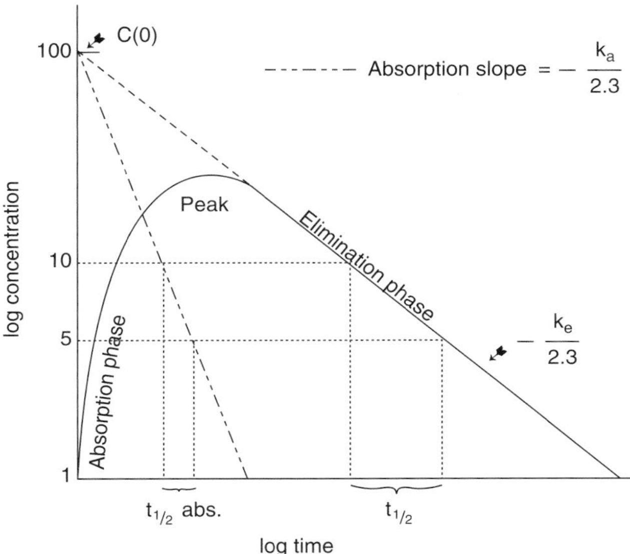

Fig. 14-7 One-compartment model blood level–time curve after extravascular administration, with monoexponential slopes for elimination, k_e, and absorption, k_a. (*From Ritschel WA:* Graphic Approach to Clinical Pharmacokinetics, *Barcelona, 1983, Prous Science.*)

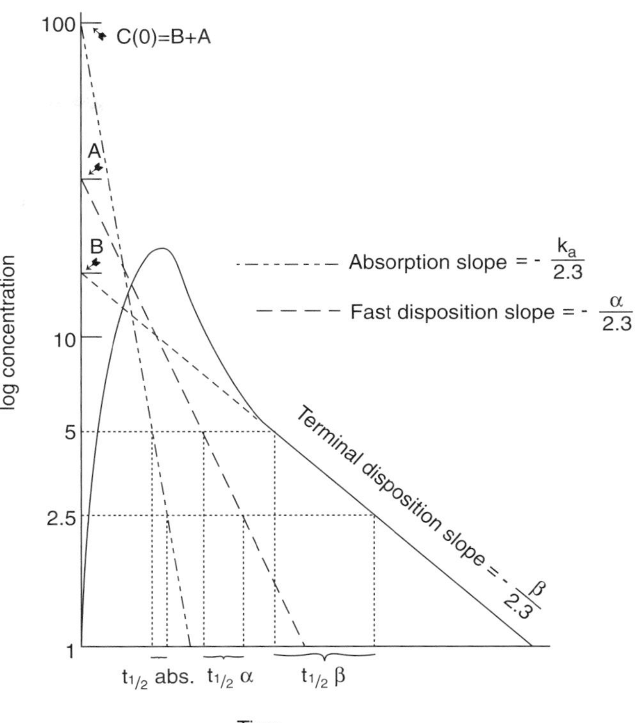

Fig. 14-8 Two-compartment model blood level–time curve after extravascular administration, with monoexponential slopes for slow disposition, β; fast disposition, α; and absorption, k_a. (*From Ritschel WA:* Graphic Approach to Clinical Pharmacokinetics, *Barcelona, 1983, Prous Science.*)

Clinically speaking, the concept of one-compartment and two-compartment models is usually satisfactory for therapeutic use. The difference between a one-compartment and a two-compartment model is that in the former, the distribution occurs instantly, whereas in the latter, the distribution process needs a measurable time before pseudoequilibrium is obtained.

Terminal Disposition Rate Constant

In the one-compartment open model, the last or terminal portion of the straight (monoexponential) slope of a semilog blood level–time curve gives the overall elimination rate constant, k_e (metabolism, renal excretion, and other pathways of elimination). In the two-compartment model, it gives β, the slow-disposition rate constant (Figs. 14-7 and 14-8).

Zero-Time Blood Level

Back extrapolation of the blood level–time curve after intravenous administration results in the **zero-time blood level,** C_0. After extravascular administration, the "fictitious" zero-time blood level, C_0, is the intercept of the k_e slope with the ordinate on a semilog plot in the one-compartment model, and the sum of the intercepts A + B of the α and β slopes in the two-compartment model (see Figs. 14-7 and 14-8).

Absorption Rate Constant

The k_e slope is extrapolated back to time zero. This yields C_0, a theoretical concentration roughly equivalent to that obtained from an intravenous injection of the same amount of drug. By subtraction of the observed drug concentration during the absorption phase from the concentrations read from the back-extrapolated k_e slope, *residual* points are obtained. When plotted on semilog paper, they are described by a straight line, the slope of which is the **absorption rate constant** k_a (see Fig. 14-7) in the one-compartment model.

Elimination Half-Life

Whenever a monoexponential straight line is obtained, a drug's half-life can be calculated. Note the line describing the terms k_e and β in Figs. 14-7 and 14-8. Other half-lives frequently used are the absorption half-life ($t_{1/2}$abs) and the distribution half-life ($t_{1/2}$).

The terms *half-time, half-life, plasma half-life, elimination half-life,* and *biological half-life* often are used interchangeably. Half-life is equal to the time required for elimination of one-half the total dose of drug from the body. The elimination half-life, or plasma half-life, is the time required for the elimination of one-half the amount of drug that is in the blood (plasma or serum). In those instances in which the decline in drug concentration in all tissues does not parallel the decline in drug concentration in plasma, blood, or serum, the half-life and the elimination half-life will be different. Most statements on drug disposition refer to the elimination half-life. In Fig. 14-8, the elimination half-life ($t_{1/2}$β) is depicted graphically.

Volume of Distribution

The volume of distribution is not a real volume and usually has no relationship to any physiological space or body fluid volume. It is simply a term to make the mass-balance equation

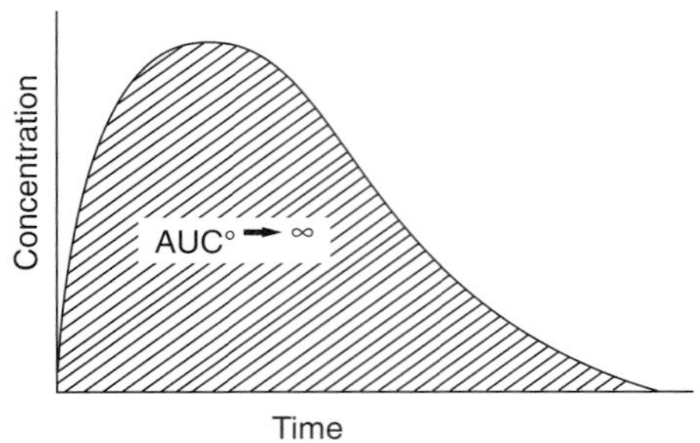

Fig. 14-9 Scheme of total area under the blood level–time curve. $AUC^{0 \to \infty}$, Area under curve from time = 0 to time = ∞. (*From Ritschel WA:* Graphic Approach to Clinical Pharmacokinetics, *Barcelona, 1983, Prous Science.*)

(see Eq. 14-4) valid. On intravenous administration, the amount of drug in the body is known; however, only the blood can be sampled. Because an amount of drug, *A*, equals the product of concentration and volume (μg/mL × mL), the volume of distribution is the hypothetical volume that would be required to dissolve the total amount of drug to achieve the same concentration as is found in blood.

The volume of distribution is expressed in milliliters. If this value is divided by the patient's body weight, the distribution coefficient, Δ′ is obtained in mL/g (or L/kg).

Area Under Blood Level–Time Curve

The integral under a blood level–time curve is a measure of the total amount of drug in the body. The area under the blood level–time curve (AUC) can be calculated from time zero to infinity. The AUC is shown in Fig. 14-9.

Total Clearance

The **total clearance** in pharmacokinetics describes how much of the volume of distribution of the drug is cleared per unit of time, regardless of the pathway for loss of drug from the body. In effect, it is the sum of all clearances by different pathways. The total clearance is the product of the apparent volume of distribution and the **terminal disposition rate constant.**

Steady State

Steady state refers to the accumulation of drug in the body in multiple dosing when input and output are equal within a dosing interval. The magnitude of accumulation depends on the drug's elimination half-life and the dosing interval. The smaller the dosing interval for a given dosage, the greater is the accumulation and the smaller is the fluctuation around the mean serum value. At steady state, the drug concentration oscillates around a mean steady-state concentration, C^{ss}_{av}, with a definite maximum steady-state concentration, C^{ss}_{max}, and a minimum steady-state concentration, C^{ss}_{min}. Only in the case of an intravenous constant rate infusion are C^{ss}_{max}, C^{ss}_{min}, and C^{ss}_{av} identical.

PHARMACOGENOMICS

Although it is now known that any two individuals are more than 99.9% identical in sequence of the human genome,[16] genetic variability can be individually important for drug absorption, drug metabolism, and drug interactions with receptors.[17] This forms the basis for slow and rapid drug absorption; poor, efficient, or ultrarapid drug metabolism; and poor or efficient receptor interactions. Furthermore, drug-drug and drug-food interactions can affect drug transport and metabolism.

Gene test–guided choice of therapy could facilitate the selection of a drug to which the patient responds best, as well as the optimal dose needed to avoid serious adverse reactions. A future goal is use of the patient's individual pharmacogenetic data as a further step toward personalized medicine. Genomic biomarkers of drug disposition have been listed by the U.S. Food and Drug Administration (FDA) and can be regarded as efficient tools for the evaluation of patient variability.[18] For all of the listed enzymes, polymorphisms have been described that are associated with changes in drug effects. The valid pharmacogenomic biomarkers listed in Table 14-2 include enzymes of phase I and II metabolism. Phase I reactions involve modifications of functional groups (e.g., oxidation, hydrolysis, reduction, *N*-desalkylation). Phase II reactions comprise conjugation reactions with endogenous substituents (e.g., glucuronidation, acetylation, methylation). A selection of drugs whose metabolism can be affected by the polymorphism of these enzymes is given in Table 14-2. Mutations that result in a loss of function of these enzymes result in an accumulation of drugs metabolized by these enzymes with the risk of adverse events. Individuals who are homozygous for such mutations are genotypically characterized as poor metabolizers (PMs). In the case of *CYP2D6*, ultrarapid metabolizers (UMs) can also occur as the result of gene duplications. The frequency of variant alleles can differ among ethnic groups (e.g., Africans, Asians, Caucasians). For all of the listed

Table 14-2 Valid Pharmacogenomic Biomarkers

Gene*	Drugs
CYP 2C9	Warfarin, celecoxib
CYP 2C19	Voriconazole, omeprazole, diazepam
CYP 2D6	Atomoxetine, risperidone, tamoxifen, fluoxetine
DPD	Capecitabine, fluorouracil
NAT	Rifampin, isoniazid
TPMT†	Azathioprine, mercaptopurine, thioguanine
UGT1A1†	Irinotecan
*HLA-B*5701*	Abacavir
VKORC1	Warfarin Phenprocoumon

Table adapted from U.S. Food and Drug Administration (FDA). Table of valid genomic biomarkers in the context of approved drug labels. Available at http://www.fda.gov/cder/genomics/genomic_biomarkers_table.htm. Accessed October 2008.

DPD, Dihydropyrimidine dehydrogenase; *NAT, N*-acetyltransferase (slow and fast acetylators); *TPMT,* thiopurine methyltransferase; *UGT 1A1,* uridine diphosphate–glucuronosyltransferase 1A1.

*CYP (cytochrome P450) isoenyzmes are a group of heme-containing enzymes that oxidize many drugs. The root nomenclature is CYP, the family number is followed by the subfamily and the gene; thus *CYP 2C9.*

†Testing recommended by FDA.

enzymes, genotyping is possible. Testing is recommended by the FDA for *TPMT* and *UGT 1A1*. For *TPMT*, in addition to genotyping, phenotyping has been successfully applied as a routine test. As an example of the necessity of pharmacogenetic testing, TPMT deficiency can be associated with azathioprine intolerance. In patients with homozygous TPMT deficiency (1 in 200), a standard therapeutic oral dosage of azathioprine results in 6-thioguanine nucleotide accumulation to toxic concentrations within 4 to 6 weeks. The consequences include severe myelosuppression leading to life-threatening pancytopenia.[19]

Drug disposition marker genotyping should be used in combination with TDM. It is an additional tool for dosage individualization and can be helpful in improving drug efficacy and safety. In a broader perspective, **pharmacogenomics** in the future may help to define subgroups of patients who will benefit from targeted therapy.[20]

KEY CONCEPTS BOX 14-3

- Pharmacokinetics is the study of drug disposition in the body via the use of mathematics, allowing the clinician to set appropriate dosing schedules for patients, while taking the biochemistry of the drug and the patient's condition into account.
- Genetic variability in enzymes necessary for the metabolism of drugs affects how different patients respond to drug therapies.
- Pharmacogenomics may allow drug therapy to be tailored to individuals particular set of genes that control the LADME system, leading to safer and more efficacious drug therapy regimens.

SECTION OBJECTIVES BOX 14-4

- List clinical indications for therapeutic drug monitoring.
- Explain why the sampling time of drug levels is vital for the proper interpretation of clinical response.
- Explain reasons why the frequency of drug monitoring varies from drug-to-drug or patient-to-patient.
- List indications for and likely drugs to be included in a STAT analysis protocol.
- List common causes for higher-than-expected or lower-than-expected drug concentrations.

APPLICATION OF PHARMACOKINETICS TO TDM

Clinical Assessment

Clinical (physician) estimation of patient response to a drug is the first and most important task in therapeutic monitoring. It must be remembered that therapy requires an approach that considers all aspects of a patient's condition, including the disease symptoms; the disease itself; other diseases present; and the patient's physical condition, age, nutritional status, and psychological aspects. Furthermore, it must be remembered that clinical pharmacokinetics is only a tool that can assist with but never substitute for clinical evaluation.

Box 14-3
Clinical Settings Requiring Therapeutic Drug Monitoring

- Suspected drug overdose*
- Lack of therapeutic effect
- Compliance problems
- Toxic effects not easily differentiated from disease-specific symptoms
- Drug interaction or multidrug therapy
- Drug used as a prophylactic
- Disease state that alters pharmacokinetic response
- Dosage optimization in the critically ill patient*
- Unknown medication (as in a comatose patient)*
- Leucovorin rescue therapy during treatment with high-dose methotrexate*

*Indications for measuring drug levels in the stat laboratory.

Application

The clinical evaluation of patient response is composed of the evaluation of vital signs and change of symptoms in response to the drug therapy, such as blood pressure, pulse rate, electrocardiogram, edema, and urinary output. Furthermore, supportive laboratory analyses, such as serum glucose and electrolyte levels, may be required. In all these cases, the pharmacological response is evaluated clinically, either as a direct measurement of pharmacological effect or as a measurement of body constituents, but not by the measurement of drug concentration in biological fluid.

Limitations

Sometimes the clinical evaluation might be difficult because of the presence of two or more disease states with similar or overlapping symptoms, polypharmacy (many drugs given simultaneously), or unexpected results. Unexpected results that might occur are that (1) the patient is not responding as expected, showing either no effectiveness or limited effectiveness of therapy; or (2) the patient may exhibit unexpected toxicity or side effects.

A drug may be less effective than expected because (1) the drug has a low bioavailability, (2) the patient is not complying with the prescribed drug regimen, or (3) a malabsorption syndrome exists and less of the drug than expected is being absorbed. A patient may exhibit unexpected toxicity or side effects because of drug interactions, enzyme induction, enzyme inhibition, renal or hepatic impairment, edema, and dehydration. In these cases, it is advisable, when possible, to request drug monitoring in biological samples (Box 14-3, Fig. 14-10).

Assessment by Drug Analysis

For those drugs for which there is knowledge of dose response and toxicity, the need for monitoring is dependent on patient clinical status. A set of guidelines for TDM services has been proposed.[21]

Clinical indications for the need to have information on drug concentrations are presented in Box 14-3. In the prophy-

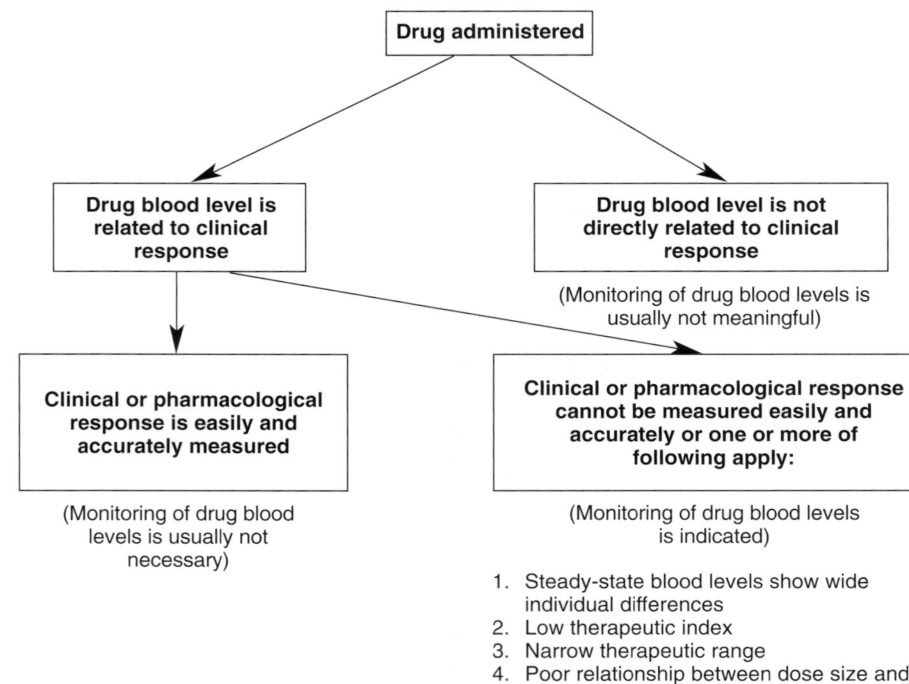
Drug administered
Drug blood level is related to clinical response
Drug blood level is not directly related to clinical response
(Monitoring of drug blood levels is usually not meaningful)
Clinical or pharmacological response is easily and accurately measured
Clinical or pharmacological response cannot be measured easily and accurately or one or more of following apply:
(Monitoring of drug blood levels is usually not necessary)
(Monitoring of drug blood levels is indicated)
1. Steady-state blood levels show wide individual differences
2. Low therapeutic index
3. Narrow therapeutic range
4. Poor relationship between dose size and blood level
5. Suspected bioavailability problem
6. Suspected malabsorption
7. Toxic effects not easily differentiated from disease symptoms
8. Drug used as a prophylactic
9. Suspected poor compliance
10. Suspected tolerance
11. Suspected drug interaction
12. Polypharmacy therapy
13. Renal impairment for drugs predominantly eliminated in unchanged form by the kidneys
14. Liver impairment for drugs that are predominantly eliminated by hepatic metabolism

Fig. 14-10 Scheme to identify cases and situations for which drug monitoring is indicated. (Modified from Pippenger CE: *Ther Drug Monit* 1:3, 1979.)

lactic application of drugs, for example, it is essential to know whether the drug concentration is in the desired therapeutic range to prevent disease symptoms. One example is determination of theophylline levels to ascertain whether they are in the range that prevents asthmatic attacks. A further example is the optimization of immunosuppressive regimens for which prophylaxis of acute rejection is required.[2]

Knowledge of drug concentrations is critical for patient management when symptoms resulting from drug toxicity and underlying disease are similar. Premature ventricular contractions, for example, can indicate either digitalis toxicity or intrinsic heart disease. High levels of quinidine or procainamide can induce ventricular arrhythmias similar to the ones controlled by these drugs. Tachycardia cannot be used in the diagnosis of a theophylline overdose because tachycardia is present in patients with severe respiratory obstruction. Toxic doses of phenytoin can cause seizures that are symptomatic of the underlying epilepsy.

Measurement of serum drug levels is required to optimize drug dosage in cases in which drug interactions are suspected, or for those drugs that have considerable interindividual pharmacokinetic variability. It must be stressed that in many severely ill patients, abnormal drug absorption, protein binding, and drug elimination can change the effective drug concentration or allow potentially active metabolites to accumulate. Determination of drug concentrations is necessary when a change in bioavailability is suspected, or when persistent adverse effects occur. Monitoring is also necessary to avoid toxicity such as that seen in patients undergoing high-dose methotrexate therapy, in whom severe adverse reactions usually are avoidable if the dosage of the antidote, leucovorin, is adjusted according to methotrexate serum concentrations.

Basis for Monitoring

For monitoring, it is essential to fulfill certain requirements. Otherwise, any evaluation will be in error[22]:

1. The dose size, dosage form, and route of administration must be known.
2. The dosage regimen must be followed.
3. The time between administration of the last dose and drawing of the blood sample must be known.
4. The blood sampling time or times must be recorded exactly.
5. The sampling times must be appropriate.

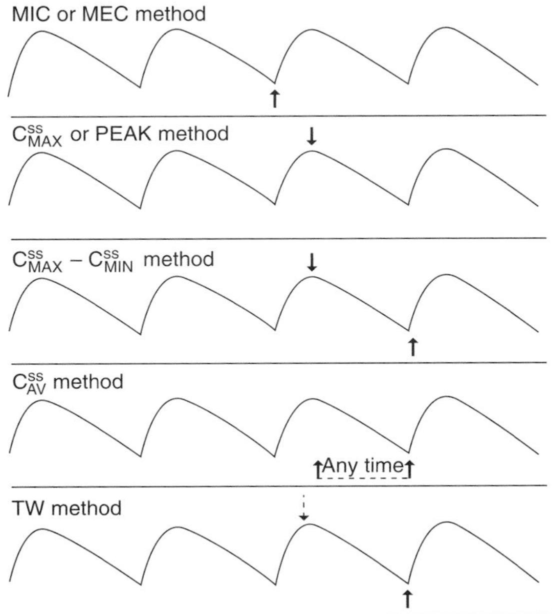

Fig. 14-11 Scheme showing optimal sampling times for monitoring for different methods used for dosage regimens.

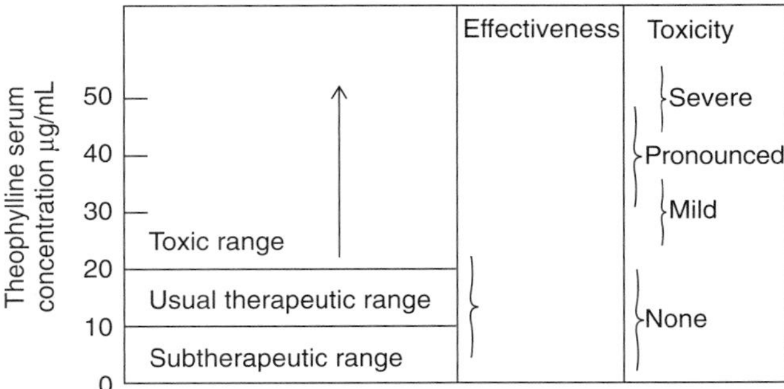

Fig. 14-12 Relationship between serum theophylline concentration and effectiveness and toxicity.

Most of the requirements listed above are self-explanatory. To understand item 5, remember that any samples taken during the absorption or distribution phase are useless for monitoring. Samples taken at peak time allow only an approximation of pharmacokinetic data. Samples taken at peak time and during the terminal elimination phase will result in an overestimation of the elimination rate constant and an underestimation of the elimination half-life.

Optimal sampling times for the various dosage regimen methods are shown in Fig. 14-11. Sampling times and therapeutic ranges of commonly monitored drugs are listed in Table 14-1.[23]

Limitations

The ability to monitor a specific drug in a blood sample sometimes can be limited because (1) accurate information about times of drug administration and blood drawing is not available, (2) a reliable assay method is not available, and (3) laboratory analysis time is not reasonable. Most difficulties experienced in monitoring are caused by limited or inaccurate information. Precision of the assay also must be considered. The coefficient of variation of an assay can be important when the drug concentration is found to be at the lower or the upper end of the therapeutic range. The therapeutic ranges reported in Table 14-1 are applicable to most patients; the therapeutic or toxic concentration may be different for a particular patient (Fig. 14-12).

Sampling

For most drugs, either plasma or serum samples are used to determine circulating levels of the drug. However, in the case of cyclosporine and tacrolimus,[1,2] whole blood is the preferred matrix. The recommended sampling times of commonly monitored drugs are presented in Table 14-1. The specimen has to be accompanied by a request form that provides demographic data on the patient and the collection date and time. Data on dose amount, dose interval, time of last dose, route of administration, and other medications also should be included.

Frequency of Drug Monitoring

In addition to the acute care cases described earlier, the frequency of monitoring will depend on the clinical situation of the patient, the experience of the physician, whether serum concentrations have reached steady state, and the half-life of the drug.

In the case of critically ill patients who are being treated with drugs that have rapid clearance changes, such as the aminoglycosides, daily modification of the drug dosage may be necessary. For other drugs such as cyclosporine, the variability in response and thus in dosage requirement means that blood level monitoring of this drug should start immediately after initiation of therapy. Monitoring of cyclosporine A in the early post-transplantation hospitalization period of liver, heart, and kidney transplants is done four to seven times per week. After intensive early monitoring, the measurement of cyclosporine blood levels can be reduced gradually, for example, in renal transplant recipients with an uncomplicated course, cyclosporine concentrations should be monitored once a month during the first year and at 1-month to 3-month intervals thereafter.[1] However, there are no hard and fast rules, and measurements should be performed if clinical signs or symptoms indicate that dosage adjustment might be necessary.

Frequent monitoring often is required when optimizing drug dosage or initiating drug therapy. For example, frequent serum digoxin measurement (daily) early in the course of therapy is desirable in patients with moderate to severe renal failure because of the variability in both volume of distribution and elimination that is associated with diminished renal function. Knowledge of drug concentrations is particularly important when a loading dose is administered (e.g., sirolimus). Frequent measurements may be necessary to monitor the appropriateness of a modified dosage regimen or to follow the course of drug interaction–induced changes.

The frequency of monitoring usually is decreased for outpatients after a course of long-term drug therapy has been completed. Frequency is in part dependent on the drug. For theophylline, the narrow therapeutic index and the relationship of serum concentration to both efficacy and toxicity make measurement of serum concentrations an essential part of patient management. Serum concentrations of theophylline should be monitored during the initial phase until the steady state has been reached and then at regular intervals (such as 6 to 12 months) thereafter. Serum concentrations of phenytoin should be measured after initiation of therapy to determine whether a therapeutic serum concentration has been achieved. Measurements can be made 2 weeks to 1 month after initiation of therapy because a steady state is generally reached by this time. In case of dosage changes, subsequent control of the drug concentration should be verified after an additional four to five half-lives have elapsed.

The measured concentration should be used with relevant clinical information to decide whether an adjustment in the daily dose is required. In patients with therapeutic failure, signs of drug overdose, or suspected noncompliance, an immediate response is indicated to obtain an appropriate measurement of serum drug concentration.

High-dose methotrexate therapy requires serial monitoring of serum concentrations during the leucovorin rescue phase because the dose of leucovorin needed depends on the serum methotrexate level. In patients with normal renal function, it is usually sufficient to measure serum methotrexate levels at 24, 48, and 72 hours.

Turnaround Times

For the drugs listed in Table 14-1, a same-day analytical service is feasible. When dosage adjustment is necessary, the results of serum or blood drug concentration measurements will be required before the next dose is administered. When aminoglycoside levels are ordered as peaks and troughs, it is more accurate and efficient to obtain both specimens during the same dosing interval. The laboratory then can measure both peak and trough levels in the analytical batch to minimize variance. This immediate response often allows the laboratory to give results to the physician on the same day, thus allowing sufficient time to establish a new regimen.

Stat Analyses

In certain clinical situations, prompt determination of serum drug levels may be necessary. Some of the most important indications for the rapid measurement of serum drug concentrations are indicated in Box 14-3, and the drugs most likely to require monitoring in the stat laboratory are listed in Box 14-4. The drugs requiring analysis in the stat laboratory can be divided into two categories depending on the urgency of the analysis. In the case of a suspected drug overdose, that is, a potentially life-threatening situation, an immediate analysis should be carried out. One example is measurement of tricyclic antidepressants that may be used in suicide attempts. Drug levels that include parent and metabolite are useful for clarification of intoxication with these drugs.

There are occasions for which analyses outside of the usual routine laboratory working hours are necessary. Examples include treatment with aminoglycosides, in which urgent determination of serum drug levels is performed in critically ill patients for whom an individual dosage adjustment is necessary; specific treatment protocols for high-dose methotrexate with leucovorin rescue, which may require the off-hour determination of serum methotrexate concentrations; and cyclosporine and tacrolimus levels, which may be required 6 to 7 days a week.

Box 14-4

Drugs for Which Analyses Should Be Available in the Stat Laboratory

Stat Analyses in Suspected Drug Overdose

- Theophylline
- Digoxin
- Phenytoin, phenobarbital, carbamazepine
- Salicylic acid, acetaminophen
- Lithium, tricyclic antidepressants, barbiturates, benzodiazepines

Other Analyses

- Tobramycin, amikacin, gentamicin, netilmicin
- Cyclosporine, tacrolimus
- Methotrexate

Critical Value Callback

It is sometimes necessary to communicate urgently a critical drug concentration to the clinician or health care provider. Critical values include high concentrations associated with enhanced risk of toxicity for that particular drug (see Table 14-1), or low concentrations that are inadequate to achieve the desired therapeutic effect. The usual practice is to exclude analytical error by checking the internal quality control used in the analytical run for the assayed specimen and to exclude possible preanalytical errors (such as inverted peak and trough values that may result from mislabeling of sample, inappropriate time of sampling, or specimen taken from same infusion line used to administer the drug) as possible causes of unexpected serum drug concentrations.

Assessment by Pharmacokinetic Calculations

To evaluate blood samples pharmacokinetically, it must be known whether the drug concentration is at steady state. To decide whether a steady state has been achieved, the dosage regimen (dose size and dosing interval) and how long this dosage regimen has been in effect must be known. Usually, it is assumed that a steady state is reached when the dosage regimen has been implemented for a time greater than four times the drug's elimination half-life. If the regimen has been in effect for less than $4t_{1/2}$, the number of doses given before the sample was obtained should be known. With the use of classic pharmacokinetic equations, what the drug concentration should be can be calculated, based on mean pharmacokinetic parameters from the literature and on patient information (age, body weight, sex, height, renal status, and so on). The purpose of drug monitoring is to compare the observed drug concentration versus the expected or desired one. The observed concentration may be equal to, smaller than, or greater than the desired one. In the latter two cases, an adjustment of the dosage regimen may be indicated and recommended.[23]

If C_x (the measured drug concentration) differs from the desired concentration (such as $C^{ss}_{av\ des}$ or $C^{ss}_{max\ des}$), a reason for the deviation should be sought. Some general and probable causes are presented here.

A concentration higher than the expected one could be associated with increased bioavailability of a drug of generally low bioavailability (e.g., cimetidine increases the bioavailability of propranolol), patient noncompliance (i.e., use of more drug or shorter dosage intervals than prescribed), decreased total clearance (as occurs with renal or liver failure and acute congestive heart failure), or increased protein binding. A concentration lower than expected could result from decreased bioavailability (possible drug interaction), insufficient drug dosing (longer dosing intervals, missed doses, or noncompliance), increased total clearance (drug interaction or enzyme induction), or decreased protein binding.

Estimates of the dose required to achieve a drug concentration in the therapeutic range have been tabulated on the basis of levels found in test populations. The use of this information is termed *population-based pharmacokinetic dosing*. These estimates, which are available in the form of tables or nomograms, allow the clinician to choose a dose based on certain features of the patient (such as age, diseases, smoking habits). Although these procedures are inexpensive, they often have a large prediction error. Therefore, prediction methods that allow estimation of drug clearance from a few drug concentration measurements on an individual have been developed to facilitate individual dosage adaptation.

Adjustment of Dosage at Steady State

Clearance is the most important parameter to be considered in designing a rational dosage regimen. At steady state, clearance can be estimated easily by dividing the dosing rate by the average steady-state serum drug concentration. For those drugs that have a clearance that is linearly proportional to dosage, a new dose (DN) to achieve the desired concentration can be calculated from the actual dosage (DA), the actual steady-state serum drug concentration (CA), and the desired serum drug concentration (CN), according to the following equation:

$$\mathrm{DN} = \frac{\mathrm{DA}}{\mathrm{CA}} \times \mathrm{CN} \qquad \text{Eq. 14-5}$$

For practical purposes, the trough concentrations rather than the average steady-state concentrations generally are employed. The use of Equation 14-5 is limited in patients whose LADME parameters are at the extremes of the usual patient range. In these cases, peak and trough levels may not change in a linear manner after a dosage adjustment, and more sophisticated methods based on a small number of consecutive serum concentration measurements are used to estimate individual pharmacokinetic parameters. These estimates are used to predict the optimal dosing scheme when measurements are made under non–steady state conditions, or when drugs are used whose elimination cannot be described by first-order kinetics.

Three-Point Method of Sawchuk

The dosage prediction method of Sawchuk requires determination of (1) a predose level, (2) a drug concentration obtained 30 minutes after the end of a constant-rate IV infusion, and (3) an additional concentration measured 1 hour before the next dose.[24] If a one-compartment model is assumed, the elimination-rate constant can be estimated from the slope of the concentration-time curve (see Fig. 14-7). The distribution volume, V_d, then can be calculated from the dosage, *D;* the duration of constant-rate infusion, *t;* the elimination-rate constant, *k;* the predose level, C_0; and the theoretical initial concentration, *C*, according to the following equation:

$$V_d = \frac{D}{t \times k} \times \frac{(1 - e^{-kt})}{(C \times e^{-kt} - C_0 \times e^{-kt})} \qquad \text{Eq. 14-6}$$

The clearance, CL, then is the product of the elimination-rate constant, *k*, and the distribution volume, V_d.

Bayesian Forecasting

The clearance and distribution volume of an individual patient can be derived through application of the Bayes formula to a pharmacokinetic parameter estimation.[25] This approach uses previously obtained information on the distribution range of pharmacokinetic parameters within the population combined with data on one or more serum drug concentrations observed in the test individual. Estimates of pharmacokinetic parameters in the individual patient are obtained from the Bayes formula. These estimates can be improved by taking into account patient-specific data (such as age, sex, disease, and medications). Given a patient data set, a best fit is obtained for possible clearance and distribution volume values. Bayesian drug-dosing programs are now available and have been applied to various drugs.[26-28] Use of clinical pharmacokinetic service recommendations has led to lower direct costs of hospitalization, including reduction in hospital stay, illustrating the cost-savings effect achieved through rational use of TDM predictive models.[29]

QUALITY ASSURANCE

Quality control programs use commercially available quality control materials and proficiency testing programs for TDM. TDM differs from other clinical chemistry testing in that the level of analyte is achieved by changing the dose. It is common practice that laboratories involved in therapeutic drug monitoring regularly participate in national and international proficiency testing schemes.

FUTURE PROSPECTS

The number of drugs that must be monitored to optimize therapy continues to grow as new agents are approved for human use.[23] Individualization of therapy based on an understanding of the patients' pharmacogenomics will complement drug monitoring.[17,20]

Finally, new biomarkers related to pharmacodynamics may serve as an adjunct to drug concentration monitoring to achieve the goal of optimal individually tailored pharmacotherapy.[30]

KEY CONCEPT BOX 14-4

- Clinical reasons for requiring TDM include when the clinical response to a drug is not easily determined, there are large inter-individual variation in response to a drug, low therapeutic index, patient has another condition that might affect FADME system.
- Proper interpretation of drug levels reported by the clinical laboratory depends on knowledge of the drug's pharmacokinetics, proper sampling time, timely analysis and reporting, and sound quality assurance practices.
- The type of drug (e.g., therapeutic index) and the clinical situation (i.e., overdose, pediatric patient) may require stat response times and physician call back of TDM results.

REFERENCES

1. Oellerich M, Armstrong VW, Kahan B, et al: Lake Louise Consensus Conference on cyclosporin monitoring in organ transplantation: report of the consensus panel, Ther Drug Monit 17:642, 1995.
2. Oellerich M, Armstrong VW: The role of therapeutic drug monitoring in individualizing immunosuppressive drug therapy: recent developments, Ther Drug Monit 28:720, 2006.
3. Mahalati K, Belitsky P, Sketris I, et al: Neoral monitoring by simplified sparse sampling area under the concentration-time curve: its relationship to acute rejection and cyclosporine nephrotoxicity early after kidney transplantation, Transplantation 68:55, 1999.
4. van Gelder T, Smak Gregoor PJH, Weimar W: Therapeutic drug monitoring of mycophenolate mofetil in transplantation, Ther Drug Monit 28:145, 2006.
5. Belitsky P, Dunn S, Johnston A, et al: Impact of absorption profiling on efficacy and safety of cyclosporin therapy in transplant recipients, Clin Pharmacokinet 39:117, 2000.
6. Matzuk MM, Shlomchik M, Shaw LM: Making digoxin therapeutic drug monitoring more effective, Ther Drug Monit 13:215, 1991.
7. Baumann P, Hiemke C, Ulrich S, et al: The AGNP-TDM expert group consensus guidelines: therapeutic drug monitoring in psychiatry, Pharmacopsychiatry 37:243, 2004.
8. Turnidge J: Pharmacodynamics and dosing of aminoglycosides, Infect Dis Clin North Am 17:503, 2003.
9. Loebstein R, Koren G: Clinical pharmacology and therapeutic drug monitoring in neonates and children, Pediatr Rev 19:423, 1998.
10. Soldin SJ, Steele BW: Mini-review: therapeutic drug monitoring in pediatrics, Clin Biochem 33:333, 2000.
11. Tenge SM, Soldin S, editors: *Guidelines for the Evaluation and Management of the Newborn Infant,* Washington, DC, 1999, NACB.
12. Oellerich M, Armstrong VW: Prodrug metabolites: implications for therapeutic drug monitoring, Clin Chem 47:805, 2001.
13. Ritschel WA, Kearns GL: *Handbook of Basic Pharmacokinetics Including Clinical Applications,* ed 7, Washington, DC, 2009, American Pharmacists Association.
14. Benet LZ, Hoener BA: Changes in plasma protein binding have little clinical relevance, Clin Pharmacol Ther 71:115, 2002
15. Ritschel WA: The effect of aging on pharmacokinetics: a scientist's view of the future, Contemp Pharm Pract 5:209,1982.
16. Venter JC, Adams MD, Myers EW, et al: The sequence of the human genome, Science 291:1304, 2001. Erratum in Science 292:1838, 2001.
17. Eichelbaum M, Ingelman-Sundberg M, Evans WE: Pharmacogenomics and individualized drug therapy, Annu Rev Med 57:119, 2006.
18. U.S. Food and Drug Administration (FDA): Table of valid genomic biomarkers in the context of approved drug labels. Available at http://www.fda.gov/cder/genomics/genomic_biomarkers_table.htm. Accessed October 2007.
19. Schütz E, Gummert J, Mohr F, et al: Azathioprine-induced myelosuppression in thiopurine methyltransferase deficient heart transplant recipient, Lancet 341:436, 1993.
20. Evans WE, McLeod HL: Pharmacogenomics—drug disposition, drug targets, and side effects, N Engl J Med 348:538, 2003.
21. Warner A, Annesley T, editors: *Guidelines for Therapeutic Drug Monitoring Services,* Washington, DC, 1999, NACB.
22. Hassan FM, Pesce AJ, Ritschel WA: Pitfalls and errors in drug monitoring: analytical aspects, Methods Find Exp Clin Pharmacol 5:567, 1983.
23. Burton ME, Shaw LM, Schentag JJ, et al, editors: *Applied Pharmacokinetics and Pharmacodynamics: Principles of Therapeutic Drug Monitoring,* ed 4, Philadelphia, 2006, Lippincott Williams & Wilkins.
24. Sawchuk RJ, Zaske DE, Cipolle RJ, et al: Kinetic model for gentamicin dosing with the use of individual patient parameters, Clin Pharmacol Ther 21:362, 1977.
25. Sheiner LB, Rosenberg B, Melmon KL: Modelling of individual pharmacokinetics for computer-aided drug dosage, Comput Biomed Res 5:411, 1972.
26. Böttger HC, Oellerich M, Sybrecht GW: Use of aminoglycosides in critically ill patients: individualization of dosage using Bayesian statistics and pharmacokinetic principles, Ther Drug Monit 10:280, 1988.
27. Pryka RD, Rodvold KA, Garrison M, et al: Individualizing vancomycin dosage regimens: one- versus two-compartment Bayesian models, Ther Drug Monit 11:450, 1989.
28. Le Meur Y, Büchler M, Thierry A, et al: Individualized mycophenolate mofetil dosing based on drug exposure significantly improves patient outcomes after renal transplantation, Am J Transplant 7:2496, 2007.
29. van Lent-Evers NA, Mathôt RA, Geus WP, et al: Impact of goal-oriented and model-based clinical pharmacokinetic dosing of aminoglycosides on clinical outcome: a cost-effectiveness analysis, Ther Drug Monit 21:63, 1999.
30. Oellerich M, Barten MJ, Armstrong VW: Biomarkers: the link between therapeutic drug monitoring and pharmacodynamics, Ther Drug Monit 28:35, 2006.
31. Morrisett JD, Abdel-Fattah G, Hoogeveen R, et al: Effects of sirolimus on plasma lipids, lipoprotein levels, and fatty acid metabolism in renal transplant patients. J Lipid Res 43:1170, 2002.

INTERNET SITES

iatdmct.org—International Association of Therapeutic Drug Monitoring and Clinical Toxicology

www.sfaf.org—Description of TDM by San Francisco AIDS Foundation

Therapeutic Drug Monitoring Lab Tests – http://www.labtestsonline.org/understanding/analytes/thdm/glance.html accessed October 2008

MedlinePlus – http://www.nlm.nih.gov/medlineplus/ency/article/003430.htm; accessed October 2008

Why do therapeutic drug monitoring? – http://www.pharmj.com/pdf/cpd/pj_20040731_pharmacokinetics03.pdf

Clinical Enzymology

David C. Hohnadel

Chapter 15

Chapter Outline

The Nature of Enzymes
- *Composition and Structure*
- *Apoenzymes and Cofactors*
- *Catalysts*
- *Reactive Sites*
- *Specificity of Reaction*
- *Subunit Structure*
- *Anabolism and Catabolism*

Enzyme Classification
- *International Union of Biochemistry (IUB) Names and Codes*
- *Enzyme Commission (EC) Classification*
- *Nonstandard Abbreviations*

Measurement of Enzymes
- *Enzyme Assays*
- *Principles of Kinetic Analysis*
- K_m *and* V_{max}
- *Determination of Enzyme Activity*

Analytical Factors Affecting Enzyme Measurements
- *pH*
- *Buffer*
- *Cofactors*
- *Activators and Inhibitors*
- *Coupling Enzymes*
- *Temperature*
- *Defining Assay Conditions*
- *Enzymes as Reagents*
- *Storage of Enzymes*

Clinical Enzyme Measurements
- *Extracellular versus Cellular Enzymes*

Factors Affecting Reference Values
- *Sampling Time*
- *Age*
- *Sex*
- *Race*
- *Exercise*

Isoenzymes
- *Nomenclature*
- *Isoforms*

Key Terms

activation energy The energy required in a chemical reaction to convert reactants to activated or transition-state species that will spontaneously proceed to products.

activators Inorganic ions that are required cofactors for an enzyme reaction.

active sites The specific areas on an enzyme where a substrate binds and catalysis takes place.

activity The amount of substrate for a particular enzymatic reaction that is converted to product per unit time under defined conditions.

allosteric sites, or **regulatory sites** The sites of an enzyme, other than an active site or sites, that bind regulatory molecules and affect the activity of the enzyme.

apoenzyme An enzyme without associated cofactors or with less than the entire number of cofactors or prosthetic groups.

auxiliary enzyme In a coupled assay system, an enzyme that links the enzyme being measured with an indicator enzyme.

binding sites The sites on the surface of the enzyme that serve to bind the substrate or the product of the reaction.

bond specificity The nature of enzyme action that causes the disruption of only certain bonds between atoms.

catalyst A substance that increases the rate of a reaction without being changed by the reaction.

catalytic site Another name for active site.

coenzymes Organic cofactor compounds, such as thiamine pyrophosphate and pyridoxyl-5-phosphate.

cofactors Nonprotein substances associated with an enzyme that are needed for catalytic activity.

competitive inhibitor An inhibitor of an enzyme reaction that competes with the substrate by binding at the active site.

constitutive enzymes Enzymes that are always present during the life of a cell.

coupled assay Assays with one or more auxilliary enzyme reaction that lead to an indicator reaction with an easily measured substance.

denaturation The loss of the biological properties of a protein, usually as a result of changes in tertiary or quaternary structure.

EC code The four-number Enzyme Commission (EC) code for the systematic classification of enzyme reactions.

ELISA Enzyme-linked immunosorbent assay.

EMIT Enzyme-multiplied immunoassay technique.

endopeptidases Protein-hydrolyzing enzymes that break bonds in the interior of a protein substrate.

enzyme kinetics The study of enzyme reaction rates and the factors that affect them.

enzyme specificity The degree to which an enzyme will catalyze one or more reactions.
enzyme-substrate complex An intermediate active complex formed between the substrate and the enzyme during the reaction.
enzymes Biological materials (usually proteins) with catalytic properties.
equilibrium constant The ratio of the concentration of product to the concentration of substrate when the reaction is at equilibrium.
exopeptidases Protein-hydrolyzing enzymes that break bonds proceeding from one end of the protein substrate toward the center of the substrate.
first order kinetic State that occurs when the rate of an enzyme reaction is proportional to the concentration of the substrate.
holoenzymes The complete enzyme-cofactor complex that gives full catalytic activity.
hydrophilic amino acids Polar, water-loving amino acids.
hydrophobic amino acids Nonpolar, water-hating amino acids.
in vitro systems Those systems outside of a living organism, that is, within a test tube.
inactivation The reversible denaturation of a protein.
indicator enzyme Enzyme that produces (or consumes) an easily measured substance.
inducible enzymes Enzymes whose cellular concentrations increase when presented with the appropriate stimulus.
inhibitors Materials that reduce the catalytic activity of an enzyme.
initial rates Enzyme measurements made at the start of a reaction just after the lag phase at zero-order kinetics.
International Unit of enzyme activity The amount of enzyme that catalyzes the conversion of one micromole of substrate per minute under defined conditions, $1 \text{ IU} = 1.67 \times 10^{-8}$ katal.
isoenzymes Different forms of an enzyme that catalyze the same reaction.
K_m The symbol for the Michaelis-Menten constant.
katal (kat, K) An enzyme unit in moles per second defined by the SI system: $1 \text{ K} = 6.0 \times 10^7$ U.
kinetic assays Assays that form increasing amounts of product with time, usually monitored by multiple data points.
labile enzymes Unstable or easily denatured proteins.
lag phase The early time in an assay when mixing occurs and temperature and kinetic equilibria are becoming established.
linear phase Time when an assay is following zero-order kinetics, producing a constant amount of product per unit of time.
metalloenzymes Enzymes that contain very tightly bound metal ions.
Michaelis-Menten constant A constant related to the rate constants of an enzyme reaction and equal to the concentration of substrate that gives one-half the maximal catalytic velocity.
noncompetitive inhibitor An inhibitor that binds to an allosteric site of an enzyme and does not compete with the substrate by binding at the active site.
optimal assay conditions Conditions for reaction concentrations of substrates, cofactors, activators, and buffer that produce the maximum rate of enzyme catalysis.
primary structure The sequence of amino acids of a protein.
prosthetic groups Cofactors that are so tightly bound that they are considered to be part of the enzyme structure.
quaternary structure The structural relationship of various enzyme subunits to one another.
reactivation The restoration of the biological properties of a protein after a temporary loss.
regulatory sites See *allosteric sites.*
secondary structure The twisting of amino acids into a semifixed steric relationship in two dimensions.
stereoisomeric specificity The specificity of an enzyme for one form of a D-,L- pair of compounds with an asymmetrical carbon atom.
substrate-depletion phase The time late in an enzyme assay when the substrate concentration is falling and the assay is not following zero-order kinetics.
substrates The materials enzymes act upon.
subunits Single protein chains from enzymes composed of two or more peptide chains in an active form.
Système International d'Unités An international system of rational and internally consistent units for all types of scientific quantities; SI units.
tertiary structure The folding of amino acid chains into a three-dimensional structure.
uncompetitive inhibitor An inhibitor that appears to bind only to the enzyme-substrate complex and not to the free enzyme.
V_{max} The maximum rate of catalysis obtained from a variation of substrate.
zero-order kinetics State that occurs when the rate of an enzyme reaction is independent of the concentration of the substrate.

Methods on Evolve Website

Angiotensin converting enzyme (ACE)
Alanine aminotransferase (ALT)
Alkaline phosphatase (ALP)
Amylase
α1-antitrypsin

Aspartate aminotransferase (AST)
Cholinesterase
Creatine kinase (CK) and creatine kinase isoenzymes
Gamma-glutamyl transferase (GGT)
Lactate dehydrogenase (LD) and lactate dehydrogenase isoenzymes
Lipase

SECTION OBJECTIVES BOX 15-1

- Describe the composition and structure of enzymes.
- Describe the properties of catalysts.
- Describe the reactive site of enzymes, and explain how an enzyme can act as a catalyst.
- Describe the specificity of enzymes.

THE NATURE OF ENZYMES

Enzymes are biological materials with catalytic properties; that is, they increase the rate of chemical reactions in cells and in **in vitro systems** that otherwise proceed very slowly. Most of the enzymes in cells are **constitutive enzymes,** that is, they are always present, performing some metabolic function. Some tissues, notably the liver, also have enzymes, called **inducible enzymes,** that are not always present but are produced in response to a stimulus. The ingestion of certain drugs causes the liver to produce enzymes capable of metabolizing the drugs to a form that is more easily excreted than the parent compound. The changes in enzyme **activity** that occur in body fluids over time have become a valuable diagnostic tool for the elucidation of various disease states and for testing organ function.

Different tissues or cellular materials contain different quantities or types of enzymes. Cellular enzymes are attached to cell walls and membranes and are dissolved in the cytoplasm or in sequestered specialized subcellular organelles, including microsomes, mitochondria, nuclei, and lysosomes. Often the determination of one or several enzymes in plasma gives a pattern of activities that is indicative of the tissue or cell type from which the enzymes have been derived. Different cells or compartments within a single cell can even contain different forms of an enzyme that catalyzes the same chemical reaction. Assays for these different forms sometimes can be performed to determine the compartment from which an enzyme has come. A few enzymes are found in plasma or other extracellular fluids, where they seem to perform a physiological function, but the physiological function of most enzymes is to catalyze reactions inside cells or within the lumen of various organs.

Composition and Structure

(See Chapter 27, Part 1, Proteins.)
For the purposes of this discussion, enzymes are large, naturally occurring proteins (see p. 508) with molecular weight usually between 13,000 and 500,000 D. Chemically, they are complex compounds that contain quantities of carbon, hydrogen, oxygen, nitrogen, and sulfur that are similar to quantities found in other protein materials. Enzymes are distinguished from other proteins by their catalytic action.

The catalytic behavior of an enzyme is dependent on the **primary, secondary, tertiary,** and **quaternary structures** of the protein molecule, which are discussed on pp. 508 and 510. Changes to the primary amino acid sequence usually result in differences in the three-dimensional structure because secondary and tertiary types of folding are different. However, changes to any one of these structures can affect the enzymatic activity of the protein, usually reducing or abolishing it.

Apoenzymes and Cofactors

An enzyme may have nonprotein substances associated with it that are needed for maximal activity. These other materials, called **cofactors,** may be bound loosely or tightly to the protein portion of the enzyme. Those that are loosely bound often can be removed by dialysis. These materials may be organic compounds such as the oxidized form of nicotinamide adenine dinucleotide phosphate ($NADP^+$) and pyridoxyl-5-phosphate, which are called **coenzymes,** or inorganic ions like chloride (Cl^-) and magnesium (Mg^{2+}), which are called **activators.** Cofactors like the heme portion of peroxidase that are so tightly bound that they are considered to be an integral part of the enzyme structure are termed **prosthetic groups.** Enzymes that have metal ions bound very tightly are called **metalloenzymes.** Two examples of metalloenzymes are ferroxidase, also called *ceruloplasmin,* which contains a large amount of tightly bound copper, and carbonate dehydratase, also called *carbonic anhydrase,* which contains a large amount of zinc.

The term *coenzyme* is often used loosely when one is referring to the compound NADH (or NADPH) in a reaction like the lactate dehydrogenase (LD) reaction.

$$\text{Pyruvate} + \text{NADH} + \text{H}^+ \underset{}{\overset{\text{LD}}{\rightleftharpoons}} \text{L-Lactate} + \text{NAD}^+ \quad \text{Eq. 15-1}$$

In a formal kinetic sense, both pyruvate and NADH are **substrates** for the enzyme reaction, and lactate and NAD^+ are the products. In this case, pyruvate and NADH react with one another on a molar basis. For historical reasons, NADH is still called a coenzyme, that is, a nonprotein organic material needed for maximal activity, although it should be more correctly called a *second substrate,* or *co-substrate.*

Because it is possible to dialyze away loosely held cofactors from some enzymes and still retain some activity, an enzyme without associated cofactors is referred to as an **apoenzyme,** and the complete enzyme-cofactor complex is termed a **holoenzyme.** In the clinical use of enzyme assays, the enzyme assay mixture must contain an excess of all activators and cofactors to ensure that the holoenzyme is the enzyme form that is being measured, rather than a mixture of apoenzyme and holoenzyme forms.

Catalysts

Catalysts have the property of accelerating chemical reactions toward equilibrium without being consumed in the process.

The Gibbs free-energy change ($-\Delta G$) is the measure of the amount of work a chemical reaction can produce. All reactions that can proceed from reactants to products have a net negative free energy ($-\Delta G$). However, the reactants do not become products directly but must absorb enough energy to pass through an activated, or transition, state, in which molecular bonds are weakened. Without a catalyst present, even with a favorable negative free energy, that is, with products that have a G lower than that of substrates, the reaction may not proceed to any appreciable extent (Fig. 15-1). The reactants must gain the energy to overcome this **activation energy** barrier to enter the transition state (activated state) and then pass on to products. Without a catalyst present, the reaction will occur only if enough heat or energy of activation can be added to the reaction system. Catalysts lower the energy required for activation to the transition state, allowing ambient temperature to serve as the activation energy.

Enzymes function as biological catalysts. The material with which the enzyme reacts is termed the *substrate,* and a simple enzymatic reaction for one substrate and one product is listed below:

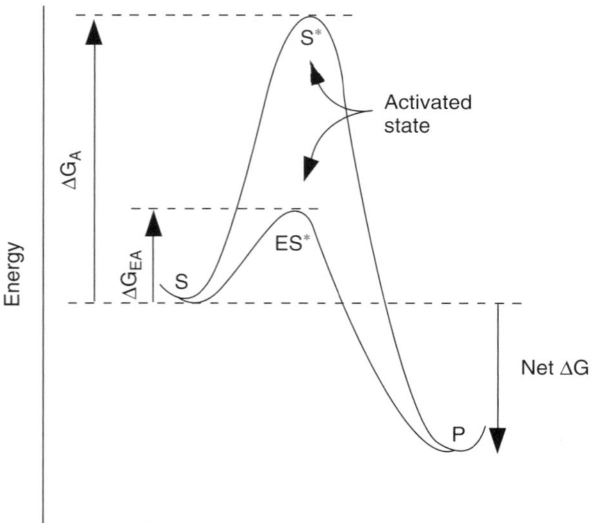

Fig. 15-1 Energy diagram showing reduction in activation energy $\Delta G_{EA} << \Delta G_A$ that occurs for same reaction with and without enzyme catalyst. *A,* Activated state (also *); *EA,* enzyme activation; *ES,* enzyme-substrate complex; *G,* Gibbs free energy; *P,* product; *S,* substrate.

$$E + S \underset{k_{-1}}{\overset{k_{+1}}{\rightleftharpoons}} \{ES\} \underset{k_{-2}}{\overset{k_{+2}}{\rightleftharpoons}} P + E \qquad \text{Eq. 15-2}$$

In this case, the enzyme is represented by *E,* the substrate on which the enzyme acts by *S,* a postulated enzyme-substrate intermediate complex by *{ES},* and the product of the reaction by *P.* The forward reaction rate constants are represented by k_{+1} and k_{+2}, whereas the reverse reaction rate constants are represented by k_{-1} and k_{-2}.

With an enzyme catalyst, the reaction may proceed easily at normal physiological temperatures. By rewriting Eq. 15-2 to account for this transition state in an enzyme-catalyzed reaction, we find that

$$E + S \underset{k-1}{\overset{k+1}{\rightleftharpoons}} \{ES \rightarrow ES^* \rightarrow EP\} \underset{k_{-2}}{\overset{k_{+2}}{\rightleftharpoons}} P + E \qquad \text{Eq. 15-3}$$

in which *ES** is the transition state form of the substrate with weakened covalent bonds, and *ES* and *EP* are enzyme-substrate and enzyme-product forms with materials bound but not activated. Substantial reductions in the activation energy requirements often are found when enzymes are used as catalysts for the process. For example, the activation energy necessary for the decomposition of hydrogen peroxide is 18,000 cal/mol, but in the presence of the enzyme catalase, the activation energy is less than 2000 cal/mol.

An example of a single-substrate enzyme reaction is the action of the enzyme urease on the substrate urea, although in this case, two products are produced:

$$\underset{\textbf{Urea}}{H_2N{-}\overset{\overset{\large O}{\|}}{C}{-}NH_2} + E \underset{k_{-1}}{\overset{k_{+1}}{\rightleftharpoons}} \{Urea - E\} \underset{k_{-2}}{\overset{k_{+2}}{\rightleftharpoons}} \underset{\textbf{Ammonia}}{2NH_3} + \underset{\textbf{Carbon dioxide}}{CO_2} + E$$

Although water is involved in this hydrolysis reaction, it usually is not considered a substrate. Enzymes are like other chemical catalysts in many respects, except that they function in biological systems. Enzyme catalysts, although they are unstable and are easily destroyed, have catalytic properties similar to those of other chemical catalysts (Box 15-1).

Because enzymes are effective in very small amounts, measurement of changes in enzyme concentrations is a very sensitive diagnostic tool for following changes that have occurred

Box 15-1
Properties of Enzymes as Catalysts

- They are effective in small concentrations.
- They are unchanged by the reaction.
- They affect the speed of attaining equilibrium at any given temperature.

but

- They do not change the final concentrations of substrates and products of the equilibrium state. They demonstrate greater specificity than the usual chemical catalysts for the reactions that they accelerate.

in various types of tissues. The amount of enzyme involved in an enzyme assay is very much smaller than the amount of glucose present in an assay for glucose. A conventional chemical assay for an enzyme would be very difficult to produce and would require large amounts of sample. Of the several thousand enzymes in plasma, the measurement of the concentration of a single enzyme, even if it is present at a very elevated value, is below the limit of detection for most chemical protein assays. What is easier to measure and is biologically related to many clinical conditions is the amount of catalytic activity of the enzyme and how it changes over time.

Another property of biological catalysts is that they accelerate the attainment of equilibrium but do not shift the final proportions of S and P in the equilibrium state. One way of considering this process is to examine the effect of lactate dehydrogenase on the conversion of pyruvate to lactate. In the presence of the enzyme LD and the coenzyme NADH, conversion of pyruvate to lactate and attainment of equilibrium occur in minutes. Without the enzyme, the process is so slow that it can hardly be demonstrated; it takes years:

$$\text{Pyruvate} + \text{NADH} + \text{H}^+ \underset{}{\overset{\text{LD}}{\rightleftharpoons}} \text{L-Lactate} + \text{NAD}^+$$

Equilibrium: achieved in minutes

$$\text{Pyruvate} + \text{NADH} + \text{H}^+ \underset{}{\overset{\text{No enzyme}}{\rightleftharpoons}} \text{L-Lactate} + \text{NAD}^+$$

Equilibrium: achieved in years

Note that this is not a one-way process but an approach to the equilibrium concentrations of pyruvate and lactate, because the same enzyme converts lactate to pyruvate with the coenzyme NAD^+. The speed of the reaction and the conditions employed are not the same in both directions, because they are related to the **equilibrium constant** (see below, p. 291). It is possible to measure the conversion from either direction, and both methods are widely used to determine LD activity in the clinical laboratory. Also note that although the times needed to achieve equilibrium greatly differ, when equilibrium is achieved, the final proportions of substrates and products will be the same under both conditions.

Reactive Sites

One of the most difficult problems that enzyme chemists had faced was to explain how an enzyme can reduce the activation energy and at the same time remain unchanged by the reaction. Our understanding is based on the knowledge that catalysts are surface-acting materials, that is, they work by adsorbing substrates onto their surfaces, where molecular interactions now can occur more easily (see ES* in Eq. 15-3). For a better understanding of the mechanisms of enzyme catalysis, an examination of the details of enzyme structure is therefore necessary.

A wide variety of nonpolar **hydrophobic** and polar **hydrophilic amino acids** are present in enzyme proteins (see Table 27-1, p. 291). The external surface of the enzyme for reasons of solubility is believed to be composed for the most part of polar but also of unreactive side chains of amino acids. The unreactive amino acid side chains may contain structures like the methyl and isopropyl groups found in alanine and leucine:

$$\text{R—CH}_3 \quad \text{and} \quad \text{R—}\underset{\displaystyle \text{CH}_3}{\underset{|}{\text{CH}}}\text{—CH}_3$$

Some areas of the enzyme surface contain amino acids with reactive side chains as a part of their structure. The reactive amino acid side chains may contain charged groups like carboxyl and amino groups (i.e., $R—COO^-$ and $R—NH_3^+$) found in aspartic and glutamic acids or lysine and arginine, respectively. Noncharged but highly polar moieties like the hydroxyl and sulfhydryl groups (i.e., R—OH and R—SH) found in serine, tyrosine, and cysteine are also reactive. Other types of reactive groups are present in amino acids, such as histidine, which has active nitrogen in a ring structure. A group of reactive amino acids that are relatively close together on the three-dimensional surface of an enzyme form part of an active **catalytic site,** attracting substrate, activator, and inhibitor molecules and adsorbing them onto the surface by ionic and hydrogen bonds. Areas on the surface of the enzyme that bind the molecules that participate in the reaction are termed **binding sites.** This adsorption process binds the substrate(s) in a specific way so as to lower the activation energy (E_A) for bond breaking, thus facilitating the breaking and forming of new bonds and causing the conversion from substrate to product. There are only a limited number of areas on the enzyme where catalysis can take place. These specific areas are called **active sites,** or active centers, and may involve only 5 to 10 amino acids out of a total of 200 to 300 in the entire enzyme.

When the substrate of an enzymatic reaction binds to the active site, it is oriented so that a particular covalent bond in the substrate interacts with the reactive side-chain moieties of other amino acids of the enzyme's active site, so that the covalent bond becomes weakened. This bond weakening decreases the activation energy needed for a chemical reaction. The weakened bond now undergoes a chemical reaction that breaks the covalent bond and allows new bonds to form. The product no longer has the same affinity for the active site as the original substrate and is released from the enzyme (see Color Plate 3).

The specific interactions between the substrate and reactive amino acids can be disrupted by such factors as heavy metals or detergents, which may bind to active groups and inactivate them, leading to loss of enzymatic activity. Changes in surface tension, that is, vigorous shaking, may cause unfolding of the protein's tertiary stucture, or **denaturation,** which can disrupt the close spatial relationships of the reactive amino acids , thus destroying the active site and preventing the usual reaction from taking place.

Enzymes, particularly those of a complex structure composed of several **subunits,** often have non-catalytic binding sites that are far removed from the amino acid sequence at the catalytic site but that nevertheless affect enzyme activity. These sites are called **allosteric sites,** or **regulatory sites.** When small molecules, often the product of the last of a series of related reactions, bind to the allosteric site, they cause a change in the three-dimensional structure of the enzyme, thereby changing (often inhibiting) the catalytic properties of the enzyme.

Changes in the amino acid sequence of a protein may produce different enzymes with different catalytic sites, or even similar proteins without any catalytic activity. Such changes, caused by genetic mutations, are often the cause of inborn errors of metabolism and other diseases of genetic origin (see Chapter 52).

Specificity of Reaction

Differences in **enzyme specificity** are believed to be related to physical differences at the active site. Some enzymes react with many related compounds and are said to have a broad substrate specificity. Acid phosphatase is one of the enzymes that exhibit a broad **bond specificity** by hydrolyzing several types of organic phosphate esters, such as β-glycerol phosphate, thymolphthalein phosphate, para-nitrophenyl phosphate, and α-naphthyl phosphate. At an acid pH, the enzyme-catalyzed reaction

$$R—O—P + H_2O \xrightarrow{\text{Acid phosphatase}} R—O—H + P_i$$

produces an organic alcohol and an inorganic phosphate.

Many enzymes that hydrolyze proteins also exhibit a broad bond specificity, hydrolyzing a large number and variety of peptide bonds within a protein substrate. If the peptide bonds of the substrate that are hydrolyzed are located on the inside of the protein chain, the enzyme is called an **endopeptidase,** such as pepsin A. Alternatively, carboxypeptidases are enzymes that act on protein substrates and cleave peptide bonds, starting from the outside carboxyl end of the substrate and moving toward the middle of the protein chain. These enzymes are termed **exopeptidases,** and they also demonstrate a broad substrate specificity.

In contrast to the broad specificity of many peptidases, other enzymes are more specific in their action; they will catalyze only a definite reaction with a few possible substrates. In extreme cases, an almost absolute specificity is demonstrated in which only a single compound will serve as a substrate, such as phosphoenolpyruvate for the pyruvate kinase reaction:

$$\begin{matrix} \text{Phosphoenolpyruvate} \\ \text{(PEP)} \\ + \\ \text{Adenosine diphosphate} \\ \text{(ADP)} \end{matrix} \overset{\text{PK}}{\rightleftharpoons} \begin{matrix} \text{Pyruvate} \\ \text{(PYR)} \\ + \\ \text{Adenosine triphosphate} \\ \text{(ATP)} \end{matrix}$$

Enzyme specificity should be described for each substrate involved in a reaction. In contrast to the absolute specificity shown for phosphoenolpyruvate in the pyruvate kinase reaction, several natural and synthetic nucleoside diphosphates, such as uridine diphosphate (UDP), inosine diphosphate (IDP), guanosine diphosphate (GDP), and cytidine diphosphate (CDP) will also serve as phosphate acceptors in the reaction in place of ADP. Thus, although an absolute specificity is shown for one substrate (PEP), an intermediate degree of specificity is shown for the other substrate (ADP).

An intermediate degree of specificity for each substrate is shown by the hexokinase reaction in which D-glucose and several other sugars may be phosphorylated, that is, D-mannose, 2-deoxy-D-glucose, and D-glucosamine. However, D-galactose and five-carbon sugars like D-xylose are not substrates. The enzyme also can use a variety of nucleoside triphosphates as phosphate donors, such as inosine triphosphate (ITP) and guanosine triphosphate (GTP), as well as adenosine triphosphate (ATP).

$$\left.\begin{matrix} \text{D-Glucose} \\ + \\ \text{Adenosine triphosphate} \\ \text{(ATP)} \end{matrix}\right\} \xrightarrow{\text{HK}} \left\{\begin{matrix} \text{Glucose-6-phosphate} \\ + \\ \text{Adenosine diphosphate} \\ \text{(ADP)} \end{matrix}\right.$$

Many enzymes demonstrate a **stereoisomeric specificity** for the L-form or the D-form of a pair of compounds. For example, hexokinase is absolutely specific for the D-form of glucose; the L-form is not a substrate. However, stereoisomeric specificity does not necessarily mean that the enzyme is absolutely specific; as was mentioned above, hexokinase functions with several D-form substrates.

Subunit Structure

Some enzymes occur in nature in several forms, that is, several forms of an enzyme all catalyze the same reaction. These are known as **isoenzymes,** or isozymes. In a few well-studied enzymes, it has been found that different forms of isoenzymes occur because the enzymes are composed of two or more different polypeptide chains, or subunits, bound into an active form. The subunits may have enzymatic activity, but alone do not have the catalytic properties of the whole enzyme. The isoenzymes may have different kinetic or other physical properties that allow the various forms to be separated or measured. Many of these features have been used to differentiate and characterize the various enzyme forms and to assay for their presence in a sample. Other types or classes of isoenzymes can occur and are considered in the section on isoenzymes (see p. 300), but clinically, the most widely used form is the subunit type of isoenzymes. See Chapter 16 for a discussion of isoenzymes.

Anabolism and Catabolism

The synthesis of all enzymes is assumed to occur by intracellular protein synthetic pathways within the tissues that contain the enzymes (see p. 299). Enzymes with an extracellular function, like those involved in the coagulation process or serum proteases, are synthesized in the liver and discharged into the plasma. In some cases, other organs, that is, the kidney, lung, and pancreas, also contribute to the extracellular enzyme pool. See further discussion on intracellular/extracellular changes in Chapter 16. The large size and complexity of the structure of enzymes result in molecular forms that are somewhat unstable and therefore are said to be **labile enzymes.** Many enzymes in vitro lose their catalytic activity with relatively slight changes in pH, temperature, or even salt concentration of the surrounding medium. It is presumed that similar processes occur intracellularly, and that constant synthesis of enzymes occurs in a steady-state fashion to maintain the required quantities of intracellular enzymes needed for intermediary metabolism.

A spontaneous loss of enzyme activity can be either reversible and temporary or irreversible and permanent. *Denaturation* is a process whereby biological properties are lost by a protein; in this case, enzyme activity is lost. It has been suggested that the denaturation process is an unfolding or "melting" of tightly coiled peptide chains, leading to loss of the organized tertiary structure that established the protein's function.

Much experimental support for this idea, including increased reactivity of side chains, changes in viscosity, and changes in the sedimentation behavior of the "melted" protein solutions, has been documented. *Irreversible denaturation* can occur when the enzyme protein chains unfold and are unable to refold to their biologically active form, or when a heavy metal ion (such as mercury or lead) or other material binds tightly at or near the active site. Many other factors and events can lead to denaturation and loss of activity, including changes in temperature, the addition of strong acids or bases, exposure to high pressure, treatment with ultraviolet rays, repeated freezing, the addition of detergents or organic solvents, or the presence of high concentrations of urea or guanidine.

A *reversible denaturation,* or loss of enzyme activity, is called **inactivation.** For example, inactivation can occur if an enzyme solution is allowed to remain for an extended time at room temperature and the enzyme partially loses activity. This temporary activity loss can have several causes, including heat instability with the breaking of hydrogen bonds or oxidation of sulfhydryl groups. In both of these cases, some loss of the natural structural form occurs. With some enzymes, reducing the temperature of the solution or adding a sulfhydryl reducing agent like dithiothreitol may allow the enzyme to refold to the original active form, with reformation of hydrogen bonds or reduction of oxidized sulfhydryl groups, thus producing a **reactivation** of the enzyme and a restoration of lost activity.

It is known that various enzymes have different half-lives (Table 15-1), an indication that several mechanisms of removal may be present. Extracellular proteases hydrolyze protein, thus inactivating enzymes that are lost from cells. The degraded inactive proteins then are removed by one of several excretory routes, that is, excretion in bile, the intestine, liver, kidney, or the reticuloendothelial system.

KEY CONCEPTS BOX 15-1

- Enzymes are proteins that act as catalysts, that is, they speed up biochemical reaction rates.
- The three-dimensional (3D) structure of enzymes forms "reactive sites," whose chemical groups bind substrates, and lowers the activation energy (E_A) of a reaction to allow the reaction rate to proceed at catalytic rates.
- The structure of protein's reactive sites can restrict the types of molecules that bind to very few substrates or a larger number; this restriction is called the specificity of an enzyme.

Table 15-1 Plasma Half-Lives for Clinically Important Enzymes

Enzymes	Half-Life, Hours (Mean ± 2 SD)
LD_1	53 to 173
LD_5	8 to 12
CK	15
AST	12 to 22
ALT	37 to 57
AMS	3 to 6
LPS	3 to 6
ALP	3 to 7 days
GGT	3 to 7 days

CK, Creatine kinase; *ALS*, alkaline phosphatase; *AMS*, amylase; *ALT*, alanine transaminase; *AST*, aspartate transaminase; *GGT*, γ-glutamyl transferase; *LPS*, lipase; *LD*, lactate dehydrogenase.

SECTION OBJECTIVES BOX 15-2

- Describe the International Union of Biochemistry (IUB) classification of enzymes and the numbering sytem used.
- List the usual names of enzymes commonly used in clinical analysis.

ENZYME CLASSIFICATION

Many enzymes were first named for their function (such as lactate dehydrogenase), but some have also been named for the type of substrate on which they act: urease hydrolyzes urea, lipase hydrolyzes lipids, and phosphatases act on organic phosphates. Many of the clinically important enzymes are still known by these trivial names, which arose from historic circumstances and will continue to pervade the literature because of their simplicity. A systematic convention for the naming of enzymes was developed by the Enzyme Commission (EC) of the International Union of Biochemistry (IUB) and is widely used.

International Union of Biochemistry (IUB) Names and Codes

The IUB systematic name describes the reaction catalyzed. The IUB also recognized that trivial names were important and assigned practical names to many enzymes but no abbreviations. For each individual enzyme, the system provides a numerical **EC code** designation, which consists of four numbers separated by periods. The first number assigns the enzyme to one of six categories of reaction. The second number denotes the subclass, which often is based on the type of group, such as amino group or hydroxyl group, that takes part in the reaction. The third number indicates the different subsubclass of reaction, often the acceptor group, and the last number is merely the serial number of the particular enzyme in this subsubgroup. For the enzyme lactate dehydrogenase (EC 1.1.1.27), the first number, *1*, indicates that the enzyme is an oxidoreductase; the second number, *1*, indicates that the

Table 15-2 Examples of Enzyme Nomenclature

EC Code	Recommended Name (trivial)	Abbreviation*	Systematic Name	Other Name or Abbreviation
Oxidoreductases				
1.1.1.27	Lactate dehydrogenase	LD	1-Lactate:NAD$^+$ oxidoreductase	LDH
Transferases				
2.3.2.2	γ-Glutamyl transferase	GGT	(5-Glutamyl)-peptide:amino acid 5-glutamyl transferase	—
2.6.1.1	Aspartate aminotransferase	AST	1-Aspartate:2-oxoglutarate aminotransferase	Serum glutamic oxaloacetic transaminase (SGOT)
2.6.1.2	Alanine aminotransferase	ALT	1-Alanine:2-oxoglutarate aminotransferase	Serum glutamic pyruvic transaminase (SGPT)
2.7.3.2	Creatine kinase	CK	ATP:creatine *N*-phosphotransferase	CPK
Hydrolases				
3.1.1.3	Triacylglycerol lipase	LPS	Triacylglycerol acyl hydrolase	Lipase
3.1.3.1	Alkaline phosphatase	ALP	Orthophosphoric-monoester phosphohydrolase (alkaline optimum)	—
3.1.3.2	Acid phosphatase	ACP	Orthophosphoric-monoester phosphohydrolase (acid optimum)	—
3.1.3.5	5′- Nucleotidase	NT	5′- Ribonucleotide phosphohydrolaste	—
3.2.1.1	α-Amylase	AMS	1,4,α,-D-Glucan glucanohydrolase	Diastase
3.4.11.1	Aminopeptidase (cytosol)	LAS†	α-Aminoacyl-peptide hydrolase (cytosol)	Arylaminadase, LAP, leucine, aminopeptidase
Lyase				
4.1.2.13	Fructose-bisphosphate aldolase	ALS	D-Fructose-1,6,bisphosphate: D-glyceraldehyde-3-phosphate-lyase	Aldolase
Isomerases				
5.3.1.9	Glucose phosphate isomerase	GPI	D-Glucose-6-phosphate: ketol-isomerase	Phosphohexose isomerase
Ligases				
6.3.1.2	Glutamine synthetase	—	L-Glutamate:ammonia ligase (ADP-forming)	—

*Baron DN et al: J Clin Pathol 24:656, 1971 and Baron DN et al: J Clin Pathol 28:592, 1975; are not recommended by the International Union of Biochemistry but are in common use.
†Baron DN et al: J Clin Pathol 28:592, 1975 incorrectly lists (EC 3.4.11.2), the microsomal form of this enzyme, as "leucine aminopeptidase."

enzyme acts on the —CHOH— group of donors; the third number, *1,* indicates that the acceptor is NAD$^+$ or NADP$^+$; and the fourth number, *27,* is merely the serial number of the enzyme in the EC 1.1.1.x group (Table 15-2).

Enzyme Commission (EC) Classification

All enzymes are divided into one of six general classes depending on the type of reaction they catalyze. A few clinically important enzymes are listed in Table 15-2, along with EC codes and systematic names.

The first class includes the **oxidoreductases,** those enzymes that catalyze electron transfer or oxidation-reduction reactions, which can be illustrated schematically as follows:

$$A_{red} + B_{ox} \rightleftharpoons A_{ox} + B_{red}$$

An example of an enzyme in this category is lactate dehydrogenase (EC 1.1.1.27). Some common names of enzymes in this category include dehydrogenases, reductases, oxidases, and peroxidases.

The second group of enzymes contains the *transferases,* those enzymes that catalyze the transfer of a group, such as an amino, carboxyl, glucosyl, methyl, or phosphoryl group, from one molecule to another. These reactions can be listed schematically as follows:

$$A{-}X + B \rightleftharpoons A + B{-}X$$

Alanine aminotransferase (EC 2.6.1.2) is an example of this group. Other common enzymes in this category include kinases and transcarboxylases.

A third group includes the *hydrolases,* which catalyze the cleavage of C—O, C—N, C—C, and some other bonds with the addition of water. These hydrolysis reactions can be illustrated as follows:

$$A{-}B + H_2O \rightleftharpoons A{-}OH + B{-}H$$

An example of this group is acid phosphatase (EC 3.1.3.2). Other common enzymes in this category include amylase, urease, pepsin, trypsin, chymotrypsin, and various peptidases and esterases.

A fourth group contains the *lyases,* which hydrolyze C—C, C—O, and C—N bonds by elimination, with the formation of a double bond, or catalyze the reverse reaction, the addition of a group to a double bond. In cases in which the reverse reaction is important, the term *synthase* is used in the name.

This type of reaction is illustrated as follows:

$$\mathrm{R{-}\overset{\displaystyle O}{\overset{\|}{C}}{-}\overset{\displaystyle O}{\overset{\|}{C}}{-}OH + H^{+} \rightarrow R{-}\overset{\displaystyle O}{\overset{\|}{C}}{-}H + CO_2}$$

An examination of the EC listing shows that this and subsequent groups contain relatively few enzymes that are used in clinical diagnosis.

The fifth group includes the *isomerases,* which catalyze structural or geometrical changes within a molecule. They are also called *epimerases* and *mutases,* depending on the type of isomerism involved. This reaction can be illustrated as follows:

$$ABC \rightleftharpoons CAB$$

An example of this group is the enzyme glucose phosphate isomerase (EC 5.3.1.9). It is not commonly used diagnostically.

A sixth and last group consists of the *ligases,* or *synthetases.* In this reaction, two molecules are joined, coupled with hydrolysis of the pyrophosphate in ATP. Many of these enzymes are involved in DNA, RNA, and protein synthesis; none is used currently in clinical diagnosis. The synthetic reaction type is illustrated as follows:

$$A + B + \mathrm{ATP} \rightleftharpoons AB + \mathrm{ADP} + \mathrm{P_i}$$

An example of this group is the enzyme glutamine synthetase (EC 6.3.1.2), which is rarely used clinically.

Nonstandard Abbreviations

A variety of simple abbreviations containing four or fewer capital letters are also used to represent the enzymes that are measured routinely. These abbreviations are widely used in practice but are not part of the IUB system. They are so popular and have become so commonly used that it would be difficult to discard them, and some are listed in Table 15-2.

KEY CONCEPTS BOX 15-2

- The numbering classification divides enzymes into six general categories of reaction; further subclasses are based on the type of group that takes part in the reaction, the acceptor group; and the last number is merely the serial number of the particular enzyme in the last subgroup.
- In clinical practice, enzymes are described by their common names and abbreviations. These include creatine kinase (CK), alanine and aspartate aminotransferases (ALT and AST), and alkaline phosphatase (ALP or AP).

SECTION OBJECTIVES BOX 15-3

- Describe the lag, linear, and substrate exhaustion phases of an enzymatic reaction with respect to substrate concentration and reaction velocity.
- Describe zero-order and first-order reaction kinetics and the substrate concentrations found in these reaction conditions.
- Write the general enzyme reaction and the equation for initial rates.
- Write the Michaelis-Menten constant, and explain its relationship to the substrate concentration needed for zero-order kinetics.
- Define the International Unit of enzyme activity, and write and use the complete equation used to calculate enzyme activity.
- Describe two ways of calculating enzyme activity with the use of automated instruments.
- Describe the most important parameters of an enzyme assay that must be controlled for best performance.

MEASUREMENT OF ENZYMES

In most enzymatic procedures, the reaction rates are not constant with time. The reaction can be followed by observing the rate of change of concentration for a substrate or product; this is usually done by monitoring the product or substrate at a specific wavelength. Initially, there is a **lag phase** with little change in absorbance per unit time when the reactants are mixed and reach thermal and kinetic equilibrium, then a **linear phase** of constant absorbance change per unit time, and finally a **substrate-depletion phase** with little change in absorbance per unit time (Fig. 15-2).

Enzyme assays must be performed during the linear phase of absorbance change at which a constant amount of activity can be determined for this period of time (see Fig. 15-2, *A*). Thus, measurements do not start at zero time but begin after the lag phase has occurred. Measurements can be made at any time during the linear phase and can continue up to the substrate-depletion phase. This is discussed in greater detail below ("Principles of Kinetic Analysis").

If the enzyme activity is too great, substrate depletion may occur before the measurements have been completed. Rather than changing the assay time, the most common way to handle samples with high activity is to dilute them to the point that the diluted activity should be within the assay's dynamic range; this is usually fivefold or tenfold dilution with saline solution or water (see Fig. 15-2, *B*). However, not all enzymes demonstrate linearity on dilution, particularly if the enzymes are active at a lipid-water interface, such as lipase (EC 3.1.1.3), or if **inhibitors** are present in the sample, such as LD (EC 1.1.1.27), when measured in urine.

One of the more convenient methods of assaying enzyme activity is based on measurement of the absorbance of the substrates or the products. Many enzyme systems involve the conversion of NAD^{+} to its reduced form NADH, or vice versa. The reduced form, NADH, has a much greater absorption at 340 nm than does the oxidized form, and consequently,

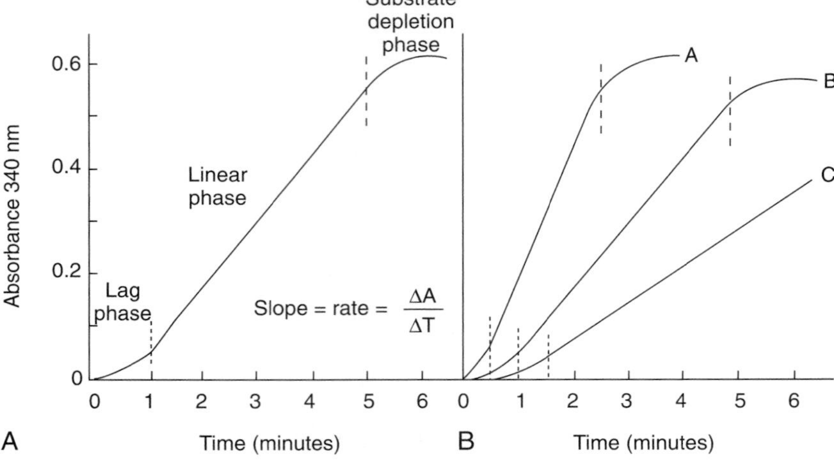

Fig. 15-2 A, Typical enzyme reaction with initial lag phase, linear change of absorbance, and final phase of substrate depletion. Enzyme activity is the slope of the linear phase. **B,** Time course of an enzyme reaction with three different amounts of enzyme present. Curve *A* has a high activity, *B* has a medium activity, and *C* has a low activity. As enzyme activity is increased in an assay system, lag phase decreases, linear phase decreases, and substrate depletion occurs sooner. ΔA, Change of absorbance; ΔT, change of time.

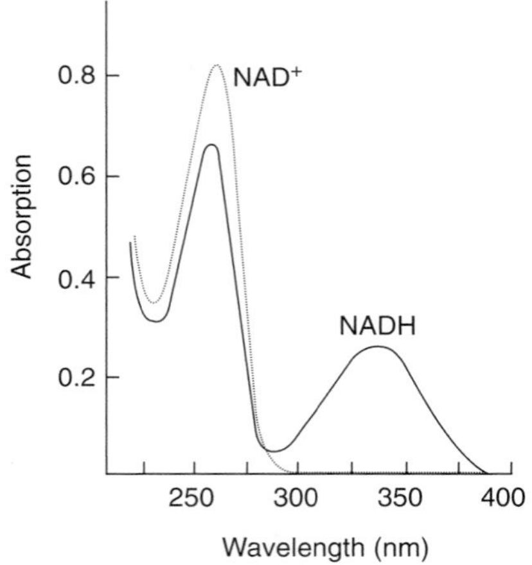

Fig. 15-3 Absorption spectrum of 5×10^{-5} M NAD^+ in 0.1 M Tris buffer, pH 7.5 *(dotted line),* and absorption spectrum of 4×10^{-5} M NADH in 0.1 M Tris buffer, pH 9.5 *(solid line).*

reactions that convert one form to the other may be followed conveniently by measuring the change in absorption at this wavelength. The difference in the absorption spectrum of reduced and oxidized compounds is shown in Fig. 15-3.

Enzyme Assays

Enzymes currently are measured by assessing their immunochemical or catalytic properties. The method most commonly used to measure their catalytic properties is the multipoint fixed-time assay, in which the rate of reaction is followed continuously or with many observation points (usually absorbance measurements) as a function of time; these assays are termed ***kinetic assays.*** Usually, the reaction time is short, that is, a few seconds to a few minutes, and there is little danger of enzyme degradation. Continuous or multiple-point assays are superior to single-point, fixed-time assays because they make it easier to demonstrate approximate linearity of the reaction over the entire measurement period.

Principles of Kinetic Analysis

Enzyme kinetics is the study of enzyme reaction rates and the factors that affect them. Initially, many experiments are performed to examine the effects of different assay conditions on measurements of enzyme activity (see below, p. 294). Eventually, a series of specific conditions are established that give rise to the maximum rate of enzyme activity.

The general enzyme reaction given previously for a *single-substrate reaction* may be rewritten slightly for **initial rates,** as in Eq. 15-4. In this case, the amount of product is very small, and the reverse reaction of *P* combining with *E* and forming *{ES}* is ignored because initial rate measurements are to be made. The initial rate is the rate at the start of the reaction, after the lag phase and during the linear phase in Fig. 15-4, *A*, but before substantial product formation.

$$E + S \underset{k_{-1}}{\overset{k_{+1}}{\rightleftharpoons}} \{ES\} \xrightarrow{k_{+2}} P + E \qquad \text{Eq. 15-4}$$

For a given quantity of enzyme, the rate of activity that is observed increases with increasing quantities of substrate, as is shown in Fig. 15-4. At low substrate concentrations, the rate is linearly dependent on the amount of substrate, that is, ***first order*** with respect to substrate concentration, but at high substrate concentrations, the rate is essentially independent of substrate concentration, that is, *zero order.* A mathematical description of this reaction must explain how the reaction can be first order at low substrate concentrations and zero order at high substrate concentrations.

If the enzyme has a limited number of active sites, at a low substrate concentration the rate will be dependent on the amount of substrate present, because there will be a large effective concentration of unfilled active sites (Fig. 15-5, *A*). However, because the total number of sites on the enzyme is limited and the amount of enzyme is constant, then, as the amount of substrate is increased, the sites will become increasingly saturated with substrate until the reaction will appear to be independent of the substrate concentration (Fig. 15-5, *B*). At these high substrate concentrations, all enzyme active sites

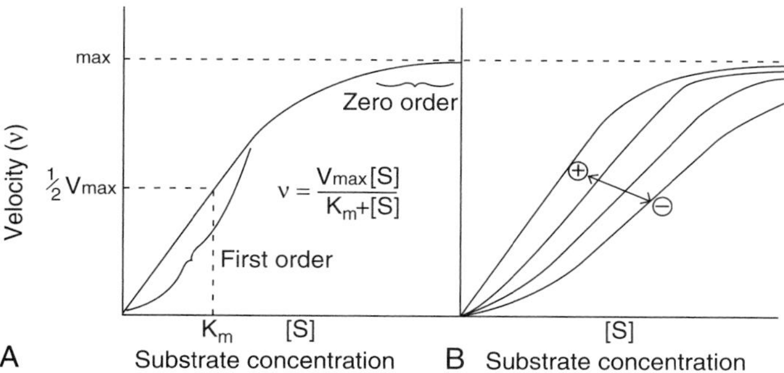

Fig. 15-4 **A,** Relationship of substrate, *S*, to velocity of reaction. At low substrate concentrations, the rate is first order (linearly dependent) with respect to substrate concentration. At high substrate concentrations, the rate becomes zero order (independent) with respect to substrate concentration. K_m, Michaelis-Menten constant; V_{max}, maximal rate of reaction. **B,** Relationship between velocity and substrate concentration for an allosteric enzyme. Presence of positive or negative effectors shifts curve toward the + or – side, respectively.

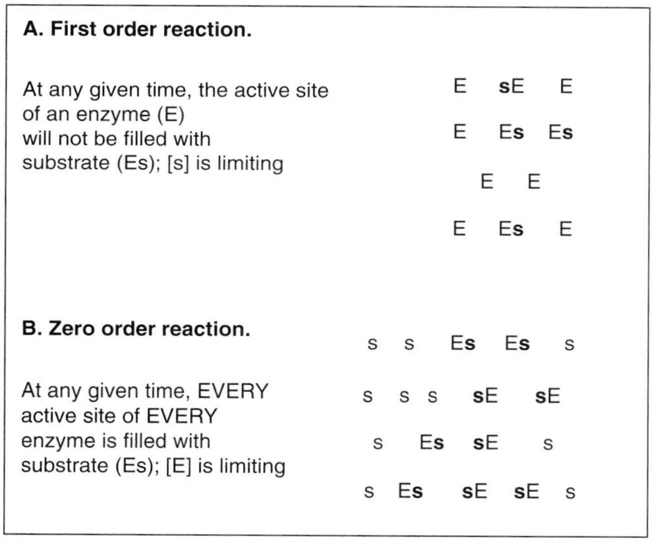

A. First order reaction.

At any given time, the active site of an enzyme (E) will not be filled with substrate (Es); [s] is limiting

E sE E
E Es Es
E E
E Es E

B. Zero order reaction.

At any given time, EVERY active site of EVERY enzyme is filled with substrate (Es); [E] is limiting

s s Es Es s
s s s sE sE
s Es sE s
s Es sE sE s

Fig. 15-5 Schematic depiction of first- and zero-order kinetics.

are filled, excess substrate is still available, and the reaction proceeds at maximal velocity. Small changes in substrate concentration after saturation will not affect the reaction rate.

The second step, product formation, is assumed to be the rate-limiting step or the one that determines the overall activity. The equilibrium for the formation of ES complex can be written as follows with the molar concentrations of all reacting species expressed in brackets:

$$K_{eq} = \frac{k_{+1}}{k_{-1}} = \frac{[ES]}{[E][S]} \qquad \text{Eq. 15-5}$$

The equilibrium constant, K_{eq}, is equal to the ratio of forward over reverse rate constants. From Eq. 15-3, it can be seen that the rate of formation of the product *P* is the amount of *[ES]* times the rate k_{+2} at which the enzyme complex is converted to $E + P$. Thus the rate of formation of product is as follows:

$$\text{Velocity, or Rate} = [ES] \times k_{+2}$$

Because the rate is the amount of product formed for some period of time (ΔT):

$$\text{Rate} = \frac{\Delta P}{\Delta T} = [ES] \times k_{+2}$$

and substituting from K_{eq} [E][S] for [ES] and rearranging yields the following:

$$\Delta P = K_{eq} \times [S] \times [E] \times k_{+2} \times \Delta T$$

That is, the amount of product formed is proportional to the amount of enzyme and substrate present, as well as the time of the assay. When a proportionality constant is substituted for the rate constants, the equation becomes

$$\Delta P = K_1 \times [S] \times [E] \times \Delta T$$

in which ΔP is the amount of product formed during the assay time, $[E]$ is the amount of enzyme, $[S]$ is the amount of substrate, ΔT is the assay time, and K_1 is a proportionality constant. The enzyme activity, or rate of product formation over time, then is given by

$$\text{Rate} = \frac{\Delta P}{\Delta T} = K_1 \times [S] \times [E]$$

Usually, enzyme assays are performed at a high substrate concentration for a short enough period that the substrate concentration can be assumed to be constant. The value of this constant substrate concentration can be combined with K_1 to produce a second proportionality constant, K_2, which is the product of K_1 times the substrate concentration. The rate then can be expressed so that it is dependent only on the amount of enzyme present, that is, a zero-order reaction, independent of substrate concentration.

$$\text{Rate} = \frac{\Delta P}{\Delta T} = K_2 \times [E]$$

This rate of reaction, or velocity, often is listed as v, or V_i, or V_o, in the enzyme kinetic literature.

K_m and V_{max}

When the amount of substrate is low relative to the amount of enzyme present in an assay, the enzyme activity is dependent on the substrate concentration. This relationship for a single substrate reaction is shown graphically in Fig. 15-4, *A*, with the same enzyme concentration assayed at many different substrate concentrations. At steady state, before much product is present, the rate of formation of the [ES] complex will equal the rate of breakdown. This can be described by the following rate equation:

Formation		**Breakdown**
$k_{+1}[E][S]$	$=$	$k_{-1}[ES]+k_{+2}[ES]$

By collecting terms and rearranging, the rate constants can be removed, and a constant, $\boldsymbol{K_m}$, the Michaelis-Menten constant, is defined (see Eq. 15-6 in Box 15-2). This constant is important for demonstrating the relationship between reaction velocity and substrate concentration. The full derivation of the **Michaelis-Menten equation** is shown in Box 15-2.

In the Michaelis-Menten equation, [S] is the concentration of substrate, v is the velocity, $\boldsymbol{V_{max}}$ is the maximal rate of reaction when the enzyme is saturated with substrate, and K_m, the Michaelis-Menten constant, is the substrate concentration that produces one-half the maximal velocity (see Fig. 15-4, *A*).

Box 15-2

Derivation of the Michaelis-Menten Equation

1. $\frac{[E][S]}{[ES]}=\frac{k_{-1}+k_{+2}}{k_{+1}}=K_m$ Eq. 15-6
2. The velocity or rate of product formation at any given time and free enzyme concentration [E] is as follows:

$$v=k_{+2}[ES]\text{ and }[E]=[ET]-[ES]$$

where *ET* is the amount of total enzyme.

3. $V_{max}=k_{+2}$ [ET], when the rate of product formation is only dependent upon [ET].

Combining the above three equations gives the following:

4. $[E]=\frac{V_{max}}{k_{+2}}-\frac{v}{k_{+2}}=\frac{V_{max}-v}{k_{+2}}$

Because from ***Eq. 15-6,***

$$[E]=\frac{K_m[ES]}{[S]}\text{ and }[ES]=v/k_{+2}$$

$$\text{then, }\frac{K_m[ES]}{[S]}=\frac{V_{max}-v}{k_{+2}}\text{ or }\frac{K_m\times v}{[S]\times k_{+2}}=\frac{V_{max}-v}{k_{+2}}$$

Rearranging and solving for v gives the Michaelis-Menten equation

$$v=\frac{V_{max}[S]}{K_m+[S]} \qquad \text{Eq. 15-7}$$

At the fixed high substrate concentration that is found in the usual clinical laboratory assays, the velocity, v, approaches V_{max} and is proportional to the amount of enzyme present, because all other factors are constant and enzyme is limiting. The reaction is said to be zero order with respect to substrate, that is, independent of the concentration of substrate. At such high substrate concentrations in which [S] >> K_m:

$$v=\frac{V_{max}[S]}{K_m+[S]}\cong\frac{V_{max}[S]}{[S]}=V_{max}$$

Thus the common condition used for assaying enzyme activity is a high substrate concentration in which [S] > 10 × K_m or higher. The following equation shows that the enzyme rate at a substrate concentration of 10 × K_m is approaching V_{max}:

$$v=\frac{V_{max}\,(10\times K_m)}{K_m+(10\times K_m)}=V_{max}\frac{10\times K_m}{11\times K_m}=0.91\,V_{max}$$

To practically estimate the optimal [S] needed to perform a clinical assay, the accurate K_m for each substrate or activator must be determined. To assist in these calculations, the Michaelis-Menten equation can be transformed in several ways. The most common of these, the Lineweaver-Burk transformation, and the resulting straight line $^1/_v$ vs $^1/_{[S]}$ curve are shown in Fig. 15-6.

Determination of Enzyme Activity

Units of Activity

The results of an enzyme determination are expressed as an *activity* unit in terms of the amount of product formed per unit of time under specified conditions for a given volume of sample. Thus one unit of enzyme activity might be the amount of enzyme that would, under certain specified conditions, cause the formation of 1 mg of the product, *P*, per minute when 1 mL of the sample was used. In older procedures, arbitrary units like these were often employed.

In 1961, the Enzyme Commission recommended the adoption of an **International Unit (IU) of enzyme activity.** The IU was defined as the amount of enzyme that would convert 1 micromole of substrate per minute under standard conditions.

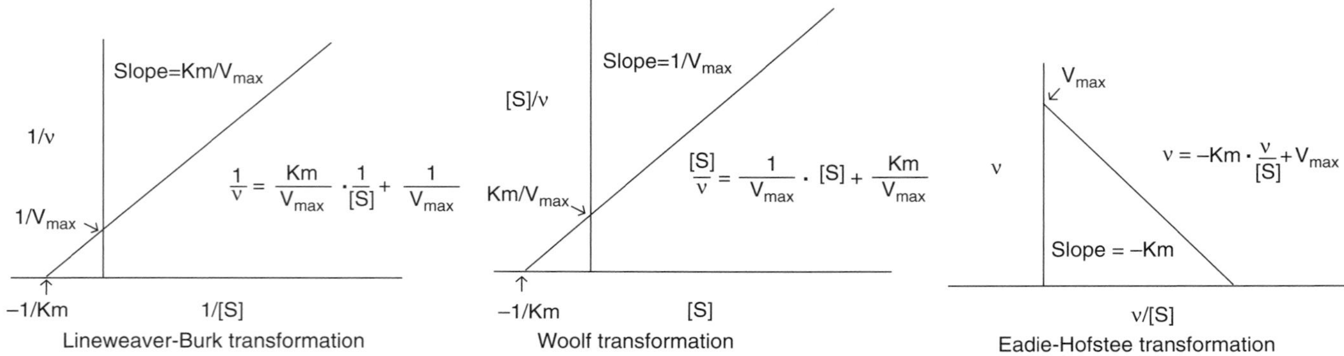

Fig. 15-6 Graphic representation of linear forms of the Michaelis-Menten equation.

$$1\,IU = micromole/minute$$

In those instances in which one molecule of substrate is transformed into two or more molecules of a product, the definition is per micromole of product formed. This unit has been widely adopted, and in some respects, it has standardized assay units. It has not reduced the number of reference intervals because if the standard conditions change, the apparent enzyme activity changes. For example, if a new buffer is used in the assay, it may affect the enzyme rate and produce a different reference interval.

The **Système International d'Unités** (SI), as originally adopted by the World Health Organization, established the unit of enzyme activity as the **katal** (K). This is defined as 1 mol/sec of substrate changed. To convert international units to katals,

$$1\,IU = \frac{\text{Micromole}}{\text{Minute}} \times \frac{10^{-6}\text{ mole}}{\text{Micromole}} \times \frac{1\text{ min}}{60\text{ sec}} = 1.67 \times 10^{-8}\text{ K}$$

Thus, 1.0 IU = 16.7nK (nanokatals). Only the IU is widely adopted by workers in the field of clinical enzymology; the katal has not gained widespread acceptance in the United States or in most of the world.

Standardization by Extinction Coefficient

(see Chapter 1, part B, p. 38)

Pure human enzyme materials are not readily available, and so enzyme assays cannot always be standardized in each laboratory by calibration with pure materials. One standardization method that is used depends on having an accurately calibrated spectrophotometer. Many enzyme assays are followed by spectrophotometric measurements that are being made at a specific wavelength. For example, with a spectrophotometric method, it is usually assumed that at 340 nm, NADH has a molar absorption coefficient, ε, of

$$A/(l \times c) = 6.22 \times 10^{3}\,\text{L} \times \text{mol}^{-1} \times \text{cm}^{-1}$$

in which A is the actual absorbance of a solution, l is the light path in centimeters through the solution, and c is the concentration in moles per liter of the absorbing substance. For a 1 cm light path, rearranging for c,

$$c = (A \times 10^{-3}/6.22)\,\text{mol/L}$$

When the concentration is expressed in micromoles per liter instead of moles per liter, the expression is as follows:

$$c = (A \times 10^{3}/6.22)\,\mu\text{mol/L}$$

From the absorbance change that was measured during an enzyme reaction and the volume of solution used, the number of micromoles of NADH formed or used up during the enzyme measurement period (Δc) can be readily calculated.

$$\Delta c = (\Delta A \times 10^{3}/6.22)\,\mu\text{mol/L}$$

For example, in the lactate dehydrogenase reaction discussed earlier, if a change in absorbance of 0.06 per minute was observed at 340 nm in a 1cm curette, and a 0.1 mL sample was used with a total assay volume of 3.0 mL, the calculation of activity would be as follows:

$$\text{International Units/L} = \frac{0.06/\text{min} \times 1000\,\mu\text{mol/mmol} \times 3.0\text{ mL}}{6.22\text{L/mmol} \times 0.1\text{ mL}}$$

This equation can be generalized to read:

$$\text{IU/L} = \frac{\text{TV} \times 10^{3}\,\mu\text{mol/mmol} \times \Delta A/\text{min}}{\varepsilon \times \text{SV} \times 1}$$

where TV is the total reaction volume, SV is the sample volume, ε is the molar extinction coefficient for the product/substrate being monitored, l is the path length, and $\Delta A/min$ is the change in absorbance per minute. Because all the bolded components in this equation are constant, the equation can be simplified as IU/L = F × ΔA/min, where the factor contains all these constants. This can be useful when calibrating automated instruments for which the pathlength is essentially constant. The F factor is multiplied by the absorbance change for each unknown sample to yield the enzyme activity of the unknown.

Standardization by a Serum Calibrator

Much of the between-laboratory variation for enzyme analysis is related to variations in methods and calibration. To control variations in calibration, serum-based enzyme calibrators have been developed with assigned values and methods traceable to primary standards developed by the International Federation of Clinical Chemistry (IFCC; see Canalias F, International Federation, and Lessinger JM for details). The enzymes for which calibrator values have been assigned include alkaline phosphatase, alanine aminotransferase, aspartate aminotransferase, γ-glutamyl transferase, creatine kinase, lactate dehydrogenase, and α-amylase. These primary serum calibrators have been used also as secondary calibrators. The calibrator is analyzed, and the assigned enzyme level and change in absorbance compared with the unknown's change of absorbance to calculate the unknown's enzyme concentration.

Other Units of Concentration

The enzyme units that have been described express the activity in terms of IUs per volume of sample. This is a particularly convenient unit of measure in the clinical laboratory to assay enzymes in biological fluids like serum and plasma. To measure an enzyme found in erythrocytes (red blood cells [RBC]) or in white blood cells (WBC), another unit of measure is needed; in these cases, the enzyme activity can be expressed as IUs per 10^{10} cells.

In biochemistry laboratories where enzyme purification is important, the enzyme activity might be expressed per milligrams of protein, per dry weight of cells, or per micrograms of DNA.

KEY CONCEPTS BOX 15-3

- The lag and linear phases of an enzyme reaction have excess substrate, while the exhaustion phase occurs with depleted substrate.
- Enzyme reaction velocity is highest during the linear, zero-order phase of the reaction when the excess substrate has all reactive sites saturated.
- The Michaelis-Menten constant can be used to estimate the amount of substrate [S] needed to maintain zero-order kinetics; generally, clinical assays have [S] $> 10\ K_m$.
- The International Unit (IU) of enzyme activity is the number of μmoles of substrate that is converted to product per minute. The basic equation used to calculate enzyme activity is as follows: IU = absorbance change /min/ε × l.
- Automated equipment calculates enzyme activity by using the extinction coefficient (ε) or by using serum calibrator material.

SECTION OBJECTIVES BOX 15-4

- Explain the major factors that may affect the rates of an enzyme reaction.
- Describe how the optimal assay conditions are determined and controlled.
- Describe the types of inhibitors of enzyme reactions, and explain how they work.
- Describe how enzyme reactions can be coupled to create a measurable enzyme assay.
- Describe how enzymes can be used as reagents to measure other analytes.
- Explain how samples should be stored before an enzyme assay is run.

ANALYTICAL FACTORS AFFECTING ENZYME MEASUREMENTS

The rate of enzyme reactions is greatly influenced by temperature, pH, concentration of substrate, and several other factors. Accordingly, all the details of a given procedure must be followed exactly to produce precise and accurate results.

Assays of enzyme activity should be performed under optimal conditions of **zero-order kinetics,** and so the measured rate is dependent only on the amount of enzyme present. To optimize an assay, such as the lactate dehydrogenase reaction given earlier, a series of assays are set up with increasing concentrations of lactate but with a high fixed NAD^+ concentration and a fixed amount of enzyme. The enzyme rates are measured, and a graph similar to that in Fig. 15-6 is constructed to determine the K_m for lactate. A second series of assays then is performed with increasing concentrations of NAD^+ but at the fixed high concentration of lactate determined from the first experiment, that is, [S] $> 10\ K_m$ for lactate, and with the same amount of enzyme present. The enzyme rates are determined again, and another graph is created to determine the K_m for NAD^+. Similar types of optimization experiments are performed for each component of the assay mixture (such as metal ions, pH, buffer) until all variables have been evaluated for the production of maximal enzyme activity. The final conditions determined from this set of experiments are the **optimal assay conditions.** Diagnostic kits are commercially available, with all materials usually at optimal concentrations.

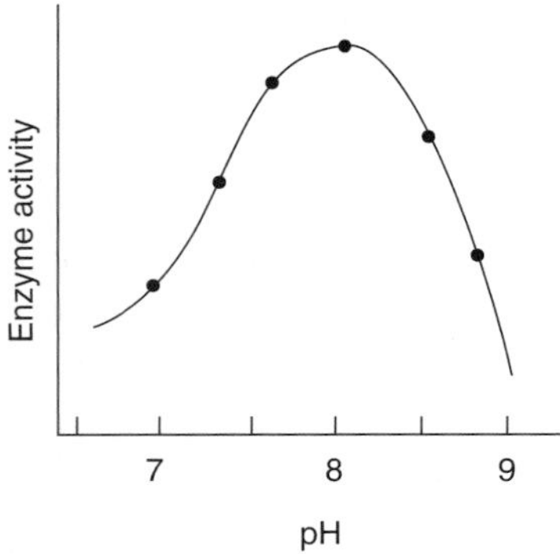

Fig. 15-7 Enzyme activity as a function of pH. Optimal pH range is 7.8 to 8.2; lower activities are observed at pH < 7.8 and pH > 8.2.

pH

Changes in pH considerably affect the enzyme reaction rate. For most enzymes, there is a definite pH range at which the enzyme is most active. A pH near the center of this range is usually specified for measurement of that particular enzyme. The optimal pH is different for different enzymes. Reduced activity is observed at pH values greater or less than the optimal.

A typical bell-shaped curve showing changes in enzyme activity versus pH is given in Fig. 15-7. Because the active site of an enzyme often contains ionizable side chains of amino acids, such as $RCOO^-$ or RNH_3^+, a significant change in pH from optimal can lead to the gain or loss of a proton. This might result in a substantial change in surface charge at the active site, which might, therefore, lose its ability to attract a substrate with an opposing charge. A similar loss of activity occurs if the change in charge is on the substrate molecule rather than on the enzyme. A change of pH might bring about an unfolding of the enzyme and loss of activity if the effect of pH change is to disrupt hydrogen bonds and other intramolecular forces that are holding the enzyme in an optimally active conformation (see Chapter 27, Part 1).

Buffer

In many cases, as the enzyme reaction proceeds, products that tend to alter the pH are produced. Most assays include a buffer to maintain the assay pH within the optimal pH range. The buffer chosen should have a pK_a within 1 pH unit of the optimal pH of the enzyme to exert effective pH control.

Buffers not only serve to regulate the pH of an assay but also may take part in the reaction. Alkaline phosphatase (ALP,

EC 3.1.3.1) assays with *p*-nitrophenyl phosphate as a substrate use the buffer 2-amino-2-methyl-1-propanol (AMP) to maintain the pH at 10.2. The enzyme hydrolyzes the substrate into *p*-nitrophenol and inorganic phosphate in a multistep process, part of which involves a temporary phosphorylation of the enzyme. The final and rate-limiting step includes hydrolysis of the enzyme-phosphate bond to regenerate free enzyme. At similar pH values, buffers that are phosphate acceptors in a transphosphorylation process with the enzyme produce rates of alkaline phosphatase activity higher than those of buffers that do not act as phosphate acceptors. Thus at pH 10.2, the AMP buffer produces rates of alkaline phosphatase activity higher than those of glycylglycine buffer because AMP is a phosphate acceptor. In the case of buffers that do not participate in the reaction, the concentration of buffer that gives maximal enzyme activity at the optimal pH also must be experimentally determined.

It has been found that the buffer and certain salts may have an unusual effect on the K_m. When the buffer-to-substrate ratio is very large, the buffer may compete with the substrate for the enzyme and may make the enzyme activity appear to be related to substrate concentration in a nonlinear way. This has been observed with NADH in the LD reaction. Here, the buffer-to-substrate molar ratio is 10^4:1, and the rate of reaction is affected by Tris, phosphate, and NH_4HCO_3 buffers and certain salts, such as NaCl and $(NH_4)_2SO_4$, which often are found in the coupling or **auxiliary enzymes** used to prepare assays. There seems to be no effect at buffer concentrations below 0.05 mol/L, which is consistent with several recommendations for optimal LD assay conditions. It would seem prudent to maintain as low a concentration of buffer as possible without compromising pH stability or enzyme rate.

Cofactors

Many enzymes require a nonprotein, often dialyzable, material for maximal activity. Some of these materials are related to vitamin structures. For example, thiamine or vitamin B_1 can be converted to thiamine pyrophosphate, a cofactor in many decarboxylation reactions. Niacin can be converted to nicotinamide adenine dinucleotide (NAD), and vitamin B_2, riboflavin, can be converted to flavin adenine dinucleotide. Both of these compounds are involved in many dehydrogenation reactions. Pyridoxine, vitamin B_6, is modified to pyridoxal phosphate, which is used in many transamination reactions.

In analytical assays of transaminase activity, pyridoxyl-5-phosphate is an example of a tightly bound cofactor that is not a substrate. The optimal concentration of a cofactor is determined in the same way as a substrate so that assay conditions can be established with a cofactor concentration of approximately 10 K_m or higher.

Activators and Inhibitors

Many enzymes require specific ions for maximal activity. All phosphate-transferring enzymes, such as hexokinase, require magnesium ions (Mg^{2+}). Other common metal ion activators include manganese (Mn^{2+}), calcium (Ca^{2+}), zinc (Zn^{2+}), iron (Fe^{2+}), and potassium (K^+). Amylase requires chloride (Cl^-) for maximal activity, and some enzymes require several ions for maximal activity, for example, pyruvate kinase requires Mg^{2+} and K^+. In each case, the optimal concentration of the activator must be determined just as the optimal pH or the concentration of substrate is determined.

Inhibitors are materials that reduce the catalytic activity of an enzyme. There are many types of inhibitors and several classes of inhibition. Inhibitors may act by removing an activator by chelation, for example, Ca^{2+} and Mg^{2+} are bound by ethylenediaminetetraacetic acid (EDTA) or oxalate to cause the inhibition of hexokinase. They also may act by binding to the active site to compete with the substrate or by forming a complex at a different site, that is, an allosteric site, which may affect the enzyme activity.

Inhibitors are classed into three main groups. **Competitive inhibitors** bind at the active site and compete with the substrate for binding sites. These materials demonstrate a reversible inhibition that often can be reduced by using a higher substrate concentration.

$$\begin{array}{ccccc} E & + S \rightleftharpoons & \{ES\} & \rightarrow P + E \\ + & & + & \\ I & & I & \\ \upharpoonleft\downharpoonright & & \upharpoonleft\downharpoonright & \\ \{EI\} & + S \rightleftharpoons & \{ESI\} & \end{array}$$

The maximum rate of reaction is not affected if enough substrate is present, because of the reversibility of the reactions. The binding of substrate is affected, and thus the apparent K_m will be higher while the V_{max} will remain the same (Fig. 15-8, *A*).

Noncompetitive inhibitors bind at an allosteric or regulatory site, which may be near or far removed from the active site. These inhibitors cannot be reversed by the addition of more substrate because they bind at a different location on the enzyme surface.

$$\begin{array}{l} \quad S \rightleftharpoons \{ES\} \rightarrow P + E \\ + \\ E \\ + \\ \quad I \rightleftharpoons [EI] \end{array}$$

Because the inhibitor does not compete with the substrate, the K_m will be unaffected, but the amount of E or ES that converts substrate to product will be reduced, and the V_{max} will be lessened (Fig. 15-8, *B*).

Uncompetitive inhibitors, a third group of inhibitors, are believed to bind to the enzyme-substrate complex and not to the free enzyme. In this case, at low substrate concentrations, the addition of more substrate increases the inhibition, because it produces more **enzyme-substrate complex** to react with the inhibitor. The result of this type of inhibition is that the V_{max} is reduced and the K_m is increased (Fig. 15-8, *C*).

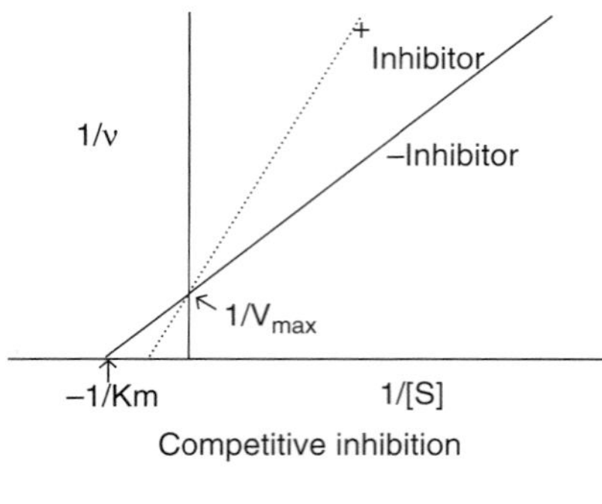

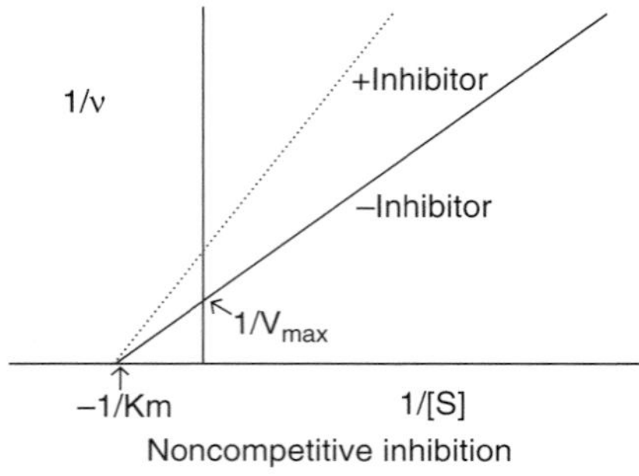

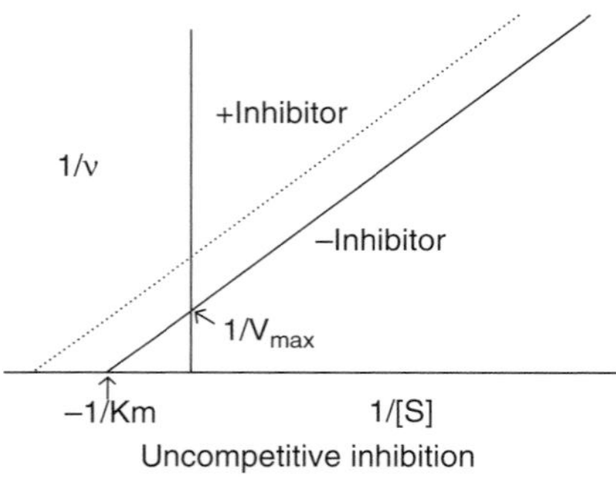

Fig. 15-8 The three types of inhibition are shown with use of the Lineweaver-Burk graphic method to demonstrate the effects of types of inhibition of K_m and V_{max}.

$$\begin{array}{c} E + S \rightleftharpoons \{ES\} \rightarrow P + E \\ + \\ I \\ \upharpoonleft\downharpoonright \\ \{ESI\} \end{array}$$

A brief summary of the effects of various types of inhibition is given in Table 15-3. The simple types of inhibition may be classified by examination of the kinetic effect on the K_m and V_{max}.

Coupling Enzymes

Some enzyme reactions of interest, such as alanine aminotransferase (ALT) and aspartate aminotransferase (AST), do not have substrates and do not form products that can be monitored directly. Using a coupled assay format, the initial enzyme reaction usually is coupled to a second, *indicating enzyme* reaction that, for example, does contain a product or substrate, such as the NAD^+/NADH conversion, to make a convenient assay. The AST enzyme reaction can be coupled to the malate dehydrogenase reaction (MD, EC 1.1.1.37) as follows.

Table 15-3 Kinetic Effects of Inhibition

Type of Inhibition	Change in K_m	Change in V_{max}
Competitive	Increased	No change
Noncompetitive	No change	Decreased
Uncompetitive	Increased	Decreased

Reaction to be measured:

$$\text{L-Aspartate} + \alpha\text{-Ketoglutarate} \xrightleftharpoons{AST} \text{L-Glutamate} + \text{Oxaloacetate}$$

Indicator reaction:

$$\text{Oxaloacetate} + \text{NADH} + H^+ \xrightleftharpoons{MD} \text{L-Malate} + NAD^+$$

This gives the following net reaction:

$$\text{L-Aspartate} + \alpha\text{-Ketoglutarate} + \text{NADH} + H^+ \rightleftharpoons \text{L-Glutamate} + \text{L-Malate} + NAD^+$$

Oxaloacetate supplied as the product of the AST reaction and the cofactor NADH serve as the substrates for the malate dehydrogenase indicator reaction. This assay would have L-aspartate, α-ketoglutarate, NADH, and the enzyme malate dehydrogenase (MD) present at large excesses so that the rate-limiting item in the assay would be the amount of AST in the sample. For other enzymes, such as creatine kinase (CK, EC 2.7.3.2), measurement of the first enzyme requires an intermediate auxiliary enzyme reaction and then an **indicator enzyme.** In the measurement of CK, hexokinase (EC 2.7.1.1) is used as an auxiliary enzyme and glucose-6-phosphate dehydrogenase (EC 1.1.1.49) is used as the indicating enzyme reaction. Both of these additional enzymes have to be present in large excesses for correct measurement of CK. It is difficult to establish optimum assays that have more than two coupled reactions because of the large number of components in the assay system and the problems associated with maximizing all components without causing inhibition of the limiting reaction.

Temperature

There is no optimal temperature for enzyme assays. Most enzymes show increasing activity as the temperature is raised over a limited temperature range, such as 10°C to 40°C; an example is shown in Fig. 15-9.

To minimize any losses of activity if the enzyme cannot be assayed immediately after collection, samples should be temporarily stored at refrigerator temperatures (2°C to 6°C) for several days or frozen if longer storage periods are needed (Table 15-4). In a few cases, some forms of enzymes, such as LD_4 and LD_5, have been found to be more stable at room temperature than at refrigerator temperatures. The repeated freezing and thawing of a specimen will often cause denaturation and loss of enzyme activity. Above 40°C, most enzymes are rapidly denatured and lose almost all activity after a short time. An exception to this general rule is amylase, which seems to be stable up to about 60°C before significant losses of activity occur.

For many enzymes, a 1 Celsius degree change in temperature produces about a 10% change in activity. A tolerance of ± 0.1 Celsius degree for temperature control of an enzyme analyzer is recommended, because this produces an approximately ± 1% change in the activity measured. This amount of variation is small enough to be ignored as an insignificant source of error for most clinical work. A recommendation of ± 0.05 Celsius degree for temperature control, which reduces the change in activity to ± 0.5%, has been suggested.

The apparent increase in activity with increasing temperature means that assays that are performed at higher temperatures, such as 37°C, will be more sensitive to slight changes in the amount of enzyme in a sample. Enzymes commonly employed for clinical diagnosis are less stable at this temperature than at 25°C to 30°C; therefore, assays carried out at 37°C must be performed with relatively short assay times, so that enzyme denaturation is minimized. The incubation temperature used for most commercial instruments is 37°C. A very accurate gallium standard melting point cell is now available to all laboratories from the National Institute of Standards and Technology. This material has a melting temperature plateau of 29.772°C and can be used to calibrate or check the assay temperature of a wide variety of instruments.

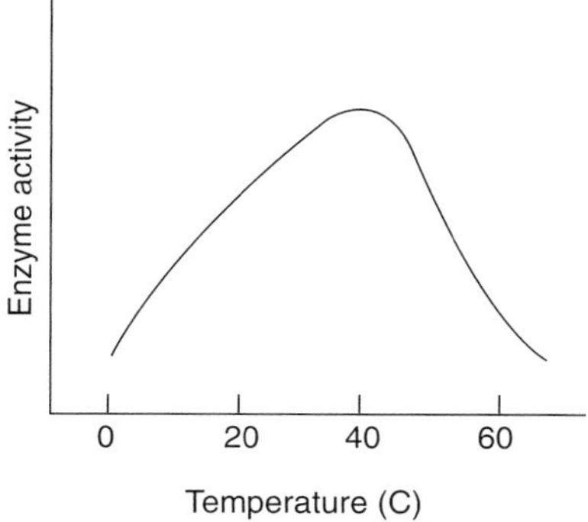

Fig. 15-9 Enzyme activity as a function of temperature of assay. Activity decreases at low temperatures. As temperature is raised, activity increases until rate of denaturation is greater than the increase in activity.

Defining Assay Conditions

Although an optimal set of conditions for the assay of an enzyme can be established, there may not be agreement as to what the optimal conditions are. At times, the differences between commercial assays may not appear to be significant, and yet the results obtained will be substantially divergent. The effects of various components of an assay upon one another, and thus the results, are even more significant in a **coupled assay.** These assays not only have the concentrations of substrates and activators of the primary reaction to consider, but they also must have excesses of the auxiliary and indicating enzymes and their associated activators.

Alanine aminotransferase (ALT) often is measured in an assay that contains an excess of lactate dehydrogenase and NADH, plus L-alanine and α-ketoglutarate and buffer. The usual commercially available kits often specify that about 500 U/L of LD are present as an indicating enzyme and perhaps the animal source of this enzyme. This is not sufficient to define the assay completely, because the K_m of pyruvate varies with the LD isoenzyme type. About four times as many units of LD_1 would be required than would be needed if LD_5 were

Table 15-4 Enzyme Stability under Various Storage Conditions (Less Than 10% Change in Activity)

Enzyme	Room Temperature (about 25°C)	Refrigeration (0°C to about 4°C)	Frozen (–25°C)
Aldolase (ALS)	2 days	2 days	Unstable*
Alanine aminotransferase (ALT)	2 days	5 days	Unstable*
α-Amylase (AMS)	1 month	7 months	2 months
Aspartate aminotransferase (AST)	3 days	1 week	1 month
Ferroxidase I (ceruloplasmin)	1 day	2 weeks	2 weeks
Cholinesterase (CHS)	1 week	1 week	1 week
Creatine kinase (CK)	1 week	1 week	1 month
γ-Glutamyl transferase (GGT)	2 days	1 week	1 month
Isocitrate dehydrogenase (ICD)	1 day	2 days	1 day
Lactate dehydrogenase (LD)	1 week	1 to 3 days†	1 to 3 days†
Leucine aminopeptidase (LAP)	1 week	1 week	1 week
Lipase (LPS)	1 week	3 weeks	3 weeks
Phosphatase, acid (ACP)	4 hours‡	3 days§	3 days§
Phosphatase, alkaline (ALP)	2 to 3 days¶	2 to 3 days	1 month

*Enzyme does not tolerate thawing well.
†Depending on isoenzyme pattern in the serum.
‡Unacidified.
§With added citrate or acetate to pH ≈ 5.
¶Activity may increase.

used to achieve an equivalent reaction rate. A crude mixture of isoenzymes would be somewhere in between these extremes. Even if the units of LD added to different commercial assays were the same, the measured enzyme rates might vary with each lot of a kit if the indicating enzyme was added without regard for the isoenzyme content. This same kind of variability would occur between manufacturers' kits that contained the same concentrations of substrates, activators, and units of LD if a different source, such as a bacterial source, of the indicating enzyme were used. Although agreement as to optimal assay parameters has increased, each laboratory must validate the reference interval for each enzyme assay, particularly when changing reagent manufacturers.

Enzymes as Reagents

It is possible to measure the serum levels of the substrate of many enzyme reactions by using many of the principles of enzyme kinetics applied in a slightly different way. The enzyme activity at low substrate concentrations is first order, that is, linear with respect to substrate concentration. To measure the concentration of pyruvate in a sample, for example, a special LD assay mixture is prepared, without substrate and with only a small amount of the sample added, so that the amount of unknown pyruvate in the assay is low, that is, less than the K_m. An assay mixture is used that contains an excess of LD, an excess of the coenzyme NADH, and a buffer. Using the millimolar absorption coefficient of NADH at 340 nm, the reduction in the amount of NADH in this assay is related to the amount of pyruvate present in the sample. Alternatively, a series of pyruvate standards could be used to calibrate the assay.

Enzymatic assays that are used commonly in the clinical laboratory involve the determination of glucose, urea, ethanol, cholesterol, triglycerides, lactate, and uric acid. Enzymes sometimes are used as components of other assays or assay systems, most commonly in immunometric assays of various designs, which are called enzyme-linked immunosorbent assay (**ELISA**) or enzyme-multiplied immunoassay technique (**EMIT**) assays (see Chapters 8 and 9). In most cases, the enzymes are used as indicators that an immunoassay reaction has taken place, by the production of a colored product.

Storage of Enzymes

Most of the enzymes that are used clinically are stable at refrigerator temperatures for 2 to 3 days to about a week and at room temperature for a shorter time. Table 15-4 summarizes data for three temperatures.

Several enzymes deserve particular comment. Acid phosphatase is unstable at all temperatures unless the pH of the serum is reduced to about 5 to 6 with citrate or acetate. Alkaline phosphatase in human serum demonstrates a linear increase in activity that is dependent on temperature and time. At 96 hours (4 days), there is a 6% increase at room temperature, a 4% increase at refrigerator temperature, and a 1% increase at –20°C. Enzymes in control materials are usually of nonhuman origin and are much more varied, with some more stable and some less stable than human serum.

KEY CONCEPTS BOX 15-4

- pH, type and concentration of buffers, cofactors and activators, and temperature all affect enzyme activity.
- By independently varying the pH and concentration of components, one can determine the value of each that provides the optimum or highest enzyme activity.
- Competitive inhibitors act on the active site, competing with the substrate for binding. Diluting out the inhibitor or adding more substrate can reverse the inhibition. Noncompetitive inhibitors active at some site distant from the active site to change enzyme structure and cause inhibition. Uncompetitive inhibitors react directly with the substrate to inhibit binding. The last two types of inhibitions cannot be reversed easily.
- If the enzyme reaction to be measured cannot itself be monitored, it can be coupled to one or more other enzyme reactions, the last of which can be monitored to give a measure of the activity of the first reaction.
- If a measurable enzyme reaction in which the substrate is limiting can be performed, the amount of measured enzyme activity is proportional to the substrate concentration (first-order reaction); this assay can be used to measure the concentration of the substrate. Example: urease reaction to measure urea.
- Enzyme levels in clinical samples tend to be more stable at refrigerated temperatures. The most stable temperature and length of storage vary from enzyme to enzyme.

SECTION OBJECTIVES BOX 15-5

- Explain the basis for measuring cellular enzymes in body fluids.
- Describe the factors that affect the reference interval for an enzyme.

CLINICAL ENZYME MEASUREMENTS

Changes in enzyme activity in the plasma or serum are followed, because it is known that enzymes are primarily intracellular constituents that are released after cell damage or cell death has taken place in a specific organ or tissue. The changes that occur with many diseases or in a particular organ often can be understood by examination of the pattern of several enzyme or isoenzyme changes in serum over a period of hours or days.

Extracellular versus Cellular Enzymes

The enzymes that are found in plasma can be categorized into two major groups. These major subdivisions consist of plasma-specific enzymes and non–plasma-specific enzymes.

Plasma-specific enzymes are those enzymes that have a definite and specific function in plasma. Plasma is their normal site of action, and they are present in plasma at higher concentrations than in most tissues. Among these are the enzymes involved in blood coagulation, as well as ferroxidase, pseudocholinesterase, and lipoprotein lipase. These enzymes are synthesized in the liver and are constantly liberated into the plasma to maintain a steady-state concentration. These enzymes are clinically of interest when their concentration decreases in plasma, and some have been used historically as estimates of liver function.

Non–plasma-specific enzymes are those enzymes with no known function in plasma. Their concentrations in plasma usually are found to be lower than in most tissues, and there may be a deficiency in plasma of the activators or cofactors necessary for maximum enzyme activity. These enzymes can be divided further into the enzymes of secretion and the enzymes of intermediary metabolism.

The enzymes of secretion are those enzymes secreted from the exocrine glands, that is, the pancreas and prostate, and some enzymes from the gastric mucosa and the bones. Enzymes in this group are clinically important when their concentrations are either higher or lower than the reference interval. Elevated values are found when the usual mode of excretion is blocked, there is gland destruction, or when the amount of enzyme produced is increased. Decreases in the amount of enzyme are found when the tissue that ordinarily produces the enzyme is damaged or necrotic. Common examples of this group are amylase, lipase, and acid and alkaline phosphatases.

The other major group of non–plasma-specific enzymes includes the enzymes of cellular metabolism. The concentrations of these enzymes in tissues are very high, sometimes thousands of times higher than in plasma. Cellular damage results in leakage of cellular constituents and allows a fraction of these proteins to escape into the plasma, causing a sharp rise in the concentration usually observed. Some common examples are creatine kinase (CK), lactate dehydrogenase (LD), lipase, alanine aminotransferase (ALT), and aspartate aminotransferase (AST).

FACTORS AFFECTING REFERENCE VALUES (see Chapters 18 and 24)

Several important factors affect the reference intervals for clinically useful enzymes. If these factors are not accounted for in the interpretation of results, a misdiagnosis is possible. In the following items, a brief comment on the problem and an example are given.

Sampling Time

Because enzymes do not undergo any significant circadian rhythm, sampling time with respect to time of day is unimportant for the determination of enzyme reference intervals. On the other hand, sampling time with respect to the onset of a clinical condition may be important for detection of a variety of acute and chronic conditions if the changes observed are sufficiently rapid. The classical average time for maximum elevation for a series of enzymes in patients with a myocardial infarction was reported to be as follows: CK-MB, 12 hours; CK, 18 hours; AST, 24 hours; and LD, 48 hours. Not all patients follow this classical pattern, and a spread of several hours is seen for the rapidly changing analytes and several days for the slower changing analytes if a variety of patients are tested.

Age

Variations in the quantities of enzymes usually present in serum may result from differences in age between various subgroups in the population. There are three principal ages to consider as a factor for determining a reference interval for an enzyme assay. These occur during the first year of life as various organs, such as liver, are becoming functional, during puberty, and in late middle age when aging changes occur.

Perhaps some of the most dramatic changes are seen with the enzyme alkaline phosphatase. With the use of an alkaline phosphatase method with AMP buffer and *p*-nitrophenyl phosphate substrate at 30°C, the following values can be found: 135 to 270 U/L for children 6 months to 10 years of age, 90 to 320 U/L for children 10 to 18 years of age, and 40 to 100 U/L for adults.

Sex

Differences between the enzyme reference intervals for male and female populations are seen with some enzymes. These differences most probably are related to muscle mass, exercise, or hormone concentration.

An example of these effects is seen with the enzyme creatine kinase; males have higher reference intervals than females, which is most likely attributable to increased muscle mass. The alcohol dehydrogenase level in gastric mucosa also is reported to be higher in males than in females, allowing males to metabolize ethanol more rapidly. An alcohol load therefore does not adversely affect males as much as it affects females.

Race

Race also may be a factor in a limited number of assays. Black populations are reported to have higher reference intervals than comparable white populations for creatine kinase, but this effect may be an indirect result of several factors other than race in the two populations.

Exercise

Exercise and movement are important variables in the consideration of reference intervals for several enzymes. Patients who have been on complete bed rest for several days are found to have 20% to 30% lower values for creatine kinase than ambulatory patients. Normal amounts of exercise also elevate creatine kinase, most often of the MM type, CK_3. The increases seen after exercise usually disappear after 12 to 24 hours, unless the exercise is extremely strenuous. In ultralong-distance runners, those who run races longer than 26 miles, the CK_2 can be up to threefold higher than the reference interval, and the total CK can be up to 40-fold higher than usual. Even when CK isoenzymes are determined, it may be difficult to distinguish a runner with chest pain from a runner with chest pain and a myocardial infarct. Total serum bilirubin also can be elevated as the result of increased destruction of red blood cells in the soles of the feet.

KEY CONCEPTS BOX 15-5

- When tissues or cells are damaged or killed, intracellular enzymes are released into the blood. The blood levels of an enzyme can be used to determine which tissue has been damaged and what the extent of the damage is.
- The age, gender, race, and level of physical activity can affect the usual, or reference, range of serum enzyme activity.
- The time of blood collection after tissue damage has occurred can affect interpretation of serum enzyme levels.

SECTION OBJECTIVES BOX 15-6

- Explain the biochemical basis for isoenzymes and isoforms.
- Describe how measurements of an isozyme can be clinically useful.

ISOENZYMES (see Chapter 16)

Nomenclature

The multiple natural forms of an enzyme that catalyze the same reaction in a single species are known as *isoenzymes,* or *isozymes.* The EC of the IUB has designated that this term is to apply only to those forms of enzymes that arise from genetically determined differences in amino acid structure, although complete agreement on this designation has not been reached. Isoenzymes can be distinguished on the basis of electrophoretic mobility and can be subscripted, with the first form having mobility closest to the anode (+). For example, CK-BB is subscripted as CK_1, CK-MB as CK_2, and CK-MM as CK_3.

Three groups of multiple enzyme forms have been defined as isoenzymes by the IUB. These include the following: genetically independent proteins, such as mitochondrial and cytosol forms of CK and malate dehydrogenase; heteropolymers of two or more different subunits, such as CK and LD; and genetic variants in protein structure, such as the glucose-6-phosphate dehydrogenases, with more than 50 varieties known in humans.

The polymeric forms of glutamate dehydrogenase and phosphorylase are not isoenzymes by the IUB definition, because they are polymers of a single subunit and do not differ in amino acid composition. Some additional forms of enzymes that do not fit the strict definition of isoenzymes are those with variations in molecular weight (or length). These forms may occur with the cleavage of different terminal segments of a protein that does not affect the enzyme activity, thus producing various isoenzymes. Hexokinase and carbonate dehydratase are examples of this type of isoenzyme.

Isoforms

An isoenzyme that is released from tissue (e.g., CK-MB) is a single unmodified isoenzyme form. As part of the normal clearance process of the body, carboxypeptidases in serum cleave the terminal lysine from the CK-M subunit and produce other isoforms of the isoenzyme with slightly different charges. High-resolution electrophoresis or isoelectric focusing can be used to demonstrate the presence of three CK-MM isoforms and two CK-MB isoforms, forming and disappearing with time. The CK-MM isoforms differ only in whether none, one, or two lysines have been removed from the CK-M subunits. The two CK-MB isoforms are the intact CK-MB and the CK-MB in which the M subunit has had a lysine removed. These are of interest as possible early diagnostic markers of acute myocardial infarction (Table 15-5). A more complete description of isoenzymes is given in Chapter 16.

Table 15-5 CK Isoforms

Isoform	Subunit	Comment
MM_3	CK-MM	Unchanged isoenzyme
MM_2	CK-MM_{-L}	End lysine removed from one M subunit
MM_1	CK-M_{-L} M_{-L}	End lysine removed from both subunits
MB_2	CK-MB	Unchanged isoenzyme
MB_1	CK-M_{-L} B	End lysine removed from M subunit

KEY CONCEPTS BOX 15-6

- Genetic differences in protein structure can give rise to different proteins with essentially the same enzyme activity.
- Often, this can occur when the protein includes multiple protein chains as part of its quarternary structure.
- Because different organs have different isoenzyme composition, the blood level of a specific isoenzyme can indicate a damaged organ.

BIBLIOGRAPHY

Cornish-Bowden A: *Fundamentals of Enzyme Kinetics,* ed 3, London, 2004, Portland Press.

Bakerman P, Strausbauch P: *Bakerman's ABC's of Interpretative Laboratory Data,* ed 4, Myrtle Beach, SC, 2002, Interpretative Laboratory Data.

Berg J, Tymoczko J, Stryer L: *Biochemistry,* New York, 2002, WH Freeman and Company.

Bowers GN Jr, Inman SR: The gallium melting-point standard: its evaluation for temperature measurements in the clinical laboratory, Clin Chem 23:733, 1977.

Bugg T: *Introduction to Enzyme and Coenzyme Chemistry,* Oxford, United Kingdom, 2004, Blackwell Publishing Limited.

Canalias F, Camprubí S, Sánchez M, Gella FJ: Metrological traceability of values for catalytic concentration of enzymes assigned to a calibration material, Clin Chem Lab Med 44:333, 2006.

Colowick and Kaplan's Methods in Enzymology Series, Philadelphia, Harcourt.

Cook PE: *Enzyme Kinetics and Mechanism,* Oxford, 2007, Routledge.

Copeland RA: *Enzymes: A Practical Introduction to Structure, Mechanism, and Data Analysis,* New York, 2000, John Wiley & Sons.

Eisenthal R, Danson M: *Enzyme Assays: A Practical Approach (The Practical Approach Series, 257),* ed 2, New York, 2002, Oxford University Press.

Enzyme Nomenclature, San Diego, 1992, Academic Press. Supplement 1 (1993), supplement 2 (1994), supplement 3 (1995), supplement 4 (1997), supplement 5, Eur J Biochem 223:1, 1994; Eur J Biochem 232:1, 1995; Eur J Biochem 237:1, 1996; Eur J Biochem 250:1, 1997; Eur J Biochem 264:610, 1999.

Fischbach FT, Dunning MB III, eds: *Manual of Laboratory and Diagnostic Tests,* ed 7, Philadelphia, 2004, Lippincott Williams & Wilkins.

Fersht A: *Structure and Mechanism in Protein Science: A Guide to Enzyme Catalysis and Protein Folding,* New York, 1998, WH Freeman and Company.

Frey PA, Hegeman AD: *Enzymatic Reaction Mechanisms,* Oxford, United Kingdom, 2007, Oxford University Press.

Garcia-Viloca M, Gao J, Karplus M, Truhlar DG: How enzymes work: analysis by modern rate theory and computer simulations, Science 303:186, 2004.

Goodrich JA, Kugel JF: *Binding and Kinetics for Molecular Biologists,* Cold Spring Harbor, 2007, Cold Spring Harbor Press.

International Federation of Clinical Chemistry and Laboratory Medicine (IFCC), Schumann G, Aoki R, Ferrero CA, et al: IFCC primary reference procedures for the measurement of catalytic activity concentrations of enzymes at 37 degrees C, Clin Chem Lab Med 44:1146, 2006.

Lessinger JM, Schiele F, Vialle A, et al: Enzyme calibrators: principle and practical use, Ann Biol Clin (Paris) 60:281, 2002.

Marangoni AG: *Enzyme Kinetics: A Modern Approach,* New York, 2003, John Wiley & Sons.

Schnell S, Turner TE: Reaction kinetics in intracellular environments with macromolecular crowding: simulations and rate laws, Prog Biophys Mol Biol 85:235, 2004.

Tousignant A, Pelletier JN: Protein motions promote catalysis, Chem Biol 11:1037, 2004.

INTERNET SITES

http://www.chem.qmul.ac.uk/iubmb/enzyme/—Enzyme nomenclature, accessed September 2007

http://www.ebi.ac.uk/thornton-srv/databases/CSA/—Accessed April-May 2007

http://tutor.lscf.ucsb.edu/instdev/sears/biochemistry/tw-enz/tabs-enzymes-frames.htm—Web tutorial on enzyme structure and function, accessed September 2007

http://www.ebi.ac.uk/thornton-srv/databases/cgi-bin/MACiE/index.pl http://metacyc.org/MetaCycOverall.shtml—Databases of enzyme reaction mechanisms, accessed September 2007

http://www.pdb.org/pdb/home/home.do—Protein structures, accessed September 2007

http://web.chemistry.gatech.edu/~williams/bCourse_Information/6521/protein/images/act_site.html—Schematics of enzyme active sites, accessed September 2007

http://www.genome.ad.jp/kegg/pathway.html#metabolism—KEGG metabolic pathways, accessed September 2007

http://www.biochem.ucl.ac.uk/bsm/enzymes/index.html—Enzyme structure database (deposited in the Brookhaven Protein Data Bank—6562 entries), accessed September 2007

http://www.expasy.ch/enzyme—ENZYME, Enzyme nomenclature database (ExPASy site, January 27, 2001—3721 entries), accessed September 2007

http://www.rcsb.org/pdb/home/home.do—RCSB protein data bank, accessed September 2007

http://video.google.com/videoplay?docid=-2634831898823939947&q=enzyme+kinetics&hl=en—online lecture, accessed September 2007

http://www.youtube.com/watch?v=lijQ3a8yUYQ—Video on protein structure, accessed September 2007

http://www.youtube.com/watch?v=BBUZbqEYwaw—Video on enzyme kinetics, accessed September 2007

Protein Isoforms: Isoenzymes and Isoforms

16 Chapter

Wendy R. Sanhai and Robert H. Christenson

Chapter Outline

Key Terms

dimer Composed of two monomers,

heterodimer A dimer composed of two different monomers.

heteropolymer A polymer composed of two or more types of monomers.

homodimer A dimer composed of two identical monomers.

homologous Similar in structure, origin, or purpose. Pertaining to different proteins or nucleic acids, either between or within species, that have similar or identical function. Homologous features are conserved genetically through evolution and result in similar or identical amino or nucleic acid sequences.

homopolymer A polymer composed of only one type of monomer.

isoelectric point (pI) The pH at which the molecule has an overall net charge of zero.

isoenzymes Multiple forms of an enzyme that catalyzes the same biochemical reaction; different isoenzymes may exist within or between species, within an organism, or within a cell. Various isoenzymes may differ chemically, physically, or immunologically.

isoforms Multiple forms of serum protein, most of which result from post-translational modifications of the gene product. They are functionally related and may differ only slightly in structure.

microenvironment The cellular level; a specific environment or location that is associated with a specific physiological function.

peptidase An enzyme that catalyzes the hydrolysis of a peptide bond; also called *protease.*

post-translational modification A series of in vivo chemical reactions whereby a newly synthesized polypeptide is converted to a functional protein. The changes occur after the protein emerges from the ribosome.

subunit The smallest definable unit of a protein; it may consist of one or more covalently linked polypeptide chains with a distinct secondary (2^0) structure. Subunits associate in a geometrically specific manner to give rise to a protein's quaternary (4^0) structure.

tetramer A protein composed of four monomers.

Methods in Evolve

Creatine kinase isoenzymes
Lactate dehydrogenase and lactate dehydrogenase isoenzymes
Troponin

SECTION OBJECTIVES BOX 16-1

- Describe the nature of protein isoforms.
- Describe the genetic basis of protein isoforms.
- List the types of post-translational modifications of proteins that result in isoforms.
- Distinguish between isoenzymes and isoforms.
- Define the structural differences between isoenzymes.
- Describe the differences between macroenvironmental and microenvironmental distributions of isoenzymes and isoforms.
- Describe changes in the developmental distribution of isoenzymes and isoforms.

FUNCTION AND CHARACTERISTICS

Protein Isoforms

Protein isoforms are different molecular forms of a specific protein. Different forms of a protein may be produced directly from different but related genes, from the same gene via alternative splicing, or by single nucleotide polymorphisms (small genetic differences between alleles of the same gene).[1,2] However, as many as 90% of protein isoforms are generated as **post-translational modifications** of the initially formed protein. These metabolic processes include glycosylation and phosphorylation, as well the formation of protein fragments by peptidases. It is important to remember that each

Box 16-1
Examples of Protein Isoforms

Alkaline phosphatase, different genes, post-translational glycation (current chapter)
Angiotensin I, protease degradation (see Chapters 28 and 30)
Apoprotein B 48 and 100, gene slicing (see Chapter 37)
Creatine kinase, multiple peptides, multiple genes, protein degradation (current chapter)
Ferritin, multiple chains, post-translational glycosylation (see Chapter 39)
Hemoglobin A1c, post-translational glycosylation (see Chapter 38)
Hemoglobin, different genes (see Chapter 40)
Lactic dehydrogenase and creatine kinase, multiple peptides/genes (current chapter)
Troponin-T, gene slicing (see Chapter 37)
Trypsin, protease degradation (see Chapter 34)

isoform retains the essential biological function of the protein form, as well as physiological functions specific to an isoform.[3,4] Many of the functionalities of protein isoforms are time dependent and appear at specific times in the life cycle of the cell or organism. Other protein isoforms perform specific functions for different organs or subcellular organelles. Examples of protein isoforms, many of which are discussed throughout this text, are shown in Box 16-1. The most well studied of the protein isoforms is hemoglobin; different hemoglobin forms normally predominate at different stages of life, presumably for different fetal and adult needs (see Chapters 5 and 40). Some of the genetic variations are associated with disease. In this chapter, specific types of protein isoforms of enzymes are discussed.

Properties of Isoenzymes and Isoforms

Enzymes are proteins that catalyze biochemical reactions (see Chapter 15). **Isoenzymes,** also termed *isozymes,* are genetic variations that arise from multiple gene loci or from allelic genes at a particular locus, giving rise to one or more forms of an enzyme. All isoenzymes possess the ability to catalyze the enzyme's characteristic reaction and share the same Enzyme Commission (EC) number. (see p. 280). Although isoenzymes of a particular enzyme usually do not differ substantially in molecular size, each isoenzyme has a distinct structure. Various isoenzymes can differ in three major ways. First, they may differ in their enzymatic properties, specifically in terms of their ability to be inhibited by specific agents, in their Michaelis-Menten constants (K_m), and their reactivity with different substrates. Secondly, they may differ in terms of their physical properties, such as heat stability or **isoelectric point (pI).** Lastly, they may differ in their biochemical properties, such as amino acid composition and immunological reactivities. The above differences may have been used for measurement of specific isoenzymes. Although isoforms can be the product of related proteins encoded by different genes, most are formed from post-translational modifications of a parent protein structure. Isoforms also may differ in structure and have distinct physical, biochemical, and sometimes biological properties.

Structural Basis

Improved techniques for analyzing mixtures of proteins show that a particular type of catalytic activity, and hence active site structure within a single species, is frequently associated with the existence of several distinct structural forms of isoenzymes. These different isoenzymes can be distinguished on the basis of differences in physical and chemical properties and three-dimensional (3D) structure. Although isoenzymes may exhibit quantitative differences in their catalytic properties, by definition they all retain the ability to catalyze a characteristic reaction. Yet, their existence as multiple forms of enzymes in human tissue has important implications in the study of human disease and in the understanding of organ-specific patterns of metabolism. For example, variations in enzyme structure may account for differences in sensitivity to drugs and differences in metabolism that manifest themselves as hereditary metabolic diseases.

The amino acid sequences of isozymes are usually **homologous,** that is, much of the amino acid sequence is similar. Dissimilarities in the amino acid sequences of isoenzymes and resulting differences in protein structure give rise to differences in catalytic properties, active site structures, pI, charge distribution, hydrophobicity patterns, K_m, and pH optima, and therefore, differences in the responses of isoenzymes to inhibitors. Such differences can serve as the basis for identification and measurement of particular isoenzymes.

The biochemical properties of an isoenzyme that consists of multiple protein chains are dependent on the number and type of constituent **subunits.** If all subunits are identical in terms of primary, secondary, and tertiary structure, as in AA, BB, AAA, or BBB, the isoenzyme is termed a **homopolymer.** If different subunits are present, as in AB, AAB, or ABBB, the isoenzyme is called a **heteropolymer.** An example of a heteropolymer is the **dimeric** isoenzymes of cytosolic creatine kinase (CK), which are formed by different paired combinations of two types of subunits, termed M (muscle) and B (brain), that differ from each other in primary, secondary, and tertiary structure. Both CK-MM and CK-BB are homopolymers **(homodimers);** the hybrid CK-MB isoenzyme is a heteropolymer **(heterodimer).**

Genetic Basis

The existence of multiple gene loci and of the protein isoforms and isozymes derived from them has presumably conferred an evolutionary advantage on the species and has become part of its natural biological pattern. Some of these adaptations are related to the differences in function between and within different types of specialized cells and tissues. Thus, similar to protein isoforms in general, the distribution of isozymes is not uniform throughout the body, and wide variations in the activity of different isoenzymes can occur between organs, between the cells that make up a particular organ, and even between the structures that constitute a single cell. The tissue-specific distribution of isoenzymes and of other multiple forms of enzymes provides the basis for organ-specific diagnosis through isoenzyme measurement.

The presence of different but highly homologous amino acid sequences suggests that some isoenzymes may have arisen through gene duplication, followed by independent mutations of the two genes, resulting in different but homologous primary sequences. In fact, a substantial number of human enzymes are determined by more than one structural gene locus. The genes that determine a particular group of isoenzymes are not necessarily closely linked on one chromosome and sometimes are located on different chromosomes. For example, the genes that code for the human salivary and pancreatic amylases both are located on chromosome 1, whereas the genes that code for mitochondrial and cytoplasmic malate dehydrogenase (MD) are carried on chromosomes 7 and 2, respectively. CK and some forms of alkaline phosphatase (ALP) are clinically important and have isoenzymes attributable to multiple gene loci.

Certain gene loci may be expressed almost exclusively in a single tissue, some at a particular stage in development. For example, in addition to the two gene loci that determine the two most common subunits (H and M) of LD, a third LD locus is active only in mature testes. Four distinct structural genes that encode for multiple forms of ALP are known. The isoenzyme of ALP that is normally detectable only in the human placenta is the product of a single structural gene locus, distinct from loci that specify the structures of the other forms of ALP.

A particularly striking example of the localized expression of multiple gene loci is provided by isoenzymes that occur exclusively in specific subcellular organs. Human mitochondria have isoenzymes (having separate gene loci, they are true isoenzymes) for aspartate aminotransferase (AST) and MD that are distinctly different from their functional counterparts in the cytoplasm. The variants are inherited in a Mendelian manner, without corresponding changes in the isoenzymes located elsewhere in the cell.

Post-Translational Modifications

Post-translational modifications of proteins can give rise to isoforms of an enzyme. These reactions include proteolytic cleavage, protein degradation, and covalent modification of amino acids, and they can occur intracellularly or after the proteins have been released from cells into the plasma.

Proteolytic cleavage, a type of protein degradation, is the most common type of post-translational modification. The reaction, which is catalyzed by **peptidases,** involves cleaving peptide chains from end termini by the action of exopeptidases, or internally by endopeptidases (see p. 286, Chapter 15). Probably all mature proteins have been modified in this way, because the proteolytic removal of their leading amino acid residue occurs shortly after assembly by the ribosome.

Protein degradation and other processing that occurs during both normal metabolism and disease are very important considerations in clinical chemistry. This is because a purified protein that is used for standardization of an assay may not necessarily reflect the analyte's degradation products present in vivo. A particular problem may arise in immunoassay measurement when the test target's amino acid epitopes on the purified protein are different than the degraded or modified in vivo analyte. In this case, the standard will be different from the compound that is to be measured. For this reason, it is important to characterize the isoforms in the biological matrix that are used for clinical measurement and then to configure the immunoassay to measure the analyte molecule as it appears in vivo, rather than in a purified or recombinant form.

The function of protein degradation is fourfold: (1) to eliminate abnormal proteins whose accumulation could be harmful to the organism or cell, (2) to remove enzymes that appear outside their normal cellular location, (3) to permit the regulation of cellular metabolism by eliminating superfluous isoenzymes, and (4) to conserve amino acids within unneeded proteins for synthesis of other proteins. A clinical example of the degradation process is seen with the dimeric homopolymer CK-MM. After release of intracellular CK-MM into plasma, the *N*-terminal lysine residue of each M subunit can be cleaved successively by an irreversible enzyme reaction catalyzed by a plasma carboxypeptidase. Because lysine residues impart a positive charge to the protein, the three CK-MM isoforms can be separated by serum electrophoresis; these three isoforms are named according to their electrophoretic mobility. CK-MM_3, which migrates closest to the cathode, is the "tissue" isoform that predominates (>95%) within the intracellular compartment; CK-MM_2 shows intermediate migration and is formed after CK-MM_3 is released from the cell by cleavage of the terminal lysine from one of the two M subunits of CK-MM_3; CK-MM_1 migrates closest to the anode and results from cleavage of the remaining intact terminal lysine from the unmodified M subunit of CK-MM_2. Similar enzymatic processing of the M subunit of CK-MB occurs to allow the formation of CK-MB_1 from the tissue isoform CK-MB_2. The B subunit of CK-MB also undergoes terminal lysine cleavage, giving rise to four CK-MB isoforms.

Covalent modification involves chemical derivatization at the protein's functional groups of side chains and/or at their end terminals. More than 150 amino acid side-chain post-translational modifications are possible, including oxidations/reductions, acetylations, glycosylations, methylations, and phosphorylations/dephosphorylations; these can alter the structural properties of isoenzymes and their catalytic properties and specificities. The result can be a large number of isoforms with different net charges and physical properties, thus allowing separation and identification of isoform activities. For example, a comparison of heat stability and catalytic properties of ALP from bone, liver, and kidney indicates that these isoforms result from different post-translational modifications of a single gene product common to them all, termed *tissue-nonspecific ALP* (*TNALP*).[5] Evidence from selective modifications of enzymes by glycosidases indicates that the differences in ALP isoforms may result from variations in carbohydrate side chains that are enzymatically added to the gene product. ALP isoforms are difficult to separate by electrophoretic methods because the carbohydrate side chains do not substantially alter the overall charge of the enzyme.

Microenvironmental Distribution

Similar to protein isoforms in general,[1-4] isoenzymes have functional significance, and their differential expression in specific subcellular organelles has led to intriguing biological questions. The fact that different isoenzymes and isoforms are compartmentalized[1,2,6] within the organelles of cells has given rise to theories of specific metabolic processes that presumably conferred an evolutionary advantage on the species. The different structures and net charges of the isoenzymes may influence their interactions with other charged molecules within the cell. For example, the mitochondrial isoenzyme of AST accounts for about 60% of this activity in the parenchymal cells of the liver and cardiac myocytes.

Microenvironmental factors are also important for ALP. All ALP isoenzymes and isoforms are attached to the membranes of cells by a COOH-terminal glycanphosphatidylinositol "anchor." Although the exact function of ALP is unknown, given the enzyme's location, it has been hypothesized that ALP may play a relatively nonspecific role in several transport processes by dephosphorylating metabolites, thereby facilitating their passage through the selectively permeable cell membrane. In addition, because of the bone ALP isoforms on the cell membrane of osteoblasts and the association of this ALP with bone mineralization, it has been suggested that ALP functions to promote mineralization by removing inhibitors of crystallization such as inorganic phosphate.

Macroenvironmental Distribution

Tissue-specific differences have been found in the distribution of isoenzymes and isoforms (Table 16-1). Although the exact reasons for differential distribution of various isoenzymes and isoforms are not known, it has been proposed that they exist to satisfy particular needs and metabolic demands that have evolved in various tissues. The isoenzymes of lactate dehydrogenase (LD), CK, and ALP are included here because they are of major clinical interest.

Table 16-1 Creatine Kinase Activity in Various Human Tissues

	ISOENZYME DISTRIBUTION IN UNITS/G OF WET TISSUE (% OF TOTAL ACTIVITY)		
Tissue	**MM**	**MB**	**BB**
Skeletal muscle	3281 (100)	0 to 623 (0 to 19)	0
Heart	313 (78)	56 to 169 (14 to 42)	0
Brain	0	0	157 (100)
Colon	4 (3)	1 (1)	143 (96)
Stomach	4 (3)	2 (2)	114 (95)
Uterus	1 (2)	1 (3)	45 (95)
Thyroid	7 (26)	0.3 (1)	21 (73)
Kidney	2 (8)	0	19 (92)
Lung	5 (35)	0.1 (1)	9 (64)
Prostate	0.3 (3)	0.4 (4)	9.3 (93)
Spleen	5 (74)	0	2 (26)
Liver	3.6 (90)	0.2 (6)	0.2 (4)
Pancreas	0.4 (14)	0 (1)	2.6 (85)
Placenta	1.4 (14)	0.2 (6)	1.4 (46)

From Chapman J, Silverman L: Bull Lab Med 60:1, 1982, National Committee for Mental Health.

Lactate Dehydrogenase

LD isoenzymes are found in different tissues, and although they all catalyze the reversible oxidation/reduction of lactate to pyruvate, they do so at different rates. The enzymes are composed of four polypeptide chains of two types, M and H, each under separate genetic control, thereby producing five isoenzymes—LD_1 (HHHH; H_4); LD_2 (HHHM; H_3M); LD_3 (HHMM; H_2M_2); LD_4 (HMMM; HM_3); and LD_5 (MMMM; M_4). A different isoenzyme, LD-X or LD-C, with four subunits of X or C is present in the postpubertal human testis.

The pH optimum for the lactate-to-pyruvate (L→P) reaction is 8.8 to 9.8; the reverse reaction (P→L) requires a pH optimum of 7.4 to 7.8. Cardiac muscle, kidneys, and erythrocytes show a predominance of H chains in LD_1 and LD_2 isoenzymes, whereas skeletal muscle and liver have a high content of the M chains in LD_4 and LD_5. The **tetramer** of H chains that make up LD_1 has an affinity for pyruvate that is 10-fold less than the affinity of LD_5, a tetramer of M chains. Thus LD_1 preferentially catalyzes the conversion of lactate to pyruvate. It has been suggested that because of its kinetic properties, the LD_1 isoenzyme predominates in tissues that receive a rich oxygen supply, such as cardiac tissue, since these tissues undergo oxidative metabolism and ordinarily do not accumulate lactate (or pyruvate) because they can use lactate as a fuel. On the other hand, the LD_5 isoenzyme is the major form in skeletal muscle, which is more dependent on anaerobic glycolysis and accumulates pyruvate under anaerobic conditions. By having the LD_5 isoenzyme, muscle cells are better able to convert P→L and to regenerate NAD^+, permitting the energy-producing reactions of the Embden-Meyerhof pathway.

Creatine Kinase (see Chapter 36 for additional details)

CK-MM (CK-3) is the predominant CK isoenzyme in adult skeletal muscle and cardiac tissue. CK-MB (CK-2) is present mainly in cardiac muscle (25% to 46% of CK activity), with only a small concentration (up to 3% of total CK activity) in most skeletal muscle. However, CK-MB is not specific for myocardium, and proportions of this isoenzyme can reach as high as 19% in some types of noncardiac muscle. The tissue distribution of CK isoenzymes is listed in Table 16-1. In brain tissue, CK is expressed primarily as the CK-BB (CK-1) isoenzyme. A fourth CK form, CK-Mt, differs from the others both immunologically and in terms of electrophoretic mobility. Mt is located between the inner and outer membranes of mitochondria, and it accounts for (e.g., in the heart) up to 15% of total CK activity. Its structure is determined by a separate gene locus on chromosome 15.

Alkaline Phosphatase (ALP)[5]

The tissue-nonspecific form of ALP is expressed in virtually all tissues. High activity is particularly noted in mineralizing bone, where ALP is located in the plasma membrane of osteoblastic cells. Placental ALP is detectable in the serum of pregnant women between 16 and 20 weeks of gestation and becomes undetectable within 3 to 6 days after delivery. Serum from adults contains many ALP isoenzymes and isoforms, although the major forms released into serum derive from bone, liver, kidney, and intestinal tissue.

Developmental Distribution

Multiple gene loci and their independent isoenzyme products provide means for the adaptation of metabolic patterns to the changing needs of different organs and tissues in the course of development. In addition, differential expression of isoenzymes over time occurs in response to environmental changes and pathological conditions. Gene activation and suppression of the different loci effect such changes. This process is very similar to the shift from the fetal form of hemoglobin to the adult form (see pp. 773-774, Chapter 40) or the expression of troponin-T isoforms over time.[4]

Changes in the relative proportions of several isoenzymes are noted during the embryonic development of skeletal muscle. The proportions of electrophoretically more cathodic isoenzymes of LD (LD-5) and CK (CK-MM) increase in this tissue, so the qualitative patterns associated with differentiated muscle are present by about the sixth month of intrauterine life. Smaller changes in isoenzyme distribution can continue to the time of birth and into early postnatal life. These patterns appear to coincide with the energy production demands of fetal tissues. Reversion to the fetal CK isoenzyme pattern is seen in Duchenne's muscular dystrophy and in some cancers (see below).

KEY CONCEPTS BOX 16-1

- Different molecular forms of the same functional protein are called *isoforms.* Isoforms of enzymes are call *isoenzymes.* Peptidase modified isoenzymes are called *isoforms.*
- Isoenzymes can exist as different gene products, combinations of gene products (multiple chains), and post-translational modifications.
- The genetic basis of protein isoforms is the need for slightly different protein functionality to fill specific macroenvironmental or microenvironmental or developmental needs of the organism.
- Protein isoforms can be created by post-translational modification, including glycosylation, phosphorylation, and peptidase activity.
- The macromolecular distribution of isoforms and isoenzymes is based on the different metabolic needs of various organs. The microenvironmental distribution of protein isoforms and isoenzymes is based on different biochemical activities in the various subcellular compartments.

SECTION OBJECTIVES BOX 16-2

- List the biological causes of changed isoenzyme patterns in tissues.
- Describe the factors that can result in changed levels of isoenzymes in serum.
- Describe the clinical significance of creatine kinase isoenzymes.

CLINICAL SIGNIFICANCE OF ISOENZYMES

Change in Isoenzyme Patterns in Pathological Processes

Certain diseases, such as the progressive muscular dystrophies, appear to involve failure of the affected tissue to mature normally or to maintain a normal state. Cancer cells show progressive loss of the structure and metabolism of the healthy cells from which they arise. Therefore, the protein isoforms and isoenzyme pattern of mature, differentiated tissue may be lost or modified if normal differentiation is arrested or reversed. The isoenzymes and protein isoforms associated with tumors often are referred to as *oncofetal tumor markers* because their expression is similar to that observed during early embryological development. Examples include α-fetoprotein (AFP) and CK-BB, which are elevated in the fetus but occur at very low concentrations in the normal adult. However, re-expression of AFP can be substantial during ongoing tissue injury, such as in hepatitis, and both AFP and CK-BB can be extremely elevated in hepatic malignancy.

Examples of changes in isoenzyme distribution can be seen with aldolase, LD, and CK in the muscles of patients with progressive muscular dystrophy, which appear to be similar to distributions in the embryological development of fetal muscle. Isoenzyme abnormalities in dystrophic muscle have been interpreted as failure to achieve or maintain a normal degree of differentiation. Isoenzyme patterns in regenerating tissues also may show some tendency to approach fetal distributions. CK-MB represents a significant proportion of the CK activity in both fetal and adult myocardium, whereas in the fetus, CK-MB is also present as a high proportion of CK activity in skeletal muscle. Thus, although increased amounts of the CK-MB isoenzyme in the sera of normal adults probably represent damage to the heart, in children, CK-MB increases may be seen in either heart or skeletal muscle.

Human tumors are found to produce increased concentrations of the placental (PL-ALP), intestinal (I-ALP), and germ cell (GC-ALP) isoenzymes and isoforms of ALP. It appears that malignant processes either activate or amplify the expression of an ALP gene that normally is repressed or expressed at a very low level.

Specific Isoenzymes

For an enzyme to be clinically useful as a marker of disease, it must have a substantial tissue-to-plasma concentration ratio and a relatively long lifetime in blood. In addition, serum isoenzyme levels after disease onset should accurately reflect the stage of disease, and the isoenzyme ideally should be tissue-specific. For all practical purposes, serum and plasma have been the only clinical specimens examined for isoenzyme and isoform markers of specific tissue abnormalities. The most important factors that affect enzyme activities in serum or plasma are those that influence the rate at which enzymes enter the circulation from cells. These factors can be divided into two main categories: (1) those that affect the rates at which enzymes are released from cells; and (2) those that reflect altered rates of enzyme production, caused by increased synthesis of a particular enzyme by individual cell types, or by proliferation of a particular type of enzyme-producing cell.

Release of isoenzymes caused by normal cell death (apoptosis) and characteristic release from living cells is responsible for the "normal" or baseline concentrations in serum that define laboratory reference intervals for isoenzymes. Levels beyond the minimum and/or maximum reference values are associated with a variety of pathological abnormalities and serve as the basis for the clinical usefulness of enzyme determinations. The purpose of this section is to discuss the major disease states associated with increased levels of isoenzymes and isoforms, and to provide a basis for interpretation of abnormal values.

Creatine Kinase (CK)

Although the CK-MM, CK-MB, and CK-BB isoenzymes are cytoplasmic, CK activity occurs in other subcellular locations, particularly in mitochondria. Although CK-BB is abundant in the brain, its 85,000-dalton molecular weight precludes its passage across the blood-brain barrier, except in cases of severe trauma. Significant increases in serum CK levels usually reflect release of CK from skeletal or cardiac muscle.

A common interpretative problem is encountered when skeletal muscle injury (Box 16-2) results in significant elevation of CK activity in serum. Because skeletal muscle contains CK concentrations that are eightfold higher per gram of wet tissue than those in cardiac tissue, small areas of skeletal muscle injury or disease can result in serum CK-MB concentrations consistent with substantial damage to the heart. Historically, calculation of a relative index, in which CK-MB concentration is the numerator and total CK is the denominator, has been helpful in elucidating the source of CK-MB. Because skeletal muscle usually consists of greater than 97% CK-MM, a low relative index is consistent with muscle damage. For cases in which both cardiac and muscle damage is suspected as the result of trauma or surgery, interpretation of CK-MB levels is more complicated. CK-MB measurements now have been virtually replaced by cardiac troponin measurements, which have become the "gold" standard for assessing cardiac injury (see Chapter 36).

As was noted previously, an increased proportion of CK-MB content is frequently associated with muscle fiber regeneration. For this reason, certain diseases of skeletal muscle, such as Duchenne's muscular dystrophy or polymyositis, often result in serum elevations of total CK and an abnormal increase in serum CK-MB concentrations, often to 5% to 15% of the total CK activity. Because most patients with these muscle diseases are not being evaluated for myocardial infarction, and because of the advent of cardiac troponin testing, misinterpretation of these CK-MB elevations is infrequent.

Earlier work on CK isoforms suggested that they might be useful in diagnosing or monitoring myocardial damage. However, the advent of troponin as the gold standard marker for cardiac damage and practical issues of isoform measurements have largely rendered isoform measurements unimportant at this time.[7,8]

More specific markers of myocardial injury, such as the protein isoform troponin-I or troponin-T, have replaced CK-MB.[8] The greatest use for CK-MB analysis by rapid immunoassay is to ensure that following a myocardial infarction, no additional myocardial damage such as reinfarction has occurred. Additional information on this subject can be found in Chapter 36.

Box 16-2

Skeletal Muscle Conditions Causing Elevations of Serum CK-MB

- Crush injury
- Duchenne's muscular dystrophy
- Extreme physical activity (e.g., marathon)
- Malignant hyperthermia
- Polymyositis
- Viral myositis

Alkaline Phosphatase (ALP)

Most often, ALP fractionation is requested to determine whether bone or liver is the source of an elevated level of total serum ALP activity. Specific ALP isoenzyme and isoform measurements, as compared with total ALP measurements, are at least twofold more sensitive for assessment of both bone and liver diseases. As a practical matter, routine differentiation between liver and bone as the possible source of an increased serum ALP is made by measuring the activity of serum γ-glutamyl transferase (GGT). Elevations of serum GGT, found in liver but not in bone, indicate liver as the likely source of the increase in APL (see Chapter 31).

In cases in which the source of increased serum ALP activity cannot be readily explained, fractionation of ALP isoenzymes can be readily performed by electrophoretic techniques.

Lactate Dehydrogenase (LD)

Because LD is found in virtually every tissue, the clinical usefulness of measuring either total serum LD or its isoenzyme is very limited. Although some tissue specificity has been noted for the various isoenzymes, considerable overlap is seen in the tissue specificity of the five isoenzyme forms commonly found in serum.

Other Isoenzymes

Rarely, isoenzyme analysis of amylase may be useful for determining the source of an elevated serum amylase—pancreatic, salivary, or ectopic.

Future of Protein Isoform and Isoenzyme Analysis

The heyday of isoenzyme analysis occurred in the 1990s, when measurement of CK and LD isoenzymes was the gold standard for determination of cardiac damage, especially myocardial infarction. Isoenzymes were measured by electrophoresis and later by immunoassay. In the current millennium, the field of proteomics has opened up the array of protein isoforms that exist in cells. Because these protein isoforms are being studied more fully, many will certainly serve as diagnostic markers for disease.

An expanding use of isoenzyme analysis reflects the burgeoning field of cell culture technology in the pharmaceutical industry. Isoenzyme analysis for malate dehydrogenase, glucose-6-phosphate dehydrogenase, nucleoside phosphorylase, lactate dehydrogenase, and others is used to authenticate and maintain cell culture lines.[9]

KEY CONCEPTS BOX 16-2

- The pattern of isoenzymes present in serum can reflect a change in the developmental state of cells or tissues, as in the case of Duchenne's muscular dystrophy, or a change that reflects the health of an organ or tissue, as in the case of myocardial infarction.
- The reference interval of an isoenzyme is based on the natural turnover of cells (death) and the normal "leakage" of cell contents. Decreased health of the cells or increased cell death increases the rates of release of cell isoenzymes into serum.
- The creatine (CK)-MB isoenzyme is useful for determining reinfarction.

SECTION OBJECTIVE BOX 16-3

- Identify the methods by which protein isoforms and isoenzymes are measured.

MODES OF PROTEIN ISOFORM AND ISOENZYME ANALYSIS (Table 16-2)

Most of the physical and catalytic differences among individual isoenzymes and isoforms have been used to determine isoenzyme concentrations in serum. All these methods depend on differences in 3D structure and post-translational modifications that impart detectable variations to the molecule of interest. More sophisticated methods using specific immunoassays, many of them employing monoclonal antibodies, can differentiate between isoenzymes and isoforms on the basis of immunological differences in subunit chains.

Protein isoform analysis can be accomplished through a variety of analytical techniques as reviewed in this textbook, including immunoassay using monoclonal antibodies (see Chapter 8) and liquid chromatography (LC)/mass spectrometry (MS) (see Chapter 4).[10-12]

KEY CONCEPT BOX 16-3

- Protein isoforms, including isoenzymes, can be measured by immunological methods, as well as by separation methods, including electrophoresis and liquid chromatography (LC)/mass spectrometry (MS).

Table 16-2 Modes of Isoenzyme (Isoform) Analysis

Technique	Principles of Analysis	Isoenzyme, Isoform
Electrophoresis	Subunits have different charges; isoenzymes are separated in an electrical field.	All
Ion-exchange chromatography	Subunits have different charges; isoenzymes are separated by differential affinity for ion-exchange resin.	CK, LD
Immunoinhibition	Antibody reacts specifically with one subunit type; this property can be used to render an isoenzyme or isoenzymes catalytically inactive, or to physically remove an isoenzyme or isoenzymes from solution.	CK, LD, acid phosphatase
Immunoassay	Antibody reacts specifically with one subunit type; extent of reaction is monitored by use of radioisotope, enzyme, or fluorescent tag.	CK, LD, acid phosphatase, alkaline phosphatase, amylase
Heat stability	Individual isoenzyme subunits are rendered catalytically inactive at different temperatures.	Alkaline phosphatase
Catalytic inhibition	Individual isoenzyme subunits bind low-molecular-weight inhibitors with different affinities; such binding results in different inhibition of each isoenzyme.	Acid phosphate (L-tartrate), alkaline phosphatase (urea and L-phenylalanine), cholinesterase (dibucaine)
Substrate specificity	Each isoenzyme subunit binds a substrate with a different affinity (K_m), giving each isoenzyme various rates of activity. Also, each isoenzyme subunit may bind various substrates with different affinities; different isoenzymes have increased catalytic rates with certain substrates, whereas others have very low activities.	CK, acid phosphatase (α-naphthyl phosphate), LD_1

CK, Creatine kinase; *LD*, lactate dehydrogenase.

REFERENCES

1. Tadokoro K, Yamazaki-Inoue M, Tachibana M, et al: Frequent occurrence of protein isoforms with or without a single amino acid residue by subtle alternative splicing: the case of Gln in DRPLA affects subcellular localization of the products, J Hum Genet 50:382, 2005.
2. Nakao M, Barrero RA, Mukai Y, et al: Large-scale analysis of human alternative protein isoforms: pattern classification and correlation with subcellular localization signals, Nucl Acid Res 33:2355, 2005.
3. Liao H, Zhang J, Shestopal S, et al: Nonredundant function of secretory carrier membrane protein isoforms in dense core vesicle exocytosis, Am J Physiol Cell Physiol 294:C797, 2008.
4. Gomes AV, Guzman G, Zhao J, Potter JD: Cardiac troponin T isoforms affect the Ca^{2+} sensitivity and inhibition of force development: insights into the role of troponin T isoforms in the heart, J Biol Chem 277:35341, 2002.
5. Moss DW: Alkaline phosphatase isoenzymes, Clin Chem 28:2007, 1982.
6. Khaïtlina SI: Mechanisms of spatial segregation of actin isoforms, Tsitologiia 49:345, 2007.
7. Hedges JR: The role of CK-MB in chest pain decision-making, J Accid Emerg Med 12:101, 1995.
8. Collinson PO, Stubbs PJ, Kessler A-C, for The Multicentre Evaluation of Routine Immunoassay of Troponin T Study (MERIT): Multicentre evaluation of the diagnostic value of cardiac troponin T, CK-MB mass, and myoglobin for assessing patients with suspected acute coronary syndromes in routine clinical practice, Heart 89:280, 2003.
9. Nims RW, Shoemaker AP, Bauernschub MA, et al: Sensitivity of isoenzyme analysis for the detection of interspecies cell line cross-contamination, In Vitro Cell Dev Biol Anim 34:35, 1998.
10. Baxevanis AD, Ouelette BFF, editors: *Bioinformatics: A Practical Guide to the Analysis of Genes and Proteins,* ed 3, Malden, Massachusetts, 2004, Wiley InterScience.
11. Westermeier R, Naven T: *Proteomics in Practice: A Laboratory Manual of Proteome Analysis,* Weinheim, Germany, 2002, Wiley-VCH.
12. Ottens AK, Golden EC, Bustamante L, et al: Proteolysis of multiple myelin basic protein isoforms after neurotrauma: characterization by mass spectrometry, J Neurochem 104:1404, 2008.

INTERNET SITES

http://www.chem.qmw.ac.uk/iubmb/misc/isoen.html—IUPAC-IUB Commission on Biochemical Nomenclature (CBN)

http://www.biologie.uni-hamburg.de/b-online/e17/17g.htm—Botany online

http://www.nlm.nih.gov/medlineplus/ency/article/003504.htm—Medline Plus. This is for CK isoenzymes. One can search for other isoenzymes described in this chapter.

Interferences in Chemical Analysis

17

Chapter

Lawrence A. Kaplan and Amadeo J. Pesce

Chapter Outline

Key Terms

Allen correction Multichromatic analysis of a reaction to correct for background absorbance. Two wavelengths, in addition to the A_{max} (maximum absorption) of the chromophore, are monitored to subtract average background absorbance.

bichromatic analysis Spectrophotometric monitoring of a reaction at two wavelengths. Used to correct for background color.

chemical interferent A compound that either produces an endogenous color or interferes directly in the reaction or process that is being monitored.

DLIF (digoxin-like immunoreactive factor) An endogenous substance that cross-reacts with antibody to digoxin.

end-point reaction Monitoring of a reaction after the reaction has been essentially completed.

HAMA Human antimouse antibody found in the serum of individuals.

hemolysis Breakage of red blood cells, either in vitro or in vivo. Hemolysis will give a plasma specimen a red color.

icteria Pertaining to the orange color imparted to a sample because of the presence of bilirubin.

in vitro interference An interference that is not caused by any in situ physiological process. Also called *exogenous interferent.*

in vivo interference An interfering process that results from physiological processes within the body. Also called *endogenous interferent.*

interferent Any chemical or physical phenomenon that can interfere in or disrupt a reaction or process. An in vivo interferent results from physiological processes within the body; also called *endogenous interferent.* An in vitro interferent is not caused by any in situ physiological process; also called *exogenous interferent.*

kinetic analysis Analysis in which *change* in the monitored parameter over time is related to concentration, such as change in absorbance per minute. Measurements are usually made very early in the reaction period.

lipemia Presence of lipid particles (usually very-low-density lipoprotein) in a sample, which gives the sample a turbid appearance.

reagent blank Reaction mixture minus the sample; used to subtract endogenous reagent color from the absorbance of the complete reaction (plus sample).

sample blank Sample plus diluent; used to correct absorbance of a complete reaction mixture for endogenous sample color.

turbidity Scatter of light in a liquid that contains suspended particles.

window Term used to denote a specific time during which reactions are monitored, a phenomenon can be observed, or a procedure can be initiated.

The Institute of Medicine (IOM) has reported that 44,000 to 98,000 people per year die in hospitals as the result of medical errors, at an annual societal cost of \$37.6 billion.[1] The burden of laboratory-generated errors may be substantial, both personally and financially, and this textbook has devoted much space discussing the sources of error and strategies for minimizing such errors. Chapter 18 reviews ways to control sources of preanalytical error—those errors that arise from sample acquisition and sample processing. Chapter 19 discusses the use of the Laboratory Information System to detect errors before an erroneous report is filed. Chapter 20 discusses automation techniques for analysis that reduce bias and random errors. Chapter 21 discusses an important alternative to laboratory testing that can remove most sources of preanalytical

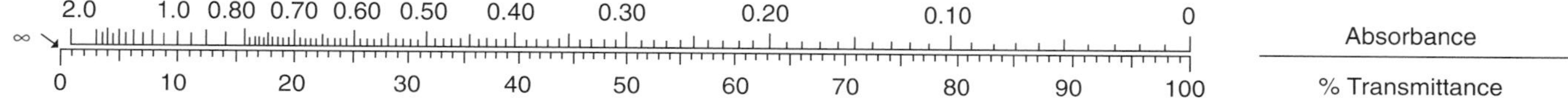

Fig. 17-1 Absorbance and percentage of transmittance scales juxtaposed.

error; the use of point-of-care testing. Chapter 26 reviews the process of evaluating analytical systems, so that the most error-free methods can be chosen.

This chapter reviews specific analytical techniques that can be used to reduce error during the analytical phase of laboratory analysis, although this phase probably is the smallest source of error.

A chemistry laboratory uses many techniques for measuring the concentration of specific biochemicals. All these techniques are subject to interferences from a variety of sources. Specific interferences that affect one technique may not be important for another. However, there are general concepts that, when understood, help to control and minimize the effects of interferences on method accuracy and precision.

Four basic types of interferences can occur in laboratory analysis: (1) those that arise from limitations of detectors; (2) chemical substances in the sample that directly interfere with the analytical method; (3) disease states or exogenous agents that modify certain physiological processes, thus changing the concentrations of an analyte in vivo; and (4) those that occur as a result of sample (blood) processing.

SECTION OBJECTIVES BOX 17-1

- Describe the relationship between transmitted light (%T) and light absorbance (A).
- Describe the errors that can arise from measuring %T, A, and fluorescence and the impact when relating these measurements to sample concentration.

LIMITATIONS OF DETECTORS

Methods that yield quantitative answers usually employ a detector, such as a spectrophotometer. In this way, it is possible to obtain a relationship between the detector response and the concentrations of analytes in various samples. In the case of absorption spectrophotometry, a complex logarithmic relationship can be seen between concentration and detector response (see Chapter 2). When fluorescence is used, a linear relationship between concentration and the fluorescence signal is observed. Similarly, when other optical properties, such as refractive index, or electrochemical properties, such as ion current from oxidation, are used by detectors, the response is also linear. Knowledge of the type of relationship that exists between concentration and detector response is important.

The first section describes errors that can occur with absorption spectrophotometry. Because the clinical chemistry laboratory quantifies most of its analytes by this technique, it is most important to understand the interference problems associated with this mode of measurement. As the nature and sophistication of the laboratory change, other types of interferences become important to consider when one is performing a laboratory analysis.

Absorption Spectrophotometer

Two interrelated types of error can occur in spectrophotometric measurement. The first is caused by the nature of the mathematical relationship between absorbancy and percentage of transmittance, and the second is related to limitations of the instrument.

Absorbance Variance

As was discussed in Chapter 2, a logarithmic relationship exists between the percentage of light transmittance (%T), which is the quantity actually measured, and the absorbance (A), which is calculated. Fig. 17-1 shows the relationship between the linear percentage of transmittance and the log absorbance scales. At very low percentages of transmittance, small changes in the percentage of transmittance result in large changes in absorbance. For example, a change in percentage of transmittance of 60% to 50% T produces only a small absorbance change of approximately 0.08 A. A change in percentage of transmittance from 15% to 5%, however, results in a change in absorbance of 0.65 A. Thus, small changes in %T at very low transmittances will result in disproportionately large changes in the calculated absorbance at this part of the scale and will lead to an increased error of analysis.

One can consider the error of a spectrophotometric measurement as a function of the total or full-scale deflection of the detection meter or its electronics. When the absorbance scale is set at 0.000 or the transmittance scale is adjusted to 100%, the maximum electronic signal is obtained. For error analysis, the variation in this measurement is presumed to be constant throughout all readings on the scale. Because percent T directly reflects the electrical signal, some simple calculations can be done using percent T. At full-scale deflection (100% T), a 1% variation in percent T means an error of ±1% T. At half-scale, a 1% variation in the 50% T value means a 2% absolute error (1/50), and at 10% T, this becomes a 10% error (1/10). However, it is not percent T that is directly proportional to concentration; it is absorbance. One can convert these percent T values into absorbance and calculate the error (Table 17-1).

Because the conversion of percent T to absorbance is a logarithmic function, both ends of the absorbance scale, low absorbance (approaching 0.000) and high absorbance (more than 1.0), have the greatest error. In simple terms, when the solution has little color, it is difficult to tell the difference between no color and some color. The relative error can be huge because this difference is so small. At high absorbances, it is not easy to record accurately a small amount of light

Table **17-1** Absorbance Error as a Function of Percentage of Transmittance

%T and Error	Absorbance	Variation in Absorbance	Percent Error of Absorbance Measurement
4 ± 1	1.398	0.22	15.8
10 ± 1	1.000	0.041	8.60
25 ± 1	0.602	0.035	5.79
35 ± 1	0.456	0.025	5.44
50 ± 1	0.301	0.017	5.78
70 ± 1	0.155	0.012	8.03
90 ± 1	0.046	0.0097	21.2

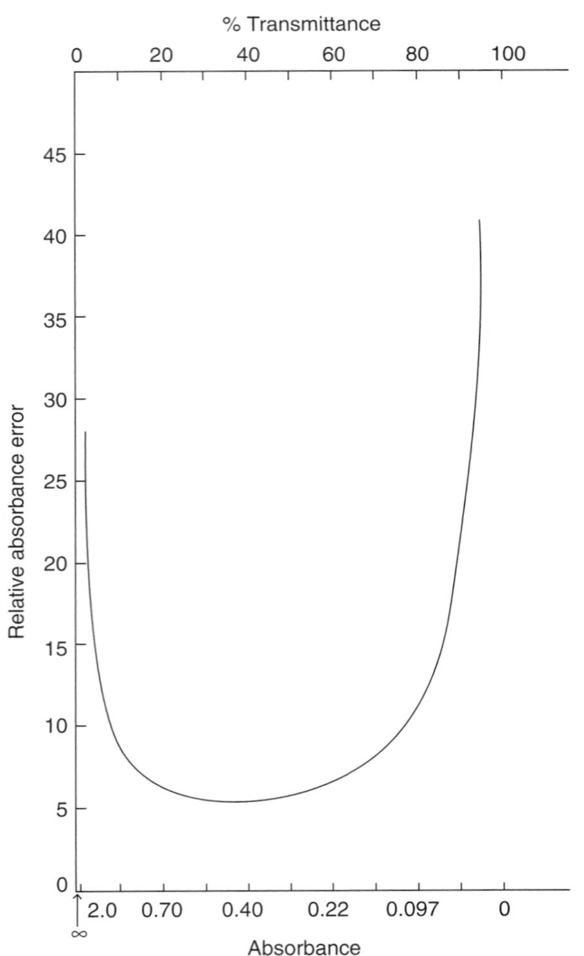

Fig. 17-2 Relative absorbance error versus absorbance (A) and percentage transmittance (%T) for a ±1% error in measurement of transmitted light. Relative error is minimum at 36.8% T, and A is 0.434.

passing through the solution. Thus, differences between the two values are minute compared with the total incident light used to calibrate 100% T, and it is difficult to measure these small changes.

The relative error of spectrophotometric measurements versus percentage of transmittance and absorbance is shown in Fig. 17-2. One should make most spectrophotometric measurements at absorbances between 0.1 and 1.1 to minimize this type of error.

Instrument Limitations

Consider how a spectrophotometer functions. At 100% T, or zero absorbance, all the light signal is converted to an electronic signal. Assume that this signal measures 1000 nanoamps (nA). If the absorbance changes by 0.010, there is a decrease to 990 nA, and the instrument must measure accurately 10/1000 nA, or a 1% change in signal. To do this accurately (1%), it must measure the signal to +0.10 nA (1% of 10). Thus, at zero absorbance, there is the difficulty of accurate measurement of 1 part in 104 of signal. In contrast, if the absorbance is 2.0, the signal to the photomultiplier is only 10 nA because only 1% of the light reaches the photodetector. To achieve the same degree of accuracy between values of absorbance of 2.00 and 2.02, the instrument must measure the difference between 10 and 9.9 nA, or 0.1 nA. To do this accurately, it must measure to within 0.001 nA (1% of 0.1). Thus, at high absorbances, limitations are caused by the inability of the detection system to accurately measure small differences between high levels of absorbance.

Thus, in analyses with relatively high levels of absorbing compound or **interferent,** a large spectrophotometric error will occur. An initial dilution used to lower total absorption *in addition to* a **sample blank** may be needed to eliminate this problem (see the discussion of **turbidity** on p. 314 for an example).

Fluorescence Spectrophotometer

Fluorescence measurements are different from those of transmission spectrophotometry in that the intensity of the fluorescence signal is linearly related to concentration. A doubling of the fluorescence signal is indicative of a twofold increase in concentration. This is true only if very little light is absorbed by the sample. If a significant portion of the light passing through a fluorescence sample is absorbed, the relationship is no longer linear; it becomes a more complex mathematical function. Thus, to minimize error, fluorescence analysis should be performed with relatively dilute solutions, the absorbance of which is less than 0.1.

Scattering of light or the presence of stray light has pronounced effects on fluorescence measurements. If the sample scatters light, some light may be observed by the detector as fluorescence. Similarly, if there is *stray light* (a term meaning that the light used to excite the sample was not pure, that is, not of a very narrow color band), this also may be recorded by the detector. Because only a small fraction of the incident light (less than 1% and often less than one part in a million of the total light input into the instrument) is detected as fluorescence, these extraneous signals have a disproportionate effect on the reading and thus on the error.

Fluorescence measurements, similar to absorption measurements, can be inaccurate or invalid because of high signals. Unlike with absorption spectrophotometry, this usually occurs because of the blanking system. If the fluorometer is adjusted to read zero for the blank, the entire detector sensitivity is adjusted for this zero reading. Assume that there is a blank solution that the instrument records as 10 units on its most sensitive scale. The instrument now is set to read this blank as zero fluorescence units. If the instrument can record accurately this zero unit to ±1 unit, and if it can also measure a full scale of 100 units in the same way, it can accurately measure a signal of 100 ± 1 units. If a different blank solution is used and this is recorded as 100 units, this new blank value can be set at zero with the use of electronic manipulation (subtraction of the signal). At this new full-scale deflection of 100, the detector is really recording 200, of which 100 is subtracted as the blank. Because the instrument is accurate to 1%, it is now accurate to 1% of the new full scale of 200 units. The inaccuracy of measurement is now ±2 units. The accuracy is therefore twice as poor as that for the first example. Similarly, if a blank records as 1000, the accuracy is one-tenth as great. Therefore, the signal strength of the blank limits the accuracy of fluorescence measurements.

This same line of argument applies to other linear measurements, as in electrochemical analysis. The background can be blanked, but this must be considered in relation to the total signal.

KEY CONCEPTS BOX 17-1

- There is a log-linear relationship between calculated A and measured %T. All spectrophotometric determinations of concentration are based on A.
- At low %T, there is greater imprecision when transmitted light is measured and very large error when the corresponding A is calculated because of the compressed nature of the log A scale.
- At high %T, the error of calculating A is large relative to the absolute value of A.
- This results in a U-shaped error curve and requires that measurements be made ay appropriate concentrations.

SECTION OBJECTIVES BOX 17-2

- List the three most likely sources of spectrophotometric interference in clinical analysis.
- Explain how these sources of interference actually cause analytical error.
- Describe the analytical techniques used to minimize the most common spectrophotometric interferences.
- Describe the interferences of immunochemical-based assays.

IN VITRO INTERFERENCES

In vitro interferences arise from the fact that biochemical analyses are performed in the complex matrices that make up biological fluids (serum, plasma, urine, cerebrospinal fluid, and so on). These fluids contain hundreds of compounds that either have chemical groups that can react to some extent with the test reagents or can mimic the physical, chromatographic, immunological, or spectral properties of the desired analyte. This situation is further complicated because the chemical composition of body fluids can vary with the nature and extent of disease processes. This variability is increased by the possible presence of a large number of drugs. Each of these factors, alone or in combination, can result in a possible interference.

The **in vitro interferences** can be subclassified into those of a spectral nature and those caused by competing chemical reactions. The most commonly observed spectrophotometric interferences are **hemolysis, icteria,** and **lipemia.** From one-fourth to one-third of samples obtained from clinic patients or hospitalized patients[2] are lipemic, icteric, or hemolyzed. A compendium listing the degree of interference by hemolysis, icterus, and lipemia on the analysis of 21 analytes on 22 different instruments is available.[2]

Spectral Interferences

Absorbance

Spectral interferences are observed when a compound causes a response in the spectrophotometer similar to that of the analyte of interest, although the interferents themselves do not necessarily undergo any chemical change during the analytical reaction. The simplest and most common example is the effect of hemoglobin (Hb) on many analytical procedures. A partial spectrum of HbO_2 (Fig. 17-3) shows significant absorption in the 500 to 600 nm portion of the visible spectrum. If one were monitoring the reaction of a colorimetric procedure in this region of the visible spectrum, significant positive interference would be evident whenever Hb was contaminating the specimen. Other molecules, such as bilirubin, cause a similar interference.

An example of hemoglobin interference can be seen when a serum total protein (TP) concentration is determined by monitoring the biuret reaction at 540 nm. A standard curve for this reaction is depicted in Fig. 17-4. If a significant concentration of hemoglobin is added to a sample, the absorption

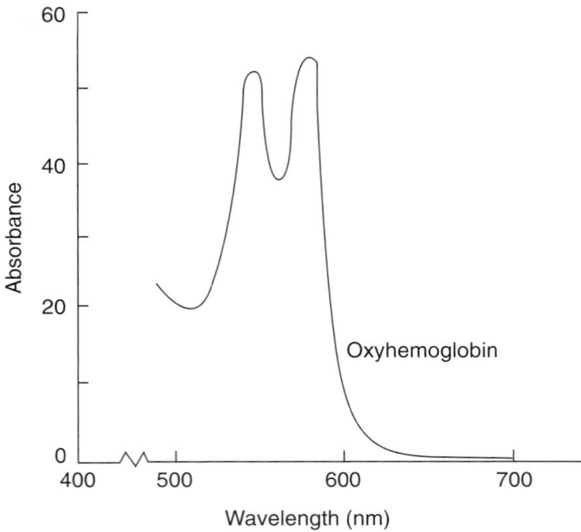

Fig. 17-3 Partial spectrum of oxyhemoglobin (HbO_2).

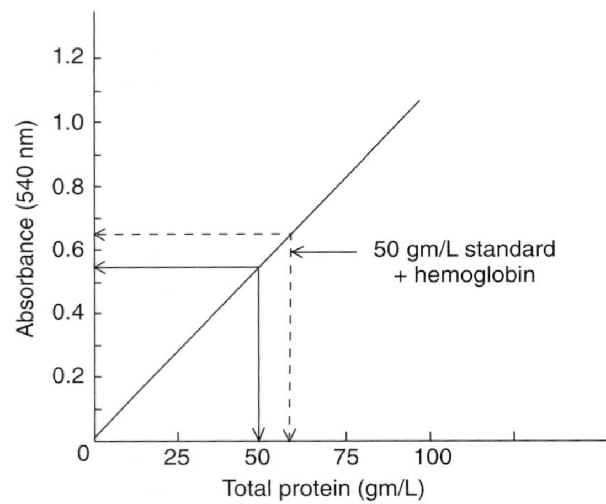

Fig. 17-4 Standard curve for measurement of total protein by the biuret reaction: A_{540} versus concentrations. *Solid arrow,* A_{540} for 50 g/L standard; *dotted arrow,* A_{540} for same standard containing hemoglobin.

Table 17-2 Effect of Turbidity on Measurement of LD Activity, U/L

	LD ACTIVITY, U/L			
	NONTURBID SAMPLE		*TURBID SAMPLE*	
Dilution (with saline)	**Uncorrected**	**Corrected**	**Uncorrected**	**Corrected**
Undiluted	440	—	28	—
1:2	245	450	32	64
1:4	136	444	30	120
1:8	62	496	26	208
1:16	30	480	25	400
1:32	14	450	13	416

at 540 nm is increased, thus giving a falsely high total protein reading. In this example, the A_{540} of a 50 g/L standard is 0.550. If small amounts of hemoglobin are added to this standard, the A_{540} is 0.650. When this solution is read from the standard curve, a higher apparent concentration of protein is calculated *(dotted line)*. Most spectral interferences give falsely elevated results in this manner.

Turbidity

A common type of spectral interference is caused by the turbidity of the sample. Turbidity is caused by large lipoprotein molecules called *very-low-density lipoproteins (VLDLs)*, which are suspended in serum. When a turbid specimen is analyzed in a colorimetric reaction, the lipoproteins cause the incident light to scatter, much as in nephelometry (see Chapter 2).

Because spectrophotometric analysis normally measures transmitted light at 180 degrees to the incident light, any light scattering tends to decrease transmitted light and therefore to increase the apparent absorbance of the specimen. This, of course, results in falsely elevated results. Sample blanks normally work poorly here, just as two-point **kinetic analysis** does (see below), because of the error resulting from the very high absorbances often encountered. The best method for eliminating the interference caused by turbidity is dilution of the specimen. The extent to which the sample can be diluted to minimize turbidimetric interference is limited by the ability of the analytical procedure to measure the diluted analyte. If possible, several dilutions should be analyzed simultaneously to determine the best response. An example of the effect and elimination of turbidimetric interference is presented in the analysis of equal amounts of lactate dehydrogenase (LD) activity in a turbid and a nonturbid specimen (Table 17-2). When the nonturbid specimen is diluted, all corrected LD activities calculate out to the same approximate value. This indicates linearity of dilution. In contrast, when the turbid specimen is diluted, the calculated LD activity changes with dilution. Only at higher dilutions that contain minimum turbidity do calculated LD activities converge with true values of the nonturbid specimen.

Fluorescence

Turbidity affects fluorescence measurements in a similar fashion. Here, some scattered light will reach the detector set at 90 degrees to the incident light, thus causing an apparent increase in fluorescence and falsely elevated concentrations. Reducing problems of turbidity in fluorescence measurements is more difficult than for absorption spectroscopy. The best approach is the elimination of the source of light scattering by filtration or centrifugation.

Correction of Spectral Interferences

Sample Blank

One can minimize spectral interferences by measuring the absorbance of the assay against a sample blank. The simplest sample blank is obtained with a mixture of the sample and diluent (instead of reagent). The correction for spectral interference is made by subtracting the absorbance value of the blank from the absorbance of the complete reaction mixture. Any significant color inherent to the sample is eliminated by this calculation. In the example of the biuret reaction discussed previously, the absorbance of the sample and the hemoglobin diluted with saline is 0.100. If this is subtracted from the absorbance of the complete reaction mixture (0.650), the true absorbance of the standard (0.550) is obtained. Such a sample blank usually can work, unless gross amounts of the interferent are present. In these cases, the very large total absorption ($A_{interferent} + A_{reaction}$) results in large spectrophotometric and calculation errors. Random access analyses (see Chapter 20) easily permit the measurement of sample blank absorbances before the addition of reagent. **Reagent blanks** (reagent plus diluent) are used in a similar fashion to correct for high absorbance of the reagent. In the case of fluorescence, the sample blank allows for the correction of nonspecific fluorescence; however, the fluorescence of this blank cannot constitute a great portion of the total fluorescence signal (see preceding text).

Kinetic Measurements

One frequently used method for the correction of spectral interference is the measurement of a typical end-point reaction as a two-point kinetic reaction. If the absorbance of a noninstantaneous, colorimetric reaction is monitored versus time, a reaction curve as shown in Fig. 17-5 will be observed. An **end-point reaction** is monitored at a single time point when the reaction is mostly completed (see Fig. 17-5, *arrow 3*). If no spectral interferences are present, the reaction curve should pass through the origin. If such interferences are present, the curve will be *parallel* to the original curve but biased high because of the endogenous color in the sample. If a sample blank was used to subtract endogenous color, a line identical to that in the sample containing no interferences would be obtained.

In a two-point kinetic assay, absorbance is measured at *two* different time points (see Fig. 17-5, *arrows 1* and *2*) when (1) the final color development has not occurred and in fact may be small, and (2) the response of absorbance versus time remains linear.

The initial absorbance reading (see Fig. 17-5, *arrow 1*) is actually taken when almost no color formation has occurred. Thus any absorbance at this time is caused primarily by endogenous spectral interferents. A second reading is taken a short time later, when only a small amount of color has formed and the response of absorbance versus time is still linear (see Fig. 17-5, *arrow 2*). This absorbance therefore includes both the original endogenous color and the color formed by the specific analytical reaction. With subtraction of the first reading from the second, the calculated *delta absorbance* (ΔA) is caused only by the specific color formed by the analytical reaction. Standard curves based on kinetic analysis have the change in absorbance (ΔA) plotted versus concentration (Fig. 17-6). In this standard curve, the presence of a *nonreacting,* endogenous, colored interferent has no effect. Thus no separate sample blank measurement needs to be made; a two-point kinetic reaction is self-blanking when there is no change in the nature of the interferent during the reaction. This is an important technique when one is performing automated chemical analysis on large numbers of specimens.

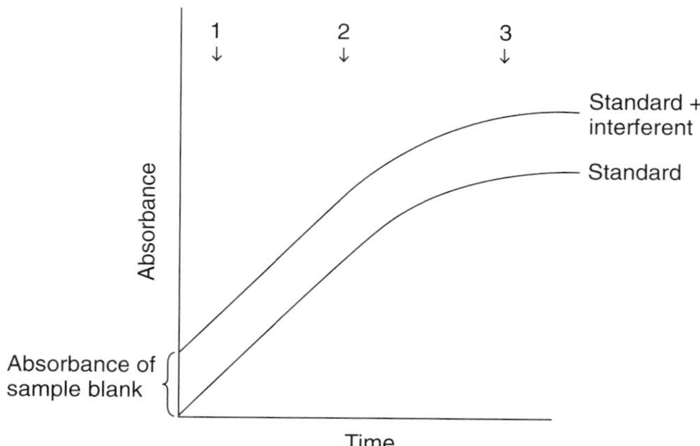

Fig. 17-5 Absorbance changes versus time for colorimetric reaction, with and without interferent present. *Arrows 1* and *2,* Time frame for kinetic analysis; *arrow 3,* end-point reading.

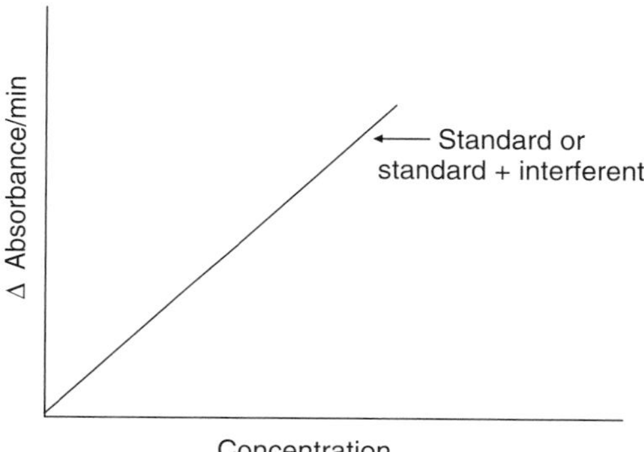

Fig. 17-6 Kinetic analysis of both reactions shown in Fig. 17-5. Change in absorbance (ΔA) per minute versus concentration during linear portion of curve of absorbance versus time between *arrows 1* and *2* in Fig. 17-5.

Biochromatic Analysis[3]

Many instruments in current use employ a different technique for correction of spectral interferences. This technique involves simultaneous measurement of the absorbance of the reaction

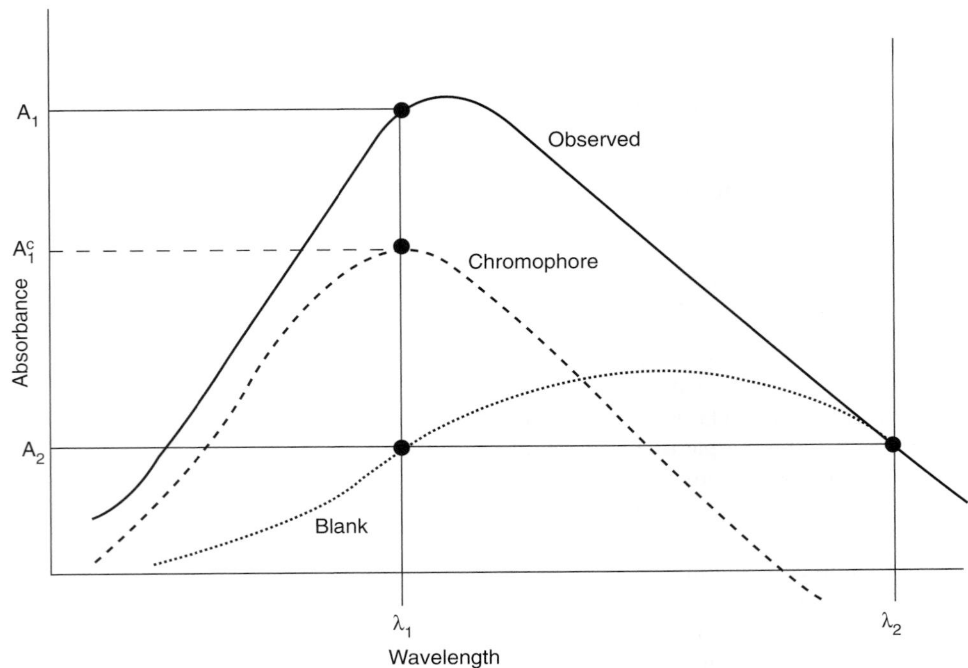

Fig. 17-7 Spectral curves for chromophore and nonreactive blank, where blank absorbance is equal at λ_1 and λ_2.

mixture at two different wavelengths. These include the primary wavelength (λ_1) and one other wavelength (λ_2) that is close by. As is shown in Fig. 17-7, λ_1 is the wavelength at which the chromogen maximally absorbs. At λ_2, there is minimum absorbance of the chromogen. Because the reaction is monitored simultaneously at two wavelengths, this is known as **bichromatic analysis.** This technique is based on the premise that although a compound may give a spectral interference, the absorbance maxima of the interferent will differ from that of the actual analytical reaction. In addition, this procedure is performed under the assumption that the absorption caused by the interfering compound is approximately the same at λ_1 as at λ_2. Although the measured absorbance at λ_1 will be caused by both the analytical reaction and the interferent, the absorbance at the second wavelength (λ_2) will be caused by only the interferent. This technique can also correct for instrument problems such as dirt on the cell, which causes light scattering or reflectance. Standard curves then are based on either $A_1 - A_2$ or the ratio of the two absorbances (A_1/A_2). Use of this procedure, which can also be run in the kinetic mode, also allows each sample to serve as its own blank for endogenous color.

Another similar method for the correction of background interference is the measurement of absorbance at the primary wavelength A_{max} and at two additional wavelengths, usually equidistant from the peak, A_1 and A_2. Absorbance readings at these last two wavelengths are averaged to give the average background absorbance in the specimen. This technique for the correction of background absorbance from interfering substances is known as the **Allen correction.**[4]

The Allen correction is valid only if the background absorbance is approximately linear with wavelength over the region

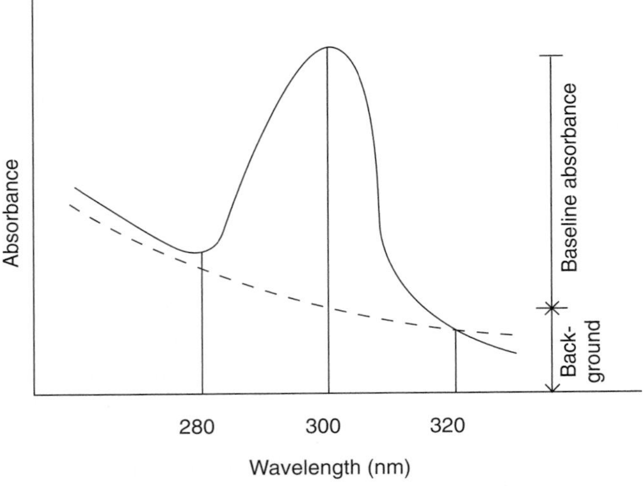

Fig. 17-8 Spectral curves of chromophore and interferent, *solid line,* and background interferents, *dotted line.* Average of A_{280} and A_{320} represents background absorbance at A_{max} for chromophore (300 nm).

in which the measurements are being taken. Thus the shape of the absorption curve for both the analyte and the interferent *(solid line)* and the interferents *(dotted line)* must be obtained as shown in Fig. 17-8. Use of the Allen correction in this example, when the wavelengths used to correct for background are equidistant from the absorbance maxima, would yield the following equation:

$$A_{300}\ \text{corrected} = A_{300} - (A_{320} + A_{280})/2 \quad \text{Eq. 17-1}$$

The "A_{300} corrected" has the average background absorbance subtracted from the absorbance maximum to give the

Table 17-3 Examples of Chemically Interfering Biochemicals

Analyte	Method	Interferences
Glucose	Reducing sugar	Uric acid (+), creatinine (+), protein (+), glutathione (+)
	Glucose oxidase–horseradish peroxidase	Uric acid (+), ascorbic acid (−), bilirubin (−)
	Glucose oxidase–O_2 consumption	Hemoglobin (−), ascorbic acid (+)
	Hexokinase	Fructose (+)
Creatinine	Alkaline picrate	Ascorbic acid (+), glucose (+), protein (+), ketones (+)
Vanillylmandelic acid	Pisano	Certain foods (such as bananas), vanilla, aspirin (+)
	High-performance liquid chromatography	Certain drugs and their metabolites (+)

−, Negative interference; +, positive interference.

actual absorbance above baseline value. The Allen correction is widely used, but improper use of the Allen correction, that is, with nonlinear background interference, can lead to even larger errors. Because the final corrected absorbance is based on three measurements, the precision of the assay is decreased.

There are many variations of this technique, including the use of one secondary wavelength as a measure of background interference. In this case, the ratio of the signals from primary and secondary wavelengths versus sample concentration is employed to create a calibration curve (see above).

Dilution

As was discussed for turbidity, dilution of a sample that contains a spectral interferent sometimes can reduce the problem. One must be careful not to overdilute the desired analyte or chromogen to a concentration below the minimum detectable level for a given assay. Several dilutions should be assayed simultaneously to determine the most effective dilution.

Chemical Interferences

All the interferences discussed so far have been spectral interferences caused by compounds that do not react in the analytical chemical reaction. However, many interferents do react with reagent chemicals in the analytical reaction. The reaction products of these interferences usually result in positive interferences, although negative interferences may be observed.

Types of nonspecific, chemically reacting interferents can vary greatly, as can be seen in the examples in Table 17-3. Uric acid produces a positive interference, and bilirubin and ascorbic acid yield negative interferences, in the glucose oxidase-peroxididase methods used for glucose measurement. The alkaline picrate reaction for the measurement of creatinine is known to have both positive (ketones, protein) and negative (bilirubin) interferences.

Correction of Chemical Interferences

Elimination of many nonspecific **chemical interferents** often is achieved by one or more of the following techniques:

- Diluting the interferent
- Increasing the specificity of the reaction
- Removing the interferent
- Monitoring an assay by kinetic measurement
- Monitoring an assay by bichromatic measurement

Dilution of the sample is an effective method in the case of interferents that do not react at the same rate or produce the same color intensity as the analyte. Interference by protein is minimized in many automated analyzers by a large specimen dilution.

Increased specificity of an analytical reaction is often achieved by the use of specific enzymes as reagents. Examples of this approach include the measurement of glucose by hexokinase or glucose oxidase, uric acid by uricase, and urea by urease. Immunochemical-based reactions also are used to increase the specificity of the analysis. An example would be the measurement of theophylline by enzyme immunoassay versus older methods, which employed ultraviolet absorbance.

Separation of an interferent from the analyte may be achieved by the use of (1) a protein-free sample, (2) liquid-liquid extraction, or (3) adsorption or partition chromatography. Protein-free samples originally were prepared by precipitation of serum proteins and separation of the protein-free sample by filtration or centrifugation. Agents used to precipitate proteins include tungstic acid (Folin-Wu procedure) and heavy-metal salts (such as barium and zinc; Somogyi-Nelson procedure).

Liquid-liquid extractions are used when the analyte and interferent or interferents can be separated into different liquid phases. Similarly, in adsorption and partition chromatography, the analyte and the interferent are separated by their differential affinity for the stationary phase (see Chapters 3 and 4).

The basis for the elimination of nonspecific chemical reactants by the use of a two-point kinetic reaction is that many interferents react at a different rate from the one at which the specific analyte of interest reacts. This is observed in the example of the Jaffe reaction with creatinine.[5]

Creatinine reacts with alkaline picrate at a finite rate (curve TC [true creatinine]) (Fig. 17-9). Many of the nonspecific interferents (such as acetone) react at a faster kinetic rate (FR), whereas some (such as protein) react at a slower rate (SR), producing a complex change in absorbance over time for the reaction of a mixture of all three species (Fig. 17-10). Therefore, by properly choosing an optimal **window** of time for the two absorbance readings for the kinetic analysis (*arrows*, see Fig. 17-9), one can minimize the effects of the fast-reacting and slow-reacting nonspecific interferents and can isolate the

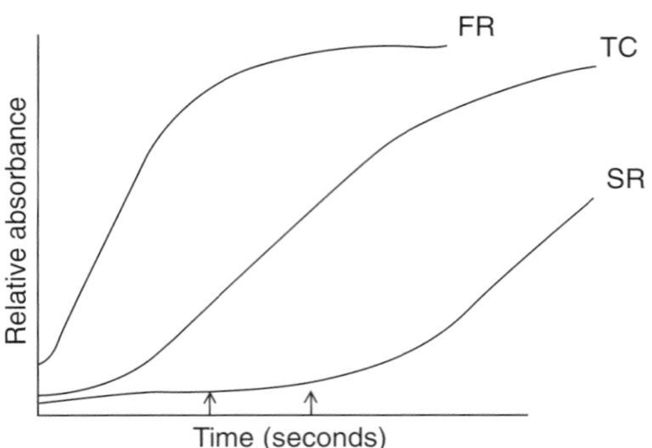

Fig. 17-9 Relative absorbance versus time curves for alkaline picrate reaction, for creatinine *(TC),* slow-reacting interferents *(SR),* and fast-reacting interferents *(FR). Arrows,* Time during which absorbance, over time, primarily reflects change attributable to the TC reaction.

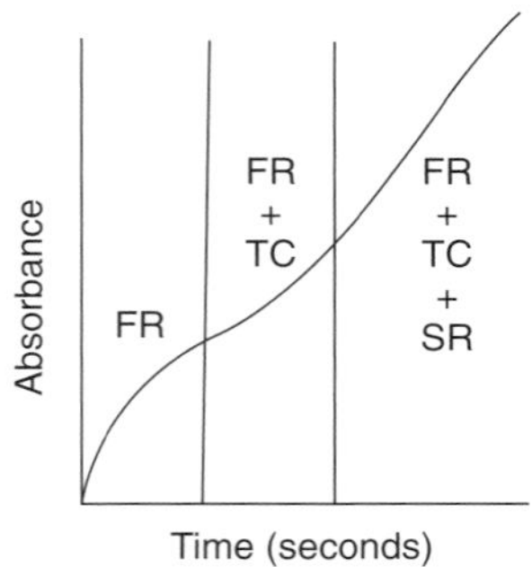

Fig. 17-10 Complex reaction of mixture containing fast-reacting *(FR)* and slow-reacting *(SR)* interferents plus creatinine *(TC).* Only by measurement of the change in absorbance over time can TC reaction be isolated and SR and FR interferences minimized.

absorbance change caused primarily by creatinine. During the window of time, the reaction of the FR interferents is essentially complete, whereas that of the SR interferents is not yet occurring (see Fig. 17-10). The ΔA during this time is caused by the analyte, that is, creatinine. This concept has also been used for the glucose oxidase reaction and is, in fact, a popular technique for increasing the specificity of reactions with many instruments.

Chromatographic Interferences

The third type of common in vitro, or methodological, interference is chromatographic interference. This often occurs when an interfering compound co-chromatographs with the compound of interest to give falsely elevated results.

Currently, many analytical procedures use chromatography to separate the analyte to be measured from interfering compounds. A chromatographic method is used under the assumption that the desired analyte is completely isolated from other compounds that may be recorded by the detection system. However, no single set of chromatography conditions can possibly prevent interferences from co-chromatographing or closely chromatographing compounds, especially when the patient may be receiving several potentially interfering drugs.

An example of this type of interference and its correction can be seen in the high-performance liquid chromatographic (HPLC) separation of catecholamines and the drug methyldopa (Aldomet), which is used in the treatment of patients with hypertension. In some HPLC assays, methyldopa is eluted from the column just before norepinephrine. Because the pharmacological dose of Aldomet is much greater than the physiological concentrations of norepinephrine, it will obliterate or be confused with the norepinephrine peak. The only way to eliminate this type of interference is to remove the source of exogenous interferent. In the case of methyldopa, removal of the drug from the patient for 2 to 10 days is required. Drug or diet restrictions before biochemical analysis are often a necessity for many compounds.

There are two primary modes of minimizing chromatographic interferents: (1) increasing the specificity of the detector, and (2) removing the interferent from the analyte. Detectors can measure compounds according to a variety of different principles. If the interferent has physical or chemical properties different from those of the analyte, it is possible to select a detector that will not respond significantly to a potential interferent. In liquid chromatography, refractive index detectors can detect almost any compound in the eluant; thus, they are very nonspecific. Fluorescence detectors have much higher specificities because not all compounds fluoresce. Through appropriate setting of excitation and emission wavelengths, the detector can be made even more specific. Electrochemical detectors also have high specificities because not all compounds are electrochemically active. Specificity can be further increased by selection of an electrode voltage at which the interferent will not react.

As was discussed earlier, separation of the analytes from potentially interfering compounds is achieved by several techniques. These techniques are based on differences in solubility or chromatographic behavior between the analyte and interferents. The techniques commonly used are single liquid-liquid extractions, multiple extractions including back-extractions, and adsorption and ion-exchange chromatography. The complexity of the procedure used depends on the nature of the interference and the required sensitivity. HPLC methods for serum theophylline, which is present in relatively large amounts, usually employ only a simple liquid-liquid extraction. In contrast, HPLC analysis of the tricyclic antidepressants present in nanogram quantities requires several extraction steps, including back-extractions. Chapter 4 discusses these types of procedures in greater detail.

A technique for detecting contaminating or co-chromatographing compounds is dual-detection analysis. This technique uses two different types of detectors or parameters, such as multiple wavelengths, to monitor the column eluate. The response of the two different detectors (D_1 and D_2) is determined for a standard, and the ratio of the responses is calculated (D_1 standard/D_2 standard). The probability that another compound will have a similar characteristic ratio is quite small. Thus, significant deviations of the ratio found in patient analyses would strongly suggest that the analyte peak contains a contaminating, co-eluting compound.

Box 17-1

Interferences Common to Immunoassays

Exogenous Interference
- Sample collection and preparation, including anticoagulants, sample storage, drugs, and serum-separating gels
- Calibration matrix
- Changes in solid-phase surface binding caused by coating molecule
- Incomplete saturation of solid-phase binding sites for antigen or antibody

Endogenous Interference
- Hyperlipidemia/turbidity
- Heterophilic anti-immunoglobulin antibodies (HAMAs)
- Iatrogenic antibodies, such as Digabind [see Methods on Evolve for digoxin]
- Rheumatoid factor
- Autoantibodies against analyte
- Complement
- Cross-reacting substance, such as DLIF
- Competing immunospecific antibodies to analyte

Modified from Pesce AJ, Michael JG: J Immunol Methods 150:111, 1992.
DLIF, Digoxin-like immunoreactive factor; *HAMAs,* human antimouse antibodies.

Often the presence of a co-chromatographing interferent is recognized because of the abnormal shape of the peak. The presence of a contaminant often causes a normally symmetrical peak to become skewed. In these cases, rerunning the chromatogram at lower flow rates sometimes will separate or partially separate the analyte from the interfering compound, allowing quantitation.

Immunochemical Interferences

Immunochemical methods are subject to the usual causes of exogenous interference (Box 17-1).[6] In addition, however, they are subject to matrix effects of the reaction solution and, in some cases, the surface where the reaction is occurring. Hyperlipidemia can greatly affect immunochemical reactions that use turbidimetric or nephelometric measurements because of the increased sample turbidity. The most difficult interference to detect is that in which the patient has antibodies to the test reagent antibodies (heterophile antibodies), or to the actual test antigen. The most frequently encountered heterophile antibodies, those against mouse antibodies **(HAMAs),** can cause interference in assays that employ mouse monoclonal antibodies. Methods for reducing these interferents include adding specific animal sera, such as mouse serum, to the test reagent to combine with the heterophile antibodies and neutralize them.[7] Often the only indication that the patient has antibodies to the test analyte is the patient history, which can indicate that test results are not consistent with clinical findings. An interesting example of the problem of endogenous antibodies can be seen in the measurement of digoxin. In acute digoxin overdoses, the patient may be treated with Digabind, an Fc fragment of immunoglobulin (Ig)G antibodies to digoxin that binds digoxin, minimizes toxicity, and increases clearance. Digabind will also react with labeled digoxin in an immunoassay and will cause apparently highly elevated digoxin levels.

Box 17-2

Interferences for Enzyme Immunoassays

Exogenous Interference
- Enzyme inhibitor
- Endogenous interference
- Endogenous enzyme
- Endogenous substrate
- Spectral: lipids, hemoglobin
- Drugs that inhibit enzyme activity

Measurement of Enzyme Activity
- Temperature
- Substrate reaction on solid phase
- Nonlinear kinetics
- Limited sensitivity
- Substrate depletion

Modified from Pesce AJ, Michael JG: J Immunol Methods 150:111, 1992.

For enzyme immunoassays, some of the interferences are the same as those observed in ordinary enzyme assays, as is shown in Box 17-2.

KEY CONCEPTS BOX 17-2

- Hemolysis, icteria, and lipemia are the most common sources of interference in spectrophotometric analyses.
- Hemolysis causes interference from the high A from hemoglobin (Hb), as well as the addition of intracellular chemicals from the breakage of blood cells.
- Icteria causes interference from the high A of bilirubin.
- Lipemia results in a high background A from light scattering off of lipoprotein particles.
- Effects of these interferences can be minimized by sample dilution, subtraction of sample blank A from the reaction A, use of bichromatic analysis, use of kinetic analysis, or combinations of all these.
- Interferences also can be minimized by the use of more specific reagents, such as enzymes or monoclonal antibodies.

SECTION OBJECTIVE BOX 17-3

- Describe the resources available for assessing the presence of interferences.

IN VIVO INTERFERENCES

Factors such as age and sex, time of day, diet, pregnancy, and menses, as well as sample processing errors, can affect the test result. These are discussed in Chapter 18. The presence of drugs in the patient is a common source of interference.

Drugs

Virtually every drug affects some laboratory procedure, and any laboratory procedure may be affected by one or more drugs. This interference may occur in vivo or in vitro. An example of a commonly encountered drug is alcohol, whose ingestion may affect glucose, lactate, urate, bicarbonate, γ-glutamyl transferase, and creatine phosphokinase levels.[8] Smoking may alter catecholamine, cortisol, and blood-gas results. Reference to source material is needed to determine the effect of any one of the huge number of drugs on a specific test.

SOURCE-REFERENCE MATERIAL

This chapter provides only a brief description of the wide variety and types of interferences in chemistry laboratory testing. Laboratories minimize errors by understanding their sources and constantly trying to control them. This requires being constantly vigilant for new interferents for old assays and new and old interferents for new assays. Many commonly interfering substances are well documented in the professional literature and in published compendiums, and an alert laboratory staff often can eliminate these as sources of interference. For example, the development of the interferogram[2] allows the laboratory to estimate the effects of hemolysis, icterus, and lipemia on analyses performed on frequently used instruments. Newer automated chemistry analyzers can be calibrated to detect increased levels of hemolysis, lipemia, and icterus (see Chapter 20). However, as the number of drugs produced by pharmaceutical companies and consumed by the public increases, the laboratory must determine both in vivo and in vitro effects exerted by each of these drugs on clinical laboratory analysis.

A list of the known effects of drugs and other interferences on chemical analysis is available.[9] Although it becomes outdated when published, this remains the best and only single listing of drug effects on laboratory tests. In one of the two major sections, possible interferents (not only drugs) are listed in alphabetical order. Listed under each interferent are those laboratory tests that may be affected by that interferent. The section that lists interferents is cross-indexed by another section that lists, in alphabetical order, laboratory tests.

A complementary issue to this listing lists the effects of disease on clinical laboratory tests.[10] The format for this volume is similar to the one just described. The first section lists each analyte and those disease states in which changes in the concentration of that analyte have been noted. The second section lists diseases and those analytes that change during the course of the disease.

Evaluation of Analytical Interference

Because virtually all clinical chemistry analytical procedures can be interfered with by the factors of preanalytical variation and the patient specimen itself (see Chapter 18), many protocols have been proposed for use in evaluating the extent of potential interference.[11-14]

Often the testing of spectral interference involves the addition of a lipid substance (Intralipid, Kabi Vitrum, Alameda, California), a hemolysate, or bilirubin.[2] In some cases, the test method is compared with a reference or definitive method that is not subject to the interference under evaluation. These techniques include isotope dilution mass spectroscopy, neutron activation, atomic absorption, and other specialized techniques. The most extensive proposal for interference testing can be found in Reference 13.

Allowable Interference

Because some interference is potentially present for every assay, clinical chemists must determine how much interference is allowable. A statistically significant interferent may not be a clinically significant one. One approach is to use the medical decision limit.[15] The concept of clinically important errors is reviewed in Chapter 25, and examples of its application are found in Chapter 26. The size of allowable error is determined through consultations with clinicians who are using the results of testing and through discussions of allowable error in the literature.

The total analytical error, E_A, of a method is the sum of its imprecision, which equals the sum of twice the standard deviation (2SD), its analytical bias (E_B), and the error resulting from interferents (E_I):

$$E_A = 2SD + E_B + E_I \qquad \text{Eq. 17-2}$$

For an assay to be clinically useful, the total analytical error, E_A, must be less than the total allowable error at the medical decision level, E_{MDL}, for each analyte. If the laboratory knows the errors SD + E_B and can estimate E_{MDL}, the allowable contribution from an interferent, E_I, can be calculated as follows:

$$E_I = E_{MDL} - 2SD - E_B \qquad \text{Eq. 17-3}$$

This discussion assumes that the total allowable error for medical decision making needs is greater than the total allowable error permitted for Clinical Laboratory Improvement Amendments (CLIA) '88—regulated analytes. These calculations can be used to determine the analytical errors permissible under these regulations (see Chapter 25).

Thus, for assays with small standard deviations and biases and E_As that are much smaller than the medical decision value, larger errors caused by interferences can be tolerated. In contrast, some measurements, such as creatinine in transplant patients, have a small allowable error (often less than 20%), which must include bias, method variability, and interference. Thus, with these methods, there is less tolerance to interference.

KEY CONCEPTS BOX 17-3

- Knowledge of possible assay interferences can be obtained from published journals and lists of known interferences.
- Investigating the source of laboratory error and reviewing a lab's "error budget" can allow lab staff to effectively control error in a clinically meaningful manner.

REFERENCES

1. http://www.quic.gov/report/errors6ver6.doc—Report to the President on Medical Errors.
2. Glick MR, Ryder KW: *Interferographs: User's Guide to Interferences in Clinical Chemistry Instruments,* Indianapolis, 1987, Science Enterprises, Inc.
3. Hahn B, Vlastelica DL, Snyder LR, et al: Polychromatic analysis: new applications of an old technique, Clin Chem 25:951, 1979.
4. Allen E, Rieman W: Determining only one compound in a mixture, short spectrophotometric method, Anal Chem 25:1325, 1953.
5. Soldin SJ, Henderson L, Hill JG: The effect of bilirubin and ketones on reaction rate methods for the measurement of creatinine, Clin Biochem 11:82, 1978.
6. Pesce AJ, Michael JG: Artifacts and limitations of enzyme immunoassay, J Immunol Methods 150:111, 1992.
7. Bjerner J, Nustad K, Norum LF, et al: Immunometric assay interference: incidence and prevention, Clin Chem 48:613, 2002.
8. Freer DE, Statland BE: The effect of ethanol (0.75 g/kg body weight) on the activities of selected enzymes in sera of healthy young adults. I. Intermediate-term effect, Clin Chem 23:830, 1977.
9. Young DS: *Effects of Drugs on Clinical Laboratory Tests,* ed 5, Washington, DC, 2000, American Association for Clinical Chemistry.
10. Young DS, Friedman KB: *Effect of Diseases on Clinical Laboratory Tests,* ed 4, Washington, DC, 2001, American Association for Clinical Chemistry.
11. Young DS: *Effects of Preanalytical Variables on Clinical Laboratory Tests,* ed 3, Washington, DC, 2007, American Association for Clinical Chemistry.
12. Büttner J, Dybkaer R, Stamm D, et al: Symposium 2: Reference methods in clinical chemistry—objectives, trends, Fresenius' Journal of Analytical Chemistry 337:633, 1990.
13. *Interference Testing in Clinical Chemistry: Proposed Guideline,* ed 2, CLSI Publication EP7-A2, Villanova, Pennsylvania, 2005, Clinical and Laboratory Standards Institute.
14. Guder WG, Narayanan S, Wisser H, Zawta B: *Samples: From the Patient to the Laboratory: The Impact of Preanalytical Variables on the Quality of Laboratory Results,* ed 3, revised, Weinheim, Germany, 2003, Wiley-VCH.
15. Castano-Vidriales JL: Interferences in clinical chemistry, J Int Fed Clin Chem 6:7, 1994.

INTERNET SITES

http://www.ahrq.gov/qual/errback.htm

http://www.fda.gov/fdac/features/2000/500_err.html

Sources and Control of Preanalytical Variation

Chapter 18

D. Robert Dufour

Chapter Outline

Key Terms

additive A chemical added to a specimen that changes one or more of its physical or chemical properties.

adsorb Attachment of a chemical substance to a solid surface.

aerosol A fine mist produced by atomization of a liquid.

analyte A substance that can be measured by an analytical technique.

anastomotic Connecting two blood vessels.

anticoagulant A substance that can suppress, delay, or prevent coagulation of blood by preventing formation of fibrin.

antiseptic A chemical that reduces the number of bacteria.

arterial Related to or derived from arteries—the vessels that deliver blood from the heart to the tissues of the body.

artifactual Changed state of a material, resulting from artificial, rather than natural, processes or conditions.

bar code A system of bars of varying widths, used as a way to provide identification information.

capillary Related to tiny blood vessels in tissues, through which nutrients are delivered and waste products are removed by the blood.

catheter A hollow plastic or rubber tube that connects a body cavity with the surface of the body.

chelation The process by which an organic molecule binds multiple metal ions.

circadian (ser-ca-de′-un) **rhythms** Changes in the concentration of analytes that occur over the course of a single day.

clot An aggregation of blood cells held together by fibrin, a polymerized protein.

cyclical variation Changes in the concentration of analytes that occur repetitively in a predictable fashion over a given period of time.

delta check Comparison of analyte concentration in one specimen from a person versus that in the previous specimen from the same person.

EDTA Ethylenediaminetetraacetic acid, a commonly used chemical that chelates calcium. It acts as an blood anticoagulant and preservative by binding calcium and other cations, which inactivates several enzymes needed for clot formation and for the breakdown of protein and lipid analytes in blood.

evaporation Transformation of water to vapor.

extracellular Outside of cells.

glycolytic Related to the process of metabolism of glucose.

hemoconcentration The process of increasing the concentrations of cells, proteins, and, occasionally, other analytes in blood through loss of water (in vitro or in vivo).

hemolysis Rupture of red blood cells that releases into the serum or plasma analytes found in blood cells.

heparin An anticoagulant that directly inhibits formation of fibrin.

infradian (infra-de′-un) Changes in the concentration of analytes that occur less frequently than once a day.

intraindividual Within a single person.

intravenous Within a vein; usually refers to intravenous fluid in which water that contains medications, glucose, or electrolytes is given to a patient through a catheter inserted into a vein.

in vitro Literally, "in glass"; occurs in an artificial situation, as in a test tube.

nonlaminar Not in an orderly, layered fashion with smooth gradations from one layer to another. With liquids, nonlaminar flow produces shearing forces whereby different layers or laminae come into contact.

phlebotomy Puncturing a vein with a needle for the purpose of obtaining a sample of blood.

plasma The liquid portion of blood in the bloodstream; obtained as a specimen by collecting blood with an anticoagulant and centrifuging the specimen.

postprandial After a meal; also postcibal.

preanalytical variation Factors that alter the results of a laboratory test and that occur before the process of performing that test.

preservatives Chemicals that prevent a change in the concentration of analytes in a sample of blood, urine, or other body fluid.

proteolysis The process of degradation of proteins, which may occur by chemical reactions or by enzymatic processes.

serum The liquid part of blood that remains after a clot has formed.

serum separator A mechanical device that physically separates sera from cells (plasma separators separate plasma from cells), thus preventing changes in the concentration of serum analytes that may result from cell metabolism.

stasis A decrease in the flow of blood to or from a part of the body.

TBEP Tris(2-butoxyethyl) phosphate, a chemical found in some types of rubber, which may leak from stoppers and bind to proteins, displacing chemicals and altering their serum (or plasma) concentrations.

tourniquet A mechanical device (such as a wide rubber band) used on the surface of an extremity to compress veins, enlarging them by preventing the return of blood to the heart and lungs.

ultradian (ultra-de′-un) Changes in the concentration of analytes that occur over a period of time much shorter than 1 day.

venous Related to veins—the vessels that return blood from the tissues to the heart and lungs.

SECTION OBJECTIVES BOX 18-1

- List available resource guides to determine and control preanalytical error.
- State the most common error in the preanalytical testing cycle.
- Discuss how cyclic biological variables and intraindividual variation may affect laboratory results.
- Discuss procedures that may be followed that can minimize patient preparation errors.
- Discuss how physical variables, such as exercise, stress, posture, and diet affect certain laboratory tests.

Laboratory testing is often thought of as a process that begins with collection of a sample from an individual and ends with reporting of the results of testing. Growing emphasis has been placed on the total testing cycle,[1] which begins and ends with the interaction between a health care provider and a patient. This cycle divides the testing process into three phases: preanalytical, which begins with the patient and ends with preparation of a sample for testing; analytical, which includes all steps involved in the actual performance of a laboratory test; and postanalytical, which begins with reporting of results to the health care provider and ends with actions being taken by the health care provider (or patient) that are based on test results. This chapter focuses almost exclusively on issues that occur in the preanalytical phase of the testing cycle, although it does discuss delta checks, a postanalytical step that is aimed primarily at reducing preanalytical variation. In research on laboratory errors, data consistently show that the preanalytical stage is the source of most laboratory errors.[2]

Laboratory tests are ordered to evaluate the status of a patient because test results are a good reflection of the physiological state of the patient, as is discussed in later chapters. Errors in the testing cycle can invalidate the link between test results and the patient's state. Just as control of temperature, wavelength, and time of incubation can limit analytical error, preanalytical error also can be controlled. The purpose of this chapter is to detail the common sources of preanalytical error and the methods that can be used to control this type of error.

Laboratories are responsible for taking steps to minimize sources of error by developing standard procedures that govern patient preparation, sample collection, methods of sample transport, and preservation of samples. Agencies that accredit laboratories, including the College of American Pathologists (CAP) and the Joint Commission, require each laboratory to provide a detailed manual that documents the proper method used for specimen collection. Such a document ideally should include procedures used to minimize errors at each of the points at which variation may develop. A number of guides to good laboratory practice are available to help laboratory scientists determine and control sources of preanalytical error. Many of these can be obtained from the Clinical and Laboratory Standards Institute (CLSI, formerly NCCLS); see Box 18-1 for a partial listing. An extensive bibliography of patient-related variables that may affect test results is available and is updated regularly.[3]

PRECOLLECTION CAUSES OF VARIATION

Procedural Errors in Test Order Processing

The processing of orders for laboratory tests is one of the most common sources of error in the testing cycle. Two large Q-probe studies were performed by CAP to look at the accuracy of order processing by laboratories in outpatient and inpatient settings. In outpatients, 3.5% of encounters had at least one

Box 18-1

Standards From the Clinical and Laboratory Standards Institute*

H1-A4, Evacuated Tubes and Additives for Blood Specimen Collection
H3-A4, Procedures for the Collection of Diagnostic Blood Specimens by Venipuncture
H4-A4, Procedures for the Collection of Diagnostic Blood Specimens by Skin Puncture
H18-A2, Procedures for the Handling and Processing of Blood Specimens
H21-A3, Collection, Transport, and Processing of Blood Specimens for Coagulation Testing and General Performance of Coagulation Assays
C38-A, Control of Preanalytical Variation in Trace Element Determinations
H11-A3, Procedures for the Collection of Arterial Blood Specimens
GP16-A2, Urinalysis and Collection, Transportation, and Preservation of Urine Specimens

*From CLSI, www.clsi.org.

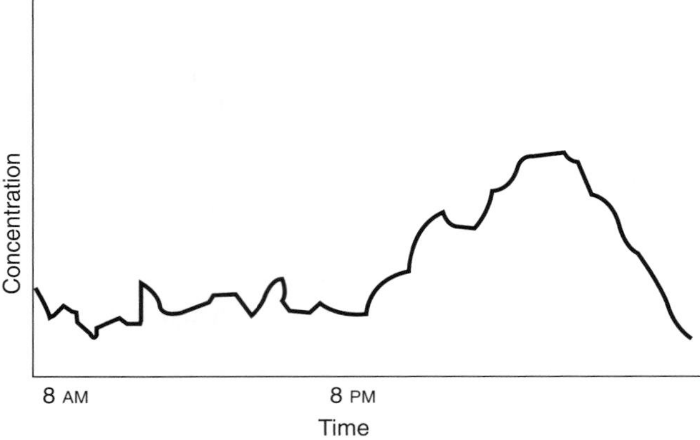

Fig. 18-1 Diurnal and ultradian pattern of hormone release. Most pituitary hormones show pronounced diurnal variation, with levels generally higher during sleep than during the day. Some, such as growth hormone (illustrated here), are released in episodic bursts during the day. A randomly obtained result is difficult to interpret because it may represent a peak, a trough, or some point between.

error, including 1.4% in which ordered tests were not performed and 1.1% in which tests not ordered were performed.[4] In inpatients, although total order errors were similar, 1.9% of ordered tests were not performed.[5] In both of these studies, almost all orders were processed manually and did not use physician order entry.

Cyclical Biological Variables

Cyclical variation refers to changes in the concentration of **analytes** that occur in a predictable fashion at certain times of the day, week, or month. The most reproducible cyclical variation is **circadian,** which occurs during the course of a single day. The blood concentration of most pituitary hormones increases at night and falls during the day. Those hormones whose concentrations are affected by pituitary stimulation show a similar diurnal variation. Diurnal changes seem to be influenced by sleeping and waking, rather than simply by the time on the clock. Individuals who work irregular shifts or who have recently arrived in a new time zone typically experience some delay in adjusting their diurnal cycle; however, eventually, the concentration of pituitary hormones will be highest during sleep and will fall gradually after awakening. Urinary excretion of most electrolytes, such as sodium, potassium, and phosphate, shows considerable circadian variation. The excretion rates of these analytes as determined in specimens obtained at different times of the day may differ by as much as 50%. Both serum and urine levels of bone turnover markers such as osteocalcin and collagen telopeptides show values that differ by 50% to 100% between highest and lowest values. For such tests, it is advisable to recommend to physicians that test specimens be collected only at certain times of the day, and reference limits should be based on those collection times.[6]

Most pituitary hormones are not released into the circulation in a constant fashion but are secreted in episodic bursts. This **ultradian** variation is typical of most pituitary hormones, as is shown in Fig. 18-1. The concentration that occurs during such a burst of secretion may be several times the basal level. A single specimen, therefore, is unlikely to be representative of total hormone production. For such tests, it may be necessary to collect multiple specimens and either analyze them separately to determine an integrated secretory rate, or pool multiple specimens to analyze the pool.

Cyclical variation over a period longer than 1 day (**infradian**) may affect laboratory test results. In women, the menstrual cycle is associated with significant changes in the concentrations of ovarian hormones. Related to this are monthly fluctuations in the concentrations of other analytes such as calcium, magnesium, cholesterol, parathyroid hormone, renin, aldosterone, and antidiuretic hormone.[7] *Circannual* variation, which has been reported for some substances, is related to seasonal changes in diet or climatic variation. For example, vitamin D concentration is higher in the summer than in the winter, and urinary oxalate is higher in the summer than in other seasons (oxalate is present in high concentrations in strawberries). Bone alkaline phosphatase also shows significant annual variation.

In addition to such predictable variability, random fluctuations can cause pronounced changes in concentration from one day to the next. Although blood levels of many analytes such as electrolytes, proteins, and alkaline phosphatase show less than 5% **intraindividual** variation, day-to-day variation may be over 20% for substances such as bilirubin, creatine kinase, and triglycerides, along with most steroid hormones. Urinary excretion of creatinine varies by approximately 10% in a given individual, but most other substances excreted in

Table 18-1 Intraindividual Variation for Common Laboratory Tests

Test Serum	Average, %	Range, %
Alanine aminotransferase	20	5 to 30
Albumin	2.5	1.5 to 4
Alkaline phosphatase	7	5 to 10
Amylase	9	5 to 12
Aspartate aminotransferase	8	5 to 12
Bilirubin, total	19	13 to 30
Calcium, total	2	1 to 3
Chloride	1.2	1.1 to 1.3
Cholesterol, total	6	5 to 9
Cholesterol, HDL	6	3 to 9
Creatinine	5	3 to 8
Ferritin	10	5 to 18
Glucose, fasting	10	5 to 13
Iron	15	10 to 25
Lactate dehydrogenase	10	8 to 13
Magnesium	4	3 to 5
Osmolality	1	1 to 2
Phosphate	8	5 to 10
Potassium	3	1 to 5
Protein, total	2	2 to 3.5
Sodium	0.6	0.5 to 1
Thyrotropin (TSH)	18	15 to 20
Thyroxine	5	4 to 7
Triglycerides	20	15 to 30
Urea (BUN)	10	5 to 17
Uric acid	7	5 to 10

From Rosen JF, Chesney RW: J Pediatr 103:1, 1983; Fraser CG: Arch Pathol Lab Med 116:916, 1992; Fraser CG: Arch Pathol Lab Med 112:404, 1988; Dufour DR, in Becker KL, editor: *Principles and Practice of Endocrinology,* ed 3, Philadelphia, 2001, Raven-Lippincott, pp. 2173-2226.
BUN, Blood urea nitrogen; *HDL,* high-density lipoprotein; *TSH,* thyroid-stimulating hormone.

the urine show fluctuations of 25% to 50% over relatively short periods.[8] Table 18-1 lists long-term biological variability for many common analytes.

Patient-Related Physical Variables

Exercise is a common, controllable cause of variation in laboratory test results. Among routine chemistry tests, potassium, phosphate, creatinine, and serum proteins are significantly altered by a brief period of exercise.[9] Regular aerobic exercise at a fairly constant level is associated with lower plasma activities of muscle enzymes (such as creatine kinase [CK], aspartate aminotransferase [AST], alanine aminotransferase [ALT], and lactate dehydrogenase [LDH]) than are seen in sedentary individuals, as well as with lower levels of inflammatory and coagulation markers linked to cardiac disease risk.[10] Strenuous exercise, such as strength training, is associated with increases in muscle enzymes, uric acid, and bilirubin (Fig. 18-2). Short-term intensive exercise, such as marathon running, produces rapid increases in potassium, uric acid, bilirubin, and muscle enzymes, whereas glucose and phosphate concentrations fall significantly. In persons who are training for distance events, serum gonadotropin and sex steroid concentrations are greatly decreased, whereas prolactin concentration is increased.

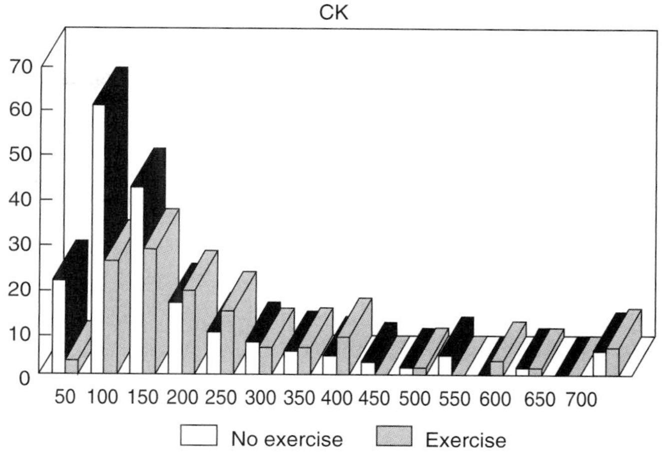

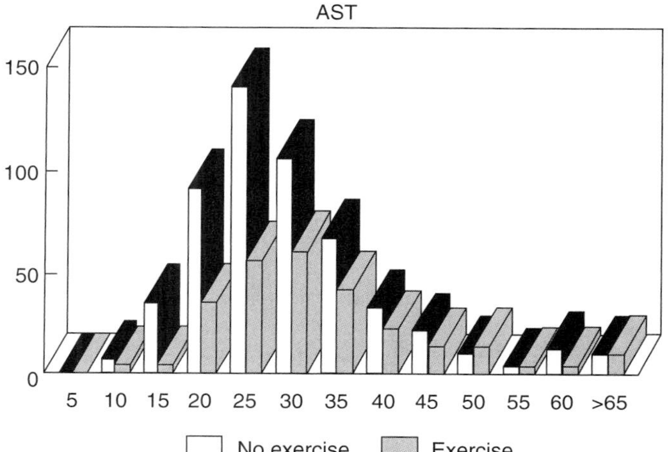

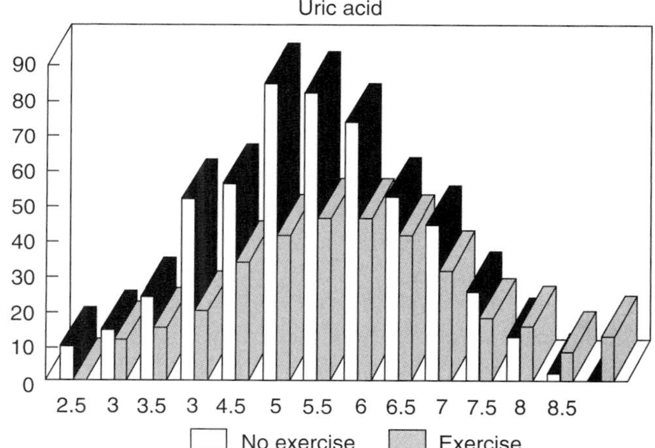

Fig. 18-2 Effect of exercise on laboratory test results. Data from 750 medical students show that exercise is associated with shifting of the distribution of results to higher values (displayed on x-axis; y-axis represents number of students).

Diet-related changes in laboratory tests are pronounced for many analytes; most are transient and are easily controlled. After food ingestion, an increase is noted in the concentration of substances absorbed from food, such as glucose and triglycerides. The increase in glucose is not marked in normal individuals because glucose is released slowly from starches present in food. In addition, sodium, uric acid, iron, and LD concentrations are significantly altered after a meal, showing a **postprandial** rise. Hormones that are secreted in response to eating, such as gastrin and insulin, also show a postprandial rise. The plasma concentration of substances such as potassium and phosphate that shift into cells under the influence of insulin falls after meals. Substances present in food may interfere chemically with test results. For example, vanillin interferes in chemical assays for vanillylmandelic acid, and dietary serotonin can increase urinary concentration of 5-hydroxy-indoleacetic acid (5-HIAA). Stool occult blood tests that detect the peroxidase activity of heme, such as guaiac, are affected by intake of meat and, in some cases, iron and horseradish. Dietary variation can induce longer-lasting changes in laboratory tests; alteration in dietary protein intake is associated with reversible changes in urine creatinine excretion and in creatinine clearance.

Stress, whether mental or physical, can reversibly alter the results of many laboratory tests. It is well known that stress induces production of adrenocorticotropic hormone (ACTH), cortisol, and catecholamines. Even mild stress, such as that associated with preparing for a driver's license exam, may be enough to cause changes.[11] More severe stress causes more profound changes. After acute myocardial infarction, cholesterol begins to fall within 24 hours and may reach a nadir of 60% of baseline value, returning to typical values for the patient after about 3 months.[12] Patients in intensive care units experience suppression of production of many pituitary hormones and aldosterone.[7] Because of these changes, unless no acceptable alternative exists, elective evaluation of endocrine function and lipid status should not be performed during a hospital admission for some other cause.

Posture is a readily controllable cause of **preanalytical variation.** In the upright position, increased hydrostatic pressure causes leakage of water and electrolytes from the intravascular fluid compartment, resulting in an increase in concentration of proteins. If **phlebotomy** is performed before a patient is seated for at least 15 minutes after a period of standing, **hemoconcentration** as great as 5% to 8% may occur.[13] This increase can also produce clinically important differences in concentrations of serum calcium, cholesterol, and lipoproteins. In the supine position, water and electrolytes return to the vascular space, resulting in a fall in protein concentrations of a similar magnitude. Differences in measured hemoglobin concentration from the time of admission to a hospital (when the patient may have had phlebotomy performed after a period of standing) to the next morning (when blood may have been drawn while the patient was lying in bed) could lead the physician to suspect that the patient has developed internal hemorrhage, or **hemolysis.**

Box 18-2

Tests Subject to Diurnal Variation

Acid phosphatase*
ACTH
Catecholamines
Cortisol (and other adrenal steroids)
Gastrin*
Growth hormone*
Glucose tolerance
Iron
Osteocalcin*
Parathyroid hormone*
Prolactin*
Renin/aldosterone
TSH*

ACTH, Adrenocorticotropic hormone; *TSH,* thyroid-stimulating hormone.
*Higher in the afternoon and evening; all others higher in the morning.

Procedures to Minimize Precollection Errors

Improving Order Processing Accuracy

A number of approaches have been developed to improve order processing accuracy. Use of physician order entry has been shown to significantly reduce errors for medications and will likely achieve similar error reduction in laboratory testing.[14] Monitoring for errors in order processing steps, having a second person review computer entries, and having a system for final check at order entry all are associated with reduced frequency of errors.[4]

Minimizing Patient Preparation Errors

Important ways to control patient variables include asking the health care provider to take a complete patient history, providing the phlebotomist or patient with clear instructions, and taking steps to determine that all protocols have been followed.

Biological Cyclical Variables

The laboratory should determine which tests have significant cyclical or food-related changes in concentration; Boxes 18-2 and 18-3 list the most important tests affected in this manner. Optimally, specimens for these tests should be collected shortly after the patient awakens, with the patient still in the fasting state. If an ultradian pattern of variation is noted, as it is for most pituitary hormones, several specimens should be collected at intervals extending over the usual cycle, to provide an accurate picture of hormone production. For example, for gonadotropins, it is advisable to collect three or four specimens, waiting at least a half hour between specimen collections, and to pool the serum before analysis. A more sophisticated method is to place an indwelling **catheter** in the patient and obtain specimens hourly over a day. Each specimen is analyzed separately, and the concentration is plotted against the time of day the specimen was obtained. The area under the curve is reported as an integrated measure of hormone production.

Box 18-3

Tests Affected by Meals

Chloride*
Gastrin
Glucagon
Glucose
Growth hormone
Insulin
Ionized calcium
Phosphate*
Potassium*
Triglycerides
Urine pH

*Lower after meals; all others higher.

Physical Variables

If samples are being collected for analytes that will be affected by exercise, it is prudent to inquire whether the patient has engaged in strenuous exercise in the past 24 to 48 hours. Any history of strenuous exercise can be noted on the requisition form and included in the final report. Alternatively, the patient may be asked to return at a later time for specimen collection. Stress before collection is difficult to control; however, physicians should be apprised of those tests that are thus affected and of the magnitude of change induced by physical and mental stress. It may be advisable for the laboratory to require special consultation before samples are collected from hospital inpatients for tests that are severely affected by patient stress, such as adrenal or pituitary function tests, catecholamine metabolites, lipids, and glucose tolerance tests. The effects of posture can be minimized if one requires ambulatory patients to be seated for at least 15 minutes before blood is drawn. For assays that are subject to pronounced dietary effects, including measurements of glucose tolerance, urine hydroxyproline, 5-HIAA, and catecholamine metabolites, it is advisable to provide the patient with specific dietary guidelines before the day that is scheduled for sample collection. If a test requires special patient preparation, such as measurement of renin and aldosterone, glucose tolerance tests, 24-hour urine analysis, or 72-hour fecal fat, it is good practice to schedule the test in advance and to give the patient a printed instruction sheet at that time.

KEY CONCEPTS BOX 18-1

- Cyclic biological variables (circadial, ultradian, infradian) and intraindividual variations affect optimal sample collection times for many laboratory analytes.
- Many laboratory tests are affected by variables, such as exercise, stress, diet, and posture.
- Knowledge of how these variables affect certain tests and means to control the variability contributes to good laboratory practice.
- There are numerous means to minimize pre-collection errors.

SECTION OBJECTIVES BOX 18-2

- Explain why adequate training in phlebotomy is essential to minimize causes of variation in blood collection.
- Explain why blood collected in a syringe, then injected into evacuated tubes, is acceptable for chemistry testing.
- Explain the differences among arterial, capillary, and venous blood.
- State why heparinized plasma is the recommended specimen for cardiac marker measurement.
- List the recommended order of collection tubes during phlebotomy.

BLOOD COLLECTION CAUSES OF VARIATION

Blood Collection Technique

The use of improper procedures for obtaining specimens can introduce significant error in the final results of laboratory tests; in the author's laboratory, collection-related errors are the most common cause of erroneous results. A number of textbooks on phlebotomy technique are currently available,[15,16] guidelines have been published by CLSI,[17] and certification programs in phlebotomy have established standards for the training and education of phlebotomists. In teaching hospitals, phlebotomy often is performed by a variety of individuals (such as nurses, physicians' assistants, and students) who have limited or no formal training in phlebotomy techniques. Data show that nonlaboratory personnel have significantly higher rates of sample rejection[18,19] and significantly lower rates of successful phlebotomy.[20] Continuing education by laboratory personnel, feedback on causes of rejected specimens, and oversight by the laboratory of phlebotomy performance have been shown to reduce the frequency of errors.

In most laboratories, specimens are collected with the use of evacuated tubes and specially designed needles that allow simultaneous puncture of the vein and the tube's stopper. Although collection tubes typically were made of glass in the past, plastic tubes are now recommended to reduce the risk of broken glass leading to bloodborne pathogen exposure for laboratory and housekeeping staff. Specimens collected in plastic and glass tubes are equally suitable for most assays. Many tubes are coated with silicone, which reduces adhesion of **clot,** allowing better separation of serum and cells. Stoppers typically are made of rubber. In older formulations, tris(2-butoxyethyl) phosphate (**TBEP**) was used as a plasticizer; this compound is capable of displacing many drugs from their transport proteins. The drugs then diffuse into red cells, lowering the serum concentration of the drug. TBEP has been removed from most currently used stoppers. Some tubes have special protective caps over the stoppers that are not in direct contact with the blood, thus lowering the risk of transmission of infectious agents.

In some cases, blood is drawn into a syringe and then is transferred to tubes for transport to the laboratory. If this

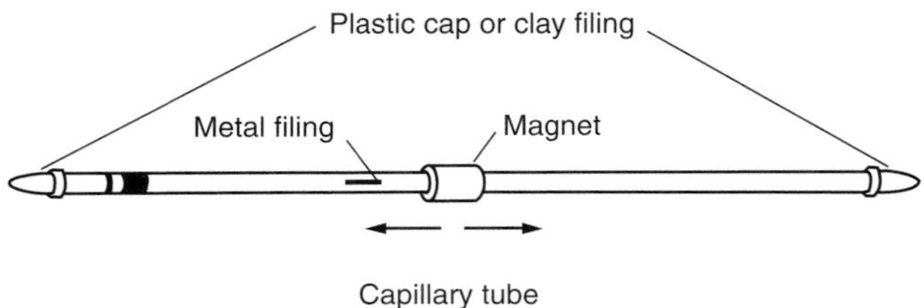

Fig. 18-3 Schematic of heparinized capillary tubes. Magnet is used to move metal filing back and forth through the sealed tube to mix the blood sample with heparin and, later, to remix the sample before analysis.

procedure is used, there is a risk of infection for the phlebotomist during specimen transfer. Injection of blood into evacuated tubes also increases the risk of skin puncture by the needle and the risk of producing a hemolyzed specimen (p. 330); therefore, this technique is *not* recommended for tubes intended to be used for chemistry testing.

In infants and in adults with poor **venous** access, skin puncture may be used to obtain specimens. Special microtubes that contain **anticoagulants** are filled by **capillary** action. If capillary tubes are to be transported to the laboratory, they should contain a small piece of metal, which can be moved through the specimen by means of a magnet to mix the blood immediately after collection and before centrifugation or analysis (Fig. 18-3). If testing is to be done immediately near the site of collection, as is typical for many point-of-care testing instruments, mixing devices usually are not needed. Contamination of the sample with fluid from tissue is a potential cause of concern in all capillary blood collection procedures. Tissue fluid contains virtually no protein and therefore no protein-bound analytes; contamination decreases the concentration of such analytes in the specimen. One may minimize tissue fluid contamination by using only freely flowing blood from puncture sites. It is therefore unacceptable to "milk" blood by applying pressure to tissue near the puncture site.

Sources of Blood Samples

Differences between **arterial,** capillary, and venous blood are an occasional cause for misleading test results. *Arterial blood,* which is the source of nutrients for all body tissues, is the best sample to use for evaluation of adequate delivery of necessary substances such as oxygen to the body tissues. *Venous blood* differs from arterial blood in that it has lower concentrations of substances used in metabolism, such as oxygen and glucose, and higher concentrations of waste products, such as organic acids, ammonia, and carbon dioxide. The extent of the difference in analyte concentration between arterial and venous blood is dependent on tissue perfusion; with poor perfusion, the difference increases, which in the case of blood gases has been used to evaluate tissue perfusion. *Capillary blood* is, in general, closer in composition to arterial than to venous blood. Specimens of capillary blood that closely resemble arterial blood are obtained by warming specific sites, such as the earlobe or the foot. In states of poor tissue perfusion and in neonates, however, there is a significant difference in the Po_2 of capillary and arterial blood. For some substances, the difference between venous and capillary blood concentrations depends on hormonal factors that affect tissue extraction. For example, in the fasting state, capillary blood glucose concentration is similar to that of venous blood. In postprandial specimens, when insulin concentration is increased, the difference between capillary and venous blood glucose concentrations may be as high as 15%.

Errors Related to Preservatives and Anticoagulants

Preservatives and anticoagulants are widely used for collecting specimens of blood, urine, and other body fluids. When blood is removed from the body and is allowed to clot, it separates into a solid clot that contains blood cells and fibrin and a liquid phase termed **serum.** If an anticoagulant such as **heparin** is added, the liquid phase is termed **plasma.**

Serum and heparinized plasma are similar in most respects; however, serum differs from plasma in that it lacks fibrinogen, lowering total protein by an average of 0.3 g/L. Platelets release potassium into serum during clot formation; plasma potassium is typically about 0.2 to 0.3 mmol/L lower than that of serum potassium. For unknown reasons, phosphate concentration is lower in plasma by an average of 0.2 mg/dL. In patients with some hematological disorders and increased numbers of white blood cells or platelets, these differences are exaggerated. With these few exceptions, serum and heparinized plasma are routinely used interchangeably for laboratory tests. The choice of specimen type is dependent on instrumentation, assay methods, and the need for rapid results.

Heparinized plasma can be separated from cells immediately after collection; thus plasma specimens are suitable for rapid analysis in emergency situations. Although heparin prevents coagulation with the high concentrations achieved in heparin-containing tubes, the amount of heparin in "serum" specimens from patients receiving heparin may only delay or inhibit clot formation; fibrin formation continues after separation, which may cause coating and plugging of sampling probes and tubing. In patients admitted for unstable angina, heparin-related fibrin formation in "serum" may trap the indicator antibody of immunoassays, causing falsely elevated CK-MB and troponin. This has led the National Academy for Clinical Biochemistry to recommend in its guidelines that heparinized plasma, rather than serum, should be used for cardiac marker measurement.[21] Heparin also displaces thyroxine from its binding proteins, causing falsely elevated free thyroxine results. The cation used in heparin salts (such as lithium or ammonium) will cause contamination of specimens used for these analytes. For these reasons, some laboratories prefer not to use heparinized blood for routine chemistry testing.

In addition to heparin, other anticoagulants and preservatives often are used for various specimens. Table 18-2 lists some of the most commonly used substances and some typical indications for the use of these **additives.** Although these

Table 18-2 Commonly Used Anticoagulants and Preservatives and Indications for Their Use

Sample	Type of Anticoagulant or Additive	Chemical Basis of Anticoagulant or Additive	Application
Whole blood	EDTA*	Binds calcium	Hematology
	Na heparin	Lead-free	Lead
Plasma	Na citrate	Binds calcium	Coagulation
	Heparin, ± separator†	Inhibits thrombin	Chemistry
	Oxalates	Binds calcium	Coagulation
Serum	None	None	Chemistry
	None	Contaminant-free	Trace elements
	Serum separator	Gel barrier	Chemistry
	Thrombin	Increased rate of clotting	Stat. Chemistries
Antiglycolytic agents			
Partial plasma	Fluoride/oxalate	Inhibits enolase	Glucose

EDTA, Ethylenediaminetetraacetic acid.
*Comes as Na^+ or K^+ salt forms.
†Comes as Na^+, Li^+, or NH_4^+ salt forms.

Box 18-4

Effects of EDTA Contamination

Increased potassium
Reduced calcium, magnesium (colorimetric assays)
Reduced alkaline phosphatase, creatine kinase

EDTA, Ethylenediaminetetraacetic acid.

compounds are essential for certain tests, they may be totally inappropriate for other tests. Ethylenediaminetetraacetic acid **(EDTA),** which is used for hematology specimens, is also used for some chemistry assays because **chelation** of divalent cations inactivates several enzymes that cause **in vitro** changes in lipids, nucleic acids, and peptide hormones. Chelation of cations such as iron, magnesium, and calcium, however, falsely lowers results in most colorimetric assays for these analytes and reduces the activity of enzymes that require cation activators (including alkaline phosphatase and creatine kinase). Coagulation specimens contaminated with EDTA may have falsely prolonged clotting times because calcium chelation is more potent than that which occurs with sodium citrate. Contamination of serum specimens with anticoagulants, especially EDTA, is a common problem in many laboratories. In the author's laboratory, approximately two or three EDTA-contaminated specimens are received each month. The pattern of abnormalities seen with EDTA contamination is shown in Box 18-4.

To avoid contamination, glass tubes without anticoagulants or preservatives should be filled first, followed by tubes for coagulation samples, plastic tubes without additives or preservatives, gel-containing tubes, and finally tubes with other preservatives and anticoagulants.[17] Because of the potential for EDTA interference in many assays, tubes that contain EDTA should be drawn last.

If liquid anticoagulants are used, it is important to ensure that the proportions of blood and anticoagulant used are constant. In specimens with inadequate blood volume ("short draw"), significant dilution of blood by the anticoagulant solution may be seen. Because most anticoagulants do not enter into cells, alterations in hematocrit will affect the ratio of anticoagulant to plasma. For example, patients with a high hematocrit will have relative excess of the anticoagulant and resulting dilution of the plasma, whereas in anemic individuals, anticoagulant may be insufficient.

Errors Related to Serum Separator Tubes

Serum and plasma separator tubes are used by many laboratories to simplify the process of separating serum (or plasma) from cellular elements. If separation does not occur, metabolism continues in the cellular phase, producing a variety of changes that are discussed later in this chapter. Serum and plasma separator tubes contain a relatively inert, impenetrable gel that has a density intermediate between that of cellular elements and normal plasma or serum. During centrifugation, the gel rises from the bottom of the tube and forms a mechanical barrier that prevents metabolic changes from affecting plasma concentrations (Fig. 18-4). Tubes that contain such gels can be centrifuged and stored without removal of the stopper, reducing the risk of producing infectious **aerosols** and preventing **evaporation.** It is critical that centrifugation of tubes that contain gels should be performed with the use of "swinging bucket" rotors (see p. 20, Chapter 1). Use of fixed-angle centrifuge rotors often leads to incomplete separation of red cells from serum or plasma and allows metabolic changes to affect the sample. Some therapeutic agents **adsorb** onto the gel, falsely lowering the concentrations of phenytoin, tricyclic antidepressants, and certain antiarrhythmic drugs, such as flecainide. A recent manufacturing change by the manufacturer of one separator gel led to unpredictable increases in total triiodothyronine and changes in some other analytes.[22] With these exceptions, most substances in plasma are unaffected by the use of separator gels. Recentrifugation of tubes with separator gels once samples reach the laboratory can lead to **artifactually** high potassium results.[23]

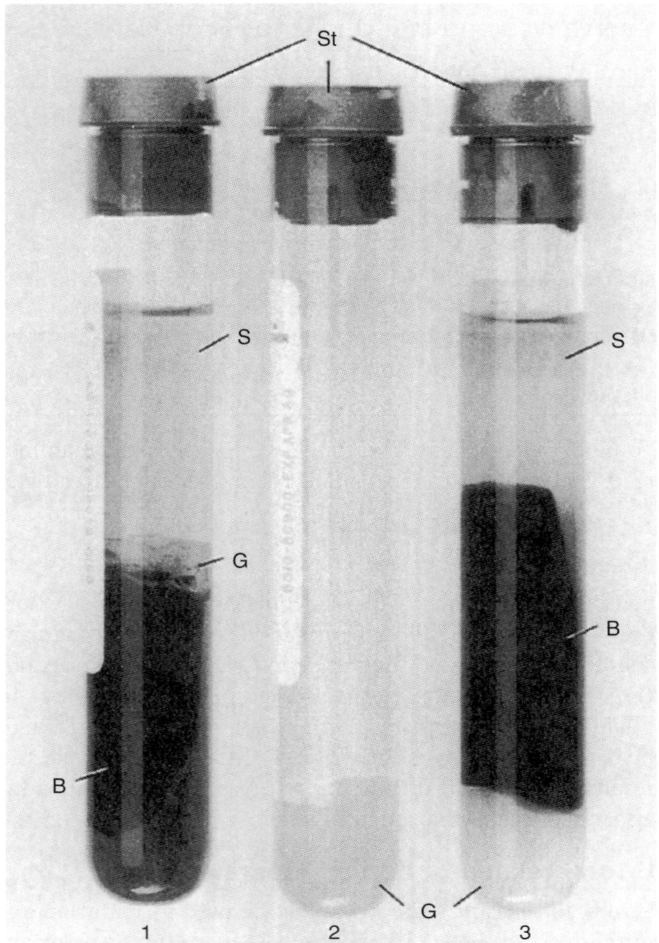

Fig. 18-4 Vacutainer phlebotomy tubes containing barrier gel *(red/gray tops). 1,* Tube filled with blood and centrifuged; *2,* unfilled tube; and *3,* tube filled with blood and not centrifuged. Note the positions of gel before *(3)* and after centrifugation *(1). B,* Clotted blood; *St,* red/gray stoppers; *G,* barrier gel; *S,* serum.

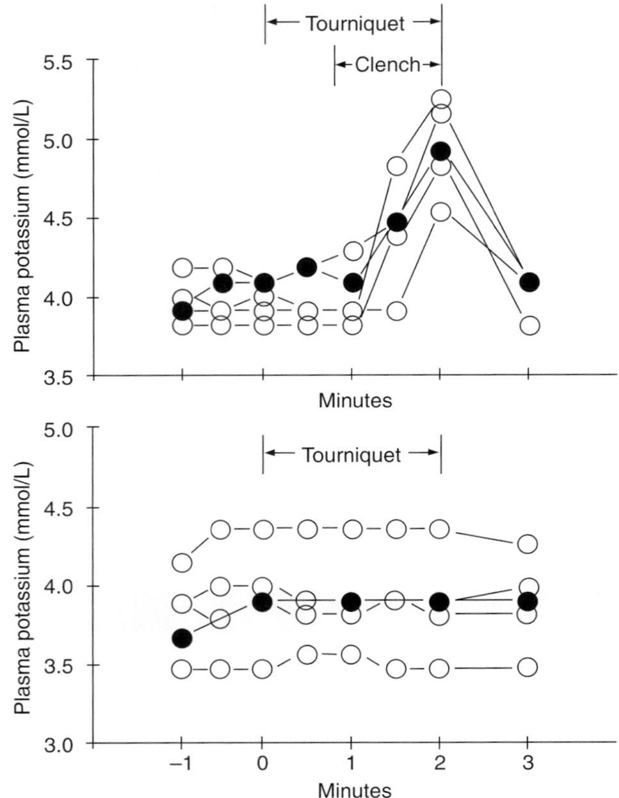

Fig. 18-5 Effects of the application of a tourniquet plus fist clenching *(upper panel)* and of a tourniquet alone *(lower panel)* on plasma potassium concentrations. *Solid circles* represent the patient, and *open circles* the control subjects. The application of a tourniquet alone had no effect on plasma potassium levels, whereas clenching of the fist as well resulted in a strong increase in these levels in both the patient and control subjects. (From Don BR Sebastian A, Cheitlin M, et al: N Engl J Med 322:1291, 1990.)

Errors Related to Faulty Collection Techniques

Tourniquets

Tourniquet use is an important, controllable cause of variation in laboratory test results. Tourniquets are widely used in phlebotomy to block venous return, causing dilation of the veins and making identification of an appropriate site for venipuncture easier. Tourniquets often are left on during the process of venipuncture, under the assumption that continued venous dilation will allow faster specimen collection and will prevent "collapse" of the vein. Although tourniquets do make the process of phlebotomy easier, the **stasis** they induce causes predictable changes in laboratory test results. Within 1 minute after application of a tourniquet, the increased pressure causes loss of water and electrolytes from the plasma to the **extracellular** fluid space, producing a rise in the concentrations of proteins, cells, and substances bound to cells and proteins. After 3 minutes, there is generally a 5% to 8% increase in concentration of proteins. If a tourniquet is left on for as long as 15 minutes, the increase in concentration may reach 15%. The magnitude of this effect may differ from the first tube to the last tube drawn, with later specimens showing greater hemoconcentration. An additional concern with tourniquet use is relative stasis of blood flow. Concentrations of metabolic by-products such as lactate increase in tissue, causing a rise in lactate concentration in collected samples. When blood is collected during use of a tourniquet, the patient often is advised to alternately clench and relax the fist to increase the speed of collection of specimens. Not only is there little evidence of the efficacy of this procedure, but it may also be the cause of artifactual hyperkalemia (Fig. 18-5).

Hemolysis

Hemolysis occurs whenever there is trauma to the relatively fragile red blood cells, either during collection or, less commonly, after phlebotomy is completed. Failure to allow drying of skin disinfectants, such as alcohol, before phlebotomy, is an uncommon cause of hemolysis. More frequently, hemolysis is

Box 18-5

Effects of Hemolysis on Chemistry Tests

Increase caused by release from red blood cells
  Potassium, magnesium, lactate dehydrogenase, aspartate aminotransferase, total protein, iron, phosphate, ammonium
Increase caused by interference in assay
  Cholesterol, triglycerides, creatine kinase, CK-MB (immunoinhibition)
Decrease caused by interference in assay
  Bilirubin (direct spectrophotometry), carotene, insulin, albumin

caused by turbulent, **nonlaminar** flow during the process of collection. Within the range of needle diameters commonly used, hemolysis is not caused by using a needle that is too small or too large. Nonlaminar flow is a common occurrence when blood moves too slowly or too rapidly through a needle. If blood is drawn with a syringe, drawing the plunger back forcefully or injecting blood into evacuated tubes by using pressure on the plunger frequently produces hemolysis. Similarly, a slow flow rate into an evacuated tube from a collapsed vein often produces a hemolyzed specimen. Turbulence in a tube that contains blood also can cause hemolysis after collection is completed; faulty mechanical transporters and centrifuges are rare causes of hemolysis, as is discussed later in the chapter.

Hemolysis is the most common reason for rejection of chemistry samples; in one large multicenter study, hemolysis leading to sample rejection occurred in 2 in 1000 samples submitted and was the cause of about 60% of rejections.[18] Hemolysis alters laboratory test results in two ways. Most important, the contents of the red blood cells are released, increasing the concentration of intracellular substances such as lactate dehydrogenase (LD), potassium, and magnesium, while lowering the concentration of extracellular solutes such as sodium. Because the activity of LD is approximately 150 times higher and the potassium concentration is 30 times higher within red blood cells, hemolysis falsely elevates the serum or plasma levels of these analytes. Because hemoglobin absorbs light over much of the visible and near-ultraviolet spectrum, hemolysis can interfere with the results of many spectrophotometric assays. Box 18-5 lists the tests most commonly affected by hemolysis and the nature of the interference in each assay. Sample hemolysis can be detected most easily at the time of analysis, when many automated instruments can measure the degree of hemolysis. At that time, decisions as to the acceptance of the sample for a particular analysis can be made on the basis of each laboratory's criteria (see p. 340).

Hemolysis is more difficult to detect in whole blood samples, where plasma cannot be observed directly. In one study, hemolysis was actually more common in whole blood samples, and to a degree that changed potassium results by >0.5 mmol/L in 8% of samples.[24] Hemolysis was much more common when sample volumes were <0.5 mL.

Intravenous Fluid Contamination

Intravenous fluid contamination can be an important cause of variation in test results. Many inpatients are given intravenous fluids, which typically have higher concentrations of glucose, drugs, and some electrolytes than are found in blood. Intravenous fluid contamination occurs when blood is drawn from a vein that is connected to the vein containing the catheter. Although it may appear that a vein in the forearm is sufficiently distant from the catheter, **anastomotic** connections are extensive. Any blood drawn from a vein on the same side of a tourniquet as a catheter runs the risk of fluid contamination. In many cases, blood is drawn through a connector or port in a catheter. It has been shown that, for most analytes, removing and discarding a volume of blood equal to the volume of the catheter is adequate for preventing contamination. In the case of drugs administered through a catheter (including heparin and potassium), it may take a volume of more than five times that of the catheter to prevent incorrect results. In patients receiving intravenous fluids on a long-term basis, a multilumen catheter is commonly used to provide a port for collection of blood. Even if blood is drawn through this separate port, contamination can still occur if intravenous fluid is being administered simultaneously through a different lumen.

The most common pattern of intravenous fluid interference is a sharp increase in the blood concentration of substances contained in the fluid. The potassium concentration of intravenous fluid can be as much as tenfold higher than that of blood, and the glucose concentration of intravenous fluid is 5000 mg/dL. Drug concentrations are typically over a hundred-fold higher than those of blood when fluid is administered as a slow infusion. Less frequently, enough fluid may be present to actually dilute the concentration of normal blood constituents, including solutes such as urea and creatinine; in most cases of fluid contamination, these are only minimally altered.

Errors Related to Patient and Sample Identification

Proper specimen identification is essential to the proper use of results in treatment of a particular individual. Accurate patient and sample identification has become a major patient safety initiative of both the Joint Commission and the College of American Pathologists. In large studies of sample acceptability, labeling errors were a cause of sample rejection in about 0.02% of samples but were two to three times as common in samples drawn by nonlaboratory personnel.[18,19] However, this may represent an underestimation of the true frequency, in that errors often are identified only when unexpected laboratory results are encountered. In data from an international study involving blood banks, inadequately labeled samples occurred in 1 of 165 submitted samples, and misidentified samples (wrong patient identification on the tube) occurred in 1 of 2000 submitted samples.[25] Another study that identified mislabeled samples through discrepancies in ABO blood group (which will not identify all

TOXICOLOGY LABORATORY

Chain of Evidence Form

SUBJECT NAME ______________ SUBJECT SOCIAL SEC. # ______________

DATE/TIME OF COLLECTION ______________ COLLECTED BY ______________

NUMBER OF SPECIMENS ____ TYPE OF SPECIMEN: ____ BLOOD ____ SERUM ____ URINE

WITNESS ______________

Sent by Name/Date/Time	Received by Name/Date/Time	Condition of Seals
1.		
2.		
3.		
4.		
5.		

Specimen Opened for Testing Name/Date/Time	Witnessed by Name/Date/Time	Condition of Seals
A. Outside Package 6.		
B. Specimen 7.		

LABORATORY ACCESSION NUMBER:

This form must remain with the specimen until line #7 is completed. At that time the form should be turned over to the laboratory supervisor or the designate for filling.

Fig. 18-6 Example of a chain-of-custody form. (From Pesce AJ, Kaplan LA: *Methods in Clinical Chemistry,* St. Louis, 1987, Mosby.)

mislabeled samples) found mislabeled samples in 1 of 3400 submitted samples.[26] Although errors can be made when one is labeling specimens from patients with similar names, in our experience, the most common cause of inaccurate specimen identification is the phlebotomist's failure to label the specimen before leaving the patient's bedside; more than 99% of mislabeled specimens occur in this setting.

Chain of Custody

In certain situations, as in forensic testing, positive specimen identification is required at every step in the process of collection, transport, and analysis. For such specimens, an appropriate chain-of-custody form (Fig. 18-6) should be used. Positive identification begins with placement of a tamperproof seal on the specimen container before it leaves the donor's sight; the label typically is initialed by the donor and sometimes by the witness. After the donor certifies on the chain-of-custody form that the specimen was obtained from him or her, each person who takes possession of the specimen signs the form and notes the date and time the specimen was transferred to the next person in the testing process. Commonly, each person certifies that the specimen was kept in a secure condition during the time it was in that person's custody. This ensures that the result will be legally admissible in court because it can be traced directly to the person from whom it was obtained.

Procedures to Minimize Phlebotomy-Related Variation

Generally, procedures to minimize collection-related variation are directly under the control of the laboratory. Therefore, the laboratory should work closely with the phlebotomy team, nursing administration, and physicians to produce clear written guidelines to help minimize all errors. Phlebotomy guidelines for *each* test that the laboratory performs should be included in the laboratory manual. Guidelines should specify the type of specimen to collect, the volume of specimen needed, and, for blood, whether arterial, capillary, or venous blood is required. The frequency of phlebotomy errors should be monitored, as is suggested by Clinical Laboratory Improvement Amendments (CLIA) '88 regulations.

Patient Identification

The initial step in preventing collection errors is accurate identification of the patient before specimen collection. When working with an outpatient, ask for a name, including the correct spelling of the last name, and any identification number needed (such as patient registration or insurance number). A hospital inpatient should be asked for a name, and identification should be confirmed by comparison with that written on the hospital wrist band. Wristband errors occur relatively commonly in hospital settings; even with continuous monitoring, approximately 2% of inpatients have missing or inaccurate wristbands. Use of policies that prohibit sample collection when wristband errors are present and nursing cooperation with replacing faulty or absent wristbands are associated with lower rates of such errors.[27]

With children or adults with neurological or mental illnesses, a more positive form of identification, such as a hospital card or picture identification, may be necessary. Handwritten specimen labels should be written clearly and legibly before the phlebotomist leaves the patient's bedside; the label should include the name and identification number of the patient and the date and time of collection.

To assist in making proper identification, laboratory computer systems usually provide preprinted labels, along with collection lists (see Chapter 22). Many hospitals have begun to use a bar-code system on these labels to increase the accuracy of positive patient identification by the computers on instruments. Use of patient **bar-code** identification bracelets or cards and portable bar-code readers at the site of collection has been shown to markedly reduce the frequency of sample identification errors.[28,29] Because of the many types of bar codes available, laboratories should carefully review manufacturers' specifications before starting to use a bar-code label system. Chapters 20 and 22 discuss the use of bar codes in greater detail.

Preservatives and Anticoagulants

Any anticoagulants or preservatives that are needed should be specified, and allowable alternatives should be itemized. Because many laboratories prefer to use plasma or serum from separator tubes for most chemistry analyses, those tests for which these *cannot* be used should be clearly listed; a short list is provided in Box 18-6. Use of a specific order of specimen collection[17] will prevent specimen contamination; glass tubes without anticoagulants or additives are always collected first, followed in order by samples for coagulation testing, plastic tubes without anticoagulants or additives, tubes with separator gels, heparin tubes, other anticoagulants, and finally EDTA.

Box 18-6

Tests for Which Separator Gels Are Inappropriate

Analyte adsorbs to gel
- Flecainide, tricyclic antidepressants, haloperidol

Whole blood needed
- Red blood cell enzymes, hemoglobin A1c, lead, cyclosporin A

Possible contaminants in gel
- Trace metals

Preservatives needed
- Most peptide hormones, renin, catecholamines

Sample Collection

Guidelines for phlebotomy procedures on patients with indwelling catheters should be included in the phlebotomy manual. If the patient has an intravenous line, blood should not be drawn from the same side of a tourniquet as the intravenous line and preferably not from the same arm. Instructions on the amount of blood to be withdrawn before sampling from an intravenous or intra-arterial line must be provided. Because removal of a volume of blood equal to the volume of the catheter is adequate for most analytes, the volume of the most commonly used catheters should be provided in the manual. Those tests that are more severely affected by fluid contamination, such as therapeutic drugs, should carry the caution not to draw specimens through an indwelling catheter.

Although many veins can be used for venipuncture, the antecubital fossa in the arm is the most widely used site. Because tourniquets are used in most instances of venipuncture, specific instructions on appropriate tourniquet use are needed. The phlebotomist can identify the phlebotomy site and clean the skin before applying the tourniquet; alternatively, the tourniquet should be released after a suitable vein has been identified. The tourniquet should be kept on for as short a period as possible, preferably less than 1 minute, before phlebotomy is actually performed. Any **antiseptic** used should be allowed to dry before specimen collection to minimize the likelihood of hemolysis. Specimens should be collected only if blood is free-flowing; otherwise venous blood samples may hemolyze, and capillary blood specimens will be diluted with tissue fluid. Because chemistry tests usually are most affected by hemoconcentration, specimens for these tests should be among the first drawn. The patient should not be advised to clench and loosen his or her fist during collection because this action will stimulate the release of muscle metabolites into the vein.

KEY CONCEPTS BOX 18-2

- Phlebotomy should be performed by trained individuals in order to reduce sample rejection rates.
- Biochemical composition differs among arterial, venous, and capillary blood.
- Laboratory tests must be collected in the correct tube, with or without additive, in order for the laboratory to produce reasonable and reliable results.
- Potential sources of contamination for laboratory testing include use of serum separator tubes, improper tourniquet use, in vitro hemolysis, and intravenous fluid contamination.
- Sample labeling errors are a cause of sample rejection and are a source of concern for patient safety.
- Chain of custody is a formal and legal way of identifying the persons who handled and stored a patient's specimen.

SECTION OBJECTIVES BOX 18-3

- Describe the cumulative effect of leaving a tourniquet on too long during phlebotomy.
- Discuss two major effects of *in vitro* hemolysis on laboratory testing, alternation of laboratory results, and spectrophotometric measurements.
- Describe typical effects on common laboratory measurements if intravenous fluid contamination is present.
- Discuss ways to minimize variations in specimens that must be transported to remote sites.
- Explain the effect on glucose, potassium, enzymes, and phosphate levels if serum is not separated as soon as possible from cells.
- Discuss potential errors that result from improper sample storage and means to minimize those errors.

POSTCOLLECTION CAUSES OF VARIATION

Postcollection causes of variation are controlled more easily by the laboratory than are phlebotomy-related variations because it is possible to develop criteria for acceptable conditions for storage and handling of specimens after collection, at a time when the specimens are usually in the laboratory's possession. Among the specimen-handling variables that may affect test results are transportation, separation of serum from cellular elements, and storage conditions.

Sample Transportation

Errors Related to Sample Transportation

Specimens usually are transported manually by phlebotomists or couriers. A reasonable delay in transportation usually is well tolerated for most analytes because metabolic changes occur relatively slowly at room temperature. In general, delays of up to an hour will not change the concentration of most analytes. Glucose, often considered one of the more labile substances in blood, falls by approximately 2% to 3% per hour at normal room temperature in tubes without **glycolytic** inhibitors, such as fluoride.[30] An arterial blood-gas sample is probably the specimen that is most subject to handling error. Table 18-3 lists common causes of changes in arterial blood-gas results and the direction and relative magnitude of changes induced. Products of metabolism (such as lactate, ammonia, and hydrogen ion) accumulate in the sample after collection unless enzymatic reactions are slowed. Other metabolic processes, such as **proteolysis,** also occur at room temperature. Peptides, which are susceptible to degradation by plasma proteases, generally will decrease in concentration; however, renin precursors (prorenin) will be converted to enzymatically active renin if plasma is allowed to cool slowly.[31]

Procedures to Minimize Sample-Transportation Errors

Sample Preservation During Transportation

To minimize postcollection variation, specimens should be delivered, processed, and stored promptly after collection. Analytes that are subject to in vitro changes in concentration at room temperature should be transported promptly to the laboratory in an ice slurry. Handling instructions should be clear; in many cases, specimens are placed improperly on top of ice, or they are transported while protruding from a container of ice or immersed in ice without water. Because a solid conducts heat less rapidly than a liquid, specimens handled in this way will not cool as rapidly and may show artifactual changes. Although cooling of samples during transport minimizes many artifactual changes in analyte concentration, cooling increases the release of potassium from cells.

For a substance whose concentration changes with in vitro metabolism, a specific time of delay that can be tolerated should be specified. The two most common techniques for preventing metabolism of glucose in unseparated blood samples are use of the glycolytic inhibitor fluoride and chilling

Table **18-3** Effects of Specimen Handling Variables on Blood-Gas Measurements

Factor Not Controlled	pH	Po_2	Pco_2
No ice slurry	Decrease of up to 0.01 in 10 minutes	Decrease of up to 5% in 10 minutes	Minimal change
Air bubbles not removed	Increase if sample agitated	Slight increase, decrease in patients with high initial Po_2	Decrease
Excess liquid heparin added	Decrease with some forms; usually no effect	Slight increase, decrease in patients with high initial Po_2	Decrease

of specimens in ice water. If plain or **serum separator** tubes are used, at least a half hour should pass before centrifugation to allow clot formation to become complete. Tubes with clot accelerators or anticoagulants can be centrifuged immediately. After centrifugation, specimen collection tubes without barrier gels should have the plasma or serum separated from the cells as quickly as possible to prevent artifacts.

Use of Mechanical Transporters

Transportation of specimens to the laboratory often significantly delays processing. A CAP Q-probe on emergency department laboratory tests showed that specimen transport by couriers adds a median of 60% to 100% to the total turnaround time for stat specimens.[32] Mechanical transport systems, typically with pneumatic tubes, are used by some laboratories to expedite specimen delivery. Carefully designed systems can greatly reduce the time needed for specimens to reach the laboratory. In contrast to the average delay of approximately 30 minutes for manual transport, the average delay with pneumatic tube systems in one hospital system was 2 minutes. Thus pneumatic tube systems have the potential to reduce the need for satellite laboratories and near-patient testing devices. However, the pneumatic tube system may produce trauma to red blood cells. The risk of hemolysis is increased by the use of specimen tubes that are less than fully filled, sudden deceleration, and sharp turns in the tube system. Lack of adequate packing can increase the number of tubes that are broken during transit. Pneumatic tube systems should be monitored periodically to ensure that tube velocity does not increase beyond acceptable limits. Monitoring of the prevalence of hemolyzed samples can be used for this purpose.

Transportation to Remote Sites

When specimens are transported to remote testing sites, such as reference laboratories or in laboratory outreach programs, changes can occur in the concentration of many substances. In general, unless the assay specifically calls for whole blood testing, it is best to separate plasma or serum physically from cells before preparing specimens for shipping. Serum or plasma separator tubes also can be used for this purpose; the collection site performs centrifugation, then sends the tube to the laboratory. When separator gels are used, the collection site must use centrifuges that have swinging buckets to avoid the problem of incomplete separation by the gel. Recentrifugation of samples collected with serum separator tubes can cause marked increases in potassium and should be prohibited.[23] To avoid breakage during transit, it is preferable to use tightly capped plastic tubes. Precautions must be taken to prevent the thawing of frozen specimens. Although most referral laboratories suggest the use of insulated containers packed with dry ice, overnight delivery services have become reliable enough that most specimens can be adequately preserved with the use of reusable "ice packs." Specimens must be packaged securely to prevent leakage and must be labeled as potentially infectious.

Sample Processing

Errors Arising from Incorrect Sample Processing

Centrifugation is the method that is commonly used for the initial separation of serum and cells. The principles of centrifugation are covered in Chapter 1. In general, centrifugation of samples for 5 to 10 minutes at 1000 to 2000 *G* is adequate for complete separation of serum and red blood cells, including specimens that contain serum or plasma separator gels. Serum specimens should not be centrifuged until clot formation is completed (at least 20 to 30 minutes after the specimen is collected). When separator gels are used, centrifuges with horizontal rotors produce better separation, as was discussed earlier. In our laboratory, we store samples with separator gels for up to 72 hours with no significant changes in the concentration of most analytes, as long as no points of contact are visible between serum and cells.

Caution should be taken to ensure that clotting has, in fact, been completed because there can be physiological reasons for extended clotting times. For example, specimens from patients undergoing dialysis or patients in cardiac care units may continue to clot for hours after collection because of heparin received by the patient. In such cases, recentrifugation, serum filters, and wooden sticks can be used to remove additional fibrin. With tubes that do not contain separator gels, an additional step is necessary to complete the separation. Before centrifugation, substances such as glass beads, plugs, or other mechanical devices may be added to tubes to perform the same function as the gel. After centrifugation, hollow cylinders that contain filters or one-way valves at one end can be inserted into the collection tube to provide a physical barrier, and pipets can be used to remove the serum manually. The serum yield when these alternative separation methods are used is often less than that achieved with gels. The use of such alternative procedures instead of serum separator gels increases the risk of spillage and concomitant infection and thus often increases laboratory costs.

As was discussed previously, serum must be separated from cells because hematological cells will continue to perform their metabolic functions and will alter specimen composition. Although this occurs most rapidly and most dramatically for blood-gas samples, more subtle changes occur with delayed separation of other specimens. At room temperature, glycolysis continues slowly, with glucose falling by an average of 3% per hour. After approximately 24 hours, the lack of glucose causes leakage of potassium and smaller proteins, such as enzymes, from the cells; in addition, breakdown of organic phosphate compounds causes a rise in inorganic phosphate. After several days, visible hemolysis becomes apparent. If specimens are refrigerated without separation, glycolysis is inhibited, but leakage of potassium and enzymes occurs.

In persons with high white blood cell or platelet counts, dramatic changes can occur in vitro following phlebotomy. Platelets release potassium from their cytoplasm during clot

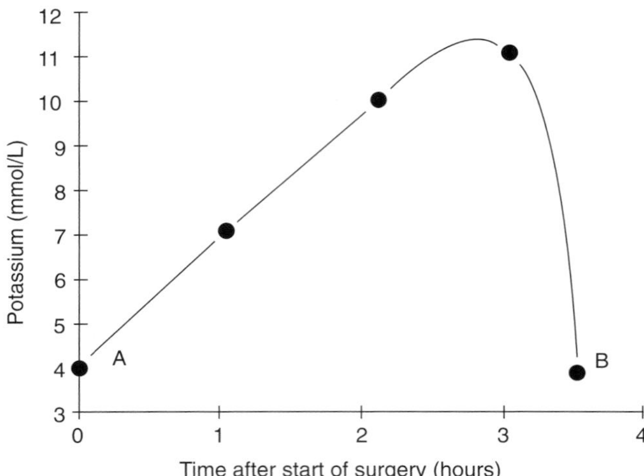

Fig. 18-7 Effect of heparin on potassium in lymphocytic leukemia. The graph represents "serum" potassium concentration obtained during surgery to remove the spleen in a patient with chronic lymphocytic leukemia and white blood count of about 350,000/mm^3. *Point A* represents preoperative serum potassium. The next three points represent specimens obtained through an arterial catheter containing heparin at 1, 2, and 3.25 hours into the surgery. *Point B* represents serum potassium obtained from the arm opposite the arterial catheter 15 minutes after the previous specimen with "serum" potassium of 11.2 mmol/L.

formation; this causes potassium concentration to be higher in serum than in plasma. Although normal individuals have a difference of 0.2 to 0.3 mmol/L between serum and plasma potassium, the difference in patients with very high platelet counts may be markedly higher (up to 1-3 mmol/L); this difference is not directly proportional to the increase in platelet count seen in those with thrombocytosis.[33] Because white blood cells are more active metabolically than are red blood cells, changes resulting from delayed separation are exaggerated in patients with leukemia. Glucose concentration may fall and potassium concentration may begin to rise in as little as 30 minutes[34] and pH may decrease by as much as 0.6 in 10 minutes if the specimen is not rapidly chilled in an ice slurry. In patients with lymphocytic leukemia, heparin appears to induce degeneration of lymphocytes in vitro, leading to rapid rises in plasma (but not serum) potassium concentration,[35] as is shown in Fig. 18-7.

Procedure to Minimize Sample-Processing Errors

The most effective way to minimize sample-processing errors is to centrifuge as soon as possible samples requiring cell separation. If plain tubes are used, centrifugation should not be performed until at least a half hour after blood collection, to allow complete clot formation. Tubes with clot accelerators or anticoagulants can be separated immediately. After centrifugation, in specimens without gels, plasma or serum should be separated from the cells as quickly as possible to prevent changes to the sample.

Sample Storage

Errors Arising from Improper Sample Storage

Once serum or plasma has been separated from cells, most substances show little change in concentration over a 2- or 3-day period when kept at 4°C. For labile analytes, including enzymes such as creatine kinase and lactate dehydrogenase, most polypeptide hormones, and some other substances, the specimen must be frozen to prevent storage-related changes. Analytes that may be intrinsically stable on storage may change in the presence of other compounds. For example, triglyceride concentration falls in "serum" obtained from patients who are taking heparin, apparently because of the activation of lipoprotein lipase. Aminoglycoside antibiotics, such as tobramycin and gentamicin, are stable when stored at refrigerator temperatures unless the serum also contains certain synthetic penicillins, most notably piperacillin; aminoglycoside concentrations can fall to less than 50% of baseline value at 72 hours when both drugs are present.

Evaporation can increase sample concentration. When a sample is uncovered, the rate of evaporation is affected by temperature, humidity, air movement, and the surface area of the sample. If humidity is low, a situation often found in air-conditioned laboratories, there is a direct linear relationship between temperature and rate of evaporation; however, at high humidities, temperature changes have a minimal effect on evaporation rate. One of the most important factors affecting evaporation is the rate of air movement over the surface of a liquid. For any given rate of air flow, increasing the height of the column of air over the specimen or decreasing the area of opening in the specimen container will decrease the rate of evaporation by decreasing air movement over the specimen. Small, fully filled sample cups may show as much as 50% loss of water in a few hours. As with any other form of hemoconcentration, this will lead to an increase in the concentration of proteins and protein-bound substances; however, evaporation also increases the concentration of other solutes.

Procedures to Minimize Storage Errors

Storage errors can be prevented by the proper selection of time, temperature, and storage conditions. Most analytes are stable when stored at refrigerator temperatures for up to 72 hours. If an analyte is not stable, specimens should be frozen until analysis. Most specimens can be stored at −70°C without affecting analyte concentrations, even when frozen for many years.[36] Alkaline phosphatase activity will increase with freezing, apparently as a result of the destruction of an inhibitor. At standard freezer temperatures of −10°C to −20°C, most substances will be stable for shorter periods. Care must be taken to prevent repeated thawing and refreezing of specimens; this is especially problematic with newer frost-free freezers, which periodically increase freezer temperature to allow the melting of frost. Analytes that are susceptible to repeated freeze/thaw cycles, such as complement, should be stored in other types of freezers. Frozen samples should be allowed to thaw slowly at room temperature or in a 37°C water bath and then should be mixed thoroughly before analysis.

To prevent specimen evaporation, specimens should be covered while stored and kept, if at all possible, away from areas of rapid air flow. Whenever possible, containers with a small surface area and a large column of air over the specimen should be used to minimize evaporation.

The identification of each sample should be confirmed every time an aliquot is made or serum is sampled, to minimize the likelihood of specimen confusion. Direct sampling from the collection tube is the best way to minimize such errors, especially if bar-coded labels and bar-code readers are available.

KEY CONCEPT BOX 18-3

- Post-collection variables for laboratory specimens include transportation, serum separation, and storage conditions.

SECTION OBJECTIVES BOX 18-4

- Summarize the similarities and differences between the effects of biological variables for urine samples versus those for blood samples.
- Summarize the different factors involved in sampling from infants and the important preanalytical factors that can affect test results in newborns.
- Explain the effect of various preservation techniques used for urine specimens.

OTHER PREANALYTICAL COLLECTION CONCERNS

Urine Collection: Sources of Variation

Biological Variables

Preanalytical variation in urine is somewhat difficult to control. Although changes in serum concentration are related primarily to the degree of hemoconcentration, urine variation can be caused by several factors. The most important variable affecting the urine concentration of a substance is the relative amount of water excreted. The body is capable of greatly altering urine concentration to meet the need for water excretion or water conservation. Because most of the solute in urine is composed of waste products such as urea and creatinine, urine osmolality is a measure of relative water excretion. Normal individuals may have urine osmolality as low as 75 mOsm/kg and as high as 1200 mOsm/kg; the relative concentration of other solutes thus may vary over a 15-fold range in concentration. As was mentioned earlier in the discussion of random variation, intraindividual variation in urinary concentration is, on average, several times higher than intraindividual variation for the same analytes in serum.[7] Controlling the hydration status of the patient during the urine collection process can minimize this source of variability.

Other causes of preanalytical variation also affect urine measurements. *Diurnal variation* independent of relative concentration is observed for many urine substances, notably protein, sodium and potassium, phosphate, and hormones. Part of the diurnal variation in protein excretion is posture related in that the relative concentration of protein compared with creatinine increases in the upright position. *Stress* increases protein excretion; both exercise and fever have been shown to cause transient increase in urinary protein. *Dietary changes* in intake of a substance often will alter urinary excretion. Creatine supplements, which are used increasingly by body-builders, also increase urine creatinine excretion.[37] Creatinine excretion often is used to evaluate the adequacy of collection of timed urine. However, short-term fluctuation in dietary protein intake alters the excretion of creatinine in urine.

Time of Collection

Variation in urine measurements can be the result of improperly collected 24-hour urine specimens. Such specimens are among the most difficult to collect properly. As was mentioned earlier, urine creatinine often is used as a measure of the completeness of urine collection, and specimens with too much or too little creatinine are considered to indicate an improperly timed collection. Because excretion of creatinine is relatively reproducible in a given individual on a stable diet (average day-to-day variation of 10% with little diurnal variation), the ratio of the concentration of the substance of interest to that of creatinine has been advocated as a means of providing an accurate estimate of total urinary excretion. This is especially important for pediatric specimens because it is often difficult to get children to cooperate with timed urine collections.

Sample Stability

Many compounds that are stable in serum are unstable in urine. Both bacterial contamination and low pH can produce in vitro changes in the concentration of many analytes. Collection of urine into containers with various preservatives, acids, or bases is often needed to prevent such variation. In general, stable substances such as electrolytes, protein, and creatinine can be measured in urine samples without the use of preservatives. The addition of concentrated acids or bases usually does not affect electrolyte or creatinine measurements; however, a specimen that contains an appropriate preservative for the measurement of one analyte may be unsuitable for use in the measurement of a different substance. Storage of urine specimens during collection also may alter analyte concentration. For example, porphyrins are unstable when exposed to light, whereas calcium may precipitate at low temperatures. Most formed elements in urine, such as cells and casts, are unstable when stored. Refrigeration often is used to prevent bacterial growth in urine specimens. Refrigeration, however, promotes the formation of crystals that would not have been found at body temperature and lowers the concentration of those substances that have precipitated.

Preanalytical Variation in Other Body Fluids

Preanalytical variation in other body fluids has not been studied extensively. Many factors that affect other samples such as hemoconcentration, tourniquet use, and stress do not affect the composition of cerebrospinal, pleural, peritoneal, and synovial fluids. A delay in transport of specimens to the laboratory usually causes little change in normal fluid composition because these specimens are virtually cell free. If measurements of unstable analytes such as lactate, glucose, or pH are requested, specimens should be transported to the laboratory in an ice slurry to prevent artifactual changes in concentration. For fluids other than cerebrospinal fluid, use of an anticoagulant is advisable to prevent the formation of fibrin clots, which can lower cell counts falsely.

Specimen Collection From Infants

Capillary Sampling

Venipuncture in infants and small children is usually not an acceptable method of obtaining blood because of the difficulty associated with finding a vein and because of the importance of preserving available veins for use in administration of intravenous fluid. Capillary blood is the specimen that is usually available for testing in these children. In neonates, the outer aspects of the sole of the foot are preferred sites for skin puncture, whereas earlobes or fingers are acceptable in older infants and small children. The skin surface often is warmed to produce "arterialized" capillary blood; as was mentioned earlier, however, agreement with arterial blood gases is poor in neonates, particularly in premature infants. It is essential to allow any topical antiseptics to dry before skin puncture because the collected blood will mix freely with any remaining liquid on the surface. Contamination with antiseptics can falsely dilute specimens and may cause hemolysis. It may be helpful to apply mild pressure after the skin is punctured, but squeezing or "milking" of the puncture site will contaminate the sample with tissue fluid.

Because of the small volume of sample obtained and, in neonates, the high hematocrit, relatively little serum or plasma is available for testing. Special capillary tubes that contain appropriate anticoagulants or preservatives are available to facilitate collection of required specimens. Use of pediatric separator tubes for serum or heparinized plasma will result in a greater amount of sample for the same amount of blood obtained. However, the small sample size often results in a relatively large surface area, making evaporation an even more important consideration for pediatric specimens. Hemoconcentration, posture, and diet-related changes are relatively less important for neonates than for older children or adults. The extent of cyclical variations in infants and children is largely unknown.

Blood Collection for Metabolic Diseases

When infants are screened for inborn metabolic errors, specimens often are collected on filter paper and are transported to a specialized laboratory as dried blood spots. Little information is available on specific preanalytical factors related to dried blood spots; however, some factors do affect the results of such tests. Because such specimens are collected as capillary blood, care must be taken to avoid contamination with antiseptics, which may interfere with the assays. The paper must be fully saturated in the area of collection to provide an adequate amount of sample. For some metabolic errors (such as galactosemia), screening must not be done until at least 24 hours after the infant has begun feeding because the metabolic product that accumulates is derived from ingested food. Obtaining specimens before this time can produce false-negative results. For tests that require measurement of enzyme activity, care must be taken to prevent exposure of the specimens to excess heat during the shipping process; if specimens are mailed, temperatures in outdoor mailboxes can be high enough to cause falsely low results. All the general precautions discussed previously must be followed carefully.

Table 18-4 Delta Checks for Analysis

Appropriate	Inappropriate
Electrolytes: Na, K, Cl	Glucose
Total protein	Phosphate
Albumin	Lactate dehydrogenase
Urea	Creatine kinase
Creatinine	Aspartate aminotransferase
Alkaline phosphatase	Alanine aminotransferase
Hemoglobin and hematocrit; mean cell volume and red blood cell distribution width index	

COMPUTER-BASED AIDS FOR ERROR DETECTION

Computer-based systems that aid in error detection can reduce the number of erroneous results that are reported. In many laboratory and hospital computer systems, it is possible to compare the results from the current specimen with those from previous samples on the same patient (see Chapter 22). Such result comparisons are termed **delta checks.** A delta check can test for results that vary by a set amount or a set percentage; with some systems, it is possible to use one type of check for values at a certain level and another for higher or lower concentrations. Tests that are particularly appropriate for monitoring with delta checks are those that normally change little from one day to the next. Some of these are listed in Table 18-4. Measuring the rate of analyte change also may add to the sensitivity of error detection.[38] Delta checks should not be used for substances that are subject to pronounced intraindividual variation (see Table 18-4). A list of delta check values used in the author's laboratory is given in Table 18-5. Although fluctuations in one test result may be seen in as many as 1% of all specimens, multiple test results that fail delta checks are usually the result of a significant change in the patient's condition or a nonrepresentative specimen. Selection of tests that typically

Table 18-5 Delta Check Values

Test	Delta Check Value
Albumin	1 g/dL
Anion gap	10 mmol/L
Calcium	1 mg/dL
Chloride	5 mmol/L
Cholesterol	±30%
CO_2 content	5 mmol/L
Creatinine	±50%
Direct bilirubin	±50%
Glucose (fasting only)	±30%
Magnesium	0.25 mmol/L
Mean corpuscular volume	4 μm^3
Mean platelet volume	1.5 μm^3
Osmolality	15 mOsm/kg
Potassium	1 mmol/L
Protein	1 g/dL
Red blood cell distribution width	2% (absolute change)
Sodium	5 mmol/L
Total bilirubin	±50%
Urea nitrogen	±50%
Uric acid	1.5 mg/dL

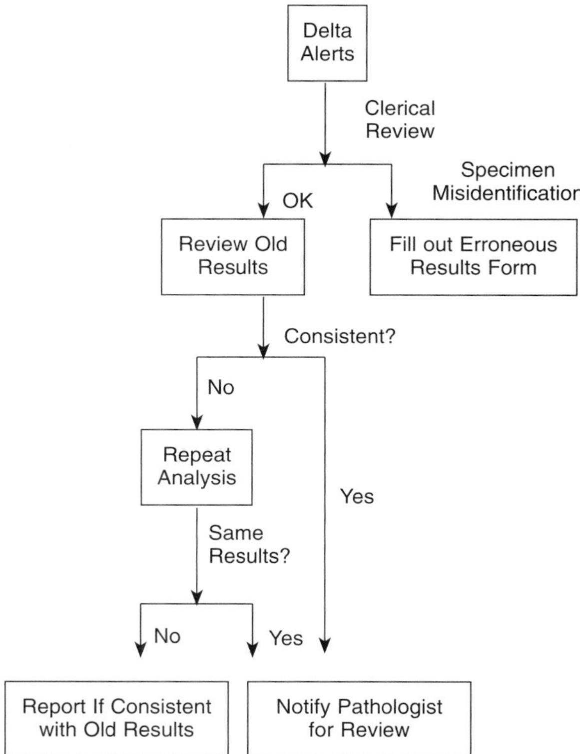

Fig. 18-8 Flow chart for delta alerts.

change in parallel, such as AST and ALT or urea and creatinine, may improve delta check utility (see Table 18-4).[39] Common causes of failed delta checks include specimens drawn above intravenous lines, contaminated specimens, and misidentified specimens. Review of such results before release can lead to a significant reduction in the reporting of erroneous results. A method that can be used for the evaluation of specimens that fail delta checks is outlined in Fig. 18-8. The laboratory information system can automatically perform the delta check review as part of autoverification routines (see Chapter 22).

Criteria for Rejection of Specimens

To prevent the reporting of misleading results, each laboratory must establish criteria for specimen rejection. A specimen must be rejected when the results obtained by analysis of that specimen will not be representative of the patient's condition. The most common cause of specimen rejection is inadequate identification. Manually accessioned specimens must have the patient's name and identification number on both the sample and the accompanying request slip. Specimens that are not drawn by laboratory personnel should be checked carefully before they are accepted by the laboratory. For specimens that require special handling, improper collection and transportation are the most common reasons for rejection. In most laboratories that process blood-gas specimens, an average of 5% of the specimens have not been collected correctly and must be rejected. Specimens often are collected in the incorrect tube for the assay requested. Each laboratory must have a list of acceptable alternative specimens for each test, for example, a laboratory manual may suggest collection of serum for a particular test, but heparinized plasma is an acceptable alternative. If the specimen contains another anticoagulant or preservative, it should be rejected (although it may be used for other analyses). For tubes that contain preservatives or anticoagulants, a proper ratio of specimen to preservative is necessary. This is most critical with liquid solutions of preservatives but may also occur with powdered anticoagulants. Tubes that do not have the appropriate ratio should not be accepted for analysis. For tests that require special patient preparation, the absence of such preparation should lead to rejection. If a test is affected by hemolysis, the amount of hemolysis may be estimated on a number of instruments; because the relationship between degree of hemolysis and extent of effect on results is unpredictable, hemolyzed specimens should be rejected and repeat testing recommended.[40] For example, in the author's laboratory, samples with hemolysis are assayed for hemoglobin concentration; if it is above the threshold where differences in results commonly affect clinical interpretation, the sample is rejected. However, if (for example) a hemolyzed sample has a low potassium result, we will report the result with a comment that the actual potassium concentration is likely to be lower and will suggest repeat testing. If a test result is affected by lipemia (and the specimen cannot be cleared by ultracentrifugation before analysis), test results should not be reported. Lipemia typically does not affect results determined by nondiluted ion-selective electrode measurements (such as those found for electrolyte measurements on whole blood analyzers). Finally, any specimens with results that fail delta checks or results that are considered unlikely to be valid (potassium over 10 mmol/L, calcium less than 4 mg/dL, and so on) should be reported to the laboratory director for review before the results are reported. Although many physicians complain when the laboratory does not report results for tests ordered, if there is any question about the validity of a result, it should not be reported. Erroneous results can lead to inappropriate treatment of the patient.

KEY CONCEPTS BOX 18-4

- Variations inherent in urine collection include biological variables, time of collection, means of preservation, and stability of analytes.
- Failed delta checks may be due to specimens drawn above intravenous lines, contaminated specimens, and misidentification of the patient.
- Each laboratory should establish criteria for specimen rejection.
- Delta checks can reduce the reporting of results from miscollected samples, but, if rules for delta checks are not judiciously selected, many false alerts will be generated.

REFERENCES

1. Lundberg G: Acting on significant laboratory results, JAMA 245:1762, 1981.
2. Bonini P, Plebani M, Ceriotti F, et al: Errors in laboratory medicine, Clin Chem 48:691, 2002.
3. Young D: *Effects of Prenalytical Variables on Clinical Laboratory Tests,* ed 3, Washington, DC, 2007, AACC Press.
4. Valenstein P, Meier F: Outpatient order accuracy: a College of American Pathologists Q-probe study of requisition order entry accuracy in 660 institutions, Arch Pathol Lab Med 123:1145, 1999.
5. Valenstein P, Howanitz P: Ordering accuracy—a College of American Pathologists Q-probe study of 577 institutions, Arch Pathol Lab Med 119:117, 1995.
6. Vesper H, Demers L, Eastell R, et al: Assessment and recommendations on factors contributing to preanalytical variability of urinary pyridinoline and deoxypyridinoline, Clin Chem 48:220, 2002.
7. Dufour D: Reference values in endocrinology. In Becker K, editor: *Principles and Practice of Endocrinology and Metabolism,* Philadelphia, 2001, Lippincott Williams & Wilkins, p. 2173.
8. Fraser C: Biological variation in clinical chemistry: an update: collated data, 1988-1991, Arch Pathol Lab Med 116:916, 1992.
9. Statland B, Winkel P, Bokelund H: Factors contributing to intra-individual variation of serum constituents. 2. Effects of exercise and diet on variation of serum constituents in healthy subjects, Clin Chem 19:1380, 1973.
10. Panagiotakos D, Pitsavos C, Chrysohoou C, et al: The associations between leisure-time physical activity and inflammatory and coagulation markers related to cardiovascular disease: the ATTICA study, Prev Med 40:432, 2005.
11. Dugue B, Leppanen E, Grasbeck R: The driving license examination as a stress model: effects on blood picture, serum cortisol and the production of interleukins in man, Life Sci 14, 2001.
12. Gore J, Goldberg R, Matsumoto A, et al: Validity of serum total cholesterol level obtained within 24 hours of acute myocardial infarction, Am J Cardiol 54:722, 1984.
13. Statland B, Bokelund H, Winkel P: Factors contributing to intra-individual variation of serum constituents: 4. Effects of posture and tourniquet application on variation of serum constituents in healthy subjects, Clin Chem 20:1513, 1974.
14. Kuperman G, Gibson R: Computer physician order entry: benefits, costs, and issues, Ann Intern Med 139:31, 2003.
15. Hoeltke L: *The Complete Textbook of Phlebotomy,* Clifton Park, NY, 2006, Thomson Delmar Learning.
16. Garza D, Becan-McBride K: *Phlebotomy Handbook: Blood Collection Essentials,* Upper Saddle River, NJ, 2004, Prentice Hall.
17. Arkin C, Bessman J, Calam R, et al: *Procedures for the Collection of Diagnostic Blood Specimens by Venipuncture, Approved Standard,* ed 5, Wayne, PA, 2004, Clinical and Laboratory Standards Institute.
18. Jones B, Calam R, Howanitz P: Chemistry specimen acceptability: a College of American Pathologists Q-probe study of 453 laboratories, Arch Pathol Lab Med 121:19, 1997.
19. Jones B, Meier F, Howanitz P: Complete blood count specimen acceptability: a College of American Pathologists Q-probe study of 703 laboratories, Arch Pathol Lab Med 119:203, 1995.
20. Dale J, Novis D: Outpatient phlebotomy success and reasons for specimen rejection: a Q-probes study, Arch Pathol Lab Med 126:416, 2002.
21. Morrow D, Cannon C, Jesse R, et al: National Academy of Clinical Biochemistry Laboratory Medicine Practice Guidelines: clinical characteristics and utilization of biochemical markers in acute coronary syndromes, Clin Chem 53:522, 2007.
22. Bowen R, Chan Y, Cohen J, et al: Effect of blood collection tubes on total triiodothyronine and other laboratory assays, Clin Chem 52:1627, 2005.
23. Hira K, Ohtani Y, Rahman M, et al: Pseudohyperkalaemia caused by recentrifugation of blood samples after storage in gel separator tubes, Ann Clin Biochem 38:386, 2001.
24. Hawkins R: Measurement of whole-blood potassium—is it clinically safe? Clin Chem 49:2105, 2003.
25. Dzik W, Murphy M, Andreu G, et al: An international study of the performance of sample collection from patients, Vox Sang 85:40, 2003.
26. Chiaroni J, Legrand D, Dettori I, et al: Analysis of ABO discrepancies occurring in 35 French hospitals, Transfusion 44:860, 2004.
27. Howanitz P, Renner S, Walsh M: Continuous wristband monitoring over 2 years decreases identification errors: a College of American Pathologists Q-Tracks study, Arch Pathol Lab Med 126:809, 2002.
28. Bologna L, Mutter M: Life after phlebotomy deployment: reducing major patient and specimen identification errors, J Healthcare Information Management 16:65, 2002.
29. Turner C, Casbard A, Murphy M: Barcode technology: its role in increasing the safety of blood transfusion, Transfusion 43:1200, 2003.
30. Sazama K, Robertson E, Chesler R: Is antiglycolysis required for routine glucose analysis? Clin Chem 25:2038, 1979.
31. Sealey J: Plasma renin activity and plasma prorenin assays, Clin Chem 37:1811, 1991.
32. Howanitz P, Steindel S, Cembrowski G, et al: Emergency department stat test turnaround times: a College of American Pathologists Q-probe study for potassium and hemoglobin, Arch Pathol Lab Med 116:122, 1992.
33. Sevastos N, Teodossiades G, Efstathiou S, et al: Pseudohyperkalemia in serum: the phenomenon and its clinical magnitude, J Lab Clin Med 147:139, 2006.
34. Ringelhann B, Laszlo E, Vajda L: Pseudohyperkalaemia in acute myeloid leukemia, Lancet 1:928, 1974.
35. Dufour D, Mesonero C, Miller K: Artifactual hyperkalemia induced by heparin in patients with extreme lymphocytosis, Clin Chem 33:914, 1987.
36. DiMagno E, Corle D, O'Brien J, et al: Effect of long-term freezer storage, thawing, and refreezing on selected constituents of serum, Mayo Clin Proc 64:1226, 1989.
37. Ropero-Miller J, Paget-Wilkes H, Doering P, et al: Effect of oral creatine supplementation on random urine creatinine, pH, and specific gravity measurements, Clin Chem 46:295, 2000.

38. Lacher D, Connelly D: Rate and delta checks compared for selected chemistry tests, Clin Chem 34:1966, 1988.
39. Lacher D: Relationship between delta checks for selected chemistry tests, Clin Chem 36:2134, 1990.
40. Lippi G, Salvagno G, Montagnana M, et al: Influence of hemolysis on routine clinical chemistry testing, Clin Chem Lab Med 44:311, 2006.

INTERNET SITES

http://library.med.utah.edu/WebPath/TUTORIAL/PHLEB/PHLEB.html

The Society for Research on Biological Rhythms—http://www.srbr.org/

CLSI Approved Guideline—Contains guidelines for patient preparation, specimen collection—www.clsi.org

Laboratory Management

Lawrence J. Crolla, Demetra Callas, Lisa Reninger, Marilyn Nelson, Anita Snodgrass, and Paul Stiffler

19

Chapter

Chapter Outline

Key Terms

CAP College of American Pathologists.

CLIA '88 Clinical Laboratory Improvement Amendments of 1988.

CMS Centers for Medicare and Medicaid Services (formerly known as HCFA).

complexity model The seven criteria used for categorizing test systems, assays, and examinations; based on assignment of a score of 1, 2, or 3 within each category.

deemed status Equivalency between accreditation/state requirements and CLIA standards.

demographics Personal data about a specific patient or specific population.

empowerment When managers create a nurturing environment in which their staff can learn, grow, improve, and function effectively.

Federal Register Provides a uniform system for making available to the public regulations and legal notices issued by federal agencies.

full-time equivalent (FTE) Full-time employee scheduled to work 8 hours per workday for 260 days, or 10 hours per workday for 208 days, or 2080 hours per year.

HHS Department of Health and Human Services.

high-complexity test One that scores 13 or higher by the complexity model categorization system described in CLIA '88.

HIPAA Health Insurance Portability & Accountability Act of 1996. Major aspects of this federal law include standardizing electronic patient health transactions; providing unique health identifiers for employers, health plans, and health care providers; and establishing security and privacy standards (www.HIPAA.org).

HIS (hospital information system) Also known as mainframe computers.

LIS Laboratory information system.

Medicaid A program sponsored by federal, state, and local governments that provides medical benefits to the medically indigent regardless of age.

Medicare A program of medical care and hospital services sponsored by the federal government for persons 65 years and older.

moderate-complexity test Test with a score of 12 or less by the complexity model categorization system.

NPSG National Patient Safety Goals set forth by the Joint Commission to promote specific improvements in safety.

patient mix The percentages of Medicare, Medicaid, private pay, and charity patients in a hospital's patient population.

productivity Production efficiency expressed as units of work divided by defined hours or defined positions.

quality assurance (QA) program Program designed to (1) monitor and evaluate the ongoing and overall quality of the total testing process and the effectiveness of its policies and procedures; (2) identify and correct problems and ensure accurate, reliable, and prompt reporting of test results; and (3) ensure the adequacy and competency of the staff.

quality control (QC) Procedures for monitoring and evaluating the quality of the analytical testing process used for each method to ensure the accuracy and reliability of patient test results and reports.

service level demands Specimen collection and test turnaround time requirements for the laboratory.

The Joint Commission An independent, not-for-profit organization, which certifies more than 15,000 health care organizations and programs in the United States.

waived test Test systems or simple laboratory examinations and procedures that are cleared by the Food and Drug Administration (FDA) for home use; they employ methods that are so simple and accurate as to render the likelihood of erroneous results negligible and pose no reasonable risk of harm to the patient if the test is performed incorrectly. See also Chapter 21.

SECTION OBJECTIVES BOX 19-1

- Describe the core regulations that govern clinical laboratories, and explain how laboratories can comply with these regulations.
- Explain what is meant by laboratory compliance and give 4 examples of an elements of a compliance program.
- Describe the purpose of the Laboratory Emergency Preparedness program.
- Discuss the basic organizational structure of hospitals and clinical laboratories.

By performing analyses on various human specimens, the personnel of a clinical chemistry laboratory provide information to physicians that they can use to diagnose and treat human diseases. The laboratory not only must comply with legal operating regulations, but must perform tests in a cost-effective manner. Balancing these requirements is the responsibility of the laboratory management staff. The production of patient results requires a complex infrastructure that comprises testing systems (e.g., analyzers, reagents, test procedures), staff to perform the analyses, administrative staff, and systems for the integration of laboratory results with a hospital or other information system.

Much of the way a laboratory must operate is delineated in great detail by federal regulations. One of the most important of these is the Clinical Laboratory Improvement Amendments of 1988 (**CLIA ’88**). The goal of these regulations is to ensure the quality of laboratory test results regardless of where the tests are performed. In addition, laboratory management must keep abreast of other federal and state regulations, including guidelines on compliance and appropriate billing, bloodborne pathogen exposure, and chemical exposure and waste disposal, as well as a growing number of employee safety regulations (see Chapter 1) and the **Health Insurance Portability and Accountability Act of 1996 (HIPAA)** (see Chapter 22). Therefore, this chapter begins by reviewing the regulatory concerns of laboratories.

REGULATIONS

A large part of managing a laboratory today involves ensuring that the laboratory is in compliance with all federal, state, and city regulations that now abound. A hospital laboratory must be certified by the Centers for Medicare and Medicaid Services **(CMS),** by a private certifying agency, or by a state regulatory agency that has received **“deemed status.”** These certifying agencies inspect laboratories to determine whether they are in compliance with federal regulations, including CLIA ’88. The College of American Pathologists **(CAP)** and **The Joint Commission** are two of the private certifying agencies that have received deemed status to act on behalf of the federal government. Blood banks may require inspections by different certifying agencies.

CLIA ’88

The CLIA ’88 regulations apply to almost every laboratory in the United States that performs laboratory testing for assessment of the health of human beings. These regulations are broken into various subparts, the most important of which include the following:

Subpart H—*Participation in Proficiency Testing* is required for laboratories that perform tests of moderate complexity (including the subcategory) or high complexity, or any combination of these tests.

Subpart I—*Proficiency Testing Programs* provide unknown samples for tests of moderate complexity or high complexity, or any combination of these tests, to laboratories that perform these tests on human specimens.

Subpart J—*Patient Test Management* deals with test requisition; patient preparation; collection, identification, transportation, and processing of samples; and reporting of test results. This subpart also specifies how long records must be kept and outlines the documentation necessary for any problems that may have occurred in the reporting process.

Subpart K—***Quality Control (QC)*** specifies how QC is to be done and how often. This also covers procedure manuals (Box 19-1) and the documentation required to bring a new test into the laboratory.

Subpart M—*Personnel* defines the responsibilities, education, training, and experience required for each of the personnel positions at a testing site where **moderate-complexity testing** or **high-complexity testing** is performed.

Subpart P—***Quality Assurance (QA) Programs*** deal with the various monitors that should be evaluated to ensure that the laboratory is producing quality work. If all monitors are evaluated in a consistent program, according to the

Box 19-1

What Every Procedure Manual Must Include

When applicable to the test procedure, the procedure manual must include the following:

1. Requirements for specimen collection and processing and criteria for specimen rejection
2. Procedures for microscopic examinations, including the detection of inadequately prepared slides
3. Step-by-step performance of the procedure, including test calculations and interpretation of results
4. Preparation of slides, solutions, calibrators, controls, reagents, stains, and other materials used in testing
5. Calibration and calibration verification procedures
6. The reportable range for patient test results as established or verified in the Clinical Laboratory Improvement Amendments (CLIA) '88, Section 493.1213
7. Control procedures
8. Remedial action to be taken when calibration or control results fail to meet the laboratory's criteria for acceptability
9. Limitations in methods, including interfering substances
10. Reference interval (normal values)
11. Imminent life-threatening laboratory results or "panic" (critical) values
12. Pertinent literature references
13. Appropriate criteria for specimen storage and preservation to ensure specimen integrity until testing is completed
14. The laboratory's system for reporting patient results, including (when appropriate) the protocol for reporting critical values
15. Description of the course of action to be taken in the event that a test system becomes inoperable
16. Criteria for the referral of specimens, including procedures for specimen submission and handling as described in CLIA '88, Section 493.1103

guidelines presented in this section, laboratories will be in compliance with most regulations and should not have to fear unannounced inspections.

Subpart Q—*Inspection* describes requirements applicable to all CLIA '88–certified and CLIA '88–exempt laboratories. Failing an inspection or failing to permit an inspection has severe consequences.

Subpart R—*Enforcement Procedures* provide for intermediate sanctions that may be imposed on laboratories that perform clinical diagnostic tests on human specimens when those laboratories are found to be noncompliant with one or more of the conditions for Medicare coverage of their services.

Subpart T—*Consultations* will be available from the federal Clinical Laboratory Advisory Committee. This committee advises and makes recommendations on technical and scientific aspects of the provisions of CLIA '88.

OSHA (see pp. 23-31, Chapter 1)

Another federal regulation that is very important to laboratories is the Occupational and Safety Health Act of 1970. This act authorizes the Occupational Safety and Health Administration (OSHA) to implement regulations that ensure the operation of a safe laboratory. OSHA covers all forms of safety, from the physical environment to working with chemicals and bloodborne pathogens. OSHA mandates that laboratories have documented plans for occupational exposure to hazardous chemicals (Chemical Hygiene Plan) or bloodborne pathogens (Exposure Control Plan), and prevention of needlestick and other "sharps" injuries. In addition, the **Department of Health and Human Services (HHS),** Centers for Disease Control and Prevention (CDC), requires laboratories to have documented Tuberculosis Control Plans. Chapter 1 discusses many aspects of OSHA regulations; additional information on these regulations can be found on the OSHA website at www.osha.gov.

Security

Security standards mandated by HIPAA require covered entities to develop plans that integrate every component of security related to privacy of patient health care information. Security plans should include contingency backup in the event of a disaster. Government regulations are in place for laboratories that handle select agents (biological or toxicological hazardous agents) or other agents of high public health and agricultural concern. Laboratories that qualify under this select agent rule are required to conduct risk assessments and develop plans to limit access to facilities and information. Although no federal government requirement currently exists for laboratories not covered by the select agent rule, it is recommended by CDC and other public health organizations that current security plans be expanded to include appropriate levels of control for biological agents or toxins, as well as other hazardous material (HAZMAT) chemicals. These measures are in place in most laboratories that apply good laboratory management practices.

National Patient Safety Goals

The Joint Commission has developed many National Patient Safety Goals (**NPSG**) designed to promote patient safety in key areas.

Among them are several on which the laboratory can have a direct impact (Table 19-1).

Laboratory Emergency Preparedness

Laboratories should have policies and procedures in place to prepare for all types of emergency situations. Proper training and documentation for staff of their roles in a disaster are essential. Laboratories should have plans such as the one outlined in the Clinical and Laboratory Standards Institute (CLSI) document, *X4-R Planning for Challenges to Clinical Laboratory Operations During a Disaster: A Report.*

During very large-scale emergencies (terrorist attacks, public health outbreaks), the laboratory may not have the capacity to handle the disaster alone. In this case, the laboratory may have to rely on the Laboratory Response Network (LRN).

Presidential Decision Directive 39 outlined national antiterrorism policies and assigned specific missions to federal

Table 19-1 The Joint Commission National Patient Safety Goals (NPSG)

Goal 1	Improve the accuracy of patient identification.
1A	Use at least two patient identifiers when providing care, treatment, or services.
1B	Prior to the start of any invasive procedure, conduct a final verification process (such as a "time-out,") to confirm the correct patient, procedure, and site using active—not passive—communication techniques.
Goal 2	Improve the effectiveness of communication among caregivers.
2A	For verbal or telephone orders or for telephonic reporting of critical test results, verify the complete order or test result by having the person who receives the information record and "read back" the complete order or test result.
2B	Standardize a list of abbreviations, acronyms, symbols, and dose designations that are not to be used throughout the organization.
2C	Measure, assess, and, if appropriate, take action to improve the timeliness of reporting and the timeliness of receipt by the responsible licensed caregiver of critical test results and values.
2E	Implement a standardized approach to "hand off" communications, including an opportunity to ask and respond to questions.
Goal 7	Reduce the risk of health care–associated infection.
7A	Comply with current Centers for Disease Control and Prevention (CDC) hand hygiene guidelines.
7B	Manage as sentinel events all identified cases of unanticipated death or major permanent loss of function associated with a health care–associated infection.
Goal 13	Encourage patients' active involvement in their own care as a patient safety strategy.
13A	Define and communicate the means by which patients and their families can report concerns about safety, and encourage them to do so.

Table from Joint Commission at http://www.jointcommission.org/PatientSafety/NationalPatientSafetyGoals/08_lab_npsgs.htm.

departments and agencies. In response to this Directive, the CDC and the HHS established the LRN.

The Laboratory Response Network is a collaborative effort between its founding partners, the CDC, the Federal Bureau of Investigation (FBI), and the Association of Public Health Laboratories, as well as many other local, state, and federal laboratories. The LRN became operational in August 1999. Its objective was to ensure an effective laboratory response to bioterrorism by helping to improve the nation's public health laboratory infrastructure, which had limited ability to respond to bioterrorism. The Network provides laboratory diagnostics and capacity to respond to chemical, biological, or other public health emergencies. More information on the LRN can be found at www.bt.cdc.gov/lrn.

Laboratory Compliance

In the August 24, 1998, ***Federal Register*** 63 FR 45076, the HHS Office of Inspector General (OIG) released Compliance Guidelines for Clinical Laboratories. These guidelines provide a framework by which hospital laboratories can develop compliance programs to help ensure acceptable ethical and legal conduct by their employees and prevent fraud, abuse, and waste. Each laboratory should develop compliance programs that are applicable to its particular configuration, taking into consideration the scope of services and available resources. The OIG guidelines highlight seven program elements that laboratories should adopt to be in compliance:

1. Written standards of conduct for employees, including policies and procedures
2. Designation of a compliance officer
3. Compliance training programs for all employees
4. Maintenance of a process such as a hotline to receive complaints while protecting the anonymity of the complainant
5. System to respond to allegations of misconduct and enforce disciplinary action against violators
6. Use of audits to monitor compliance
7. Investigation and remediation of identified problems and policies regarding nonemployment of sanctioned individuals

More information on laboratory compliance can be obtained by reviewing the *Federal Register.*

Several organizations have issued guidelines regarding the length of time that laboratory records must be retained (Table 19-2). Because the agencies that issue these guidelines also accredit hospitals and laboratories, these guidelines have the force of law.

Laboratories should devote time to these compliance issues. Severe fines can be levied for violation of any of the federal CLIA '88 or OSHA regulations, as well as for any identified fraudulent billing practices. CLIA '88 certification is also required for Medicare reimbursement, providing strong motivation for compliance.

One of the most important actions the laboratory can take to ensure compliance with regulations is to obtain copies of the regulations and make them available to laboratory personnel. Forming a regulatory committee made up of representatives from each laboratory section also helps to ensure that a laboratory is in compliance with all regulations. The committee can help formulate needed policies and procedures for compliance issues and conduct in-service education and inspections to keep the laboratory aware of

Table **19-2** Suggested Laboratory Records Retention Schedule

Type of Record	Length of Record Retention, Years	Sources and Notes
General	Always check State requirements to see if they are more rigorous.	Always check with your risk management dept.
Test requisitions	2 years	1, 2, 3
Test printout/worksheets	2 years	1, 2
Patient laboratory results and sendouts	2 years	1, 3 from date of report
Pathology test reports	20 years	1 from date of report
Accession logs	2 years	1
Bone marrow reports	20 years	1
Controlled substances	3 years	DEA
Radioactive materials	3 years	NRC
Quality control	2 years	1, 2, 3
Test procedure	2 years	1, 2, 3 after discontinuance and date of initial use
Proficiency tests	2 years	1, 2 from date of performance
Proficiency test failure—corrective action	2 years	1
Instrument maintenance	2 years after life of instrument	
Environmental exposure measurement	30 years	5 postemployment
Training records	3 years	5
Specimens		
Blood/body fluid smears	7 days	1
Bone marrow smears	20 years	2
Microbiology—stained smears	7 days	1
Blood Bank	Because of patient look-backs it has been suggested that blood bank records be kept indefinitely.	
Autologous donor records	10 years	4
Unit disposition records/logbooks	10 years	4
Records of employee signatures	5 years	4
Test records	5 years	1, 2
Test reports	5 years	1, 2
Quality control/maintenance	Indefinitely	1, 2
Permanently deferred donors	10 years	4
Patient transfusion record	10 years	4
HCV/HIV look-back records	10 years	4
Therapeutic phlebotomy records	10 years	4
Investigation of transfusion transmitted disease reports	10 years	4

1, College of American Pathologists (CAP); *2,* Clinical Laboratory Improvement Amendments of 1988 (CLIA '88); *3,* American Hospital Association (AHA); *4,* American Association of Blood Banks (AABB); *5,* Occupational Safety and Health Administration (OSHA).
DEA, Drug Enforcement Agency; *NRC,* Nuclear Regulatory Commission.

its responsibilities. Managers can achieve compliance with regulations only by having everyone involved.

HOSPITAL MANAGEMENT STRUCTURE

Organization of a Hospital

The size, **patient mix,** market, and affiliations of a hospital affect its organizational structure. Fig. 19-1 illustrates a common organizational structure for many hospitals. Hospital vice presidents each have several departments that report to them. Because they cannot be experts in all areas, they must work closely with the managers in each reporting department. Each department has its own internal structure, depending on its specific functions. In general, the flow of responsibility is from least senior managers to more senior managers and then to the department head. The importance of fiscal concerns is so great that most departments have a real or assumed line of responsibility to the finance department to manage billings, research funds, and purchasing.

A discrete computer section usually is located within both the hospital and the laboratory. The hospital information system consists of mainframe computers. The hospital computer section processes patient demographic and billing information, whereas the laboratory computer processes laboratory data. Ideally, these systems are interfaced for maximum efficiency and billing accuracy (see Chapter 22).

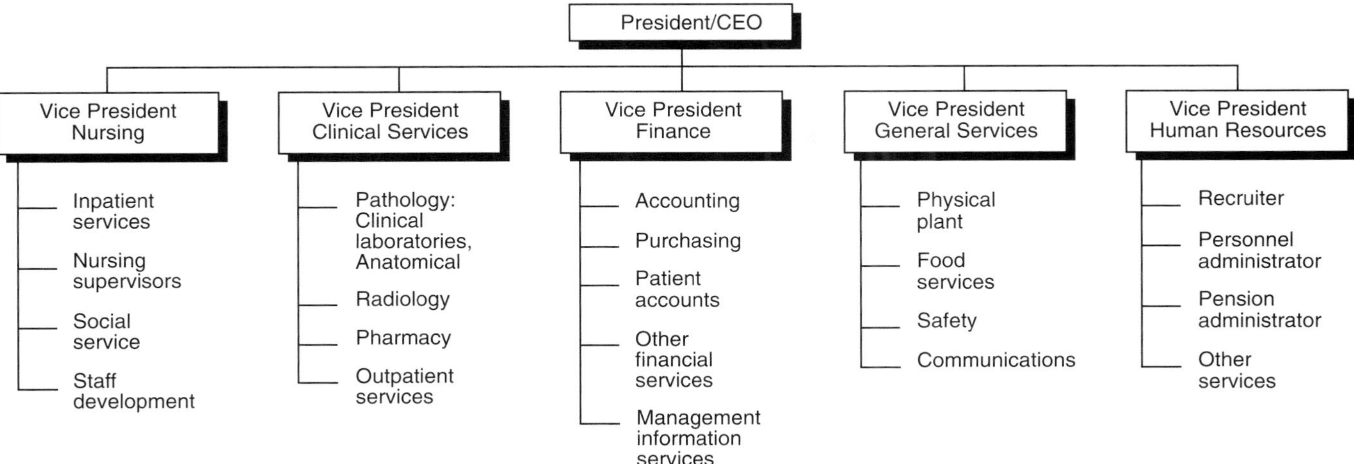

Fig. 19-1 Chart of a hospital organizational structure.

Organization of a Clinical Chemistry Laboratory

Pathology departments should have a generalized organizational chart that shows the reporting relationship between staff member positions in each laboratory or section. This helps everyone involved to understand the chain of command (authority). This organizational chart should show the lines of "courtesy" reporting as well as direct reporting; it also should show any outside factors that strongly affect the organizational reporting structure. A typical schema of a department of pathology is illustrated in Fig. 19-2.

Each clinical laboratory also should have a detailed organizational chart that depicts the way each laboratory section is structured. A schema of a "typical" chemistry laboratory is shown in Fig. 19-3. Subdividing a clinical laboratory into departments, sections, or units, and then into shifts, should be done in a manner that enables the individual laboratory to use space, equipment, reagents, and personnel efficiently and flexibly to meet its expected service demands. Therefore, the laboratory is not likely to be made up of departments that correspond to the specialties and subspecialties described in the final regulations for CLIA '88 published in the *Federal Register.* All laboratory testing must be performed and supervised by qualified and properly trained employees (see the Personnel Management section on p. 352).

CLIA '88 explicitly delineates the education, certification, and experience requirements for the *laboratory director* of a laboratory that performs moderately and highly complex testing (sections 493.1405, 493.1406, and 493.1443). These requirements are summarized in Figs. 19-4 and 19-5. A state-licensed MD, DO, DPM Doctor of Podiatric Medicine, or a board-certified PhD, may serve as the laboratory's clinical consultant, who can interpret both moderate- and high-complexity testing laboratory data for the clinical staff. If the laboratory performs only moderate-complexity testing, it must have a staff technical consultant and testing personnel. If high-complexity testing is performed, the laboratory must also have a designated technical supervisor and a general supervisor. CLIA '88 defines a technical supervisor as one who acts as the principal laboratory supervisor, whereas a general supervisor acts as the immediate bench supervisor, reviewing daily work and QC. Personnel requirements under CLIA '88 are being modified constantly. The reader should consult the most current regulation for personnel requirements before making any personnel decisions.

KEY CONCEPTS BOX 19-1

- Federal regulations, such CLIA '88 and the Occupational Health and Safety Act of 1970, have had a significant impact on the development of new policies and procedures in the clinical laboratory. There are government-mandated quality and safety procedures that must be followed in order for the laboratory to legally operate.
- Laboratories must ensure that there is an emergency preparedness plan.
- Compliance guidelines for clinical laboratories have been developed by the HHS department in order to ensure ethical and legal conduct, as well as to prevent fraud.

SECTION OBJECTIVES BOX 19-2

- Discuss how managerial tools can be applied to the operation of the laboratory.
- Discuss how technical and financial resources can be managed.
- Discuss the pros and cons of standard versus non-standard work schedules and cross-training versus specialization of work knowledge.
- Describe the functions of test utilization and turn-around reports.
- Discuss the utility of an "empowered" employee.

GOOD MANAGEMENT SKILLS AND PERSONAL CHARACTERISTICS

The management skills and personal characteristics of the laboratory manager determine the day-to-day work environ-

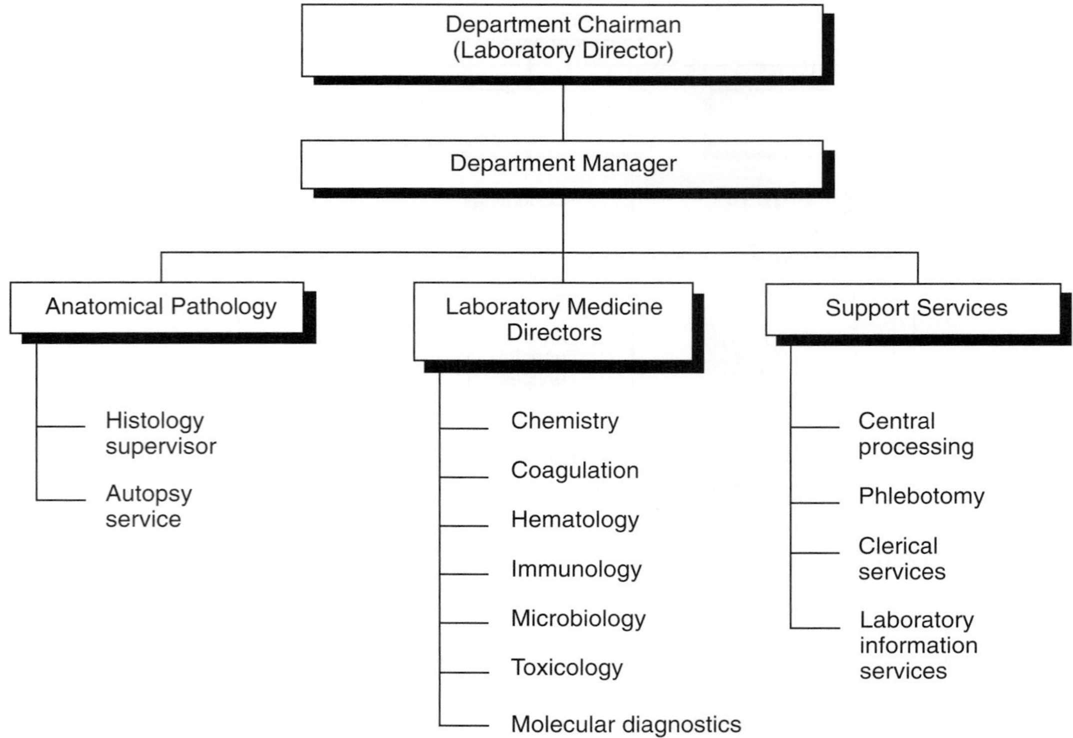

Fig. 19-2 Organizational chart for a department of pathology.

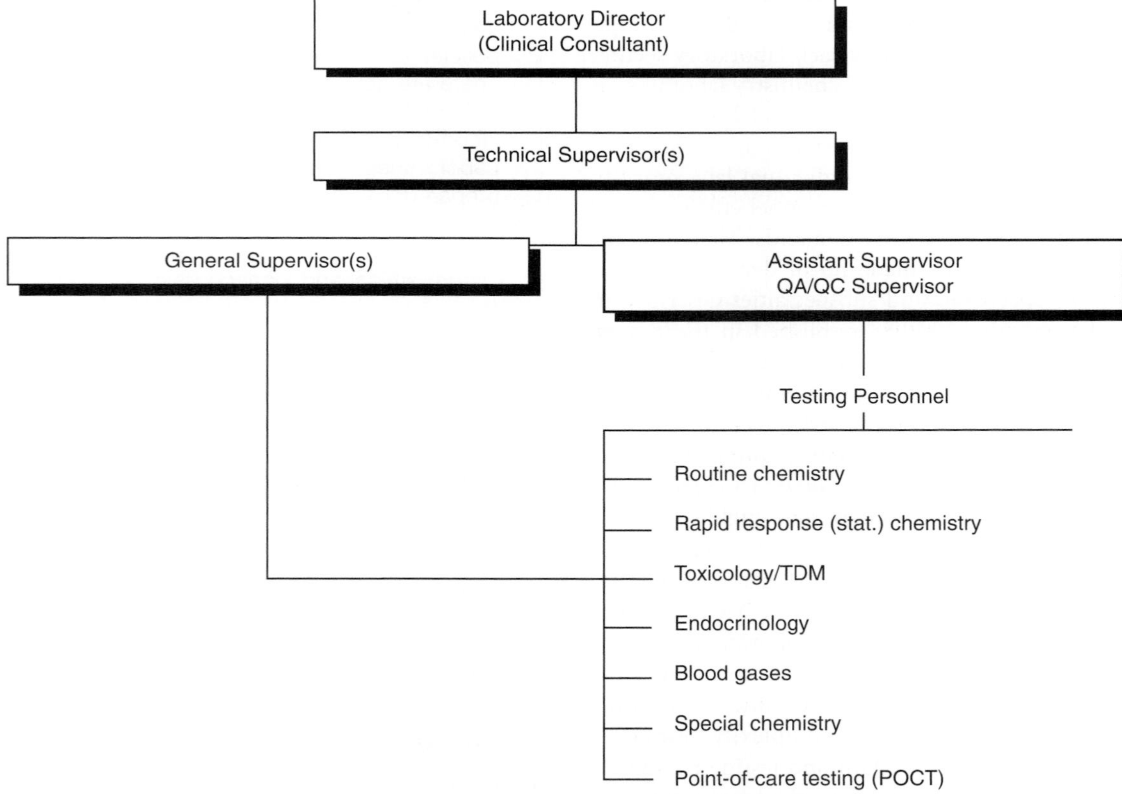

Fig. 19-3 Organizational chart for a chemistry laboratory.

Personnel Qualifications
Laboratory Director
Moderate Complexity Testing
42 CFR 493.1405

A qualified laboratory director must meet the requirements stated in one of the boxes below.

MD or DO and certified by ABP or AOBP or MD or DO or DPM and one of the following: • 1 year directing or supervising nonwaived lab testing • As of 1/19/93, 20 CMEU in lab practice • Lab training in Medical Residency equivalent to 20 CMEU	PhD in chemical, physical, biological, or clinical lab sciences and 1 of the following: • Certified by ABMM, ABCC,ABB, or the ABMLI • 1 year directing or supervising nonwaived lab testing	Master's degree in chemical, physical, biological, or clinical lab sciences, or medical technology and 1 year of lab training or experience or both and 1 year supervisory lab experience
This chart is a paraphrased and abridged version of the Code of Federal Regulations, Chapter 42, Section 493. Please consult the Code of Federal Regulations for exact wording. See *Federal Register* for job responsibilities and more detailed information.	Bachelor's degree in chemical, physical, or biological science or medical technology and 2 years of lab training or experience, or both and 2 years of supervisory lab experience or be serving as a laboratory director and meet qualifications on or before 2/28/92 as laboratory director under CFR 493.1406 or be qualified on or before 2/28/92 under state law to direct a lab in state in which lab is located	MD or DO or DPM always needs to be licensed in the state in which the lab is located. State may require other degrees and experience to be licensed. All degrees must be from an accredited institution.

Fig. 19-4 Summary chart of Clinical Laboratory Improvement Amendments (CLIA) '88 personnel qualifications for a laboratory director for moderate-complexity testing.

ment of the clinical laboratory. The success of a laboratory's operation is dependent upon the manager's leadership abilities in forming a capable and participative management team. This motivated professional team not only is able to provide the level of service expected by the medical staff, hospitalized patients, and patients from outpatient and outreach services, it also is able to establish and accomplish its strategic goals.

Many positive management skills and personal characteristics are listed in Box 19-2. Laboratory managers should concentrate on those skills and characteristics that fit their own personalities and the personalities of their employees.

In addition to working with their strengths, good laboratory managers must identify their weaknesses, so that these, in turn, can be strengthened by formal education and training or by finding the resources (plans and people) to balance these weaknesses. Although the technical staff members of laboratories receive training for the specific tasks they perform, laboratory managers rarely receive management training in advance. They should be provided both formal and on-the-job training. The laboratory manager's personal style, which is the result of the integration of management skills and personal characteristics, strongly determine how easily and how well the laboratory achieves its goals.

The mix of management skills and personal characteristics differs for each successful laboratory manager for three basic reasons. The first is that each hospital's administration, management team, and laboratory staff have unique personalities. The second is that each hospital has a different strategic plan that provides specific goals for the laboratory, in addition to maintaining its established service level. The third reason is that the amount and type of resources allocated to the laboratory for maintaining its day-to-day operations vary from institution to institution.

COMMUNICATION MANAGEMENT

Communication within the Total Organization

The laboratory manager must communicate effectively and frequently with appropriate departmental and hospital administrators, hospital departments, hospital committees,

Personnel Qualifications
Laboratory Director
High Complexity Testing
CFR 493.1443

A qualified laboratory director must meet the requirements stated in one of the boxes below.

MD or DO and certified by ABP or AOBP or MD or DO or DPM and one of the following: • 2 years directing or supervising high-complexity testing • 1 year of lab training during medical residency	PhD in chemical, physical, biological, or clinical lab sciences and one of the following: • Certified by ABMM, ABCC, ABB, or the ABMLI • 1 year directing or supervising nonwaived lab testing	Be serving as a lab director and must have previously qualified or been eligible to qualify under 42CFR 493.1415 (published 3/14/90 at 55 FR 9538) on or before 2/28/92 or On or before 2/28/92 be qualified under state law to direct a lab in the state in which the lab is located

This chart is a paraphrased and abridged version of the Code of Federal Regulations, Chapter 42, Section 493. Please consult the Code of Federal Regulations for exact wording. See *Federal Register* for job responsibilities and more detailed information.

MD or DO or DPM always needs to be licensed in the state in which the lab is located.

State may require other degrees and experience to be licensed.

All degrees must be from an accredited institution.

Fig. 19-5 Summary chart of Clinical Laboratory Improvement Amendments (CLIA) '88 personnel qualifications for a laboratory director for high-complexity testing.

and medical staff to keep them informed of the laboratory's role in achieving the hospital's goals. Frequent and effective communication is also a good way for the laboratory manager to keep laboratory staff informed of any changes in the strategic plan or goals or in the priority of those goals. All interdepartmental communications regarding problem resolution should be documented formally. When a problem exists, the laboratory manager should gather the facts and assess the relative effect of the problem on patients and service level. Then the manager weighs possible solutions and develops a plan of corrective action. The problem, action plan, and outcome must be documented. After an appropriate time, everyone involved must review and reevaluate the original problem and solution, to ensure that the action plan has resulted in improved outcomes.

In addition to solving problems as they arise, the lab manager should use frequent, formal communication modes to maintain a professional, cooperative relationship with the medical staff. Modes of communication can include participation in daily medical rounds, participation in departmental and hospital grand rounds, and publication of newsletters. One tool that may be used to periodically assess physician satisfaction with laboratory services and to identify physician expectations is a survey. These devices allow the laboratory to keep the medical staff apprised of changes in the field of laboratory science and in the laboratory itself (such as new methods, new tests, or test availability) and, ideally, allow the medical staff to have input into prospective changes. When a change in laboratory policy is made without appropriate medical staff review and input, the change is at risk for failure. It is important to provide physicians with feedback as their issues are addressed and their suggestions are implemented.

The laboratory manager must be adept at using political skills to represent the interests and concerns of the laboratory staff to the entire hospital, especially when resources are limited and additional supplies, space, and staff are needed. Political skill is required to negotiate agreements and promote understanding and cooperation in the total organization. The laboratory manager must be an advocate for the laboratory, while at the same time, a loyal member of the administrative staff.

Communication within the Laboratory

As health care evolves in complexity, and as competing demands for resources increase, one's ability to manage a changing environment plays a key role in maintaining a

Box 19-2

Desirable Management Skills and Personal Characteristics for Laboratory Managers

Analytical
Communicative
Fair
Understanding
Objective
Accurate
Visionary
Competent
Articulate
Informed
Political
Punctual
Providing leadership
Resourceful
Compassionate
Giving feedback
Considerate
Listening
Responsible
Rational
Credible
Trustworthy
Financially astute
LIS literate
Organized
Respectful
Able to delegate
Goal setting

LIS, Laboratory information system.

thriving laboratory. Today's successful laboratory manager fosters a staff of "knowledge workers," that is, **empowered** staff members who participate in management decisions. This manager combines empowerment and participative management with the added value that comes from experience and judgment gained as information is gathered and distributed. When staff combines experience and judgment with information, information becomes knowledge. Therefore, to develop and maintain empowered knowledge workers, the laboratory manager provides accurate and timely information to staff, so they can use this information to participate in planning and implementation (participative management). This process is especially helpful in setting and implementing the short-term and long-term goals of the strategic plan. In addition, staff must be valued for their experience and judgment, which is based, in part, on their performance and **productivity,** competency, entrepreneurial skills, risk taking, and creativity.

For laboratory staff to be empowered, they must have a clear understanding of the human and financial resources necessary to meet service level expectations (based on workload, test mix, and turnaround time goals) and customer service expectations (based on the need to satisfy both the customer and the patient). With this information, the empowered laboratory staff can participate in helping the laboratory manager set objectives and plan the implementation process needed to reach the short-term and long-term goals of the strategic plan, while solving daily problems. Because the perspective of the technical staff, supervisors, and nontechnical staff is clearly different from that of a laboratory manager, each can contribute uniquely to the overall planning process. Their input also helps ensure that the process of planning the objectives and the process of reaching laboratory goals are reasonable and effective. To prevent overwhelming the staff when implementing plans to achieve higher levels of technical and customer service, the manager should prioritize goals and select one goal at a time as the focus. By empowering the laboratory staff and having them participate in the management of the laboratory, the laboratory manager establishes visibility, accessibility, and credibility. The staff gains trust and respect for its manager. Also, when the manager gives and receives feedback, both positive and negative, this helps focus the laboratory staff to stay on-target to achieve goals.

The laboratory manager should not assume that the laboratory staff has unlimited capacity and no burnout threshold. With the use of positive feedback on a regular basis, dedicated staff members occasionally can achieve Herculean goals under unusual circumstances. However, a good manager recognizes that routinely operating a laboratory this way does not work. The good manager knows that a laboratory that is operating with the appropriate number of knowledge workers plus the necessary reagents and equipment to process the routine workload is more likely to achieve the technical and customer service goals of the laboratory's strategic plan. Regular feedback from employees related to their needs—such as, Do they have the tools to do their jobs? Are morale issues appearing? Do they feel that any information is lacking?—allows a listening manager to proactively prevent burnout or negativity among staff.

There is no limit to the amount of communication that should be provided, nor in the number of ways that it can be provided. Adequate communication is the single most important factor in ensuring that staff members have a clear understanding of their role in the lab and where it fits into the larger picture, from the most repetitive of their tasks to creating new strategies together as a team. The manager needs to stay in constant touch with the staff, either directly or through the supervisory staff, to monitor the progression of assigned tasks. This may take the form of informal meetings in the laboratory or formal meetings with one or more staff members. Formal meetings should always have an agenda. The laboratory manager also can communicate with the staff by memorandum, bulletin board postings, computer mailboxes, e-mail, telephone, or facsimile transmission. Minutes should always be taken when meeting with personnel, either individually or in groups. The minutes should clearly state the purpose and the outcome of the meeting, including goals that have been set and/or actions that need to be taken. Meeting minutes should be distributed to everyone who attended or usually attends a meeting and often should be provided to others on a need to know basis. Frequent communication shortens the period of time that the staff or manager is "off target" in achieving goals and allows constant reassessment of the suitability and effectiveness of the plan of action.

Lastly, although the successful laboratory manager strives to implement positive changes to maintain the laboratory as a strong, viable entity within the organization, it is important for the manager to understand that change often is not easy to implement, nor for many to accept. By adhering to the practices and behaviors of empowerment and effective communication, the laboratory manger can create and maintain a culture wherein change is accepted and even welcomed.

PERSONNEL MANAGEMENT

Staff

CLIA '88 has created job categories for all clinical laboratory technical and testing positions. It has also established uniform requirements that include the minimum education and experience a person must have to direct, consult, supervise, or perform each specific test on human specimens. Under CLIA '88, the education and experience requirements for each job category depend on the complexity rating of the tests being performed in the laboratory. The test **complexity model** assigns all tests to one of four categories: waived, physician-performed microscopy, moderately complex, or highly complex. The Centers for Medicare & Medicaid Services (CMS) classifies each test by method, instrument, reagent, and complexity. These test classifications change and are published periodically in the *Federal Register.* Laboratory managers must keep abreast of changes in test complexity to assign staff appropriately. Until a test is classified, it is considered highly complex. No education or experience requirements are needed for personnel who perform and report the results of **waived tests.**

If tests performed by the laboratory are classified as moderately complex (with no highly complex tests being performed), the laboratory must have a laboratory director, a technical consultant, a clinical consultant, and testing personnel. The requirements for education, experience, and training for each of these positions are less stringent than for the positions required when highly complex tests are performed.

If highly complex testing is performed (regardless of whether moderately complex tests are performed too), the laboratory must have a laboratory director, a technical supervisor, a clinical consultant, a general supervisor, and testing personnel. Laboratory managers must review additions, changes, and deletions to personnel qualifications for each of these positions as HCFA makes them.

The laboratory manager must identify each test performed in the laboratory as waived, moderately complex, or highly complex, so that adequately trained and supervised personnel can perform the tests. The test mix, test volume, and service level, including test frequency and turnaround time, then determine the actual number and types of supervisory and testing personnel positions needed to be in compliance with CLIA '88 and to provide adequate service.

Box 19-3

Useful Information to Keep in Each Employee's Personnel File

- Performance standards
- Employee application, including work experience
- Relevant education and certification
- Level of Clinical Laboratory Improvement Amendments (CLIA) '88 test complexity that the employee can perform
- Whether the employee requires direct supervision
- Areas of the laboratory the employee is competent to staff
- Periodic evaluations for competency
- In-service education record
- Record of training in health and safety measures
- Training courses attended
- Record of vaccinations, such as for hepatitis B, or a signed statement declining the vaccination

Job or Position Description

Every technical and testing staff position should have a clearly written job or position description. The job description should state, at a minimum, the education and experience or training required by CLIA '88 for the position, along with any additional requirements formulated by the laboratory. It also should indicate the specific job functions the laboratory worker is expected to perform. CLIA '88 requires that technical and testing personnel should be evaluated against the requirements for moderate- or high-complexity testing and found to meet the qualifications of those duties. CLIA '88 and other accrediting bodies also mandate that specific information be maintained in an employee's personnel file. Box 19-3 lists the information that should be kept in each analyst's personnel file.

Work Scheduling

The actual staff schedule for a particular laboratory may not conform to the standard three 8-hour shifts per day, with staff members working five 8-hour days per week. Alternative scheduling formats include the use of 10-hour shifts, flex time, and staggered shifts. Many laboratories use a combination of all these formats to achieve complete coverage. This provides overlap between shifts and enhances intershift communication and continuity of workflow.

Laboratory managers must take into account the strengths and weaknesses of individual technologists when planning a work schedule, including the balance of weaker and stronger technologists in each shift. By carefully reviewing workload statistics, the laboratory manager can determine whether the workload is distributed equitably (within a shift, as well as between shifts) and can schedule staff accordingly. Some work areas, such as an intensive care laboratory, are "fixed" positions, that is, they do not depend on productivity or volume and must always be staffed.

Laboratory staffing must take into account the number of days off allowed for sick leave, personal leave, holiday leave, and vacation leave. Therefore, for one "fixed" position, between

1.5 and 2.0 individuals must be hired for each shift to provide coverage 7 days a week.

Because the largest single cost for a laboratory is labor, most laboratories attempt to increase productivity (billable tests/**full-time equivalents** [FTE]) by using automation or by combining workstations to enhance efficiency (see Chapter 20). Further discussion of productivity is found on p. 354 (Resource Management).

Continuing Education and Employee Competency

Continuing Education

The final regulations of CLIA '88 state that the laboratory director or technical consultant in a moderately complex testing laboratory and the laboratory director or technical supervisor in a highly complex testing laboratory must identify needs for remedial training or continuing education to improve skills. Managers must also identify the training needs for each workstation and must ensure that each individual who is performing tests receives regular in-service training and education appropriate for the type and complexity of laboratory services performed. Therefore, the laboratory should maintain and post a current list of the continuing education programs available both in-house and through professional organizations that meet these needs for laboratory personnel.

The laboratory can offer programs on general topics such as laboratory management, laboratory information systems, government regulations for laboratories, OSHA, safety, and technology of the future, as well as on specific technical topics such as pathophysiology, current in-house testing, and instrumentation. Attendance at state, regional, and national meetings should be encouraged when topic and exhibits are pertinent. Attendance at all continuing education programs must be documented and a record of attendance maintained in the employee's personnel file.

Employee Competency

The laboratory director has the ultimate responsibility for ensuring the competency and continuing education of all testing personnel under the final regulations of CLIA '88. The February 28, 1992, *Federal Register* states that the director (493.1407 and 493.1445), technical consultant (493.1413), technical supervisor (493.1451), or general supervisor (493.1463) is

> Responsible for: (8) evaluating the competency of all testing personnel and assuring that the staff maintain their competency to perform and report test results promptly, accurately, and proficiently. The procedures for evaluation of the competency of the staff must include, but are not limited to (i) Direct observations of routine patient test performance, including patient preparations, if applicable; specimen handling, processing and testing; (ii) Monitoring the recording and reporting of test results; (iii) Review of intermediate test results or worksheets, quality control records, proficiency testing results, and preventive maintenance records; (iv) Direct observation of performance of instrument maintenance and function checks; (v) Assessment of test performance through testing previously analyzed specimens, internal blind testing samples or external proficiency testing samples; and (vi) Assessment of problem solving skills; and (9) Evaluating and documenting the performance of individuals responsible for moderate-complexity testing (technical consultant) and high-complexity testing (technical supervisor) at least semiannually during the first year the individual tests patient specimens. Thereafter, evaluation must be performed at least annually unless test methodology or instrumentation changes, in which case, prior to reporting patient test results, the individual's performance must be reevaluated to include the use of the new test methodology or instrumentation.

The frequency of reviews may be greater, according to local regulations. Besides evaluating employee competency under CLIA '88, the manager needs to discuss with each individual employee routine assessments for productivity, professionalism, and general goal achievement. Personnel should know why they have performed less well than, as well as, or better than expected, and each should be given positive ways to achieve better performance. The employee must be given an opportunity to comment on the review. The entire assessment process must be documented, with copies sent to the employee and the employee's file. Documentation of fair and frequent assessments is important for the development of the employee (see discussion later in this chapter) and as a framework for necessary disciplinary actions.

Alternative Positions

The process of continuously training and motivating the laboratory staff is a significant part of the manager's job. Routine technical work coupled with limited opportunity for advancement can lead to high staff turnover. The use of a system of alternative positions can help overcome these obstacles to staff retention. With this system, the credentials and experience required to advance to another position are clearly delineated.

New positions with responsibilities that are intermediate between those of a technologist and those of a supervisor may have to be created. In addition, whenever possible, the laboratory manager should promote from within. This type of practice tends to produce dedicated and loyal employees who can move both horizontally and vertically within the organization.

The final regulations of CLIA '88 state that anyone with at least a high school diploma or equivalent can be trained to perform moderately complex tests (493.1423). Appropriate training and proficiency must be documented before the staff member is permitted to analyze patient specimens. This allows certain nontesting personnel such as phlebotomists and aides to be trained to function as testers. Criteria should be established for the promotion of testing personnel to supervisory positions within the laboratory. Similarly, management positions or ancillary positions such as laboratory information systems coordinator, phlebotomy trainer, outreach programs coordinator, and off-site or off-shift supervisor should be identified. The education and training requirements and job responsibilities for all positions must be recorded in writing. The benefits of promotion for the employee include greater job satisfaction, additional education, recognition of achievement by feedback, a basis for a more objective performance appraisal, and monetary compensation.

Cross-training, which allows staff members to be rotated into several departments, is another option for alternative positions. Cross-training helps relieve the monotony of specialization, whereby an analyst performs the same job function day after day. Cross-training can broaden and sharpen a worker's skills, allowing that staff member to work with more people and to develop a better understanding of the entire laboratory operation. In some laboratories, cross-training may be a necessity, providing increased staffing flexibility so that the laboratory can meet service demands. A specialist in an area can promote continuity and can competently train new staff members. However, specialization can cause staffing problems by decreasing laboratory flexibility.

RESOURCE MANAGEMENT

The laboratory manager is responsible for managing laboratory resources, which include laboratory staff, reagents, supplies, and capital equipment. All these are crucial in providing various laboratory services for patients, as defined in the strategic plan. The laboratory's service level expectations should be developed during discussions with the hospital's or system's management and laboratory users and should be based on available laboratory resources.

The laboratory manager must accept the hospital's or the system's strategic plan on behalf of the laboratory and must use all laboratory resources to fulfill the laboratory's goals within the plan. The laboratory manager must be able to look at the hospital's or system's strategic plan as a whole and must understand how the laboratory is interconnected to the other departments/services and the effect that each component has on the whole. Competent managers motivate and empower the laboratory staff to plan and implement the tasks necessary to achieve the laboratory's goals within the strategic plan. Therefore, the manager must promote an atmosphere of freedom and creativity that values employee involvement. In addition to introducing new diagnostic tests to maintain service levels at the highest possible standards, the laboratory manager, when appropriate, seeks new business for the laboratory. If successful, the manager must motivate laboratory staff to realize that these opportunities are in their best professional interest.

Practically speaking, resource management is used to carry out the day-to-day laboratory operation. To manage these responsibilities successfully, the laboratory manager must prepare one set of agenda for the short term (day-to-day) operation plan and a second set of agenda for the long-term (strategic) plan, which sets goals for the next 5 years. These plans should be updated yearly.

Resources must be allocated on the basis of current data, historical data, and predictions regarding the effects of current trends on the laboratory's operation. In the short term, sudden increases in workload can be accommodated if the laboratory has equipment with the capacity to handle higher volumes or backup equipment and cross-trained staff. Using overtime, reassigning work to another workstation, or sending low-volume testing to a reference laboratory also may help. Moving work to another shift that has the capacity to absorb the extra work is another option. If the trend is sustained and permanent increases in the routine workload are seen, appropriate measures must be taken to obtain additional staff, reagents and supplies, and equipment if necessary. If the workload suddenly decreases, workstations can be shut down or consolidated with other workstations that have the capacity to handle additional work. Laboratory staff members also can be encouraged to use earned vacation time, take personal time off, or cut back on hours.

Long-term planning is concerned with the laboratory's operation a year or more into the future. The laboratory manager must review short-term plans and closely follow the current day-to-day operation of the laboratory, predicting the effects of current trends on laboratory operations in the future. Specifically, the effects of projected changes in test volume and test mix on staffing, reagents, supplies, and equipment must be evaluated so that future **service level demands** can be adequately met. When planning for the future, the manager should consider the following significant factors:

- The possibility of new government regulations
- The opportunity for reimbursement
- The need for cost control
- Cost accounting
- The existence of markets for laboratory services
- Customer satisfaction
- Employee satisfaction
- Existing competition

In addition, the laboratory manager must be aware of technological advances that have the potential to increase the laboratory's productivity while reducing costs and improving test result turnaround times.

The laboratory manager must communicate regularly with the laboratory staff about changes that strongly influence the day-to-day operation of the laboratory, as well as changes that may influence the laboratory in the future. All staff members should participate in the process of making provisional or final plans to accommodate these changes.

FINANCIAL MANAGEMENT

Budgeting

The laboratory manager is responsible for preparing the laboratory's operating budget and ensuring that the laboratory operates within that budget. Supervisors and section heads should participate in preparing the budget by taking responsibility for the budgets of their respective sections.

The budget is prepared by using actual figures from the laboratory's current operating expenses, revenues, utilization data, and patient **demographics.** Any factors that may have a material effect on the financial operation of the laboratory during the current and next budget years must be taken into account during budget preparation. The greater the service level demands, the greater are the basic operating expenses because more personnel, reagents, and equipment are needed. Increases in basic expenses must be considered during analysis of the profitability of increasing testing volume. After the budget has been approved by the administration, the laboratory manager must verify that all provisions are accurate. The actual verification of the budget should be done by those in the laboratory most familiar with each component of the operation. Supporting detailed documents used to prepare the budget are also used for this process.

The budget should be easy to read and understand so that it can be regularly monitored and variations beyond established limits can be readily identified and investigated. The expense, revenue, and utilization line items for each laboratory unit should be defined individually so they can be closely monitored to ensure that the budget is being followed. The line items for each financial and operational laboratory unit may include labor and benefits, testing supplies, nontesting supplies, reagents, equipment rental and lease contracts, service contracts, repairs and maintenance, payment for tests sent to reference laboratories, individual test utilization, inpatient/outpatient/other charges and revenue (billed and collected), and bad debt.

The records used to prepare the current budget should be retained so that variations within each line item can be readily investigated. Monthly reports should compare each unit's actual performance versus that predicted in the budget. The laboratory should establish criteria for investigating variances from the budget. Explanations for each unacceptable line item variance should describe the variance as a trend, a random fluctuation, or an actual change caused by periodic ordering or payment patterns, changes in workload, personnel-related matters, or operational changes. The explanation should include any corrective actions to be taken. Notes kept during the corrective action investigation help in preparation of the next budget.

Comparisons of year-to-date actual performance with both budget predictions and the previous year's actual figures show trends in specific line items. Sometimes these trends are evident only in the budget of a particular item and not in the budget of the entire laboratory. Monthly and year-to-date comparison studies allow the laboratory manager to review each unit's specific variances and to take corrective action to adjust the budget for the individual unit or total laboratory. An understanding of the reasons for the variances from budget enables the laboratory manager to prepare future budgets that more accurately reflect revenue and expense items.

Two types of budget analysis can be done—static and flexible. A comparison of the current month's actual dollars spent versus the budgeted dollars is a static one. This comparison excludes variances attributable to increases or decreases in test volume. A comparison of the current month's actual dollars spent per test versus the budgeted dollars per test is a flexible reporting system. This comparison allows for budget variances related to volume changes. See the example in Table 19-3.

At first glance, the manager would see the static negative variance of $40 and might be tempted to justify it by noting

Table 19-3 Static versus Flexible Budget Analysis

	Actual	Budget	Variance
Test supply costs	$960	$1000	($40)
Billable tests	90	100	(10)
Supply cost/test	$10.60	$10.00	$.60

the number of billable tests. However, a look at the supply cost per test would show that further investigation is required because the supply cost per test is $.60 per test unit over budget.

Capital Justification

Most laboratories require capital justification for one-time purchases costing more than a designated amount. The amount can be as low as $500 or as high as $100,000. The level of detail required to justify a purchase may vary with the cost of the purchase. If equipment is purchased for laboratory testing, the justification must clearly detail the costs of the item, installation, supplies, reagents, controls, standards, and a service contract. The laboratory manager should calculate the cost per reportable result, taking into account the frequency and size of runs, the frequency of calibrations, whether the equipment will be used for urgent or routine testing (or both), whether single or duplicate samples will be tested, and the numbers of repeat, control, and standard samples analyzed per run. The labor cost per test must also be accurately calculated. An operational and financial comparison of the proposed method versus the existing method should underscore and substantiate the capital justification. The formal financial justification is called a *proforma.* A proforma is financial analysis of a future condition. The proforma is made up of the elements listed in Box 19-4.

The proforma uses the concept of discounted cash flow, a system that evaluates a purchase by considering the future value of money. The yearly return on investment is the value obtained by subtracting expenses from revenues. Essentially, if positive discounted cash flow remains after expenses, the investment is positive. The proforma calculation employs data on the cost of capital, which can be obtained from the institution's finance department. Please see Table 19-4 for an example of the proforma calculation.

When acquiring a piece of capital equipment, the laboratory manager may wish to maximize flexibility for obtaining "state of the art" technology by minimizing the time that the laboratory is obligated to use a specific instrument. Therefore, the laboratory manager must carefully evaluate the costs of purchasing, leasing, renting, or reagent renting an instrument. When an instrument is acquired through a reagent rental plan, the laboratory is billed for the reagents only (the vendor includes the equipment price in the reagent pricing) at an agreed price. The laboratory contracts to purchase a minimum quantity of testing materials, based on current and future needs. Table 19-5 compares reagent rental costs versus outright purchases. The types of buying decisions described in

Box 19-4

Elements of a Proforma

- Expenses
  - Capital
  - Indirect
  - Direct
- Other costs (to be included with expenses)
- Revenues
  - Existing
  - Future
- Savings

Table 19-5 are based on cash flow. If lump sum capital dollars are not available, reagent rental can be used to acquire a piece of equipment. However, buying capital equipment through reagent rental programs may cost the hospital more real dollars than a lump sum purchase. If cash flow is an issue, a true lease can be used. In this vehicle, a monthly capital cost is billed, along with the reagent cost.

Manufacturers sometimes offer additional incentives when more than one unit is to be obtained. As was stated previously, the manager must perform a cost analysis for each test being considered and must prepare a proforma financial statement for the equipment being acquired. Managers also need to take into account the costs of evaluating and setting up the method

Table 19-4 Example of a Financial Proforma Calculation

5 Years Cash Flow Analysis for Capital Budgeting

PROJECT *PROFORM IT SE, VERSION 1.3*

Project Name	Initial Capital Investment	Year 1	Year 2	Year 3	Year 4	Year 5	Total Years 1 to 5
Income Statement							
Test Revenues							
Inpatient test revenue		$9,500,000	$9,785,000	$10,078,550	$10,380,907	$10,692,334	$50,436,790
Outpatient test revenue		$2,350,000	$2,420,500	$2,493,115	$2,567,908	$2,664,946	$12,476,469
Gross Patient Test Revenue		$11,850,000	$12,205,500	$12,571,665	$12,948,815	$13,337,279	$62,913,259
Contractual allowances for tests		$5,925,000	$6,102,750	$6,285,833	$6,474,407	$6,668,640	$31,456,630
Net patient test revenue		$5,925,000	$6,102,750	$6,285,833	$6,474,407	—	—
Revenue from sale of existing equipment		—	—	—	—	—	—
Residual value of capital investment		—	—	—	—	—	—
Net Revenue		$5,925,000	$6,102,750	$6,285,833	$6,474,407	$6,668,640	$31,456,630
Operating Expenses to Perform Tests							
Wages and salaries		$740,000	$769,600	$800.384	$832,399	$865,695	$4,008,079
Employee benefits		$148,000	$153,920	$160,077	$166,480	$173,139	$801,616
Supplies, consume., reagents, expend.		$3,115,000	$3,208,450	$3,304,704	$3,403,845	$3,505,960	$16,537,958
Equipment service contract		—	—	—	—	—	—
Equipment depreciation		$200,000	$200,000	$200,00	$200,00	$200,000	$1,000,000
Construction depreciation		$1,600	$1,600	$1,600	$1,600	$1,600	$8,000
Software/Interface depreciation		$1,200	$1,200	$1,200	$1,200	$1,200	$6,000
Other test-related expenses		$10,000	$10,000	$10,000	$10,000	$10,000	$50,000
Indirect expenses		$1,303,500	$1,342,605	$1,382,883	$1,424,370	$1,467,101	$6,920,459
Total operating expenses for tests		$5,519,300	$5,687,375	$5,860,847	$6,039,893	$6,224,695	$29,332,111
Net operating cash flow		$405,700	$415,375	$424,985	$434,514	$443,945	$2,124,519
Depreciation add-back		$202,800	$202,800	$202,800	$202,800	$202,800	$1,014,000
Net cash flow	$(1,014,000)	$608,500	$618,175	$627,785	$637,314	$646,745	$3,138,579
Cumulative cash flow		$608,500	$1,226,675	$1,854,460	$2,491,774	$3,138,519	
Discounted Cash Flow		***$563,426***	***$529,985***	***$498,356***	***$468,445***	***$440,164***	***$2,500,376***

Financial Analysis					
Total capital investment	$(1,014,000)		Discounted payback period versus	1.9	Years
Total discounted cash flow	2,500,376		Depreciated life of equipment	5.0	Years
Net present value @8.00%	$1,486,376	Acceptable			
Internal rate of return	54%	Acceptable			
Hurdle rate	11%				
Return on investment	68%				

Table 19-5 Comparison of Outright Purchase* versus Reagent Rental

Outright Purchase	Reagent Rental
a instrument price	Reagent cost/test†‡ × Test volume/year × 5 years
b Lost interest on money for 5 years	= Total rental cost for 5 years
c Service contract for 4 years	
= Total instrument cost for 5 years	
a instrument cost for 5 years	
b Reagent cost†/test × Test volume/year × 5 years	
= Total purchase cost for 5 years	

*Add individual lines to sum up costs.
†Includes volume of calibrators and controls.
‡Assumes service is included for 5 years.

chosen. Some of the items to be considered in the evaluation and setup costs are environmental retrofits (space, plumbing, power supplies, temperature and humidity controls, noise buffers), materials, labor (for validation studies, for writing procedures, for training and competency assessments), proficiency testing subscriptions, and data management (IT resources and support in the form of labor, services, hardware and software, including interfaces). In all cases, the test cost analysis and the proforma financial statement must be clearly written and carefully documented with supporting data attached to the written report. A copy of the manufacturer's contract should be included.

Purchasing

Supplies, reagents, and equipment are purchased with funds allocated in the department budget. To stay within this budget, the laboratory manager, staff, IT support, and the purchasing department must work as a team, securing the lowest prices available from vendors, national contractors, and various buying groups. Price, location of distribution centers, availability of items, and a vendor's customer service should be evaluated before a specific or standing order is placed. The laboratory may have to purchase a more expensive reagent or supply instead of a lower-price generic item to be certain that test results are accurate and that test systems function properly. The purchasing department should aid in negotiating volume discounts and in obtaining the same lot numbers over time for longer consistency of results.

One of the biggest problems that most hospitals face is cash flow—that is, collecting sufficient funds in time to pay expenses. For this reason, alternative purchasing options have become common in the laboratory setting. However, when making these transactions, management and the purchasing department must always consider the cost of borrowing money.

Cost Accounting

Cost accounting is a method by which all costs associated with the production or acquisition of a particular item are identified. In the clinical laboratory, this is applied primarily to calculation of the cost per billable test result. The more detailed and complete the analysis, the more accurate and useful is the cost determination. Box 19-5 supplies a list of costs to be included in the analysis. A complete analysis may highlight overlooked cost factors that significantly influence the true cost per reportable result. A significant advantage lies in understanding which factors have the greatest effect on test costs and which factors are affected by equipment or methods within the manager's laboratory. This type of analysis is also advantageous when a new test method or procedure is compared with an existing one, to calculate more accurately the true cost per reportable test result. The ultimate goal of cost accounting is the determination of the actual cost for a billable test. This allows the laboratory manager to set the price of tests appropriately in a competitive marketplace. The simplest way to perform cost accounting is to use software which is designed specifically for laboratory cost accounting.

Box 19-5 Direct versus Indirect Costs

Direct Costs
Reagents
Labor
Equipment costs
Service costs
Collection supplies
Testing supplies
Quality control material
Depreciation

Indirect Costs
Building depreciation
Hospital overhead
Laboratory overhead
Accounting expenses
Regulatory expenses
Management labor
LIS expenses

LIS, Laboratory information system.

Overview of Reimbursement Issues

Reimbursement in a hospital setting refers to the process by which payments are received from payers such as **Medicare** and **Medicaid,** private insurance companies, health maintenance organizations, and patients. Private patient billing is the smallest billing component at most institutions and the only one whereby payment for the full amount of the hospital bill is expected. Most other payers negotiate a discount rate with the hospital or laboratory.

Medicare reimbursement is broken into two categories: Part A and Part B. Most simply stated, Part A billings provide payment for inpatient hospital services, whereas Part B billings pay for physician services and outpatient laboratory tests. For inpatients, Medicare pays a flat rate per diagnosis. This flat rate is based on a 1983 system called the Diagnosis Related Group (DRG). The flat payment is fixed for each diagnosed disease and covers all inpatient services, including laboratory tests performed during a patient's hospital stay. If outpatient laboratory tests are performed within 72 hours of admission, hospitals are required to include them for coverage under the DRG payment rather than bill for them separately. All outpatient tests are reimbursed according to a code number. These numbers, called Common Procedure Terminology (CPT) codes, are constantly updated and modified. The laboratory must always have a current copy of CPT codes for billing.

Reimbursement plans such as Medicare's have the effect of forcing a laboratory to operate more like a business. Medicare reimbursements are based on a capital payment of approximately $420 per discharge.

INFORMATION MANAGEMENT

Chapter 22, Laboratory Information Systems, reviews the use of a **laboratory information system (LIS)** to manage information and increase a laboratory's productivity. Financial and utilization reports generated by the LIS or the **hospital information system (HIS)** are some of the tools used to manage information. Table 19-6 lists many of the utilization reports that a laboratory manager should review routinely. A list of work production reports can be found on p. 396 in Chapter 22.

When setting up a management system to evaluate laboratory performance, the manager should ensure that the system, at a minimum, gathers data that can be used to monitor the laboratory's financial performance, productivity, utilization, and test result turnaround time.

Table 19-6 Examples of Laboratory Management Reports Provided by an LIS

Type of Report	Function
Total workload	Monitors adequacy of the total number of personnel in the laboratory Monitors workload trends
Shift workload	Monitors adequacy of the number of staff on each shift
Employee workload	Monitors the workload of one analyst; compares productivity with others on the shift and between shifts
Routine quality control	Monitors short-term accuracy and precision
Turnaround time	Monitors the adequacy of service

The following section briefly summarizes several key indicators for each of the monitors. The management system should be able to evaluate these monitors for each section (such as chemistry, hematology, and microbiology) and for the laboratory as a whole.

Financial Performance

Financial reports by the LIS and/or the HIS should provide accurate, up-to-date, detailed information about the way actual laboratory expenses compare with those in the budget. However, these financial reports do not inform the laboratory manager about how well the laboratory is performing compared with laboratories of similar size, patient acuity (a measurement that indicates how sick the patient is), location, and service level. Subscribing to a commercially available database system such as Labtrends (Health Care Development Services, Northbrook, IL, www.hcdsinc.com) or LMIP (College of American Pathologists, Northfield, IL) allows such comparisons to be made. Specific laboratory areas can be compared and significant differences evaluated so that corrective action can be taken to improve productivity, expenses, and revenue. The average cost per performed test is an exceptionally important measure of operational performance. Because labor and supplies usually constitute about 70% to 75% of most laboratories' budgets (including employee benefits, depreciation expense, and pathologist compensation), these elements must be monitored closely. Repair, preventative maintenance, and referred testing usually represent 3% to 10% of most hospital laboratory budgets. Monitors for these costs are shown in Box 19-6.

Productivity

Measuring the overall productivity of the laboratory and of each laboratory section should be part of any operational performance system that is developed. The following indicators should be included in the review of productivity:

- Number of performed tests/testing FTE (including supervisor time) assigned to an individual workstation
- Number of performed tests/total FTE
- Number of performed tests/worked hour
- Worked hours as a percentage of paid hours

Using these parameters and comparing the laboratory with a database such as Labtrends or LMIP, the laboratory manager can see how efficient the laboratory is compared with similar laboratories. This comparison then can be used to help justify

Box 19-6

Financial Performance Monitors

- Cost/on-site billed test
- Compensation and benefit expense/billed test
- Compensation and benefit expense/hour
- Supply expense/billed test
- Cost/referred test
- Repair and preventive maintenance expense/billed test
- Pathologist compensation as a percentage of total laboratory expense

additional personnel if the laboratory is operating with insufficient staff (higher than average productivity) compared with the mean of the comparative database.

Test Utilization

A medical staff's use of laboratory tests varies greatly from hospital to hospital and is not driven exclusively by patient acuity or programmatic demands. Laboratory test use at hospitals with similar inpatient acuity and programs (such as organ transplant or acquired immunodeficiency syndrome [AIDS]) can differ substantially. Systems used to monitor operational performance should include the following key utilization indicators:

- Number of inpatient performed tests/patient day
- Number of inpatient performed tests/patient discharge

Some hospitals may perform test utilization reviews for individual areas or for individual physicians in an attempt to control overuse of laboratory resources.

Turnaround Time

Test result turnaround time (TAT) statistics can help laboratory managers better understand and evaluate operational performance. Because service demands can greatly affect staffing patterns, instrumentation choice, and labor costs, managers should measure actual TATs to determine whether the TAT expectations of the hospital's medical staff are met. The TAT monitoring system should include the 20 to 30 tests most commonly performed in the laboratory, as well as those requiring an especially short TAT (such as urgent [stat.] tests and pregnancy tests).

Several approaches are available for monitoring TAT by test name. A common method identifies and tracks the distribution of TATs based on the length of time elapsed from the time the test was ordered until the result was available. Evaluation of TAT should take into account its three time components: the preanalytical, analytical, and postanalytical phases. To monitor TAT in this manner, LIS software needs to identify specimen collection time, specimen accession time (or time that the specimen is received in the laboratory), and the time the result was available to a physician.

KEY CONCEPTS BOX 19-2

- In order to be effective, it is essential that a laboratory manager continually foster good management skills, such as keeping communication flowing between the hospital and laboratory staff and assuring that there is adequate, competent staff to perform the work.
- A good laboratory manager also must manage available resources adequately, both for day-to-day operation of the laboratory and for fulfilling long-term goals of the hospital management. Operating within budgetary constraints is crucial.
- The type of information management selected by the laboratory manager should be adequate to not only facilitate laboratory test reporting, but be able to generate financial reports, productivity, test volumes, and turnaround time.

SECTION OBJECTIVES BOX 19-3

- Outline quality monitors that can be used for laboratory improvement.
- Discuss how a medical technologist can help improve laboratory services.

PERFORMANCE IMPROVEMENT

Performance improvement is a method of measuring and improving a laboratory's total effectiveness and contribution to the organization. Although performance improvement can be approached in many ways, the following core elements are always present:

- Planning
- Process design
- Performance measurement
- Performance assessment
- Performance improvement

An organization may follow several models for performance improvement that incorporate these elements, all equally acceptable. A few performance improvement models that are commonly used are the PDCA (Plan, Do, Check, Act), LEAN, Six Sigma, and the DMAIC (Define, Measure, Analyze, Improve, Control) models.

The laboratory should evaluate its core processes and should develop performance measures that support the strategic plan or mission of the hospital. Performance measures also may be chosen as the result of an identified problem (risk management activities) or as the result of customer (physician) feedback. Measures may include but are not limited to QA or operational excellence monitors, customer service goals (e.g., TAT), financial performance goals (such as cost per procedure), human resource goals (retention or decreased turnover rates of workers), and compliance monitors (billing accuracy).

After choosing the measures, the manager next must decide how often to examine them. Some (such as TAT) might be evaluated monthly until the target time is repeatedly met.

The next step is to establish target goals for the measures through a system of internal or external benchmarking. With these benchmarks, the laboratory can begin not only to measure but also to assess the process in a routine, continuous manner. If the results of the monitor are stable but do not meet the target goal, the manager can put a plan of action into place to correct the deficiency. Measurement of the monitor again determines whether the process has been improved. If not, a new plan and audit are put in place until the performance of the indicator is satisfactory.

In addition to performance improvement monitors, CLIA '88 demands that, at a minimum, the monitors listed in its Quality Assurance Monitors be evaluated. An example of a form for performance monitoring is found in Fig. 19-6. The reader can obtain copies of the *Federal Register* for a complete description of the QA process under CLIA '88.

Name of Institution: Sunland Hospital
Name of Laboratory or Section: Chemistry

Quality Assurance Monitor Report

Test Name: Stat. pregnancy test, serum
Monitor: Turnaround time
Evaluation criteria and/or threshold:

95% of stat. serum pregnancy tests are completed within:
(a) 30 minutes within receipt in the laboratory.
(b) 90 minutes from the time of collection.

Time period of monitor: Month, Year: July, 1995 OR
Quarter: 1st 2nd 3rd 4th

Status of monitor: MET NOT MET (underline)

Data for monitor:

(a) 96.3% of all requests completed within 30 minutes of receipt in laboratory.
(b) 95.9% of all requests completed within 90 minutes of collection.

Review of action: There was 1 outlier that was completed 2 hours after collection. Sample lost in accessioning area, clerk was advised.

Further action or comments: Three samples outside laboratory turnaround times. Samples entered laboratory during lunch periods. Will speak with supervisor about maintaining coverage during this time.

Comparison with previous monitors: Give % within limits

Previous:
Date:________ %: ________

Two previous:
Date:________ %: ________

Laboratory Director: ____________
Technical supervisor: ____________

Fig. 19-6 Forms for quality assurance monitoring.

Quality Assurance Monitors

QA is a process that the laboratory uses to ensure the correct result for the right patient at the right time. The following monitors should be included in a QA program.

Patient Test Management

Based on the results of its evaluations, the laboratory must monitor, evaluate, and revise (if necessary) the following elements:

1. Criteria established for patient preparation and for specimen collection, labeling, preservation, and transportation
2. Information solicited and obtained on the laboratory's test requisition for its completeness, relevance, and necessity for testing patient specimens
3. Use and appropriateness of the criteria established for specimen rejection
4. Completeness, usefulness, and accuracy of the test report information necessary for the interpretation or use of test results
5. Timely reporting of test results based on testing priorities (e.g., stat., routine), as well as accuracy and reliability of test reporting systems, appropriate storage of records, and retrieval of test results

Quality Control Assessment

The laboratory must have an ongoing QC mechanism to evaluate the corrective actions taken under the Remedial Actions section of CLIA '88 (493.1219). The outcome of the evaluation determines which ineffective policies and procedures must be revised. The mechanism must reevaluate and review the effectiveness of corrective actions taken for the following:

1. Problems identified during the evaluation of calibration and control data for each test method
2. Problems identified during the evaluation of patient test values for the purpose of verifying the reference range of a test method
3. Errors detected in reported results

Statistical quality control (QC) is critically important in laboratories today to ensure the quality of the test results produced by any measurement procedure. The almost universal applicability of statistical QC to quantitative measurement procedures provides laboratories with a quality management tool that can be deployed whenever and wherever needed. It also allows laboratories to independently verify and validate the ongoing performance of in vitro diagnostic device manufacturers' built-in quality control measures and monitors.

The Clinical and Laboratory Standards Institute (CLSI, formerly the National Committee on Clinical Laboratory Standards [NCCLS]) has recently published a new edition of the document, *Statistical Quality Control for Quantitative Measurement Procedures: Principles and Definitions; Approved Guideline—Third Edition* (C24-A3). This guideline addresses the purpose of statistical quality control for quantitative measurement procedures; describes an approach for planning quality control for a particular measurement procedure; addresses the use of quality control material and quality control data, including the use of data in quality assurance and interpretation; and provides detailed examples that demonstrate a practical QC planning process for clinical laboratories.

Proficiency Testing Assessment

Under Subpart H of the Proficiency Testing part of CLIA '88, the corrective actions taken for any unacceptable, unsatisfactory, or unsuccessful proficiency testing result(s) must be evaluated for effectiveness.

Comparison of Test Results

If a laboratory performs the same test using different methods or instruments, or performs the same test at multiple testing sites, it must have a system in place to evaluate and define the relationship between test results using different methods, instruments, or testing sites; this evaluation should be performed twice a year. If a laboratory performs tests that are not included under Subpart I of the Proficiency Testing part of CLIA '88, the laboratory must have a system for verifying the accuracy of its test results at least twice a year.

Relationship of Patient Information to Patient Test Results

For internal QA, the laboratory must have a mechanism by which to identify and evaluate patient test results that appear inconsistent with clinically relevant criteria. These include patient age; gender; diagnosis or pertinent clinical data, when provided; distribution of patient test results when available; and relationship with other test parameters, when available within the laboratory.

Personnel Assessment

The laboratory must have an ongoing mechanism for evaluating the effectiveness of its policies and procedures to ensure employee competence and, if applicable, consultant competence.

Communications

The laboratory must have a system in place to document problems that occur as a result of breakdowns in communication between the laboratory and the individual authorized to order or receive the results of test procedures or examinations. Corrective actions must be taken to resolve the problems and minimize communication breakdowns.

Complaint Investigation

The laboratory must have a system for documenting all complaints and problems reported to the laboratory. Investigations of complaints must be made and corrective actions instituted as necessary and appropriate.

QA Review with Staff

The laboratory must have a mechanism for documenting and assessing problems identified during QA reviews and discussing them with the staff. The laboratory must take any corrective actions necessary to prevent recurrences.

QA Records

The laboratory must maintain documentation of all QA activities, including problems identified and corrective actions taken. All QA records must be available to the HHS and maintained for 2 years.

KEY CONCEPTS BOX 19-3

- It is essential that a clinical laboratory continue to evaluate its effectiveness. Several models exist that may be followed in this process.
- CLIA '88 mandates ten quality assurance monitors that are collectively designed to assist the clinical laboratory in producing the highest quality of patient care.

BIBLIOGRAPHY

General

Davidson JP: Are you entrepreneurial material? Clin Lab Manage Rev 4:192, 1990.

Fritz R: I'm your new boss . . . why are you laughing? Clin Lab Manage Rev 6:162, 1992.

Harty-Golder B: Lab portion of OSHA exposure control plan for bloodborne pathogens, MLO 10:June 2001.

Holland C, Lien J: Systems thinking: managing the pieces as part of the whole, Clin Leadersh Manag Rev 15:157, 2001.

Leebov W: How to help your staff strengthen customer service: a do-able approach, Clin Leadersh Manag Rev 15:192, 2001.

Snyder JR: Managing knowledge workers in clinical systems, Clin Leadersh Manag Rev 15:120, 2001.

Regulations

Federal Register 56(235):64175-64182, Dec 6, 1991.

Federal Register 57(40):7001-7186, Feb 28, 1992.

Federal Register 58(11):5211-5237, Jan 19, 1993.

Federal Register 58(139):39154-39156, July 22, 1993.

Federal Register 60(78):20035, Apr 24, 1995.

Federal Register 60:25944-25976, May 15, 1995.

Security

American Biological Safety Association: ABSA biosecurity task force white paper: understanding biosecurity, Mundelein, Illinois, 2003, The Association.

U.S. Department of Health and Human Services, Public Health Services, Centers for Disease Control and Prevention and National Institutes of Health: *Biosafety in Microbiological and Biomedical Laboratories,* ed 5, Washington, DC, 2007, USDHHS.

Casagevall A, Pirofski L: *The Weapon Potential of a Microbe,* Bethesda, MD, 2005, The National Institutes of Health.

Laboratory Biosafety Manual, ed 3, Geneva, 2004, World Health Organization.

Possession, use and transfer of select agents and toxins, 42 C.F.R., Part 73, 2005.

Possession, use and transfer of biological agents and toxins, 7 C.F.R., Part 331, 2005.

Possession, use and transfer of biological agents and toxins, 9 C.F.R., Part 121, 2005.

Richmond JY, Nesby-O'Dell SL: Laboratory security and emergency response guidance for laboratories working with select agents, MMWR Recomm Rep 51:1, 2002.

Hospital Management Structure

Communication management

Baytos LM: Launching successful diversity initiatives, HR Magazine 37:91, 1992.

Haynes ME: How to conduct quality meetings, Clin Lab Manage Rev 4:29, 1990.

Hunt LB: Here's how you can harness the positive energy of conflict, Clin Lab Manage Rev 6:456, 1992.

Ketchum SM: Overcoming the four toughest management challenges, Clin Lab Manage Rev 5:246, 1991.

Lussier RN: Assigning tasks effectively using a model, Clin Lab Manage Rev 6:150, 1992.

Miner FC: If two heads are better than one, why do I have bruises on my forehead? Clin Lab Manage Rev 5:386, 1991.

Pfeiffer IL, Dunlap JB: Empowered employees—a good personnel investment, Clin Lab Manage Rev 6:154, 1992.

Rinke WJ: Establishing a shared vision in your organization, Clin Lab Manage Rev 3:95, 1989.

Veninga RL: Crisis management: strategies for building morale in uncertain times, Clin Lab Manage Rev 6:449, 1992.

Young S: Developing your political skills, Clin Lab Manage Rev 3:100, 1989.

Personnel management

Comer DR: Improving group productivity by reducing individual loafing, Clin Lab Manage Rev 6:232, 1992.

Dawson KM, Dawson SN: The cure for employee malaise—motivation, Clin Lab Manage Rev 5:296, 1991.

Fritz R: How to keep your best people for the '90s, Clin Lab Manage Rev 4:306, 1990.

Petrick JA, Manning GE: Work morale and assessment and development for the clinical laboratory manager, Clin Lab Manage Rev 6:141, 1992.

Surber JA, Wallhermfechtel M: A comprehensive career ladder for the clinical laboratory, Clin Lab Manage Rev 4:441, 1991.

Resource management

Hinterhuber HH, Popp W: Are you a strategist or just a manager? Harvard Bus Rev 70:105, 1992.

Reeves PN: Strategic planning for every manager, Clin Lab Manage Rev 4:272, 1990.

Financial management

Brase SJ, Matysik MK: Laboratory manager's financial handbook, Clin Lab Manage Rev 6:164, 1992.

Carpenter RB: Laboratory cost analysis: a practical approach, Clin Lab Manage Rev 4:168, 1990.

Getzen TE: Laboratory manager's financial handbook: what is value? Clin Lab Manage Rev 6:237, 1992.

Kisner HJ: Laboratory manager's financial handbook: expense management—supplies, Clin Lab Manage Rev 6:341, 1992.

Melbin JE: One for all, MT Today, p. 8, Dec 7, 1992.

Patterson PP: Cost accounting in hospitals and clinical laboratories: part II, Clin Lab Manage Rev 3:26, 1989.

Portugal B: Factors influencing relative financial performance of hospital laboratories, Clin Lab Manage Rev 3:81, 1989.

Continuous quality improvement

Bull G, Maffetone MA, Miller SK: As we see it: implementing TQM, Clin Lab Manage Rev 6:256, 1992.

Clark GB: Quality assurance, an administrative means to a managerial end, Clin Lab Manage Rev 6: Part I, 4:7, 1990; Part II, 4:224, 1991; Part III, 5:463, 1991; Part IV, 6:426, 1992.

Westgard JO, Barry PL, Tomar RH: Implementing total quality management (TQM) in health-care laboratories, Clin Lab Manage Rev 5:353, 1991.

General Resources

Lifshitz MS, De Cresce RP: *Understanding, Selecting, and Acquiring Clinical Laboratory Analyzers,* New York, 1986, Alan R. Liss.

Martin BG, editor: *The CLMA Guide to Managing a Clinical Laboratory,* Malvern, Pennsylvania, 1991, Clinical Laboratory Management Association.

Rubenstein NM: *Handbook of Clinical Laboratory Management,* Rockville, MD, 1986, Aspen Publishers.

Sattler J, Smith A: *A Practical Guide to Financial Management of the Clinical Laboratory,* ed 2, Oradell, NJ, 1986, Medical Economics Books.

Snyder JR, Senhauser DA, editors: *Administration and Supervision in Laboratory Medicine,* Philadelphia, 1989, JB Lippincott.

INTERNET SITES

http://www.ascp.org—ASCP
http://www.asm.org—ASM
http://www.bt.cdc.gov/lrn—Laboratory Response Network
http://www.cap.org—CAP
http://www.cdc.gov—CDC
http://www.cms.hhs.gov—CMS
http://www.cms.hhs.gov/clia—CLIA '88
http://www.clma.org—CLMA
http://www.fda.gov—FDA
http://www.gpoaccess.gov/cfr/index.html—Federal Register
http://www.jointcommission.org
http://www.clsi.org/—CLSI (formerly NCCLS)
http://www.nist.gov—NIST
http://oig.hhs.gov—OIG
http://www.osha.gov—OSHA
http://www.hipaa.org—HIPAA
http://www.ascld.org—American Society of Crime Laboratory Directors (ASCLD), a nonprofit professional society devoted to the improvement of crime laboratory operations through sound management practices

Laboratory Automation

Chapter 20

Michael A. Pesce

Chapter Outline

Key Terms

analog A measurement derived directly from an instrument's continuous signal (such as voltage) and usually presented in graphic form.

automation Use of a machine designed to follow repeatedly and automatically a predetermined sequence of individual operations.

autoverification Automatic reporting of test results without technologist review if they fall within a predetermined set of parameters.

bar-code label A computer-driven sample-recognition system that identifies both the specimen and the analyses to be performed and relays this information to the automated analyzer.

bulk reagents Those that must be measured before being added to a reaction mixture to attain the desired proportion. Usually, a reservoir contains the reagents for more than one analysis.

carryover Contamination of a specimen by the previous one.

computation Calculation of a desired result from the signal or readout of an instrument; it can be electronically automated by the use of either digital or analog conversion.

dead volume The volume in a sampling container that must be present for proper sample aliquot measurement but is not consumed.

digital Related to data available in the form of discrete units or to the calculations that use such data.

discrete Term applied to instruments that compartmentalize each sample reaction.

dwell time The minimum time required for an instrument to obtain a result, calculated from the initial sampling of the specimen.

incubation time The time allowed for a chemical reaction or process to proceed to completion.

middleware Software that resides between the analyzer and the LIS.

mixing Process by which individual components of a chemical assay are formed into a homogeneous solution.

proportioning Addition of individual components of a chemical assay in proper ratios or amounts.

random access instrument An instrument capable of performing multiple tests on a sample. Instead of performing all possible tests on each sample, these instruments are capable of performing only those tests that are programmed.

readout Written or computer display of the result of an analysis performed on an instrument.

sensor A system or device that monitors changes in the reaction mixture that are related to analyte concentration.

test menu The number of different tests available on an instrument at one time without changes in reagents or components.

test repertoire All the different tests that are available on an instrument, including those that can be made available by changing reagents or instrument components.

throughput The maximum number of individual samples or test analyses that can be practically performed per hour by an assay system, with the required dwell time taken into account.

total laboratory automation Automating all the steps involved in laboratory testing from specimen processing to storage, to retrieval and disposal of specimens.

unit test reagents Premeasured reaction chemicals packaged so that only one package (unit) is used per sample test.

SECTION OBJECTIVES BOX 20-1

- State the reason for the shortage of qualified medical technologists.
- Outline the steps that should be taken before an automated laboratory system is selected.
- List the goals of laboratory automation.

In this chapter, the reasons for laboratory automation and the ways to achieve it are considered. Examples of major automated instrument categories are examined.

In the 1990s, health care costs became an important issue for the United States. Reductions in reimbursement rates by the government and the proliferation of managed care contracts have resulted in a significant change in the laboratory environment. Cost containment or reduction has become a primary goal for the laboratory. The laboratory now is considered a cost center rather than a source of revenue. At the same time, the laboratory was asked to improve the turnaround time for reporting of test results, and to provide a more comprehensive service. For example, immunosuppressant drug monitoring for transplant patients, screening for inborn errors of metabolism, testing for neural tube defects and Down syndrome, maternal human immunodeficiency virus (HIV) testing, tumor and cardiac marker analysis, and ultrasensitive C-reactive protein (CRP) measurements for evaluation of neonatal sepsis or for assessment of patients who may be at cardiac risk must be performed as quickly as possible for physicians to treat patients in a timely fashion.

Another issue faced by clinical laboratories in the United States is the shortage of qualified medical technologists that has resulted from the closure of medical technology schools. From 1980 to 2006, the number of medical technologist programs decreased from 638 to 229, and the number of medical technology graduates dropped by 70%.[1] In addition, the current pool of medical technologists is getting older, and these individuals are getting ready to retire while the volume of laboratory testing is increasing.[2] The lack of qualified medical technologists will continue to be a major problem for the laboratory. Laboratories had to come up with a plan to do more with fewer resources. Laboratories are being asked to reduce costs, improve turnaround time, expand the **test menu,** reduce laboratory errors, and deal with the shortage of qualified medical technologists. To meet these demands, the laboratory has to be on the cutting edge of technology, and automation is the key to achieving these goals.

LABORATORY PROCESSES

Automation in a hospital must be viewed as a global process. The entire testing sequence begins when a physician examines a patient and a decision is made to obtain specific laboratory information. The overall process is shown in Fig. 20-1 and can be broken down into the following components: test ordering, sample acquisition (phlebotomy), sample transport, front-end

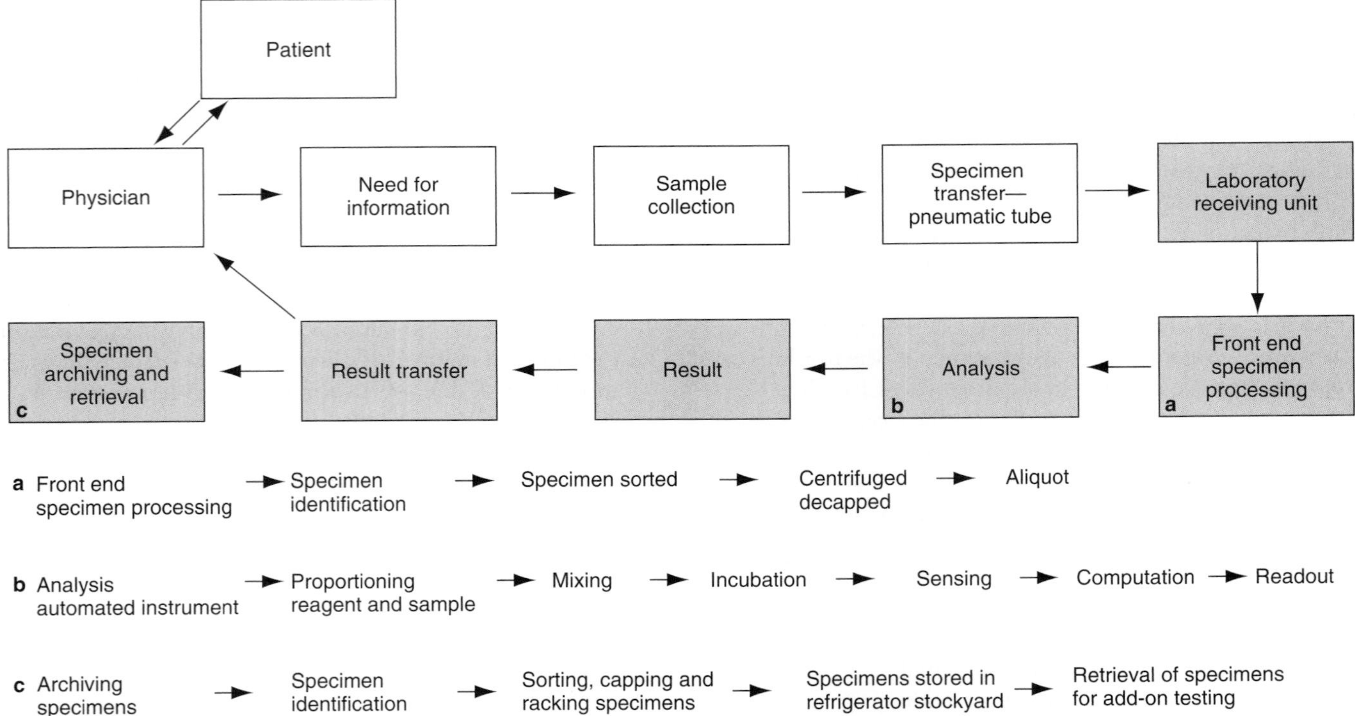

Fig. 20-1 Diagram illustrating specimen and information flow between physician and laboratory. The shaded area is that portion of the system that usually is considered part of the laboratory. The lower portion amplifies steps involved in sample processing and analysis.

sample processing, sample analysis, result acquisition, result reporting, sample archiving and retrieval, and disposal of samples. Laboratorians must be aware of each step in this process and of what can cause a breakdown in these steps, resulting in longer turnaround times or an increase in the error rate from any cause (see below). In general, laboratory automation has focused on analysis of the specimen in the laboratory and transfer of information back to the requesting physician. Interest in automating the process of transferring the sample to the laboratory, preanalytical sample processing, and archiving and retrieval of specimens is increasing.

Laboratory Error

The Institute of Medicine (IOM) reported that 44,000 to 98,000 people die in hospitals each year from medical errors at a societal cost of $37.6 billion per year.[3] Hospital medical errors are the eighth leading cause of death among Americans, exceeding motor vehicle accidents, breast cancer, and AIDS. Although documentation is available to identify ≈1.5% of adverse medical events and 6% of adverse drug events, it is also believed that incident reports generally capture only 5% to 30% of adverse surgical events.

The error rate in clinical laboratories has been studied and has been estimated to range from 0.1% to 2.5%, with only 10% to 32% of these errors occurring in the analytical portion.[4,5] Several studies have estimated that the preanalytical testing phase has an error rate of 68% to 87%.[4,6] A laboratory department that controls patient phlebotomy might want to provide automation solutions to this part of the laboratory process. The manual phlebotomy process is susceptible to error, which results in mislabeled samples, and unacceptable transfusion errors[7] and errors in reading patient wristbands[8] have been documented. Automation of the phlebotomy process can greatly reduce these errors (see p. 374).

The seminal IOM report has highlighted one of the important goals of laboratory automation: the need to reduce hospital-associated errors.

Goals of Laboratory Automation

The goals of laboratory **automation** include the following: (1) reduction in costs, (2) expansion of laboratory testing to generate more revenue, (3) reduction in turnaround time, (4) reduction in laboratory errors, and (5) improvement in laboratory safety. The primary driving force for automation is still the reduction of costs; laboratories that have consolidated workstations have seen a reduction in their labor costs and reagent and supply budgets. This is so because labor accounts for most of the costs in laboratory testing, and successful justification for automation usually is based on staff reductions. However, a careful cost analysis must be developed because the time it takes to recover the capital investment ("payback time") for the automated equipment depends on many factors. Comparing payback time with that of other laboratories can be misleading because it depends on the baseline value, which is different for each laboratory. For example, if the laboratory is not very efficient and has high staff salaries, the payback period will be more rapid and the savings will be greater than for a laboratory with lower salaries.

However, staff reductions resulting from automation rarely mean that these workers will become unemployed. They usually are redeployed for other laboratory functions, such as to assist in the measurement of new, often esoteric, tests that have been sent to commercial laboratories, or to help with quality or regulatory processes. Alternatively, they can use their expertise as medical technologists in the point-of-care section of the laboratory, or they may be transferred to other departments, for example, molecular diagnostics.

The volume of work performed also has a significant effect on cost and must be accurately determined to optimize the type of automation needed to process the current workload and to allow for future increases in volume. The volume of work must be determined both from a global viewpoint, that is, the total number of samples or analyses in a day or week, and from a local viewpoint, that is, the number of samples at peak work flow. The laboratory also must have an estimate of the clinicians' expectations for turnaround time. The laboratory must work with vendors to develop a realistic financial and equipment plan. A usual result of laboratory automation is a reduction in turnaround time for reporting test results as the number of steps in the testing process is reduced. This is especially true if the front-end sample-handling process becomes automated.

Most laboratory errors occur during phlebotomy and front-end processing of the samples (see above). The most common errors include misordering and mislabeling of the sample (4.8% of outpatient samples were associated with such errors[9]), incorrect preparation of aliquot samples (pouring from the wrong sample), mislabeling of the aliquot tube, and misplacement of samples in the laboratory. Automation of sample processing will eliminate most of these errors.

Laboratory safety is an important issue. Staff members who handle specimens are subject to exposure to potentially infectious biological fluids as the result of spills, aerosols, breakage of tubes, and removal of stoppers from primary tubes to prepare aliquots or for analysis. Automation of sample processing will help protect staff from these hazards. With proper planning by hospital administrators and laboratory staff, improved safety goals can be achieved.

KEY CONCEPTS BOX 20-1

- Obtaining an automated laboratory system is a complicated and time-consuming process that requires input from the laboratory director and from medical technologists, hospital administrators, medical staff, and the information technology department.
- Goals of automation should be to automate every step of the testing process and to reduce the errors encountered in each step.
- Automation of phlebotomy and sample processing is needed to reduce large error rates of these processes.

Box 20-1

General Considerations for Laboratory Automation

Union issues
Power and cooling requirements
Inventory management
Cross-training of staff
Laboratory information system (LIS) interface needs
Autoverification and Middleware software
Peak volume testing
Staff involvement
Stat. testing
Centralized customer service area
Site visit

SECTION OBJECTIVES BOX 20-2

- Describe total laboratory automation, modular integrated systems, and stand-alone processing systems.
- List the benefits and drawbacks of these automated systems.
- Define Middleware software.

AUTOMATED LABORATORY SYSTEMS

General Considerations

Although several approaches have been used to maximize the degree of automation in a laboratory, several general, nontechnical issues should be considered before the laboratory chooses an automated system. These are listed in Box 20-1. Union issues can be important, and if they are not addressed, they can reduce potential labor savings and improvements in laboratory efficiency. For example, policies that affect seniority, overtime, time off, and job responsibilities can significantly affect laboratory operations. In addition, a significant increase in efficiency may reduce the need for manpower—a critical union concern. These issues must be discussed and resolved with the union before an automated system is implemented.

The air conditioning system must have enough capacity to cool the laboratory with present and future equipment. Sufficient emergency power outlets should be present in the laboratory, along with enough emergency lighting to operate the laboratory in case of a power failure.

The automated laboratory system should be able to review reagent inventory and, when needed, automatically order reagents and supplies from the vendor. This will reduce the possibility that the laboratory will have to temporarily suspend testing because of lack of reagents or consumables.

Cross-training of the staff, for example, in chemistry and hematology, is important if maximum laboratory efficiency is to be achieved because this provides the laboratory manager with flexibility in staff scheduling. Cross-training also benefits the staff because technologists who are cross-trained in more than one laboratory section usually receive higher salaries and are more marketable if they need to look for another position.

The laboratory information system (LIS, see Chapter 22) should interface with all components of the automated system. If the LIS is not compatible, significant delays in implementation may occur as software is written.

Autoverification of sample results, an essential part of laboratory automation, is the automatic reporting of test results without review by the technologist. This process allows the laboratory to verify results if they fall within a predetermined set of parameters (see result reporting section, p. 372, for a detailed discussion of autoverification). Autoverification can be implemented with an LIS (see p. 401, Chapter 22) or with the use of **middleware** software. The middleware concept offers some advantages over the LIS. Middleware systems can be connected to a number of analyzers and provide a central workstation in the laboratory at which quality functions can be monitored. This may allow reduction of staff assigned to instruments. Information flows from the analyzers to the software, where decision rules are applied. Test results are validated against a computer-generated algorithm, and if they pass, the results are sent to the LIS. For example, middleware systems can be used for autoverification, delta checking, reflex testing, defining samples with critical values, monitoring serum indices on all samples, quality control monitoring, and tracking specimens, and they can provide user-defined comments for patient results. Although some LIS systems may be able to perform most of these functions, a significant advantage of middleware over an LIS system is that the rules are written and managed by the laboratory staff, thus reducing the influence of the information technology department.

In a hospital laboratory, specimens arrive throughout the day, but peak volumes usually occur in mid to late morning, late afternoon, and early evening. The laboratory must carefully calculate the peak volume. The automated system should be able to handle at least twice the peak load to anticipate future growth.

Staff involvement is an important part of any automation project. Committees that include laboratory staff and hospital administrators should be established for all aspects of the process, such as site coordination, stat testing, instrumentation selection, and specimen processing. For example, sample-tube standardization is important because some automated systems use only one tube size. If a tube of a different size comes into the laboratory, it has to be manually processed, which reduces laboratory efficiency and can result in processing errors. The staff must be convinced that automation improves patient care and makes their work more efficient, and that there is some job security.

A centralized customer service area must be established to receive calls regarding laboratory testing. This area should be staffed on the day and evening shifts and should be located close to the laboratory. The customer service area handles, for example, calls for add-on tests, types of tubes needed for specimen drawing, and reference ranges. Some service centers will process all laboratory test results that must be called to physicians, such as critical values. Any technical or clinical information that is requested should be directed to the appropriate individual.

A critical part of the decision-making process is visiting laboratories that have the automated system. Vendors should arrange for the laboratory staff to visit several sites that have a similar mix of inpatient and outpatient testing, stat testing, and a similar volume of chemistry, immunochemistry, hematology, and coagulation testing. The laboratory director should contact other hospitals that have the automated system but were not recommended by the vendor. These sites can be a valuable source of information.

Whatever an automated system is chosen, careful planning for all steps is required. It is crucial that the laboratory fully list all costs that will be needed for complete implementation of a fully automated laboratory, including automation of the steps outside the analytical area. The laboratory must be able to justify costs by achieving the goals of automation listed above. Hospital administrators, laboratory directors, laboratory managers, and staff must be convinced that the automated system will meet the needs of the laboratory and the hospital. Success or failure usually depends on the cooperation of all individuals involved in the laboratory automation process.

Laboratory Automation

The different types of laboratory automated solutions that are available include (1) **total laboratory automation** (TLA), (2) modular integrated automation, and (3) modular or stand-alone systems for front-end sample processing and archiving and sample retrieval.

Total Laboratory Automation

TLA employs an integrated track system that links all the laboratory's workstations (front-end processing, instrumentation, and archiving systems) together to create a continuous, comprehensive network that automates almost all the steps involved in clinical laboratory testing. TLA systems usually automate the chemistry, immunochemistry, hematology, and coagulation sections of the laboratory. TLA systems are important choices for laboratory automation for larger laboratories because of the potential for substantial cost savings.

TLA systems are usually turnkey systems that contain the components for each step in the process, including sample sorters, aliquoters, centrifuges, and analyzers that are interconnected by the track system. Bar-coded labeled specimens are brought to an inlet station, where the bar-code reader scans the bar code to check its integrity and to query the host computer for test selection. Specimens that have an unreadable bar code or that have the label facing the wrong direction are placed in an exception rack for manual processing. Specimens with an acceptable **bar-code label** are machine-sorted into racks and transported to the hematology workstation for analysis, or to a centrifuge station.

The capacity of the centrifuge can be the rate-limiting step in specimen processing. For high-volume laboratories, at least two refrigerated centrifuges should be attached to the track. Some samples may continue to be centrifuged manually because of special needs, such as tube type or stat. status.

After centrifugation, the decapper module uncaps the specimens, which are sorted, placed in analyzer specific racks, and transported to the chemistry or coagulation workstations. If aliquots are required, the sample is sent to the aliquoting workstation, which usually can create the required number of bar code–labeled aliquot tubes per specimen. At this station, sample clots are detected, and a liquid level **sensor** identifies samples of insufficient quantity for the tests that have been ordered; these are also sent for manual processing. The aliquot tubes are sent by the track to the appropriate workstations. After the analysis has been completed, the specimens are transported to the archiving workstation, where they are unloaded from the sample carriers, scanned, placed in racks, recapped, and stored in a refrigerated stockyard for sample retrieval. If the sample is needed for repeat or add-on testing, the system locates the sample in the stockyard, removes the cap, and sends the sample to the appropriate analyzer workstation for testing. However, for large-volume laboratories, the capacity of the refrigerated stockyard may be too small to store 1 week's volume of specimens. In this case, the racks must be manually removed from the stockyard and placed in a long-term storage refrigerator. Some TLA systems also dispose of the samples.

Major drawbacks of TLA systems include the substantial financial investment and the considerable amount of open space required for these systems. For example, the cost of some TLA systems can range from $2 million to $5 million, not including the costs of space rennovation. To justify this investment, a careful financial assessment must be performed. The major cost savings from automation involves reduction in labor. One must carefully balance any projected reduction in technolgists who are manning instruments versus the additional personnel needed to maintain the TLA. In addition, the volume of testing performed has a significant impact on cost, and a large test volume is required to justify TLA. In one analysis, it was estimated that the laboratory needed to process more than 2500 tubes per day and to assay more than 2 million tests per year to justify TLA. In many cases, when laboratories calculate the return on investments based on current and future workloads, the anticipated increase in testing never comes to fruition. This results in increased time for the laboratory to recoup its initial investment and a laboratory with large quantities of unused testing capacity.

Laboratory space is an important issue when TLA systems are considered. TLA requires a considerable amount of open space, which is at a premium in most hospitals; a typical TLA system requires anywhere from 3000 to 5000 square feet. TLA systems can use existing space in the laboratory, or they can be set up in another area of the hospital or placed in a centralized laboratory off-site but relatively close to the sending hospitals. However, because of the large quantities of instrumentation and components and the additional structural support needed to bear the weight of the systems, installation of a TLA system usually requires extensive renovations, sometimes requiring building permits, which usually delays construction. If the TLA system is to be put into the same area as the existing laboratory, removal of counters and walls is usually required, which may cause havoc in the laboratory. If possible, TLA systems should be configured into a new area within the hospital.

Other factors besides cost and space must be considered before a TLA system is obtained. Although a TLA system is purchased from a single vendor, some laboratories may want to integrate instruments sold by different vendors on the same line. This can present a significant challenge in interfacing the analyzers to the LIS. Companies must be willing to work together to resolve any interface or troubleshooting issues. Because of the complex nature of TLA, it may be necessary to have an on-site biomedical engineer troubleshoot the system and dedicated supervisors and staff ensure its day-to-day operation. TLA also requires standardization of the sample tubes, usually into one size. Plastic tubes are preferred over glass because they are less apt to break and shatter.

TLA systems, which are available from Roche Diagnostics, Beckman-Coulter, and Siemens, have been placed in large hospitals and some commercial laboratories. TLA systems have been shown to decrease labeling errors by 27%, reduce turnaround time by 17% to 23%, and reduce full-time equivalents (FTEs) staff by 15% to 24%.[10-14] TLA has been shown to decrease the number of turn-around outliers from the Emergency Department from 18% to 5% for potassium and from 29% to 9% for troponin-I.[15]

Modular Integrated Systems (MIS)

Modular integrated systems offer an alternative to TLAs. MIS link together multiple laboratory disciplines into a single testing platform that is interconnected by a track. This approach allows for configuration of different modules, such as chemistry and immunochemistry, and consolidates, into a single area, sample loading and unloading and reagent loading and unloading. Modular systems have a two-lane track system to facilitate rapid processing of stat. specimens and samples that require repeat or reflex testing. The second lane allows these samples to be sent directly to the analyzer without disrupting the high-volume routine testing. Front-end automated specimen-processing systems also can be interconnected to the chemistry-immunochemistry module. MIS automate part of what TLA offers but provide flexibility because different types of modules can be added readily, depending on work flow or change in test patterns.

Compared with TLA systems, the modular approach is significantly lower in cost, requires less laboratory space, is quicker to install, and is easier to interface with the LIS. A limitation of this approach is that when a front-end sample-processing system is linked to a workstation, it can process specimens only for that workstation. Studies have shown that MIS can decrease mean turnaround time by 50 minutes to 2 hours, reduce staff, and result in a 30% increase in productivity.[16,17] Modular automated systems are available from Roche, Beckman-Coulter, Ortho, and Siemens.

Stand-Alone Systems: Sample Processing and Archiving

Another approach to laboratory automation is to automate specific sections of the process that are still manual operations. These sections include specimen processing and sample archiving.

Sample Processing

Front-end sample processing is usually a manual procedure in which samples are sorted, centrifuged, uncapped, and divided into aliquots if tests for more than one workstation have been requested. It is usually the rate-limiting step in providing rapid and accurate test results. In some laboratories, labor required for manual front-end sample processing accounts for about 60% of the testing cost. Manual sample processing is responsible for about 40% of the turnaround time and for most of the laboratory errors and lost specimens.[11,18]

Various approaches have been employed to automate the manual steps of front-end sample processing. There are modular systems that automate the entire process and stand-alone systems that automate one portion of front-end processing. A modular system consists of a sorting station, a decapping station, a centrifuge, an aliquot station, and a loading station for workstation-specific sample racks, all of which are linked by a track system.

Bar code–labeled primary tubes are placed on the system, and the host computer is queried for test selection. Tubes are sorted by test and placed into racks. Samples with processing issues, such as clots, unreadable bar codes, and insufficient samples, are placed in an exception rack for manual intervention. If no further processing is required, for example, in assays that use whole blood (complete blood count [CBC], hemoglobin A1c), samples are placed in sample racks and are distributed manually to the appropriate workstation. Tubes for serum or plasma analyses are sent to a refrigerated centrifuge. The tubes are weighed and are selectively loaded into the sample tube holders to balance the centrifuge. The centrifuge should have the capacity to handle the peak load of samples that come into the laboratory and should be able to accommodate more than one tube size. For optimum efficiency, laboratories should standardize the size of the blood drawing tube that is sent to the laboratory. However, this may be a challenge for hospitals with many outpatient locations. Most front-end processing systems are not able to process pediatric microtainers and may not be able to handle urine and fluid specimens. After centrifugation, the primary tubes are uncapped and placed into racks. If no further processing is required, samples are manually transported to the appropriate workstations.

If an aliquot is needed, the tube is is automatically decapped and sent to the aliquot workstation, where the host computer is queried for test and sample volume requirements. The aliquoting station should have the capability of producing the required number of aliquot tubes and generating the appropriate bar-code labels for each tube. An aliquot may be needed for sending tests to commercial laboratories, or for sending

Table 20-1 Automated Features of Some Specimen Processing and Archiving Systems

Manufacturer	Abbott	Beckman-Coulter	Olympus	Ortho Clinical Labs	Roche Diagnostics Corp	Siemens Medical Solutions	Siemens Medical Solutions
System name	Accelerator, APS	Power Processor	Olympus OLA 2500	enGen Laboratory Automation System	Modular Pre-Analytics	ADVIA Automation Systems	Stream Lab II Analytical Workcell
Sorting*	600	500	1200	450	500	400	600
Centrifuge*	320	300	NA	400	250	220	80
Decapping*	300	600	1200	400	400	600	600
Aliquoting*	NA	140	650	Approx. 150	400	NA	In development
Recapping or sealer*	300	500	1200	450	500	In development	600
Interfaced with LIS system	GE, Misys, Cerner, Nexus, MIPS, Labmaster, Meditech, Connectivity to LIS through middleware	SCC, Siemens, Philips, MISYS, Cerner, McKesson, Meditech	Cerner, Meditech, SCC, Misys, Data Innovations, Atlas, McKesson	Cerner, Misys, SCC, Connectivity to LIS through middleware	Misys, Cerner Millenium, Soft, Data Innovations, Meditech, McKesson	Siemens, Misys, Cerner, Meditech, SCC, Data Innovations, NetLab	Cerner, Meditech, SCC, Misys
Specimen Storage/ Retrieval‡	15,000	3,060	NA	In development	In development	1000	NA

*Specimens processed per hour.
‡Specimen capacity.
NA, Not Available.

specimens to distant workstations for molecular and special chemistry testing. Disposable pipette tips should be used to eliminate **carryover,** and the system should have clot detection and liquid level-sensing capabilities. The samples then are recapped and brought to the appropriate workstation. Automatic recapping or foil-based sealing of specimens is important because it eliminates a repetitive function and reduces the possibility of stress injury. The rate-limiting step in front-end sample **throughput** is usually the capacity of the centrifuge or aliquoting system. These modular systems provide some flexibility and may have the capability of adding another centrifuge. Some modular systems can also store and retrieve specimens.

Stand-alone systems can be used to automate part of the front-end sample processing and to archive specimens.[19] Stand-alone systems automate the sample sorting, sample uncapping, and aliquot functions of the front-end sample processing. If a centrifuge is not included in the stand-alone systems, the sample must be manually brought to the centrifuge for tests that require serum or plasma. Table 20-1 compares the operational parameters for some of the front-end specimen-processing and archiving systems.

Archiving

Archiving and retrieval of specimens is a labor-intensive process that accounts for up to 20% of a technologist's time. Sample retrieval occurs when a test needs to be repeated, for reflex testing, or when the physician requests that additional tests be performed on that sample. Specimen retrieval is a very time-consuming and frustrating process because the technologist has to manually sort through a large number of specimen racks to find the required specimen.

With automated sample-archiving systems, bar-coded specimens are automatically unloaded from the sample carriers and are scanned and placed in numbered positions in numbered racks. Retrieval of specimens is initiated by entering the patient's sample accession number or medical record number into the archival system database, which then displays the rack number and identifies the row and column where the specimen was placed in the rack. With this system, technologists can retrieve referigerated specimens in minutes. In addition, some archiving systems provide for automatic disposal of samples at predetermined times established by the laboratory. The ability of laboratory personnel to quickly retrieve primary and aliquot tubes automates a tedious function and reduces the time and stress associated with locating specimens within the laboratory.

Stand-alone systems have a relatively small footprint (i.e., floor or counter space) and provide maximum flexibility in placing the units in the laboratory. They are less costly and easier to set up than the modular front-end processing systems.

Studies have shown that automating front-end specimen processing decreased sample-processing time by 2 to 6 hours, reduced labor cost by 30% to 40%, decreased daily phone calls from physicians waiting for stat. results from 28 to fewer than 5 per day, reduced specimen pour-off and labeling errors by almost 98%, and reduced specimen sorting and routing errors by almost 95%.[11,20,21]

KEY CONCEPTS BOX 20-2

- Available space, volume of work in the laboratory, and costs of the automated system are the major issues that should be addressed before an automated laboratory system is obtained.
- Automated laboratory systems have been shown to decrease turnaround time and reduce costs and laboratory errors.

SECTION OBJECTIVES BOX 20-3

- Define sample carryover, and explain how it can be detected and eliminated.
- Define autoverification.
- Describe how the reporting of critical laboratory values can be automated.

AUTOMATION OF CHEMICAL ANALYSIS

To understand how patient samples are processed by automated procedures, the process of analysis must be divided into a series of stages or steps, as might be performed in a manual assay. Commonly, the following steps are performed during the course of an analysis: (1) **mixing** an aliquot of the sample with a series of reagents in an ordered sequence with defined amounts, (2) incubating the reaction mixture at a specified temperature for a specified length of time, (3) monitoring or sensing the result of the reaction, (4) quantitating the extent of the reaction, and (5) providing an appropriate **readout** of the permanent record. The automation of each one of these steps is now discussed in some detail.

Reagent Preparation

Although **bulk reagents** can be prepared manually, almost all laboratories use ready-to-use liquid reagents or lyophilates. Reconstitution of the lyophilized reagent may be performed automatically on board the instrument; however, a few instruments may require mixing of reagent with diluent before the reagent is placed on the instrument. This simple step can lead to analytical errors caused by improper processing. **Unit test reagent** preparation, in which sufficient reagent is present for the performance of a single test, has been automated in two ways. The first is the dry-film or impregnated-paper technique. The dry-chemical techniques use either paper or a series of thin films impregnated with the desired reagent. The analytical reactions take place when the sample is placed on the dry reagent. In this type of reagent, preparation consists of wetting the reagent with water, buffer, or sample. The second kind of unit test reagent is a container or test tube that contains premeasured liquids or powders to which water, buffer, or sample is added. Unit test reagents tend to be more consistent on a long-term, within-lot basis. However, unit test reagents also tend to be more expensive than bulk reagents—a consideration that can be important for many laboratories.

Proportioning of Samples and Reagents

Most chemical reactions require the combining of reagent and sample in exact amounts to yield specific, final concentrations of analyte and reagents. Because the reagents, as just described, are prepared in predetermined amounts, the ratio, or proportion, of reagent to sample must be kept constant to achieve reproducible and accurate final reagent concentrations. Thus the addition of sample to reagent is termed **proportioning.** The case of unit test reagents is considered first. In these systems, the reagents are already proportioned in the required amounts; therefore, only the sample must be proportioned. The dry-film reagent may have the sample added volumetrically or by saturation addition. The latter technique requires some explanation. The film is exposed to an excess of the sample, and the pores of the film allow only a fixed amount of the sample to be absorbed. This fixed amount of sample required to wet the film represents the proportioning mechanism. In some cases of saturation addition, the rate of diffusion of the sample into the film may also affect the proportioning step. In the case of bulk reagents, proportioning is always accomplished by volumetric addition.

Three automated volumetric dispensing methods are in common use. Syringes or volumetric overflow devices are used in random access test analyzers, in which sample and reagents are volumetrically added to a test tube or container. The second mechanism is the continuous-flow technique, in which sample and reagents are proportioned by their relative flow rates. Typically, peristaltic pumps are used to move the reagents through tubing, and the cross-sectional area (diameter) of the pump tubing controls the flow rate. Usually, the sample and reagent streams are allowed to flow continuously through the tubing, where mixing and incubation are also accomplished. The third type uses electrical valves to control the time reagents can flow. The flow rate is controlled by the air pressure applied to the reagent container and the flow resistance in the tubing that is connected to the reaction vessel.

In almost all systems, the sample is introduced into the analyzer with a thin, stainless steel probe. This probe passes into a sample by direct penetration of a stopper or after the stopper is removed from the specimen tube. The probe aspirates a defined quantity of sample and moves from the sample to a probe washing station, and then to dispense the aliquot into an appropriate vessel. A potential problem with these probes is the risk of clots; this risk is directly related to sample size. As the amount of sample that is pipetted decreases, the diameter of the probe decreases and the risk of clots increases. Some sample probes are designed to detect clots specifically and to reject clotted samples. Many sample probes have an associated level-sensing device that permits the tip of the probe to go a specified distance below the level of the sample to detect short samples.

Because the same probe is used repeatedly for sequential samples, there is the potential for contamination of a specimen by a preceding one. This is called *sample carryover.* Various techniques have been used, often in combination, to minimize the interaction between samples. These include (1) aspiration of a wash liquid (such as saline solution or water) between sample aspirations, and (2) a back flush of the probe. In the latter technique, the wash liquid flows through the probe in a direction opposite to that of the aspiration, into a waste container. This procedure has the advantage of minimizing the risk of pulling a small clot farther into the system.

The degree of sample carryover can be determined by immediately assaying four identical high-level samples followed by four identical low-level samples. Carryover is calculated by using the following equation:

$$\text{Percent carryover} = \frac{L1-(L3+L4)/2}{\frac{(H3+H2)}{2}-\frac{(L3+L4)}{2}} \times 100$$

in which $L1$, $L2$, $L3$, and $L4$ are the consecutive low samples, and $H1$, $H2$, $H3$, and $H4$ are the consecutive high samples.

Carryover affects the test results by contaminating the current sample with a proportional part of the previous sample. The amount of contamination attributable to carryover that is permitted affects the instrument's throughput. If less carryover is permitted, a longer time must be allowed for the previous sample to be flushed out, reducing the number of samples that are processed per hour. Some immunoassay instruments eliminate carryover by using disposable pipet tips.

Mixing

Those instruments that use the dry-film technique mix sample and reagents by diffusion of sample into the reagents. Most dry-film reagents are premixed during manufacturing, although some are mixed by diffusion, which becomes possible only when the film is wet. The **random access instruments** can mix the reagent and sample by (1) motion of a test tube or container, (2) stirring by paddle or stick, (3) agitation by air bubbles or ultrasonic waves, or (4) convection resulting from the forceful addition of sample into the container.

Incubation

Automated incubation is merely a programmed time delay in the analysis during which the test mixture is allowed to react. This is performed, in most cases, under the conditions of a specified, constant temperature, which is achieved most frequently by the use of heating blocks or air or water baths. These constant temperature devices are monitored electronically by thermocouples. Random access analyzers accomplish incubation by allowing the reaction mixture to dwell in a chamber (test tube or cuvette) for a specified time. A similar approach is used for dry-film analyzers. It should be noted that many test methods require the addition of a second reagent, possibly followed by additional **incubation time.** The automated means for doing this are similar to those just discussed.

Sensing

The techniques of automation do not depend on the method of sensing, whether optical, thermal, or electrical. There are two major approaches to automated sensing: in situ and external. The term *in situ* refers to measurement in the vessel where the reaction has taken place, for example, in the reaction cuvette. The term *external* is applied to systems of measurement in which the sample is transferred from its original incubation position in the reaction vessel to the sensing device. The dry-film tests are measured in situ by reflectance photometry (see Chapter 2) or by integral electrodes (electrometric; see Chapter 12). Random access instruments use both in situ and external sensing mechanisms. External sensing generally exposes the sensing chamber to many samples, and so care must be taken to eliminate carryover from one sample to the next. Optical or electrode surfaces also may be contaminated by components from the samples. On the other hand, in situ sensing makes special demands on the test chamber or requires an elaborate, automated washing procedure. If the test container is disposable, it is impractical to calibrate it for optical or electrical characteristics. Such containers, therefore, must be manufactured with very good reproducibility. However, disposable containers are meant to eliminate the mechanical complexity required to wash and recertify the sensing chamber; these are used most often in immunoassay instruments. Most sensing is done in situ because this approach decreases the mechanical complexity of the instrument. Chemical reactions can be monitored at one time point or at many. Commonly, single-point monitoring is used for end-point analyses in which the reaction has gone to completion. Multiple-point monitoring is used for kinetic analyses. Random access analyzers are easily adapted for multiple time-point monitoring.

Spectrophotometric instruments often have the capability of automatically sensing the presence of common interferents, such as icterus, hemolysis, and lipemia. An "index" of the presence of these interferents, closely related to the actual concentrations of bilirubin, hemoglobin, and triglycerides, is printed with test results. This helps to automate the technologist's review of results and to alert the technologist that a result may not be accurate.

Computation

Automated **computation** has taken two forms: **analog** and **digital**. Analog computations use an electrical signal such as a voltage or current from a sensor (such as a phototube) and quantify the signal by comparing it with a reference signal. For example, a "blank" reaction mixture will give a 100% T (blank transmittance), resulting in a certain electronic signal. A test standard will give a lower percentage of T and thus a decreased electronic signal. The analog computer compares the two signals and takes the logarithm of the result. The final result is related to the quantitation of the reaction.

Some reaction signals by their very nature are in the form of **discrete** numbers. Two examples are individual photon-counting events and counting of radioactive decay. These signals, which consist of a number of individual events, can be monitored by a digital computer that can process the signal. Digital processing is restricted to certain arithmetical functions (such as subtraction or addition) unless the computer is programmable.

For a digital computer to process signals from many types of sensing devices in automated instruments (such as the spectrophotometer and ion-selective electrodes), an analog-to-digital converter is necessary. This converts the voltage or current signal into a digital form, which can be processed by the digital computer.

There are no straightforward rules as to which is the best form of computation. The decision usually is based on economics. However, if any part of the signal processing is done digitally, virtually all the processing is done digitally. Perhaps the major exception is the analog conversion of transmittance to absorbance, which is performed to improve analytical performance.

Readouts and Result Reporting

Readouts

The simplest method that can be used to visualize an instrument readout is the use of light-emitting diodes (LEDs) or a television monitor (cathode-ray tube) to report the data in numerical form. These devices allow the technologist to review the data before accepting the results. The instrument readout may be converted to a hard copy, such as a paper printout. If the data must be transferred manually to laboratory slips or other permanent records, transcription errors may occur. More sophisticated, automated computer systems usually are used to collate all test results for each patient and to print the results directly on the report form. When results are transferred into a laboratory computer, the instrument readout is interfaced directly to the computer. Although analog connections are possible, most connections are digital. Chapter 22 discusses the use of computer interfaces for automation of the process of reporting results.

Autoverification

However, in laboratories with very large workloads, it is not practical for technologists to carefully review data for each patient. LIS have the capability for data autoverification, which is defined as the process whereby the computer performs the initial review and verification of test results. Data that fall within a set of parameters or rules established by the laboratory are verified automatically in the LIS and transferred to the patients' files. The technologist must review all data that fall outside of the set of parameters or rules established by the laboratory. Criteria for automatic data verification can include results that fall within a specified range (typically, the reference range), the absence of common interferences, and delta checks (see Chapters 18 and 22). This process speeds up the result verification process for routine results and permits the technologist to perform a more careful review of results with potential problems.

Results Reporting

There is usually a delay between the time when a result is entered into the LIS and becomes available to a physician and the time when a physician actually sees the result. This delay occurs because a physician never knows exactly when a result will be available and either must waste time looking for a result that is not yet in the LIS or must delay looking for that result. This delay is often a very large component of the overall turnaround time for a sample result. For example, reporting of critical values to a physician is required by all regulatory agencies and is a time-consuming process. Software systems are available that automate the delivery of critical values to the physician, without intervention by the laboratory. The LIS receives the critical value directly from the laboratory instrument, transmits the verified data to the physician's pager, and documents receipt of the critical value. These systems streamline reporting of critical values and reduce the risk for adverse patient outcomes.

Troubleshooting and Training

Medical technologists intervene to correct problems encountered when an instrument fails (see p. 470). This process, called *troubleshooting,* is limited by a technologist's training and by the availability of in-laboratory resources, such as instrument manuals. These resources have been greatly expanded by the application of electronic technology, such as on-line modems connected to the instrument manufacturer, Internet help sites, and CD-ROMs.

Modems allow electronic information to be rapidly transferred over normal telephone lines. Sophisticated computers that are part of new laboratory instruments can detect an instrument problem, often before a technologist has become aware of it, and automatically transmit data about that problem to the instrument manufacturer. The manufacturer's technicians can provide the laboratory technologist with detailed instructions for resolving the problem.

KEY CONCEPTS BOX 20-3

- Sample carryover can be a significant problem, especially for analytes like markers for infectious diseases and cancers that can have a wide range of values.
- Autoverification improves work flow in the laboratory and reduces turnaround time.

SECTION OBJECTIVE BOX 20-4

- Define test repertoire, random access and batch analyzers, and dwell time.

CONCEPTS OF AUTOMATION: DEFINITIONS

Test Repertoire

Economic priorities require that instruments perform more than one kind of test. Once an investment has been made in an automated instrument, increasing the number of tests performed on each sample reduces the cost and labor required to produce each result. Following this logic to an extreme would require that an instrument be capable of performing every conceivable kind of test. This has not been possible. However, six chemistry tests account for 50% of the workload in the average chemistry laboratory, and 14 tests account for another 40% of the total workload. Thus automated instruments have been designed to perform the most frequently ordered tests. Automation, although usually not essential, is desirable for rarely ordered tests as well.

The automation of tests may be done on the basis of type of analysis rather than test volume (number of samples), that is, an automated immunoassay instrument will perform immunoassays for many different analytes, regardless of the numbers of specimens per analysis.

The *immediate* **test repertoire** of an instrument therefore can be defined as the number of tests that can be performed by that instrument at any one time, without the need to change reagents. The total test repertoire includes the total number of different tests that can possibly be performed on the instrument by changing reagents and a few components. Improvements in techniques and changes in economic priorities have led to *workstation consolidation.* This involves increasing the immediate test repertoire of random-access analyzers (see later discussion) and having many high-volume tests on the least number of instruments. The automation of immunoassays on traditional chemistry analyzers has further stimulated this movement.

Random Access

Instruments that are capable of performing multiple tests are random access if different test combinations can be performed for each individual sample, and if no sample and no reagent are consumed by tests that are not requested. For example, the SMAC (Sequential Multiple Analyzer Computer) was not a random-access instrument because all tests in the immediate repertoire were performed on each sample, regardless of the exact tests requested. Random-access analyzers have replaced almost all non–random-access (batch) chemistry instruments.

Discrete

Instruments that compartmentalize each test reaction are discrete analyzers. Typically, the sample aliquot and the reagent for each test are contained in a single cuvette that is physically separated from all other cuvettes.

Batch Analyzer

Instruments that perform the same tests simultaneously on all samples presented to it are termed *batch analyzers.* The type of test can vary widely, but usually only a limited number of samples are processed per analysis. A blood-gas instrument is a batch analyzer.

Dwell Time

The **dwell time** is the minimum time required to obtain a result after initial sampling of the specimen. Some instruments can give results in as little as 15 seconds for single tests such as glucose. Commonly, instruments that perform multiple tests on a single sample have longer dwell times, ranging from 60 seconds to 15 minutes. Certain test procedures, such as kinetic analyses for enzyme activity or immunoassays, that require long incubations have longer dwell times. Dwell time is extremely important when significant or life-threatening physiological changes can take place rapidly. Thus blood-gas determinations (pH, Pco_2, and Po_2) need instruments with dwell times on the order of seconds. On the other hand, a dwell time of several days for a vitamin assay is clinically acceptable.

Throughput

The throughput is the maximum number of samples or tests that can be processed in an hour. For similar analyzers, the total test throughput can be calculated by multiplying the number of samples processed per hour by the number of tests performed on each specimen. For discrete analyzers, the sample throughput obviously depends on the number of different tests requested on each sample. In addition, the time required per test can vary widely (i.e., from less than 30 seconds to more than 10 minutes). In general, the more tests that are ordered per sample, the slower is the sample throughput on a discrete analyzer. Thus it is more difficult to give a simple, accurate value for the sample throughput for a discrete analyzer. The calculation for throughput does take into account the dwell time, that is, the fact that no results are produced until the dwell time has elapsed. The desired throughput of an instrument usually is matched to the number of samples that need to be processed in a given time period. For example, a higher-throughput (and more costly) instrument may be required to process samples from a clinic, so results can be made available before the patient's return home. In general, an automated analyzer is chosen on the basis of its ability to process the bulk of the routine workload in time for routine clinical decision making.

Stat. Testing

The word *stat.* is an abbreviation of the Latin word "statim," meaning "immediately." Stat. tests account for a large portion (up to 30% to 50% in many laboratories) of the laboratory workload. Stat. tests must be analyzed before less urgent test samples, resulting in the interruption of the normal work flow of the laboratory. Unfortunately, many stat. requests are ordered for reasons other than a medical emergency.

The acceptable within-laboratory turnaround time (TAT, beginning when the sample is received in the laboratory and ending when the result is reported) must be defined for each stat. test, usually after consultation with the appropriate clinical staff. The Clinical Laboratory Improvement Amendments of 1988 (CLIA '88) require that the laboratory's ability to achieve the target TATs must be monitored routinely. TATs usually are kept well within 60 minutes for most stat. tests but may be greater for tests that are needed quickly but not immediately (see p. 359). Point-of-care instruments are also available for the performance of stat. tests at the patient's bedside. These devices improve turnaround time in critical areas of the hospital (see Chapter 21). A test result that is needed in less than 10 minutes can be obtained through the use of whole blood samples for measurement of blood gases, glucose, urea nitrogen, hematocrit, electrolytes, hemoglobin, prothrombin time, human chorionic gonadotropin (hCG), and cardiac markers.

Instruments that are to be used for stat. testing need not necessarily have a high throughput but should have a short dwell time. Many stat. instruments are dedicated instruments that analyze no more than a half dozen high-frequency tests simultaneously.

KEY CONCEPTS BOX 20-4

- Turnaround time is dependent on the dwell time of the assay.
- The dead volume in the sample cup should be small to accommodate samples from pediatric patients.

SECTION OBJECTIVES BOX 20-5

- Outline the steps that can be taken to automate phlebotomy.
- Define workstation consolidation.

AUTOMATED CLINICAL CHEMISTRY INSTRUMENTS

This section summarizes the data for a number of instruments that are used for routine chemistry testing in the hospital laboratory, or that illustrate a category of instrument type. The demand for analyzers with a high throughput and a comprehensive test menu has led to the development of systems that can perform both chemistry and immunochemistry testing. Hormones, specific proteins, and traditional chemistry analytes now can be measured using a single platform, making workstation consolidation a reality in the clinical laboratory. Many chemistry instruments can automatically determine the degree of hemolysis, lipemia, and icterus present in a sample and can "flag" the results to indicate the possibility of significant interference with an assay. A comparison of operational parameters for some automated instruments is shown in Table 20-2. Obviously this table is not meant to be all-inclusive but rather to demonstrate the features available for common types of instruments.

AUTOMATED IMMUNOCHEMISTRY INSTRUMENTS

During the past several years, the number of immunochemistry systems available for use in the clinical laboratory has increased greatly, and the laboratory director is able to select the optimal systems for the laboratory. The immunochemistry system that best fits into a laboratory depends on the number and type of analytes to be measured, and on the size and work flow of the laboratory. Requirements for turnaround time, throughput, degree of automation, data management system, and cost all must be considered when an immunochemistry system is chosen. Many laboratories will have more than one type of immunoassay analyzer—one type to rapidly handle large daily loads with a smaller test menu, and a second type to batch lower-volume tests of a more esoteric nature. Many of the immunochemistry systems employ chemiluminescent assays, which improves analytical sensitivity and extends the dynamic range of the assay. Many immunochemistry systems, such as COBAS Vitros and AU3000i use disposable tips to pipet each sample, thus eliminating carryover, which can be a problem for tumor markers assays. Immunochemistry systems usually have liquid level sensing, clot detection capabilities, and an extensive test menu, which promotes workstation consolidation.

Multiplex Testing

Multiplex testing, which is defined as the measurement of multiple analytes in a single sample well, has been introduced into the clinical laboratory and has the potential to perform disease-specific panel analysis. This immunoassay technology is based on the principle of flow cytometry. Microspheres in a sample cuvette are tagged precisely with different ratios of red and orange fluorochromes. The ratio of the two fluorochromes identifies the analyte that the spheres in the sample well will be measuring. Each sphere in the well is also coupled with a target molecule—either an antigen or an antibody. Within each well are many spheres that are tagged with different antigens or antibodies. Sample that contains the analytes to be measured is added to the well, and this is followed by a green fluorescent tagged conjugate to form an immune complex. For detection, spheres from a single well pass through the instrument's two laser beams. A red laser identifies each sphere; therefore, the analyte that is being measured and a green laser determine the amount of fluorescent product, which is related to the concentration of the analyte that is being measured. Currently, the U.S. Food and Drug Administration (FDA) has approved this technique for a number of tests including extractable nuclear antigens (ENA), antinuclear antibody (ANA), antineutrophil cytoplasmic antibodies (ANCA), rheumatoid factor (RF), and antithyroid-peroxidase antibody (TPO), in addition to some infectious disease markers. Expansion of the test menu to include celiac disease, hepatitis, and human immunodeficiency virus (HIV) panels and syphilis testing is under development. Multiplex testing also has been used for genetic disease screening for cystic fibrosis and for HLA and DNA typing.

A comparison of some of the operational features of some immunochemistry systems is shown in Table 20-3.

TRENDS IN AUTOMATION

The ideal scenario for the clinical laboratory is the automation of all steps involved in collecting, processing, and analyzing the specimen and reporting laboratory results. This scenario begins with the phlebotomist who uses a hand-held wireless device for positive patient identification and subsequent specimen labeling at the patient's bedside.

Order entry is logged into the LIS, and the information is seamlessly linked to the hand-held device. The phlebotomist scans the bar code on the patent's wristband to identify the patient, views the drawlist, which lists the needed specimen containers and the correct order of draw, and collects the blood. Bar-coded labels are printed using a lightweight portable printer and are affixed to the tubes at the bedside, thus preventing mislabeling of specimens. These labels also identify the phlebotomist and the collection time, which allows the laboratory to track specimens and calculate turnaround time. After the blood is drawn, the patient and test information is sent via the hand-held device to the LIS. The specimens are placed in a pneumatic tube, which transfers the specimens to the laboratory or to a central processing area, significantly decreasing the amount of time it takes for specimens to reach the laboratory. The arrival time of samples in the laboratory is recorded automatically by means of the bar-coded labels.

For those areas that require the most rapid turnaround time, two options are available. Whole blood can be used as the sample because some analyzers can perform analyses on whole blood, thus obviating the need for sample processing and greatly reducing turnaround time. Alternatively, point-of-care instruments can be used at the bedside (see Chapter 21).

Table 20-2 Comparison of Operational Features for Some Chemistry Analyzers

Manufacturer	Abbott	Beckman-Coulter	Olympus	Ortho-Clinical Diagnostics	Roche Diagnostics /Hitachi	Siemens Medical Solutions	Siemens Medical Solutions
System name	Architect c8000	Unicell DxC 800 PRO	AU2700	Vitros 5.1 FS	COBAS c501 Analyzer	ADVIA 1800	Xpand Plus/HM
Assay principle(s)	Photometric, potentiometric, turbidimetric	Photometric, potentiometric, turbidimetric	Photometric kinetic rate, potentiometric fixed rate	Potentiometric, photometric, immuno-rate, turbidimetric	Photometric, potentiometric	Photometric, potentiometric, turbidimetric	Photometric, Integrated Medisense Technology, EMIT, Petinia, Acmia
Calibration frequency	8 hrs-60 days	1-90 days	30 days, median	Reagent lot change, except for caffeine which is 7 days	ISE's once every 24 hr. Most chemistry tests calibrated once per lot	Daily for ISE, 14-45 days for chemistries	30-90 days
Sample type	Serum, plasma, urine,CSF	Serum, plasma, urine, CSF, whole blood hemolysate	Serum, plasma, urine, CSF	Serum, plasma, urine, CSF	Serum, plasma, whole blood, urine, CSF	Serum, plasma, urine, CSF	Serum, plasma, urine, CSF and whole blood for select assays
Tube type/sizes	Primary tubes, diameter 8.25-16.1 mm, pediatric tubes and sample cups	Primary tubes, diameter 10.25 × 64 mm, 13 × 75 mm, 13 × 100 mm, 16 × 75 mm, 16 × 100 mm	Primary tubes 3, 5, 7, 10 mL pediatric cups, and nested cups	Primary tubes 2, 5, 7 and 10 mL, microsample cups	Primary tubes, diameter 13 × 75, 13 × 100, 16 × 75, 16 × 100 Hitachi standard cup, Hitachi micro cup, false-bottom tubes	Primary tubes 5, 7 or 10 mL, sample cups, microtainers	Primary tubes 3, 5, 7, 10 mL and sample cups
Clot detection capability	Clot and bubble detection	Yes	Yes	Clot and bubble detection	Yes	Yes	No
Disposable pipets	No	No	No	Not needed with microtip technology	Not needed	No	No
Disposable cuvettes	No	No	No	Yes	No	No	Yes
Sample volume (μL)*	2-35 μL	3-40 μL	1-25 μL	2-20 μL	Minimum 1.5 μL, maximum 35 μL, average 2-4 μL	2-58 μL	2-60 μL
Dead volume (μL)ǿ	50 μL	40-175 μL	100 μL	35-500 μL	50-70 μL	50 μL	30 μL
Reagent type and preparation	Liquid, ready to use	Liquid, ready to use	Liquid, ready to use	Microslides or liquid, no reagent preparation ready to use	Liquid, ready to use	Liquid, ready to use	Liquid or tablet, no preparation
Temperature control of reagent compartment, °C.	2-8	2-8	4-12	13-23	18-32	Refrigerated	2-8
Mixing of sample and reagents	Piezoelectric mixers	Ultrasonic	Mix bars	Not required for microslides	Ultrasonic	Rotational and reciprocating mixer assemblies	Ultrasonic
Optical characteristics of lamp	Tungsten-halogen lamp	Pulse xenon lamp	Tungsten-halogen lamp	Reflectometer lamp	Tungsten-halogen lamp	Tungsten-halogen lamp	Halogen lamp
Wavelength range, nm	340-804	340, 380, 410, 470, 520, 560, 600, 650, 670, 700 and 940	340, 380, 410, 450, 480, 520, 540, 570, 600, 660, 700, 750 and 800	340, 400, 460, 540, 600, 630, 670 and 680	340, 376, 415, 450, 480, 505, 546, 570, 600, 660, 700 and 800	340-884	293-700
Test menu	General chemistry, proteins, TDM, DAU, toxicology and cardiac	General chemistry, TDM, DAU, Specific proteins	General chemistry special chemistry, TDM, DAU, Thyroid	General chemistry, TDM, DAU, Specific proteins	General chemistry, DAU, TDM	General chemistry, Specific proteins, TDM, DAU	General chemistry, TDM/ DAU, plasma proteins, cardiac and endocrine
User defined methods	Yes	Yes	Yes	Yes	Yes	Yes	Yes
Hemolysis, turbidity, icterus detection	Yes	Yes	Yes	Yes	Yes	Yes	Yes
Test repertoire§	65	70	51	125	88	55	47
Total repertoire≠	>100	>200	125	125	78	80	96
Stat. capability	Yes	Yes	Yes	Yes	Yes	Yes	Yes
Dwell time (min)¶	3-10 minutes	Photometric: 3-5 min	STAT 3 min, 53 sec; Routine 8 min, 20 sec	5-20 min	All test results in 10 min. STAT application from 3-7 min	10 min	Varies by method
Throughput (tests/hr)#	1200	1,440	1600	981	1,000 (600 photometric, 400 ISE's)	1800	800

DAU, drugs of abuse; TDM, therapeutic drug monitoring.
*Sample volume needed to perform a test or simultaneous profile.
ǿ Dead volume in sample cup.
§The number of tests available at one time, without a change of reagents or instrument module.
≠Total number of analytes for which reagents are commercially available.
¶Approximate time between sampling and availability of test.
#Calculated by multiplication of maximum number of tests per sample available, times number of samples capable of being processed per hour.

Table 20-3 Comparison of Operational Features for Some Immunochemical Analyzers

Manufacturer	Abbott	Beckman-Coulter	Olympus	Ortho-Clinical Diagnostics	Roche Diagnostics/Hitachi
System name	Architect I2000SR	Unicell Dxl 800	AU3000i	VITROS ECIQ	COBAS e601
Assay principle (s)	Chemiflex (enhanced chemiluminesence)	Dioxetane-based chemiluminescent detection with magnetic particle separation	Magnetic particle separation, chemiluminescence	Enhanced chemiluminescence	ECL (electro-chemiluminescence)
Calibration frequency	30 days or with lot change	Average 28 days	28 days, (median)	28 days or with lot change	Once every 28 days or if test is not run in 7 days
Sample type	Serum, plasma, whole blood, urine	Serum, plasma, urine, amniotic fluid, whole blood	Serum, plasma, urine, other (CSF, RBC)	Serum, plasma, urine, CSF	Serum, plasma, whole blood, urine, CSF
Tube type/sizes	Primary tubes 8.25-16.1 mm in diameter, pediatric and false-bottom tubes and sample cups	Primary tubes, 13 × 75, 16 × 100, 16 × 75 16 × 85 mm in diameter, and sample cups	Primary tubes: 11.5-16 mm in diameter. Pediatric tubes and nested cups	Primary tubes 5, 7 and 10 mL, pediatric microtainers and sample cups	Primary tubes 13 × 75, 13 × 100, 16 × 75, 16 × 100 mm in diameter, Hitachi standard cup, false-bottom tubes
Clot detection capability	Clot and bubble detection	Yes	Yes	Clot and bubble detection	Yes
Disposable pipets	No	No	Yes	Yes	Yes
Disposable cuvettes	Yes	Yes	Yes	NA	Yes
Sample volume (μL)*	Average 50 μL	<50 μL	10-100 μL	10-80 μL	8-40 μL
Dead volume (μL)ǿ	50 μL	160 μL	250 μL (primary tubes); 90 μL (nested cups)	80 μL	100 μL
Reagent type and preparation	Liquid, ready to use	Self-sealing, bar-coded reagent packs, liquid, ready to use	Liquid, ready to use	Liquid, ready to use	Liquid, ready to use
Temperature control of reagent compartment, °C.	2-10	4-10	4-12	2-8	20+/-3
Mixing of sample and reagents	Vortex	Ultrasonic mixing	Vortex	Vibration	Not required
Test menu	Cancer, cardiac, fertility, hepatitis, infectious disease, and thyroid markers, anemia profile, retrovirus, TDM and immunosuppressant Drugs	Cancer, cardiac, fertility, infectious disease and thyroid markers, anemia profile, maternal screen profile for Down syndrome	Thyroid, fertility, others in development	Hormones, TDM, cardiac, tumor, fertility, thyroid, hepatitis and infectious disease markers	Cardiac, fertility, thyroid, cancer markers, anemia profile
User defined methods	No	3 Open channels	No	No	No
Hemolysis, turbidity, icterus detection	No	No	No	No	Yes
Test repertoire§	25	50	24	20	25
Total repertoire≠	31	>50	10	20	39
Stat. capability	Yes	Yes	Yes	Yes	Yes
Dwell time (min)¶	15.6-25 min	15 min	16 min (STAT), 26.5 min (routine)	24 min	18 min (27 min for B_{12} and Folate)
Throughput (tests/hr)#	200	400	240	90	170

Anemia profile,(vitamin B12, folate, and ferritin); DAU, drugs of abuse; TDM, therapeutic drug monitoring.
*Sample volume needed to perform a test or simultaneous profile. Varies by test.
ǿ Dead volume in sample cup, that is the minimum value that must remain in the sample cup for proper sampling.
§The number of tests available at one time, without a change of reagents or instrument module.
≠Total number of analytes for which reagents are commercially available.
¶Approximate time between sampling and availability of test result.
#Calculated by multiplication of maximum number of tests per sample available, times number of samples capable of being processed per hour.

			Multiplex Systems	
Siemens Medical Solutions	Siemens Medical Solutions	Siemens Medical Solutions	BioRad Laboratories	Luminex Corp/Zeus Scientific/Sias Corp.
IMMULITE 2500 Luminescence	ADVIA Centaur XP Chemiluminescence, magnetic particle separation	Dimension Vista®1500 Photometric, integrated microsence technology, EMIT, petinia, acmia	BioPlex 2200 Multiplex flow immunoassay/ magnetic particle	AIMS Multiplexed, fluorescent microbead and ELISA
1-4 weeks	Median, 28 days	30-90 days	14-30 days, kit dependent	Assay dependent
Serum, plasma, urine	Serum, plasma	Serum, plasma, urine, CSF, and whole blood	Serum, plasma, urine, (kit dependent)	Serum
Primary tubes 12-16 mm in diameter	Primary tube sampling	Primary tubes 2, 3, 5, 7, 10 mL and sample cups	Primary tubes 10-16 mm in diameter	Primary tubes 10-16 mm in diameter
Yes	Yes	Yes	Yes	Yes
No	No	No	No	No
Yes	Yes	Yes	Yes	Multiplexed uses a flow cell. ELISA uses disposable microtiter plate
5-100 μL	10-200 μL	2-20 μL	5 μL	10 μL for Multiplex. For ELISA it is kit dependent (usually 10 μL)
200 μL	50 μL	10 μL	70 μL	200 μL
Liquid, ready to use	Liquid, ready to use	Liquid and tablet/No preparation	Liquid, ready to use	Liquid, ready to use
4-8	4	2-8	2-8	No on board refrigeration
Mixing in incubator/shaking	On board rotation	Electromagnetic pulse mix	Agitation, incubation	Microbead suspension needs offline mixing
Hormones, cardiac, cancer, infectious disease markers, anemia profile, TDM	Thyroid, cancer, cardiac, hepatitis, fertility, and infectious disease markers, TDM, anemia profile	General chemistry, immunosuppressant drugs, specific proteins, anemia profile, and TDM, cardiac, fertility, endocrine, cancer and thyroid markers	ANA Screen (12 results), EBV IgG (3 results) and IgM (2 results), Syphilis IgG (1 composite result)	ANA qualitative, dsDNA, SSA, SSB, SM, RNP, Scl-70, Jo-1, Centromere and Histone, ANCA MPO and PR3, EBV VCA IgG, EBNA IgG, EA IgG and VCA IgM, Immune Status: Measles, Mumps, Rubella, and VZV, TPO and TG, RF
No	No	10 Open channels	No	Yes, system is open on Multiplex side and ELISA side
No	No	Yes	No	Corrected for internal calibration on Multiplex side
24	30	100	18	23
72	65	100	18	23
Yes	Yes	Yes	Yes	No
15-60 min	18 min	Varies by method, up to 17.4 min	45 min	Approximately 70 min
200	240	1500	100 samples/hr, kit dependent (up to 2200 results/hr theoretical)	Approximately 475

Once the specimen arrives in the laboratory or in the central processing area, all the steps that are required for processing and analyzing the sample should be automated. Medium-sized and large hospitals use some type of automated front-end specimen-processing system in their laboratories. Many hospitals use the core laboratory concept, in which all automated laboratory analyses, including chemistry, immunochemistry, therapeutic drug monitoring, drugs of abuse, hematology, urinalysis, and coagulation, are performed in one workspace. Tests that are time critical for patient care and are required 24 hours a day (stat. testing) also are performed here. Tests that are manual, not highly automated, or that are performed infrequently usually are run in workspaces that are peripheral to the core laboratory. Closed tube sampling, which eliminates splashing of biological fluids when the tube is uncapped, can be used for tests that require a single workstation for analysis.

Critical to the core laboratory concept is *workstation consolidation*—performing as many tests as possible on the fewest instruments—which is also essential for the efficient operation of any clinical laboratory. The ideal situation is to use instrumentation from one vendor for all testing. Recent advances in technology have allowed several vendors to combine the majority of chemistry and immunochemistry testing using a single instrument. Expansion of the immunochemistry menu to include HIV, syphilis, chlamydia, and other infectious disease and autoimmune markers would be helpful. Workstation consolidation that uses a single platform to measure the majority of chemistry and immunochemistry testing would significantly improve the management of the laboratory.

Implementing these concepts of automated specimen processing and archiving of specimens and workstation consolidation, and automating as many of the laboratory tests as possible using the least number of instruments, will be the top priority of laboratories if they are to survive and prosper as independent, economically viable departments.

KEY CONCEPTS BOX 20-5

- The Core Laboratory concept can be applied to the automation of hematology, special coagulation, clinical chemistry, immunology, infectious disease testing, and urinanalysis.
- Most testing in the clinical laboratory can be performed by using analyzers from two or three vendors.

REFERENCES

1. Laboratory industry report, Washington G2 Reports X1:1, 2007.
2. Rodriques S: Guidelines for implementing automation in a hospital laboratory setting, Part 1, Clin Leadersh Manag Rev 21:E2, 2007.
3. *To Err Is Human: Building A Safer Health System*. Available at http://www.quic.gov/report/errors6ver6.doc
4. Bonini P, Plebani M, Ceriotti F, et al: Errors in laboratory medicine, Clin Chem 48:691, 2002.
5. Khoury M, Burnett L, Mackay MA: Error rates in Australian chemical pathology laboratories, Med J Aust 165:128, 1996.
6. Astion ML, Shojania KG, Hamill TR, et al: Classifying laboratory incident reports to identify problems that jeopardize patient safety, Am J Clin Pathol 120:18, 2003.
7. Pandey P, Chaudhary R, Tondon T, et al: Predictable and avoidable human errors in phlebotomy area—an exclusive analysis from a tertiary health care system blood bank, Transfusion Medicine 17:375, 2007.
8. Howanitz PJ, Renner SW, Walsh MK: Continuous wristband monitoring over 2 years decreases identification errors: a College of American Pathologists Q-Tracks study, Arch Pathol Lab Med 126:809, 2002.
9. Novis DA: Detecting and preventing the occurrence of errors in the practices of laboratory medicine and anatomic pathology: 15 years' experience with the College of American Pathologists' Q-PROBES and Q-TRACKS programs, Clin Lab Med 24:965, 2004.
10. Parsons V: Navigating to lab automation: a lesson in identifying challenges, opportunities and solutions, Adv Admin Lab 14:27, 2005.
11. Stat YT: Laboratory automation—boon or bust? Lab Med 31:369, 2000.
12. The effects of total laboratory automation on the management of a clinical chemistry laboratory: retrospective analysis of 36 years, Clin Chim Acta 329:89, 2003.
13. Seaberg RS, Stallone RO, Statland BE: The role of total laboratory automation in a consolidated laboratory network, Clin Chem 46:751, 2000.
14. Lamb DA, Lopinski R, Sun DH, et al: Operational effects of total laboratory automation, Clin Leadersh Manag Rev 14:173, 2000.
15. Holland LL, Smith LL, Blick KE: Total laboratory automation can help eliminate the laboratory as a factor in emergency department length of stay, Am J Clin Pathol 125:765, 2006.
16. Foreback C: Making modular automation pay, Adv Admin Lab 9:70, 2000.
17. Auerbach HE, Durr K: Integrated automated task targeted analyzer systems, MLO Med Lab Obs 35:38, 2003.
18. Mooney B: Front-end automation in the mid-sized clinical lab, Adv Admin Lab 13:18, 2001.
19. Orsulak PJ: Stand-alone automated solutions can enhance laboratory operations, Clin Chem 46:778, 2000.
20. Dadoun R: Case study: automation's impact on productivity and turnaround time, MLO Med Lab Obs 34:36, 2002.
21. Holman JW, Mifflin TE, Felder RA, et al: Evaluation of an automated preanalytical robotic workstation at two academic health centers, Clin Chem 48:540, 2002.

BIBLIOGRAPHY

Hawker C: Laboratory automation: total and subtotal, Clin Lab Med 27:749, 2007.

Hawker CD, Schlank MR: Development of standards for laboratory automation, Clin Chem 46:746, 2000.

Melanson SEF, Lindeman NI, Jarolim P: Selecting automation for the clinical chemistry laboratory, Arch Pathol Lab Med 131:1063, 2007.

Point-of-Care (Near-Patient) Testing

21 Chapter

James H. Nichols

Chapter Outline

Key Terms

diagnostic test An examination of a human body or materials derived from the human body for the purpose of providing information for the diagnosis, prevention, or treatment of a disease or impairment, or for the assessment of the health of human beings.

ex vivo test A diagnostic test performed on a specimen that is temporarily removed from a living organism for analysis and then returned to the organism.

in vivo test A diagnostic test in which the analyte is measured in fluids that are still located within the body.

point-of-care testing (POCT). Diagnostic testing performed at or near the site of patient care, outside a central laboratory.

quality system essentials A set of coordinated management activities designed to direct and control an organization with regard to quality.

SECTION OBJECTIVES BOX 21-1

- Differentiate point-of-care testing (POCT) and testing within a centralized laboratory.
- List agencies that regulate the quality of POCT.

Point-of-care testing (POCT) is clinical laboratory testing that is conducted close to the site of patient care.[1,2] POCT is typically performed by clinical personnel whose primary training was not completed in the clinical laboratory sciences, or it is performed by patients (self-testing). POCT refers to any testing performed outside of the traditional core or central laboratory.

POCT is referred to by many names (Box 21-1). Each has a slightly different context within the delivery of testing. *Near-patient* simply means performing the test close to the patient; *bedside* assumes that the test will be conducted at the patient's bedside. Satellite laboratory testing, on the other hand, involves collecting a specimen from the patient and carrying the sample to a location away from the patient such as to a satellite laboratory for analysis. Although the terminology can be confusing, *POCT* is the more encompassing term that includes variations of test delivery outside of a centralized laboratory.

One feature of POCT is that testing is conducted by nonlaboratory clinical personnel or by patient self-testing. These individuals are not trained in clinical laboratory sciences, nor do they have experience in detecting preanalytical variation and other common sources of laboratory error. Because of this difference in training, result quality is a primary concern with POCT, and manufacturers have designed POCT devices to be simple with a reduced possibility of error.

As with all laboratory testing, numerous regulatory guidelines have been put forth to address training, quality control, and documentation, so as to ensure the quality of POCT results; these include, among others, the International Organization for Standardization (ISO)[3] guidelines and the U.S. Clinical Laboratory Improvement Amendments of 1988 (CLIA '88).[4] Before they can be marketed, devices must demonstrate truth in package labeling and must conform to general production standards that ensure patient safety (e.g., U.S. Food and Drug Administration [FDA][5] approval in the United States, Conformité Européne [CE mark] of the European Union).[6] Regional, state, and private accreditation agencies like the College of American Pathologists (CAP),[7] the Joint Commission,[8] and the Commission on Office Laboratory Accreditation (COLA)[9] have separate guidelines that also cover the quality of POCT.

Management of POCT quality is complicated by the numbers of sites, devices, and operators involved in the testing process. In a centralized laboratory, the bulk of tests are performed on a few analyzers, run by a small set of skilled technologists who are focused on laboratory analysis for the entire day. POCT may involve dozens of locations with hundreds of devices and thousands of operators who are clinically

Box 21-1

Names for Point-of-Care Testing

Alternate site testing
Ancillary testing
Bedside testing
Decentralized testing
Distributed testing
Near-patient testing
Patient-focused testing
Satellite laboratory testing
Value-added testing

trained and focused on patient care, not on device maintenance and control. Even small clinics may have an extensive menu of tests with several operators who manage training, competency, and device performance. Ensuring quality in a larger institution requires formal organization, policies, and a tiered approach to test supervision. Computerization of newer POCT devices can automate much of the required documentation, assist in staff and device management, and ensure that results get documented in the patient's electronic medical record. With increasing demand for faster turnaround of test results, the management of POCT quality will become ever more complicated in the future.

KEY CONCEPTS BOX 21-1

- Point-of-care testing (POCT) is that testing that occurs near the patient being tested.
- POCT encompasses a wide variety of diagnostic tests.
- In a major change in clinical practice, this method of testing is performed most often by nonlaboratory personnel.

SECTION OBJECTIVES BOX 21-2

- List potential benefits of POCT.
- Discuss the Johns Hopkins study concerning real versus perceived benefits of POCT.
- List laboratory tests that are included in critical care profiles in POCT.
- Explain why hemoglobin A1c, creatinine, and fingerstick prothrombin times performed by POCT has improved patient care.
- Discuss four limitations of POCT: cost, different methodologies used than the central laboratory, availability of results in patient's record, and quality.

USE OF POINT-OF-CARE TESTING

Driving Forces and Potential Benefits

Increasing pressure on health care services to provide better patient care at lower cost with fewer available resources is driving reliance on POCT. Hospitalized patients are being discharged more quickly to turn over the limited number of beds to the most acutely ill patients. Increasingly, patients are presenting to patient care facilities with more severe levels of illness. It is estimated that more than 70% of patient care decisions are based on laboratory testing,[10,11] and many of these facilities may not have the stat. laboratories to provide the necessary patient support. POCT testing can provide many of the acutely needed laboratory tests. Clinics, home nursing programs, and outpatient surgery centers all require test results to make management decisions. To enhance efficiency, these facilities no longer wait for results from a regional laboratory; they perform POCT onsite.

Table 21-1 Potential Benefits of Point-of-Care Testing

For physicians:	Improved turnaround time for lab results
	Better and more immediate patient care
	Less labor in result follow-up
For patients:	Less traumatic (for fingerstick systems)
	Improved convenience
	Less blood withdrawn
	Patient-focused system
For laboratory:	Decreased preanalytical errors
	Improved visibility
	Collaboration with clinicians
	Direct patient involvement
	Team management system
For administration:	Shorter intensive care unit (ICU) stays
	Decreased overall length of stays
	Financial savings

POCT provides potential benefits for clinicians, patients and laboratorians that address these health care pressures (Table 21-1). For the clinician, POCT provides faster turnaround of test results by eliminating the need to transport specimens to a central laboratory for analysis. Labor is reduced because test results are immediately available without the need for staff to look up these results in a computerized record, to call for results, or to sort through faxed results on a printer. POCT results can be available while the physician is still examining the patient, allowing for more immediate patient care. Having laboratory results, such as lipid and hemoglobin A1c, available at the time of an office visit allows for timely patient counseling, including patient diet and exercise regimens. This can possibly eliminate the need for subsequent phone calls and office visits. For patients, POCT at the bedside and during an office visit provides improved convenience, less trauma (fingerstick vs. venous phlebotomy), and a sense of patient-focused care. For the laboratory, participation in POCT management allows greater visibility and improved collaboration with clinicians and more direct patient involvement than occurs with central laboratory testing. POCT also offers the potential for a reduction in preanalytical errors, particularly in terms of patient identification and delays in transportation.

Perception versus Reality

Although POCT has great potential, realized outcomes often fall short of predicted benefits. This is because testing must be integrated into patient care strategies. The perceived failure of traditional, central laboratory testing to keep pace with changing clinical needs depends on the capacity of hospitals to maintain modern facilities. Pneumatic tubes and electronic mechanisms designed to facilitate return of results to clinicians have achieved significant improvement in turnaround of results over couriers and manual communication methods. Yet, facility upgrades are expensive and take time. Clinical needs change rapidly, and the laboratory is often a scapegoat for blamed inefficiencies in patient management. The ability to provide testing on the medical unit is a convenience that places the responsibility of result availability solely on the shoulders of the clinical staff. The POCT process is simple and flexible enough to adapt to changing medical treatment protocols on the unit, placing the responsibility for improved patient care in the hands of the clinical staff. So once POCT is adopted, clinicians can no longer blame the laboratory for delays in patient care. They must instead reflect on the efficiency of the overall patient care pathways that are under their control.

The perceived benefits of POCT were examined in a study conducted in the Interventional Radiology setting at Johns Hopkins.[12] Delays in laboratory results for coagulation and renal function were thought to be the source of procedural hold-ups and operating room postponements. POCT was viewed as an optimal solution, since fast test results would allow improved patient triage. However, the implementation of POCT did not result in the predicted outcomes and only complicated an already flawed system by adding one more task that staff had to maintain. After implementation of POCT, fewer patients actually met scheduled procedure times compared with before implementation of POCT. Only after changes were made in the patient care pathway to reduce inefficiencies and improve communication between patient reception and operating room staff were significant improvements in meeting scheduled procedure times achieved.[12] POCT was a tool that unveiled other operational inefficiencies but was not the sole means of improving care. This emphasizes that faster test results alone do not necessarily achieve better patient care unless practice changes to better utilize the faster results.

The National Academy of Clinical Biochemistry (NACB) conducted a systematic review of the scientific literature and has developed practice guidelines for POCT.[1,2] Recommendations are divided into various disease states (e.g., cardiac, diabetes, infectious disease, reproduction), and general guidelines for maintaining quality results are provided.[1,2] These guidelines emphasize several important conclusions about POCT. First, there are few randomized controlled trials in laboratory diagnostics, and most of the evidence is based on cohort, case description, and peer consensus evidence. Unfortunately, most POCT has been adopted without rigorous evaluation of patient outcomes. Second, patient outcomes are dependent on specific clinical applications, sites, and devices. The conclusions of one study cannot be generalized easily to other patient care settings without consideration of staff training, motivation, and other quality requirements. Finally, optimal patient outcomes can be achieved with POCT only when the medical practice changes simultaneously to better utilize the POCT results.

Immediate Medical Management Benefits

Ideally, POCT can be predicted to have the greatest impact in the management of critically ill patients with unstable conditions. Analytes like blood gases, electrolytes (Na^+, K^+, Ca^{++}, Mg^{++}), glucose, coagulation, and hemoglobin/hematocrit that demonstrate rapidly changing levels—faster than the turnaround time for results from a central laboratory—are important tests to be considered for POCT (Table 21-2). With POCT, results are available so that medical action can be taken while the patient's test results are still most physiologically valid.

Table 21-2 Critical Care Profiles

Physiological Function	Diagnostic Measures
Energy	Glucose, hemoglobin, hematocrit, Po_2, O_2 saturation
Conduction	K^+, Na^+, Mg^{++}, Ca^{++}
Contraction	Mg^{++}, Ca^{++}
Perfusion	Lactate
Acid-base	pH, Pco_2, TCO_2, HCO_3^-
Osmolality	Calculated as 1.86 ([Na] + [K]) + gluc/18
Hemostasis	PT, PTT, platelets, hematocrit, ACT, platelet function
Renal function	Creatinine, BUN
Cardiac ischemia	Myoglobin, CK-MB, troponin-T or -I

ACT, Activated clotting time; *BUN*, blood urea nitrogen; *CK-MB*, creatine kinase-MB fraction; *PT*, prothrombin time; *PTT*, partial thromboplastin time.

Other rapidly changing metabolites are also targets for consideration for POCT (see Table 21-2). These tests can be performed individually or as profiles, that is, in logical groups of physiological indicators that are diagnostic for specific vital functions. These tests all have maximum turnaround time requirements in the 5- to 60-minute time frame. For these tests, faster results may translate to decreased morbidity and mortality in the management of trauma, surgical, and critically ill patients. Lactate is a marker of perfusion that is important in the diagnosis of sepsis and hypoxia in patients with decreasing organ function. POCT assessment of coagulation status is important for patients undergoing cardiac surgery and catheterization, patients who require close heparin management. Similarly, POCT assessment of cardiac markers can be useful in the evaluation of chest pain in the emergency room. Analysis of parathyroid hormone has become a standard component of the minimally invasive surgeries performed on the parathyroid gland. Intraoperative levels can indicate surgical success while the operation is in progress and can enhance success rates and postoperative recovery. These tests all have maximum turnaround time requirements in the 5- to 60-minute time frame. For this group of tests and for the management of trauma, surgical, and critically ill patients, faster results may translate into decreased morbidity and mortality.

Other tests can be performed at the point of care, more for reasons of convenience when a central laboratory result cannot be obtained within a medically useful time frame. Many of the outpatient physician office and home nursing tests fall into this category. Hemoglobin A1c, for instance, is a stable analyte whose concentration depends on average blood sugar levels and red blood cell turnover. Although hemoglobin A1c levels are constant for about 3 months, POCT performed in the physician's office has been demonstrated to enhance patient counseling, decrease hemoglobin A1c levels, and improve patient and physician satisfaction.[13-16] More importantly, offering the hemoglobin A1c POCT helps the physician's office meet health care recommendations of the Health Quality Institute and the American Diabetes Association regarding monitoring of every diabetic patient at least every 3 to 6 months. Other tests, like creatinine, may be useful in monitoring renal function for oncology patients; offering creatinine POCT can reduce patient wait times for chemotherapy.[17] Fingerstick coagulation prothrombin testing is a rapidly growing strategy for coumadin monitoring that has improved patient and physician satisfaction over venous phlebotomy for monitoring patients on anticoagulation therapy.[18,19] Virtually any test can be offered in the physician's office in which the clinical need is sufficient to balance the costs of maintaining the quality of testing, and a patient management strategy is used, leading to faster test results and improved patient outcomes.

POCT Limitations

POCT is not without limitations. Cost is one disadvantage. POCT analyzers tend to have higher disposable and reagent costs compared with traditional laboratory systems. Although POCT does not require permanent space, indirect costs, including labor, training and competency, quality control, method validation, maintenance, documentation of results, and performance of external quality control/proficiency testing, are associated with managing the quality of test results. Thus, POCT systems are more expensive to operate on a per test basis than are automated chemistry analyzers that operate with bulk liquid reagents.

POCT testing methodology may differ from central laboratory testing. Therefore, results from POCT devices may not match central laboratory results for the same test. Calibration, whole blood vs. plasma samples, interferences, and matrix effects will have different effects on POCT devices and on central laboratory instrumentation. Such differences are apparent when results of the same sample are compared between glucose meters from different manufacturers and central laboratory methods. Recent comparisons reveal a unique bias for each glucose meter in the high, normal, and low areas of the reportable range that differ between manufacturers and models of a device.[20] Clinicians should take these diffferences into account when treating patients on the basis of POCT versus central laboratory test results. Treatment algorithms developed from central laboratory results may have to be modified when they are applied to POCT.[1,17]

The rapid availability of POCT results creates a quality dilemma. Results can be seen and acted upon before any control checks or other external mechanisms of ensuring test result reliability can be applied to the result. Reagents and other aspects of testing can be compromised by operator technique, storage conditions, and the environment in which the test is being used. Therefore, POCT devices require built-in quality control systems that automatically check the function of the device and the viability of the chemical reagents with each test. These automatic functions keep faulty instruments from being used and prevent erroneous results from being given to and acted on by the clinician. Quality of test results is a major concern with POCT. While POCT look deceptively simple, there are many preanalytical, analytical, and postanalytical errors possible with any POCT device. Because POCT is performed by a large number of staff members with varying levels of aptitude, shortcuts and inadvertent errors may occur. The performance of POCT by staff members with minimal or no laboratory training and experience suggests that the quality of the result should be considered when POCT results are interpreted. The performance of any laboratory test requires a defined sequence of steps if an accurate result is to be attained. As more staff with less experience become involved in the testing process, the probability increases that errors may be generated and results may be incorrect. Incorrect results can compromise patient care by leading the physician to an incorrect diagnosis and generating follow-up testing and diagnostic procedures that increase the cost of care. More complaints about self-monitoring blood glucose meters have been filed with the U.S. Food and Drug Administration than any other medical device; more than 3200 incidents, including 16 deaths, have been reported. Even very simple devices carry some risk. POCT devices may be shared between patients and in this way can be a source of nosocomial infection. Failure to properly clean the device, change gloves, and thoroughly decontaminate lancet holders has led to the transmission of hepatitis B infection between patients at nursing homes in three states.[21]

Most POCT errors are unintentional. Staff members simply do not understand and may not have the experience to predict how patient-specific factors, reagent conditions, and operator technique can affect test results. In a recent survey of physician office practices by U.S. inspectors, numerous alarming POCT quality issues, including the following, were noted in more than half the laboratories inspected: staff not following manufacturers' instructions, failure of staff members to identify incorrect results, untrained staff, lack of quality controls, poor equipment, poor storage of reagents, poor record keeping, and failure of staff to understand regulatory requirements.[22] When approached with these issues, staff did not recognize that these problems could lead to test errors. Staff wanted the best for patient care but just did not understand the fundamentals of good laboratory practice. After education was provided, follow-up surveys demonstrated significant improvement in most of the laboratories upon reinspection.[22] This survey shows that education, experience, and ongoing supervision, along with regular inspections, are important components of POCT quality that should be integrated into all POCT programs during implementation.

KEY CONCEPTS BOX 21-2

- Rapid availability of POCT results may counter increased POCT results.
- Potential benefits of POCT may not be realized, especially if clinical setting is inappropriate.
- Staff using POCT must be taught pitfals of POCT to avoid errors.

SECTION OBJECTIVES BOX 21-3

- Explain what is meant by "waived" tests, according to CLIA '88.
- List United States regulations that govern POCT.
- Describe the interdisciplinary coordination required to properly manage POCT.

IMPLEMENTATION AND MONITORING OF POCT

Regulations (see also Chapter 19)

Despite its relative simplicity, the use of POCT is subject to the various regulations associated with clinical laboratory testing. In the United States, the CLIA '88 amendments[4] subject virtually all clinical laboratory testing to federal regulation and inspection. State and city governments may enact regulations that are more, but not less, stringent than federal regulations. Furthermore, these government agencies and nonprofit accrediting organizations, such as the Joint Commission[8] and the College of American Pathologists (CAP),[7] may apply for "deemed" status, by which their laboratory inspections and accreditation are accepted by the federal government.

Test procedures are grouped into one of four categories: waived testing, provider-performed microscopy, moderate-complexity testing, or high-complexity testing.[23] Test complexity is determined by seven criteria that assess knowledge, training, reagent and material preparation, operational technique, quality assurance/quality control characteristics, maintenance and troubleshooting, and interpretation and judgment. Originally, only nine waived tests were available, but many more tests and devices have been added to the waived category since the adoption of CLIA '88 (Box 21-2). Any analytical system approved by the FDA to be sold as an over-the-counter test, that is, in a store or pharmacy without the need for a prescription, is automatically placed into the waived category. Waived tests are thought to be so simple that the chance of an erroneous result leading to medical harm is negligible. However, no device is used without risk, and the literature describes many cases in which unintentional misuse and erroneous results have led to patient harm and increased cost of care. Federal regulations and inspections of laboratories that perform only waived tests are minimal. Waived laboratories need only to enroll in the CLIA '88 program, pay the biennial fees, and follow manufacturers' instructions. These laboratories, primarily physicians' offices, account for more than 50% of all laboratories enrolled in the CLIA '88 program. Point-of-care tests fall within the waived or the moderate-complexity category, with one exception: gram stains sometimes are performed as a POCT and are classified as high-complexity testing. A separate category of testing, provider-performed microscopy, consists of tests performed by clinicians on their own patients using samples that are so fragile that it is not practical to send them to a central laboratory. Nine provider-performed microscopy tests are available (Box 21-3).

Laboratories that perform moderate-complexity POCT also may perform waived tests but must fulfill all the requirements for higher personnel training and competency, proficiency testing, quality assurance and quality control, patient test management, and inspections required for moderately complex tests. Personnel standards for the performance of waived tests are minimal. However, in several states, California and Florida for example, training and/or licensure is required even for waived testing. When personnel documentation is reviewed, the following criteria must be satisfied:

- Staff members responsible for testing, direction, and supervision are identified.
- Adequate training to perform the test, specific to the device, is provided.
- Competency is checked at least annually.

The laboratory must document that these requirements are met. In addition, written policies and procedures must be established to encompass preanalytical, analytical, and post-analytical steps of the testing process (Box 21-4).

Regulations in several states, including New York, New Jersey, and Pennsylvania, and CAP dictate that the central laboratory must supervise hospital-based POCT, and that the laboratory director is responsible for standards of performance in all areas, including quality control, quality assurance, and test utilization in patient care.

Each laboratory or testing site that performs nonwaived POCT must establish written policies regarding total quality assurance. The POCT quality program should be integrated into the institution's quality improvement program for hospital testing under the Joint Commission and CAP (see Chapter 25, Quality Control). An ongoing system must be in place to monitor and evaluate quality control and proficiency testing data. Quality control specimens at two or three different analyte concentrations must be analyzed on a daily basis. Corrective action should be taken for all quality controls that fail acceptable limits before patient testing is performed. The reportable range should be verified before devices are initially put into use, and then every 6 months. Calibration must be verified initially, when significant changes are made to the reagent or major instrument maintenance is performed, and then every 6 months. Split sample studies or correlation with other testing systems should be performed for each POCT device that is initially placed into use, and every 6 months thereafter. Federal CLIA '88 standards require proficiency testing several times a year against each testing method so that individual site results can be compared nationwide with those from other laboratories that are performing the same test.

An integral component of patient test management and a laboratory quality assurance (QA) system is proper record keeping. The information in Box 21-5 must be recorded and documentation kept for a minimum of 2 to 3 years, for the life of the device, or as required by state and federal law.

Training

POCT is performed primarily by clinical staff, and this represents a major paradigm shift. Nurses, physicians, respiratory therapists, operating room technologists, physician assistants, medical office assistants, and emergency medical technicians are among those who may perform POCT. Qualifications for

Box 21-2

CLIA '88 Waived Tests*

General Chemistry

Alanine aminotransferase (ALT)
Albumin (whole blood and urine)
Alkaline phosphatase (ALP)
Amylase
Aspartate aminotransferase (AST)
Bilirubin, total
Calcium, total
Carbon dioxide, total
Cholesterol, total
Creatine kinase (CK)
Creatinine
Electrolytes (Na, K, Cl bicarbonate)
Fructosamine
Gamma-glutamyl transferase (GGT)
Glucose
Glucose monitoring devices (FDA approved for home use)*
Glucose, fluid (continuous monitoring)
Glycated hemoglobin, total
HDL cholesterol
Hemoglobin A1c
Ketones, blood or urine
Lactate
LDL cholesterol
Microalbumin
pH, gastric and other body fluids
Protein, total
Triglycerides
Urea (BUN)
Uric acid
Vaginal pH

Cardiac Marker, Tumor Marker, and Other

B-type natriuretic peptide (BNP)
Bladder tumor–associated antigen
Fecal occult blood*
Gastric occult blood

Endocrinology

Collagen type 1 cross-link, N-telopeptides
Estrone-3 glucuronide
Fern test, saliva
Follicle-stimulating hormone (FSH)
Luteinizing hormone (LH)
Thyroid stimulating hormone (TSH)
Urine pregnancy tests (hCG) (visual comparison of color)*
Urine pregnancy tests (hCG) (instrument-read)
Ovulation tests (LH) (visual comparison of color)*

Toxicology and Therapeutic Drug Monitoring

Alcohol, saliva
Amphetamines
Barbiturates
Benzodiazepines
Cannabinoids
Cocaine metabolites
Ethanol
Lead, blood
Lithium
Methadone
Methamphetamine
Methamphetamine/amphetamine
Methylenedioxymethamphetamine (MDMA)
Morphine
Nicotine and/or metabolites
Opiates
Oxycodone
Phencyclidine (PCP)
Propoxyphene
Tricyclic antidepressants

Urinalysis

Dipstick or tablet reagent urinalysis for bilirubin, glucose, hemoglobin, ketones, leukocytes, nitrites, pH, protein, specific gravity, and urobilinogen (nonautomated)*
Dipstick or tablet reagent urinalysis for ascorbic acid, bilirubin, creatinine, glucose, hemoglobin, ketones, leukocytes, nitrites, pH, protein, specific gravity, and urobilinogen (automated)

Hematology

Erythrocyte sedimentation rate, nonautomated*
Hematocrit
Hematocrit, spun*
Hemoglobin
Hemoglobin (automated using single-analyte instrument)*
Hemoglobin (copper sulfate)*
Platelet aggregation
Prothrombin time
Semen analysis

Infectious Disease

Adenovirus
Aerobic/anaerobic organisms–vaginal
Amines
Catalase, urine
Helicobacter pylori
Helicobacter pylori antibodies
HIV antibodies
HIV-1 and HIV-2 antibodies
HIV-1 antibody
Infectious mononucleosis antibodies
Influenza A, B, or A/B
Lyme disease *(Borrelia burgdorferi)* antibodies
Rapid strep A antigen
Respiratory syncytial virus
Streptococcus, group A (direct from throat swab)
Trichomonas

From http://www.accessdata.fda.gov/scripts/cdrh/cfdocs/cfCLIA/analyteswaived.cfm.
This list based on data as of February 2009.
BUN, Blood urea nitrogen; *CLIA,* Clinical and Laboratory Improvement Amendments; *hCG,* human chorionic gonadotropin; *HDL,* high-density lipoprotein; *HIV,* human immunodeficiency virus; *LDL,* low-density lipoprotein; *LH,* luteinizing hormone.
*Nine originally waived tests.

Box 21-3

CLIA '88 Provider-Performed Microscopy

Wet-mount preparations of vaginal, cervical, or skin specimens
Semen analysis, limited to presence or absence of sperm and motility
Urine sediment examination
Potassium hydroxide preparations
Fern testing
Postcoital direct, qualitative examinations of specimens from vagina or cervix
Pinworm preps
Nasal smears for eosinophils
Fecal leukocyte examination

CLIA, Clinical and Laboratory Improvement Amendments.

Box 21-4

Policies and Procedures Needed for POCT

Method validation
Patient preparation
Specimen collection and preservation
Instrument calibration
Quality control and remedial actions
Equipment maintenance
Test performance, result reporting, and recording

POCT, Point-of-care testing.

Box 21-5

Record Keeping of POCT Information

- Time and date of test
- Patient results
- Operator performing testing
- Quality control results
- Maintenance performed
- Actions taken to correct unacceptable quality control
- Initial training and competency checks of personnel
- Initial and 6-month method validations (reportable range, calibration verification, correlation studies)
- Proficiency testing results and actions for unacceptable results
- Dates when devices were implemented and retired from clinical use
- Policies and procedures (initial, revisions, and annual reviews)

POCT, Point-of-care testing.

performing bedside testing are defined by state/local and federal requirements, as well as by the laboratory director. The minimum educational and experience requirement for personnel performing POCT ranges from a high school degree with no experience to a bachelor of science with 2 years of experience. In specific cases, other health care professionals may qualify by state-defined scope of practice to perform select testing, for example, a certified respiratory therapist is allowed to conduct blood-gas analysis. In addition, all POCT personnel must undergo documented training and annual review of skill competency that are specific by the manufacturer and for the device.

Box 21-6

POCT Training Form Agenda

Device theory of operation
Specimen collection/preservation
Instrument maintenance
Quality control procedures
Patient testing procedure
Sources of common errors
Clinical significance of results

POCT, Point-of-care testing.

The depth of training depends on the background and experience of the individuals involved, as well as the type of analytical system used and the complexity of the operation. Seven main areas of focus should be included in the training program (Box 21-6). In addition to teaching the specific sequence of steps required to perform the test, trainers must address quality control and overall QA of the device and the test result. Most errors in POCT occur before analysis, in the preanalytical phase. Poor clinical and analytical correlations and erroneous results most often derive from a poor specimen. Factors that affect the specimen include collection problems (interstitial fluid contamination, skin surface contamination; see Chapter 18), interference from circulating metabolites (drugs, uremia, lipemia, icterus, hematocrit), source of the specimen (arterial, venous, fingerstick, ancillary sites like arms or legs), and the patient's physiological status (hypervolemia and/or hypovolemia, poor peripheral circulation). These factors should be addressed thoroughly by the training program.

The training program should include written examination of the staff for comprehension of key issues, as well as supervised demonstration of acceptable performance for specimen collection, quality control, and analysis. Other key aspects of training and competency as recommended by CAP include reporting and recording test results, maintaining instruments, obtaining correct results (by testing previously analyzed specimens or proficiency samples of known value), and exhibiting problem-solving skills. Annual competency of testing personnel should include all aspects of skill competency that are applicable to the specific POCT device.

Management of training and competency is facilitated by the use of newer devices that provide electronic lockout of staff based on their training and current competency levels. These devices require an operator to enter an identification number before the device can be used for patient testing. If the operator identification does not match a list of trained operators with current competency, then the device will lock out the operator and prevent testing. These features provide a means of managing multiple operators and ensuring that only skilled staff members perform POCT.

Box 21-7

Total Quality Management for POCT

Multidisciplinary team approach
Focus on entire system, rather than on individual performance
Continuous quality improvement (CQI)
Quantitative benchmarks and assement of ongoing performance

POCT, Point-of-care testing.

Coordination of Central Laboratory Testing and POCT

The decentralization of testing away from traditional, central laboratories has increased the direct involvement between the laboratory and other members of the patient's health care team. One of the goals of POCT is to implement a system that will improve the delivery of critical laboratory results. To achieve this goal, the clinician must view POCT as part of a larger plan or pathway of care. POCT is not just a faster alternative to central laboratory testing but must be seen as an integral component of an overall scheme that requires rapid test results for immediate management of changes in patient care. Clinical staff members find the notions of quality control and device maintenance challenging and believe that these are more laboratory functions than clinical functions. However, once POCT is introduced, clinicians must have the resources to support all of its functions, including quality control and documentation, as required to ensure quality results. Because quality management is so important, POCT must be integrated into the total quality management (TQM) plans of the institution (Box 21-7). Because POCT implementation crosses many boundaries within a hospital, an interdepartmental approach is required for establishing goals, addressing compliance issues, and setting future directions of the program.

An interdisciplinary POCT committee should be established with representation from all participating areas, including physician, nursing, laboratory, respiratory therapy, infection control, materials management, information systems, and administration. Laboratory participation is essential for a successful committee. Laboratorians can contribute their technical expertise, scientific perspective, and familiarity with the demands of laboratory regulatory issues. In addition, the clinical laboratory staff can help evaluate new technology, design training programs, and identify potential weaknesses in new systems. Working in partnership with clinicians, who bring their own understanding of clinical and patient needs and priorities, the committee can forge a dynamic relationship that enhances the clinical effectiveness of POCT. The POCT committee should determine institutional policies, define levels of service, evaluate and select equipment, and establish staff responsibilities that will meet the various regulatory requirements (Table 21-3). The committee should review all requests for new POCT and should approve which devices should be used and how the test will be applied to patient care. Five questions should be addressed in the request for POCT; see Box 21-8 for a list of these.

Table 21-3 Point-of-Care Testing Committee Responsibilities

Implementation Phase	Oversight Phase
Define the operation.	Review quality control records.
Define what documentation is required.	Monitor compliance.
Select method.	Review test utilization.
Assign staff responsibility for test and control performance.	Assess impact/outcomes.
	Approve expansion and additional testing.

Box 21-8

Questions to Be Asked Before Implementation of New POCT

1. What is the medical and/or financial justification for the testing?
2. What is the anticipated frequency and volume of testing?
3. Why are current laboratory services insufficient?
4. Who, and how many individuals, will perform the testing?
5. Who will be the key person who will supervise testing on the medical unit?

Another critical component of a POCT program is the opportunity for staff to respond to what is working and is not working. This feedback can be provided by an end-user committee (one for each type of testing), which is different from the interdisciplinary committee that establishes and oversees POCT. Staff also can be invited to attend the interdisciplinary committee meeting when new tests are being reviewed or compliance issues discussed, or whenever the committee can benefit from hearing staff responses. Some institutions have a POCT contact on each medical unit, and periodic meetings of these POCT contacts can provide a connection between issues arising on the medical unit and the discussions of the interdisciplinary POCT committee. Typically, POCT contacts meet on a monthly basis, and the interdisciplinary POCT committee should meet at least every other month to review new test requests, monitor compliance, and set future program goals.

The ultimate responsibility for POCT resides with the laboratory director named on the CLIA certificate. This individual can delegate responsibilities to other qualified staff but must ensure that device validations are performed before they are placed into service; the director is responsible for enrollment in proficiency testing, performance of quality control, analysis of control trends, staff training, compliance with documentation, and technical guidance. If more than one POCT device and test is in use, a POCT coordinator can assist in oversight and coordination of the entire POCT program. The POCT coordinator can assume the following responsibilities as delegated by the laboratory director:

- Ensurance that all POCT systems are in compliance with accreditation requirements
- Review and analysis of quality control data
- Preparation of periodic compliance reports for individual units and overall institutional performance

- Coordination and supervision of POCT personnel
- Development and coordination of training for staff involved in POCT

KEY CONCEPTS BOX 21-3

- CLIA '88 regulation specify laboratory tests in terms of overall complexity.
- Waived tests, the least complex, require the least regulatory oversight and include most POCT tests, including over-the-counter tests.
- Additional POCT regulatory oversight may come from individual states and private agencies with "deemed status" (Joint Commission, CAP).
- Good POCT programs coordinate activities with lab staff, physicians, nurses, and hospital administrators, often through formal committees.

SECTION OBJECTIVES BOX 21-4

- List three means to manage the sources of error in POCT.
- Compare and contrast the advantages and disadvantages of internal and external quality control in POCT instruments.
- Describe the characteristics of non-instrument based POCT systems, including specimens used, testing methodologies employed, examples of tests performed, advantages, and disadvantages.

COMPLIANCE MONITORING

Sources of error in POCT can be managed in three ways, one technical and the others part of the quality assurance plan. The first requires manufacturers to design the device so that errors are improbable or easy to detect. This can be accomplished by engineering internal systems that can check device functionality, automate calibration, encode (via bar code or microchip) reagent expiration dates and quality information on test packages, monitor the testing process, and provide lockout functions for failure of any internal checks. Second, errors in POCT can be detected through recovery of expected results from external quality control solutions of known concentration intended to mimic the patient sample matrix. The third way that sources of error can be managed is by warning staff of likely errors through product labeling and training, for example, by ensuring that staff members are aware of potential errors that can result from various patient conditions (such as fingerstick, capillary specimens in patients with hypovolemia or poor peripheral circulation due to shock) or analytical interferences (such as lipemia or drugs).

The purpose of quality assurance is to manage the residual risk of errors that have not been controlled by the instrument itself. Quality assurance of POCT devices requires an understanding of how the device functions, the probability and medical consequences of residual errors, and recommended management strategies for ensuring consistent and reliable test results. Total quality management is accomplished through a combination of appropriate training, external quality control, proficiency testing, competency assessment, and validation of devices before they are used in patient care.

Table 21-4 Compliance Monitoring of Point-of-Care Testing

Frequency	Task
Daily	Temperature monitoring
	Quality control performance
	POCT staff provides troubleshooting.
Weekly	Reagent inventory and reordering
Monthly	POCT coordinator makes compliance rounds of test sites.
	Quality assurance reports are distributed.
	POCT contact committee meets for unit feedback.
Bimonthly	Interdisciplinary committee meeting is held.

POCT, Point-of-care testing.

Box 21-9 Compliance Reports Indicators

Daily control performance
Corrective actions for failed controls
Reagent storage
Refrigerator temperature monitoring
Maintenance performance
Proficiency testing
Patient identification errors
Critical value confirmations
Quality indicators that are unique to each testing system

All medical units and clinical settings experience noncompliance with regulatory requirements at one time or another. The degree of noncompliance is directly related to the size and complexity of the POCT program. Many of these problems occur because staff members do not know the regulatory requirements, do not understand the function of quality control testing, or do not recognize the causes of erroneous results. External pressures of patient care in a busy intensive care unit or emergency department may lead to staff shortcuts, sporadic documentation, and other compliance problems.

Identifying compliance issues requires close supervision of POCT and an understanding of the individual staff roles involved in the overall POCT program—from test operator, staff educator, unit POCT contact, nurse manager, and physician to POCT coordinator and laboratory director (Table 21-4). Nursing or unit managers are responsible for work performance and compliance with policies and procedures on a daily basis, with laboratory POCT coordinator and personnel providing troubleshooting and guidance as needed. Weekly and monthly reviews of system operations by POCT personnel and unit nurse managers ensure continuous compliance. Once a month, the POCT coordinator should generate a compliance report on each medical unit's degree of compliance with various quality indicators. This report can include a variety of indicators but at a minimum should review the indicators listed in Box 21-9. The compliance report should include both a numerical/statistical and a narrative

Box 21-10

Quality System Essentials

Documents and records
Organization
Personnel
Equipment
Purchasing and inventory
Process control
Information management
Occurrence management
Assessment
Process improvement
Service and satisfaction
Facilities and safety

analysis of individual medical unit compliance and systemwide tests and volumes.

When compliance is deemed to be below established thresholds, the unit nurse managers should investigate and develop a corrective action plan. Periodically, the laboratory director or his or her designee (the POCT coordinator) and a representative from nursing management should perform compliance rounds. In addition to serving as a second level of review, these rounds focus on staff awareness of policies and of how staff would respond to an external inspector. Regular compliance rounds keep staff aware of key issues and make staff members comfortable when speaking with accreditation program inspectors. These compliance rounds may involve review of physician orders versus testing performed and documentation of patient results in the medical record. Compliance rounds provide another feedback channel for staff and send a clear signal of the program's importance and the institution's commitment to quality.

International standards have been developed by both the ISO and the CLSI to help hospitals and physician offices manage the quality of POCT. These standards encourage a quality systems approach to testing whereby multiple aspects of the testing process are controlled and documented to ensure traceability of records and reliability of results. For POCT, the core set of 12 **quality system essentials** provide a framework for delivery of quality test results (Box 21-10).

QUALITY CONTROL OF UNIT-USE DEVICES

Quality control has traditionally been mandated by U.S. regulatory agencies with each analytical run, or every 24 hours for most laboratory tests (every 8 hours for coagulation and blood-gas testing, see Chapter 25). Quality control is different for unit-use POCT with single test cartridges or strips. Quality control in a unit-use system destroys the test that is in the process of performing the analysis. External controls do not indicate performance characteristics of the next test or the next box of tests from the same lot because each test is an individual, self-contained unit. These systems must rely on internal control processes to manage common sources of error such as sample clots, bubbles, reagent degradation, and device electronics. Internal controls may enhance detection of random errors because they are performed with each test. Internal controls can only address those aspects of the testing process that the manufacturer predicted as a potential source of error. However, not all errors can be predicted in advance of device implementation and use of the test in a real-world setting. This is the advantage of external controls—they detect the sum of all processes in the testing system and do not require prior knowledge of a potential error.

Three standards are being developed by the Clinical Laboratory Standards Institute: EP-18, *Risk Management Techniques to Identify and Control Laboratory Error Sources*[24]; EP-22, *Presentation of Manufacturers' Risk Mitigation Information for Users of* In Vitro *Diagnostic Devices*[25]; and EP23, *Laboratory Quality Control Based on Risk Mananagement.*[26] EP-18 presents the principles of failure mode and effects analysis (FMEA) and describes how FMEA can be used to predict the frequency and consequences of potential errors and to develop processes that can mitigate residual risk of error. Manufacturers conduct an extensive FMEA before submission is made to the FDA for approval to market laboratory **diagnostic tests.** Laboratories can learn to conduct a similar FMEA when implementing new devices; EP-18 includes an appendix table with a comprehensive list of potential preanalytical, analytical, and postanalytical errors for consideration. EP-22 is a document directed toward manufacturers that describes how to present validation studies conducted by the manufacturer that prove that internal control mechanisms are effective, and how to present residual risk information to the laboratory director and the user of diagnostic tests. EP-23 describes a process for developing a customized quality control plan that is based on manufacturer-provided information, local regulations, and the laboratory's unique environment (the staff and clinical application of the test). Together, these documents help laboratory directors develop a quality control plan that balances external control frequency with internal control processes for optimal quality of the test result.

DATA MANAGEMENT AND CONNECTIVITY

One concern of POCT is the volume of data that must be managed. Regulations mandate documentation of method validation before patient testing is performed for each individual device. Reagent shipments must be validated upon arrival and lot numbers tracked. Operators must document training and competency at defined intervals. Quality control results must be recorded and reviewed for trends. Patient results must be recorded in the medical record. For accreditation, a documentation trail must link each patient result to the operator (and his or her training and competency records), the reagent lot (and shipment validations), and the device serial number (and its validation and maintenance). For large health care systems with dozens of sites, hundreds of devices, and thousands of operators, the volume of data becomes enormous. Therefore, POCT devices have electronic data management features that enable them to automatically document required information during the testing process to meet accreditation requirements, later downloading this information to a computerized database for storage, review, and management. Some of these systems are proprietary, making change difficult. To overcome this issue, a communication standard, called POCT1-A, was developed. It has been transferred to the Clinical Laboratory Standards Institute for maintenance and revision.[27] This standard sets the communication specifications for devices that transfer control data and patient results from an individual POCT device to a computerized database or data manager. The patient data is then transfered to a laboratory or hospital information system where it is entered into the permanent medical record.

TECHNOLOGY USED IN POCT

Clinical personnel involved with POCT are oriented to obtaining results rapidly for immediate use for patient care and may not fully understand the need to comply with all the procedural and regulatory requirements associated with the test.To aid in compliance, a number of desirable characteristics are incorporated into many POCT devices; these are similar to, but also distinct from, those of laboratory-based diagnostic systems (Box 21-11). Significant differences include instrument portability and ease of use (i.e., no venipuncture or volumetric pipetting required), minimal technique dependence, and automated documentation functions that fulfill regulatory requirements.

Box 21-11

"Ideal" Point-of-Care System Testing Characteristics

Self-contained and portable
Flexible test menu
Minimal training
Ease of use; simple to operate
Accepts whole blood or urine
Accuracy and precision comparable with those of central laboratory systems
Minimum maintenance
Bar-coded test packs and controls to track lot and expiration dates
Room temperature stability
Able to print results
Interfaceable with laboratory and hospital information systems
Provides automatic calibration, system lockouts, and data management

Non–Instrument-Based Systems

The predominant forms of POCT consist of non–instrument-based systems that use a manual, visually read end point (Table 21-5). A variety of specimen types, including whole blood,

Table 21-5 Noninstrumental Technology Employed in POCT

Types of Assays	Assay Principle	Format	Specimen	Analytes
Qualitative	Chemical reactions	Impregnated paper strips	Feces	Occult blood
	Immunoconcentration	Dry reagent cartridges—single use	Urine and serum	hCG, Strep A
	Microparticle capture immunoassay	Dry reagent cartridges—single use	Urine	Drugs of abuse
	Latex agglutination	Dry reagent cartridges—single use	Amniotic fluid	Fetal lung maturity
			Blood	Therapeutic drugs Myoglobin
	Latex agglutination inhibition slides	Dry reagent cartridges—single use	Urine	Drug of abuse
	Immunochromatographic	Dry reagent cartridges—single use	Blood, plasma, and serum	CK-MB, troponin-I, troponin-T, myoglobin
		Dry reagent cartridges—single use	Urine	hCG
		Dry reagent cartridges—single use	Swabs	Chlamydia, Strep A, herpes
	Optical immunoassay	Dry reagent cartridges—single use	Swabs	Strep A, Strep B, influenza
Semiquantitative	Chemical/enzymatic reactions	Impregnated paper strips	Blood, urine	Glucose, urine chemistries
		Dry reagent cartridges—single use	Saliva	Ethanol
	Latex agglutination	Dry reagent cartridges—single use	Serum	Myoglobin
Quantitative	Chemical/enzymatic reactions	Dry reagent cartridges—single use	Blood	Lipids
	Immunochromatography	Dry reagent cartridges—single use	Blood, serum, and plasma	Therapeutic drugs, CK-MB

CK, Creatine kinase; *hCG,* human chorionic gonadotropin; *POCT,* point-of-care testing.

serum or plasma, urine, amniotic fluid, saliva, and feces, can be analyzed with the use of non–instrument-based POCT systems. Qualitative assays with a positive or negative indicator represent the predominant form of non–instrument-based POCT. Systems based on competitive or noncompetitive immunoassays are used to detect a variety of analytes, including human chorionic gonadotropin, drugs of abuse, indicators of fetal lung maturity, cardiac markers, and markers for infectious diseases. Other major qualitative assays include occult fecal blood testing and visually read blood glucose reagent strips. The glucose concentration can be semiquantified through visual comparison of color development on glucose reagent strips versus a color chart. Urine dipstick systems are also semiquantitative and use chemical and enzymatic reactions to generate a colored product that can be interpreted via comparison with a color chart printed on the side of the reagent bottle. A few non–instrument-based quantitative POCT systems employ chemical or enzymatic reactions and immunochromatographic techniques to determine concentrations of lipids, cardiac markers, and therapeutic drugs. These tests have the advantages of being inexpensive, requiring no instrumentation, and being easy to use in terms of training and interpretation. However, non–instrument-based systems require visual acuity and accurate timing. Overdevelopment can produce false-positive results, and underdevelopment can generate false-negative results. Non–instrument-based systems also have the major disadvantage of being completely manual, so there is no way to ensure compliance with performance of quality control or documentation of test results.

Instrument-Based Systems

Instrument-based POCT systems can be very sophisticated and highly automated, using a small sample size, requiring minimal routine and preventive maintenance, and eliminating calibration functions. This functionality is made possible by advances in reagent stabilization; by development and miniaturization of electrodes and biosensors; by the ability to produce relatively inexpensive, precise, disposable devices; and by the development of microcomputers and microelectronics. These advances in engineering and technology have allowed the incorporation of real-time process control and the encoding (through microchips and bar codes) of information (such as calibration data, lot number, and test name) into reagents and controls. Through the application of these technologies and processes, the manufacturer has engineered and automated into the device the major portion of quality assurance for laboratory test results.

Most POCT instruments require a minimum amount of technical support because they are relatively maintenance free. The devices are easy to operate and retain accuracy and precision with automatic periodic calibration. In addition, these instruments incorporate a number of characteristics of ideal POCT software that facilitates quality assurance (Box 21-12). Automatic documentation of patient results, quality control results, and device maintenance with attached comments and operator identification is a feature of several systems. Some analyzers have quality assurance software that allows automatic lockout of unauthorized users. Lockout features can be customized to prevent patient testing when quality control has not been performed or is out of range, when a valid or trained operator identification is not entered, or when a patient ID is not entered. Integration of data generated from POCT into the medical record is important for providing legal documentation for medical action and for billing.

Box 21-12
Ideal POCT Analyzer QA/QA Software

System lockouts that prevent patient testing when
- Quality control is not performed
- Quality control is out of range
- Patient identification is not entered
- Valid/trained operator identification is not entered

Calibration
  Automatic
  Slope/offset adjustments
Security access at several levels
Device location
User defined reportable/reference/quality control ranges
Alert value flagging
Delta checking
Data entry
Bar-code scanners
Touchscreens
Magnetic card readers
Data management
Patient result logs
Quality control logs
Maintenance logs

POCT, Point-of-care testing; *QA,* quality assurance.

POCT devices generally require only a few microliters of whole blood or urine. Internally, these instruments may test the analyte directly in the whole blood matrix, or the sample may be processed within the device by filtration or centrifugation so the red cells are removed to allow analysis of the analyte in the separated plasma. Many different technologies are currently employed in instrument-based POCT systems (Table 21-6). The most common instrument-based systems use reflectance photometry or biosensors. Some POCT systems employ new analytical concepts, such as optodes, paramagnetism, optical immunoassays, and centrifugal separation with optical signature analysis. Other POCT instruments are miniaturized versions of traditional laboratory analyzers, often using the same chemistries and incorporating ingenious techniques to internally generate plasma for analysis.

The ability to perform analytical processes with only a few microliters of blood prevents iatrogenic blood loss and is a major benefit of POCT. Newer alternatives eliminate all blood loss through the use of **ex vivo testing.** Ex vivo devices remove blood from the body, analyze it, and then reinfuse it. Two main approaches may be used with ex vivo monitoring systems: (1) flow-through sensors, similar to those found in the extracorporeal loop on a heart-lung bypass pump or

Table 21-6 Current Technology Employed in Instrument-Based POCT

Technology	Format	Sample Type	Precise Pipetting	Sample Volume, µL	Representative Systems	Testing
Photometry, reflectance	Dry reagent strip—single test	Whole blood	No	10-45	Glucose meter	Glucose
		Serum/plasma	Yes	10	Ektachem (Johnson and Johnson)	Chemistry and TDM
Photometry, transmittance	Wet reagent cartridges—single test	Whole blood Serum/plasma	No	≈20	Vision (Abbott)	Chemistry and drugs
	Dry reagent cartridges—single test	Whole blood	No	10	HemoCue (Hemocue)	Glucose and hemoglobin
			No	≈120	Careside (Careside)	
	Dry reagent cartridges—multiple tests	Whole blood Serum/plasma	No	≈90	Picolo (Abaxis)	Chemistry
Fluorometry	Dry reagent cartridges—multiple tests	Serum	No	20	IOS (Biocircuits)	Hormones
	Wet reagent cartridges—multiple tests	Whole blood Serum	No	3 mL draw tube	Alpha DX (Sigma) Stratus CS (Dade)	CK-MB, myoglobin, cTnI
Optodes	Dry reagent cartridges—multiple tests	Whole blood	No	80	AVL Opti (Roche)	Blood gases/electrolytes
				95	NPT7 (Radiometer)	
	Dry reagent cartridges—multiple tests, multiple use	Whole blood	No	80	AVL OptiR (Roche)	Blood gases/electrolytes
Potentiometry/ electrochemistry	Biosensor strips—single test	Whole blood	No	10	Precision PCX (Medisence)	Glucose
	Biosensor chips—multiple tests	Whole blood	No	≈70	PCA (i-Stat)	Chemistry/blood gases
				125	IRMA (Diametrics)	
	Miniature electrodes—multiple tests, multiple uses	Whole blood	No	150	Gem Premier (Instrumentation Labs)	Chemistry/blood gases
				180	ABL 77 (Radiometer)	
Immunochromatography	Dry reagent cartridges—single test	Whole blood	Yes	140	Triage (Biosite)	CK-MB, myoglobin, cTnI, BNP
				150	CardiacT Quant (Roche)	
Turbidimetry—latex agglutination inhibition	Dry coated latex particles cartridges—single use	Whole blood	No	10	DCA2000 (Bayer)	Hemoglobin A1c
	Dry paramagnetic particles motion reagent card—single use	Whole blood	No	1 large drop	Rapidpoint (Bayer)	ACT, PT, PTT
					CoaguChek (Roche)	PT
	Dry sample motion cartridges—single use	Whole blood	No	1 large drop	Biotrack (Roche), Hemochron Jr (International Technidyne)	ACT, PT, PTT
	Dry reagent tubes—single use	Whole blood	No	2 mL	Hemochron Response (International Technidyne), Hepcon (Medtronics)	ACT, PT, PTT Heparin, protamine
Luminescence/fiberoptic	Intra-arterial catheter	Not applicable	Not applicable	Not applicable	PB3300 (Puritan Bennett), Paratrend Sensor (Agilent Technologies)	Blood gases
Centrifugal separation—optical signature analysis	Single-use capillary tube	Whole blood	No	250	QBC Autoread (Becton Dickinson)	Hct, HgB, platelets, granulocytes, lymphocytes/monocytes

ACT, Activated clotting time; *BNP*, brain natriuretic peptide; *CK-MB*, creatine kinase-MB fraction; *cTnI*, cardiac troponin I; *Hct*, hematocrit; *HgB*, hemoglobin; *PT*, prothrombin time; *PTT*, partial thromboplastin time; *TDM*, therapeutic drug monitoring.

plasmapheresis machine, and (2) withdrawal, in which blood is removed from the body, analyzed, and then reinfused (e.g., Via Medical devices for analysis of pH, blood gases, electrolytes, hematocrit, and glucose). Other approaches that may be used to reduce blood loss employ intravascular **in vivo** monitoring. With in vivo blood-gas and pH monitors, the sensors are located on or near the tip of a single fiberoptic probe that is inserted through a catheter, typically into the radial artery. Probe placement is essential for proper functioning and does not impede blood flow.

The major advantage of instrument-based POCT systems is their ability to automate data management, maintenance, and calibration functions while testing a wide menu of analytes, quantitatively, in a small amount of sample. Unfortunately, instrument-based POCT systems are more expensive than non–instrument-based technologies, are more complicated to operate, and require more staff training.

Noninvasive/Minimally Invasive Technology

Minimally invasive and noninvasive POCT reduces or eliminates the need for specimen withdrawal. Many minimally invasive technologies have focused on glucose measurements. With the requirement of only 0.3 to 1.5 μL of blood, sampling can be done at sites where fewer pain receptors are present than in capillary fingerstick (e.g., the forearm). Diabetic patients complain about the pain of repeated fingersticks, and alternative site testing ensures better patient compliance with frequent glucose self-monitoring. Interstitial fluid analysis is another mechanism for providing minimally invasive glucose monitoring. Interstitial fluid is different from plasma in that glucose levels in plasma precede levels in interstitial fluid by 15 to 20 minutes—the time required for glucose to diffuse from the intravascular to the extravascular space. This lag time may change, depending on the patient's condition and how rapidly glucose levels are changing. Several continuous glucose meters that use interstitial fluid for analysis are currently available or are under development. These devices are calibrated every few days against a fingerstick glucose meter result and can provide an interstitial glucose level every few minutes for up to 4 or more days. The term *continuous* is somewhat of a misnomer, in that all of the continuous devices sample only every few seconds to minutes, and the software in the device averages several levels over time to produce a smoothed trending curve. Although continuous glucose monitors are not as accurate or precise as glucose meters or laboratory analyzers, the software algorithms can provide a rate of change, in addition to an absolute level. This trend can estimate the magnitude of glucose change over time and can predict hypoglycemic events before they occur, allowing intervention to prevent the event.

In addition to minimally invasive devices, several noninvasive systems are currently available on the market: pulse oximeters for O_2 saturation, end-tidal CO_2 measurements for Pco_2, transcutaneous and conjunctival Po_2/Pco_2 measurements, and transcutaneous bilirubin measurements. These systems do not provide exact measurements but are used as trend indicators, providing continuous monitoring of analyte level. Similar to continuous glucose monitors, these devices have the ability to rapidly recognize a change in status. The use of noninvasive devices results in fewer infection control problems and better self-monitoring compliance rates produced by elimination of the discomfort of multiple fingersticks.

KEY CONCEPTS BOX 21-4

- POCT errors can be managed by strict compliance with regulations, a tight quality control (QC) program, and good data management.
- Whereas external QC tests both sample processing and testing functions, internal POCT can only test the latter.
- Non-instrumental POCT devices are manual systems, more prone to sample ID, testing, and interpretation errors. Instrument POCT devices are much less susceptable to these errors but are often more costly.

REFERENCES

1. Nichols JH, Christenson RH, Clarke W, et al: *National Academy of Clinical Biochemistry Laboratory Medicine Practice Guidelines: Evidence Based Practice for Point of Care Testing,* Washington, DC, 2006, AACC Press.
2. Nichols JH, Christenson RH, Clarke W, et al: Evidence based practice for point of care testing: an NACB laboratory medicine practice guideline, Clin Chim Acta 379:14, 2007.
3. International Organization for Standardization. Available at http://www.iso.org/iso/home.htm.
4. Code of Federal Regulations (10/98) Part 493 Laboratory Requirements. Available at http://www.fda.gov/cdrh/CLIA/CLIAfedregin.html.
5. U.S. Food and Drug Administration Centers for Devices and Radiologic Health. Available at http://www.fda.gov/cdrh/.
6. Conformite Europene Council Directive Concerning Medical Devices, 93/42 EEC 14, June 1993. Available at http://www.thequalityportal.com/q_cemark.htm.
7. College of American Pathologists. Available at http://www.cap.org/apps/cap.portal?_nfpb=true&_pageLabel=home.
8. The Joint Commission. Available at http://www.jointcommission.org/.
9. COLA (formerly Commission on Office Laboratory Accreditation). Available at http://www.cola.org/.
10. Forsman RW: Why is the laboratory an afterthought for managed care? Clin Chem 42:813, 1996.
11. Becich MJ: Information management: moving from test results to clinical information, Clin Leadersh Manage Rev 14:296, 2006.
12. Nichols JH, Kickler TS, Dyer KL, et al: Clinical outcomes of point-of-care testing in the interventional radiology and invasive cardiology setting, Clin Chem 46:543, 2000.
13. Cagliero E, Levina E, Nathan D: Immediate feedback of HbA1c levels improves glycemic control in type 1 and insulin-treated type 2 diabetic patients, Diabetes Care 22:1785, 1999.
14. Thaler LM, Ziemer DC, Gallina DL, et al: Diabetes in urban African-Americans, XVII: availability of rapid HbA1c measurements enhances clinical decision-making, Diabetes Care 22:1415, 1999.
15. Miller CD, Barnes CS, Phillips LS, et al: Rapid A1c availability improves clinical decision-making in an urban primary care clinic, Diabetes Care 26:1158, 2003.
16. Grieve R, Beech R, Vincent J, et al: Near patient testing in diabetes clinics: appraising the costs and outcomes, Health Technol Assess 3:1, 1999.

17. Nichols JH, Bartholomew C, Bonzagi A, et al: Evaluation of the IRMA TRUpoint and i-STAT creatinine assays, Clin Chim Acta 377:201, 2007.
18. Ansell J, Hirsh J, Poller L, et al: The pharmacology and management of vitamin K antagonists: the Seventh ACCP Conference on Antithrombotic and Thrombolytic Therapy, Chest 126 (3 suppl):204S, 2004.
19. Choudry R, Scheitel SM, Stroebel RJ, et al: Patient satisfaction with point-of-care international normalized ratio testing and counseling in a community internal medicine practice, Managed Care Interface 17:44, 2004.
20. Chen ET, Nichols JH, Duh SH, et al: Performance evaluation of blood glucose monitoring devices, Diabetes Technol Ther 5:749, 2003.
21. Webb R, Currier M, Weir J, et al: Transmission of hepatitis B virus among persons undergoing blood glucose monitoring in long-term care facilities—Mississippi, North Carolina, and Los Angeles County, California, 2003-2004, MMWR 54:220, 2005.
22. U.S. Department of Health and Human Services, Office of Inspector General: *Enrollment and Certification Processes in the Clinical Laboratory Improvement Amendments Program,* Washington, DC, 2001, U.S. Department of Health and Human Services. Available at http://oig.hhs.gov/oei/reports/oei-05-00-00251.pdf (October 2007).
23. Centers for Medicaid and Medicare Services: *Certificate of Waiver and Provider Performed Microscopy Procedures Pilot Project,* Washington, DC, 2003, U.S. Department of Health and Human Services. Available at http://www.cms.hhs.gov/CLIA/downloads/ppmpfr2001.pdf (October 2007).
24. Clinical Laboratory Standards Institute: *EP-18, Risk Management Techniques to Identify and Control Laboratory Error Sources,* Wayne, PA, CLSI, 2007.
25. Clinical Laboratory Standards Institute: *EP-22, Presentation of Manufacturer's Risk Mitigation Information for Users of* In Vitro *Diagnostic Devices,* Wayne, PA, CLSI, in press.
26. Clinical Laboratory Standards Institute: *EP23, Laboratory Quality Control Based on Risk Management,* Wayne, PA, CLSI, in press.
27. Dubois JA, Dunka L, Allred T, et al: *POCT1-A2, Point-of-Care Connectivity, Approved Standard,* ed 2, Wayne, PA, 2006, CLSI, pp. 1-306.

INTERNET SITES

http://www.aacc.org/members/divisions/cpoct/pages—AACC Division of Point-of-Care Testing (for members only)
www.diabetes.org—American Diabetes Association
www.cap.org—College of American Pathologists
www.cola.org—Commission on Office Laboratory Accreditation
www.iso.org—International Organization for Standardization
www.jointcommission.org—The Joint Commission
www.pointofcare.net—Medical Automation Systems POCT Information Site
www.aacc.org/members/nacb/pages/default.aspx—National Academy of Clinical Biochemistry
www.guideline.gov—National Guideline Clearinghouse
www.tmf.org—TMF Health Quality Institute

Chapter 22

Laboratory Information Systems

David Chou

Chapter Outline

Key Terms

ADT (admissions/discharge/transfer) Administrative and demographic patient information provided by a central computer covering patient admissions, transfers, and discharges.

archived data Patient data that have been placed in a form that is not immediately accessible by the user without intervention by a computer operator.

backup A procedure, usually performed daily, by which operational data on disks are transferred to a secondary medium, usually magnetic tape. Normally, data on these tapes will be restored to disk only in the event that the disk fails.

bar code A series of parallel lines or squares of varying thickness, printed in a fashion to represent numbers or numbers and letters, that can be read by automated equipment.

bidirectional interface A program that allows electronic communications between an instrument and a laboratory information system (LIS), permitting the interchange of information in both directions.

central processing unit (CPU) The part of the computer responsible for executing programs and making decisions (i.e., the brains of the computer).

client A locally networked computer that accesses data from other remotely networked computers, called *servers.* Data on the client also may be sent to the server for processing and/or storage.

CPOE (computerized provider order entry) CPOE allows clinical providers to order laboratory tests and other procedures electronically rather than by paper.

cumulative report A report designed to display results over a period of time for a single patient in a tabular fashion.

data structure The organization of data as they are stored in the computer.

database manager A program designed to manage the storage and retrieval of data to and from computer storage media such as disks and/or tapes.

delta check A method of quality control by which the current patient result is compared with a previous patient result.

EMR (electronic medical record) An electronic database and computer system designed to replace the paper medical record; it includes results reporting, order entry, image storage and retrieval, and administrative activities.

Ethernet A common family of electrical, wiring, and physical connection standards used for connecting computers into local networks and the Internet.

firewall A term used for an electronic device that controls the type of information that can enter or leave a local network. Most often, firewalls are designed to prevent unwanted intrusions into a computer system.

hardware The physical parts of a computer. After manufacturing, hardware updates and changes occur much less frequently than changes to software.

HIPAA (The Health Insurance Portability and Accountability Act of 1996) A federal law that addresses health insurance reform, mandates the use of standardized electronic data interfaces, and sets standards for the privacy of medical records and data security.

The Joint Commission A private voluntary organization that sets standards for, performs inspections of, and accredits hospitals and other health care organizations. Joint Commission inspections may serve in lieu of federal and state inspections.

inbox or physician inbox A means by which an EMR provides new laboratory results to the ordering physician or to another specified provider for review.

incomplete list An LIS report listing specimens that have not yet been processed. Different incomplete lists may be printed for each task performed in the laboratory.

informatics Informatics studies the representation, processing/transformation, and communication of information in natural and artificial systems by organisms or artifacts such as computers.

interpretive reports Reports generated to provide information to the clinician that differs depending on the results; these reports describe possible treatments or diagnostic possibilities for a given set of results.

intranet Web, file sharing, and other Internet-like services provided for an institution's or organization's private internal use.

middleware Software and hardware inserted between an instrument and an LIS to facilitate management of the instrument, validation of results, and reporting.

network or digital computer network The use of cable television, microwave, fiberoptic, or telephone lines to permit communications between computers in a group.

online Data that are kept in a computer in a manner that allows immediate access.

operating system Software designed to supervise the orderly execution of programs and provide support for basic functions used by most programs.

order entry The action of entering test orders into a computer system. This order process may occur on the LIS or on a remote computer linked to the LIS.

patient demographics Pertinent clinical and administrative patient information collected at the time of patient admission. These include patient number, name, sex, age, and birth date, as well as other information related to the patient.

personal computer A small desktop computer designed to be used by a single user in the office or home environment and costing between $500 and $5,000.

privacy The need to ensure that data are accessed only by authorized individuals and parties.

program A series of instructions that direct computer hardware to perform specified actions.

run As defined by the Clinical Laboratory Improvement Amendments of 1988 (CLIA '88), a run is an interval within which the accuracy and precision of a testing system are expected to be stable but cannot be greater than 24 hours.

security The need to protect data from being unintentionally accessed and altered. Also, see "privacy".

server A networked computer, which may be remote, that acts as a data storage center for data generated by clients (see client).

software Collectively, the programs that operate the computer.

software maintenance Changes in software intended to fix problems, to improve functionality, or to provide new capabilities.

specimen number A number assigned to a sample by the LIS for identification purposes. This number may be reused periodically and must not duplicate the number of any specimen that is still being processed.

table maintenance Activities that update commonly changed information in an LIS, such as test names, reference ranges, patient locations, reagent lot numbers, and so forth.

unidirectional interface A program that permits electronic communication between an LIS and an instrument, permitting the instrument to send or upload information to the LIS.

Uniform Resource Locator (URL) A unique name assigned to an Internet resource that is translated to a single numerical address that identifies a computer. URLs make it convenient for users to access specific websites.

validation The process whereby a technologist reviews one or more analyses and releases the results to the patient file for reporting.

virus A software program, often destructive in nature, that is designed to embed itself into the operating system or other commonly available software.

work flow Refers to those processes, human or automated, that are associated with the collection and generation of data and how an information system captures them (e.g., specimen receipt by a laboratory).

worklist A list of specimen numbers generated by a technologist before performing a specified task, such as an analytical run or a specimen collection.

The laboratory information system, or LIS, can be defined as the applications software and associated **operating systems,** other **software,** and **hardware** needed to run **programs** that support the operational and management needs of a clinical laboratory. To handle laboratory variations, the software and hardware used and the functions of an LIS can differ significantly as it is implemented from one laboratory to another. The LIS structures tasks, or the **work flow,** and assists in the management of data produced by the laboratory. *Work flow* broadly refers to how the work received by the laboratory is processed and analyzed. An LIS, therefore, must be closely attuned to the needs of each laboratory and its organization. Likewise, the LIS requires reconfiguration as instrumentation and testing change. The computer can be a powerful tool for improving productivity and quality; unlike an automated instrument, which most affects testing and analysis, the LIS also affects the preanalytical and postanalytical parts of the laboratory. For example, physicians may request changes to the way an LIS reports results to assist them in their practice.

LIS vendors, similar to most software developers, depend on technologies provided by others in the computer industry. The development of an application, such as the LIS, depends on other software and tools such as the **database manager,** the programming language(s) and their associated libraries, and the operating system. To operate, software requires hardware, the physical computer itself. This multi-vendor technology chain presents complications, as well as benefits. For example, a problem with an LIS program may be related to a defect in the operating system developed by another vendor, who is unable to correct the problem. On the other hand, vendors of applications software usually finds it easier and cheaper to develop software tools and hardware received from others than to develop similar software and hardware themselves. Most hardware today is comparatively inexpensive. Software development and personnel for support and implementation account for most of the cost of systems purchased today.

SECTION OBJECTIVES BOX 22-1

- Briefly summarize how LIS support functions affect preanalytical, analytical, and postanalytical functions of the laboratory.
- Describe the three analytical functions of LIS.
- Explain the various laboratory uses of barcodes.

Box 22-1

Laboratory Information System (LIS) Functions

Preanalytical

Test ordering
Preparation of phlebotomy draw lists
Phlebotomy (labels, collection times)
Specimen accessioning and aliquoting
Specimen tracking

Analytical

Manual worklist
Instrument worklist
Manual results entry
Automated results entry through interfaces
Patient delta check
Quality control
Results validation
Interfaces to laboratory automation systems

Postanalytical

Noncumulative patient chart reports
Cumulative patient chart reports
Immediate remote report printing
Electronic results inquiry
Historical patient archiving
Workload recording
Results correction
Billing
Results interfaces with other systems

LIS CHARACTERISTICS

Overall Functions

An LIS supports functions that allow a laboratory to control and monitor the execution of critical actions (Box 22-1). These functions include those servicing (1) preanalytical steps, including phlebotomy, specimen collection labels and lists, specimen tracking, and **order entry;** (2) testing and analysis steps, including manual results entry, results verification, and interfaces to automated instrumentation, and (3) postanalytical steps for results reporting, intersystem computer interfaces, management reporting, and financial and billing functions. An LIS may operate as a module of an integrated system or may operate as a stand-alone system that is connected to other systems through interfaces. An integrated environment offers the benefits of simplifying support because users need to work with only a single vendor. Larger LISs, however, are more complex to maintain, and coordination is required when changes are needed; in addition, customization may be difficult unless the change is desired by a large number of users. Stand-alone LISs allow greater autonomy but require interfaces when information is required from or must be sent to another system. Some packaged systems are stand-alone systems that are interfaced to other systems from the same vendor.

For marketing purposes, vendors may subdivide the LIS into modules. Typically, these modules include one for the general laboratory supporting high-volume hematology and chemistry testing, a microbiology module, a blood bank module, and an anatomical pathology module. Rarely will institutions use separate vendors for the general laboratory and specialty laboratory areas, such as blood bank, anatomical pathology, or customer billing. Most of the following sections discuss features of an LIS that supports the general laboratory.

LIS ROLE IN PREANALYTICAL ACTIVITIES

Patient Demographics

Before a test can be requested, the patient must be entered into the system with an identifying number and other patient-specific information, called **patient demographics.** Most hospitals assign a permanent patient identifier for this purpose. Systems that service reference laboratories or outreach programs may define patients under the auspices of the **client** who is sending the test. A clerk can manually enter demographic information into the LIS. Alternatively, an interface between an LIS and an **ADT** (for admissions, discharge, and transfer) administrative computer system allows the information to be transmitted to the LIS as needed during test request processing, upon admission of the patient to the hospital, or when a patient is scheduled for an outpatient visit. ADT interfaces significantly reduce data entry errors and data entry time. Demographic information entered at this time includes (1) patient number or other identifier, (2) patient name, (3) sex, (4) age or birth date, (5) referring or attending physician who should receive reports, and (6) admitting diagnosis. Most systems also capture patient information such as height and weight and billing/accounting information. If a patient number cannot be determined, such as when an unconscious patient is handled in an emergency room, the laboratory may assign a temporary pseudo number and pseudo name. These pseudo data must be changed later and merged into a record with the proper patient information.

Box 22-2

Data Acquired During Order Entry Process

1. A patient identifier, such as a patient number and a patient name
2. One or more ordering physicians or providers
3. One or more physicians receiving reports, along with their reporting locations
4. Test request time and date
5. Time the specimen was collected or will be collected
6. Person entering the request
7. Tests to be performed
8. Priority of the test request (e.g., stat, now, routine)
9. Diagnosis (e.g., ICDA9 code) or other medical reason for the test
10. Any special comments or instructions pertaining to the request

Order Entry

Following admission of the patient, the next LIS interaction usually involves processing a test request, also known as *order entry.* Orders may be received by the LIS through a computer-to-computer interface, for example, by an **electronic medical record (EMR),** from which nursing personnel or physicians can directly perform the test request. This is called **CPOE,** or **computerized provider order entry.** Alternatively, the laboratory may receive a paper requisition from a clinical area, and laboratory personnel can enter the test request into the LIS. Typically, order entry requires the entry, or acquisition, of the information listed in Box 22-2. In some cases, such as with CPOE, the information may be implicitly provided as part of the work flow. For example, the system will know which provider is ordering the test by knowing the logged-in user. Data collected during order entry identify the patient, the person(s) ordering the tests, the tests themselves, and the reasons for ordering the tests. Information collected at this time is used for administrative/billing/legal, as well as medical, purposes.

The LIS may automatically perform validity checks on entered data. Most systems have internal tables with lists of valid entries such as laboratory and nursing personnel, ordering physicians, patient locations, available laboratory tests, and reasonable test order dates (e.g., a specimen received today should not have been collected two months ago). These tables prevent the entry of erroneous information but also require updates; this is referred to as **table maintenance.** Institutions also incorporate a check-digit as part of the patient number. This is usually a single digit added to the patient number that is computed during data entry from other digits in the patient number. If the computed number does not match the check-digit, the data entry is rejected. For example, assume that the patient number is 12345676 and the last digit is the check-digit. If a user types 22345676 and the check-digit calculation results in a 7, the computer rejects the patient number because it is expecting a 6. Check-digits do not guarantee accuracy, but they do help reduce errors.

Test requesting in the order entry process appears deceptively simple, but numerous details complicate the process.[1] Even checking for duplicate orders by computer can be complicated, in that a check for a single test must include situations in which it is ordered as a single test or as a component of a test panel. The allowable interval between duplicate test orders will depend on a number of factors, such as the ordering physician, the patient's location, the test, and the cost of performing the test. For example, two electrolyte panels ordered in an intensive care unit within an hour would be reasonable, but a similar order from an outpatient clinic would be unreasonable. A daily testosterone level, however, is rarely needed for an inpatient or an outpatient. For most tests, determining the appropriateness of a test order requires knowledge of the clinical situation, and such information may not be available at the time tests are ordered, even with physician order entry. Determination of the appropriate duplicate test interval can be formidable, and checks can add overhead to the order entry process. Most often, the LIS checks for duplicate orders and leaves it to the operator to decide whether an order is appropriate. In general, ordering rules are difficult to implement, and they are relatively ineffective in changing ordering behavior and reducing the frequency of test ordering.

The order entry process itself can be a source of substantial errors. One study of nearly 115,000 requisitions reported that 4.8% had at least one error associated with the process, and 10% of institutions reported that 18% or more of requisitions had errors.[2] Errors may result from clerical errors in the laboratory or nursing unit. CPOE reduces some clerical errors,[3] but it requires that the physician spend time entering orders and may introduce physician-generated errors.

Phlebotomy

When the specimen is collected, laboratory personnel log it into the LIS as it is about to be collected or is being received. With automated equipment linked to the LIS, the receiving

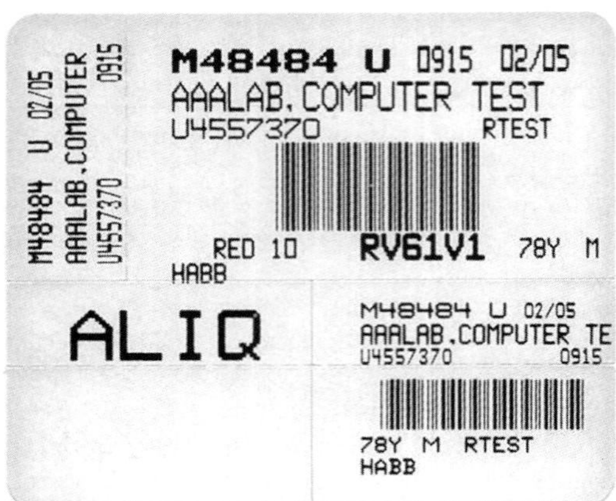

Fig. 22-1 An example of a bar-coded specimen label. The specimen number (M48484) is bar-coded. The patient number, patient demographics, time/date, and test are written in human readable form. The label is perforated, so it can be applied to both the primary specimen tube and its aliquoted (ALIQ) samples.

step can be automated (see Chapter 20). Otherwise, the computer places the test requisition onto a collection list for future collection. In either case, the LIS then creates a specimen label containing collection information, such as patient name, number, location, sex, and age or birth date, as well as tests ordered and collection container type to be used (Fig. 22-1). Most specimen labels also include a specimen, or accession, number, which is a tracking number that allows the computer to reference that sample back to a specific test request and patient. **Specimen numbers** may be assigned for each phlebotomy transaction or, less commonly, for each orderable test. Another approach, which is used by larger laboratories, requires separate specimen numbers for different processing areas or for many of the larger laboratory automation systems. To keep numbers short, the LIS sometimes recycles specimen numbers. Systems that reuse specimen numbers must check to see whether a number is inactive before reassigning it. Some systems assign a permanent specimen number by combining a date code with a number. Although this offers the advantages of a permanent specimen number, the larger number adds to the work associated with manual data entry. In most cases, the LIS assigns a specimen number at the time of test requisition, but for tests ordered for the future, this assignment may occur later. Some systems allow users to reserve specimen numbers for manual assignment. Although this is convenient under conditions such as computer failure, manual assignment of specimen numbers greatly increases errors, especially if the same specimen number is assigned accidentally to multiple patients.

Bar Codes

Bar codes consist of a series of lines or squares of varying widths that represent numbers, or letters and numbers, and are readable by automated equipment. A number of bar-code formats may be used. Most bar codes used in the laboratory are linear, constructed from parallel lines. The most common of this format are Code 39 and Code 128. Code 39 can represent numbers and uppercase alphabets. Code 128 can represent numbers, uppercase/lowercase letters, and some special symbols. For the labeling of blood products, ISBT-128, a special variant of Code 128, is used.[4] Two-dimensional bar codes consist of squares of varying sizes ordered in rows that can store much more information, such as calibration data for reagents.

Bar codes are also used to identify reagents and other products used by the clinical laboratory. Bar-coded reagents can be used to efficiently monitor inventory and reagent use on instruments. Through the use of devices connected to suppliers and instrument vendors, reagent use can be monitored automatically and replacement reagents supplied as depleted.

Specimen label bar coding decreases errors in specimen handling and increases productivity. For maximum benefit, specimen bar coding must be carefully coordinated with automated instrumentation; preferably, the instrument will have the ability to automatically read bar-coded labels applied to the tube. Misapplication of the specimen label on the specimen tube can cause instruments to misread bar codes. Mechanical limitations of instruments and the use of small venipuncture tubes (for pediatric purposes) may impose limitations on the use of bar codes. Larger bar codes read more reliably but compete for label space with valuable human readable information.

The patient number usually is not included in the specimen bar code because it is not unique to a given test request. Only the specimen number or a part of the specimen number is typically bar-coded. Standards have been developed for bar codes used on specimen containers handled by instruments.[5]

For samples to be collected for future scheduled phlebotomy procedures, the LIS prints up a collection list and specimen collection labels (Fig. 22-2). These specimen labels can also serve as the phlebotomy list. The LIS often prints additional labels for aliquots or other purposes, either as part of the initial test request or on demand. After specimen collection, the phlebotomist or a clerk verifies collected samples and deletes or reschedules uncollected requests in the LIS. To further increase accuracy, specimen collection may occur with portable computers, or PDAs (for portable data assistants), portable bar-code printers, and bar-code readers connected to the LIS via wireless network. Coupled with bar-coded patient armbands and wireless connections to the LIS, the system can verify that the correct patient is being drawn. These systems allow bar codes to be applied to the specimen at the point of collection and significantly reduce errors, but their costs are high.[6] Bar coding reduces many errors, but errors are still possible. For example, a phlebotomist can apply a specimen label to a tube from the wrong patient.

Following collection, the specimen must be prepared for transport or analysis If processing occurs at a satellite, the LIS can track the sample, schedule required transportation, determine specimen location, and help locate lost specimens. Automated specimen tracking can provide labor-saving benefits in a larger laboratory, where clinicians frequently add extra tests to samples presumed to be in the laboratory. In such

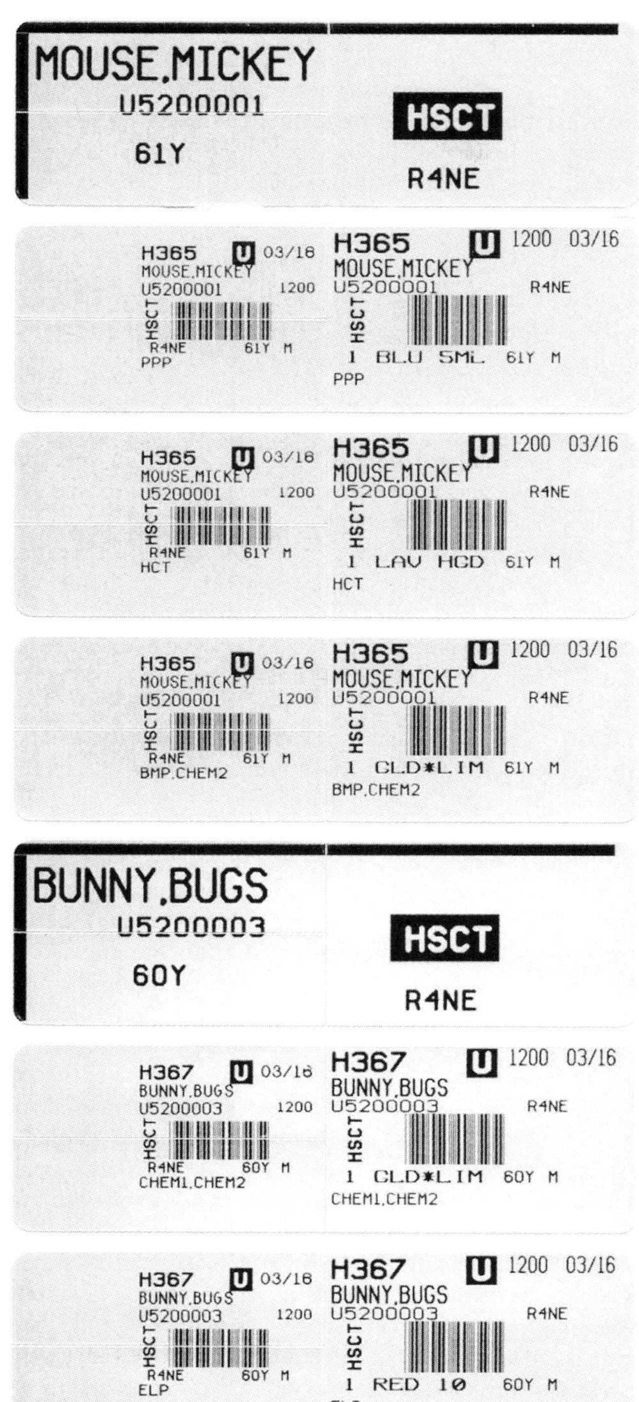

Fig. 22-2 A draw list using bar-coded specimen labels. The labels bar-code the specimen number—one for each collection tube type. Aliquot labels are available on the left of the bar-coded specimen label.

cases, the technologist must locate a sample, enter the add-on test into the LIS, and print a new specimen label. If one cannot be found, a test request must be entered into the LIS for re-collection by a phlebotomist or nurse. The complexity of the process for handling add-on testing frequently results in errors. Tracking specimens, however, adds complexity to the installation of an LIS because the LIS must have knowledge of anticipated paths for specimens, and some manual steps are needed in the handling process to inform the LIS of the specimen status.

KEY CONCEPTS BOX 22-1

- The laboratory information system (LIS) controls and monitors the preanalytical, analytical, and postanalytical phases of testing.
- The LIS may exist as a complete stand-alone system or as part of a larger integrated system in which the LIS manufacturer provides all necessary computer functions for an institution.
- Patient information must be entered correctly into the admissions, discharge, and transfer (ADT) system before any testing can occur.
- An order for lab testing can be made with the use of paper requests or can be entered directly into the laboratory information system (LIS) by physicians. Direct ordering is more rapid and produces fewer errors.
- Phlebotomy orders are created by the LIS, which also can be used to reduce the errors associated with the blood collection.
- *Specimen numbers* identify and track specimens.
- *Bar codes* provide a way to perform some of these tasks automatically.

SECTION OBJECTIVES BOX 22-2

- Explain the difference between a unidirectional and a bidirectional interface.
- Describe three ways by which a worklist may be created.
- Explain why a data manager is used for point-of-care LIS.
- Describe the role of LIS in autoverification.

LIS ROLE IN TESTING AND ANALYSIS

Instruments and Interfaces

Because automated instruments perform most high-volume testing, interfacing these instruments to an LIS greatly improves productivity and decreases errors. Before an instrument can be interfaced, however, two conditions must be satisfied. First, the LIS and the instrument must be linked by a physical connection. Today, most such connections are made through a point-to-point **Ethernet** connection over a network. Second, interface software must be made available on the LIS to allow it to receive data from and transmit data to the instrument. The Clinical Laboratory Standards Institute (CLSI) has developed standards to facilitate the interfacing of instruments to an LIS.[7] Standards do not always guarantee easy compatibility, but they can significantly decrease problems with incompatibilities. Most instrument manufacturers do provide LIS vendors with interface specifications before instruments are introduced into the marketplace, to allow time for interface software development. Interfaces, however, often are customized for each instrument, and different interfaces may be needed for different versions of the same instrument or specific needs of a laboratory.

In an interfaced instrument, each specimen must be linked to its specific test request, typically through a bar-coded specimen number. The instrument reads the bar-coded specimen label and transmits the number to the LIS, along with the analytical results. An interface is **unidirectional** if the instrument only transmits or uploads results to the LIS computer; the interface is **bidirectional** if the LIS simultaneously transmits or downloads information to and receives uploaded information from the instrument. The most common information downloaded to an instrument from the LIS is a list of tests requested for the specimen. A bidirectionally interfaced instrument first transmits the specimen number to the LIS; the LIS then returns the information on which tests have been ordered, and finally, the instrument sends the results to the LIS. Communications and interactions between the host LIS computer and the instrument can be complex. Adding to this complexity is that many instruments reject specimens if they do not receive a response from the LIS after sending a bar-coded specimen number, making processing slow or impossible if the LIS becomes unavailable.

If the instrument cannot identify the specimen automatically through the interface, the operator must manually enter specimen numbers and tests performed into the instrument and/or the LIS. The order in which the LIS processes specimens for a specified instrument is called a **worklist** or a loadlist. At least three ways are used to create the worklist. The first and most laborious method is to have the operator manually create ("build") a worklist on the LIS containing the specimen numbers and instrument position. For example, position 1 on the instrument contains specimen A, position 2 contains specimen B, and so forth. The second method simplifies this by having the operator enter only the specimen number, with the tray position implicitly provided by the worksheet position. This method requires that results are released from the instrument in the order that specimens are processed. These first two approaches can be simplified by entering patient specimen numbers with a bar-code scanner interfaced to an LIS. The third approach is to have the computer automatically build a worklist, typically in the order that specimens are received or in sample number order, and to have the operator load the instrument in that order. This frees the operator from entering the information needed for the worklist but requires him or her to locate specimens and load them in the specified order. For the smaller laboratory, the computer-generated worklist will be more efficient in that the receiving area often can place the specimens in computer-specified order. In the larger laboratory, multiple receiving areas complicate the specimen receipt order, making it easier for the operator to specify explicitly the worklist by one of the first two approaches, rather than searching for a specific specimen.

Some instruments, such as blood-gas analyzers, process samples on a one-at-a-time basis. Test ordering frequently occurs at the time of analysis, rather than in advance. For such instruments, the interaction between the analyzer, the LIS, and the operator will be greater and more labor intensive than for other instruments. The test request, result reporting, and **validation** processes are similar to those of instruments mentioned earlier but occur serially and manually for each sample. Some older hematology analyzers also operate in this fashion.

Total Laboratory Automation

(See also Chapter 20.)

Total laboratory automation (TLA) refers to a highly automated laboratory environment where robotics, conveyors, other mechanical devices, and computer systems significantly decrease the human handling of samples. A front-end automation device usually performs many steps associated with preanalytical sample handling, such as centrifugation, decapping, aliquoting, and sorting. Specimen handlers, conveyors, and robotic arms transfer specimens to and from parts of the laboratory, the automation devices, and instrumentation. Once analysis has been performed, specimens are sorted and routed to storage and refrigeration, if needed, where they can be retrieved.

TLAs most often require the LIS to be modified significantly; these modifications have been designated as a third-generation design.[8] For example, although the LIS often generates a single specimen number for each patient contact, which may include several collection tubes, most TLAs require that each tube possess a unique specimen number, so that it can be properly routed. An LIS may be interfaced to the TLA through a separate laboratory automation system (LAS), a computer system specially designed for managing the automation devices and directing specimens. In such cases, the LIS often treats the TLA as an automated instrument.

The LIS usually interacts with the analytical instruments in a TLA in a conventional manner. LIS validation of results also is likely to be similar to that of conventional automated instruments, whereby an operator reviews results before they are released for general use. In most TLAs and with most high-volume instruments, manual verification may be replaced or supplemented with some form of autoverification algorithm to increase the accuracy and efficiency of verifying results. Autoverification is an approach whereby an LIS uses a defined set of parameters, such as the reference range value, in releasing results (see section on data verification).

Integrating Off-Site Testing

(See Chapter 21.)

Changes in microchip technology have led to improved LIS interfacing of point-of-care testing (POCT) devices. This is very important in that users of these devices may fail to document the testing event or the test results in the patient's chart, especially the electronic record, both of which are legally required. Increasingly, point-of-care instruments support the electronic uploading of results into an LIS. In such cases, the laboratory is typically responsible for this uploading.

In an attempt to address the problems of documenting results from off-site testing, POCT vendors have developed interface standards.[9] POCT devices, such as glucose meters, sell for less than $100. Because most LIS instrument interfaces cost 10 to 100 times this amount, LIS and POCT vendors and users all have avoided interfacing LISs and POCT instruments. To make interfacing costs acceptable, a point-of-care data manager is used; this is usually a **personal computer** with special software. The data manager acts as an intermediary by receiving data from one or more portable devices through a plug-in cradle and transmitting through preexisting wires, or through an infrared transmitter. Once the data have been uploaded into the data manager, it makes an LIS test request or finds an existing one, uploads the result through an interface along with other pertinent patient information, documents and checks devices for proper maintenance, and ensures proper operational procedures. Because both the LIS/data manager and the POCT instrument/data manager interfaces are standardized, it is possible for a single data manager to service many POCT instruments.

Results Entry

Automated

The interaction between a technologist and automated instrumentation has been discussed previously. With an interfaced instrument, the results entry process proceeds automatically, usually after the specimen has been received by the laboratory. Most LISs place unverified results in a pending area to await the technologist, who manually reviews and validates the entered results (see previous section). This holding area limits results access to those in the laboratory. Upon validation, results are released for reporting to external users. A number of LIS features may be available to help the technologist during the review process. Typically, these include the display of flags signifying results outside reference ranges, life-threatening results (critical or "panic" values), results outside technical ranges, or other checks described under Quality Assurance. Most LISs also can display previous results for the same tests, allowing the operator to do a **"delta check,"** for discrepant results that may suggest a misanalysis or a sample misidentification. Most instruments produced today for the clinical laboratory support automated interfaces.

Manual

The laboratory must perform manual results entry for specimens analyzed manually and for tests performed on instruments that are not interfaced. Most instruments that are not interfaced are low volume or perform specialized testing. For such instruments, an interface may require highly complex and idiosyncratic software, forcing the LIS vendor to price it prohibitively high for most users, or it may have such a low volume that it is not cost-effective. Manual results entry also may be used when interfaces have failed, or under special conditions such as abnormal tests being reanalyzed on a different instrument. For instruments designed for batched testing, the operator first generates a manual worklist, similar to that described for an instrument, and prints a worksheet. The printed worksheet usually will contain a list of specimen numbers with patient demographics and blank spaces on which the user can write results. This worksheet is a guide for the specimen-processing order and provides a place on which results can be manually transcribed, so they can be later entered at an LIS terminal.

As the technologist manually enters results into the computer terminal, most systems will check the data for technical credibility, life-threatening conditions, abnormal limits, and other conditions specified by the site, as is done by automated systems. Most LISs compare the patient's current result with his or her previous result and will alert the technologist to large changes ("delta check"). In addition, the LIS will alert the technologist to a value outside of a specified range. To assist in the data entry process, software can perform automatic calculations, and terminals can be set up so that keyboards perform special functions. For example, programs can convert the numerical pad on a data entry terminal to a differential counter. To support the urinalysis area, the computer can translate the single keystroke "m" into the word "many." After results are entered, a validation report similar to that generated for an automated instrument is printed. This report is similar to the initial worklist, with test results replacing blank lines. Normally, the technologist who performs the test will also validate the worklist in a manner similar to that for automated instruments. In some areas, a second technologist may be required to validate critical results in addition to, or in lieu of, the first technologist. Even with computer assistance, manual data entry can be tedious and error prone, particularly if more than 100 tests are performed daily. For efficiency, manual data entry usually occurs at the end of the workday or at the end of a **run,** but this delays results reporting if completed results are held for data entry.

Data Verification

Whether results are generated by an interfaced instrument or are entered manually, the operator reviews and approves, or verifies, test results before they are released for patient reporting. Verification may be performed individually, in batch with a worklist, or automatically by computer rules. In the simplest form, usually on single sample instruments, the technologist validates one specimen at a time on a computer screen. If the operator detects a sample or a condition that he/she believes can affect the results, the sample is reanalyzed, often on a second analyzer, or other actions are taken to remediate the condition.

Batch verification is similar to individual verification but results in the release of a group of specimens at a time. This usually starts with review of a printed verification report, followed by exclusion of results by the technologist (for additional investigations), then validation of the entire worklist, or batch. Batch verification may be more efficient for the operator but delays reporting. For most systems, the verification review occurs in the specimen order in which the worksheet was created, or by numerical ordering of specimen

Box 22-3

Some Rules Used in Autoverification

1. Accept results within the *reference range.*
2. Accept results within the *release range.*
3. Reject results from a sufficiently *hemolyzed, lipemic,* or *icteric* specimen.
4. Reject results if system detects *insufficient sample volume.*
5. Reject results if there is an *instrument error (flag).*
6. Accept abnormal results from *specific clinical areas,* for example, a low platelet count from a patient in an oncology clinic or a high creatinine from a patient in a dialysis clinic.
7. Reject results if *concordance of paired results* is not sufficiently close, for example, AST activity > 100 U/L but ALT < 50 U/L.

ALT, Alanine aminotransferase; *AST,* aspartate aminotransferase.

numbers. If results exceed predetermined parameters, the operator must perform specified activities, such as a dilution or a repeat analysis. Frequently, the LIS displays both initial and reanalyzed results and allows the operator to validate or reject one or both results.

Autoverification

In autoverification, the computer assists in the data verification process and performs many of the more routine steps in the review. The simplest approach is to release results within the reference range. For hospitals with severely ill patients, however, only a small number of results are released automatically, in keeping with this rule. An LIS, therefore, may use a release range defined for the purposes of autoverification. The release range offers flexibility by allowing the release of results above or below the reference range. Other common capabilities in autoverification include blocking the release of clinically related results if any one result is out of autoverification range. For example, both creatinine and blood urea nitrogen (BUN) are blocked only if the creatinine value is out of range. Another example is blocking the release of the white blood cell (WBC) differential if the WBC count is below 1000. Autoverification also may review instrument flags. For example, if the sample volume is insufficient, or if analytical reagents are exhausted, all results in that sample are blocked. Autoverification algorithms may also use clinical information. A platelet count of 20,000 is acceptable for patients in an oncology clinic, for example, but would be unacceptable for others. Some rules for autoverification are shown in Box 22-3.

Autoverification rules typically are customized by institutions to meet their own needs. These rules may be created in LIS tables and/or through **middleware.** Middleware describes software, typically supplied by an instrument vendor, the LIS vendor, or a third party, that allows the user to manipulate data between the LIS and the instrument. Because the LIS and the instrument have different information, release rules may be required in both LIS and middleware systems to achieve the desired behavior. For example, the instrument may have information regarding instrument status and reagents, while the LIS has information about the patient's previous results. Sophisticated autoverification rules can be a powerful tool for improving both productivity and quality. All autoverification rules must be tested thoroughly before implementation and on a periodic basis to ensure that they are working as intended. Complex rules, however, will make testing and validation more challenging.

Some LISs provide for the release of verified results directly to physicians' pagers or office faxes. Release parameters can include the nature of the physician's service, the need for critical values, or service-specific test results (e.g., creatinine to the dialysis service). In addition, results can be released to a call center, which has the responsibility to telephone a provider or patient. These can include critical results, results that exceed parameters specified by individual physicians, or results that cannot be reported because of sample-related problems. These automated LIS-dependent processes greatly increase the efficiency of testing personnel.

KEY CONCEPTS BOX 22-2

- *Instrument interfaces* automatically download test requests and upload test results and greatly improve the accuracy and efficiency of the laboratory.
- *Autoverification* uses rules in the LIS or middleware to assist in the verification of results.
- Both interfaces and autoverification are critical to the success of *total laboratory automation,* whereby instruments are linked to operate as a unit.

SECTION OBJECTIVES BOX 22-3

- Describe types of LIS results reporting.
- Describe the role of LIS in a quality control support function.
- Discuss the support role of LIS in areas of quality assurance, such as monitoring turnaround time, identifying sources of error, and integrated patient care with other health care departments.

LIS ROLE IN POSTANALYTICAL ACTIVITIES

Results Reporting

The end product of any clinical laboratory is its results, provided in the form of paper reports or via an information system. Although paper reports often are required for the patient chart and remain important, especially for private physician offices, electronic transmittal via an interfaced EMR is becoming more common and convenient. EMRs have reduced to seconds the delays associated with test result availability; delivery of paper reports may take hours to days. Computer reporting and retrieval of laboratory results have virtually replaced the paper report, greatly reducing personnel time and errors associated with telephone and manual transmission of results.

Regulations require that paper and electronic reports contain the information listed in Box 22-4. Federal regulations,[10] accreditation requirements,[11] and common sense

Box 22-4

Required Patient Report Information

1. Patient demographics (name, number, age, etc.)
2. Time of report generation
3. Name of lab reporting and performing the test
4. Test name(s)
5. Collection time(s) and date(s) for test(s)
6. Results with abnormal flags as needed
7. Reference range
8. Result and order comments
9. Ordering physician or other provider

dictate that LISs have the capability to reprint paper reports or resend electronic results easily on demand. For inpatients, reports usually are presented in a tabular format, displaying current and past results. This report also may be called a **cumulative report** because results are accumulated. Most commonly, tests appear as a column on paper (Fig. 22-3) or on a computer screen (Fig. 22-4), with test result dates displayed in rows horizontally. An alternative format is to have the dates appear in columns and tests in rows. With a tabular format, a very high density of results can appear on a screen. Typically, the report will accumulate results for an entire inpatient stay or some other predetermined interval. On patient discharge, a final summary report may be generated. For outpatients, a simpler line-by-line presentation may be used. For these patients, each result is printed or displayed on a single line, usually in a reverse chronological order, and is grouped by date of service (Figs. 22-5 and 22-6). Most EMRs provide an **inbox**, a facility in which the ordering physician or another specified provider can review laboratory results in a manner akin to email. Inboxes deliver new results to providers as soon as they are available and highlight patients with abnormal and critical results.

Interpretive reports, reports that contain comments to explain one or more results, also may assist physicians with uncommonly ordered tests. Sending interpretations requires sensitivity to the receiving audience. For example, too many interpretations for a frequently ordered test may be viewed as being repetitive, while comments on complex testing results sent to those who infrequently order them can be valuable. Therefore, the laboratory must use these reports selectively. In some cases, an LIS can store and report graphics or images, but it is not unusual for such graphics or images to be lost when they are transmitted to another system such as an EMR.

Of particular importance are the handling and reporting of critical results, or results considered to be life threatening. In our institution, only about 50 tests out of a total menu of thousands have critical values defined. Typically, the laboratory has rules that direct the technologist to take steps to ensure that the result is not related to analytical error. If the critical value is confirmed, most laboratories will attempt to notify the ordering clinician. Tasks performed by the LIS to facilitate this might include automatic faxing of the critical result to the provider or to a laboratory call center. A call center is a special area of the laboratory that is dedicated to calling results and receiving inquiries. For inpatients, the action typically is directed toward notifying the inpatient ward; for outpatients, the notification process is directed to the provider clinician. Although technology exists whereby a provider can be paged or telephoned whenever critical results are obtained, most institutions have avoided this practice because it has significant implications for intruding into the private life of care providers, and it may be difficult to transfer this notification to another provider when patients are transferred.

Quality Control

(See also Chapter 25.)

The LIS can contribute greatly to improved efficiency of technologists and laboratory managers by supporting quality control (QC) and quality assurance (QA) procedures (see below). These activities include maintaining desired precision and accuracy of results and monitoring critical laboratory functions, such as turnaround time. QA and QC procedures tend to be consistent among most laboratories, because regulatory requirements under Clinical Laboratory Improvement Amendments of 1988 (CLIA '88)[10] require strict adherence to specified guidelines (see Chapter 19). These regulations require laboratories to retain QC information associated with any released test result, and most LISs capture these data and automatically or manually link QC results to patient data.

CLIA '88 defines a run as an interval for which the accuracy and precision of a testing system are expected to be stable, but this interval cannot be longer than 24 hours. Most LISs allow users to define a run that matches an instrument's physical sample tray or to perform continuous analyses between controls. These runs, however, may not meet CLIA requirements if they do not include proper control samples. Most LISs evaluate the status of controls in real time and provide the instrument operator with immediate feedback if QC results are out of the expected range. Most instruments have built-in computers, and it is uncommon for an LIS to support the derivation of standard curves from calibration samples. Although the LIS can allow release of results for runs after automatic review of control data and calibration data, as well as other checks (see above, p. 401), most systems leave critical decisions to the operator. Usually, the LIS will provide a warning to the analyst and will require the operator to document corrective action.

Numerous QC calculations are easily and commonly performed by an LIS. These include routine checking for controls that deviate by more than a specified number from an expected mean, or that deviate from expected values determined by established rules such as Westgard rules.[12] Delta checking a patient value against his or her own previous result can also assist in identifying a QC or specimen identification problem.[13] In larger laboratories, inter-instrument, inter-method, and test level comparisons of controls and calibrations help ensure result consistency. Most LIS systems typically provide such QC

08/23/2001
16:54

UNIVERSITY OF WASHINGTON MEDICAL CENTER
INCLUDING LABORATORIES AT UWMC, HMC AND SCCA

CUMULATIVE SUMMARY
PAGE 1

Name: AAALAB, COMPUTER TEST
Pt #: U4557370

Age: 25Y
Loc: TEST

Sex: F
Room: RTEST

**************************** BLOOD ELECTROLYTES AND COMMON CHEMISTRIES ****************************

TEST:	NA	K	CL	CO2	ANION GAP	GLU	WHOLE BLOOD GLU	BUN	CREAT
UNITS:	mEq/L	mEq/L	mEq/L	mEq/L		mg/dL	mg/dL	mg/dL	mg/dL
LO-HI:	136-145	3.7-5.2	98-108	22-32	5-20	62-125	62-125	8-21	0.3-1.2
01/21/01									
1130	135*	4.3	103	22	15	156*		23*	1.3*
1140	143	3.5*	105	20*	10	156*		23*	1.4*
RCV1712		3.5*							
02/01/01									
RCV0834	139	4.3	109*	19*	11	83		54*	2.1*
RCV0924	145	4.0	105	20*	NOT DONE				
04/05/01									
RCV1039						100			

= = = = = = = = = = = = = = = = = = BLOOD ELECTROLYTES AND COMMON CHEMISTRIES = = = = = = = = = = = = = = = = = =

TEST:	ALB
UNITS:	g/dL
LO-HI:	3.5-5.2
01/21/01	
1005	3.5
1145	2.3*
RCV1247	2.4*
1303	2.3*
01/23/01	
1300	2.3*

**************************** CALCIUM METABOLISM ****************************

TEST:	SERUM CALCIUM	CALCIUM SERUM IONIZED	SERUM PO4	SERUM MG	PTH
UNITS:	mg/dL	mmol/L	mg/dL	mg/dL	pg/mL
LO-HI:	8.9-10.2	1.18-1.38	3.0-4.5	1.8-2.4	10-65
01/21/01					
1005	8.8*		4.5	1.3*	
1145	7.0*		8.5*	2.0	
RCV1247	7.5*		6.0*	1.3*	
1303	8.1*		2.3*	1.3*	
01/23/01					
1300	8.8*		1.5*	1.2*	
04/04/01					
0800	10.8*				<1* NREF8

- - - FOOTNOTES - - -
NREF8 Note new reference range effective 8/3/99

AAALAB, COMPUTER TEST
4-55-73-70

PAGE 1
INPATIENT CUMULATIVE SUMMARY
08/23/2001

Fig. 22-3 A tabular patient report, printed by the Sunquest LIS. (Courtesy University of Washington Medical Center, Seattle, WA.)

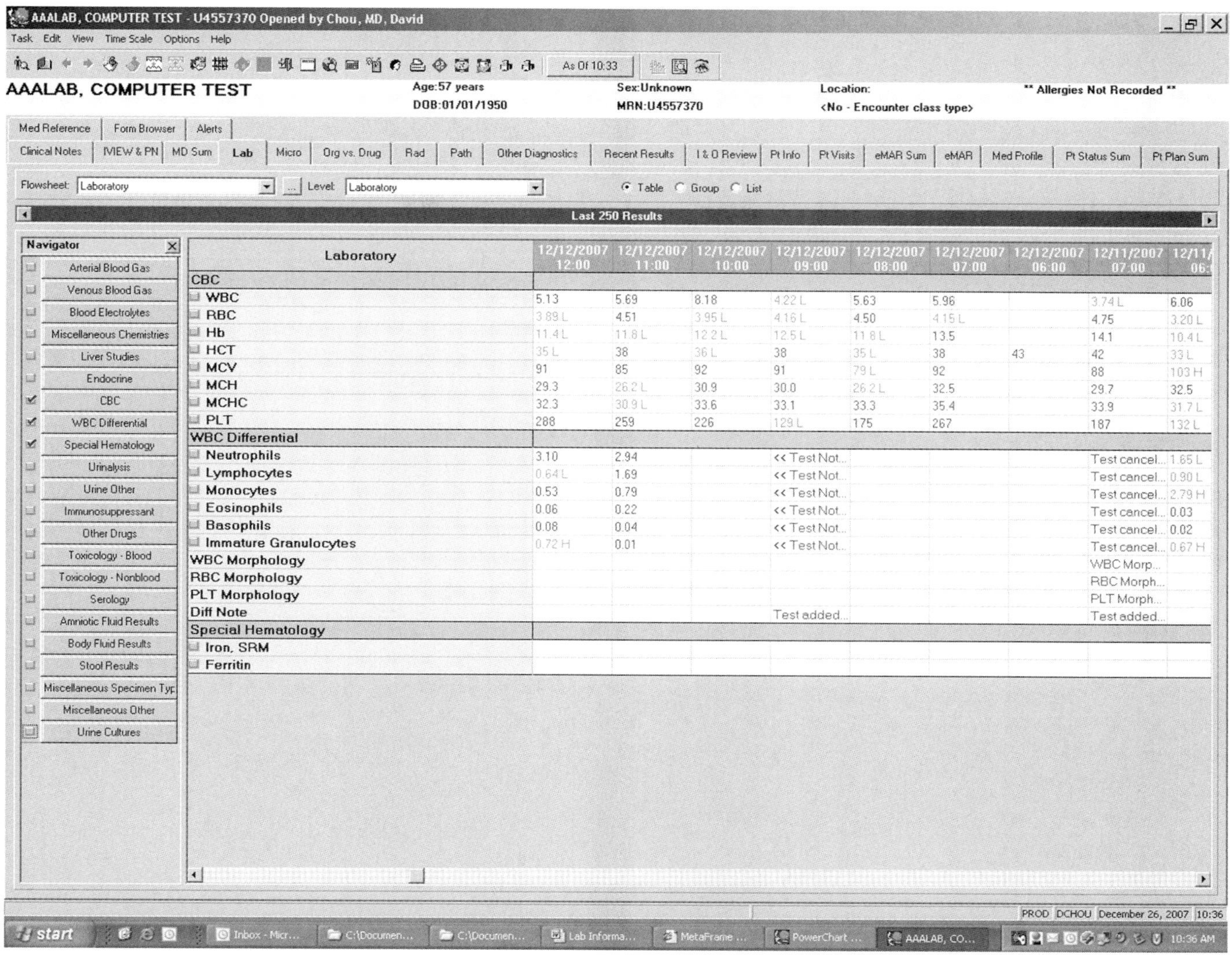

Laboratory	12/12/2007 12:00	12/12/2007 11:00	12/12/2007 10:00	12/12/2007 09:00	12/12/2007 08:00	12/12/2007 07:00	12/12/2007 06:00	12/11/2007 07:00	12/11/ 06:
CBC									
WBC	5.13	5.69	8.18	4.22 L	5.63	5.96		3.74 L	6.06
RBC	3.89 L	4.51	3.95 L	4.16 L	4.50	4.15 L		4.75	3.20 L
Hb	11.4 L	11.8 L	12.2 L	12.5 L	11.8 L	13.5		14.1	10.4 L
HCT	35 L	38	36 L	38	35 L	38	43	42	33 L
MCV	91	85	92	91	79 L	92		88	103 H
MCH	29.3	26.2 L	30.9	30.0	26.2 L	32.5		29.7	32.5
MCHC	32.3	30.9 L	33.6	33.1	33.3	35.4		33.9	31.7 L
PLT	288	259	226	129 L	175	267		187	132 L
WBC Differential									
Neutrophils	3.10	2.94		<< Test Not...				Test cancel...	1.65 L
Lymphocytes	0.64 L	1.69		<< Test Not...				Test cancel...	0.90 L
Monocytes	0.53	0.79		<< Test Not...				Test cancel...	2.79 H
Eosinophils	0.06	0.22		<< Test Not...				Test cancel...	0.03
Basophils	0.08	0.04		<< Test Not...				Test cancel...	0.02
Immature Granulocytes	0.72 H	0.01		<< Test Not...				Test cancel...	0.67 H
WBC Morphology								WBC Morp...	
RBC Morphology								RBC Morph...	
PLT Morphology								PLT Morph...	
Diff Note				Test added...				Test added...	
Special Hematology									
Iron, SRM									
Ferritin									

Fig. 22-4 A tabular laboratory results screen on the Cerner EMR.

08/23/2001 16:53

UNIVERSITY OF WASHINGTON MEDICAL CENTER
INCLUDING LABORATORIES AT UWMC, HMC AND SCCA

INTERIM REPORT
PAGE 1

Name: AAALAB, COMPUTER TEST   Age: 25Y   Sex: F   *** PATIENT ***
Pt #: U4557370   Loc: TEST   Room: RTEST   *** DISCHARGED ***

X54 783   COLL: 01/21/2001 10:05   REC: 01/21/2001 12:10

Chemistry Panel 2			
Albumin	3.5	[3.5-5.2]	g/dL
Magnesium	*1.3	[1.8-2.4]	mg/dL
Calcium	*8.8	[8.9-10.2]	mg/dL
Phosphate	4.5	[3.0-4.5]	mg/dL

X54052   COLL: 01/21/2001 11:30   REC: 01/21/2001 12:23

Chemistry Panel 1			
Sodium	*135	[136-145]	mEq/L
Potassium	4.3	[3.7-5.2]	mEq/L
Chloride	103	[98-108]	mEq/L
Carbon Dioxide	22	[22-32]	mEq/L
Ion Gap	15	[5-20]	
Glucose	*156	[62-125]	mg/dL
Urea Nitrogen	* 23	[8-21]	mg/dL
Creatinine	* 1.3	[0.3-1.2]	mg/dL

[ ] = Reference Range
AAALAB, COMPUTER TEST   END OF REPORT   PAGE 1

Fig. 22-5 A nontabular patient report, printed by the Sunquest LIS. (Courtesy University of Washington Medical Center, Seattle, WA.)

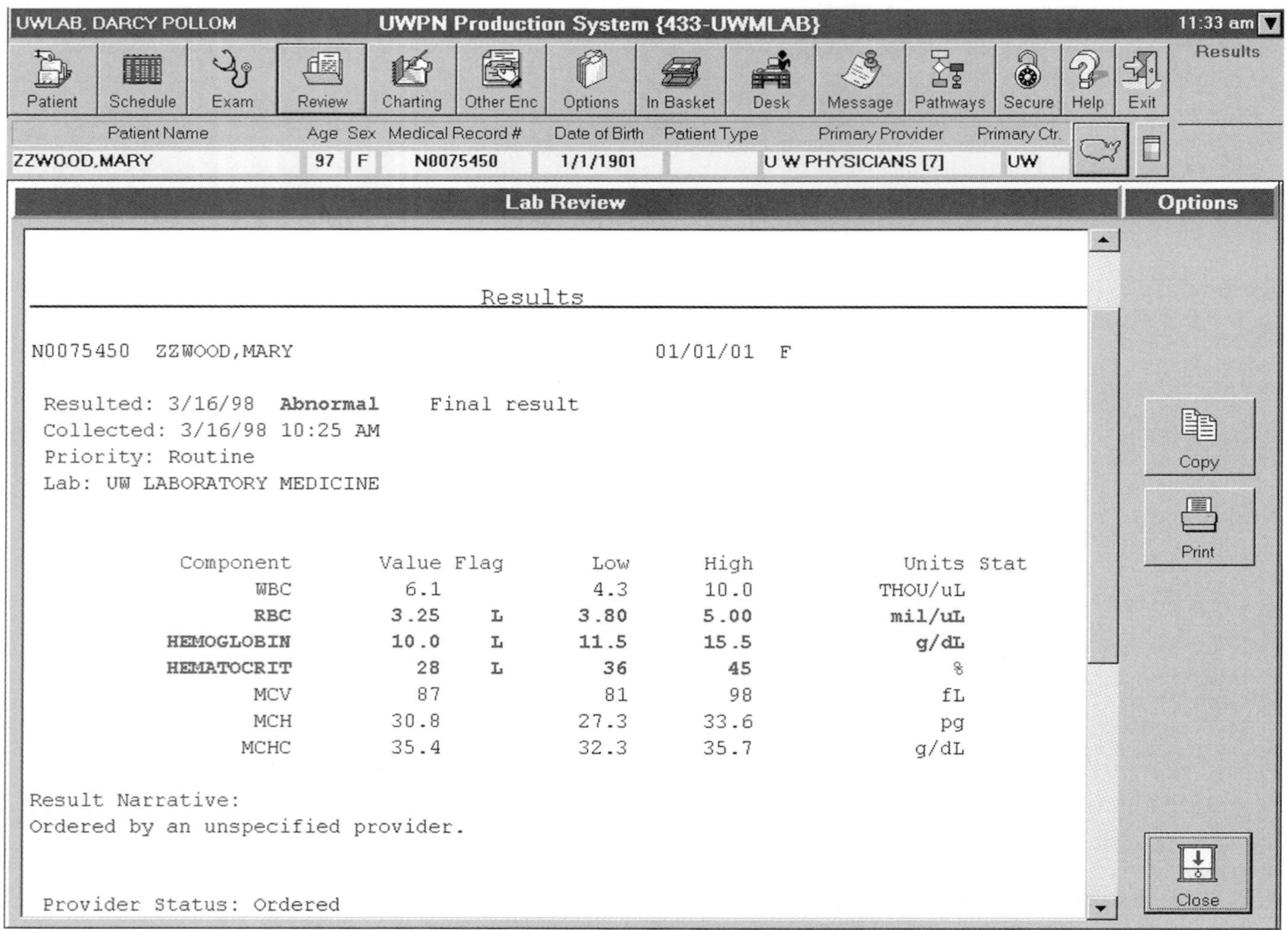

Fig. 22-6 A nontabular laboratory results screen on the EpicCare EMR.

information both in summary format and as the analysis is performed. Levy-Jennings plots are popular for following and displaying such information. Typically, the LIS collects control statistics by instrument, by methodology, and by analyte and allows comparisons of controls at multiple levels.

Quality Assurance and Management Reporting

(See also Chapters 18, 19, and 25.)

The LIS can collect and provide much quality assurance and management information as part of its daily activities. QA differs from QC in that it monitors more global and less quantifiable parameters about the quality of work produced by the laboratory rather than only the accuracy and precision of the testing. The ability of the LIS to perform 100% sampling of laboratory activities with little effort encourages a level of laboratory monitoring that is not possible with a manual system. Examples follow.

First, turnaround time has become an important indicator of the overall average quality of service for high-acuity areas of the hospital. Coupled with specimen tracking and **incomplete lists** to identify slow or lost specimens, such information assists the manager in identifying operational bottlenecks by looking at samples exceeding predetermined parameters and at the overall average service quality. This helps the manager to properly staff work areas, improve workflow, and provide corrective staff training during low and peak work periods.

Second, management reports can assist the manager in identifying sources of error. Errors can occur during preanalytical processing, during test analysis, or after analysis. The most frequent error in the preanalytical process is misidentification of the patient or specimen. Preanalytically and postanalytically, manual data entry can have as much as a 3% error rate, most of which is unlikely to be detected even with tools such as delta checking or supervisor validation. One way of evaluating errors is to compare the data entered into the computer automatically versus data expected to be entered manually. Although this comparison can be tedious, it can be useful in identifying systematic problems associated with data entry of results or requisitions. The computer can provide information regarding test results that have been corrected. Summarizing this information assists in identifying causes.

Most information systems provide a way to change results after they have been validated. Depending on the laboratory, the responsibility for correcting results may be limited to a few individuals. Changing of results may have an unpredictable impact on patient reports. When reports are reprinted, older reports often remain in the chart and are potentially confusing. Likewise, revised reports sent electronically should be handled in such a way that both revised and older reports are available, making it unclear which report is the most current. Most federal and other regulatory agencies require that corrected results be indicated as such.

Third, the laboratory can monitor the quality of patient care by combining data from other hospital computer systems, such as a pharmacy system. Adverse effects associated with gentamicin, for example, can be reduced by coupling drug dispensation records with drug levels, renal function tests, and antimicrobial sensitivity patterns. This information then can be used to warn a clinician of drug toxicity or ineffective dosing.

Fourth, reports of patients with grossly abnormal results provide interesting teaching cases and help in detection of possible problems.

Most LISs produce epidemiology reports that support quality assurance, accreditation, CLIA, and public health. Usually, these reports are customized to retrieve or report information on infectious disease results of interest to public health, such as hepatitis, human immunodeficiency virus (HIV), and sexually transmitted diseases. For example, the prevalence of methicillin-resistant *Staphylococcus aureus* (MRSA) can be compiled in the LIS and sent to hospital and public health agencies, so that actions can be taken to identify and eradicate sources of infection. Likewise, a hepatitis result may trigger an immunization program for those exposed individuals. In some metropolitan areas, public health systems aggregate regional information to act as an early warning system for biosurveillance activities.

Although these activities can be performed on other computers, the amount of patient information contained in most LISs allows more complete reporting. Many other examples exist, and unfortunately, most information systems are capable of generating far more data than can be reviewed. Often, requesters of QA data also fail to realize the extent of human resources and computer time needed to generate useful reports. For example, a programmer may be asked to retrieve historical patient data that have been stored haphazardly and inconsistently, requiring repeated searches of patient records. Such situations translate to intensive computer searches that last weeks, followed by manual examination of collated data. Because few sites have spare computers available to perform such data analyses, these searches can interfere with daily laboratory activities by slowing down response time and consuming labor.

Management reports may be viewed as a by-product of an LIS, but when used effectively, they can become a principal benefit. At the organizational level, management information provided by information systems may not prove useful until trends have been established after several years. Information collected for QC and QA also may be used in managing operations. One of the more commonly used reports from any LIS consists of the ordering frequency of all laboratory tests. This information may be used from an operational perspective to project the need for instrumentation, personnel, and other resources. Another common report is a list of billing transactions, which usually is generated nightly. With the use of computer statistics, workload monitoring can provide information regarding appropriate personnel staffing and can help in rescheduling of employees as test ordering patterns change. Workload information also helps to identify inefficient work areas or individuals.

KEY CONCEPTS BOX 22-3

- *Results reporting* often occurs through the interfacing of electronic medical records (EMRs) with the laboratory information system (LIS). Paper reporting is decreasing as EMRs gain in prominence.
- Technologists can review daily and long-term QC results on LIS, assisted by LIS rules and algorhythms.
- *Management and quality assurance reports* are critical components in the operation of the laboratory.

SECTION OBJECTIVES BOX 22-4

- Explain the following terms: central processing unit (CPU), operating system, and database manager.
- List advantages and disadvantages of the use of the Internet and intranet in the laboratory.
- Describe the maintenance activities of a computer system: backup and software maintenance.
- Discuss privacy challenges introduced by the use of computer systems in the health care industry.
- List four ways that computer systems may be successfully compromised, leading to security and privacy problems.
- Explain how CLIA '88, the FDA, and HIPAA regulations have influenced the design and functionality of LISs.

LIS TECHNOLOGY AND ITS MANAGEMENT

Hardware refers to the physical parts of a computer, which typically are mass produced. *Software* collectively refers to a series of instructions, called *programs,* which direct the behavior of a computer. Software may be mass produced or may be customized for a specialized application. Both hardware and software often are updated after their delivery. Because of this, the initial purchase price for an LIS represents significantly less than half of its total lifetime cost. Programming is an intellectual activity that requires large amounts of time and effort. Increasing software complexity has driven costs up dramatically. More than 95% of the cost of an LIS will involve software and its operation and support.

Over the past 30 years, computer technology has made significant advances in disk and silicon microchip technology. Competition and improved production techniques have greatly reduced computer costs. Larger and more powerful computers often include clusters of smaller computers. At the heart of any computer lies the **central processing unit,** or **CPU,** which usually is manufactured from a single piece of silicon. A CPU is responsible for making logical decisions, performing computations, and translating program instructions into actions. A CPU requires RAM, or random access memory, which is analogous to short-term memory in humans. Data that require longer-term storage are moved to disks and tapes. Disks store data in magnetic or optical form on rotating media. Optical media have higher density, that is, they can store more data in a given area. Optical media frequently are used for historical data, and in CD-ROM format, they can be used for data distribution. Old data may be migrated to magnetic tape, which is slower than disk technology but is often used to **backup** disks because of its low cost. Disk backups of LIS data must be performed regularly, so that data can be recovered after disk failure, or a disk crash. Other ways to protect against disk crashes include disk shadowing, whereby two or more devices duplicate the same data, and RAIDs (redundant array of independent disks), in which a series of small disks work together as a large disk but are protected against any single device failure.

An operating system is a program that supervises the orderly execution of programs and supports the basic functions commonly performed by all programs. Some of these functions include management of disks and disk files, support for terminals and printers, and computer networking (see following section). Microsoft Windows, Unix, and Linux are common operating systems. For applications such as those performed in the laboratory, *real-time capability* is necessary. This term refers to the need to capture input data and process them immediately. For example, a high-volume instrument requires that an LIS respond with the tests to be performed within 5 seconds after sending a specimen number.

Computers are synonymous with data management and data processing. Programs generally operate on data within the program itself, or on data acquired from sources external to the program, such as patient data. In either case, such data and their organization are called the **data structure,** and the organized data are stored on disks, tapes, and other devices in files referred to as a *database.* A *database manager* refers to software that is responsible for handling the physical storage and retrieval of data. Examples of database managers include Intersystems Cache (or M), IBM's DB2, Oracle, Sybase, and Microsoft SQL. From a monetary perspective, the database manager can represent a significant portion of the cost of the LIS. Although files and data structures may contain explicit information about the purpose and type of data stored, the context of the data may be implicit. For example, an accounting system may omit the dollar sign ($) and the decimal point, so that $15.25 appears as 1525. The data context holds significance in that those who use the data must understand them. In addition, contextual information can reduce the number of keystrokes required to input the data.

The purpose of a database design is to ensure that data are stored in such a fashion as to permit their retrieval in a sufficiently fast manner. Although it is possible to store data in an unorganized way and to attempt their retrieval sequentially, computers will reach practical limits despite their speed. To make retrieval practical, data usually are stored in a manner that reflects the way they will be used. The design of the data structure may impose limitations on stored information. For example, a search of the database for selected abnormal results may fail if the search forces the computer to review results on all patients. One solution is to create a separate database of abnormal results; however, multiple copies of data introduce other problems, particularly if data are changed. Despite the performance of modern hardware, a proper and efficient database design is still important when one is working with very large data sets.

Computer Networks, the Internet, and Intranets

A computer **network** is any interconnection between computer systems or computerized devices that supports the interchange of data. In the 1970s, the Advanced Research Projects Agency of the Department of Defense (DARPA) sponsored the development of a nationwide network that became the Internet. Most computers today include a network port as an integral part of the hardware and require networks to communicate with other computers for tasks such as ADT and billing functions. Interchanging of data between different computers requires software that can support a common protocol, or an agreed upon way to interchange data. On a network, computer systems interact with each other as a client or as a server. The server computer stores data from which the desktop client computer retrieves and processes data. In a large system, hundreds of clients can access a single server computer. A single client allows a user to transparently access one or more servers.

The Internet Browser[14]

The Internet browser integrates a number of existing network protocols into a user friendly interface with graphics capabilities. Internet browsers are clients that support the hypertext transport protocol (HTTP) and the hypertext markup language (HTML), and that interact with Internet Web servers to enable users to perform familiar "Web surfing" activities. These browsers also may interact with traditional information systems modified to support Internet protocols. Browsers, because of their prevalence and ease of use, are used frequently as an interface into LISs and other information systems. Internet computers often register a unique name, or **URL (Uniform Resource Locator),** so that they can be referenced conveniently by users for email, as a browser, or for other services. Service bureaus also may provide access to a patient information database, LIS, or billing system through the Internet. These providers are called *application service providers,* or ASPs. Useful websites on the Internet that contain information on medical **informatics** and clinical chemistry, along with their URLs, are listed in Table 22-1.

The fluidity of the Internet, however, remains both its primary asset and its largest liability. Important information may be introduced rapidly and easily with the use of Web browsers. Such information, however, also disappears rapidly if the person(s) or organization(s) that is supporting the website loses interest or declares bankruptcy. Archiving Web information can be difficult. Documents can be distributed in electronic format instantly without mailing and other

Table 22-1 Popular Internet URLs

http://www.google.com	Possibly the most popular search engine for the Web
http://www.aacc.org	Website of the American Association for Clinical Chemistry, a professional organization of clinical chemists
http://www.cap.org	College of American Pathologists website (laboratory accreditation checklists)
http://www.clsi.org	Website for Clinical Laboratory Standards Institute, an organization that develops laboratory standards
http://www.cms.gov	Website for Centers for Medicare and Medicaid Services
http://en.wikipedia.org	Web encyclopedia written by users (English site)
http://www.yahoo.com	Popular Web portal that contains a variety of news, video, and other materials

distribution costs. Web search engines, such as Google (www.google.com) and Yahoo (www.yahoo.com), are computers that systematically search the Internet and index the content of websites. Search engines permit users to find websites that contain desired information. Because of ease of presentation, it may be difficult to ascertain the accuracy of information on the Internet, making fraud and abuse relatively easy.

Organizations can build **intranets,** which are similar to the Internet but limit access to private internal use. Intranets provide information, such as a telephone directory, policy and procedure manuals, or quality assurance data, that an institution does not want public but that is needed by many individuals. Intranets are more convenient than paper for disseminating constantly changing data. To ensure **privacy,** access to intranets may be limited physically by the network, and/or users may be required to identify themselves through a login process.

Satellite, cellular telephone, wifi, and other radio frequency systems support mobile computing activities, such as handheld phlebotomy collection devices, mentioned previously, which promote accurate collection times and enhance patient identification. Many hospitals support a wifi network by which mobile devices can be connected to an intranet. The impact of all these network technologies is to allow connection to the LIS from physically diverse locations. Networks are critical for supporting laboratory facilities by allowing remote locations to have access to patient data, and by promoting the creation of a regional health care delivery system.[15,16] Such satellite operations become increasingly important as laboratories expand through the creation of health care alliances.

Maintenance

Following the installation of a computer system, the user must perform certain routine housekeeping activities, often referred to as *maintenance.* These activities are necessary to sustain proper functions and to allow for data recovery in case of failure. Backup, or making a copy of files, is one such activity. Most operating systems and databases allow housekeeping activities to occur with the system still available to users. Ultimately, disk space will be limited by design or by physical constraints. As a result, inactive patient information must be archived, or transferred to storage tapes or optical disks, periodically and purged from the active disk. Programs usually are available that restore the **archived data** for reprinting of reports or for other purposes, or that allow the direct processing of archived data. Users who wish to access archived data may incur delays while waiting for an operator to load the appropriate tape or optical disk. Magnetic tape and disks are not permanent in that data may "fade" in 5 to 10 years. Optical disks appear to have greater permanence and are likely to satisfy legal definitions for archiving.

Software maintenance refers to the processes associated with updating software after installation. Updates may include repair of software defects or design problems, enhancements, support for new hardware or operating systems, and changes in the user environment. Because updates occur as often as several times a year, software updates usually cause more downtime than is caused by unanticipated failures. Users often are tempted to skip updates in an LIS that is operating satisfactorily, but these deferrals must be balanced by other considerations. Vendors refuse to provide support for older software, and new software may not operate properly when combined with older software. Maintenance charges remain a significant source of revenue for software vendors, often amounting to 1.5% per month of the original purchase price. Conversely, maintenance charges represent a significant expense for users. Skilled users may terminate software support to save expenses, especially when they perceive that they are getting little benefit. Vendors often will entice users to continue software support by offering enhancements. Maintenance also includes updates dictated by local changes, such as the introduction of new automated instrumentation or the replacement of a financial system with which the LIS interfaces. Locally mandated changes can easily add another 25% to maintenance costs.

Privacy and Data Security

Privacy is defined as those activities designed to protect information from being accessed by unauthorized individuals or parties. **Security** refers to activities designed to ensure that data are not accessed or altered unintentionally. Balancing privacy, data security, and access to medical information challenges computer systems, especially as computerized databases increase in use and systems are exposed to external Internet activities. The LIS keeps information directly accessible throughout the laboratory and, in many cases, throughout the hospital. As technology for the EMR improves, the availability of prepaid medical care increases, and national health care progresses; privacy, security, and the need for information come into even greater conflict when demands for greater information are increased.[17] Computers can provide ready access to information and can be used to control ordering, but they can achieve this only at the risk of reducing privacy and possibly security.

Federal legislation under **the Health Insurance Portability and Accountability Act (HIPAA)**[18-21] sets standards and imposes significant penalties for health care providers for violations of patient privacy and data security. Privacy concerns are now very important, in that electronic storage of increasing amounts of patient data increases the likelihood of exposing sensitive information. Unfortunately, most systems in use today are not designed to resist systematic and determined attacks at gaining access.

To control access into the LIS, most current systems require the use of a username and password. Passwords should be of sufficient length and complexity to prevent guessing. Even long passwords based on common dictionary words can be guessed by systematic attacks at an LIS. Systems or laboratory procedures should force the changing of passwords at regular intervals. Most systems limit access of users to system functions and test results, as required by HIPAA under the minimum necessary privileges requirement. For example, physicians might have access only for test results inquiry, laboratory technologists might have access to ordering, resulting, and inquiry functions, and order entry clerks may have access only to test ordering functions. A special access privilege might be needed for accessing data such as HIV results. Systems should automatically disconnect inactive terminals to prevent inappropriate access. Managing access rights in a large institution can be an extraordinarily difficult problem, in that residents, interns, and students change services frequently, and information regarding their role can be difficult to obtain. Personal information implied by data such as home address, patient location, appointments, and billing transactions also affects privacy but is difficult to block because of the large number of people who require access to such data.[22]

New technologies have introduced substantial challenges for piracy and security. Most computers are connected to data networks, and these networks are connected to the Internet, allowing access to confidential information from physically remote sites. Infrequently, malicious intruders destroy or alter data. More often, intruders steal computer resources for illicit purposes or for information of financial value, such as social security numbers. Technical complexity and resource limitations often prevent vendors and users from responding. Widespread use of computer systems by health care institutions and insurance carriers increases the risk. Networks and microcomputers are exposed to computer **viruses**—computer programs that embed themselves into the operating system programs. Many viruses remain dormant and are not destructive, but some destroy or steal data. Security and privacy issues require dealing with conflicting laws and diversified medical practices without inhibiting convenience of access. Users must be educated and encouraged to take steps to guard privacy. Networks and computers must be designed with data security considerations as a fore-thought rather than an after-thought. Patient care computers may require the use of **firewalls**—electronic devices designed to control traffic into and out of the network. Messages sent over a public network should be encrypted, or scrambled, so that they can be read only by their intended recipients. Messages sent over the Internet can be encapsulated through a virtual private network, or VPN, in which all conversations between computers are encrypted. Internet websites and Web-based software operating over the Internet are particularly vulnerable to malicious activities because the Web **server** and the user client operate on a network that is open to the public. The tight integration of popular desktop software (word processors, spreadsheets, and presentation graphics) with Web browsers and email systems provides opportunities for malicious tampering of the LIS database via Web pages, email messages, and documents.

In spite of their complexity, most systems are compromised successfully because of failures in basic practice. Common problem areas include user accounts left active for employees who have left or changed jobs, missing or trivial passwords, failure to perform backups or to test backup procedures, and failure to patch vulnerabilities in systems.

Regulatory Requirements, Software Validation, and Disaster Recovery

Federal regulations and accreditation agencies have greatly influenced the design and functionality of the LIS from both vendor and user perspectives. Most significant are those that cover laboratory and information systems requirements under CLIA '88[10]; the U.S. Food and Drug Administration's (FDA) ruling on LISs, especially blood bank systems as a medical device; and regulations on billing, patient privacy, and data security mandated under HIPAA. Lesser impacts on the LIS, but not necessarily on the laboratory, include requirements for the laboratory to collect diagnosis codes from the ordering provider on testing reimbursed by Medicare—a requirement under the Balanced Budget Act of 1997.

CLIA '88 specifies regulations for managing record keeping, including the capture of quality control data, technologist workload, and technologist proficiencies, as well as the proper operation of information systems. The major impact of CLIA '88 on the LIS lies in data retention requirements. Records of test requests and results must be retained in a conveniently retrievable manner for 10 years for anatomical pathology and cytology results, 5 years for blood bank and immunohematology (HLA typing) results, and 2 years for all other results. Although it may be possible to retain data **online** in computer systems for this length of time, most laboratories archive the data to microfiche or optical disks for greater permanence.

In 1988, the FDA ruled that blood bank laboratory information systems are medical devices[23] that require validation procedures similar to those of other medical devices, such as patient monitors. Because such software influences the quality of blood products produced by a blood center, it is a part of the manufacturing process and therefore is subject to FDA review. The FDA exempts other laboratory areas from detailed validation because LIS data are reviewed by a clinician before use, but other accreditation organizations and good practices

Box 22-5

Areas of Testing for Software Validation

1. Basic functions (phlebotomy, order entry, results entry, results reporting, etc.)
2. Instrument interfaces
3. External results and orders interfaces to/from foreign systems
4. Known problem areas (system and software release dependent)
5. Calculations (calculated results, indices, etc.)
6. Rules for autoverification
7. Custom reports
8. Any area where custom or nonstandard software is being used

require that users perform some form of system validation at least annually. Validation requires testing, verification, and documentation.[24] Validation reduces exposure to software errors and user training problems but requires time and personnel resources. Software validation is a critical activity in the management of the LIS. Some areas for validation are listed in Box 22-5. Ideally, the laboratory should test the full spectrum of activity from specimen collection to patient reports. Other testing should include known problem areas such as those that have been noted in previous upgrades.

Calculations and autoverification rules require initial testing and periodic retesting. It is important that these functions are carefully tested, so they behave as intended. Calculations are used to (1) perform mathematical computations for results or for quality control purposes, and (2) assist in taking some action associated with a condition or value. Errors in computation result most often when a mathematical expression is mistranslated into the LIS. For example, the international normalized ratio (INR) calculation requires division and exponentiation and can result in an unfamiliar computer representation. Complex autoverification rules are particularly difficult to test because they involve so many variables and cover unusual situations. Simulations (e.g., creating situations by artificially generating test values) are mandatory because these abnormal situations are encountered infrequently. Accreditation agencies, such as the College of American Pathologists (CAP) and **The Joint Commission,** provide suggestions for compliance with federal and state regulations. Typical testing requirements for data processing include user procedures for documenting and validating software, documentation of software and hardware maintenance, and documentation of standard operating procedures.[11] CAP laboratory inspection checklists have added requirements for review of computerized verification of results, security, and privacy procedures.

With the increasing dependence of hospitals on information systems, disaster recovery and activities related to the continuation of laboratory and hospital operations during and following a disaster have become increasingly important. For information systems, protection from computer failure should include at least three aspects: (1) The LIS system should be designed so that common failures do not affect routine operations. Examples include redundant disk drives and a second system that is operating in a standby mode, ready to take over should the primary system fail. (2) In addition, recovery of data should be possible should the system be destroyed following a disaster. Copying disks to backup tapes and storing them off-site typically play an important role in this recovery. Rotating backup tapes may be kept protected in a secure off-site location for weeks to months. Tapes should be restored regularly to ensure that backup procedures are satisfactory.

Third and last, manual procedures must be developed so the laboratory can operate in the absence of the LIS. Many data centers are remote to hospitals, and major disasters will likely result in the failure of computer networks that connect the laboratory with the LIS. Disaster recovery plans should distinguish between short-term minor outages and long-term major failures because the procedures for each are different. Sophisticated plans are difficult to develop and are even more difficult to test. At a minimum, planning should be detailed enough that laboratory personnel can operate the laboratory during scheduled outages.

MISCELLANEOUS

Role of the LIS With Other Hospital Computers

LISs are expected to send and receive routine information to and from other systems. In a hospital setting, an administrative computer typically maintains patient demographic information, which is communicated to the LIS through an ADT system. Likewise, laboratory test requests and results are received through an EMR. After the analysis is performed, the LIS may send a transaction to a financial system of services performed by the laboratory. The financial system then performs billing and accounting functions, translating the LIS transactions into charges, Current Procedural Terminology (CPT) codes, and other information required by insurance carriers. If the LIS performs its own billing and accounting, it must send similar information to an insurance carrier either through an EDI (electronic data interchange) or, more rarely, through paper claims. These complex interchanges between computers occasionally may fail and may require updates as regulations change (e.g., HIPAA has changed the procedures for EDI). Updates of test definitions in the laboratory require coordination with financial computer systems and require adherence to strict protocols in larger organizations. Patient locations, test definitions, and other information must be coordinated with the EMR and with other clinical systems. In most institutions, the LIS participates as one member in a complex quilt of unrelated and interconnected computerized information systems (Fig. 22-7).

Integration of information and sharing of data with other patient information systems increase in importance as clinicians and hospitals attempt to improve patient care and reduce costs. To achieve these goals, informaticians distinguish data, the laboratory result by itself, from information that is data

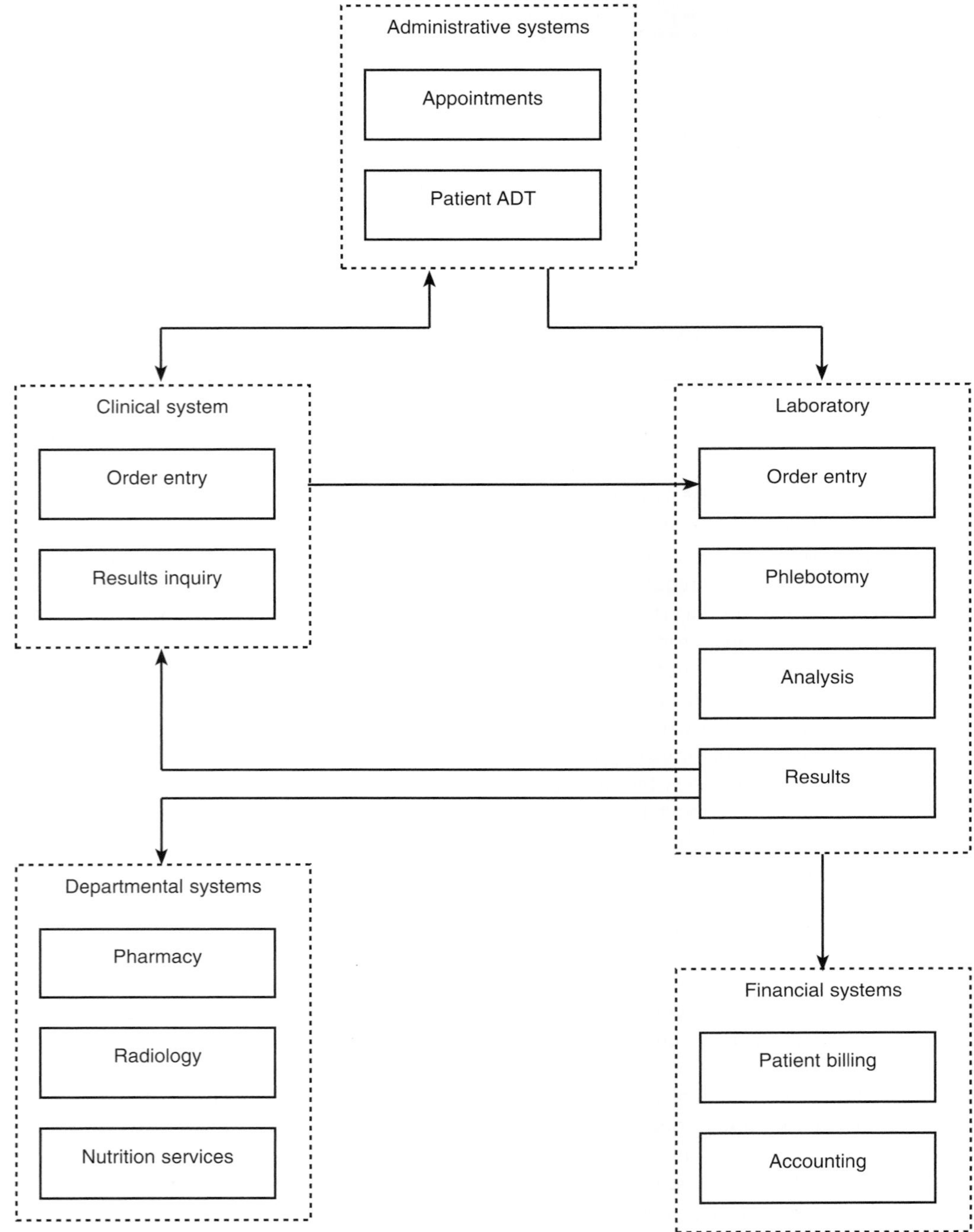

Fig. 22-7 The interchange of information between computer systems in a hospital environment. Most laboratory computer systems today are expected to interact with hospital administrative, financial, nursing, and other departmental systems. In an integrated system environment, blocked functions are modules. In an interfaced environment, blocks represent individual systems.

aggregated and applied to decision making. For example, the report of a drug level—data—to a physician becomes information when it is coupled with the clinical context of the data (e.g., peak or trough level) and data associated with adverse drug reactions, dosing, and drug toxicity. In a broader context, the integration of ancillary and nursing data allows a hospital to make decisions that can decrease the costs of patient care.

The LIS plays a key role in a matrix of computer systems designed to support the delivery of patient care. Coordinating information in such an environment with many different systems, each with different requirements, can be complex. To address the high cost of software development and the lack of coordination between various information systems, the health care computer industry (LIS and EMR users) and the federal government have created voluntary groups to set standards, particularly for the interconnection between information systems and between an information system and computerized equipment. For the clinical laboratory, standards address the interchange of data (1) with bedside monitoring systems; (2) with administrative systems, including those associated with insurance payers and government agencies; and (3) between laboratory systems. Of particular importance are those functions that cover the interchange of laboratory test requests and results. The voluntary groups responsible for standards in the laboratory informatics arena include the CLSI and HL7.

HL7 has become the de facto language for interfaces between different hospital systems, such as an EMR and an LIS.[25] Just as instrument interfaces have improved laboratory efficiency and accuracy, HL7 interfaces provide similar benefits for the laboratory through increased accuracy and efficiencies for order entry and results. Interface standards have improved the ability to share medical information through standardized medical terminology such as SNOMED for medical terminology and its LOINC subset[26,27] for test names and nomenclature used in the clinical laboratory. Unfortunately, HL7 interfaces can be expensive, and implementing them is still time consuming and labor intensive.

Future Directions

Computerizing patient records is the most effective way to decrease costs and reduce errors.[28] Coupled with order entry and medical practice guidelines, this can structure patient care for maximum benefit.[3] Unfortunately, the lack of common medical terminologies and language syntaxes, the differences in medical practices and workflow, the politics associated with complex projects, and the high cost and challenge of developing complex software make this goal formidable. Individuals with skills in both medicine and programming are required but are often difficult to find. Creating an effective EMR continues to be both a challenge and a solution to medical care problems.[29]

U.S. and U.K. governments have promoted implementation of EMRs to reduce costs and improve patient care as evidenced by successes with the Veterans Administration's VistA System.[30] The National Health Information Network (NHIN), sponsored by the U.S. Health and Human Services Agency, is promoting standards and certifying systems for the interchange of medical records. Standards for laboratory interchange for the personal health record and biosurveillance are two of the three first "use cases" released.[31,32] Successes in these efforts will likely be linked to the ability to limit and manage vocabulary and include sufficient context in the information exchanged. Within the United States, the absence of a universal patient identifier has also made it difficult to link patients seen at multiple institutions, especially if they move across regional boundaries. The future success of information systems in health care will result from continued improvements and subtle application of new and existing technologies. Ultimately, these will lead to better information systems that have a positive impact on health care.

KEY CONCEPTS BOX 22-4

- *Maintenance* includes those activities associated with a laboratory information system (LIS) that ensure that privacy, security, and disaster recovery details are handled. Maintenance also includes activities designed to keep software and hardware updated to meet laboratory requirements.
- The Health Insurance Portability and Accountability Act *(HIPAA)* has set legal requirements for the LIS in the areas of privacy and security.
- *Validation* of LIS functions must be performed periodically to ensure that an LIS is performing properly and to meet accreditation requirements.

REFERENCES

1. Aarts J, Ash J, Berg M: Extending the understanding of computerized physician order entry: implications for professional collaboration, workflow and quality of care, Int J Med Inform 76(suppl 1):4, 2007.
2. Valenstein P, Meier F: Outpatient order accuracy: a College of American Pathologists Q-Probes study of requisition order entry accuracy in 660 institutions, Arch Pathol Lab Med 123:1145, 1999.
3. Kohn LT, Corrigan JM, Donaldson MS, eds: *To Err is Human: Building a Safer Health System,* Washington, DC, 2000, National Academy Press.
4. Aandahl GS, Knutsen TR, Nafstad K: Implementation of ISBT 128, a quality system, a standardized bar code labeling of blood products worldwide, electronic transfusion pathway: four years of experience in Norway, Transfusion 47:1674, 2007.
5. Mountain PJ, Callaghan JV, Chou D, et al: *AUTO2-A2—Laboratory Automation: Bar Codes for Specimen Container Identification; Approved Standard,* ed 2, Wayne, PA, 2006, Clinical Laboratory Standards Institute.
6. Hayden RT, Patterson DJ, Jay DW, et al: Computer-assisted barcoding system significantly reduces clinical laboratory specimen identification errors in a pediatric oncology hospital, J Pediatr 152:219, 2008.
7. Laboratory Automation Standards: Auto3-A (Communications with Automated Clinical Laboratory Systems, Instruments, Devices, and Information Systems), Auto4-A *(Systems Operational Requirements, Characteristics, and Information Elements)* and Auto5-A (*Electromechanical Interfaces*), Wayne, PA, 2001-2007, Clinical Laboratory Standards Institute.
8. Hoffman GE: Concepts for third generation of laboratory systems, Clin Chim Acta 278:203, 1998.
9. Dunka L, et al: *POCT1-A2: Point of Care Connectivity, Approved Standard,* ed 2, vol 26, Wayne, PA, Clinical Laboratory Standards Institute, 2006.
10. U.S. Department of Health and Human Services, Health Care Financing Organization, U.S. Department of Health and Human Services: 42 CFR part 405, Clinical Laboratory Improvement Amendments of 1988, Final Rule [CLIA '88]. Fed Register 57:7001, 1992.
11. Commission on Laboratory Accreditation: *Inspection Checklist, Section 1, Laboratory General—Computer Services,* Northfield, IL, April 2006, College of American Pathologists (CAP). Available online at http://www.cap.org/
12. Westgard JO, Barry PL, Hunt MR, et al: A multi-rule Shewhart chart for quality control in clinical chemistry, Clin Chem 27:493, 1981.
13. Ladensen JH: Patients as their own controls: use of the computer to identify "laboratory error," Clin Chem 21:1648, 1975.

14. Schatz BR, Hardin JB: NCSA Mosaic and the World Wide Web: global hypermedia protocols for the Internet, Science 265:895, 1994.
15. Aller RD: Creating integrated regional laboratory networks, Clin Lab Med 19:299, 1999.
16. Connelly DP: Integrating integrated laboratory information into health care delivery systems, Clin Lab Med 19:277, 1999.
17. Huston T: Security issues for implementation of e-medical records. Communications of the ACM 44:89, 2001.
18. Health Insurance Reform: Standards for Privacy of Individually Identifiable Health Information, Final Rule (45 CFR, parts 160 and 164) [HIPAA, Part 1], Fed Register 65:82461, 2000.
19. Health Insurance Reform: Security Standards, Final Rule (45 CFR, parts 160, 162, and 164) [HIPAA, Part 2]. Fed Register 68:8334, 2003.
20. Health Insurance Reform: Standards for Electronic Transactions; Announcement of Designated Standard Maintenance Organizations; Final Rule and Notice (45 CFR Parts 160 and 162) [HIPAA, Part 3]. Fed Register 65:50312, 2000.
21. Health Insurance Reform: Modifications to Transactions and Code Set Standards for Electronic Transactions; Final Rule (45 CFR Part 162), Fed Register 68:8381, 2002.
22. McGilchrist M, Sullivan F, Kalra D: Assuring the confidentiality of shared electronic health records, BMJ 335:1223, 2007.
23. Parkman PD: FDA letter to registered blood banks on recommendations for implementation of computerization in blood establishments, April 6, 1988.
24. Cowan DF, Gray RZ, Campbell B: Validation of the laboratory information system, Arch Pathol Lab Med 122:239, 1998.
25. HL7 v2.x: *An Application Protocol for Electronic Data Interchange in Health Care Environments,* Ann Arbor, MI, 2004, Health Level Seven, Inc.
26. Nachimuthu SK, Lau LM: Practical issues in using SNOMED CT as a reference terminology, Medinfo 12(Pt 1):640, 2007.
27. Khan AN, Griffith SP, Moore C, et al: Standardizing laboratory data by mapping to LOINC, J Am Med Inform Assoc 13:353, 2006.
28. Dick RS, Steen EB, Detmer DE, eds: *The Computer-Based Patient Record: An Essential Technology for Health Care, Revised Edition,* Washington, DC, 1997, National Academy Press.
29. Kaplan L: *Connecting the Laboratory to the Electronic Medical Record, National Academy of Clinical Biochemistry Symposium, September 15-16, 2000,* Philadelphia [CD], 2001, Pesce Kaplan Publishers. Available through AACC.
30. Brown SH, Lincoln MJ, Groen PJ, et al: VistA*/U.S. Department of Veterans Affairs national scale HIS, Int J Med Informatics 69:135, 2003.
31. Harmonized Use Case for Electronic Health Records (Laboratory Result Reporting), March 19, 2006, HHS.gov: Health Information Technology. Available at http://www.hhs.gov/healthit/
32. Harmonized Biosurveillance (Visit, Utilization, and Lab Result Data) Use Case, March 19, 2006, HHS.gov: Health Information Technology. Available at http://www.hhs.gov/healthit/.

Laboratory Statistics

Mark A. Jandreski and Stephen E. Kahn*

23 Chapter

Chapter Outline

Key Terms

accuracy Estimate of nonrandom, systematic **error** or bias between samples of data or between a sample of data and the true population value.

ANOVA (ANalysis Of VAriance) Statistical method for comparison of three or more means.

central tendency The value about which a population is centered. The mean, the median, and the mode all are used to describe the central tendency of a population.

chi-square (χ^2) A test statistic that measures the difference between the observed and expected frequencies of occurrences in two or more populations.

coefficient of variation (CV) A relative standard deviation in which the standard deviation is divided by the mean and multiplied by 100%.

confidence interval A range around an experimentally determined statistic that has a known probability of including the true parameter.

correlation coefficient A statistic that measures the distribution of data about the estimated linear regression line.

degrees of freedom *(df)* The number of independent observations in a data set. This is the number of observations minus the number of restrictions for a set of data.

***F*-test** A statistical test used to determine whether there are differences between two variances.

gaussian distribution *See* normal distribution.

histogram A graphic display of data in which the frequency of a certain value (or range of value or values) is plotted against a scale of all values.

Mann-Whitney test A nonparametric statistical test based on the ranks of data and used to test the null hypothesis that the central tendencies of two independent populations are identical.

mean Arithmetic average of a set of data.

median A value or interval of a population that occurs in the middle of a population, of which half falls above and half falls below the median.

mode The value or interval of a population that occurs with the greatest frequency.

nonparametric statistics Statistics employed when the assumption of a normal or symmetrical (i.e., gaussian) distribution of data is not valid.

normal distribution A population of data that has a tendency to cluster symmetrically around a central value such that the mean, median, and mode of the data are the same; also known as a *gaussian distribution.*

null hypothesis The working hypothesis of a statistical test that states that there is no difference between the statistics of two different populations.

outlier A result or data point that lies far outside the range of all other results or data points. The outlier is not considered to be from the population that has been sampled.

parametric statistics Statistics employed when the assumption that a population has a symmetrical distribution of data (such as gaussian or log-normal) is valid.

precision A descriptor of the random variation in a population of data.

random error Error that affects the reproducibility of a method (precision). Also called random variation.

*With acknowledgment to the previous authors, Carl C. Garber and R. Neill Carey.

range The difference between the highest and lowest values in a population.
sign test A nonparametric statistical test used to assess differences between population medians.
standard deviation Square root of a variance.
standard error A descriptor of the variability that results from sampling data from a population.
statistic A number that describes a property of a set of data or other numbers.
statistics The plural of *statistic*; also the science that deals with the use and classification of numbers or data.
systematic error Nonrandom error that affects the mean of a population of data and defines the bias between the means of two populations (*see* accuracy).
***t*-test** A statistical test that is used to determine whether there are differences between two means or between a target value and a calculated mean in populations that have a normal distribution.
variance A statistic used to describe the distribution or spread of data in a population.

Generating test results, using effective quality control procedures, monitoring the performance of existing methods, and assessing the utility of new test methods are routine analytical activities that are performed in the clinical laboratory. All analytical techniques and methods are subject to several types of error, or variation, that create a degree of uncertainty in the quantitative test results that a laboratory produces. The clinical laboratorian must be able to apply basic statistical techniques in order to evaluate the validity of test results. Statistics, therefore, are an important laboratory tool.

Webster[1] defines *statistics* as "(1) a branch of mathematics dealing with the collection, analysis, interpretation, and presentation of masses of numerical data, and (2) a collection of quantitative data."

A **statistic** (singular) is a number that describes some property of a set of other numbers. In the clinical laboratory, statistical descriptions of data sets can be useful in many ways:

1. To identify how a population of data is distributed
2. To assess random variation in a population of data
3. To compare the amounts of random variation within populations of data
4. To analyze which parameters are significant components of variance
5. To test for a systematic difference between populations of data
6. To assess the degree of correlation between populations of data

This chapter describes each of these uses of statistics and illustrates how each can be applied effectively in laboratory situations.

A basic and theoretical knowledge of appropriate statistical methods is critically important in the clinical chemistry laboratory. Equally important, however, is the correct application of statistical methods to relevant laboratory problems. Students are encouraged to refer to basic statistics textbooks (see, for example, references 2 to 8, as well as the general references) for information on statistics beyond that presented in this chapter.

SECTION OBJECTIVES BOX 23-1

- Explain the difference between populations and samples, including desirable attributes of a sample.
- Recognize the following distribution characteristics on diagrams: gaussian (normal), skewness, and kurtosis.

POPULATION DISTRIBUTIONS

Populations and Samples

The term *population* usually refers to a number of animate creatures or persons, such as the inhabitants of the United States. However, in statistics, *population* also may refer to a collection of objects, events, procedures, or observations. For example, all the serum glucose values for all the people living in Chicago on a given day could be considered a population of glucose values. As a second example, if the glucose concentration of a single blood specimen were measured 10,000 times, a population of slightly different glucose results would be obtained; no chemical measurement is exact because of the random variation inherent in all laboratory measurements.

The number of observations in these glucose examples is too large to be studied conveniently; therefore, a representative sample must be drawn from the population for investigational purposes. Before the sample is drawn, the population from which it comes must be carefully described. Once the attributes of the population are known, sample criteria for such variables as age, sex, occupation, family history, disease state, or any other parameter that might be relevant to the study can be applied. For example, if a serum glucose reference range analysis were carried out, serum samples from diabetic patients could not be used. The number of individual data points needed must be defined as well. If the number is too large, the study may be too difficult to carry out. If the number is too small, the sample may not be a statistically significant representation of the population. The sample must be chosen in such a way that true inferences can be made about the population under study from results obtained from the sample. Most of the concepts and applications discussed in this chapter focus on statistical evaluations of samples of data obtained from a population.

Frequency Distributions

Conceptually, perhaps the simplest way to describe a population of data is to construct a **histogram,** also called a *frequency distribution diagram.* A histogram shows the frequency, or the number of times, a particular value or range of values is obtained versus the scale of all values. Fig. 23-1, *A*, is a histogram of 20 glucose results obtained by repeated measurement of an individual blood specimen. The horizontal axis is glucose concentration divided into small convenient ranges,

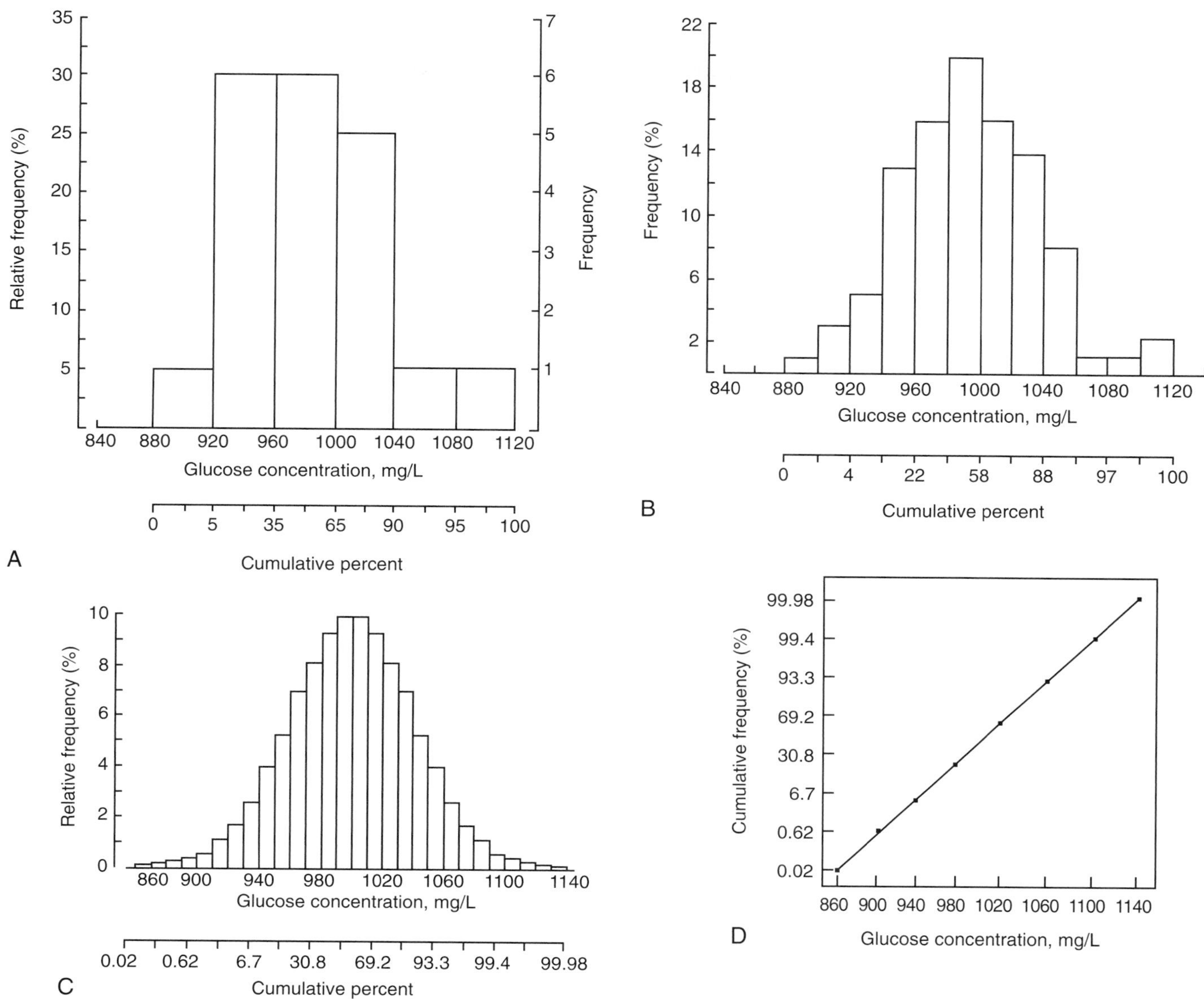

Fig. 23-1 A, Histogram (frequency distribution) of glucose results obtained from 20 repetitive measurements of the same specimen using bin width 40 mg/L. **B,** With $N = 100$ and bin width = 20 mg/L. **C,** With infinite N and bin width = 10 mg/L. **D,** Normal probability plot of glucose results obtained as described in **C.**

or *bins.* The vertical axis is the frequency (or relative frequency) with which results from each bin are obtained, such as the number of patients having a given range of glucose values. When relative frequencies are used, each bin frequency is presented as a percentage of the total number of samples. The histogram's horizontal axis can also represent cumulative percentiles (cumulative percentage of the population up to and including each bin), as well as concentration units. When the number of observations, N, is small, and the bins are relatively wide, the histogram has a choppy appearance (see Fig. 23-1, *A*). As N increases and the bins are made narrower, the shape of the histogram becomes smoother, and the histogram becomes more truly representative of the population (Fig. 23-1, *B*). As N increases further, the histogram takes on the appearance of a continuous function (Fig. 23-1, *C*). In the histogram of hypothetical glucose data in Fig. 23-1, *C,* one can see that the population is centered around 1000 mg/L, with few observations less than 920 mg/L and few greater than 1080 mg/L. The general spread of the data also can be assessed.

If enough data are represented in the histogram and the data are truly random (i.e., each result was affected by random processes alone), the histogram can be used to predict the probability of obtaining future results above or below a certain value. Fig. 23-1, *C,* shows that there is about a 2.3% chance that a future glucose result from this population will be less than 920 mg/L, and a 2.3% chance that a future glucose result will be greater than 1080 mg/L.

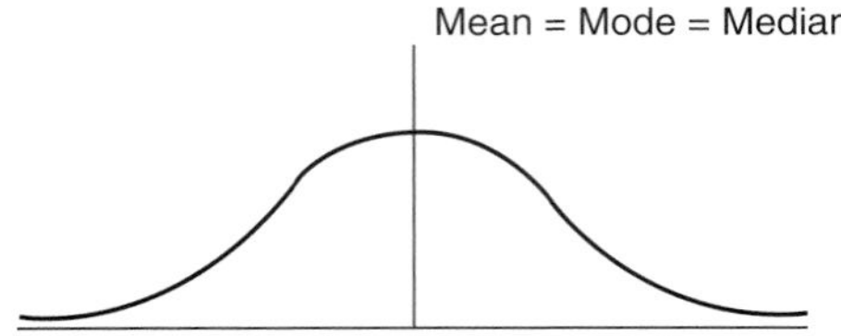

Fig. 23-2 Normal (gaussian) distribution, symmetrical about the mean.

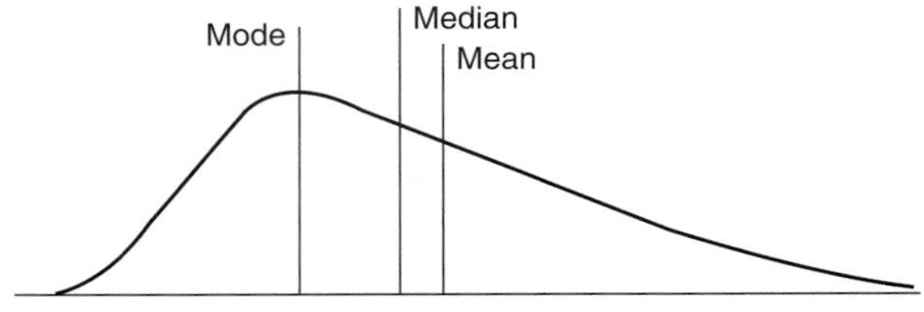

Fig. 23-3 Non-normal distribution.

The curve approximated by the glucose histogram in Fig. 23-1, *C*, is a smooth, "bell-shaped" curve called a *gaussian*, or *normal*, distribution, which is depicted in Fig. 23-2. This symmetrical curve was first described by the French mathematician Abraham de Moivre in 1733 and was further developed by the astronomer-mathematician Karl Friedrich Gauss during the 1800s. The portion of the curve on the right is usually referred to as the *upper tail*, and the portion on the left is called the *lower tail*. Many random variables of interest in medicine and health care, such as reference ranges, have distributions similar to **normal distributions.**

The *parametric* statistical tests discussed in this chapter are used under the assumption that the population being tested is distributed in a gaussian fashion. Before we proceed with parametric statistical comparisons, it is important to establish whether the population is distributed normally. A graphical analysis using *normal probability paper* can be used to test for a normal distribution. However, this method requires a visual evaluation of the sample data for deviation from a straight line and therefore can be very subjective. The graph is constructed by plotting the bin values, such as glucose concentration, along a linear x-axis and the cumulative frequency of the distribution on a nonlinear y-axis, the mathematical function of which is based on a normal distribution. Fig. 23-1, *D*, shows a normal probability plot for 600 glucose values drawn from a group of normal healthy volunteers.

The *Kolmogorov-Smirnov test* can be used to test for normally distributed data. This analysis measures vertical distances between the cumulative distribution and the straight line on normal probability paper. Critical values for the statistically significant difference are obtained from a statistical table.

Another way to measure how well data fit a normal distribution is to calculate skewness and kurtosis coefficients. Skewness measures the asymmetry of the data distribution. Values greater than zero indicate that the upper tail of the curve is longer than the lower tail. Negative values indicate that the lower tail is longer. Kurtosis measures how steep or flat the distribution is with respect to a true normal distribution. Kurtosis coefficients greater than zero indicate that the curve is steep in the center, and that the tails are relatively long. Values less than zero indicate that the curve is flat in the center, and that the tails are short. For data that follow a reasonably **gaussian distribution,** the skewness and kurtosis coefficients should be between 1 and −1. Different types of coefficients called *standard skewness* and *kurtosis coefficients* test for significant deviations from the normal distribution and, analogous to standard deviation, should be between 2 and −2 for normally distributed data.[6] These calculations are usually done with computer software.

When a nonsymmetrical or nongaussian distribution is observed, one option is to *transform* the nongaussian distribution into one that is more normally distributed. This can be accomplished by converting the population values into another form. Transformation techniques include taking the logarithm (base 10, or natural) of the data, taking the reciprocal of the data, and raising the numbers exponentially. After one of these methods is used, the resulting data set often is distributed in a gaussian fashion. If the data still are not normally distributed, *nonparametric* statistical tests are used to analyze the data. In the medical and health care fields, nonparametric distributions usually are either *skewed* or *bimodal.* As alluded to previously, a skewed distribution is one in which the upper or lower tail of the distribution is longer than the other (Fig. 23-3). Serum gamma-glutamyl transferase reference interval data obtained from healthy individuals usually are skewed to the right. A bimodal distribution is seen when data are composed of two related populations (Fig. 23-4). Combined serum uric acid reference interval data obtained from healthy males and females typically demonstrate the appearance of a bimodal distribution when plotted appropriately. This type of distribution often indicates that separate, sex-based reference ranges should be established for the analyte under study.

KEY CONCEPTS BOX 23-1

- A *population* is a large collection of all objects, events or observations under study, whereas a *sample* is a smaller but statistically valid representative subset of the population that can be used to determine statistical data that describes the population.
- The population data can be plotted as a histogram or a probability plot; the shape of the plots can allow conclusions to be drawn about the nature of the distribution.
- A "normal," or *gaussian,* distribution has an even distribution about the center of the population; a *skewed* population has more data in the lower or upper values.
- Tests can be used to determine if an untransformed or transformed sample set is a gaussian distribution.

SECTION OBJECTIVES BOX 23-2

- List three measures of central tendency and the calculations necessary to determine their values.
- Interpret values for mean, median, and mode in order to determine if the distribution is normal or non-normal.
- List three measures of variation and the calculations necessary to determine their values.
- Explain advantages and limitations of the use of coefficient of variation in evaluating variation in methods.
- Apply statistical equations and *t*-tables to determine 95% confidence intervals.
- Differentiate the definitions of accuracy and precision and the statistical calculations that are used to assess each.
- Evaluate diagrams of data in order to assess accuracy and precision.

BASIC DISTRIBUTION STATISTICS

In the previous section, plotting a histogram or frequency distribution was identified as a simple method for visually describing a population of data to assess, at least initially, whether the data set is distributed in a gaussian or a nongaussian fashion. Two general categories of statistics can also be used to describe the distribution of data. These two categories include measures of central tendencies and measures of variation.

Measures of Central Tendencies

Measures of central tendencies are statistics that represent some central value around which the data are distributed. Three measures of central tendencies that often are calculated for clinical laboratory applications are the mean, the median, and the mode.

The **mean** is probably the most widely used statistic and is a simple *arithmetic average.* One calculates the mean by adding up all the observations and dividing by the number of observations, *N*. For a sample of data, calculation of the mean, designated as $\bar{x}$, is illustrated by Eq. 23-1, wherein x_i is an individual observation:

$$\bar{x} = \frac{\sum x_i}{N} \qquad \text{Eq. 23-1}$$

If the entire population of data is used to calculate the mean, the calculated mean is the actual mean of the population, indicated by the symbol "μ." For clinical laboratory applications, it is usually impossible to have the entire population of data collected (i.e., one can always make another measurement unless the population is defined restrictively). For these applications, use of the symbol for the sample mean, $\bar{x}$, is appropriate. This convention indicates that a subset of data from the population was used to calculate $\bar{x}$, which is an estimate of the true population mean.

If the sample data are distributed symmetrically about the mean, the arithmetic mean is actually representative of the

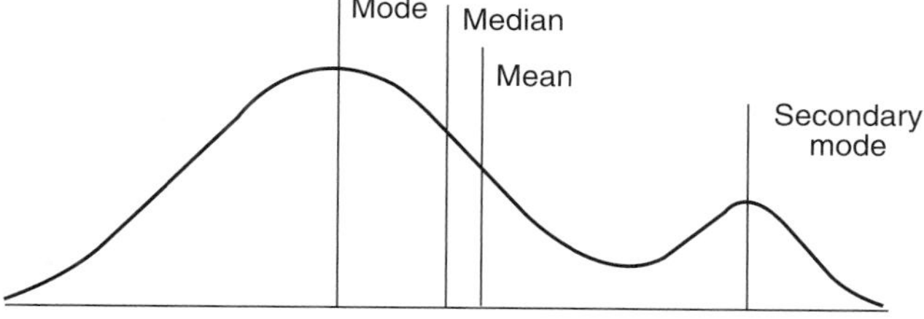

Fig. 23-4 Bimodal distribution.

central tendency of the sample. This feature is illustrated in Fig. 23-1, *D*, which depicts a *normal,* or *gaussian,* distribution. However, any sample of data from a population would have a mean value, whether the distribution was gaussian or nongaussian.

A second measure of central tendency is the **mode.** The mode of a sample of data is that value that is observed most frequently in the sample. It is the value at the peak of the frequency distribution (see Fig. 23-3). If a frequency distribution of data has two peaks, the distribution is *bimodal.* An example of a bimodal distribution is illustrated in Fig. 23-4. For practical applications in the laboratory, each frequency distribution has a minimum of one mode (i.e., the distribution is at least unimodal).

A third measure of central tendency is the **median.** The median is the middle value in a sample of data when all values in the distribution are ranked individually from lowest to highest (or vice versa). Unlike the mean and the mode, the median value describes a true central tendency for all types of distributions, because half of the observations are greater than the median and half of the observations are less than the median.

One characteristic of a perfect normal distribution is that the arithmetic average is the value observed most frequently, and it is also the middle value observed in the sample when values are ranked from lowest to highest. As is illustrated in Fig. 23-1, *D,* this fact results in the same values for mean, median, and mode. All three of these statistics are true measures of central tendency in a true gaussian, or normal, distribution.

In contrast, in a non-normal distribution, such as that depicted in Fig. 23-3, the mean, median, and mode are all different values. The mean does not accurately describe the center of the distribution (although it is still an arithmetic average of the data). It is also apparent that the mode of this distribution does not describe a true central tendency of the sample of data. The median is the only value that can be considered a true measure of this distribution's central tendency. For those non-normal distributions for which the mean and median might be considerably different, it may be more appropriate to use both values or the median value alone to describe central tendencies of the distribution.

There is a significant and often overlooked limitation to using mean values to describe samples of data, even for those samples that are normally distributed. Means can be influenced strongly by values in the data that lie at the extremes of the data range. This feature indicates that when calculating a mean value for a sample of data, one should be critical in evaluating which values may not be representative of the data set, that is, which values are outliers that should be excluded by the use of appropriate techniques (see below). The median is less affected than the mean by extreme values in the data set.

Measures of Variation

In addition to measures of central tendency, other kinds of statistical data are required to characterize effectively a sample of data or a distribution. Measures of central tendency do not provide sufficient information on how close together or far apart the values in a sample of data are. Statistics that indicate the degree to which observed values vary, or the spread of the distribution, are measures of variation. Three measures of variation that often are calculated for clinical laboratory applications are range, variance, and standard deviation.

The **range** is simply the difference between the largest and smallest values in the sample of data. The range is useful for indicating the spread of data when N is small, but when one is using the range, no assumptions can be made concerning the shape of the distribution. However, a limitation of the range as a measure of variation is the fact that it is based on only two values in the sample of data.

More useful measures of variation are the **variance** and **standard deviation.** Variance is calculated by first determining the mean of the sample of data and then subtracting the mean from each value to get N differences. The squares of the differences between the individual values (x_i) and the mean are added. The sum of the squared differences is divided by $N - 1$, which yields the variance (Eq. 23-2, A):

$$\text{Variance} = s^2 = \frac{\sum (x_i - \bar{x})^2}{N-1} \qquad \text{Eq. 23-2A}$$

The *standard deviation (s)* is the square root of the variance, which often is represented as *SD*. The denominator of Eq. 23-2, A, is $N - 1$ rather than N because there are only $N - 1$ **degrees of freedom *(df)*** for the variance once $\bar{x}$ has been used to calculate the variance. The concept of degrees of freedom is explained more fully later in this chapter.

Although s is normally calculated by using the results of single analyses, one frequently needs to know the imprecision of replicate analyses. To calculate this estimate of variation, use the following equation:

$$s_{rep} = \left(\frac{\sum d^2}{N} \right)^{1/2} \qquad \text{Eq. 23-2B}$$

where d is the difference between the replicate measurements. This calculation can be useful for determining whether duplicate analyses can help to achieve a desired level of within-run imprecision for an assay.

Another statistic that is often calculated in laboratory applications is the **coefficient of variation (CV)**. The CV indicates what percentage of the mean is represented by the standard deviation, as is illustrated in Eq. 23-3:

$$\%\text{CV} = \frac{100\%\, s}{\bar{x}} \qquad \text{Eq. 23-3}$$

One advantage of using the CV to express the variation of analytical methods is that the variation is reported in units that are independent of the particular analytical method. Keep in mind, however, that the magnitude of the CV of an analytical method is not completely independent of concentration. In certain instances, routine statistics on two levels of quality control materials may indicate a larger CV at the lower level simply because the numerator of the CV calculation, the mean, is a smaller number than the mean of the higher level of control material. Example 1 depicts the calculation of basic measures of central tendency and basic measures of variation using data from a single level of quality control material.

Example 1. Calculation of basic statistics using a sample of data from repeated cholesterol measurements on one level of quality control material.

Calculate the mean, mode, median, variance, standard deviation, and coefficient of variation.

Sample x_i (mg/L)	$x_i - \bar{x}$	$(x_i - \bar{x})^2$
2080	−1.4	1.96
2090	8.6	73.96
2110	28.6	817.96
2100	18.6	345.96
2010	−71.4	5097.96
2090	8.6	73.96
2040	−41.4	1713.96
2140	58.6	3433.96
2070	−11.4	129.96
2070	−11.4	129.96
2100	18.6	345.96
2110	28.6	817.96
2030	−51.4	2641.96
2090	8.6	73.96
2080	−1.4	1.96
2060	−21.4	457.96
2170	88.6	7849.96
2060	−21.4	457.96
2130	48.6	2361.96
2090	8.6	73.96
2080	−1.4	1.96
2100	18.6	345.96
2000	−81.4	6625.96
2090	8.6	73.96
2040	−41.4	1713.96
2070	−11.4	129.96
2100	18.6	345.96
2080	−1.4	1.96
$\sum x_i = 58{,}280$		$\sum (x_i - \bar{x})^2 = 36{,}142.88$

Mean

$$= \overline{x} = \frac{\sum x_i}{N} = 2081.4 \text{ mg/L}$$

*Median**

$$= 2085 \text{ mg/L}$$

Mode

$$= 2090 \text{ mg/L}$$

Measures of Variance

$$s^2 = \frac{\sum (x_i - \overline{x})^2}{N-1}$$
$$= 36{,}142.88/27 = 1338.6 \text{ mg/L}$$
$$s = 36.5 \text{ mg/L}$$
$$\%CV = 100\% \; s/\overline{x}$$
$$= \frac{36.5 \text{ mg/L} (100\%)}{2081.4 \text{ mg/L}}$$
$$= 1.75\%$$

*When even-numbered samples of data are collected, the two middle values are averaged to obtain the median. For an N of 28, the two middle values are the 14th and 15th values, 2090 mg/L and 2080 mg/L, respectively.

Confidence Intervals

Use of mean and standard deviation values for the purposes of assessing quality control results and determining reference ranges is an important laboratory application. To use the mean and standard deviation values for these applications, the data in the sample must be distributed normally. In a normal distribution, the standard deviation and the mean (which are in the same units) can be used to describe the proportion of values falling in a given area under the normal curve.

The total area under the normal curve theoretically represents all the values in the given population. As is illustrated in Fig. 23-5, the area under the perfect normal distribution from $+1s$ to $-1s$ represents 68.3% of the values, from $+2s$ to $-2s$ represents 95.4% of the values, and from $+3s$ to $-3s$ represents 99.7% of the values. These intervals that contain a stated percentage of the data are called **confidence intervals.** For samples of data that are distributed normally, confidence intervals calculated using the mean and standard deviation can form the basis of statistical quality control rules for acceptance and rejection decisions concerning specific analytical runs (see Chapter 25).

If the results obtained by analyzing the quality control material discussed in Example 1 were perfectly distributed, it would be expected that the range between the mean plus $2s$ and the mean minus $2s$ (2008.4 to 2154.4 mg/L) would exclude 4.6% of the data. In reality, this range excludes 7.1% of the data (2 of 28 values, 2000 mg/L and 2170 mg/L, are outside the $2s$ range). For this sample of data, the $\pm 2s$ range should not be expected to include exactly 95.4% of the values. It was known that the distribution was not perfectly normal once different results for the mean, median, and mode were obtained.

The measurement of cholesterol levels in Example 1 is characterized by a certain degree of imprecision (the %CV is 1.75%). Because the error of the mean measurement of the set of values is smaller than that of a single measurement, the more times a measurement is made, the more certain you can be of its true value. If several means are calculated from different groups of measurements of this quality control specimen, the individual means are distributed about the actual population mean. The random variation in this group of means is described by the **standard error** of the mean ($S_{\overline{x}}$) in Eq. 23-4:

$$s_{\overline{x}} = \frac{s}{\sqrt{N}} \qquad \text{Eq. 23-4}$$

Suppose that for the cholesterol QC measurements discussed in Example 1, you wished to determine the $s_{\overline{x}}$ and the likelihood that the population mean is within a certain range. Putting the appropriate values into Eq. 23-4:

$$s_{\overline{x}} = \frac{36.5 \text{ mg/L}}{\sqrt{28}} = 6.9 \text{mg/L}$$

It then would be expected that 68.3% of the various sample means (with Ns of 28) would be within $\pm 1 \times 6.9$ mg/L of the population mean (2074.5 to 2088.3 mg/L), 95.4% of the means would be within $\pm 2 \times 6.9$ mg/L of the population mean (2067.6 to 2095.2 mg/L), and 99.7% of the means would be within $\pm 3 \times 6.9$ mg/L of the true population mean (2060.7 to 2102.1 mg/L). Therefore, it can be assumed with 95% confidence that the *true* population mean lies within the range of 2067.6 to 2095.2 mg/L. This is termed the *95% confidence interval.*

The true mean cholesterol concentration of the quality control material in Example 1 cannot be determined exactly unless an infinite number of measurements are made. In practice, the population is sampled by obtaining groups of quality control values such as those shown in Example 1. The mean obtained therefore is not the true mean but is an estimate of the true mean. The standard error of the experimentally derived mean, $\overline{x}$, can be used to develop a more exact *confidence interval* that has a known probability of including the true population mean, μ. This interval is described in Eq. 23-5:

$$\mu = \overline{x} \pm t \times s_{\overline{x}} \qquad \text{Eq. 23-5}$$

The t-value is obtained from a t-table (Table 23-1). The t-value depends on the number of degrees of freedom ($N-1$) and the desired probability, p, that the true mean is outside the confidence interval because of chance alone. A probability of $p = 0.05$ implies 95% confidence [$100 \times (1-p)\%$] that the interval includes the true mean.

The t-values describe the same probability distribution depicted in Fig. 23-5, but the distribution in Fig. 23-5 should be used under the assumption that the true population mean and the standard deviation are known. Use of the t-table makes allowances for decreasing confidence in the estimated values of specific parameters as N decreases. Therefore,

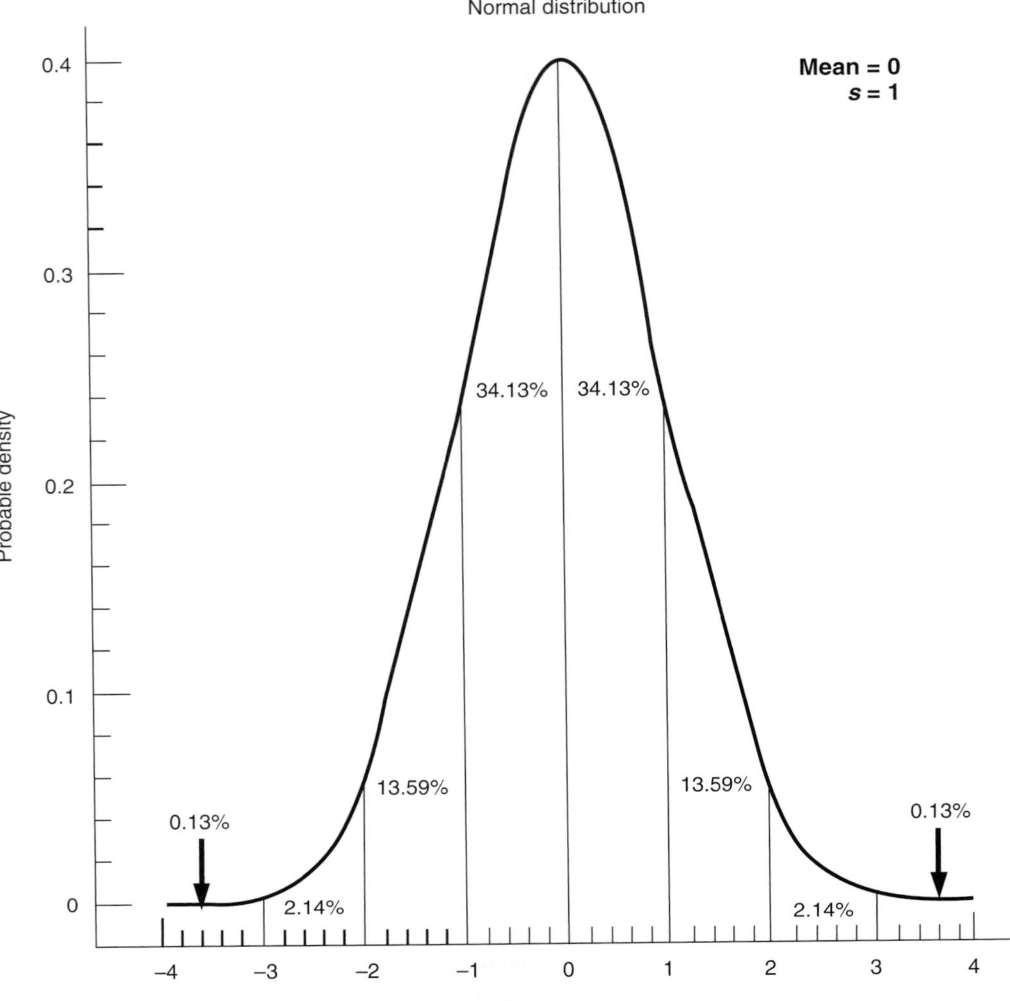

Fig. 23-5 Perfect normal distribution, with a mean = 0, indicating the percentage of results that are in each standard deviation interval between –4 and +4 standard deviations.

an appropriate use of *t*-values is to calculate more accurate confidence intervals for statistics obtained from small samples. An illustration of this is given in Example 2. To construct a confidence interval that includes a true mean, one should be sure that the 0.05 probability that the true mean may be beyond the calculated limits is spread over both ends or tails of the distribution, as is shown in Fig. 23-6. For these purposes, a two-sided, $p = 0.05$, *t*-value is used. To state that the true mean is greater than some single limit, use a one-sided *t*-value. Note that the *t*-value for a two-sided interval for $p = 0.05$ is the same as the *t*-value for a one-sided limit of $p = 0.025$. The practical application of confidence limits is demonstrated on pp. 501-505.

Example 2. Calculating 95% confidence intervals for the mean of a small sample.

Calculate the 95% confidence interval for the mean value of the lactate dehydrogenase (LD) activity of a stable control material after performing only 15 daily determinations.

Sample: All LD values are in IU/L: 324, 337, 350, 295, 284, 322, 339, 350, 309, 322, 348, 320, 298, 345, 335.

The calculated mean and standard deviation of the sample are 325 and 21 IU/L, respectively.

The standard error of the mean (SEM) is calculated as follows:

$$s_{\bar{x}} = s/\sqrt{N} = 21/\sqrt{15} = 5.42\,\text{IU/L}$$

Using the *t*-table in Table 23-1, find the two-sided *t*-value for p = 0.05 and $N - 1$ degrees of freedom ($df = 14$). The *t*-value of 2.14 is the factor used to adjust the SEM so that the correct lower and upper limits of the 95% confidence interval for the mean can be determined for this small sample. Using Eq. 23-5,

$$\mu = \bar{x} \pm t \times s_{\bar{x}}$$

Lower limit of confidence interval: 325 – (2.14) (5.42) = 313.4 IU/L

Upper limit of confidence interval: 325 + (2.14) (5.42) = 336.6 IU/L

There is a 95% probability that the mean LD activity of this sample of quality control measurements is between 313.4 and 336.6 IU/L.

Table 23-1 Critical Values of *t* for Selected Probabilities, *p,* and Degrees of Freedom, *df*

	TWO-SIDED INTERVALS OR TESTS		
	p = 0.10	*p* = 0.05	*p* = 0.01
	ONE-SIDED LIMITS OR TESTS		
df	*p* = 0.05	*p* = 0.025	*p* = 0.005
1	6.31	12.70	63.70
2	2.92	4.30	9.92
3	2.35	3.18	5.84
4	2.13	2.78	4.60
5	2.01	2.57	4.03
6	1.94	2.45	3.71
7	1.89	2.36	3.50
8	1.86	2.31	3.36
9	1.83	2.26	3.25
10	1.81	2.23	3.17
12	1.78	2.18	3.05
14	1.76	2.14	2.98
16	1.75	2.12	2.92
18	1.73	2.10	2.88
20	1.72	2.09	2.85
30	1.70	2.04	2.75
40	1.68	2.02	2.70
60	1.67	2.00	2.66
120	1.66	1.98	2.62
∞	1.64	1.96	2.58

Condensed from Davies OL, Goldsmith PL: *Statistical Methods in Research and Production*, ed 4, New York, 1972, Longman.

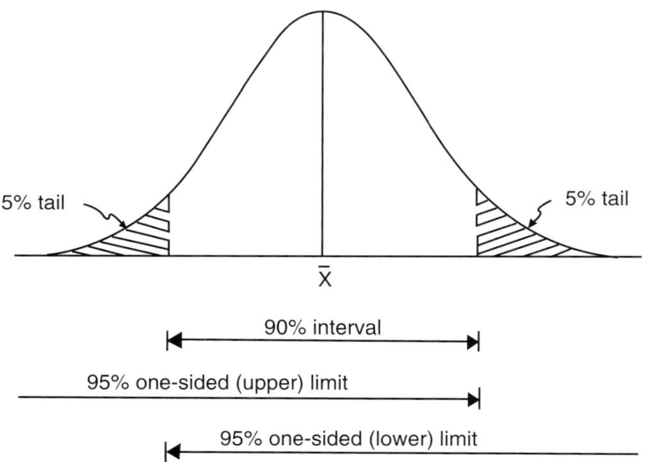

Fig. 23-6 One-sided versus two-sided *t*-values. *t*-values used to calculate 90% interval and 95% one-sided limits are the same.

Measures of Accuracy and Precision

In previous sections, the mean and standard deviation of a normally distributed population were described. When a new analytical method is evaluated by the laboratory, these parameters are used to describe the accuracy and precision of the method (see Chapter 26). **Accuracy** describes the ability of an analytical method to obtain the "true" or correct result after a number of replicate analyses are performed. The closer the mean of *N* replicate analyses of a sample comes to the "true" or known value of that sample, the more accurate is the method. **Precision** (also called **random error**) describes the reproducibility of a method. The narrower the distribution of results, that is, the smaller the standard deviation, after a number of replicate analyses, the better is the precision of a method.

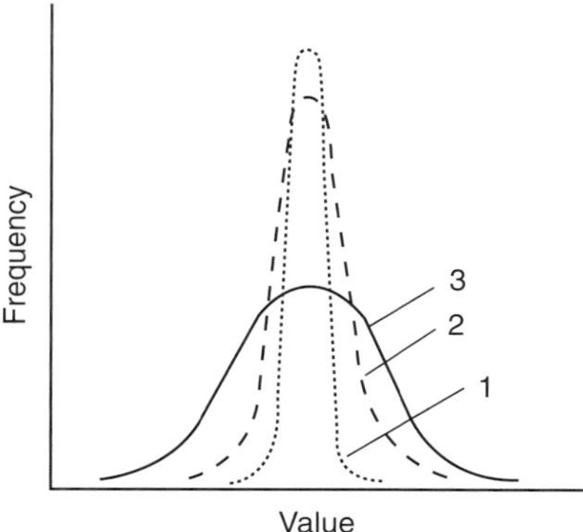

Fig. 23-7 Frequency distributions for three methods using the same means, but different distributions. *1* has the narrowest distribution, whereas the distribution of *3* is wider than that of *2*.

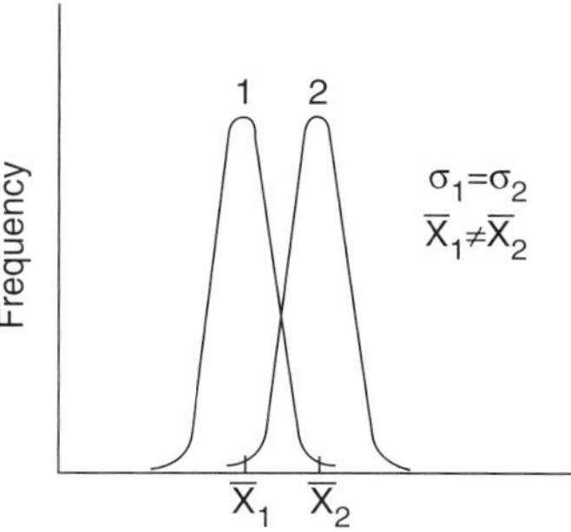

Fig. 23-8 Frequency distribution for replicate analysis by two different methods, *1* and *2*. These two methods are equally precise ($\sigma_1 = \sigma_2$) but are biased in relationship to each other ($\bar{x}_1$ does not equal $\bar{x}_2$).

Fig. 23-7 shows the results of replicate analyses of the same sample performed by three different methods. All three methods have a similar mean and thus similar accuracy. However, the distributions or standard deviations of the results are different for each method. Method 1 has the narrowest distribution or smallest standard deviation and hence has the best precision of the three methods. Method 3 has the widest distribution or largest standard deviation and thus has the poorest precision.

Fig. 23-8 shows the results of replicate analyses of the same sample performed by two different methods. The two methods have a similar distribution of data or similar standard deviations; therefore, their precision is about the same. The means, however, are not equal, and the relative accuracies for the two methods are not the same, which indicates a nonrandom bias, or **systematic error,** between the methods. Determining which method has the better accuracy will depend on which mean

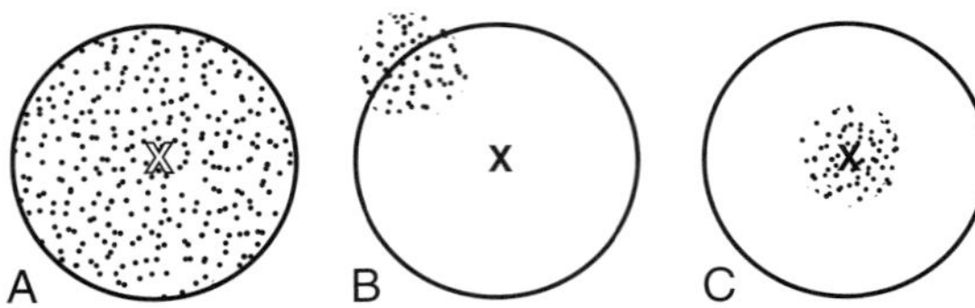

Fig. 23-9 Xs on these targets each denote the true value for a sample. The dots shown on each of the circles **A** to **C** denote the results of three replicate analyses by three different methods: **A,** imprecise but accurate; **B,** precise but inaccurate; **C,** accurate and precise.

is closer to the "true" value of the analyte examined in the sample.

Although the terms are sometimes used interchangeably, accuracy and precision are two distinctly different concepts and must never be interchanged. This is shown in Fig. 23-9. Repeated attempts to hit the middle of the target, the true value, are indicated by dots. A method can be accurate but not very precise, as is shown in Fig. 23-9, *A*. Inaccuracy but good precision is shown in Fig. 23-9, *B*, where the values fall close together but are grouped far from the middle, or "true," value. Fig. 23-9, *C*, shows the goal of all good analytical methods—excellent accuracy *and* precision.

KEY CONCEPTS BOX 23-2

- For a "normal" population, the *mean,* or *average,* best describes the central tendency of a population; for a skewed, or non-normal population, the *median* should be used.
- The statistic that is used to describe the range of data in the population is the *standard deviation* (SD); the coefficient of variation (%CV) normalizes the SD against the mean of the population. The narrower the distribution, the smaller is the SD.
- The confidence interval includes a certain percentage of the data falling within that interval. A 95% confidence interval would include 95% of the data, or almost all of the data within ±2 SD around the mean.
- *Accuracy* is the degree to which the mean of a population differs from the true value; *precision* describes the reproducibility of a repeated measurement.

SECTION OBJECTIVES BOX 23-3

- State the null hypothesis.
- Explain why degrees of freedom are calculated using $n - 1$, or the sample size minus the number of estimated parameters.
- Explain the usefulness of the *F*-test, the *t*-test, the unpaired *t*-test, the paired *t*-test, and the gap test.
- Interpret calculated *t*-statistics to determine the overlap of probability distributions.
- Explain the advantage of ANOVA rather than individual *t*-test calculations in the clinical laboratory.

PARAMETRIC COMPARISONS OF POPULATIONS

The Null Hypothesis and Statistical Significance

When a comparison is made between two samples from two populations, invariably a difference between the means $(\bar{x})$ and standard deviations (s) is observed. These observed differences may or may not reflect a true difference between populations. Therefore, it is necessary to test the **null hypothesis,** which states that there is no difference between the true means (μ) or the true standard deviations (σ) of the two populations. The corresponding calculated values, $\bar{x}$ or s, are used for this purpose.

Two Hypotheses

$$s_1^2 = s_2^2 \quad \text{or} \quad \bar{x}_1 = \bar{x}_2 \quad \text{Null hypothesis}$$

$$s_1^2 \neq s_2^2 \quad \text{or} \quad \bar{x}_1 \neq \bar{x}_2 \quad \text{Alternative hypothesis}$$

Many different statistical tests can be used to generate a test *statistic* that indicates whether the null hypothesis should be accepted or rejected. If the statistical test result indicates that the null hypothesis should be accepted, the possibility still exists that the calculated test statistic that forms the basis for the test results does not reflect the truth, and the null hypothesis may be incorrectly accepted. The level of significance or the chance of this occurring is defined by the value p, where $100\% \ (1 - p)$ is the percentage of confidence that the test results are statistically significant. A minimum value of $p = 0.05$ is customarily used to test for significance. This value means that there is a 95% chance that the results of a statistical test are significant or, conversely, that there is a 5% chance that accepting the statistical test result is the wrong decision.

For many applications in clinical chemistry, a difference that is only statistically different may still be acceptable for routine applications. It is of course important to identify differences that *are* medically significant or that do not meet regulatory requirements (see Chapters 25 and 26).

Degrees of Freedom

The term *degrees of freedom* usually is defined as the number of ways in which a group of numbers can vary independently. This is often a difficult idea to explain or define. It is calculated by subtracting the number of estimated parameters from the sample size. For example, consider 20 bilirubin measurements; the sample size is 20, and for this series, the number of degrees of freedom is 20. Any one of these 20 values can be altered, and this change will not affect the value of any of the other measurements in the series. However, if the mean of the 20 values is calculated, the mean has only 19, or $n - 1$, degrees of freedom. It is possible to change 19 values without changing the mean, but the 20th value will have to be a specific number, so that the mean remains the same. Therefore, for the calculation of the mean, the degrees of freedom are calculated as $n - 1$. The number of degrees of freedom is an important parameter used in the calculation of many statistical tests, for example, the *t*-test.

Table 23-2 Critical Values of F for $p = 0.05$ and Selected Degrees of Freedom, *df*

	DEGREES OF FREEDOM FOR NUMERATOR						
***df* for Denominator**	**5**	**10**	**15**	**20**	**30**	**60**	**∞**
1	230.00	242.00	246.00	248.00	250.00	252.00	254.00
2	19.30	19.40	19.40	19.40	19.50	19.50	19.50
3	9.01	8.79	8.70	8.66	8.62	8.57	8.53
4	6.26	5.96	5.86	5.80	5.75	5.69	5.63
5	5.05	4.74	4.62	4.56	4.50	4.43	4.36
6	4.39	4.06	3.94	3.87	3.81	3.74	3.67
7	3.97	3.64	3.51	3.44	3.38	3.30	3.23
8	3.69	3.35	3.22	3.15	3.08	3.01	2.93
9	3.48	3.14	3.01	2.94	2.86	2.79	2.71
10	3.33	2.98	2.85	2.77	2.70	2.62	2.54
15	2.90	2.54	2.40	2.33	2.25	2.16	2.07
20	2.71	2.35	2.20	2.12	2.04	1.95	1.84
30	2.53	2.16	2.01	1.93	1.84	1.74	1.62
60	2.37	1.99	1.84	1.75	1.65	1.53	1.39
∞	2.21	1.83	1.67	1.57	1.46	1.32	1.00

Modified from Barnett RN: *Clinical Laboratory Statistics*, ed 2, Boston, 1979, Brown & Co.

Comparison of Random Variation (Precision)—The *F*-Test

The **t-test** often is used to compare the means ($\overline{x}$) of two groups of observations so one can test whether there is a significant difference between the two group means (see p. 426). Two assumptions are made with the *t*-test: that the groups are *normally* distributed and that there is no significant difference between the group variances. It is not possible to tell simply by observation of the data how different the variances in the two groups must be before the *t*-test cannot be used. However, the null hypothesis that there is no significant difference between the variances can be tested by use of the ***F*-test.**

The *F*-test, or variance ratio test, is used to determine whether an observed difference between the standard deviations *(s)* of two sets of data is statistically significant. One calculates the *F*-test statistic by dividing the larger variance (s_1^2) by the smaller variance (s_2^2), as is shown in Eq. 23-6:

$$F = \frac{s_1^2}{s_2^2} \qquad \text{Eq. 23-6}$$

The calculated *F*-value is compared with a critical *F*-value obtained from an *F*-table (Table 23-2) by using the number of degrees of freedom from each group at a specified level of *p*, such as $p = 0.05$. If the calculated *F*-value is less than the critical value, the null hypothesis is accepted as true. If the calculated *F*-value is greater than the critical value, the alternative hypothesis is accepted as true.

Example 3. *F*-test.

A comparison between folate levels in two groups is needed, but the standard deviations look considerably different. The data below show folate levels from 21 laboratory workers and 16 individuals suspected of having dietary anemia.

	Serum Folate, μg/L	
	Workers ($n = 21$)	**Patients ($n = 16$)**
	13	5
	18	15
	14	2
	16	21
	19	6
	15	7
	12	16
	17	4
	13	3
	16	5
	15	18
	17	2
	18	6
	20	1
	17	4
	13	16
	21	
	15	
	16	
	19	
	16	
Average	16.2	8.2
Standard deviation	2.44	6.59

$$F = \frac{(6.59)^2}{(2.44)^2} = \frac{43.43}{5.95} = 7.30$$

Use the F-table (see Table 23-2) to find a critical F-value. Scan across the F-table to the column that corresponds to $n - 1$ degrees of freedom in the numerator (15) and down to the row that corresponds to $n - 1$ degrees of freedom in the denominator (20), and note a critical value of 2.20. Because the calculated value exceeds this value, the difference in the calculated SDs is significant with $p < 0.05$.

The results of this test indicate that the t-test should *not* be used to compare the two means. The **Mann-Whitney test** may be a better alternative; this test is discussed later in this chapter.

Comparison of Means (Accuracy or Bias)—The *t*-Test

The t-test is used to check for statistically significant differences between two experimental means, or between an experimental mean and a stated value.

Hypothesis Testing

Testing the difference between an experimental mean and a stated or known value involves testing to see whether the stated value is included in the confidence interval around the experimental mean. If it is not, the null hypothesis is rejected, and there appears to be a difference between the stated value and the experimental mean value. In this case, Eq. 23-7 and 23-8 are used to calculate the paired t-statistic, which is used to determine whether the null hypothesis will be accepted or rejected.

$$t = \frac{\text{Sample mean} - \text{Hypothesized mean}}{\text{Standard error of sample mean}} \qquad \text{Eq. 23-7}$$

$$t = \frac{\bar{x} - \mu}{s/\sqrt{n}} \qquad \text{Eq. 23-8}$$

For example, assume that the glucose concentration in a quality control specimen obtained from the National Institute of Standards and Technology is stated to be 1120 mg/L. This material is used as a quality control sample for 30 consecutive days.

For these data, the mean is 1110 mg/L, and the s is 25 mg/L. Is the mean of the data significantly different from the stated value?

$$t = \frac{1110 - 1120}{\frac{25}{\sqrt{30}}} = -2.19$$

The critical t-value for $p = 0.05$ and 29 df (rounded to 30 in Table 23-1) is 2.04. Thus this month's mean of 1110 mg/L is significantly different from the assigned glucose concentration of 1120 mg/L. See also p. 494 for an application of the t-test to assess bias in a methods comparison experiment.

Testing the statistical significance between two measured means using the t-test involves testing the degree of overlap of their respective probability distributions. If there is little or no overlap, the populations are considered to be different. If significant overlap exists, you cannot be sure that there is any difference. A t-value is calculated from the data and compared with a critical t-value. Table 23-1 gives many of the critical values from the t-distributions. If the absolute value of the calculated t-value does not exceed the critical t-value, the null hypothesis is accepted, and such acceptance indicates that a statistically significant difference between the two distributions does not exist, that is, the means are the same.

Two different t-tests are available for comparing the means of different sample populations: the *unpaired t-test* and the *paired t-test.*

Unpaired t-Test

The unpaired t-test is used when the difference between the means of two independent populations is being analyzed. One example is the comparison of the means of patients' glucose values from two different hospitals. When the unpaired t-test is used, it is assumed that the variances of the two populations are equal, and this must be verified first with the F-test. If there is no statistically significant difference between the variances, it is proper to proceed with the t-test. The *pooled sample variance* (s_p^2) is first calculated as shown in Eq. 23-9:

$$s_p^2 = \frac{(n_1 - 1)s_1^2 + (n_2 - 1)s_2^2}{n_1 + n_2 - 2} \qquad \text{Eq. 23-9}$$

where s_1 and s_2 are the standard deviations of the two groups of sizes n_1 and n_2. With use of $\bar{x}_1$ and $\bar{x}_2$ for the means of the two groups, the *unpaired t-statistic* is calculated as shown in Eq. 23-10:

$$t = \frac{\bar{x}_1 - \bar{x}_2}{s_p\sqrt{1/n_1 + 1/n_2}} \qquad \text{Eq. 23-10}$$

where s_p is the pooled standard deviation. Each group contributes to the degrees of freedom associated with s_p, so that the calculated unpaired t-statistic has $(n_1 - 1) + (n_2 - 1)$ or $n_1 + n_2 - 2$ degrees of freedom. The critical t-value is found from a t-table using the calculated degrees of freedom and comparing with the calculated t-value.

Example 4. Equal variance unpaired t-test.

A reference laboratory begins to use a new method for serum immunoglobulin A. Samples are received from two regions of the country. Random samples from healthy patients from each region are tested to find out whether the reference ranges for these two regions are the same.

	Region A	**Region B**
Mean ($\bar{x}$) (mg/L)	2260	2650
Standard deviation (s) (mg/L)	584	473
Number of samples (n)	33	29

The unpaired t-test is used to determine whether the observed differences between the two means are significant. The F-test is first performed to ensure that the variances are statistically the same.

$$F = \frac{(584)^2}{(473)^2} = \frac{341{,}056}{223{,}729} = 1.52$$

Use the F-table (see Table 23-2) to find a critical F-value. Scan across the F-table to the column that corresponds to $n - 1$ degrees of freedom in the numerator (32) and down to the row that corresponds to $n - 1$ degrees of freedom in the denominator (28), and note a critical value of 1.84. (You can interpolate the table to obtain the exact value for $n_1 = 32$ and $n_2 = 28$ or round off to 30, as shown in this example.) Because the calculated value is less than the critical value, the difference in precision is insignificant with $p < 0.05$. The result of this test indicates that the t-test can be used to compare the two mean values.

To calculate the t-statistic, first calculate s_p:

$$s_p^{\,2} = \frac{(33-1)(584)^2 + (29-1)(473)^2}{33+29-2}$$

$$s_p^{\,2} = 286{,}303$$

$$s_p = \sqrt{286{,}303} = 535$$

Then calculate the t-statistic:

$$t = \frac{2260 - 2650}{535 \times \sqrt{1/33 + 1/29}} = -2.86$$

Use the t-table (see Table 23-1) to find a critical t-value. Scan down the t-table to the column that corresponds to $n_A + n_B - 2$, or 60 degrees of freedom, and note a critical value of 2.00. Because the absolute value of the calculated t-value $|-2.86| = 2.86$, and this is greater than 2.00, the difference in the means is significant with $p < 0.05$. Thus the sample distributions for the two regions do not overlap enough to declare them the same. The laboratory would need separate regional reference ranges for the samples it is testing.

Suppose that $s_1 \neq s_2$, but you are reasonably certain that the two populations are normally distributed. In this case, the pooled estimate of the variance, $s_p^{\,2}$, cannot be used. However, another form of the unpaired t-test, sometimes called the *separate-variance t-test,* can be used. The formula in Eq. 23-11 approximates a student's t-distribution for normally distributed response variables and does not require that the population variances be equal:

$$t = \frac{\bar{x}_1 - \bar{x}_2}{\left(s_1^{\,2}/n_1 + s_2^{\,2}/n_2\right)^{1/2}} \qquad \text{Eq. 23-11}$$

The number of degrees of freedom can be found by using the formula shown in Eq. 23-12. The answer is rounded down to the next lowest integer. For example, 7.6 becomes 7 degrees of freedom.

$$df = \frac{(w_1 + w_2)^2}{w_1^{\,2}/(n_1 - 1) + w_2^{\,2}/(n_2 - 1)} \qquad \text{Eq. 23-12}$$

where df = degrees of freedom and $w_1 = s_1^{\,2}/n_1$ and $w_2 = s_2^{\,2}/n_2$.

Example 5. Separate variance unpaired t-test.

In a study of chronic hepatitis, serum alkaline phosphatase levels were reported for 9 patients with inactive disease and 25 patients with active disease. Use the unpaired t-test to test the hypothesis that there is a difference between the alkaline phosphatase means for the active-disease and the inactive-disease populations.

	Serum Alkaline Phosphatase (IU/L)	
	Inactive	**Active**
	65	103
	72	210
	84	92
	68	225
	89	110
	110	286
	77	96
	95	216
	81	94
		150
		195
		208
		95
		163
		184
		89
		238
		99
		116
		224
		124
		135
		201
		92
		176
$\bar{x}$	82	157
s	14.2	58.5
n	9	25

The F-statistic for the sample variances is $(58.5)^2/(14.2)^2 = 16.74$, which is much greater than the critical value of 3.12 (see Table 23-2). Because the variances are very different, the separate-variance t-test is used.

$$t = \frac{82 - 157}{\left[(14.2)^2/9 + (58.5)^2/25\right]^{1/2}}$$

$$t = -75/12.6 = -5.95$$

The degrees of freedom are as follows:

$$w_1 = (14.2)^2/9 = 22.4$$

$$w_2 = (58.5)^2/25 = 136.9$$

$$df = \frac{(w_1 + w_2)^2}{w_1^{\,2}/(n_1 - 1) + w_2^{\,2}/(n_2 - 1)}$$

$$df = \frac{(22.4+136.9)^2}{(22.4)^2/(9-1)+(136.9)^2/(25-1)}$$

$$df = 25376/843 = 30.1 \simeq 30$$

For 30 degrees of freedom from Table 23-1, the critical t-value at $p = 0.05$ is 2.04.

Because the absolute value of the calculated t-value $|-5.95| = 5.95$, and this is greater than 2.04, the difference in the means is significant with $p < 0.05$. Thus the sample distributions for the two disease groups do not overlap enough for them to be declared the same.

Paired t-Test

A special case of comparison of means is the paired-sample t-test. Paired-sample testing (also called "split" sample testing) is used to minimize the effects of sample variations, which can lead to ambiguous results. For example, if you were comparing the blood-gas Po_2 method x with the blood-gas Po_2 method y, and specimens were drawn from different random patient populations for each method, extraneous variations in the populations could mask true methodological differences. To eliminate this variance, analyze the same specimens using both methods (see Example 6). The equation used to calculate the paired t-statistic is as follows:

$$t = \frac{\bar{x}_1 - \bar{x}_2}{s_d/\sqrt{n}} \qquad \text{Eq. 23-13}$$

where $\bar{x}_1$ and $\bar{x}_2$ are the means of the two paired populations, s_d is the standard deviation of the *difference* between the populations, and n is the number of samples. There are $n - 1$ degrees of freedom. To calculate s_d, find the standard deviation of the differences between each pair of results, or between each result and a known or stated value. Example 6 shows the calculation of a paired t-test between two groups of data.

Example 6. Paired t-test.

A laboratory examines a new method for Po_2 by running 40 samples in a paired fashion on the old and new instruments. Using a paired t-test, compare the data to determine whether any bias exists between the methods.

	Po_2 (mm Hg)		
	Old	**New**	**Difference**
	88	88	0
	118	121	−3
	115	119	−4
	189	198	−9
	36	36	0
	123	123	0
	123	118	5
	200	203	−3
	60	62	−2
	86	86	0
	61	62	−1
	81	87	−6
	33	31	2
	223	232	−9
	47	48	−1
	38	36	2
	140	142	−2
	67	67	0
	87	90	−3
	218	225	−7
	79	80	−1
	56	56	0
	228	224	4
	65	67	−2
	86	88	−2
	327	334	−7
	59	62	−3
	36	36	0
	100	101	−1
	146	140	6
	112	106	6
	218	212	6
	95	94	1
	67	68	−1
	71	72	−1
	102	100	2
	92	91	1
	106	105	1
	64	60	4
	105	114	−9
Avg	108.7	109.6	−0.93
s	64.1	65.3	3.86

First, the variances must be checked by using the F-test to verify that there is no significant difference between the SDs of the methods. The F-statistic for the sample variances is $(65.3)^2/(64.1)^2 = 1.04$, which is less than the critical F-value of 1.69 (see Table 23-2) for $p = 0.05$ at 39 degrees of freedom. Because the variances are not significantly different, the t-test can be used.

$$t = \frac{\bar{x}_1 - \bar{x}_2}{s_d/\sqrt{n}}$$

$$t = \frac{-0.93}{3.86/\sqrt{40}}$$

$$t = -1.52$$

The critical t-value for $p = 0.05$ at 39 degrees of freedom is 2.02. Because the absolute calculated t-value $|-1.52| = 1.52$, which, according to Table 23-1, is less than the critical value, 2.02, the means are not significantly different. The methods are yielding results that are not statistically biased from each other.

One-Way Analysis of Variance (ANOVA)

ANOVA is a method used for testing the hypothesis that several different groups (three or more), the distributions of which are normal, all have the same mean. A logical approach to this problem might be to perform a t-test on each difference, beginning with the largest, until the null hypothesis is rejected for one test. For example, if three population means were compared by testing of the hypothesis that all three population means are equal, it would be necessary to carry out three t-tests: a test of the hypothesis that $\bar{x}_1 = \bar{x}_2$, a test of the hypothesis that $\bar{x}_1 = \bar{x}_3$, and a test of the hypothesis that $\bar{x}_2 = \bar{x}_3$. However, this approach would become increasingly inefficient as the number of populations increased. Also, when many comparisons are being performed, some may fail because of chance alone.

In ANOVA, k means (where $k \geq 3$) are compared by testing with the null hypothesis that $\bar{x}_1 = \bar{x}_2 = \bar{x}_3 = \ldots \bar{x}_k$. An F-statistic is calculated, and if this statistic is less than a specified value, the null hypothesis is accepted, and the means for all groups are not significantly different from one another. The alternative hypothesis is always that at least one sample mean does not equal another sample mean. If the null hypothesis is rejected, it cannot be stated that all the sample means are different. It can be concluded only that one of the sample means does not equal one other sample mean. Because ANOVA analysis cannot tell which of the means is significantly different from the others, alternative methods, such as the Bonferroni method for multiple comparisons,[6] are used to determine which of the means is different.

A major advantage of ANOVA compared with the use of individual t-tests is that ANOVA deals with the larger overall sample population. By using as many data as possible, ANOVA is essentially calculating the best estimate of the true population variance. Differences among the group means then are tested with reference to this best estimate of the population variance. This decreases the possibility that random differences in the variances within individual groups will obscure true findings. In the clinical chemistry laboratory, ANOVA can be a useful statistical tool.

Testing a Sample for Outliers Using the Gap Test

(see also p. 426)

When results or data points are distributed in gaussian fashion, graphing a frequency plot of the data allows them to be assessed visually. It is possible that during this assessment, the investigator may identify an **outlier,** which is a result or data point that is so far outside the range of all other results or data points that it is considered unlikely that the result is from the population that has been sampled. Unfortunately, although the experienced investigator might feel comfortable with this assessment, a visual inspection of a frequency distribution or histogram is subjective in nature.

Certain samples of data can be evaluated for the presence of outliers through the use of more rigorous criteria established by the investigator, for example, exclusion of data points that exceed a given percentage of the mean or median value. A statistical technique that allows the investigator to test a sample for outliers is the *gap test.*[9]

Use of the gap test provides valid statistical evidence that justifies the exclusion of an outlier from a particular sample. To use the gap test on a sample, you must arrange the series of results in order, from the lowest to the highest value. Then assign the results particular values of x in one of the following two ways:

$x_1 < x_2 < \ldots < x_n$ when testing an extreme high value

$x_n < x_{n-1} < \ldots < x_1$ when testing an extreme low value

In the first case, the smallest value is designated as x_1, whereas in the second, the largest value is x_1. Particular sample test quotients are then selected from standard statistical tables comparing different values of n and varying levels of significance.[9] A sample test quotient is a ratio of two different equations that describes the relationship of x to the overall range of data. Once the sample test quotient is calculated, it is possible to determine whether there is a statistically unacceptable "gap" between this x and the rest of the data. If so, the x can be justifiably discarded from the data set as an outlier. Because there are different levels of significance and different values of n, different sample test quotients can be used. Texts that provide these tables indicate which sample test quotient should be used, given the value of n, the level of significance selected, and the value (extremely high or extremely low value) that is to be tested. Tests of an extremely high value require the use of a table that is different from that used for the test of extremely low values.

Use of the sample test quotient allows for calculation of a gap using specific data points in the ordered list. As an example, the sample test quotient used for an n of 15 when an extremely high value is tested would require a gap calculation based on the ordered results designated as follows:

$$\frac{x_n - x_{n-2}}{x_n - x_3}$$

The recommended gap then is calculated on the basis of n of the sample and is compared with the value listed in the statistical table in the significance column of choice (for example, $p < 0.05$). If the calculated gap is greater than the value listed in the table (at the desired probability level and n value), the investigator is justified in discarding this value as an outlier with the significance limit selected in the table.

KEY CONCEPTS BOX 23-3

- The "null hypothesis" assumes that there is no difference between two statistics that are being compared. A statistical test is used to prove or disprove that hypothesis.
- For a "normal" population, the *F-test* is used to compare the variability, or variances (*s* or *SD*), of two populations.
- For a "normal" population, the *t*-test is used to compare the means of two populations.
- The *t*-test can be used to determine whether there is a difference between a population mean and a target value for that mean.
- The *t*-test also can be used to test the null hypothesis for two means when the data are gathered from two separate populations *(unpaired t-test),* or when two observations are collected on the same sample *(paired t-test).*

SECTION OBJECTIVES BOX 23-4

- Contrast parametric and nonparametric statistics.
- Explain the purpose, process, and interpretation of the sign test, the Mann-Whitney rank sum test, and chi-square analysis.

NONPARAMETRIC COMPARISONS OF POPULATIONS

Nonparametric Distribution Statistics

The statistical tests described above are termed **parametric statistics** because they assume a gaussian, or normal, distribution of the data. Many populations do not meet this criterion, and the analyst needs techniques for describing and comparing these populations statistically. **Nonparametric statistics** require no assumptions about the distribution and thus can be considered more general than parametric statistics.

The simplest nonparametric procedure is to rank the data in order from the lowest (value = 1) to the highest (value = n). The range of the data set is the difference between the lowest and highest values, and the median value indicates the central tendency of the data set. The ranked data can be used, for example, to determine the limits of reference intervals for those analytes whose distributions are not gaussian. The lower 2.5 percentile and the upper 97.5 percentile of the ranked data usually are selected as the lower and upper limits of a reference interval; this is analogous to ± 2 SDs of a Gaussian distribution. The central 95% of the data are within the reference interval limits.

Sign Test

One of the simplest nonparametric tests for the comparison of two nongaussian populations is the **sign test,** which is analogous to the t-test. The sign test essentially uses the median rather than the mean of a data set. In one application, all the data in a single data set can be compared with some stated (critical) value. Data points higher than the stated value are assigned a plus value (+), lower points are assigned a minus value (−), and zeros are assigned to those values equal to the critical value. The sign test also can be used to compare the results of two methods (A with B) using paired samples. If the B value is higher than A for a given sample, the sample is assigned a plus value. If the B value is less than A, it is assigned a minus value, and zeros are assigned to those samples in which A = B. A hypothesis is assumed that there is no difference between the median of the sample data set and the critical value, or between the two samples in each pair, depending on how the test is used. If this hypothesis is correct, the median difference (A − B) should be zero, and there should be approximately equal numbers of positive and negative differences.

The investigator performs the test by designating the difference between each data pair as negative, positive, or zero, with the actual numerical difference being unimportant, and then tabulating the results. The number of negative results then is compared with a critical range from a table of "exact" confidence limits for Np (Table 23-3), with the table entered at the level of the number of nonzero differences observed between the two populations. Np is a short-term designation for the sample size, N, and the significance level of probability, p. So, Table 23-3 can be said to describe exact confidence limits for a given sample size at a given probability. If the negative difference value (the number of negative results) is outside the critical range, the difference between the median values of the two populations is considered significant. Example 7 demonstrates the use of the sign test.

Example 7. Sign test.

To determine whether there is a significant difference between plasma and serum potassium concentrations (mmol/L), investigators obtain for analysis both types of samples from 18 volunteers.

Table **23-3** Exact Confidence Limits for Np (Binomial Distribution), $p = 0.05$; $N = 0$ to 99

N	0	1	2	3	4	5	6	7	8	9
0	—	—	—	—	—	—	0-6	0-7	0-8	1-8
10	1-9	1-10	2-10	2-11	2-12	3-12	3-13	4-13	4-14	4-15
20	5-15	5-16	5-17	6-17	6-18	7-18	7-19	7-20	8-20	8-21
30	9-21	9-22	9-23	10-23	10-24	11-24	11-25	12-25	12-26	12-27
40	13-27	13-28	14-28	14-29	15-29	15-30	15-31	16-31	16-32	17-32
50	17-33	18-33	18-34	18-35	19-35	19-36	20-36	20-37	21-37	21-38
60	21-39	22-39	22-40	23-40	23-41	24-41	21-42	25-42	25-43	25-44
70	26-44	26-45	27-45	27-46	28-46	28-47	28-48	29-48	29-49	30-49
80	30-50	31-50	31-51	32-51	32-52	32-53	33-53	33-54	34-54	34-55
90	35-55	35-56	36-56	36-57	37-57	37-58	37-59	38-59	38-60	39-60

Condensed from Lenter C: *Geigy Scientific Tables*, vol 2, *Introduction to Statistics, Statistical Tables, Mathematical Formulae*, ed 8, Allschwil, Switzerland, 1982, Ciba-Geigy.

Table 23-4 Acceptance Region for the Rank Sum *T* (Mann-Whitney-Wilcoxon 2-Sample Test), $p = 0.05$

N_1 / N_2	1	2	3	4	5	6	7	8	9	10	11	12	13	14	15
1	—	—	—	—	—	—	—	—	—	—	—	—	—	—	—
2	—	—	—	—	—	—	—	36-52	45-63	55-75	66-88	79-101	92-116	106-132	121-149
3	—	—	—	—	15-30	22-38	29-48	38-58	47-70	58-82	69-96	82-110	95-126	110-142	125-160
4	—	—	—	10-26	16-34	23-43	31-53	40-64	49-77	60-90	72-104	85-119	99-135	114-152	130-170
5	—	—	6-21	11-29	17-38	24-48	33-58	42-70	52-83	63-97	75-112	89-127	103-144	118-162	134-181
6	—	—	7-23	12-32	18-42	26-52	34-64	44-76	55-89	64-104	79-119	92-136	107-153	122-172	139-191
7	—	—	7-26	13-35	20-45	27-57	36-69	46-82	57-96	69-111	82-127	96-144	111-162	127-181	144-201
8	—	3-19	8-28	14-38	21-49	29-61	38-74	49-87	60-102	72-118	85-135	100-152	115-171	131-191	149-211
9	—	3-21	8-31	14-42	22-53	31-65	40-79	51-93	62-109	75-125	89-142	104-160	119-180	136-200	154-221
10	—	3-23	9-33	15-45	23-57	32-70	42-84	53-99	65-115	78-132	92-150	107-169	124-188	141-209	159-231
11	—	3-25	9-36	16-48	24-61	34-74	44-89	55-105	68-121	81-139	96-157	111-177	128-197	145-219	164-241
12	—	4-26	10-38	17-51	26-64	35-79	46-94	58-110	71-127	84-146	99-165	115-185	132-206	150-228	169-251
13	—	4-28	10-41	18-54	27-68	37-83	48-99	60-116	73-134	88-152	103-172	119-193	136-215	155-237	174-261
14	—	4-30	11-43	19-57	28-72	38-88	50-104	62-122	76-140	91-159	106-180	123-201	141-223	160-246	179-271
15	—	4-32	11-46	20-60	29-76	40-92	52-109	65-127	79-146	94-166	110-187	127-209	145-232	164-256	184-281

Condensed from Lenter C: *Geigy Scientific Tables*, vol 2, *Introduction to Statistics, Statistical Tables, Mathematical Formulae*, ed 8, Allschwil, Switzerland, 1982, Ciba-Geigy.

Plasma	Serum	Difference
4.0	4.2	–
3.8	3.8	0
3.6	3.7	–
3.9	3.8	+
4.4	4.5	–
4.6	4.4	+
4.8	4.9	–
4.5	4.7	–
4.3	4.5	–
4.0	3.9	+
4.1	4.1	0
4.0	4.1	–
3.5	3.6	–
3.7	3.7	0
3.6	3.7	–
4.2	4.2	0
4.1	4.0	+
4.5	4.5	0

The null hypothesis assumes that there is no difference between the medians of the two samples, and if this hypothesis is correct, the difference between the median of the plasma samples and the median of the serum samples should be zero. There should be approximately equal numbers of positive and negative differences.

Negatives 9
Positives 4
Zeros 5

Take the number of negative differences to a table of "exact" confidence limits for *Np*. Enter the table at $N =$ (total number of data pairs) – (number of zero differences). (See Table 23-3.)

$$N = 18 - 5 = 13$$

The critical range for an adjusted sample size of 13 is 2 – 11. Because the observed number of negative differences, 9, does not fall outside this range, the median difference between the paired plasma and the serum samples is not significantly different from zero at the 5% level.

Mann-Whitney Rank Sum Test

(See Example 8.)

Another alternative to the *t*-test is the *rank sum test*. There are two forms of this test, one by Wilcoxon, the other by Mann and Whitney. The test is commonly called the *Mann-Whitney test* to avoid confusion with the paired test also developed by Wilcoxon.

The test is performed by taking sample data from the two populations being compared, ranking them as if the data belonged to one population, and then calculating the sum of the ranks of each group. The sum of the smaller *N* is designated *T* and is used in a table of *acceptance regions for the rank sum T* (Table 23-4); the larger *N* is designated in the table as N_2. If the *T*-value is outside the acceptance range for the number of values in each sample, the difference in the median values of the two populations is taken to be significant at a chosen *p* value.

If the populations were identical, an even distribution among the ranks of the two samples would be expected. An extremely large or extremely small rank sum in one of the samples should not be observed when the populations are the same. The rank sum table gives the limits for these extremes, and if these limits are exceeded, it makes sense to reject the null hypothesis of equality between the two populations.

Example 8. Mann-Whitney rank sum test.

A comparison is conducted to determine whether there is any difference between the blood urea nitrogen (BUN) concentrations in renal transplant recipients with stable graft function and those in a group of patients with urinary tract infection (UTI). The following results in milligrams per liter are observed in the two groups:

UTI ($n_1 = 14$)		Transplant ($n_2 = 12$)	
Rank	BUN	Rank	BUN
1	150		
2	170		
3	180		
*4.5	190		
		*4.5	190
**7	200		
**7	200		
		**7	200
9.5	210		
		9.5	210
12	220		
		12	220
		12	220
14	230		
16.5	240		
16.5	240		
		16.5	240
		16.5	240
		19	250
20.5	260		
		20.5	260
		22	270
23	280		
24	290		
		25	310
		26	320
Sum = 160.5		Sum = 190.5	

$$*4.5 = \frac{4+5}{2}$$

$$**7 = \frac{6+7+8}{3}$$

The smaller of the two sums ($T = 160.5$) is taken to a table of acceptance ranges for the rank sum T (see Table 23-4) at a level of $p = 0.05$ for $n_1 = 14$, $n_2 = 12$. The range of acceptance is 150 to 228. The calculated T-value falls within this range, and the difference in the median values of BUN between these two populations is not considered significant at the 5% level.

χ^2 (Chi-Square) Analysis

When populations contain a continuum of numbers, regression analysis and **correlation coefficients** usually can be used to measure their association. However, when the values of two populations are discrete, with few possible values, such as yes/no, or positive/negative, **chi-square** (χ^2) analysis is used to test whether the populations are related. The analysis is based on the difference between the observed frequency of the values in a population and the expected frequency of the values of a population.

Often, the results obtained with real samples do not agree exactly with the theoretical results expected according to the rules of probability. For example, if a fair coin is tossed 100 times, 50 heads and 50 tails would be the expected result. However, these exact results are rarely obtained. A statistical method would be needed to determine whether the observed frequencies, say 47 heads and 53 tails, differ significantly from the expected frequencies (50 heads and 50 tails). The χ^2 statistical method provides a measure of the chance discrepancy that may exist between the observed and expected frequencies of the results of an analysis. The formula for the calculation of χ^2 is shown in Eq. 23-14:

$$\chi^2 = \frac{(o_1 - e_1)^2}{e_1} + \frac{(o_2 - e_2)^2}{e_2} + \ldots \frac{(o_k - e_k)^2}{e_k} \quad \text{Eq. 23-14}$$

where o = the observed frequency result and e = the expected frequency result. If $\chi^2 = 0$, the observed and expected frequencies agree, whereas if $\chi^2 > 0$, they do not agree exactly. The larger the value for χ^2, the greater is the discrepancy between the observed and expected frequencies.

In medical and health care research, chi-square analysis often is used to answer questions about the relationship between sex, age, race, or hormonal status and some laboratory test result or physical condition of a patient (such as diabetes or hypertension).

Example 9. χ^2 (chi-square analysis).

In a study designed to determine whether there was a significant difference in estrogen receptor positivity between breast tumors resected from premenopausal and postmenopausal women, the following frequencies of positive results were observed:

Premenopausal women:	ER+	308/581
Postmenopausal women:	ER+	648/1079

Is the observed difference in ER (estrogen receptor) positivity between the two groups significant?

	Pos	Neg	Total
Observed			
Pre	308	273	581
Post	648	431	1079
Total	956	704	1660
Expected			
Pre	335	246	581
Post	621	458	1079
Total	956	704	1660

Table 23-5 Critical Values for Chi-Square

Level	0.10	0.05	0.01
df			
1	2.706	3.841	6.635
2	4.605	5.991	9.210
3	6.251	7.815	11.345
4	7.779	9.488	13.277
5	9.236	11.070	15.086
6	10.654	12.592	16.812
7	12.017	14.067	18.475
8	13.362	15.507	20.090
9	14.684	16.919	21.666
10	15.987	18.307	23.209

Condensed from Lenter C: *Geigy Scientific Tables*, vol 2, *Introduction to Statistics, Statistical Tables, Mathematical Formulae*, ed 8, Allschwil, Switzerland, 1982, Ciba-Geigy.

$$\chi^2 = \frac{(308-335)^2}{335} + \frac{(648-621)^2}{621} + \frac{(273-246)^2}{246} + \frac{(431-458)^2}{458}$$

$$\chi^2 = 7.90$$

The critical value $\chi^2_{0.05}$ for 1 degree of freedom is 3.84 (Table 23-5). Because 7.90 > 3.84, the hypothesis that there is no difference between the groups is rejected, and the hypothesis that there is a significantly higher estrogen receptor rate of positivity in breast tumors resected from postmenopausal women is accepted.

When a comparison is made between one sample and another, as in this estrogen receptor sample, an easy rule for the degrees of freedom is that they equal:

$$(\text{Number of variables in columes} - 1) \times (\text{Number of vaiables in rows} - 1)$$

Sample: (Pos + Neg −1) × (Pre + Post − 1) = 1

Example 10. A continuation of χ^2 (chi-square analysis).

The numbers in the previous chi-square table are represented by variables in the chart below. The expected values are calculated under the assumption that the percentage of distribution between positive and negative values should be equal for both premenopausal and postmenopausal populations. This is true with any 2 × 2 chi-square table.

	Pos	**Neg**	**Total**
Observed			
Pre	a_1	a_2	N_a
Post	b_1	b_2	N_b
Total	N_1	N_2	N_T
Expected			
Pre	$N_1\ (N_a/N_T)$	$N_2\ (N_a/N_T)$	N_a
Post	$N_1\ (N_b/N_T)$	$N_2\ (N_b/N_T)$	N_b
Total	N_1	N_2	N_T

There are simple formulas for computing χ^2 that use only the observed frequencies. The following give results for the 2 × 2 contingency table used in the previous estrogen receptor example.

$$\chi^2 = \frac{N(a_1b_2 - a_2b_1)^2}{(a_1+b_1)(a_2+b_2)(a_1+a_2)(b_1+b_2)} = \frac{N\Delta^2}{N_1N_2N_aN_b}$$

$$\chi^2 = \frac{1660(132{,}748-176{,}904)^2}{956\times704\times581\times1079} = 7.67$$

KEY CONCEPTS BOX 23-4

- Statistical tests used to determine differences between populations when NO assumption is made about the shape of the distributions, or when it is known that the distributions are non-normal, are called *nonparametric* tests.
- The most common nonparametric tests are the sign test, the Mann-Whitney rank sum test, and the χ^2 test.

SECTION OBJECTIVES BOX 23-5

- Explain the purpose, process, and interpretation of simple linear regression analysis.
- List four clinical laboratory applications of simple linear regression analysis.
- Explain how to calculate regression parameters, the y-intercept, slope of the regression line, standard deviation about the regression line, and the Pearson correlation coefficient.
- Discuss potential limitations of simple linear regression analysis.

LINEAR-REGRESSION AND CORRELATION

For a wide variety of clinical laboratory applications, it is useful to determine the relationship between two variables, *x* and *y*. If *x* can be considered a "fixed," or an *independent,* variable and *y* can be considered a "not fixed," or a *dependent,* variable, then it is mathematically valid to describe *y* as a *function* of *x*. A widely used, and sometimes misused, statistical procedure for assessing this relationship or describing this function is regression analysis.

Simple "linear" regression analysis can be used when the relationship between the independent *x* and dependent *y* variables is a linear one. This type of regression analysis is termed "simple" because there is one independent variable. The simplest model for a relationship between two variables would be a straight line. Linear-regression analysis can be graphed on a rectilinear *x,y* plot, where each pair of values is a point on the graph. Once all the *x,y* pairs are plotted, a straight line of "best fit" can be drawn manually through the points. If the straight-line model appears to be a valid depiction of the relationship between *x* and *y*, the line is termed the *regression line,* and its calculation is referred to as "regressing *y* on *x*."

Simple linear regression analysis is used to answer this question: If you know what one variable *(x)* is, can you calculate what the other variable *(y)* would be under certain conditions? Here is another way to ask this question: Can changes in *x* be used to predict changes in *y*? In consideration of this question,

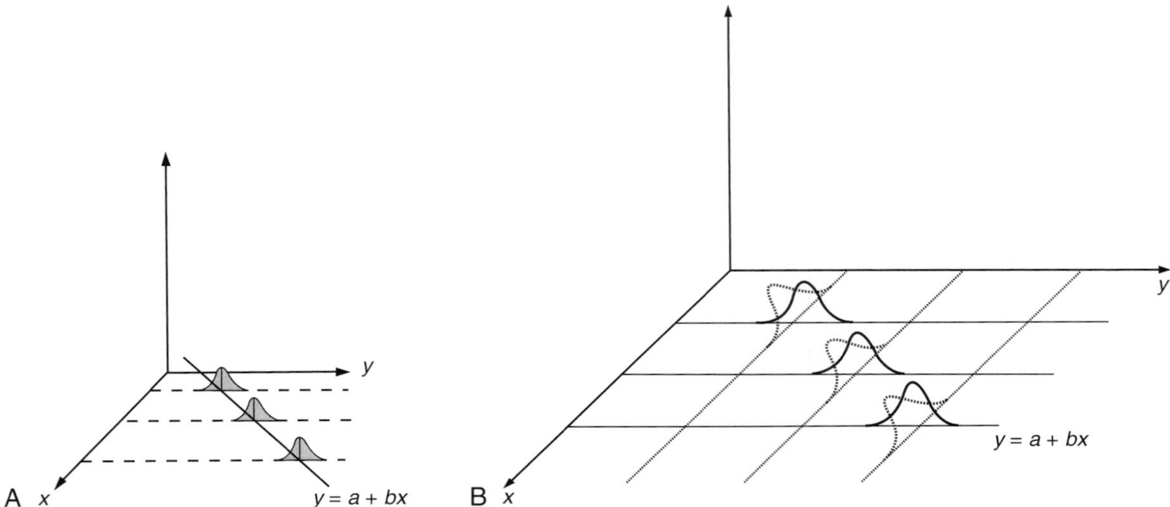

Fig. 23-10 A, Gaussian distributions of y values around simple linear-regression line. **B,** Gaussian distribution around Deming regression.

the x variable can also be termed the "predictor" variable, and the y variable can be called the "response" variable.

In simple linear regression analysis, the equation that describes the linear relationship between x and y also can be said to describe y as a function of x, that is, $y = f(x)$. This function is described in Eq. 23-15:

$$y = \alpha + \beta x + \varepsilon \qquad \text{Eq. 23-15}$$

where α is the true value of the intercept of the regression line and β is the true value of the slope of the regression line. When this function is used, x can be used to make a prediction of y.

In practice, the values of α and β in Eq. 23-15 are unknown and must be estimated as a and b, respectively. It is also expected that most of the data points will not fall precisely on the regression line. The term ε is included in Eq. 23-15 to describe the distance between any observed value of y and the corresponding value of y that would be predicted or expected for y, which is denoted as $\hat{y}$. This value of ε is also termed the *residual* and exists because variability is expected in y for any fixed, accurately known value of x. This basic assumption for using simple regression analysis is that for every known value of x, there is a corresponding normal distribution of y values. This assumption is illustrated graphically in Fig. 23-10, *A*. Note that the regression line passes through the means of the distributions.

Use of the simple linear regression model for appropriate applications requires that the two variables x and y satisfy several conditions.

1. The x values are considered fixed, and any random error in the measurement of x can be considered "negligible."
2. For every value of x, there is a normal distribution of y values, as illustrated in Fig. 23-10, *A*.
3. The distribution of y values for every value of x has the same variance, that is, the variance around the line is independent of the value of x.
4. The expected values of y for each x generally fit the straight-line model.
5. The straight-line model that is estimated is not horizontal (i.e., β does not equal 0). If the straight line were horizontal, the values of y on the regression line would not be a better predictor of y than the mean y value, or $\bar{y}$.

If these conditions are met, use of the simple linear-regression model will allow correct estimates of expected y values for each fixed value of x to be inferred.

The above conditions for simple linear-regression should be satisfied for most clinical laboratory applications. However, in certain instances, the x values cannot be considered "fixed" or "invariable," as defined in condition 1. The most common misuse of simple linear regression analysis involves the false assumption that values of x are fixed, or that x is an independent variable, when, in fact, it is not. For example, in a typical comparison of two methods, the results of one method will be considered to be the "x," independent variable (see pp. 495-496). Although this may be the current method, each "x" result cannot be considered "fixed" but is reported with a certain error. In this instance, it is appropriate to consider using a different type of regression analysis. Although several types of regression techniques are described in the literature, the technique that may be most appropriate to apply when variability exists in the values of x and in the values of y is the *Deming regression* technique (Fig. 23-10, *B* and p. 436).[10,11]

In a simple linear regression analysis, an investigator could attempt to determine values for a and b using the manual plot of the data and the "best-fit" regression line (see p. 433). Conventionally, however, the method used to determine the correct regression parameters is the *method of least squares*. Using this method, the analyst mathematically minimizes the sum of the squares of the residuals of all the y values. Predicting expected y values based on the actual x,y data points by this method and calculating the subsequent regression statistics, for either the simple or the Deming model, are accomplished most easily with the use of a calculator or software program that can generate the appropriate statistics automatically.

The method of least squares is valid if the residuals are random (i.e., independent of values of x and y) and have a gaussian distribution with a mean of 0 and a standard deviation, $S_{y,x}$.[11] The standard deviation of the residuals, or *standard error of the estimate,* should be constant at every x value (see Eq. 23-19). It has been reported that within the range of measurement commonly encountered in most clinical laboratory applications, the method of least squares also correctly calculates a regression line when $S_{y,x}$ is proportional to x.[11]

Appropriate clinical laboratory applications for simple linear regression analysis, when x can legitimately be considered a fixed or independent variable, are as follows:

1. Comparison of results from a new procedure versus results from an established procedure
2. Comparison of a technique versus a reference method (see Chapter 26 for these two applications)
3. Comparison of paired results for the same test or analyte collected from two different analytical systems in current use. This application could be used to validate test systems secondarily with a test system that has been validated by external proficiency testing. This application would satisfy the Clinical Laboratory Improvement Amendments of 1988 regulations for proficiency testing.
4. Comparison of results from the same analytical system collected during two different analytical runs

In simple linear or Deming regression analysis, a relationship exists between the x and y variables, although the mathematical description of this relationship would be somewhat different for each type of regression technique. When a linear relationship exists between two variables, these variables can be considered to have a *correlation* with each other. If increasing values of x are related in a linear fashion to increasing values of y, there is a *positive correlation* between these variables. If increasing values of x are related in a linear fashion to decreasing values of y, a *negative correlation* is seen between these variables (see p. 436).

It is, of course, possible that the relationship between two variables is a nonlinear relationship. If this is the case, the computation of basic linear regression parameters may reflect this relationship. For example, determination of the correlation coefficient, r, may indicate a value much closer to 0 than either 1 or −1. It is also likely that a nonlinear relationship would be reflected in an increased value $S_{y,x}$. If this were the case, the application of simple linear-regression or Deming regression analysis would be inappropriate and other regression techniques would be used.[4-8] Of course, it is also true that a nonlinear relationship or an increased amount of scatter may be apparent upon visual inspection of the regression plot.

Basic Statistics of Simple Linear Regression and Correlation

With the two methods of linear regression described above, the line of best fit would be determined by the method of least squares or the method of Deming. In either case, once the correct line to fit the appropriate model has been identified, this line can be described by Eq. 23-16:

$$y = bx + a \qquad \text{Eq. 23-16}$$

where b is the estimated slope of the regression line, and a is the estimated intercept of the regression line on the y-axis.

Although the "best fit" of the regression line may appear obvious on visual examination of the graphed scatterplot, this method is not recommended. More appropriately, calculation of the regression parameters, a and b, with the use of a calculator or software program, allows for an exact prediction of any additional value of y once the x value is known. Automatic calculation of the regression parameters and the subsequent determination of two predicted y values from two different x values would allow for the correct graphical placement of the regression line, because two points determine the location of a straight line.

In simple linear regression, the statistical parameters, a and b, the y-intercept, and the slope of the regression line, respectively, can be calculated by the use of Eq. 23-17 and 23-18:

$$a = \bar{y} - b\bar{x} \qquad \text{Eq. 23-17}$$

$$b = \frac{\sum(x-\bar{x})(y-\bar{y})}{\sum(x-\bar{x})^2} \qquad \text{Eq. 23-18}$$

To measure the variability of the data points about the regression line, the investigator must determine the standard deviation about the regression line of the differences between the observed and predicted values of y (i.e., the residuals). This variability, termed the *standard error of the estimate,* is calculated by the use of Eq. 23-19:

$$S_{y,x} = \left(\frac{\sum(y-\bar{y})^2}{N-2}\right)^{1/2} \qquad \text{Eq. 23-19}$$

Use of (N − 2) degrees of freedom in the denominator is appropriate because two regression coefficients, a and b, had to be determined from the data in order to calculate the predicted values of y, that is, two restrictions are placed on the N observations.

The variability of the estimated slope, b, of the simple linear regression line is determined by first calculating the standard deviation of the slope, s_b, using Eq. 23-20:

$$s_b = S_{y,x} \Big/ \left[\sum(x_i-\bar{x})^2\right]^{1/2} \qquad \text{Eq. 23-20}$$

and then determining a $100(1 - p)\%$ confidence interval for the true slope, β, using Eq. 23-21:

$$\beta = b \pm t \times s_b \qquad \text{Eq. 23-21}$$

where t is obtained from a two-sided t-table for $N - 2$ degrees of freedom and the desired level of significance.

The variability of the estimated intercept, a, of the simple linear regression line is determined in a similar manner. The estimated standard deviation of a, s_a, is calculated by the use of Eq. 23-22:

$$s_a = S_{y,x}\left[\sum x_i^2 / N\sum(x_i - \bar{x})^2\right]^{1/2} \qquad \text{Eq. 23-22}$$

and then by determination of a $100(1-p)\%$ confidence interval for the true intercept, a, by the use of Eq. 23-23:

$$\alpha = a \pm t \times s_a \qquad \text{Eq. 23-23}$$

where t is, again, obtained from a two-sided t-table for $N-2$ degrees of freedom and the desired level of significance.

The statistic that provides a measure of how closely the data points lie to the regression line is r, or the Pearson correlation coefficient. This correlation coefficient, r, is a measure of the degree to which two variables are linearly related. The calculation of r is illustrated in Eq. 23-24:

$$r = \frac{\sum(x_i - \bar{x})(y_i - \bar{y})}{\{\sum[(x_i - \bar{x})^2][\sum(y_i - \bar{y})^2]\}^{1/2}} \qquad \text{Eq. 23-24}$$

Essentially, r describes the strength of correlation between the x and y variables.

The correlation coefficient, r, can range in value from -1 to 1. If r is equal to 1, there is a perfect positive correlation between the variables. If r is equal to -1, there is a perfect negative correlation between the variables. The farther the correlation coefficient is from 0, the stronger the correlation is, positive or negative, between the variables. If the correlation coefficient is equal to 0, there is no *linear* relationship between the variables. This should not be interpreted to mean that there is no relationship between the two variables; it is possible that these two uncorrelated variables are strongly related in *nonlinear* fashion (this would be apparent from a visual inspection of the x,y scatterplot).

At what value of r can one assume that there is not a linear relationship between the x and y variables? From an empirical perspective, an r value between -0.7 and 0.7 would indicate that the probability that the relationship between x and y is linear is less than 50%. As r approaches zero, this probability also approaches zero. If the data collected for analysis by linear regression are obtained from routine laboratory methods, a practical consideration is that a low r value can be caused by very poor precision in the method used to obtain x values, y values, or both variables.

An example of the use of Eq. 23-17 to 23-24 to calculate the basic statistics of simple linear regression analysis is illustrated in Example 11. This example shows the use of simple linear regression analysis and Deming regression analysis for the comparison of two potassium methods. Equations for the calculated Deming regression statistics are given elsewhere.[10]

Example 11. Linear-regression analysis.

In an initial method-comparison study, 42 pairs of potassium measurements are obtained from an established method (old) and an experimental method (new). Calculate regression statistics, first assuming there is negligible variability in the old method (use simple linear regression analysis) and then assuming that there is variability in the established method (using Deming regression equations, as cited in references 10 and 11).

Assuming that there is negligible variability in the established method, calculate the standard error of the estimate, the variability of the estimated slope and intercept, and the 95% confidence intervals for the actual slope and intercept for the population.

All x,y (old, new) potassium results are expressed in millimoles per liter:

3.9, 3.9	3.9, 3.9	3.4, 3.4	5.4, 5.2	4.0, 4.0
4.6, 4.5	4.2, 4.2	4.3, 4.1	4.3, 4.3	4.8, 4.7
3.7, 3.6	4.4, 4.3	4.4, 4.4	4.5, 4.4	3.9, 3.9
4.3, 4.3	3.8, 3.7	3.8, 3.7	3.9, 3.8	4.0, 3.9
4.6, 4.5	3.4, 3.4	4.2, 4.1	3.8, 3.8	3.6, 3.6
4.3, 4.3	4.1, 4.0	3.5, 3.4	4.6, 4.8	4.1, 4.2
3.7, 3.1	4.1, 4.1	4.8, 4.7	3.3, 3.2	5.4, 5.4
4.0, 3.9	4.5, 4.4	3.5, 3.6	3.7, 3.7	4.1, 4.1
3.6, 3.5	3.0, 3.1			

	Simple linear-Regression Analysis	Deming Regression
Slope *(b)*	0.99	0.98
Intercept *(a)*	−0.03	0.22
$S_{y,x}$	0.12	0.09
r	0.97	0.98

For 95% confidence intervals and $N-2$ degrees of freedom (40), the t-value from a two-sided table = 2.021.

Variability of estimated slope:

Standard deviation of estimated slope (b) =

$$s_b = S_{y,x}\Big/\left[\sum(x_i - \bar{x})^2\right]^{1/2} = 0.12/3.24 = 0.04$$

Confidence interval for the true slope (β) =

$$\beta = b \pm t \times s_b = 0.99 \pm 2.021(0.04) = 0.99 \pm 0.07$$

Variability of estimated intercept:

Standard deviation of estimated intercept (a) =

$$s_a = S_{y,x}\left[\sum x_i^2 / N\sum(x_i - \bar{x})^2\right]^{1/2} = 0.12(1.28) = 0.15$$

Confidence interval for the true intercept (α) =

$$\alpha = a \pm t \times s_a = -0.03 \pm 2.021(0.15) = -0.03 \pm 0.30$$

Testing for Outliers Using Residual Analysis

Simple linear regression analysis can be used to identify outliers, or extreme paired values, in the x,y data points. This procedure involves the plotting of the residuals, or ε, against the independent variable x.[8] It may then be appropriate to exclude any data points that generate residuals greater than 4 $S_{y,x}$. The plot of residuals can be evaluated against the independent variable x for assessment of the equality of variances. If the variances are equal, the plotted residuals will be seen as a horizontal band of points independent of x (one of the conditions necessary to apply simple linear regression to a pair of variables).

Additional information can be obtained by plotting the residuals against the predicted values of y. If there is truly a linear relationship between the x and y variables, the residuals would be randomly scattered, in horizontal fashion, around zero.

Limitations of Simple Linear Regression Analysis

When paired data spanning a limited range are analyzed by the simple linear-regression method, an acceptable level of random error can still result in inaccurate estimates of the slope and intercept of the regression line. This problem is magnified if the x variable really should not be considered fixed or independent. In this instance, an unacceptably large standard error of the slope and intercept, as well as an unacceptably low correlation coefficient, may be calculated, and it is appropriate to use Deming regression analysis instead of simple linear-regression analysis.

Other considerations may suggest that Deming regression should be used instead of simple linear-regression analysis. An initial assessment of this question can be made by plotting one variable on the x-axis in a first x,y plot and generating regression statistics. The procedure then is repeated with the second variable plotted on the x-axis. If the two least-squares regression lines are substantially different from each other, the Deming regression should be used. The Deming method will yield one regression line between x and y that takes into account the error in measuring both variables. A characteristic of the Deming regression technique is that switching the variables and recalculating regression statistics will yield statistics identical to the initial calculation.

Finally, it must be noted that the value of r in simple linear-regression analysis is sensitive to both the scatter of the data points and the range of data points. The scatter of the data points is a characteristic of the dependent method being evaluated, but it is possible to increase the value of r by simply extending the range of data. Extension of the range of data by one single point farther away from most of the data points where this single point coincidentally happens to demonstrate close agreement between x and y will dramatically increase the value of r. This characteristic is described in Eq. 23-25:

$$r = (1/s_x)(s_x^2 + S_{y,x}^2)^{1/2} \quad \text{Eq. 23-25}$$

where s_x is the standard deviation of the x population, an indication of the spread in the x data. As s_x becomes very large relative to $S_{y,x}$, r approaches 1.0. Because of this characteristic, it is always wise to visually evaluate an x,y plot, examining the simple linear-regression line generated from the data. It may be obvious that a point lying far above or below the regression line is an outlier, but a more insidious outlier might be the point that lies exactly on the regression line but is considerably removed from the range of the remaining data points used to generate the regression statistics.

KEY CONCEPTS BOX 23-5

- The two variables of a simple linear-regression analysis are the dependent (y) and independent (x) variables. In practice, the latter variable is the "known," or current, variable.
- The equation for simple linear regression is $y = bx + a$, where b is the estimated slope of the regression line and a is the estimated intercept of the regression line on the y-axis. If r is very high ($r > 0.95$), it is assumed that there is good correlation between the two data sets; that is, y changes similarly to the way x changes. Regression analysis can be used to compare two methods, such as validating a new method versus a current one.
- Regression analysis may be difficult to interpret when there are outlier values, when very poor precision (large scatter) is seen with one of the methods, or when data are collected in a nonlinear portion of the assay.

REFERENCES

1. *Merriam-Webster's Collegiate Dictionary*, ed 11, Springfield, MA, 2003, Merriam-Webster, Inc.
2. Lenter C: *Geigy Scientific Tables*, vol 2, *Introduction to Statistics, Statistical Tables, Mathematical Formulae*, ed 8, Allschwil, Switzerland, 1982, Ciba-Geigy.
3. Spiegel MR: *Schaum's Outline Series: Theory and Problems of Statistics*, ed 2, New York, 1988, McGraw-Hill.
4. Mason RL, Gunst RF, Hess JL: *Statistical Design and Analysis of Experiments With Applications to Engineering and Science*, New York, 2003, Wiley-Interscience.
5. Snedecor GW, Cochran WG: *Statistical Methods*, ed 8, Ames, Iowa, 1989, Iowa State University Press.
6. Shott S: *Statistics for Health Professionals*, Philadelphia, 1990, Saunders.
7. Altman DG: *Practical Statistics for Medical Research*, ed 2, New York, 2006, Chapman & Hall/CRC.
8. Dowdy S, Wearden S, Chilko D: *Statistics for Research*, ed 3, New York, 2004, Wiley-Interscience.
9. Lenter C: *Geigy Scientific Tables*, vol 2, *Introduction to Statistics, Statistical Tables, Mathematical Formulae*, ed 8, Allschwil, Switzerland, 1982, Ciba-Geigy. Significance limits for testing extreme values of a sample, p. 60.
10. Wallers PJM, et al: Applications of statistics in clinical chemistry—a critical evaluation of regression lines, Clin Chem Acta 64:173, 1975.
11. Cornbleet PJ, Gochman N: Incorrect least-squares regression coefficients in method-comparison analysis, Clin Chem 25:432, 1979.

BIBLIOGRAPHY

Barnett RN: *Clinical Laboratory Statistics*, ed 2, Boston, 1979, Little, Brown & Co.

Barnett V, Lewis T, Rothamsted V: *Outliers in Statistical Data* (Wiley Series in Probability and Mathematical Statistics. Applied Probability and Statistics), ed 3, New York, 1994, John Wiley & Sons Ltd.

Draper NR, Smith H: *Applied Regression Analysis* (Wiley Series in Probability and Statistics), ed 3, New York, 1998, Wiley-Interscience.

Fisher LD, Van Belle G: *Biostatistics: A Methodology for the Health Sciences*, New York, 1993, Wiley Press.

Freedman D, Pisani R, Purves R: *Statistics,* ed 4, New York, 2007, Norton Press.

Hahn GJ, Meeker WQ: *Statistical Intervals: Guide for Practitioners,* New York, 1991, Wiley-Interscience.

Hollander M, Wolfe DA: *Nonparametric Statistical Methods,* ed 2, New York, 1999, Wiley-Interscience.

Jones RG, Bayne RB: *Clinical Investigation and Statistics in Laboratory Medicine,* London, 1997, ACB Ventures Publications.

Sheskin DJ: *Handbook of Parametric and Nonparametric Statistical Procedures,* Boca Raton, FL, 1996, CRC Press.

Snedecor GW, Cochran WG: *Statistical Methods,* ed 8, Ames, IA, 1989, Iowa State University Press.

Strike PW: *Measurement in Laboratory Medicine—A Primer on Control and Interpretation,* Oxford, England, 1996, Butterworth-Heinemann.

INTERNET SITES

www.math.yorku.ca/SCS/StatResource.html—York University Mathematics Department, Statistics and Statistical Graphics Resources, Statistical resource links from their Statistical Consulting Service area (checked January 2, 2008).

http://www.stat.ufl.edu/vlib/statistics.html—The University of Florida's Department of Statistics, The World Wide Web Virtual Library: Statistics. Comprehensive list of statistical resources (checked January 2, 2008).

Reference Intervals and Clinical Decision Limits

24

Chapter

Paul S. Horn*

Chapter Outline

Key Terms

abnormal Test results outside of reference intervals, most often observed in people with disease or in less than good health.

cutoff values Those limits above or below which the patient is considered abnormal or positive for a condition such as substance abuse.

decision analysis Strategy comparing risks and benefits of predicting the true diagnosis or outcome.

gaussian A particular symmetrical statistical distribution; also called the *normal distribution*.

healthy A relative term that must be defined for each reference population.

log normal A symmetrical gaussian population distribution obtained by a distribution plot of the logarithm of the data.

log-normal distribution A sample of values with a long tail to the right can often be made to act as a gaussian distribution when the logarithms of values are used.

medical decision limits The values or changes in values that result in immediate medical intervention or a change in medical management.

negative predictive value The probability that a laboratory result falling within the reference interval reflects the true absence of disease; defined as true negatives divided by the sum of true negatives and false negatives, or as the predictive value of a negative result.

normal A term with many meanings, including those persons in the nondiseased population and an equivalent term for a gaussian distribution (see later discussion).

observed value The quantitative value (test result) obtained for a test subject (such as a patient) for comparison with reference values, distributions of reference values, reference limits, or reference intervals.

outlier An observation that arises from a population that is different from the reference population. The outlier can be an erroneous result or an observation on a subject that does not conform to the characteristics of a reference individual.

partitioning of reference values The process of separating reference intervals of subjects on the basis of such criteria as age, sex, and race, as well as statistical analysis showing significant differences between the populations.

positive predictive value The probability that a laboratory result outside the reference interval actually reflects the presence of disease; defined as true positives divided by the sum of true positives and false positives.

predictive value Probability that a laboratory result accurately reflects the true presence or absence of disease. It is dependent on the actual prevalence of the disease.

prevalence The number of persons who have a disease in a given population at any one point in time, or more often, the rate of such disease, which is also called *disease frequency*.

receiver-operating characteristic (ROC) curve A graphical presentation of discrimination of disease from nondisease by plotting sensitivity (the true-positive rate) of the test versus 1.0 minus specificity (the false-positive rate).

reference individual An individual selected for a reference interval study on the basis of well-defined criteria. It is usually important to define the individual's health, age, sex, and race.

reference interval (Listed in the Clinical Laboratory Improvement Amendments of 1988 [CLIA '88] as a

*The author wishes to acknowledge the efforts of the previous author Edward Sasse and members of the CLSI Subcommittee on Reference Intervals, who prepared the new C28-P Guideline: Gary L. Horowitz, James C. Boyd, Ferruccio Ceriotti, Uttam Garg, Sousan Altaie, Harrison E. Sine, Jack Zakowski.

reference range.) The interval between and including two reference limits. It is designed as the central interval of values bounded by the lower reference limit and the upper reference limit at certain designated percentiles. For example, for fasting glucose, the central 95th percentile reference interval is 65 to 110 mg/dL (3.6 to 6.1 mmol/L), that is, 95% of the apparently healthy population will have a fasting glucose value of 65 to 110 mg/dL.

reference limit A numerical value or values derived from the distribution of reference values and used for descriptive purposes. It is common practice to define a reference limit so that a stated fraction of the reference values will be less than or equal to, or greater than or equal to, the respective upper or lower limit.

reference population A group that consists of all the reference individuals. The reference population usually includes an unknown number of members and therefore is a hypothetical entity.

reference range The entire range (actual minimal to maximal measured values) of laboratory values of people without disease.

reference sample group An adequate number of reference individuals selected to represent the reference population.

reference value The value (test result) obtained through the observation or measurement of a particular analyte for a reference individual. Reference values are obtained from a reference sample group.

sensitivity A term used to describe the probability that a laboratory test is positive (i.e., outside of the reference interval) in the presence of disease; defined as true positives divided by the sum of true positives and false negatives.

specificity A term used to describe the probability that a laboratory test will be negative (i.e., within the reference interval) in the absence of disease; defined as true negatives divided by the sum of true negatives and false positives.

standard deviation (SD) A measure of variability. In the gaussian distribution, two standard deviations above and below the mean encompass the central 95% of the population data, and one standard deviation above and below encompasses 68.3% of the data.

SECTION OBJECTIVES BOX 24-1

- Define and contrast of the following terms: reference limit, reference interval, reference sample group, reference population, and reference range.
- Discuss inherent ambiguities in using the terms "health" and "normal range."
- Outline the 12-step federally-defined protocol for obtaining reference values and reference intervals.
- Describe criteria that should be considered when selecting reference individuals.
- Describe how to assess whether age-related differences in analyte concentration are medically significant.
- Differentiate a priori and a posteriori methods of selecting reference individuals.

DEFINITION OF REFERENCE INTERVAL

The medical interpretation of clinical laboratory data is a comparative decision-making process in which a laboratory test result for an individual is compared with a **reference interval** derived from **reference values.** Therefore, reliable reference values are required for all tests in the clinical laboratory and must be provided by clinical laboratories and diagnostic test manufacturers. The reference intervals most commonly used (often known as normal values, and sometimes expected values) are often poorly defined.

Reference intervals should be determined in a systematic and scientific manner that provides an acceptable degree of confidence for the clinical decision-making process, which includes consideration of the significant factors and variables introduced by the specific individual's reference sample or by the analytical process itself. An understanding of the process used to establish a reference interval yields a better understanding of the limitations of the defined reference interval.

To facilitate the generation of reliable reference intervals, the Clinical and Laboratory Standards Institute (CLSI, previously the National Committee for Clinical Laboratory Standards [NCCLS]) has published a document entitled C28-A Defining, Establishing, and Verifying Reference Intervals in the Clinical Laboratory; Approved Guideline-Third Edition, Villanova, PA, 2008,[1] which establishes guidelines and procedures for determining valid reference values and reference intervals for quantitative clinical laboratory tests. The CLSI document catalogs the significant factors and variables that may affect the reference interval and is based on the recommendations of the Expert Panel on the Theory of Reference Values (EPTRV) of the International Federation of Clinical Chemistry (IFCC).[2-7] The recommendations given in the CLSI guideline are intended to constitute a standard protocol for determining reference intervals that meet the minimum, mandatory requirements for reliability.

Consequently, reference interval determination should follow the guidelines of the CLSI protocol. However, there are instances, particularly for geriatric and pediatric populations, when it is difficult to collect data from the recommended number of **reference individuals.** In these instances, the proper and well-defined selection of reference individuals becomes preeminent. These reference values, with their limitations, are still useful to the practice of medicine in these particular patient categories.

Reference values may be associated with good health or with specific physiological or pathological conditions and may be used for different reasons. For example, to establish the **sensitivity** and **specificity** of a laboratory test, the laboratory must carefully define the population. In all cases, the reference values allow comparison of observed data versus reference data for a defined population of subjects. This comparison then becomes part of the medical decision-making process.

TERMINOLOGY

Specific definitions for terms permit relatively unambiguous description and discussion of the subject of reference values. The definitions listed in the key terms have been proposed by the EPTRV of the IFCC[2] and the International Council for Standardization in Hematology and have been endorsed by the World Health Organization (WHO) and other organizations worldwide.

The following scheme[2] demonstrates the relationships between the defined terms.

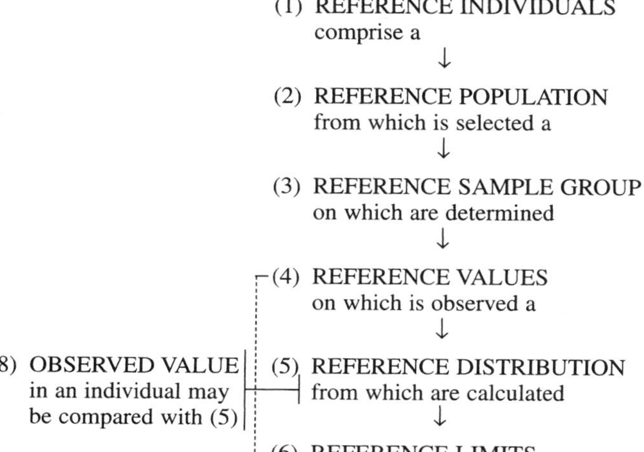

The **reference limits** and associated reference intervals usually are estimated by a statistical method. Reference limits serve only to describe the **reference sample group** or **reference population** and are strictly a function of the characteristics of the designated population.

The term **reference range** has commonly been used as a substitute for *reference interval;* however, such a term should be avoided. *Range* should be reserved for describing a set of values defined by the actual minimal and maximal measured values, that is, the entire range of values of the measured set.

The reference intervals most commonly used to describe **healthy** individuals have been known as *normal values,* referring to reference values that have been observed in **normal,** or healthy, persons. Therefore, test results outside of these reference intervals may be observed in individuals with disease or in states of less than good health and consequently have been termed **abnormal.** There is often an overlap of normal and abnormal values in disease because most disease processes and associated biological analytes change in a continuous fashion. Consequently, normal values do not always indicate a lack of disease (Figs. 24-1 to 24-3), nor does a value exceeding a defined limit always indicate disease. The use of the term *normal* in this context is now considered to be ambiguous.

The word *normal* has several different connotations in laboratory medicine that can cause confusion. Values often are described as normal if their observed distribution seems

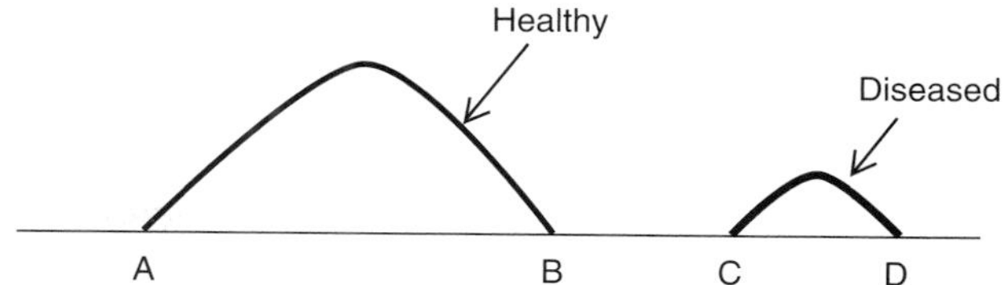

Fig. 24-1 Perfectly separated test result distributions of healthy and diseased populations. This clear separation rarely occurs in reality.

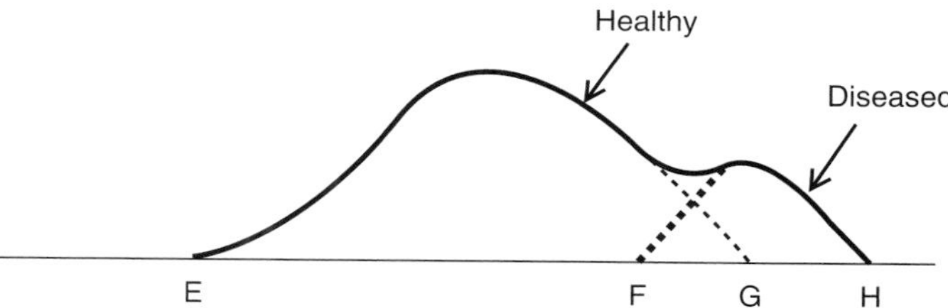

Fig. 24-2 Usual test result distributions of healthy and diseased populations in which an overlap between the two occurs.

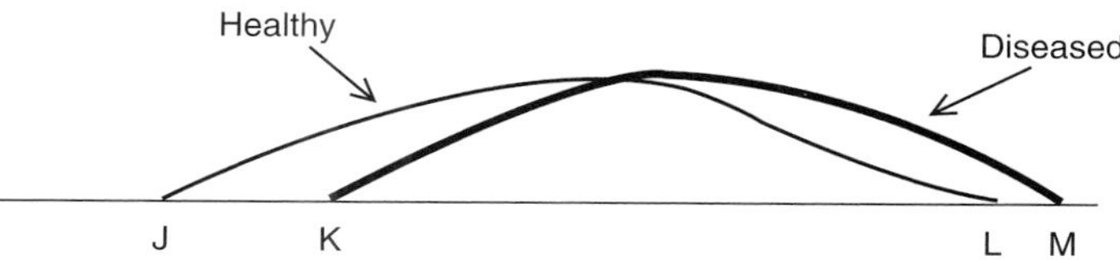

Fig. 24-3 Degree of test result overlap does not permit differentiation between healthy and diseased populations.

to follow the theoretical **gaussian** ("normal") distribution. However, biological data from a reference sample group often are not gaussian, and the use of *normal* may be misleading by implying that the data are symmetrical or bell-shaped in distribution. Other meanings of *normal* are *common, frequent, usual,* and *typical,* which also may be used in statements referring to biological or clinical values. Therefore, it is more precise and less confusing to avoid the term *normal values* and replace it with *reference values* (or *reference interval*) *obtained from healthy individuals, health-associated reference values* (or *reference intervals*), or, colloquially, *healthy reference values (intervals).* As was previously mentioned, reference intervals also can be established for physiological conditions other than good health.

PROTOCOL OUTLINE FOR OBTAINING REFERENCE VALUES AND ESTABLISHING HEALTH-ASSOCIATED REFERENCE INTERVALS[1]

The collection or verification of reference values from healthy subjects and the subsequent estimation of the reference interval for a given analyte is a requirement of CLIA '88 regulations (§493.1213), *Federal Register* 57(40), Feb 28, 1992, and must be carried out in accordance with a well-defined protocol. This involves following the sequence of operations listed in Box 24-1.

Box 24-1

Protocol Outline for Obtaining Reference Values and Reference Intervals

The procedure manual must include the following, when applicable to the test procedure:

1. Consult the medical and scientific literature, and list possible biological variations and analytical interferences. (In the case of a totally new analyte, a laboratory may need to perform its own studies.)
2. Establish selection (or exclusion) and partition criteria and an appropriate questionnaire designed to reveal these criteria in potential reference individuals.
3. Categorize potential reference individuals on the basis of questionnaire findings and the results of other appropriate health assessments.
4. Exclude individuals from the reference sample group on the basis of exclusion criteria or other assessments indicating a lack of good health.
5. Select the appropriate reference individuals.
6. Prepare reference individuals properly and consistently for specimen collection in keeping with specific requirements for the analyte and consistent with routine practice for patients.
7. Collect and process biological specimens properly and uniformly and consistent with routine practice for patient specimens.
8. Determine reference values by analyzing the specimens according to the respective analytical methodology under well-defined conditions.
9. Inspect reference value data and prepare a histogram.
10. Identify data errors and values that are outliers.
11. Analyze the reference values, that is, select a statistical method of estimation, and estimate reference limits and the reference interval (include partitioning into subclasses for separate reference intervals, if appropriate).
12. Document all of the above steps and procedures.

Box 24-2

Examples of Possible Exclusion Criteria

Alcohol consumption
Recent illness
Abnormal blood pressure
Lactation
Blood donor, frequent
Obesity
Drug abuse
Occupation
Prescription drugs
Oral contraceptives
Over-the-counter drugs
Pregnancy
Environment
Recent surgery
Fasting or nonfasting
Tobacco use
Genetic factors
Recent transfusion
Current/recent hospitalization
Vitamin abuse

From Clinical Laboratory Standards Institute: Defining, Establishing, and Verifying Reference Intervals in the Clinical Laboratory; Approved Guideline, ed 3, Villanova, PA, 2008, CLSI.

It is sometimes acceptable to transfer a previously established reference interval that is based on a valid reference value study from a donor laboratory or manufacturer to a receiving laboratory without performing a new, full-scale study. Such a transfer is acceptable only if the test subject population and the entire methodology, from preparation of the test individual to the analytical measurement in the receiving laboratory, are the same as or appropriately comparable with those of the donor laboratory (see following text). The comparability of the analytical measuring system can be validated with the techniques discussed in CLSI Document EP9-A, *Method Comparison and Bias Estimate Guideline.*[8] It may be necessary to carry out an abbreviated reference value study, as described later, to validate the transferred reference interval.

SELECTION OF REFERENCE INDIVIDUALS

Health is a relative condition that lacks a universal definition. Defining what is to be considered healthy becomes the initial problem in any study, and establishing the criteria used to exclude nonhealthy subjects from the reference sample is the first step in selecting reference individuals. Frequently, it can be determined only that a particular individual is apparently "disease free," that is, does not have a specific medical condition that might affect the reference interval study. In some cases, individuals with minor illnesses or "unrelated" conditions may be used as reference individuals. However, it is often difficult to estimate the potential physiological and pharmacological influences in these subjects, and appropriate caution is required.

The selection of reference individuals for a reference value study is important and should be systematic.[1,3,9] Each institution or investigator may have different criteria for health; these criteria should be defined *before* selection proceeds. As a minimum, it is recommended that the investigator establish lists of selection, exclusion, and potential partition criteria (examples are shown in Boxes 24-2 and 24-3) and use a questionnaire to evaluate these criteria in potential reference individuals. The use of designed questionnaires is one of the best ways to consistently implement the exclusion and partitioning criteria. Forms should be simple and nonintimidating, requiring only *yes* or *no* responses to questions. The questionnaire may be used with simple measurements, such as blood pressure, height, and weight, and with an interview during which it is appropriate to ask individuals if they consider themselves to be in good health. Name, address, and phone number and any additional information, such as a patient identification number, should be included to facilitate contacting the reference individual when abnormal results are obtained. Certainly there is an obligation to notify the individual or the individual's physician in such cases. In some situations, anonymous questionnaires may be a better vehicle for obtaining the required information. In these instances, a numbering system can be used. (The reference individual is then responsible for contacting the laboratory to determine whether the testing showed any

Box 24-3

Examples of Possible Partitioning Factors

Age
Posture when sampled
Blood group
Race
Circadian variation
Sex
Diet
Stage of menstrual cycle
Ethnic background
Stage of pregnancy
Exercise
Time of day when sampled
Fasting or nonfasting
Tobacco use
Geographical location

From Clinical Laboratory Standards Institute: Defining, Establishing, and Verifying Reference Intervals in the Clinical Laboratory; Approved Guideline, ed 3, Villanova, PA, 2008, CLSI.

problems that require follow-up study.) In all cases, the usual policy for patient confidentiality must be enforced.

Informed consent should be obtained from reference individuals for specimen collection and testing. In some cases, protocol review and approval by an institutional research committee (human use committee) may be necessary. A sample questionnaire is provided in the CLSI C28-A3 document.[1] Determination of the health status of the individual by medical examinations and laboratory testing is not considered to be essential. However, if these assessments are performed, they will, of course, strengthen the reliability of the reference interval determination. All criteria and assessments used should be documented so that others can evaluate the health status of the reference sample group.

Reference individuals used for the determination of a health-associated reference interval do not have to be young, healthy adults but should closely resemble the patient population in the specific hospital or practice that will be using the results. However, for some particular analytes, a "standard" population of young, healthy adults may be appropriate. For others, age-related sets of reference intervals may be more appropriate. In the elderly population, it may be particularly important to rule out disease through the use of additional diagnostic assessments. Patient populations should not be used as disease-free reference individuals unless it is absolutely essential, as in certain instances for pediatric or geriatric populations.

It is necessary to determine for each analyte whether there are age-related differences, whether these differences are clinically important, and whether the use of age subgroups for reference intervals will be clinically appropriate. For certain biological constituents, age-related differences are consistent with good health and are part of a normal process of growth or maturation, such as alkaline phosphatase levels in children versus those in adults. However, for levels of other substances, such as cholesterol, or possibly growth hormone in the elderly, the use of different levels to reflect age differences may not be medically suitable when developing health-associated reference intervals. Consequently, determination of the need for separate reference intervals for age subgroups at specified age-group intervals is a rather complex medical decision. Review of the literature can be very helpful in making this evaluation.

The terms *a priori* and *a posteriori* are used to describe two general methods of selecting reference individuals from the reference population. *A priori* sampling is a method that is best used for well-studied, established laboratory procedures. Well-defined exclusion and partitioning criteria are established before the reference individuals are selected. For established methods, a thorough search of the literature should allow identification of known sources of biological variation, enabling researchers to establish exclusion and partitioning criteria and to develop an appropriate questionnaire. Reference individuals are then selected and are partitioned into subclasses, if necessary. This process should take place *before* any blood samples are collected. The number of reference individuals selected for analysis must closely match the number required to be statistically valid.

The *a posteriori* approach is especially appropriate for new or poorly studied laboratory procedures for which the literature contains little information. In *a posteriori* sampling, the process of exclusion and partitioning takes place after sampling and analyte testing rather than before. Because the factors defining a subclass usually are not known, the questionnaire for this approach should be more detailed than the one designed for the *a priori* sampling process. Generally, the *a posteriori* approach requires large numbers of subjects and substantial computing power to be implemented effectively.

KEY CONCEPTS BOX 24-1

- The reference interval (RI) describes percentiles of a healthy population, and thus, by design, a specified percentage of a non-diseased population will be outside the RI.
- Selected individuals from the entire *reference population* will be used as *reference individuals* on which analytical values are obtained. From the distribution of these reference values the *reference limits* (the upper and lower limit values) will be calculated.
- While the word "normal" infers *a non-diseased state*, it has many other ambiguous meaning and a better description of a reference population is "healthy."
- Reference individuals must be carefully selected to produce an unbiased reference sample group; exclusion and partitioning of the reference values can be made at the beginning of the testing (a priori method) or after values have been gathered (a posteriori method).

SECTION OBJECTIVES BOX 24-2

- List characteristics of the analytical method that must be considered in determining reference intervals.
- Explain why a minimum of 120 reference values is recommended if a nonparametric method is used to determine reference intervals.
- Discuss how nonparametric and parametric statistics may be used to determine reference intervals.

Box 24-4

Examples of Preanalytical Variables

Subject Preparation
Prior diet
Fasting versus nonfasting
Abstinence from pharmacological agents
Drug regimen
Synchronization in analysis
Relation to biological rhythms
Physical activity
Rest period before collection
Stress

Specimen Collection
Environmental conditions during collection
Time of day
Body posture
Specimen type
Collection site analysis
Site preparation
Blood flow promotion
Equipment
Technique

Specimen Handling
Transport
Clotting
Separation of serum/plasma
Storage
Preparation for analysis

From Clinical Laboratory Standards Institute: Defining, Establishing, and Verifying Reference Intervals in the Clinical Laboratory; Approved Guideline, ed 3, Villanova, PA, 2008, CLSI.

PREANALYTICAL AND ANALYTICAL VARIABLES

Analytical results from reference populations are affected by preanalytical and analytical variables. Therefore, all these variables must be considered and controlled consistently when reference intervals are determined.[10-15] In addition, it is important that reference subjects and samples be handled in an approved manner[16-22] and in exactly the same manner as patients and patient samples will be handled in the actual clinical analysis situation. All the preanalytical variables discussed in detail in Chapter 18 and reviewed in Box 24-4 must be carefully considered, controlled if necessary, and documented.

ANALYTICAL METHOD CHARACTERISTICS

The validity of information provided by the laboratory is critical for establishment of an accurate reference interval. The methods chosen for specimen analysis must be described in detail, clearly stating accuracy, precision, minimum detection limit, linearity, recovery, and interference characteristics.[10-12] Other factors that affect analytical performance also require control and documentation. These include equipment or instrumentation, reagents (including water), calibration standards, and calculation methods.

Reagent lot-to-lot and technologist variability, as well as instrument-to-instrument variability (if the test will be performed on more than one instrument), must be determined. Thus the use of more than one technologist and more than one lot of reagent should be incorporated into the study protocol.

It is important to document the validity of data generated during the reference interval study. Therefore, during the determination of reference intervals, quality control materials are routinely analyzed in the same format used for patient samples. This not only monitors the analytical protocol used during the process but also ensures equivalence of results over the long term.[13] Ideally, data will be gathered by analyzing specimens over several days, resulting in values that reflect average run-to-run variation (see Chapter 25). In addition, an assessment of the interference from naturally occurring constituents is essential.

ANALYSIS OF REFERENCE VALUES

Statistical Methods

The reference interval is defined here as the interval between and including two numbers, an upper and lower reference limit. These two numbers are estimated to enclose a specified percentage (usually 95%) of the values for a population from which reference subjects have been drawn. For most analytes, the lower and upper reference limits are assumed to demarcate the estimated 2.5th and 97.5th percentiles, respectively, of the underlying distribution of values. In some cases, only one reference limit is of medical importance, usually an upper limit, say, the 97.5th percentile.

Two general statistical methods for determining such limits include nonparametric and parametric procedures (see Chapter 23). A third method based on robust statistics will be discussed at the end of this section. Detailed presentations of the nonparametric and parametric procedures have been published by Solberg.[6,9] The nonparametric method of estimation makes no specific assumption concerning the mathematical form of the probability distribution represented by observed reference values. The parametric method, as applied in practice, is used under the assumption that the **observed values,** or some mathematical transformation of those values, follow a gaussian (i.e., "normal") probability curve. Because the reference values of many analytes do not follow the gaussian form, use of the parametric method requires that they be transformed to some other measurement scale that will "normalize" them. This requires selecting the most suitable transformer (such as log, power, or some other function of the original scale) and then testing whether, on this new scale, the reference values do indeed appear to conform to a gaussian distribution. When the log function is used to transform the data to gaussian, the data are considered to have a **log-normal distribution.** The Shapiro-Wilk test and the Kolmogorov-Smirnov nonparametric test of the cumulative distribution may be used to determine whether the reference values have a gaussian distribution. This may involve some moderately complex statistical theory and corresponding computer programs.

Table 24-1 Frequency Distributions of Calcium Levels in 240 Medical Students, by Sex

	FREQUENCY		
Analyte, (mg/dL)	Women	Men	Combined
8.8	1	0	1
8.9	2*	0	2
9.0	1	0	1
9.1	3	2	5*
9.2	11	1*	12
9.3	11	8	19
9.4	8	6	14
9.5	16	11	27
9.6	16	12	28
9.7	26	13	39
9.8	8	16	24
9.9	7	14	21
10.0	3	7	10
10.1	2	10	12
10.2	3†	11	14
10.3	2	7†	9†
10.4	0	1	1
10.6	0	1	1
Total	120	120	240

From Clinical Laboratory Standards Institute: Defining, Establishing, and Verifying Reference Intervals in the Clinical Laboratory; Approved Guideline, ed 3, Villanova, PA, 2008, CLSI.
*2.5th percentile.
†97.5th percentile.

The CLSI Guideline document[1] recommends that the reference interval be estimated by the nonparametric method, and that a minimum of 120 reference values be used for reference interval determination. The nonparametric method is simple, depending only on the ranks of reference data arrayed in order of increasing value. As an example, the frequency distribution for calcium reference values is shown in Table 24-1. The rank of the percentile observation is the percentile $\times (n + 1)$ where n is the sample size. Thus for 120 values, the rank of the 2.5th percentile observation is 3, that is, $0.025 \times 121 = 3.025$; and the rank for the 97.5th percentile observation is 118, that is, $0.975 \times 121 = 117.975$. These are indicated in Table 24-1 by * and †, respectively. Using these rank values to estimate upper and lower reference limits, we obtain the following 95% reference intervals: 8.9 to 10.2 mg/dL for women and 9.2 to 10.3 mg/dL for men, or 9.1 to 10.3 mg/dL for the combined population.

Using the nonparametric method, it is impossible to distinguish between two percentiles of a distribution unless the number of observations, n, equals or exceeds $(100/P) - 1$. Consequently, the nonparametric method requires an absolute minimum of 39 measurements to distinguish the 2.5th percentile from the 5th percentile or the 95th percentile from the 97.5th percentile, $n = (100/2.5) - 1 = 39$. Reed, Henry, and Mason[23] have suggested that a minimum of 120 observations be secured, one from each reference group, allowing 90% confidence limits to be computed nonparametrically for each reference limit at the 2.5th and 97.5th percentiles. To estimate the reference limits for these same percentiles with 95% confidence, 153 reference values are needed; for 99% confidence, 198 reference values are needed. Lott et al,[24] using a Monte Carlo simulation technique and large numbers of samplings of a medical student population, found that increasing the size of the sample had a stabilizing effect on the 2.5th and 97.5th percentiles. At about 200 individuals, the lower and upper reference limits for seven tests (Na, K, Cl, glucose, hemoglobin, erythrocytes, hematocrit), as determined by the nonparametric method, became stable. This experimental finding agrees with the 198 subjects required by strictly statistical criteria to define the same limits with a 99% confidence level. Linnet[25] has proposed that up to 700 observations should be obtained for highly skewed distributions. Clearly, a greater number of observations will improve the statistical accuracy of the estimation.

The minimum number of 120 samples is made under the assumption that no observations have been deleted from the reference set. If aberrant or outlying observations have been deleted, additional subjects should be selected, until at least 120 acceptable reference values have been obtained for each determination of a reference interval. Moreover, if separate intervals are needed for different subclasses (e.g., for sex or age class), each such interval should be determined using the recommended number (at least 120) of reference observations.

If it is not possible to obtain 120 reference observations, then a reference interval based on robust statistics may be used. The robust reference interval is based on robust quantile estimators first proposed by Horn.[26,27] These estimators mimic the parametric estimators by using robust estimators of location (e.g., population mean or median) and spread instead of the mean and standard deviation. Whereas the mean and standard deviation give equal weight to every observation, the robust estimators assign weights depending on how far an observation is from the general bulk of the data. The robust reference interval uses data transformation to estimate the lower reference limit but may use the raw, untransformed data to estimate the upper reference limit. As a result, the robust reference interval is able to reasonably estimate the needed percentiles without requiring the assumption of an underlying gaussian distribution, nor the minimum sample size of 120. The robust reference interval may be derived for samples as small as 20, although caution must be used in such cases. See Horn and Pesce[28] for details. By way of comparison, the robust reference intervals for the data in Table 24-1 range from 9.0 to 10.1 mg/dL for females, from 9.2 to 10.4 mg/dL for males, and from 9.1 to 10.3 mg/dL for the combined sample. However, the robust procedure can be used for samples as small as 20 observations. For example, a random sample selected from the 120 female Ca measurements produced a robust reference interval from 9.0 to 10.2 mg/dL.

Confidence Intervals (see p. 421, Chapter 23)

Reference limits computed from a sample of selected subjects are estimates of the corresponding percentiles in the population of individuals studied. Confidence intervals are useful for two reasons. First, they remind the investigator of the variability of estimates and provide a quantitative measure of this vari-

Table 24-2 90% Confidence Intervals for Lower and Upper 95% Reference Limits

Analyte	Lower Reference Limit	Upper Reference Limit
Calcium (mg/dL)		
Women (n = 120)	8.8 to 9.1	10.1 to 10.3
Men (n = 120)	9.1 to 9.3	10.3 to 10.6
Combined (n = 240)	8.8 to 9.1	10.3 to 10.6

From Clinical Laboratory Standards Institute: Defining, Establishing, and Verifying Reference Intervals in the Clinical Laboratory; Approved Guideline, ed 3, Villanova, PA, 2008, CLSI.

ability. Second, confidence intervals narrow as the size of the sampling increases. Therefore, the investigator can get an idea of the improved precision in an estimated 95% reference interval that would be obtained from a larger sampling of reference individuals. Table 24-2 demonstrates 90% confidence intervals for the lower and upper 95% reference limits for calcium.

For robust reference interval end points, confidence intervals may be derived using bootstrap technology. The bootstrap[29] is a resampling procedure whereby a sample is selected with replacement from the data set. For each of these "pseudo" samples, the robust reference limits are derived. This process is repeated a large number of times, producing a large number of robust reference interval end points. From this large number of estimates, the 90% confidence interval is estimated by taking the upper and lower 5th percentiles of these generated values. For example, the 90% confidence intervals for the female Ca data in Table 24-1 range from 8.9 to 9.1 mg/dL and from 10.0 to 10.2 mg/dL for the upper and lower robust reference interval end points, respectively.

Treatment of Outlying Observations
(see also p. 429, Chapter 23)

An important implicit assumption in the estimation of reference limits is that the set of measured reference values represents a "homogeneous" collection of observations. This means that all values come from the same underlying probability distribution.

It may be that this condition is satisfied by almost all reference values, but that one or two arise from a probability distribution that is different from that of the others. When such values fall within the expected distribution, they are practically impossible to identify unless the individual performing the biochemical analysis happens to know that these observations represent atypical analytical conditions or are the result of some arithmetic or procedural mistake. Often, however, such "aberrant" values lie outside the range of the remaining measurements and can be identified as **outliers** requiring special attention.

Unless outliers are known to be aberrant observations, that is, the result of a mistake in the analysis or a lapse in the preanalytical controls applied to remaining subjects, emphasis should be placed on retaining rather than deleting them. Nonparametrically estimated reference limits based on at least 120 observations would be only slightly changed, or not changed at all, if an extreme value were deleted. Many statistical techniques are available for testing the atypicality of outlying observations.[30] A test proposed by Dixon[31] uses the ratio D/R, in which D is the absolute difference between an extreme observation (large or small) and the next largest (or smallest) observation, and R is the range of all observations, including extremes, used to evaluate outlying observations. Reed, Henry, and Mason[23] have suggested the use of $^1/_3$ as a **cutoff value** for the ratio D/R, that is, if the observed value of D is equal to or greater than one-third of the range R, the extreme observation is deleted. For sample sizes as large as 120, this criterion is rather conservative,[23] that is, it often would fail to reject outliers that really are not part of the distribution. However, in the absence of evidence that an outlier is indeed an aberrant observation, and given that the underlying distribution often will not be exactly gaussian in form, the one-third rule for the ratio D/R seems appropriate, especially when reference intervals are determined by the nonparametric method. Therefore, the CLSI guideline supports the use of this test and the cutoff value of one-third suggested by Reed, Henry, and Mason when statistically significant outliers are sought in a set of observed reference values.

When two or three outliers are present on the same side of the distribution (i.e., all are extremely large or extremely small), the one-third rule (or any similar D/R rule) can fail to label the most extreme outlier as statistically significant and thereby can mask the presence of other outliers that are just slightly less extreme. Common sense indicates that, in such a case, the one-third rule should be applied to the least extreme outlier as if it were the only outlier. If the rule leads to rejection of this outlier, the more extreme observations naturally should be rejected as well. If the rule does not reject the least extreme value, either all the extreme values should be accepted, or, alternatively, a test that considers all the outliers together should be applied. Such a test is called a *block procedure;* examples are given by Barnett and Lewis.[30] When any outlier is rejected, it is appropriate to test the remaining data for an additional outlier or outliers.

PARTITIONING OF REFERENCE VALUES

The possibility that separate reference intervals will be required for subclasses of subjects should be considered before the process of securing and analyzing subject specimens is begun. However, the use of separate reference intervals for men and women or for different age groups, for example, may not be justified unless these separate intervals will be clinically useful or are well grounded physiologically. When necessary, at least 120 subjects of each sex or age or other subclass should be sampled. The information necessary to decide whether **partitioning of reference values** is needed may not be available in advance for a new analyte.

Generally, it has been assumed that when the difference between the observed means of two subclass populations is statistically significant (at the 5% or 1% probability level), each subclass warrants its own reference interval. However, any observed difference, no matter how unimportant clinically, will become statistically significant if the sample sizes are large enough. It is important to consult with an appropriate clinician to define what a *clinically significant* difference is. If the difference between subgroups is *not clinically significant*, the reference values should not be partitioned, even if there is a statistically significant difference between the means (as determined by a *t*-test).

Research by Harris and Boyd[32] has shown that differences between subclass means or differences in **standard deviations (SDs)** of the subclasses, even when the means are identical, can lead to deviations in sensitivity and specificity for disease detection. These investigators found that at times there is a statistical need for separate reference intervals, which, if ignored, could potentially hamper the interpretation of laboratory results as part of the diagnostic process. An approach suggested by Harris and Boyd[1,32] tests the *statistical* significance of the difference between subclass means by the standard normal deviate test (*z*-test), beginning with a pilot sample of 60 subjects in each subclass. If the calculated statistic z exceeds a "critical" z value, separate reference intervals should be calculated for each subclass. In addition, if the larger SD of the two subclasses exceeds 1.5 times the smaller SD, regardless of the z value, separate reference intervals should be calculated.

For two subclasses, such as men and women, or two age groups, the statistical significance of the difference between subclass means should be tested by the standard normal deviate test:

$$z = \frac{[\bar{x}_1 - \bar{x}_2]}{[(s_1^2/n_1) + (s_2^2/n_2)]^{1/2}} \quad \text{Eq. 24-1}$$

in which $\bar{x}_1$ and $\bar{x}_2$ are the observed means of the two subgroups, s_1^2 and s_2^2 are the observed variances, and n_1 and n_2 are the number of reference values in each subclass, respectively. If at least 60 subjects are assumed in each subclass, the *z*-test is essentially a nonparametric test that may be applied to the original data, whether or not the values represent a gaussian distribution. The calculated statistic z should be compared with a "critical" value z^*:

$$z^* = 3(n_{\text{average}}/120)^{1/2} = 3[(n_1 + n_2)/240]^{1/2} \quad \text{Eq. 24-2}$$

In addition, the larger standard deviation, for example s_2, should be checked to see whether it exceeds $1.5s_1$, or, equivalently, whether $s_2/(s_2 - s_1)$ is less than 3 (Box 24-5).

For example, suppose that at the end of the first stage of sampling, the average number of reference values in each subclass is 60. Then, if the calculated z exceeds a z^*, that is, $3(60/120)^{1/2} = 2.12$, or if the larger standard deviation exceeds 1.5 times the smaller standard deviation, sampling should be continued to obtain at least 120 subjects in each subclass. The *z*-test and SD comparisons should be repeated. If the average number of subjects in each subclass is now 120, $z^* = 3$.

At this point, if the calculated z value exceeds z^*, or if the larger standard deviation exceeds 1.5 times the smaller, regardless of the z value, separate reference intervals should be calculated for each subclass, under the assumption that the difference between the two reference intervals is likely to be of importance in medical practice. If these conditions do not hold, a single reference interval for the combined group of reference subjects should be calculated for general use. Box 24-5 gives an example of this calculation.

When more than two subclasses are being compared, the problem is more complicated. A statistically significant difference found when the means of all subclasses are compared may, in fact, be attributable only to a difference between two means, such as the mean of one subclass versus the mean of the other subgroups combined. For three or more subclasses, the common statistical analysis of results would be the analysis of variance, if it is assumed that all subclasses have equal standard deviations. In this case, a critical *F*-statistic that is comparable with the z^* value defined earlier (and therefore dependent on the sample sizes in each subclass) would have to be defined. It is suggested that in this situation, the aid of a statistical consultant should be sought.[33]

The statistical tests and criteria recommended earlier may also be applied to the question of whether reference intervals determined in one laboratory should be transferred without change for use in another laboratory (see the discussion of transference).

In the preceding examples, the differences in calcium values between men and women, although statistically significant, are small and may not be clinically significant. The *z*-test in this case is certainly sensitive. When the imprecision of the assay and the 90% confidence intervals calculated previously for calcium are considered, a laboratory may choose to provide only a single reference range of 9.1 to 10.3 mg/dL for both men and women in this age group. The final decision may be

Box 24-5

Calculation of a z Statistic to Test for Subclass Difference

Example: To test for subclass difference between the calcium reference values for men and women, the means and standard deviations of each group are needed:
Calcium (mg/dL), $n_1 = n_2$

$\bar{x}$, *men*	$\bar{x}$, *women*	*SD, men*	*SD, women*
9.80	9.57	0.331	0.29

Inserting these statistics into the formula given above for z (Eq. 24-1), the results are as follows:
Calcium:

$$z = \frac{|9.80 - 9.57|}{\left[\frac{(0.331)^2}{120} + \frac{(0.29)^2}{120}\right]^{1/2}} = 5.94$$

The z value exceeds the critical value $z^* = 3$ for n = 120, indicating that separate reference intervals for men and women should be considered. The SD of the male population is not greater than 1.5× the SD of the female group and thus does not indicate a subclass difference on this basis.

made on the basis of the clinical relevance of the statistically significant difference.

TRANSFERENCE

Because the determination of reliable reference intervals can be a major and costly task, it is cost-effective to transfer a reference interval from one laboratory to another by a convenient process of validation. As new tests and methods are introduced into laboratories, it is unrealistic to expect each laboratory, large or small, to develop its own reference intervals. Consequently, clinical laboratories rely on other laboratories or on manufacturers of diagnostic tests to provide adequate reference value data that can be transferred. To transfer reference values properly, certain conditions must be fulfilled. For example, the original reference value study must meet the minimum requirements of a valid study as outlined by CLSI C28-A3. Preanalytical and analytical procedural details, analytical performance, the complete set of reference values, and the method of estimating the reference interval must be stated.

If it is assumed that the original reference value study was performed properly, the transference of a reference interval from one testing agency to another involves two problems: the comparability of the two analytical systems, and the comparability of the two test subject populations. If both testing agencies do not use the same closed analytical system, the comparability of the two systems can be assessed as outlined by the CLSI Approved Guideline EP09-A2.[8] In addition, all preanalytical procedures used during the reference value study, such as preparation of test subjects and specimen collection and handling procedures, must be the same as those used by the receiving laboratory. The factors that must be considered before a reference interval is transferred are reviewed in Box 24-6. If, in the judgment of the laboratorian, these factors are consistent with the receiving laboratory's operation and test subject population, the reference interval may be transferred.

The CLSI approved guideline[1] provides two alternative procedures for the transference protocol that use either n = 20 or n = 60. Both shorter protocols require the same considerations as are required by the larger protocol (see Box 24-6).

KEY CONCEPTS BOX 24-2

- In order to obtain accurate reference values, all the known preanalytical and analytical variable of the testing method must be controlled.
- To understand the error associated with the calculated reference limits, the confidence limits about these values should be calculated.
- The most accurate reference intervals are obtained with the largest sampling number (N) possible. While an N of 120 is preferable, fewer numbers may be more realistic.
- The actual calculation of the reference interval may be accomplished with parametric and non parametric statistics; the latter is preferred, especially when N may be less that optimal.

Box 24-6

Factors to Consider for Transference of Reference Intervals

1. Appropriateness of donor laboratory reference interval (i.e., selection of reference individuals, exclusions and partitions, number of reference values, method of estimation, and valid reference interval determination according to CLSI C28-A3 requirements)
2. Comparability of preanalytical factors (i.e., subject preparation and specimen collection and handling and other items listed in Box 24-4)
3. Comparability of analytical method (i.e., same [closed method] or different [use CLSI EP09-A2] method)
4. Comparability of test subjects in terms of factors listed in Box 24-2
5. Validation study, if necessary

From Clinical Laboratory Standards Institute: Defining, Establishing, and Verifying Reference Intervals in the Clinical Laboratory; Approved Guideline, ed 3, Villanova, PA, 2008, CLSI.

SECTION OBJECTIVES BOX 24-3

- Explain the difference between clinical decision limits and reference intervals.
- Define the following terms: diagnostic sensitivity/specificity, true positives/negatives, predictive value of a positive test/negative test, and efficiency.
- Evaluate diagnostic sensitivity, diagnostic specificity, and predictive values in order to assess clinical utility of laboratory test.

PRESENTATION OF REFERENCE INTERVALS

Every quantitative clinical result should be accompanied by an appropriately presented *reference interval.* Reference intervals should reflect the subclass partitions that have been determined to be significant for that laboratory's particular reference population. Reports that include the results of many tests should clearly highlight those results that are not within the reference interval. It is helpful to indicate the relationship of a patient's results to those of the reference interval. Printing *high* or *low* adjacent to a result is an acceptable option.

When forms with preprinted reference intervals are used, reference intervals for all appropriate subclasses should be included. This can result in a confusing report. A better approach is for the computer or instrument to print the reference interval that is appropriate for the particular patient. In most cases, the age and sex of the patient will determine the subclass reference intervals. Any report that uses subclass reference intervals should include the patient's partitioning factors in the heading or in the demographics portion of the report.

Ideally, detailed information describing the reference population and the details of the reference interval study should be available to all users of a laboratory service. This information should be updated any time a change is made in the laboratory that affects the reference intervals in use. A memo addressing changes in a reference interval should be sent to all users of the laboratory.

INTRAINDIVIDUAL REFERENCE INTERVALS

The National Institutes of Health (NIH) has shown that even healthy individuals studied over several weeks under standardized conditions exhibited a range of values for numerous analytes.[34,35] (See Tables 26-2 and 26-3, pp. 486 and 497, for examples of intraindividual variations.) For the same analyte, some individuals had analyte values that fell within a narrow range, whereas for others, the variability was large. The larger component of variability in some analytes was the preanalytical and analytical variation, whereas in others, it was biological variation. In the NIH study, the spread of results obtained in any one individual was consistently less than the population-based reference interval. Thus an intraindividual abnormal result for a particular individual could fall within the so-called healthy population–based reference interval. Variability of results also means that a healthy individual occasionally might have test results that fall outside a reference interval derived from a central 95% population–based interval; this individual might be falsely categorized as having abnormal test results. Another individual might have a result that is abnormal for his or her specific range but that falls within the population-based reference interval; this individual would have a falsely normal result.

These studies show that it is clearly impossible to develop a reference interval from 120 healthy individuals that is appropriate for every individual. They also show that it is impractical to develop a series of reference intervals that consider each and every possible variable that might affect the concentration of an analyte. Consequently, laboratorians are left with the compromise of the population-based reference interval that is developed under those conditions that can be controlled, and that is reasonably consistent with patient testing conditions. D.S. Young[36] discusses this in detail.

Many clinicians are unaware of the preanalytical and analytical factors that may affect the interpretation of test results. It is important for all clinicians to understand that all results within the reference interval are not always considered healthy, nor are all results outside the reference interval considered abnormal. Thus it is essential that clinical laboratories interact with the clinicians who use their services to ensure the proper interpretation of test values in patients.

Table 24-3 Purposes for Which Laboratory Tests Are Ordered and the Importance of Reference Intervals in Interpretation of their Results

Purpose	Reference Interval
Diagnosis of disease	++
Screening for disease	+++
Determination of severity of disease	+
Monitoring progress of disease	+
Monitoring response to therapy	+
Monitoring therapy	+++
Monitoring drug toxicity	++
Predicting response to treatment	+
Predicting prognosis	+
Reassurance of patient	++

From Young DS: Determination and validation of reference intervals, Arch Pathol Lab Med 116:704, 1992.
+, Minor importance; ++, moderate importance; +++, great importance.

CLINICAL DECISION LIMITS

Predictive Value Theory

Clinical decision limits are different from reference intervals because they are based on medical information related to a specific medical condition. They may be "critical values," describing limits of analyte concentrations that demand immediate medical intervention or change in management, they may be diagnostic cutoff values with a high association for a disease or a clinical condition, or they may be therapeutic window limits for pharmaceutical agents (Table 24-3).

Decision analysis is a practical strategy for considering the risks and benefits of decision making based on the quantitative probability of predicting the true diagnosis or outcome. The respective quantitative approaches used by the laboratorian or clinician in evaluating clinical laboratory measurements and data have been well described[37,38] and generally have been accepted. The concepts of sensitivity, specificity, and **predictive values** of test results are fundamentally important to these probabilistic approaches. These concepts are now being applied more frequently in the clinical laboratory, not only to establish clinical decision limits, but also to assist in determining the relative clinical merits of a given test (Fig. 24-4).[36]

The *diagnostic sensitivity* of a test is the probability of obtaining a positive result for a patient with a given disease, that is, the percentage of individuals with the disease who test positive. In contrast, the *diagnostic specificity* of a test is the probability of obtaining a negative result for a patient without the disease, that is, the percentage of individuals without the disease who test negative. The true positives (TP) are the individuals with the disease who are correctly classified by the test, that is, individuals with the disease who have positive test results. The false positives (FP) are the individuals without the disease who are incorrectly classified by the test, that is, healthy individuals who have positive test results. The false negatives (FN) are the individuals with the disease who are incorrectly classified by a negative test result. The true negatives (TN) are the individuals without the disease who correctly test negative. Because sensitivity is the true-positive rate, the complement, 100% minus sensitivity, is the false-negative rate. For example, if the sensitivity is 75%, the false-negative rate will be 25%. Accordingly, because specificity is the true-negative rate, 100% minus specificity is the false-positive rate.

The *predictive value of a positive test*, or the **positive predictive value,** is the probability that the patient with a positive test result has the given disease, that is, the fraction obtained when the number of true-positive results is divided by the total number of positive test results. The *predictive value of a negative result*, or the **negative predictive value,** is the probability that the patient with a negative result does not have the

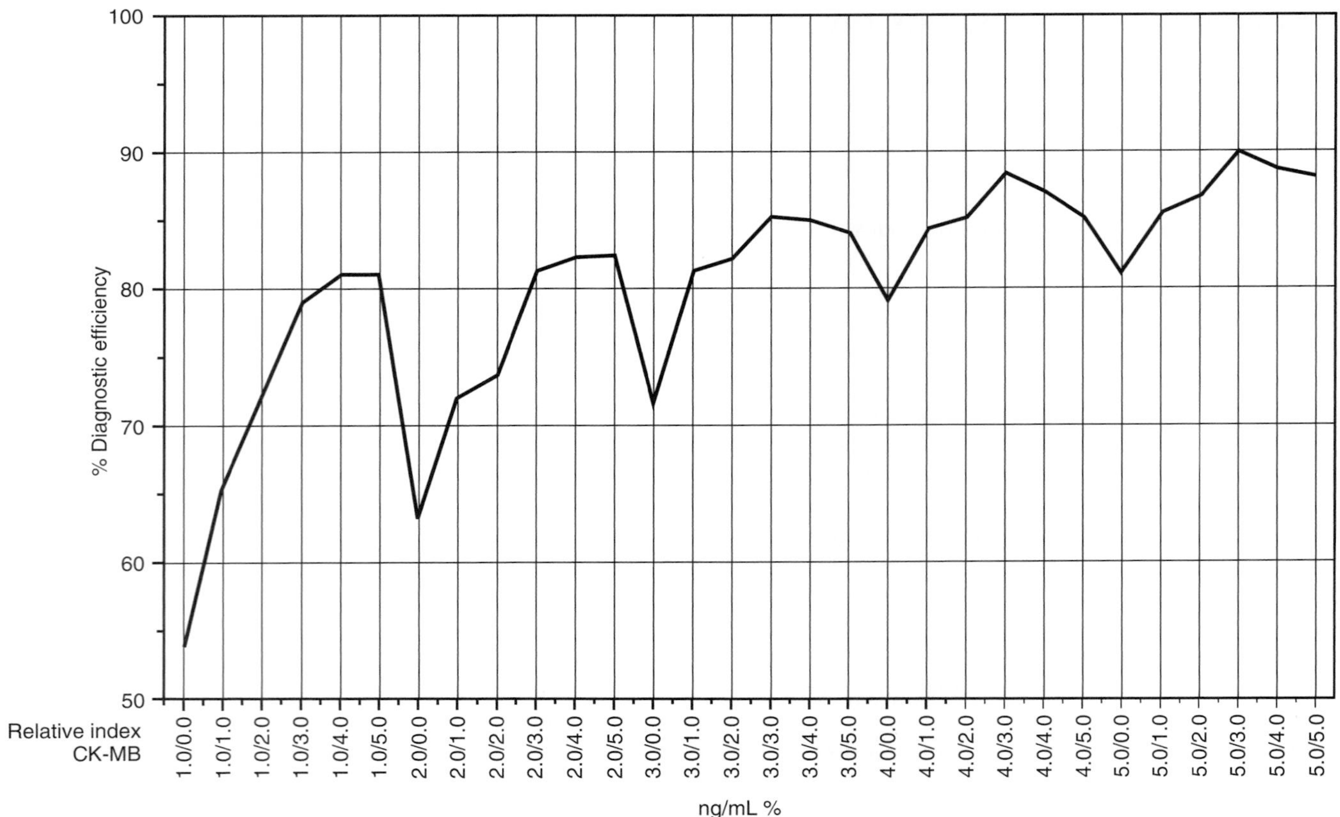

Fig. 24-4 Percent diagnostic efficiency versus combined cutoff levels of creatine kinase (CK)-MB in ng/mL (lower set of values on x-axis) and percent relative index (upperset of values on x-axis), expressed as (CK-MB/total CK) × 100. Combining these two tests at different respective cutoff levels produced the highest diagnostic efficiency, 90%, at a cutoff of 5 ng/mL for CK-MB and 3% for the relative index. (Courtesy D. Obzansky, Du Pont Co., Wilmington, Delaware.)

disease, that is, the fraction obtained when the number of true-negative results is divided by the total number of negative test results. The *efficiency* of the test is the fraction of all tested individuals who were correctly classified as having or not having the disease. These probabilities often are converted to and discussed as percentages.

Predictive values and diagnostic efficiency are greatly influenced by false-positive and false-negative rates and by the **prevalence** of the disease in the population being tested (Table 24-4). The importance of prevalence in determining the predictive value (expressed as a percentage) can be seen by rearrangement and substitution of the terms for the predictive value of a positive result (PV+) to give the following equivalent equation:

$$PV+ = \frac{[\text{Prevalence} \times \text{Sensitivity}] \times 100\%}{[\text{Prevalence} \times \text{Sensitivity}] + [(1 - \text{Prevalence})(1 - \text{Specificity})]} \quad \text{Eq. 24-3}$$

Thus, for a test with a diagnostic sensitivity of 95% and a diagnostic specificity of 95%, the predictive value for a positive result in a population with a prevalence of the disease of 50% is 95%. However, if the prevalence is 5%, the PV+ is 50%, or, for a prevalence of 1%, the PV+ is only 16.1%. When the PV+ is 50%, the predictive value of the test is no better than chance; thus a coin may be tossed to decide whether a patient with a positive test result actually has the disease.

It is clear that although a test has high sensitivity and specificity and is a good diagnostic test in a defined population of patients, it will perform less well in another population, in which the prevalence is very low. For example, a positive creatine kinase-MB (CK-MB) result is more significant (has a higher PV+) in a population of patients in a cardiac care unit (with prevalence of myocardial infarction at 30% to 50%) than in an emergency unit (with prevalence of myocardial infarction at ≈5%).

The sensitivity of a specific laboratory test can vary as the disease progresses through various stages in the continuum of disease development over a relatively long term. This variability is seen, for example, with atherosclerosis, cancer, and diabetes. Thus a tumor marker test may have low sensitivity for very early cancer but a much higher sensitivity for detecting advanced stages of the same cancer. On the other hand, certain tests can be so sensitive as to detect or predict disease before there are symptoms. The predictive value of the test in a population will also be dependent, in part, on the relative

Table 24-4 Sensitivity, Specificity, Predictive Value

	Number of Subjects With Positive Test Result	Number of Subjects With Negative Test Result	Total
Number of subjects with disease	TP	FN	TP + FN
Number of subjects without disease	FP	TN	FP + TN
TOTALS	TP + FP	FN + TN	TP + FP + TN + FN

From Statland BE et al: Quantitative approaches used in evaluating laboratory measurements and other clinical data. In Henry JB, editor: *Clinical Diagnosis and Management by Laboratory Methods,* Philadelphia, 1979, Saunders.
TP, True positives, or number of diseased patients correctly classified by the test; *FP,* false positives, or number of patients without the disease misclassified by the test; *FN,* false negatives, or number of diseased patients misclassified by the test; *TN,* true negatives, or number of patients without the disease correctly classified by the test.

$$\text{Diagnostic sensitivity} = \frac{TP}{TP + FN}$$

$$\text{Diagnostic specificity} = \frac{TN}{FP + TN}$$

$$\text{Predictive value of positive test, PV+} = \frac{TP}{TP + FP}$$

$$\text{Predictive value of negative test, PV−} = \frac{TN}{TN + FN}$$

$$\text{Efficiency of the test (number fraction of patients correctly classified), that is, } \frac{TP + TN}{TP + FP + TN + FN}$$

$$\text{Prevalence} = \frac{TP + FN}{TP + FP + TN + FN}$$

proportion of patients with disease that has advanced to a detectable level.

As a general rule, tests that are used for the screening of occult disease in the general population (low disease prevalence) should have as high a diagnostic sensitivity as possible, consistent with an acceptable level of false-positive results (specificity). Generally, maximal sensitivity and specificity are desired. In the example above of a test with 95% sensitivity and specificity, if the test is used to screen for a disease that is present in a population at 1% prevalence, 83.9% of persons who have a positive test result will *not* have the disease. If this rate of false-positive values is unacceptable, the specificity of the test will have to be increased at the expense of the sensitivity. Alternatively, if the diagnostic sensitivity and the positive predictive value are not mutually acceptable, the test should not be used for screening but should be applied only to populations with a higher prevalence of the disease.

Galen and Gambino[38] have suggested the following guidelines for deciding whether a test should have the highest sensitivity, the highest specificity, the highest positive predictive value, or the highest efficiency. Please note that it is not possible to have all these attributes at the same time.

The highest sensitivity (preferably 100%) is desired in the following diagnostic situations:

1. The disease is serious and should not be missed.
2. The disease is treatable.
3. False-positive results do not lead to serious physical, psychological, or economic trauma to the patient.

Example. Pheochromocytoma.

This disease can be fatal if missed, but if diagnosed, it is nearly 100% curable. Other examples include phenylketonuria, venereal disease, and other treatable infections.

The highest specificity (preferably 100%) is desired in the following diagnostic situations:

1. The disease is serious but is not treatable or curable.
2. The knowledge that the disease is absent has psychological or public health value.
3. False-positive results can lead to serious psychological or economic trauma to the patient.

Example. Multiple sclerosis and most occult cancers.

These diseases are serious but generally are not treatable or curable.

A high predictive value for a positive result is essential in the following diagnostic situation:

1. Treatment of a false-positive individual might have serious consequences.

Example. Occult cancer of the lung, in which the treatment of lobectomy or radiation has significant morbidity.

The highest efficiency is desired in the following diagnostic situations:

1. The disease is serious but treatable.
2. False-positive results and false-negative results are essentially equally serious or damaging.

Example. Myocardial infarction.

The disease may be fatal but is treatable. Other examples include lupus erythematosus, some forms of leukemia and lymphoma, and diabetes mellitus.

It is apparent that the predictive value or efficiency estimation for a given test is highly dependent on the population of patients tested. Comparisons of the predictive value or efficiency of different tests or different methodologies are valid only if the populations studied are the same. Unless the patient populations studied are carefully defined, sufficiently large, and very similar, predictive values from different studies may be misleading if the relative merits of the tests are judged. For example, as was suggested earlier, a study of the predictive value or efficiency of a CK-MB assay for diagnosing myocardial injury in a patient population that consists of patients in the cardiac intensive care unit most certainly will yield different results from those that would be obtained for a population of patients with chest pain in the emergency room. Caution must even be used in comparing predictive values between different studies of critical care unit patients from different institutions because the institutions may treat different patient populations and may use different specific criteria for admission to the unit or for making a final diagnosis.

Medical Decision Limits

Another important use of the concepts of sensitivity, specificity, and predictive value is seen in the determination of an optimal cutoff value or **medical decision limit** for a clinical laboratory test. Diagnostic sensitivity and specificity are dependent on the cutoff value selected. When a relatively low medical decision limit is used for CK-MB, the diagnostic sensitivity of the test may approach 100% for the diagnosis of myocardial injury (few or no false-negative results); however, the diagnostic specificity may decrease to a range of 50% to 60% (a large number of false-positive results). When a higher cutoff value is used, the specificity will improve but the sensitivity will decrease. Whenever a medical decision limit is changed, there is a tradeoff between the diagnostic sensitivity and the specificity of the test. The perfect test, if it were to exist, at a perfect cutoff value would have a sensitivity and a specificity of 100% and a diagnostic efficiency of 100%.

Certainly, laboratories and clinicians have to collaborate and agree on the balance of false positives versus false negatives for each diagnostic situation. Some knowledge of the distributions of test results for diseased versus nondiseased populations can be very helpful when medical decision limits (see Figs. 24-1, 24-2, and 24-3) are chosen. As is illustrated in Figs. 24-2 and 24-3, test result distributions of healthy and diseased populations commonly overlap. For some diseases and certain tests, not all individuals with a particular disease will ever have a test result for a particular test outside the healthy reference interval. Also, test results may be affected by more than one disease. In addition, test results distribution can reflect the continuum from good health to the diseased condition or the stage of a given disease. For example, knowledge of the distribution of prostate-specific antigen (PSA) levels in men with benign prostate hyperplasia (BPH), in men with prostate cancer, and in men with normal prostates has led to the adoption of four decision limits: 0 to 4 ng/mL associated with normal prostates; 4 to 10 ng/mL normally associated with BPH but rarely with prostate cancer; 10 to 20 ng/mL often associated with prostate cancer; and >20 ng/mL associated almost always with prostate cancer. Thus, as the concentration of PSA increases, the likelihood of disease increases, and the specificity of the assay increases. Most experienced clinicians have a practical feel for such medical decision limits, using a relative high (or low) analyte level as an inclusion level to conclude confidently that a patient is included in the population with the disease, or vice versa, to exclude the patient from the population with the disease. The medical decision limit helps the clinician make choices regarding diagnosis, follow-up care, and the need for adjunct diagnostic testing.

The intended clinical use of a test will also be a factor in selecting the best cutoff value. In a given clinical setting, the consequences of a false-negative result may be far more serious than those of a false-positive result. False negatives are entirely unacceptable in testing for human immunodeficiency virus (HIV) infection among blood donors and organ transplant donors. Alternatively, less harm may be caused by classifying a patient as having myocardial injury by CK-MB test results when the patient in fact did not have a myocardial infarction (MI) (a false positive) than by classifying a patient with an MI as negative (a false negative). Clearly, discharge of a patient with an MI from the emergency department or clinic could be catastrophic for that patient. On the other hand, needlessly subjecting a patient with a falsely positive test result to other diagnostic procedures or interventions associated with a certain amount of risk is also not desirable. In addition, it could be prohibitively expensive to admit too many patients who have not had an MI to the cardiac intensive care unit. Galen and Gambino[38] have suggested that the best cutoff value that can be used for classifying a patient as having had an MI is the value that produces the greatest diagnostic efficiency.

There is no simple way to select the optimum combination of sensitivity and specificity. This choice, as discussed earlier, depends on the nature of the disease, the clinical population, and the relative cost of a false-positive or false-negative result. Additional sequential, supplemental, or confirmation testing can compensate for a test with a high rate of false-positive results and can minimize the associated undesirable consequences.

Receiver-Operating Characteristic Curve

The ability of a test, using a specific analyte concentration, to discriminate disease from nondisease can be graphically portrayed by use of **receiver-operating characteristic (ROC) curve** analysis. By plotting several ROC curves on the same graph, the laboratory staff can compare the merits of two different tests or the performance of one test under different conditions, such as different cutoff values or different patient populations. An example of such curves in Fig. 24-5 shows discrimination between subjects with and without coronary

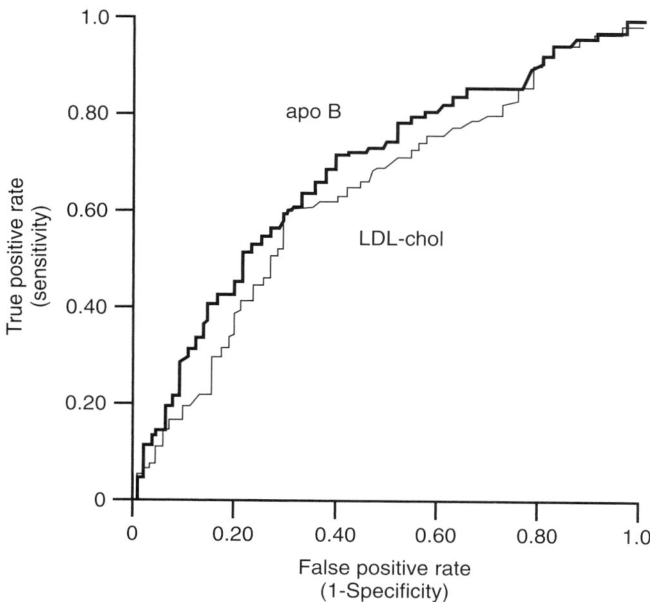

Fig. 24-5 Receiver-operating characteristic (ROC) curves showing discrimination between subjects with and without any coronary artery disease as measured by cardiac catheterization for two different biochemical indicators. (From Zweig MH, Broste SK, Reinhart RA: ROC curve analysis: an example showing the relationships among serum lipid and apolipoprotein concentrations in identifying patients with coronary artery disease, Clin Chem 38:1425, 1992.)

artery disease at different decision levels for apolipoprotein B and low-density lipoprotein (LDL) cholesterol. Refer to the article by Zweig, Broste, and Reinhart[39] and the review by Zweig and Campbell[40] for a good discussion of the use of ROC curves.

An ROC curve is derived by plotting the sensitivity (the true-positive rate) of the test versus 1.0 minus specificity (the false-positive rate). The multiple points on a curve represent the true-positive rate and the false-positive rate with different cutoff values used for the diagnosis or differentiation of illness versus nonillness. The point on the curve that is closest to the upper left-hand corner of the plot represents the cutoff value or decision limit that provides the greatest diagnostic accuracy, that is, the efficiency of the test. The area under the curve represents the overall accuracy of the test.

Other useful ways can be employed to represent and examine the relative diagnostic value of different cutoff values. One example is the modified Gerhardt plot,[41] which was used in a study of the relative utility of serum total amylase, total lipase, pancreatic amylase isoenzyme, and a lipase isoform in the diagnosis of acute pancreatitis.[42] These four tests were used on the same population of 81 patients with suspected acute pancreatitis. In this population, 41 of the patients did have pancreatitis, and 40 did not. In Fig. 24-6, the open bars in the plots above the zero line represent patients with pancreatitis, and the striped bars, below the line, represent patients without pancreatitis. Using these graphs, investigators could judge the

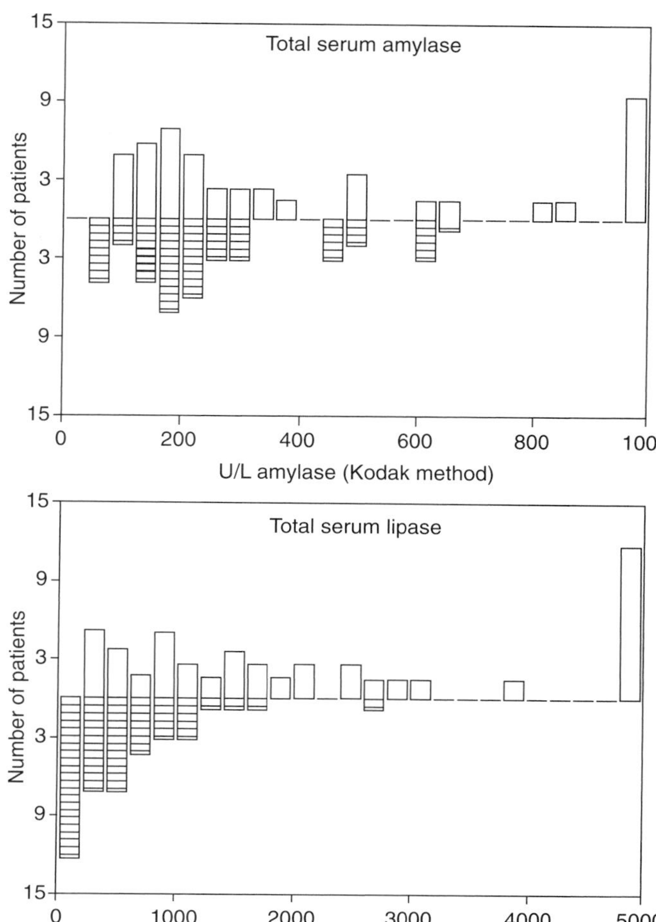

Fig. 24-6 Modified Gerhardt plots for serum amylase, lipase, and in the diagnosis of acute pancreatitis. See text for details. (From Gerhardt W: The Bayes approach: systematic graphic evaluation of diagnostic tests. In Keller H, Trendelenburg CH, editors: *Data Presentation, Interpretation,* New York, 1989, Walter de Gruyter.)

best discrimination or cutoff point for maximizing the sensitivity or specificity of each test. They concluded that, at least in this set of study patients, total amylase was a poor test for evaluating patients with an "acute abdomen," and a better test choice would be total lipase.

Other representations of cutoff values, such as those shown in Figs. 24-4 and 24-7, are also useful when a hypothetical immunochemical CK-MB assay is applied in the diagnosis of myocardial injury.[43] When diagnostic efficiency is the goal, a simple plot of the percent efficiency versus the diagnostic cutoff values is helpful. The highest efficiency at the lowest cutoff is the most appropriate, because increasing the cutoff value produces a greater number of false-negative results. Fig. 24-4 is interesting in that the diagnostic efficiency is plotted as a function of the combination of two cutoff values: the CK-MB in ng/mL and the percent relative index of CK-MB to total CK. The maximum diagnostic efficiency for this patient population for these specific CK-MB and CK assays appears to be 90% at a CK-MB cutoff of 5 ng/mL and a relative index of 3%:

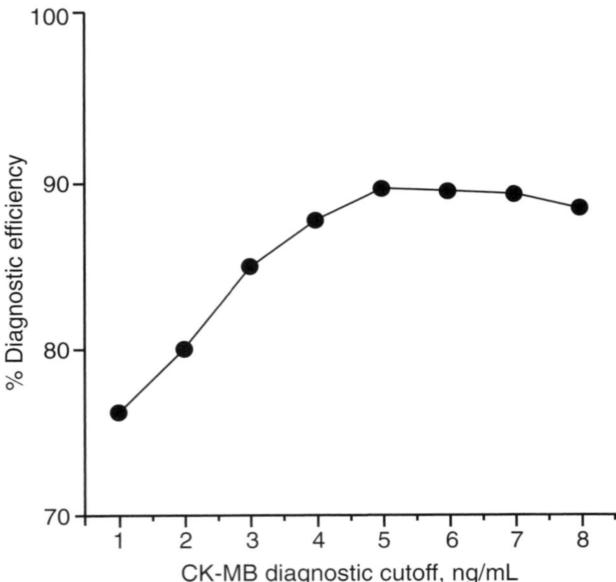

Fig. 24-7 Percent diagnostic efficiency plotted versus different diagnostic cutoff levels in nanograms per milliliter for a hypothetical immunochemical serum creatine kinase (CK)-MB assay. The highest diagnostic efficiency, 90%, at the lowest cutoff, 5 ng/mL, for CK-MB is the optimal decision level. (Courtesy D. Obzansky, Du Pont Co., Wilmington, Delaware.)

$$\text{relative index} = \frac{\text{CK-MB } (\mu g/L)}{\text{CK-MB } (U/L)} \times 100$$

Decision analysis involving multiple testing or combination testing may be similar to the concepts presented here for the measurement of a single variant value and is discussed in Galen and Gambino's text.[38] This process can be complex regarding the sequential or simultaneous assessment of multiple variate values according to the Bayes theorem, as discussed by Statland et al.[37]

KEY CONCEPTS BOX 24-3

- An effort should be taken to detect outliers that are present in a reference population study, as these may adversely affect accurate estimation of the RI.
- An alternative way of presenting reference intervals is to establish reference limits, or cut-offs, that are based on the ability to differentiate between healthy and diseased populations. These are called clinical decision limits.
- A test's ability to detect diseased individuals is its clinical sensitivity; clinical specificity defines the ability to detect healthy individuals.
- The likelihood that a positive result or a negative result will actually be associated with a sick or healthy individual is based on the prevalence of the disease and is calculated as the test's positive and negative predictive value, respectively.

REFERENCES

1. Clinical Laboratory Standards Institute: *Defining, Establishing, and Verifying Reference Intervals in the Clinical Laboratory, Approved Guideline,* ed 3, Villanova, PA, 2008, CLSI.
2. Solberg HE: Approved recommendation (1986) on the theory of reference values. Part 1. The concept of reference values, Clin Chem Acta 167:111, 1987; J Clin Chem Clin Biochem 25:337, 1987; Ann Biol Clin 45:237, 1987; Labmedica 4:27, 1987.
3. PetitClerc C, Solberg HEL: Approved recommendation (1987) on the theory of reference values. Part 2. Selection of individuals for the production of reference values, J Clin Chem Clin Biochem 25:639, 1987; Clin Chem Acta 170:S1, 1987.
4. Solberg HE, PetitClerc C: Approved recommendation (1988) on the theory of reference values. Part 3. Preparation of individuals and collection of specimens for the production of reference values, Clin Chem Acta 177:S1, 1988.
5. Solberg HE, Stamm D: Approved recommendation on the theory of reference values. Part 4. Control of analytical variation in the production, transfer and application of reference values, Eur J Clin Chem Clin Biochem 29:531, 1991.
6. Solberg HE: Approved recommendations (1987) on the theory of reference values. Part 5. Statistical treatment of collected reference values: determination of reference limits, J Clin Chem Clin Biochem 25:645, 1987; Clin Chem Acta 170:S13, 1987.
7. Dybkaer R, Solberg HE: Approved recommendations (1987) on the theory of reference values. Part 6. Presentation of observed values related to reference values, J Clin Chem Clin Biochem 25:657, 1987; Clin Chem Acta 170:S33, 1987; Labmedica 5:27, 1988.
8. CLSI EP09-A2 (Electronic Document) *Method Comparison and Bias Estimation Using Patient Samples; Approved Guideline,* ed 2, Villanova, PA, 2002, CLSI.
9. Solberg HE: Establishment and use of reference values. In Burtis CA, Ashwood ER, and Bruns DE, editors: Tietz Textbook of Clinical Chemistry and Molecular Diagnostics, ed 4, Philadelphia, 2006, Elsevier/Saunders.
10. Schultz EK, Aliferis C, Aronsky D: Clinical Evaluation of Methods. In Burtis CA, Ashwood ER, and Bruns DE, editors: Tietz Textbook of Clinical Chemistry, ed 4, Philadelphia, 2006, Elsevier/Saunders.
11. Linnet K, Boyd JC: Selection and evaluation of methods-with statistical techniques. In Burtis CA, Ashwood ER, Bruns DE, editors: Tietz Textbook of Clinical Chemistry and Molecular Diagnostics, ed 4, Philadelphia, 2006, Elsevier.
12. Harris EK, Boyd JC: Statistical Basis of Reference Values in Laboratory Medicine. New York, 1995, Marcel Dekker.
13. Westgard JO: Statistical Quality Control for Quantitative Measurement Procedures: Principles and Definitions; Approved Guideline—CLSI document, ed 3, (C24-A3) *2006,* Villanova, PA, 2004.
14. Irjala KM, Gronroos PE: Preanalytical and Analytical factors affecting laboratory results, Ann Med 30:267-272, 1998.
15. Felding P[1]; Rustad P[2]; Mårtensson A[3]; Kairisto V[4]; Franzson L[5]; Petersen H[6]; Uldall A[7]: Reference individuals, blood collection, treatment of samples and descriptive data from the questionnaire in the Nordic Reference Interval Project 2000, Scandinavian Journal of Clinical and Laboratory Investigation, 64(4):327-342(16), 2004.
16. Clinical Laboratory Standards Institute (CLSI): *Procedures for the Collection of Diagnostic Blood Specimens by Venipuncture: Approved Standard,* ed 5, CLSI document H3-A5, Villanova, PA, 2003, CLSI.
17. Clinical Laboratory Standards Institute (CLSI): *Procedures and Devices for the Collection of Diagnostic Capillary Blood Specimens: Approved Standard,* ed 5, CLSI document H4-A5, Villanova, PA, 2004, CLSI.

18. Clinical Laboratory Standards Institute (CLSI): *Percutaneous Collection of Arterial Blood for Laboratory Analysis: Approved Standard,* CLSI document H11-A4, ed 3, Villanova, PA, 2004, CLSI.
19. Clinical Laboratory Standards Institute (CLSI): *Collection, Transport, and Preparation of Blood Specimens for Coagulation Testing and Performance of Coagulation Assays: Approved Guideline,* ed 4, CLSI document H21-A4, Villanova, PA, 2003, CLSI.
20. Clinical Laboratory Standards Institute (CLSI): *Analysis of Body Fluids in Clinical Chemistry: Approved Guideline,* CLSI document C-49-A, Villanova, PA, 2007, CLSI.
21. Clinical Laboratory Standards Institute (CLSI): *Collection, Transportation, and Preservation of Timed Urine Specimens: Approved Guideline,* ed 2, CLSI document GP16-A2, Villanova, PA, 2001, CLSI.
22. Clinical Laboratory Standards Institute (CLSI): *Procedures for the Handling and Processing of Blood Specimens: Approved Guideline,* ed 3, CLSI document H18-A3, Villanova, PA, 2004, CLSI.
23. Reed AH, Henry RJ, Mason WB: Influence of statistical method used on the resulting estimate of normal range, Clin Chem 17:275, 1971.
24. Lott JA, Mitchell LC, Moeschberger ML, et al: Estimation of reference ranges: how many subjects are needed, Clin Chem 38:648, 1992.
25. Linnet K: Two-stage transformation systems for normalization of reference distributions evaluated, Clin Chem 33:381, 1987.
26. Horn PS: A biweight prediction interval for random samples, Journal of the American Statistical Association 83:249, 1988.
27. Horn PS: Robust quantile estimators for skewed populations, Biometrika 77:631, 1990.
28. Horn PS, Pesce AJ: *Reference Intervals: A User's Guide,* Washington, DC, 2005, American Association of Clinical Chemistry Press.
29. Efron B: *The Jackknife, the Bootstrap, and Other Resampling Plans,* Philadelphia, PA, 1982, Society for Industrial and Applied Mathematics.
30. Barnett V, Lewis T: *Outliers in Statistical Data,* New York, 1978, Wiley & Sons.
31. Dixon WJ: Processing data for outliers, Biometrics 9:74, 1953.
32. Harris EK, Boyd JC: On dividing reference data into subgroups to produce separate reference ranges, Clin Chem 36:265, 1990.
33. Harris EK: Personal communication.
34. Cotlove E, Harris EK, Williams GZ: Biological and analytical components of variation in long-term studies of serum constituents in normal subjects, III: physiological and medical implications, Clin Chem 16:1028, 1970.
35. Young DS, Harris EK, Cotlove E: Biological and analytical components of variation in long-term studies of serum constituents in normal subjects, IV: results of a study designed to eliminate long-term analytic deviations, Clin Chem 17:403, 1971.
36. Young DS: Determination and validation of reference intervals, Arch Pathol Lab Med 116:704, 1992.
37. Statland BE, et al: Quantitative approaches used in evaluating laboratory measurements and other clinical data. In Henry JB, editor: *Clinical Diagnosis and Management by Laboratory Methods,* Philadelphia, 1979, Saunders.
38. Galen RS, Gambino SR: *Beyond Normality: The Predictive Value and Efficacy of Medical Diagnoses,* New York, 1975, Wiley & Sons.
39. Zweig MH, Broste SK, Reinhart RA: ROC curve analysis: an example showing the relationships among serum lipid and apolipoprotein concentrations in identifying patients with coronary artery disease, Clin Chem 38:1425, 1992.
40. Zweig MH, Campbell G: Receiver-operating characteristic (ROC) plots: a fundamental evaluation tool in clinical medicine, Clin Chem 39:561, 1993.
41. Gerhardt W: The Bayes approach: systematic graphic evaluation of diagnostic tests. In Keller H, Trendelenburg CH, editors: *Data Presentation, Interpretation,* New York, 1989, Walter de Gruyter.
42. Lott JA, Lu CJ: Lipase isoforms and amylase isoenzymes: assays and application in the diagnosis of acute pancreatitis, Clin Chem 37:361, 1991.
43. Obzansky D: Personal communication, Wilmington, Del.

INTERNET SITES

http://www.analyse-it.com/products/clinical/diagnostic-testing.htm—Trial software that works with Microsoft Excel, Analyse-It Software, Leeds, United Kingdom.

http://www.cche.net/usersguides/decision.asp—Centres for Health Evidence: How to use a clinical decision analysis.

http://www.westgard.com/essay8.htm—Medical decision limits by Westgard.

http://www.pubmedcentral.nih.gov/articlerender.fcgi?artid=1994109—Prerequisites for Use of Common Reference Intervals Ferruccio Ceriotti accessed 11/15/08.

Quality Control for the Clinical Chemistry Laboratory

Kenneth E. Blick and Richard B. Passey*

25

Chapter

Chapter Outline

Key Terms

action limits Ranges set for quality control pools that, if exceeded, signal possible deterioration of the quality of the testing system and require an investigation by a technologist. (*See* out of control.)

autoverification Verification and release of patient results using software-based algorithms with decision-making logic on the laboratory information system.

certified reference material (CRM) "A reference material that has one or more property values certified by a technically valid procedure and is accompanied by, or traceable to, a certificate or another document issued by a certifying body."[1] The material has high purity for the specified compound. Certified reference materials are used in preparing calibrators or specimens of known concentration.

CLIA compliance The term used to describe the laboratory program and plan intended to ensure that all aspects of the Clinical Laboratory Improvement Amendment (CLIA) regulations are followed.

CMS Center for Medicare and Medicaid Services.

control limits Numerical limits (expressed in test units) within which the assay values of control samples must fall for the assay results to be considered valid or in control.

definitive method An analytical method that has been subjected to thorough investigation and evaluation for sources of inaccuracy, including analytical nonspecificity. The magnitude of the definitive method's final imprecision and bias, as expressed in the uncertainty statement, is compatible with the definitive method's stated end purpose. The assay value obtained by a definitive method is taken as the true value.[2]

electronic quality control Type of quality control available on selected point-of-care instruments provided that manufacturer's claims are verified and the system is tested periodically with liquid quality control (QC) materials.

error budget A testing system's total allowable error, which must be determined by each laboratory on the basis of medical or regulatory requirements. The error expenditure comprises all sources of error, including imprecision, bias, interference, and other errors.

external quality control A program in which an external agency provides unknown samples for analysis. (*See*

*Special thanks to Bradley E. Copeland, MD, for his previous authorship of this chapter, much of which is retained.

survey or proficiency testing specimen.) Results are returned to the participant with an evaluation of "acceptable" or "not acceptable" performance. Under the Clinical Laboratory Improvement Amendment (CLIA) '88, this process is called *proficiency testing.*

false rejection Incorrect rejection of an analytical run because quality control results suggest that analytical problems are present.

inherent variability Repeated measurements on the same material vary around an average value. The standard deviation measures the magnitude of this variability.

internal quality control An analysis program that uses quality control samples to verify the acceptability and stability of laboratory results.

Levey-Jennings plot A visual tool for evaluating quality control (QC) data in the context of previous QC results whereby data are plotted relative to the mean ± a specified number of standard deviations (SD) on the vertical (y) axis versus days on the horizontal (x) axis.

method The methodological principles used in the performance of a laboratory test; must include the chemical or physical basis of the test.

monthly average Daily quality control values averaged over a period of 1 month.

monthly standard deviation Standard deviation calculated by using daily quality control values over a period of 1 month.

out of control A circumstance in which a testing system has been shown, by quality control results or other indicators, to be unusable for patient care. This circumstance must be formally declared by the laboratory director or technical supervisor because this decision implies that specified actions need to be taken under the Clinical Laboratory Improvement Amendment (CLIA) '88 regulations (*see* §493.1219, Remedial Actions, and §493.1705, Quality Assurance of Quality Control). Routine responses to quality control results that exceed set limits should be documented; *see* action limits.

patient running mean An approach to real-time quality control that is based on 20 or more patient laboratory results for a particular analyte. Significant shifts and trends noted in patient running means can be an early signal of problems in the analytical testing process.

peer group Term that, when used in proficiency testing programs, indicates a group of laboratories that use the same or similar methods. Commercial quality control suppliers also provide monthly peer group comparisons.

performance specifications Numerical limits established by each laboratory for each analyte and each testing system to delineate acceptable performance. Performance specifications for accreditation and good laboratory practice often include accuracy, precision, analytical sensitivity (minimum reportable amount), analytical specificity (interfering substances), the reportable range of patient test results (or AMR, for analytical measurement range), and the reference intervals or normal values.

power curves Plots of the magnitude of the error detected by a control system versus the probability of detecting an error of that size under various control rules.

primary standard Chemicals of the highest known purity that can be used to produce calibrators for analytical systems.

procedure A set of instructions for using a particular method that, when followed, will produce an analytical test value.

proficiency testing *See* external quality control.

proficiency testing specimen A sample that is prepared by an independent agency and submitted to a laboratory that is participating in an external quality control program.

quality control pool A quantity of stable material (such as serum, plasma, or urine) that is used in an internal quality control program to evaluate the acceptability and stability of a testing system.

reference method "A thoroughly investigated method in which exact and clear descriptions of the necessary conditions and procedures are given for the accurate determination of one or more property values; the documented accuracy and precision of the method are commensurate with the method's use for assessing the accuracy of other methods, for measuring the same property values, or for assigning reference method values to reference materials."[3]

regional quality control A group of laboratories that jointly purchase a large amount of quality control material so that target values and data can be shared.

results verification The final step of the testing process whereby an analyst with both clinical and analytical expertise verifies and releases patient results for clinical use purposes.

run "An interval within which the accuracy and precision of a testing system are expected to be stable but cannot be greater than 24 hours." (CLIA '88 §493.1218[b])

shift An abrupt and sustained change (in one direction) in control values. A shift usually indicates a problem (or change) with the analytical system or the control material.

significant difference A difference that is statistically shown to be outside the expected variability limit; medically, it is a difference that is large enough to influence a medical decision; operationally, it is a statistically significant difference that testing personnel and supervisors believe to be large enough to require investigation.

systemic bias Systemic bias can be constant or proportional. Constant systemic bias denotes a constant difference between the true analyte value and the observed value, regardless of the concentration level. Proportional systemic bias denotes a difference between the true value and the observed value, which changes proportionately as the concentration level changes.

target value The established mean value for an analyte in a quality control pool. Target values for both method and instrument types are often used for peer group comparison purposes.

testing system The combination of the following: an analytical method; a procedure for using the method; reagents, calibrators, and supplies; and an instrument for measurements.

trend A gradual change over time in the test results obtained from control material that is suggestive of a progressive problem with the testing system or control material; also termed *drift.*

true rejection The correct rejection of an analytical run because the control specimens indicate that a problem exists.

usual standard deviation (USD) The average of 3- to 6-month average standard deviation values based on consecutive quality control values. This estimates the usual precision that a laboratory's testing system is capable of achieving.

Westgard Multirule System Warning and rejection rules developed by James Westgard to evaluate quality control data more effectively. These rules are used on many computerized quality control programs found on laboratory information systems (LIS) and laboratory instruments.

SECTION OBJECTIVES BOX 25-1

- List five primary analytical goals of a clinical laboratory's quality control system.
- Explain the calculation and interpretation for total allowable error.
- Explain how medical usefulness criteria influence the total error specifications for a clinical laboratory.

This discussion of quality control, as practiced in clinical laboratories, is designed to provide a practical guide for establishing and maintaining quality in laboratory practice.[1,2,3] We will present quality control as it is handled manually in laboratories with the knowledge that computerized quality control is now commonplace in many clinical laboratories. Breitenberg[4] identified 10 quality ensuring items from the International Organization for Standardization series 9000 standards that are common to all quality control systems: (1) having an effective quality system; (2) ensuring valid and timely measurements; (3) using calibrated measuring and testing equipment; (4) using appropriate statistical techniques; (5) developing a product identification and traceability system; (6) maintaining adequate record-keeping systems; (7) ensuring adequate product handling, storage, packaging, and delivery systems; (8) maintaining an adequate inspection and **testing system;** (9) establishing processes for dealing with nonconforming items; and (10) ensuring adequate personnel training and experience. It should be the goal of quality control procedures to meet all 10 of these standards. Careful examination of the rules delineated by the Clinical Laboratory Improvement Amendment of 1988 (CLIA '88) shows that all these items must be included by law in a laboratory's quality control system.

The primary analytical goals of a clinical laboratory's quality control program should include the following:

1. Establishing and maintaining accurate and precise **methods**
2. Determining the level of precision needed by the laboratory and maintaining that level of reproducibility
3. Ensuring that analytical systems are stable and are operating according to established **performance specifications.** This increases the reliability of both short- and long-term medical decisions.
4. Ensuring that all regulatory requirements relative to **CLIA compliance** are followed
5. Providing objective analytical benchmarks for methods and instruments so that continuous improvement of existing methods is achievable

To achieve these analytical goals, a laboratory must (1) meet the 10 quality-assuring goals; (2) institute policies that govern patient preparation; (3) reduce preanalytical errors (see Chapter 18); and (4) maximize the effective use of the laboratory's resources, personnel, equipment, supplies, and physical facilities. Accordingly, a laboratory's quality control program must be designed to evaluate and document how well these analytical goals are being met.

GOALS FOR A QUALITY CONTROL PROGRAM

Setting Goals

The first step in establishing a laboratory quality control program is to develop criteria for acceptable laboratory performance. How accurate and precise *should* the laboratory be? How precise and accurate *must* it be? These considerations include the determination of what constitutes acceptable analytical error based on the use of the test result in clinical care.[5,6] Control beyond that required for medical purposes can waste time and materials, hence it is important to evaluate whether error reduction improves medical diagnosis, treatment, or prognosis.

Several bases exist upon which performance criteria can be formulated. The first is the body of regulatory standards, for example, the precision and accuracy demanded by CLIA '88 regulations. Second is the precision and accuracy that appear to be attainable by most laboratories. This information can be obtained through communications with other laboratory professionals or from data derived from proficiency surveys, such as that of the College of American Pathology (CAP). Third and probably most important, it is essential to determine the precision and accuracy required by the clinical staff, the users of data produced by the laboratory. In general, a testing system's analytical error should be much smaller than the allowable error in the regulatory requirements. Otherwise, the laboratory may not meet its regulatory and perhaps medical requirements. The following section will review the medical criteria used to establish and evaluate performance.

Total Allowable Error

The total allowable error of a testing system is composed of individual components. In general, each component of a testing system can be a source of imprecision or bias. If the total error can be likened to an **error budget,** the individual components of the total allowable error make up the total error expenditure of that budget. When the error budget is exceeded, more error than can be tolerated exists in the testing system. The more completely one can identify the components of error, the better one can adjust the testing system to reduce these errors. Medical and CLIA '88 requirements are not based on whether the error is introduced by imprecision or bias; rather it is the combination that determines the effect of the total error. Therefore, the laboratory staff must know what roles imprecision and **systemic bias** play in the error expenditure because the resolution processes for these errors are often different. The systemic bias between testing systems can be constant or proportional, depending on whether the error is constant with changes in analyte concentration or varies proportionately with changes in concentration (see Chapter 26).

Total error[7] is estimated from imprecision and bias as follows:

$$\text{Total error} = \text{Sum of bias errors} + 1.96 \times \text{SD (standard deviation)} \quad \text{Eq. 25-1}$$

Notice that 1.96 is the 95% confidence limit (often rounded to 2.0 for convenience) for a normally distributed set of results (see Chapter 23).

Example

If your medical requirements for glucose require that the total error be less than 6 mg/dL at a concentration of 120 mg/dL, and you know that your imprecision is ±2 mg/dL, the maximum bias that your method can have is calculated as follows:

$$6\ \text{mg/dL} = x\ \text{mg/dL} + 1.96 \times 2\ \text{mg/dL}$$

$$\text{Maximum bias} = x = 6 - (1.96 \times 2) = 2.08\ \text{mg/dL}$$

If the bias of the assay is too large, it can often be reduced by more accurate calibration **procedures** and materials. Imprecision is often increased by poor mechanical and electronic components in the analyzer or measurement device. Thus the state of instrument calibration and maintenance can affect both bias and imprecision. An accuracy-based quality control system can provide information on both accuracy and precision.

Table 25-1 contains analytical data from the Oklahoma University Medical Center showing the total error for each listed test. The total errors are large because they include error contributions from all the instruments used to report the test values. Accurate error budgeting must include the bias introduced by the use of multiple testing systems. The problem of bias between different testing systems is one that can affect the medical use of test results because a test is often performed by more than one testing system. Currently, CLIA '88 requires that laboratories periodically document the correlation of results when two or more testing systems are in use. The real-time use of **patient running mean** data to ensure that multiple platforms performing the same test are harmonized and thus are essentially free of significant bias appears to have promise.

Table 25-1 Performance Specifications for Total Error (%)*

Test	Analytical†	Medical‡	CLIA '88§
Albumin	13 to 15	—	10
Alkaline phosphatase	10 to 15	—	30
Aspartate aminotransferase (AST)	5 to 20	14 to 26	20
Bilirubin, total	12 to 16	5 to 28	20% or 4 mg/L
Blood urea nitrogen (BUN)	18 to 33	12 to 25	9% or 20 mg/L
Calcium	5.5 to 6.4	5 to 7	10 mg/L
Chloride	5	—	5
Cholesterol	11 to 14	9¶	10
Cholesterol, high-density lipoprotein	5	—	30
Creatine kinase (CK)	8 to 10	—	30
Creatinine	15 to 47	—	30
Glucose	5 to 11	11 to 16	10% or 60 mg/L
Iron	—	17	20
Lactate dehydrogenase (LD)	7 to 8	—	20
Phosphorus	4 to 10	14 to 17	NA
Potassium	10 to 12	5 to 10	0.5 mmol/L
Protein, total	7 to 8	8	10
Sodium	5 to 6	2 to 3	4 mmol/L
Triglycerides	10 to 16	16	25

CLIA, Clinical Laboratory Improvement Amendment; *NA,* not applicable.
*Total analytical error calculated by: T.E. = Bias + 1.96 × standard deviation.
†Data from Oklahoma Medical Center, University of Oklahoma. Testing systems include Beckman CX3 and Kodak 700XRC; bias differences between these two systems are important sources of the high total error. The difference between these systems accounts for part of the error in a patient's results when different systems are used interchangeably.
‡Rounded to the nearest whole percentage. (From Skendzel LP, Barnett RN, Platt R: Am J Clin Pathol 83:200, 1985.)
§Tests and acceptable performance are from the *Federal Register,* February 28, 1990, p. 7158.
¶Cholesterol medical goals are now set at 3% bias and 3% imprecision. (From NCEP: NIH Pub. No. 90-2964, 1990.)

Performance Required for Proficiency Testing

The federal government has set allowable error criteria for 154 tests in 13 laboratory disciplines plus cytology (**proficiency testing** rules of CLIA '88 *Federal Register,* February 28, 1990, pp. 7152-7162). The CLIA criteria for common chemistry tests are listed in Table 25-2. These allowable error criteria define

Table 25-2 CLIA Required Performance on Proficiency Testing (*Federal Register*, February 28, 1992)

Analyte or Test	Criteria for Acceptable Performance
Immunology Tests	
α_1-Antitrypsin	Target value ± 3 SD
α-Fetoprotein (tumor marker)	Target value ± 3 SD
Antinuclear antibody	Target value ± 2 dilutions or positive or negative
Antistreptolysin O	Target value ± 2 dilutions or positive or negative
Anti–human immunodeficiency virus	Reactive or nonreactive
Complement C3	Target value ± 3 SD
Complement C4	Target value ± 3 SD
Hepatitis (HBsAg, anti-HBc, HBeAg)	Reactive (positive) or nonreactive (negative)
IgA	Target value ± 3 SD
IgE	Target value ± 3 SD
IgG	Target value ± 25%
IgM	Target value ± 3 SD
Infectious mononucleosis	Target value ± 2 dilutions or positive or negative
Rheumatoid factor	Target value ± 2 dilutions or positive or negative
Rubella	Target value ± 2 dilutions or immune or nonimmune or positive or negative
Chemistry Tests	
Alanine aminotransferase (ALT/SGPT)	Target value ± 20%
Albumin	Target value ± 10%
Alkaline phosphatase	Target value ± 30%
Amylase	Target value ± 30%
Aspartate aminotransferase (AST/SGOT)	Target value ± 20%
Bilirubin, total	Target value ± 4 mg/L or ± 20% (greater)
Blood-gas Po_2	Target value ± 3 SD
Pco_2	Target value ± 5 mm Hg or ± 8% (greater)
pH	Target value ± 0.04
Calcium, total	Target value ± 10 mg/L
Chloride	Target value ± 5%
Cholesterol, high-density lipoprotein	Target value ± 30%
Cholesterol, total	Target value ± 10%
Creatine kinase	Target value ± 30%
Creatine kinase isoenzymes	MB elevated (presence or absence) or target value ± 3 SD
Creatinine	Target value ± 3 mg/L or ± 15% (greater)
Glucose (excluding glucose performed on monitoring devices cleared by FDA for home use)	Target value ± 60 mg/L or ± 10% (greater)
Iron, total	Target value ± 20%
Lactate dehydrogenase (LD)	Target value ± 20%
LD isoenzymes	LD_1/LD_2 (±), or target value ± 30%
Magnesium	Target value ± 25%
Potassium	Target value ± 0.5 mmol/L
Sodium	Target value ± 4 mmol/L
Total protein	Target value ± 10%
Triglycerides	Target value ± 25%
Urea nitrogen	Target value ± 20 mg/L or ± 9% (greater)
Uric acid	Target value ± 17%
Endocrinology	
Cortisol	Target value ± 25%
Free thyroxine	Target value ± 3 SD
Human chorionic gonadotropin	Target value ± 3 SD positive or negative
Thyroid-stimulating hormone	Target value ± 3 SD
Thyroxine	Target value ± 20% or 10 mg/L (greater)
Triiodothyronine	Target value ± 3 SD
Triiodothyronine uptake	Target value ± 3 SD
Toxicology	
Alcohol, blood	Target value ± 25%
Blood lead	Target value ± 10% or 40 mg/L (greater)

Table 25-2 CLIA Required Performance on Proficiency Testing (*Federal Register,* February 28, 1992)—cont'd

Analyte or Test	Criteria for Acceptable Performance
Carbamazepine	Target value ± 25%
Digoxin	Target value ± 20% or ± 0.2 ng/mL (greater)
Ethosuximide	Target value ± 20%
Gentamicin	Target value ± 25%
Lithium	Target value ± 0.3 mmol/L or ± 20% (greater)
Phenobarbital	Target value ± 20%
Phenytoin	Target value ± 25%
Primidone	Target value ± 25%
Procainamide (and metabolite)	Target value ± 25%
Quinidine	Target value ± 25%
Theophylline	Target value ± 25%
Tobramycin	Target value ± 25%
Valproic acid	Target value ± 25%
Hematology	
Cell identification	90% or greater consensus on identification
White blood cell differential	Target ± 3 SD based on the percentage of different types of white blood cells in the samples
Erythrocyte count	Target ± 6%
Fibrinogen	Target ± 20%
Hematocrit (excluding spun hematocrits)	Target ± 6%
Hemoglobin	Target ± 7%
Leukocyte count	Target ± 15%
Partial thromboplastin time	Target ± 15%
Platelet count	Target ± 25%
Prothrombin time	Target ± 15%

FDA, U.S. Food and Drug Administration; *HBc,* hepatitis B core antigen; *HBeAg,* hepatitis e antigen; *HBsAg,* hepatitis B surface antigen; *IgA,* immunoglobulin A; *IgE,* immunoglobulin E; *IgG,* immunoglobulin G; *IgM,* immunoglobulin M; *SD,* standard deviation; *SGOT,* serum glutamic oxaloacetic transaminase; *SGPT,* serum glutamic pyruvic transaminase.

the total amount of error a proficiency testing value can have. The **target value** used to determine bias is defined by the proficiency testing service with use of the overall mean, a **peer group** mean, or the value established by a definitive or **reference method.** It is noteworthy that CLIA '88 error windows (budgets) are too large for routine quality **control limits** because imprecision errors this large cause frequent proficiency testing failure.[8]

Compare the total errors listed in Table 25-1 versus the suggested allowable medical errors and the maximum error windows specified by CLIA '88. Note that several tests in Table 25-2 show potential problems with proficiency testing because of unacceptably high total errors when the analysis is performed by more than one testing system. This would be the case if proficiency testing truly mimicked laboratory practice. However, as currently practiced, proficiency testing usually compares testing systems only with instrument peer grouping.

Medical Decision Limits

For true control of quality, it is necessary to evaluate, from the customer's perspective, the performance required for each aspect of the clinical laboratory's operation.[8-11] The elements of a good quality control program include establishment of analytical accuracy and precision with performance criteria based on medical usefulness requirements.[7,12-17]

In Table 25-1, the total analytical error for several analytical instruments is compared with the allowable error suggested by medical requirements and with the CLIA '88 mandated allowable error. An example of medically defined criteria for precision and accuracy are the guidelines formulated by the National Institutes of Health (NIH) for cholesterol analysis.[18,19] To minimize errors in diagnosing hyperlipidemias, the NIH established a target of 3% for the limits of imprecision and 3% for an acceptable degree of bias (inaccuracy). Documents from professional organizations can provide estimates based on review of accepted practice (e.g., National Academy of Clinical Biochemistry, www.nacb.org). Each laboratory should consult the appropriate users or clinicians to obtain their estimate of allowable error based on their particular medical practice.[20-23] If their suggestions are reasonable and would not place the laboratory in conflict with regulatory requirements, the laboratory should try to attain these limits of error. If no information is available about the precision and accuracy targets needed for medical decision making, one can estimate a theoretical error based on the degree of intraindividual and interindividual variation noted for each analyte.[24,25] Chapter 26 (p. 483) lists equations that relate total analytical imprecision with these biological variabilities. Table 26-2 lists examples of the intrapersonal variability of certain analytes.

Once the allowable total error based on medical requirements has been decided, the methods and testing systems chosen must be capable of producing values that consistently meet those requirements. In addition, the quality control program must be designed to ensure that the testing system maintains these limits over time.

Reference intervals for laboratory tests describe the expected values for carefully selected groups of individuals, determined by testing systems that are assumed to be performing appropriately (see Chapter 24). Increased bias will cause a **shift** in test values and thus will invalidate the medical usefulness of the established reference intervals and may in fact lead to inappropriate patient care.

Meeting Medical Usefulness Criteria by Calculating the Significant Change Limit

The day-to-day medical usefulness of clinical laboratory tests depends on maintaining the accuracy and precision of the testing system. Physicians make many clinical decisions on the basis of day-to-day differences in patient test values, assuming that day-to-day accuracy and precision are maintained at the same level from month to month and from year to year. Thus the actual accuracy and precision of the measurement procedure directly influence the medical interpretation of these day-to-day changes in test values. One key element in interpreting the medical usefulness of a test result is an estimate of the magnitude of an analytically significant change in concentration. This estimate is called the *significant change limit (SCL)*.

The significant change limit is a decision-making tool that helps physicians distinguish day-to-day changes in results that are caused by the **inherent variability** of the analytical procedure from changes that are caused by modifications in the patient's physiology and pathology. The significant change limit is based on the assumption that the **usual standard deviation (USD)** represents day-to-day method variability. The theoretical standard deviation of the difference (SD_{diff}) between two separate analyses of the same material on different days is related to the USD of the procedure by the following formula:

$$SD_{diff} = \sqrt{2(USD)^2} = 1.4\ USD \qquad \text{Eq. 25-2}$$

The SCL then represents the 95% confidence limits (or $\pm 2\ SD_{diff}$) that define the extent of the inherent method variability:

$$\begin{aligned} SCL &= \text{Mean value} \pm 2\ SD_{diff} \\ &= \text{Mean value} \pm 2.8\ USD \end{aligned} \qquad \text{Eq. 25-3}$$

As an approximation, the significant change limit is three times the USD (Table 25-3). Changes greater than the significant change limit are likely to represent a real change in the patient. For example, if the usual standard deviation for cholesterol is 5 mg/dL, the significant change limit is 2.8 times 5, or 14 mg/dL. A change from 200 to 220 mg/dL would exceed the significant change limit and would represent a real change in the patient. A change from 200 to 190 mg/dL would not exceed the SCL and could be the result of the method's imprecision. Clearly, in order to facilitate consistent decision making by the attending physician, it is important to maintain a consistent level of precision from month to month and from year to year.

KEY CONCEPTS BOX 25-1

- Quality control is designed to ensure reproducible accurate results. Documentation is an essential component.
- Acceptable laboratory performance is determined after goals are set. Some goals are set by CLIA.
- Medical decision limits define the amount of change the physician will accept before intervening in patient care.

SECTION OBJECTIVES BOX 25-2

- Differentiate with examples the activities associated with, and personnel responsible for, each of the three levels of the quality control process.
- State CLIA '88-mandated quality control requirements for analytical runs of routine analyses and special requirements for blood gas analyses.
- Outline a seven-step method to establish temporary quality control target values.
- Discuss potential problems associated with using target ranges based on ±2 standard deviations, based on ±2.5 or 3 standard deviations, and based on medical usefulness criteria.
- Discuss the following aspects of the Westgard rules: definition of each rule, what type of error each rule is designed to detect, and advantages for this system.

CONTROL OF QUALITY (PROCESS CONTROL) AND ERROR DETECTION

Once a laboratory's performance criteria have been established, a process control system must be put into place. The purpose of this system is to allow continuous monitoring of the testing process (including preanalytical and postanalytical testing) to ensure that the performance goals are met, or that steps are taken to achieve these goals. It is important to recognize the key role of laboratory personnel in the quality process.

Levels of Activity in the Control Process

The control process that we call quality control (QC) is designed to detect error in the measurement system. This process consists of three levels, each of which is the responsibility of a different individual. For the control process to be most effective, active communication among the individuals within each level of responsibility is crucial.

The first level of the process involves the responsibility of the bench medical technologist and the supervisors. At this

Table 25-3 Calculation of Quality Control Parameters

Test/method: Potassium by ion-selective electrode
Analyst: RBP
Start/finish date: 3/15/02-3/26/02
Control source and level: Superior control–elevated
Manufacturer's target value: 6.02 mEq/L
How determined: By National Reference System for the Clinical Laboratory (NRSCL) definitive method
Manufacturer's typical standard deviation for users: 0.15 mEq/L

	VIAL 1		*VIAL 2*	
Day	**Sample A**	**Sample B**	**Sample A**	**Sample B**
1	6.1	6.1	6.2	5.9
2	6.2	6.2	6.0	6.0
3	5.7	5.8	6.0	6.0
4	5.9	5.8	5.9	5.8
5	6.0	6.0	6.0	6.0
6	5.9	6.0	6.0	6.0
7	5.9	6.0	6.0	6.0
8	5.9	5.8	6.0	5.9
9	6.0	6.1	6.1	6.2
10	6.0	6.1	6.1	6.1

Grand total (sum of all observations) = 239.7; n = 40 observations.
Average initial target value = 239.7/40 = 5.99 mEq/L.
Temporary standard deviation = 0.12 mEq/L.

Calculation of average final target and usual standard deviation (USD) values

Data	Average Target Value (mEq/L)	Standard Deviation
Initial Target Value	5.990	0.12 mEq/L
1 April	6.070	0.13 mEq/L
2 May	6.020	0.11 mEq/L
3 June	6.010	0.13 mEq/L

Average final target = 6.02 (average of 5.99, 6.07, 6.02, and 6.01)
Usual standard deviation (USD) = 0.12 mEq/L (average of 0.12, 0.13, 0.11, and 0.13)
Medically allowable error = 0.3 mEq/L (set by the medical staff, Jan. 14, 2002)
Number of USDs in the medically allowable error = 0.3/0.12 = 2.5
Significant change value = 2.8 × USD = 2.8 × 0.12 = 0.34 mEq/L
Chosen control range is the average final target value ± 2.5 USD, or 6.02 ± 2.5(0.12) = 6.02 ± 0.3 mEq/L, or 5.72 to 6.32 mEq/L.
If the chosen control range is the average final target value ± 3 USD, range = 6.02 ± 3(0.12) = 6.02 ± 0.36, or 5.66 to 6.38 mEq/L (larger than the medical requirements).
Also be careful when less than 2.5 SD is contained in the medically allowable error because the imprecision may be too large to show medically required changes in test results.

level, the control process includes the daily analysis of QC specimens (discussed in this section) and the review and verification of patient results (**results verification**) and reports. The technologist is responsible for performing QC analyses at appropriate intervals and for determining that, during any given **run,** there is no significant systematic error. Technologists and the supervisor are responsible for reviewing patient data to ensure that no excessive random error exists.

The second level of control ensures that minimal systematic bias enters into the system over a relatively short period of weeks to months. The responsibility for this level of error control usually is shared by supervisors and the laboratory director, although technologists often contribute greatly. The control process at this level requires timely review of QC data and proficiency testing results that have accumulated during that review period.

The third level of the control process ensures that the analytical systems are as precise and accurate as possible. This is the responsibility of the laboratory director or technical consultant. The control process at this level requires review of proficiency testing results, knowledge of the levels of precision and accuracy achievable by other laboratories, and, when applicable, the use of accuracy-based standards to verify or correct errors. This level of quality control review occurs over a longer period of time, from months to years. Discussion of proficiency testing is provided in a later section.

Quality control of the *entire* testing system (i.e., from the physician order to phlebotomy to generating a patient report) requires additional process control measures. Many of these measures include regulatory-mandated monitors of individual steps in the testing process, which are reviewed in Chapter 18. One important factor that is rarely formally recognized includes the complaints of physicians about perceived problems. Physicians' complaints very often are based on real deficiencies in one part of the testing system. These errors may not be known to the laboratory until they are revealed by the laboratory staff's investigation of a complaint. Monitoring physicians' complaints and their resolution is thus important in helping to control the overall quality of the testing system. Accreditation standards such as ISO9001:1987, ISO9001:1994, and ISO9001:2000 also have been implemented by some clinical laboratories for error and incident detection in the testing process. It is noteworthy that a new version of ISO9001 was published on November 15, 2000.

Testing Quality Control Specimens—Daily Decision Making

The daily preparation and analysis of quality control samples is a regular responsibility of the analyst. The **quality control pools** are analyzed as "known" controls during analysis of patient samples. The values are considered "known" because some attempt has been made to determine the actual level of each constituent using the procedures employed for routine analysis. The laboratory can estimate the target values of the control samples by repeated analysis (the "true value" being estimated as the mean), can use the manufacturer's estimates of the values, or, ideally, can determine the values by definitive or reference methods (see p. 474). The frequency of analysis of the QC material is established by each laboratory for each method. CLIA '88 requires the analysis of at least two controls of different values for each run (defined as up to 24 hours of stable operation for most analytes), as do other accrediting bodies with deemed status from CLIA.

Most laboratories use two different pools—one normal and one abnormal. A normal pool contains constituents at concentrations within the nondiseased reference interval, whereas an abnormal pool contains analytes at concentrations outside the reference interval. Some laboratories may employ three pools—low abnormal, normal, and high abnormal—especially when medically significant decisions are made at each level. CLIA allows each laboratory to set its own protocols for chemistry testing of assay control samples as long as at least two control samples of different concentrations are assayed every 24 hours. Some states mandate three pools for certain tests. CLIA mandates special rules for blood gases, requiring as a minimum the analysis of one QC sample every 8 hours of testing and the use of a combination of QC samples and calibrators that includes samples with both high and low concentrations each day of testing. CLIA also requires the use of one calibrator or control each time a patient sample is analyzed, unless the blood-gas instrument is calibrated at least every 30 minutes (§493.1243). Because of this complexity of blood-gas quality control, some manufacturers have included QC reagents as part of the reagents resident on blood-gas analyzers and thus have assumed a more active role in the QC process. More commonly, however, the manufacturer of a testing system recommends the testing frequency that should be used as a basis for a laboratory's QC policy.

Testing personnel must use the data from each QC analysis to make a decision about the validity of patients' test data generated during a run. Generally, if the results for a QC sample are within the accepted target range, technologists may assume that the patients' results obtained during the same run are equally valid and the run can be "accepted." On the other hand, if results for the QC pool are unacceptable, the run is not acceptable (see pp. 467 and 468). The decision to accept or reject an analytical run must be documented and should include the decision (either *accept* or *reject*), the analyst's name (or code number), and the date on a worksheet, in a separate log book, on a data sheet, or in the laboratory information system (LIS) (see Chapter 22). Usually, the process of verification of patient data in the LIS by technologists is regarded as implied acceptance of the associated QC data included in the run. Although the term *run* implies a batch process, current laboratory practice usually has the measurements continuously performed in real time on automated analyzers, that is, the run is more generally associated with the 8-hour work shift.

Although daily bench-level quality control testing is most useful for detecting systematic errors, it can also be used to detect consistent increases in imprecision. However, random errors, which occur unpredictably, are not usually detectable by a quality control system. Random errors can be detected by review of reported problems and patients' results (see pp. 468-470).

Quality Control Mechanics

How to Choose a Quality Control Pool

Quality control material should have a matrix that closely matches that of the specimens in the analytical run. This means that if the run includes cerebrospinal fluid, serum, and urine, then controls composed of cerebrospinal fluid (CSF), serum, and urine must also be included in the analytical run.

Because the quality control material is analyzed in every run along with patients' specimens, large amounts of control material are needed each year. Several sources currently exist from which a laboratory can obtain sufficient quantities of quality control material: (1) commercial lyophilized pool material; (2) commercial stabilized liquid pools; and (3) frozen, pooled patient specimens (serum or plasma). Frozen liquid or pools that have been clarified (with materials that reduce turbidity) generally show smaller standard deviations than do lyophilized pools.[26] The smaller imprecision errors of the liquid pools derive, in part, from the absence of errors involved with the lyophilization and reconstitution processes. However, the liquid pools may experience greater instability errors associated with shipping batches of a lot to the customer. Some characteristics of three sources of quality control material are listed in Table 25-4. It is important to select a pool with a matrix that interacts least with the methods employed in the laboratory. Certain characteristics of a control

Table 25-4 Comparison of Quality Control Materials

Criteria	Frozen	Lyophilized	Low-Temperature Liquid
Cost	Low, if not manipulated* Medium, if manipulated	High	Highest
Clarity	Clear, if carefully collected	Turbid	Clear
Stability	12 months	18 to 24 months	18 to 24 months
Validation	Compare with accurately measured materials (NIST and CAP)	Regional and manufacturer's peer group analysis available, or by NIST and CAP	Regional and manufacturer's peer group analysis available
Lyophilization error	Absent	Present	Absent

CAP, College of American Pathologists; *NIST,* National Institute of Standards and Technology.
*That is, if additional analyte is added.

pool, including turbidity or chemical constituents, can render it unusable.

Notice that control pools prepared in the laboratory from pooled patient samples (serum, plasma, urine, and CSF) can be contaminated with viruses; thus it is essential to test each specimen or group of specimens and the final pool for harmful viruses. Therefore, the following statements apply to all specimen pools used for quality control. First, all pooled human material should be monitored for the human immunodeficiency virus (HIV) and the hepatitis B virus. No pools should be used if evidence of either virus is found. Second, all control material requires refrigerator or freezer space for storage of a 1- to 2-year supply. Alternatively, commercial distributors may supply quantities from a single lot number of stored material on a monthly or quarterly basis so that the laboratory can use the same lot number over 1 to 2 years. This helps bring long-term stability to the quality control process, although the possibility of shipment-to-shipment variations within the lot must be considered.

Some professional groups and manufacturers offer participation in **regional quality control** programs in which laboratories use the same batch of pooled serum. This offers both scientific advantages and cost benefits. The comparison between laboratories can help predict how similar testing systems (peer groups) will perform in proficiency testing. This comparison becomes more valuable when the accuracy of the quality control pool is established by reference or by **definitive methods** (see p. 474).[1-3,27-29]

Preliminary Considerations for Estimating Limits for Quality Control Pools

Unless the true value of a pool is established by definitive or reference methods, the target values are only averages of repeated measurements of the pool. The average temporary or average final target values of the quality control pool are the estimated concentrations of each analyte within the pool. Each laboratory usually establishes its own average target values for the analytes by performing the laboratory's test procedures on each pool. CLIA '88 allows the pool's manufacturer to establish target values, with the laboratory confirming that each target value is applicable to its testing system.

Laboratories must resolve a dilemma regarding target limits that result from CLIA's rules. On one hand, the need exists to optimize a testing system's calibration according to the manufacturer's instructions, but on the other hand is the need to meet proficiency testing requirements. The Centers for Medicare and Medicaid Services (**CMS**) allows each proficiency testing provider to determine how the program will establish the target values that will be used to judge acceptable performance. If the target value is calculated from peer group means for each testing system, it is better to establish the laboratory's QC system target values by using the manufacturer's recommendations for both calibration and QC. However, if the target values for proficiency testing are set by the mean of all participants or by the true target values established by definitive methods, optimizing assays to the manufacturer's specifications may result in problems with the proficiency testing results if a bias is present as a result of those specifications.

Part of the problem with establishing a quality control program using manufacturers' recommendations is the effect of lyophilization (which causes matrix changes) on various constituents, resulting in method-specific interference or bias (e.g., as a result of the turbidity of these specimens). The dilemma, then, arises from the fact that if a laboratory adheres to the requirement of CLIA '88 and follows the manufacturer's instructions, failure in proficiency testing may result. However, a laboratory can, by the rules of CLIA '88, modify the manufacturer's instructions if the laboratory has data validating a method based on these changes.

When new target values are established for a new lot of quality control material, it is important to ensure that, during the data collection period, the analytical systems perform according to normal performance specifications. The new lot of quality control material should be tested in parallel with the current lot of quality control material. If analytical data from the current quality control material indicate satisfactory performance of the methods, the data for the new lot can be assumed to be valid. When a quality control system is being set up for the first time, the current methodology is accepted as valid if the method meets performance specifications. As was mentioned earlier, the choice of the laboratory's testing method (or testing system) is based on experience with medical usefulness, significant change limits, **external quality control** and accuracy comparisons, and quality control performance.

Three approaches can be used to establish the limits of acceptable values for a control pool. One method is to use the medically allowable error for choosing the range. Another, more usual approach is to estimate the target value and usual standard deviation (SD) for the method and use some number of SDs to establish the range. The third technique is to employ the more statistically accurate method of **power curves.** These approaches are described in the following pages.

A Simple Method for Establishing Average Temporary Target Values for Quality Control Pools

1. Procure a minimum of a 1-year supply of quality control test material.
2. If possible, plan a 6-week lead time before changing control pools to allow for (a) comparative analyses of old and new lots of control materials (3 weeks); (b) data reduction and calculation and evaluation of control limits (1 week); and (c) a buffer of 2 additional weeks because not all planning is perfect. It is also advisable to retain 20 or 30 vials of each expiring pool for use in evaluating problems that may result from system changes. Clearly identify the expiring pool to ensure that it is not used beyond its expiration date and that it is not mistaken for the current lot of control materials. CLIA prohibits a laboratory from using out-of-date reagents, solutions, controls, calibrators, or culture media (§493.1205[e][1]). Any exception must be specifically granted by the U.S. Food and Drug Administration (FDA).
3. Always reconstitute the lyophilized material carefully, while following the label's directions. Mixing too quickly or too vigorously may interfere with the solubilization of the lyophilized material or may denature its protein constituents. Denatured enzymes have reduced activity. The date, time, and technologist's initials should be recorded on each vial of control material after reconstitution. If a frozen liquid pool is used, after thawing, mix the sample six times by inversion because the protein and other compounds become concentrated at the bottom of the vial during freezing.
4. Test duplicate samples from two separate vials (20 vials, 40 measurements) each day for 10 days. An alternative procedure is to reconstitute one vial per day and perform the tests in duplicate on each of 20 consecutive days (20 vials, 40 measurements). See Table 25-3 for an example of these calculations.
5. Determine temporary target values for each constituent by calculating the mean of these 40 analytical values ($n = 40$). This temporary target value is replaced after 2 months with a final average target value (see #7).
6. Calculate the standard deviation of the 40 values. Note that this calculated standard deviation is a hybrid between within-run and total imprecision because the tests are done both in single runs and over several days. Set the range of allowable control values around the average temporary target by using the newly calculated standard deviation multiplied by the laboratory's control limit, expressed as the number of standard deviations (such as 2.5 or 3.0). The number of standard deviations for the control range can also be set according to the size of the USD and the test's allowable error (see the following text and Table 25-3). If the allowable error for glucose at 120 mg/dL is ±6 mg/dL, the control range should fit within these boundaries. In other words, the testing system's full control range (such as ±3 SD) should fit within the allowable ±6 mg/L. For this example, a single standard deviation can be as large as 2 mg/L. Alternatively, if the usual standard deviation is 1.5 mg/dL, then ±4 standard deviations can fit within the allowable window. For the next 3 months, use the temporary average target and range of allowable control values for routine quality control in the laboratory.
7. After the third month, use 4 values to calculate the average final target value: the temporary target value and 3 **monthly averages** (see Table 25-3). If the control material is slightly unstable over time (e.g., alkaline phosphatase activity often changes over time), the process used to change the target value must include evidence that the test value of the control material changed while the testing system remained constant. Such evidence can be provided by the use of additional stable materials with known values (such as a different control, excess proficiency testing material, or additional calibrator materials). The decision process for changing the target value must be well documented. It is best to avoid unstable control material.

Calculation of the Usual Standard Deviation

Every method has a characteristic inherent variability termed the *usual standard deviation.* The USD is calculated from a series of three to six consecutive **monthly standard deviations** that are obtained during a time when the testing instrument is assumed to be stable. The USD is a valid estimate of the usual day-to-day variability of individual measurements. The USD can be used eventually instead of the temporary SD to establish the daily control limits around the average final target value. Table 25-3 shows how the USD can be used to calculate the allowable number of standard deviations for control values that will still maintain the medical usefulness of the testing system. The medically allowable error is divided by the USD to calculate the number of USDs in the medically allowable error. This calculation assumes no significant bias. If significant bias is present, first subtract the bias from the total medically allowable error, and then divide the result by the USD. This calculated number of standard deviations should be equal to or greater than the number of standard deviations used for the laboratory's control range. Otherwise, the test will be persistently out of control, or its medical usefulness will be compromised.

The USD can also be used to establish the statistical significance of the difference between two values from the same patient. The latter is often referred to as the significant change limit (see p. 462).

Setting the Action Control Limits for Each Level of the Control Pool

The limits of acceptable results are used to determine the **action limits** of the control range. Historically, a QC result that exceeded the set limits was known as an out-of-control value. However, CLIA regulations now specifically define the term ***out of control*** as a situation in which a testing system cannot be used for reporting patients' results. Thus the term *exceeding action limits* is now used to designate the less serious condition in which the result of a routine QC analysis exceeds the set limits. The documented response of a medical technologist to a QC result that exceeds action limits (see following text) does not include shutting the procedure down. This occurs only when the laboratory director formally declares that a testing system is out of control, and the laboratory begins a formal remedial process to correct this more serious situation (see following text). A laboratory will be best served by designating in their laboratory manual the conditions that will define these two situations.

Historically, the action limits were ±2 standard deviations around the target value and covered 95% of expected control values. However, this means that 5% of results for control pools are expected to exceed action limits even when the method is working perfectly. A **false rejection** of a run results in excessive rerunning of samples and necessitates performing the documentation required under CLIA regulations. Therefore, limits other than ±2 SDs have been suggested for establishing control limits. Currently, many laboratories use 2.5 or 3 standard deviations for the acceptable limits in an attempt to reduce false-run rejection time and unnecessary retesting.

However, the use of 2.5 or 3 standard deviations to set error limits may not result in error detection that is sufficient for medical and CLIA requirements.[8,10,15] Thus a second approach is to establish daily quality control ranges that are based on the considerations discussed earlier. The target range must be equal to or less than the total allowable error (see p. 459), which, in turn, is equal to or less than the allowable medical and legal (CLIA) error. The target control limits will therefore be some multiples of the USD or temporary SD that will fulfill these requirements. The number of multiples chosen will be based on the need to detect true cases of inaccurate measurement while minimizing false rejections of acceptable runs (see following text).

Another approach is to set the allowable range only on the basis of medical usefulness criteria. The range is expressed as plus or minus the medically allowable error window around the target value. This process does not require that the laboratory use ±2 or more standard deviations. The control window is as wide as medical use will allow. An "action limit" situation is demonstrated when the test value of the control material exceeds the error limits. One should determine that this approach will not place the laboratory at risk for failure of proficiency testing. For all these approaches, the final control range must not be so large that the testing system will fail to detect true instances of failure of the method.

Setting Quality Control Limits by Power Curves

Among the main questions in quality control are the following: "How much quality control testing is enough?" "Am I sure that I am detecting appropriately small errors?" and "Is my error detection sensitive enough to show whether the testing system is appropriate for the medical needs?" If a laboratory has adequately set allowable errors for medical needs, the second question is of academic interest only because detection of the smallest errors is costly and time-consuming.

A more scientific approach to answering these questions uses power curves to determine how many controls should be run, how frequently controls should be run, and what control rules should be used. Power curves are plots of the size of the error detected by a control system versus the probability of detecting an error of that size by various control rules. The power curve rules can calculate the probability of falsely rejecting a valid test run, the probability of **true rejection** (detection of a significant error in the run), the probability of error detection, and the average number of control observations required to identify a given error.[7,30-36] The design of specific control rules for a laboratory requires a five-step process[35] that includes (1) defining total allowable analytical error, (2) estimating the method's actual standard deviation and bias at the medical decision concentrations, (3) determining size of the systematic and random error that must be detected by the control system, (4) determining the probability level used for error detection (i.e., do you want to detect 90%, 95%, or 99% of errors?), and (5) plotting and inspecting the power curves to determine the number of control specimens that should be tested per run. In general, the most difficult part of these evaluations is determining how much error is allowable.

Westgard[37-39] (www.westgard.com) used these power curves to develop a series of specific control guidelines, popularly called the "Westgard rules" or the **"Westgard Multirule System."** These rules, which are used to determine whether an analytical run is out of control, are written in shorthand as follows: (1) 1_{2s}, $1_{2.5s}$, and 1_{3s} mean one control value exceeding two, two and one half, or three standard deviations; (2) 2_{2s} means two control values exceeding two standard deviations; and (3) R_{4s} means that the range of two control specimens exceeds four standard deviations. For many testing situations, the sequential application of the $1_{3s}/2_{2s}/R_{4s}$ set of control rules allows two control specimens to give sufficient error detection for a single run.[40] These rules mean that the run is rejected (action limits are exceeded) if any of the following happen: (1) 1_{3s}, if one control value differs by more than three standard deviations from the mean value; (2) 2_{2s}, if two control values differ by more than two standard deviations from the mean value; and (3) R_{4s}, if the range between two controls in the same run exceeds a combination of four standard deviations (i.e., one control ≥1.5 SD from mean and the other >–2.5 SD from mean). The first two rules will detect excessive bias, whereas the last rejects the run because of excessive imprecision. With use of these rules, the data in Fig. 25-1 for

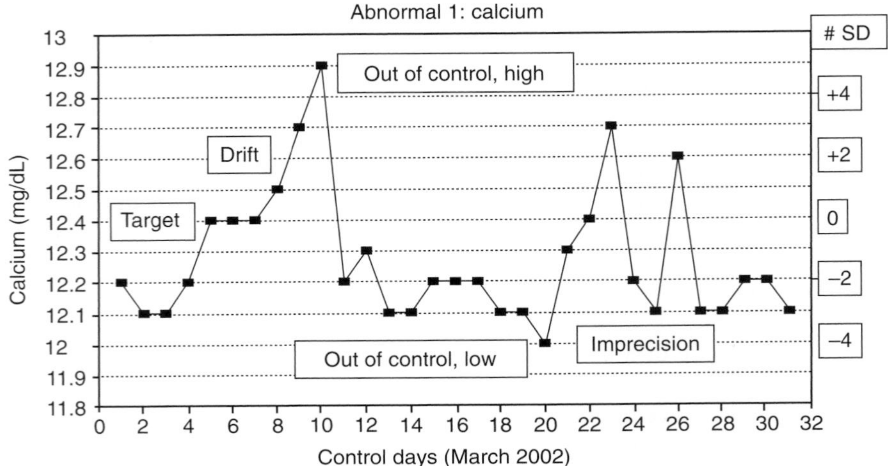

Fig. 25-1 Levey-Jennings plot of quality control values. Quality control (QC) actions (testing personnel documentation of how all out-of-control values were resolved): Days 5 through 7 represent a shift from the target value (monitor carefully). Days 6 through 10 demonstrate a gradual trend toward higher values. Day 10 patient results were not reported—an unresolved problem (one control >3 standard deviations [SD]), probably need a new bottle of calibrator. On day 11, recalibrated using new bottle of calibrator. Control values are now in control range; patient specimens from day 9 were retested. Day 13 begins a shift to lower values. This shift was investigated on day 20 when one control was low by more than 3 SD. Recalibration on day 21 resolved the problem because values were nearer to the target value. Days 23 through 26 showed increased imprecision. On day 27, cleaning the flow cell resolved the problem; however, the low bias was still present. General note: When this method shows acceptable imprecision, the values are below the target. It was subsequently determined that the manufacturer's target value for this QC pool was inaccurate. Proficiency results from testing performed on March 16 were within 0.01 mg/dL from all participants' target values. After this documentation, the laboratory director approved a new target value for this QC pool.

one control show values that exceed the action limits on days 10 (1_{3s}) and 20 (1_{3s}). Notice that, for rejection, the control value should exceed the control limit, not just be equal to that value. For many chemistry tests, power curves allow cost-effective detection of significant total errors (based on clinical usefulness) when two controls are used and the limits are set somewhere between 2.5 and 3.5 standard deviations.[7] For this reason, many use 3.0 usual standard deviations as a generalized control limit. For best implementation of Westgard rules, the LIS or the analyzer must have the proper software present to support this level of quality control checks. A more sophisticated approach to quality control will minimize run rejection and, at the same time, ensure the quality of patient results. Accordingly, some version of the Westgard approach is a useful feature of most LIS QC applications.

KEY CONCEPTS BOX 25-2

- Quality control is an analytical way to detect measurement errors in the analytical system.
- Quality control values are set by the laboratory or by verifying manufacturer's values. Detecting bias to prevent proficiency failure is important.
- If control values are exceeded, decisions are made to accept or reject the patient values in the run.

SECTION OBJECTIVES BOX 25-3

- Describe the format of a typical Levey-Jennings quality control plot.
- Define "trend" and "shift" and how these would be identified on a Levey-Jennings plot.
- Discuss the usefulness of delta checks in the clinical laboratory.
- Describe a sequential, 14-step corrective scheme for quality control that exceeds action limits.
- Apply concepts in this section to evaluate quality control results and implement appropriate corrective action.

DETECTION AND RESOLUTION OF QUALITY PROBLEMS

The Out-of-Control Decision

A testing system is designated as "out of control" when the validity of the results is not considered to be appropriate. Grossly out-of-control testing systems are usually unsuitable for medical purposes. This determination is made by the director or the technical supervisor.

Conditions for an out-of-control determination should be set by each laboratory; at a minimum, the criteria for an out-of-control decision include the following elements:

1. Control values exceed predetermined out-of-control limits within a specified period. Technologists must be directed to document their response to every control value that exceeds the established limits.
2. A method is determined to have an inappropriate reference interval; if the range is not immediately correctable, the method is "out of control."
3. A method demonstrates unacceptable imprecision, nonlinearity, or interferences. Interferences usually are limited to specific specimen types or substances.
4. A pattern of inappropriate patient results with large numbers of abnormal values is observed, or individual patient results exceed "delta" checking against previous results.
5. The laboratory director, section director, or technical supervisor declares the method out of control for other reasons.

Techniques for detecting and resolving out-of-control situations are discussed in the following text.

Detection of Quality Problems

Computer Assistance

The target values and limits for acceptable results that are established for each control pool are used in daily practice to detect analytical problems. A control result can be reviewed in a variety of ways by a technologist to evaluate acceptability. The technologist can simply compare the result with the posted range. This limits the technologist's ability to employ the Westgard rules or to evaluate the **trend** of previous results. More complex selection rules are now available as part of some computer programs, either on the instrument or as part of the laboratory's information system (LIS, see Chapter 22). Computer assistance allows real-time review of control results, early detection of QC problems, and better documentation of the quality control process.

Levey-Jennings Plots[41,42]

Current quality control data are best interpreted in the context of previous QC results as described above. To facilitate this goal, the data obtained from daily analysis of quality control pools can be plotted to create a visual presentation of the data. The most common visual analysis is the **Levey-Jennings plot.** The expected analyte concentrations, the established target value, and the desired number of standard deviations are drawn on the y-axis, and the days of the month (typically 31) are indicated on the x-axis (see Fig. 25-1). A large piece of graph paper can be used to show the data for several months. Thus cumulative information from quality control results can be observed simultaneously. Levey-Jennings plots are usually available on the LIS (see Chapter 22) or on the instrument that is performing the assays, obviating the need to plot these QC results manually.

Fig. 25-1 shows an example of a Levey-Jennings plot. The sudden change in control values (days 1 to 4 vs. days 5 to 7) from one average to a new average is called a *shift.* The increasing deviation from the target value, seen from day 8 to day 10, is called a *trend.* Changes in the precision of the testing system are shown on days 21 to 26, that is, a greater dispersion of data points is shown than is shown for days 13 to 19. This system was judged as unacceptable for the reasons documented at the bottom of Fig. 25-1. On day 32, the laboratory director reevaluated the target value and concluded that it had been set too high. A lower value was set, and QC results for the next month were closely monitored to assess this change.

All positive or negative trends (or drifts) or shifts from the target value represent biases that should be evaluated. Levey-Jennings plots should be routinely evaluated by technologists and supervisory personnel who are looking for trends or shifts in the data that could indicate problems in the testing system. Normally, a trend or a shift is noticed within 6 to 10 days after it begins. A shift or a trend that occurs during this period is usually a nonrandom, permanent change in the assay system.

Using Patients' Data in Decision Making

Pattern of Patients' Results

The results of most patients' sample analyses fall within reference (healthy) intervals established for each analyte.[51] Thus, for an analytical run of patients' samples, the results fall into a familiar pattern, that is, most results are within the nondiseased patient reference interval, and a few results are abnormal. The distribution of abnormal results, that is, the percentage of high or low results, will vary from test to test and even from hospital to hospital. Deviations from the usual pattern of cumulative patient results should alert testing personnel that a shift in the system's performance may be occurring, and that the patient analyses may be invalid. For example, a series of patient results for potassium greater than 5 should alert a technologist to a possible bias problem (Table 25-5). The example in Table 25-5 shows a typical set of potassium

Table 25-5 Use of Patient Data in Daily Quality Control

Sample Number	Patient Set A	Patient Set B
Control I	4.4—in control	4.4—in control
Control II	6.9—in control	6.8—in control
1	3.8	4.1
2	4.6	3.9
3	5.0	5.7
4	4.3	6.1
5	4.2	6.5
6	3.6	5.8
7	4.7	6.4
8	4.0	6.2
9	4.6	5.1
10	3.9	4.7
Control I	4.3—in control	4.6—in control (at +2 SD)
Control II	6.8—in control	7.0—in control (at +2 SD)

Would you wait until the quality control samples after the tenth sample to make a judgment about the system? No. After about the third or fourth patient sample with an extremely high or low value, quality control could be moved ahead, and trouble detection should begin. Keep in mind that occasionally, by chance, a series of specimens from very ill patients may fall in consecutive order. Repeated testing usually will solve the problem.

values (patient set A) and a clearly abnormal series (patient set B). The technologist should, of course, evaluate special circumstances. For example, a workload that includes a larger number than usual of patients' specimens from renal dialysis or cancer chemotherapy clinics will abnormally skew the otherwise typical pattern of test results. Clearly, verification of patient results by the technologist serves as a critical final check of quality control, especially when results are reviewed as part of a batch of results from the same run.

Newer LIS quality control applications and some real-time middleware applications provide for patient running mean monitoring. Thus real-time shifts and trends in the running mean of patient data can be included in the rules-based **autoverification** software to alert technologists that the method may be out of control. The technologist usually is prompted by the software to run a quality control specimen at that time to ensure that the method is in control and that patient results can be reported.

The Delta Check

Another important quality control check is the pattern of consecutive results for an individual patient. For most analyses, it is unlikely that a consecutive series of two or three test values from one patient will show large differences unless a major medical change has occurred. Unexpected changes from a single patient's serial specimens are called *delta changes,* meaning that a value for a single patient changed from the previous results to a greater degree than the laboratory's delta limit allows. Delta limits are set primarily to detect misidentified specimens or other errors (see p. 31 in Chapter18). When these types of changes are noted, the analyst must determine whether the change is real, or whether problems exist that are not identified by analysis of quality control specimens. Delta checks are usually part of an autoverification program (see pp. 401-402 in Chapter 22).

Specimen Indices and Instrument Flags

Because many measurements are routinely influenced by interferences from hemolysis, lipemia, and icteria, it is now essential that automated instruments measure and quantitate the degree of such potential interfering factors. Often, more than one of these factors occurs simultaneously. In addition, many newer automated instruments provide instrument flags along with patient results—flags that often indicate significant problems with the measured result. Newer autovalidation software often includes serum indices (indicating degrees of hemolysis, icteria, or lipemia), delta check ranges, instrument flags, and even patient running mean data in the real-time validation and release of patient data. When the software encounters a pre-programmed rules-based data event, the technologist is alerted in real time that there may be a problem. Appropriate corrective action is often included in the technologist alert message. These newer approaches to analytical system monitoring better ensure that consistent corrective action is employed, especially regarding (1) the adequacy of the specimen for the test that is being performed, (2) specimen-specific problems with the analytical system, and (3) the verification and release of individual patient results.

Actions to Bring a Testing System Back Into Control

When analytical problems are found, it is best to have a plan of action that is executed sequentially until the problem is resolved. For CLIA '88, it is necessary to document the problem, the investigation, the problem resolution, and any data that indicate that the problem is actually resolved (so-called corrective action). In a manual QC system, this documentation is kept in a separate "action limits" or "out-of-control" log book. A good LIS system also allows the analyst to point and click on a specific QC point on a displayed Levey-Jennings plot and list comments regarding the point such as associated corrective action. A list of actions follows that are among the sequential actions that might be taken to identify a problem. After each step is taken, the routine QC pools are analyzed; if the results are now within limits, it is assumed that the problem has been resolved, and patient results can be retested and then released. If the QC results are still not satisfactory, the next step is taken.

1. Repeat assays on control specimens using fresh aliquots of QC pools.
2. Repeat assays on control specimens using a separate or newly reconstituted set of controls. A set of controls can be mishandled, resulting in changed analyte concentrations caused by possible enzyme deterioration, evaporation, precipitation, or other causes.
3. Look for obvious problems such as clots, reagent levels, and mechanical fault.
4. Recalibrate the instrument for the out-of-control analyte; then reassay all controls.
5. Install a new bottle or a new lot number for one or all of the reagents, recalibrate, and reassay all the controls.
6. Perform periodic maintenance, recalibrate, and reassay all the controls.

If any of these responses results in acceptable QC data, patient results can be released if and only if at least three (or the entire run, whichever is less) patient specimens taken from the last run are reassayed, and the differences between previous and new results are found to be within the performance specification for precision (see p. 467). If the differences exceed performance specifications, further action must be taken (see example below). This requirement is established by CLIA, which states (§493.1219[b]) that "all patient test results obtained in the unacceptable test run or since the last acceptable test run must be evaluated to determine if patient test results have been adversely affected and the laboratory must take the remedial action necessary to ensure the reporting of accurate and reliable patient test results."

Technologists should be encouraged to perform all the above steps by themselves before requesting help from a supervisor. However, in a critical testing area, time limits for instrument downtime should be set. For an instrument in a stat. area, probably no more than 15 to 20 minutes should be spent in problem solving before supervisors are notified.

Example

At the start of the day, the laboratory's method for potassium produced results for controls that were elevated by more than five standard deviations. This change coincided with a change in the potassium ion-selective electrode (ISE). A new potassium ISE was installed, the instrument was recalibrated, and the controls were retested; they then were back in control. Three patient samples from the last run were retested to see whether the problem affected reported values. Potassium results reported for the previous runs were 3.9, 4.6, and 5.3 mmol/L; when repeated, the results were 4.1, 4.5, and 5.3 mmol/L. The method's performance specification for potassium precision is 1 SD = 0.11 mmol/L. The patients' potassium results each changed by <0.22 mmol/L. This is less than a 2 SD change; therefore, the old report does not have to be changed. This reevaluation of a patient's results should continue until a **significant difference** is seen, or the previously accepted quality control sample is reached.

When reevaluation of previous patient results shows unacceptable differences, all patient specimens that were tested after the last in-control QC sample was taken must be reassayed. If problems persist, the test may have to be performed on an alternative system or sent to a reference laboratory. If a sufficient quantity (or quantity not sufficient, QNS) of a patient's specimen is not available for reevaluation, the laboratory should request that another specimen be collected. It is inappropriate to report a result when the assay quality is in question.

7. Assay a different control of a similar known concentration to determine whether the original control material is at fault. In such situations, it is good policy to include some alternative control materials that are different from the QC materials that are routinely used, possibly with previously established, reliable assay values. The determination of a shift in the control material's assay value (which requires resetting of the target value) is to be made only by the director or the technical supervisor. If the values for a routine QC pool have changed slightly, assuming a new, stable pattern, but the test system appears stable (as judged by values from separate QC materials), then the target values of the routine QC pool may be changed. The laboratory director, with concomitant documentation of the decision process, must authorize such changes. If only one of the controls is showing the slight shift while a material of similar concentration continues to give a stable value and the test system shows stable performance, the initial estimation of the control material's target value was probably incorrectly set. In this case, the target value should be modified. If both controls and additional controls show similar shifts or trends, the problem is probably in the testing system.
8. Call the manufacturer to help determine the cause of the problem. Follow the manufacturer's instructions, and then reassay all controls.
9. Have the instrument serviced by the manufacturer, recalibrate, and reassay all controls, if necessary, to resolve the problem.
10. Use commercial accuracy-based materials to evaluate the quality specifications of the analytical system by checking linearity (reportable range), accuracy, bias, precision, analytical sensitivity, and minimal detectable change (smallest concentration change that is significant). Careful evaluation of these data should help reveal the cause of the control problem. Performing parallel testing on patient samples on a second instrument can also be very helpful at this point.
11. Determine whether the testing system has changed by reevaluating the reference interval. You can do this by obtaining data on the last 100 patients who have near-normal chemistry profiles with two or fewer slight abnormalities (acceptable patients are determined by the director or the technical supervisor). Estimate the reference interval by excluding 2.5% of the values from the tails of the distribution. This interval should agree (within ±1 SD) with the laboratory's established reference interval. This procedure will demonstrate only gross changes in the system. The director or the technical supervisor should determine whether a significant shift in the reference interval has occurred.
12. Reestablish the method's linearity[44] using the Clinical Laboratory Standards Institute (CLSI) (formerly the National Committee on Clinical Laboratory Standards [NCCLS]) protocols EP6-A (ISBN: 1-56328-498-8; 2003) to P2 (2004). If the method is linear over the reporting range, and the reference interval has not changed, the method is probably usable with adjustments to the appropriate target values for control specimens.
13. Consult the director or the technical supervisor to declare the method out of control if the above steps fail.
14. A final action involves replacement of the method or instrument with one that will allow the laboratory to meet its medical and proficiency testing goals.

Every quality control decision should be recorded in a permanent record. To meet the requirements of CLIA '88, quality control records should state acceptable limits and should include written documentation of the actions taken in response to out-of-range values. These responses must include date, analyte, complete testing system (i.e., source of reagents, instrument, calibrators, and controls), description of the problem, problem resolution, and names of the persons performing the test and approving the final actions. It may be convenient to prepare check-off forms or graphs for each control and analyte (Fig. 25-2). These records are also useful for predicting the need for maintenance, repair, or replacement of deteriorating reagents and instrument components, as indicated by the circled check marks in Fig. 25-2. Computerized records can greatly simplify and speed the documentation process.

Actions to Be Taken When a Method Is Out of Control

1. The decision that a testing system is out of control and must be suspended is communicated to all laboratory personnel, including the director, technical consultant, technical supervisor, clinical consultant, general supervisor,

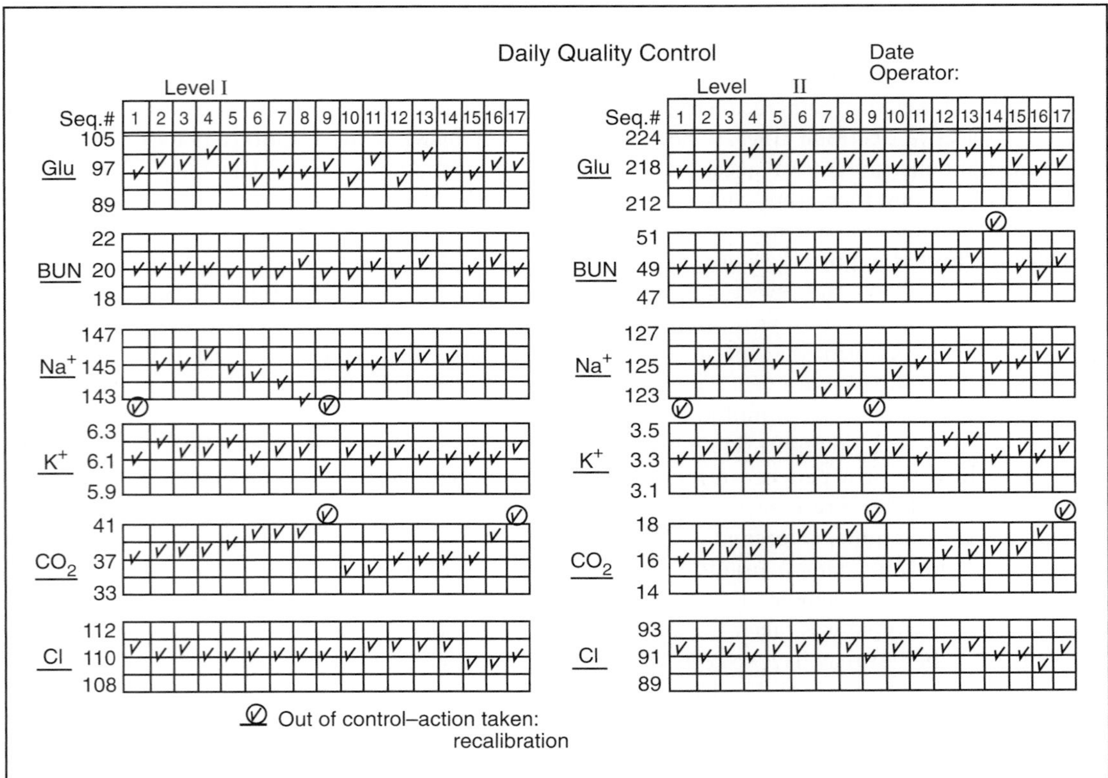

Fig. 25-2 Multiple analyte daily quality control check-off record. As each control is reported, it is quickly logged on a data sheet. Notes on out-of-control values and actions taken are included. A daily value for quality control calculation is selected through the use of a random number table basis. (Form developed by Rosvoll RV: In Copeland BE, Rosvoll RV, Casella JM, editors: *Quality Control Workshop Manual,* Chicago, 1978, American Society of Clinical Pathologists Commission on Continuing Education.)

and all appropriate testing personnel. As previously stated, the time frame for making this problem known will vary from section to section and should be stated in the laboratory's manual.

2. Suspension of a testing system means that no additional patient test results are to be released until the out-of-control condition is corrected and the director or the technical supervisor approves resumption of the testing.
3. Steps must be taken to have the test performed by an alternative method or by a reference laboratory. The alternative procedure must be listed in the laboratory manual. Notify the appropriate clinicians if the alternative method will have any adverse influence on test results or turnaround times.
4. An out-of-control condition that cannot be dealt with by the use of alternative methods or testing systems must be communicated within a reasonable time to the medical staff and any other authorized persons (such as senior administrative staff).
5. Supervisory personnel may define, for medical or analytical reasons, out-of-control conditions that differ from those stated in the general policy. These special conditions must be defined in the QC manual as well as in the test method's procedure manual.
6. Bringing a suspended test back into production requires the following actions at a minimum. The method must be recalibrated, or a calibration verification must be performed. Two levels of controls and at least one other material, such as proficiency testing materials of known or established value, must be used. This method can be used when the results of known specimens are within the expected mean ±2 times the appropriate usual standard deviation (established at a concentration close to the control value that was out of control). The method's reuse must be authorized by the technical supervisor or director. This authorization must be entered into the laboratory's problem log and formally signed and dated.

Procedures to Follow During a Testing System Failure

An out-of-control condition that is not immediately correctable can constitute a laboratory emergency. These emergencies can be managed by (1) using a suitable backup method, (2) sending the test to a reference laboratory, or (3) temporarily discontinuing the test. A laboratory must list an alternative or backup method of analysis for each test in the procedure manual. Laboratory policy should define how much time the technologist can spend troubleshooting a method before using the alternative system. Other factors that affect the decision include the medical requirements of the test (stat. vs. routine), laboratory staffing, and the laboratory's workload. For example, a stat. potassium analysis would be treated very differently from a 72-hour fecal fat determination. In the case of a potassium test, a delay of longer than 30 minutes in providing a backup result may affect a critical medical decision, whereas several days' delay in the fecal fat analysis may not be crucial to patient care. Decisions about processing of patient samples during a testing system failure should be made in consultation with the laboratory technical supervisor/consultant and the laboratory director, as specified by laboratory policy.

KEY CONCEPTS BOX 25-3

- "Out of control" values may be detected by data plots such as Levy-Jennings or by examining patient data.
- A system of responding to "Out of control" values must be in place.

SECTION OBJECTIVES BOX 25-4

- Discuss uses of calibrators in the clinical laboratory.
- Explain how proficiency testing may be used to validate internal quality control or to estimate system bias.
- Differentiate the following terms: definitive method, reference method, and field method.

CALIBRATION AND QUALITY CONTROL

Use of Calibrators

Controls may not be used as calibrators. Controls and calibrators must be different because each has a separate and important function. Calibrators set the reported values accurately, whereas controls verify the stability and accuracy of the calibration and of the testing system. However, for those tests for which suitable controls are not available, CLIA '88 allows calibration materials to be used as controls. For evaluation of system stability in these cases, it is best to find calibrator materials other than those used for calibration of the testing system.

A commercially available calibrator has an assigned value that the manufacturer establishes by using a definitive or reference method or by using reference materials traceable to **primary standards.** The calibrator is used to set the value reported by the laboratory's method or instrument. This process establishes correspondence of the instrument output signal with known concentrations. Differences between an aqueous and serum matrix can affect the transfer of known concentrations to a reported patient result. These matrix differences include turbidity, surface tension, which can affect sample pipetting, interactions between analytes and proteins, and the effect of the volume fraction occupied by protein or other large molecules (especially lipoproteins) on the actual concentration of analytes.

Calibrators are usually purchased in lots large enough to last 12 months or longer. It is recommended that a new lot of calibrator material be tested 6 weeks before it is used. This delay allows the laboratory to detect any systematic bias between values of the current calibrator and the new calibrator. Bias in a new lot of calibrators is detected when changes are seen in the mean values of quality control pools or patient test results. Some testing systems do not allow calibrators (especially calibrators from other systems) to be run as an unknown because of matrix mismatch. Often a calibrator will have assigned values that do not represent actual analyte values. These assigned-value calibrators are designed to calibrate testing systems to produce accurate test values when patient samples are used. Although the FDA requires manufacturers to use reference methods to assign calibrator values, significant differences between calibrator lots are frequently seen. Because of matrix effects, errors can be introduced into the calibration process when calibrators are used that are not specifically designed for the analytical system. Under CLIA '88, any modification of the manufacturer's instructions for the analytical portion of an FDA-cleared procedure requires documentation of the validity of the change. A laboratory that wishes to change a manufacturer's calibration set point must document that the change does not adversely affect the method's performance specifications. Some of the newer analyzers employ a two-dimensional bar code with a specific calibration associated with the particular lot of reagents. In this case, the manufacturer provides one or two point "adjusters" or calibrator-like reagents to refine the calibration curve when the reagents are placed into use. Of course, controls are subsequently run to verify the accuracy of such factory calibrations.

A Practical System for New Calibrator Verification

1. Use a 10-day verification period.
2. If the manufacturer allows the assay of calibrators as unknowns, each day insert two aliquots from one vial of new calibrator as an unknown into the regular daily run (n = 10 vials; 20 values). Calculate the average for each analyte. Compare each average with the value assigned by the manufacturer. Any difference between assigned and measured values will allow you to predict the average change expected in the quality control pool's target value (and also in patients' test values) when the new calibrator is introduced. A change in the quality control pool's target value greater than 1.0 USD is statistically significant, and a decision must be made as to which calibrator value is truly accurate. This decision must include consideration of CLIA's requirements (especially those that concern proficiency testing) and consultation with the manufacturer.

CLIA '88 requires that, when control values demonstrate significant changes (defined by each laboratory), the laboratory must establish, through calibration verification, that calibration has not been changed. Calibration verification requires that three specimens with high, low, and normal analyte concentrations be run to verify the quality of the test results. These specimens can be controls, calibrators, or other specimens with known values. If the manufacturer has specified a calibration verification protocol, you may follow it (§493.1217). CLIA rules do not set the quantity of allowable error, except as judged by proficiency testing. By setting an allowable error that is too large, however, a laboratory increases the danger of failing proficiency testing and may compromise patients' test values. Performance specifications can be used to judge excessive change (see Table 25-3).

Quality Control of Reagent Changes and Instrument Maintenance

Each lot of reagent or separate shipment of the same lot must be evaluated for quality before it is put into use. The laboratory can show that new lots or shipments of reagents (including calibrators and quality control pools) are acceptable if, after their use, the control values do not change significantly. It is also a good practice, after any maintenance has been done, to test a set of controls and run several patient samples from a previous batch before testing is resumed. Maintenance problems can lead to an "action-limits" situation because operating parameters may be changed. A chronological record of all reagent changes, instrument repairs, and maintenance procedures, along with any calibration-verification tests performed, must be kept.

Table 25-6 Partial List of CMS (HCFA)-Approved Providers of Proficiency Testing Programs for CLIA '88

Provider	Telephone Number
Accutest	800-356-6788
American Academy of Family Physicians	800-274-2237
American Association for Bioanalysts	800-234-5315
American Association of Pediatrics	800-433-9016
American Osteopathic Association	800-621-1773
American Proficiency Institute	800-333-0958
American Society of Internal Medicine	800-338-2746
American Thoracic Society	212-315-8789
California Thoracic Society	714-730-1944
College of American Pathologists/Excel	800-323-4040
College of American Pathologists/Surveys	800-323-4040
State of Idaho	208-334-2235
State of New York	518-485-5378
State of Ohio	614-466-2278
Wisconsin State Laboratory of Hygiene	800-462-5261

From the American Association for Clinical Chemistry, Clinical Laboratories Improvement Act, Fax No. 800-254-2329.
CLIA, Clinical Laboratory Improvement Amendment; *CMS (HCFA),* Center for Medicare and Medicaid Services (formerly Health Care Financing Administration).

EXTERNAL QUALITY CONTROL PROGRAMS AND OTHER TOOLS FOR ACCURACY CONTROL

Accuracy Control Is Required by CLIA '88

CLIA '88 requires that all laboratories holding a certificate that allows testing of moderately or highly complex tests must participate successfully in proficiency testing. Proficiency testing (PT) specimens are used to evaluate the adequacy of laboratory performance in all laboratory specialties. The analyst must test these specimens in the same manner in which patients' specimens are tested. Historically, PT has been part of a volunteer peer review and educational process. Proficiency testing is now regulatory, and failure in PT has serious penalties. However, the value of proficiency testing is the provision of independent validation of **internal quality control** programs.[45] Some of the providers of proficiency testing programs approved by the CMS are listed in Table 25-6. Because the analyst does not know the target value of the PT sample, it is difficult for the operator to influence the results. These programs, if properly used, can provide an estimation of the inherent accuracy of a system, at least as compared with a peer group or with the overall mean.[19] Continued or significant deviations from PT target levels, even if there is no failure, should alert the laboratory to a possible accuracy problem. If a method's USD is not significantly smaller than the SD of the comparative group, that method is at increased risk for PT failure.

An *estimation* of a system's bias can be made from proficiency testing performance. To do this, evaluate the specific test method's observed values against a comparison value, which may be the mean value reported for all similar methods (peer group mean), the mean value for all methods, or the definitive method value. Bias is calculated by subtracting the comparison value from the method's value. The algebraic sign shows whether the method's value is higher (positive bias) or lower (negative bias) than the group mean. Notice that comparison versus a peer group mean or even versus the mean of all participants does not establish accuracy. These comparisons show bias only from the comparison value. Accuracy is determined only when the comparison value is the true value. Certainly, repeated bias on proficiency tests must raise the suspicion of a true bias and will require that additional steps be taken to prove or disprove a real bias.

Definitive and Reference Methods

Definitive and reference methods are established by the National Reference System for the Clinical Laboratory (NRSCL) through applications by groups of interested persons representing different disciplines and organizations from professional societies (such as the International Federation of Clinical Chemistry) or practitioners, industrial companies, and governmental agencies. The NRSCL is a part of the CLSI. Definitive and reference methods are used to establish accuracy-based reference materials (see below).

A *definitive method*[2,46-47] is the most accurate way that a particular chemical substance can be measured. Analysis by definitive methods usually involves instrumentation of the most sophisticated type and performance of a separation procedure to purify the analyte before its concentration is measured. These methods are available in institutions such as the National Institute of Standards and Technology (NIST), the

Table 25-7 NRSCL Definitive and Reference Methods

Document Number	Analyte
Definitive Methods	
CLSI/NCCLS RS1-A	Glucose
CLSI/NCCLS RS3-A	Cholesterol
CLSI/NCCLS RS7-P	Sodium
CLSI/NCCLS RS8-P	Potassium
CLSI/NCCLS RS9-P	Calcium
CLSI/NCCLS RS10-P	Chloride
CLSI/NCCLS RS11-P	Urea
Reference Methods	
CLSI/NCCLS RS1-A	Glucose
CLSI/NCCLS RS2-A	Aspartate aminotransferase (AST)
CLSI/NCCLS RS3-A	Cholesterol
CLSI/NCCLS RS4-A	Alanine aminotransferase (ALT)
CLSI/NCCLS RS5-A	Total protein
CLSI/NCCLS RS6-A	Total bilirubin
CLSI/NCCLS RS7-P	Sodium
CLSI/NCCLS RS8-P	Potassium
CLSI/NCCLS RS9-P	Calcium
CLSI/NCCLS RS10-P	Chloride
CLSI/NCCLS RS11-P	Urea
CLSI/NCCLS RS12-P	Creatinine*
CLSI/NCCLS RS13-P	Rubella antibody*
CLSI/NCCLS RS14-P	Creatine kinase
CLSI/NCCLS RS15-P	Hemoglobin*
CLSI/NCCLS RS16	Antimicrobial susceptibility testing
CLSI/NCCLS RS17	Gamma-glutamyl transferase
CLSI/NCCLS RS18	Uric acid*

A, Approved; *NRSCL,* National Reference System for the Clinical Laboratory; *P,* proposed.
*In development.

Centers for Disease Control and Prevention (CDC), and large reference laboratories. Table 25-7 lists seven definitive and 18 reference methods defined by the NRSCL.

A *reference method*[3] is less rigorously proved than a definitive method, but it is well accepted because there is considerable evidence of its analytical ability. Thus the reference method has a demonstrated record of transferability of accuracy. The equipment and methodology are such that these methods are usually available at a university hospital–level laboratory. If a definitive method is not available for comparison, the reference method is established by consensus among authorities in the field. Some examples of reference methods credentialed by the NRSCL are listed in Table 25-7. The NRSCL is also involved in designing specifications for designated comparison methods that could be readily used by many laboratories.

A *field method* is one that is in common use. It is not classified as a reference or definitive method. It has been compared with a reference method and has been shown to yield comparable results that are acceptable to the user. Information on these method comparisons and evaluations is available in the medical literature and often from the manufacturer of a testing system.

Reference Materials

Commercially available aqueous and protein-based materials may be used as calibrators or controls in determining or monitoring the accuracy of assays. Each of these reference materials is useful for investigating the accuracy of a method. True target concentrations are assigned by the use of definitive or reference methods, and these can be certified by a certifying body to produce **certified reference materials (CRMs).** Alternatively, reference material is prepared at a specific concentration with the use of known quantities of high-purity analytes. These true target values are the most accurate values obtainable by state-of-the-art technology and thus are preferable when they are available. An example of such a reference material is the lyophilized human serum product, SRM909, produced by the NIST. A number of constituents in this material have levels measured by reference and definitive methods.

Other materials (similar to quality control materials) are available that have consensus values established by thousands of laboratories. These values are reported as overall average values or average values of methods performed by a specific testing system. The College of American Pathologists (CAP) produces survey-validated sera that have values established by thousands of individual assays from laboratories that participate in proficiency testing.[48] Some systems will show matrix effects caused by the lyophilization process or by the presence of interfering compounds, and so one must be careful when using these materials as the sole judge of a testing system's bias.[49]

Primary standards are always required for definitive and reference methods. The NIST provides a number of standard reference materials (SRMs) that may be used to prepare primary liquid standards. These include albumin, angiotensin, anticonvulsant drugs, aspartate aminotransferase, bilirubin, blood gases, calcium, chloride, cholesterol, cortisol, creatinine, electrolytes for ion-selective electrodes, fat-soluble vitamins, glucose, hydrogen ion, inorganic ions in bovine serum, iron, lead, lithium, magnesium, potassium, phosphorus, sodium, trace metals in serum, tripalmitate, urea, and uric acid. Aqueous materials in sealed vials prepared from these NIST primary standards are available from CAP. When NIST reference materials are used for calibration, a method's accuracy may be said to be "traceable to NIST reference materials." It is essential that the matrix of the prepared calibrator is consistent with the requirements of the testing system. Some testing systems require inclusion of protein or other constituents in the calibrator before it will behave appropriately in the testing system. A catalog of reference materials (NIST Special Publication 260) can be obtained from NIST at 1-301-975-6776 or at www.nist.gov/srm.

Selection of a Reference Laboratory for Assistance in Accuracy Control

One procedure that a laboratory can use to confirm the accuracy of a method is to send aliquots of patients' samples to a reliable reference laboratory. This is required by CLIA when no proficiency testing material is available for a test.

It is important, however, for the laboratory to be completely confident of the quality of the reference laboratory's analytical work. Always obtain information on the accuracy and precision of the laboratory's analytical methods. The laboratory should request a list of the methods and performance specifications used by the reference laboratory, as well as the results of their proficiency testing. The laboratory should evaluate all data carefully to determine whether the methods are appropriate for its needs. The laboratory's method is considered accurate if its results are not significantly different from those of the reference laboratory.

Manufacturer's Responsibility in the Control of Testing Systems

The responsibility for solving systematic and random bias problems does not belong solely to the user but should also be shared by the manufacturer of equipment and reagents. Manufacturers should provide performance specifications so that the laboratory can determine whether the system can be used appropriately to meet its medical and CLIA requirements. After the laboratory chooses a testing system, the technical supervisor must determine (often with the manufacturer) that the manufacturer's performance specifications are met by laboratory operation. Careful perusal of national proficiency surveys quickly reveals instrument systems and reagent systems that show the presence of significant systematic bias in the analysis of **proficiency testing specimens.** Proficiency testing specimens are the same or very similar to the specimens used for quality control evaluation. However, some bias may be apparent only because of the difference in the matrix of the control materials.[50] These matrix-specific biases are not seen when fresh patients' specimens are tested. The presence of matrix bias is shown by testing fresh human specimens and control materials using the laboratory's test method and a different method that does not show the matrix bias. Any differences noted between these methods may be the result of the matrix effect. Analytical problems that cannot be resolved after consultation with the manufacturer should be reported through the FDA's reporting system, administered by the U.S. Pharmacopeia, at 1-800-638-6725.

Automated Quality Control Initiatives

Manufacturers are playing an ever-increasing role in the quality control of new instruments and, in some cases, are taking over some of the traditional roles of the analyst. This is especially true for point-of-care testing (or decentralized testing, see Chapter 21),[37,51] for which, in many cases, the operator of the testing device is much less knowledgeable about issues of quality control than are the technologists and scientists in the central laboratory. New blood-gas instruments, for example, have included quality control material in test packs that allow the user to program when quality control is to be performed. A one-point calibration in some blood-gas instruments is performed automatically after each patient sample is taken; some manufacturers have included plans to automatically generate maintenance procedures and other corrective actions in response to out-of-control results. Such automated QC systems use expert software tools and automatically document QC and maintenance activities in computer files for CLIA requirements (§42 CFR 492.801.01.3000). The concept of a reagent lot–specific factory calibration stored on two-dimensional bar codes with "adjusters" to refine the factory calibration onsite is becoming more common in the laboratory industry. Given that the FDA is becoming more involved in the traditional oversight of medical devices, one might regard built-in, automated quality control features on laboratory instruments as a requirement, to ensure accuracy and reliability of generated test results. In this regard, it is not surprising that many newer chemistry analyzers have features that allow quality control materials to be stored on the system and run periodically without operator intervention. Many vendors of chemistry analyzers provide continuous real-time monitoring of their customers' instrument functions and quality control via Web initiatives and modem communications. Use of modem access allows the vendor to assume remote control of the instrument for testing and troubleshooting without having to go onsite, greatly speeding the response time needed to correct a testing problem. In addition, one manufacturer of quality control materials is providing real-time evaluation of quality control results generated at customer sites, again using modem and Web communication tools. As automated instruments improve in terms of reliability, stability, redundancy of components, remote QC and QA monitoring, and self-diagnostics/expert software tools, defects in the analytical system often will be detected before any change in testing accuracy and precision becomes observable by testing personnel. In addition, as vendors obtain real-time access to QC results, they will be empowered to possibly identify problems with field-installed instruments before requesting assistance from the local analyst.

Frequency of Calibration, Reagent Systems, and QC

Clearly, one goal of the laboratory must be to minimize the number of assays required to produce a patient result. Manual calibration in lieu of factory calibration, frequent recalibration resulting from out-of-control QC, and frequent reanalysis of QC and patients are characteristics of older, poorly designed analyzers and QC programs. Newer analyzers tend to be much more stable, with reagents stored "onboard" in temperature-controlled, refrigerated compartments and calibrations lasting for at least 30 to 60 days. If a method is entirely in control over this period of time, then theoretically, one can compute the costs of performing quality control. An example of such a computation, shown in Table 25-8, assumes that calibration is part of quality control expense, and that the only controls that would be repeated would be outliers or those 5% beyond the ±2 SD limits. The theoretical achievable test performed to reportable test ratio (TRR)[52] for a hypothetical laboratory test would be in the 1.02 to 1.46 range, or 2% to 46% of QC overhead cost. Of course, dilutions on patient assays beyond linear range would increase the TRR slightly; however, new analyzers have expanded the linear range on most of their assays to minimize this occurrence. Extending the shelf-life of reagents

Table 25-8 Theoretical Test to Reportable Ratios on an Automated Chemistry/Immunochemistry Analyzer Based on 31-Day Onboard Reagent and Calibration Stability*

Patient Assays per Day	Control Assays per Month (2/Day) +5% Outlier Repeats	Factory Calibration Verification Assays	Theoretical Test to Reportable Ratio (TRR)	Theoretically Achievable QC Overhead
100	65	6	1.02	2%
10	65	6	1.23	23%
5	65	6	1.46	46%

QC, Quality control.
*Assumptions: A totally in-control, stable method for 31 days with no recalibrations required, manufacturer's factory calibration with two "verifiers" run in triplicate, no patient dilution reruns due to expanded linear range on the assay, and no reagent or control lot number changes during the 31-day period.

minimizes waste and tends to lower the TRR; vendors have accomplished this, as was described earlier. All of the design features now available on new analyzers have markedly increased the overall efficiency and cost-effectiveness of the laboratory, as demonstrated by TRRs in the 1.2 to 1.3 range on some well-designed instruments. On the other hand, analyzers for immunoassay are still being manufactured that operate with TRRs in the 2 to 3 range. Note that these are instruments with which reagents must be manually calibrated (six calibrators or more in duplicate) or frequently recalibrated because of reagent or calibration instability, with packaging of as few as 50 assays per calibration and daily controls set at two to three levels with frequent repeats. Also, as can be seen in Table 25-8, higher TRRs and thus higher QC costs will be seen in lower-volume esoteric assays like prostate-specific antigen (PSA) and troponin-I, which may be performed only once or twice daily in a smaller hospital laboratory. Clearly, instruments with high TRRs are much more expensive to operate. These days, instrument vendors are highly motivated to achieve the lowest TRRs possible in the U.S. market because many of them are paid on a per reportable patient result system (CRR, Cost per Reportable Result), with the vendor supplying the required instruments, reagents, calibrators, and expendable supplies. A high TRR, therefore, will be expensive for the manufacturer, as well as for the hospital.

Electronic Quality Control

(see also p. 388, Chapter 21)

For most of the previous quality control discussion, we have assumed that laboratory testing is being performed in the traditional manner, that is, in the central laboratory (or core laboratory), and that QC has been performed on liquid materials similar to the patient sample. However, as computer chip and biosensor technology allows for more testing to be conveniently and cost-effectively performed at the patient's bedside, one can anticipate the need for a more sophisticated approach to quality control. Hand-held testing devices that employ **electronic quality control** have already demonstrated a high level of success in the marketplace. Indeed, CLIA rules accept the concept of electronic controls with the provision that the manufacturer's claims are verified and liquid control materials are assessed periodically, as required by the Joint Commission and the College of American Pathologists (CAP).

 **KEY CONCEPTS BOX 25-4**

- Controls and calibrators serve different functions and cannot be used interchangeably.
- Proficiency testing results can be used for evaluating accuracy.

REFERENCES

1. National Committee for Clinical Laboratory Standards: *Development of Certified Reference Materials for the National Reference System for the Clinical Laboratory, Approved Guideline,* CLSI/NCCLS publication NRSCL3-A, Villanova, PA, 1991, CLSI/NCCLS.
2. National Committee for Clinical Laboratory Standards: *Development of Definitive Methods for the National Reference System for the Clinical Laboratory, Approved Guideline,* CLSI/NCCLS publication NRSCL1-A, Villanova, PA, 1991, CLSI/NCCLS.
3. National Committee for Clinical Laboratory Standards: *Development of Reference Methods for the National Reference System for the Clinical Laboratory, Approved Guideline,* CLSI/NCCLS publication NRSCL2-A, Villanova, PA, 1991, CLSI/NCCLS.
4. Breitenberg M: *Questions and Answers on Quality, the ISO 9000 Standard Series, Quality Systems Registration, and Related Issues,* U.S. Department of Commerce, National Institute of Standards and Technology Publication NISTIR 4721, Gaithersburg, MD, 1991, USDC.
5. Dorsey DB: Evolving concepts of quality in laboratory practice: a historical overview of quality assurance in clinical laboratories, Arch Pathol Lab Med 113:1329, 1989.
6. Harris EK: Statistical principles underlying analytic goal-setting in clinical chemistry, Am J Clin Pathol 72:374, 1979.
7. Koch DD, Oryall JJ, Quam EF, et al: Selection of medically useful quality-control procedures for individual tests done in a multitest analytical system, Clin Chem 36:230, 1990.
8. Ehrmeyer SS, Laessig RH, Leinweber JE, et al: Medicare/CLIA final rules for proficiency testing: minimum intralaboratory performance characteristics (CV and bias) needed to pass, Clin Chem 36:1736, 1990.
9. Barnett RN: Analytic goals in clinical chemistry: the pathologist's viewpoint. In *Analytical Goals in Clinical Chemistry,* Northfield, IL, 1977, College of American Pathologists.
10. Ehrmeyer SS, Laessig RH: The relationship of intralaboratory bias and imprecision on laboratories' ability to meet medical usefulness limits, Am J Clin Pathol 89:14, 1988.

11. Tonks DB: A study of the accuracy and precision of clinical chemistry determination in 170 Canadian laboratories, Clin Chem 9:217, 1963.
12. Barnett RN: *Clinical Laboratory Statistics,* ed 2, Boston, 1979, Little, Brown & Co.
13. Douville P, Cembrowski GS: An approach to the use of clinical limits for quality control, Lab Med 406, June 1989.
14. Gilbert RK: Progress and analytic goals in clinical chemistry, Am J Clin Pathol 63:960, 1975.
15. Goals for allowable analytical error better based on medical usefulness criteria, Am J Clin Pathol 85:391, 1986.
16. Skendzel LP, Barnett RN, Platt R: Medically useful criteria for analytic performance of laboratory tests, Am J Clin Pathol 83:200, 1985.
17. Turcotte G, Bourget C, Talbot J, et al: Analytic clinical chemistry precision and medical needs: the Canadian interlab program (CID), Am J Clin Pathol 74:336, 1980.
18. National Cholesterol Education Program: *Recommendations for Improving Cholesterol Measurements,* NIH Publication No. 90-2964, Bethesda, MD, 1990, U.S. Department of Health and Human Services, National Institutes of Health.
19. Oxley DK: Cholesterol measurements: quality assurance and medical usefulness interrelationships, Arch Pathol Lab Med 112:387, 1988.
20. Cotlove E, Harris EK, Williams GZ: Biological and analytic components of variation in long-term studies of serum constituents in normal subjects: III. Physiological and medical implications, Clin Chem 16:1028, 1970.
21. Elion-Gerritzen WE: Analytic precision in clinical chemistry and medical decisions, Am J Clin Pathol 73:183, 1980.
22. Linnet K: Choosing quality-control systems to detect maximum clinically allowable analytical errors, Clin Chem 35:284, 1989.
23. Kaplan LA: Determination and application of desirable analytical performance goals: the ISO/TC 2121 approach, Scand J Clin Lab Invest 59:479, 1999.
24. Fraser CG: The application of theoretical goals based on biological variation data in proficiency testing, Arch Pathol Lab Med 112:404, 1988.
25. Ricós C, Alvarez V, Cava F, et al: Current databases on biological variation: pros, cons, progress, Scand J Clin Lab Invest 59:491, 1999.
26. Hardin E, Passey R, Gillum RL, et al: The use of "clear" enzyme control materials, Am J Med Technol 45:183, 1979.
27. Bowers GN Jr: Clinical chemistry analyte reference systems based on true value, Clin Chem 37:1665, 1991.
28. Castañeda-Méndez K: Chemometrics: measurement reliability, Clin Chem 34:2494, 1988.
29. Lasky FD: Proficiency testing linked to the National Reference System for the Clinical Laboratory: a proposal for achieving accuracy, Clin Chem 38:1260, 1992.
30. Carey RN: Implementation of multi-rule quality control procedures, Lab Med, 393, June 1989.
31. Groth T, Falk H, Westgard JO: An interactive computer simulation program for the design of statistical control procedures in clinical chemistry, Comput Programs Biomed 13:73, 1981.
32. Parvin CA: Comparing the power of quality-control rules to detect persistent systematic error, Clin Chem 38:358, 1992.
33. Parvin CA: Comparing the power of quality-control rules to detect persistent increases in random error, Clin Chem 38:364, 1992.
34. Westgard JO, Groth T, Aronsson T, et al: Performance characteristics of rules for internal quality control: probabilities for false rejection and error detection, Clin Chem 23:1857, 1977.
35. Westgard JO, Groth T: Power functions for statistical control rules, Clin Chem 25:863, 1979.
36. Westgard JO, Oryall JJ, Koch DD: Predicting effects of quality-control practices on the cost-effective operation of a stable multitest analytical system, Clin Chem 36:1760, 1990.
37. Westgard J, Qia E, Barry T: *Basic QC Practices—Training in Statistical Quality Control for Healthcare Laboratories,* Madison, WI, 1998, Westgard Quality Corp, www.westgard.com.
38. Carroll TA, Pinnick HA, Carroll WE: Brief communication: probability and the Westgard rules, Ann Clin Lab 33:113, 2003.
39. Westgard JO: Internal quality control: planning and implementation strategies, Ann Clin Biochem 40:593, 2003.
40. Westgard JO, Barry PL, Hunt MR, Groth T: A multi-rule Shewhart chart for quality control in clinical chemistry, Clin Chem 27:493, 1981.
41. Levey S, Jennings ER: The use of control charts in the clinical laboratory, Am J Clin Pathol 20:1059, 1950.
42. Shewhart WA: *Economic Control of Quality of the Manufactured Product,* New York, 1931, Van Nostrand Co.
43. Ladenson JH: Patients as their own controls: use of the computer to identify "laboratory error," Clin Chem 21:1648, 1975.
44. Jhang JS, Chang CC, Fink DJ, et al: Evaluation of linearity in the clinical laboratory, Arch Pathol Lab Med 128:44, 2004.
45. Ehrmeyer SS, Lassig RH: Has compliance with CLIA requirements really improved quality in US clinical laboratories? Clin Acta 346:37, 2004.
46. Gilbert RK: Accuracy of clinical laboratories studied by comparison with definitive methods, Am J Clin Pathol 70:450, 1978.
47. Velapoldi RA, Paul RC, Schaffer R, et al: *A Reference Method for the Determination of Potassium in Serum,* NBS Special Publication, No. 260-63, Washington, DC, 1979, National Measurement Laboratory, National Bureau of Standards.
48. Hartmann AE, Naito HK, Burnett RW, et al: Accuracy of participant results utilized as target values in the CAP Chemistry Survey Program, Arch Pathol Lab Med 109:894, 1985.
49. Miller GW: Specimen materials, target values and commutability for external quality assessment (proficiency testing) schemes. Lin Chim Acta 327:25, 2003.
50. Uldall A: Quality assurance within clinical chemistry—a brief review emphasizing "good laboratory practice," Scand J Clin Lab Invest 47(suppl 187):507, 1987.
51. Ehrmeyer SS: U.S. legislation for decentralized testing, Blood Gas News 8:20, 1999, CFR Part 493, CLIA Laboratory Requirements, *Federal Register,* October 1, 1997.
52. Blick KE: Cost effective workstation consolidation using the Chiron ACS:180 and valuanalysis, J Clin Ligand Assay 43:908, 1997.

BIBLIOGRAPHY

CLAS 19th National Meeting, Complying with CLIA '88, Wayne, MI, 1993, Clinical Spring Ligand Assay Society.

CLIA '88 final rules, Northfield, IL, 1992, College of American Pathologists. (The titles listed are CLSI guidelines, Wayne, PA, www.nccls.org.)

Statistical Quality Control for Quantitative Measurement Procedures: Principles and Definitions (C24-A3), 2006, Clinical and Laboratory Standards Institute, Wayne, PA, Catalog 2009-2009, CAT-0908, www.clsi.org.

Evaluation of Precision Performance of Quantitative Measurement Methods (EP5-A2), 2004, Clinical and Laboratory Standards Institute, Wayne, PA, Catalog 2009-2009, CAT-0908, www.clsi.org.

Method Comparison and Bias Estimation Using Patient Samples (EP9-A2), 2002, Clinical and Laboratory Standards Institute, Wayne, PA, Catalog 2009-2009, CAT-0908, www.clsi.org.

Preliminary Evaluation of Quantitative Clinical Laboratory Measurement Procedures (EP10-A3), 2006, Clinical and Laboratory Standards Institute, Wayne, PA, Catalog 2009-2009, CAT-0908, www.clsi.org.

Evaluation of Matrix Effects (EP14-A2), 2005, Clinical and Laboratory Standards Institute, Wayne, PA, Catalog 2009-2009, CAT-0908, www.clsi.org.

User Verification of Performance for Precision and Trueness (EP15-A2), 2005, Clinical and Laboratory Standards Institute, Wayne, PA, Catalog 2009-2009, CAT-0908, www.clsi.org.

Risk Management Techniques to Identify and Control Laboratory Error Sources (EP18-P2), August 2007, Clinical and Laboratory Standards Institute, Wayne, PA, Catalog 2009-2009, CAT-0908, www.clsi.org.

Estimation of Total Analytical Error for Clinical Laboratory Methods (EP21-A), 2003, Clinical and Laboratory Standards Institute, Wayne, PA, Catalog 2009-2009, CAT-0908, www.clsi.org.

INTERNET SITES

Clinical Laboratory Standards Institute—www.CLSI.org (formerly NCCLS)

www.iso.org—International Organization for Standardization

www.cap.org—College of American Pathologists (CAP)

www.jcaho.org—Joint Commission on Accreditation of Healthcare Organizations (JCAHO)

www.cms.gov/—Centers for Medicare and Medicaid Services

http://www.multiqc.com/—Multivariate QC in clinical laboratories

http://www.itl.nist.gov/div898/handbook/pmc/section3/pmc31.htm/, accessed 7/4/08—Description of control charts by the NIST National Institute of Standards and Technology

http://www.sqconline.com/six-sigma-control-charts.html/, accessed 7/4/08—Includes a control chart calculator

http://www.westgard.com/, accessed 7/4/08—Describes the Westgard rules

http://www.cms.hhs.gov/clia/, accessed 7/4/08—Describes the role of quality control in CLIA compliance, CLIA, Wayne, PA

Evaluation of Methods

Chapter 26

Carl C. Garber and R. Neill Carey

Chapter Outline

Key Terms

accuracy The agreement between the mean estimate of a quantity and its true value.[1] Closeness of agreement between a measured quantity value and a true quantity value of a measurand.[2]

allowable error (E_A) The amount of error that can be tolerated without invalidating the medical usefulness of the analytical result, or the maximum amount of error defined for successful performance in proficiency testing.[3]

analytical measurement range (AMR) The concentration range of a method over which the analytical performance (i.e., imprecision and inaccuracy) has been determined and judged to meet medical application requirements. Also known as reportable range. Applies only to quantitative tests.

assigned value The value assigned either arbitrarily (as by convention) or from preliminary evidence (as in the absence of a recognized reference method).[1]

bias A systematic component of analytical error, estimated from a comparison-of-methods experiment.[4] Also known as the difference between two quantities. A measure of inaccuracy (*see* trueness).

coefficient of variation (CV) The standard deviation expressed as a percentage of the mean.

comparative method The analytical method against which the test method is compared in the comparison-of-methods experiment. This term makes no inference about the quality of the comparative method.[5]

comparison-of-methods experiment An evaluation experiment in which a series of patient samples are analyzed by both the test method and the comparative method. The results are assessed to determine whether differences exist between the two methods.[4,5]

confidence interval The numerical interval that contains the population parameter with a specified probability.

constant systematic error (CE) An error that is always in the same direction and of the same magnitude, even as the concentration of analyte changes.[5]

demonstration A minimum evaluation needed for a laboratory to show that it is able to obtain expected results by following the manufacturer's instructions. This is appropriate for test systems whose performance characteristics have been well studied and documented.[6]

error The difference between a single estimate of a quantity and its true value. If a good estimate of the true value is not available, the difference may have to be expressed as the deviation from an assigned value.[1] Measured quantity value minus a reference quantity value (measurement error).[2]

establish To perform studies to determine performance specifications that provide evidence that the accuracy, precision, analytical sensitivity, and analytical specificity over the analytical measurement range of the procedure are adequate to meet stated quality goals or intended use. This applies to laboratory-developed tests and FDA cleared or approved tests that the laboratory has modified.

evaluation Determination of the analytical performance characteristics of a new method.

ideal value The value of a parameter under conditions of zero error.

imprecision The standard deviation or coefficient of variation of the results in a set of replicate measurements. The mean value and the number of replicates must be stated, as well as the particular type of imprecision, such as between-laboratory, within-day, or between-day imprecision.[1]

inaccuracy The systematic error estimated by the difference between the mean of a set of data and the true value known or estimated from other approaches.

interference The effect of any component of the sample on the accuracy of measurement of the desired analyte.[1]

interference experiment An evaluation experiment that is used to estimate the systematic error in a method which results from interference or lack of specificity.[5,7]

limit of blank (LOB) The highest measurement result that indicates that the analyte is not present in the sample.[8]

limit of detection (LOD) The lowest amount of analyte in a sample that can be detected with (stated) probability. Also called *lower limit of detection,* or *minimum detectable concentration* (or dose or value), and sometimes used to indicate "sensitivity."[8] The minimum concentration of analyte whose presence can be qualitatively detected under defined conditions.

limit of quantitation (LOQ) The lowest amount of analyte in a sample that can be quantitatively determined with (stated) acceptable precision, under stated experimental conditions. Also called *lower limit of determination* and *lower end of the measuring range.*[8]

linear range The range over which results of a testing system are acceptably linear, that is, where nonlinear error is less than the error criterion.[9]

linear regression An approach that is used to choose a single line through a data set that "best" describes the relation between two subsets or two methods. This approach is used under the assumption that there are no errors in the data obtained by the X method. (Also see Chapter 23.)

measurand Quantity intended to be measured.[2]

medical decision level (X_C) A concentration of analyte at which some medical action is indicated for proper patient care. There may be several medical decision levels for a given analyte. (Also see Chapter 24.)

parameter A number that describes a feature of a population. This is in contrast to a statistic that is an estimate of a parameter derived from a sample of the population.

precision The agreement among replicate measurements.[1]

proficiency testing A program in which specimens are periodically sent to laboratories for analysis for the purpose of assessing overall analytical performance. Participation in proficiency testing is required under CLIA '88.[3] (Also see Chapter 25.)

proportional systematic error (PE) An error that is always in one direction, the magnitude of which is a percentage of the concentration of the analyte being measured.[5]

random analytical error (RE) An error, either positive or negative, the direction and exact magnitude of which cannot be predicted; imprecision.[5]

recovery experiment An evaluation experiment that estimates proportional systematic error.[5] The determination of recovery is based on the measurement of added analyte. Percent recovery is the ratio of the measured amount to the added amount. Deviation of percent recovery from 100% is one example of proportional systematic error.

replication experiment An evaluation experiment that estimates random analytical error.[5,10] Measurements are made on aliquots of a stable sample over specified periods, as within a run, within a day, or over a period of days.

sample The appropriately representative part of a specimen used in analysis. This sample should be called a *test sample* when it is necessary to avoid confusion with the statistical term *random sample from a population.*[1]

standard deviation (SD) Square root of the variance. A measure of imprecision.

standard deviation of differences The standard deviation of the differences (s_d) between observed y-values and corresponding x-values for a group of samples in which each sample is measured by the x-method and the y-method. This is a measure of the dispersion of differences around the average difference.

standard error of the estimate The standard deviation of the differences, $s_{y,x}$, between observed y-values and y-values predicted by the regression line for a given x. This statistic measures the dispersion or spread of data around the regression line.

systematic analytical error (SE) An error that is always in one direction; inaccuracy.[5]

test method In this chapter, the method that is chosen for experimental testing or study by means of method evaluation.[5]

total error (TE) A combination of random and systematic analytical errors; an estimate of the magnitude of error that might occur in a single measurement.

true value A term considered to have self-evident meaning requiring no definition. In practice, the true value is approximated closely by the definitive (method) value and somewhat less closely by the reference (method) value.[1]

trueness (of measurement) Closeness of agreement between the average of an infinite number of replicate measured quantity values and a reference quantity value.[2] *Note:* The measure of trueness is usually expressed in terms of bias.[6]

validation Confirmation by examination and provision of objective evidence that the particular requirements for a specific intended use of an analytical procedure can be consistently fulfilled (21 CFR Section 820.3, Definitions).[11]

variance A statistic used to describe the distribution or spread of data in a population (see Chapter 23).

verification Confirmation by examination of objective evidence that specified requirements have been fulfilled (21 CFR Section 820.3, Definitions).[11]

Over the past several decades, the quantitative analytical methods used in clinical laboratories have become more reliable and more standardized. Commercial manufacturers supply most analytical procedures. The emphasis of the clinical chemist has shifted away from methods development to the selection and **evaluation** of those commercially available methods that best suit a particular laboratory situation. Since implementation of the Clinical Laboratory Improvement Amendments of 1988[3] (CLIA '88), this selection and evaluation process has taken on greater significance because these regulations require, among other things, successful performance of **proficiency testing** for any laboratory to continue to perform tests in a particular specialty, subspecialty, or test procedure.

The process of method evaluation has been evolving.[12] It is critical to recognize that a method's performance can be objectively judged as acceptable only if its **errors** are small enough to be acceptable for medical use and to pass proficiency testing. The protocols developed by Westgard et al[5] and the Clinical and Laboratory Standards Institute (CLSI, formerly the National Committee on Clinical Laboratory Standards [NCCLS])[4,6-10,13,14] measure error in terms of analyte (**measurand**) concentration units but present different criteria for assessment of error. Westgard et al[5] take a quality management approach and include an error budget for the operation of the quality control (QC) procedure when they compare derived estimates of error to medically allowable error. CLSI protocols provide procedures for comparing observed errors to manufacturers' claims or to an allowable error specified in terms of a statistical **parameter** (such as allowable **standard deviation** or allowable **bias**). This chapter describes the Westgard and CLSI approaches.

SECTION OBJECTIVES BOX 26-1

- List the purposes of method evaluation experiments.
- Relate the relative amount of allowable error for a particular test to medical decision levels for that test.

PURPOSE OF METHOD EVALUATION

Laboratory Requirements

New analytical methods usually are developed to improve **accuracy** or **precision** over existing methods, to allow automation, to reduce reagent or labor cost, or to measure a new analyte. In any case, the method's analytical performance in a clinical laboratory setting must be verified experimentally, even if the new method is believed to be an improvement over all previous methods. Beyond scientific and medical reasons for performing an evaluation are regulatory (CLIA '88) and accreditation requirements for evaluating new methods.

The process of evaluating a method is different from the process of performing routine QC of a method after it has been introduced into daily use. Routine (daily) QC (see Chapter 25) is a process established to detect increases in the analytical errors of a method, to avoid the release of incorrect patient data. Routine QC detects errors only when they significantly exceed the error that was present in the method when the control ranges were established. The use of routine QC does not enable the investigator to determine the magnitude of the inherent errors of the method or to decide whether they are acceptable. Method-evaluation experiments are required to assess the inherent analytical errors of the method and relate them to medical or regulatory requirements, and to select effective QC procedures.

The scope of a method evaluation depends on who is doing the evaluation and what is already known about the analytical performance of the method. In order of decreasing amounts of effort, the scope of different evaluations can be described by the terms in Box 26-1. The scope of evaluations is also described in several CLSI documents, such as *Guideline EP15-A2: User Verification of Performance for Precision and Trueness.*[6]

Manufacturer Requirements

When a manufacturer develops a new method and prepares to market it, the manufacturer is required by the U.S. Food

Box 26-1

Scope of Method-Evaluation Studies

Establish refers to studies conducted to determine performance specifications that provide evidence that the accuracy, precision, analytical sensitivity, and analytical specificity over the analytical measurement range of the procedure are adequate to meet stated quality goals or intended use. This applies to laboratory-developed tests and FDA cleared or approved tests that the laboratory has modified.

Evaluation is the determination of analytical performance characteristics of a new method.

Validation is confirmation by examination and provision of objective evidence that the particular requirements for a specific intended use can be fulfilled consistently (21 CFR Section 820.3, Definitions).[11]

Verification is confirmation by examination of objective evidence that specified requirements have been fulfilled (21 CFR Section 820.3, Definitions).[11]

Demonstration, a form of verification, is a minimum evaluation for a laboratory to use to show that it is able to obtain expected results by following the manufacturer's instructions. This is appropriate for test systems whose performance characteristics have been well studied and documented.

and Drug Administration (FDA) to make claims about the analytical performance of the method, specifically about its precision and accuracy.[11,15] In addition, the FDA has provided a number of guidance documents for industry to ensure that appropriate testing standards have been followed, and that the data provided support the labeling information in the appropriate premarket submission by the manufacturer.[16] All claims must be supported by experimental method-evaluation data. It is essential that these claims be realistic and conservative. The level of performance of the method in most laboratories must be consistent with that claimed by the manufacturer. Extensive experimental data are required for the manufacturer to develop defensible claims. CLSI has developed evaluation protocols that enable manufacturers to produce defensible performance claims that can be verified by the laboratory.

Laboratory personnel in hospital and commercial laboratories perform most method evaluations. These evaluations are performed to determine whether the performance of a method meets, primarily, the requirements for medical applications intended by the user and, secondly, the quality goals specified by CLIA '88 for successful performance in proficiency testing. The method may be a commercial method, a laboratory-developed test, a method that uses analyte-specific reagents (ASR),[17] or a method that the user has seen in the literature and is setting up in his or her own laboratory. The user needs to perform the evaluation as efficiently as possible and should determine with a minimum of experimental work whether the method's performance is acceptable as each experiment is completed. If performance is not acceptable at any stage of the evaluation, the user can "repair" or reject the method without performing all the time-consuming studies required for acceptance.

Medical Requirements

The decision to accept or reject a candidate laboratory method should be based on the ability of the method to meet the requirements of the final user—the physician who is using the results of a laboratory test for patient care (see Chapter 25). The error of the test result is excessive if it causes a misdiagnosis. The greatest chance for misdiagnosis caused by an analytical error in a test result occurs at the concentration at which a medical diagnosis is made; this concentration is termed the **medical decision level** (**X_C**) concentration. For example, a fasting glucose concentration below 70 mg/dL may be diagnostic of hypoglycemia.[18] For each decision-level concentration, a performance standard consisting of the decision-level concentration, X_C, and the **allowable error, E_A,** may be formulated. Allowable error is stated in concentration units so that errors of the **test method** may be judged by comparison with clinically allowable error. The method-evaluation data are interpreted by using the data to estimate the error of the method at the medical decision level of concentration and then comparing this estimate with the allowable error. If the method's error exceeds allowable error, performance is not acceptable. If the error is less than the allowable error, performance is acceptable.

The amount of error present in the single measurement of an analyte is different each time the analyte is measured because a portion of the error is purely random. Thus the magnitude of error for a measurement on a given patient specimen cannot be known exactly, and the absolute maximum error that a method could ever make on the analysis of a single patient specimen cannot be predicted. However, an estimate of the upper limit of the error can be calculated such that there is only a 5% or 1% chance that the actual error would exceed the upper limit and possibly cause a misdiagnosis.

Exact performance standards for allowable error based on medical criteria have not been defined for most analytes. Performance standards have been proposed for those analytes that are measured most often, but generally, professional judgment and input from clinicians must be used to establish the performance standard for a particular analyte. Barnett[19,20] presented a summary of medically allowable standard deviations. Tonks[21] proposed that allowable error should be either one fourth of the reference range or 10%, whichever is less. For enzymes, the limit is expanded to 20%.[22] Cotlove, Harris, and Williams[23] recommended a "tolerable analytical variation" based on one-half the combined individual and group biological variation. The 1976 Aspen Conference[24] sponsored by the College of American Pathologists (CAP) provided the basis for the use of intraindividual and interindividual biological variations for determining the goals for the precision of a method used for group testing. The analytical **coefficient of variation** (**CV**) is denoted as CV_A,

$$CV_A = \tfrac{1}{2}\sqrt{CV_{Intra}^2 + CV_{Inter}^2} \qquad \text{Eq. 26-1}$$

in which CV_{Intra} is the biological variation observed within an individual and CV_{Inter} is the biological variation observed between individuals. To enable the physician to monitor intraindividual changes, the method must be even more precise:

$$CV_A = \tfrac{1}{2}\sqrt{CV_{Intra}^2} \qquad \text{Eq. 26-2}$$

A similar equation has been written to specify allowable bias (B_A) based on the biological CVs, as described below. Note that "A" is subscripted "B_A."

$$B_A = \tfrac{1}{4}\sqrt{CV_{Intra}^2 + CV_{Inter}^2} \qquad \text{Eq. 26-3}$$

Fraser extended the application of the biological variability model to define three levels of performance as indicated in Table 26-1.[25,26]

Fraser and associates[25,27-29] and Ricós et al[30] reviewed and summarized various approaches that have been used to establish quality goals, concluding that biological variation can serve as a key consideration for establishing allowable error specifications for many analytes. For therapeutic drugs, quality goals were based on pharmacokinetic theory. Professional organizations have made recommendations; these include the National Academy of Clinical Biochemistry, which provided recommendations for cardiac markers,[31] and the National

Table 26-1 Three-Tiered Analytical Performance Specifications

Level of Quality	Analytical Imprecision	Analytical Bias
Minimum quality	$CV_A < 0.75 \times CV_{intra}$	$B_A < 0.375\sqrt{CV_{intra}^2 + CV_{inter}^2}$
Desirable quality	$CV_A < 0.50 \times CV_{intra}$	$B_A < 0.250\sqrt{CV_{intra}^2 + CV_{inter}^2}$
Optimum quality	$CV_A < 0.25 \times CV_{intra}$	$B_A < 0.125\sqrt{CV_{intra} + CV_{inter}^2}$

Glycohemoglobin Standardization Program, which has implemented quality goals for hemoglobin A1c.[32]

Other factors, such as turnaround time, may affect the medically allowable error. Clinicians sometimes may accept increased error if turnaround time is short.

Performance Standards Based on Proficiency Testing

The government specifies allowable error for proficiency testing for many analytes, the most notable of which are contained in the CLIA '88 regulations.[3] The Occupational Safety and Health Administration (OSHA) has specified allowable errors for monitoring of heavy metals.[33] CAP has specified allowable errors for many nonregulated analytes[34] (see the participant summary of a recent CAP survey for current allowable errors). A laboratory must select, evaluate, and then monitor (by statistical QC; see Chapters 23 and 25) the test method, so that when it is in routine use, the laboratory will have confidence that the method will meet proficiency testing requirements. These requirements are given as (1) fixed limits, such as an absolute limit on the amount of variability or a limit expressed in terms of a fixed percentage of concentration or activity, or (2) three–standard deviation limits, which are based on the overall or peer groups standard deviation, or (3) plus or minus two dilutions for assays reported in units of titers. Ehrmeyer et al[35] showed that if the internal laboratory standard deviation (SD) for a procedure is less than one third of the fixed-limit criteria, and the assay's bias is "small," the likelihood for passing proficiency testing is greater than 99%. Westgard and Burnett,[36] using error budget analysis, found that the assay's **total error**, calculated as "bias + 4 × SD," should be less than the specified limit. In practice, this indicates that the internal SD should be less than 25% of the limit. Table 26-2 lists the CLIA '88 proficiency testing requirements. The fifth column shows the maximum allowable within-laboratory SD (using the 4 × SD criterion and zero bias). For comparison, maximum internal SDs derived from recommendations based on biological variation[25,27-30] are listed. Note that for some analytes, the SD derived from proficiency testing and from biological variation are similar, whereas they are different for other analytes. A laboratory method must be able to pass proficiency testing and provide medically useful test results.

Westgard[37] relates laboratory performance to the Six Sigma model as defined by Motorola in the 1980s and subsequently adopted by many manufacturing and service industries.[38] This model states that if the process SD is less than one sixth of the allowable total error (E_A), the process is said to be Six Sigma capable. Even in the presence of small undetectable shifts or drifts of less than one fourth of the allowable error,[39] the potential defect rate for such a Six Sigma process is 3.4 defects per million tests, where a defect is a result that includes an error that exceeds the allowable error (E_A).

KEY CONCEPTS BOX 26-1

- Allowable errors have been suggested for many commonly tested analytes. The user can derive allowable errors when necessary from biological variation or based on CLIA '88 needs.
- The analytical errors of a method must be less than the specified *medically allowable error*.
- The quality of a method is determined by comparing its errors to allowable error.
- *Bias (trueness)* and *imprecision* must be minimized to maintain maximum quality.
- *Six Sigma* methods are capable of maintaining a defect rate of 3.4 defects per million tests.

SECTION OBJECTIVES BOX 26-2

- Outline the four general steps in method selection.
- List examples of application characteristics to be considered in method selection.
- List characteristics of an "ideal" method that should be applied to a candidate method before selecting that method for consideration in the laboratory.
- List analytical performance characteristics to be considered in method selection.

SELECTION OF METHODS

Evaluation of Need

The quality of service achievable by a laboratory is determined by selection of personnel, equipment, and analytical methods. The process of method selection is complex, and unless this process is well organized, method selection can be a traumatic and costly experience. Box 26-2 provides a logical sequence to be followed in method selection.

Often the decision to set up a new method or instrument is based on a medical or economic requirement for the laboratory to provide a new test onsite. Advances in laboratory practice also may dictate a change in the methodology of a presently offered test. The need for a new method or device

Table 26-2 Comparison of Allowable Error as Specified by CLIA '88 vs That Recommended by Fraser et al Based on Biological Variability

Analyte	Acceptable Performance Criteria, CLIA '88	Decision Level (X_C[a])	Allowable Error (CLIA '88[b])	Maximum SD (CLIA '88[c])	Biological CV-Based Maximum SD (Fraser[d])
Routine Chemistry					
Albumin	±10%	3.5 g/dL	0.35	0.09	0.06
Bilirubin	±0.4 mg/dL or ±20%	1.0 mg/dL	0.40	0.10	0.13
		20 mg/dL	4.0	1.0	2.6
Calcium	±1.0 mg/dL	7.0 mg/dL	1.0	0.25	0.07
		10.8 mg/dL	1.0	0.25	0.10
		13.0 mg/dL	1.0	0.25	0.12
Chloride	±5%	90 mmol/L	4.5	1.1	0.54
		110 mmol/L	5.5	1.4	0.66
Cholesterol	±10%	200 mg/dL	20	5.0	6.0
Creatinine	±0.3 mg/dL or ±15%	1.0 mg/dL	0.30	0.08	0.02
Glucose	±6 mg/dL or ±10%	70 mg/dL	7.0	1.75	2.0
		126 mg/dL	12.6	3.15	3.6
		200 mg/dL	20	5.0	5.7
Hemoglobin A1c		7.0% GHB	0.85%[e] GHB	0.21% GHB	0.07% GHB
Iron	±20%	150 mg/dL	30	7.5	20
Magnesium	±25%	2.0 mg/dL	0.50	0.12	0.036
pH	±0.04	7.35	0.04	0.01	0.01
Pco_2	±5 mm Hg or ±8%	35 mm Hg	5.0	1.2	0.84
		50 mm Hg	5.0	1.2	1.2
Po_2	±3 SD_g	30 mm Hg	3 SD_g	0.75 SD_g	
		80 mm Hg	3 SD_g	0.75 SD_g	
Potassium	±0.5 mmol/L	3.0 mmol/L	0.50	0.12	0.07
		6.0 mmol/L	0.50	0.12	0.14
Protein, total	±10%	7.0 g/dL	0.70	0.18	0.10
Sodium	±4 mmol/L	130 mmol/L	4.0	1.0	0.52
		150 mmol/L	4.0	1.0	0.6
Triglycerides	±25%	160 mg/dL	40	10	18
Urea nitrogen	±2 mg/dL or ±9%	27.0 mg/dL	2.4	0.6	1.7
Uric acid	±17%	6.0 mg/dL	1.0	0.25	0.25
Enzymes					
Alkaline phosphatase	±30%	150 U/L	45	11	4.8
ALT	±20%	50 U/L	10	2.5	6.8
Amylase	±30%	100 U/L	30	7.5	3.7
AST	±20%	30 U/L	6.0	1.5	1.8
		70 U/L	14	3.5	4.2
CK	±30%	200 U/L	60	15	23
LD	±20%	300 U/L	60	15	13
Endocrinology					
Cortisol	±25%	5 μg/dL	1.25	0.3	0.2
		30 μg/dL	7.5	1.8	3.1
Free thyroxine	±3 SD_g	2.3 ng/dL	3 SD_g	0.75 SD_g	0.1
hCG	±3 SD_g or positive/negative	25 IU/L	3 SD_g	0.75 SD_g	
T_3 uptake	±3 SD_g	25%	3 SD_g	0.75 SD_g	0.6
Triiodothyronine	±3 SD_g	100 ng/dL	3 SD_g	0.75 SD_g	4.0
		200 ng/dL	3 SD_g	0.75 SD_g	8.0
TSH	±3 SD_g	0.1 mIU/L	3 SD_g	0.75 SD_g	0.025
		5.0 mIU/L	3 SD_g	0.75 SD_g	0.4
Thyroxine	±1.0 μg/dL or ±20%	3 μg/dL	1.0	0.25	0.1
		13 μg/dL	2.6	0.65	0.45
Toxicology					
Alcohol, blood	±25%	0.10 g/dL	0.025	0.006	
β_2-microglobulin, urine		300 μg/L	45.0	11.25[e]	
		750 μg/L	112.5	28.1[e]	
		1500 μg/L	225.0	56.2[e]	

Continued

Table 26-2 Comparison of Allowable Error as Specified by CLIA '88 vs That Recommended by Fraser et al Based on Biological Variability—cont'd

Analyte	Acceptable Performance Criteria, CLIA '88	Decision Level (X_C[a])	Allowable Error (CLIA '88[b])	Maximum SD (CLIA '88[c])	Biological CV-Based Maximum SD (Fraser[d])
Cadmium, blood		5 µg/L	1.0	0.25[f]	
		10 µg/L	1.5	0.375[f]	
		15 µg/L	2.2	0.505[f]	
Cadmium, urine		3 µg/L	0.45	0.11[f]	
		7 µg/L	1.05	0.26[f]	
		10 µg/L	1.5	0.375[f]	
Carbamazepine	±25%	8 mg/L	2.0	0.5	0.8
		12 mg/L	3.0	0.8	1.2
Digoxin	±0.2 µg/L or ±20%	0.8 µg/L	0.2	0.05	0.04
		2.0 µg/L	0.4	0.10	0.10
Ethosuximide	±20%	40 mg/L	8.0	2.0	2.0
		100 mg/L	20.0	5.0	4.9
Gentamicin	±25%	10 mg/L	2.5	0.6	
Lead, blood	±4 µg/dL or ±10%	10 µg/dL	4.0	1.0	
Lithium	±0.3 mmol/L or ±20%	0.5 mmol/L	0.3	0.08	0.06
		1.5 mmol/L	0.3	0.08	0.18
Phenobarbital	±20%	15 mg/L	3.0	0.75	1.3
		40 mg/L	8.0	2.0	3.6
Phenytoin	±25%	10 mg/L	2.5	0.6	0.7
		20 mg/L	5.0	1.2	1.3
Primidone	±25%	5 mg/L	1.2	0.3	0.56
		12 mg/L	3.0	0.75	1.36
		4 mg/L	1.0	0.25	
		20 mg/L	5.0	1.25	
Quinidine	±25%	7 mg/L	1.8	0.45	
Theophylline	±25%	10 mg/L	2.5	0.6	0.7
		20 mg/L	5.0	1.2	1.4
Valproic acid	±25%	50 mg/L	12	3.0	3.3
		100 mg/L	25	6.2	6.7

ALT, Alanine aminotransferase; *AST,* aspartate aminotransferase; *CK,* creatine kinase; *CLIA,* Clinical Laboratory Improvement Amendments; *CV,* coefficient of variation; *GHB,* glycohemoglobin; *hCG,* human chorionic gonadotropin; *IU,* international units; *LD,* lactate dehydrogenase; *SD,* standard deviation; SD_g, proficiency testing peer group standard deviation; T_3, triiodothyronine; *TSH,* thyroid-stimulating hormone; *U,* units; X_C, concentration of ***x*** analyte to indicate medical intervention.

[a]Medical decision levels, most of which are based on Barnett.[19,20]

[b]Allowable error based on CLIA '88 performance requirements at the respective medical decision level (see column 3 for units).[3]

[c]Maximum internal SD based on criteria that 4 SD is less than the allowable error[36] (see column 3 for units).

[d]Maximum internal SD based on biovariability criteria (Fraser et al[25,27-30]) (see column 3 for units).

[e]No CLIA criterion. Maximum allowable SD calculated from National Glycohemoglobin Standardization Program (NGSP) requirement. "95% of results must be within target ±0.85% GHB units," which is in effect a specification for allowable total error.[32] Also in 2007, the College of American Pathology (CAP) revised its specification for acceptable performance as reference method target ±12% of the target value. At a glycosylated hemoglobin (HbA1c) value of 7% GHB, the allowable error (E_A) would be 0.84% GHB, showing the same requirement at 7% GHB as required by NGSP.

[f]No CLIA criterion. Allowable error is from Occupational Safety and Health Administration (OSHA) regulations on cadmium monitoring.[33] Actual medical decision level for cadmium in urine is in terms of µg Cd/g creatinine. Similarly for β_2-microglobulin (µg/g creatinine). However, for the purposes of this table, we assumed a urinary creatinine concentration of 1 g/L.

Box 26-2

Steps in the Selection Process

Determine need
Define requirements
- Application
- Methodological
- Performance

Review literature
Select candidate methods

may be dictated by the age and lack of operational reliability of the present method.

Application Characteristics

After the need for a new method or analyzer has been determined, all the practical features required of the method are defined. These are termed *application characteristics* (Box 26-3). Emphasis may be placed on **sample** size for pediatric

Box 26-3

Application Characteristics

Sample size
Turnaround time
Sample throughput rate
Specimen type
Automated calibration
Online quality control review
Self-diagnostics
Laboratory space required
Reagent storage facilities required
Availability and skill of laboratory staff
Time available for training
Cost per test
Safety and environmental hazards

applications, on turnaround time and interrupt features for stat. applications, and on the sample throughput rate for high-volume screening applications. It is essential that a candidate method meet these fundamental requirements before it is considered further.

Cost per test is an important application characteristic because cost can be considered separately in light of the present emphasis on reducing medical costs. The factors that affect direct cost should be considered when candidate methods are compared. These include the depreciated capital cost, reagent (including water for many analyzers) and supplies costs, service and repair costs, computer interface cost, and labor cost. Much of this information, including initial equipment cost, estimated reagent and supplies consumption and costs, and estimated productivity and service costs (by contract or per visit), is available from the manufacturer. Other information, such as expected workload and anticipated modifications in productivity based on internal QC procedures, is available from within the laboratory. Users must adjust this information to their own laboratory situations. By far, the largest cost component is labor, which usually accounts for more than 75% of the total. If the laboratory wishes to add new tests in a way that minimizes added overall cost, new tests that have the smallest labor component should be considered for evaluation, given that other attributes are acceptable.

Method Characteristics

The next step in the selection process is the definition of ideal methodological characteristics that will enable the selected method to have a good chance for success in the user's laboratory. These characteristics include preferred methodology that potentially will have the necessary chemical specificity (freedom from **interferences**) and chemical sensitivity (ability to detect small quantities or changes in analyte concentration). The ability to use primary aqueous standards for calibration (freedom from matrix effects) is also important. Reagents, temperature, reaction time, measurement time, and measurement approach (such as end-point, two-point, or multipoint kinetic methods) are all characteristics of a method and should be defined. A source of recommended principles for clinical chemistry methods has been developed by the National Reference System for the Clinical Laboratory (NRSCL).[40]

Analytical Performance Characteristics

The method should also be defined in terms of its analytical performance capabilities. Overall goals for analytical performance have been discussed in terms of allowable error based on the medical application of the test and on proficiency testing requirements. Other aspects of performance that must be defined include working range of the method (**analytical measurement range,** which may or may not be the same as the linear range), stability of the reagents and calibration materials, ability of the analyzer to detect reagent depletion in the case of enzyme substrates, expected reference range, amount of error caused by interfering substances, precision (within-run, between-run, between-day, and total), and accuracy of the method (determined by comparison of results vs. those obtained by a reference or standard method). Although the manufacturer is required to provide information about precision and accuracy, the selected method must be evaluated experimentally to determine whether the method's actual performance in the user's laboratory is good enough to meet the medical application needs of the user's institution. The manufacturer's claimed performance should be considered as a starting point for determining actual performance in the user's laboratory setting.

Next, the technical and professional literature and proficiency testing data should be reviewed to determine what methods are available and to obtain some information about their application and methodological and performance characteristics. It is also very useful to confer with colleagues about their experiences and recommendations.

The final step in the selection process involves putting all the information together to arrive at a final choice. The use of a rating scheme enables a more objective overall ranking of candidate methods.[41,42] This rating scheme can be customized by the use of appropriate weighting factors for the characteristics that are more important. The final choice may include several candidate methods that meet the desired criteria. These methods then can be subjected to the evaluation process described later, so the method with the best analytical performance characteristics is selected.

KEY CONCEPT BOX 26-2

New methods are selected as candidates for evaluation based on how well their application, method, and performance characteristics match the needs of the laboratory.

SECTION OBJECTIVES BOX 26-3

- Define "random analytical error," and list five factors that contribute to it.
- List causes of within-run variation; within-day variation, between-run variation; and between-day variation.
- Define the following terms: systematic analytical error, constant systematic error, and proportional systematic error.
- Evaluate graphs of comparison-of-methods experiments to identify constant or proportional systematic error.
- List causes of both constant and proportional systematic error.

LABORATORY EVALUATION OF A METHOD

Usually a method-evaluation study is performed not to test all methods to determine the method with the smallest error, but to determine whether the selected method yields acceptably small analytical error. The process of method evaluation involves estimation of the magnitude of analytical error for a single patient specimen. Laboratory experiments performed to obtain data for estimating errors are chosen because they result in quantitative estimates of random and systematic errors with a minimum of experimental work. The error estimates obtained may be invalid, however, if certain underlying assumptions are not true. These assumptions include operator familiarity with the method's procedure; the stability of calibrators, controls, and reagents; and linearity of response throughout the working range.

Familiarization

It is essential that operators of the method become thoroughly familiar with the details of the method and of instrument operation before data that will be used to characterize the method's performance are collected. This familiarization period has been addressed by CLSI[4,7,9,10] and may include training by the manufacturer. It should be of sufficient duration that, at its completion, operators can comfortably perform all aspects of the method or instrument operation. Obviously, time needed for device familiarization varies with the complexity of the method or analyzer.

Stability

Verification of the stability of reagents, calibrators, and control materials, especially those prepared in-house, can be a lengthy procedure. The matter is simplified considerably for commercially prepared materials. The manufacturer's expiration date can be used during the method evaluation because serious stability problems will be detectable through unacceptable analytical performance of the method. For in-house preparations, it is necessary to document these characteristics. Preliminary studies should be performed with crossover analyses that compare the results of patient samples analyzed using both fresh calibrators and old calibrators and fresh reagents to test the stability of calibrators. This should be done several times, and the differences for each specific age of calibrator should be averaged to reduce the effects of different preparations. Similarly, the stability of reagents can be tested by periodically (daily, weekly, or monthly, depending on the anticipated decay rate) preparing new reagents and testing them against the older reagents by analyzing patient samples under both configurations of reagents. The older reagents should be stored under specified conditions for subsequent measurements. Observed differences between the old and new reagents can be tested with the use of a *t*-test (see pp. 426 and 494).

Analytical Measurement Range (Linearity)

The International Federation of Clinical Chemistry has defined the analytical range in a qualitative sense, stating that it is "the range of concentration or other quantity in the specimen over which the method is applicable without modification."[1] CLIA '88 regulations do not explicitly require that a "linearity" experiment be performed but instead discuss "verification" of the reportable range,[3] which is the range defined by a minimum (or zero) value and maximum-value calibration material. The College of American Pathologists (CAP) uses the term *analytical measurement range,* or AMR, to mean the same as the reportable range. When the limits of linearity are studied experimentally, the range of concentrations included should at least encompass the limits claimed by the manufacturer. The absolute minimum number of different concentrations that must be measured for linearity verification is three. Replicate measurements, at least in duplicate, should be made on each concentration sample.

Random and Systematic Error

In general, errors that affect the performance of analytical procedures are classified as either random or systematic. Factors that contribute to **random analytical error (RE)** are those that affect the reproducibility of the measurement. These include (1) instability of the instrument; (2) variations in temperature; (3) variations in reagents and calibrators (and calibration curve stability); (4) variability in handling techniques such as pipetting, mixing, and timing; and (5) variability in operators. These factors superimpose their effects on each other at different times. Some cause rapid fluctuations, and others occur over a longer time. Thus RE has different components of variation that are related to the actual laboratory setting. The *within-run* component of variation (σ_{wr}) is caused by specific steps in the procedure, such as sampling and pipetting precision, and by short-term variations in the temperature and stability of the instrument. Within-day, between-run variation (σ_{br}) is caused by instability of the calibration curve or by differences in recalibration that occur throughout the day, longer-term variations in the instrument, small changes in the condition of the calibrator and reagents, changes in the condition of the laboratory during the day, and fatigue of the laboratory staff. The between-day component of variation (σ_{bd}) is caused by variations in the instrument that occur over days, changes in calibrators and reagents (especially if new vials are opened each day), and changes in staff from day to day. Although it is not a truly

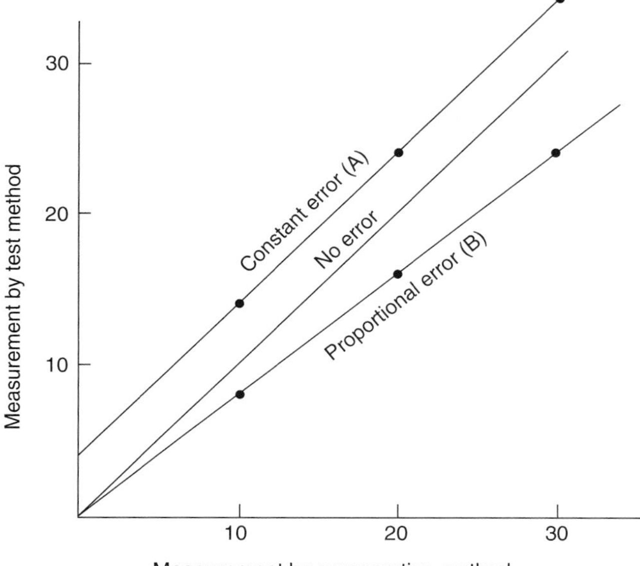

Fig. 26-1 Constant and proportional errors. (From Westgard JO, et al: Concepts and practices in the evaluation of laboratory methods. I. Background and approach, Am J Med Technol 44:290, 1978.)

random component of variation, any drift in the stability of the calibration curve over time greatly affects the between-day component of variation as well. These components can be combined in such a way as to produce an estimate of the total **variance** of a method (σ_t^2).

$$\sigma_t^2 = \sigma_{wr}^2 + \sigma_{br}^2 + \sigma_{bd}^2 \qquad \text{Eq. 26-4}$$

Terms used to indicate RE include *precision,* ***imprecision,*** *reproducibility,* and *repeatability.* In each case, these terms refer to the random dispersion of results or measurements around some point of central tendency.

Systematic analytical error (SE), or **trueness,** describes error that is consistently low or high. If the error is consistently low or high by the same amount, regardless of the analyte concentration, it is called **constant systematic error** (CE) (Fig. 26-1). If the error is consistently low or high by an amount proportional to the concentration of the analyte, it is called **proportional systematic error** (PE).

Factors that contribute to CE are independent of the analyte concentration, and the magnitude of this error is constant throughout the concentration range of the analyte. CE is caused by an interfering substance in all samples or in reagents that gives rise to a false signal. The error can be positive or negative. A reaction between an interfering substance and the reagents that is caused by a lack of specificity is an example of a CE. Another cause of systematic error is an interfering substance that interferes in the reaction between the analyte and the reagents. This type of error is seen in enzymatic methods that use oxidase-peroxidase–coupled reactions, in which the hydrogen peroxide intermediate is destroyed by endogenous reducing agents, such as ascorbic acid. An interfering substance also may inhibit or destroy the reagent, causing it to remain at suboptimal quantities for the reaction with the analyte. A nonchemical source of CE is the error caused by improper blanking of the sample or the reagents.

PE most often is caused by incorrect assignment of the amount of substance in the calibrator. If the calibrator has more analyte than is labeled, all unknown determinations will be low; less analyte than is labeled will result in a positive error. The error will be proportional to the original calibration error. PE also may be caused by a side reaction of the analyte. The percentage of analyte that undergoes a side reaction will be the percentage of error in the method.

KEY CONCEPTS BOX 26-3

- Linearity (analytical measurement range) is evaluated by replicate testing of a series of materials in which the relationship of increasing analyte concentrations is known.
- Random error (imprecision) is evaluated by replicate testing of stable materials within a single day and over many days. The total standard deviation quantifies random error. Its components are the within-run, between-run, and between-day standard deviations.
- Constant error is evaluated by testing the effects of potential interfering substances.
- Proportional error is evaluated by testing the amount of pure analyte recovered when it is added to patient samples.

SECTION OBJECTIVES BOX 26-4

- Explain the purpose, process, and interpretation of replication experiments, interference studies, recovery experiments, and linearity studies,
- Explain what is meant by "limit of detection" and "limit of quantitation" and how they are determined experimentally.

EXPERIMENTS TO ESTIMATE MAGNITUDE OF SPECIFIC ERRORS

In designing experiments that will be used to determine the analytical errors of a method, it is imperative that the experiments be carefully conceived to avoid ambiguous conclusions. The aim of this section is to describe specific experiments that will enable estimation of the magnitude of a specific error. The size of the error then can be compared with the allowable error to determine the acceptability of the method. This approach is used for all types of errors described previously. Each type of error is considered individually before combinations of errors are considered. Fig. 26-2 presents an organization of experiments to be performed for specific error determinations, arranged in such a way that the easy experiments can be done first. The more extensive (and expensive) final studies are performed only if the errors estimated by these preliminary experiments are acceptable.

Type of Analytical Error	Evaluation Experiments	
	Preliminary	Final
Random error	Replication within-run Pure materials Real samples	Replication run-to-run Real samples
Constant error	Interference	Comparison with comparative method
Proportional error	Recovery	
Other systematic errors	Linearity Limit of detection	

Fig. 26-2 Specific evaluation experiments for estimating specific types of analytical error. (From Westgard JO, et al: Concepts and practices in the evaluation of laboratory methods. I. Background and approach, Am J Med Technol 44:290, 1978.)

Random Error Estimated from Replication Studies

The within-run **replication experiment** is the simplest type of study and should be one of the first performed to assess the performance of a new method. Because it allows assessment of precision over a very short time, the results cannot be extrapolated to indicate long-term performance. The short-term performance must be judged acceptable before the long-term performance of the method is studied.

The replication study should be performed with samples whose matrix is as similar as possible to that of the intended patient samples. The concentrations to be studied should be at or near the medical decision concentrations for the analyte. This is where the laboratory data will be interpreted most critically; thus the method's performance at these concentrations must be ensured.

An estimate of RE is developed by consideration of repeated analyses of the same specimen. Sixty-eight percent of the results are within ±1.0 SD of the test mean, and 95% of the results are within 1.96 SD of the mean (see p. 422). Using the error budget approach recommended by Westgard and Burnett,[36] we define the RE as four times the SD. If the estimate of RE is less than the allowable error, the RE is acceptable. An example of the calculation of RE is shown on p. 501.

CLSI EP5-A2 is designed for evaluation of precision and verification of manufacturers' precision claims.[10] It requires duplicate measurements on sample pools that contain at least two different levels of the analyte in a run, two runs per day, for 20 days. An analysis of variance calculation is used to determine within-run, within-day, and day-to-day components of variance. These are combined to estimate the total SD.

Constant Error Estimated from Interference Studies

The **interference experiment** measures the CE caused by the presence of a substance suspected of interfering with the test method. To perform the study, a sample that is spiked with the interferent is used. The volume of this addition should be small, less than 10% of the sample volume, so that disruption of the matrix is minimal. To compensate for the dilution of the spiked sample, a baseline sample should be prepared by adding to another aliquot of the sample an equal amount of the solvent that was used for the interferent. The two samples should then be analyzed, at least in duplicate. The difference between results in the two samples is attributable to an interference caused by the added substance.

A scheme for studying the effects of hemolysis involves taking two blood samples. One is centrifuged and analyzed directly (baseline sample), and the red blood cells in the other blood tube are physically traumatized to rupture the cell membranes to yield an elevated amount of serum hemoglobin. After centrifugation, this hemolyzed sample is analyzed. The difference between the two samples is attributable to the effects of hemolysis. Mild, moderate, or severe hemolysis may be simulated, depending on the volume of red blood cells traumatized. This approach is more consistent with the actual problems encountered in the laboratory than is the approach in which pure hemoglobin is added to a sample. However, this procedure is not valid if red blood cells contain the analyte.

The effects of lipemia may be studied by dividing a lipemic sample into two portions and analyzing one directly while centrifuging the other with an ultrahigh-speed centrifuge to remove the lipoproteins before analysis. The difference in results is attributable to the effects of lipemia. Alternatively, turbid specimens may be prepared for each decision-level concentration by adding small quantities of lipid-containing materials (e.g., IntraLipid [Baxter Healthcare Corporation, Deerfield Park, IL], Lyposin [Abbott Laboratories, Abbott Park, IL]) to nonlipemic specimens of appropriate analyte concentrations to obtain slightly, moderately, and grossly lipemic samples. Baseline concentrations are prepared by adding equal volumes of water to the original specimens.

Pools with increased amounts of unconjugated bilirubin are produced from a stock solution of bilirubin prepared by dissolving pure bilirubin in dimethylsulfoxide to 250 mg/dL. Clear, nonicteric patient sera are spiked to the desired bilirubin concentration. Baseline specimens are prepared as already described. This technique does not test the effect of the more water-soluble conjugated bilirubin on the analysis.

The choice of substances to be tested is almost infinite. For all spectrophotometric methods, the effects of hemolysis, icterus, and lipemia should be determined. Other substances that have been reported to affect methods similar to the one under review should be tested (see CLSI guideline EP7-A2).[7]

Pipetting should be (1) precise so that baseline and spiked samples reflect the same extent of dilution and (2) accurate so that a known amount of interfering substance is added. Again, it is important that the concentration of the analyte in the sample be near medical-decision levels. A substance that is a possible interferent should be added so that its final concentration is at the maximum physiologically expected concentration. If no errors are caused at this high concentration, it can be assumed that lower concentrations will not adversely affect the performance of the method. If an error is too large at the maximum concentration of interfering substance, it is appropriate to test the interference at lower concentrations. A slightly icteric sample may be acceptable, but a grossly icteric one may not. It is recommended that these interference studies be conducted on the **comparative method** (see later discussion) at the same time, as a way of checking on the experimental technique.

An example of the calculation of CE from data obtained from an interference experiment is shown on p. 502. The overall average difference (bias) is called a *constant error* because it is independent of the analyte concentration. This CE is compared directly with the allowable error budgeted for an interference for the appropriate decision level, $E_{A,I}$, where $E_{A,I}$ is some fraction of E_A. If the CE is less than $E_{A,I}$, the CE caused by the interference is judged acceptable. This decision is based on clinical limits instead of on a statistical test of significance (see p. 483), and the SD of the interference values is a measure of the uncertainty of the estimated CE.

CLSI guideline EP7-A2 presents two approaches for interference testing in the clinical chemistry laboratory.[7] The first one is similar to that already discussed. The second describes the determination of interferences with increasing concentrations of interferent (dose-response method). This guideline also presents extensive lists of exogenous and endogenous interferents and recommended testing concentrations.

Proportional Error Estimated from a Recovery Experiment

Another preliminary study is the **recovery experiment.** This procedure involves the addition of a known amount of analyte to an aliquot of sample. As in the interference experiment, the sample is divided into two aliquots. One aliquot is spiked with a stock solution that contains the analyte. An equal volume of diluent is added to the second; this is the baseline sample. The two samples are then analyzed. The baseline sample provides the original amount of analyte. The difference between the results of analyses of the spiked sample and the baseline sample indicates the amount of added analyte that is "recovered." The amount of analyte added to the sample is calculated from the concentration of the stock solution of the analyte and the volume added. The volume of analyte added to the sample should be less than 10% to avoid major disruption of the sample matrix. Pipetting accuracy is critical because the amount of added analyte is calculated from the volume. The concentration of the sample and the amount added should be such that they test the performance of the method near the medical decision levels of the analyte. In some instances, a very small amount of analyte is added to the sample, and the amount recovered is lost in the randomness of the method. Thus it is advisable to make two to four measurements on each sample to reduce the effects of the imprecision of the method. Analysis of these samples with the comparison method is recommended as a check on the experimental technique.

The calculation of recovery is illustrated with an example on p. 503. *Recovery* is defined as the ratio of the amount of analyte recovered to the amount added and is given as a percentage. The difference between the calculated percentage of recovery and 100% recovery is the percentage of PE. The SD of the percentage of recovery is a measure of the uncertainty of the percentage of PE. The percentage of PE cannot be directly compared with E_A to decide acceptability because the percentage of PE is not given in concentration units. PE can be converted to concentration units at the medical-decision level, as shown on pp. 503 and 504. If the PE is less than $E_{A,R}$ (where $E_{A,R}$ is some fraction of E_A), then PE is acceptable. Again, the decision is based on medical requirements rather than on statistical tests of significance.

Error Caused by Nonlinearity

An initial linearity study could use aqueous standards to identify the capabilities of the method in an ideal specimen matrix. This should be followed by analysis of the analyte in a dilution series of samples containing the biological matrix,[9] such as serum or urine, that will be used for patient tests. Each sample should be tested at least in duplicate. The aqueous and matrix samples will provide important information about the influence of the biological matrix on the method.

It may be difficult to prepare specimens in a biological matrix with a range of analyte concentrations from zero to the limit of linearity. For analytes not normally present in the matrix, such as drugs, the analyte is simply added to an analyte-free specimen to obtain the desired maximum concentration, and a dilution series is prepared using analyte-free serum or urine. Diluting stock aqueous pools of analyte with human serum albumin or enzyme-inactivated serum can also approximate serum matrices. A patient specimen that contains the analyte at a concentration known to exceed the linearity of the method can also be used, and then a dilution series can be constructed using analyte-free materials. The accuracy of the volumetric dilutions is very important, and serial dilutions are not recommended because errors are propagated through subsequent samples. Rather, each sample should be prepared by direct dilution from the original high sample or pool. For commonly measured analytes, linearity materials are available from commercial sources and proficiency testing providers.

Finally, all data points should be plotted for visual inspection of linear performance. The actual result of analysis of each dilution is plotted against the percentage of high pool present in each dilution (or against known concentrations). The straight portion of the resulting curve represents the

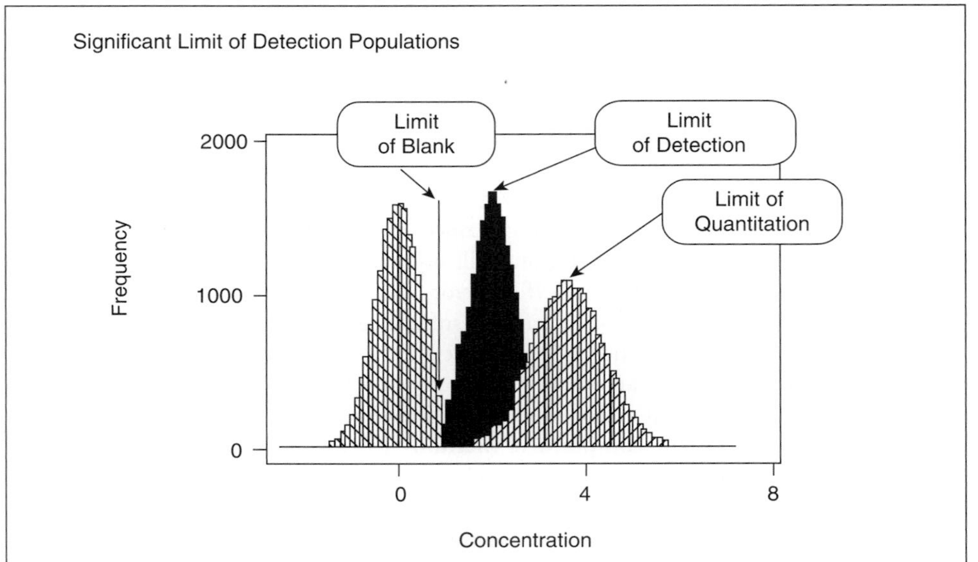

Fig. 26-3 Illustration of different aspects of analytical sensitivity or detection limits.

linear portion of the assay. In the case of methods with curvilinear response, such as enzyme immunoassay (EIA) procedures, results obtained from the recommended curve-straightening algorithms should be plotted to show linearity of final results. If linearity is not certain on visual inspection, the significance of the degree of nonlinearity can be tested statistically.[9,43] If the statistical test shows that the degree of nonlinearity is statistically significant (calculations are described in detail in CLSI EP6-A[9]), the error (measured in terms of concentration) caused by nonlinearity can be determined at the concentration of each material tested in the experiment. The concentration error due to nonlinearity then can be compared with a stated allowable error budgeted for nonlinearity $E_{A,L}$, where $E_{A,L}$ is some fraction of E_A. If the concentration error due to nonlinearity is less than $E_{A,L}$, the degree of nonlinearity is acceptable.

Sensitivity (Limit of Detection)

Several terms describe the different aspects of the minimum analytical sensitivity of a method.[8] These terms are demonstrated graphically in Fig. 26-3. The **limit of blank (LOB)** is the highest value of a zero sample. Typically, a specimen with zero concentration, or blank, is tested repeatedly, and the limit of blank is taken as an upper confidence limit of the resulting population of blank values. It is calculated from the mean and SD of the blank values.

$$\text{Limit of Blank} = \overline{Y}_{blank} + z \times SD_{blank} \quad \text{Eq. 26-5}$$

When the limit of blank is calculated using typical values for "z" of 2 or 3, it represents the upper 97.72% or 99.87% confidence limit of the blank. If the method under evaluation reports negative results as zero, it may be necessary to collect data in terms of raw signal units and convert them into concentration units before performing this calculation. *Note:* This threshold can be viewed as a qualitative definition of analytical sensitivity, providing an indication as to whether analyte is *absent* or *present* (a no/yes response based on the result compared with this value). This threshold also may be determined nonparametrically (see CLSI EP17-A[8]).

The **limit of detection (LOD)** is the minimum concentration of analyte whose presence can be qualitatively detected under defined conditions; it is also the concentration at which an observed value will be very likely to exceed the limit of the blank. It is the mean of the population in the center of Fig. 26-3 and is calculated as the upper confidence limit of the blank ($\overline{Y}_{blank} + z \times SD_{blank}$) plus two or three times the SD of the result of a spiked sample whose concentration is close to this value.

$$\text{Limit of Detection} = \overline{Y}_{blank} + z \times SD_{blank} + z \times SD_{spike} \quad \text{Eq. 26-6}$$

Often, the standard deviation of a sample with concentration near zero is equal to the standard deviation of the blank, and Equation 26-6 becomes

$$\text{Limit of Detection} = \overline{Y}_{blank} + 2 \times (z \times SD_{blank}) \quad \text{Eq. 26-6, A}$$

Defined in this manner, limit of detection is 4 to 6 SD_{blank} above the average value for a zero sample.

The **limit of quantitation (LOQ)** is the minimum concentration of analyte whose presence can be quantitatively measured reliably under defined conditions. It is the lowest actual concentration at which the precision performance of the measurement is less than the allowable error. Determining the LOQ involves testing method precision at several low concentrations until the concentration with the desired precision is determined. The limit of quantitation can be as low as the limit of detection, but not lower.

KEY CONCEPTS BOX 26-4

- Interference should be evaluated for all commonly encountered interferents, especially including hemolysis, lipemia, and icterus. The effect of interference is expressed as "constant" error in analyte concentration units and is compared with allowable error allocated to interference.
- Proportional error, estimated by a recovery experiment, detects problems with calibration and side reactions. Proportional error is expressed in concentration units and is compared with allowable error allocated to proportional error.
- Error due to nonlinearity is quantified by differences between the observed value and the value predicted from a straight line and is compared with allowable error allocated to nonlinearity.
- Three terms define the analytical sensitivity of a method at low concentrations: limit of blank, limit of detection (lowest concentration that can be detected as present), and limit of quantitation (lowest reportable concentration).

SECTION OBJECTIVES BOX 26-5

- Explain why the between-day replication experiment must be over a period of at least twenty days.
- Explain the purpose and process of the comparison-of-methods experiment.
- List at least three requirements for patient specimens used in the comparison-of-methods experiment.
- Evaluate the application of *t*-test statistics and correlation coefficients to determine the degree of difference between the test and comparison methods.
- Evaluate linear-regression statistics to determine proportionality, random variation, and systematic error between the test and comparison methods.

FINAL-EVALUATION EXPERIMENTS

Final-evaluation experiments take the most time to perform and potentially yield the most definitive information about the test method's day-to-day performance on real patient specimens.

Between-Day Replication Experiment

The between-day replication experiment is an expansion of the within-run experiment over many days, usually 20. This period must be long enough to allow the random effects that occur over several days to influence the long-term estimate of RE. This experiment and the comparison-of-methods experiment described next usually are combined in the study for better efficiency.

A material known to be stable for the time of the experiment is used, usually a frozen serum or plasma pool or a lyophilized control product. Aliquot-to-aliquot variation of the material must be minimal because it will appear to be day-to-day variance of the test method.

RE is estimated as four times the total SD and is compared with E_A, as was described previously for the within-run study.

Comparison-of-Methods Experiment

The **comparison-of-methods experiment** determines the systematic error of the test method, using real patient specimens. A group of patient specimens are analyzed by both the test method and a comparative method, a method known to be accurate and precise. Systematic differences between the two methods are interpreted as errors of the test method if results of the comparison method are known to have little or no error (negligible random and systematic errors). Thus the comparative method should be of the highest quality possible so that errors will not be erroneously assigned to the test method.

Quality of the Comparative Method

Through a process of "traceability," the quality of a laboratory method can be documented back to an internationally recognized reference method, analogous to an animal's pedigree.[44-46] A system of credentialing reference materials and reference methods has been established by the International Union of Pure and Applied Chemistry and the International Federation of Clinical Chemistry, called the Joint Committee for Traceability in Laboratory Medicine, to form the basis for defining the accurate measurement of specific analytes. Accuracy is transferred from the reference materials and reference methods down to routine test methods at several different stages. Accuracy is transferred from reference material to secondary standards and national reference methods, to working standards and standard methods within a manufacturing organization, which, in turn, may serve as the basis for commercial reagents and calibrators that are used in the clinical laboratory. Although it is expected that most general chemistry tests are amenable to this traceability scheme, most immunoassays do not lend themselves to this traceability model because of the existence of matrix effects that affect commutability and different specificities of antibody reagents when reference method reagents are compared with routine method reagents.[45,46]

Awareness has increased regarding standardization of laboratory testing to better serve the needs of a worldwide mobile society and to improve patient safety. An example of the traceability of creatinine methods is shown in Fig. 26-4.

Accuracy or trueness (based on traceability to reference materials and reference methods when they exist) is more important than "relative accuracy," based on comparison of a new method to another routine method. On the other hand, it is important to predict for customers how results from the test method compare with those of the routine method being replaced, although differences between the two methods should be interpreted cautiously unless the comparative method is known to be of high quality.

At least 40 and preferably 100 or more patient specimens should be analyzed. These should include the variety of disease states that will be encountered by the test in routine use. Analyte concentrations of the specimens should be distributed evenly throughout the analytical range; otherwise, regression analysis of the comparison data will be inaccurate. However, even distributions are not always practical.

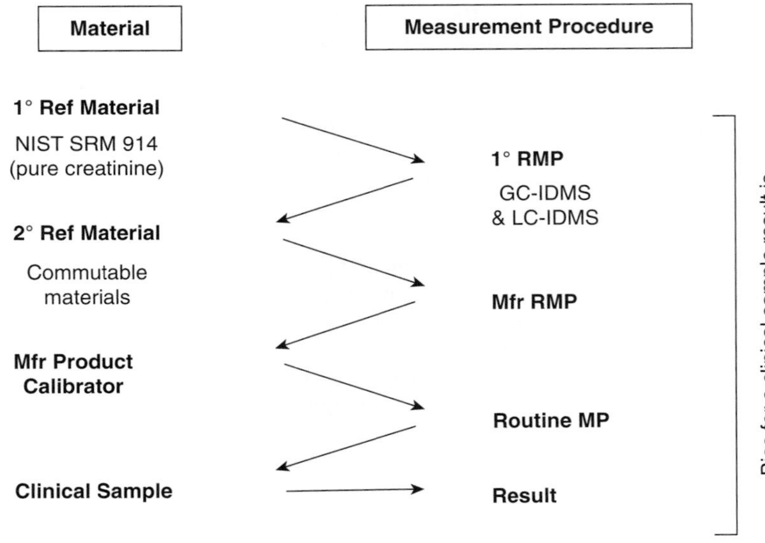

Fig. 26-4 Traceability of creatinine methods proposed by the National Kidney Foundation. (Adapted from ISO: *17511, In Vitro Diagnostic Medical Devices—Measurement of quantities in biological samples—Metrological Traceability of Values Assigned to Calibrators and Control Materials,* Geneva, Switzerland, 2003, International Standards Organization.)

CLSI guideline EP9-A2[4] for comparison of methods suggests some alternative distributions of patient sample concentrations. Hemolyzed, lipemic, and icteric specimens should be included if they are not proscribed by the manufacturer of the test method, and if they do not cause errors in the comparative method. If included in the study, they should be identified. Specimens must be carefully selected from the routine workload to serve as an efficient representation of the patient mix and of the AMR; preanalysis by the routine method is usually necessary. Specimens are analyzed in duplicate by each method to facilitate checks for outliers. Results should be examined carefully and plotted daily. Any specimen with large differences between results for duplicate pairs within a method or between paired results between methods should be reanalyzed in duplicate by both methods in the next run. A large difference (outlier) is defined as being greater than four times the average difference (using the within-assay difference or the between-assay difference as appropriate).[4] If the large between-method difference is confirmed for a given specimen, the patient should be investigated for disease(s) present that might affect one of the methods, and the specimen should be checked for other analytes (possible interferents) to determine the cause of the large difference. An immediate follow-up examination is essential to avoid later unanswerable questions about outliers.

Specimens should be tested on the test method and the comparative method at the same time, or as close in time to each other as possible. If this is not possible, specimens must be stored in a manner that guarantees analyte stability.

The comparison-of-methods experiment usually is combined with the between-day replication experiment. Patient specimens should be spread evenly over at least five runs, preferably all 20 runs, to ensure that day-to-day effects have a chance to influence the data and to ensure that day-to-day effects are "fully confounded" (in statistical parlance). Both methods must be maintained with acceptable QC during the period.

t-Test Statistics: Bias, S_d

Systematic differences between the test and comparative methods are estimated most easily with the comparison-of-methods data by the bias. The bias is the difference between the average result by the test method and the average result by the comparative method. Bias can indicate the magnitude of the systematic error between the two methods. (Each patient specimen must be analyzed by both methods for bias to be valid.) Bias is calculated by Eq. 26-7, in which y_i and x_i are the analyte concentrations of individual specimens by the test method and the comparative method, respectively, and N is the number of paired results compared.

$$\text{Bias} = \frac{\sum (y_i - x_i)}{N} \qquad \text{Eq. 26-7}$$

The standard deviation about the bias, called the *standard deviation of the difference,* s_d, is calculated in a manner analogous to that used to calculate the SD in the replication experiment. The s_d may be viewed as an indicator of random variation between the two methods.

$$s_d = \sqrt{\frac{\sum (y_i - x_i - \text{Bias})^2}{(N-1)}} \qquad \text{Eq. 26-8}$$

The statistical significance of the bias, that is, whether it really differs from zero, or no bias, is determined by use of the t-test. A t-value is calculated according to the following formula:

$$t = \frac{\text{Bias}\sqrt{N}}{s_d} \qquad \text{Eq. 26-9}$$

The t-value is the ratio of a systematic error term (bias) to a random error term (s_d). If the bias increases relative to the **standard deviation of differences,** there is less of a probability that the observed bias is caused by random variations and more of a probability that there really is a systematic difference

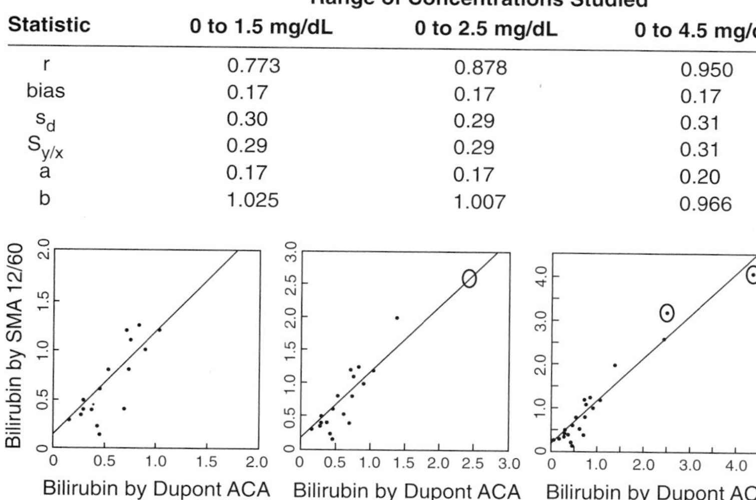

Statistic	Range of Concentrations Studied 0 to 1.5 mg/dL	0 to 2.5 mg/dL	0 to 4.5 mg/dL
r	0.773	0.878	0.950
bias	0.17	0.17	0.17
s_d	0.30	0.29	0.31
$S_{y/x}$	0.29	0.29	0.31
a	0.17	0.17	0.20
b	1.025	1.007	0.966

Fig. 26-5 Effect of range of data on correlation coefficient, *r.* (From Westgard JO, et al: Concepts and practices in the evaluation of laboratory methods. III. Statistics, Am J Med Technol 44:552, 1978.)

between the test and comparative method mean values. For example, in a comparison of glucose methods, there were 101 specimens, the bias was 3 mg/dL, and the *t*-value was 2.11. The critical *t*-value for $p = 0.05$ and for 100 degrees of freedom (obtainable from a statistics textbook) is 1.99. (The two-sided critical *t*-value is used because the bias could be either positive or negative.) The calculated *t*-value exceeds the critical *t*-value; therefore, a statistically real bias exists between the two methods (see also p. 426).

The acceptability of the systematic error, as estimated by the bias, is judged by comparison with $E_{A,MD}$, where $E_{A,MD}$ is some fraction of E_A budgeted for allowable error for method difference. If bias is less than $E_{A,MD}$, the systematic error is acceptable. If bias exceeds $E_{A,MD}$, the systematic error is not acceptable. Decisions about acceptability should never be based on the *t* value alone. A large bias and a large s_d may combine to yield an insignificant *t*-value, even though the bias is unacceptably large. Also from this equation, it can be seen that if *N* is very large, the value of *t* can become statistically significant for some ratio of bias to s_d, indicating a statistically significant bias even though that bias may be medically unimportant.

Westgard and Hunt[47] have shown that bias can result in inaccurate estimates of systematic error if a PE is present, because both proportional and constant errors are combined in the bias. PE also increases s_d. Bias should not be used as an estimator of systematic error unless PE is absent, or unless the mean analyte concentration as measured by the comparative method is very near the decision-level concentration (X_C) and the data are well distributed around X_C. Otherwise, the bias will be weighted toward the side of X_C that has the greatest number of samples with large individual biases.

Correlation Coefficient

The statistic most frequently cited in reports of comparison-of-methods experiments is the correlation coefficient (*r*). An *r*-value of zero indicates that there is no correlation between methods. A value of +1 indicates perfect positive correlation. See Chapter 23 for a more extensive discussion of the calculation of **linear-regression** statistics and their interpretation.

The correlation coefficient is misused frequently in method-evaluation reports. Westgard and Hunt[47] demonstrated that the correlation coefficient is extremely sensitive to the range of analyte concentrations of patient specimens in the comparison-of-methods experiment. In a comparison of bilirubin methods over a range of 0 to 4.5 mg/dL, a correlation coefficient of 0.950 was obtained. When data pairs with bilirubin concentrations above 1.5 mg/dL were eliminated, the correlation coefficient dropped to 0.773. This is shown in Fig. 26-5.

The correlation coefficient is simply a way of looking for a correlation, not agreement, between pairs. Thus, if the values for one population were twice those of the other, then as one population's value doubled, the other population's value would double as well. The correlation between the two methods would be excellent (high *r*). Thus decisions about the acceptability of the analytical performance of a method should never be based on the value of the correlation coefficient alone.

Linear-Regression Statistics

If the test method and the comparative method do correlate with each other, an *x*:*y* plot of results resembles a straight line, which can be described by the linear-regression expression

$$Y_i = a + bx_i \qquad \text{Eq. 26-10}$$

in which Y_i is the calculated value on the straight line corresponding to the actual comparative method result, x_i. The proportionality between the methods is given by the slope, *b*, the **ideal value** of which (no proportional error) is 1.00. CE is indicated by the *y* intercept, *a*. Random variation between the methods is indicated by the standard error of the regression, $s_{y,x}$, also called the **standard error of the estimate,** or the *standard deviation of the residuals.*

An estimate of systematic error at X_C, the decision-level concentration, may be obtained from the linear-regression statistics by substitution of X_C for x_i in Eq. 26-10, to calculate Y_C, the concentration the test method would measure for a specimen whose true analyte concentration is designated as X_C. The systematic error, SE, is calculated by subtraction of X_C from this Y_C:

$$SE = |Y_C - X_C| = |a + bX_C - X_C| \qquad \text{Eq. 26-11}$$

SE is acceptable if the absolute value is less than the allowable error budgeted for method differences, $E_{A,MD}$, which is some fraction of the allowable error, E_A. This estimate of error will be valid only if the following limitations of linear regression are observed.

The data used to calculate the regression equation (see Eq. 26-10) must first be plotted and carefully examined for nonlinearity, and the data used for the final calculation must be limited to data in the **linear range.** Nonlinearity at higher concentrations will lower the slope, increase the y-intercept, and increase $s_{y,x}$.

The importance of daily examination and plotting of comparison-of-methods data cannot be overemphasized, and the data must be examined carefully for outliers. A commonly used definition of an outlier from a regression line is a specimen for which the absolute difference between the test method result, y_i, and the corresponding value on the line Y_i, exceeds $4 \times s_{y,x}$, ($|y_i - Y_i| > 4 \times s_{y,x}$) (see Chapter 23). As was stated before, outlier specimens must be detected immediately and reanalyzed by both methods so the data can correct or confirm the outlier. The linear regression line is "pulled" toward the outlier, with the greatest effects caused by outliers at extreme ranges of the data. Confirmed outliers should be investigated for their causes. A confirmed outlier really is representative of the true analytical performance of the method. The SE of the test method should be calculated both with the outlier included in the data set and with it excluded. If errors are acceptable with the outlier excluded and excessive with it included, extreme caution should be exercised. Other statistical tests can be used for removal of an outlier,[48] but no more than one outlier should be excluded in a set of 40 patient comparisons. If the outlier discrepancy is less than the E_A, do not exclude it, even though it may be a statistically significant outlier. If more than one clinically significant outlier is present per 40 patient comparison samples, the test method should be rejected until a cause for the outliers can be found and corrected.

The range of analytical concentrations must be wide. The effects of a narrow range of data on the least-squares statistics are seen in Fig. 26-6. Methods-comparison data often fail to meet one additional assumption of linear-regression calculations. This assumption requires that the x data (comparison) be known without error. Actually, in a methods-comparison experiment, random errors do affect the results of the comparison method. When the range of data is sufficiently large, the effect of failure to know the x values without error becomes negligible.[49,50]

Wakkers et al[49] have suggested that the correlation coefficient should be used to decide whether the range of data is sufficient for using traditional least-squares calculation. If the correlation coefficient is greater than 0.99, calculation by the traditional least-squares approach will produce a slope whose mathematical error will be less than 1%. If the correlation coefficient is less than 0.99, the slope will be falsely low, and the y intercept will be too high. Cornbleet and Gochman[50] have suggested another decision limit. If the ratio of the

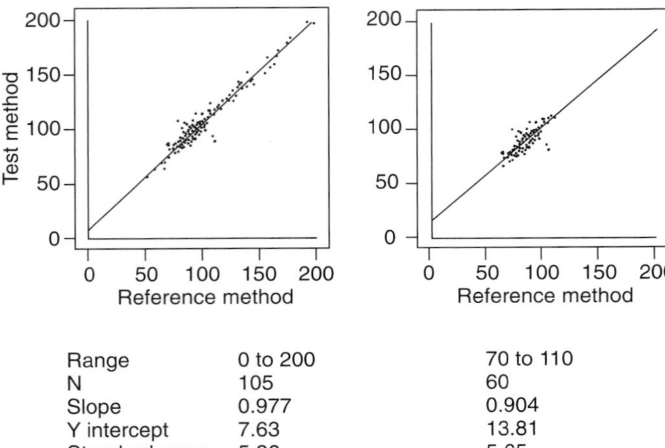

Range	0 to 200	70 to 110
N	105	60
Slope	0.977	0.904
Y intercept	7.63	13.81
Standard error	5.36	5.65

Fig. 26-6 Effect of range of data on linear-regression statistics. (From Westgard JO, Hunt MR: Use and interpretation of statistics in method-comparison studies, Clin Chem 19:49, 1973.)

analytical SD of the comparative (x) method, S_{CM}, to the SD of the x-method population, S_x, is less than 0.2, the least-squares calculation will be appropriate. If these tests on the data fail, more robust regression approaches should be used to calculate regression coefficients, such as those discussed by Cornbleet and Gochman[50] (see also Chapter 23).

One robust regression method, the Deming regression,[49,50] is based upon minimizing the sum of squares of residuals determined perpendicularly from the line (as opposed to only in the y direction by the traditional least-squares method). The Deming approach is much more robust and provides a good estimate of the slope, even when the data are not precise, or when the data are limited to a narrow range (see also p. 434). Another approach, the method of Passing-Bablock,[51] involves drawing a straight line between each pair of data points and then ranking the slopes and selecting the median slope as the best nonparametric estimate of the slope. This approach makes no assumption about the distribution of the data.

Calculation of the SE by the use of linear-regression statistics is demonstrated on p. 504.

KEY CONCEPTS BOX 26-5

- Reliable estimates of long-term random error require 20 or more days of replicate testing. To maintain quality, the standard deviation must be less than one fourth times allowable error, and preferably less than one sixth times allowable error.
- In the comparison-of-methods experiment, a wide range of patient sample concentrations must be obtained to obtain a reliable estimate of systematic error. If this is not possible, ordinary least squares is not accurate; consider using alternative statistical techniques.
- Never use the correlation coefficient alone to judge the equivalence of two methods.
- Avoid making decisions on the acceptability of systematic error on the basis of the t-test alone. Consider the magnitude of the systematic error compared with the allocated allowable error.

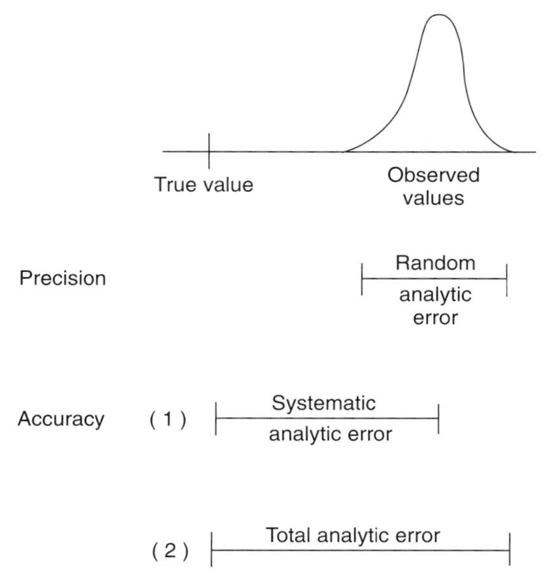

Fig. 26-7 Total analytical error. (From Westgard JO, Carey RN, Wold S: Criteria for judging precision and accuracy in method development and evaluation, Clin Chem 20:825, 1974.)

SECTION OBJECTIVES BOX 26-6

- Evaluate total error and allowable error values to determine if the comparison method's performance is acceptable.
- Interpret medical decision charts to ascertain how complex a quality control procedure should be to ensure acceptable allowable error.
- Discuss the purpose of confidence-interval criteria for random error, constant, proportional, systematic, and total error.
- List two other evaluation protocols that may be used for preliminary evaluation of errors between methods.

ESTIMATION OF TOTAL ERROR

Estimates of RE and SE are combined to estimate the total error (TE) of the test method. This is the most severe criterion for the test method to meet. The rationale for the TE concept is shown in Fig. 26-7. The horizontal line is the error in concentration units, and the vertical line is located at the true value concentration, the medical decision-level concentration, or zero error. The vertical distance from the horizontal line represents the probability of obtaining a test method result at any given amount of error (difference from X_C). The bell-shaped curve shows the distribution of test method data obtained from repeated analyses of a patient specimen whose true analyte concentration is designated as X_C. The distance from the mean of that curve to the **true value** (or **assigned value**) is the SE. The dispersion around the mean of the data is the RE, which is defined as four times the SD. There will be (1) instances in which the combined error will be exactly equal to the SE, (2) other times when the combined error for a given result will be less than the average SE by some amount because of the RE of the method, and (3) other times when the combined error will be greater than the SE, again by some amount caused by the RE of the method. The physician has no way of knowing what the various components of error are, or when they will cause a larger error. Therefore, it is essential to consider the worst-case combination and to define this as total error (TE):

$$TE = RE + SE \qquad \text{Eq. 26-12}$$

If TE is less than E_A, the method's overall performance is acceptable. Calculation of TE is demonstrated on pp. 504-505.

Equations for estimating the magnitude of the various errors and the criteria for judging their acceptability are summarized in Table 26-3.

Table 26-3 Point Estimate Criteria for Acceptable Performance

Type of Error	Criteria
Random (RE)	$4 \times S_{TM} < E_A$
Constant (CE)	$\lvert Bias \rvert < E_{A,I}$
Proportional (PE) in concentration units	$\frac{\lvert \bar{R} - 100 \rvert}{100} \times X_C < E_{A,R}$
Systematic (SE)	If $\bar{X} = X_C, \lvert \bar{Y} - \bar{X} \rvert < E_{A,MD}$ Or $\lvert a + b \times X_C - X_C \rvert < E_{A,MD}$
Total (TE)	$RE + SE = 4 \times S_{TM} + \lvert a + b \times X_C - X_C \rvert < E_A$

where $E_{A,I} = 1/2 \times E_A$, where $E_{A,R} = 1/4 \times E_A$, and where $E_{A,MD} = 1/2 \times E_A$.

Medical Decision Charts

A graphic aid can best illustrate the relationship between method performance (determined in the method-evaluation studies) and QC. If a method's inherent errors are small relative to allowable error, large deviations from the method's usual performance are required for total error to exceed allowable error. Relatively insensitive QC procedures will be able to detect errors before they are large enough to exceed E_A. If a method's inherent errors are larger, smaller deviations from routine performance cause TE to exceed E_A, and more sensitive QC procedures are necessary to ensure adequate error detection. When a method's inherent errors are so large that they frequently exceed E_A (e.g., over 5% of the time), no QC procedure can maintain acceptable performance.

The Medical Decision Chart (also called OpSpecs QC chart) developed by Westgard[37] shows the interrelationship between SD, bias, and E_A (Fig. 26-8). This chart shows that the combination of RE (some multiple of SD) and SE (bias) must be less than the allowable (total) error defined for the assay. The chart is divided into regions according to the magnitude of the SD. From right to left on the chart, these include *Unacceptable, Marginal, Fair, Good,* and *Six Sigma,* according to the complexity of the QC procedure required to maintain the method's errors below the E_A. The lines on the chart are defined by the following equations:

- TE = 2 SD + bias (crosses *y*-axis where SD = 0, or bias = E_A and crosses *x*-axis where bias = 0, hence, 2 SD = E_A, or SD = 50% E_A)

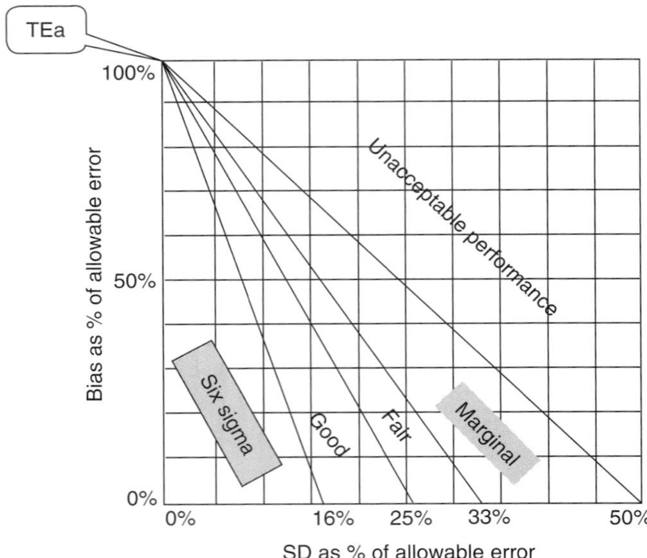

Fig. 26-8 Medical decision chart. In the unacceptable performance region, the standard deviation (SD) exceeds 50% of allowable error (E_A), and precision errors alone will exceed E_A more than 5% of the time, regardless of bias and quality control (QC) procedure. In the marginal performance region, the SD is so large (between 33% and 50% of E_A) that the method's total error is very close to E_A. Only QC procedures with unacceptably high rates of false rejection could maintain errors below E_A. This means many rejected runs. In the fair performance region, QC procedures must be developed carefully to maintain errors below E_A. This can be done with four to six QC measurements per run. In the Good performance region, ordinary multirule QC procedures will detect unacceptable method performance. This will involve two to three QC measurements per run. In the Six Sigma region, relatively weak QC procedures will be sufficient to detect errors that might exceed the E_A. Only one or two QC measurements per run are required. See Chapter 25 for a discussion of QC procedures. (From Westgard JO: *Six Sigma Quality Design and Control,* Madison, WI, 2001, Westgard QC.)

- TE = 3 SD + bias (crosses *y*-axis where SD = 0, or bias = E_A and crosses *x*-axis where bias = 0, hence, 3 SD = E_A, or SD = 33.3% E_A)
- TE = 4 SD + bias (crosses *y*-axis where SD = 0, or bias = E_A and crosses *x*-axis where bias = 0, hence, 4 SD = E_A, or SD = 25% E_A)
- TE = 6 SD + bias (crosses *y*-axis where SD = 0, or bias = E_A and crosses *x*-axis where bias = 0, hence, 6 SD = E_A, or SD = 16.7% E_A)

CONFIDENCE INTERVAL CRITERIA FOR JUDGING ANALYTICAL PERFORMANCE

To this point, it has been assumed that the error estimated by each of the previous equations is absolutely accurate. However, if the same experiment were repeated in as identical a manner as possible, a slightly different estimate of error would probably be obtained. Exact measurements of random and systematic errors cannot be obtained from the limited numbers of specimens analyzed in the procedures recommended previously.

Table 26-4 Factors for Computing One-Sided Confidence Limits for Standard Deviation

Degrees of Freedom (N – 1)	$A_{.05}$	$A_{.95}$
1	.5103	15.947
5	.6721	2.089
10	.7391	1.593
15	.7747	1.437
20	.7979	1.358
25	.8149	1.308
30	.8279	1.274
40	.5470	1.228
50	.8606	1.199
60	.8710	1.179
70	.8793	1.163
80	.8861	1.151
90	.8919	1.141
100	.8968	1.133

From Natrella MG: Experimental Statistics, National Bureau of Standards Handbook 91, Washington, DC, 1963, U.S. Government Printing Office; also published by Wiley & Sons, 1966.

In the approach developed by Westgard, Carey, and Wold,[52] 95% upper and lower limits of error are calculated. If the 95% upper limit of an error is smaller than the E_A, there is at least a 95% certainty that estimated error is acceptable. If the 95% lower limit is greater than the E_A, there is at least 95% certainty that the error (and thus the method's performance) is not acceptable, and no further testing is indicated. The method should be rejected or modified to improve its analytical performance. When the lower 95% limit is less than E_A, and the 95% upper limit of error exceeds E_A, no decision can be made about whether the method is unacceptable or acceptable, and more data are required to make a definitive decision.

Calculations of confidence interval estimates of each type of error are demonstrated on pp. 502-505. For additional discussion of confidence limits, see p. 421.

Confidence Interval Criterion for Random Error

In the calculation of RE, the true value of the SD is not known. The upper and lower confidence limits of the SD can be estimated by multiplying the observed SD by the appropriate one-sided 95% factors. These factors (Table 26-4) are referenced to $N - 1$ degrees of freedom.

$$s_{TM_u} = s_{TM} \times A_u \qquad \text{Eq. 26-13, a}$$

and

$$s_{TM_l} = s_{TM} \times A_l \qquad \text{Eq. 26-13, b}$$

in which A_u and A_l are the factors for computing the upper and lower one-sided limits of the SD.[52,53] The upper confidence limit of RE is four times the upper confidence limit of

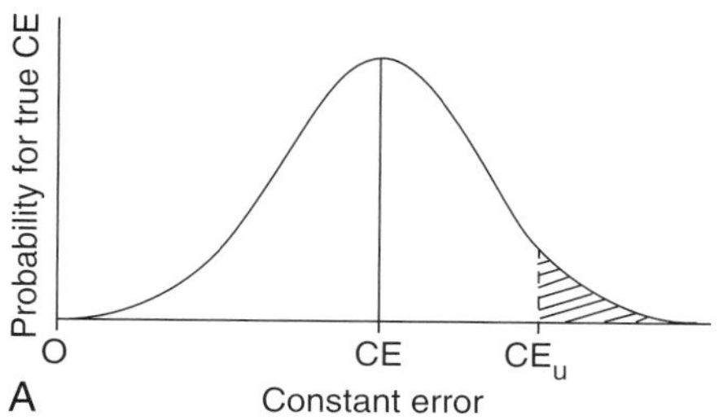

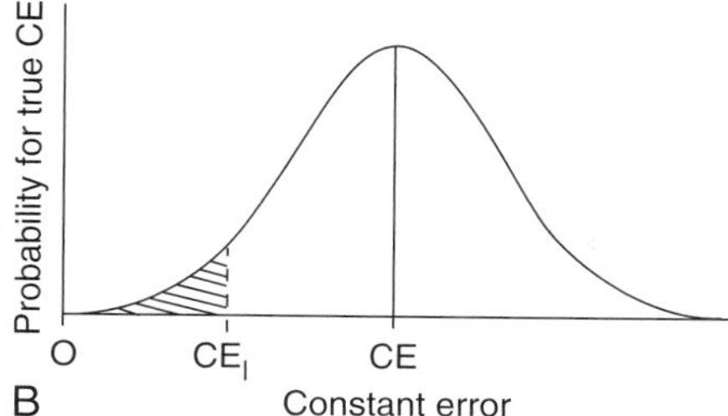

Fig. 26-9 A, One-sided 95% upper limit of constant error, CE_u. **B,** One-sided 95% lower limit of constant error, CE_l.

the SD, and the lower confidence limit of RE is four times the lower confidence limit of the SD.

$$RE_u = 4 \times s_{TM_u} \quad \text{Eq. 26-14, a}$$

And

$$RE_l = 4 \times s_{TM_l} \quad \text{Eq. 26-14, b}$$

Confidence Interval Criteria for Constant Error and for Proportional Error

Upper (E_u) and lower (E_l) confidence limits for constant and proportional error can be derived from the point estimates ($\bar{E}$) of constant and proportional error calculated above, and their SD, using the following general equations:

$$E_u = \bar{E} + \frac{t \times s}{\sqrt{N}} \quad \text{Eq. 26-15, a}$$

and

$$E_l = \bar{E} - \frac{t \times s}{\sqrt{N}} \quad \text{Eq. 26-15, b}$$

Fig. 26-9, *A*, shows the upper 95% limit of constant error, leaving only a 5% chance that the error exceeds this upper limit, CE_u. Similarly, Fig. 26-9, *B*, shows the lower 95% limit of constant error, CE_l. A one-sided *t*-value is used only when there is interest in an upper limit on the error without regard to how small the error is, and vice versa for a lower limit. (A two-sided *t* is used to answer the question, "Is there a difference?" without regard for whether the difference is positive or negative, as in the *t*-test used in the comparison-of-methods experiment.)

Confidence Interval Criterion for Systematic Error

Fig. 26-10 shows the profile of a **confidence interval** around a least-squares regression line. The expression for the limits, *w*, of this interval is given as

$$w = t \times s_{y,x}\sqrt{\frac{1}{N} + \frac{(X_C - \bar{X})^2}{\sum(x_i - \bar{X})^2}} \quad \text{Eq. 26-16}$$

This equation is similar to those used to calculate the limits for constant and proportional errors in terms of the component $t \times s_{y,x}$. The component under the square root sign becomes $1/N$ if X_C equals the mean of patient data by the comparative method. As X_C moves away from the mean, the right term begins to contribute to widening of the limits. The denominator of this second term can be calculated from the SD of the patient population by the comparative method (s_x) as follows:

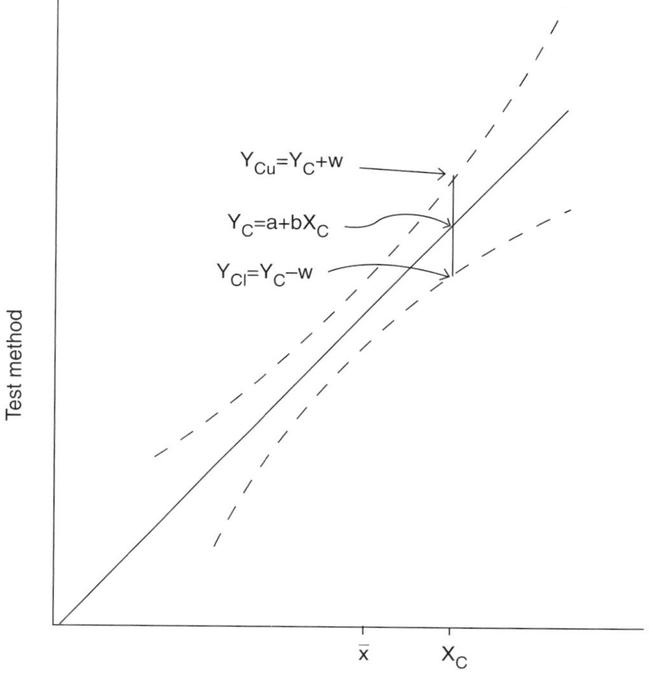

Fig. 26-10 Confidence interval around regression line. (From Westgard JO, et al: Concepts and practices in the evaluation of laboratory methods. IV. Decisions on acceptability, Am J Med Technol 44:727, 1978.)

$$\sum(x_i - \bar{X})^2 = s_x^2(N-1) \quad \text{Eq. 26-17}$$

In this situation, the regression line cannot be known exactly, and for a given X_C, the corresponding Y_C could be as large as ($Y_C + w$) or as small as ($Y_C - w$). The limit that is farther from the ideal value is used to estimate the upper limit of SE, and the limit closer to the ideal value is used to estimate the lower limit of SE:

$$SE_u = |(Y_C \pm w) - X_C|_u \quad \text{Eq. 26-18, a}$$

and

Table 26-5 Confidence Interval Criteria for Unacceptable Performance and Acceptable Performance

Type of Error	Criteria for Unacceptable Performance	Criteria for Acceptable Performance
Random (RE)	$RE_l = 4 \times S_{TMl} > E_A$	$RE_u = 4 \times S_{TMu} < E_A$
Constant (CE)	$CE_l = \left[\lvert Bias \rvert \pm t \times \frac{s}{\sqrt{N}} \right]_l > E_{A,l}$	$CE_u = \left[\lvert Bias \rvert \mp t \times \frac{s}{\sqrt{N}} \right]_u < E_{A,l}$
Proportional (PE)	$PE(\text{conc. units})_l = \left[\frac{\lvert \bar{R} - 100 \rvert}{100} \times X_C \pm t \times \frac{s_R}{\sqrt{N}} \right]_l > E_{A,R}$	$PE(\text{conc. units})_u = \left[\frac{\lvert \bar{R} - 100 \rvert}{100} \times X_C \mp t \times \frac{s_R}{\sqrt{N}} \right]_u < E_{A,R}$
Systematic (SE)	$SE_l = [\lvert a + b \times X_C - X_C \rvert \pm w]_l > E_{A,MD}$	$SE_u = [\lvert a + b \times X_C - X_C \rvert \mp w]_u < E_{A,MD}$
Total (TE)	$TE_l = \sqrt{RE_l^2 + w^2} + \lvert a + b \times X_C - X_C \rvert > E_A$	$TE_u = \sqrt{RE_u^2 + w^2} + \lvert a + b \times X_C - X_C \rvert < E_A$

where $E_{A,l} = \frac{1}{2} \times E_A$, where $E_{A,R} = \frac{1}{4} \times E_A$, and where $E_{A,MD} = \frac{1}{2} \times E_A$.

$$SE_l = \lvert (Y_C \pm w) - X_C \rvert_l \qquad \text{Eq. 26-18, b}$$

Eq. 26-16 may not provide a valid estimate of the confidence limits of the linear-regression line if the precision of the test method is not reasonably constant throughout the concentration range of the patient specimens included in the comparison-of-methods experiment.

Confidence Interval Criterion for Total Error

As was described before, TE is the worst-case combination of random and systematic errors. Because both random and systematic errors include variances in the equations used to calculate them, they must be combined vectorially. Their variances are combined as shown:

$$TE_u = \sqrt{RE_u^2 + w^2} + SE \qquad \text{Eq. 26-19, a}$$

and

$$TE_l = \sqrt{RE_l^2 + w^2} + SE \qquad \text{Eq. 26-19, b}$$

If the upper 95% limit of the TE is less than the E_A, there is 95% certainty that the method performs acceptably. If the lower 95% limit of the TE exceeds E_A, there is 95% certainty that the method does not perform acceptably and should be modified or rejected.

It should be noted that whenever the ideal value (zero error condition) is between the upper and lower limits of the estimated error, there is a chance that the true error might be zero. Thus in these situations the lower limit of error is simply zero. The upper limit of error remains as just calculated. This situation can arise for the constant, proportional, or systematic error estimates but not of course for RE. If the lower limit of SE is zero, the lower limit of the estimate of TE is equal to the lower limit of the estimate of RE because an SE may not be present. Equations for calculating the confidence intervals of various errors and the criteria for judging their acceptability are summarized in Table 26-5.

Confidence limits for the calculated SD and SE (bias) can be used along with the method decision chart to define the confidence interval of the operating point. Appropriate QC procedures should be used that take into account the worst-case limits for SD and for bias when the method is put into routine use. See the example on pp. 504-505.

OTHER EVALUATION PROTOCOLS

A protocol for user verification of precision and accuracy is described in CLSI EP15-A2.[6] This protocol assumes that the method's performance is already well documented, and that the user believes it will perform acceptably in his laboratory. Its purpose is for the user to demonstrate that he can obtain performance similar to that claimed by the manufacturer, as required by CLIA.[3] Precision is estimated in a replication experiment of a minimum of 5 days. Accuracy is estimated by a comparison-of-methods experiment with 20 patient specimens, or by analysis of materials with known analyte concentration such as proficiency testing specimens or materials recommended by the manufacturer. This protocol is appropriate for use when the user is evaluating an FDA-approved method and believes that the method's performance has been well characterized in previous studies. It has relatively low power to detect performance that deviates from that claimed by the manufacturer, so its use should be limited to situations in which the user believes the method will perform as claimed, and the user intends to demonstrate that the method performs consistently with the manufacturer's claims.

Multifactor experimental designs have been proposed to study several method characteristics at the same time.[54] A special example of this approach is given in CLSI guideline EP10-A3, *Preliminary Evaluation of Quantitative Clinical Laboratory Methods.*[13] This protocol enables the estimation of imprecision, **inaccuracy**, nonlinearity, carryover, and drift in one series of studies over 5 days, using three levels of analyte. Samples must be measured in a specific sequence for a total of three readings each day, as well as two "primer" samples of the midlevel sample, for a total of 11 analyses per day, or 55 for the whole study. If unusual effects are observed, each effect should be investigated more thoroughly with a specific study performed for each factor separately, as described in this chapter, or, if the method was obtained from a commercial manufacturer, the manufacturer should be contacted for help. As its name states, EP10 is intended for use as a preliminary, quick screen to estimate several errors simultaneously and to determine possible interactions among these performance characteristics.

CLIA regulations require that duplicate instruments within a laboratory should demonstrate concordance with each other. In addition, a single health care system might find it desirable to show that similar instruments within the system are reporting concordant patient results. CLSI C54-A[55] addresses this comparability requirement for multiple devices after each one has been previously validated. This approach considers the range of results (or range of instrument averages) for each of up to 10 different instruments, where the range may be related to a stated allowable error. The inherent precision of each instrument is taken into account to determine how many replicate measurements are to be made for each instrument to determine the instrument-specific average value.

KEY CONCEPTS BOX 26-6

- Total error can be calculated and compared with allowable error to judge a method's acceptability.
- The graphical method decision chart shows the relationships of random, systematic, and total error.
- Confidence interval criteria allow for the uncertainty of error estimates caused by limited numbers of data.
- Confidence interval criteria enable accept/reject decisions to be made with a stated level of confidence (e.g., 95%).
- CLSI EP15 is intended for a user to demonstrate that a method's performance in the user laboratory is consistent with performance claimed by the manufacturer.
- CLSI EP10 is intended for use as a preliminary test of performance by assessing several characteristics simultaneously in one "multifactor" experiment and by determining the possibility of interactions among these factors.

DISCUSSION

In some situations, as in the study of different enzyme methods, suitably close agreement is not expected or possible because of different reaction conditions or different definitions of enzyme units. In these cases, rather than concluding that the method is unacceptable, a new clinical baseline of information is necessary, and a new reference interval is needed (see Chapter 24). Specific disease-related data should be obtained to provide new clinical information for interpretation of test method results.

Evaluation of a method for a "new" analyte previously not measured in the user's laboratory is an analogous situation. Because no comparative method is available on site, accurate estimates of SE are harder to obtain. Reliance on published evaluation reports increases. The conclusions of these reports must be reviewed cautiously after analysis of a laboratory's own experimental data has been completed. If an analyte is not usually measured, the emphasis of the laboratory should shift to experiments conducted to estimate specific errors. Accurate recovery studies are essential. Interference studies are expanded to include a broader range of chemicals that could interfere with measurement reactions. Patient specimens that have been analyzed in another laboratory may be analyzed for comparison purposes, but specimen instability and lack of user control of the other laboratory's procedure may reduce the reliability of the SE estimate. However, if the other laboratory is the reference laboratory to which the user has previously referred specimens for measurement of this analyte, the comparison is really being made to present practice.

Smaller laboratories often do not have the resources for exhaustive method-evaluation studies, but fortunately, these usually are not among the first to evaluate a new method. Usually, some evaluation reports have been published. Even when a method's performance has been well documented by published evaluation studies, the user should still evaluate RE and perform the comparison-of-methods experiment to verify acceptable performance in his or her own laboratory. The experiments described in CLSI EP15-A2 are appropriate here.[6] A reference interval study should be performed (see Chapter 24).

Using the decision-making approaches and tools that have been described in this chapter, it is possible to perform evaluations of methods efficiently and objectively. Conducting a method evaluation enables the laboratory scientist to understand the capabilities and quality of an assay before it is used routinely for patient testing, regardless of whether an evaluation is required by government regulation.

AN EXAMPLE PERFORMANCE EVALUATION FOR GLUCOSE

1. **Estimation of random error from replication data**
   a. **Statistics calculations.** (y_i = Results from the method being tested)

Mean:

$$\bar{y} = \frac{\sum y_i}{N}$$

SD:

$$s_{TM} = \sqrt{\frac{\sum (y_i - \bar{y})^2}{N-1}}$$

or

$$s_{TM} = \sqrt{\frac{\sum y_i^2 - (\sum y_i)^2/N}{N-1}}$$

Coefficient of variation:

$$CV = \frac{s_{TM}}{\bar{y}} \times 100\%$$

Example

For 20 replicate measurements of a sample, the mean was 128.3 mg/dL, with a standard deviation of 1.43 mg/dL (%CV = 1.1%).

b. Point estimate of random error

$$RE = 4 \times s_{TM}$$

If RE < E_A, performance is acceptable.

Example

For glucose, E_A = 10% of 128.3 = 12.83 mg/dL.

$$\bar{y} = 128.3\,mg/dL$$

$$s_{TM} = 1.43\,mg/dL$$

RE = 4 × 1.43 = 5.72 mg/dL; RE is acceptable.

c. Confidence interval estimate of random error (RE_u, RE_l)

$$s_{TM_u} = s_{TM} \times (A_{0.95})\ldots \text{(see Table 26-4)}$$

$$s_{TM_u} = 1.43 \times 1.358 = 1.94\,mg/dL$$

$$s_{TM_l} = s_{TM} \times (A_{0.05})$$

$$s_{TM_l} = 1.43 \times 0.7979 = 1.14\,mg/L$$

$$RE_u = 4 \times s_{TM_u} = 4 \times 1.94\,mg/dL = 7.8\,mg/dL$$

$$RE_u < E_A\,(7.8\,mg/dL < 12.83\,mg/dL)$$

We can be at least 95% certain that random error is acceptable because the upper limit of the confidence interval for random error is less than the allowable error.

2. Estimation of constant error from an interference study for a glucose method

a. Sample preparation

(1) 1.00 mL of serum A + 0.10 mL of water

(2) 1.00 mL of serum A + 0.10 mL of 30 mg/dL of creatinine standard

(3) 1.00 mL of serum A + 0.10 mL of 100 mg/dL of creatinine standard

b. Results

	Creatinine Added (mg/dL)	Glucose Measured (mg/dL)	Interference (mg/dL)	Average Interference (CE) (mg/dL)
(1)	—	120, 122, 119 (mean = 120.3)	—	—
(2)	2.73	124, 124, 123	+4, +2, +4	+3.3
(3)	9.09	131, 134, 129	+11, +12, +10	+11.0

c. Formulas for calculations

Concentration added =

$$\text{Concentration of standard} \times \frac{\text{Volume standard}}{\text{Total volume}}$$

Interference =

Concentration (test) − Concentration (baseline)

d. Point estimate of constant error (CE)

$$CE = \text{Interference}$$

If CE < $E_{A,I}$, performance is acceptable.

Example

For glucose, E_A = 10% of 120.3 mg/dL, = 12.0 mg/dL.

Let's define $E_{A,I} = {}^1/_2 \times E_A$ = 6.0 mg/dL.

With the addition 2.73 mg/dL of creatinine, CE = 3.3 mg/dL; CE is acceptable.

With the addition of 9.09 mg/dL of creatinine, CE = 11.0 mg/dL; CE is not acceptable. This assay should not be used for patients with renal disease.

e. Confidence-interval estimate of constant error (CE_u, CE_l)

(1) With the addition of 2.73 mg/dL of creatinine, CE = 3.3 mg/dL, s = 1.15 mg/dL, N = 3, and t for (N − 1), or 2 degrees of freedom; 95% one-sided limit is 2.92 (see p. 423).

$$CE_u = CE + \frac{t \times s}{\sqrt{N}}$$

$$CE_u = 3.3 + \frac{2.92 \times 1.15}{\sqrt{3}} = 5.2\,mg/dL$$

$$CE_l = CE - \frac{t \times s}{\sqrt{N}}$$

$$CE_l = 3.3 - \frac{2.92 \times 1.15}{\sqrt{3}} = 1.4\,mg/dL$$

$CE_u < E_{A,I}$ (5.2 mg/dL < 6.0 mg/dL). The interference effect on the measurement of glucose caused by the addition of 2.73 mg/dL creatinine is acceptably small because the upper confidence limit of the interference due to creatinine is less than the error allowed (or budgeted) for interferences.

(2) With the addition of 9.09 mg/dL of creatinine, CE = 11.0, s = 10 mg/dL, and N = 3.

$$CE_u = 11.0 + \frac{2.92 \times 10}{\sqrt{3}} = 12.7\,mg/dL$$

$$CE_l = 11.0 - \frac{2.92 \times 10}{\sqrt{3}} = 9.3\,mg/dL$$

$CE_l > E_{A,I}$ (93 mg/L > 6.0 mg/L). We are at least 95% certain that the creatinine interference for this glucose method in the presence of high concentrations of creatinine is not acceptable because the lower confidence limit of the interference exceeds the error allowed for interferences. This assay should not be used to measure glucose for patients with end-stage renal disease. This assay may be acceptable for general testing of other types of patients.

3. Estimation of PE from a recovery study for a glucose method

a. Sample preparation

(1) 2.0 mL of serum A + 0.1 mL of water
(2) 2.0 mL of serum A + 0.1 mL of 1000 mg/dL of glucose standard
(3) 2.0 mL of serum B + 0.1 mL of water
(4) 2.0 mL of serum B + 0.1 mL of 1000 mg/dL of glucose standard

b. Results (mg/dL)

Sample	Glucose Added	Glucose Measured	Glucose Recovered (Test – Baseline)	Percentage Recovery*
(1) Baseline	—	51, 53, 54	—	—
(2) Spike	47.6	97, 100, 98	46, 47, 44	96.6%, 98.7%, 92.4%
(3) Baseline	—	124, 120, 121	—	—
(4) Spike	47.6	169, 166, 164	45, 46, 43	94.5%, 96.6%, 90.3%

*Average recovery ($\bar{R}$) = 94.8%; SD of recovery (s_R) = 3.09%; SD of average recovery = 1.26%.

c. Formulas for calculations

$$\text{Concentration added} = \text{Concentration of standard} \times \frac{\text{Volume standard}}{\text{Total volume}}$$

$$\text{Concentration recovered} = \text{Concentration (test)} - \text{Concentration (baseline)}$$

$$\%\ \text{Recovery} = \frac{\text{Concentration recovered}}{\text{Concentration added}} \times 100$$

d. Point estimate of proportional error

$$(\text{PE})\% = |\bar{R} - 100|$$

$$\text{PE (concentration units)} = \left|\frac{|\bar{R} - 100|}{100}\right| \times X_C$$

If PE < $E_{A,R}$, recovery is acceptable.

Example

For glucose, E_A = 10% of 126 mg/dL, = 12.6 mg/dL.

Let's define $E_{A,R} = {}^1/_4 \times E_A = 3.2$ mg/dL

$$\bar{R} = 94.8\%$$

$$\text{PE}(\%) = |94.8\% - 100| = 5.2\%$$

or

$$\text{PE(units)} = \left|\frac{|94.8 - 100|}{100}\right| \times 126\,\text{mg/L} = 6.6\,\text{mg/dL}$$

PE is not acceptable (6.6 mg/dL > 3.2 mg/dL).

e. Confidence-interval estimate of proportional error (PE_u, PE_l)

$\bar{R} = 94.8\%$, $s = 3.09\%$, $N = 6$, and t for $(N - 1)$, or 5 degrees of freedom, and the 95% one-sided limit is 2.02.

$$\bar{R}_u = \bar{R} + \frac{t \times s}{\sqrt{N}}$$

$$\bar{R}_u = 94.8\% + \frac{2.02 \times 3.09}{\sqrt{6}} = 97.4\%$$

$$\bar{R}_l = \bar{R} - \frac{t \times s}{\sqrt{N}}$$

$$\bar{R}_l = 94.8\% - \frac{2.02 \times 3.09}{\sqrt{6}} = 92.3\%$$

The limit that deviates more from the ideal recovery of 100% is used to estimate the upper limit of proportional error, PE_u%.

$$PE_u\,\% = |92.3 - 100| = 7.7\%$$

and for the lower limit

$$PE_l\,\% = |97.3 - 100| = 2.7\%$$

To relate PE_u% and PE_l% to E_A, convert them to concentration units at X_C.

$$PE_u = \frac{PE_u}{100} \times X_C$$

$$= \frac{7.7\%}{100} \times 126\,\text{mg/dL} = 9.7\,\text{mg/dL}$$

$$PE_l = \frac{PE_l}{100} \times X_C$$

$$= \frac{2.7\%}{100} \times 126\,\text{mg/L} = 3.4\,\text{mg/dL}$$

$PE_l > E_{A,R}$ (3.4 mg/dL > 3.2 mg/dL)

We can be 95% certain that PE (recovery) is not acceptably small for this glucose method because the lower confidence limit of the recovery error exceeds the error allowed for recovery. The accuracy of the glucose calibrator should be investigated.

4. Estimation of SE from a comparison-of-methods study for glucose

a. In a comparison of an automated glucose oxidase method (y) versus the manual glucose national

reference method (x), the following statistics were obtained by linear-regression analysis:
$y = 0.973 \times x - 6$ mg/dL, $s_{y,x} = 37$ mg/dL, $N = 82$, $\overline{x} = 172.3$, $\overline{y} = 167$, $s_x = 57.1$ mg/dL (in which s_x is the SD of the x values for the 82 samples), and $r = 0.9941$.

b. Point estimate of SE

Consider bias:

$$\text{Bias} = |\overline{y} - \overline{x}| = 5.3\,\text{mg/dL}$$

Let's define the allowable error for method differences, $E_{A,MD} = {}^1\!/_2 \times E_A$. If bias < $E_{A,MD}$, the difference between the two methods at the mean of the data is acceptable. At $\overline{x} = 172.3$ mg/dL, E_A = 10% = 17.2 mg/dL; $E_{A,MD} = {}^1\!/_2 \times E_A$ = 8.6 mg/dL. Because the bias < $E_{A,MD}$ (5.3 mg/dL < 8.6 mg/dL), the difference between the two methods around the mean of the data is acceptably small.

The bias provides an estimate of SE at the mean of the data. However, if $\overline{x}$ is not equal to the X_C of interest, there must be no PE between methods for the bias to provide an accurate estimate of SE at these other concentrations. If PE is present, use linear-regression statistics or calculate the bias using only those samples whose analyte concentrations are close to X_C.

Consider linear regression:

$$\text{SE} = |Y_C - X_C|$$

in which $Y_C = a + b \times X_C$

For

$$X_C = 126\,\text{mg/dL glucose,}$$

Then

$$Y_C = 0.973 \times 126 - 0.6\,\text{mg/dL}$$

$$Y_C = 122\,\text{mg/dL}$$

and

$$\text{SE} = |122 - 126| = 4.0\,\text{mg/dL}$$

At a concentration of 126 mg/dL, E_A = 10% = 12.6 mg/dL. As above, let's define $E_{A,MD} = {}^1\!/_2 \times E_A$ = 6.3 mg/dL.

Because SE < $E_{A,MD}$ (4.0 mg/dL < 6.3 mg/dL), the systematic error is acceptable at this concentration.

c. Confidence interval estimate of systematic error (SE_u, SE_l)

$$Y_{C_u} = Y_C + w$$

and

$$Y_{C_l} = Y_C - w$$

in which

$$w = t \times s_{y,x}\sqrt{\frac{1}{N} + \frac{(X_C - \overline{X})^2}{\sum (x_i - \overline{X})^2}}$$

in which

$$\sum (x_i - \overline{X})^2 = s_x^2(N-1)$$

in which w is the width of the confidence interval around the regression line (see Fig. 26-10). The value for t, obtained from a 95% one-sided t-table and $N - 2$ degrees of freedom, has the value of 1.66.

$$w = 1.66 \times 3.7\sqrt{\frac{1}{82} + \frac{(126 - 116.2)^2}{57.1^2 \times 81}} = 0.7\,\text{mg/dL}$$

thus

$$Y_{C_u} = 122 + 0.7 = 122.7\,\text{mg/dL}$$

$$Y_{C_l} = 122 - 0.7 = 121.3\,\text{mg/dL}$$

The limit that deviates more from the ideal value for Y_C (ideally, $Y_C = X_C$) will be used to estimate the upper limit of SE.

$$\text{SE}_u = |(Y_C \pm w - X_C)|_u$$

$$\text{SE}_u = |121.3 - 126| = 4.7\,\text{mg/dL}$$

and

$$\text{SE}_l = |(Y_C \pm w - X_C)|_l$$

$$\text{SE}_l = |122.7 - 126| = 3.3\,\text{mg/dL}$$

Because SE_u < $E_{A,MD}$ (4.7 mg/L < 6.3 mg/dL), we can be 95% sure that the SE between these methods is acceptable at this concentration, X_C. The upper confidence limit of the systematic error is less than the allowable error for method differences.

5. Estimation of TE

a. Point estimate of TE

$$\text{TE} = \text{RE} + \text{SE (see Fig. 26-7)}$$

$$\text{TE} = 4 \times s_{TM} + |Y_C - X_C|$$

$$\text{TE} = 5.7\,\text{mg/dL} + 4.0\,\text{mg/dL} = 9.7\,\text{mg/dL}$$

Because TE < EA, the TE of the new glucose method is acceptable.

b. Confidence interval estimate of total error (TE_u, TE_l)

$$\text{TE}_u = \sqrt{\text{RE}_u^2 + w^2} + \text{SE}$$

and

$$\text{TE}_l = \sqrt{\text{RE}_l^2 + w^2} + \text{SE}$$

Note that the variance of the uncertainty in repetitive measurements and the uncertainty of the regression line are added and the square root of the sum is taken, to estimate the overall uncertainty, which then is combined with the point estimate of SE to yield the appropriate limit for TE. Thus

$$TE_u = \sqrt{7.8^2 + 7^2} + 4.0 = 11.8\,mg/dL$$

and

$$TE_l = \sqrt{4.6^2 + 0.7^2} + 4.0 = 8.7\,mg/dL$$

$$TE_u < E_A\,(11.8\,mg/dL < 12.6\,mg/dL)$$

We can be 95% sure that the TE is acceptable at the concentration, X_C, because the upper confidence limit for total error is less than the allowable error.

6. Method decision chart analysis of point estimates of precision and bias

a. Express SD as percentage of E_A.
At X_C = 126 mg/dL, s_{TM} = 1.43 mg/dL, E_A = 12.6 mg/dL, or SD = 11.3% of E_A.

b. Express bias as percentage of E_A.
At X_C = 126 mg/dL, SE = 4.0 mg/dL, E_A = 12.6 mg/dL, or SE = 31.7% of E_A.

c. Plot percent bias and SD on the medical decision chart.

The operating point is in the region of Good performance.

d. Calculate the upper and lower confidence limits of SD as percentages of E_A.

$$s_{TM_u} = 1.94\,mg/dL = 15.4\%\text{ of }E_A.$$

$$s_{TM_l} = 1.14\,mg/dL = 9.0\%\text{ of }E_A.$$

e. Calculate the upper and lower confidence limits of bias (SE by regression) as percentages of E_A.

$$SE_u = 4.7/12.6\,mg/dL = 37.3\%\text{ of }E_A.$$

$$SE_l = 3.3/12.6\,mg/dL = 26.2\%\text{ of }E_A.$$

f. Plot confidence limits of percent bias and percent SD on the medical decision chart (the arrows mark the confidence limits).

The uncertainty limits indicate that the method's performance could be either Good or Six Sigma.

The QC rules that are selected for this assay should accommodate the worst-case SD of 15.4% of E_A and an inaccuracy of 37.0% of E_A. For example, a simple, single-rule QC procedure could be the $1_{2.5s}$ rule, with three controls in the run. This would yield a probability for error detection (P_{ed}) of 80% and a probability for false rejection (P_{fr}) of 3%. (For more discussion on probability for error detection and probability for false rejection, and for QC rules, see Chapter 25.)

If the inaccuracy were reduced to near zero (method is in the Six Sigma zone), the $1_{2.5s}$ rule could be used with only one control per run. This would yield a P_{ed} of >94% and a P_{fr} of 1%.

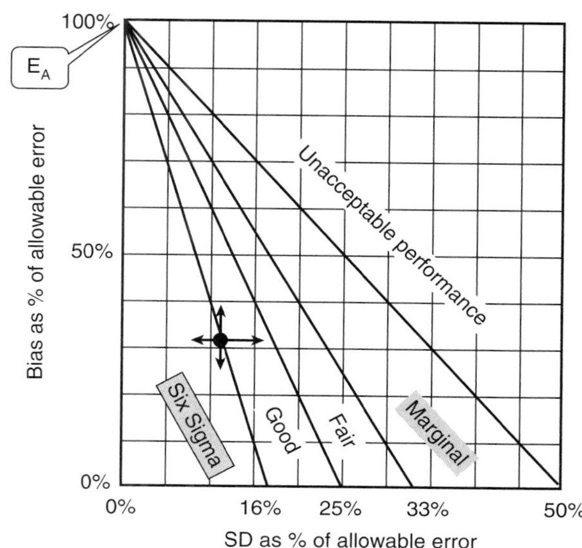

REFERENCES

1. Büttner J, Borth R, Boutwell JH, et al: IFCC approved recommendations on quality control in clinical chemistry. Part 1. General principles and terminology, Clin Chim Acta 98:129F, 1979.
2. ISO/IEC: *Guide 99, International Vocabulary of Metrology—Basic and General Concepts and Associated Terms (VIM 3),* Geneva, Switzerland, 2008, International Standards Organization.
3. Health Care Financing Administration (42 CFR Part 493, et al), the Public Health Service, U.S. Department of Health and Human Services: Clinical Laboratory Improvement Amendments of 1988, Final Rule, Federal Register 57:7003, 1992.
4. CLSI: *Approved Guideline EP9-A2, User Comparison of Quantitative Clinical Laboratory Methods Using Patient Samples,* Wayne, PA, 2002, Evaluation Protocols Area Committee.
5. Westgard JO, de Vos DJ, Hunt MR, et al: Concepts and practices in the selection and evaluation of methods, Am J Med Technol: Part I, Background and approach, 44:290, 1978; Part II, Experimental procedures, 44:420, 1978; Part III, Statistics, 44:552, 1978; Part IV, Decision on acceptability, 44:727, 1978; Part V, Applications, 44:803, 1978.
6. CLSI: *Approved Guideline EP15-A2, User Verification of Performance for Precision and Trueness,* Wayne, PA, 2006, Evaluation Protocols Area Committee.
7. CLSI: *Approved Guideline EP7-A2, Interference Testing in Clinical Chemistry,* Wayne, PA, 2005, Evaluation Protocols Area Committee.
8. CLSI: *Approved Guideline EP17-A, Protocols for Determination of Limits of Detection and Limits of Quantitation,* Wayne, PA, 2004, Evaluation Protocols Area Committee.
9. CLSI: *Approved Guideline EP6-A, Evaluation of the Linearity of Quantitative Analytical Methods,* Wayne, PA, 2003, Evaluation Protocols Area Committee.
10. CLSI: *Approved Guideline EP5-A2, Guidelines for User Evaluation of Precision Performance of Clinical Chemistry Devices,* Wayne, PA, 2004, Evaluation Protocols Area Committee.
11. Definitions, 21 Code of Federal Regulations (CFR) Section 820.3 (CFR website, updated April 1, 2007).
12. Westgard JO: Precision and accuracy: concepts and assessment by method evaluation testing, CRC Crit Rev Clin Lab Sci 13:283, 1981.
13. CLSI: *Approved Guideline EP10-A3, Preliminary Evaluation of Quantitative Clinical Laboratory Methods,* ed 2, Wayne, PA, 2006, Evaluation Protocols Area Committee.

14. CLSI: *Approved Guideline EP21-A, Estimation of Total Analytical Error for Clinical Laboratory Methods,* Wayne, PA, 2003, Evaluation Protocols Area Committee.
15. Labeling requirements and standards development for in-vitro diagnostic products, 21 CFR 809.10 (CFR website, updated April 1, 2007).
16. www.fda.gov/cdrh/devadvice/ (FDA website, updated February 21, 2008).
17. Analyte Specific Reagents, 21 CFR 809.30 and 21 CFR 864.4020 (CFR website, updated April 1, 2007).
18. Cryer PE: American Diabetes Association Workgroup on Hypoglycemia: Defining and reporting hypoglycemia in diabetes, Diabetes Care 28:1245, 2005.
19. Barnett RN: Medical significance of laboratory results, Am J Clin Pathol 50:671, 1968.
20. Barnett RN: Analytic goals in clinical chemistry: the pathologist's viewpoint. In Elevitch FR, editor: *Proceedings of the 1976 Aspen Conference on Analytic Goals in Clinical Chemistry,* Skokie, IL, 1977, College of American Pathologists.
21. Tonks D: A study of the accuracy and precision of clinical chemistry determinations in 170 Canadian laboratories, Clin Chem 9:217, 1963.
22. Tonks D: A quality control program for quantitative clinical chemistry estimations, Can J Med Technol 30:38, 1968.
23. Cotlove E, Harris E, Williams G: Biological and analytic components of variation in long-term studies of serum constituents in normal subjects. III. Physiological and medical implications, Clin Chem 16:1028, 1970.
24. Elevitch FR, editor: *CAP Aspen Conference 1976: Analytical Goals in Clinical Chemistry,* Skokie, IL, 1977, College of American Pathologists.
25. Fraser CG: *Biological Variation: From Principles to Practice,* Washington, DC, 2001, AACC Press.
26. Garber CC, Kaufman HK: Quality systems for the clinical laboratory in the 21st century. In Ward-Cook KM, Lehmann CA, Schoeff LE, Williams RH: *Clinical Diagnostic Technology—The Total Testing Process,* vol 3, *The Post-Analytical Phase,* Washington, DC, 2003, AACC Press, Chapter 1, pp. 1-36.
27. Fraser CG: The application of theoretical goals based upon biological variation in proficiency testing, Arch Pathol Lab Med 112:404, 1988.
28. Fraser CG: Desirable standards of performance for therapeutic drug monitoring, Clin Chem 33:387, 1987.
29. Fraser CG, Hyltoft PP, Ricos S, et al: Quality specifications. In Haeckel R, editor: *Evaluation Methods in Laboratory Medicine,* New York, 1993, VCH.
30. Ricós C, Alvarez V, Cava F, et al: Current databases on biological variation: pros, cons, and progress, Scand J Clin Lab Invest 59:491, 1999.
31. Morrow DA, Cannon CP, Jesse R, et al: National Academy of Clinical Biochemistry practice guidelines: clinical characteristics and utilization of biochemical markers in acute coronary syndromes, Clin Chem 54:552, 2007.
32. National Glycohemoglobin Standardization Program. Available at http://web.missouri.edu/~diabetes/ngsp.html
33. OSHA regulations on cadmium surveillance, 29 CFR 1910.1027 (CFR website, updated January 1, 2007).
34. Ross JW: A theoretical basis for clinically relevant proficiency testing evaluation limits: sensitivity analysis of the effect of inherent test variability on acceptable method error, Arch Pathol Lab Med 112:421, 1988.
35. Ehrmeyer SS, Laessig RH, Leinweber JE, et al: 1990 Medicare/CLIA final rules for proficiency testing: minimum intralaboratory performance characteristics (CV and bias) needed to pass, Clin Chem 36:1736, 1990.
36. Westgard JO, Burnett RW: Precision requirements for cost-effective operation of analytical processes, Clin Chem 36:1629, 1990.
37. Westgard JO: *Six Sigma Quality Design and Control,* Madison, WI, 2001, Westgard QC.
38. Pande PS, Neuman RP, Cavanaugh RR: *The Six Sigma Way: How GE, Motorola, and Other Top Companies Are Honing Their Performance,* New York, 2000, McGraw/Hill.
39. Garber CC: Six Sigma: its role in the clinical laboratory, Clinical Laboratory News, AACC, April:10-14, 2004.
40. National Reference System for the Clinical Laboratory: *NRSCL6-T, Development of Methodological Principles Documents for Analytes in the Clinical Laboratory: Tentative Guideline,* Villanova, PA, 1989, NRSCL.
41. Tremblay MM: Evaluation of instruments in biochemistry, Can J Med Technol 41:65, 1979.
42. Shaikh AH: A systematic procedure for selection of automated instruments in the clinical laboratory, Am J Med Technol 45:710, 1979.
43. Kroll MH, Emancipator K: A theoretical evaluation of linearity, Clin Chem 39:405, 1993.
44. Joint Committee on Traceability in Laboratory Medicine. Available at www.bipm.org/en/committees/jc/jctlm
45. ISO: ISO 17511, In Vitro Diagnostic Medical Devices—Measurement of Quantities in Biological Samples—Metrological Traceability of Values Assigned to Calibrators and Control Materials, Geneva, Switzerland, 2003, International Standards Organization.
46. CLSI: *Report X5-R, Metrological Traceability and Its Implementation,* Wayne, PA, 2006, Evaluation Protocols Area Committee.
47. Westgard JO, Hunt MR: Use and interpretation of common statistical tests in method-comparison studies, Clin Chem 19:49, 1973.
48. American Society for Testing and Materials: *ASTM Standard E178-68: Standard Recommended Practice for Dealing With Outlying Observations,* Philadelphia, 1968, ASTM.
49. Wakkers PJ, Hellendoorn HB, Op de Weegh GJ, et al: Applications of statistics in clinical chemistry: a critical evaluation of regression lines, Clin Chim Acta 64:173, 1975.
50. Cornbleet PJ, Gochman N: Incorrect least-squares regression coefficients in method-comparison analysis, Clin Chem 25:432, 1979.
51. Passing H, Bablock W: Comparison of several regression procedures for method comparison studies and determination of sample sizes, J Clin Chem Clin Biochem 22:431, 1984.
52. Westgard JO, Carey RN, Wold S: Criteria for judging precision and accuracy in method development and evaluation, Clin Chem 20:825, 1974.
53. Natrella MG: *Experimental Statistics, National Bureau of Standards Handbook 91,* Washington, DC, 1963, U.S. Government Printing Office; also published by Wiley & Sons, 1966.
54. Krouwer J: A multifactor experimental design for evaluating random access analyzers, Clin Chem 34:1984, 1988.
55. CLSI: *Approved Guideline C54-A, Verification of Comparability of Patient Results Within One Healthcare System,* Wayne, PA, 2008, Evaluation Protocols Area Committee.

INTERNET SITES

www.access.gpo.gov—Use this site for the latest updates to Code of Federal Regulations (CFR) information.

www.asq.org

www.clsi.org

www.cms.gov

www.dgrhoads.com

www.fda.gov

www.krouwerconsulting.com

www.westgard.com

Classifications and Descriptions of Proteins, Lipids, and Carbohydrates

Chapter 27

Lawrence A. Kaplan, Herbert K. Naito, and Amadeo J. Pesce

Chapter Outline

Key Terms

aldose The chemical form of monosaccharides in which the carbonyl group is an aldehyde.

apoprotein Polypeptide chain not yet complexed to its specific prosthetic group.

carbohydrates Chemicals with the general formula of hydrated carbon $(CH_2O)_n$, which are aldehyde or ketone derivatives of polyhydric alcohols. Commonly called *sugars.*

compound (conjugated) proteins Polypeptide chain complexed with other chemical classes such as lipids (lipoproteins), carbohydrates (glycoproteins), or nucleic acids (nucleoproteins).

conjugated lipids Esters of fatty acids and alcohols containing additional chemical moieties. Group includes phospholipids, sphingolipids, sterols, and bile acids.

denaturation Unfolding the tertiary structure of a protein that often renders it insoluble, causing it to precipitate out of solution; also, "melting" of DNA.

derived lipids Lipids derived from the hydrolysis of simple and conjugated fats; these include the fatty acids.

furanose Five-membered rings of monosaccharides formed by intramolecular reaction between the carbonyl group and a hydroxyl group; present in α- or β-stereoisomeric form.

ketose The chemical form of a monosaccharide in which the carbonyl group is a ketone.

nucleosides Purine or pyrimidine bases linked to the 5′-carbon sugar molecule ribose or deoxyribose through a β–*N*-glycosidic bond to the 1 position of the pyrimidine ring or the 9 position of the purine ring.

nucleotides Nucleosides with phosphate groups attached at the 3′ and/or 5′ position of the sugar molecule.

peptide bond The covalent amide bond between a primary amino group of one amino acid and the carboxylic acid group of a second amino acid.

primary structure The linear sequence of amino acids in a protein, defined by the genetic code resident in DNA or RNA.

prosthetic group A nonprotein chemical group that is bound to a protein and is responsible for the biological activity of the protein. The functional complex between protein and a prosthetic group is called a *holoprotein,* and the protein without the prosthetic group is called an *apoprotein.*

pyranose Six-membered rings of monosaccharides formed by intramolecular reaction between a carbonyl group and a hydroxy group, present in an α- or β-stereoisomeric form.

quaternary structure The three-dimensional spatial arrangement of polypeptide chains, resulting from the combining of more than one polypeptide chain into a larger, stable complex.

Schiff's base Covalent complex between a primary amine and the carbonyl function of an aldose.

secondary structure The spatial arrangement of a linear chain of amino acids in a polypeptide; common structures include the β-pleated sheet, the α-helix, and random coil.

sialic acids *N*-acetyl derivatives of neuraminic acid that are covalently linked to many proteins.

simple lipids Esters of fatty acids with various alcohols, including the triglycerides and some steroids.

simple proteins Polypeptide chain consisting only of amino acid groups.

tertiary structure The intramolecular folding of a polypeptide chain onto itself, resulting from interactions between side-chain groups of individual amino acids.

zwitterion (pronounced tsvit″-er-i′-on) Molecule that contains two ionized groups of opposite charge

This chapter is not intended to provide a complete biochemical review of the analytes measured in the chemistry laboratory. (For this, refer to the excellent biochemistry texts listed in the bibliography.) Instead, this chapter focuses on those properties of proteins, lipids, carbohydrates, and nucleic acids that affect how the analytes may be measured.

SECTION OBJECTIVES BOX 27-1

- Describe how proteins are classified, and name six types of proteins.
- List the four types of protein structures, and describe how they are formed.
- List the chemical properties of proteins that serve as the basis for measuring total protein.
- Define *isoelectric point* and *denaturation.*
- List the physical properties of proteins used by analytical techniques.
- Outline some of the biological properties of proteins.

PART 1: Proteins

Lawrence A. Kaplan

DEFINITION AND CLASSIFICATION

Proteins are linear polymers of α-amino acids. There are 20 natural amino acids with the general structure shown in Fig. 27-1. These exist as the L-stereoisomeric form with the amino group placed on the α-carbon atom next to the carboxylic acid group. The pK_a of the carboxylic acid group is approximately 1.8 to 2.4, whereas the pK_a of the α-amino group is approximately 8.53 to 10.53. This means that at pH less than 2.53, the carboxylic acid will be in nonionized form (COOH), whereas the α-amino group will remain ionized at pH values less than 9.53 (Fig. 27-2). At physiological pH (approximately 7.4), both groups are ionized. A compound (such as an amino acid) with two opposite charges is called a ***zwitterion*** ("hybrid ion" or "hermaphrodite ion").

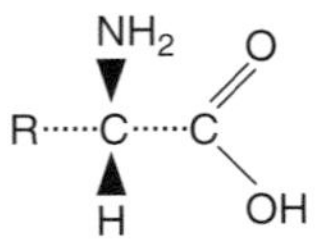

The side-chain groups of the 20 amino acids are listed in Table 27-1, along with the pK_a values of all ionizable groups. These side-chain groups can interact with one another to determine the overall chemical, physical, and biological properties of the polypeptide chain. The amino acids are covalently linked together by the protein-synthesizing machinery of cells. The actual order or sequence of amino acids in a protein chain is predetermined by the genetic code within the cell. The sequence of genetic information in DNA is transcribed into messenger RNA, which is translated in the cytoplasm into protein (Fig. 27-3). The specific sequence of amino acids for protein is called its **primary structure.**

Amino acids are linked together by the **peptide bond.** As shown in Fig. 27-4, this bond has a specific arrangement in three-dimensional space. The linear polypeptide chain can exist in three possible conformations—α-helix, β-pleated sheet, and random coil (see Color Plate 1). These conformations make up the **secondary structure** of the protein.

When a polypeptide chain is in solution, it is flexible enough for the molecule to bend, allowing the side-chain groups to interact with one another. The types of interactions are listed in Table 27-2. Although the interaction energy of each side group is small, the net energy of all these interactions is great enough to stabilize proteins in a folded, convoluted, three-dimensional spatial arrangement called the ***tertiary structure*** (see Color Plates 1 and 2). Each protein's unique tertiary structure confers on it specific biological properties.

NH2 O R C C H OH

Fig. 27-1 General structure of amino acid of L-stereoisomeric form. *Heavy lines,* bonds coming out of plane of page; *dotted lines,* bonds extending behind plane of paper.

NH+3 O R—C—C H OH <pH 2.5 >pH 3.5 NH+3 O R—C—C H O− >pH 10.5 <pH 9.5 NH2 O R—C—C H O−

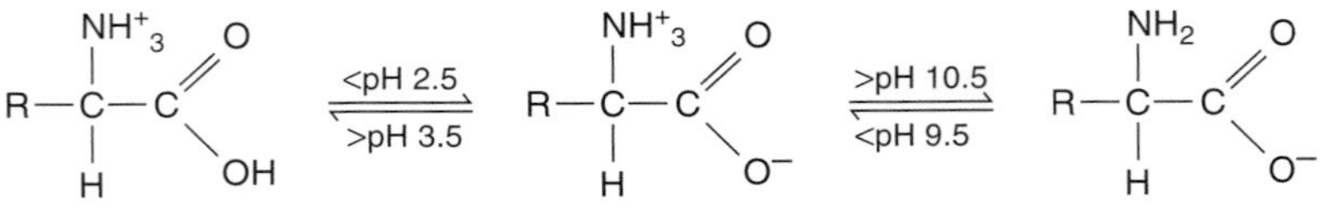

Zwitterion

Fig. 27-2 Various ionized and nonionized forms of amino acids present at various pH levels. When two opposite charges are present on the same molecule, the molecule is called a *zwitterion.*

Table 27-1 Classification and Properties of Side Chains (R Groups) for Naturally Occurring Amino Acids

R Group (R—CH(NH_2)COOH)	L-Amino Acid (Symbol)	Amino Acid Molecular Weight	pK_A* (25° C) Primary —COOH	Primary —NH_2	Secondary Groups
Nonpolar (Hydrophobic)					
H—	Glycine (gly), G	75.07	2.34	9.60	—
CH_3—	Alanine (ala), A	89.09	2.34	9.69	—
$(CH_3)_2CH$—	Valine (val), V	117.15	2.32	9.62	—
$(H_3C)_2CH—CH_2$—	Leucine (leu), L	131.18	2.36	9.60	—
$CH_3CH_2—CH(CH_3)$—	Isoleucine (ile), I	131.18	2.36	9.68	—
C_6H_5—CH_2—	Phenylalanine (phe), F	165.19	1.83	9.13	—
$H_2C—CH_2$, H_2C CH_2, N H (ring)	Proline (pro), P	115.13	1.99	10.60	—
$CH_3—S—CH_2CH_2$	Methionine (met), M	149.21	2.28	9.21	—
Neutral Polar (Hydrophilic)					
$OHCH_2$—	Serine (ser), S	105.09	2.21	9.15	—
$CH_3CH(OH)$—	Threonine (thr), T	119.12	—	—	—
$NH_2—C(=O)CH_2$—	Asparagine (asp), N	132.12	2.02	8.80	—
$NH_2—C(=O)CH_2CH_2$—	Glutamine (gln), Q	146.15	2.17	9.13	—
$HSCH_2$—	Cysteine (cys), C	121.16	1.96 (30°)	10.28	8.18 (SH)
HO—C_6H_4—CH_2—	Tyrosine (tyr), Y	181.19	2.20	9.11	10.07 (OH)
(indole) C—CH_2—, CH, N H	Tryptophan (trp), W	204.23	2.38	9.39	—
Acidic Polar (Hydrophilic)					
$HOOCCH_2$—	Aspartic acid (asp), D	133.10	1.88	9.60	3.65 (COOH)
$HOOCCH_2CH_2$—	Glutamic acid (glu), E	147.13	2.19	9.67	4.25 (COOH)
Basic Polar (Hydrophilic)					
$H_2NCH_2CH_2CH_2CH_2$—	Lysine (lys), K	146.19	2.18	8.95	(10.53) (ε—NH_3)
$H_2N—C(=NH)—NH—CH_2CH_2CH_2$—	Arginine (arg), R	174.20	2.17	9.04	12.48 (guanidinium)
HC=—CH_2—, N NH, C H (imidazole)	Histidine (his), H	155.16	1.82	9.17	6.00 (imidazolium)

From Cohn EJ, Edsall JT: *Proteins, amino acids and peptides,* New York, 1943, Reinhold Co.

*The pK_a values will be slightly different in a protein molecule.

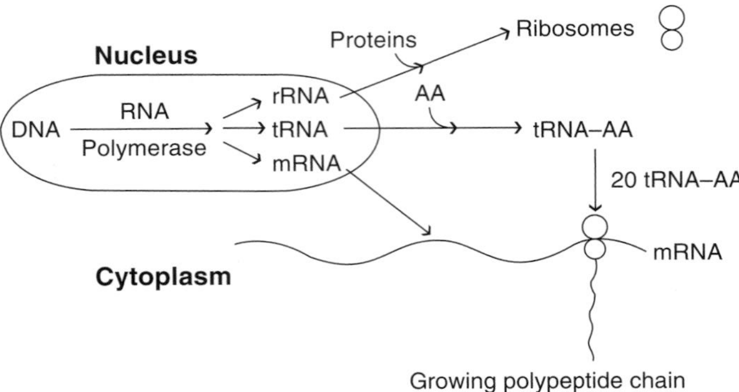

Fig. 27-3 Scheme of synthesis of proteins. *AA,* amino acid; *DNA,* deoxyribonucleic acid; *mRNA,* messenger ribonucleic acid; *rRNA,* ribosomal ribonucleic acid (18S and 28S forms); *tRNA,* transfer ribonucleic acid; *tRNA-AA,* activated amino acid covalently bound to amino acid–specific tRNA.

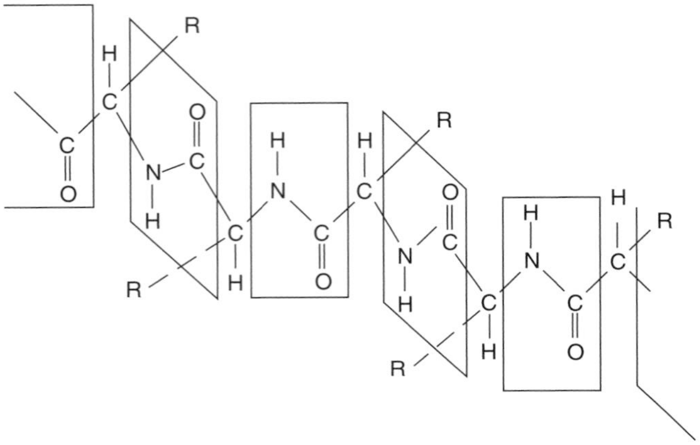

Fig. 27-4 Spatial relationships of a polypeptide bond. *C,* carbon atom; *H,* hydrogen atom; *N,* nitrogen atom; *O,* oxygen atom. (From Orten JM, Neuhaus OW: *Human Biochemistry,* ed 10, St Louis, 1982, Mosby.)

Table 27-2 Types of Intramolecular Side-Chain Interactions of Protein R-Groups

Type of Bond	Schematic*
Covalent	
Disulfide (cystine)	—S—S—
Lysinonorleucine (in collagen)	$-(CH_2)_3-CH_2-\overset{H}{N}-(CH_2)_4-$
Noncovalent	
Electrostatic	$C(=O)O^{\ominus}$ … $^{\oplus}NH_3$
Hydrogen	O—H···O=C—O^-
Hydrophobic	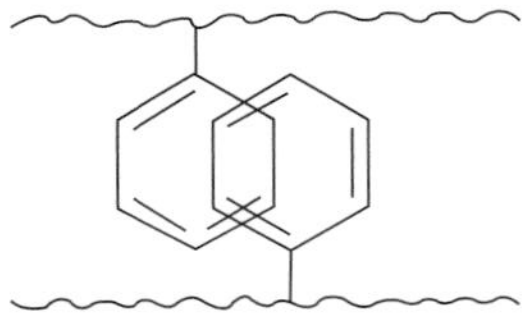
Van der Waals	CH_2OH … CH_2OH

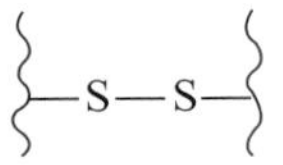

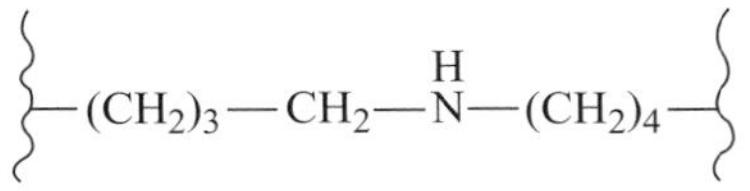

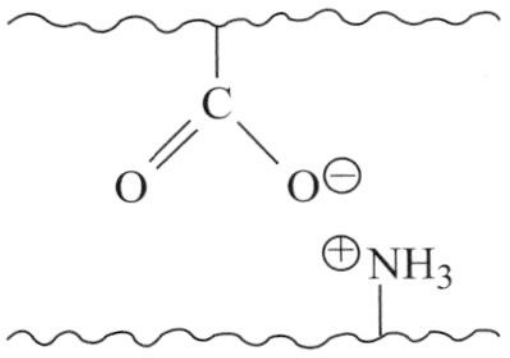

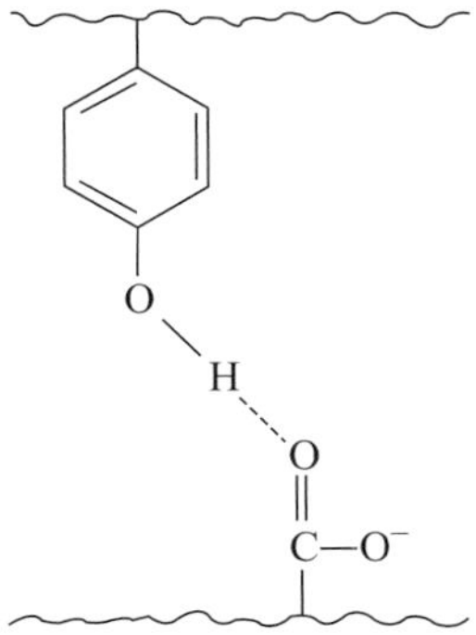

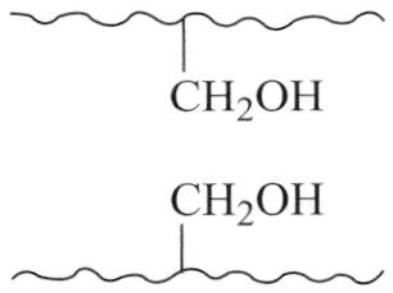

**Wavy line,* Polypeptide chain.

The folded polypeptide chains often are organized as aggregates with identical or different polypeptides. The specific number and type of these polypeptide chains determine the specific properties of the entire complex. The spatial arrangement of these multi-chain proteins is called the ***quaternary structure*** of the protein (see Color Plates 1 and 2). Usually, the biological properties of such quaternary proteins consisting of subunit chains are the sum of the properties of each individual chain.

Proteins generally are classified into two major groups—**simple proteins** and **compound (conjugated) proteins,** with several subdivisions within each group. This classification scheme is based on the physical properties and chemical composition of the protein.

I. Simple proteins—Generally not associated with other major chemical classes
   A. Globular proteins—Relatively symmetrical water-soluble or saline-soluble proteins
      1. Albumin—Major serum protein
      2. Globulins—Most other serum proteins
      3. Histones—Basic proteins found associated with nucleic acids
      4. Protamines—Strongly basic proteins found associated with nucleic acids
   B. Fibrous proteins—Asymmetrical proteins that are insoluble in water or dilute salts; highly resistant to most proteolytic enzymes
      1. Collagens—Major proteins of connective tissue; high in hydroxyproline content
      2. Elastins—Found in elastic tissue such as tendon and arteries
      3. Keratins—Major proteins in animal hair, nails, hooves, and elsewhere

II. Compound (conjugated) proteins—Combined with other non–amino acid biochemicals; considered to consist of two components: the protein, called the **apoprotein,** and the nonprotein **prosthetic group,** with the ability of the prosthetic group and the apoprotein to dissociate varying from group to group
   A. Nucleoproteins—The prosthetic groups are the nucleic acids (DNA or RNA)
   B. Mucoproteins—Contain large quantities (more than 4% by weight) of complex carbohydrates covalently linked to the protein
   C. Glycoproteins—Also contain covalently linked carbohydrate residues but usually less than 4% by weight
   D. Lipoproteins—Contain cholesterol, triglycerides, and phospholipids associated with highly water-insoluble apolipoproteins
   E. Metalloproteins—Include proteins that contain metals strongly bound to the protein, either as the ion or as complex metals, such as flavoproteins and hemoproteins
   F. Phosphoproteins—Contain high concentrations of phosphate groups covalently linked to protein

The biological functions of the proteins are extraordinarily varied, but many functions (see later discussion) are specific for only one or two of these classes of proteins.

CHEMICAL PROPERTIES

The chemical properties of proteins are based on the sum of their parts, that is, the constituent amino acids and prosthetic groups. The peptide bond is chemically reactive and serves as the basis for the most popular, specific method for quantifying total protein in serum. This is the biuret reaction. The amino acid side-chain groups are also chemically reactive, although only a few of these reactions are used in the chemistry laboratory. The amino groups at the *N*-terminus of the polypeptide chain and those of lysine and the guanidino groups of arginine can react with several compounds to produce an intense fluorescence. These same groups can react with ninhydrin to give a blue color. Both of these reactions have been used to quantify total protein. The phenolic group of tyrosine and the indole group of tryptophan react with the oxidizing reagent of the Folin-Wu or Lowry reactions to form a blue color. This method is employed with dilute solutions or microanalysis.

PHYSICAL PROPERTIES

The aromatic amino acids (tryptophan, phenylalanine, and tyrosine) give most proteins an absorption spectrum with the unique absorption maximum at 278 to 280 nm. The absorption at 280 nm is used to estimate the concentration of proteins in solution. In addition, complex proteins, such as hemoglobin, which have prosthetic groups with unique absorption properties, can be quantitated individually without extensive purification on the basis of their specific absorption spectra. The Soret absorption band of hemoglobin at 415 nm is used extensively to quantitate the concentration of hemoglobins.

Polypeptide chains vary widely in molecular size. The smallest polypeptides, such as the endorphins or the hypothalamic hormones, contain 5 to 25 amino acids, whereas the largest proteins, which contain several subunits, can have molecular weights in the millions of daltons. Although separation of protein on the basis of different molecular weights can be done, it is a method that is rarely used in the chemistry laboratory.

The density of most proteins falls within a fairly narrow range, averaging about 1.33 g/mL. Lipoproteins represent an important exception because the lipid content of these proteins gives them an unusually low density, allowing the various classes of lipoproteins to be separated from each other and from other proteins on the basis of their density. This technique is used mainly in specialized laboratories.

An important physical property of proteins is the net charge on the protein molecule. The net charge on a protein is the sum of all ionic charges of the amino acids and the carbohydrate and the prosthetic groups of the protein. Because the various chemical groups are ionized at different pH levels, the net charge of a protein varies with pH. The pH at which a protein carries no net charge is called *the isoelectric point (pI);* the isoelectric point of a protein is the point at which the number of positively charged groups equals the number of negatively charged groups. At a pH greater than the pI, the protein will be negatively charged, whereas at a pH less than the pI, it will be more positively charged. At physiological pH, most serum proteins are negatively charged.

Because proteins differ in the number and type of constituent amino acids, they also differ in their pIs. Therefore, at different pH levels, proteins will carry different net charges. This difference in net charge serves as the basis of many procedures for separating and quantifying classes of proteins or individual proteins. The most common procedures are electrophoresis, ion-exchange chromatography, and isoelectric focusing. After separation, individual proteins are detected spectrophotometrically, by their specific biological activity, or by use of specific stains.

Proteins found in body fluids are readily water soluble but can become insoluble in the presence of a wide range of denaturing or precipitating agents. These include organic solvents (such as acetone and acetonitrile), heavy metals (such as tungstic acid), certain salts (such as zinc hydroxide and ammonium sulfate), and strong acids (such as sulfosalicylic acid, trichloroacetic acid, and mineral acids). The **denaturation** of proteins from solution by the use of one or more of these chemicals forms the basis for a few routine clinical analyses. Cerebrospinal fluid and urine protein measurements are commonly performed by turbidimetric analysis. In addition, protein precipitation steps are often included as part of purification schemes for analytes before analysis.

BIOLOGICAL PROPERTIES

All proteins fulfill some physiological or biological function. The known functions of proteins cover a wide range of activities and are listed in Table 27-3. Often the known biological

Table 27-3 Biological Functions of Proteins

Function	Examples
Transport of small molecules	Transcortin (cortisol), thyroxine (thyroxine-binding globulin [TBG])
Receptors	Estriol receptors (cytoplasmic), insulin receptors (surface)
Catalytic	All enzymes
Structural	Collagen
Nutritional (source of calories and amino acids)	Albumin
Oncotic pressure	Albumin
Host defense vs. foreign antigens	Antibodies (all classes)
Hormonal function	Thyroid-stimulating hormone (TSH)
Coagulation	Fibrinogen

property of a protein forms the basis of a method for its detection and quantification.

Of the important physiological functions of proteins, the most important to the clinical chemistry laboratory are the transport, receptor, and catalytic functions. Many serum proteins function as specific transporters of small molecules. Most transport proteins are globular proteins. Examples include thyroid-binding globulin (TBG), which binds thyroxine; transcortin, which binds cortisol; and albumin, which transports free fatty acids, unconjugated bilirubin, calcium, and many other endogenous and exogenous compounds. The specific binding properties of these transport proteins have been used as the basis for procedures to measure the serum concentrations of cortisol, TBG saturation, and other analytes. The lipoproteins function as transporters of lipids in serum (see Chapter 37). The ability for many proteins, especially albumin, to act as non-specific binding agents is the basis for the quantitation of serum albumin and urinary total protein. Bromophenol blue binds rapidly to albumin and serves as the basis for the most commonly used serum albumin assay.

Many cellular proteins act as intermediary information processors for hormone molecules. Each protein, called a *receptor,* binds a specific hormone and then acts to transmit the hormonal message to the cell. Receptor proteins are usually glycoproteins. Assays for specific receptors, such as estrogen and progesterone receptors, are valuable for the management of breast cancer.

An important property of some proteins is their ability to catalyze biochemical reactions. The serum concentrations of these proteins, called *enzymes,* are important in determining the nature of a disease process. Most proteins that exhibit catalytic properties are globular proteins or metalloproteins. An enzyme most often is measured by monitoring the biochemical reaction that it catalyzes. The conditions of the enzyme assay are defined so as to attain maximum enzymatic activity and sensitivity of analysis (see Chapter 15).

One of the most important biological properties of proteins is their ability to act as antigens (see Chapter 7). An antigen inserted into an immunologically competent host will stimulate the synthesis of antibodies. Antibodies are also globular proteins. An antibody raised against a specific antigen will be able to bind specifically to that antigen. This antibody-antigen interaction is the basis of many assays for the sensitive and specific measurement of proteins and other molecules that cannot be detected by other means.

Proteins play a major role both intracellularly and in tissues. For example, connective tissue is composed primarily of collagen and mucoproteins. The proteins that form the cytoplasmic endoskeleton also fall into this group.

KEY CONCEPTS BOX 27-1

- The linear chains of L-amino acids constitute proteins, which can be categorized as globular, fibrous, and compound proteins.
- Chemical reaction with the peptide bond (biuret reaction) is the most common method of measuring total serum protein. Reaction by ninhydrin with free amino groups and the reaction of the Folin-Wu reagent with tyrosine and tryptophan are other reactions that can be used to quantitate protein. The ability of proteins, especially albumin, to bind dyes serves as the basis for quantifying serum albumin and urine protein.
- The absorption of light by peptide bonds (280 nm) or by prosthetic groups (e.g., heme group of hemoglobin) is an important basis for detecting proteins.
- The net charge on a protein can serve as the basis for separating and detecting proteins by electrophoresis or ion-exchange chromatography.
- The ability of proteins to act as antigens is the basis of immunological assay for many proteins.
- Important biological functions of proteins include structural, informational (receptors and hormones), catalytic (enzymes), blood carriers of small molecules, and their participation in the coagulation process.

SECTION OBJECTIVES BOX 27-2

- Describe how lipids are classified.
- Briefly describe the structures of triglycerides, phosphatidic acid, lecithins, cephalins, and steroids.
- List the chemical or physical properties of lipids that serve as the basis for their measurement.
- Outline some of the biological properties of lipids and their locations in specific tissues.

PART 2: Lipids

Herbert K. Naito

DEFINITION AND CLASSIFICATION

Lipids (fats) consist of a wide range of organic compounds that differ greatly in their chemical and physical properties and in their physiological roles. These include a variety of substances, such as fatty acids, sterols, triacylglycerides (more commonly called *triglycerides*), phosphorus-containing compounds (phospholipids), fat-soluble vitamins, bile acids, waxes, and other complex fats. As a consequence, it is difficult to provide a uniform and clear-cut definition of lipids that is broad enough to encompass all of these diverse compounds. In general, however, one can say that lipids are substances that are insoluble in water but soluble in organic solvents such as alcohol, chloroform, ether, acetone, hexane, and benzene. Even with this general definition, there are some exceptions, such as phospholipids, that are somewhat insoluble in acetone. In addition, some phospholipids, such as phosphatidyl serine, phosphatidyl inositol, and phosphatidyl ethanolamine, have a limited but significant ability to dissolve in water. There is no generally agreed-on system for the classification of lipids, but for simplicity, the following commonly used classification of lipids may be used.

Simple Lipids

Simple lipids are esters of fatty acids with various alcohols.

Neutral Fats

Neutral fats are esters of fatty acids and glycerol (triglycerides). Because they are uncharged, cholesterol and cholesterol esters are also called *neutral lipids.* However, structurally they are steroids and not neutral fats. The neutral fats contain mixtures of triglycerides such as stearic, palmitic, or oleic acid. The general formula for such a fat is

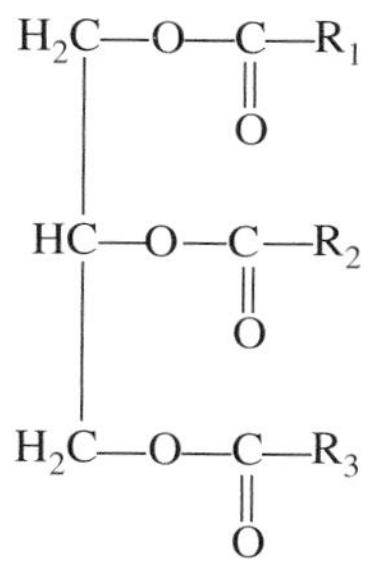

$$\begin{array}{l} H_2C—O—\overset{\displaystyle O}{\overset{\|}{C}}—R_1 \\ \ \ | \\ HC—O—\overset{\displaystyle O}{\overset{\|}{C}}—R_2 \\ \ \ | \\ H_2C—O—\overset{\displaystyle O}{\overset{\|}{C}}—R_3 \end{array}$$

If $R_1 = R_2 = R_3$ (where R = fatty acid), then the fat is a simple triglyceride. If the Rs are not equivalent, the fat is a mixed triglyceride. Naturally occurring fats usually exist as mixtures of mixed triglycerides.

The fats then are triesters of trihydric alcohol (glycerol) and of certain but not all organic acids. Because all three glycerol alcohol radicals are esterified, they are termed *triacylglycerides,* or more commonly, *triglycerides.* A simple ester would be formed by the combination of an acid and an alcohol as follows:

$$CH_3COOH + C_2H_5OH \rightarrow CH_3COOC_2H_5 + H_2O$$

A fat is formed by the combination of a fatty acid (usually of relatively high molecular weight) with the alcohol glycerol.

Because they are esters, the fats are readily hydrolyzed:

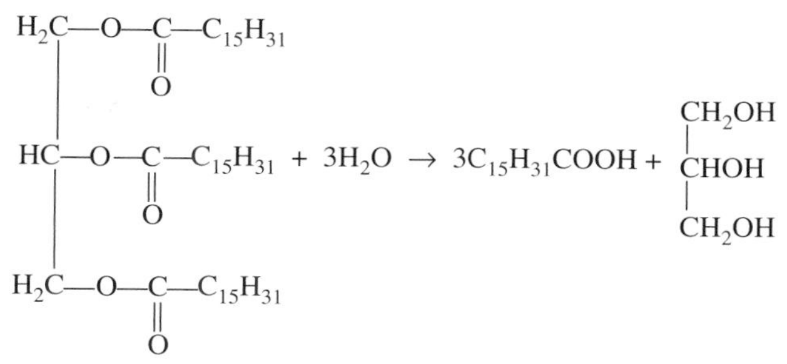

$$\begin{array}{l} H_2C—O—\overset{\displaystyle O}{\overset{\|}{C}}—C_{15}H_{31} \\ \ \ | \\ HC—O—\overset{\displaystyle O}{\overset{\|}{C}}—C_{15}H_{31} + 3H_2O \rightarrow 3C_{15}H_{31}COOH + \begin{array}{l} CH_2OH \\ | \\ CHOH \\ | \\ CH_2OH \end{array} \\ \ \ | \\ H_2C—O—\overset{\displaystyle O}{\overset{\|}{C}}—C_{15}H_{31} \end{array}$$

Tripalmitin **Palmitic acid** **Glycerol**

This hydrolysis is accomplished by the use of acid, alkali, superheated steam, or an appropriate enzyme (such as pancreatic lipase). In acid hydrolysis, the free fatty acid is liberated. When alkali is used, a soap is formed, and the process is called saponification:

$$\underset{\textbf{Stearin}}{C_3H_5(O—CO—C_{17}H_{35})_3} + 3NaOH \rightarrow \underset{\substack{\textbf{Sodium stearate} \\ \textbf{(a soap)}}}{3C_{17}H_{35}COONa} + \underset{\textbf{Glycerol}}{C_3H_5(OH)_3}$$

The fats that we eat are made up mostly of triglycerides that contain even-numbered fatty acids because of their mode of biosynthesis. These range from butyric (C_4) to lignoceric (C_{24}) and probably higher fatty acids (Table 27-4). Odd-numbered fatty acids do occur naturally.

Waxes

Waxes are esters of fatty acids with higher-molecular-weight alcohols than glycerol. Examples include carnauba wax, wool wax, beeswax, and sperm oil. Industrially, these are used in the manufacture of lubricants (sperm oil), polishes (carnauba wax), ointments (lanolin, which contains wool wax), candles (spermaceti), and so forth. Aside from cholesterol, the common alcohols found in waxes are cetyl alcohol ($C_{16}H_{33}OH$), ceryl alcohol ($C_{26}H_{53}OH$), and myricyl alcohol ($C_{30}H_{61}OH$).

Conjugated Lipids

Conjugated lipids are esters of fatty acids and an alcohol, plus additional chemical groups such as alcohols, phosphate, and sugars (Table 27-5).

Phospholipids

Phospholipids are lipids that have, in addition to fatty acids and glycerol, a phosphoric acid residue, nitrogen-containing bases, and other constituents. These lipids include phosphatidyl choline (lecithin), phosphatidyl ethanolamine, phosphatidyl inositol, phosphatidyl serine, sphingomyelins, and plasmalogens. Phosphatidyl ethanolamine, phosphatidyl serine, and phosphatidyl inositol (lipositol) are also known as cephalins. This class of complex lipids is also referred to as *glycerophosphatides, phosphoglycerides, glycerol phosphatides,* or, more commonly, *phospholipids.* Keep in mind that not all phosphorus-containing lipids are phosphoglycerides, that is, sphingomyelin is a phospholipid because it contains phosphorus, but it is better classified as a sphingolipid because of the nature of the backbone structure to which the fatty acid is attached. In phospholipids, one of the primary OH groups of glycerol is esterified to phosphoric acid; the other OH groups are esterified to fatty acids. The parent compound of the phospholipids is phosphatidic acid, which contains no polar alcohol group. The phospholipids are constituents of all animal and vegetable cells. They are present in abundance in brain, heart, kidney, eggs, soybeans, and so forth. In addition to carbon, hydrogen, and oxygen, the compounds contain the elements nitrogen and phosphorus. In lecithin and cephalin, the nitrogen-phosphorus ratio is 1:1; in sphingomyelin, it is 2:1.

$$
\begin{array}{l}
H_2{-}C{-}O{-}\overset{\overset{\large O}{\|}}{C}{-}R_1 \\
\quad\;| \\
H{-}C{-}O{-}\overset{\overset{\large O}{\|}}{C}{-}R_2 \\
\quad\;| \\
H_2{-}C{-}O{-}\overset{\overset{\large O}{\|}}{\underset{\underset{\large OH}{|}}{P}}{-}OH
\end{array}
$$

Phosphatidic acid

Phosphatidic Acid

Phosphatidic acid is important as an intermediate in the synthesis of triglycerides and phospholipids, but it is not found in any quantity in tissues. Phosphatidic acid is the simplest type of phospholipid. Phosphatidic acid is derived from glycerophosphoric acid by esterification of the two remaining OH groups with fatty acids.

Lecithins

On hydrolysis, a typical lecithin forms glycerol, 2 mol of fatty acids, phosphoric acid, and the nitrogenous base, choline. Most lecithins have a saturated fatty acid in the C-1 position and an unsaturated fatty acid in the C-2 position. The structural formula may be written as follows:

$$
\begin{array}{l}
H_2{-}C{-}O{-}\overset{\overset{\large O}{\|}}{C}{-}R_1 \\
\quad\;| \\
H{-}C{-}O{-}\overset{\overset{\large O}{\|}}{C}{-}R_2 \\
\quad\;| \\
H_2{-}C{-}O{-}\overset{\overset{\large O}{\|}}{P}{-}O^- \\
\qquad\qquad\;| \\
\qquad\qquad O{-}CH_2{-}CH_2{-}\overset{+}{N}(CH_3)_3
\end{array}
$$

Lecithin (phosphatidyl choline)

The lecithins, like cholesterol, are common cell constituents that occur principally in animal tissue, having both structural (as part of cell membranes) and metabolic functions. Although not found in depot fat, they make up a considerable proportion of the liver and brain lipids. They also occur in the plasma as part of the lipid-protein complexes called *lipoproteins;* thus they are important for the formation of these macromolecules, which play an important role in fat transport. Lecithins play an important role in the esterification of free cholesterol to form cholesterol ester. Lecithins are an important constituent of functional lung surfactant.

Table 27-4 Common Unsaturated Fatty Acids, Number of Double Bonds, and Length of Carbon Chain

Fatty Acid	Number of Double Bonds	Number of Carbons
Palmitoleic	1	16
Oleic	1	18
Linoleic	2	18
Linolenic	3	18
Arachidonic	4	20

Table 27-5 Classification of Phosphatides and Glycolipids

Name	Main Alcohol Component	Other Alcohol Components
Glycerophosphatides		
Phosphatidic acid	Diglyceride (= glycerol diester)	
Lecithin	Diglyceride (= glycerol diester)	Choline
Cephalin	Diglyceride (= glycerol diester)	Ethanolamine, serine
Inositide	Diglyceride (= glycerol diester)	Inositol
Plasmalogens (acetyl phosphatides)	Glycerol diester and enol ether	Ethanolamine, choline
Sphingolipids		
Sphingomyelins	*N*-Acylsphingosine	Choline
Cerebrosides	*N*-Acylsphingosine	Galactose,* glucose*
Sulfatides	*N*-Acylsphingosine	Galactose*
Gangliosides	*N*-Acylsphingosine	Hexoses,* hexosamine,* neuraminic acid*

*These components are not present as phosphoric esters but rather in glycosidic linkage; for this reason, cerebrosides, sulfatides, and gangliosides are called *glycolipids.*

Cephalins

The cephalins resemble the lecithins in structure except for the chemical component that replaces choline. The three main types of cephalins are the ethanolamine cephalins, the serine cephalins, and the inositol cephalins. The cephalins differ from lecithins in their insolubility in ethanol or methanol.

Phosphatidyl Ethanolamine

Phosphatidyl ethanolamine differs from lecithins in that ethanolamine replaces choline. Both α- and β-cephalins are known. This is one of the more abundant cephalins found in higher plants and animals.

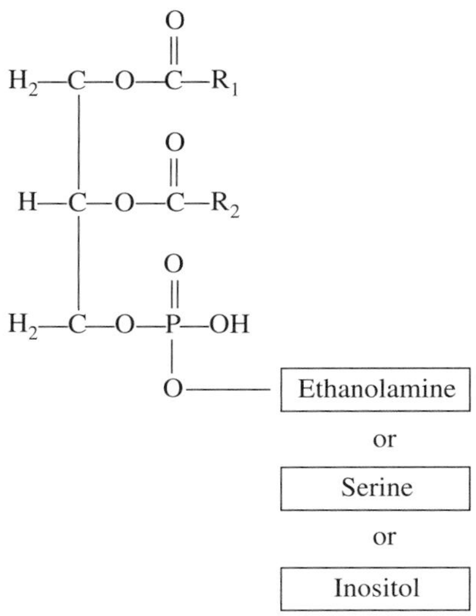

$$
\begin{array}{l}
H_2-C-O-\overset{\overset{O}{\|}}{C}-R_1 \\
\quad\;| \\
H-C-O-\overset{\overset{O}{\|}}{C}-R_2 \\
\quad\;| \\
H_2-C-O-\overset{\overset{O}{\|}}{\underset{\underset{O}{|}}{P}}-OH
\end{array}
$$

O—— Ethanolamine or Serine or Inositol

Phosphatidyl Serine

Phosphatidyl serine, which contains the amino acid serine rather than ethanolamine, has been found in tissues such as the brain.

Phosphatidyl Inositol

Phosphatidyl inositol is found in phospholipids of brain tissue and of soybeans and in other plant phospholipids as well. The inositol is present as the stereoisomer myoinositol.

Plasmalogens

Plasmalogens constitute as much as 10% of the phospholipids of the membranes of nerves and muscles. They are also found in the liver and other organs. Structurally, the plasmalogens resemble lecithins and cephalins, but they give a positive reaction when tested for aldehydes with Schiff's reagent (fuchsin-sulfurous acid) after pretreatment of the phospholipid with mercuric chloride. These phospholipids contain long-chain fatty aldehydes in place of fatty acids. Thus the basic units of this class of compounds include glycerol, phosphorus, fatty aldehyde, and ethanolamine.

Sphingolipids

The amino dialcohol group *sphingosine* characterizes all sphingolipids. The amino and the alcohol groups serve as a structural unit for substitution, just as the trihydroxyalcohol glycerol does in glycerides. Sphingosine is a long-chain C_{18} compound that contains a trans-double bond, an NH_2 group on C-2, and two OH groups (on C-1 and C-3). Sphingolipids are especially abundant in the brain. Some storage diseases are characterized biochemically by the accumulation of certain sphingolipids. There are four major categories (see Table 27-5): sphingomyelins, cerebrosides, sulfatides, and gangliosides.

Sphingomyelins

Sphingomyelins are found in the brain and other organs. Stearic, lignoceric, and nervonic acids are the sole fatty acids present in brain sphingomyelins, whereas palmitic and lignoceric acids are the fatty acids in lung and spleen sphingomyelins. A typical formula is shown below.

Sphingomyelin

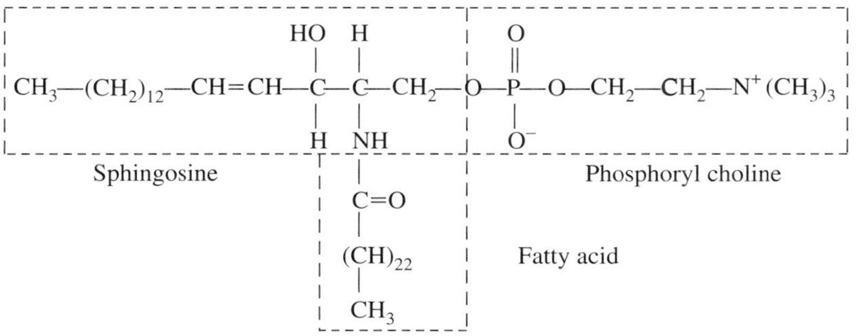

$$
CH_3-(CH_2)_{12}-CH=CH-\underset{\underset{H}{|}}{\overset{\overset{HO}{|}}{C}}-\underset{\underset{\underset{\underset{\underset{\underset{\underset{CH_3}{|}}{(CH)_{22}}}{|}}{C=O}}{|}}{NH}}{|}}{\overset{\overset{H}{|}}{C}}-CH_2-O-\underset{\underset{O^-}{|}}{\overset{\overset{O}{\|}}{P}}-O-CH_2-CH_2-N^+(CH_3)_3
$$

Sphingosine | Fatty acid | Phosphoryl choline

and its two important constituents are:

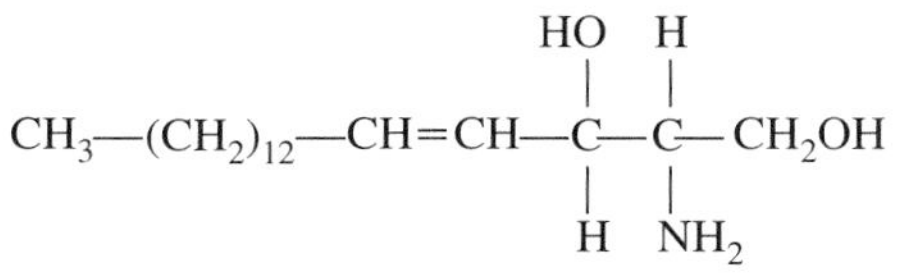

$$
CH_3-(CH_2)_{12}-CH=CH-\underset{\underset{H}{|}}{\overset{\overset{HO}{|}}{C}}-\underset{\underset{NH_2}{|}}{\overset{\overset{H}{|}}{C}}-CH_2OH \qquad CH_3(CH_2)_{22}-COOH
$$

Sphingosine 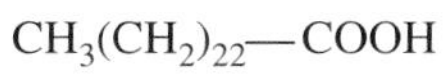 **Lignoceric acid**

Cerebrosides

Cerebrosides contain galactose or glucose, a high-molecular-weight fatty acid, and sphingosine. Thus cerebrosides have the following basic structure:

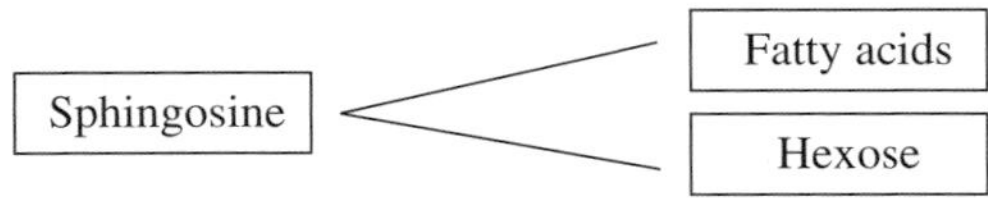

Cerebrosides are structurally similar to sphingomyelins. They also may be classified with the sphingomyelins as sphingolipids. Individual cerebrosides are differentiated by the type of fatty acid in the molecule: kerasins contain lignoceric acid; cerebrons contain a hydroxylignoceric acid (cerebronic acid); nervons contain an unsaturated homologue of lignoceric acid called *nervonic acid;* and oxynervons apparently contain the hydroxyl derivative of nervonic acid as a constituent fatty acid.

$$CH_3\text{—}(CH_2)_{22}\text{—}COOH$$

Lignoceric acid

$$CH_3\text{—}(CH_2)_{21}\text{—}CH(OH)\text{—}COOH$$

Cerebronic acid

$$CH_3\text{—}(CH_2)_7\text{—}CH{=}CH\text{—}(CH_2)_{13}\text{—}COOH$$

Nervonic acid

$$CH_3\text{—}(CH_2)_7\text{—}CH{=}CH\text{—}(CH_2)_{12}\text{—}CO(OH)\text{—}COOH$$

Oxynervonic acid

Cerebrosides are found in many tissues other than the brain. In Gaucher's disease, the cerebroside content of the reticuloendothelial cells (as in the spleen) is very high. The cerebrosides occur in much higher concentration in myelinated than in nonmyelinated nerve fibers.

Sulfatides

Sulfatides are sulfate derivatives of the galactosyl residue in cerebrosides.

Gangliosides

Gangliosides are glycolipids that occur in the brain (in ganglionic cells). The main components are sphingosine, fatty acids, and branched chain carbohydrates with as many as seven sugar residues. The construction of gangliosides is similar to that of cerebrosides, but the carbohydrate moiety is far more complex. The various gangliosides are different primarily in terms of the number of sugar residues.

Derived Lipids

Derived lipids are compounds derived from the hydrolysis of simple and conjugated fats. These include the compounds described below.

Fatty Acids

Fatty acids are straight-chain carboxylic acids (both saturated, containing no double bonds, and unsaturated, containing one or more double bonds). More than 100 different kinds of fatty acids have been isolated from various lipids of animals, plants, and microorganisms. All possess a long hydrocarbon chain and a terminal carboxyl group. Fatty acids are obtained from the hydrolysis of fats or can be synthesized from two carbon units (acetyl radicals). Fatty acids that occur in naturally occurring fats usually contain an even number of carbon atoms (because they are synthesized from two carbon units) and are straight-chain derivatives.

Some generalizations may be made about the fatty acids present in lipids of higher plants and animals. Nearly all have an even number of carbon atoms and have chains that are between 14 and 22 carbon atoms long; those that have 16 or 18 carbons are by far the most abundant. In general, unsaturated fatty acids predominate over the saturated type, particularly in the neutral fats and in cells of poikilothermic (cold-blooded) organisms living at lower temperatures. Unsaturated fatty acids have lower melting points than saturated fatty acids. Most neutral fats rich in unsaturated fatty acids are liquid down to 5° C or lower. In most unsaturated fatty acids in higher organisms, a double bond is present between carbon atoms 9 and 10; additional double bonds usually occur between C-10 and the methyl end of the chain. In fatty acids containing two or more double bonds, the double bonds are never found in conjugation but are separated by one methylene group. The double bonds of nearly all naturally occurring unsaturated fatty acids are in the cis configuration. The most abundant unsaturated fatty acids in higher organisms are oleic, linoleic, linolenic, and arachidonic acids (see Table 27-4).

Alcohols

Straight-chain alcohols and cyclic alcohols (such as the sterols) are a subclass of derived lipids.

These compounds are widely distributed in plant and animal tissues, either in the free state or in the form of esters (in combination with higher fatty acids). Chemically, the sterols are known as phenanthrene derivatives, or, more correctly, cyclopentanoperhydrophenanthrene derivatives.

Steroids

The best known steroid is cholesterol. It is present in all animal cells and is particularly abundant in nervous tissue and liver. Varying quantities of this steroid are found admixed in animal fats but not in vegetable fats. The structure of a cholesterol molecule is illustrated in Fig. 27-5.

Steroids may be classified into the following groups:

- Sterols
- Bile acids
- Substances obtained from cardiac glycosides
- Substances obtained from saponins
- Sex hormones

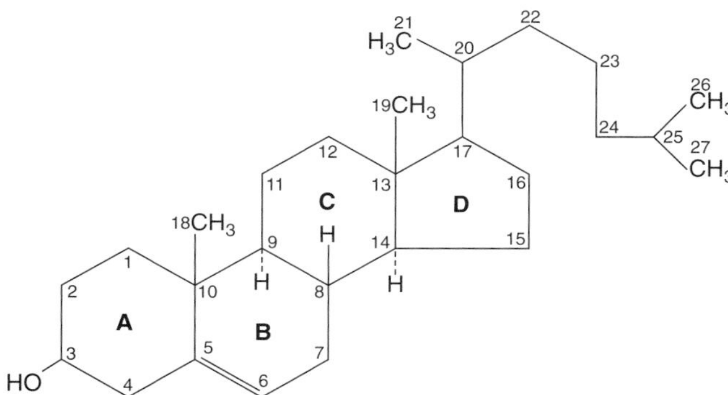

Fig. 27-5 Structure of cholesterol molecule, a C_{27} hydrocarbon sterol.

- Adrenocorticosteroids
- Vitamin D

Cholesterol is the precursor of many other steroids in animal tissues, including the bile acids, detergent-like compounds that aid in emulsification and absorption of lipids in the intestine; the androgens, or male sex hormones; the estrogens, or female sex hormones; the progestational hormones; and the adrenocortical hormones.

Cholesterol, a member of a large subgroup of steroids called *the sterols,* is a steroid alcohol that contains a hydroxyl group at carbon 3 of ring A and a branched aliphatic chain of eight or more carbon atoms at carbon 17. Sterols occur either as free alcohols or as long-chain fatty acid esters of the hydroxyl group at carbon 3; all are solids at room temperature. Cholesterol melts at 150° C and is insoluble in water, but it is readily extracted from tissues with chloroform, ethyl ether, or hot alcohol. Cholesterol occurs in the plasma membranes of animal cells and in the lipoproteins of blood. Cholesterol is found only in animal tissues and fluids, never in plants.

Other similar steroids are phytosterols, which are steroids derived from plants. Among these are stigmasterol, campesterol, and sitosterol. Fungi and yeasts contain still other types of sterols, the mycosterols. Among these is ergosterol, which is converted to vitamin D.

Bile Acids

Bile acids (C_{24} steroids) are digestion-promoting constituents of bile. They are surface-active agents, which means that they lower surface tension and thus can emulsify fats—an important step in the formation of micelles. Bile acids also activate gastrointestinal lipases. For these reasons, bile acids play an important physiological role in the digestion and absorption of fats.

The major primary bile acids are cholic acid and chenodeoxycholic acid, which are made in the liver by the enzymatic cleavage of the terminal three carbons on the cholesterol molecule (a C_{27} hydrocarbon). Thus the bile acids are one of the end products of the metabolism of cholesterol; however, it should be noted that bile acid constitutes the acidic sterol fraction of the bile, which is about 50% to 60% of the total steroid excreted. The remainder of the steroid output in the bile is in the form of neutral steroids, such as cholesterol.

Hydrocarbons

The hydrocarbons are both aliphatic and cyclic compounds.

Vitamins

Vitamins and their structures are presented in Chapter 43.

Other Compound Lipids

Sulfolipids, aminolipids, and lipoproteins also may be placed in this category.

CHEMICAL AND PHYSICAL PROPERTIES

Melting Point

The melting point of fatty acids is influenced by the chain length and the degree of chain unsaturation. Increasing the chain length and decreasing the number of unsaturated double bonds will increase the melting point of fatty acids. The melting points of fatty acids and other lipids can be used to identify the compound, but this property is not used routinely in analysis.

Solubility

The relative insolubility of lipids in aqueous solutions is an important property of lipids. The major consequence of this insolubility is that analyses of lipids often require treatment of the sample to extract the lipid into a more lipid-soluble medium, such as methanol, chloroform, or ethyl ether.

Specific Gravity

The specific gravity of all fat is less than 1 g/mL. Consequently, all fats float in water, and refrigerated serum samples that contain increased amounts of lipid-containing lipoproteins often will have a distinct fat layer floating on top of the aqueous serum. This characteristic has made it possible for lipoproteins to be selectively separated from more dense proteins, and for individual lipoproteins to be separated from one another, on the basis of varying proportions of lipid content.

Alcohol Groups of Steroids

The chemically reactive alcohol group of steroids forms the basis of many assays for quantitating cholesterol. The hydroxyl group can be specifically oxidized by the enzyme cholesterol oxidase. Monitoring of this reaction serves as the basis for enzyme assays for cholesterol.

Triglyceride Composition

The chemical composition of triglycerides (i.e., glycerol esterified by three fatty acids) is the basis of all methods of quantitating triglycerides. These techniques are based on the quantitation of glycerol released from triglycerides after chemical or enzymatic hydrolysis of the fatty acid esters. The glycerol can be oxidized chemically or enzymatically to form measurable chromogens.

BIOLOGICAL PROPERTIES

The most important biological properties of lipids are structural, nutritional, and hormonal (see Chapter 48). Almost all classes of lipids are used as structural components of membranes. The triglycerides are essential components in the formation of the bimolecular protein-lipid–lipid-protein membranes. Cell membranes also contain varying quantities of steroids, phospholipids, and other complex lipids.

Triglycerides also function as an important source of calories and as a source of carbon atoms for the synthesis of other macromolecules.

KEY CONCEPTS BOX 27-2

- Lipids usually are classified as neutral lipids (triglycerides); conjugated, and derived lipids, such as steroids.
- Triglycerides are the products of three esterification reactions between one molecule of glycerol and three molecules of fatty acids to form the neutral triacyl compounds.
- The conjugated phospholipids are formed from phosphatidic acid, in which the last hydroxyl group on glycerol reacts with phorphoric acid. The phosphate groups of phosphatidic acid can react with choline to form the charged lecithin molecule, or with ethanolamine, serine, or inositol to form the cephalins.
- Steroids are highly insoluable lipids derived from cholesterol; the C-3 alcohol group can be esterified with fatty acids.
- Important biological functions of fats include structural (cell membranes), nutritional (triclycerides), and hormonal (steroids) functions.
- Lipids can be separated and measured by their size or density and by reactions with metabolic enzymes.

SECTION OBJECTIVES BOX 27-3

- Describe how carbohydrates are classified, and give an example of each.
- List the primary functions of carbohydrates in human biology.
- Explain how the chemical and physical properties of carbohydrates are related to their biological properties.
- List the properties of the carbohydrates that serve as the basis of laboratory measurements.

PART 3: Carbohydrates

Lawrence A. Kaplan

DEFINITION AND CLASSIFICATION

The earliest **carbohydrates** were found to have the empirical formula of $(CH_2O)_n$. Thus these chemicals were defined simply as compounds consisting of hydrated (H_2O) carbon, hence the name *carbohydrate.* Subsequently, the existence of complex carbohydrates containing other chemical moieties was noted. Thus carbohydrates can be linked covalently to proteins, lipids, and nucleic acids. The various classes of carbohydrates are discussed below.

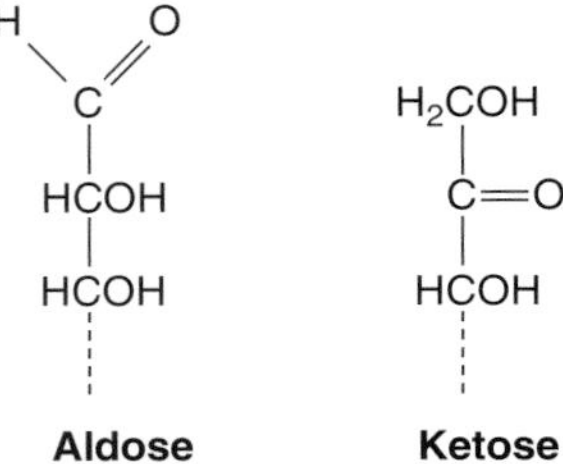

Fig. 27-6 Structural differences between aldoses and ketoses, which are aldehydes and ketones, respectively.

Simple Monomeric Carbohydrates (Saccharides)

Saccharides are also known as sugars, and their common names all end with the suffix "-ose," meaning "sugar." The smallest sugar units are monosaccharides, in which the *n* in the formula $(CH_2O)_n$ is valued from 3 to 8. If n = 3, the sugar is a triose; if n = 4, a tetrose; and so forth. The monosaccharides are straight carbon chains in which each carbon atom except one carries a hydroxyl group (–OH); the one remaining carbon atom has a carbonyl group. If the carbonyl group is on the first or the last carbon atom, the carbonyl group is an aldehyde and the monosaccharide is called an **aldose**. If the carbonyl group is on an internal carbon atom, it is a ketone, and the monosaccharide is called a **ketose** (Fig. 27-6). Thus a 4-carbon aldose is an aldotetrose, a 6-carbon ketose is a ketohexose, and so forth.

The monosaccharides found in nature are all stereoisomers. Stereoisomerism is physically defined by the ability of a molecule to rotate the plane of incident polarized light. The physical and chemical properties of, for example, all eight aldohexoses (6-carbon chain) are exactly the same, except for their different actions on polarized light. All the monosaccharides in human biochemistry are of the dextroisomeric (D) form. Examples of some monosaccharides are given in Fig. 27-7.

The pentose and hexose monosaccharides also have the ability to form ring structures by intramolecular reaction of the terminal hydroxyl group with the carbonyl function. The six-membered ring forms of the sugars are called **pyranoses,** whereas the five-membered rings are called **furanoses.** The aldohexoses, such as D-glucose, form six-membered rings, whereas an aldoketose, such as D-fructose, forms a five-membered ring (see Fig. 27-7).

Glucose can form two types of six-membered rings. These rings differ in how the hydroxyl group at the number 1 carbon atom is positioned with respect to the plane of the ring. If the hydroxyl group is on the same side of the molecule as the ring oxygen (see Fig. 27-7), the isomer is known as the α-D-glucose isomer, whereas if the hydroxyl group is on the opposite side

α-D-Glucose (α-D-glucopyranose) ⇄ D-Glucose (aldehyde form) ⇄ β-D-Glucose (β-D-glucopyranose)

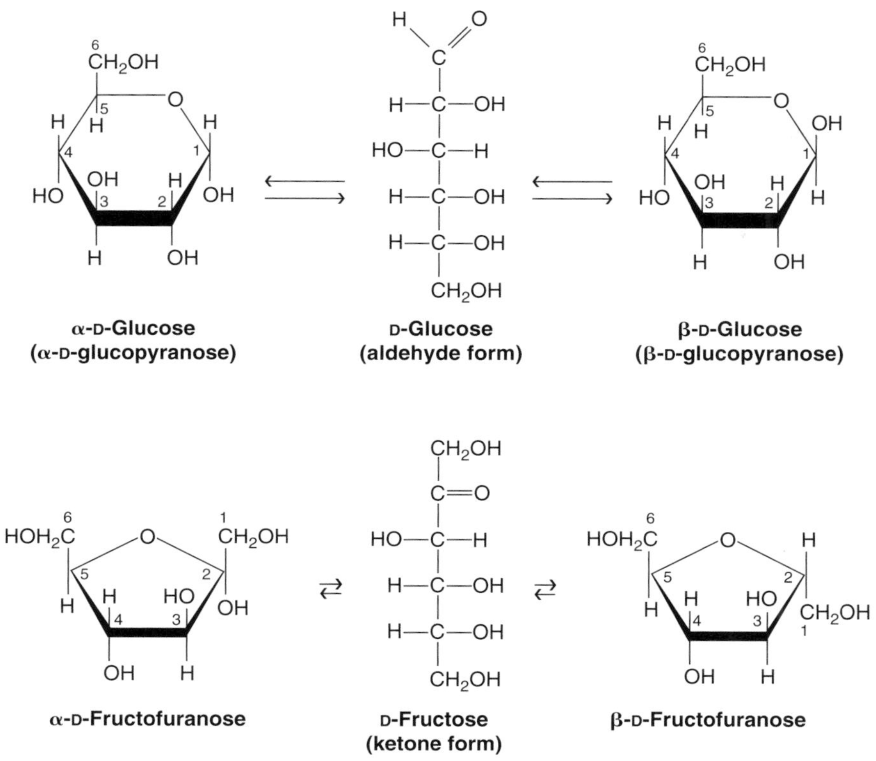

α-D-Fructofuranose ⇄ D-Fructose (ketone form) ⇄ β-D-Fructofuranose

Fig. 27-7 Interrelationships between straight-chain and ring forms of D-glucose and D-fructose, which form pyranose and furanose rings. (From Orten JM, Neuhaus OW: *Human Biochemistry,* ed 10, St Louis, 1982, Mosby.)

of the ring oxygen, then this isomer is known as the β-D-glucose. Enzymes that act on carbohydrates usually have a specificity directed toward one of the isomers, usually the most common one found, such as β-D-fructose.

Derived Monosaccharides

Derived monosaccharides are formed by the reduction or oxidation of the carbonyl groups. The products of reductive reactions are polyols (polyalcohols), such as D-sorbitol or D-mannitol, whereas the products of oxidation are acids, such as D-glucuronic acid (from D-glucose). Many acid forms of monosaccharides are important constituents of more complex carbohydrates, such as mucopolysaccharides.

An important group of derived monosaccharides is the result of the replacement of a hydroxyl group by an amino group. The term ***sialic acid*** is used to describe the important *N*-acetyl derivatives of neuraminic acid, which often are found covalently linked to proteins (Fig. 27-8).

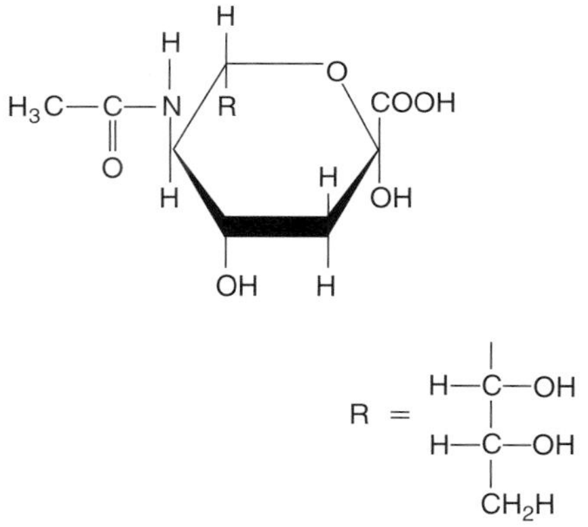

N-Acetylneuraminic acid

Fig. 27-8 Structure of *N*-acetylneuraminic acid ("sialic acid"). (From Orten JM, Neuhaus OW: *Human Biochemistry,* ed 10, St Louis, 1982, Mosby.)

Complex Carbohydrates

These molecules are formed by linking two or more monosaccharides through a glycosidic linkage (Fig. 27-9). The simplest disaccharides, which are important nutritionally, are maltose (two glucose), lactose (milk sugar, one galactose and one glucose), and sucrose (one fructose and one glucose). *Oligosaccharides* often are defined as carbohydrates that contain two to ten monosaccharide subunits. Polysaccharides are larger polymers of up to 100 million daltons. All three of the most important polysaccharides contain glucose as the monomeric subunit. Cellulose, a structural component of plant walls, consists of glucose units linked by a β-(1→4) glycosidic bond to form long, unbranched chains. Starch, a storage form of glucose in plants, consists of glucose residues connected by α-(1→4) glycosidic linkages, which, unlike the β-(1→4) linkages of cellulose, are amenable to degradation by human hydrolytic enzymes (such as amylase). Starch also differs from cellulose in that it is a branched molecule. Branching points are scattered throughout the molecule formed by α-(1→6) bonds. The two forms of starch therefore are called *amylose* (the straight-chain fraction) and *amylopectin* (the highly

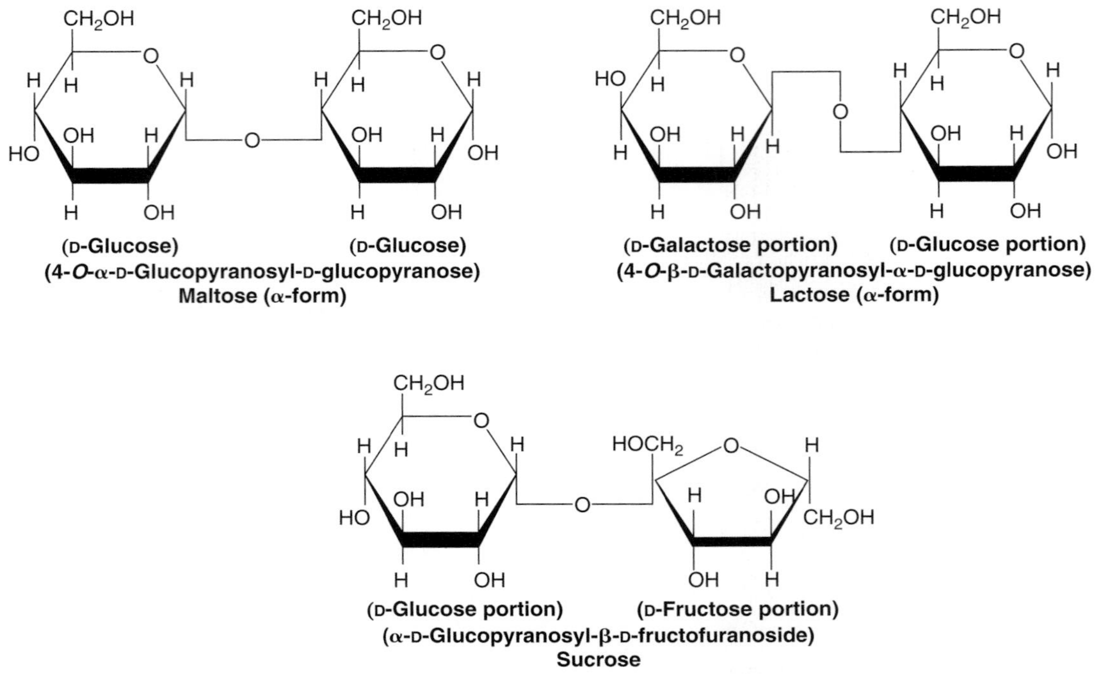

(D-Glucose) (D-Glucose)
(4-*O*-α-D-Glucopyranosyl-D-glucopyranose)
Maltose (α-form)

(D-Galactose portion) (D-Glucose portion)
(4-*O*-β-D-Galactopyranosyl-α-D-glucopyranose)
Lactose (α-form)

(D-Glucose portion) (D-Fructose portion)
(α-D-Glucopyranosyl-β-D-fructofuranoside)
Sucrose

Fig. 27-9 Common disaccharides linked by α-glycosidic bonds. (From Orten JM, Neuhaus OW: *Human Biochemistry,* ed 10, St Louis, 1982, Mosby.)

branched fraction). Glycogen is the glucose-storage molecule found in animal cells. Glycogen more closely resembles amylopectin than amylose because of its highly branched nature (see Fig. 38-4).

Complex polysaccharides that contain hyaluronic acid, chondroitin-4-sulfate, and keratin sulfates as the repeating subunits are important constituents of synovial fluid and connective tissue. Heparin is a complex negatively charged, polysaccharide that contains D-glucuronic acid-2-sulfate-*N*-acetyl-D-glucosamine-6-sulfate as the repeating subunit.

CHEMICAL PROPERTIES

The monosaccharides (pentoses and larger) can undergo dehydration in the presence of hot mineral acids to form the cyclic furfural derivatives. Glucose can be dehydrated in this manner to form 3-hydroxymethylfurfural—a reaction that forms the basis for a colorimetric assay for glycosylated proteins.

An important chemical property of the monosaccharides is the ability of these compounds to be oxidized or reduced, and in turn to reduce or oxidize some other compounds. The ability of reducing aldoses, such as glucose, to be oxidized to the acid form has been the historical basis for chemical assays for glucose. The glucose in turn reduced such compounds as Cu^{++} or $Fe(CN_6)^{-3}$ with the formation of colored complexes of the reduced forms of these compounds (such as Cu^+ and Cu_2O), which is the basis for a confirmation test for the presence of urine glucose.

The enzymatic oxidation of glucose by glucose oxidase forms the basis of many of the current glucose assay procedures, whereas the oxidation of glucose-6-phosphate is the basis of the hexokinase assay for glucose.

Aldoses, such as glucose, can react with primary amines to form **Schiff's base.** This nonenzymatic condensation is the mechanism for the formation of glycoproteins, such as glycosylated hemoglobin, in blood.

PHYSICAL PROPERTIES

The commonly measured monosaccharides and disaccharides are highly water-soluble compounds. Assays for these analytes thus do not require prior extraction or purification. Separation of the monosaccharides by adsorption chromatography is possible, although this process is usually performed by specialized metabolic laboratories. The simple monosaccharides, disaccharides, or polysaccharides are not readily distinguished by their spectral or electrophoretic properties.

BIOLOGICAL PROPERTIES

The monosaccharides and the disaccharides are the major sources of calories for the human body and as such serve as a primary form of energy nutrition. Polymeric forms of glucose, such as glycogen, provide storage for glucose in liver and muscle cells. Complex polysaccharides are found in body fluids and connective tissue.

KEY CONCEPTS BOX 27-3

- Carbohydrates are classified as simple monosaccharides such as glucose, derived carbohydrates that contain other functional groups such as an amino group in glucosamine, and complex, or polymerized, carbohydrates. The latter can contain two subunits, such as galactose or fructose, or thousands of subunits, such as glycogen or starch.
- The primary function of carbohydrates is nutritional; glucose is the body's primary energy source.
- The monosaccharides are all polyols, that is, they contain multiple hydroxyl groups, and contain an aldehyde or ketone group, and these carbonyl groups are very reactive and allow the monosaccharides to react freely with primary amines of proteins.
- The enzymes used in the metabolism of carbohydrates have been used for measurement of the carbohydrates. The sugars can act directly, as glucose does in the glucose oxidase or glucose dehydrogenase assays, of after release from larger molecules, as does glucose following its release from glycogen.

SECTION OBJECTIVES BOX 27-4

- Describe the basic structure of the predominant purine and pyrimidine bases.
- Describe how nucleosides and nucleotides are defined.
- Outline the polymeric structure of DNA and RNA.
- What is the primary function of DNA? RNA?
- List the steps that result in a synthesized protein, and explain where in the cell each of those steps takes place.

PART 4: Nucleic Acids

Amadeo J. Pesce

DEFINITION AND CLASSIFICATION

Purine and Pyrimidine Bases

The building blocks of the nucleic acids are the purine and pyrimidine bases. They are part of the structure of adenosine triphosphate (ATP) and guanosine triphosphate (GTP), which function as immediate sources of energy, coenzymes (such as NAD), intracellular messenger molecules, and core components of DNA and RNA. The general structures of purines and pyrimidines are shown in Fig. 27-10. The structures of the most commonly observed bases are found in Fig. 27-11. The structure of 5-methylcytosine formed by methylation of cytosine is also presented in Fig. 27-13. These molecules usually are found linked to the 5-carbon sugar molecule ribose or deoxyribose through a β–*N*-glycosidic bond to the

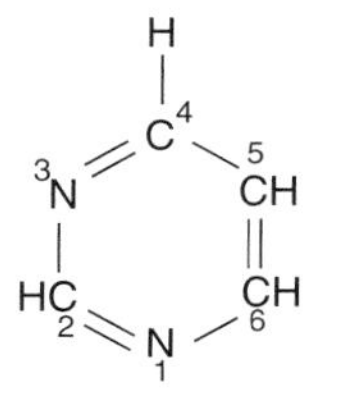

Pyrimidine

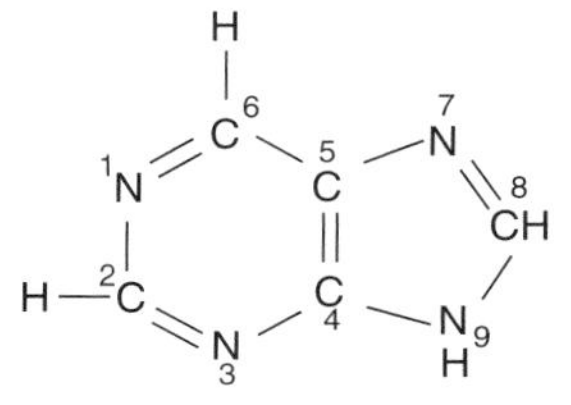

Purine

Fig. 27-10 General structures of pyrimidine and purine bases and the International Union of Pure and Applied Chemistry (IUPAC) numbering of the ring positions.

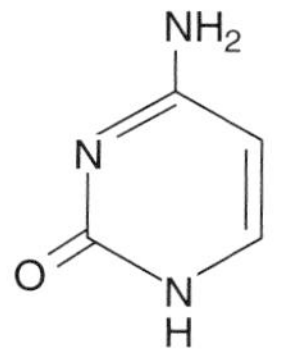

Cytosine (C) (2-oxy-4-aminopyrimidine)

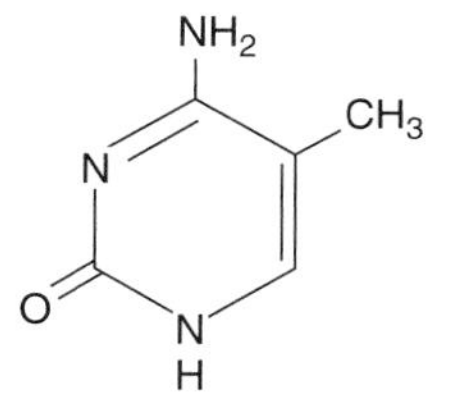

5-Methylcytosine

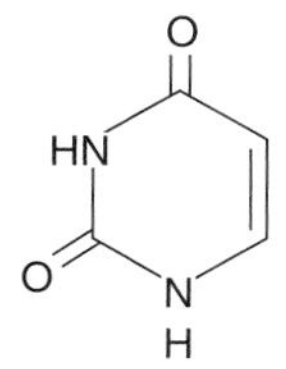

Uracil (U) (2,4-dioxypyrimidine)

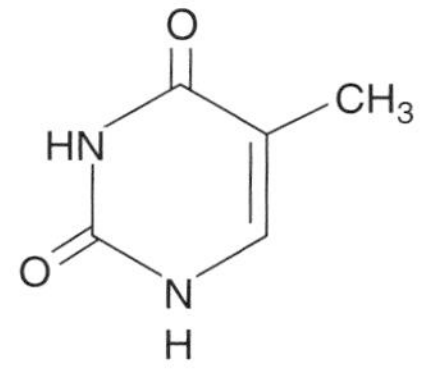

Thymine (T) (2,4-dioxy-5-methylpyrimidine)

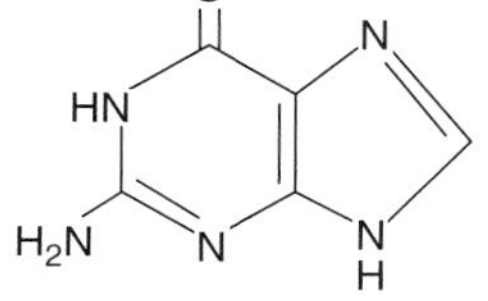

Guanine (G) (2-amino-6-oxypurine)

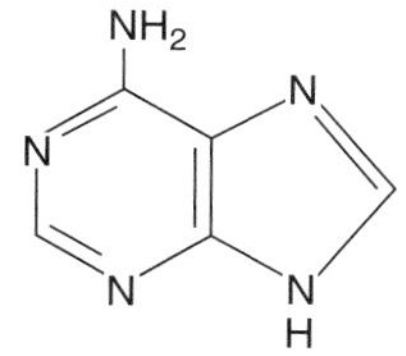

Adenine (A) (6-aminopurine)

Fig. 27-11 Structures of the most common pyrimidine and purine bases.

1 position of the pyrimidine ring or the 9 position of the purine ring (Fig. 27-12); as such, they are termed **nucleosides.** When the sugar molecules can have phosphate groups attached at the 3′ and/or 5′ position (Fig. 27-13), these structures are termed **nucleotides.** The nucleotides can exist as the monophosphate, diphosphate, and triphosphate forms (Fig. 27-14). The triphosphate forms have regulatory properties and serve as the chemical energy reservoir of the cell. The adenosine and guanosine monophosphate nucleotides can exist in cyclic forms, in which the phosphate is linked to both 3′ and 5′ positions (Fig. 27-15).

Nucleoside **(Deoxy) nucleoside**

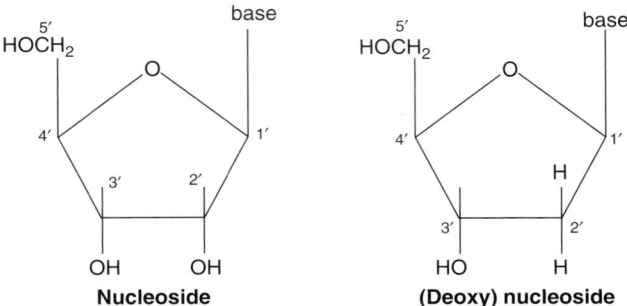

Fig. 27-12 General structures of the ribonucleosides and deoxyribonucleosides and the International Union of Pure and Applied Chemistry (IUPAC) numbering of the sugar positions.

DNA AND RNA

DNA and RNA are linear polymers of nucleotide bases. Four natural nucleotides constitute DNA, and four nucleotides constitute RNA. These nucleotides are linked through phosphate glycoside bonds at the 3′ and 5′ positions of the 5-carbon ribose or deoxyribose when these molecules are polymerized (Fig. 27-16). The order or sequence of nucleotides in the DNA chain is the genetic code present within the cell. The sequence of information in the DNA is transcribed into messenger RNA, which then is translated into protein (see Fig. 27-3).

The DNA polymer chain has a specific arrangement in three-dimensional spaces. Each chain of the DNA polymer has an opposite or complementary chain. These chains are noncovalently bound to each other through hydrogen bonds, forming a double helix. The bonding is specifically paired, with adenosine hydrogen-bonded to the thymidine molecule and the cytosine molecule hydrogen-bonded to the guanosine molecule (Fig. 27-17). The DNA polymers combine with groups of polycationic proteins termed *histones,* which contain high concentrations of lysine and arginine amino acids. The histones assist in the regulation of DNA transcription. The resulting nucleosome fibers (Fig. 27-18) form very compact structures called *chromosomes.*

5′ Ribonucleotide **3′ Ribonucleotide**

Fig. 27-13 General structures of the 3′ and 5′ nucleotides.

Nucleotide diphosphate

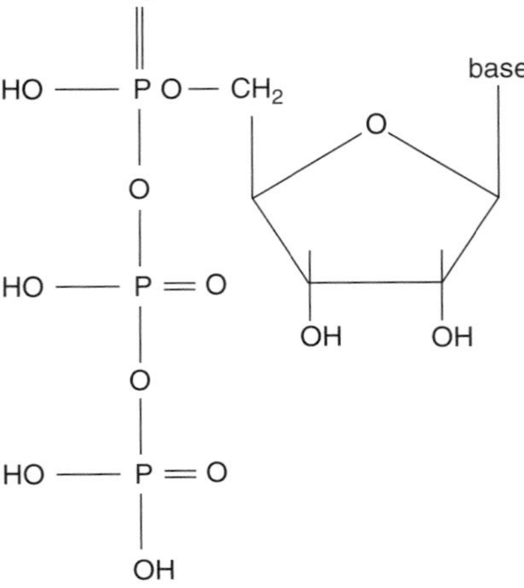

Fig. 27-14 5′ nucleotide diphosphate and triphosphate structures.

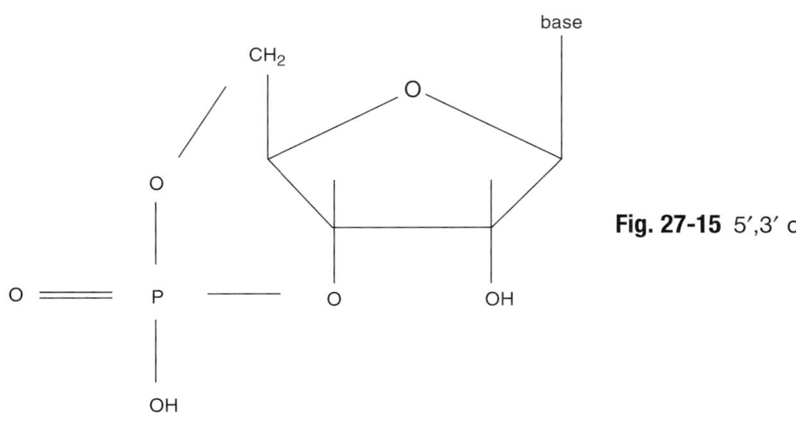

Fig. 27-15 5′,3′ cyclic nucleotide structure.

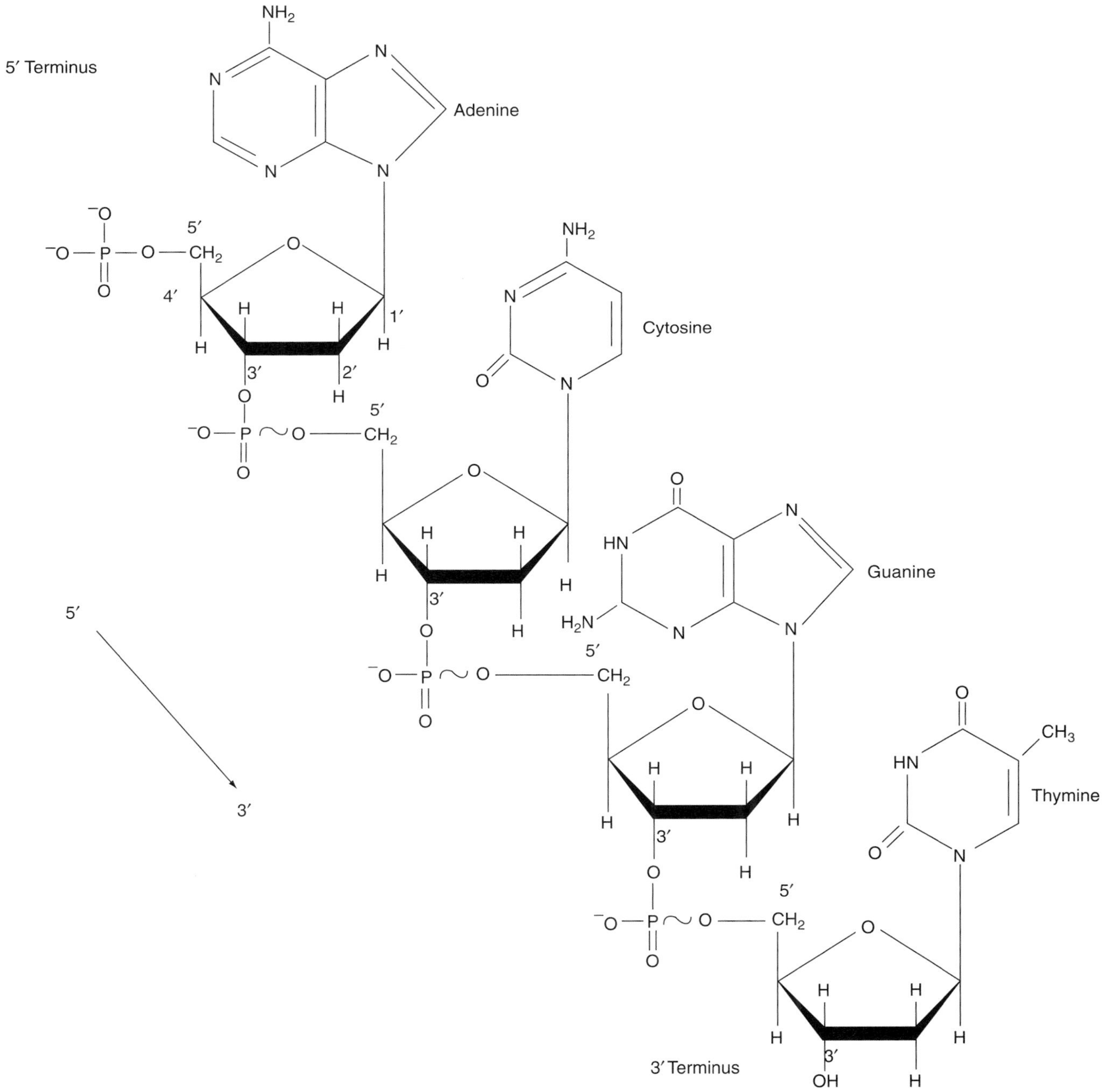

5′ Terminus

Adenine

Cytosine

Guanine

Thymine

5′

3′

3′ Terminus

Fig. 27-16 Covalent structure of a single DNA (deoxyribonucleic acid) strand. The polarity of the molecule is shown in the 5′ to 3′ direction by the arrow. (Reproduced with permission from Roskoski R Jr: *Biochemistry,* Philadelphia, 1996, Saunders.)

Cytosine-guanine
Thymine-adenine
Deoxyribose
Deoxyribose
Deoxyribose
Deoxyribose

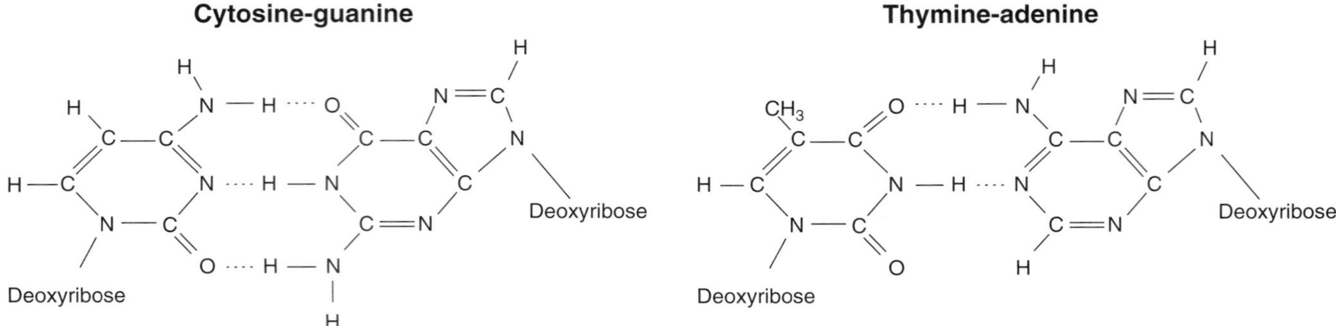

Fig. 27-17 Illustration of complementary base pairing. (Reproduced with permission from Roskoski R Jr: *Biochemistry,* Philadelphia, 1996, Saunders.)

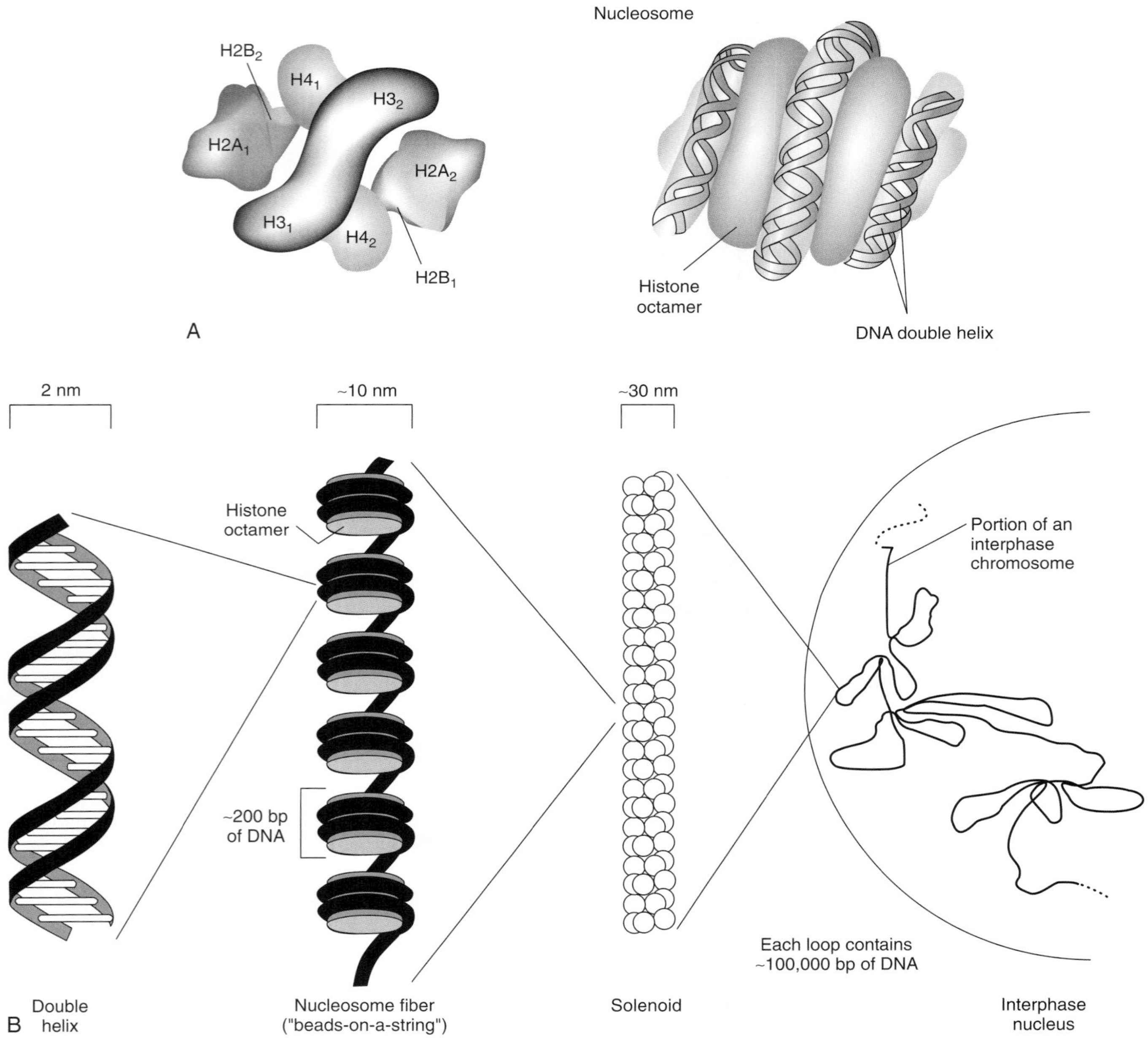

Nucleosome
H2B₂
H4₁
H3₂
H2A₁
H2A₂
H3₁
H4₂
H2B₁
A
Histone octamer
DNA double helix
2 nm
~10 nm
~30 nm
Histone octamer
Portion of an interphase chromosome
~200 bp of DNA
Each loop contains ~100,000 bp of DNA
B
Double helix
Nucleosome fiber ("beads-on-a-string")
Solenoid
Interphase nucleus

Fig. 27-18 Packaging of human DNA. **A,** Structural organization of the nucleosome. Nucleosomes consist of two turns of a DNA duplex coiled around a histone octamer. The histone octamer of the nucleosome consists of two molecules of each histone H2A, H2B, H3, and H4. (Reproduced with permission from Garrett RH, Grisham CM: *Biochemistry,* Fort Worth, 1995, Saunders College Publishing. Reprinted with permission of Brooks/Cole, an imprint of the Wadsworth Group, a division of Thompson Learning [Fax 800-730-2215].) **B,** Progressive levels of DNA condensation. (Reproduced with permission from Thompson MW, McInnes RR, Willard HF: *Thompson and Thompson Genetics in Medicine,* ed 5, Philadelphia, 1991, Saunders.)

DNA and RNA Binding Affinity

The binding affinity of one DNA strand for another is very high, and laboratory conditions can be modified such that the complementary sequences must be exact for the binding of one DNA strand to its complementary strand. This is termed *very stringent binding*. Similarly, the binding between the DNA and its RNA replicate can be very stringent. These properties are used for a number of nucleic acid assays, as described in Chapter 13.

KEY CONCEPTS BOX 27-4

- Pyrimidine and purine, the nucleoside building blocks of nucleic acids, are multi-ringed structures that contain nitrogen atoms.
- When they react with the pentoses ribose or deoxyribose to form the nucleotide bases, they can be polymerized to form strands of RNA or DNA, respectively.
- The nucleoside bases in DNA and RNA have the ability to form complementary pairs: G and C, and A and T (replaced by U, uracil, in RNA). When long stretches of RNA or DNA pair up with their complementary bases on another strand of nucleic acid, this heteroduplex structure is very stable.
- When DNA binds with specific proteins—histones—the complex structure called a *chromosome* is formed.
- The primary function of DNA is informational, that is, it contains the triplet base code for each amino acid and thus contains the information needed to synthesize proteins. RNA also serves as the informational compound for viruses, but in mammalian cells, it serves to transfer the information from DNA in the nucleus in the cytoplasm, where transfer RNAs line up specific amino acids to synthesize a protein on ribosomes (RNA and proteins).

BIBLIOGRAPHY

General

Berg JM, Tymoczko JL, Stryer L: *Biochemistry,* ed 6, New York, 2006, WH Freeman.

Devlin TM: *Textbook of Biochemistry With Clinical Correlations,* ed 5, New York, 2002, John Wiley & Sons.

Lodish H, Berk A, Matsudaira P, et al: *Molecular Cell Biology,* ed 5, New York, 2004, WH Freeman.

Murray RK, Granner DK, Rodwell VW: *Harper's Illustrated Biochemistry,* ed 27, New York, 2006, McGraw Hill.

Nelson DL, Cox CT: *Lehninger's Principles of Biochemistry,* ed 4, New York, 2004, WH Freeman.

Voet D, Voet JG: *Biochemistry,* ed 3, New York, 2004, John Wiley & Sons.

Proteins and Amino Acids

Branden C, Tooze J: *Introduction to Protein Structure,* ed 2, New York, 1998, Garland Press.

Creighton TE: *Protein Structure: A Practical Approach,* ed 2, New York, 1997, Oxford Press.

Kyle J: *Structure in Protein Chemistry,* New York, 1995, Garland Press.

Petsko GA, Ringe D: *Protein Structure and Function,* Malden, MA, 2004, Blackwell.

Lipids

Cave G, Paltauf F, editors: *Phospholipids: Characterization, Metabolism, and Novel Biological Applications,* Champaign, IL, 1995, AOCS Press.

Fahy E, Subramaniam S, Brown HA, et al: A comprehensive classification system for lipids, J Lipid Res 46:839, 2005.

Gurr M, Harwood J, Frayn K: *Lipid Biochemistry,* ed 5, Malden, MA, 2003, Blackwell.

Moffatt RJ, Stamford B, editors: *Lipid Metabolism and Health,* London, 2005, Taylor & Francis.

Sebedio JL, Perkins EG, editors: *New Trends in Lipid and Lipoprotein Analysis,* Champaign, IL, 1995, AOCS Press.

Spiller GA, editor: *Handbook of Lipids in Human Nutrition,* Boca Raton, FL, 2006, CRC Press.

Vance DE, Vance JE: *Biochemistry of Lipids, Lipoproteins and Membranes,* St Louis, 2008, Elsevier Science.

Carbohydrates

Brinkley RW: *Modern Carbohydrates Chemistry,* New York, 1988, Marcel Dekker.

Chaplin MF, Kennedy JF, editors: *Carbohydrate Analysis,* ed 2, New York, 1994, Oxford University Press.

Garg H, Cowman M, Hales C: *Carbohydrates Chemistry, Biology and Medical Applications,* St Louis, 2008, Elsevier.

Sinnott M: *Carbohydrate Chemistry and Biochemistry,* London, UK, RSC Publishing, 2007.

Stick R: *Carbohydrates: The Essential Molecules of Life,* ed 2, St Louis, 2008, Elsevier.

Nucleic Acids

Blackburn M, Gait M, Loakes D, et al, eds: *Nucleic Acids in Chemistry and Biology,* Cambridge, UK, 2006, The Royal Society of Chemistry.

Bloomfield VA, Crothers DM, Tinoco I, et al: *Nucleic Acids: Structures, Properties, and Functions,* Sausalito, CA, 2000, University Science Books.

Calladine CR, Drew H, Luisi B, et al: *Understanding DNA: The Molecule and How It Works,* ed 3, Amsterdam, Elsevier Academic Press, 2004.

Neidle S: *Nucleic Acid Structure and Recognition,* New York, 2002, Oxford University Press.

INTERNET SITES

Proteins

www.friedli.com/herbs/phytochem/proteins.html

http://www.umass.edu/microbio/chime/pe_beta/pe/atlas/atlas.htm
http://www.uwsp.edu/chemistry/pdbs/#PEPTIDES%20&%20PROTEINS

http://www.wiley.com/legacy/college/boyer/0470003790/animations/animations.htm

http://resources.schoolscience.co.uk/Unilever/16-18/proteins/

http://www.pdb.org/pdb/home/home.do protein structures

http://www.proteinatlas.org/ Human Protein Atlas

Lipids

www.cyberlipid.org/cyberlip/desc0004.htm

http://www.lipidmaps.org/

http://www.lipidlibrary.co.uk/

Carbohydrates

http://www.chem.qmw.ac.uk/iupac/2carb/

http://ull.chemistry.uakron.edu/genobc/Chapter_17/

http://www2.ufp.pt/~pedros/bq/carb_en.htm

Nucleotides

http://www.genome.gov/glossary.cfm?key=nucleotide

http://biostudio.com/c_%20education%20mac.htm neat automation

http://www.genome.gov/glossary.cfm?key=deoxyribonucleic%20acid%20

http://molvis.sdsc.edu/dna/index.htm (DNA)

Physiology and Pathophysiology of Body Water and Electrolytes

28 Chapter

John M. Lorenz

Chapter Outline

Key Terms

acidosis Abnormally low body fluid pH. Respiratory acidosis is caused by an abnormally high P_{CO_2}; metabolic acidosis is caused by an abnormally low bicarbonate concentration.

active transport The passage of ions or molecules across a cell membrane by an energy-consuming process. This energy is generated by cellular metabolism.

aldosterone A mineralocorticoid hormone secreted by the adrenal cortex, which influences sodium and potassium metabolism.

alkalosis Abnormally high body fluid pH. Respiratory alkalosis is caused by an abnormally low P_{CO_2}; metabolic alkalosis is caused by an abnormally high bicarbonate concentration.

angiotensin A vasoconstrictive polypeptide produced by the enzymatic action of renin on **angiotensinogen.** A converting enzyme from the lung removes two C-terminal amino acids from the inactive decapeptide angiotensin I to form the biologically active octapeptide angiotensin II.

angiotensinogen A serum globulin produced in the liver that is the precursor of angiotensin.

anion An ion that carries a negative charge.

anorexia Diminished appetite for food.

antidiuretic hormone A peptide hormone of the neurohypophysis that acts on the collecting tubule of the kidneys to allow increased water reabsorption and therefore decreased free water excretion by the kidney. Also known as *vasopressin.*

arrhythmia Irregularity of the heartbeat.

ascites The accumulation of fluid in the peritoneal cavity.

asphyxia Interference with lung ventilation, and oxygen delivery to and carbon dioxide removal from the tissue.

atrial natriuretic peptide (ANP) A natriuretic peptide hormone secreted primarily by the cardiac atria that produces vasodilation, diuresis, and natriuresis.

baroreceptor A nerve ending that responds to change in pressure.

Bartter's syndrome A rare inherited defect of renal tubular chloride reabsorption; associated with hypokalemia, metabolic alkalosis, and normal to low blood pressure.

brain natriuretic peptide (BNP) A natriuretic peptide hormone secreted primarily by the cardiac ventricles that produces vasodilation, diuresis, and natriuresis.

cation An ion that carries a positive charge.

cirrhosis Progressive disease of the liver characterized by damage to hepatic parenchymal cells.

colloid As used in this chapter, this term applies to the large molecules in the body to which the capillary endothelium and the cell membrane are impermeable.

colloid osmotic pressure The effective osmotic pressure of plasma and interstitial fluid across the capillary endothelium; it is largely the result of the presence of protein.

C-type natriuretic peptide (CNP) A natriuretic peptide produced locally in the vascular endothelium, which acts locally to produce venodilation, but not natriuresis.

dehydration Abnormal decrease in total body water (see Table 28-4). Hypernatremic dehydration is a net loss of sodium and water from the body, with net water loss exceeding net sodium loss. Hyponatremic dehydration is the net loss of sodium and water from the body, with net sodium loss exceeding net water loss. Normonatremic dehydration is the net loss of sodium and water from the body in equal extracellular proportions. Simple dehydration is the net loss of body water alone with no net sodium loss.

diabetes insipidus The chronic excretion of very large amounts of hyposmotic urine caused by an inability to concentrate urine because of the lack of antidiuretic hormone (ADH) production, secretion, or effect. The pituitary (or central) form is caused by inadequate ADH synthesis or secretion; the nephrogenic form is caused by unresponsiveness of the renal tubules to ADH.

distension receptor A nerve ending that responds to stretch.

edema An increase in interstitial fluid volume.

extracellular water (ECW) Water external to cell membranes. Anatomical ECW is all body water external to cell membranes; physiological ECW is plasma and body water into which small solutes can freely diffuse; excludes the transcellular portion of anatomical extracellular water; includes the plasma and interstitial fluid (see Fig. 28-1).

free water Water that contains no solute.

Gibbs-Donnan equilibrium The steady-state distribution of permeable ions and transmembrane potential that results across a semipermeable membrane when an impermeant ion exists in unequal amounts on the two sides of the membrane. At this equilibrium, solvent movement across the semipermeable membrane is exactly opposed by osmotic forces (see Fig. 28-9).

hyperaldosteronism A disorder caused by excessive secretion of aldosterone and characterized by hypokalemic alkalosis, muscular weakness, hypertension, polyuria, polydipsia, and normal or elevated plasma sodium concentration.

hyperchloremia An abnormally high plasma chloride concentration.

hyperkalemia An abnormally high plasma potassium concentration.

hypernatremia An abnormally high plasma sodium concentration.

hyperosmotic Denoting an effective osmotic pressure higher than that of normal plasma.

hypertonic Denoting a theoretical osmotic pressure higher than that of normal plasma.

hypochloremia An abnormally low plasma chloride concentration.

hypokalemia An abnormally low plasma potassium concentration.

hyponatremia An abnormally low plasma sodium concentration. Dilutional hyponatremia is caused by an excess of water (relative to sodium) in the extracellular compartment.

hyposmotic Denoting an effective osmotic pressure lower than that of normal plasma.

hypothalamus Portion of brain beneath the thalamus and connected to the pituitary gland (see Chapter 48).

hypotonic Denoting a theoretical osmotic pressure lower than that of normal plasma.

hypovolemia An abnormally low blood volume.

insensible water loss Evaporation of water through the skin or from the respiratory tract.

interstitial fluid (ISF) Extravascular, extracellular water (see Fig. 28-2).

intracellular water (ICW) Water inside the cells of the body; water within cell membranes.

juxtaglomerular cells Smooth muscle cells that synthesize and store renin and release it in response to decreased renal perfusion pressure, increased sympathetic nerve stimulation of the kidneys, or decreased sodium concentration in fluid in the distal tubule.

macromolecule A molecule of colloidal size; e.g., proteins, nucleic acids, and polysaccharides.

natriuretic peptides A family of peptides secreted in response to intravascular volume expansion that reduce blood pressure and plasma volume through coordinated actions on the brain, vasculature, adrenal glands, and kidneys.

osmolarity Osmotic concentration expressed as osmoles or milliosmoles of solute per liter of solvent (see Chapter 11).

osmotic pressure The force necessary to exactly oppose the movement of water across a semipermeable membrane from a solution with low solute particle concentration to a solution with high solute particle concentration.

paresthesia An abnormal spontaneous sensation, such as burning, pricking, numbness, and so forth.

plasma The extracellular, intravascular fluid of the body (see Fig. 28-2).

polyanionic Possessing multiple negative charges.

polydipsia Excessive fluid intake as the result of extreme thirst. Psychogenic polydipsia is secondary to a psychiatric disorder, without a demonstrable organic lesion.

polyuria Excessive urine output, that is, more than 1 to 2 L/day in the adult.

pseudohyperkalemia Abnormally high plasma potassium concentration in a sample obtained from a patient in the absence of true elevation of plasma potassium concentration in that patient.

renin An enzyme produced, stored, and secreted by the juxtaglomerular cells of the kidney, which metabolizes circulating angiotensinogen to form angiotensin I.

semipermeable Permeable to certain molecules but not to others; usually permeable to water.

syndrome of inappropriate antidiuretic hormone secretion (SIADH) A group of findings, including hypotonicity of the plasma, hyponatremia, and hypertonicity of the urine with continued sodium excretion, that is produced by excessive ADH secretion, and that improves with water restriction.

total body water (TBW) All water within the body, both inside and outside the cells, including that contained in the gastrointestinal and genitourinary systems.

transcellular water That portion of extracellular water that is enclosed by an epithelial membrane, the volume and composition of which are determined by the cellular activity of that membrane.

urodilatin A natriuretic peptide similar in structure to ANP that is peptide produced locally in the kidneys.

water intoxication An increase in free water in the body; results in dilutional hyponatremia.

Methods on Evolve

Anion gap
Chloride
Osmolality
Sodium and potassium

Water is the most abundant constituent of the human body, accounting for approximately 60% of the body mass in a normal adult. Water is important not only because of its abundance but also because it is the medium in which body solutes, both organic and inorganic, are dissolved and metabolic reactions take place. The discussion in this chapter focuses on (1) a description of the dynamic steady-state compartmentalization of body fluid and its inorganic solutes, (2) the physiological mechanisms involved in maintenance of this compartmentalization, and (3) pathophysiological events that occur during certain clinical states that alter the composition of body fluids.

SECTION OBJECTIVES BOX 28-1

- Define the compartments into which total body water is divided.
- List the electrolyte composition of the two main compartments of total body water.
- Define *anion gap,* and state its clinical significance; calculate and interpret anion gap results from given data.

BODY WATER COMPARTMENTS

Total body water (TBW) includes water both inside and outside of cells and water that is normally present in the gastrointestinal and genitourinary systems (Fig. 28-1). TBW can be theoretically divided into two main compartments. The anatomical **extracellular water (ECW)** includes all water external to cell membranes; it constitutes the medium through which all metabolic exchange occurs. **Intracellular water (ICW)** includes all water within cell membranes and constitutes the medium in which chemical reactions of cell metabolism occur (Fig. 28-2). This compartment is heterogeneous and discontinuous; the interior of each cell is separated from the ECW and from the interior of every other cell by the **semipermeable** cell membrane.

The anatomical ECW is functionally subdivided into **physiological extracellular water** and **transcellular water.** The physiological ECW is that portion of the anatomical ECW whose volume is accessible to direct measurement; it includes **plasma** (intravascular water) and **interstitial fluid (ISF).** The ISF, which includes extravascular, extracellular water into which ions and small molecules diffuse freely from plasma, is the fluid that directly bathes the cells of the body. In addition,

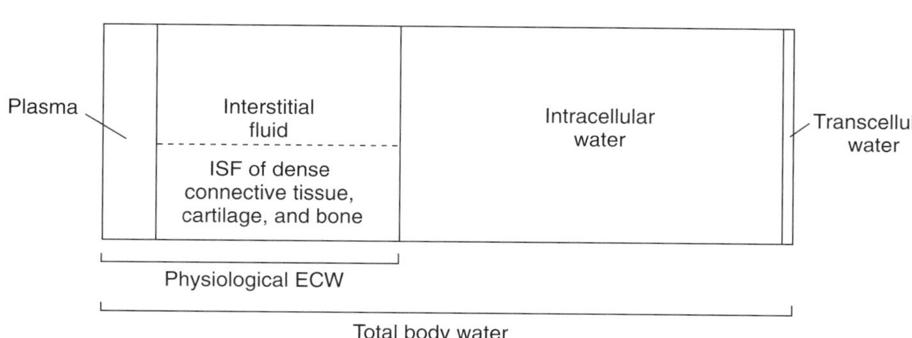

Fig. 28-1 Body water compartments. Note that anatomical extracellular water (ECW) includes physiological extracellular water and transcellular water. *ISF,* Interstitial fluid.

there are potential spaces in the body (pericardial, pleural, peritoneal, and synovial, see Chapter 46) that are normally empty except for a few milliliters of viscous lubricating fluid and are considered to be part of the ISF compartment. Transcellular water includes water in extracellular compartments enclosed by an epithelial membrane, the volume and composition of which are determined by the cellular activity of that membrane. These heterogeneous compartments include the aqueous humor in the eye, the cerebrospinal fluid, and the water within the gastrointestinal, genitourinary, and nasorespiratory systems. The volume of the transcellular water portion of the anatomical ECW is not included in conventional measurements of extracellular water.

Volume of Body Water Compartments

TBW is 65% of body weight in average adult men and 55% of body weight in women (Table 28-1). This difference between men and women is largely the result of differences in body fat. As a percentage of total body weight, TBW varies inversely with body fat content, from approximately 70% in very thin persons to 50% in very obese persons.

Physiological ECW volume is approximately 20% of body weight and one third of TBW in the average adult. In contrast to TBW, neither physiological nor anatomical ECW volumes can be measured accurately. Plasma volume can be accurately measured and is approximately 5% of body weight. ISF volume is calculated as the difference between the ECW and plasma volumes. It is approximately 15% of body weight and one fourth of TBW. ICW is calculated as the difference between TBW and ECW volumes. It is equal to 40% of body weight and two thirds of TBW in the average adult. ICW volume calculated in this manner includes transcellular water, which has been estimated to account for 1% to 3% of body weight.

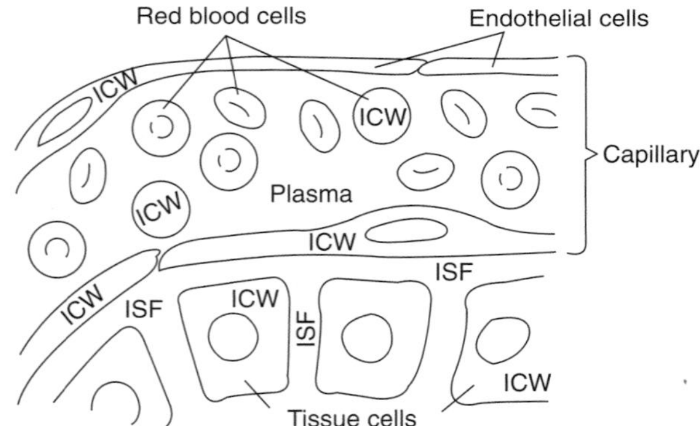

Fig. 28-2 Diagram of plasma, interstitial fluid (ISF), and intracellular water (ICW) in tissue at the microscopic level.

Maturational Changes in Body Water Compartment Volumes

The fraction of body weight that is water and the proportions of TBW that are ECW and ICW do not remain constant during growth (Fig. 28-3). When expressed as a percentage of body weight, TBW gradually decreases during intrauterine gestation and early childhood, reaching a value approximating that found in the adult by about 1 year of age. During this time, ECW (expressed as a percentage of body weight) decreases and ICW (expressed as a percentage of body weight) increases. Thus, ECW becomes a lesser and ICW a greater proportion of TBW. Plasma volume remains constant at 4% to 5% of body weight throughout life. Of course, the absolute volumes of TBW, ECW, ICW, and plasma all increase with growth.

Composition of Body Water Compartments

Plasma Compartment

The plasma compartment is the only compartment in which the composition is directly measurable. Note that the concentration of ions in the plasma is lower than that in plasma water (Table 28-2). The reason is that plasma is composed of water, ions, and macromolecules. Ions are present only in the water phase. The term *plasma water* is used to indicate this aqueous fraction as distinct from the remainder, which is composed of protein, lipid, and other **macromolecules.** The concentration of ions in plasma is lower than that in plasma water because plasma contains both the plasma water (in which plasma ions are dissolved) and the macromolecule fraction (in which no ions are dissolved). Plasma water represents only 93% of total plasma volume. Consequently, the concentration of ions in plasma is 93% of that in plasma water (see p. 531). Whether a laboratory detects the concentration of ions in plasma or in plasma water depends on the method of measurement used (see Sodium, in Evolve Methods). However, it is the concentration of ions in plasma water that affects the distribution of ions across the capillary endothelium. If plasma contains an greatly increased quantity of macromolecules (such as lipids), the measured concentration of ions in plasma will be low, even though the concentration of ions in plasma water and the resultant chemical activities of these ions may be normal. In addition to protein, plasma contains high concentrations of sodium and chloride, moderate concentrations of bicarbon-

Table 28-1 Compartment Volumes

	Percentage of Body Weight	Pecentage of Total Body Water	Volume in 70 kg Adult
Total body water	60		42 L
Extracellular water	20	33	14 L
Plasma	5	8	3.5 L
Interstitial fluid	15	25	10.5 L
Intracellular water	40	67	28 L

ate, and low concentrations of calcium, magnesium, phosphate, sulfate, and organic acids.

The sum of all the charges of positively charged ions (**cations**) must be equal to the sum of all the charges of negatively charged ions (**anions**) for electrical neutrality to be maintained in the plasma. Most often in clinical medicine, however, the plasma concentrations of only sodium, potassium, chloride, and bicarbonate are measured. The sum of these measured cations exceeds that of the measured anions. Therefore, the sum of unmeasured plasma anions must be greater than that of unmeasured cations. The difference between the sum of measured cations and the sum of measured anions is known as the *anion gap* and is calculated as $[Na^+] + [K^+] - [Cl^-] - [HCO_3^-]$ or as $[Na^+] - [Cl^-] - [HCO_3^-]$ (see Anion gap in Methods on Evolve). The latter is used frequently because the plasma potassium concentration is relatively constant and may be spuriously elevated because of hemolysis (see pp. 330-331). Because total plasma cation concentration must equal total plasma anion concentration, and because decreases in unmeasured cations have little effect on the calculation, an increased anion gap is usually indicative of an increase in concentration of one or more of the unmeasured anions (Fig. 28-4). A decrease in the anion gap is suggestive of the opposite possibility. The most frequent use of the anion gap clinically is in the differential diagnosis of metabolic **acidosis** (see Chapter 29).

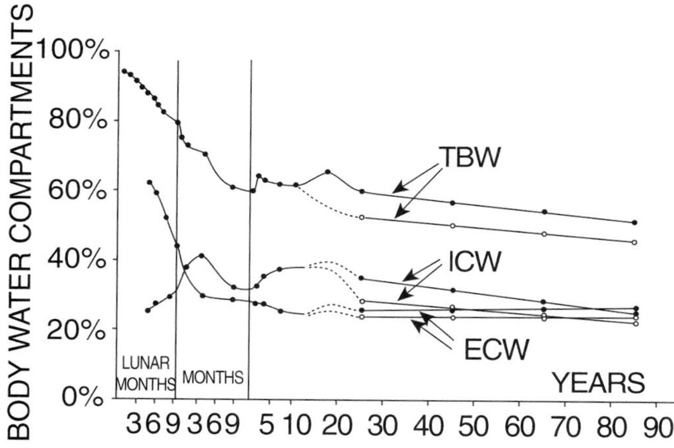

Fig. 28-3 Changes in body water and distribution with age, expressed as a percentage of body weight. (From Friss-Hansen B: Hydrometry during growth and aging. In Brozek J, editor: *Human Body Composition: Approaches and Applications,* Oxford, 1965, Pergamon Press.)

Interstitial Fluid Compartment

The ISF cannot normally be sampled in amounts sufficient for chemical analysis. The major difference between the ISF and plasma is the presence of protein in the plasma and its relative absence in the ISF. Although concentrations of freely diffusible solute in ISF might be expected to be equal to those in plasma water, this is true only for uncharged solutes. The presence of **polyanionic** protein molecules in plasma, which cannot cross semipermeable membranes, leads to the Gibbs-Donnan equilibrium (see p. 536). This equilibrium results in plasma water cation concentrations slightly greater than those in ISF and plasma water anion concentrations slightly less than those in ISF. Values for ISF ion concentrations given in Table 28-2 are theoretical approximations that are based on Gibbs-Donnan equilibrium calculations.

Intracellular Water Compartment

Solute concentrations in cell water cannot be determined directly. The ICW compartment is heterogeneous; there are important differences in intracellular solute concentrations between different cell types. However, certain features of most cell fluids are quantitatively similar and distinguish ICW from ECW. The major cations of ICW are potassium and magnesium, and the concentration of sodium is always low; the major anions of cell fluids are protein, organic phosphates, and sulfates, whereas chloride and bicarbonate concentrations are low. The profile presented in Table 28-2 is for muscle cells.

Osmotic Pressure and Osmolarity of Body Fluids

Osmotic pressure is an important factor that determines the distribution of water among body water compartments.

Table 28-2 Composition of Body Water Compartments

	Plasma (mmol/L)	Plasma Water (mmol/L)	Interstitial Fluid (mmol/L H_2O)	Intracellular Water (mmol/L H_2O)
Cations	153	164.6	153	195
Na^+	142	152.7	145	10
K^+	4	4.3	4	156
Ca^{++}	5	5.4	(2 to 3)	3.2
Mg^{++}	2	2.2	(1 to 2)	26
Anions	153	164.6	153	195
Cl^-	103	110.8	116	2
HCO_3^-	28	30.1	31	8
Protein	17	18.3	—	55
Others	5	5.4	(6)	130
Osmolarity (mOsm/L)		296	294.6	294.6
Theoretical osmotic pressure (mm Hg)		5712.8	5685.8	5685.8

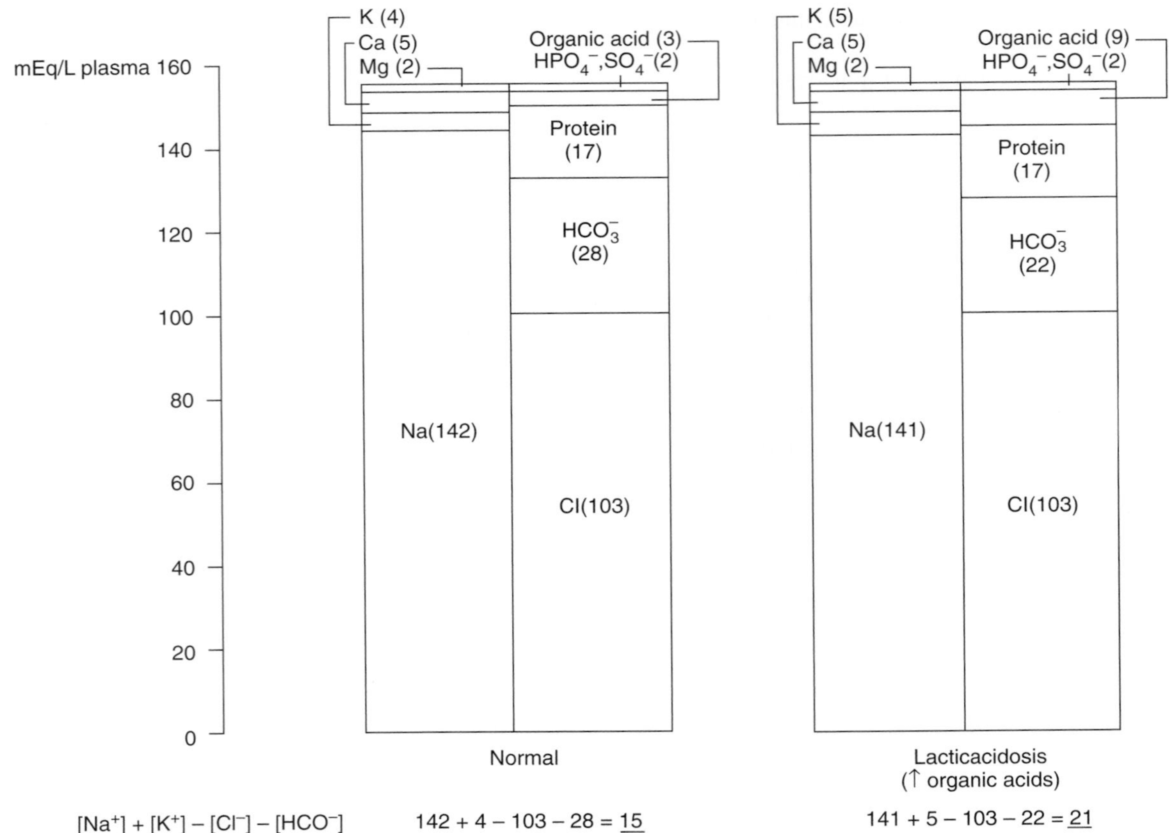

Fig. 28-4 Increased anion gap caused by an increase in unmeasured anions. Numbers in parentheses, concentration of ions in units of mEq/L plasma. Note that the sum of cations (left-hand side of each bar graph) is always equal to the sum of anions (right-hand side of each bar graph), both under normal conditions and in the presence of lactic acidosis. The sum of concentrations of unmeasured anions (organic acids, HPO_4^{2-}, SO_4^{2-}, and proteins) is larger than the sum of concentrations of unmeasured cations (Ca^{2+} and Mg^{2+}). During lactic acidosis, the difference between unmeasured anions and cations becomes greater because production of lactic acid increases the concentration of organic acids.

(See Chapter 11 for a description of colligative properties that determine osmotic pressure.) The theoretical osmotic pressure (and water attractability) of a solution is proportional to its **osmolarity.** The theoretical osmotic pressure of a solution at body temperature is calculated as follows:

$$\text{Theoretical osmotic pressure (mm Hg)} = 19.3\,(\text{mm Hg/mOsm/L}) \times \text{Osmolarity (mOsm/L)} \qquad \text{Eq. 28-1}$$

Note that the solute permeability of specific biological membranes is not considered in this calculation. The osmolarity and theoretical osmotic pressure of each of the body water compartments are listed in Table 28-2.

Osmotic pressure can be seen simply as the force that tends to move water from dilute solutions to concentrated solutions. When a membrane is permeable to a solute, the solute exerts no osmotic pressure across the membrane—it does not contribute to the effective osmotic pressure of the solution. The effective osmotic pressure of a solution thus depends on the total number of solute particles in solution and the permeability characteristics of the particular membrane in question. The higher the permeability of a membrane to a solute, the lower is the effective osmotic pressure of a solution of that solute at any given osmolarity. For example, cell membranes are much more permeable to urea than to sodium and chloride. Therefore, the effective osmotic pressure of a solution of urea across the cell membrane would be much less than that of a solution of NaCl of the same osmolarity. Measurement of the osmolarity of body compartment water is a measure of only its theoretical, not effective, osmotic pressure.

A solution with a theoretical osmotic pressure greater than plasma is said to be **hypertonic.** A solution with an effective osmotic pressure greater than that of plasma is said to be **hyperosmotic** with respect to plasma. **Hypotonic** and **hyposmotic** solutions are those with effective and theoretical osmotic pressures, respectively, less than those of plasma.

The capillary endothelium that separates the plasma and ISF is freely permeable to most solutes. These solutes contribute to theoretical, but not to effective, osmotic pressure because the capillary endothelium is impermeable only to large protein molecules **(colloids)** under usual circumstances. It is these colloids that are responsible for the effective osmotic pressure of plasma and ISF. Therefore, the effective osmotic pressure of plasma and ISF across the capillary endothelium is referred to as their **colloid osmotic pressure.**

KEY CONCEPTS BOX 28-1

- Total body water (TBW) includes water both inside and outside of cells and water normally present in the gastrointestinal and genitourinary systems.
- TBW can be theoretically divided into two main compartments: extracellular water (ECW) includes all water external to the cell membranes; intracellular water (ICW) includes all water within the cell membranes.
- ECW includes plasma (intravascular water) and interstitial fluid (extravascular, extracellular water).
- The principal cation and anion in ECW are sodium and chloride, respectively.
- Changes in the calculated plasma anion gap, $[Na^+] + [K^+] - [Cl^-] - [HCO_3^-]$, can indicate changes in unmeasured anions.
- The composition of interstitial fluid (ISF) is similar to that of plasma, except for the absence of large protein molecules (colloids), which are restricted to the plasma by the semipermeable capillary endothelium that separates ISF and plasma.
- The ICW compartment is heterogeneous; differences exist in intracellular solute concentrations between different cell types. However, in general, the major cations of ICW are potassium and magnesium, and the major anions are proteins and organic phosphates and sulfates.
- Osmotic pressure is an important factor for determining the distribution of water among body water compartments.
- Osmotic pressure is the force that moves water across a membrane that is impermeable to a solute from a compartment with a lower concentration of that solute to one with a higher concentration of that solute.

SECTION OBJECTIVES BOX 28-2

- Outline the homeostatic regulation of body water, sodium, potassium, and chloride.
- Describe the responses of the body to increased and decreased plasma osmolarity.
- Describe the role of the renin-angiotensin system in regulating total body water and total body sodium.

REGULATION OF BODY FLUID COMPARTMENT OSMOLARITY AND VOLUME

Extracellular Compartment

Regulation of ECW osmolarity and volume depends on the independent control of each of these variables by the **hypothalamus,** the renin-angiotensin-aldosterone system, atrial natriuretic factor, and the kidney.

Water Metabolism and Hypothalamus

The regulatory centers for water intake and water output are located in separate areas of the hypothalamus in the brain (Fig. 28-5). Neurons in each of these areas respond to increases in ECW osmolarity, to decreases in intravascular volume, and to **angiotensin** II. Increased ECW osmolarity stimulates these neurons directly by causing them to shrink (increased osmolarity of ISF bathing any cell will cause water to move out of the cell into the ISF; see p. 536). A decrease in intravascular volume causes a reduction in activity of **distension receptors** located in the atria of the heart, the inferior vena cava, and the pulmonary veins and a reduction in activity of blood pressure receptors in the aorta and the carotid arteries. Relay of this information to the central nervous system stimulates neurons in the water-intake and water-output areas of the hypothalamus. Circulating angiotensin II seems to act directly to stimulate neurons located in these water-control areas of the hypothalamus. Stimulation of neurons located in the water-intake area produces the conscious sensation of thirst and thereby stimulates water intake. Stimulation of neurons

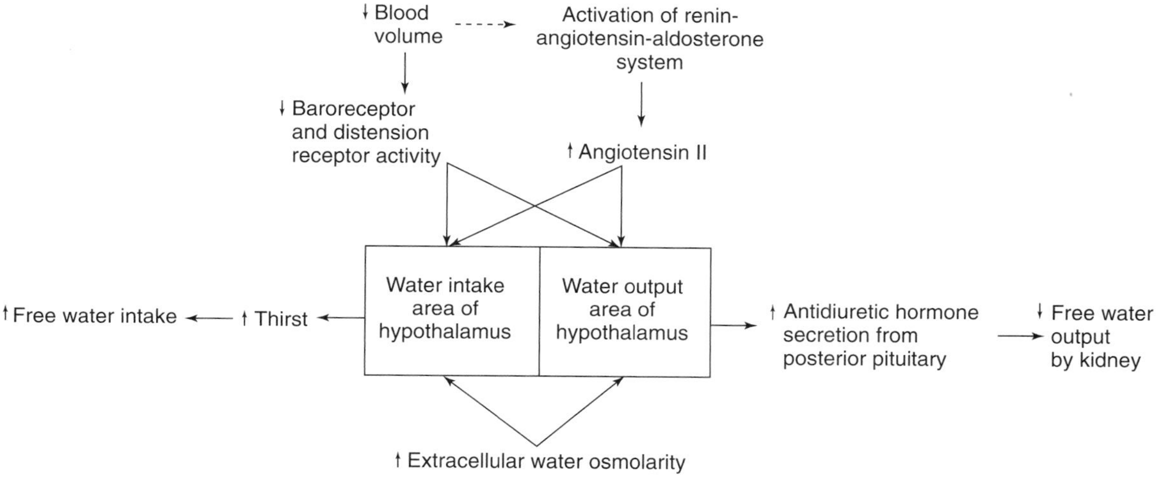

Fig. 28-5 Hypothalamic regulation of water balance.

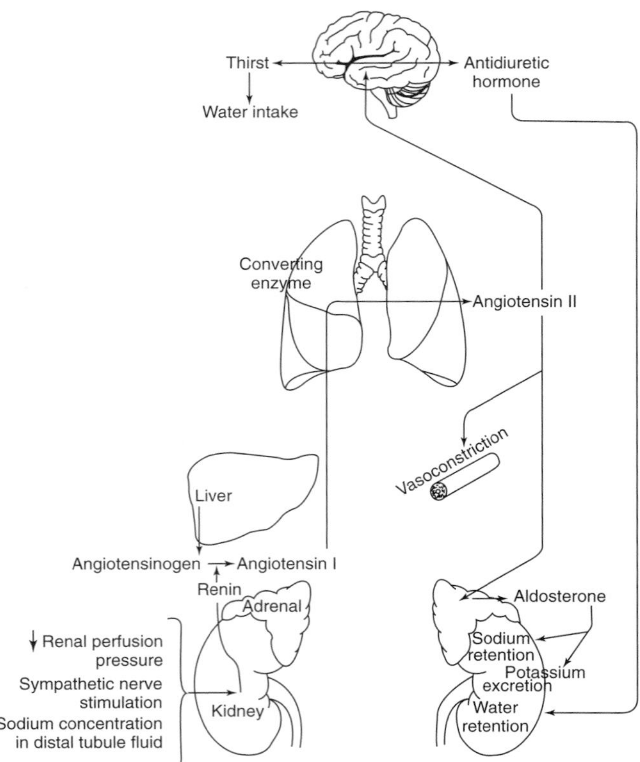

Fig. 28-6 Renin-angiotensin-aldosterone system.

located in the water-output area results in the release of **antidiuretic hormone** (**ADH**) from the posterior pituitary gland. Antidiuretic hormone stimulates water reabsorption in the collecting ducts of the kidney, which results in the formation of hypertonic urine and decreased output of **free water** (water without solute). The integration of all these control mechanisms governing water intake and output ensures maintenance of appropriate water balance.

Water and Sodium Metabolism and Renin-Angiotensin-Aldosterone System

The **renin**-angiotensin-**aldosterone** system (Fig. 28-6) functions as a neurohormonal regulating mechanism for body sodium and water content, arterial blood pressure, and potassium balance. Renin is a proteolytic enzyme that is synthesized, stored, and secreted by cells in the **juxtaglomerular cells** of the kidney. Renin secretion is increased by decreased renal perfusion pressure, stimulation of sympathetic nerves to the kidneys, and decreased sodium concentration in the fluid of the distal tubule. Renin converts **angiotensinogen** (a polypeptide synthesized in the liver) to angiotensin I. Angiotensin I is converted to angiotensin II in the lung and kidney. Angiotensin II is a potent vasoconstrictor. In addition, angiotensin II stimulates aldosterone secretion by the adrenal cortex, thirsting behavior, and ADH secretion. Aldosterone stimulates sodium reabsorption in the distal nephron. As a consequence of this sodium reabsorption, the body retains water.

Water and Sodium Metabolism and the Natriuretic Peptides

Natriuretic peptides are a family of peptides that have reciprocal effects to the renin-angiotensin-aldosterone system. They include **atrial natriuretic peptide (ANP), brain natriuretic peptide (BNP), C-type natriuretic peptide (CNP),** and urodilatin. Each is tissue specific and independently regulated. Increased secretion of these natriuretic peptides in response to intravascular volume expansion reduces blood pressure and plasma volume through coordinated actions on the brain, vasculature, adrenal glands, and kidneys. Natriuretic peptides are important in defending against salt-induced hypertension and in mitigating congestive heart failure.

ANP is a hormone that is produced primarily in the cardiac atria; it is released in response to stretching of the atrial cavity. It relaxes venous capacitance of blood vessels by suppressing sympathetic nervous system activity. This reduces the increase in venous pressure that occurs with a given increase in blood volume. ANP also increases vascular permeability and promotes natriuresis (renal loss of sodium) and diuresis. The latter results from direct effects of ANP on renal hemodynamics (which increase glomerular filtration rate), suppression of the renin-angiotensin-aldosterone system (which inhibits tubular sodium reabsorption), and antagonization of the effect of ADH in the collecting ducts (which inhibits water reabsorption). In the brain, ANP inhibits salt appetite, water intake, and secretion of ADH and corticotropin.

BNP is a hormone that is produced primarily in the left cardiac ventricles in response to left ventricular pressure overload. It has cardiovascular, natriuretic, and diuretic effects similar to those of ANP.

CNP is produced and secreted by vascular endothelial cells. Little, if any, is found circulating in the plasma. Thus it seems to act at the local level. BNP and, to a much lesser extent ANP stimulate CNP secretion. Secretion is also stimluated by local growth factors and cytokines. It is the most potent venous dilator of the four natriuretic peptides, but it has no natriuretic effects. The venodilation action of CNP is mediated via receptors in vascular smooth muscle cells.

Urodilatin is similar in structure to ANP but is formed directly in the kidney from the same precursor protein as ANP is in the atria. Its regulation is unclear, and its diuretic and natriuretic effects are more potent than those of ANP.

Measurement of circulating natriuretic peptide concentrations to classify and predict mortality in patients with congestive heart failure might reduce the need for more expensive and invasive evaluations (see Chapter 36). Although BNP is a routinely measured analyte, several analytical problems must be resolved for ANP. In addition, more work is required to refine the diagnostic accuracy and the prognostic relevance of these assays.

Control of Extracellular Water Osmolarity

ECW osmolarity is regulated by hypothalamic control of water intake (regulatory thirst) and renal excretion of free water (see Fig. 28-5). Increased ECW osmolarity stimulates water intake and ADH secretion. ADH secretion decreases renal water excretion. Increased water intake and decreased renal water excretion result in a positive water balance, that is, water gain in excess of water loss. Positive water balance decreases ECW osmolarity to normal. The opposite occurs with decreased ECW osmolarity: thirst and ADH secretion are inhibited. This causes a negative water balance (water loss exceeds water gain), and ECW osmolarity is restored to normal.

Control of Extracellular Water Volume

Control of ECW volume depends on the integrated control of water and sodium balance by the water-intake and -output areas of the hypothalamus, the renin-angiotensin-aldosterone system, atrial natriuretic factor, and the kidney. When output of water and sodium exceeds intake (water and sodium balance are negative), the ECW volume contracts. The associated decrease in plasma volume results in decreased venous blood return to the heart and decreased cardiac output. These cardiovascular changes produce the following effects:

1. Stimulation of the water-intake area of the hypothalamus and thirst center (see Fig. 28-5)
2. Stimulation of the water-output area of the hypothalamus and ADH secretion (see Fig. 28-5)
3. Stimulation of the renin-angiotensin-aldosterone system and increase in angiotensin II (see Fig. 28-6)
4. Inhibition of release of atrial natriuretic factor
5. Retention of sodium and water by the kidney

The net result of these effects is that water and sodium balance become positive and ECW volume is restored to normal.

Expansion of ECW volume results in the opposite sequence of events, with net loss of water and sodium and restoration of ECW balance to normal.

Plasma and Interstitial Fluid Compartments

Water and solute distribution between the plasma and ISF compartments depends on an intact capillary endothelial surface and is controlled passively by the interaction of hydrostatic, osmotic, and electrochemical forces. The capillary endothelium functions as a continuous tube, with numerous intercellular channels measuring 4 to 5 nm in diameter. It is freely permeable to water and small solutes and is relatively impermeable to protein.

Water Distribution

Water distribution across the capillary endothelial surface is controlled by the balance of forces that tend to move water from the plasma to the ISF (filtration forces) and forces that tend to move water from the ISF into the plasma (reabsorption forces). The major filtration force is plasma hydrostatic pressure in the capillary. A much weaker filtration force is the ISF colloid osmotic pressure. Because the protein concentration in ISF is negligible, colloid osmotic pressure is low. Another weak filtration force is a small negative ISF hydrostatic pressure. The major reabsorption force is the colloid osmotic pressure exerted across the capillary endothelium by plasma proteins. As a broad generalization, plasma hydrostatic pressure (which tends to drive water out of the capillary) exceeds plasma colloid osmotic pressure (which tends to draw water into the capillary) at the arteriolar end of the capillary, so that net filtration occurs. As plasma moves along the capillary and as filtration occurs, plasma hydrostatic pressure decreases and plasma protein concentration (and therefore, plasma colloid osmotic pressure) increases along the course of the capillary, resulting in net reabsorption toward the venous end of the capillary. This is depicted schematically in Fig. 28-7. Overall, filtration exceeds reabsorption; therefore, water must be returned to the plasma from the ISF compartment by way of the lymphatic system to prevent **edema** (defined as an abnormal increase in ISF volume).

Solute Distribution

Small differences in the concentrations of various extracellular solutes across the capillary endothelium are the result of the presence of polyanionic protein molecules (i.e., having multiple negative charges) in plasma to which the capillary endothelium is relatively impermeable. This is the result of the **Gibbs-Donnan equilibrium** (Fig. 28-8): the presence of impermeant polyanionic macromolecules restricted to one side of a membrane permeable to solvent and small ions establishes a characteristic distribution of the permeable ions. At electrochemical equilibrium, the concentrations of diffusible cations are slightly higher and the concentrations of diffusible anions slightly lower in the compartment containing the impermeant polyanionic macromolecule.

In the cases of calcium and magnesium, the larger differences between plasma water and ISF concentrations reflect the fact that approximately 45% of plasma calcium and 25% of plasma magnesium is protein bound and therefore nondiffusible.

Intracellular Compartment

Water and solute distribution across the cell membrane between ISF and ICW depends on the integrity of the cell membrane and on osmotic and electrochemical forces; all these factors are sustained by cell metabolism. The cell membrane behaves as though it were an oil film with numerous 0.7-nm-diameter pores. This membrane is highly permeable to water but differentially permeable to solutes. The permeability of the cell membrane to a solute is directly related to the

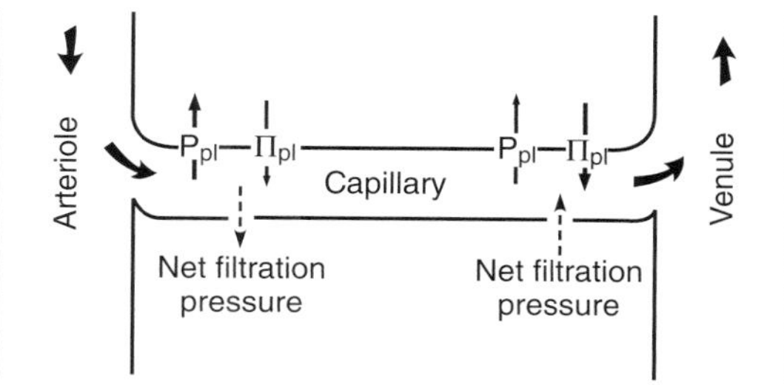

Fig. 28-7 Starling's hypothesis of water distribution between plasma and interstitial fluid compartments. Thickness of arrows representing plasma hydrostatic pressure, P_{p1}, and plasma oncotic pressure, Π_{p1}, indicate their relative magnitudes. *Dashed arrows,* Direction of net filtration pressure.

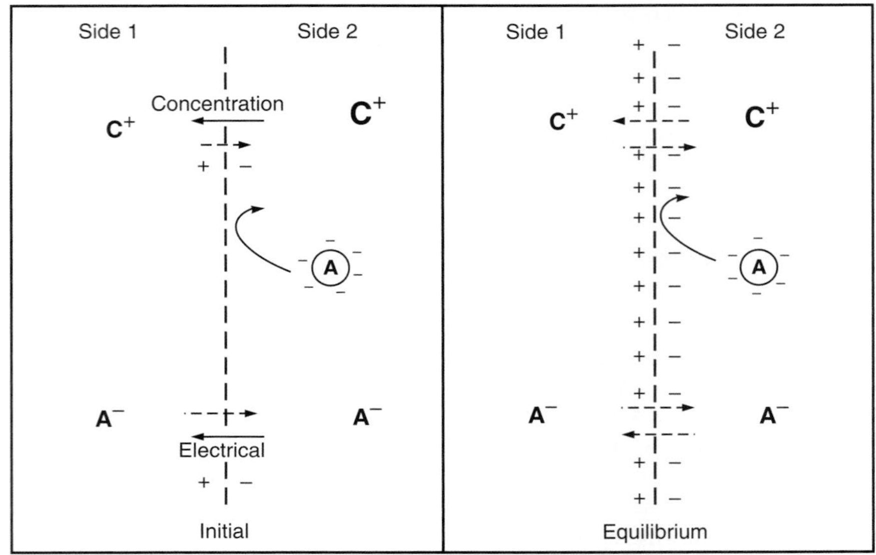

Fig. 28-8 Gibbs-Donnan equilibrium. Distribution of diffusible and nondiffusible ions and development of an electrical potential gradient across a membrane when a nondiffusible, polyvalent anion (Ⓐ) with a diffusible cation (C^+) is added to one side of a membrane in solution of diffusible cation (C^+) and anion (A^-). Initially, a diffusible cation moves down its concentration gradient from side 2 to side 1. This movement generates an electrical potential gradient across the membrane (side 2 negative with respect to side 1). The diffusible anion moves down this electrical potential gradient from side 2 to side 1. At equilibrium, the concentration of diffusible cation will be greater on side 2 than side 1 (as indicated by size of symbols), whereas the concentration of diffusible anion will be greater on side 1 than on side 2. No *net* movement of diffusible ions occurs across the membrane because no net electrochemical gradients exist. The concentration gradient for each ion is balanced by an equal but oppositely directed electrical gradient.

Table 28-3 Water Balance in Average Adult Under Various Conditions

INTAKE (mL/day)				OUTPUT (mL/day)			
	Normal	Hot Environment	Strenuous Work		Normal	Hot Environment	Strenuous Work
Drinking water	1200	2200	3400	Urine	1400	1200	500
Water from food	1000	1000	1150	Insensible water			
Water of oxidation	300	300	450	Skin	400	400	400
				Lung	400	300	600
				Sweat	100	1400	3300
				Stool	200	200	200
Total	2500	3500	5000	Total	2500	3500	5000

lipid solubility of the solute and is inversely related to its hydrophilicity (water attractability) and molecular size. Other factors being constant, membrane permeability is greater to anions than to cations.

Cell Volume

Cell volume is controlled by ISF osmolarity. Osmolarity inside the cell must equal osmolarity outside the cell because the cell membrane is highly permeable to water, and no hydrostatic pressure gradient can be maintained across animal cell membranes. The osmotic content of the intracellular compartment is kept relatively constant by cell metabolism. Therefore, osmotic equilibrium across the cell membrane can be maintained acutely in the face of changes in ISF osmolarity only by movement of water between the intracellular compartment and the interstitial space. A decrease in ISF osmolarity causes movement of water into cells and an increase in intracellular volume. Conversely, an increase in ISF osmolarity causes movement of water out of cells and a decrease in intracellular volume.

Cell Solute Content

The ionic composition of the intracellular fluid is shown in Table 28-2. This composition is largely the result of an energy-dependent ion-transport pump (Na^+,K^+-ATPase) found in the cell membrane that extrudes sodium from the cell in exchange for potassium. In addition, the intracellular solute composition depends on the intracellular production of nonpermeable polyanionic macromolecules. The cellular content of the other, permeable ions results from (1) electrochemical gradients produced by Na-K exchange and nonpermeable intracellular polyanionic macromolecules (Gibbs-Donnan effect) (see Fig. 28-8), (2) the specific permeability characteristics of the cell membrane to the various ions, and (3) other energy-dependent ion-specific transport pumps. The latter two factors vary from cell type to cell type and are responsible for the differences in ionic content among various cell types. All factors that influence cell solute content depend on normal cellular metabolism. When cellular metabolism is disrupted, as during **asphyxia,** solute and water enter the cell, causing it to swell.

KEY CONCEPTS BOX 28-2

- Regulation of extracellular water (ECW) volume and osmolarity depends on independent control of each by the renin-angiotensin-aldosterone system, atrial natriuretic factor, the hypothalamus, and the kidney.
- The renin-angiotensin-aldosterone system functions as a neurohormonal regulating mechanism for body sodium and water content (and thereby ECW volume) and arterial blood pressure. Stimulation of this system causes sodium and water retention.
- Natriuretic peptides are a family of peptides that have reciprocal effects to those of the renin-angiotensin-aldosterone system.
- ECW osmolarity is regulated by the hypothalamic control of water intake and renal excretion of free water.
- Water distribution across the capillary endothelial surface is controlled by the balance of forces that tend to move water from the plasma to the interstitial fluid (principally, plasma hydrostatic pressure) and forces that tend to move water from the interstitial fluid (ISF) into the plasma (principally, plasma colloid osmotic pressure).
- Water and solute distribution across the cell membrane between ISF and ICW depends on the integrity of the cell membrane and on osmotic and electrochemical forces.

SECTION OBJECTIVES BOX 28-3

- Describe the sources of body water loss.
- List several types of dehydration, and relate them to water and sodium balance.

WATER METABOLISM

Water Balance

Extracellular water osmolarity is maintained constant at 285 to 298 mOsm/L, as a consequence of the dynamic balance between water intake and water excretion, which is controlled by the mechanisms discussed previously. Average daily water turnover in the adult is approximately 2500 mL; however, the range of water turnover possible is great and depends on intake, environment, and activity (Table 28-3).

Under normal conditions, approximately one-half to two-thirds of water intake is in the form of oral fluid intake, and approximately one-half to one-third is in the form of oral intake of water in food. In addition, a small amount of water (150 to 350 mL/day) is produced by oxidative metabolism. Oral fluid intake is the only source of water that is regulated in response to changes in ECW volume and osmolarity.

Routes of water excretion include urinary water loss, **insensible water loss,** sensible perspiration (sweating), and gastrointestinal water loss. The kidney is the principal organ regulating the volume and composition of body fluids. Urine volume varies over a wide range in response to changes in ECW volume and osmolarity. Solute excretion is regulated independently.

Loss of water by diffusion through the skin and through the respiratory tract is known as insensible water loss because it is not apparent. This is the only route by which water is lost without solute. Normally, half of insensible water loss occurs through the skin and half through the respiratory tract. The magnitude of cutaneous insensible water loss is a function of body surface area; therefore, it is disproportionately greater in infants and children in relation to their weight. Insensible water loss varies directly with ambient temperature, body temperature, and activity, and inversely with ambient humidity.

Sensible perspiration is negligible in a cool environment but may be substantial with increases in ambient temperature, body temperature, or physical activity. Sodium and chloride are the major ionic components of sweat, but sweat is almost invariably hypotonic to plasma. An increase in ECW osmolarity causes a decrease in the rate of sensible perspiration.

Net water loss from the gastrointestinal (GI) tract is normally small, approximately 150 mL/day. However, the flux of water and electrolytes between the gastrointestinal tract and the ECW compartment is large. Therefore, if reabsorption from the GI tract is impaired, water and electrolyte losses from the GI tract can be great, as with diarrhea. Except for saliva, which is hypotonic, the total solute concentration of most GI secretions is similar to that of ISF.

Disorders of Water Imbalance

Disorders of water balance (**dehydration** and overhydration) result from an imbalance of water intake and output or sodium intake and output (Table 28-4).

Table 28-4 Changes in Total Body Water Volume and Distribution, Total Body Sodium Content, and Plasma Sodium Concentration With Dehydration and Overhydration

	Total Body Water	Extracellular Water	Intracellular Water	Total Body Sodium	Plasma Sodium Concentration
Dehydration					
Hypernatremic	↓	sl↓	↓	nl or sl↓	↑
Normonatremic	↓	↓	nl	↓	nl
Hyponatremic	↓	↓↓	↑	↓↓	↓
Overhydration					
Water intoxication	↑	↑	↑	nl	↓
Normonatremic ECW volume expansion	↑	↑	nl	↑	nl
Hyponatremic ECW volume expansion	↑	↑	↑	sl↑	↓

sl, Slight; *nl*, normal.

Dehydration

Deficit of Water

Simple dehydration, defined as a decrease in total body water with relatively normal total body sodium, may result from failure to replace obligatory water losses or failure of the regulatory or effector mechanisms that promote conservation of water by the kidney (Box 28-1). Simple dehydration is by definition associated with **hypernatremia** and hyperosmolarity because water balance is negative and sodium balance is normal. The increase in ECW osmolarity as water is lost from the body results in movement of water out of the ICW compartment. Therefore, simple dehydration results in contraction of both the ECW and ICW compartments (see Table 28-4).

Deficit of Water and Sodium

More often, dehydration results from a net negative balance of water and sodium. In this case, water balance may be more negative than, equal to, or less negative than sodium balance (see Table 28-4). If water balance is more negative than sodium balance, the result is hypernatremic or hyperosmolar dehydration; if it is equally negative, normonatremic or isomolar dehydration results; and if it is less negative, hyponatremic or hyposmolar dehydration results. Hypernatremic dehydration is most common. Some causes of water and sodium deficits are listed in Box 28-1.

The degree of extracellular volume contraction for a given sodium deficit and the associated change in intracellular volume are different for each of these types of dehydration (see Table 28-4). The degree of extracellular volume contraction is least with hypernatremic dehydration because the increase in ECW osmolarity causes water to move out of the cell; contraction of ICW volume occurs. Thus the total body water deficit is "shared" by the extracellular and intracellular compartments. The degree of extracellular volume contraction is intermediate with normonatremic dehydration; no water moves out of or into cells because there is no change in ECW osmolarity. There is also no change in ICW volume. The degree of ECW volume depletion is greatest with hyponatremic dehydration because the decrease in ECW osmolarity causes water to move into cells. Intracellular water volume is actually increased.

Box 28-1

Causes of Dehydration (Water and Sodium Deficits)

Hypernatremic Dehydration
Water and food deprivation
Excessive sweating*
Osmotic diuresis (with glucosuria)
Diuretic therapy*

Normonatremic Dehydration
Vomiting, diarrhea
Replacement of losses in the above conditions with low-sodium liquids

Hyponatremic Dehydration
Diuretic therapy†
Excessive sweating
Salt-wasting renal disease
Adrenocortical insufficiency

*If free water intake is inadequate.
†If free water intake is excessive.

Symptoms of Dehydration

The signs and symptoms of dehydration include thirst, dry mucous membranes, decreased skin turgor, decreased urine output and increased urine osmolarity (except when caused by failure of the kidney to conserve free water), increased blood urea nitrogen, and increased hematocrit. With increasing severity, weakness, lethargy, hypotension, and shock may occur.

Overhydration

Excessive Water

Water intoxication is defined as an increase in TBW with normal total body sodium. It rarely results from excessive water consumption **(polydipsia).** More often, water intoxication results from impaired renal free water excretion caused by ADH secretion in excess of that required to maintain

Box 28-2
Causes of Water Intoxication

Polydipsia
- Psychogenic—secondary to a psychiatric disturbance
- Organic—secondary to an anterior thalamic lesion

SIADH
Increased secretion of ADH by hypothalamus secondary to decreased venous return to heart with no decrease in total blood volume
- Asthma
- Pneumothorax
- Bacterial or viral pneumonia
- Positive-pressure ventilation
- Chronic obstructive pulmonary disease
- Right-sided heart failure
- Disease of spinal cord or peripheral nerves (Guillain-Barré syndrome, poliomyelitis)

Increased secretion of ADH by hypothalamus in absence of appropriate osmolar or volume stimuli
- Central nervous system disorders (intracranial hemorrhage, hydrocephalus, skull fracture, severe asphyxia, brain tumors, cerebrovascular thrombosis, meningitis, encephalitis, seizures, acute psychoses, and cerebral atrophy)
- Hypothyroidism
- Pain, fear
- Anesthesia or surgical stress
- Drugs such as morphine, barbiturates, cyclophosphamide, vincristine, and carbamazepine

Ectopic, Autonomous Secretion of ADH
- Bronchogenic carcinoma
- Adenosarcoma of pancreas
- Lymphosarcoma
- Duodenal adenocarcinoma
- Pulmonary tuberculosis
- Pulmonary abscess

ADH, Antidiuretic hormone; *SIADH*, *syndrome of inappropriate antidiuretic hormone secretion.*

normal ECW osmolarity (syndrome of inappropriate ADH secretion, SIADH; Box 28-2). With water intoxication, dilutional **hyponatremia** and hyposmolarity of the ECW result in water movement into the cells. Therefore, water intoxication produces expansion of the ECW and ICW compartments (see Table 28-4).

Symptoms of water intoxication are related to the degree and rate of fall in sodium. With an acute fall in serum sodium to 120 to 125 mmol/L, nausea, vomiting, seizures, and coma can occur.

Excessive Water and Sodium

Expansion of the extracellular compartment usually results from retention of sodium and water. This occurs with oliguric renal failure, nephrotic syndrome, congestive heart failure, **cirrhosis,** and primary **hyperaldosteronism.** In these conditions TBW excess is associated with normal or low serum sodium and osmolarity (see Table 28-4). Hypernatremia is rare with water excess. If the serum sodium is normal, the increase in TBW will be limited to the ECW. With hyponatremia, the increase in TBW will be shared by the ECW and ICW compartments.

KEY CONCEPTS BOX 28-3

- Total body water (TBW) is a reflection of the balance of water intake and water output.
- Routes of water excretion include urinary water loss, insensible water loss, sensible perspiration (sweating), and gastrointestinal water loss.
- Dehydration results from a net negative balance of water with or without a net negative balance of sodium.
- Overhydration, or water intoxication, results from an increase in TBW usually without a large change in total body sodium.

SECTION OBJECTIVES BOX 28-4

- Describe the factors that control body sodium loss.
- List and briefly describe the symptoms and at least two causes or clinical conditions associated with increased and decreased amounts of total body water and electrolytes in several types of dehydration, and relate them to water and sodium balance.

SODIUM METABOLISM

Sodium Balance

In a normal adult, the total body sodium is about 55 mmol/kg of body weight; about 30% is tightly bound in the crystalline structure of bone and thus is nonexchangeable. Thus, only 40 mmol/kg is exchangeable among the various compartments and accessible to measurement. Exchangeable sodium is distributed primarily in the extracellular space (Fig. 28-9). About 97% to 98% of the exchangeable sodium is found in the ECW space and only 2% to 3% in the ICW space. Approximately 16% of exchangeable sodium is found in plasma, 41% is in ISF that is readily accessible to the plasma compartment, 17% is in ISF of dense connective tissue and cartilage, 20% is in ISF of bone, and 3% to 4% is found in the transcellular water compartment. Total bone sodium (exchangeable and nonexchangeable) accounts for 40% to 45% of total body sodium. Concentrations of sodium in the various fluid compartments are displayed in Table 28-2. As was discussed previously, the difference in sodium concentration between plasma and ISF reflects the Gibbs-Donnan equilibrium. The difference in sodium concentration between ISF and ICW results from the **active transport** of sodium out of the cell in exchange for potassium.

The amount of sodium in the body is a reflection of the balance between sodium intake and output. Sodium intake depends on the quantity and type of food intake. Under

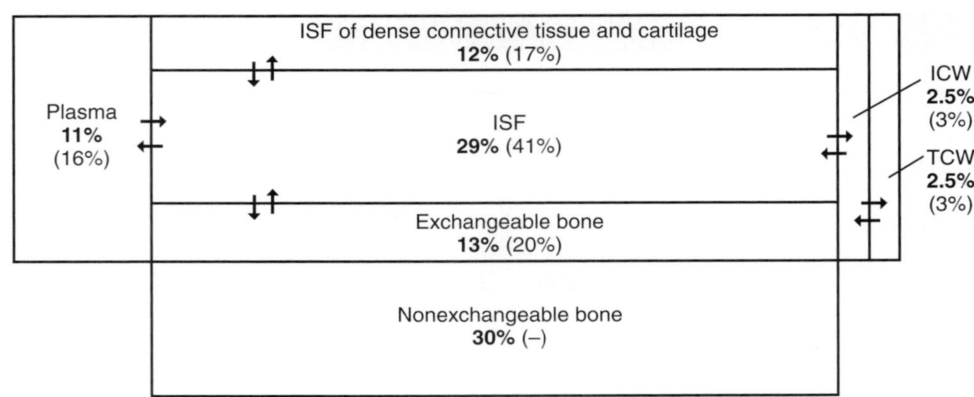

Fig. 28-9 Distribution of sodium among body compartments. Bold numbers, percentages of total body sodium in various compartments; numbers in parentheses, percentages of exchangeable sodium in various compartments; *ICW,* Intracellular water; *ISF,* interstitial fluid; and *TCW,* transcellular water.

Table 28-5 Electrolyte Composition and Volume of Various Gastrointestinal Secretions in a Normal Adult

		ELECTROLYTE CONCENTRATION (mmol/L)			
Fluid	**Volume Secreted (mL/Day)**	**Na^+**	**K^+**	**Cl^-**	**HCO_3^-**
Gastric juice*	2500	8 to 120	1 to 30	8 to 100	0 to 20
Bile	700 to 1000	134 to 156	4 to 6	83 to 110	38
Pancreatic juice	>1000	113 to 153	2 to 7	54 to 95	110
Small bowel	3000	72 to 120	3.5 to 7	69 to 127	30
Ileostomy	100 to 4000	112 to 142	4.5 to 14	43 to 122	30
Cecostomy	100 to 300	116 to 480	11 to 28	35 to 70	15
Feces	100	<10	<10	<15	<15

From Lockwood JS, Randall HT: Bull NY Acad Med 25:228, 1949.
*Electrolyte composition of gastric juice varies, depending on acidity. The higher the acidity, the lower is the sodium concentration, the higher is the chloride concentration, and the lower is the bicarbonate concentration. The average sodium concentration is approximately 100 mmol/L.

normal conditions, the average adult takes in about 50 to 200 mmol of sodium/day. Sodium output occurs through three primary routes: the gastrointestinal tract, the skin, and the urine.

Under normal circumstances, loss of sodium through the gastrointestinal tract is very small. Fecal water excretion amounts to only 100 to 200 mL/day for a normal adult, and fecal sodium excretion only 1 to 2 mmol/day. However, it should be borne in mind that although fecal losses of water and electrolytes are normally small, the total volume of gastrointestinal fluid secreted is large, averaging about 8 L/day. Almost all this volume is normally reabsorbed. However, with impaired gastrointestinal reabsorption, losses of water and electrolytes are large. The volume and electrolyte content of various gastrointestinal secretions are shown in Table 28-5. Note that most of the secretions have sodium content much greater than that of the feces. Thus, with severe diarrhea or with gastric or intestinal drainage tubes, sodium losses through the gastrointestinal tract may exceed 100 mmol/day.

The sodium content of sweat averages about 50 mmol/L, but is somewhat variable. The sweat sodium concentration is decreased by aldosterone and increased in cystic fibrosis. The rate of sweat production is highly variable, increasing in hot environments, during exercise, and with fever. Under extreme conditions, sweat production can exceed 5 L/day, accounting for a loss of more than 250 mmol of sodium. Under normal conditions, in a cool environment, sodium losses from the skin are small. With extensive burns or exudative skin lesions, great loss of sodium and water can occur.

The major route of sodium excretion is through the kidney. Furthermore, the urinary excretion of sodium is regulated carefully to maintain body sodium homeostasis, which, in turn, is critical to the control of extracellular volume. Details of the mechanisms and regulation of renal sodium excretion are discussed in Chapter 30. Sodium is filtered freely by the glomerulus. Approximately 70% of filtered sodium is reabsorbed by the proximal tubule, along with about 15% by the loop of Henle, about 5% by the distal convoluted tubule, 5% by the cortical collecting tubule, and another 5% by the medullary collecting duct; thus normally, less than 1% of filtered sodium is excreted.

Disorders of Sodium Balance

Sodium Excess

Sodium accumulates in the body when sodium intake exceeds sodium output because of an abnormality in sodium homeostatic mechanisms. Some of the major clinical causes of sodium retention are shown in Box 28-3.

Box 28-3

Clinical Conditions Resulting in Excess Body Sodium

- Cardiac failure
- Liver disease
- Renal disease—nephrotic syndrome
- Hyperaldosteronism
- Pregnancy

Because sodium is distributed in the extracellular space, an increase in total body sodium usually is accompanied by an increase in ECW volume. An abnormal increase in ECW volume, particularly an increase in the interstitial space, produces tissue swelling known as *edema.* Thus those clinical conditions that are associated with sodium retention are frequently characterized by the presence of edema. Clinically, edema is characterized by swelling and puffiness of the body.

Congestive Heart Failure

When the heart begins to fail as a pump, a series of pathophysiological mechanisms occur, leading to retention of sodium. The failing heart does not pump as much blood to the kidney, resulting in less sodium filtration, greater reabsorption, and, consequently, less excretion. The greater venous back-pressure generated from the failing heart causes fluid to move from the vascular space to the interstitial space, thereby decreasing the effective plasma volume and cardiac output. These factors stimulate the secretion of angiotensin II, aldosterone, and ADH and decrease the release of atrial natriuretic factor. These hormone responses further enhance salt and water retention.

Liver Disease

Some liver diseases are accompanied by venous obstruction, which results in increased sinusoidal and portal venous pressure. These in turn lead to leakage of fluid out of the vascular space into the peritoneal space **(ascites),** which lowers the effective plasma volume. The lowered plasma volume leads to salt and water retention by mechanisms similar to those described for heart failure.

Renal Disease

If the kidneys are damaged to such a degree that the glomerular filtration rate is greatly reduced and sodium excretion is thereby compromised, sodium retention will occur (see Chapter 30). Sodium retention can also occur through another mechanism, the nephrotic syndrome. This syndrome is characterized by proteinuria and decreased serum albumin levels, which result in low plasma colloid osmotic pressure and therefore a shift of fluid from the vascular space to the ISF space. This in turn results in **hypovolemia** with consequent salt and water retention, as was previously discussed.

Box 28-4

Clinical Conditions Resulting in Deficits of Body Sodium

- Gastrointestinal losses—vomiting, diarrhea, fistulas, drainage tubes
- Excessive sweating—exercise, fever, hot environment
- Renal disease
- Adrenal insufficiency—hypoaldosteronism
- Diuretic therapy
- Osmotic diuresis—diabetes mellitus
- Burns
- SIADH (syndrome of inappropriate antidiuretic hormone secretion)

Pregnancy

The reasons for sodium accumulation during pregnancy are still unclear, but there is no question that most women accumulate between 500 and 800 mmol of sodium during a normal pregnancy. Some suggest that this sodium accumulation may reflect a resetting of the normal homeostatic mechanisms that regulate body sodium and water.

Sodium Depletion

Sodium depletion occurs when the output of sodium exceeds the intake (Box 28-4). As was discussed previously, only small amounts of sodium are lost in the feces under normal conditions. However, under conditions of severe diarrhea or drainage of gastrointestinal secretions, gastrointestinal sodium excretion can be large. If this is not replaced by increased intake, sodium depletion will result. Moreover, because the gastrointestinal route may not be available, the intravenous replacement of water and electrolytes may be necessary. Similarly, losses of sodium through the skin are normally relatively small. However, when the volume of sweat becomes large, when the concentration of sodium in sweat is abnormally high (as with cystic fibrosis), or when there is abnormal exudation of fluid and electrolytes from the surface of the body (as occurs with extensive burns), the amount of sodium lost from the skin may be substantial, and sodium depletion may occur.

When the tubules of the kidney are unable to reabsorb sodium because of disease or hormonal abnormalities, sodium loss can be excessive (see Chapter 30). For example, aldosterone deficiency, caused by disease of the adrenal gland or abnormalities in the aldosterone-regulating system, leads to decreased reabsorption of sodium in the distal nephron and total body sodium depletion. Inhibition of tubular sodium reabsorption by a diuretic also may lead to body sodium depletion.

SIADH (see p. 539) occurs with water retention and hypotonic expansion of the ECW and ICW spaces. This in turn inhibits sodium reabsorption in the proximal nephron and also perhaps in the distal nephron, leading to body salt depletion.

Abnormalities of Plasma Sodium Concentration

Changes in total body sodium are not necessarily associated with similar changes in plasma sodium concentration, that is, with salt retention, plasma sodium concentration is not necessarily increased. In fact, plasma sodium is frequently decreased in sodium-retentive states. Similarly, salt depletion is not necessarily associated with decreased plasma sodium concentrations. Plasma sodium concentration reflects the relative balances of extracellular sodium and water.

Hyponatremia (low plasma sodium) occurs when there is a greater excess of extracellular water than of sodium or a greater deficit of sodium than of water. Some causes of hyponatremia are listed in Box 28-5. Note that in many cases, there is an excess of total body sodium.

The symptoms of hyponatremia depend on the cause, magnitude, and rate of fall of serum sodium. With acute, pronounced hyponatremia caused by water intoxication, nausea, vomiting, seizures, and coma may occur. Symptoms are less fulminant with chronic hyponatremia caused by salt depletion in excess of water depletion. With progressively severe degrees of chronic hyponatremia, constant thirst, muscle cramps, nausea, vomiting, abdominal cramps, weakness, lethargy, and finally delirium and impaired consciousness may occur.

Box 28-5

Clinical Conditions Associated With Hyponatremia

Water excess greater than sodium excess*
- Inappropriate ADH secretion
- Glucocorticoid deficiency
- Hypothyroidism
- Psychogenic polydipsia (excessive water intake)
- Heart failure†
- Liver disease†
- Renal failure†
- Nephrotic syndrome†

Sodium deficit greater than water deficit
- Certain gastrointestinal losses—vomiting, diarrhea, fistulas, and intestinal obstruction
- Burns
- Diuretic therapy
- Adrenal insufficiency—hypoaldosteronism
- Salt-losing nephropathy
- Renal tubular acidosis
- Osmotic diuresis
- Bicarbonaturia, ketonuria

Movement of sodium from extracellular to intracellular water space
- Adrenal insufficiency—hypoaldosteronism
- Sick cell syndrome—shock

Pseudohyponatremia—hyperglycemia, hyperlipidemia, hyperglobulinemia

ADH, Antidiuretic hormone.
*Hyponatremia is dilutional, that is, secondary to excessive water retention.
†Total body sodium is increased.

Hypernatremia (high plasma sodium) occurs when there is a greater deficit of extracellular water than of sodium. A greater excess of sodium than of water rarely occurs. Causes of hypernatremia are listed in Box 28-6. Note that in many cases, there is actually a deficit of total body sodium.

Hypernatremia usually occurs as a chronic process that follows loss of water in excess of sodium. Symptoms therefore are those of dehydration.

Measurement of urine sodium and urine osmolarity can be useful in the diagnosis of abnormalities of serum sodium concentration (Tables 28-6 and 28-7). However, it is critical to

Box 28-6

Clinical Conditions Associated With Hypernatremia

Sodium excess greater than water excess
- Ingestion of large amounts of sodium
- Administration of hypertonic NaCl or $NaHCO_3$
- Primary hyperaldosteronism

Water deficiency greater than sodium deficiency
- Excessive sweating*—exercise, fever, hot environment
- Burns*
- Hyperventilation
- Diabetes insipidus
  - Pituitary—ADH deficiency
  - Nephrogenic—kidney unresponsive to ADH
- Osmotic diuresis*—diabetes mellitus, mannitol infusion
- Diminished fluid input—diminished thirst
- Essential hypernatremia—reset "osmostat"
- Certain diarrheal states and vomiting*

ADH, Antidiuretic hormone.
*Total body sodium is decreased. Serum sodium concentration is increased because the magnitude of water loss exceeds the magnitude of sodium loss.

Table 28-6 Urine Sodium Concentration and Osmolarity in the Differential Diagnosis of Hyponatremia

Urine Osm (mOsm/L)	Urine [Na] (mmol/L)	Etiology
Greater than serum Osm	<20	SIADH Glucocorticoid deficiency Hypothyroidism
<200	Variable	Psychogenic polydipsia
Greater than serum Osm	<10	Heart failure Liver failure Nephrotic syndrome
Greater than serum Osm	<15	Gastrointestinal losses Burns
~300	>20	Renal failure
Greater than serum Osm	>20	Diuretic therapy Adrenal insufficiency Salt-losing nephropathy Renal tubular acidosis Osmotic diuresis Bicarbonaturia, ketonuria

SIADH, Syndrome of inappropriate antidiuretic hormone.

Table 28-7 Urine Sodium Concentration and Osmolarity in the Differential Diagnosis of Hypernatremia

Urine Osm (mOsm/L)	Urine [Na] (mmol/L)	Etiology
>400	>20	Excessive sodium intake Primary hypoaldosteronism
>400	<10	Burns Excessive sweating Diarrhea in children
>400	Variable	Hyperventilation Thirst deficit
<300	Low	ADH deficiency
≈300	Low	Nephrogenic diabetes insipidus

ADH, Antidiuretic hormone.

interpret these values in light of the clinical picture, particularly assessment of ECW volume. Interpretation of these measurements may be misleading in cases of coexisting abnormalities. Failure to find the expected values when the clinical picture is otherwise consistent with a given clinical condition should lead to consideration that one or more abnormalities may coexist.

KEY CONCEPTS BOX 28-4

- Total body sodium content is a reflection of the balance of sodium intake and output.
- Sodium intake depends on the quantity and type of food intake.
- Sodium output occurs by way of the gastrointestinal tract, the skin, and the urine.
- Under normal conditions, the major route of regulated sodium excretion is the kidney.
- Sodium accumulates in the body when sodium intake exceeds sodium output because of some abnormality of sodium homeostatic mechanisms.
- An increase in total body sodium usually is accompanied by an increase in extracellular water (ECW) volume.
- Sodium depletion (dehydration) occurs when the output of sodium exceeds the intake.
- Changes in total body sodium are not necessarily associated with similar changes in plasma sodium concentration.
- Plasma sodium concentration reflects the relative balance of extracellular sodium and ECW.
- The difference in sodium concentration between interstitial fluid (ISF) and intercellular water (ICW) is the result of the active transport of sodium out of the cell in exchange for potassium.

SECTION OBJECTIVES BOX 28-5

- Describe the factors that control body potassium loss.
- List the primary factors that regulate serum potassium.
- Describe causes of hypokalemia and hyperkalemia.

POTASSIUM METABOLISM

Potassium Balance

Total body potassium (K) is influenced by age, sex, and, very importantly, muscle mass because most of the body's potassium is contained in muscle; an adult male has a total body K of about 50 mmol/kg of body weight. Approximately 98% of the total body K is found in the intracellular fluid (ICF) space at a concentration of 100 to 150 mmol/L, depending on the cell type. Concentrations of potassium in the various fluid compartments are listed in Table 28-2. This high intracellular [K^+] is essential for many basic cellular processes. In plasma water, the concentration of K is only 3.5 to 5 mmol/L, although in interstitial fluid water, with which ICF K is in equilibrium, it is 7% to 8 % higher as a result of the Gibbs-Donnan equilibrium. This steep K gradient from the ICF to ECF compartment is maintained by active transport of K into the cell in exchange for sodium, which is mediated by a sodium-potassium-triphosphatase (Na^+,K^+-ATPase) in the cell membrane. This gradient is the major determinant of the resting membrane potential across the cell membrane; thus it affects muscle excitability and contractility.

Total body K homeostasis requires appropriate internal distribution of K and maintenance of an appropriate external K balance. Regulation of internal K balance refers to regulation of the critical concentration K gradient across cell membranes. Regulation of external K balance refers to the regulation of total body K content. Although maintenance of total body K balance is dependent on excretion of K, predominantly by the kidney, this is a relatively slow process. In the adult, daily K intake (≈100 mmol/day) exceeds total K content of the ECF, and only ≈50% of an oral K load is excreted in the following 4 to 6 hours. Of the retained K, 80% to 90% is rapidly transported from the ECF to ICF space. Life-threatening **hyperkalemia** would result were it not for the temporary, but rapid, extracellular-to-intracellular translocation of the transient excess of K.

Internal Potassium Balance

Uptake of K into cells in exchange for Na is an active process that is driven by Na^+,K^+-ATPase, whereas the efflux of K from the cell is passive and depends on the type and density of K-specific channels in various cell types, as well as the probability that these channels will be open. Increased plasma [K^+] decreases the concentration gradient against which the Na^+,K^+-ATPase pump must operate and thereby favors cellular uptake of K. Decreased plasma [K^+] decreases cellular K uptake by increasing this concentration gradient. Insulin stimulates the cellular uptake of K by hepatocytes and muscle cells, independent of its effects on glucose transport, by inducing an increase in Na^+,K^+-ATPase activity. Beta-adrenergic stimulation promotes K uptake by hepatocytes and skeletal and cardiac muscle via beta-2 receptors. Conversely, beta-adrenergic blockade impairs cellular uptake of K. Insulin and the beta-adrenergic system are important components of the extrarenal defense against hyperkalemia, and they act in both physiological and pathological concentrations.

Alpha-adrenergic receptor stimulation promotes efflux of K from hepatocytes. The role of aldosterone in modulating the internal K balance is uncertain.

Acute metabolic acidemia (see Chapter 29) caused by an acid with an associated anion to which the cell membrane is relatively impermeable (e.g., hydrochloric acid, ammonium chloride, endogenous ketoacidosis, acidosis of uremia) promotes K efflux from cells, increasing the plasma [K^+]. In this situation, K exits cells in exchange for the excess ECF protons, which are buffered intracellularly. However, with metabolic acidemia with an associated anion to which the cell is relatively permeable (e.g., lactic acidemia), the associated anion diffuses into the cell more freely; this type of acidemia is not associated with K efflux. During respiratory acidemia, the increase in plasma [K^+] for any given change in pH is greater than with acidemia associated with a permeable anion, but less than with acidemia associated with an impermeable anion. Increased diffusion of bicarbonate (HCO_3^-) into cells as the result of increased plasma [HCO_3^-], independent of ECF pH, may be associated with the concomitant uptake of K. Respiratory **alkalosis** does not promote much shift of K across cell membranes.

The shift of water out of cells with severe ECF hyperosmolarity increases the intracellular [K^+], promoting K efflux from cells. Impairment of Na^+,K^+-ATPase activity by hypoxia (or loss of Na^+,K^+-ATPase activity with cell death) results in the movement of K out of the cell down its concentration gradient.

External Potassium Balance

The amount of potassium in the body is a reflection of the balance between potassium intake and output. Potassium intake depends on the quantity and type of food intake. Under normal conditions, the average adult takes in about 50 to 100 mmol of potassium/day—about the same amount as sodium.

Potassium output occurs through three primary routes: the gastrointestinal tract, the skin, and the urine. Under normal conditions, loss of potassium through the gastrointestinal tract is very small, amounting to less than 5 mmol/day for an adult. The concentration of potassium in the sweat is less than that of sodium; therefore, potassium losses through the skin are usually small. Potassium is excreted primarily by the kidney. The kidney is capable of regulating the excretion of potassium to maintain body potassium homeostasis. Details of the mechanisms of renal potassium excretion are discussed in Chapter 30.

Disorders of External Potassium Balance

Potassium Excess

Potassium accumulates in the body when the intake of potassium exceeds output because of some abnormality of potassium homeostatic mechanisms. Some of the major conditions that may cause potassium retention are presented in Box 28-7.

Box 28-7

Causes of Potassium Retention

- Increased potassium intake
  - High-potassium diet
  - Oral potassium supplementation
  - Intravenous potassium administration
  - Potassium penicillin in high doses
  - Transfusion of aged blood
- Decreased potassium excretion
  - Renal failure
  - Hypoaldosteronism—adrenal failure
  - Diuretics that block distal tubular potassium secretion: triamterene, amiloride, spironolactone
  - Primary defects in renal tubular potassium secretion

It should be noted that under most conditions, the healthy kidney is capable of excreting a great deal of potassium; a high potassium intake leads to potassium retention only when kidney function is compromised.

Potassium Depletion

Potassium depletion occurs when potassium output exceeds intake. As was discussed previously, only small amounts of potassium are lost in the feces under normal conditions. As is the case for water and sodium, however, gastrointestinal potassium loss during diarrhea or drainage of gastrointestinal secretions can be large (see Table 28-5). Some of the major clinical conditions that may cause potassium depletion are presented in Box 28-8. Note that alkalosis results in total body potassium depletion. With alkalosis, potassium moves from the extracellular to the intracellular space. In cells of the distal nephron of the kidney, this increase in intracellular potassium stimulates potassium secretion and, therefore, increases renal excretion of potassium.

Abnormalities of Plasma Potassium Concentration

Abnormalities in plasma potassium concentration can occur, not only because of abnormalities in total body potassium, but also because of shifts of potassium between the extracellular and intracellular compartments. Although similar shifts may occur with sodium, the effect of intracellular-to-extracellular shifting on plasma concentration is more pronounced for potassium because 98% of the total potassium is intracellular. For example, if only 2% of the intracellular potassium were to shift to the extracellular space, plasma potassium concentration would double. Fortunately, the plasma potassium concentration is held fairly constant despite large fluctuations in potassium intake. An increase in potassium intake stimulates insulin secretion, which shifts potassium from the ECF space to the ICF space and directly stimulates aldosterone secretion by the adrenal cortex. Increased aldosterone stimulates potassium secretion in the distal nephron, thereby increasing

Box 28-8

Causes of Potassium Depletion

Decreased potassium intake
- Low-potassium diet
- Alcoholism
- Anorexia nervosa

Increased gastrointestinal losses
- Vomiting
- Diarrhea
- Fistulas
- Gastrointestinal drainage tube
- Malabsorption
- Laxative or enema abuse

Increased urinary losses
- Increased aldosterone
  - Primary aldosteronism
  - Adrenal hyperplasia
  - Bartter's syndrome
- Adrenogenital syndrome
- Renal disease
  - Renal tubular acidosis
  - Fanconi syndrome
- Diuretics
  - Thiazides
  - Loop diuretics—ethacrynic acid, furosemide
  - Carbonic anhydrase inhibitors—acetazolamide
- Alkalosis

Box 28-9

Causes of Hypokalemia (see Box 25-8)

Extracellular-to-intracellular potassium shift
- Alkalosis
- Increased plasma insulin*

Loop or thiazide diuretic administration
Decreased potassium intake
Increased gastrointestinal losses
Increased urinary losses

*May be associated with total body potassium excess.

Box 28-10

Causes of Hyperkalemia

Pseudohyperkalemia
- Hemolysis
- Leukocytosis

Intracellular-to-extracellular shift
- α-Adrenergic stimulation
- β-Adrenergic blockade
- Metabolic acidosis (depending on the associated anion)*
- Crush injuries
- Tissue hypoxia*
- Insulin deficiency*
- Digitalis overdose*

High potassium intake (see Box 28-7)
Decreased potassium excretion (see Box 28-8)

*May be associated with total body potassium depletion.

urinary potassium output. Increased insulin secretion has the effect of buffering the acute increase in plasma potassium comcentration until an increase in urinary potassium excretion reestablishes zero potassium balance. The opposite effect occurs with decreased potassium intake.

Hypokalemia

Low plasma potassium concentration can be caused by movement of potassium into the cell from the extracellular water space, or it may be caused by increased output or decreased intake (Box 28-9).

Hypokalemia caused by potassium shift into the cell may in fact be associated with increased total body potassium (e.g., with increase in plasma insulin in response to increased glucose intake). Hypokalemia caused by increased excretion or decreased intake is associated with total body potassium depletion.

Signs and symptoms of hypokalemia are numerous and include **anorexia,** nausea, vomiting, abdominal distension, muscle cramps or tenderness, **paresthesias,** electrocardiographic changes, **arrhythmias,** inability to concentrate the urine with resultant **polyuria** and polydipsia, lethargy, and confusion. For methods of analysis, see Sodium and Potassium Methods in the Evolve.

Hyperkalemia

Clinical conditions associated with elevated plasma potassium are listed in Box 28-10. Actual plasma potassium may be normal, but measured plasma potassium may be artifactully elevated (**pseudohyperkalemia;** see Chapter 18) if the blood sample is hemolyzed, or if there is leakage of potassium from white blood cells when there is leukocytosis (elevated white blood cell number). In addition, vigorous arm exercise, tight application of the tourniquet, or squeezing of the area around the venipuncture site may result in cellular potassium release and spurious elevation of plasma potassium concentration.

True hyperkalemia can result from movement of potassium out of the cell into the extracellular water space, increased intake, or decreased output. Hyperkalemia caused by potassium shift out of the cell may in fact be associated with total body potassium depletion (e.g., in diabetic ketoacidosis). Hyperkalemia caused by increased intake or decreased output is associated with total body potassium excess.

The clinical signs and symptoms of hyperkalemia include changes in the electrocardiogram, cardiac arrhythmia, muscular weakness, and paresthesias. The greatest danger associated with hyperkalemia is life-threatening cardiac arrhythmia or arrest.

Urine Potassium

Urine potassium concentration can be useful in the differential diagnosis of hypokalemia. As with urine sodium concentration, it is important to interpret these values in light of the clinical picture. A urine potassium concentration <20 mmol/L with hypokalemia is consistent with inadequate intake of potassium or nonurinary losses; a urine potassium level >20 mmol/L is consistent with urinary loss. On the other hand, urine potassium is of little help in the differential diagnosis of hyperkalemia.

KEY CONCEPTS BOX 28-5

- Approximately 98% of total body K is found in the intracellular fluid (ICF) compartment.
- Total body K homeostasis requires regulation of internal distribution of K and external K balance.
- Regulation of internal distribution refers to maintenance of the steep K concentration gradient across cell membranes by active transport of K into the cell in exchange for sodium.
- Factors that affect the distribution of K between extracellular water (ECW) and intracellular water (ICW) include plasma [K^+], insulin levels, adrenergic activity, and pH.
- Regulation of external K balance refers to the regulation of total body K content.
- Total body K content is a reflection of the balance of K intake and K output.
- Potassium intake depends on the quantity and type of food intake.
- Potassium output occurs by way of the gastrointestinal tract, the skin, and the kidney.
- Under normal conditions, the major route of regulated K excretion is the kidney.
- An excess of total body K occurs when the intake of K exceeds K output. This usually occurs when renal K excretion is compromised.
- Depletion of total body K occurs when K output exceeds K intake.
- Abnormalities in plasma [K^+] can occur because of abnormalities in total body K content and because of shifts of K between extracellular and intracellular compartments.
- Hypokalemia can result from movement of K into the cell from the extracellular water space, increased output, or decreased intake.
- Hyperkalemia can result from movement of potassium out of the cell into the extracellular water space, increased intake, or decreased output.

SECTION OBJECTIVES BOX 28-6

- Describe the factors that control body chloride levels.
- List the primary factors that regulate serum chloride.
- Describe causes of hypochloridemia and hyperchloridemia.

CHLORIDE METABOLISM

Chloride Balance

Chloride is the major anion in the ECW space. In a normal adult, total body chloride is about 30 mmol/kg of body weight. Approximately 88% of chloride is found in the ECW space and 12% in the ICW space. Approximately 14% of total body chloride is in the plasma, 27% in ISF that is readily accessible to plasma, 17% in ISF of dense connective tissue and cartilage, 15% in ISF of bone, and 5% in the transcellular space. Concentrations of chloride in the various fluid compartments are listed in Table 28-2. Note that the concentration of chloride in ISF is greater than that in plasma water, whereas the concentrations of sodium and potassium in ISF are less than those in plasma water. These differences between plasma and ISF are caused by the Gibbs-Donnan equilibrium. Chloride is passively distributed across the cell membrane. The difference in chloride concentration between ISF and ICW is caused by the electrical potential difference across the cell membrane. Because the inside of the cell is negative in contrast to the outside, the concentration of chloride outside the cell is higher than that inside.

The amount of chloride in the body is a reflection of the balance between chloride intake and output. Chloride intake depends on quantity and type of food intake. The chloride content of most foods parallels that of sodium. Under normal conditions, the average adult takes in about 50 to 200 mmol of chloride/day. Chloride output occurs by way of three primary routes: the gastrointestinal tract, the skin, and the urinary tract.

Under normal circumstances, loss of chloride through the gastrointestinal tract is very small. Fecal chloride excretion for a normal adult measures only 1 to 2 mmol/day. Concentrations of chloride in gastrointestinal secretions are shown in Table 28-5. With severe diarrhea or with gastric or intestinal drainage tubes, chloride loss through the gastrointestinal tract may exceed 100 mmol/day.

The chloride composition of sweat averages about 40 mmol/L but is somewhat variable. As in the case of sodium, the concentration of chloride in sweat is decreased by aldosterone and increased in cystic fibrosis. Under conditions of excessive sweating, chloride losses through the skin can exceed 200 mmol/day. However, under normal conditions, chloride losses through the skin are small.

The major route of chloride excretion is through the kidney. Details of the mechanisms of renal chloride excretion are discussed in Chapter 30.

Disorders of Chloride Balance

Chloride Excess

Chloride accumulates in the body when the intake of chloride exceeds output because of some abnormality in a chloride homeostasis mechanism. For the most part, the causes of chloride retention are much the same as those of sodium retention. Therefore, the pathophysiology of chloride excess in most cases is similar to that of sodium excess (see Box 28-3). However, there is one clinical condition in which chloride excess may not be associated with sodium excess: certain types of metabolic acidosis. The two major extracellular anions are chloride and bicarbonate. Extracellular bicarbonate is consumed by the reaction with hydrogen ions produced in metabolic acidosis. If no organic anions are produced with H^+, chloride ions are needed to replace the consumed bicarbonate ions to maintain electrical neutrality. The increase in chloride concentration is caused by the reabsorption of a relatively greater proportion of sodium with chloride than with bicarbonate by the tubules of the kidney.

Chloride Depletion

Chloride depletion occurs when the output of chloride exceeds intake. For the most part, the causes of chloride depletion are the same as those of sodium depletion (see Box 28-4). However, in one clinical condition, hypochloremic metabolic alkalosis, chloride depletion may occur without sodium depletion. Hypochloremic metabolic alkalosis may result from loss of chloride in excess of sodium loss, usually from abnormal loss of gastric fluid. Bicarbonate must be retained to maintain electrical neutrality, leading to a base-excess alkalosis. Hypochloremia also may be associated with other disorders that involve bicarbonate retention, such as renal compensation for chronic respiratory acidosis (see Chapter 29).

Abnormalities of Plasma Chloride Concentration

As for sodium, changes in total body chloride are not necessarily associated with similar changes in plasma chloride concentration; that is, with body chloride retention, the plasma chloride concentration will remain normal if there is a proportional increase in ECW and will decrease if there is a relatively greater increase in ECW. Similarly, plasma chloride concentration may remain normal or even increase with chloride depletion, depending on the concomitant change in ECW.

In most cases, the causes of **hypochloremia** and **hyperchloremia** are the same as those of hyponatremia and hypernatremia (see p. 542). The major clinical exceptions to the usual parallel changes in plasma sodium and chloride concentrations occur during chronic metabolic acidosis and alkalosis. With metabolic acidosis, hyperchloremia may not be associated with hypernatremia; with metabolic alkalosis, hypochloremia may not be associated with hyponatremia. The reasons for this are those previously discussed for chloride excess and depletion.

Symptoms are not directly attributable to hypochloremia or hyperchloremia. Rather, symptoms that occur in patients with an abnormal serum chloride concentration are caused by the associated abnormality in serum sodium or pH. A summary of the plasma electrolyte changes that occur in metabolic acidosis and alkalosis is presented in Fig. 28-10.

Urine Chloride Concentration

The concentration of chloride in the urine is important in the differential diagnosis of metabolic alkalosis (see Chapter 29). Metabolic alkalosis that results from contraction of the ECW volume is associated with a urine chloride concentration of less than 15 mmol/L. Metabolic alkalosis can be corrected with saline administration. Metabolic alkalosis with a normal ECW volume is associated with a urine chloride concentration of greater than 15 mmol/L and may be resistant to saline administration.

Urine chloride concentration can be used to distinguish surreptitious diuretic abuse and vomiting (which is sometimes used by young women to induce weight loss) from **Bartter's syndrome.** All of these entities produce hypokalemia, metabolic alkalosis (see p. 563), hyperreninemia, and hyperaldosteronism; urinary concentrations of sodium and potassium are elevated in all these situations. With chronic diuretic abuse (in the absence of diuretic intake in the previous 24 to 48 hours) or protracted vomiting, urinary chloride concentration is usually below 20 mmol/L. Patients with Bartter's syndrome always have elevated urinary chloride concentrations even in the face of volume contraction. Note, however, that with recent diuretic intake, urinary chloride concentration may exceed 20 mmol/L, even in the face of chronic diuretic abuse; in this case, the diagnosis of surreptitious diuretic abuse is made by testing urine for diuretics.

KEY CONCEPTS BOX 28-6

- Total body chloride content is a reflection of the balance between chloride intake and output.
- Chloride intake depends on the quantity and type of food intake.
- Chloride output occurs by way of the gastrointestinal tract, the skin, and the urine.
- Under normal conditions, the major route of chloride excretion, and the only route of loss that is regulated, is the kidney.
- Total body chloride content occurs when intake of chloride exceeds output because of some abnormality in a chloride homeostasis mechanism.
- For the most part, the causes of chloride retention are the same as those of sodium retention. However, with hyperchloremic metabolic acidosis, chloride excess may not be associated with sodium excess.
- Chloride depletion occurs when output of chloride exceeds intake.
- For the most part, the causes of chloride depletion are the same as those of sodium depletion. However, with hypochloremic metabolic alkalosis, chloride depletion may not be associated with sodium depletion.
- As for sodium, changes in total body chloride are not necessarily associated with similar changes in plasma chloride concentration.
- In most cases, the causes of hypochloremia and hyperchloremia are the same as those of hyponatremia and hypernatremia. However, with chronic metabolic acidosis, hyperchloremia may not be associated with hypernatremia; with chronic metabolic alkalosis, hypochloremia may not be associated with hyponatremia.

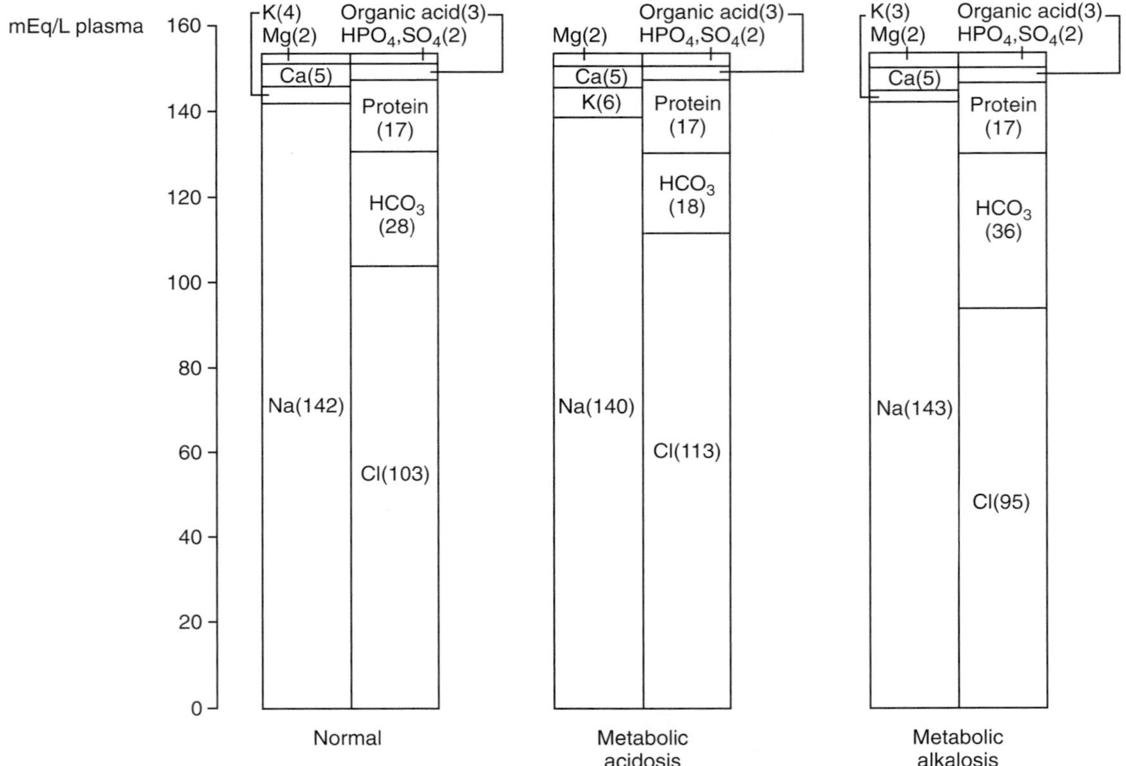

Fig. 28-10 Concentrations of electrolytes in plasma (mEq/L) with metabolic acidosis and metabolic alkalosis compared with normal. In the example of metabolic acidosis shown, there is no increase in organic acids—only loss of bicarbonate. Metabolic acidosis may be attributable to an increase in organic acids (see Fig. 28-4). In these cases, chloride may not be increased. Note that the extracellular potassium concentration is elevated in metabolic acidosis and lowered in metabolic alkalosis. Under all conditions, the concentration of anions equals the concentration of cations.

BIBLIOGRAPHY

Adler SM, Verbalis JG: Disorders of body water homeostasis in critical illness, Endocrinol Metab Clin North Am 35:873, 2006.

Ellison DH, Berl T: Clinical practice: the syndrome of inappropriate antidiuresis, N Engl J Med 356:2064, 2007.

Han DS, Cho BS: Therapeutic approach to hyponatremia, Nephron 92(suppl 1):9, 2002.

Kang SK, Kim W, Oh MS: Pathogenesis and treatment of hypernatremia, Nephron 92(suppl 1):14, 2002.

Kim GH, Han JS: Therapeutic approach to hypokalemia, Nephron 92(suppl 1):28, 2002.

Kim GH, Han JS: Therapeutic approach to hyperkalemia, Nephron 92(suppl 1):33, 2002.

Moe OW, Fuster D: Clinical acid-base pathophysiology: disorders of plasma anion gap: best practice and research, Clin Endocrinol Metab 17:559, 2003.

Oh MS: Pathogenesis and diagnosis of hyponatremia, Nephron 92(suppl 1):2, 2002.

Schrier RW: Body water homeostasis: clinical disorders of urinary dilution and concentration, J Am Soc Nephrol 17:1820, 2006.

Schrier RW: The sea within us: disorders of body water homeostasis, Curr Opin Invest Drugs 8:304, 2007.

Stoupakis G, Klapholz M: Natriuretic peptides: biochemistry, physiology, and therapeutic role in heart failure, Heart Dis 5:215, 2003.

Strange K: Cellular volume homeostasis, Adv Physiol Educ 28:155, 2004.

Williams GH: Aldosterone biosynthesis, regulation, and classical mechanisms of action, Heart Fail Rev 10:7, 2005.

INTERNET SITES

http://mcb.berkeley.edu/courses/mcb135e/kidneyfluid.html—Water and sodium balance

http://oneweb.utc.edu/~sprtnutr/fluids.html—Sports nutrition, fluids

http://www.anaesthesiamcq.com/FluidBook/—Fluid and electrolyte physiology; online text

http://www.liv.ac.uk/~petesmif/teaching/1bds_mb/notes/fluid/text.htm—Body fluid compartments

http://www.merck.com/mmpe/sec12/ch151/ch151h.html—Central diabetes insipidus

http://www.merck.com/mmpe/sec12/ch153/ch153f.html—Primary hyperaldosteronism

http://www.merck.com/mmpe/sec12/ch156/ch156b.html—Water and sodium balance

http://www.merck.com/mmpe/sec12/ch156/ch156c.html—Disorders of fluid balance

http://www.merck.com/mmpe/sec12/ch156/ch156d.html#sec12-ch156-ch156d-713—Hyponatremia

http://www.merck.com/mmpe/sec12/ch156/ch156e.html—Hypernatremia

http://www.merck.com/mmpe/sec12/ch156/ch156f.html—Disorders of potassium balance

http://www.merck.com/mmpe/sec17/ch237/ch237b.html—Bartter's syndrome

http://www.merck.com/mmpe/sec17/ch237/ch237d.html—Nephrogenic diabetes insipidus

http://www.merck.com/mmpe/sec17/ch237/ch237f.html—Renal tubular acidosis
http://www.merck.com/mmpe/sec19/ch291/ch291c.html—Fanconi syndrome
http://www.physioviva.com/movies/gibbs-donnan/index.html—Ion diffusion, Gibbs-Donnan equilibrium; animation
http://www.wisc-online.com/objects/index_tj.asp?objID=NUR1203—Fluids and electrolytes, animation
http://www.wisc-online.com/objects/index_tj.asp?objID=NUR2903—Alterations in fluid balance, animation
http://www.wisc-online.com/objects/index_tj.asp?objID=NUR4004—Osmotic pressure

Acid-Base Control and Acid-Base Disorders

29 Chapter

John E. Sherwin

Chapter Outline

Key Terms

acidemia A condition of decreased pH of the blood.

acidosis A pathological condition that results from accumulation of acid in the blood or loss of base from the blood.

alkalemia A condition of increased pH of the blood.

alkalosis A pathological condition that results from accumulation of base or loss of acid from the body.

allergen Any substance that serves as an *antigen* that is recognized by the body immune system (see Chapters 7 and 8) as foreign and causes the production of imunnoglobulin E directed against that substance (the *allergic reaction*).

alveoli Small outpouchings of walls of alveolar space through which gas exchange takes place between alveolar air and pulmonary capillary blood.

anion gap The concentration of undetermined anions, calculated as the difference between measured cations and measured anions.

apnea Cessation of breathing.

base excess or deficit The difference between the titratable bicarbonate of a blood sample and that of a normal blood sample at a pH of 7.4, a P_{CO_2} of 40 mm Hg, and a temperature of 37°C.

bradycardia Slowing of the heartbeat to a rate of less than 60 beats per minute.

carbamino group A stable, protein-bound form of CO_2 that results from the covalent chemical reaction between CO_2 and the primary amino group ($-NH_2$) of a protein.

carbonic anhydrase An enzyme that catalyzes the reaction between CO_2 and water to form carbonic acid (H_2CO_3).

chloride shift Exchange of Cl^- in serum for HCO_3^- in red blood cells in peripheral tissues as a response to increased P_{CO_2} of the blood. The shift reverses in the lungs.

conjugate base Unprotonated anionic form of a corresponding weak acid.

Henderson-Hasselbalch equation Describes the relationship among pH, the pK_a of a buffer system, and the ratio of the conjugate base to a weak acid.

hypercapnia A condition of excess carbon dioxide in the blood.

hypochloremic alkalosis A metabolic alkalosis that results from increased blood bicarbonate following loss of chloride from the body.

hypoxia A condition of low oxygen content in tissues.

isohydric shift The series of reactions in red blood cells in which CO_2 is taken up and oxygen is released without the production of excess hydrogen ions.

metabolic acidosis Pathological loss of base in the body.

metabolic alkalosis Pathological accumulation of base in the body.

metabolic component The bicarbonate concentration of plasma.

oxygen saturation The fraction of total hemoglobin (Hb) in the form of HbO_2 at a defined P_{O_2}. Percentage of saturation = $100(HbO_2)/(HbO_2 + Hb)$.

P_{50} The partial pressure of oxygen at which hemoglobin is half-saturated with bound oxygen.

partial pressure The pressure exerted by a gas, whether it is alone or mixed with other gases. The partial pressure of a gas is denoted by the letter *P* preceding the symbol for that gas (usually in small capital letters); for example, the partial pressure of CO_2 is P_{CO_2}.

pH The negative logarithm of the hydrogen-ion concentration.

relative base deficit Lowered HCO_3^-/H_2CO_3 ratio caused by an increase in P_{CO_2}. The HCO_3^- (base) is low relative to the P_{CO_2}.

relative base excess Elevated HCO_3^-/H_2CO_3 ratio caused by a decrease in P_{CO_2} (respiratory acidosis). As in the relative base deficit, the HCO_3^- (base) is elevated relative to the P_{CO_2}.

respiration The exchange of gases between the alveoli air and blood.

respiratory acidosis Pathological retention of CO_2 in the body caused by changes in respiration or ventilation.

respiratory alkalosis Pathological decrease in CO_2 caused by ventilation change.

respiratory component The "αP_{CO_2}" or acid component, which is immediately modified by respiratory status; "α" is the solubility (or Bunsen) coefficient of CO_2.

surfactant An agent that decreases surface tension. Applies to agents that coat pulmonary alveolar surfaces.

ventilation The mechanical process of moving air in and out of the lungs.

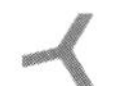

Methods on Evolve

Anion gap
Blood gas analysis and oxygen saturation
Carbon dioxide and bicarbonate
Henderson-Hasselbalch calculating algorithm
Ketones
Lactic acid
Oximetry
Pyruvic acid

SECTION OBJECTIVES BOX 29-1

- Describe clinically important physiological acids and their buffers.
- Outline the blood-buffering mechanism of the bicarbonate and hemoglobin buffering systems.
- State the Henderson-Hasselbalch equation, and identify the respiratory and metabolic components.
- Describe the process of gas exchange and ventilation.
- Define oxygen saturation and P_{50}, and describe the effects of specific biochemicals on the dissociation of oxygen from hemoglobin.
- Explain acid-base balance regulation by the kidney.

ACID-BASE CONTROL

Acids and Bases

Definitions

Using the simplest definition, an *acid* is a substance that releases protons or hydrogen ions (H^+), whereas a *base* is defined simply as a substance that accepts protons or H^+. Both acids and bases are defined further by their degree of affinity for H^+. A strong acid has little affinity for H^+ and so readily dissociates H^+, whereas a weak acid has some affinity for H^+ and thus less readily dissociates H^+. A strong base has a high affinity for H^+; a weak base has low affinity for H^+. If one molecule differs from another by only a proton, the two are called a conjugate acid-base pair. Physiological examples of a weak acid and its **conjugate base** are carbonic acid (H_2CO_3) and bicarbonate (HCO_3^-). The equilibrium mixture contains all three componants, as is shown in the following reaction:

$$H_2CO_3 \rightleftharpoons H^+ + HCO_3^- \qquad \text{Eq. 29-1}$$

Dietary and Metabolic Sources of Acids and Bases

Two types of acids are dealt with in physiological states: fixed acids and volatile acids. Fixed acids are nongaseous acids such as phosphate (HPO_4^{2-}) and sulfate (SO_4^{2-}) ions or organic acids such as lactic acid, acetoacetic acid, and β-hydroxybutyric acid. The physiologically important volatile acid is carbonic acid (H_2CO_3). The volatility of carbonic acid arises from its ability to dissociate into water and carbon dioxide (CO_2), which can be released as a gas. The reaction scheme for carbonic acid is as follows:

$$CO_2\,(\text{gas}) \rightleftharpoons CO_2\,(\text{dissolved}) \underset{-H_2O}{\overset{+H_2O}{\rightleftharpoons}} H_2CO_3 \rightleftharpoons H^+ + HCO_3^- \qquad \text{Eq. 29-2}$$

At one end of the equilibrium is carbon dioxide, which can be considered the anhydrous form of H_2CO_3, and at the other end is HCO_3^-, the conjugate base of H_2CO_3. Thus CO_2 is in equilibrium with $H^+ + HCO_3^-$. Although the reaction of CO_2 and water to form H_2CO_3 will occur spontaneously, the enzyme **carbonic anhydrase** facilitates this reaction in vivo.

Carbohydrates, lipids, and proteins are metabolized by oxidation reactions that generate fixed acids, which must be neutralized in order to maintain constant cellular and blood **pH.** Under anaerobic conditions (low tissue P_{O_2}) such as those produced by disease or strenuous exercise, carbohydrates are metabolized to lactic and pyruvic acids, which accumulate until normal tissue oxygenation is achieved. These acids can be metabolized further to the ultimate oxidation product, carbon dioxide, when aerobic metabolism is resumed. Triglycerides are metabolized to fatty acids, which can be further metabolized to ketone bodies (acetoacetic acid and β-hydroxybutyric acid); ultimately, these lipid metabolites are further oxidized to carbon dioxide. Proteins are hydrolyzed to amino acids, which then are converted to carbon dioxide. Those proteins that are composed of sulfur-containing amino acids are catabolized in part to the salt of sulfuric acid. Nucleic acids and some lipids contain phosphorus and are metabolized to salts of phosphoric acid. The overwhelmingly major metabolic acid produced by our cells is CO_2.

Table 29-1 Physiologically Important Buffers and their Concentration, pK_a, and Buffering Capacity

Buffer	pK_a	Concentration (mmol/L)	Relative Buffering Capacity (mEq/L)
Bicarbonate	6.33	25	1
Hemoglobin	7.2	53	40
Phosphate	6.8	1.2	0.3
Protein	—	—	8

pH, Hydrogen Ion, and Buffers

Please review the discussion of pH and buffer calculations in p. 37 in Chapter 1. Remember, the accepted convention is to describe the concentration of H^+ in terms of pH (the negative logarithm of the concentration of H^+) rather than in moles per liter (M).

Physiological Buffers

Normal human whole blood is buffered at a slightly alkaline pH in a range of 7.35 to 7.45, which corresponds to an H^+ concentration of 4.5×10^{-8} M to 3.5×10^{-8} M. Buffering capacity depends on the concentration of the buffer and the relationship between the pK_a of the buffer and the desired pH. A buffer is considered most effective within ±2 pH units of its pK_a; it has maximum buffering capacity when its pK_a equals the pH. For maximum blood buffering, the pK_a of buffers therefore should be near physiological pH, that is, pH 7.4, and should have equal amounts of weak acid and conjugate base. The physiologically important buffers that maintain this narrow pH range observed in the body are hemoglobin, bicarbonate, phosphate, and proteins. Table 29-1 lists the pK_a and concentrations of these buffer systems and their relative buffering capacities.

Bicarbonate buffer system

The **Henderson-Hasselbalch equation** for the bicarbonate–carbonic acid buffer system is as follows:

$$pH = pK_a + \log\frac{[HCO_3^-]}{[H_2CO_3]} \quad \text{Eq. 29-3}$$

The measured pK_a is 6.33 at 37°C. Instead of being at the maximum buffer capacity with a 1 : 1 ratio of HCO_3^- to H_2CO_3, the bicarbonate–carbonic acid buffer system at blood pH of 7.4 is at a ratio of about 20 : 1. This 20 : 1 ratio is maintained primarily by the lungs, which expel CO_2 produced during the metabolism of nutrients.

$$pH = pK_a + \log\frac{[HCO_3^-]}{[H_2CO_3]} = 6.33 + \log 20 = 7.6 \quad \text{Eq. 29-4}$$

This pH is higher than normal blood pH because Eq. 29-3 does not exactly describe physiological bicarbonate buffering. Eq. 29-3 includes three unknowns: pH, $[HCO_3^-]$, and $[H_2CO_3]$. Although pH is measurable, there is no direct measure of $[HCO_3^-]$ or $[H_2CO_3]$. To use this equation, replace the term H_2CO_3 with an analyte that is measurable. Because the concentration of H_2CO_3 is proportional to the amount of dissolved CO_2 (see Eq. 29-2), you can replace $[H_2CO_3]$ with the term for dissolved CO_2, αP_{CO_2}, where α (the Bunson coefficient) is the solubility coefficient of CO_2. The pK_a term in the Henderson-Hasselbalch equation is modified to reflect the equilibrium between the weak acid, the dissolved CO_2, and the conjugate base, HCO_3^-. The modified Henderson-Hasselbalch equation that describes the equilibrium in Eq. 29-2 is as follows:

$$pH = pK_a' + \log\frac{[HCO_3^-]}{\alpha P_{CO_2}} \quad \text{Eq. 29-5}$$

The apparent pK_a' in human plasma is 6.1 at 37°C. The solubility coefficient for CO_2 in plasma at 37°C is 0.031 mmol $\times L^{-1} \times mm\ Hg^{-1}$. *Remember: The pH of blood is only dependent upon the* $[HCO_3]/\alpha P_{CO_2}$ *ratio.* The concentration of bicarbonate base greatly exceeds that of acid in this plasma buffer system, reflecting the demands put on the body by metabolism, which primarily produces acids. This buffer system is designed to immediately neutralize fixed acids and to process the primary metabolic waste product, CO_2. The CO_2 component of the buffer system is eliminated by the lungs.

The total CO_2 content (T_{CO_2}) of plasma is described as follows:

$$T_{CO_2} = CO_2\,(\text{dissolved}) + [HCO_3^-] + [H_2CO_3] \quad \text{Eq. 29-6, A}$$

The $[H_2CO_3]$ term can be disregarded because it is so small (one-twentieth the $[HCO_3^-]$), and CO_2 (dissolved) can be replaced with the term αP_{CO_2}. Thus the equation can be reduced to

$$T_{CO_2} = \alpha P_{CO_2} + [HCO_3^-] \quad \text{Eq. 29-6, B}$$

Two of the three unknowns are readily determined, allowing calculation of the T_{CO_2} (see Fig. 29-7).

Hemoglobin

The major buffer of blood is hemoglobin, which is localized in the red blood cells (RBCs). Hemoglobin (Hb) takes up free H^+ so that the following reaction proceeds to the right:

$$CO_2 + H_2O \rightleftharpoons H_2CO_3 \rightleftharpoons HCO_3^- + H^+$$

$$H^+ + HbO_2 \rightarrow HHb^+ + O_2 \quad \text{Eq. 29-7}$$

Hemoglobin and serum proteins have high concentrations of histidine residues. The imidazole group of histidine (Fig. 29-1) has a pK_a of approximately 7.3. It is this combination of high concentration and appropriate pK_a that makes hemoglobin the dominant buffering agent of blood at physiological pH. The bulk of CO_2 formed in peripheral tissues is transported in the plasma portion of blood as HCO_3^- with the H^+ bound to hemoglobin within the erythrocyte (Fig. 29-2). The CO_2 of carbonic acid accounts for about 2 mmol/L of CO_2 in venous blood but accounts for only about 1 mmol/L in arterial blood.

Significant amounts of CO_2 are transported as a protein-bound moiety. CO_2 reacts nonenzymatically with the accessible amino groups of proteins to form a **carbamino group:**

$$O{=}C{=}O + H_2N\text{–Protein} \rightarrow {}^{-}O\text{–}\overset{O}{\overset{\|}{C}}\text{–N–Protein} + H^+ \qquad \text{Eq. 29-8}$$

Carbamino group

Approximately 0.5 mmol/L of CO_2 is transported in this fashion.

The observed arteriovenous difference in total CO_2 content is almost entirely the result of formation of bicarbonate in red blood cells. In the lungs, as deoxygenated hemoglobin becomes oxygenated and CO_2 is expelled, the H^+ is released from hemoglobin because oxygenated hemoglobin (HbO_2) is a stronger acid than deoxyhemoglobin (HbH). In the lungs, then, the reaction in Eq. 29-7 proceeds to the left. H^+ is released and reacts with transported HCO_3^- to form CO_2, which the lungs can now release (see Fig. 29-2). The overall equation linking the oxygenation process to buffering is

$$H^+ + HbO_2 \rightleftharpoons HHb^+ + O_2 \qquad \text{Eq. 29-9}$$

The forward reaction occurs in tissues in which there is a relatively high H^+ and a relatively low O_2 concentration, whereas the reverse reaction occurs in the lungs, where the O_2 concentration is relatively high.

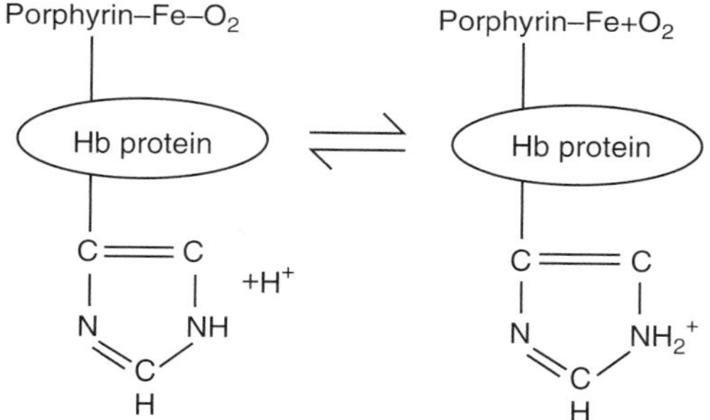

Fig. 29-1 Effects of hemoglobin oxygenation on buffering action of imidazole group of histidine. Oxygen binding affects the pK_a of the imidazole ring, making the ring more acidic with release of an H^+.

Phosphate and Proteins

Phosphate is a minor buffering component of the blood, with the following equilibrium reaction occurring:

$$H_2PO_4^- \rightleftharpoons H^+ + HPO_4^{2-} \qquad \text{Eq. 29-10}$$

The pK_a of this reaction is 6.8. Phosphate buffer is an important buffer in urine, which has relatively little protein, hemoglobin, or bicarbonate. Phosphate buffers in the blood are inorganic phosphates, but both inorganic and organic phosphates act as intracellular buffers.

Plasma proteins also act as buffers in the blood, although their buffering effect is minor compared with that of the bicarbonate system or the hemoglobin system (see Table 29-1).

Oxygen and Carbon Dioxide Homeostasis

Partial Pressure

Blood-gas analysis allows measurement of the **partial pressures** of oxygen and carbon dioxide (Po_2 and Pco_2, respectively). Historically, units of Po_2 and Pco_2 have been expressed as millimeters of mercury (mm Hg), or torr, and these units are still used by most laboratories in the United States. The international unit for partial pressure is the pascal, or Pa (1 mm Hg = 133.3224 Pa).

Table 29-2 shows the composition of atmospheric air, alveolar air (air inside the lung), and expired air. Humidity makes a substantial contribution to the composition of air in the lungs, thus altering the partial pressures of the other gases. A correction for the gas volume contributed by water vapor is therefore essential; at 37°C, the P_{H_2O} of blood is approximately 47 mm Hg.

Two terms used in discussing the oxygen content of blood are **oxygen saturation** and $\mathbf{P_{50}}$. *Oxygen saturation* is the percentage of the total hemoglobin present as oxygenated hemoglobin. P_{50} denotes that partial pressure of oxygen at which the hemoglobin is 50% saturated with oxygen.

Ventilation

Ventilation is differentiated from respiration in that *ventilation* is the mechanical process of moving air into and out of

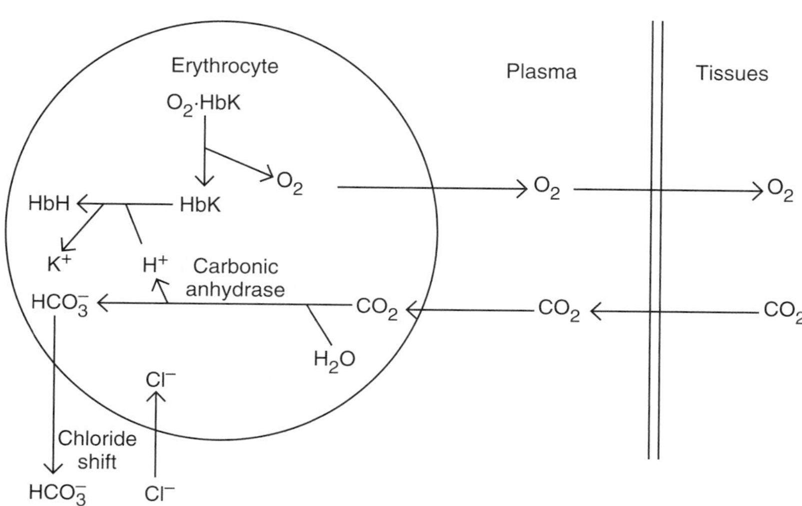

Fig. 29-2 Hemoglobin buffering action in peripheral tissues. *HbK,* Potassium salt of hemoglobin; *HbH,* protonated form of hemoglobin.

Table 29-2 Composition of Air (Partial Pressure Expressed in mm Hg)

Air	N_2	O_2	CO_2	H_2O	Total Pressure
Atmospheric air	598.0	158.0	0.3	3.7	760
Alveolar air	573.0	100.0	40.0	47.0	760
Expired air	566.0	115.0	32.0	47.0	760

Table 29-3 Reference Values for Adult Blood-Gas Parameters in Arterial and Venous Blood

Parameters	Arterial	Venous
pH	7.35 to 7.45	7.33 to 7.43
P_{CO_2}	35 to 45 mm Hg	38 to 50 mm Hg
P_{O_2}	80 to 100 mm Hg	30 to 50 mm Hg
HCO_3^-	22 to 26 mmol/L	23 to 27 mmol/L
Total CO_2	23 to 27 mmol/L	24 to 28 mmol/L
O_2 saturation	94% to 100%	60% to 85%
Venous anion gap	5 to 14 mmol/L	5 to 14 mmol/L
Base excess	−2 to +2 mEq/L	−2 to +2 mEq/L

the lungs, and *respiration* is the exchange of gases between the atmosphere and the capillaries of the pulmonary circulation; it occurs in the **alveoli.** The normal respiration rate is 13 to 16 times per minute.

The walls of the lung contain elastic connective tissues that would collapse the lung were it not for the surface tension between the wall of the lung and the wall of the thoracic cavity. The surface tension of the inner walls of the alveoli, in contrast, has a tendency to collapse the alveoli after expiration, when the alveoli are deflated. This surface tension is reduced by the presence of a phospholipid-lipoprotein complex, a **surfactant** that lines the alveolar walls in a thin film and allows the alveolar walls to be inflated easily. Premature babies without sufficient surfactant lining the alveolar walls can have respiratory difficulties because of the tendency of their alveoli to collapse. It is for this reason that the levels of surfactant (e.g., lecithin/sphingomyelin ratio) in amniotic fluid are determined for assessment of fetal lung development (see below and Chapter 44).

Gas Exchange

Gas transfer in the alveoli is a concentration-dependent phenomenon. Inspired (room) air has a relatively high P_{O_2} (158 mm Hg) and a low P_{CO_2} (0.3 mm Hg). Pressures of oxygen and carbon dioxide in capillary blood in the lungs are 50 and 40 mm Hg, respectively. Because the P_{O_2} of blood is lower than that of inspired air, and the P_{CO_2} of blood is higher than the P_{CO_2} of room air, the gases diffuse from higher to lower concentration areas, that is, CO_2 gas moves from the capillaries to the alveolar air space, whereas O_2 moves from the alveoli to the capillaries. Reference values for adult blood-gas parameters in arterial and venous blood are summarized in Table 29-3. Because of its greater water solubility, CO_2 exchanges more rapidly and more efficiently than O_2 does. In some cases of **respiratory acidosis,** this phenomenon of differential gas diffusibility can result in low blood P_{O_2} but relatively normal P_{CO_2}.

Control of Ventilation

Ventilatory control regulates the carbonate-bicarbonate buffer system but is in turn regulated by the resulting pH of cerebrospinal fluid and plasma. Control of ventilation is localized in a respiratory center of the brain where chemoreceptors are influenced by the pH of the cerebrospinal fluid. Other chemoreceptors influenced by the changes in pH of arterial blood are located in the carotid and aortic vessels. A rise in P_{CO_2} of arterial blood will result in a fall in pH. This in turn will stimulate the chemoreceptors, initiating a rise in the respiration rate that will result in the release of more CO_2 from blood in the lungs.

Acid-Base Balance

Maintenance of a constant pH is important because changes in pH will alter the functioning of enzymes and biological structural components, the cellular uptake and use of metabolites and minerals, and the uptake and release of oxygen.

In the body, physiological buffers act to maintain a constant pH in the following manner. Fixed acids enter the blood and are immediately neutralized by the bicarbonate buffering system.

$$H^+A^- \text{ (fixed acid)} + HCO_3^- \rightleftharpoons H_2CO_3 + A^- \text{ (unmeasured anions)}$$
$$H_2CO_3 \rightleftharpoons H_2O + CO_2 \quad \text{Eq. 29-11}$$

However, the volatile acid, CO_2, is neutralized by the hemoglobin buffering system because all the buffering systems are at equilibrium with one another. Although the bicarbonate buffering system has relatively low buffering capacity (see Table 29-1), it plays a large role in maintaining blood pH because it acts as the *immediate* buffer when fixed acids enter the blood.

Changes in ventilation rate will alter the bicarbonate–carbonic acid ratio and pH. To understand this process, one must reconsider Eqs. 29-2 and 29-5. A decrease in the ventilation rate will cause a decrease in release of CO_2 from the blood in the lungs. Increased blood CO_2 will result in the formation of more bicarbonate (shifting Eq. 29-2 to the right), although the increase in bicarbonate will be less than the increase in P_{CO_2}. Thus there will be a decrease in the bicarbonate/αP_{CO_2} ratio and a decrease in pH (see Eq. 29-5). If the ventilation rate were to remain constant and the metabolic release of fixed acid were to increase, the same effect would be observed. In this case, H^+ reacts with HCO_3^- to form CO_2, which is released in the lungs. There is an immediate decrease in the concentration of bicarbonate with essentially no change in P_{CO_2}, resulting in a decreased bicarbonate/αP_{CO_2} ratio and a decreased pH. If the ventilation rate increases, more CO_2 is released from the blood at the lungs, lowering the $[HCO_3]/\alpha P_{CO_2}$ ratio and causing the blood pH to increase. The ventilation rate can

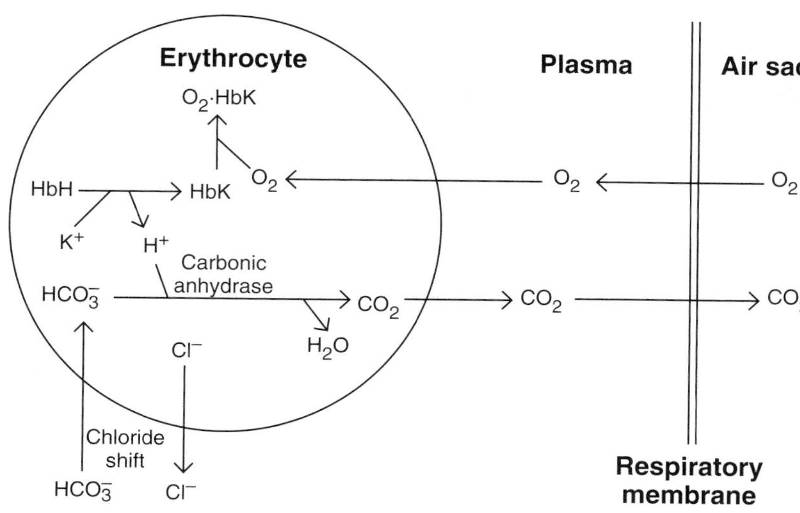

Fig. 29-3 Transfer of CO_2 in lungs from erythrocytes to air sacs. *HbK,* Potassium salt of hemoglobin; *HbH,* protonated form of hemoglobin.

range from zero to 15 times normal, allowing a significant degree of regulation of the bicarbonate–carbonic acid ratio. Thus when the rate of ventilation is increased, excess acid in the form of CO_2 is removed quickly. Similarly, when the rate of ventilation is decreased, acid (CO_2) is added to neutralize excess alkali (HCO_3^-).

Hemoglobin, which is vital for the buffering of blood pH, buffers the CO_2 produced by the tissues. The major function of hemoglobin is the transport of oxygen through the blood to the cells of the body. The relationship between the degree of oxygenation of hemoglobin and the pH, P_{CO_2}, and total CO_2 (T_{CO_2}) of blood is complex. Oxygenated hemoglobin is a stronger acid than deoxygenated hemoglobin; therefore in the lungs, RBC hemoglobin will release H^+ as it becomes oxygenated (Fig. 29-3, Eqs. 29-7 and 29-12), thus decreasing the RBC bicarbonate level and increasing the levels of blood carbonic acid and its anhydrous form CO_2, and increasing blood P_{CO_2} as well. In the lungs, ventilation will eliminate this increased P_{CO_2} by releasing CO_2 from the blood, thereby maintaining the ratio of bicarbonate to carbonic acid at 20. The rate at which this reaction proceeds is enormously increased by the presence in the red blood cells of the enzyme carbonic anhydrase. It is the action of this enzyme that allows the rapid transfer of CO_2 into and out of red blood cells, with consequent buffering by hemoglobin. This process is summarized by the following series of reactions and by Fig. 29-3.

$$\text{Gas exchange in the lungs } \underset{(\text{gas})}{CO_2} \rightleftharpoons \underset{(\text{dissolved})}{dCO_2} \overset{\text{Carbonic anhydrase}}{\rightleftharpoons} H_2CO_3 \rightleftharpoons H^+ + HCO_3^-$$

$$T_{CO_2} = dCO_2 + HCO_3^- \text{ or } T_{CO_2} = \alpha P_{CO_2} + HCO_3^- \qquad \text{Eq. 29-12}$$

Oxygenated hemoglobin is transported in the blood to peripheral cells that have relatively low P_{O_2} tension and that are releasing metabolic products such as CO_2 and organic acids into the blood, thus raising blood P_{CO_2} and T_{CO_2} and lowering its pH. The relatively low P_{O_2} causes the dissociation of O_2 from HbO_2 and the consequent delivery of O_2 to the cells. The high CO_2 pressure in the cells drives the CO_2 along a concentration gradient into the red blood cells. Carbonic anhydrase rapidly converts CO_2 into H^+ and HCO_3^- (see Fig. 29-2). Deoxygenated hemoglobin is a weaker acid than oxygenated hemoglobin. It neutralizes the H^+ to maintain pH and causes the dissociation reaction of carbonic acid to proceed to the right to increase the level of RBC bicarbonate and decrease the P_{CO_2}.

The dissociation of oxygen from hemoglobin as a function of the P_{CO_2} is shown in Fig. 29-4, which presents a graph of the percentage of O_2 saturation of hemoglobin versus P_{O_2}. The sigmoidal shape of the curve indicates that at critical levels of P_{O_2} near the P_{50}, a strong increase or decrease is seen in the percentage of O_2 saturation, with a minimal shift in P_{O_2}. In an area of the body in which there is a drop in P_{O_2} to below that of P_{50} on the sigmoid curve, the hemoglobin will release a larger portion of O_2 than at a P_{O_2} level above the P_{50}. Similarly, in areas of high O_2, such as the lungs, the hemoglobin will be essentially saturated with O_2.

Another factor that has an effect on the position of the oxygen dissociation curve is 2,3-diphosphoglycerate (2,3-DPG), an intermediate in glycolysis (see Chapter 38) whose blood levels increase during anaerobic glucose metabolism. By covalently binding to the N-terminal amino groups of the hemoglobin molecule itself, 2,3-DPG induces the release of oxygen from hemoglobin. This is reflected in the shift to the right of the O_2 dissociation curve (see Fig. 29-4). With a shift to the right, the critical P_{O_2} level that will cause 50% saturation of hemoglobin by oxygen is increased, so that areas of active glucose metabolism, which contain increased 2,3-DPG levels, release O_2 from hemoglobin at significantly lower P_{O_2} levels than do those areas without increased 2,3-DPG levels. See Chapter 40 for additional details on factors that may affect oxygen binding by hemoglobin.

As more oxygen is released in response to increased levels of P_{CO_2} and H^+, more deoxyhemoglobin, which acts as a buffer, is formed. Increased Pco_2 leads to formation of bicarbonate (HCO_3^-). Most H^+ ions are bound by deoxygenated hemoglobin, and the rest are buffered by proteins and phosphate buffer in the plasma. Because all the H^+ usually formed is buffered, essentially no change occurs in the pH. This buffering phenomenon is referred to as the **isohydric shift.** The HCO_3^- formed in red blood cells as a result of uptake of H^+ by hemoglobin diffuses out of the cells into the plasma. To preserve the electrical neutrality of the red blood cell, as HCO_3^- diffuses out of the cell, Cl^- diffuses into erythrocytes from the plasma. This increase in the erythrocyte Cl^- is termed the **chloride shift.** Thus the plasma chloride concentration of venous blood (where HCO_3^- is formed in red blood cells) is slightly *lower* than that of arterial blood. When CO_2 is expelled from the lungs, Cl^- again shifts out of red blood cells into plasma (see Figs. 29-2 and 29-3). As anion charges on the polyvalent hemoglobin molecule are replaced by diffusing monovalent chloride anions, the osmolality of the erythrocyte increases, leading to diffusion of water into the erythrocyte, slightly increasing the mean volume of venous red blood cells over the mean cell volume (MCV) in arterial blood.

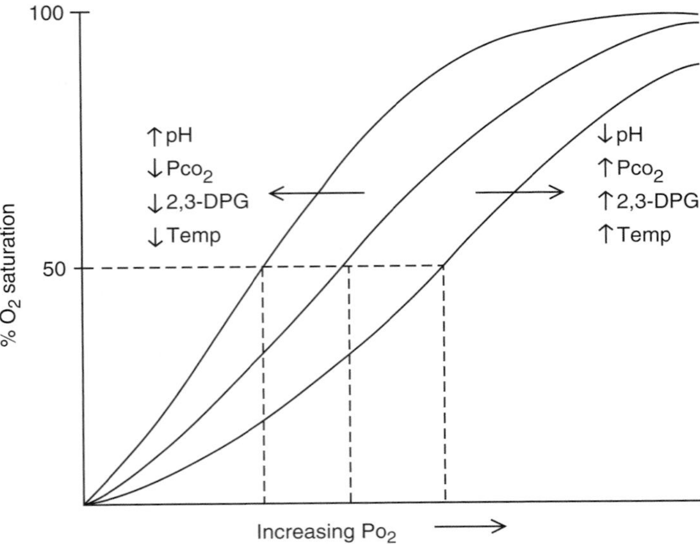

Fig. 29-4 Hemoglobin-oxygen dissociation curves and factors that shift the curve right and left. A shift of curve right or left changes the level of Po_2 at which hemoglobin is 50% saturated (P_{50}).

Although the intact respiratory system acts as an immediate regulator of the $HCO_3^-/\alpha Pco_2$ system, long-term control is exerted by renal mechanisms (see Chapter 30 for details). The kidneys excrete nonvolatile acids such as sulfuric, hydrochloric, phosphoric, and some organic acids into the urine. Hydrogen ions are excreted by the kidneys into the urine and are buffered by HPO_4^{2-} and ammonia, which is derived from deamidation of the amino acid glutamine. Sodium is the cation exchanged for excreted hydrogen ions by the kidney. The kidney also affects the bicarbonate–carbonic acid buffer system by regulating the excretion of bicarbonate (Fig. 29-5). The kidney reabsorbs almost all filtered bicarbonate at plasma bicarbonate concentrations below 25 mEq/L. Only when bicarbonate levels become elevated above 25 mEq/L will bicarbonate be excreted into the urine. The reabsorbed bicarbonate is neutralized electrically by the reabsorbed sodium ions, which have been exchanged for the hydrogen ions excreted in urine (see Fig. 29-5).

KEY CONCEPTS BOX 29-1

- CO_2, the primary metabolic acid, is buffered by hemoglobin but is carried in plasma as HCO_3^-.
- Fixed acids are neutralized by bicarbonate, which is in equilibrium with CO_2.
- By the Henderson-Hasselbalch (HH) equation, blood pH is directly related only to the ratio of $HCO_3/\alpha Pco_2$.
- The **HH equation** describes the bicarbonate/CO_2 buffering system and the metabolic (bicarbonate) and respiratory (αPco_2) components.
- There is a relationship between oxygen saturation and CO_2 buffering by hemoglobin.
- Acid-base balance is achieved through renal and respiratory means.

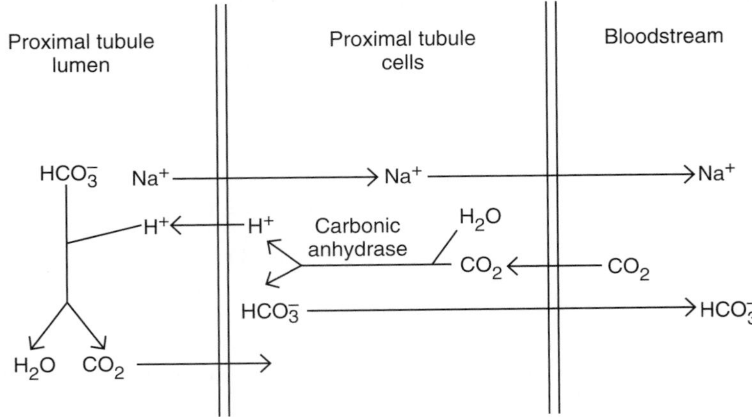

Fig. 29-5 Kidney reabsorption of bicarbonate with excretion of H^+.

SECTION OBJECTIVES BOX 29-2

- Define the measured laboratory parameters that describe acid-base status: base excess, oxygen saturation, and anion gap, as well as the calculated blood-gas parameters.
- Differentiate between base-deficient and base-excess disorders and the pH associated with these disorders.
- Using the Henderson-Hasselbalch equation, describe the laboratory changes associated with respiratory acidoses and alkaloses.
- Using the Henderson-Hasselbalch equation, describe the laboratory changes associated with metabolic acidoses and alkaloses.

ACID-BASE DISORDERS

Definitions

Acid-base disorders are classified most readily in terms of their immediate cause. Thus acidoses and alkaloses are described as being of respiratory or metabolic origin.

These classifications should always be considered in terms of the modified Henderson-Hasselbalch equation:

$$pH = pK'_a + \log\frac{[HCO_3^-]}{\alpha P_{CO_2}} \quad \text{Eq. 29-13}$$

The term αPco_2 represents the acid component that is directly and immediately modified by the respiratory rate. Thus the term αPco_2 is called the **respiratory component.** The concentration of bicarbonate is most immediately affected by changes in the hydrogen-ion concentration caused by production of fixed metabolic acids and by physiological processes that directly change the concentration of serum bicarbonate. Thus the bicarbonate concentration of plasma is called the **metabolic component** of acid-base status. Keep in mind that the pH of plasma depends on the *ratio* of the concentration of bicarbonate to αPco_2 rather than on the absolute concentration of these components (see Eq. 29-13).

Base Excess

Base excess is a calculated parameter that is used to assess the metabolic component of the patient's acid-base disturbance. The term *base excess* is used to describe clinical situations in which there is an excess of bicarbonate (positive base excess) or a deficit of bicarbonate (negative base excess). We use the term *base deficit* for a negative base excess because this is a more accurate description of the physiological condition. Base excess in the blood at pH of 7.40, Pco_2 of 40 mm Hg, hemoglobin concentration of 150 g/L, and temperature of 37°C is zero. The hemoglobin concentration is important because the blood-buffering capacity is greatly dependent on this quantity. The addition of a base, such as bicarbonate, results in a positive base excess. The loss of base, as occurs in diarrhea or with the addition of acids, results in a base deficit. Calculation of the **base excess or deficit** is useful in the management of patients with acid-base disturbances because it permits estimation of the number of milliequivalents of sodium bicarbonate or ammonium chloride that should be administered to correct the patient's pH to ≈7.4. In practice, the base excess is only a crude estimate because as the patient's condition improves, changes in respiration and metabolism will invalidate the original calculation. It is for this reason that blood-gas status is monitored closely through analysis of sequential blood specimens.

$$\text{Base excess} = (1.0 - 0.0143\ \text{Hgb})(HCO_3^-) - (9.5 + 1.63\ \text{Hgb})(7.4\ \text{pH}) - 24 \quad \text{Eq. 29-14}$$

where Hgb is the hemoglobin concentration in g/dL.

Oxygen Saturation

Oxygen saturation indicates the amount of oxygen bound to hemoglobin and is used to determine the effectiveness of respiration or oxygen therapy. Oxygen saturation is calculated by using the measured parameters of pH and Po_2 and the equation for a standard oxygen dissociation curve. A nomogram to derive O_2 saturation from pH and Po_2 values is presented in Fig. 29-6. By using the differences in the wavelengths of maximum absorbance for oxyhemoglobin and deoxyhemoglobin, oxygen saturation also is measured directly with a cooximeter. Table 29-3 contains reference values for the calculated blood-gas parameters.

Anion Gap

Plasma is electrically neutral, and the sum of its anions must equal the sum of its anions. However, if the total measured anions are subtracted from the total measured cations, the difference is the **anion gap,** or the quantity of measured cations in excess of the measured anions, as is shown by the following equation:

$$\text{Anion gap} = [Na^+] + [K^+] - [Cl^-] - [HCO_3^-] \quad \text{Eq. 29-15}$$

Usually, the only serum electrolytes measured are sodium, potassium, chloride, and bicarbonate (as total CO_2). However, other anions, such as phosphates, ketones, lactic acid, proteins, and sulfates, are found in blood. These other anions are not measured, whereas their counterions are, resulting in an apparent excess, or gap, of measured cations over measured anions. Increases in the quantities of these unmeasured anions and of the accompanying Na^+ ions will increase the apparent gap. Usually, the anion gap averages 12 mEq/L. The anion gap increases with production of organic acids. Diabetic ketoacidosis is the most common cause of an elevated anion gap. If diabetes is ruled out, other causes of acidosis, such as lactic acidosis, dehydration, renal tubular acidosis, sepsis, and toxic acidosis, must be sought.

Base-Deficient Disorders

Any condition associated with a lower-than-normal blood pH **(acidemia)** is referred to as an **acidosis.**

Metabolic Acidosis

In base-deficient disorders, the bicarbonate/αPco_2 ratio is decreased, and the pH is below the reference interval.

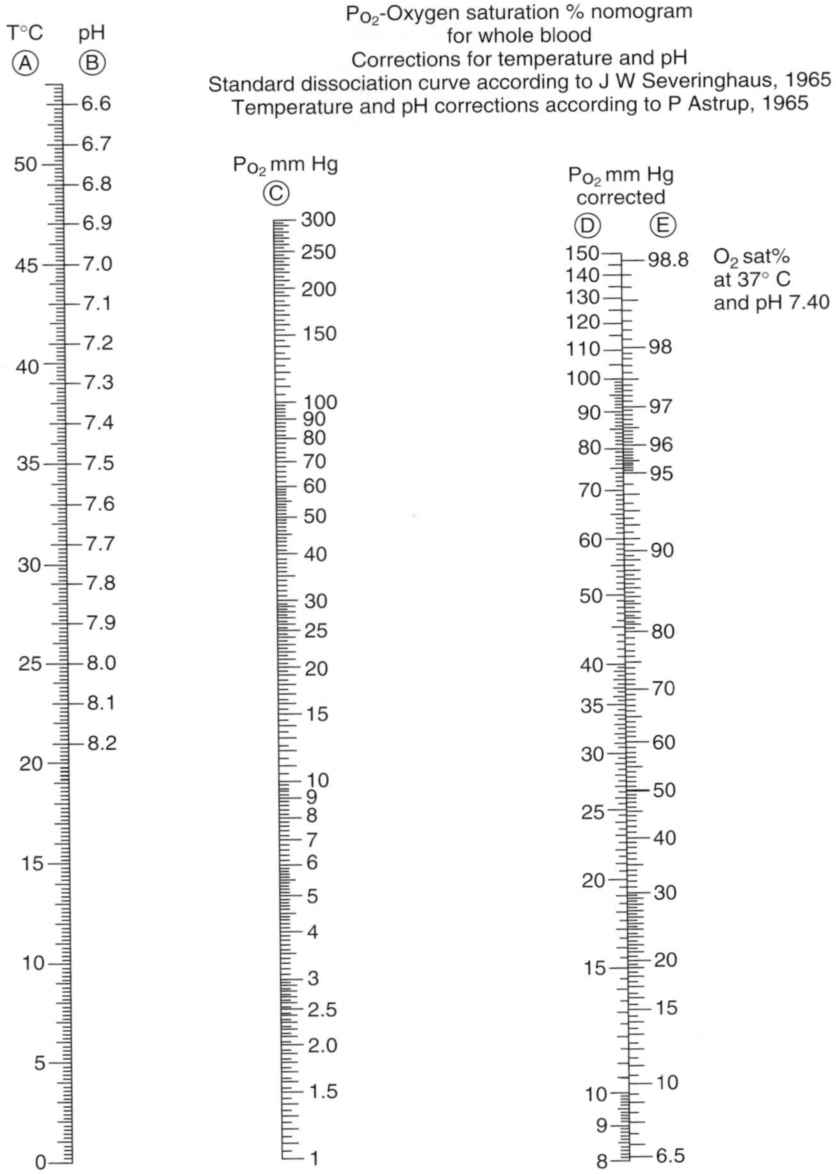

P_{O_2}-Oxygen saturation % nomogram
for whole blood
Corrections for temperature and pH
Standard dissociation curve according to J W Severinghaus, 1965
Temperature and pH corrections according to P Astrup, 1965

T°C (A) — pH (B) — P_{O_2} mm Hg (C) — P_{O_2} mm Hg corrected (D) — (E) O_2 sat% at 37° C and pH 7.40

Fig. 29-6 Nomogram of relationship among pH, P_{O_2}, and O_2 saturation. A straight line through a value of pH and of P_{O_2} will connect with a calculated value of O_2 saturation at 37°C. (Courtesy Radiometer Medical ApS, Copenhagen, Denmark.)

Such disorders occur when metabolic processes result in the accumulation of abnormal quantities of organic acids. Examples of acids that accumulate are lactic acid, β-hydroxybutyric acid, and acetoacetic acid. Metabolic organic acids that enter plasma react with plasma bicarbonate to form H_2CO_3; this is immediately converted to CO_2 gas, which, in turn, is rapidly eliminated from the body by the lungs. The net result is an immediate decrease in bicarbonate concentration with essentially no loss of P_{CO_2}. This leads to a lowered bicarbonate/αP_{CO_2} ratio and a lowered pH, or **metabolic acidosis.**

In contrast to this accumulation of acids is the pathological loss of base from the body. In severe diarrhea, bicarbonate ion is lost as part of the watery stool, resulting in a base deficit (↓[HCO_3^-], ↓ bicarbonate/αP_{CO_2} ratio). These types of disorders are termed metabolic acidoses.

Respiratory Acidosis

A relative base-deficient disorder can result from a decrease in the bicarbonate–carbonic acid ratio, which may result from an increase in P_{CO_2}. This occurs if the lungs are not able to expel CO_2 from the blood. This disorder is termed **respiratory acidosis.** The increase in P_{CO_2} (**hypercapnia**) results in an increase in the concentration of bicarbonate as the CO_2 is buffered by hemoglobin. However, the rise in bicarbonate is less than the increase in P_{CO_2}, resulting in a **relative base deficit** and a decrease in the bicarbonate/αP_{CO_2} ratio, which results in a blood pH below the reference interval.

Base-Excess Disorders

Any condition associated with a blood pH above the reference interval (**alkalemia**) is called an **alkalosis.**

Metabolic Alkalosis

In base-excess disorders, the bicarbonate/αP_{CO_2} ratio is increased, and the pH is above the reference interval. If the disorder is caused by an increase in bicarbonate, with little or no change in P_{CO_2}, the disorder is termed **metabolic alkalosis.** Such a disorder occurs when excess amounts of bicarbonate of soda are ingested or administered, or when renal reabsorption of bicarbonate is increased, as in **hypochloremic alkalosis.**

Respiratory Alkalosis

If the disorder is caused by a decrease in P_{CO_2}, as when respiration is overly stimulated, the disorder is termed **respiratory alkalosis.** In this condition, rapid ventilation greatly decreases the P_{CO_2} of blood, with minimal change in bicarbonate concentration. This results in a relative excess of bicarbonate, a **relative base excess,** so that the bicarbonate/αP_{CO_2} ratio increases. This increased ratio yields a higher plasma pH.

Instrumentation

(See also pp. 228-229 and 233 and the Evolve website.)

The traditional laboratory blood-gas analyzer includes a pH electrode, a P_{O_2} electrode, and a P_{CO_2} electrode. As point-of-care testing has gained acceptance, the use of noninvasive electrodes, applied directly to the patient's skin, has expanded. Current technology permits reliable assessment of both P_{O_2} and P_{CO_2} using noninvasive techniques but not blood pH. These are widely used in neonatal intensive care units because they do not require blood collection from small infants. It is common practice to verify the performance of these noninvasive instruments by periodically performing a traditional blood-gas analysis.

With the development of disposable microelectrodes and fully automated analyzers that are reliable, blood-gas analysis now is being done in the surgery suite and other nonlaboratory settings, resulting in shortened turnaround times for results and permitting more rapid medical intervention.

The central laboratory usually is responsible for maintaining the devices, whereas the operator, physician, or respiratory therapist is responsible for performing quality control. Documentation of operator training is required.

Calculated Parameters

The remainder of blood acid-base parameters are not measured but instead are calculated using Eqs. 29-6, *B,* and 29-13. One of the parameters is bicarbonate, which is calculated by using the measured parameters pH and P_{CO_2} in the Henderson-Hasselbalch equation:

$$HCO_3^- = [\alpha P_{CO_2}]\,\text{antilog}\,[pH - pK_a'] \quad \text{Eq. 29-16}$$

Nomograms have also been developed to derive bicarbonate levels from pH and P_{CO_2} measurements (Fig. 29-7 and the Henderson-Hasselbalch calculating algorithm on Evolve). Bicarbonate levels are useful for assessing the degree to which metabolic and renal control is involved in the acid-base status of the patient.

KEY CONCEPTS BOX 29-2

- Bicarbonate is the metabolic function and P_{CO_2} the respiratory component of the modified Henderson-Hasselbalch equation. The ratio of these two terms defines pH.
- Base excess can be positive or negative absolute gain or loss of bicarbonate, or relative to an excess or deficit of the respiratory component, P_{CO_2}.
- Metabolic acidoses can be caused by an increase in fixed acids or a loss of bicarbonate.
- Respiratory acidoses are caused by an excess of P_{CO_2}.
- Metabolic alkalosis is caused by an excess of bicarbonate; respiratory alkalosis is caused by a deficit of P_{CO_2}.

SECTION OBJECTIVES BOX 29-3

- Describe the origin of metabolic acidoses and the laboratory results associated with them.
- Describe the physiological response to metabolic acidoses.
- Describe the origin of respiratory acidoses and the laboratory results associated with them.
- Describe the physiological response to respiratory acidoses.

ACIDOSIS

Metabolic Acidosis

Etiology

Increased organic acid production resulting in metabolic acidosis can have many causes; some of these are listed in Box 29-1. Uncontrolled diabetes results in accumulation of acetoacetic and hydroxybutyric acids, which are produced by excessive oxidation of fatty acids (see Chapter 38). Fasting and fad diets also lead to increased levels of these acids. Acidosis in a newborn may be associated with an inborn error of metabolism (see Chapter 52), requiring an extensive laboratory workup to identify the metabolic and genetic defects.

Lactic acid increases as a result of increases in anaerobic metabolism caused by strenuous muscular exercise or systemic infection. Lactic acidosis also results from local tissue **hypoxia** (low tissue P_{O_2}), which is caused by dehydration, poor perfusion that results from circulatory collapse, respiratory failure, poor oxygen binding by modified hemoglobins, or cardiac failure.

Renal tubular acidosis (RTA, type 2) results from failure of the kidney to acidify urine by exchanging H^+ for Na^+. This renal insufficiency may be acquired as a result of infection or may be congenital, as in cases of severe de Toni-Fanconi syndrome. Liver disease that impairs the formation of urea and ammonia also results in metabolic acidosis caused by retention of H^+.

Salicylate intoxication initially induces respiratory alkalosis as a result of hyperventilation, which is caused by a

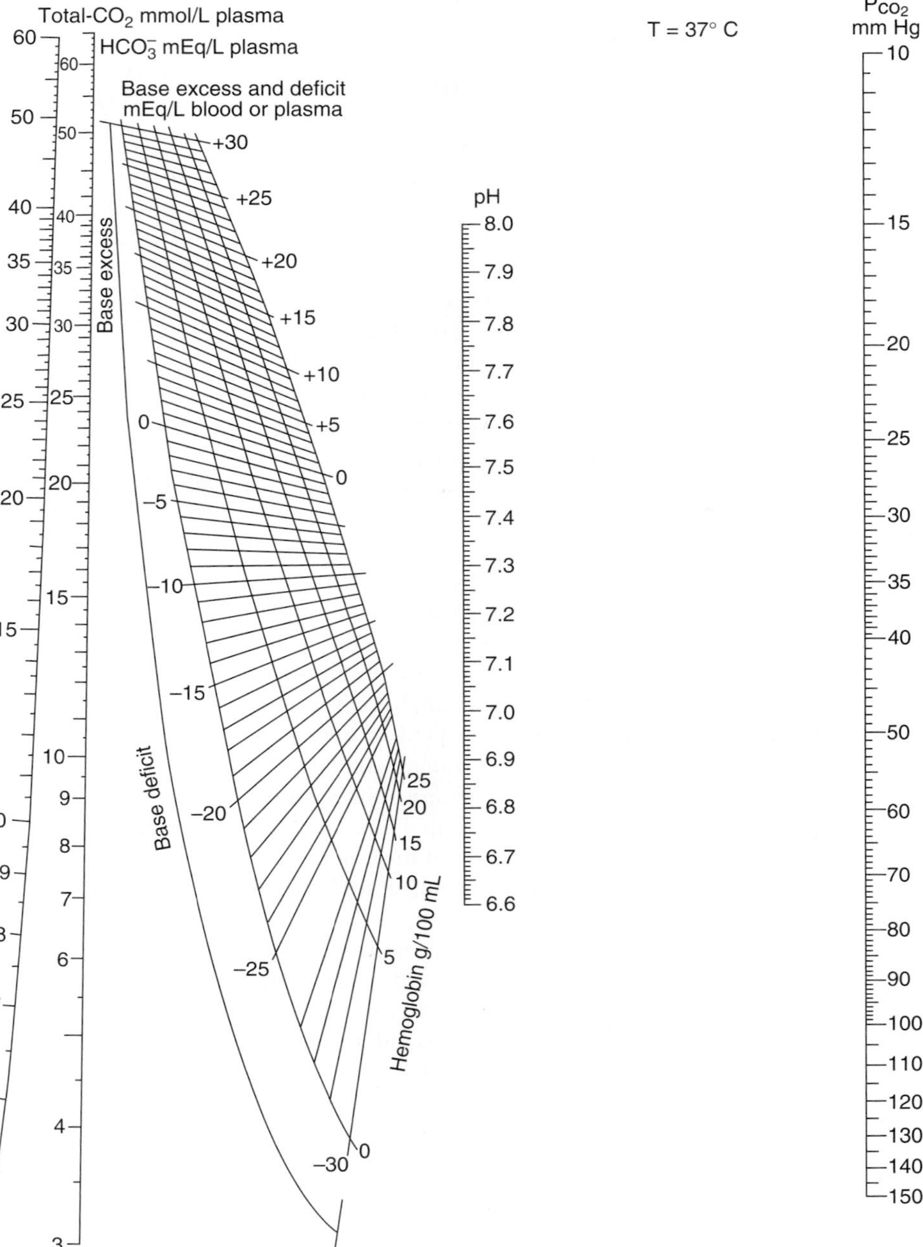

Fig. 29-7 Nomogram of relationship among P_{CO_2}, pH, base excess, hemoglobin, bicarbonate, and total CO_2. A straight line through a value of pH and of P_{CO_2} will connect with a calculated value of HCO_3^- and total CO_2. Base excess or deficit can be derived from that straight line if the hemoglobin level is known. (Courtesy Radiometer Medical ApS, Copenhagen, Denmark.)

stimulatory effect of the drug on the respiratory center. The ingested drug is converted to an acid before excretion, and the large quantities of acid formed ultimately result in metabolic acidosis. Other poisons are ingested as acids or as compounds that will lead to acid metabolites (e.g., methanol [converted to formic acid], ethylene glycol [converted to oxalic acid], paraldehyde, ammonium chloride). Infusion of large quantities of isotonic sodium chloride results in a metabolic acidosis because the high sodium load competes with hydrogen ions for renal excretion. Metabolic acidosis is also caused by ingestion of carbonic anhydrase inhibitors, such as acetazolamide sulfonamides, which interfere with the formation of bicarbonate in the erythrocyte and in renal tubule cells (see Figs. 29-2, 29-3, and 29-5).

Metabolic acidosis also may be caused by loss of bicarbonate in body fluids. Diarrhea and colitis lead to losses of intestinal fluids, which contain high concentrations of bicarbonate; RTA type 1 leads to loss of bicarbonate in urine. Both result in reduction of the $HCO_3^-/\alpha P_{CO_2}$ ratio, thereby causing acidemia.

Box 29-1
Origin of Acidoses

Respiratory Causes
Apnea
Asthma
Bradycardia
Bronchoconstriction
Emphysema
Pneumonia
Pulmonary edema
Respiratory distress syndrome (RDS, ARDS)
Toxins and drugs (e.g., barbiturate, morphine)

Metabolic Disorders
Increased Fixed Acids
Carbonic anhydrase inhibitors (acetazolamide sulfonamides)
Isotonic NaCl infusion
Ketosis
- Diabetes
- Fasting, starvation, or fad diets
- Inborn errors of metabolism

Lactic acidosis
- Cardiac failure
- Circulatory collapse
- Dehydration
- Modified hemoglobins and reduced arterial Po_2 (HbCO, HbMet, HbS)
- Strenuous muscular exercise
- Systemic infection

Liver disease
Renal tubular acidosis (RTA) 2
Toxins
- Alcohols (e.g., methanol, ethylene glycol)
- Salicylate

Bicarbonate Loss
Colitis
Diarrhea
RTA 1

Physiological Response

When acidemia occurs as a result of acute metabolic acidosis, the body attempts to correct this acidemia immediately by hyperventilation (Kussmaul breathing). Hyperventilation lowers the Pco_2 (and to a smaller extent the HCO_3) and at least partially increases the ratio of $HCO_3^-/\alpha Pco_2$, thereby returning the pH toward 7.4. This mechanism of correcting the pH during acidosis is known as *compensatory respiratory alkalosis.* The result is a decrease in Pco_2 level, a a small decrease in the HCO_3^- concentration, and a pH value closer to the reference interval.

In a metabolic acidosis that does not involve renal dysfunction, the kidney will excrete organic acids, will exchange H^+ for Na^+ in the distal region of the tubule, will excrete ammonium ions, and will retain any lost bicarbonate, all of which result in a more acidic urine. This renal compensatory mechanism becomes effective over time and eventually will correct both the blood pH and the bicarbonate toward the reference interval. This correction can take place only when the underlying cause of the acidosis has been eliminated. Part of the renal response to chronic acidosis is the excretion of ammonium ions by renal tubular cells. This excretion of ammonia into the presumptive urine allows additional H^+ to be excreted, thus reducing the H^+ load in the blood.

Table 29-4 Comparison of Acid-Base Disorders With Corresponding Effects On Selected Blood-Gas Parameters

Disorder	pH	Po_2	Pco_2	HCO_3^-	Base Excess	Anion Gap
Metabolic acidosis	↓	N	↓N	↓	↓	↑
Respiratory acidosis	↓	↓	↑	↑N	↑N	↑N
Metabolic alkalosis	↑	N	↑N	↑	↑	N
Respiratory alkalosis	↑	↑	↓	↓N	↓N	N

N, Iinitially normal (within the reference interval).

Laboratory Findings

Findings commonly seen in most metabolic acidoses, as summarized in Table 29-4, include decreased pH, total CO_2, and HCO_3^-, as well as a base deficit (negative base excess) and an increased anion gap. Initially, the Pco_2 may be within the reference interval, but it will decrease as a result of the respiratory response to acidemia.

Depending on the cause of the acidosis (see Box 29-1), additional laboratory findings may include increased lactate and decreased O_2 saturation (the hemoglobin saturation curve is shifted to the right) causing poor tissue oxygenation, the presence of a modified hemoglobin (e.g., carboxyhemoglobin, methemoglobin), the presence of ketone bodies (diabetic ketoacidosis), increased potassium, increased blood urea nitrogen (BUN) and creatinine (renal failure), or the presence of a toxic drug. Increased potassium results from shifting of excess H^+ into the cells, with a concomitant shift of K^+ out of the cells into plasma.

In cases of toxic drug ingestion, such as methanol, ethylene glycol, or paraldehyde poisoning, an increased anion gap, caused by the ingested poisons or their metabolites, and an increased osmolar gap (see pp. 216-217, 220) may be present.

Treatment

Initially, if possible, the cause of the acidemia is corrected, for example, by insulin treatment for diabetes. If the pH falls to below 7.2, the risk for cardiovascular failure is increased, and the base deficit may have to be corrected immediately. This is accomplished frequently by the administration of bicarbonate, which corrects the base deficit by raising the HCO_3^-/H_2CO_3 ratio. In all cases, the cause of the metabolic acidosis ultimately must be corrected.

Respiratory Acidosis

Etiology

Respiratory acidoses are caused by disorders (see Box 29-1) that interfere with the usual ability of the lungs to expel CO_2. This may result from decreased ventilation (breathing) caused by mechanical failure, a depressed breathing center, or physical blockage of the airways, or it may result from decreased respiration (gas exchange) caused by an inability to inflate the alveoli or by damage to the alveoli or the presence of alveolar fluid. All causes result in increased blood Pco_2, along with reduced a $HCO_3^-/\alpha Pco_2$ ratio and blood pH.

Respiratory distress syndrome (RDS), which is common (≈5%) in high-risk, premature infants, results in a respiratory acidosis because these infants lack sufficient levels of surfactant in their lungs to allow the alveoli to expand in the usual manner. Poorly expanding alveoli thus prevent sufficient respiration. Respiratory distress is also seen in some adults (adult respiratory distress syndrome [ARDS]) who experience systemic septic shock or oxygen toxicity. The incidence of ARDS in the United States is ≈150,000 to 200,000 cases per year, with risk of death between 40% and 70%. Observed blood-gas parameters in respiratory acidosis include decreased pH, increased Pco_2, decreased Po_2, and decreased oxygen saturation. Base excess, bicarbonate, and anion gap are initially within normal limits.

Asthma is a chronic respiratory condition that affects more than 20 million Americans and is one of the leading causes of absence from school and work. Asthma attacks are associated with episodes of air flow obstruction in the bronchial tubes; respiratory symptoms of asthma are listed in Box 29-2. As in other cases of physical obstruction of the air pathway, acute asthmatic attacks tend to result in respiratory acidosis and often require hospitalization.

Although asthma affects both adults and children, more than half of cases occur in children between the ages of 2 and 17 years. A wide variety of agents may initiate an episode of asthma. The most common causes are allergens, physical irritants, viral respiratory infections, and physical exertion. **Allergens** are substances to which susceptible individuals may become allergic. A partial list of common allergens is provided in Box 29-3. Inner-city children have very high rates of asthma and are especially susceptible to a number of common indoor allergens, including cockroaches, dust mites, and cats.

Normally, the body produces an immune response, in this case with immunoglobulin (Ig)E (see p. 174), to allergens in the respiratory and gastrointestinal tracts or allergens on the skin. An allergic response is an abnormal reaction, or overreaction, of the body to one or more substances from the outside environment to which a person has become sensitized. IgE stimulates a response from mast cells, which results in the production of histamine and other inflammatory response chemicals that produce many of the symptoms (see Box 29-2) associated with an allergic response. Laboratory assays (still called the radioallergosorbent test [RAST]; see p. 174) are available to detect the presence of IgE specific for an allergen that may be the cause of an allergy.

Box 29-2

Symptoms Associated With Allergy

Respiratory
Asthma
Bouts of sneezing
Bronchitis
Coughs, frequent sore throats
Frequent colds
Nasal or chest congestion
Recurrent ear infections
Respiratory acidosis
Runny nose or eyes
Sinus headaches, postnasal drip
Swelling (lips, eyes)
Wheezing and shortness of breath

Gastrointestinal
Abdominal cramps
Diarrhea
Nausea
Vomiting

Dermatological
Eczema
Itching
Hives (urticaria)

Box 29-3

Common Allergens

Cockroaches
Foods
House dust mites
Household animal dander (dog, cat)
Industrial dust (e.g., coal)
Latex (see p. 31)
Molds
Mouse or rat droppings
Plant pollen (tree, grass, and weed)
Tobacco smoke

Physiological Response

The physiological response to respiratory acidosis includes increased renal excretion of acids, retention of sodium and bicarbonate, and if possible, hyperventilation. If a response compensates for the respiratory acidosis and results in its correction, the acidosis is referred to as *compensated respiratory acidosis.* This response may be viewed as the development of a metabolic alkalosis that compensates for the respiratory acidosis. When the acute respiratory disorder is corrected, the usual respiratory response to the acidosis removes the excess CO_2, and a transient metabolic alkalosis may result. In chronic respiratory acidosis, the pH becomes essentially normal, but a base excess remains.

Laboratory Findings

Respiratory acidoses are associated with decreased Po_2, increased plasma CO_2 concentration with a smaller increase in HCO_3^-, and a concurrent decrease in the ratio of $HCO_3^-/\alpha PCO_2$, which causes the acidosis. However, as a result of low oxygen levels in the tissue, a coexisting metabolic lactic acidosis may develop (see p. 559). Depending on the extent of the metabolic acidosis, findings may include a normal to increased anion gap, a normal to decreased bicarbonate level, and a small base deficit. Table 29-4 provides a review of these findings.

As a result of the renal compensatory response, very elevated concentrations of HCO_3^- with almost normal pH are often seen. In chronic respiratory disease, the concentration of HCO_3^- may be elevated, pH near normal, and the PO_2 may be somewhat depressed.

Medical Treatment

Medical treatment is aimed primarily at correcting the underlying respiratory disorder and ventilating the patient with gases that contain higher PO_2 and lower PCO_2 through the use of mechanical respirators. Rapid correction of the acidemia may be achieved by injecting sodium bicarbonate.

KEY CONCEPTS BOX 29-3

- Metabolic acidoses are caused by production of metabolic fixed acids, such as acetoacetic and hydroxybutyric acids (diabetes) and lactic acid; toxins, such as salicylate; and low-molecular-weight alcohols, such as methanol and ethylene glycol, that are metabolized to acids.
- Although all of the above involve an excess of fixed acids, loss of bicarbonate from diarrhea or renal tubular acidosis (RTA) type 1 causes a metabolic acidosis.
- All of the above are associated with decreased serum bicarbonate and PCO_2, decreased pH, and a base deficit. Except for the bicarbonate-losing diseases, all are associated with an increased anion gap.
- Respiratory acidoses are caused by impaired respiratory or ventilatory function, resulting in low blood PO_2 (hypoxia, cardiac disease, dysfunctional hemoglobins).
- All respiratory acidoses are associated with low pH, elevated bicarbonate and PCO_2, and base excess.

SECTION OBJECTIVES BOX 29-4

- Describe the origin of metabolic alkaloses and the laboratory results associated with them.
- Describe the physiological response to metabolic alkaloses.
- Describe the origin of respiratory alkaloses and the laboratory results associated with them.
- Describe the physiological response to respiratory alkaloses.

ALKALOSIS

Metabolic Alkalosis

Etiology (see Box 29-4)

Occasionally, excessive chronic ingestion of bicarbonate of soda for gastrointestinal distress results in an increased concentration of blood bicarbonate and a resultant metabolic alkalosis. Similarly, treatment of peptic ulcer by ingestion of large quantities of alkali antacids also will produce metabolic alkalosis. More commonly, metabolic alkalosis arises from the loss of chloride. Prolonged diarrhea, vomiting, or aspiration of gastric fluids leads to loss of gastric hydrochloric acid. This in turn raises the pH of the blood because loss of the chloride anion results in increased renal retention of bicarbonate to counter reabsorption of sodium by the proximal tubule. The raised serum bicarbonate levels increase the $HCO_3^-/\alpha PCO_2$ ratio and the blood pH. This condition is known as *hypochloremic alkalosis.*

Corticosteroid administration and diseases such as hyperaldosteronism and Cushing's syndrome, which affect the ability of the kidney to regulate electrolyte balance, also raise the blood pH. In the distal tubule, Na^+ is retained at the expense of K^+ and H^+. In conditions of excess corticosteroids, resultant hypokalemia causes the release of K^+ by cells into the blood and concurrent balanced movement of H^+ from blood into the cells, thereby leading to a rise in pH of the blood.

Physiological Response

To compensate for an increased $HCO_3^-/\alpha PCO_2$ ratio during metabolic alkalosis, the respiratory system slows, raising the PCO_2 and the bicarbonate concentration of the blood. The PCO_2 rises more rapidly than the HCO_3^-, thereby decreasing the $HCO_3^-/\alpha PCO_2$ ratio and blood pH. This mechanism of readjusting the pH during metabolic alkalosis is termed *compensatory respiratory acidosis.* The result is a pH that is closer to the reference interval in the presence of an elevated concentration of HCO_3^-. If alkalosis persists, the body will attempt to correct the condition by increasing the renal excretion of excess bicarbonate.

Laboratory Findings

During metabolic alkalosis, the ratio of $HCO_3^-/\alpha PCO_2$ increases as a result of a rise in the concentration of blood bicarbonate. Because of the physiological response to alkalemia, additional laboratory findings include an increased PCO_2 and an alkaline urine that contains titratable bicarbonate (see Table 29-4).

Treatment

Treatment of metabolic alkalosis involves administration of chloride ions, either as NaCl or KCl depending on the degree of hypokalemia, and perhaps also administration of NH_4Cl if the alkalosis is severe and persistent. The Cl^- anion compensates for the chloride deficit, which may have led initially to excessive retention of bicarbonate. This permits the kidney to begin to excrete the excess bicarbonate to correct the alkalosis.

Respiratory Alkalosis

Etiology

Hyperventilation, which decreases blood Pco_2 levels, raises the $HCO_3^-/\alpha Pco_2$ ratio, causing respiratory alkalosis. Conditions that may result in hyperventilation are listed in Box 29-4.

Physiological Response

The kidneys respond to the alkalosis by excreting increased amounts of bicarbonate under the conditions of lower Pco_2 that occur during respiratory alkalosis. In response to the alkalosis, the proximal tubules of the kidney decrease the reabsorption of bicarbonate. This renal response to respiratory alkalosis is termed *compensatory metabolic acidosis.*

Laboratory Findings

Hyperventilation leads to increased loss of CO_2 from the blood at the alveolar surface, which causes the $HCO_3^-/\alpha Pco_2$ ratio to increase as carbonic acid is lost. Because of the physiological response to the alkalemia, additional laboratory findings include decreased Pco_2 and an alkaline urine that contains titratable bicarbonate (see Table 29-4).

Box 29-4

Origin of Alkaloses

Respiratory Causes

Asthma
Excessive respiration rate
- Excessive crying
- Excessive use of a mechanical respirator
- Fever
- Hysteria
- Pain

Impairment in central nervous system control of the respiratory system
Pregnancy
Pulmonary embolism
Salicylate intoxication

Metabolic Causes

Alkali antacid treatment
Excess mineralocorticoids or corticosteroids
Loss of chloride
- Diarrhea
- Gastronasal tube suction of stomach/duodenal chloride
- Vomiting

Treatment

Respiratory alkalosis is corrected by lowering the respiration rate with drugs such as sedatives, or by having the patient breathe air with higher CO_2 content. This can be accomplished easily by having the patient breathe in a restricted environment, for example, into a paper bag, which raises the Pco_2 of the air and the blood. Increased Pco_2 returns the $HCO_3^-/\alpha Pco_2$ ratio to within the reference interval and corrects the respiratory alkalosis. Table 29-4 summarizes the changes in blood-gas parameters that are seen in several diseases.

KEY CONCEPTS BOX 29-4

- Metabolic alkaloses are caused by an excess of bicarbonate. This can result from ingestion of bicarbonate or other alkali, or from the loss of chloride to produce hypochloremic metabolic alkalosis.
- All of the above are associated with increased serum bicarbonate and increased pH, as well as a base excess.
- The physiological response is slower breathing to increase Pco_2 and to decrease pH; over the long term, the kidney excretes bicarbonate and eventually restores bicarbonate levels and pH to normal.
- Respiratory alkaloses are caused by hyperventilation resulting from physiological or disease states.
- All respiratory alkaloses are associated with increased pH, decreased Pco_2, and base deficit. An alkaline urine may be produced.
- The immediate response is to slow the respiration rate, often with drugs.

SECTION OBJECTIVE BOX 29-5

- Describe the more common causes of acidoses and alkaloses and the laboratory data associated with these conditions.

CHANGE OF ANALYTE IN DISEASE

(Table 29-5)

Diabetic ketoacidosis in patients with uncontrolled diabetes is an example of metabolic acidosis. Laboratory findings include

Table 29-5 Common Disorders of Acid-Base Balance and Effects on Selected Blood-Gas Parameters

Disorders	pH	Pco_2	Po_2	HCO_3^-	Base Excess	Anion Gap	O_2 Saturation
Respiratory distress syndrome	↓	↑	↓	N*	N	N	↓
Lactic acidosis	↓	N*	N, ↓	↓	↓	↑	↓
Diabetic ketosis	↓	N*	N	↓	↓	↑	↓
Emphysema	↓	↑	↓	N*	N	N	↓
Methanol poisoning	↓	N*	N	↓	↓	↑	↓
Renal failure	↓	N*	N	↓	↓	↑	↓

*N**, Initially normal; *N,* always normal (within the reference interval).

Table 29-6 Examples of Lung Disease With a Known Genetic Basis

Disease	Gene	Protein	Gene Locus
Interstitial pneumonitis	*SFTPC*	Surfactant protein	8p21
Respiratory distress syndrome	*ABCA3*	Transporter protein	16p13.3
Lung carcinoma	*PLCL1*	Phospholipase C	2q33
Cystic fibrosis	*CF*	Cell membrane transporter	19q13.1, 7q31.2
Pulmonary fibrosis, idiopathic	Several	Polymorphism	10q22-q23, 8p21, 4q31.1
Surfactant, pulmonary—associated Protein D	*SFTPD*	Surfactant protein	2p12-p11.2
Surfactant, pulmonary—associated Protein B	*SFTPB*	Surfactant protein	10q23.3

decreased pH, acidemia, decreased P_{CO_2}, normal P_{O_2}, decreased O_2 saturation (see Evolve for blood-gas methods), decreased bicarbonate and total CO_2 (see Methods on Evolve, T_{CO_2}), increased anion gap, negative base excess, and increased serum potassium, ketones (see Evolve), and lactic and pyruvic acids (see Evolve) caused by disturbed carbohydrate and fat metabolism. An unexplained acidosis with an increased anion gap requires laboratory data to rule out a lactic acidosis, a toxin-induced acidosis, or an inborn error of metabolism in newborns.

Emphysema is a disease of impaired respiration that frequently results in respiratory acidosis. Laboratory findings include decreased pH and P_{O_2}, increased P_{CO_2} and potassium, and decreased oxygen saturation. Initially, the anion gap, base excess, bicarbonate, and T_{CO_2} are within the reference interval. As the body compensates for the acidosis, the bicarbonate and T_{CO_2} rise. As in RDS, the low P_{O_2} may result in a metabolic acidosis caused by a rise in blood lactate due to increased anaerobic metabolism.

Modified hemoglobins, such as carboxyhemoglobin, methemoglobin, and sulfhemoglobin, have decreased oxygen binding, and patients with significant amounts of these hemoglobins have low P_{O_2} levels and tissue hypoxia, which leads to lactic acidosis. Hemoglobinopathies, such as sickle cell anemia, can lead to unusual oxygen-saturation kinetics caused by the abnormal hemoglobin molecule. Laboratory findings associated with hemoglobinopathies include decreased oxygen saturation and P_{O_2} levels, which result in increased anaerobic metabolism and thereby metabolic (lactic) acidosis. Persistence of hypoxemia results in decreased bicarbonate and total CO_2, an increased anion gap (see Evolve) and blood lactate, and a negative base excess. The respiratory response to this acidosis is hyperventilation, which decreases the P_{CO_2}. The renal response to this acidosis is an increase in the reabsorption of bicarbonate, which tends to return the $HCO_3^-/\alpha P_{CO_2}$ ratio to normal.

Renal failure leads to metabolic acidosis with associated laboratory findings of decreased pH, initially normal P_{CO_2} and P_{O_2}, decreased oxygen saturation, increased potassium level, and decreased bicarbonate level and T_{CO_2}. As the anion gap increases because of organic acid production and retention, the base excess becomes negative. Respiratory compensation for metabolic acidosis eventually will lead to decreased P_{CO_2}.

Many of these diseases have a genetic basis; examples of these are given in Table 29-6.

BIBLIOGRAPHY

Arieff AI, DeFronzo RA: *Fluid, Electrolyte and Acid-Base Disorders,* ed 2, New York, 1995, Churchill Livingstone.

Busse WW, Lemanske RF: Asthma: a review, *N Engl J Med* 344:350, 2001.

Cohen JJ, Kassirer JP: *Acid-Base,* Boston, 1982, Little, Brown & Co.

Davenport HW: *The ABC of Acid-Base Chemistry,* ed 6, Chicago, 1974, University of Chicago Press.

Haber RJ: A practical approach to acid-base disorders, West J Med 155:146, 1991.

Hennessey I, Japp A: *Arterial Blood Gases Made Easy*, St Louis, 2007, Churchill Livingstone.

Kurtz I: *Acid-Base Case Studies,* Victoria, BC, Canada, 2004, Trafford Publishing.

Malley WJ: *Clinical Blood Gases: Assessment & Intervention,* ed 2, Philadelphia, 2004, Saunders.

Rosenstreich DL, Eggleston P, Kattan MM: The role of cockroach allergy and exposure to cockroach allergen in causing morbidity among inner-city children with asthma (The National Cooperative Inner-City Asthma Study), N Engl J Med 336:1356, 1997.

Soloway HB: How the body maintains acid-base balance, Diagn Med 32-41, Feb 1979.

Wilkins RL, Stoller JK, Kacmarek RM: *Egan's Fundamentals of Respiratory Care,* ed 9, St Louis, 2009, Mosby.

INTERNET SITES

Asthma

http://www.cdc.gov/MMWR/preview/mmwrhtml/ss5101a1.htm
www.niaid.nih.gov
www.foodallergy.org
www.aaaai.org
http://www.asthmainamerica.com/

Respiratory Diseases (Chronic Obstructive Respiratory Disease, COPD, CO Poisoning)

http://www.lef.org/protocols/respiratory/copd_01.htm
http://www.lung.ca/diseases-maladies/copd-mpoc_e.php
http://www.medicinenet.com/chronic_obstructive_pulmonary_disease_copd/article.htm
http://www.osha.gov/OshDoc/data_General_Facts/carbonmonoxide-factsheet.pdf

Acidoses

http://www.emedicine.com/med/topic1253.htm—Lactic acidoses
http://www.medstudents.com.br/terin/terin5.htm—Metabolic acidoses

General

www.acid-base.com—Acid-base balance
www.madsci.com/manu/indexgas.htm—Blood gases manual
http://www.lakesidepress.com/pulmonary/ABG/MixedAB.htm
http://www.fpnotebook.com/
http://cjasn.asnjournals.org/cgi/content/full/2/1/162#T1

Chapter 30

Renal Function

Joshua M. Kaplan and Martin Roy First

Chapter Outline

Key Terms

albuminuria The presence of albumin in urine.

aldosterone A steroid hormone produced in the adrenal cortex that acts on the distal tubules to stimulate sodium reabsorption and potassium and hydrogen excretion.

antidiuretic hormone (ADH) Also called *vasopressin;* a pituitary hormone that acts at the collecting duct to increase reabsorption of free water, resulting in the formation of a more concentrated urine.

anuria A condition in which no urine is formed.

ascending limb The straight portion of the loop of Henle in which the presumptive urine flows up toward the convoluted distal tubule. Osmolality of urine decreases because of loss of chloride (plus Na^+).

bladder A sac used to collect formed urine before voiding.

Bowman's capsule A structure that consists of glomeruli and extended opening of the proximal tubule.

carbonic anhydrase The enzyme at the brush border of the proximal tubule that catalyzes the reaction $H_2O + CO_2 \rightarrow H_2CO_3$.

casts Protein aggregates, outlined in the shape of renal tubules, secreted into the urine.

clearance A theoretical concept expressing that volume of plasma filtered at the glomeruli per unit of time from which an analyte would be completely removed and placed in final urine. It usually is expressed as milliliters of plasma per minute.

collecting tubule The last portion of the nephron, which connects the distal convoluted tubule and the larger collecting ducts; these in turn empty into the ureter. The final concentrating processes under the influence of ADH occur here.

countercurrent mechanism The process by which 2 streams flowing in opposite directions exchange material. In the kidney, urine and blood form opposing flows, and this mechanism allows reabsorption of substances.

creatinine clearance An estimate of the glomerular filtration rate obtained by measuring the amount of creatinine in the plasma and its rate of excretion into the urine.

descending limb The straight portion of the loop of Henle in which forming urine flows down from the convoluted proximal tubule. This portion of the loop of Henle is freely permeable to water, which leaves the presumptive urine.

distal convoluted tubule The convoluted tubule that connects the ascending loop of Henle with the collecting tubule. It has secretory and reabsorptive functions as part of the final urine formation and acidification process.

diuretic A drug that promotes the increased excretion of salt and water, thus increasing the flow of urine.

filtered load The amount of a substance presented to the tubules for reabsorption.

glomerular filtration rate (GFR) The rate in milliliters per minute at which substances in plasma are filtered through the glomeruli into the proximal tubule.

glomerulus Cluster of small blood vessels in the kidney that projects into the expanded end (capsule) of the proximal tubule and functions as a filtering mechanism for the nephron.

hematuria The presence of blood or red blood cells in the urine.

loop of Henle A U-shaped tubule that connects the proximal and distal convoluted tubules. It reduces the volume of tubule fluid.

microalbuminuria Abnormal, but low levels of albumin in urine that is undetectable by standard urine dipstick measures.

nephron The functional unit of the kidney that contains Bowman's capsule, the proximal and distal convoluted tubules, the ascending and descending limbs of the loop of Henle, and the collecting tubules.

oliguria The formation of small amounts of urine.

proteinuria The presence of protein in urine.

proximal tubule The convoluted tubule that begins at the glomeruli and connects to the descending loop of Henle. It has secretory and reabsorptive functions as part of the mechanism for urine formation.

pyuria The presence of leukocytes in the urine.

reabsorption (active and passive) The process of uptake of substance from the tubular lumen into tubular cells or blood. Active absorption requires the expenditure of energy to move substances against a concentration gradient, whereas, in the case of passive absorption, substances move from higher to lower concentrations.

renal cortex The outer part of the kidney that contains mostly glomeruli and convoluted tubules.

renal medulla The inner part of the kidney that contains mostly collecting ducts and the loops of Henle.

renal threshold The plasma concentration of a substance above which it will be present in urine.

renin An enzyme formed by the juxtaglomerular apparatus in the kidney. It converts plasma angiotensinogen to angiotensin I.

SIADH Syndrome of hyponatremia caused by excess antidiuretic hormone secretion.

specific gravity The ratio of the weight in grams per milliliter of body fluid compared with water.

titratable acid The combination of hydrogen ion with phosphate present in final urine.

urethra A membranous tube through which urine passes from the bladder to the exterior of the body.

urine The aqueous liquid and dissolved substances excreted by the kidney.

Methods on Evolve

Albumin
Anion gap
Creatinine
Creatinine clearance algorithm
Electrolytes (sodium, potassium, calcium, magnesium, phosphate)—serum and urine
Urea
Uric acid
Urine protein, total

ANATOMY OF KIDNEY

Gross Anatomy

The kidneys are paired organs located in the posterior part of the abdomen on either side of the vertebral column. Underneath the capsule of fibrous tissue that encloses the kidney lies the **renal cortex,** which contains the glomeruli and renal tubules. The inner portion of the kidney, the **renal medulla,** contains the tubules and collecting ducts. A vertical section through the kidney is shown on the left-hand side of Fig. 30-1.

The urinary system is illustrated on the right-hand side of Fig. 30-1. The renal pelvis rapidly diminishes in caliber and merges into the ureter. Each ureter descends in the abdomen alongside the vertebral column to join the bladder. The **bladder** provides temporary storage for **urine,** which eventually is voided through the **urethra** to the exterior.

Microscopic Anatomy

Each kidney is made up of approximately 1 million functional units, or nephrons. The component parts of the **nephron** are illustrated in Fig. 30-2. The nephron begins with the **glomerulus,** which is a tuft of capillaries that is formed from the afferent (incoming) arteriole and is drained by a smaller efferent (outgoing) arteriole. The glomerulus is surrounded by **Bowman's capsule,** which is formed by the blind, dilated end of the renal tubule. The proximal convoluted tubule runs a tortuous course through the cortex, entering the medulla and forming first the **descending limb** of the **loop of Henle** and then the **ascending limb** of the loop of Henle. The thick

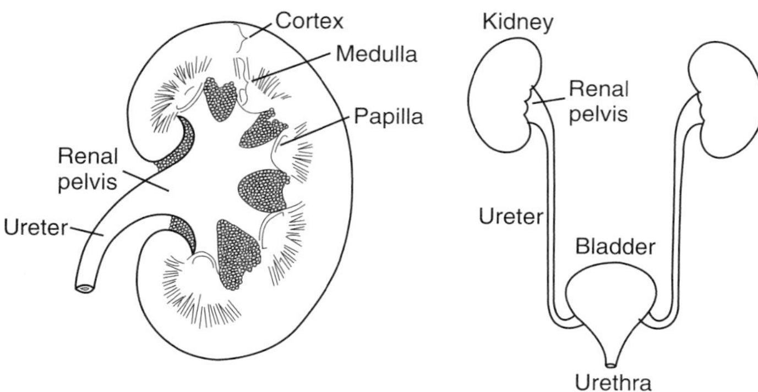

Fig. 30-1 Gross anatomy of kidney and urinary system.

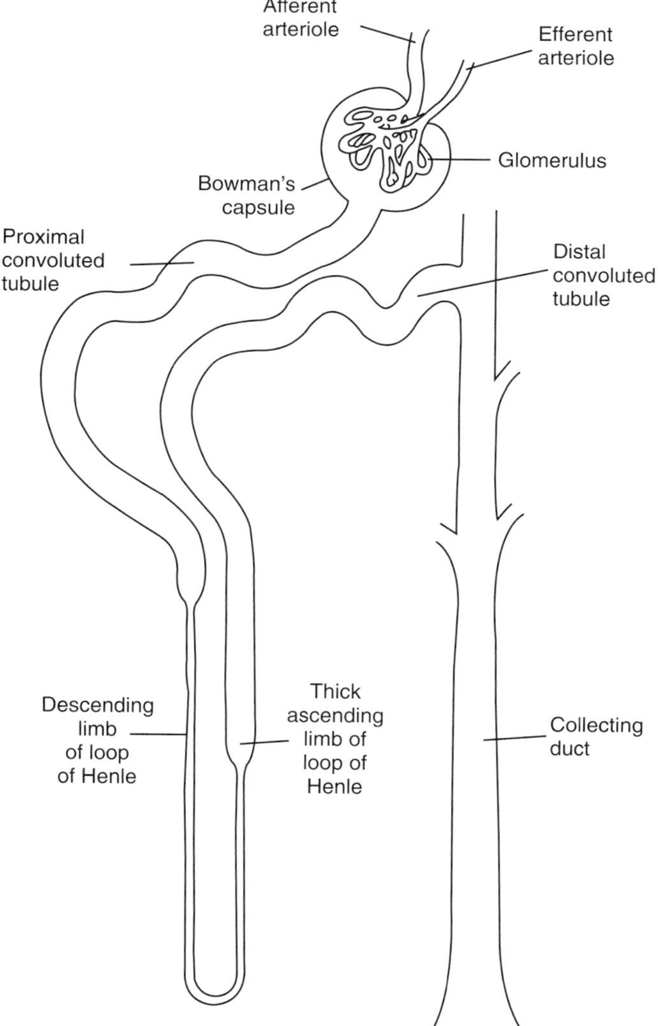

Fig. 30-2 Components of the nephron.

section of the ascending limb of the loop of Henle reenters the cortex, forming the **distal convoluted tubule.** The merging of 2 or more distal tubules marks the beginning of a collecting duct. As the collecting duct descends through the cortex and medulla, it receives the effluent from a dozen or more distal tubules. The collecting ducts join and increase in size as they pass down the medulla. The ducts of each pyramid coalesce to form a central duct, which empties through the papilla into a minor calyx, eventually draining into the renal pelvis.

SECTION OBJECTIVES BOX 30-1

- List 6 main functions of the kidney.
- Discuss the proximal convoluted tubule according to: its primary activity, a listing of substances that are reabsorbed, and the concept of the renal threshold.
- Differentiate the mechanisms of active reabsorption, passive reabsorption, and tubular secretion, listing substances that are reabsorbed or secreted according to each mechanism in the proximal convoluted tubule.
- Explain how the kidney is able to concentrate or dilute urine in order to regulate body water.
- Explain how the 4 mechanisms the kidney employs to maintain acid-base balance operate.

RENAL PHYSIOLOGY

The kidney is the chief regulator of all body fluids and is primarily responsible for maintaining homeostasis, or equilibrium of fluid and electrolytes in the body. The kidney has 6 main functions, as follows:

1. Urine formation
2. Regulation of fluid and electrolyte balance
3. Regulation of acid-base balance
4. Excretion of waste products of protein metabolism
5. Hormonal function
6. Protein conservation

The kidney is able to carry out these complex functions because approximately 25% of the volume of blood pumped by the heart into the systemic circulation is circulated through the kidneys; therefore, the kidneys, which constitute about 0.5% of total body weight, receive one-fourth of the cardiac output.

Urine Formation

The removal of potentially toxic waste products is a major function of the kidneys and is accomplished through the formation of urine. The basic processes involved in the formation of urine are filtration, **reabsorption,** and secretion. The kidneys filter large volumes of plasma, reabsorb most of what is filtered, and leave behind for elimination from the body a concentrated solution of metabolic wastes called *urine.* In healthy individuals, the kidneys, which are highly sensitive to fluctuations in diet and fluid and electrolyte intake, compensate for any changes by varying the volume and consistency of the urine.

Glomerular Filtration

Each minute, 1000 to 1500 mL of blood passes through the kidneys. The glomerulus has a semipermeable basement membrane that allows free passage of water and electrolytes but is relatively impermeable to larger molecules. The architecture of the human glomerular capillary wall is illustrated

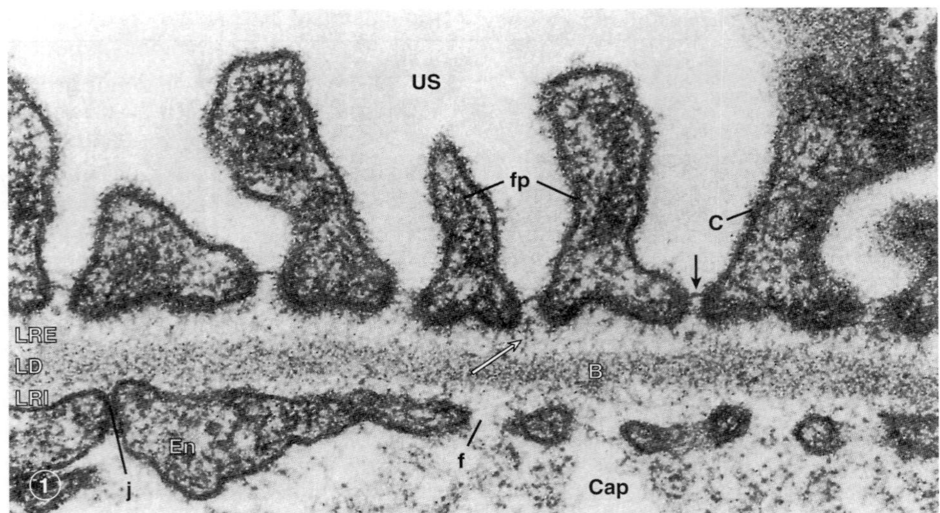

Fig. 30-3 Portion of a glomerulus showing a peripheral region of a capillary loop cut into a healthy section. The filtration surface consists of the endothelium (En) with its open fenestrae (f) lacking diaphragms, the glomerular basement membrane (B), and the epithelial foot processes (fp), between which are the filtration slits, bridged at their base by slit membranes *(short arrow).* Notice that the glomerular basement membrane (GBM) consists of 3 layers—a central dense layer, the lamina densa (LD), and 2 adjoining layers of lower density—the lamina rara interna (LRI) and externa (LRE). A thick cell coat (C) is visible on the membrane of the foot processes. The lamina densa is composed of a fine (≈ 3 nm) filamentous meshwork, and wispy filaments are seen extending from the lamina densa to the endothelial and epithelial *(long arrow)* membranes on either side. *Cap,* Capillary lumen; *j,* junction between 2 endothelial cells; *US,* urinary spaces; 80,000×. (From Farquhar MG, Kanwan YS: In Cummings NB, Michael AF, Wilson CB, editors: *Immune mechanisms in renal disease,* New York, 1983, Plenum Medical Books.)

in Fig. 30-3. In the process of transfer from capillary lumen (CL) to Bowman's space, or urinary space (US), water, solutes, and macromolecules must traverse 3 layers: (1) the endothelial wall cytoplasm (En), which contains numerous fenestrae with a mean diameter of 70 nm; (2) the basement membranes (B), with a mean thickness of 320 nm; and (3) the layers of the foot process (F), which are separated 25 to 60 nm from each other by slit pores. In glomerular capillaries, the hydrostatic pressure is approximately 3 times greater than the pressure in other capillaries. As a result of this high pressure, substances are filtered through the semipermeable membrane into Bowman's capsule at a rate of approximately 130 mL/min; this is known as the ***glomerular filtration rate (GFR).*** Cells and large plasma proteins are unable to pass through the semipermeable membrane. Therefore, the glomerular filtrate is essentially plasma without the proteins. The GFR is an extremely important parameter in both the study of kidney physiology and the clinical assessment of renal function. In the average healthy person, more than 187,000 mL of filtrate is formed per day. Normal urine output is around 1500 mL per day, which is only about 1% of the amount of filtrate formed; therefore, the other 99% must be reabsorbed.

Proximal Tubule

The proximal tubular cells perform a variety of physiologic tasks. Approximately 80% of salt and water is reabsorbed from the glomerular filtrate in the **proximal tubule.** All filtered glucose and most of the filtered amino acids are normally reabsorbed here. Low-molecular-weight proteins, urea, uric acid, bicarbonate, phosphate, chloride, potassium, magnesium, and calcium are reabsorbed to varying degrees. A variety of organic acids and bases, as well as hydrogen ions and ammonia, are secreted into the tubular fluid by tubular cells. Under normal conditions, no glucose is excreted in the urine; all that is filtered is reabsorbed. As the plasma concentration of glucose is increased above some critical level, termed the *renal plasma threshold,* the tubular maximum for glucose reabsorption is exceeded, and glucose appears in the urine. The higher the plasma concentration of glucose, the greater is the quantity excreted in the urine. Renal plasma thresholds also exist for phosphate and bicarbonate ions.

Most of the metabolic energy consumed by the kidney is used to promote active reabsorption. Active reabsorption can produce net movement of a substance against a concentration or electrical gradient and therefore requires energy expenditure by the transporting cells. Active reabsorption of glucose, amino acids, low-molecular-weight proteins, uric acid, sodium, potassium, magnesium, calcium, chloride, and bicarbonate is regulated by the kidney according to the levels of these substances in the blood and the body's needs. Passive reabsorption occurs when a substance moves by simple diffusion as the result of an electrical or chemical concentration gradient, and no cellular energy is involved in the process. Water, urea, and chloride are reabsorbed in this way.

Tubular secretion, by which substances are transported into the tubular lumen (i.e., in the direction opposite to tubular reabsorption), may also be an active or passive process.

Table 30-1 Filtration, Reabsorption, and Excretion by Kidney

Component	Amount Filtered per Day	Amount Excreted per Day	Percentage Reabsorbed
Water	180 L	1.5 L	99.2
Sodium	24,000 mEq	100 mEq	99.6
Chloride	20,000 mEq	100 mEq	99.5
Bicarbonate	5000 mEq	2 mEq	99.9
Potassium	700 mEq	50 mEq	92.9
Glucose	180 g	0	100
Albumin	360 mg	18 mg	95

Substances that are transported from the blood to the tubules and are excreted in the urine include potassium, hydrogen ions, ammonia, uric acid, and certain drugs, such as penicillin. Table 30-1 gives an idea of the magnitude and importance of these reabsorptive mechanisms.

Loop of Henle

The descending limb of the loop of Henle is highly permeable to water. In the medulla, the loop of Henle descends into an environment that is increasingly hypertonic as the papilla is approached. Passive reabsorption of water occurs in response to this osmotic gradient, leaving the presumptive urine highly concentrated at the bottom of the loop. The ascending limb is relatively impermeable to the passage of water but actively reabsorbs sodium and chloride. This segment of the nephron is often called the *diluting segment,* because removal of salt with little water from the tubular contents lowers the salt and osmotic concentrations, in effect diluting the tubular fluid. The ascending thick limb of the loop of Henle transfers sodium chloride actively from its lumen into the interstitial fluid (ISF). The tubular fluid in its lumen becomes hypotonic, and the ISF becomes hypertonic. This phenomenon is known as the **countercurrent mechanism.** A series of successive steps results in the trapping of sodium chloride in the ISF of the medulla. As the isotonic fluid in the descending limb reaches the area into which the ascending limb is pumping out sodium, it becomes slightly hypertonic because of the movement of water into the hypertonic interstitium. The first step repeats itself, and again, as more sodium and chloride are added to the interstitium by the ascending limb, more water is drawn out of the descending limb.

Distal Convoluted Tubule

A small fraction of the filtered sodium, chloride, and water is reabsorbed in the distal convoluted tubule. The distal tubule responds to the **antidiuretic hormone (ADH),** and so its water permeability is high in the presence of the hormone and low in its absence. Potassium can be reabsorbed or secreted in the distal tubule. **Aldosterone** stimulates both sodium reabsorption and potassium secretion in the distal tubule. Hydrogen, ammonia and ammonium ions, and uric acid secretion and bicarbonate reabsorption occur, but there is little transport of organic substances. This segment of the nephron has a low permeability to urea.

Collecting Duct

ADH controls the water permeability of the **collecting tubule** throughout its length. In the presence of the hormone, the hypotonic tubular fluid entering the duct loses water. Sodium and chloride are reabsorbed by the collecting tubule, with the transport of sodium stimulated by aldosterone. The collecting duct also reabsorbs potassium, hydrogen, and ammonia. When ADH is present, the rate of water reabsorption exceeds the rate of solute reabsorption, and the concentration of sodium and chloride in the presumptive urine rises. The collecting duct is relatively impermeable to urea.

Regulation of Fluid and Electrolyte Balance (see also Chapter 28)

Water

Water is the most abundant component of the human body, accounting for approximately 60% of body weight. The primary purpose of regulating body water is to maintain serum osmolality. Regulation of body water is only a secondary tool in the maintenance of body volume (see Sodium, below). Serum osmolality remains fairly constant from day to day in normal persons, despite wide fluctuations in fluid and salt intake.[1,2] One of the most remarkable properties of the human kidney is its ability to elaborate urine that is more concentrated or more dilute than the plasma from which it is derived. When the human body needs to conserve water, as in dehydration, the concentrating mechanism operates maximally, and urine osmolality increases to about 1200 mOsm/kg. Conversely, when there is excess water in the body, urine flow increases, and the diluting mechanism reduces urine osmolality to as low as 50 mOsm/kg. The capacity of the kidney to form urine of greatly varying osmolality enables it to regulate the solute concentration and hence the osmolality of body fluids within narrow physiologic limits, despite wide fluctuations in intake of salt and water.[1,2] Water balance is controlled primarily through voluntary intake (which is regulated through the thirst center in the hypothalamus) and urinary loss of water. The control of urinary water loss is the major automatic mechanism by which body water is regulated. In dehydrated states, the urine is concentrated when the kidney reabsorbs water without solute. Conversely, urine is diluted when the kidney reabsorbs solute without water.

Sodium

Sodium is the main cation found in extracellular fluid; therefore, regulation of sodium is the critical factor in the maintenance of total body water. Sodium is freely filtered through the glomerulus and is actively reabsorbed by the tubules. Sodium reabsorption is very important because it affects the regulation of several other electrolytes. Active reabsorption of the sodium ion in the proximal tubule results in passive transport of chloride and bicarbonate as counterions and in the passive reabsorption of water. In normal persons, daily urinary sodium excretion fluctuates widely according to dietary intake, thereby keeping the body sodium content remarkably constant. In the normal person, the kidneys reabsorb more than 99% of the **filtered load** of sodium. Sodium reabsorption by the nephron is controlled by the renin-angiotensin-aldosterone system (see Chapters 28 and 51).[3,4]

Chloride

The concentration of chloride in the extracellular fluid parallels that of sodium and is influenced by the same factors. However, chloride reabsorption is passive in the proximal tubule and probably is active in the distal tubule and collecting duct.

Potassium

Potassium is the chief cation of the intracellular fluid. Maintenance of a normal potassium level is essential to the life of the cells. The distribution of potassium is such that 98% of total body potassium is intracellular, and only 2% is extracellular. The high intracellular-to-extracellular potassium ratio is maintained by the Na^+,K^+-ATPase pump.[5] The healthy person maintains potassium balance by excreting daily an amount of potassium equal to the amount ingested minus the small amount eliminated in the feces and sweat. Renal function is the major mechanism by which body potassium is regulated. Potassium is filtered freely at the glomerulus, and active tubular reabsorption occurs throughout the nephron, except in the descending loop of Henle. Only about 10% of filtered potassium enters the distal tubule. The distal tubule and collecting ducts are able to both secrete and reabsorb potassium, thus regulating potassium excretion.[6] The hormone aldosterone, which stimulates tubular sodium reabsorption, simultaneously enhances potassium secretion in the distal tubule.[6,7]

Calcium

Calcium reabsorption in the proximal tubule parallels that of sodium and water. The maintenance of calcium homeostasis depends on the balance between calcium intake and calcium loss. The body loses calcium in the urine, through the gastrointestinal tract, and in sweat. Calcium balance is achieved largely by the control of calcium absorption into, and release from, bone stores and absorption from the gastrointestinal tract, rather than by the regulation of calcium excretion. The percentage of ingested calcium absorbed decreases as the dietary calcium content increases, and so the amount absorbed can remain relatively constant. The slight increase in absorption that occurs on a high-calcium diet is reflected in increased renal excretion.[8]

Phosphorus

Over a wide range of dietary intakes, roughly two-thirds of ingested phosphorus is absorbed into the bloodstream. Maintenance of the phosphorus balance is achieved largely through renal excretion.[9] Proximal tubular reabsorption of inorganic phosphate is normally about 90% of the filtered load. Parathyroid hormone depresses the renal tubular reabsorption of inorganic phosphate. In progressive chronic renal failure, there is a progressive increase in the serum phosphorus level.[10]

Magnesium

The filtration of magnesium at the glomerulus and its reabsorption from the proximal tubules parallel those of calcium and occur through the influence of parathyroid hormone. Moderate elevation of the plasma magnesium concentration occurs in patients with advanced chronic renal failure.[11]

Acid-Base Balance

Each day, acid waste products are produced in the body. If they were not disposed of efficiently, they would accumulate and cause cellular damage. Body pH is controlled by 3 systems: acid-base buffers, the lungs, and the kidneys (see Chapter 29).

Excretion of Hydrogen Ions

In subjects on a normal diet, about 50 to 100 mEq of hydrogen ions is generated each day. To prevent a progressive metabolic acidosis, these hydrogen ions are excreted in the urine.[12] Hydrogen ions are generated in the cells of the proximal and distal tubules and in the collecting duct as a result of the formation of carbonic acid by the enzyme **carbonic anhydrase (CA).** The cells secrete these hydrogen ions into the lumen[13]:

$$H_2O + CO_2 \overset{CA}{\rightleftharpoons} H_2CO_3 \rightleftharpoons H^+ + HCO_3^- \qquad \text{Eq. 30-1}$$

The role of the kidneys in the maintenance of the acid-base balance centers on the generation of bicarbonate. Hydrogen ions are excreted into the urine while newly generated bicarbonate ions pass from the tubular cells into the blood at the same rate as bicarbonate is consumed by the metabolic processes.[13] Four mechanisms are in place to handle the hydrogen ions that have been secreted into the tubular fluid.

Reaction With Filtered Bicarbonate Ions

Bicarbonate is completely filterable at the glomerulus. In the tubular lumen, the excreted hydrogen ion combines with the filtered bicarbonate to form carbonic acid, which, with CA attached to the apical membrane of the tubular cell and in contact with tubular fluid, decomposes to water and carbon dioxide, the latter then diffusing into the cell, where it can be converted by cellular CA to carbonic acid to generate another hydrogen ion. One bicarbonate ion is regenerated for every hydrogen ion that is secreted into the tubular lumen. The bicarbonate ion is reabsorbed into the blood as sodium bicarbonate, thus conserving most of the filtered bicarbonate. The **renal threshold** for bicarbonate is 28 mM; at a plasma level below this, all filtered bicarbonate is reabsorbed.

Reaction With Filtered Buffers to Form Titratable Acids

Inorganic monohydrogen phosphate is present in the tubular lumen as the disodium salt. Secreted hydrogen ions react with the filtered phosphate, releasing sodium that combines with the bicarbonate; the sodium bicarbonate is reabsorbed, and dihydrogen phosphate is excreted as follows:

$$
\begin{aligned}
&Na_2HPO_4 + H^+ \rightarrow NaH_2PO_4 + Na^+\\
&Na^+ + HCO_3^- \rightarrow NaHCO_3 \text{ (reabsorbed)}
\end{aligned}
\qquad \text{Eq. 30-2}
$$

Hydrogen ions combine with phosphate to form **titratable acid.** The rate of excretion of titratable acid is limited by the filtered load of buffer and cannot increase greatly in acidosis. The lowest possible pH of urine is 4.4.

Reaction With Secreted Ammonia to Form Ammonium Ion

The glomerular filtrate does not contain ammonium ions. Ammonia is synthesized in renal tubular cells by deamination of glutamine in the presence of glutaminase.[13] The ammonia diffuses freely into the tubular fluid, where it reacts with a secreted hydrogen ion to form an ammonium ion, which, because of its charge, is trapped within the lumen. Once again, this results in the addition of an H^+ to urine. The most important renal adaptation to acidosis is the increased excretion of ammonium ions[13]:

$$
\begin{aligned}
&\text{Glutamine} \xrightarrow{\text{Glutaminase}} \text{Glutamic acid} + NH_3\\
&NH_3 + H^+ \rightarrow NH_4^+
\end{aligned}
\qquad \text{Eq. 30-3}
$$

Excretion as Free Hydrogen Ions

Only negligible quantities of hydrogen ions are handled in this way by the kidneys. The amount of H^+ excreted as ammonium ions is much more important than the amount excreted as free H^+; ammonium in acid urine is 90 mM, and the concentration of H^+ in urine with pH of 4.5 is 30 μM (0.03 mM).

Nitrogenous Waste Excretion

One of the major functions of the kidney is the elimination of nitrogenous products of cellular catabolism. The enormous reserves of the kidney for excretion of the products of cellular catabolism are indicated by the fact that the blood concentrations of these products are not elevated in renal failure until renal function is reduced to less than one-half of normal.[14]

Urea

As amino acids are deaminated, ammonia is produced. The development of toxic levels of ammonia in the blood is prevented by the conversion of ammonia to urea. This takes place in the liver. Urea in the blood is reported as the blood urea nitrogen (BUN). Urea production and BUN are increased when a greater number of amino acids are metabolized in the liver.[15] This can occur with a high-protein diet, tissue breakdown, or decreased protein synthesis. In contrast, urea production and BUN are reduced in the presence of low protein intake and severe liver disease. Urea production exceeds renal urea excretion in healthy persons. The remaining urea is degraded to ammonium ions by intestinal bacteria. Urea is readily filtered, but approximately 40% to 50% of filtered urea is normally reabsorbed by the proximal tubules. Because many factors may influence the BUN level while the GFR remains constant, BUN is a less specific indicator of renal function and should not be relied on for that purpose.

Creatinine

Serum creatinine levels and urinary creatinine excretion are a function of muscle mass in normal persons and show little response to dietary changes.[16] Creatinine is derived from the nonenzymatic dehydration of creatine in skeletal muscle:

$$
\begin{array}{ccc}
CH_3\text{—}NCH_2\text{—}COOH & & CH_3\text{—}N\text{—}CH_2\\
C{=}NH & \longrightarrow & C{=}O + H_2O\\
NH_2 & & HN{=}C\text{—}NH\\
\textbf{Creatine} & & \textbf{Creatinine}
\end{array}
\qquad \text{Eq. 30-4}
$$

The amount of creatine per unit of muscle mass is constant, and thus the rate of spontaneous breakdown of creatine is also constant. As a result, the plasma creatinine concentration is highly stable, varying by less than 10% per day in serial observations in normal subjects. Because the serum creatinine concentration is a direct reflection of muscle mass, the serum level is higher in males than in females. Creatinine is filtered freely at the glomerulus and is not reabsorbed by the tubules. A small amount of creatinine in the final urine is derived from tubular secretion. Because of these properties of creatinine, the **creatinine clearance** can be used to estimate the GFR (see Tests of glomerular function, p. 578).

Uric Acid

Uric acid is derived from the oxidation of purine bases. Plasma levels of uric acid are variable and are higher in males than in females. Plasma urates are completely filterable, and both proximal tubular resorption and distal tubular secretion may occur. Advanced chronic renal failure is associated with a progressive increase in the plasma uric acid level.

Hormonal Function

The kidneys have important metabolic and endocrine functions. The kidney as an endocrine organ is discussed in this section.[17]

Vitamin D Metabolism

In vitamin D metabolism, the kidney produces the major biologically active hormone 1,25-dihydroxycholecalciferol.[18] The enzyme responsible for the production of 1,25-dihydroxycholecalciferol is present almost exclusively in the mitochondria of the renal cortex (see Chapter 33).

Renin

The kidney releases **renin** in response to a decrease in afferent arteriolar pressure or an increase in sympathetic nervous system activity. This results in stimulation of the renin-angiotensin-aldosterone axis, with production of aldosterone and angiotensin[2] and subsequent sodium conservation[4] (see Chapters 28 and 51).

Erythropoietin

The kidneys play a major role in the production and release of erythropoietin, a hormone that stimulates red blood cell production. The central role of the kidneys in erythropoietin production explains the anemia associated with chronic renal failure.[19]

Protein Conservation

Under normal physiologic conditions, the kidney helps to maintain the homeostasis of body proteins. In humans, 180 L of plasma, with each liter containing 70 g of protein, is filtered each day by the glomerulus.[20] Without an efficient conservation mechanism, body protein stores would be depleted very rapidly. Yet normal urine contains less than 200 mg of protein per day—only a minute percentage of the 12,600 g passing through the glomerulus daily.[20] Most of the filtered proteins are absorbed by the proximal tubules and are returned to the circulation. Most plasma proteins, except those of very high molecular weight, have been found in the urine. Albumin excretion is less than 20 mg/day.[20] Many of the proteins of nonserum origin are also found in the urine. One of these, uromucoid or Tamm-Horsfall mucoprotein, is the predominant protein in normal urine, with about 40 mg excreted daily. This high-molecular-weight mucoprotein is excreted by the cells of the distal tubule and collecting ducts. Commercially available dipsticks are in widespread use and are accurate for rapid assessment of urinary protein concentration.

KEY CONCEPTS BOX 30-1

- The functional parts of the kidney's excretory functions are the glomerulus, proximal tubule, distal tubule, and collecting ducts. Each has a different role in regulating the amount and composition of urine formed.
- The kidneys regulate the chemical composition of serum and volume status by controlling the excretion of
  - Electrolytes (e.g., sodium, potassium, phosphorus)
  - Acids and alkali
  - Water
- The kidneys also have important hormonal functions, such as synthesizing renin to control Na and water balance; erythropoietin to stimulate RBC production; and vitamin D_3 to control calcium balance.
- The kidneys excrete nitrogen wastes while conserving protein.

SECTION OBJECTIVES BOX 30-2

- Discuss acute glomerulonephritis according to definition, typical laboratory and clinical findings, and the pathognomonic urine microscopic finding.
- Explain why proximal renal tubular defects result in acidosis, hyperkalemia, hypo- or hyperuricemia, hypophosphatemia, aminoaciduria, and glucosuria.
- Discuss the abnormalities in renal function during the course of diabetes mellitus.
- Differentiate the causes and associated laboratory results in prerenal, renal, and postrenal acute renal failure.
- Discuss chronic renal disease according to the etiology of symptoms, the importance of the GFR, and the importance of staging the disease.

PATHOLOGIC CONDITIONS OF KIDNEY

Many syndromes singly or in combination indicate possible renal disease.[21]

Acute Glomerulonephritis

Acute glomerulonephritis is an acute inflammation of the glomeruli that may result in oliguria, hematuria, increased BUN and serum creatinine levels, decreased GFR, edema formation, and hypertension. The presence of red blood cells in the urine (**hematuria**) alone is insufficient evidence of acute glomerulonephritis, for blood can originate elsewhere in the kidney or in the urinary tract. The presence of red blood cell **casts** in the urine indicates glomerular inflammation and is a finding of great importance, although it is difficult to detect in the laboratory, given the speed with which cellular casts degenerate into granular casts. Other abnormalities present in acute nephritis include **proteinuria** and anemia.

Nephrotic Syndrome

The nephrotic syndrome has been classically defined as a clinical entity characterized by massive proteinuria, edema, hypoalbuminemia, hyperlipidemia, and lipiduria.[20] This syndrome, which can have many causes, is characterized by increased glomerular membrane permeability that results in massive proteinuria and excretion of fat bodies. Protein excretion rates usually are greater than 2 to 3 g/day in the absence of a depressed GFR. Hematuria and oliguria may be present. The causes of the nephrotic syndrome are listed in Box 30-1. As a result of the massive loss of serum proteins, primarily albumin, into urine, the plasma protein concentration is decreased, with

Box 30-1
Causes of Nephrotic Syndrome

- Associated with various forms of glomerulonephritis
- Associated with generalized disease processes
  - Amyloidosis
  - Carcinoma
  - Systemic lupus erythematosus
  - Diabetic glomerulosclerosis
  - Polyarteritis nodosa
- Associated with mechanical or circulating disorders
  - Renal vein thrombosis
  - Constrictive pericarditis
- Associated with infection
  - Syphilis
  - Malaria
  - Subacute bacterial endocarditis
- Associated with toxins and allergens
  - Penicillamine
  - Gold salts
  - Bee sting
  - Serum sickness
- Miscellaneous
  - Severe preeclampsia
  - Transplant rejection

a concomitant reduction in plasma oncotic pressure. This results in fluid movement from the vascular to interstitial space with consequent edema formation.

Tubular Disease

In some disorders of renal tubular function, depressed renal function cannot be explained by a reduction in GFR. Defects of tubular function may result in depressed secretion or reabsorption of specific biochemicals or impairment of urine concentration and dilution mechanisms. Renal tubular acidosis (RTA), the most important clinical disorder of tubular function,[22] occurs in 2 main types: (1) proximal RTA, which results from reduced proximal tubular bicarbonate reabsorption and causes hyperchloremic acidosis; and (2) distal RTA, in which there is an inability of the tubular cells to create and maintain the usual pH difference between tubular fluid and blood. Failure of the proximal or distal secretory mechanisms occurs in several disease states. Failure of the proximal tubule to reabsorb bicarbonate causes acidosis because more bicarbonate is passed on to the low-capacity distal mechanism than it can reabsorb. Loss of alkali in the urine causes the blood to become acidotic. Defects in potassium and uric acid secretion may result in elevations of serum potassium and uric acid levels beyond that explained by the reduction in GFR. Reabsorptive disorders of the proximal tubules may result in hypouricemia, hypophosphatemia, aminoaciduria, and renal glucosuria.

The Fanconi syndrome is a group of renal tubular defects that results in glucosuria, aminoaciduria, hypophosphatemia, and renal tubular acidosis. Tubular proteinuria may occur as the result of a tubular defect in the handling of proteins. In tubular proteinuria, less than 2 g/day of protein is excreted. Disorders of urine concentration and dilution occur in all renal disease as the GFR falls appreciably, but occasionally, these disorders may become extreme and dominate the clinical presentation.[21]

Interstitial Nephritis

Inflammation of the interstitial space of the kidneys is another cause of depressed renal function. This disorder is characterized by **pyuria** and white blood cell casts in the absence of infection, moderate proteinuria, and depressed GFR. Interstitial nephritis can be a primary, idiopathic (no known cause) disease, but it usually occurs as a reaction to medications. This reaction can be allergic, in response to any medicine, or nonallergic, in response to nonsteroidal antiinflammatory medicines. Secondary acute interstitial nephritis classically appears 7 to 10 days after exposure to the causative agent; fever, rash, and eosinophilia also may be present.[23]

Urinary Tract Infection

Infection of the urinary tract may occur in the bladder (cystitis) or may involve the kidneys (pyelonephritis). The presence of a urine bacterial concentration of greater than 100,000 colonies/mL in women or greater than 10,000 colonies/mL in men is diagnostic of urinary tract infection. In a urinary tract infection, the number of white blood cells in the urine is increased. The presence of white blood cell casts indicates pyelonephritis. An increased number of red blood cells also may be present in the urine.

Vascular Diseases

Hypertension

Long-standing and severe hypertension can result in progressive renal damage and chronic kidney disease (hypertensive nephrosclerosis). In contrast, hypertension can be caused by the sodium and water retention that occurs in chronic renal failure, acute glomerulonephritis, and the nephrotic syndrome (volume-dependent hypertension), or it can occur as a result of increased renin release from chronically damaged kidneys (renin-dependent hypertension).

Arteriolar Disease

Disease of the small arteries of the kidneys (arteritis) may occur in association with generalized disease processes that affect the kidney, such as systemic lupus erythematosus, polyarteritis nodosa, malignant hypertension, and progressive systemic sclerosis (scleroderma). These diseases may result in the clinical and biochemical abnormalities seen in acute glomerulonephritis, the nephrotic syndrome, or chronic renal insufficiency.

Renal Vein Thrombosis

Thrombosis of the renal veins results in massive proteinuria and the nephrotic syndrome. Hypertension, edema, hematuria, and impaired renal function may accompany the proteinuria.

Diabetes Mellitus (see Chapter 38)

Diabetes mellitus results in a wide variety of abnormalities in kidney function. The name of the disease comes from the Greek for sweet polyuria, reflecting the glucosuria caused by the filtered glucose exceeding the renal threshold of glucose and the resultant osmotic diuresis; the molecules of glucose are dissolved in water and bring it into the urine. The progressive loss of kidney function from diabetic nephropathy is the leading cause of morbidity and mortality in type 1 diabetes and the leading cause of end-stage renal disease in adults with type 2 diabetes mellitus.[24] In the juvenile diabetic patient, overt proteinuria develops approximately 17 years after the diagnosis has been made, hypertension develops 1 to 2 years later, and chronic renal insufficiency is seen after another year; in type 2 diabetics, hypertension often precedes proteinuria, which can occur within 5 years of diagnosis of diabetes mellitus.[25] Early in the course of diabetic nephropathy, protein excretion, particularly **albuminuria** and immunoglobulin (Ig)G, is increased. A urinary albumin excretion in the range of 50 to 200 mg/24 hr is usually predictive of diabetic nephropathy.[26] The level of albumin excretion has been shown to be increased with age and disease duration after 10 years in patients with type I diabetes mellitus.[27] A significant link also was noted with declining renal function and elevation of blood pressure. In recent years, attention has been focused on abnormal, but low levels of albumin in urine that cannot be detected by dipstick analysis, or **microalbuminuria.** This latent disease phase has been shown to be predictive of clinical nephropathy and eventual renal failure in patients with type 1 diabetes mellitus as well as worse clinical outcomes overall.[28,29]

Urinary Tract Obstruction

Lower urinary tract obstruction is characterized by residual urine in the bladder after urination or urinary retention, whereas the presence of upper tract obstruction is established by the demonstration of a dilated collecting system above a constricting lesion.[14] Lower urinary tract obstruction is characterized by a slow urinary stream, difficulty in emptying the bladder, hesitancy in initiating urination, and dribbling. Chronic renal damage may result from obstruction and incomplete bladder emptying, and symptoms of chronic renal insufficiency may develop. With complete obstruction, **oliguria** or **anuria** will occur. Symptoms of urinary tract infection also may be seen. Urinary tract obstruction may occur as a result of congenital disorders of the lower urinary tract, neoplastic lesions (benign prostatic hyperplasia, carcinoma of the prostate or bladder, or lymph nodes compressing the ureters), or acquired disorders (retroperitoneal fibrosis, renal calculi, or urethral strictures).

Renal Calculi

Renal calculi, or stones, are seen in combination with renal colic (flank pain associated with stones), hematuria, and symptoms of urinary tract infection or obstruction. Kidney stones may form after recurrent urinary tract infection by urease-producing organisms, or when the urine is supersaturated by large quantities of calcium, uric acid, cystine, or xanthine.

Acute Renal Failure

Acute renal failure (ARF) is marked by an abrupt deterioration in renal function, defined as decreased GFR and/or urine output. The latest classification system, called the *RIFLE criteria,* is defined in Fig. 30-4.[30] Acute renal failure can be classified as follows:

1. Prerenal (occurring before blood reaches the kidney) because of hypovolemia or poor perfusion that results from cardiovascular failure
2. Renal (occurring in the kidney) because of acute tubular necrosis, which is the most frequently observed cause of acute renal failure, or because of other renal diseases that may cause rapid deterioration in renal function, including arterial or venous obstruction
3. Postrenal (occurring after urine leaves the kidney) because of obstruction

The causes of acute renal failure are listed in Box 30-2. Acute renal failure usually is accompanied by oliguria or anuria; in addition, nonoliguric acute tubular necrosis can occur. Acute renal failure is associated with varying degrees of proteinuria and hematuria, and with the presence of red blood cell casts or other casts in the urine. Serum urea nitrogen and creatinine levels increase rapidly, and metabolic acidosis becomes evident. Depending on the cause, acute renal failure can progress to chronic renal insufficiency or failure, or it can be followed by recovery of renal function. Most patients with acute tubular necrosis recover once the offending cause has been treated or removed. Acute renal failure is associated with a great elevation in mortality risk.[31]

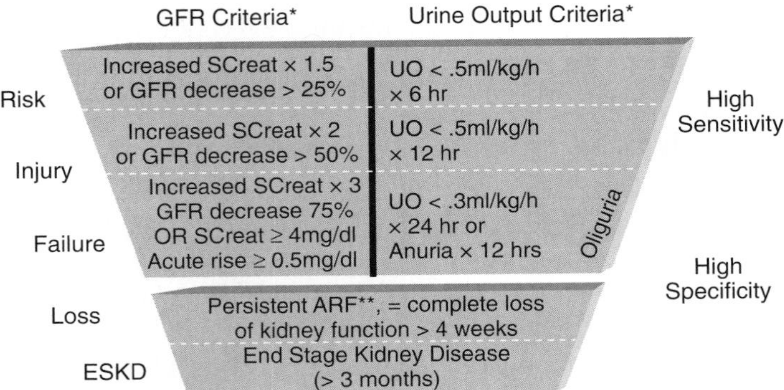

Fig. 30-4 RIFLE criteria for acute kidney injury. *ARF,* Acute renal failure; *dec,* decrease; *ESKD,* end-stage renal disease; *GFR,* glomerular filtration rate; *UO,* urine output. (From Bellomo R, Ronco C, Kellum JA, et al: Acute renal failure: definition, outcome measures, animal models, fluid therapy and information technology needs: the Second International Consensus Conference of the Acute Dialysis Quality Initiative (ADQI) Group, Crit Care 8:R204, 2004.)

Box 30-2

Causes of Acute Renal Failure

- Prerenal
  - Hypovolemia
  - Cardiovascular failure
- Renal
  - Acute tubular necrosis
  - Glomerulonephritis
  - Vasculitis
  - Malignant nephrosclerosis
  - Vascular obstruction
    - Arterial
    - Venous
- Postrenal
  - Obstruction of lower urinary tract
  - Rupture of bladder

Chronic Kidney Disease

Chronic kidney disease (CKD) is a clinical syndrome that results from progressive loss of renal function. Symptoms of chronic renal failure result not only from simple excretory failure but also from the onset of regulatory failure—the kidney's failure to regulate certain substances, such as sodium and water; from biosynthetic failure, such as the kidney's inadequate production of erythropoietin, resulting in anemia; and from excessive production of certain normal substances in response to the chemical derangements that occur in chronic

Box 30-3

Classification of Causes of Chronic Renal Failure

- Primary glomerular diseases
  - Chronic glomerulonephritis of various types
  - Systemic lupus erythematosus
  - Polyarteritis nodosa
- Renal vascular diseases
  - Malignant hypertension
  - Renal vein thrombosis
- Inflammatory diseases
  - Chronic pyelonephritis
  - Tuberculosis
- Metabolic diseases with renal involvement
  - Diabetes mellitus
  - Gout
  - Amyloidosis
- Nephrotoxins
  - Aminoglycosides
  - Analgesic nephropathy
  - Chronic heavy metal poisoning
- Obstructive nephropathy
  - Calculi
  - Prostatic hyperplasia
  - Congenital anomalies of lower urinary tract
- Congenital anomalies of kidneys
  - Hypoplastic kidneys
  - Polycystic kidney disease
- Miscellaneous
  - Chronic radiation nephritis
  - Balkan nephropathy

renal failure, such as the excessive production of parathyroid hormone.[14]

Chronic kidney disease consists of 5 stages:

Stage 1: GFR is greater than 90, but laboratory signs indicate kidney damage, either hematuria or proteinuria.

Stage 2: Laboratory signs of kidney damage are evident, and the GFR is between 60 and 90.

Stage 3: GFR is between 30 and 60.

Stage 4: GFR is between 15 and 30.

Stage 5: GFR is less than 15, or renal replacement therapy (dialysis or transplant) is required.[32]

A classification of the causes of chronic renal failure is shown in Box 30-3. Determining the GFR in CKD, and to a lesser extent in ARF, is important for several reasons. First, many drugs are cleared by the kidneys, and dosing is modified according to the GFR of the patient. Determining and reporting the estimated GFR, as opposed to creatinine and BUN alone, will allow for proper drug dosing in the presence of depressed GFR with creatinine and BUN levels that may be unremarkable. Second, CKD stages are associated with clinical outcomes. Patients with CKD stage 3 or greater have increased morbidity and mortality with almost any disease or procedure, and recognizing CKD will allow doctors to emphasize risk factor modification and optimization of therapy.[33] Finally, as CKD progresses to stage 3 and beyond, certain laboratory parameters must be monitored as metabolic and hormonal derangements arise.

KEY CONCEPTS BOX 30-2

- Kidney disease can affect any or all physiologic parts of the kidneys, including glomeruli, interstitium, tubules, collecting system, and vascular components.
- Acute kidney disease is the sudden decline in renal function.
- Chronic kidney disease is the slow, sustained loss of renal function and is associated with changes in clinical outcomes, as well as in drug metabolism.
- Calculation of glomerular filtration rate (GFR) is an important part of staging chronic kidney disease (CKD).

SECTION OBJECTIVES BOX 30-3

- List 4 characteristics of an ideal substance to measure the glomerular filtration rate (GFR).
- State the procedure and the formula for the creatinine clearance test.
- Discuss the value of the equations to calculate estimated creatinine clearance for both males and females.
- List 2 tests that are used as measures of the concentrating and diluting ability of the renal tubules.
- Explain the clinical usefulness of urinalysis testing.

RENAL FUNCTION TESTS

The kidney performs many physiologic and excretory functions. By performing a relatively small number of tests, a physician can deduce accurately the functional state of the kidney.[34] The clinician first determines whether any significant impairment of renal function exists and then assesses a particular renal function to make a specific diagnosis. In this section, evaluation of glomerular and tubular function and urinalysis are discussed.

Tests of Glomerular Function

The optimal substance for measurement of GFR would be nonmetabolized, excreted only by the kidney, freely filtered by the glomerulus, and neither reabsorbed nor secreted by the renal tubules.

Inulin Clearance

Inulin clearance therefore is the method of choice when precise determination of the GFR is required.[16] The glomerular capillary wall is freely permeable to inulin, and inulin is not reabsorbed, secreted, or metabolically altered by the renal tubule. The main disadvantages in the measurement of inulin clearance are the need for its intravenous administration and the technical difficulty of the analysis. Therefore, it is rarely done outside of research settings.

Cystatin C Clearance

Measurement of a small, endogenous nonglycosylated peptide, cystatin C (molecular weight [MW] ≈ 13,000 D), in serum has been proposed as an alternative way of assessing glomerular function.[35,36] Cystatin C is produced at a steady rate from most body tissues and is freely filtered by the glomerulus. Levels of cystatin C rise more quickly in acute renal failure than creatinine levels do. However, although elevated cystatin C has been shown to correlate well with decreased GFR, it also can be caused by an inflammatory state,[37] and thus it is not specific for renal failure. For this reason, cystatin C may be less useful as a surrogate for GFR but still may prove useful in providing prognostic information for increased risk for short-term mortality.

Creatinine Clearance

Glomerular function is measured most conveniently by the creatinine clearance test. Clearance is defined as that volume of plasma from which a measured amount of substance can be completely eliminated into the urine per unit of time. This depends on the plasma concentration of the substance and its excretory rate, which, in turn, depends on the GFR and renal plasma flow. Creatinine clearance is a renal function test that is based on the rate of excretion by the kidneys of metabolically produced creatinine. The amount of creatinine produced by endogenous creatine metabolism is relatively constant and directly proportional to the body surface area. The amount of creatinine present in the urine depends on renal excretion. Creatinine is filtered freely at the glomerulus and is not reabsorbed by the tubules. Therefore, creatinine clearance can be used to estimate GFR.

Generally, a 24-hour urine collection is performed. However, shorter collection periods are acceptable. Precise timing is critical for this test. The bladder is emptied at the beginning of the test period and the urine discarded; all urine passed subsequently during the timed collection is kept in a single container. A sample of blood is drawn during the urine collection period; a sample drawn within 24 hours of the collection period is acceptable if renal function is stable. Creatinine clearance is calculated from the following formula:

$$\text{Creatinine clearance (mL/min)} = UV/P \qquad \text{Eq. 30-5}$$

in which U is urinary creatinine (mg/dL), V is volume of urine excreted per time (mL/min), and P is plasma creatinine (mg/dL). The healthy reference interval for creatinine clearance corrected to a surface area of 1.73 m^2 is 90 to 120 mL/min (see Creatinine method on Evolve). Creatinine clearance usually parallels true GFR but overestimates it because of tubular secretion of creatinine (the clearance of endogenous creatinine may exceed that of inulin by up to 30% in healthy individuals). Moreover, at low filtration rates, when the tubular secretion of creatinine accounts for a higher percent of urinary creatinine, creatinine clearance becomes increasingly inaccurate.[16] This difficulty can be lessened by giving patients cimetidine (used for acid reflux), which blocks tubular secretion of creatinine. Creatinine clearance is lower in women, the elderly, and smaller persons, unless corrected for body surface area.

Urea clearance also may be employed as a measure of GFR. Urea is filtered freely at the glomerulus, and approximately 40% is reabsorbed in the tubules. Thus, as with creatinine, urea clearance values will parallel the true GFR. Contrary to creatinine clearance, urea clearance underestimates GFR because of tubular reabsorption. Therefore, some clinicians estimate GFR by using the average of creatinine and urea clearances.

Estimated Creatinine Clearance (e-C_{cr})

Measurement of creatinine clearance by collection of a timed (24-hour) urine specimen is burdensome to the patient and frequently is difficult to perform. Inaccurate results caused by incomplete bladder emptying, failure to collect the entire specimen, and wide intraindividual variation impair the usefulness of this procedure.[16] Numerous formulas and nomograms have been developed for estimating creatinine clearance from the serum creatinine concentration, thereby bypassing the need for urine collection. The simplest and most widely used for many years is the formula described by Cockcroft and Gault.[38]

$$C_{cr}\ (\text{males}) = \frac{[140 - \text{Age (years)}] \times \text{Weight (kg)}]}{[72 \times \text{Serum creatinine (mg/dL)}]}$$

$$C_{cr}\ (\text{females}) = \text{Above equation result} \times 0.85\ (\text{based on 15\% lower muscle mass on average}) \qquad \text{Eq. 30-6}$$

Estimated Glomerular Filtration Rate (e-GFR)

The Cockroft-Gault equation has significant bias and relatively poor accuracy. Recently, an equation was generated by analysis of patients in the Modification of Diet in Renal Disease (MDRD) study. These patients underwent extensive laboratory studies, including ^{125}I-iothalamate clearances. After analyzing which variables predicted GFR, the authors generated an equation that has been shown to be relatively accurate and bias-free for adults, known as the MDRD equation. Similarly derived equations, known as the Schwartz formula and the Counahan-Barratt formula, are available for use in children.[39,40]

Two MDRD equations have been put forth: Equation 1 assumes traditional standards used to calibrate creatinine measurements, and Equation 2 is derived from International Federation for Clinical Chemistry (IFCC) standards based on isotope dilution mass spectrometry (IDMS)-traceable standardization. In both, serum creatinine is expressed in standard units (mg/dL):

Eq. 1: $\text{GFR (mL/min/1.73 m}^2) = 186 \times (\text{Scr}) - 1.154 \times (\text{Age}) - 0.203 \times (0.742 \text{ if female}) \times (1.210 \text{ if African American})$.

Eq. 2: $\text{GFR (mL/min/1.73 m}^2) = 175 \times (\text{Scr}) - 1.154 \times (\text{Age}) - 0.203 \times (0.742 \text{ if female}) \times (1.210 \text{ if African American})$.

These equations have some limitations:

- These equations were derived from people with chronic kidney disease, so they are less well proven with GFRs within the reference interval.

- The accuracy of the e-GFR depends on proper standardization of creatinine methods run with greatest precision (see Creatinine method on Evolve).
- As with all prediction equations, these equations are accurate only in people in a steady state of creatinine excretion (e.g., excluding patients with acute renal failure).

The accuracy of these equations in certain subgroups, including the following, has not been established:

- Extremes of age and body size
- Severe malnutrition or obesity
- Disease of skeletal muscle
- Paraplegia or quadriplegia
- Vegetarian diet

Because of poor analytic precision for measurement of creatinine at higher GFRs, it has been recommended that e-GFRs greater than 60 mL/min be reported simply as >60 mL/min.

From a practical point of view, the easiest means of estimating GFR is via the use of prediction equations, particularly the MDRD equation in adults. Predicted GFR now is reported routinely by many laboratories as one of the results of a metabolic profile, and this is clearly increasing the early diagnosis of CKD in patients with relatively normal creatinine; it also is enhancing clinicians' awareness of the severity of CKD in all patients. Clinicians must be made aware of the limitations of these prediction equations, however, to prevent their misuse and to understand when direct measurement of clearances may be helpful. It is important for clinicians to understand that a large margin of reserve characterizes renal function; more than two-thirds of the GFR may be lost in the course of chronic renal disease with few clinical symptoms and biochemical abnormalities.[28] For a person whose usual serum creatinine is 0.7 mg/dL, an increase to 1.4 mg/dL, which still is defined as within the reference interval for healthy individuals for serum creatinine, is indicative of a fall in GFR to 50% of normal.

In addition to these measures of GFR, new analytes are under investigation for use in the early detection of acute kidney injury. As opposed to cystatin-C, which rises a day after renal injury occurs, and creatinine, which is delayed even further, these molecules are elevated in the urine as early as 2 hours after kidney tubule injury. These molecules still are being validated for clinical use but may enter clinical practice within a few years.[41]

Tests of Tubular Function

Concentration-Dilution Studies

Assessment of the concentrating and diluting abilities of the kidney can provide the most sensitive means of detecting early impairment in renal function because the ability to concentrate urine and conserve water requires an adequate GFR, renal plasma flow, and tubular mass, as well as healthy tubular cells that are able to pump salt against a sizable electrochemical gradient.[34] Urinary **specific gravity** and osmolality are used as measures of the concentrating and diluting abilities of the tubules. As long as the urine does not contain appreciable amounts of protein, sugar, or exogenous material such as contrast dye, specific gravity is proportional to osmolality, and a specific gravity of 1.032 will correspond to an osmolality of 1200 mOsm/kg.[34]

Impairment of renal concentrating ability is a relatively early manifestation of chronic renal disease and becomes evident before changes in other function tests appear. However, it is a nonspecific test for reduced renal function, and any disease that results in chronic renal failure, diabetes insipidus, or the use of **diuretics** may impair renal concentrating ability. The test is performed after 15 hours of fluid deprivation, and urine then is collected on the hour for 3 hours. Dehydration maximally stimulates endogenous ADH secretion. Under these conditions, the urine osmolality should be at least 3 times that of plasma (286 mOsm/kg). A specific gravity of 1.025 or more or an osmolality of 850 mOsm/kg or above in 1 of the specimens is accepted as evidence of concentrating ability within the healthy reference interval. A patient within the healthy reference interval of concentrating ability is unlikely to have a serious kidney malfunction of any type.[34] As chronic renal disease progresses, tubular ability to concentrate urine slowly decreases until the urine has the same specific gravity as the plasma ultrafiltrate—1.010. Clinically, the loss of concentrating ability is manifested by nocturia and polyuria.

To test urinary diluting capacity, the following procedure is used. The patient empties the bladder and is given 1000 to 1200 mL of water. Urine specimens then are collected every hour for the next 4 hours. Under these circumstances, urinary specific gravity should fall to 1.005 or less, or osmolality should measure less than 100 mOsm/kg. In the patient with chronic renal disease who is unable to dilute the urine, a danger of fluid overload is associated with this test.

In diabetes insipidus (DI), which can arise from inadequate ADH production (pituitary, or central DI) or from insensitivity of the renal tubules to ADH (nephrogenic DI), the distal tubular walls are impervious to water. As sodium is reabsorbed, the fluid left behind may be very dilute. In this disease, the baseline urine might have a specific gravity of less than 1.005 and an osmolality of 50 mOsm/kg. DI is diagnosed by an inability to concentrate the urine despite dehydration from water restriction, as documented by an elevation in serum osmolality. Patients with central DI will concentrate their urine after administration of synthetic ADH, and patients with nephrogenic DI will have no increase in their urine osmolality with synthetic ADH.

Urinalysis

(see Urinalysis section of Evolve)

Urinalysis is an indispensable tool for assessing renal disease. It may reveal disease anywhere in the urinary tract. Observations that can be made in standard urinalysis include appearance of the specimen, pH, specific gravity, protein semiquantitation, presence or absence of glucose and ketones, and microscopic examination of the centrifuged urinary sediment. The importance of urinalysis is indicated in Table 30-2. Microscopic examination of the centrifuged urinary sediment for cells, crystals, and casts should be done on a freshly voided specimen.

Table 30-2 Association of Pathologic Conditions Affecting the Kidney and Clinical and Biochemical Abnormalities

	AGN	NS	TD	UTI	HT	RVT	DM	UTO	RC	ARF	CRF
Hypertension	++	+	0	0	++	±	±	0	0	+	+
Edema	+	++	0	0	0	+	+	0	0	+	+
Oliguria or anuria	+	±	0	0	0	±	0	+	0	+	+
Polyuria	0	0	+	0	0	0	+	0	0	0	0
Nocturia	0	±	+	±	0	0	+	±	0	0	0
Frequency	0	0	0	+	0	0	0	±	±	0	0
Loin pain	0	0	0	+	0	+	0	+	+	0	0
Anemia	+	0	0	0	0	0	0	0	0	0	++
↑Blood urea nitrogen	+	0	0	0	±	±	±	±	0	+	+
↑Serum creatinine	+	—	—	—	±	±	±	±	0	+	+
↓GFR	+	0	0	0	±	±	±	±	0	+	+
Serum potassium	±	±	0	0	0	0	0	0	0	+	+
Serum phosphorus	±	0	0	0	0	0	0	0	0	+	+
Serum calcium	0	+	0	0	0	0	0	0	0	+	+
Serum uric acid	0	0	+	0	±	0	±	0	±	+	+
Acidosis	0	0	+	0	0	0	0	0	0	+	+
Proteinuria	+	++++	+	±	±	++	+	0	0	±	±
Hematuria	++	+	±	+	0	+	0	0	++	+	±
RBC casts	+	0	0	0	0	0	0	0	0	±	0
Pyuria	±	0	0	++	0	0	0	±	±	0	0
WBC cast	0	0	0	+	0	0	0	+	0	0	0
Glucosuria	0	0	+	0	0	0	++	0	0	0	0

AGN, Acute glomerulonephritis; *ARF,* acute renal failure; *CRF,* chronic renal failure; *DM,* diabetes mellitus; *GFR,* glomerular filtration rate; *HT,* hypertension; *NS,* nephrotic syndrome; *RBC,* red blood cells; *RC,* renal calculi; *RVT,* renal vein thrombosis; *TD,* tubular disease; *UTI,* urinary tract infection; *UTO,* urinary tract obstruction; *WBC,* white blood cells. *0,* Absent; ±, variable; +, present.

Table 30-3 Characteristic Urine Microscope Findings in Renal Disease

Condition	Protein	Red Blood Cells (per high-power field)	White Blood Cells (per high-power field)	Bacteria	Casts (per low-power field)
Normal	0 to trace	0 to 3	0 to 5	0	Hyaline, occasionally
Glomerulonephritis	1 to 2+	>20	0 to 10	0	Granular red blood cells
Nephrotic syndrome	4+	0 to 10	0 to 5	0	Oval fat bodies; hyaline
Pyelonephritis	0 to 1+	0 to 10	>30	++	Granular white blood cells

Casts are protein conglomerates that outline the shape of the renal tubules in which they were formed. Hyaline casts are composed almost exclusively of protein. Cellular elements may be trapped within hyaline casts, resulting in the formation of granular casts. When heavy proteinuria occurs, accumulation of protein within tubular cells leads to fatty degeneration of the cells and desquamation of cells into the urine; these appear in the urine as oval fat bodies. In acute pyelonephritis, white blood cells may aggregate in the tubules to form pus casts. Red blood cell casts are important markers of glomerular inflammation and should be searched for diligently when any form of glomerular nephritis is suspected. Because white blood cell casts and red blood cell casts degenerate rather quickly into granular casts, if nephritis is suspected, clinicians should be asked to provide fresh urine samples in a timely fashion (within an hour of voiding).

Microscopic examination of the urinary sediment is completed by a search for bacteria and crystals. The presence of crystals in the urine may be a clue to the diagnosis of a specific type of renal calculus. Characteristic urine microscopic findings in healthy individuals and in those with renal disease are provided in Table 30-3. (See Urinalysis section on Evolve.)

KEY CONCEPTS BOX 30-3

- Glomerular filtration rate (GFR) reflects overall kidney function but is not measured directly in clinical practice.
- GFR can be estimated by various methods, including the Modification of Diet in Renal Disease study (MDRD) equation and other related equations, the Cockroft-Gault equation, and timed urine creatinine clearance.
- Tubular function can be assessed by testing the ability to concentrate and dilute urine.
- Urinalysis by dipstick and microscopy is essential in the diagnosis of many renal diseases.

SECTION OBJECTIVES BOX 30-4

- State expected serum concentrations of urea nitrogen, creatinine, and uric acid in renal insufficiency.
- Explain why abnormal blood levels of calcium and phosphorus occur in renal disease, according to alterations in filtration, parathyroid hormone release, and production of active Vitamin D.
- Interpret urine sodium levels in order to diagnose volume depletion, acute renal failure, sodium-retaining states, or the syndrome of inappropriate ADH secretion.
- Explain why the anion gap is increased in patients in renal failure.
- Differentiate glomerular and tubular proteinuria according to what proteins are detected in the urine.
- Outline a laboratory diagnostic strategy to evaluate patients with chronic renal failure.

CHANGE OF ANALYTE IN DISEASE

The changes that occur in analytes are discussed in the section on pathologic conditions of the kidney and are summarized in Table 30-2. In this section, the following question is examined from a different perspective: What does the finding of a biochemical abnormality or group of abnormalities mean in the diagnosis of a pathologic condition in the kidney?

Serum Electrolytes

(see also pp. 539-548)

Sodium

Sodium is the major cation in the extracellular fluid; it usually has a serum concentration of 136 to 145 mmol/L. Sodium and its attendant anions are the major contributors to serum osmolality.[42]

Hyponatremia

Hyponatremia with hypo-osmolality can occur in renal disease because of increased extracellular fluid volume resulting from the kidney's inability to excrete water. This state occurs in chronic renal insufficiency, hypothyroidism, and adrenal insufficiency, and in states that cause increased levels of ADH, such as volume depletion, nephrotic syndrome, cirrhosis, congestive heart failure, and syndrome of inappropriate antidiuretic hormone secretion **(SIADH).**

Hypernatremia

Hypernatremia, by definition a relative water deficit, most frequently occurs in hospitalized patients who cannot access enough electrolyte-free water to replace insensible losses. Hypernatremia also occurs in diabetes insipidus whenever oral fluid intake cannot keep pace with urinary losses.

Chloride

The concentration of chloride in extracellular fluid parallels that of sodium and is influenced by the same factors. Chloride imbalances occur concurrently with sodium imbalances. Hyperchloremia occurs in association with renal tubular acidosis.

Potassium

Potassium is the major cation of intracellular fluid.

Hypokalemia

Hypokalemia usually is associated with overt potassium depletion that results from excessive losses of potassium-rich fluids. Potassium loss may be renal or extrarenal. Increased renal excretion of potassium occurs with diuretic agents, prolonged use of corticosteroids, primary or secondary aldosteronism, and Cushing's syndrome. Hypokalemia from extrarenal potassium losses usually occurs in the gastrointestinal tract and is seen with prolonged vomiting, diarrhea, fistulas of the intestinal tract, and villous adenomas of the colon.

Hyperkalemia

Hyperkalemia, an acute medical emergency, usually is caused by increased cellular breakdown that exceeds the normal renal excretory capacity or by impaired renal excretion.[42] Hyperkalemia may result from (1) increased intake of potassium, as occurs with dietary excess or intravenous potassium administration in the patient with compromised renal function; (2) cellular breakdown, as occurs with extensive burns or rhabdomyolysis (acute muscle necrosis); (3) decreased potassium excretion, as occurs in acute or chronic renal failure, following the use of potassium-sparing diuretics or in adrenal insufficiency or hypoaldosteronism; or (4) transcellular redistribution of potassium, as occurs with acute acidosis, diabetic ketoacidosis, familial hyperkalemic periodic paralysis, and certain drugs (see p. 545, Chapter 28 for specific details).

Creatinine, Urea, and Uric Acid

Progressive renal insufficiency is characterized by retention in the blood of urea, creatinine, and uric acid. In healthy persons, the ratio of serum urea nitrogen to serum creatinine is between 10:1 and 20:1. In the usual case of renal failure caused by intrinsic kidney disease, a similar ratio is seen. Ratios higher than 20:1 occur in renal disease resulting from decreased renal perfusion, such as volume depletion or cardiac failure, but also with gastrointestinal bleeding, excessive protein intake, or protein catabolism. In contrast, urea production and BUN are reduced in the presence of low protein intake and in severe liver disease, thus reducing the BUN-to-creatinine ratio. Ratios also can be elevated because of reduced creatinine resulting from significant muscle loss, from muscle wasting, or from amputation. Uric acid concentration in the blood rises in advanced chronic renal failure, but this rarely results in classical gout.

Calcium and Phosphorus

(see Chapter 33)

Chronic renal failure results in impaired excretion of phosphate and with progressive hyperphosphatemia. This results in a fall in the plasma calcium concentration (hypocalcemia) and secondary hyperparathyroidism. The elevated parathyroid hormone level causes calcium resorption from bone, and normocalcemia or hypercalcemia may result. However, hypocalcemia is more prevalent in uremia, both as a result of the reciprocal fall in plasma calcium concentration as the plasma phosphate level rises and because of reduced calcium absorption in the gut that results from impaired production of 1,25-dihydroxycholecalciferol (vitamin D_3).[10,18] Hypocalcemia is also present in nephrotic syndrome as a result of hypoalbuminemia. However, the ionized serum calcium level remains normal in this condition.

Urinary Electrolytes

Sodium

Urinary sodium determinations are diagnostically useful in 3 clinical settings. First, in volume depletion, the measurement of urinary sodium excretion is helpful in determining the route of sodium loss. A low urinary sodium concentration (less than 10 mEq/L) indicates an extrarenal sodium loss, whereas the presence of a high concentration of sodium in the urine indicates renal salt wasting or adrenal insufficiency. Second, in the differential diagnosis of acute renal failure, urinary sodium excretion will be less than 10 mEq/L in patients with volume depletion who have no intrinsic renal disease and usually will be greater than 30 mEq/L in patients with acute tubular necrosis.[43] In volume depletion, a urine-to-plasma osmolality ratio of more than 1.1 and a urine-to-plasma urea ratio of more than 10 are observed, compared with values of less than 1.05 and less than 10, respectively, in acute tubular necrosis.[43] Third, in hyponatremia, a low urinary sodium concentration (less than 10 mEq/L) indicates avid renal sodium retention, which may be attributable to severe volume depletion or to sodium-retaining states seen in cirrhosis, the nephrotic syndrome, and congestive heart failure. When hyponatremia is associated with urinary sodium excretion that equals or exceeds dietary sodium intake, it is likely that SIADH is present.[42] In these 3 situations, a random urinary sodium concentration can rapidly supply valuable diagnostic information (see p. 542, Chapter 28 for additional details). Calculating a fractional excretion of sodium (FENa) can be more precise than using a random urine sodium concentration, in that it accounts for urine concentration.

$$\text{FENa} = (100\% \times [\text{urine Na/serum Na}] / [\text{urine creatinine/serum creatinine}])$$

A FENa of less than 1% is consistent with a prerenal disease caused by decreased renal perfusion or avid renal sodium retention.

Patients receiving diuretics who are suspected of having prerenal azotemia will not necessarily have a low FENa because of sodium wasting caused by diuretics. Calculating a fractional excretion of urea (FEUrea) thus can be useful in these patients:

$$\text{FEUrea} = (100\% \times [\text{urine urea/serum urea}] / [\text{urine creatinine/serum creatinine}])$$

A FEUrea less than 30% is consistent with a prerenal state.[44]

Chloride

The measurement of urinary chloride is of clinical value only in patients with persistent metabolic alkalosis who are not receiving diuretics (see Chapter 28 for additional details).[42]

Potassium

Urinary potassium levels are helpful in the evaluation of patients with unexplained hypokalemia.[42] The finding of a urinary potassium concentration greater than 10 mEq/L indicates that the kidney is responsible for the potassium loss, whereas a urinary potassium concentration of less than 10 mEq/L in the presence of hypokalemia is strongly suggestive that the gastrointestinal tract is the route of potassium loss (see Chapter 28 for additional details). The trans-tubular potassium gradient (TTKG) can be more precise in the localization of potassium loss. If TTKG ([urine K/serum K]/[urine osms/serum osms]) is less than 7 in the presence of hyperkalemia or greater than 3 in hypokalemia, the potassium abnormality is the result of renal abnormalities.

The urine net charge, or urine anion gap (UAG), is calculated as follows:

$$\text{UAG (mmol/L)} = (\text{UNa} + \text{UK}) - \text{UCl}$$

The UAG can be useful in evaluating patients with non–anion gap metabolic acidoses; a urine net charge that is highly positive, reflecting unmeasured anions, mainly bicarbonate, suggests a type 2 renal tubular acidosis (RTA), and a highly negative urine net charge, reflecting unmeasured cations, mainly ammonium, reflects extrarenal losses of bicarbonate, as occur in diarrhea.

Anion Gap (Serum)

An increased anion gap occurs in renal failure because of the retention of sulfate, phosphate, and organic acid anions (see Chapters 28 and 29).

Proteinuria

Proteinuria of 2 types may occur. In glomerular proteinuria, large quantities of high-molecular-weight protein enter the glomerular filtrate and ultimately appear in the urine. Heavy proteinuria (more than 2 g/day) results from increased glomerular permeability, and the protein loss may be great enough to result in the nephrotic syndrome.[20] In tubular proteinuria, the amount of protein filtered by the glomeruli is not increased, but the low-molecular-weight proteins, which normally are filtered, appear in larger quantities in the final urine because tubular reabsorption is incomplete. Impaired tubular reabsorption of filtered proteins results in modest increases (1 to 3 g/day) in the urinary excretion of low-molecular-weight proteins and albumin.[20] Physiologic increases in protein excretion occur during maintenance of an upright posture, after strenuous exercise, and in normal pregnancy.[20]

The traditional method used for measuring proteinuria is to collect all urine for a 24-hour period. The first voided specimen of the morning is discarded; all urine then is saved for the next 24 hours, ending at the same time on the next morning with the last voided urine saved. Quantitation of 24-hour protein and creatinine excretion is performed. In any given patient whose diet, renal function, and muscle mass remain constant, 24-hour urine creatinine excretion also remains fairly constant. Because of this, creatinine excretion serves as a measure of completeness of the 24-hour collection. The average man excretes 16 to 26 mg, and the average woman excretes 12 to 24 mg, of creatinine per kilogram of ideal body weight. With aging, this value drops to 8 to 15 mg/kg of ideal body weight. Because a timed 24-hour urine specimen is inconvenient to collect, and because difficulties often are associated with assessing the completeness of collection, the concept of measuring the protein-to-creatinine ratio of "spot" urine samples has developed.[45] A value greater than 3 mg protein/mg creatinine indicates nephrotic range proteinuria. The degree of proteinuria determined by this method correlates with the rate of loss of renal function and is a risk factor for progression to end-stage renal disease.[46]

The first sign of renal glomerular disease often is microalbuminuria, a leakage of small amounts of albumin into the urine, too little to be detected with a urine dipstick. Microalbuminuria has significant prognostic implications, including progressive renal failure and worse outcomes with cardiac and other diseases.[47-50] Treatment of patients with microalbuminuria with agents such as angiotensin-converting enzyme (ACE) inhibitors can improve outcomes.[51,52] Therefore, screening patients with a predisposition to renal disease, especially diabetes and hypertension, for microalbuminuria is recommended.[53] The presence of microalbuminuria is established by testing a spot urine sample, preferably obtained from the first void in the morning, for albumin and creatinine. An albumin-to-creatinine ratio greater than 30 μg/mg establishes the diagnosis of microalbuminuria.

Hemoglobin and Hematocrit

Anemia is a common feature of chronic renal failure, and its severity reflects the extent of renal impairment.[19] Progressive anemia usually occurs when the GFR falls below 25 mL/min. The anemia of chronic renal failure is attributable to (1) reduced erythropoietin production as renal mass decreases, (2) inhibitors of erythropoiesis present in the serum of the uremic patient, (3) reduced red blood cell survival in advanced renal failure, and (4) iron deficiency caused by blood loss as a result of the hemostatic defect characteristic of renal failure.[19]

Laboratory Screening and Evaluation of Chronic Kidney Disease

Patients with any of several risk factors for CKD, particularly hypertension, diabetes, or family history of renal disease, should be screened for CKD by testing blood pressure, serum creatinine, and MDRD e-GFR; using urine dipstick to determine the presence of hematuria, pyuria, or proteinuria; and determining the albumin-to-creatinine ratio in a random or early morning urine sample to assess for microalbuminuria.

Patients with CKD stage 3 or worse should undergo specific lab testing to monitor the progression of CKD and to detect the presence of related diseases. Creatinine and MDRD e-GFR should be checked to monitor progression of CKD, hyperkalemia associated with CKD should be ruled out by measuring serum potassium, and serum bicarbonate should be measured to rule out type 1 or 4 RTA. Serum phosphorus and parathyroid hormone (PTH) should be measured to rule out hyperphosphatemia and secondary hyperparathyroidism, and hemoglobin should be measured to assess for anemia of chronic kidney disease. If anemia is present, iron (Fe), total iron-binding capacity (TIBC), and ferritin should be measured to rule out iron deficiency anemia. Albumin generally is monitored to follow nutritional status, which often decreases as a patient reaches the need for renal replacement therapy.

KEY CONCEPTS BOX 30-4

- Serum and urine parameters can assist in identification of numerous renal and non-renal disease states.
- Chronic kidney disease is commonly associated with a constellation of metabolic derangements that should be monitored with regular laboratory testing.

REFERENCES

1. Kapoor M, Chan GZ: Fluid and electrolyte abnormalities, Crit Care Clin 17:503, 2001.
2. Schrier RW: *Manual of nephrology,* ed 6, Philadelphia, 2005, Lippincott Williams & Wilkins.
3. Wagner C, Kurtz A: Regulation of renal renin release, Curr Opin Nephrol Hypertens 7:437, 1998.
4. Singh I, Grams M, Wang WH, et al: Coordinate regulation of renal expression of nitric oxide synthase, renin, and angiotensinogen mRNA by dietary salt, Am J Physiol 270:F1027, 1996.
5. Rajasekaran SA, Barwe SP, Rajasekaran AK: Multiple functions of Na,K-ATPase in epithelial cells, Semin Nephrol 25:328, 2005.
6. Giebisch G, Wang W: Potassium transport: from clearance to channels to pumps, Kidney Int 49:1624, 1996.
7. Mount DB, Yu ASL: Transport of inorganic solutes: sodium, chloride, potassium, magnesium, calcium, and phosphate. In Brenner BM, editor: *Brenner and Rector's The kidney,* Philadelphia, 2008, Saunders Elsevier.
8. Lambers TT, Bindels RJ, Hoenderop JG: Coordinated control of renal calcium handling, Kidney Int 69:650, 2006.
9. Slatopolsky E, Rutherford WE, Rosenbaum R, et al: Hyperphosphatemia, Clin Nephrol 7:138, 1977.
10. Slatopolsky E, Brown A, Dusso A: Role of phosphorus in the pathogenesis of secondary hyperparathyroidism, Am J Kidney Dis 37:S54, 2001.
11. Mountokalakis TD: Magnesium metabolism in chronic renal failure, Magnes Res 3:121, 1990.
12. Androgue HJ, Madias NE: Management of life-threatening acid-base disorders, N Engl J Med 338:26, 1998.
13. Alpern RJ, Preisig PA: Renal acid-base transport. In Schrier RW, editor: *Diseases of the kidney and urinary tract,* Philadelphia, 2007, Lippincott Williams and Wilkins.
14. First MR: *Chronic renal failure,* Garden City, NY, 1982, Medical Examining Publishing.
15. Fouque D, Aparicio M: Eleven reasons to control the protein intake of patients with chronic kidney disease, Nature Clin Pract Nephrol 3:383, 2007.
16. Greenberg A, Cheung AK, National Kidney Foundation: *Primer on kidney diseases,* ed 3, San Diego, 2001, Academic Press.
17. Peart WS: The kidney as an endocrine organ, Lancet 2:543, 1977.
18. Kovesdy CP, Mehrotra R, Kalantar-Zadeh K: Battleground: chronic kidney disorders mineral and bone disease—calcium

obsession, vitamin D, and binder confusion, Clin J Am Soc Nephrol 3:168, 2008.
19. Nangaku M, Eckdardt KU: Pathogenesis of renal anemia, Semin Nephrol 26:261, 2006.
20. Pesce AJ, First MR: *Proteinuria: an integrated review,* New York, 1979, Marcel Dekker.
21. Saxena R, Toto R: Approach to the patient with renal disease. In Brenner BM, editor: *Brenner and Rector's The kidney,* Philadelphia, 2008, Saunders Elsevier.
22. Perazella M, Rastegar A: Disorders of potassium and acid-base metabolism in association with renal disease. In Schrier RW, editor: *Diseases of the kidney and urinary tract,* Philadelphia, 2007, Lippincott Williams and Wilkins.
23. Markowitz GS, Perazella MA: Drug-induced renal failure: a focus on tubulointerstitial disease, Clin Chim Acta 351:31, 2005.
24. U.S. Renal Data System: *USRDS 2007 Annual data report: atlas of chronic kidney disease and end-stage renal disease in the United States,* Bethesda, MD, 2007, National Institutes of Health, National Institute of Diabetes and Digestive and Kidney Diseases.
25. Jawa A, Kcomt J, Fonseca VA: Diabetic nephropathy and retinopathy, Med Clin North Am 88:1001, 2004.
26. William J, Hogan D, Batlle D: Predicting the development of diabetic nephropathy and its progression, Adv Chronic Kidney Dis 12:202, 2005.
27. Wiegmann TB, Chonko AM, MacDougall ML, et al: The role of disease duration and hypertension in albumin excretion of type I diabetes mellitus, J Am Soc Nephrol 2:1587, 1992.
28. Keane WF, Zhang Z, Lyle PA, et al: Risk scores for predicting outcomes in patients with type 2 diabetes and nephropathy: the RENAAL study, Clin J Am Soc Nephrol 1:761, 2006.
29. The Diabetes Control and Complications Trial Research Group: Effect of intensive therapy on the development and progression of diabetic nephropathy in the DCCT, Kidney Int 47:1703, 1995.
30. Bellomo R, Ronco C, Kellum JA, et al: Acute renal failure—definition, outcome measures, animal models, fluid therapy and information technology needs: the Second International Consensus Conference of the Acute Dialysis Quality Initiative (ADQI) Group, Crit Care 8:R204, 2004.
31. Weisbord SD, Chen H, Stone RA, et al: Associations of increases in serum creatinine with mortality and length of hospital stay after coronary angiography, J Am Soc Nephrol 17:2871. 2006.
32. Eknoyan G, Levin NW: K/DOQI clinical practice guidelines for chronic kidney disease: evaluation, classification, and stratification, Am J Kid Dis 39:S1, 2002.
33. Choudhury D, Luna-Salazar C: Preventive health care in chronic kidney disease and end-stage renal disease, Nat Clin Pract Nephrol 4:194, 2008.
34. Bagshaw SM, Gibney RTN: Conventional markers of kidney function, Crit Care Med 36:S152, 2008.
35. Coll E, Botey A, Alvarez L, et al: Serum cystatin C as a new marker for noninvasive estimation of glomerular filtration rate and as a marker for renal impairment, Am J Kidney Dis 36:29, 2000.
36. Rule AD: Understanding estimated glomerular filtration rate: implications for identifying chronic kidney disease [Epidemiology and prevention], Curr Opin Nephrol Hypertens 16:242, 2007.
37. Knight EL, Verhave JC, Spiegelman D, et al: Factors influencing serum cystatin C levels other than renal function and the impact on renal function measurement, Kidney Int 65:1416, 2004.
38. Cockcroft DW, Gault MH: Prediction of creatinine clearance from serum creatinine, Nephron 16:31, 1976.
39. Schwartz GJ, Haycock GB, Edelmann CM Jr, et al: A simple estimate of glomerular filtration rate in children derived from body length and plasma creatinine, Pediatrics 58:259, 1976.
40. Counahan R, Chantler C, Ghazali S, et al: Estimation of glomerular filtration rate from plasma creatinine concentration in children, Arch Dis Child 51:875, 1976.
41. Zhou H, Hewitt SM, Yuen PST, et al: Acute kidney injury biomarkers: needs, present status, and future promise, NephSAP 5:63, 2006.
42. Kamel KS, et al: Interpretation of electrolyte and acid-base parameters in blood and urine. In Brenner BM, editor: *Brenner and Rector's The kidney,* Philadelphia, 2008, Saunders Elsevier.
43. Anderson RJ, Barry DW: Clinical and laboratory diagnosis of acute renal failure, Best Pract Res Clin Anaesthesiol 18:1, 2004.
44. Carvounis CP, Nisar S, Guro-Razuman S: Significance of the fractional excretion of urea in the differential diagnosis of acute renal failure, Kidney Int 62P:2223, 2002.
45. Morales JV, Weber R, Wagner MB, et al: Is morning urinary protein/creatinine ratio a reliable estimator of 24-hour proteinuria in patients with glomerulonephritis and different levels of renal function? J Nephrol 17:666, 2004.
46. Suzuki H, Kanno Y, Nakamoto H, et al: Decline of renal function is associated with proteinuria and systolic blood pressure in the morning in diabetic nephropathy, Clin Exp Hypertens 27:129, 2005.
47. Basi S, Fesler P, Mimran A, et al: Microalbuminuria in type 2 diabetes and hypertension: a marker, treatment target, or innocent bystander? Diabetes Care 31:S194, 2008.
48. Keane WF, Brenner BM, de Zeeuw D, et al: The risk of developing end-stage renal disease in patients with type 2 diabetes and nephropathy: the RENAAL study, Kidney Int 63:1499, 2003.
49. Klausen K, Borch-Johnsen K, Feldt-Rasmussen B, et al: Very low levels of microalbuminuria are associated with increased risk of coronary heart disease and death independently of renal function, hypertension, and diabetes, Circulation 110:32, 2004.
50. Gerstein HC, Mann JF, Yi Q, et al: Albuminuria and risk of cardiovascular events, death, and heart failure in diabetic and nondiabetic individuals, JAMA 286:421, 2001.
51. Brenner BM, Cooper ME, de Zeeuw D, et al: Effects of losartan on renal and cardiovascular outcomes in patients with type 2 diabetes and nephropathy, N Engl J Med 345:861, 2001.
52. Ibsen H, Olsen MH, Wachtell K, et al: Reduction in albuminuria translates to reduction in cardiovascular events in hypertensive patients: losartan intervention for endpoint reduction in hypertension study, Hypertension 45:198, 2005.
53. National Kidney Foundation: K/DOQI clinical practice guidelines for chronic kidney disease: evaluation, classification, and stratification, Am J Kidney Dis 39:S1, 2002.

INTERNET SITES

www.kidney.org—National Kidney Foundation (US)

www.kidney.ca—Canadian Kidney Foundation

www.kidney.org.au—Australian Kidney Foundation

http://www.fpnotebook.com/Renal/index.htm

http://www.epodiatry.com/education_sub3.asp?topic=General%20Medicine%20and%20Surgery&sub1=Learning%20resources&sub2=Nephrology—a nice assortment of informative articles about nephrology

http://www.kcl.ac.uk/teares/gktvc/vc/lt/rtg/sbdl18.pdf—Some illustrative cases with answers

www.isn-online.org—International Society of Nephrology

www.asn-online.org—American Society of Nephrology

http://www.bertholf.net/rlb/Lectures/Lectures/Cardiac%20Markers%20and%20Renal%20Function.pps works. Or try http://www.bertholf.net/rlb/Lectures/Lectures/Cardiac—Microsoft PowerPoint lecture by Robert L. Bertholf, PhD, Associate Professor of Pathology, Chief of Clinical Chemistry and Toxicology

http://www.emedicine.com/med/topic3437.htm—Nephrolithiasis: Acute Renal Colic, May 3, 2007

http://www.kidney.org/professionals/kdoqi/—KDOQI guidelines for treatment of kidney disease

http://www.usrds.org—A wealth of statistics on CKD in the United States

http://www.nature.com/isn/literature/index.html—A monthly digest of nephrology literature

http://www.emedicine.com/med/topic1596.htm—Nephritis, Interstitial, October 10, 2006

The Liver: Function and Chemical Pathology

Chapter 31

D. Robert Dufour

Chapter Outline

Key Terms

AFP-L3 A lectin-reactive glycosylated isoform of alpha-fetoprotein (AFP) used as a biomarker for hepatocellular carcinoma (HHC).

canaliculi Fine channels that run between liver cells, which eventually merge to form bile ductules. They form the initial portion of the bile duct drainage system.

cholestasis Accumulation of normal excretory products of the liver (bile acids, cholesterol, bilirubin, metabolites of drugs) due to impaired drainage through the bile duct (biliary) system.

cirrhosis A liver disorder characterized by replacement of normal liver architecture by regenerative nodules surrounded by bands of fibrous tissue. Cirrhosis is usually a complication of chronic hepatitis but also may result from chronic biliary tract obstruction and congestive heart failure.

Crigler-Najjar syndrome A familial form of nonhemolytic jaundice caused by the absence (type 1) or reduction (type 2) of glucuronyl transferase activity in the liver, leading to unconjugated hyperbilirubinemia and, in type 1, central nervous system damage.

cytochrome P-450 A family of cellular enzymes containing heme groups that absorb light at 450 nm. These enzymes are involved in the metabolism of drugs and other xenobiotics.

detoxification The process of changing the chemical structure of a compound to make it more water soluble and, therefore, more readily eliminated.

Dubin-Johnson syndrome A familial form of chronic, nonhemolytic jaundice caused by a defect in the hepatic excretion of conjugated bilirubin.

Gilbert's syndrome A common familial form of nonhemolytic unconjugated hyperbilirubinemia that is associated with mutations of the promoter region of the gene coding for glucuronyl transferase. It universally has a benign clinical course but may cause jaundice during fasting or times of stress.

gluconeogenesis The formation of glucose from lactate or amino acids by means of the Cori cycle.

glycogenesis The biochemical formation of glycogen from glucose.

glycogenolysis The biochemical degradation of glycogen to form glucose.

hemochromatosis Systemic accumulation of excess iron (mainly in liver, heart, pancreas) most commonly resulting from inherited disorders in iron-sensing genes.

hepatitis Inflammation of the liver produced by a variety of infections, toxins, and other causes, with damage primarily affecting hepatocytes.

hepatocellular disease Any disease in which the liver cells (hepatocytes) are destroyed.

hepatocyte A liver cell that performs virtually all the functions ascribed to the liver.

jaundice A syndrome characterized by hyperbilirubinemia to an extent that causes yellow discoloration of skin and mucous membranes (also called *icterus*).

kernicterus Literally "nuclear jaundice," resulting from deposition of unconjugated bilirubin in the basal ganglia of the brain, which causes cell destruction and encephalopathy.

parenchymal A general term referring to components, such as parenchymal organs (referring to the internal organs of the body) or the functioning cells of an organ (*see* hepatocyte).

periportal fibrosis The deposition of fibers or fibrous material within the portal triads of the liver.

portal triad An anatomic structure in sections of the liver that contains branches of the hepatic artery, portal vein, and bile ducts.

portal vein A large vein that carries blood from 1 organ to another; most commonly, refers to the vein that carries blood from the intestinal tract to the liver, along with products of digested food.

Wilson's disease Also called *hepatolenticular degeneration,* an inherited disease caused by mutations in an ATPase that cause a defect in copper metabolism; associated with excessive copper accumulation in liver, basal ganglia of brain, and eye, and with low plasma ceruloplasmin.

xenobiotic Any organic compound that is foreign to the body, such as drugs and organic poisons.

Methods on Evolve

Alanine aminotransferase
Albumin
Alkaline phosphatase, total
Alpha$_1$-antitrypsin
Ammonia
Aspartate aminotransferase
Bilirubin
Gamma-glutamyl transferase
Lactate dehydrogenase and lactate dehydrogenase enzymes

SECTION OBJECTIVES BOX 31-1

- Describe the gross anatomy of the liver, including the 2 sources of oxygenated blood.
- List at least 4 important functions of the liver.
- Explain the processes in the normal formation of bilirubin, including the importance of its binding to albumin, not only for transport to the liver, but to prevent toxicity.
- Describe the 2 mechanisms for metabolism and detoxification of endogenous and exogenous substances.
- Explain why blood urea levels fall and blood ammonia levels rise in diseases that affect the liver's metabolism and detoxification mechanism.

ANATOMY AND NORMAL FUNCTION OF LIVER

The liver is the largest internal organ of the body, usually weighing 1 to 1.5 kg. It is located in the upper right part of the abdominal cavity, just below the diaphragm. The structure of the liver and its vascular and arrangements is illustrated in Fig. 31-1. The liver is supplied by 2 major sources of oxygen-containing blood: the hepatic artery and the **portal vein.** The portal vein also carries nutrients from the intestinal tract to the liver for further metabolism and synthesis into needed body compounds. The bile duct leaves the liver as 2 separate ducts from the right and left lobes, or as a common hepatic duct. The bile duct carries bile from the liver to the gallbladder for storage; the gallbladder is attached to the inferior surface of the liver. When stimulated by cholecystokinin, the gallbladder contracts and releases bile through its duct, termed the *cystic duct,* which joins the common hepatic duct to form the common bile duct. This structure carries bile to the intestine, passing through the head of the pancreas before entering the duodenum at the ampulla of Vater.

Microscopically, the liver is separated into numerous small functional units, termed *acini,* centered around **portal triads,** which are interconnecting loose bands that contain branches of the portal vein, hepatic artery, and bile duct. Blood from the portal vein and blood from the hepatic artery mix together and enter a network of small, capillary-like blood vessels lined with perforated (fenestrated) endothelial lining, termed *sinusoids,* before reaching the central veins, which fuse to form the hepatic vein. This joins the inferior vena cava just before it crosses the diaphragm. The fenestrated endothelium allows free passage of molecules from the blood into the space surrounding the most important liver cells, the **hepatocytes.** Hepatocytes perform almost all of the functions of the liver, including metabolism, synthesis of critical components, formation of bile, and endocrine functions. Small grooves are present between adjacent hepatocytes, termed **canaliculi.** These small passages coalesce and eventually enter into small bile ducts within the portal triads. Several other cell types are found within the acini. Kupffer cells, part of the phagocytic system of the body, are randomly distributed along the sinusoids; they ingest any bacteria that may arrive via the portal vein; they also remove any antigen-antibody complexes that reach the liver. Stellate cells lie in the space between the sinusoids and the hepatocytes. Under normal circumstances, stellate cells serve to regulate blood flow through the liver; they also store fat-soluble vitamins, particularly vitamin A. When they are stimulated by injury, stellate cells transform into collagen-forming cells, which are the source of fibrous tissue in chronic **hepatitis** and cirrhosis. Oval cells are found near the portal region; they represent a reservoir for regenerating bile duct cells; when the liver is severely injured, these cells also serve as hepatic stem cells for regenerating hepatocytes.

The liver is the primary organ responsible for the metabolism of carbohydrates, proteins, lipids, porphyrins, and bile

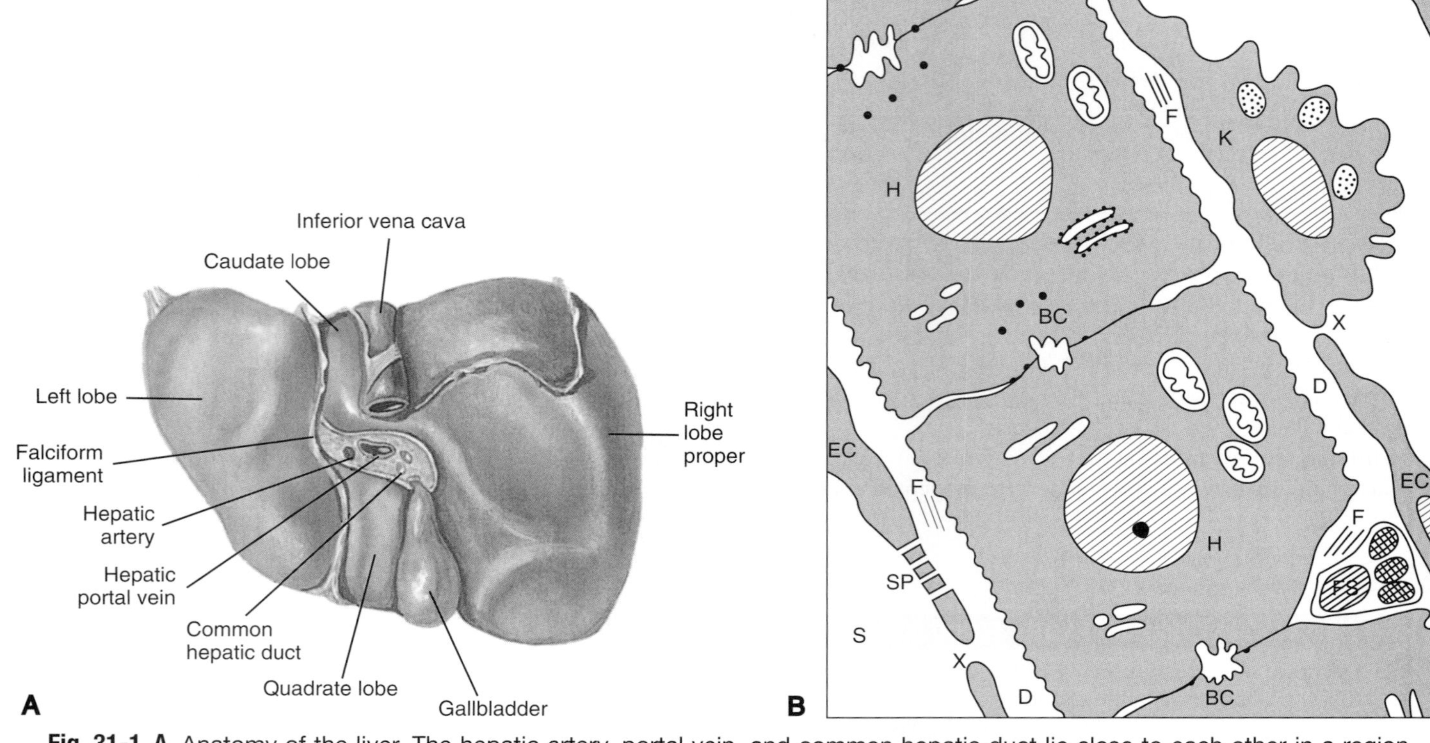

Fig. 31-1 A, Anatomy of the liver. The hepatic artery, portal vein, and common hepatic duct lie close to each other in a region known as the *porta hepatis.* The gallbladder is close to the bottom surface of the liver and stores bile within it. Its small duct (termed the *cystic duct*) joins with the common hepatic duct to form the common bile duct, which (as illustrated in Fig. 34-1) passes through the head of the pancreas before draining into the duodenum at the ampulla of Vater. **B,** Schema of structures with lobules. *BC,* Bile canaliculis; *D,* space of Disse; *E,* erythrocyte; *EC,* endothelial cell; *F,* reticulum fibers; *FS,* fat-storing (stellate) cell; *H,* hepatocyte; *K,* Kupffer cell; *N,* nerve fiber; *S,* sinusoid; *SP,* fenestrae of endothelial cell forming a sieve plate; *X,* intercellular gap. (**A,** From Mahan LK, Escott-Stump S: *Krause's food, nutrition, and diet therapy*, ed 11, St Louis, Saunders, 2004. **B,** From Tanikawa K, editor: *Ultrastructural aspects of the liver and its disorders,* ed 2, Tokyo, 1979, Igaku-Shoin.)

acids. It is responsible for synthesizing most plasma proteins except the immunoglobulins, which are produced by the lymphocytic plasma cell system. The liver is also the principal site for storage of iron, glycogen, lipids, and vitamins. Furthermore, the liver plays an important role in the **detoxification** of **xenobiotics** and the excretion of metabolic end products such as bilirubin, ammonia, and urea. Laboratory tests for evaluation of liver disease are based, in part, on evaluation of these normal functions of the liver. The usefulness of these tests has been evaluated in guidelines developed by the National Academy of Clinical Biochemistry (NACB).[1,2]

Bilirubin

Bilirubin is the product of heme metabolism. Heme, mainly found in hemoglobin but also present in myoglobin and cytochromes, is degraded by heme oxygenase to carbon monoxide and biliverdin, which is futher converted to bilirubin (Fig. 31-2). Approximately 250 to 300 mg of bilirubin is generated daily, about 85% from aging red blood cells. Bilirubin is highly insoluble in water and must be transported by albumin to the liver for further metabolism. Albumin binding prevents lipid-soluble bilirubin from crossing cell membranes and accumulating in cells. Extremely high levels of bilirubin can exceed albumin-binding capacity and allow unbound bilirubin to cross the immature blood-brain barrier in neonates, resulting in toxic damage to cells in the basal ganglia, this condition is termed **kernicterus.** However, exposure to light (in vivo or in vitro) can isomerize the *trans* forms of bilirubin to a *cis* configuration, creating a more water-soluble product that can be excreted in the urine without further metabolism. This is the basis for the use of phototherapy to treat neonatal jaundice, but it also explains why exposure of blood samples to light can increase direct reacting bilirubin in the laboratory.

In the liver, bilirubin diffuses into the space surrounding the sinusoids and binds to transport proteins to cross the cell membranes; it is bound to ligandin in hepatocytes (Fig. 31-3). Bilirubin then is modified by sequential attachment of 1 or 2 molecules of glucuronic acid, catalyzed by the enzyme uridine diphosphate (UDP)-glucuronyl transferase 1, to produce water-soluble conjugated bilirubin. An active transport mechanism moves monoconjugated and diconjugated bilirubin into the canaliculi, and eventually, bile containing conjugated

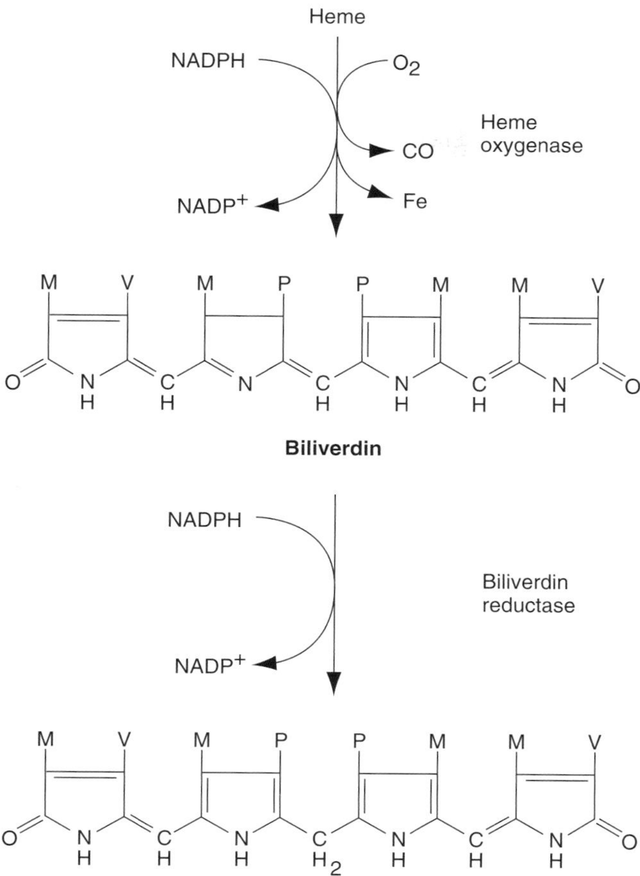

Fig. 31-2 Formation of bilirubin from heme. *M,* Methyl; *P,* propionyl; *V,* vinyl.

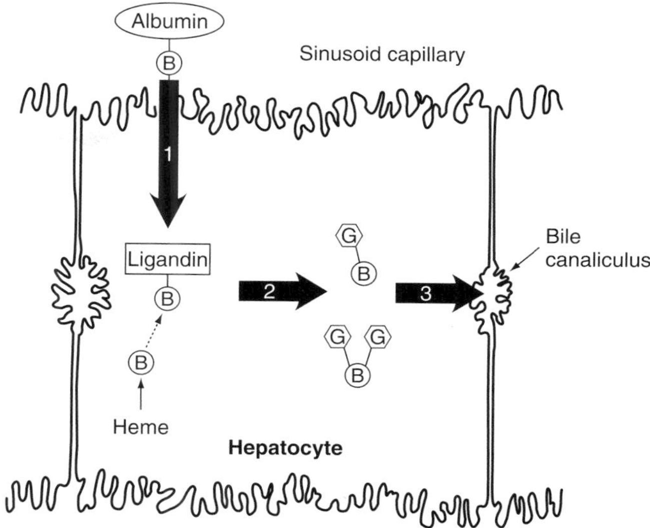

Fig. 31-3 Hepatic metabolism of bilirubin. The indicated steps are *(1)* uptake, *(2)* conjugation, and *(3)* excretion. A small amount of bilirubin is produced by breakdown of heme-containing proteins within hepatocytes. *B,* Bilirubin; *G,* glucuronic acid.

bilirubin reaches the intestinal tract. About 85% of bile bilirubin is in the diconjugate form, and about 15% is monoconjugated. This active transport of conjugated bilirubin is the rate-limiting step in the metabolism of bilirubin and is highly efficient in normal individuals, so that only trace quantities of conjugates reach plasma. Within the intestine, intestinal bacteria reduce bilirubin to colorless, water-soluble urobilinogen, which eventually is oxidized to stercobilins, the major pigments in stool. Urobilinogen can also be reabsorbed from the intestine and returned to the liver through the portal vein; urobilinogen is then extracted by hepatocytes and re-excreted into bile. Blood urobilinogen is also filtered into urine. An increase in urine urobilinogen indicates either increased production of bilirubin and delivery of conjugates to the intestine, as occurs in hemolysis or other states of increased heme turnover, or it suggests decreased clearance by the damaged liver, most often seen in cirrhosis but also in recovery from liver damage. Measurement of urinary bilirubin or urobilinogen provides little additional information in the evaluation of individuals with suspected liver disease.[1]

When disease prevents the excretion of conjugated bilirubin into bile, it enters plasma, is filtered by the kidneys, and is excreted in urine. Some monoconjugated bilirubin can become covalently bound (through a nonenzymatic process) to lysine residues on proteins, particularly albumin. This protein-bound form of bilirubin has been variously termed *biliprotein* or *δ-bilirubin.* Although the half-life of conjugated bilirubin in blood appears to be about 24 hours, the half-life of biliprotein is that of albumin, which is about 20 days. The presence of biliprotein thus can cause prolonged jaundice in persons recovering from liver disease. The function of biliprotein is unknown.

Protein Metabolism

Most plasma proteins are synthesized in the liver; major exceptions are the immunoglobulins. Table 31-1 lists some of the major liver proteins found in plasma along with their properties. The liver has extensive reserve capacity for protein synthesis, so decreased plasma protein levels are not an early indicator of liver dysfunction. Several factors affect hepatic protein synthesis. The ability of amino acids (most often derived from ingested food and from catabolism of other body proteins) to reach the liver through the portal vein is a critical first step in protein production. A number of humoral factors affect hepatocyte synthesis of proteins in a differential fashion, for example, certain cytokines, such as interleukin (IL)-6, stimulate production of so-called acute-phase response proteins, while estrogens, androgens, and glucocorticosteroids have more selective effects on various liver-produced proteins. Decreased plasma oncotic pressure also increases liver protein synthesis in a nonselective fashion. When synthesis of protein is impaired, plasma levels decrease at a rate related to the half-

Table 31-1 Major Liver-Produced Plasma Proteins

Protein	Electrophoretic Migration	Approximate Concentration (g/L)	Functions
Transthyretin	Prealbumin	1.4	Reserves binding of thyroxine; transports retinol/retinol-binding protein complex
Albumin	Albumin	37-50	Oncotic pressure; transports organic molecules, cations; amino acid reservoir
α_1-Antitrypsin	α_1	1-3	Major protease inhibitor
Orosomucoid	α_1	0.5-1	Inflammatory response modifier; transports acidic drugs
High density	α_1	3-6	Reverse transport of cholesterol
Haptoglobin	α_2	1-3	Binding of free hemoglobin
α_2-Macroglobulin	α_2	3-5	Protease inhibitor
Ceruloplasmin	α_2	0.2-0.4	Oxidizes ferrous to ferric ion to allow transferrin binding; contains most of serum copper (not transport)
Transferrin	β	2-4	Transports iron from GI tract, macrophages
Low-density lipoprotein	β	4-10	Delivery of cholesterol to tissue
C3 component of complement	β	0.5-1	Major component of innate immune system
Fibrinogen	β-γ	2-4	Precursor to fibrin, major component of clot
C-reactive protein	γ	1-5	Component of innate immune system

life of the proteins, which is long for albumin but very short (6 hours) for coagulation factor VII.

Because of the short half-life of coagulation factors, prothrombin time represents a very sensitive test of liver protein synthetic function, although it is nonspecifically affected by other factors (such as use of anticoagulants, vitamin K deficiency, and consumptive coagulation disorders). Because of variation in reagents, laboratories often use the international normalized ratio (INR) to standardize prothrombin time results for persons receiving vitamin K antagonists such as warfarin. This correction leads to marked differences in INR results among persons with liver disease, which can create problems for evaluating the severity of liver dysfunction using the MELD score[3] (discussed later). Studies suggest that the use of samples from persons with liver disease to create a liver-specific INR can eliminate these differences.[4,5]

Carbohydrate Metabolism

The liver is the major organ regulating blood glucose levels, as is discussed more fully in Chapter 38. The liver directly responds to both insulin and glucagon, the 2 major glucose regulatory hormones, which alter the activity of several processes in the liver. Insulin increases hepatocyte uptake of glucose and promotes the production of glycogen, a polymer of glucose used for energy storage. Glucagon increases **glycogenolysis,** making glucose available for entry into plasma; it also stimulates **gluconeogenesis,** the production of glucose from amino acids. The liver's ability to perform these processes is retained until very late in liver disease, but hypoglycemia may be a problem in cases of severe acute and chronic liver failure.

Lipid Biosynthesis and Transport

Lipids, for the sake of this discussion, include only free fatty acids, triglycerides, glycerophosphatides, sphingolipids, cholesterol, and cholesterol esters. General chemical structures for these lipids and their metabolism are discussed in Chapters 27 and 37. The liver, which is the major organ involved in lipid metabolism, is the major source for circulating cholesterol; it (along with diet) provides triglycerides to the blood as well. All of the major lipoproteins, with the exception of chylomicrons, are produced in the liver, and lipoprotein remnants are removed by the liver. Cholesterol is also used to synthesize bile acids, which are needed for normal digestion of dietary fat. Decreased levels of lipids and bile acids are commonly seen in advanced chronic liver failure. With obstruction to biliary drainage, abnormalities in plasma lipid and bile acid levels are common. An abnormal lipoprotein, termed *lipoprotein X,* composed of cell membrane fragments bound to albumin, often accumulates in states of **cholestasis.**[6] Although not atherogenic, it often is measured incorrectly in laboratory assays for low-density lipoprotein cholesterol.[7]

Metabolic End-Product Excretion and Detoxification

Two basic mechanisms are involved in the metabolism of endogenous and exogenous compounds to make them more water soluble and available for excretion. The first, termed *phase I reactions,* involves modification of the compound by oxidation or hydroxylation; it often is mediated by 1 or more enzymes in the **cytochrome P-450** system. The second, termed *phase II reactions,* involves conjugation of the compound to other chemical groups such as glucuronic acid, sulfate, or amino acids. A number of tests have been developed to evaluate these metabolic steps, most commonly involving metabolism of exogenous agents such as caffeine, lidocaine, aminopyrine, or galactose.[8] Although these tests may be more sensitive than more commonly used tests, metabolism may be affected by other drugs that affect the P-450 system, and such tests of xenobiotic metabolism have not found widespread acceptance. One of the major functions of the liver is the metabolism of amine remnants of protein metabolism through the hepatic urea cycle. When this process is defective, blood urea (nitrogen) levels fall, and levels of ammonia increase. Although brain accumulation of ammonia is involved in the pathogenesis of hepatic encephalopathy,[9] blood ammonia levels do not correlate to degree of encephalopathy[10]; NACB guidelines do not recommend their use for monitoring of liver disease but suggest that they may be helpful in evaluating persons with encephalopathy of unknown origin.[2]

KEY CONCEPTS BOX 31-1

- The liver is the body's primary storage and metabolic organ for carbohydrates, lipids, and bile pigments.
- The liver produces most plasma proteins, affecting serum oncotic pressure and coagulation.
- The liver is responsible for end-product metabolism of many endogenous compounds and is responsible for excretion and detoxification of exogenous compounds like drugs or poisons.
- Bilirubin, produced as a breakdown product of heme, is taken up by the liver and conjugated to more water-soluble forms. Conjugated bilirubin is excreted into the intestines where it is metabolized to urobilinogen.

SECTION OBJECTIVES BOX 31-2

- Define jaundice, and describe the various pathologic states associated with jaundice.
- List pathologic liver conditions, and describe serum biochemical alterations associated with these diseases.
- Discuss chronic hepatitis according to definition, 2 major changes to the liver that occur, importance of monitoring ALT levels, clinical course, 3 common causes, and typical associated laboratory results.
- Discuss how autoimmune hepatitis and hemochromatosis cause chronic hepatitis.
- Discuss the etiology of and associated laboratory tests for the diagnosis of Wilson's disease and alpha-1-antitrypsin deficiency.
- Correlate laboratory results for total, conjugated, and unconjugated bilirubin; urobilinogen; AST; ALT; ALP; GGT; LDH; anti-mitochondrial and anti-smooth muscle antibodies; alpha-fetoprotein; and des-gammacarboxy prothrombin with the associated liver disease.

CLINICAL PATTERNS OF LIVER DISEASE

Jaundice

Jaundice (or icterus), a yellowish discoloration of the sclera and skin, is the clinical manifestation of increased serum bilirubin concentration. Although normal values are usually less than 1 mg/dL, increased bilirubin can typically be detected as jaundice when serum bilirubin reaches 3 (in adults) to 5 (in neonates) mg/dL. Because of this dramatic physical finding, jaundice has been recognized as a key sign of liver disease since at least the time of ancient Egyptian medical writings. Increased bilirubin typically results from 1 of 3 major causes: overproduction, decreased conjugation, or decreased excretion (Fig. 31-4); the first 2 lead to increases in unconjugated bilirubin, and the last causes increased conjugated bilirubin.

Increased production of bilirubin is usually the result of increased red blood cell breakdown. The most common mechanism is hemolysis; however, ineffective erythropoiesis (as often occurs in thalassemia major and pernicious anemia) and breakdown of hemoglobin in large hematomas can also be responsible. Rarely, increased release of myoglobin from extensive skeletal muscle injury can cause overproduction of bilirubin. Chronic, increased bilirubin production leads to markedly increased bilirubin delivery to bile, which can lead to development of bilirubin-containing gallstones.

Defective conjugation of bilirubin is probably the most common cause of unconjugated hyperbilirubinemia. In neonates, the glucuronyl transferase enzymes are not fully active, so jaundice is extremely common in the newborn period. Usually, this resolves spontaneously by about 7 to 10 days of life. In adults, the most common cause of chronic increases in bilirubin is **Gilbert's syndrome.** All individuals with this syndrome have a mutation in the upstream promoter region for the gene for UDP-glucuronyl transferase 1 *(UGT1)*, which inserts an extra TA sequence into the TATA box region of the gene, resulting in reduced production (about 30% less) of the enzyme[11] (Table 31-2). This particular mutation is found in about 15% of all adults, but not all develop hyperbilirubinemia. Because the enzyme also metabolizes the chemotherapeutic agent irinotecan, testing for mutations in the *UGT1* gene has been recommended for all who are to receive this drug, to decide whether its dosage should be reduced. Cirrhosis is often associated with impaired hepatic conjugation, leading to increased unconjugated bilirubin. Rare mutations in the *UGT1* gene itself give rise to more severe reductions in enzymatic activity; this is the cause of **Crigler-Najjar** (CN) **syndrome.**[12] In the rare CN type I disorder, an autosomal recessive trait, almost complete absence of enzymatic activity leads to severe unconjugated hyperbilirubinemia and kernicterus. The autosomal dominant CN type II form has milder, chronic hyperbilirubinemia.

Decreased excretion of conjugated bilirubin leads to predominantly conjugated hyperbilirubinemia. The most common cause of increased conjugated bilirubin is impaired liver function, either caused by damage to hepatocytes (hepatitis) or by obstruction of biliary drainage. Occasionally, drugs such as sex steroids may impair bilirubin excretion, causing conjugated hyperbilirubinemia. In sepsis, possibly resulting from impaired hepatic energy generation, increased conjugated bilirubin also develops. When excretion of conjugated bilirubin is significantly impaired, stools often lose their normal brown color because of lack of bilirubin-derived pigments; in contrast, urine becomes brown because of the water-soluble conjugated bilirubin. These findings often precede the development of detectable jaundice. With recovery of function, the colors of urine and stool typically return to normal

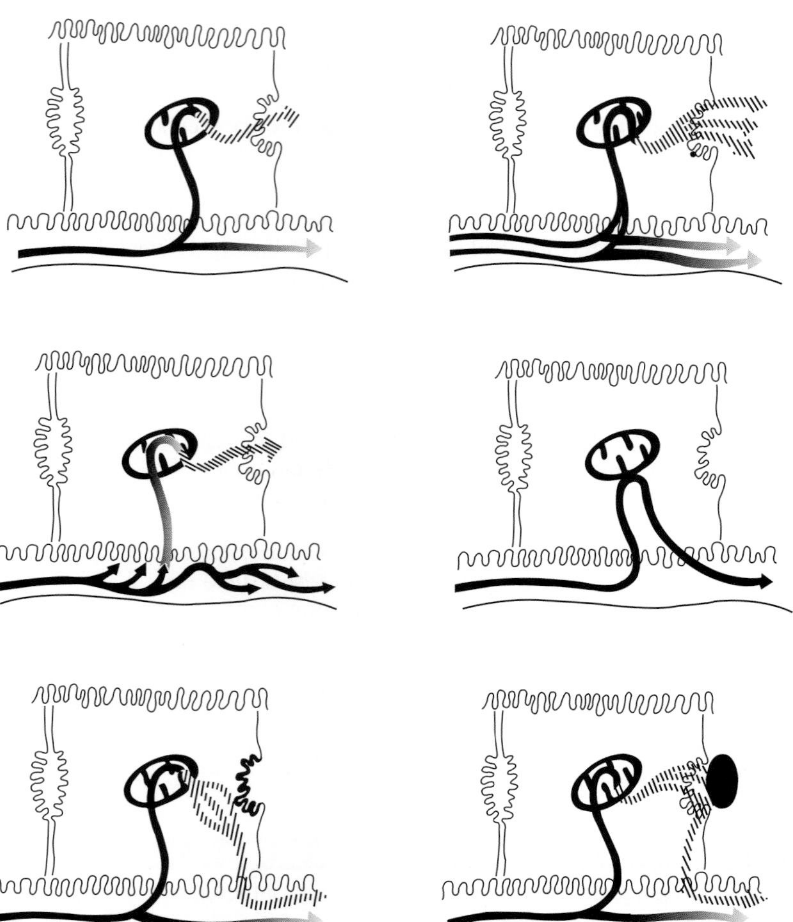

Fig. 31-4 Mechanisms of hyperbilirubinemia. **A,** Normal bilirubin metabolism with hepatocyte uptake of unconjugated bilirubin *(dark arrow)* and microsomal conjugation and excretion of conjugated bilirubin *(striped arrow)*. **B,** Hemolytic jaundice, in which increased bilirubin production results in increased excretion of conjugated bilirubin and a rise in excess (exceeding liver capacity) unconjugated bilirubin in blood. **C,** Gilbert's disease, in which decreased hepatic uptake results in a large increase in blood levels of unconjugated bilirubin. **D,** Physiological jaundice, in which microsomal conjugating system is not functional, resulting in a large increase in unconjugated bilirubin. Congenital deficiency is called *Crigler-Najjar syndrome*. **E,** Dubin-Johnson syndrome, in which there is a biochemical defect preventing secretion of conjugated bilirubin, resulting in a backflow into blood. **F,** Intrahepatic or extrahepatic obstruction in which a physical block prevents secretion of conjugated bilirubin. Hepatocellular disease results in a pattern similar to a combination of **C** and **D.** (From Leevy CM, editor: *Evaluation of liver funciton*, ed 2, Indianapolis, 1974, Lilly Research Laboratories.)

long before jaundice resolves because of the long half-life of δ-bilirubin.

Rarely, congenital defects in bilirubin excretion may cause conjugated hyperbilirubinemia. The most common of these is the **Dubin-Johnson syndrome,** wherein an autosomal recessive trait leads to impaired levels of an adenosine triphosphate (ATP)-binding cassette protein, which causes reduced ability to excrete bilirubin and other pigments from the liver, leading to accumulation of black-brown lipofuchsin in the liver, as well as to conjugated hyperbilirubinemia. Rotor syndrome, a rare autosomal recessive trait similar to Dubin-Johnson syndrome, produces conjugated hyperbilirubinemia, but without the liver pigmentation; the exact cause of this syndrome has not yet been determined.

Acute Hepatitis

The term *acute hepatitis* refers to a disorder in which damage to the liver (specifically to hepatocytes) occurs over a relatively short period of time. In contrast to the typical picture of acute inflammation seen in most organs, in which damage begins within hours of injury onset and inflammatory cells are predominantly granulocytes, acute hepatitis is a disorder that often develops gradually, persists for several weeks, and is characterized by predominantly lymphocytic inflammatory infiltrates. The most common causes of acute hepatitis are usually thought to be viruses, particularly hepatitis A (HAV), hepatitis B (HBV), and hepatitis C (HCV) (see Chapter 32); however, with development of vaccines for HAV and HBV, and with reduced transmission of sexually transmitted and transfusion-transmitted disease, acute viral infection has become an uncommon cause of acute hepatitis.[13] The most common causes of acute hepatitis are drugs (most commonly by eliciting an immune response, less commonly by direct toxicity of the drug or its metabolites[14]), ethanol, and ischemia (typically resulting from shock). In 1 study of hospitalized patients, ischemic injury and drug toxicity were responsible for the overwhelming majority of cases of acute hepatitis.[15] The most common cause of acute liver failure is ingestion of acetaminophen, which is responsible for about half of cases. Chronic disorders such as autoimmune hepatitis and Wilson's disease sometimes have an acute presentation.

Although jaundice is often the primary symptom of acute hepatitis, it is actually absent in most cases. When present, it is characteristically accompanied by dark urine (conjugated

Table 31-2 Genetic Diseases of the Liver

Disorder	Gene	Protein Product
α_1-Antitrypsin deficiency	*SERPIN1* (Pi)	α_1-Antitrypsin (serine protease inhibitor)
Crigler-Najjar syndrome	*UGTA1*	UDP-glucuronyl transferase 1
Dubin-Johnson syndrome	*COMOAT*	Canalicular multispecific organic transporter
Gilbert's syndrome	*UGTA1* (promoter)	UDP-glucuronyl transferase 1
Hemochromatosis	*HFE*	HFE protein (cell membrane protein involved in regulating iron metabolism)
Wilson's disease	*ATP7B*	ATPase, Cu(2+)-transporting beta polypeptide

UDP, Uridine diphosphate; *ATP,* adenosine triphosphate; *Cu,* copper.

Table 31-3 Typical Laboratory Findings in Acute Hepatitis of Various Causes

Feature	Viral	Alcoholic	Ischemic/Toxic	Drug Induced	Autoimmune
Peak AST	300-800	100-300	1000-10,000	300-800	300-1000
Peak ALT	400-1200	50-125	800-6000	400-1200	400-1200
AST/ALT ratio	<1	>1, usually >2	>1 for 1-2 d, then <1	<1	<1
Duration ALT	4-5 weeks	4-5 weeks	10-12 days	1-3 weeks	2-6 months
Peak ALP	<3 URL	<3 URL	<1.5 URL	>3 URL	>3 URL
Prothrombin time	Nl-sl INC	Nl-sl INC	INC	Nl-sl INC	Nl-INC
Other	Viral serologies	None	None	None	Autoimmune markers; low albumin, INC globulins

ALP, Alkaline phosphatase; *ALT,* alanine aminotransferase; *AST,* aspartate aminotransferase; *INC,* increased; *URL,* upper reference limits; *Nl,* normal; *sl,* slightly.

bilirubin). Weakness, loss of appetite, and/or nausea and vomiting may be the only symptoms in many cases. Acute hepatitis is often recognized because of a rapid, pronounced rise in the hepatocyte enzymes aspartate aminotransferase (AST) and alanine aminotransferase (ALT). Typically, AST is higher than ALT for the first day or two of disease, but the longer half-life of ALT causes this enzyme to become higher in most cases. When the ratio of AST to ALT in the hepatocyte is altered (as occurs with alcohol abuse, in cirrhosis, and with pyridoxine deficiency), AST may remain higher than ALT. Alkaline phosphatase (ALP) is usually normal or minimally (<3 × the upper reference limits) increased; greater elevations usually indicate cholestasis or cholestatic hepatitis (discussed later). The pattern and duration of laboratory abnormalities differ according to the cause of acute hepatitis, as shown in Table 31-3 and Figs. 31-5 and 31-6; this pattern may provide a clue to the origin of acute hepatitis.

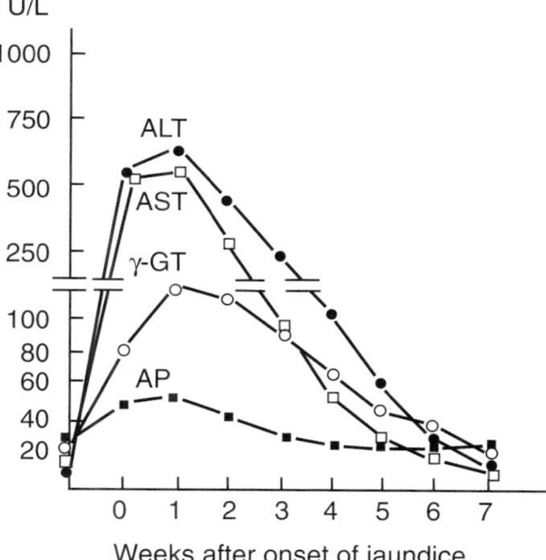

Fig. 31-5 Course of serum enzyme activities in acute viral hepatitis. (From Schmidt E, Schmidt FW: *Brief guide to practical enzyme diagnosis,* Houston, 1977, Boehringer Mannheim Diagnostics.)

Prognosis in acute hepatitis is generally good, and recovery is usually complete; however, a small percentage of those with acute hepatitis develop acute liver failure, often clinically apparent by decreased mental awareness; confusion progressing to coma in the most severe cases. Laboratory tests are often used to help evaluate prognosis; the most widely used criteria include the King's College criteria and the MELD score (discussed in detail later), although it is not clear which (if either) of these indices is more reliable.[16] Serum bilirubin, prothrombin time, and creatinine seem to be independent predictors of outcome[17] and should be monitored regularly as long as they continue to worsen. In contrast, changes in serum enzymes are not prognostically important in acute hepatitis, and no relationship of degree of enzyme elevation or duration of increased enzymes to outcomes has been detected. Recently, low levels of Gc-globulin (vitamin D–binding protein), and more specifically, of its actin-free form, have been shown to provide prognostic information similar to the King's College criteria and the MELD score.[18]

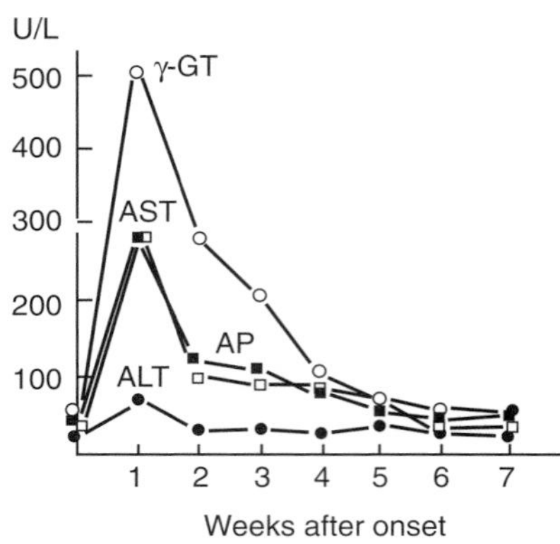

Fig. 31-6 Course of serum enzyme activities in acute alcoholic hepatitis. (From Schmidt E, Schmidt FW: *Brief guide to practical enzyme diagnosis,* Houston, 1977, Boehringer Mannheim Diagnostics.)

Table 31-4 Laboratory Tests to Establish Cause of Chronic Hepatitis

Cause	Screening Tests	Confirmatory Tests
Hepatitis B virus	HBsAg	HbeAg, HBV DNA
Hepatitis C virus	Anti-HCV	HCV RNA
NAFLD	Ultrasonography	Biopsy
Hemochromatosis	Serum iron, iron-binding capacity, ferritin	*HFE* gene analysis
Wilson's disease	Ceruloplasmin, serum/urine copper	Liver biopsy; genetic studies
Autoimmune hepatitis	ANA, anti–smooth muscle antibody	Liver biopsy

HbeAg, Hepatitis B e antigen; *HBsAg,* hepatitis B surface antigen; *HBV DNA,* hepatitis B virus deoxyribonucleic acid viral load; *HCV,* hepatitis C virus; *NAFLD,* nonalcoholic fatty liver disease; *RNA,* ribonucleic acid viral load.

Chronic Hepatitis

Chronic hepatitis is typically defined as inflammatory damage to the liver that persists for longer than 6 months. Because of its persistence, chronic hepatitis is a much more commonly encountered disease than is acute hepatitis. Chronic hepatitis has 2 major components: inflammatory damage to the liver parenchyma, and healing by fibrosis. Inflammatory damage is best reflected in plasma activities of the hepatocyte enzymes AST and, particularly, ALT; in fact, there is a correlation between the extent of inflammatory damage and serum ALT.[19] However, not all of those with chronic hepatitis have elevated ALT, for example, as many as 15% of those with chronic HCV have normal ALT,[20] and many individuals with fatty liver disease have normal ALT.[21] Other laboratory tests, including those of liver function, are typically normal, and symptoms are nonspecific or absent.

Chronic hepatitis is associated with both destruction of hepatocytes and replacement of damage by scar tissue. Damaged hepatocytes are replaced by regeneration of hepatocytes from progenitor cells. Accumulation of scar tissue initially occurs in the portal tracts of the liver (**periportal fibrosis**) and may lead to bands of fibrous tissue that distort the normal liver architecture (termed *bridging fibrosis*); over time, extension of bridges can lead to the development of cirrhosis. Recognition of the extent of fibrosis generally is based on liver biopsy, but it would be advantageous to have laboratory tests that can detect the accumulation of fibrous tissue within the liver. Direct measurement of substances deposited in scar tissue, such as hyaluronate, has a reasonable correlation with degree of fibrosis. A number of predictive algorithms that use routine or nonroutine laboratory tests have been proposed; these also have reasonable correlation with extent of fibrosis. These indices have good negative predictive value, identifying individuals with little or no fibrosis with good accuracy, and their use has helped to reduce the number of biopsies in counties where these indices have been widely used.[22,23] They appear less reliable for predicting presence of or degree of fibrosis.

Common causes of chronic hepatitis include nonalcoholic fatty liver disease (NAFLD), HBV, and HCV; together, these 3 disorders are probably responsible for more than 95% of cases, although specific data are lacking. A summary of laboratory tests useful for determining the cause of chronic hepatitis is provided in Table 31-4.

Nonalcoholic fatty liver disease is defined as the presence of increased fat in hepatocytes in a person with minimal or no alcohol intake; its most severe histologic form, termed *nonalcoholic steatohepatitis (NASH),* histologically resembles acute alcoholic hepatitis but exhibits the clinical course of chronic hepatitis. NAFLD most commonly occurs in individuals with features of the metabolic syndrome, such as insulin resistance, obesity, hypertension, and dyslipidemia (particularly increased triglycerides and low high-density lipoprotein [HDL] cholesterol).[24] Although the diagnosis (as well as recognition of the more severe form, NASH) can be established only by liver biopsy, the presence of NAFLD is often suspected by the combination of fat in the liver seen on imaging studies (especially ultrasound) with no other obvious cause for identified increased liver enzymes. Several biomarkers are under study, but none has been found to be reliable at this time.[25]

Less commonly, autoimmune hepatitis and **hemochromatosis** are causes of chronic hepatitis. Autoimmune hepatitis is a relatively common autoimmune disease that primarily affects the liver. In contrast to other forms of chronic hepatitis, it is typically characterized by increased immunoglobulins and the presence of autoantibodies (antinuclear antibody [ANA] and anti-actin [smooth muscle] antibodies in type 1, anti–liver kidney microsomal antibodies in type 2, and anti–soluble liver antigen antibodies in type 3) and rapid progression to cirrhosis if untreated.[26]

Hemochromatosis is an inherited disorder that is associated with iron accumulation in **parenchymal** organs such as the liver, heart, pancreas, and endocrine glands (see Chapter 39). It is most often due to mutations in the *HFE* gene on chromosome 6.[27] Although all individuals with a specific mutation (C282Y, representing replacement of cysteine by tyrosine at amino acid 282) appear to have higher serum iron levels than those lacking the mutation (higher in homozygotes than in heterozygotes), iron overload develops in less than half of homozygotes, and the disease hemochromatosis may occur in as few as 10% of homozygotes (about 25% of males, <5% of females).[28] Mutations in other genes involved in iron metabolism have also been associated with hemochromatosis.[27] Hemochromatosis is the most common genetic cause of liver dysfunction, so testing for this disorder is appropriate in those with chronic liver disease. Initial testing is usually based on transferrin saturation ([serum iron × 100%]/total iron-binding capacity) or unsaturated iron binding capacity; a high level of transferrin saturation (>45% in females, >50% in males) or low unsaturated iron-binding capacity on a fasting sample is an indication for genetic testing.[29] Ferritin levels correlate better with the likelihood of liver damage; those with ferritin levels <300 ng/mL almost never incur liver damage, while the likelihood of progressive liver fibrosis is high if ferritin is >1000 ng/mL.[28] Hemochromatosis is usually managed by therapeutic phlebotomy of up to 1 unit of blood per week until serum ferritin is <50 ng/mL; this allows mobilization of iron for use in hematopoiesis and reduces iron accumulation in tissue. Maintenance phlebotomy then is done periodically as needed.

Two other inherited traits can also cause chronic hepatitis. **Wilson's disease** is a rare disorder (1 in 30,000) that results from mutations in an adenosine triphosphatase (ATPase) coded for by the *ATP7B* gene on chromosome 13, which is involved in the transport of copper into the Golgi apparatus for incorporation into ceruloplasmin and into the bile for excretion. More than 400 different mutations in this gene have been linked to the development of Wilson's disease. Most affected individuals are compound heterozygotes for different mutations, making genetic testing difficult; however, because certain mutations are common in specific populations, a small number of mutations can identify a large fraction of affected individuals through the use of population-specific probes.[30] Recently, a novel approach that included testing for 5 known mutations and 3 single-nucleotide polymorphisms detected most affected individuals, suggesting that genetic screening may be feasible.[31]

Wilson's disease leads to accumulation of copper in tissues, most prominently in the liver, the basal ganglia of the brain, and the eye (producing Kayser-Fleischer rings). In the liver, increased copper can lead to acute or chronic hepatitis. In the acute form, copper is rapidly released from damaged hepatocytes, often causing hemolytic anemia and acute renal failure as well. Laboratory findings in chronic Wilson's disease include decreased ceruloplasmin, decreased total but increased free plasma copper, and increased urine copper. Because ceruloplasmin is an acute-phase reactant, it may not be decreased in acute forms of Wilson's disease, and plasma copper is often increased in any form of acute hepatitis, as is urine copper. Because these laboratory tests may not be diagnostic in acute presentations of Wilson's disease, other laboratory findings (such as low alkaline phosphatase activity, hemolysis, and acute renal failure) may be needed for suspicion of the diagnosis.[32]

α_1-Antitrypsin is the most important plasma inhibitor of serine proteases (serpins); it is coded for by the *SERPINA1* gene on chromosome 14 (formerly called the *Pi* gene). The most important mutation involves a single amino acid substitution, which produces a variant with markedly retarded electrophoretic mobility, termed the *ATZ variant*. This mutation impairs protein folding, preventing release of the protein from the liver, and markedly reduces plasma protease inhibition.[33] In addition, the abnormally folded protein polymerizes, producing inclusions of ATZ within hepatocytes. Although homozygosity for this variant is common (estimated 1:1000 to 1:2000 individuals of northern European ancestry), a minority of affected individuals develop liver disease; in fact, evidence suggests that even those heterozygous for ATZ may have an increased risk of liver damage when exposed to other factors that can damage the liver, such as HCV infection.[34] Thus, the exact role of deficiency in liver disease remains unclear. Because α_1-antitrypsin is an acute-phase reactant, NACB guidelines suggest that phenotyping (usually with isoelectric focusing) to identify variants of α_1-antitrypsin that are present rather than quantitative levels should be used to detect the disorder.[1]

Cholestatic Disorders

Failure to excrete waste products from the hepatocyte into the biliary tract and intestine is referred to as *cholestasis*. Obstruction of biliary drainage can occur from many causes. In some cases, functional obstruction of the canaliculi, often with coexisting hepatocyte damage (cholestatic hepatitis), is evident; this often occurs as an adverse reaction to drugs, but it can occur with infectious agents such as HAV, HBV, and HCV. Obstruction may affect small ducts within the liver because of space-occupying lesions (such as primary or metastatic tumors and granulomas), infiltrative processes (such as amyloidosis or leukemias/lymphomas), or damage to small intrahepatic bile ducts. Finally, cholestasis may be caused by obstruction of large bile ducts within the liver or between the liver and pancreas. In this latter situation, dilatation of bile ducts proximal to the point of obstruction can often be seen on imaging studies.

Laboratory tests are helpful in detecting the presence of cholestasis but often are not helpful in determining its cause. With cholestasis, a gradual increase in canalicular enzymes such as ALP and gamma-glutamyl transferase (GGT) is generally seen; ALP often lags behind GGT (Fig. 31-7). With acute cholestasis, especially that due to gallstones, only a mild increase is often seen in ALP, but a transient increase in AST and ALT (often to levels seen in acute hepatitis) along with a rapid decrease to within the reference interval even if obstruction persists may cause diagnostic confusion. As obstruction persists, AST and ALT decrease and ALP and GGT rise to a plateau. It is generally not possible to distinguish intrahepatic from extrahepatic causes of cholestasis by laboratory testing alone. When AST and ALT increases are persistent, the cause

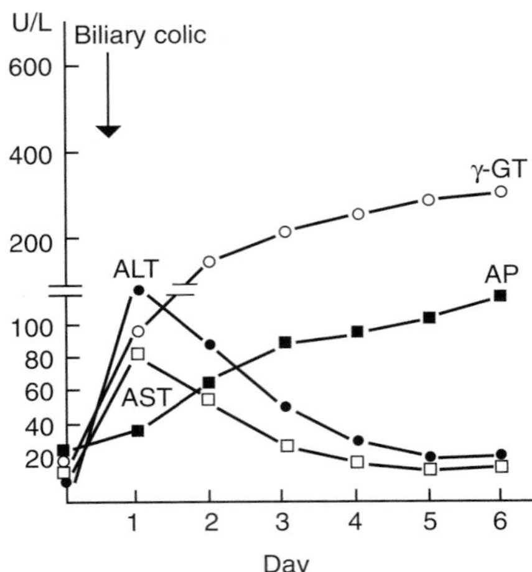

Fig. 31-7 Course of serum enzyme activities in obstructive jaundice. (From Schmidt E, Schmidt FW: *Brief guide to practical enzyme diagnosis,* Houston, 1977, Boehringer Mannheim Diagnostics.)

is more likely to be intrahepatic, but this distinction is not absolute.

Two presumably autoimmune diseases target the bile ducts. Primary biliary cirrhosis (PBC) is the more common of the two. It occurs predominantly in women, with peak incidence during middle age, and causes progressive damage to and loss of intrahepatic bile ducts. The disease is usually associated with antibodies to the pyruvate decarboxylase enzyme complex in mitochondria, often detected as mitochondrial antibodies. This disease is slowly progressive over time, and cirrhosis typically does not develop until after 10 or 20 years of disease, if at all. PBC is often associated with other autoimmune processes, particularly Sjögren's syndrome. Primary sclerosing cholangitis (PSC) typically causes patchy damage primarily affecting the extrahepatic bile ducts, although in some cases, intrahepatic ducts are also involved. It occurs most commonly in young to middle-aged males and is often (80% of cases) associated with ulcerative colitis. Although these are seldom used to help make the diagnosis, about 50% of PSC cases are associated with atypical perinuclear antineutrophil cytoplasmic antibodies (ANCAs).

Cirrhosis

Over time, scarring of the liver by disease may so distort the architecture that nodules of hepatocytes are completely surrounded by fibrous tissue; this is the pathologic definition of ***cirrhosis.*** Any cause of chronic hepatitis or chronic cholestasis can progress to cirrhosis. In its early stages, cirrhosis produces no signs or symptoms; however, over time, a number of complications may develop, including portal hypertension (often manifested by bleeding from dilated veins in the esophagus and stomach or elsewhere in the GI tract, and by recurrent ascites), hepatic encephalopathy (brain dysfunction due to accumulation of chemicals normally cleared by the liver), hepatorenal syndrome (renal dysfunction due to shunting of blood away from the renal cortex), and liver failure. Cirrhosis also markedly increases the risk of development of hepatocellular carcinoma, which is discussed in greater detail below.

Table 31-5 Laboratory Findings in Progression of Chronic Hepatitis to Cirrhosis

Laboratory Parameter	Change	Early, Mid, or Late Finding
Platelet count	Decrease	Early
Prothrombin time	Increase	Early
AST/ALT ratio	>1	Early-Mid
Albumin	Decrease	Early-Mid
Globulins	Increase	Early-Mid
AFP	Increase	Early-Mid
ALP	Increase	Mid
Cholesterol	Decrease	Late
BUN/Urea	Decrease	Late
Ammonia	Increase	Late

AFP, α-Fetoprotein; *ALP,* alkaline phosphatase; *ALT,* alanine aminotransferase; *AST,* aspartate aminotransferase; *BUN,* blood urea nitrogen.

Laboratory tests that assess fibrosis (discussed earlier) may allow recognition of advanced fibrosis but usually cannot separate cirrhosis from less advanced stages. As liver scarring worsens, several routinely measured laboratory parameters display changes that often can allow recognition of cirrhosis before the clinical features mentioned earlier become apparent (Table 31-5). Routine laboratory tests are also used to evaluate prognosis in persons with cirrhosis through calculation of the MELD (model for end-stage liver disease) score, which is determined as follows:

$$\begin{aligned}\text{MELD} &= 6.43 + 9.57 * \ln(\text{creatinine [mg/dL]}) \\ &\quad + 3.78 * \ln(\text{bilirubin [mg/dL]}) + 11.2 \ln(\text{INR}) \\ &\quad (\text{maximum creatinine 4.0 mg/dL})\end{aligned}$$

Scores greater than 15 are generally considered the point at which liver transplantation may be considered, with scores over 20 suggesting high risk of short-term mortality without transplantation. Variation in score is based on interlaboratory differences in creatinine measurement, and especially in INR, which can lead to different priorities for transplantation.[3] The recent effort to harmonize creatinine values will likely improve standardization of evaluation of patient risk, but the use of alternatives to the INR (as discussed earlier) will likely be needed to produce maximal similarity between institutions in evaluating the need for transplantation.

Liver Tumors

The liver is one of the organs that is most commonly involved by tumors, especially tumors that have metastasized from other organs. A number of benign tumors can also occur in the liver, most commonly hemangiomas, but laboratory tests are usually not helpful in their recognition or differential diagnosis. Occasionally, especially with multiple tumors (as often occur with metastatic malignancies), increased levels of canalicular enzymes such as GGT and ALP may lead to imaging studies that detect the presence of tumor. The 2 important primary liver malignancies are hepatocellular carcinoma and cholangiocarcinoma.

Hepatocellular carcinoma (HCC) is a common tumor throughout the world, although it is relatively uncommon in North America and Europe. The incidence of HCC has been increasing in recent years, mainly because cirrhosis develops in persons infected with HCV. Almost all cases of HCC in North America and Europe affect individuals with cirrhosis, although HBV infection can lead to HCC without cirrhosis. The risk of HCC once cirrhosis is present is estimated to be 3% to 5% per year.

When detected clinically, HCC has a dismal prognosis (less than 10% 1-year survival). This has led to interest in screening individuals with cirrhosis for HCC. Although no clinical guidelines have been put forth to recommend screening, it is a common practice among physicians who care for those with cirrhosis, based on data from high prevalence areas (such as Taiwan) that indicate that screening leads to improved survival from HCC. Common approaches to screening involve the use of serum biomarkers and imaging studies to look for mass lesions. α-Fetoprotein (AFP) is the most commonly used biomarker; depending on the cutoff value used, sensitivity of AFP may be as high as 90% (at the upper reference limit), but specificity and positive predictive value are poor at these values. Much higher values of AFP (>20 to 50× the upper reference limits) have high specificity for HCC but poor (50% to 60%) sensitivity. Other biomarkers, notably **AFP-L3** and des-gammacarboxyprothrombin (also called *PIVKA-II*), have been approved as diagnostic tests and are used by some centers to screen high-risk patients.[35]

Cholangiocarcinoma is much less frequent than HCC. Although most cases arise without recognized risk factors, PSC and certain parasitic infections of the biliary tract markedly increase the risk of its development. Cholangiocarcinomas tend to arise from larger bile ducts and often present with cholestasis because of bile duct obstruction. CA 19-9 is often elevated in persons with cholangiocarcinoma and can be used as a tumor marker.

Liver Transplantation

Liver transplantation is becoming increasingly common, and between 85% and 90% of patients survive their first transplant for at least 1 year. It is important to monitor these patients for liver function, as well as early signs of rejection (see Chapter 54). The calcineurin (protein phosphatase 2B) inhibitors cyclosporin A and FK-506 (tacrolimus) are widely used as immunosuppressive agents to aid in graft acceptance, although other immunosuppressive agents such as sirolimus and mycophenolate mofetil may also be used alone or in combination with a calcineurin inhibitor. Monitoring of whole blood concentrations of these drugs is important for maintaining effective drug concentrations; levels considered "therapeutic" are often lower at longer times after transplantation, because the risk of rejection is lower with liver transplantation than with transplantation of many other organs.

Maintenance of post-transplantation liver status can be assessed by measurement of the traditional liver enzymes such as ALT, lactate dehydrogenase (LD), GGT, and ALP, in conjunction with other tests, such as prothrombin time. Findings of these tests in post-transplantation patients should be interpreted in the same manner as those in other patients. A rise in liver-associated enzymes often provides evidence of either recurrence of liver disease (especially with hepatitis C and autoimmune hepatitis) or rejection of the transplant. In transplant patients whose initial liver injuries typically do not recur after transplantation, increased enzymes are often considered a sign of rejection; however, in those patients in which recurrence of disease is common, biopsy is usually needed to distinguish recurrent disease from rejection.

CHANGE OF ANALYTE IN DISEASE

Bilirubin

As is discussed in the NACB guidelines on liver disease,[2] a variable relationship has been noted between the measurement of conjugated and unconjugated bilirubin and the actual amounts present (see Evolve method). Direct-reacting bilirubin assays measure most (but not all) conjugated and δ-bilirubin, typically in the range of 70% to 90%.

Serum bilirubin analysis is helpful in differentiating the causes of jaundice. Prehepatic jaundice results in a large increase in unconjugated bilirubin because of the increased release and metabolism of hemoglobin after hemolysis. However, because the transport of bilirubin into the liver and the formation of the glucuronide conjugate become rate-limiting in prehepatic jaundice, no increase or only a slight increase in serum conjugated bilirubin is observed. Additionally, because of increased levels of conjugated bilirubin excreted by the liver, urinary urobilinogen and fecal urobilin concentrations are elevated, but urinary bilirubin (the freely soluble, conjugated form) is absent.

In contrast, cholestatic disorders and hepatitis are characterized by large increases in serum-conjugated bilirubin. δ-Bilirubin (bilirubin covalently bound to albumin) also increases in these disorders; however, the measurement of delta bilirubin as a diagnostic tool has not achieved widespread acceptance. Hepatic excretion of bilirubin metabolites is low in posthepatic obstructive jaundice, and urinary bilirubin can usually be demonstrated.

Enzymes

Hepatocytes contain a large number of enzymes that allow them to perform their metabolic functions. With injury to cells, these enzymes may be released into plasma, where their activity can be measured as an indicator of liver damage. Although a variety of these have been investigated as markers of liver injury, 4 enzymes are most widely used: aspartate (EC 2.6.1.1) and alanine (EC 2.6.1.2) aminotransferases (AST and ALT, respectively), alkaline phosphatase (ALP, EC 3.1.3.1), and gamma-glutamyl transferase (GGT, EC 2.3.2.2). Another commonly measured enzyme, lactate dehydrogenase (LDH, EC 1.1.1.27), is also present in hepatocytes but is not as helpful as the other 4. The ability of these enzymes to aid in the differential diagnosis of liver disease can be explained by their relative abundance within hepatocytes and their subcellular locations.

The aminotransferases AST and ALT catalyze the conversion of aspartate and alanine to oxaloacetate and pyruvate, respectively. (See Methods on Evolve for discussion of measurement of activity of the aminotransferases.) AST and ALT are not specific to the liver; they are found in skeletal and cardiac muscle (AST activity is similar in muscle and liver; ALT activity in muscle is only about 20% to 30% of that in liver). Lesser amounts of AST and ALT are also found in the kidney, and small amounts are present in red blood cells. In tissues that contain these enzymes, aminotransferases are each present as 2 different isoenzymes in the cytoplasm and in mitochondria, although the amount of mitochondrial ALT is small compared with the cytoplasmic form. For AST, a large amount of mitochondrial isoenzyme is found within hepatocytes, but it is seldom released into the circulation.

Within the hepatocyte cytoplasm, normally more AST than ALT is found by a factor of about 1.5; however, the amount of cytoplasmic ALT declines with alcohol abuse, pyridoxine deficiency, and, in cirrhosis, increasing the intracellular ratio of AST to ALT. In plasma, the cytoplasmic forms of the 2 enzymes have markedly different half-lives, with that of AST being about 16 to 18 hours and that of ALT being about 42 to 48 hours. With most causes of hepatocyte injury, therefore, AST is typically higher than ALT at onset, but after a short time (usually 1 to 2 days), ALT becomes higher because of its slower clearance. Although LD is also a cytoplasmic enzyme whose level within hepatocytes is similar to that of AST and ALT, its normal plasma level is only about 10% to 20% that of AST and ALT and the half-life of the liver-dominant isoenzyme 5 is only about 4 to 6 hours. In very early liver injury, therefore, such as that seen following episodes of shock or toxin ingestion, LD may be increased to levels similar to those of AST and ALT, but these levels rapidly fall toward normal.

Alkaline phosphatase (ALP) is actually a family of enzymes that hydrolyze monophosphate esters at an alkaline pH (≈ 10). Four major genes code for production of ALP, but most serum alkaline phosphatase is coded for by the tissue-nonspecific ALP gene on chromosome 1, which produces a polypeptide found in both bone and liver isoenzymes. These differ in their carbohydrate content, mainly in their degree of sialation. (See Methods on Evolve for discussion of measurement of activity of ALP and its isoenzymes.) Other genes code for production of intestinal, placental, and germ cell isoenzymes.

Within the liver, ALP is bound onto inner canalicular surfaces of the hepatocyte by a lipid linkage. With obstruction of bile duct drainage, bile acids can dissolve the lipid linkage, as well as small fragments of cell membrane with attached ALP, causing a progressive rise in plasma activity. Increased ALP of liver origin thus is usually an indication of obstruction of biliary drainage, but it does not identify the level of obstruction. ALP is also a sensitive marker of obstructive disease caused by tumors. In contrast, ALP is not normally released into plasma with hepatocyte injury. Membrane-bound ALP migrates more rapidly than the non–lipid-bound form and is often identified as the "fast liver," "macrohepatic," and "alpha-1" isoenzyme in descriptions of electrophoretic separation; however, identifying its presence does not seem to be a matter of clinical importance.

Gamma-glutamyl transferase, like ALP, is a membrane-bound enzyme; it plays a major role in glutathione metabolism and resorption of amino acids from the glomerular filtrate and from the intestinal lumen. Because the prostate contains significant GGT activity, serum activity is higher in healthy men than in women. Measurement of GGT activity is discussed in Methods on Evolve. Although GGT activity is highest in renal tissue, serum GGT generally reflects release of enzyme from liver.

Liver production of GGT is increased by medications that induce microsomal enzymes, particularly ethanol, many anticonvulsant agents, and histamine receptor blockers. As for ALP, obstruction of biliary drainage leads to disruption of the lipid linkage for GGT, thus increasing plasma activities; the membrane fragments described above have GGT, as well as ALP, attached to them. In contrast to ALP, however, no increase in GGT is noted with bone disease. GGT, which is strongly correlated with body mass index, has been found to be an independent predictor of kidney damage (microalbuminuria) in diabetic and hypertensive individuals[36]; these associations (along with others described in the next paragraph) limit the usefulness of GGT as a routine test for liver disease, and NACB guidelines recommend against its routine use.[2]

A number of other factors affect interpretation of levels of the liver enzymes described above (see Table 31-6). It has proved difficult to determine appropriate reference limits for enzymes in adults; it is not clear whether some of the factors that affect plasma levels are actually physiologic (e.g., body mass index) or pathologic, because high body mass index increases the likelihood of NAFLD (discussed in detail earlier). NACB guidelines recommend that laboratories have separate reference limits for men and women for each of these enzymes, and it is clear that separate reference limits are needed for children and adults, with values changing throughout the childhood period. It is likely that reference samples should not include persons with obesity,[37] although some have questioned the cost-effectiveness of this approach.[38] Even when such an approach is used, however, 1 study showed that for ALT, persons with values in the highest tertile of the reference interval had a significantly higher risk of developing fatty liver disease over a short follow-up period.[21] It is unclear whether it will ultimately be necessary to report ALT (and AST) reference limits with information on quartile or tertile cutoff points, as is done for high-sensitivity C-reactive protein (CRP) measurements.

Autoantibodies

Several autoantibodies have been found to be helpful in the recognition of specific liver diseases. The most commonly used of these are anti-mitochondrial antibodies and anti–smooth muscle (or anti-actin) antibodies, which are the major laboratory tests involved in recognition of their associated autoimmune diseases. Mitochondria contain a number of enzymes, and the anti-mitochondrial antibodies seen in primary biliary cirrhosis react with the dihydrolipoamide acyltransferase component of the pyruvate decarboxylase complex (so-called M2 type of anti-mitochondrial antibodies). Autoimmune hepatitis is associated with a number of autoantibodies, the most important of which are anti–smooth muscle antibodies,

Table 31-6 Factors Affecting Interpretation of Plasma Levels of "Liver" Enzymes

Factor	AST	ALT	ALP	GGT
Age	Levels in children 20% higher than in adults, reach adult levels by age 20	Levels in children less than half those in adults; gradually INC to adult levels by age 25	Levels in children 3-4 times those in adults, gradually DEC to adult levels by age 25	Levels in children 20% of those in adults. In men, reach adult level by age 25; in women, continue to increase throughout life
Gender	40% higher in men than in women	40% higher in men than in women	10% higher in men than in women until after menopause, then 10% higher in women	In adults, twofold higher in men than in younger women, similar after age 50
Race	15% higher in men of African ancestry	No effect	10%-15% higher in those of African ancestry	Twofold higher in those of African ancestry
Food ingestion	No effect	No effect	INC as much as 30 IU/L after meals in those of blood groups O, B (intestinal isoenzyme)	DEC after meals
Body mass index	40%-50% higher in obese	40%-50% higher in obese	25% higher in obese	25% higher in overweight, 50% higher in obese
Exercise	INC with strenuous exercise	INC with strenuous exercise, less than for AST	No effect	No effect
Diurnal variation	No effect	15% lower at night	No effect	No effect

ALP, Alkaline phosphatase; *ALT,* alanine aminotransferase; *AST,* aspartate aminotransferase; *DEC,* decrease; *GGT,* gamma-glutamyl transferase; *INC,* increase.

seen in type 1 autoimmune hepatitis (the only variant commonly seen in the United States). Although these autoantibodies were initially detected by their reaction with tissue sections (stomach was often used, as smooth muscle and mitochondria-rich parietal cells were both present), many assays now use purified antigens, particularly actin—the major target of smooth muscle antibodies. Other types of autoimmune hepatitis may have other autoantibodies, such as antibodies to liver-kidney microsomes (anti-LKM1) in type 2 and antibodies to soluble liver antigen (SLA) in type 3.

Other Analytes

α-Fetoprotein (AFP) is one of the major proteins produced during fetal life; fetal plasma levels during the second trimester of pregnancy are approximately 1 million times higher than those in healthy adults. AFP is also produced by a number of tumors and falls under the category of oncofetal antigen. Similar to other oncofetal antigens, AFP is produced by benign cells during regeneration after injury. Therefore, AFP levels are often increased in recovery from acute hepatitis and in persons with chronic hepatitis and cirrhosis. Hepatocellular carcinomas and hepatoblastomas also produce AFP, and AFP can be used as a tumor marker for these malignancies. Several isoforms of AFP are present in serum; one, termed the *L3 variant,* is able to bind to lectin derived from lentils (lens culinaris), while other isoforms cannot. The presence of increased amounts of the L3 variant (>10% of total AFP) is more specific for hepatocellular carcinoma than is total AFP.[35]

As was mentioned earlier, warfarin works by blocking the activation of clotting factors II, VII, IX, and X; the inactive forms are collectively termed *proteins induced by vitamin K antagonists* (or absence), or *PIVKA;* in the case of factor II (prothrombin), PIVKA-II is also called des-gammacarboxy prothrombin (DCP). Although DCP typically is not found in persons with liver disease, it is present in increased amounts in those with acute hepatitis and with hepatocellular carcinoma. DCP has been used extensively in Japan in screening for HCC and is often positive in cases where AFP is negative. Similar to AFP, it may be slightly increased in cirrhosis without the presence of AFP. An assay for measuring DCP is now approved for use in the United States; it appears to add to the usefulness of AFP in recognizing hepatocellular carcinomas.[39]

KEY CONCEPTS BOX 31-2

- Hyper-unconjugated bilirubinemia can be caused by increased red blood cell (RBC) destruction or by the liver's inability to take up or to conjugate bilirubin.
- Hyper-conjugated bilirubin can be caused by hepatocellular disease or by blockage of the biliary tract.
- Drugs and pathogens are the primary causes of acute hepatitis; chronic hepatitis is caused primarily by nonalcoholic fatty liver disease (NAFLD), hepatitis B virus (HBV), and hepatitis C virus (HCV).
- Wilson's disease is caused by a genetic inability to metabolize copper, leading to elevations in body and serum levels.
- Measurement of serum bilirubin fractions (conjugated and unconjugated) can help determine the presence and cause of liver disease.
- Aspartate aminotransferase (AST) and alanine aminotransferase (ALT) are the most useful liver enzymes for the detection of liver disease. Alkaline phosphatase (ALP) is a useful test for detecting obstructive disease, especially that related to tumors.

REFERENCES

1. Dufour D, Lott J, Nolte F, et al: Diagnosis and monitoring of hepatic injury. II. Recommendations for use of laboratory tests in screening, diagnosis, and monitoring, Clin Chem 46:2050, 2000.
2. Dufour D, Lott J, Nolte F, et al: Diagnosis and monitoring of hepatic injury. I. Performance characteristics of laboratory tests, Clin Chem 46:2027, 2000.
3. Trotter J, Brimhall B, Arjal R, et al: Specific laboratory methodologies achieve higher model for endstage liver disease (MELD) scores for patients listed for liver transplantation, Liver Transpl 10:995, 2004.
4. Bellest L, Eschwege V, Poupon R, et al: A modified international normalized ratio as an effective way of prothrombin time standardization in hepatology, Hepatology 46:528, 2007.
5. Tripodi A, Chantarangkul V, Primignani M, et al: The international normalized ratio calibrated for cirrhosis (INR [liver]) normalizes prothrombin time results for model for end-stage liver disease calculation, Hepatology 46:520, 2007.
6. Narayanan S: Biochemistry and clinical relevance of lipoprotein X, Ann Clin Lab Sci 14:371, 1984.
7. Herzum I, Giehl C, Soufi M, et al: Interference in a homogeneous assay for low-density lipoprotein cholesterol by lipoprotein X, Clin Chem Lab Med 45:667, 2007.
8. Gao L, Ramzan I, Baker A: Potential use of pharmacological markers to quantitatively assess liver function during liver transplantation surgery, Anaesth Intensive Care 28:375, 2000.
9. Shawcross D, Jalan R: Dispelling myths in the treatment of hepatic encephalopathy, Lancet 365:431, 2005.
10. Shawcross D, Wright G, Olde Damink S, et al: Role of ammonia and inflammation in minimal hepatic encephalopathy, Metab Brain Dis 22:125, 2007.
11. Hsieh T, Shiu T, Huang S, et al: Molecular pathogenesis of Gilbert's syndrome: decreased TATA-binding protein binding affinity of UGT1A1 gene promoter, Pharmacogenet Genomics 17:229, 2007.
12. Costa E: Hematologically important mutations: bilirubin UDP-glucuronosyltransferase gene mutations in Gilbert and Crigler-Najjar syndromes, Blood Cells Mol Dis 36:77, 2006.
13. Waley A, Miller J, Finelli L: Surveillance for acute viral hepatitis—United States, 2005, MMWR Morb Mortal Wkly Rep 56:1, 2007.
14. Lee W: Medical progress: drug-induced hepatotoxicity, N Engl J Med 349:474, 2003.
15. Whitehead M, Hawkes N, Hainsworth I, et al: A prospective study of the causes of notably raised aspartate aminotransferase of liver origin, Gut 45:129, 1999.
16. O'Grady J: Prognostication in acute liver failure: a tool or an anchor? Liver Transpl 13:786, 2007.
17. Dhiman R, Jain S, Maheshwari U, et al: Early indicators of prognosis in fulminant hepatic failure: an assessment of the Model for End-Stage Liver Disease (MELD) and King's College Hospital Criteria, Liver Transpl 13:814, 2007.
18. Schiodt F, Bangert K, Shakil A, et al: Predictive value of actin-free Gc-globulin in acute liver failure, Liver Transpl 13:1324, 2007.
19. Haber M, West A, Haber A, et al: Relationship of aminotransferases to liver histological status in chronic hepatitis C, Am J Gastroenterol 90:1250, 1995.
20. Puoti C, Castellacci R, Montagnese F, et al: Histological and virological features and follow-up of hepatitis C virus carriers with normal aminotransferase levels: the Italian prospective study of the asymptomatic C carriers (ISACC), J Hepatol 37:117, 2002.
21. Chang Y, Ryu S, Sung E, et al: Higher concentrations of alanine aminotransferase within the reference interval predict nonalcoholic fatty liver disease, Clin Chem 53:686, 2007.
22. Poynard T, Munteanu M, Imbert-Bismut F, et al: Prospective analysis of discordant results between biochemical markers and biopsy in patients with chronic hepatitis C, Clin Chem 50:1344, 2004.
23. Mukherjee S, Sorrel M: Noninvasive tests for liver fibrosis, Semin Liver Dis 26:337, 2006.
24. Raman M, Allard J: Non-alcoholic fatty liver disease: a clinical approach and review, Can J Gastroenterol 20:345, 2006.
25. Wieckowska A, McCullough A, Feldstein A: Noninvasive diagnosis and monitoring of nonalcoholic steatohepatitis: present and future, Hepatology 46:582, 2007.
26. Czaja A, Freese D: Diagnosis and treatment of autoimmune hepatitis, Hepatology 36:479, 2002.
27. Swinkels D, Janssen M, Bergmans J, et al: Hereditary hemochromatosis: genetic complexity and new diagnostic approaches, Clin Chem 52:950, 2006.
28. Allen K, Gurrin L, Constantine C, et al: Iron-overload–related disease in HFE hereditary hemochromatosis, N Engl J Med 358:221, 2008.
29. Tavill A: Diagnosis and management of hemochromatosis, Hepatology 33:1321, 2001.
30. Schmidt H: Introducing single-nucleotide polymorphism markers in the diagnosis of Wilson disease, Clin Chem 53:1568, 2007.
31. Gupta A, Maulik M, Nasipuri P, et al: Molecular diagnosis of Wilson disease using prevalent mutations and informative single-nucleotide polymorphism markers, Clin Chem 53:1601, 2007.
32. Ala A, Walker A, Ashkan K, et al: Wilson's disease, Lancet 369:397, 2007.
33. Stoller J, Aboussouan L: Alpha$_1$-antitrypsin deficiency, Lancet 365:2225, 2005.
34. Teckman J, Lindblad D: Alpha-1-antitrypsin deficiency: diagnosis, pathophysiology, and management, Curr Gastroenterol Rep 8:14, 2006.
35. Sterling R, Jeffers L, Gordon F, et al: Clinical utility of AFP-L3% measurement in North American patients with HCV-related cirrhosis, Am J Gastroenterol 102:2196, 2007.
36. Lee D, Jacobs D, Gross M, et al: Serum gamma-glutamyltransferase was differently associated with microalbuminuria by status of hypertension or diabetes: the Coronary Artery Risk Development in Young Adults (CARDIA) study, Clin Chem 51:1185, 2005.
37. Prati D, Taioli E, Zanella A, et al: Updated definitions of healthy ranges for serum alanine aminotransferase levels, Ann Intern Med 137:1, 2002.
38. Kunde S, Lazenby A, Clements R, et al: Spectrum of NAFLD and diagnostic implications of the proposed new normal range for serum ALT in obese women, Hepatology 42:650, 2005.
39. Carr B, Kanke F, Wise M, et al: Clinical evaluation of lens culinaris agglutinin-reactive alpha-fetoprotein and des-gamma-carboxy prothrombin in histologically proven hepatocellular carcinoma in the United States, Dig Dis Sci 52:776, 2007.

INTERNET SITES

www.aasld.org—American Association for the Study of Liver Disease (AASLD), particularly see tab on guidelines, which contains links to all published guidelines (including the NACB guidelines on liver disease tests)

www.childliverdisease.org—Children's Liver Disease Foundation, particularly see tab on education programs

www.liverfoundation.org—American Liver Foundation, many useful brochures available as PDF's with explanations in lay terms

http://digestive.niddk.nih.gov/—National Institute of Diabetes and Digestive and Kidney Diseases page on digestive and liver disease, extensive information on many liver disorders

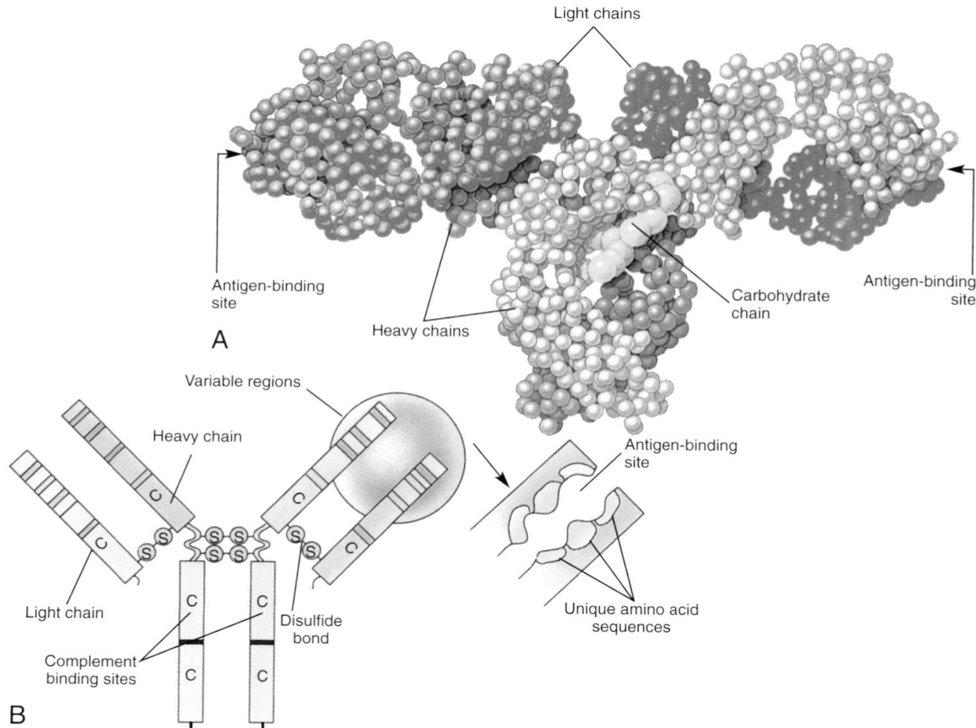

Color Plate 1 Structure of the antibody molecule. **A,** In this molecular model of a typical antibody molecule, the light chains are represented by strands of red spheres (each represents an individual amino acid). Heavy chains are represented by strands of blue spheres. Notice that the heavy chains can complex with a carbohydrate chain. **B,** This simplified diagram shows the variable regions, highlighted by yellow bars that represent amino acid sequences unique to that molecule. Constant regions of the heavy and light chains are marked *C.* The inset shows that the variable regions at the end of each arm of the molecule form a cleft that serves as an antigen-binding site. (From Thibodeau GA, Patton KT: Anatomy & Physiology, ed 6, St. Louis, 2007, Mosby.)

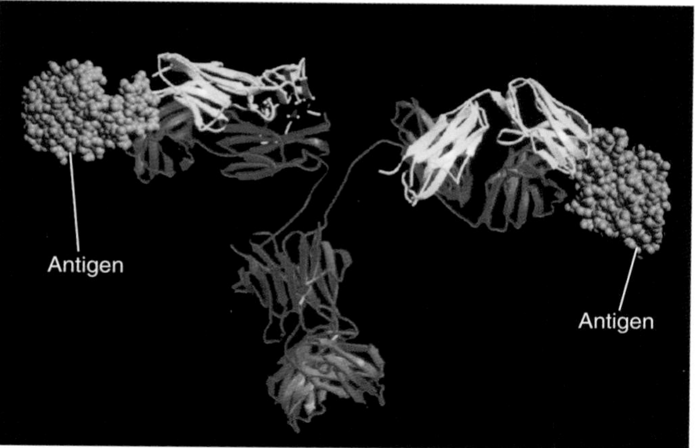

Color Plate 2 Binding of antigen by an antibody. This ribbon model of an antibody shows the heavy chains in red and the light chains in yellow. Note the blue antigen molecules bound to each antigen-binding site. (Courtesy Dr. Dan Vaughn, Cold Spring Harbor Laboratory. From Abbas AK et al: Cellular and Molecular Immunology, ed 6, Philadelphia, 2007, Saunders.)

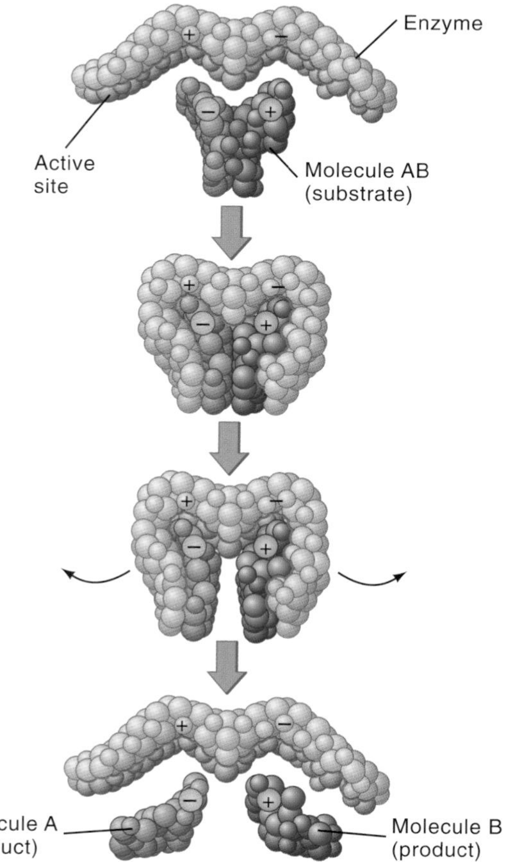

Color Plate 3 Model of enzyme action. Enzymes are functional proteins whose molecular shape allows them to catalyze chemical reactions. Substrate molecule AB is acted on by a digestive enzyme to yield simpler molecules A and B as products of the reaction. Notice how the active site of the enzyme chemically fits the substrate—the lock-and-key model of biochemical interaction. Notice also how the enzyme molecule bends its shape in performing its function. (From Thibodeau GA, Patton KT: Anatomy & Physiology, ed 6, St. Louis, 2007, Mosby.)

Color Plate 4 Three ways to visualize the same folded protein molecule. Three common types of protein models are shown. The *ribbon model* shows the areas where alpha helices and folded sheets form within the molecule. The *space-filling model* shows each atom as a "cloud" filing up the space occupied by that atom. The *surface-rendering model* shows the three-dimensional boundaries of the whole protein molecule, often also color-coding for charge regions on the surface of the protein. (From Thibodeau GA, Patton KT: Anatomy & Physiology, ed 6, St. Louis, 2007, Mosby.)

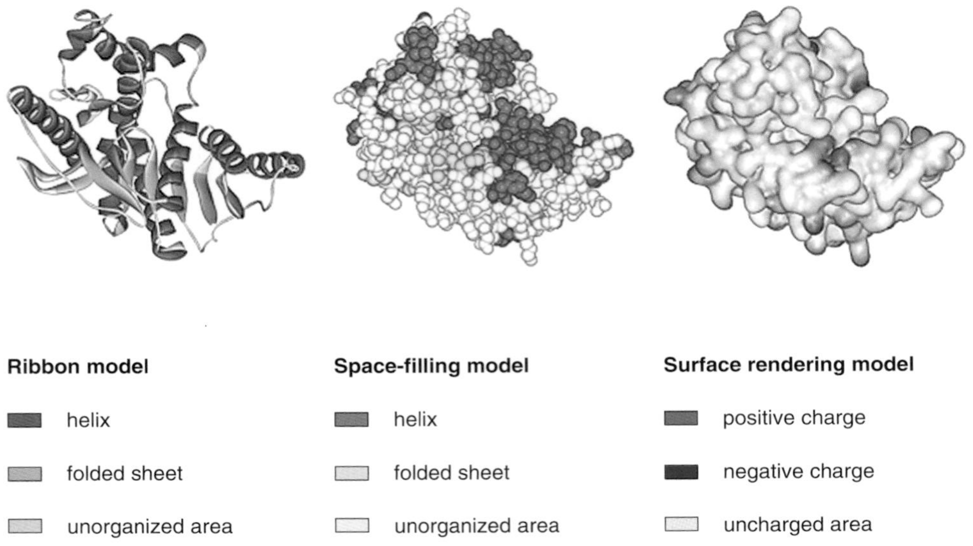

Ribbon model

- helix
- folded sheet
- unorganized area

Space-filling model

- helix
- folded sheet
- unorganized area

Surface rendering model

- positive charge
- negative charge
- uncharged area

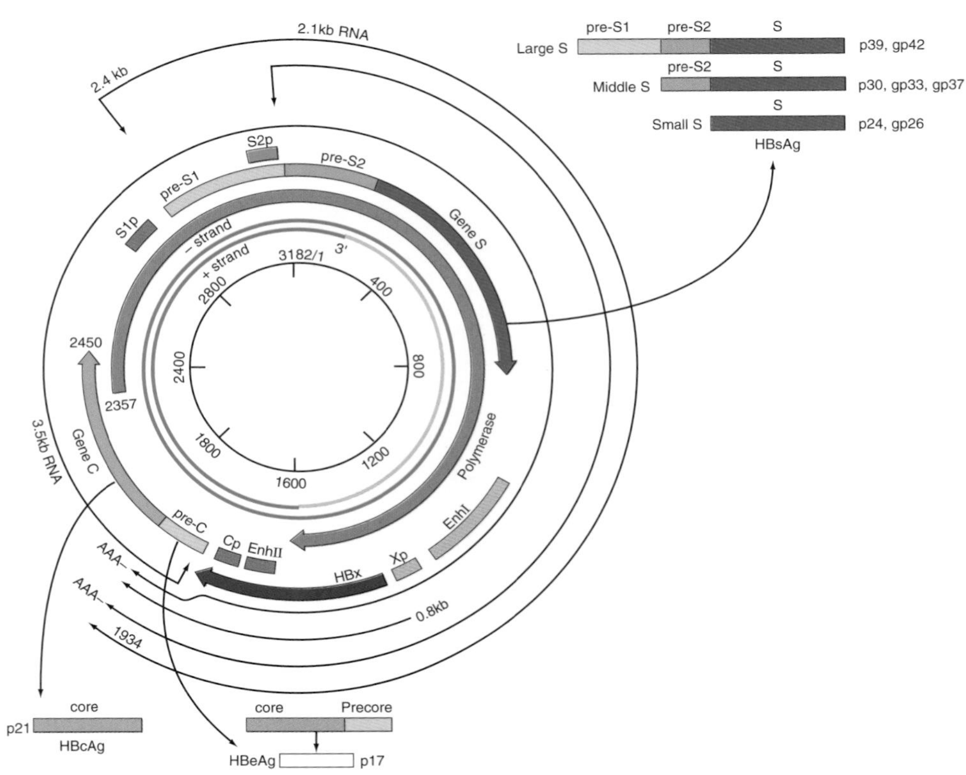

Color Plate 5 Hepatitis B virus (HBV) genome organization, map of viral transcripts, and proteins. The partially double-stranded 3.2-kb viral DNA is shown in the inner circle. The single-stranded *(ss)* region is indicated in yellow-orange. Viral transcripts are indicated in the outermost circles *(thin lines)*. The three forms of HBsAg, HBcAg, and HBeAg (surface, core, and early antigen) polypeptides are also shown. (From Mandell GL, Bennett JE, Dolin R: Principles and practice of infectious diseases, ed 6, Philadelphia, 2005, Churchill Livingstone.)

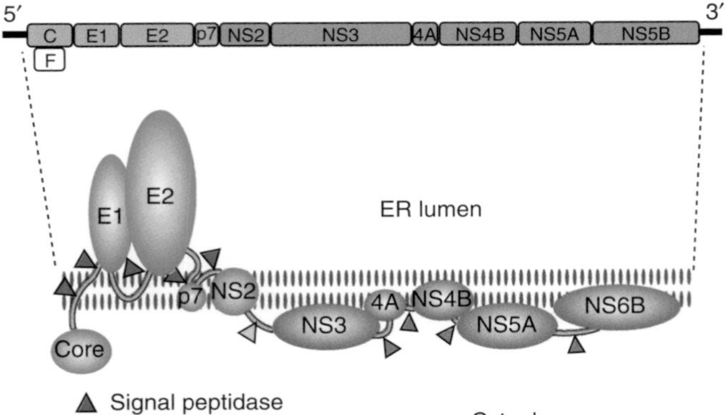

Color Plate 6 Organization of HCV genome and viral proteins. (From Mandell GL, Bennett JE, Dolin R: Principles and practice of infectious diseases, ed 6, Philadelphia, 2005, Churchill Livingstone.)

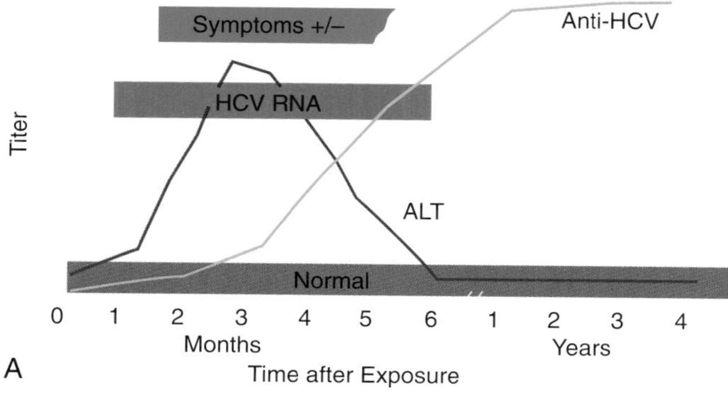

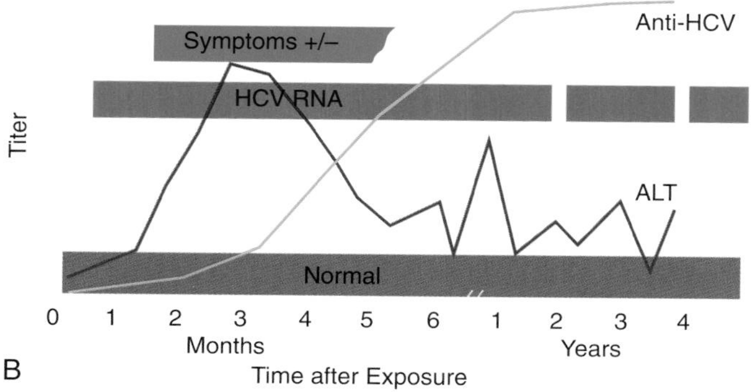

Color Plate 7 Clinical, virological and serological events associated with hepatitis C. **A,** Acute HCV infection. **B,** Acute HCV infection with progression to chronic HCV infection.

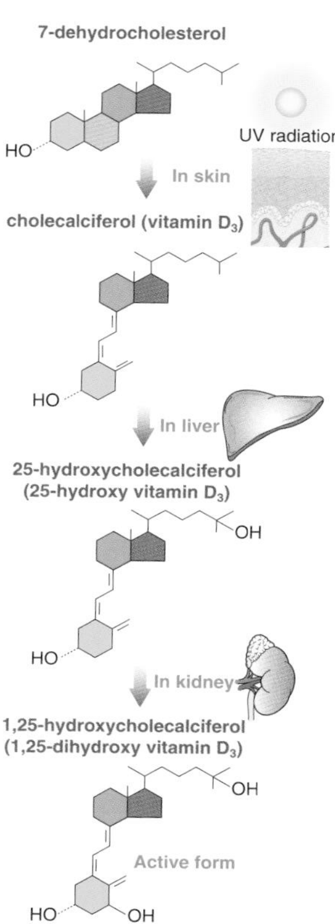

Color Plate 8 Conversion of 7-dehydrocholesterol to activated vitamin D by ultraviolet (UV) light and by liver and kidney. (From Thibodeau GA, Patton KT: Anatomy & Physiology, ed 6, St. Louis, 2007, Mosby.)

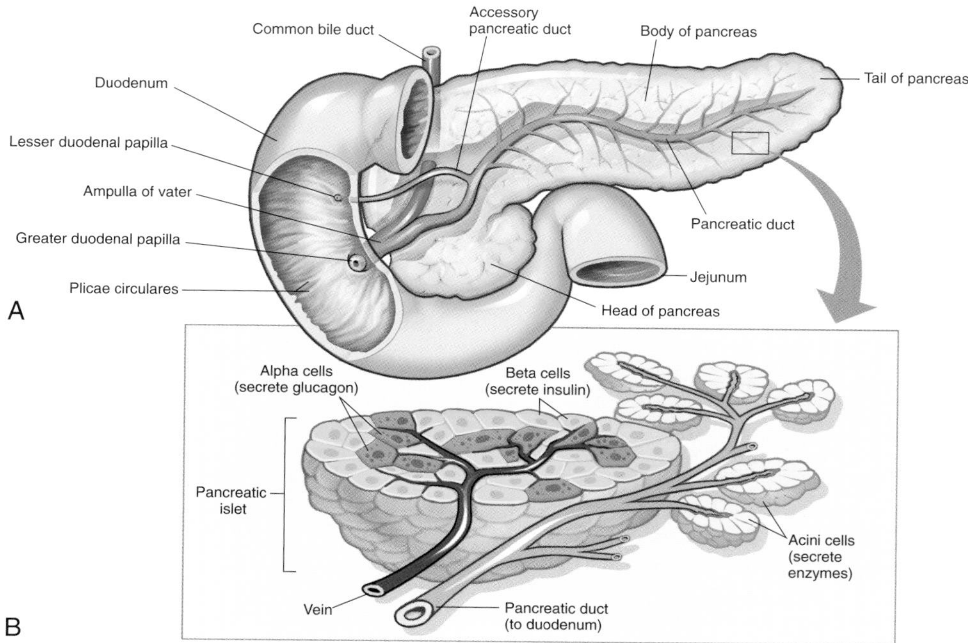

Color Plate 9 Pancreas. **A,** Pancreas dissected to show the main and accessory ducts. The main duct may join the common bile duct, as shown here, to enter the duodenum by a single opening at the major duodenal papilla, or the two ducts may have separate openings. The accessory pancreatic duct is usually present and has a separate opening into the duodenum. **B,** Exocrine glandular cells (around small pancreatic ducts) and endocrine glandular cells of the pancreatic islets (adjacent to blood capillaries). Exocrine pancreatic cells secrete pancreatic juice, alpha endocrine cells secrete glucagon, and beta cells secrete insulin. (From Thibodeau GA, Patton KT: Anatomy & Physiology, ed 6, St. Louis, 2007, Mosby.)

Color Plate 10 Wall of the small intestine. Note folds of mucosa are covered with villi and each villus is covered with epithelium, which increases the surface area for absorption of food. (From Thibodeau GA, Patton KT: Anatomy & Physiology, ed 6, St. Louis, 2007, Mosby.)

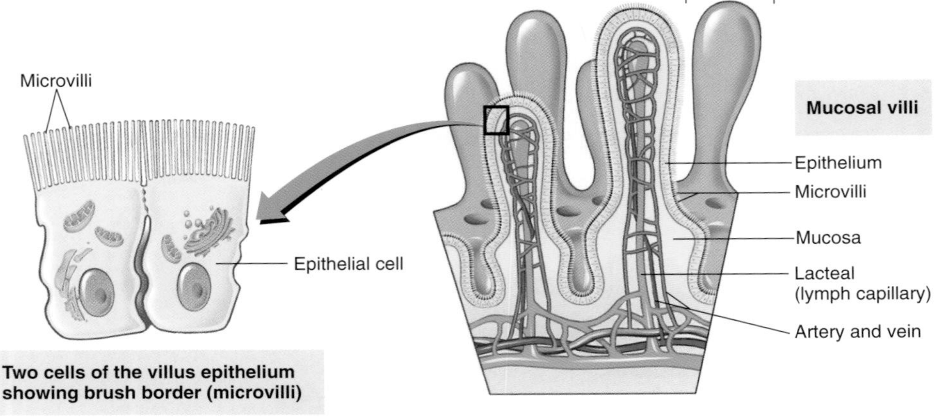

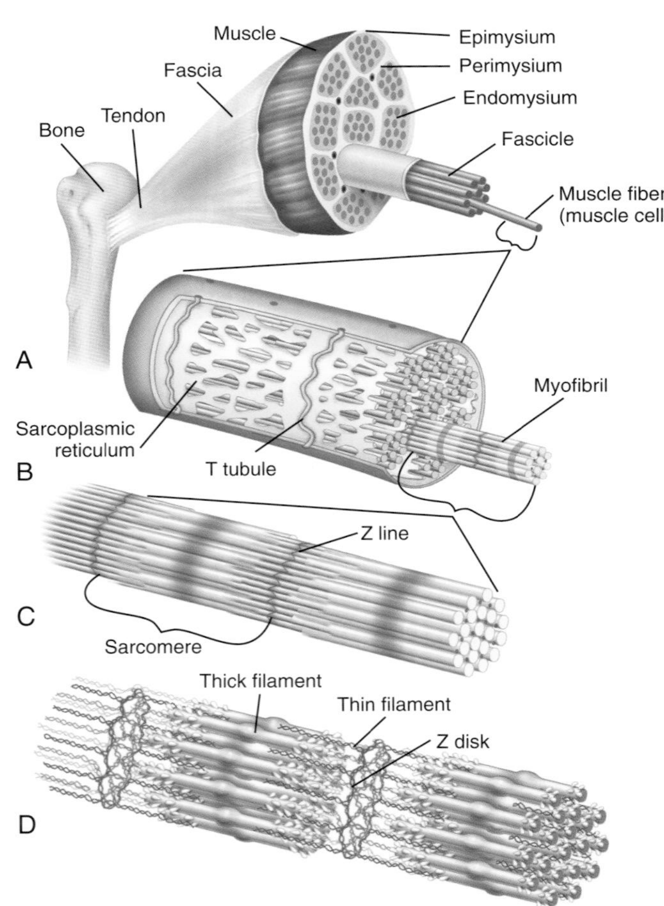

Color Plate 11 Structure of skeletal muscle. **A,** Skeletal muscle organ composed of bundles of contractile muscle fibers held together by connective tissue. **B,** Greater magnification of a single fiber showing smaller fibers—myofibrils—in the sarcoplasm. Note the sarcoplasmic reticulum and T tubules forming a three-part structure called a *triad*. **C,** Myofibril magnified further to show a sarcomere between successive Z lines (Z disks). Cross striae are visible. **D,** Molecular structure of a myofibril showing thick myofilaments and thin myofilaments. (From Thibodeau GA, Patton KT: Anatomy & Physiology, ed 6, St. Louis, 2007, Mosby.)

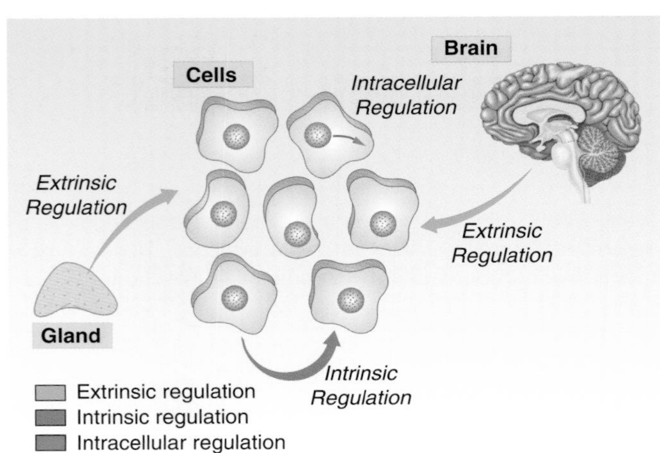

Color Plate 12 Levels of control. The many complex processes of the body are coordinated at many levels: intracellular (within cells), intrinsic (within tissues/organs), and extrinsic (organ to organ). (From Thibodeau GA, Patton KT: Anatomy & Physiology, ed 6, St. Louis, 2007, Mosby.)

Viral Hepatitis: Diagnosis and Monitoring

32 Chapter

Dan Chen

Chapter Outline

Key Terms

antisense RNA genome The RNA genome has the complementary sequence for the mRNA used for protein translation.

escape mutant A point mutation in a highly antigenic determinant of HBsAg that allows the person infected with this viral genotype to "escape" passive or active immunization against hepatitis B.

HBIG A preparation of anti–hepatitis B immunoglobulin G that is used to treat the patient passively.

NAT Nucleic acid testing; consists of any methods used to detect genetic material of a target pathogen, such as polymerase chain reaction (PCR) and sequencing tests.

neutralization test A confirmatory test used to confirm the initial reactive HbsAg result. It is based on a significant reduction of assay reaction signal when neutralizing antibody (anti-HBsAg) is added to the patient sample before confirmatory analysis. Significant reduction in signal, usually ≥50%, allows the reporting of a "confirmed reactive."

open reading frame (ORF) The segment of an organism's genome that consists of the coding for one or more proteins, including the start and stop signals for producing messenger RNAs.

recombinant immunoblot assay (RIBA) A version of the "Western blot" technique (see Chapter 8) that is used to confirm the presence in a patient's serum of antibodies to hepatitis C virus.

stop codon mutant A mutation of one or two nucleotides in the protein coding sequence or pre-coding sequence, which results in the appearance of a stop codon (UAA, UAG, or UGA) that leads to abnormal cessation of translation of messenger RNA.

Abbreviations

aHBcIgM IgM antibody against Hepatitis B core antigen
aHBc Total Antibody against Hepatitis B core antigen
aHBs Antibody against Hepatitis B surface antigen
HBsAg Hepatitis B surface antigen

Methods on CD-ROM

HBsAg
aHBs
aHBcIgM

Table 32-1 Composition of Hepatitis Viruses

Hepatitis Virus	Viral Classification	Presence of Viral Envelope	Incubation Time (Days)*	Route of Transmission	Genome	Size of Genome (kbases)
A	Picornaviridae	A	10-50	Oral/enteral	Positive ssRNA	7.5
B	Hepadnaviridae	P	30-150	Blood, fluids	Partial dsDNA	3.2
C	Flaviviridae	P	15-160	Blood, fluids	Positive ssRNA	9.6
D	Deltaviridae	P†	21-50	Blood, fluids	Particle G–negative ssRNA	1.7
E	Caliciviridae	A	28-40	Oral/enteral	Positive ssRNA	7.5

A, Absence of viral envelope; *ds*, double-stranded RNA; *P*, presence of viral envelope; *ss*, single-stranded RNA.
*Days to clinical symptoms.
†Delta virus uses hepatitis B surface antigen (HBsAg) as its envelope protein.

SECTION OBJECTIVE BOX 32-1

- Compare and contrast the characteristics that are similar among the hepatitis viruses.
- Describe the common clinical symptoms and biochemical changes seen in acute viral hepatitis.
- For each hepatitis virus, give the prevalence of disease and the primary route of transmission.
- List the hepatitis viruses that have genetic variants, and describe the clinical significance of these variants.

INTRODUCTION TO VIRAL HEPATITIS

Hepatitis A, B, C, D, and E are the main viral causes of hepatitis in humans. They have very little in common besides the fact that their primary infection site is the liver. They are further grouped by their primary route of transmission: the fecal-oral route or the blood-fluid route. Hepatitis A (HAV) and hepatitis E (HEV) are transmitted through the fecal-oral route, and hepatitis B, C, and D (HBV, HCV, and HDV) are transmitted through the blood-fluid route (Table 32-1). All five types can cause an acute viral hepatitis, which is marked by necrosis and inflammation of the liver. Although hepatitis A and E usually cause only acute hepatitis infection, hepatitis B, C, and D can cause both acute and chronic forms of infection.

Symptoms of Acute Viral Hepatitis

In general, an acute symptomatic viral hepatitis infection goes through four phases: incubation, pre-icteric, icteric, and convalescence. The length of the incubation phase, during which the infected individual is usually without symptoms, ranges from a couple of weeks to several months, depending on the type of viral infection (see Table 32-1). Pre-icteric symptoms include malaise, joint and muscle pain, fatigue, anorexia, nausea, vomiting, and a vague dull, right upper quadrant pain produced by the swollen, tender liver. A quarter of symptomatic viral hepatitis patients also have flulike symptoms, including fever, which lasts 3 to 10 days.

The icteric phase is marked by increasing levels of jaundice, which become apparent in the yellowing of the sclera of the eye at a serum bilirubin concentration of about 3 mg/dL (see Chapter 31). The decreased ability of the injured liver to clear conjugated bilirubin into the bile duct results in increasing serum levels of conjugated bilirubin. Conjugated bilirubin spills into the urine, producing dark yellow urine 1 to 7 days after jaundice is first observed. The decreased clearance of conjugated bilirubin into the intestinal tract can result in pale stools. The icteric phase may last 1 to 3 weeks. On average, patients start to feel better after the onset of jaundice and after the transition to the convalescence phase begins.

During the convalescence phase, all symptoms gradually improve, jaundice is resolved, and patients recover from the viral hepatitis. The convalescence phase lasts up to several months.

It is important to remember that asymptomatic hepatitis is very common in acute viral hepatitis. Asymptomatic hepatitis is 10 to 30 times more common than symptomatic infection and is recognizable only by serum viral markers and liver function tests.

Symptoms of Chronic Viral Hepatitis

Chronic viral hepatitis is defined as an abnormality in liver function caused by persistent production of hepatitis virus for longer than 6 months. Clinically, a prolonged and indolent pre-icteric phase usually indicates the development of chronic hepatitis caused by the B, C, and D viral infections. Patients with B, C, or D chronic hepatitis may have mild or strong symptoms of fatigue, jaundice, and right upper quadrant discomfort, depending on the severity or stage of the hepatitis. Patients with delta hepatitis virus–induced chronic infection often have more severe symptoms, and those with hepatitis C virus (HCV) chronic hepatitis have fatigue as the most common feature.

General Laboratory Changes in Viral Hepatitis

The hallmarks of acute hepatitis include a rise in serum bilirubin and elevation in the serum transaminases aspartate aminotransferase (AST) and alanine aminotransferase (ALT) (Fig. 31-5; see Chapter 31). The rise in serum AST and ALT is observed during the late incubation phase and peaks in the early icteric phase. Peak values of AST and ALT are usually

Table 32-2 Prevalence of Hepatitis Viruses

Hepatitis Viruses	Prevalence Worldwide	Area or Group With High Prevalence
A	20% to 90%*	Asia, Africa, South America
B	<2% to 20%*	Southeast Asia, China, Sub-Saharan Africa
C	1% to 2%	Egypt, Japan, Taiwan, and Italy, adults >40 yr
D	5% of HBV infection	HBV-infected patients
E	1% to 28%†	Adults

HBV, Hepatitis B virus.
*Geographically dependent; see specific virus section for details.
†Region dependent; see Hepatitis E section for details.

more than 8 times the upper limits of their reference intervals, and the AST-to-ALT ratio is usually <1 (see Table 31-3). Serum bilirubin is elevated above 2.5 mg/dL, serum ALT is elevated for 4 to 5 weeks, and hyperbilirubinuria lasts 1 to 3 weeks. Alkaline phosphatase (ALP) may become moderately elevated as well (see Table 31-3). In parallel with these biochemical changes is the appearance of serological markers of the virus that is responsible for the observed hepatitis. These markers serve as critical criteria for the differential diagnosis of viral hepatitis. Serological markers of each hepatitis viruses are discussed in later sections of this chapter.

The persistence of abnormal serum levels of the liver enzymes AST and ALT for longer than 6 months indicates chronic hepatitis, although AST levels may fluctuate. The serological markers associated with chronic hepatitis are seen too. See later sections for individual viruses.

Prevalence of Viral Hepatitis (Table 32-2)

The annual incidence of acute viral hepatitis in the United States is 0.1% to 0.2 %. Worldwide, the prevalence of hepatitis A varies geographically from ≈20% in North America to near 100% in Asia. The prevalence of hepatitis B is 5% to 6% worldwide and 2% in the United States. The prevalence of hepatitis C infection is 1% to 2% worldwide and in the United States. Although the HAV infection rate is almost 100% in parts of Asia, Africa, and South America, the rate in Scandinavian countries is very low. See each virus section for details.

Common Genetic Variants

The DNA or RNA sequence homology of the hepatitis viruses determines the viral genotypes, and the serological determinants (epitopes) on the viral particle surface establish the serotype. Genotype variants of each hepatitis virus have been identified. The impact of genotypes on disease outcome varies for each virus (Table 32-3). The genotype variation of Hepatitis A and E has no impact at all on disease outcome and immunity; hepatitis B virus (HBV) and HCV genotypes have a significant impact on choice of treatment.

Table 32-3 Common Genetic Variants of Hepatitis Virus Genotypes

Hepatitis Virus	Genotypes	Clinical Significance
A	I-VII	None
B	A-H	Affects treatment
C	1-6	Affects treatment
D	Types 1-3	Not clear
E	Five major types	None

KEY CONCEPTS BOX 32-1

- The hepatitis viruses all reproduce in the liver and cause liver disease. They differ with respect to the presence of a viral envelope, the route of transmission (food/water, blood/sexual), the chemical type of genome (RNA or DNA, single- or double-stranded), and genomic and serological variants.
- Common clinical symptoms of a viral hepatitis infection include malaise, joint and muscle pain, fatigue, anorexia, nausea, vomiting, jaundice, and a vague dull, right upper quadrant pain produced by the swollen, tender liver. Jaundice is noted by hyper-conjugated bilirubinemia and bilirubinuria.
- The worldwide prevalences of the hepatitis viruses are: HVA, 20-90%; HVB, 2-20%; HVC, 1-2%; HVD, <1-2%; and HEV, 1-28%. HAV and HEV are primarily transmitted through contaminated food and water while HBV, HCV, and HDV are transmitted by contaminated body fluids.
- Hepatitis viruses B and C are the only ones with clinically significant genotype variants. The response of individuals to specific treatments varies with the variants.

SECTION OBJECTIVES BOX 32-2

- Describe lab tests used to diagnose different viral hepatitis infections.
- Describe how to determine the stage of a viral disease by using laboratory tests.
- Describe how to differentiate between an HBV infection and an HBV vaccination.
- Describe the limitations of serology tests for hepatitis B virus (HBV) and hepatitis C virus (HCV), while discussing false positives and false negatives.

HEPATITIS A

Clinical Background

Approximately 25% of the worldwide cases of acute hepatitis are caused by HAV; more than 32,000 new hepatitis A cases are reported per year in the United States alone. Although seven genotypes of HAV have been identified, four of which can infect humans, they are so closely related to each other antigenically that there is only one serotype.[1] This means that infection by *any* of the genotypes will produce immunity against all, resulting in lifelong immunity to HAV. Hepatitis A

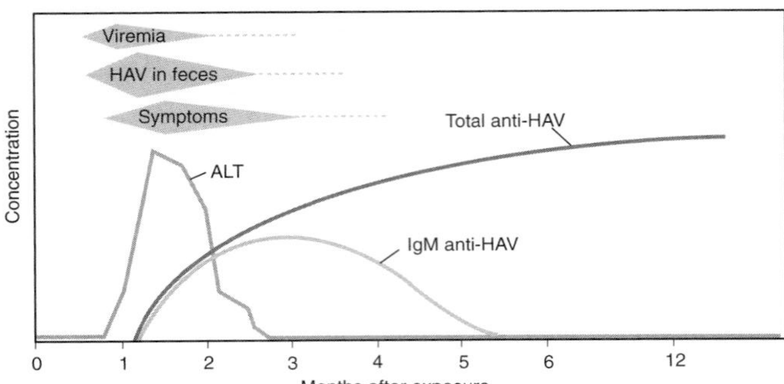

Fig. 32-1 Clinical, virological, and serological events associated with hepatitis A virus (HAV) infection. *ALT*, Alanine aminotransferase. (From Mandell GL, Bennett JE, Dolin R: *Principles and Practice of Infectious Diseases*, 6th ed, Philadelphia, 2005, Elsevier Churchill Livingstone.)

is transmitted by person-to-person contact or by ingestion of feces-contaminated food or water. HAV replicates only in the liver, which excretes the virus via the biliary tract into the intestines. High concentrations of HAV can then be found in the stool.

The peak of HAV infectivity occurs during the 2 weeks before the onset of symptoms. Hepatitis A infection can be asymptomatic; only 7% of children younger than 5 years old have symptoms of jaundice when infected by HAV. The rate of jaundice increases to 70% in infected adolescents and adults. Hepatitis A is a self-limiting disease with a very low incidence of fulminant hepatic failure, which occurs at the rate of 0.14% to 0.35% of all hepatitis A cases.

Prophylactic treatment with immune globulin (Ig) against HAV has been recommended after exposure to HAV. The Advisory Committee on Immunization Practices (ACIP) recommends that HAV single-antigen vaccine be administered as soon as possible after HAV exposure, especially in those from 12 months to 40 years of age. For other age groups, the ACIP still recommends Ig as the preferred choice for prophylaxis.[2] Vaccination to prevent HAV infection is effective; the HAV infection rate has decreased by 89% since HAV vaccination became available in 1995.

Laboratory Changes Associated With HAV Infection

Serum ALT levels peak 2 to 3 weeks post infection and remain abnormal for longer than 5 weeks (Fig. 32-1). Anti-HAV IgM is usually detectable by 4 weeks after infection and is undetectable after 6 months. Anti-HAV IgG usually appears in serum several weeks after the appearance of IgM, and it persists, resulting in lifelong immunity.

Diagnosis of HAV Infection

The earliest diagnostic marker of current HAV infection is the presence of anti-HAV (aHAV) IgM. Past infection is detected when the combination of the absence of anti-HAV IgM and the presence of aHAV IgG (indicated by a positive aHAV total result) is evident.

The presence of aHAV IgG antibody can result from past infection or from HAV vaccination. Currently, no assay is available to distinguish between these two situations, because there will be a positive aHAV total and a negative aHAV IgM result in both situations. HAV can be detected in the stools of patients 1 to 2 weeks before symptoms develop, but it is not used for routine clinical diagnosis. Nucleic acid testing **(NAT),** such as PCR, can be used to detect environmental contamination by HAV.[3,4]

Monitoring HAV Infection

Serum ALT and bilirubin levels or aHAV IgM can be used to monitor the HAV infection process. Usually, ALT levels will return to within the reference interval 5 to 7 weeks after the initial elevation. aHAV IgM becomes undetectable several months after normalization of the serum ALT level.

HAV Assays

Both enzyme immunoassay (EIA) and chemiluminescent immunoassay formats are available for aHAV IgM and aHAV total tests. The sensitivity of aHAV IgM assays is set in such a way that a positive (reactive) result implies an acute or recent infection. aHAV IgM assays can yield a reactive aHAV IgM result as early as 10 days post infection.

Anti-HAV total assays, which measure both IgM and IgG antibodies against HAV, can detect seroconversion as early as 4 weeks post vaccination.

False-positive aHAV IgM results are seen in some assays. The aHAV total assay can be used to confirm the positive result of aHAV IgM and to reduce the reporting error; a negative result in the aHAV total assay suggests that a positive aHAV IgM may be false.

HEPATITIS B

Clinical Background

The fatality rate following hepatitis B infection is 0.5% to 1.5%, and most patients infected with HBV will recover completely. More than 10% of HBV-infected patients will become chronic carriers. More than a million people in the United States and 350 million persons worldwide are HBV chronic carriers. The risk for becoming a chronic carrier is much higher if infection occurs in childhood, especially in infancy, than if an individual is infected as an adult. Approximately 90% of infants infected by HBV will become chronic carriers, in contrast to a 6% to 10% carrier conversion rate for infected adults. Approximately 25% of chronic HBV carriers infected perinatally will die from cirrhosis or liver cancer.

Immunization with hepatitis B surface antigen vaccine is very efficient at preventing HBV infection. Anti–hepatitis B immunoglobulin G (**HBIG**) given to HBV-exposed newborns is also very effective.[5] Current World Health Organization (WHO) guidelines suggest that individuals with a level of anti-HBs above 10 mIU/mL should have lifelong immunity to HBV.

Acute HBV Infection

Symptoms for hepatitis B acute infection are similar to those seen with the other hepatitis viruses. It is rare for children younger than 1 year to develop symptoms, and the likelihood of developing icteric illness is inversely proportional to age.

Chronic HBV Infection

Chronic hepatitis is defined by the persistence of HBV for longer than 6 months. Patients may be asymptomatic or may have nonspecific symptoms of fatigue, nausea, and anorexia. If the chronic infection progresses to cirrhosis, patients may develop jaundice, splenomegaly, ascites, encephalopathy, and pedal edema.

Hepatitis Genotypes

The HBV genome contains four **open reading frames (ORF)** that code for proteins that make up the HBV viron or are involved with viral DNA transcription. These include C, encoding for the core (HBcAg) and e (HBeAg) proteins; P, encoding for RNA polymerase; S, encoding for three envelope proteins (S ORF; large [L], middle [M], and small [S]); and X, encoding for a transcriptional trans-activator protein.[6] See Color Plate 5.

Hepatitis B has an intergroup DNA sequence divergence of more than 8% in the complete genome sequence and more than 4% within the S ORF, resulting in eight genotypes, A to H.[7] Some of the genotypes have a specific geographic distribution; genotype A is found mainly in Europe, North America, and Africa, genotypes B and C are found in Asia and Oceanea, and genotype D is found in the Mediterranean region.[8]

The genotypes are also associated with different clinical outcomes for HBV infection. Among the eight genotypes, type A is associated with better disease outcomes and better long-term survival.[9] The type B genotype is associated with an increased risk for development of hepatocellular carcinoma.[10]

The response to treatment for HBV infection varies with the genotype. The type A variant responds better to interferon treatment than does type D, when HBeAg seroconversion is used as the standard.[11] Patients infected with the type B variant respond better to lamivudine treatment than do patients infected with the type C variant[12] and may respond better than those with type D to interferon treatment.[13]

HBeAg-Negative Mutations

Stop codon mutants in the pre-core region of the C gene ORF of the HBV genome abolish the production of HbeAg. A stop codon mutation in the core promoter region or the signal peptide of core antigen results in diminished production of HbeAg. Although these types of mutations do not stop HBV DNA replication, they are associated with a more severe type of acute infection.[14,15]

Hepatitis B Surface Antigen (HBsAg) Escape Mutants

The most common **HBsAg** escape mutation is the result of a glycine-to-arginine substitution at codon 145 (G145R) coding for an HbsAg epitope. This mutation greatly decreases the binding of antibody to HBsAg. Infants can develop an infection with this mutant HBV, the so-called escape infection, even after passive-active vaccination. It was also found that hepatitis B viruses with this mutation are able to infect liver transplant patients who already have been given HBIG prophylaxis.[16-18] It has been reported that mutations in the S ORF region may result in false-negative HBsAg test results in patients who are infected by the HBV that carries this mutation.

Laboratory Changes Associated With HBV Infection

Laboratory findings in the acute phase of the infection include the typical profile of HBV serological markers (see below) and elevations in serum ALT and AST; serum bilirubin may be within the reference interval or elevated. A long prothrombin time indicates fulminant liver failure, which occurs in 0.1% to 0.5 % of acute HBV infections. The serum AST level will return to normal within 4 months if the patient recovers from the infection.

Elevations in serum ALT lasting longer than 6 months indicate a transition into chronic hepatitis. Serological markers associated with chronic HB hepatitis are discussed below. HB viral DNA usually is detected in serum by **NAT** testing. Cirrhotic patients may have hypoalbuminemia, hyperbilirubinemia, and decreased platelet count.

Serological Markers

The serological markers of HBV infection are listed in Box 32-1. With the exception of HBcAg, all HBV markers can be measured by commercially available assays. Fig. 32-2 illustrates the correlation between serological markers and the stage of hepatitis B infection. The combination of test results for the HBV serological markers (Table 32-4) can be used to identify carrier status or vaccination status, to differentiate the stage of an active infection, and to estimate the clinical outcome of the disease. Occasionally, the profile of a patient sample can have multiple interpretations. In these cases, additional tests, such as nucleic acid analyses, may have to be ordered to differentiate between outcomes.

Diagnosis of HBV Infection

The detection of serum HBsAg is used as the diagnostic marker for current infection of hepatitis B. Its appearance in blood is the earliest serological marker that can be detected after hepatitis B infection; it usually occurs less than 4 weeks post infection. Typically, serum levels of HBsAg peak around 8 to 12 weeks post infection, fall during the recovery phase, and generally become undetectable within 6 months of the onset of acute infection.

Serum HBsAg levels usually are reported qualitatively as "reactive" (positive result) or "nonreactive" (negative result).

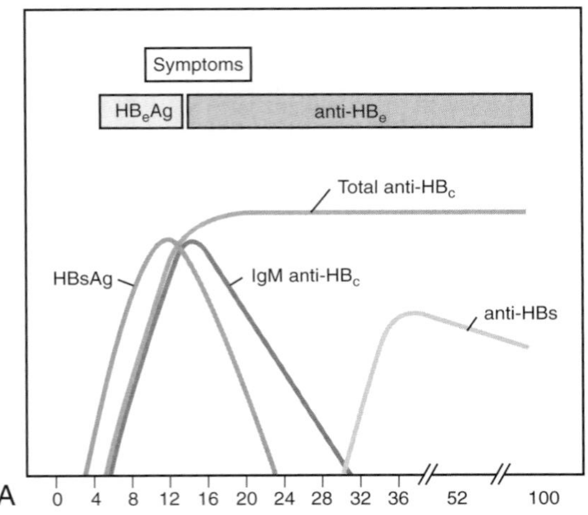

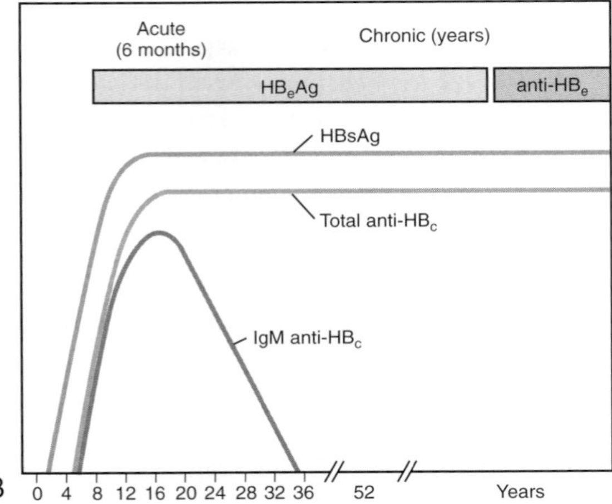

Fig. 32-2 Serological events associated with hepatitis B virus (HBV) infection. **A,** Serological profile of acute hepatitis B infection with complete recovery; time in weeks. **B,** Serological profile of chronic hepatitis B infection; time in weeks, up to 52. (From Mandell GL, Bennett JE, Dolin R: *Principles and Practice of Infectious Diseases*, 6th ed, Philadelphia, 2005, Elsevier Churchill Livingstone.)

Box 32-1

Serological Markers of HBV Infection

Antibody (IgG) against surface antigen (aHBs)
Antibody (IgG) against HBeAg (aHBe)
e antigen (HBeAg)
Core antigen (HBcAg)
IgM antibody against core antigen (aHBcIgM)
Surface antigen (HBsAg)
Total antibody against core antigen (aHBc Total)

The typical format is a one- or two-step immunometric assay (see Evolve). Initially reactive samples often are reflexed to a confirmatory test. The HBsAg confirmatory test, also called the **neutralization test,** is based on a significant reduction of assay reaction signal when neutralizing antibody (anti-HBsAg) is added to the patient sample before confirmatory analysis. Significant reduction in signal, usually ≥50%, allows the reporting of a "confirmed reactive" result. A few commercial HBsAg assays (Siemen's Centaur and Ortho's ECI) allow a result to be reported as "HBSAg positive" without a confirmatory test if the assay signal is greater than a specific "hot zone" cutoff; false positives are very rare for samples with signals in this zone. HBsAg results from certain types of patient samples, such as pregnant women, may continue to require the confirmatory test, regardless of whether or not they fall into the hot zone.[19,20]

The acute phase of the infection will be associated with the presence of **aHBcIgM,** while findings from a patient with chronic HB status will include a positive **aHBc total,** negative **aHBs,** and detectable HB DNA (see Fig. 32-2, *A* and *B*).

Table 32-4 Interpretation of Hepatitis B Serology Profiles

Test*	Results	Interpretation
HBsAg aHBcT aHBs	Negative Negative Negative	Susceptible
HBsAg aHBcT aHBs	Negative Positive Positive	Immune owing to natural infection
HBsAg aHBcT aHBs	Negative Negative Positive	Immune owing to vaccination
HBsAg aHBcT aHBcIgM aHBs	Positive Positive Positive Negative	Acutely infected
HBsAg aHBcT aHbcIgM aHBs	Positive Positive Negative Negative	Chronically infected
HBsAg aHBcT aHBs	Negative Positive Negative	Multiple interpretations†

aHBcIgM, Immune globulin (Ig)M antibody against hepatitis B core; *aHBcT*, both IgG and IgM antibodies against hepatitis core; *aHBs*, antibody against hepatitis B surface antigen; *HBsAg*, hepatitis B surface antigen.

*For abbreviations, see the Glossary.

†Multiple possibilities include recovering from acute hepatitis B (HB) infection; very old immunity with very low aHBs titer; false + result aHBc (antibody against hepatitis B core); chronically infected HB.

Monitoring the Development of HBV Infection and the Treatment

Serum AST and ALT levels, viral serological markers, and HBV DNA levels ("viral load") are useful indicators for monitoring the infection process and recovery. In chronic infection, HBsAg will stay detectable for the rest of the patient's life in most cases, although the levels will vary.

IgG antibody against HBsAg (aHBs) becomes detectable approximately 6 months after infection, and its appearance usually correlates with serum levels of HBsAg becoming undetectable. Occasionally, aHBsAg will test positive while HBsAg is still at a very high titer. The reason for this phenomenon is that although IgG aHBs is present in the circulation as early as 3 months after the infection begins, it remains undetectable until HBsAg is totally cleared from circulation since assays of aHBs do not detect the antigen-bound aHBs. However, occasionally, small amounts of aHBs may escape binding by circulating HbsAg. This free aHBs is detected, resulting in a false positive result while HBsAg is still in excess. An uninfected individual who has been vaccinated against HBV also will test positive for aHBs, because the vaccination material is composed of recombined hepatitis B surface antigen fragments.

Test results for aHBs are reported as "positive," "negative," and "indeterminate." The indeterminate zone cutoff usually is barely below the cutoff for positive, and this result should be followed by analysis of a second sample several weeks later. Analysis for aHBs occurs by a one- or two-step immunometric assay. The cutoff for aHBs positive, generally ≥10 mIU/mL, is also the generally accepted protective level of immune response after vaccination.

IgM antibody against hepatitis B core antigen (aHBcIgM) is first detected at about 6 weeks post infection and remains positive for 3 to 4 months before becoming undetectable. aHBc IgM is usually measured by a two-step immunometric assay in which the aHBcIgM is captured by anti-human IgM antibody. The assay signal is developed with the use of labeled HBV core antigen. Results are reported as "negative," "positive," or "indeterminate"; indeterminate results usually require analysis of a follow-up sample taken several weeks later.

Total antibody against hepatitis B core antigen (aHBcT) assay detects the presence of both IgM and IgG directed against hepatitis B core antigen. The earliest time for detection of aHBcT is similar to that of aHBcIgM, and the levels peak around the same time HBsAg reaches its peak. In contrast to aHBcIgM, aHBcTotal stays positive, regardless of whether a patient is in the acute phase or the chronic phase of HBV hepatitis, because IgG antibody levels remain positive for years post infection. The presence of aHBcT indicates a past or current infection of hepatitis B. A negative aHBcT result reveals that a patient has never been infected by, or has been vaccinated against, HBV. aHBcT results are reported as "negative," "positive," or "indeterminate"; indeterminate results may require retesting with a sample drawn several weeks later. aHBcT assays usually are performed by immunometric assay.

The e antigen of hepatitis B (HBeAg) is translated off of RNA transcribed from the same ORF region of the HBV genome that codes for part of the core antigen. HBeAg is detected in serum at the same time as, or shortly after, the detection of HBsAg. The presence of HBeAg correlates with the highly contagious stage of HBV infection. Clinically false negative results may arise from infections by HB viruses that contain mutations in codon 28 of the pre-core ORF or other pre-core sequence areas that prevent the synthesis of HBeAg.[21] HBeAg is detected by immunometric assay, and results are reported as "negative" or "positive."

Serum IgG antibody against hepatitis B e antigen (aHBe) is detected when patients are recovering from acute hepatitis B infection. Patients with chronic hepatitis stay HBeAg positive or convert to an HBeAg-negative state. Seroconversion from HBeAg positive to HBeAg negativity and aHBe negativity to aHBe positivity usually indicates decreased infectivity and impending recovery; both assays are used to make a prognosis for recovery. aHBe is detected by immunoassay and is reported as "negative" or "positive."[22,23]

An assay for HB core antigen (HBcrAg) has been developed that uses a chemiluminescence enzyme-immunometric assay (CLEIA). This assay detects both HBcrAg and HBeAg because monoclonal antibodies against both antigens are employed as the capture antibody. HBcr-related antigens detected by this assay correlate well with HBV DNA level,[24,25] but its use as a replacement for DNA assays is yet to be determined.

Frequently Encountered Issues in the Interpretation of HBV Serology Tests

Most of the HBV serology tests yield qualitative results. Inherent variations of these assays may result in inconsistent consecutive results if the true value is close to the assay's cutoff point. An HBsAg assay's high background signal about the cutoff value and relatively poor precision can lead to a poor separation of positive and negative results.[26] Consequences of false-negative results include a delay in or absence of treatment and continued spread of the virus. Consequences of releasing false-positive results of HBsAg include unnecessary isolation of the patient in hemodialysis treatment, unnecessary HBIG injection for the newborn baby, and general emotional stress for patients. To minimize this problem, the laboratory should clearly define an "equivocal zone," in which most false-negative and false-positive results occur. Samples whose results fall in the equivocal zone should require additional follow-up tests whose results will allow clarification of the patient's status. Reflex testing to additional tests can be used to differentiate between vaccination and early infection. Repeat testing of consecutive samples in 1 or 2 weeks should be recommended if it is still necessary to monitor the development of an infection.[27]

Molecular Tests of HBV (see Chapter 13)

HBV Viral Load

The HBV viral load test can be used to determine the status of HBV replication in cases when HBsAg is undetectable, such as in fulminant hepatitis or certain aHBcIgG positive–only cases. The HBV viral load test is most useful for selecting a treatment strategy and monitoring the treatment's effectiveness. Patients with high pretreatment levels of HBV DNA respond poorly to interferon treatment, and clearance of HBV DNA from blood is used as a criterion for successful treatment.

HBV DNA viral loads usually are determined with real-time polymerase chain reaction (PCR)-based assays, such as the COBAS TaqMan HBV test (Roche Diagnosis, Indianapolis IN). Assay sensitivity can be as low as 6 IU/mL, and the detection range can be as high as 1.1×10^8 IU/mL.[28]

HBV Genotyping

The clinical characteristics of the different HBV genotypes make identification of them critical for optimizing treatment procedures. The most frequently used genotyping methods, the INNO-LiPA and PCR/sequence assays, can identify all eight genotypes according to their sequences. The pre-S1/pre-S2 region is one of the most widely targeted areas for sequencing-based genotyping. The sequencing results are aligned with gene bank sequences to determine the genotypes.[29]

The INNO-LiPA genotyping assay involves two steps: first, one or more specific regions of the HBV genomes are amplified by PCR; second, the labeled amplicons are hybridized with known genotype-specific oligonucleotides immobilized on nylon strips to establish the patient's HBV sequences and genotype. Real-time PCR methods have also been used to identify genotypes B and C.[30] HBV mutations, such as YMDD mutants that decrease response to lamivudine and pre-core mutations that result in HBeAg-negative serology, can also be determined by sequencing and by line probe assays.

HEPATITIS D

Clinical Background

Hepatitis delta virus (HDV) consists of an **antisense RNA genome** and 70 copies of a nucleocapsid protein—the hepatitis delta antigen (HDAg) (see Table 32-1). The genome and the HDAgs are enveloped by the surface antigens of HBV, HDV's helper virus, which is absolutely required for HDV infection. The prevalence of HDV co-infection in the HBV-infected population is estimated to be 5% to 10%; epidemiologically, the distribution of HDV infection is not parallel to that of HBV infection. Regions of highest HDV prevalence include the Mediterranean basin, North Africa, and South America.

Type I is the most common HDV genotype worldwide; type II is found mainly in Asia. Type II is associated with a milder hepatitis form, and type III, which is distributed in South America, is associated with the most severe form of HDV infection.[31]

HDV infection occurs either through simultaneous infection (co-infection) by both HBV and HDV or through superinfection of a patient chronically infected with HBV. The former type of infection is usually acute and self-limiting, and the latter type is more severe. Chronic hepatitis occurs in 1% to 3% of patients co-infected with HDV/HBV, while 70% of hepatitis B carriers superinfected with HDV develop chronic hepatitis.[32]

The clinical features of HDV infection range from benign acute hepatitis to fulminant liver disease that is usually more severe than other types of viral hepatitis. The rate of conversion to fulminant hepatitis in HDV infection is 10 times higher than that seen with other types of viral hepatitis. More than 60% of patients chronically infected with HDV will develop cirrhosis, and overall, the mortality rate associated with HDV infection is 2% to 10%—ten times higher than that for hepatitis B.

Laboratory Changes Associated With HDV Infection

Fig. 32-3 shows the typical pattern of laboratory tests associated with type D hepatitis infection. In the case of acute HDV/HBV hepatitis, whether by co-infection or superinfection, HDV RNA and HDAg will become detectable in blood after HBsAg appears and will become undetectable about the same time that HBsAg is cleared. IgM antibodies against HDAg stay detectable only during the early part of the infection; IgG antibodies against HDAg develop in the late stage of the acute infection and may stay detectable for years. An HDV superinfection of an HBV carrier that results in a chronic hepatitis will be characterized by the persistence in blood of HDV RNA and HDAg, together with detectable levels of HBsAg.[33]

Diagnosis of HDV Infection

The diagnosis of acute type D hepatitis is based on the presence of HDAg and HDV RNA in HBV-infected patients Chronic HDV hepatitis is usually associated with high levels of anti-HDAg IgG, together with the presence of HDV RNA and HDAg. The presence of anti-HDV IgG can indicate a past or current acute HDV infection, or chronic HDV infection.

Vaccination against HBV effectively prevents HDV infection. No cases of HDV reinfection have been reported, so it is assumed that long-term immunity occurs after acute HDV infection.

Monitoring HDV Infection

HDV RNA and HDAg can be used to monitor the status of the HDV infection.

HDV Assays

Enzyme-linked immunosorbent assay (ELISA) microtiter plate assays are available for anti-HDV IgM, anti-HDV IgG

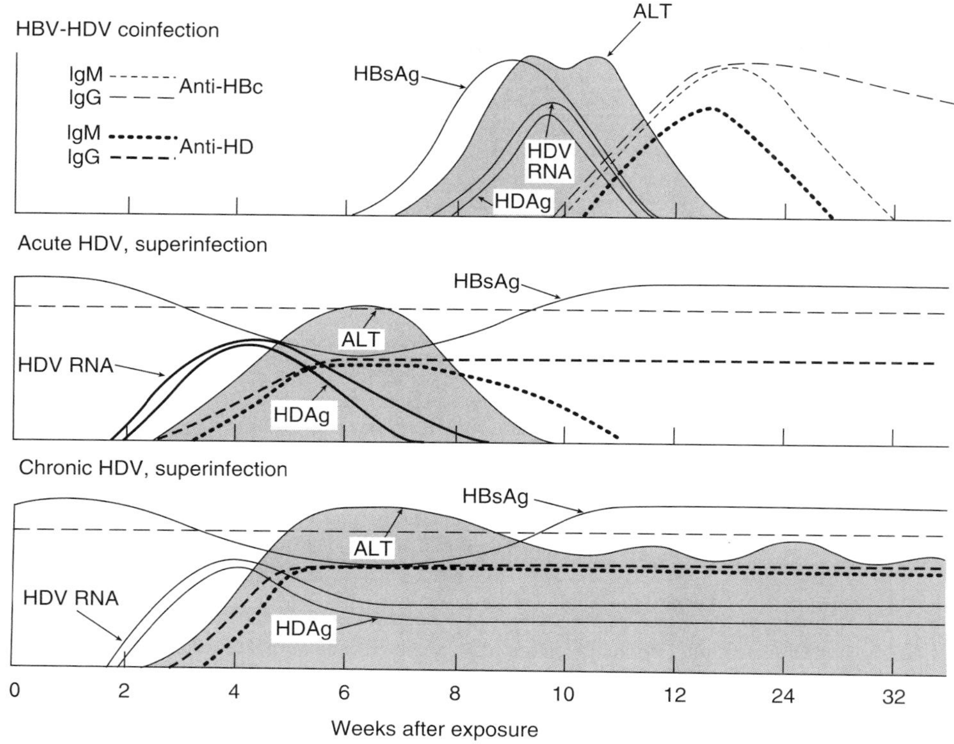

Fig. 32-3 Clinical and serological events associated with hepatitis D virus (HDV). Diagrammatic illustration of clinical and serological events in typical cases of type D hepatitis resulting from acute hepatitis B virus (HBV) and HDV co-infection *(top)*, acute HDV superinfection of a hepatitis B surface antigen (HBsAg) carrier *(middle)*, and HDV superinfection progressing to chronic type D hepatitis in an HBsAg carrier *(bottom)*. (From Lennette EH, Lennette DA, Lennette ET: Diagnostic procedures for viral, rickettsial, and chlamydial infections, ed 7, Washington DC, 1995, American Public Health Association.)

antibodies, and HDAg. Results are reported as "positive" or "negative."[34-36]

HEPATITIS C

Clinical Background

It is estimated that 170 million individuals worldwide and approximately 4 million Americans are infected by HCV. HCV infection is the third highest cause of liver infection after infection by HAV and HBV, and it is responsible for one of every six cases of acute viral hepatitis. HCV is transmitted through blood transfusion, needle sharing, IV drug use, and sexual transmission, and by maternal blood contamination of the newborn during birth.[37] It is estimated that 50% to 85% of HCV-infected patients will become chronic carriers, and approximately 5% to 20% of all chronically infected HCV individuals eventually develop chronic liver disease. In the United States, HCV infections are the primary cause of chronic liver disease such as cirrhosis; ≈25% of cirrhotic patients progress into hepatocellular carcinoma or other end-stage liver disease. Symptoms of HCV infection are similar to those of the other hepatitis viruses, although most HCV-infected patients (80%) are asymptomatic. A vaccine against HCV is not currently available.

Six major genotypes of HCV are based on genome sequencing heterogeneity. Very little is known regarding the extent of serotypical variation among HCV strains. Although no evidence of genomic-based differences in transmissibility or infectivity has been found, HCV-genomic differences in patients' response to interferon-based treatment have been noted.

The 9.0 kb HCV genome encodes at least 10 proteins, including the nucleocapsid protein (core protein), envelope proteins E1 and E2, nonstructural proteins comprising the viral RNA replicase complex (NS3, NS4A, NS4B, NS5A, and NS5B), and the nonstructural proteins NS1 (p7) and NS2. See Color Plate 6.

Laboratory Changes Associated With HCV Infection

Antibodies against HCV are detected in the blood of infected patients as early as 8 weeks post exposure, and HCV RNA can be detected as early as 2 to 3 weeks post exposure (see Color Plate 7). As for other viral hepatitis infections, serum ALT and AST are elevated during the acute phase of infection. During the chronic phase of HCV infection, HCV RNA blood levels are fairly constant, anti-HCV IgG is elevated, and serum ALT levels fluctuate independently of the symptoms.

Diagnosis of HCV Infection

The diagnosis of an HCV infection is based on the detection of IgG antibodies against HCV (aHCV) in blood. Because false positives are associated with aHCV assays, a positive aHCV result should be confirmed either by the **recombinant immunoblot assay (RIBA)** or by measurement of HCV RNA. A positive aHCV result does not distinguish between past and present infections. The presence of HCV RNA in blood is evidence of a current infection.

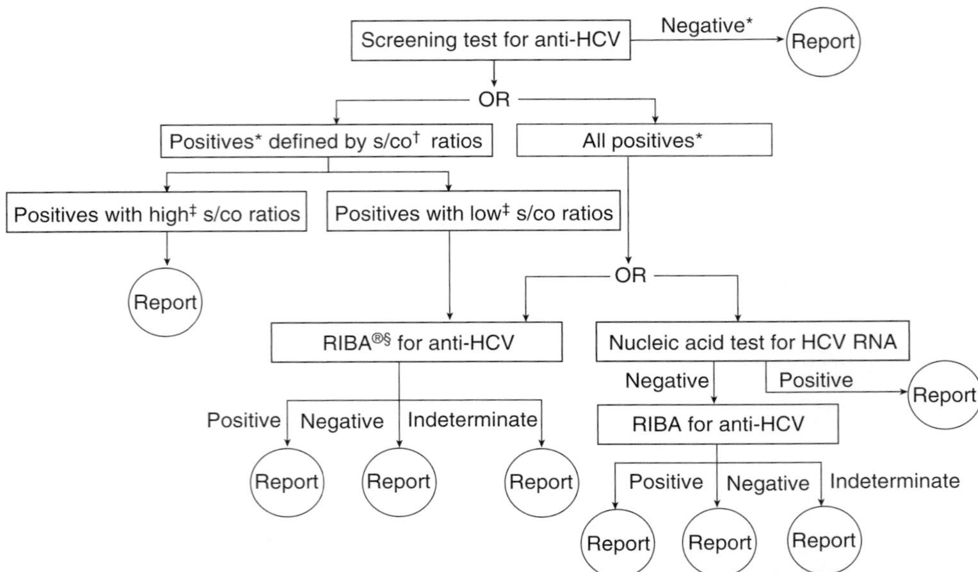

* Interpretation of screening immunoassay test results based on criteria provided by the manufacturer.
† Signal-to-cut-off.
‡ Screening-test-positive results are classified as having high s/co ratios if their ratios are at or above a predetermined value that predicts a supplemental-test-positive result ≥ 95% of the time among all populations tested; screening-test-positive results are classified as having low s/co ratios if their ratios are below this value.
§ Recombinant immunoblot assay.

Fig. 32-4 Laboratory algorithm for antibody to hepatitis C virus (HCV) testing and result reporting. (From CDC: MMWR 52:RR-3, 2003.)

HCV Diagnosis Test Algorithms

To minimize the effects of false-positive and false-negative HCV tests, the Centers for Disease Control and Prevention (CDC) has recommended a laboratory testing algorithm (Fig. 32-4) that describes what to test, how to verify positive aHCV results, and how to interpret the HCV laboratory results. A positive immunoassay test result for aHCV must be confirmed by RIBA testing unless the aHCV assay signal is above the high signal/cutoff that the CDC has established for each commercial aHCV assay.[39] After a positive aHCV result is confirmed, an HCV RNA assay is still required to differentiate between current and past infection. A positive result for the presence of HCV RNA can also be used to confirm aHCV results without the RIBA step, or to directly determine a patient's infectious status. Each laboratory should establish its own algorithm for aHCV testing and result reporting on the basis of its physicians' needs.

Monitoring HCV Infection

HCV RNA Viral Load

The treatment goal of HCV infection is the inhibition of HCV replication. The combination of pegylated interferon alpha and ribavirin seems to be the most effective treatment. Response to treatment is monitored by measuring the blood level of HCV RNA. A "sustained virologic response" (SVR) is defined as an undetectable level of HCV RNA at the end of the treatment and 6 months after it. An individual who achieves an SVR usually has a two $\log_{10}$ decrease in viral RNA ("viral load") within 12 weeks of treatment.[40]

HCV genotyping. HCV genotyping and viral load measurement play an important role in determining treatment and in monitoring a patient's response to therapy. Genotypes I and IV are much less responsive to treatment than are types II and III.[41] Patients with higher initial viral loads and advanced hepatic fibrosis are also less responsive to treatment. Because adverse reactions (e.g., anemia, thrombocytopenia, neutropenia) to treatment with both interferon alpha and ribavirin are not insignificant, it is important to select patients who will respond to this treatment. Genotype and viral load must be determined before treatment is provided, and viral load must be monitored during and at the end of the treatment period so the SVR can be determined.

HCV Assays

aHCV

This test detects IgG antibodies against HCV proteins of the NS3, NS4, NS5, and core regions. With the use of recombinant HCV proteins, the third generation of EIA aHCV assays exhibits 97% sensitivity and can detect the presence of aHCV as early as 6 to 8 weeks post exposure. Chemiluminescence immunoassays have a similar sensitivity and improved specificity.[42,43]

Hepatitis C RIBA

The U.S. Food and Drug Administration (FDA) licensed this test to confirm a positive result of an aHCV by EIA or chemiluminescence immunoassay. RIBA detects the presence of antibodies against the four HCV antigens listed above that are fixed on an immunoblot membrane. A test result is aHCV positive if two or more antigens are recognized, it is indeterminate if only one antigen is recognized, and it is negative if none of the antigens on the membrane is recognized. The test's specificity is very high, but its sensitivity is lower than that of the aHCV EIA and chemiluminescence immunoassays.

Qualitative HCV RNA Assay

HCV RNA can be directly detected by reverse transcriptase (RT)-PCR transcription–mediated amplification (TMA) and branched DNA (b-DNA) assays (see Chapter 13). In 2008, two FDA-approved qualitative RT-PCR tests became available. The Roche assay (Roche Molecular Systems, Branchburg, NJ) has a detection limit of 50 IU/mL of HCV RNA in plasma; the TMA assay (Versant HCV RNA Qualitative Assay, Bayer Diagnostics, Tarrytown, NY) has a detection limit of 10 IU/mL.

Genotyping Assays (see Chapter 13)

Three different methods have been used to determine the genotypes of HCV: direct sequencing, the INNO-LiPA assay,[44] and the Invader assay (Third Wave Molecular Diagnositcs, Madison, WI). The sequence at the 5′UTR end of the HCV genome is the primary target area for all three assays. Sequencing the genome is labor intensive but yields accurate results. INNO-LiPA, a reverse hybridization–based method, is the only FDA genotyping assay for HCV approved by 2008. The Versant HCV Genotype 2.0 assay (Bayer Health Care, Eragny, France) significantly improved its characterization of Genotype 1 by adding a probe for the core region.[44]

Quantitative HCV RNA Test

Quantitative HCV RNA tests can be accomplished by b-DNA–based or RT-PCR techniques. Roche's COBAS Amplicor HCV Monitor test (Roche Molecular Systems, Branchburg, NJ), version 2.0, is an RT-PCR–based assay that has an HCV RNA detection limit of 600 IU/mL. The target region for the amplification of HCV RNA is within the highly conserved 5′-UTR of the HCV genome present in all known genotypes.

HEPATITIS E

Clinical Background

HEV was first described as an independent clinical entity in the 1980s, and its 7 kb genome, cloned in the 1990s, encodes three ORFs. HEV is usually transmitted by water contaminated by human feces that contain HEV.[45] HEV has a relatively high incidence in Southeast and Central Asia, the Middle East, and North and West Africa. Although five major HEV genotypes have been identified, all the genotypes appear to belong to one serotype. The prevalence of HEV infection is highest in young adult males. HEV causes a self-limiting, mild hepatitis, with clinical symptoms similar to those of the other viral hepatitis infections. HEV is responsible for less than 4% of new hepatitis infections each year. Although HEV infection does not result in chronic liver disease such as cirrhosis, a relatively high proportion of HEV-infected pregnant women will develop fulminant liver disease; in one study, 6 of 10 HEV-infected pregnant women developed fulminant hepatitis.[46]

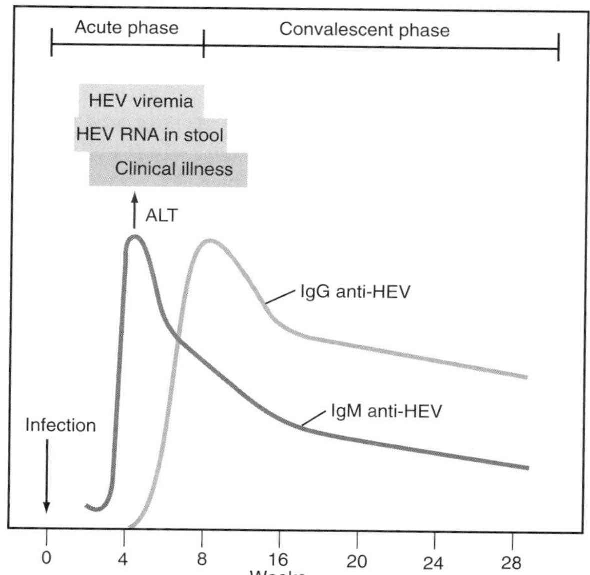

Fig. 32-5 Clinical, virological, and serological events associated with hepatitis E. (From Mandell GL, Bennett JE, Dolin R: *Principles and Practice of Infectious Diseases*, 6th ed, Philadelphia, 2005, Elsevier Churchill Livingstone.)

Mortality from HEV infections in pregnant women increases with each succeeding trimester.[47]

Laboratory Changes Associated With HEV Infection

The incubation time from exposure to development of symptoms in an HEV infection is about 4 to 6 weeks. Serum ALT levels peak approximately 4 weeks after exposure to HEV, and HEV viremia can be detected as early as 3 weeks post exposure by RT-PCR. Serum IgM antibody to HEV can be detected at about the same time that jaundice is observed—approximately 30 days post exposure. HEV infection is usually resolved within 2 to 6 months of infection (Fig. 32-5).

Diagnosis of HEV Infection

The presence of antibody against HEV (aHEV) establishes HEV as the cause of an acute hepatitis. The presence of aHEV IgM suggests that the patient is acutely infected by HEV, but the presence of aHEV IgG indicates only a past HEV infection. Immunoassays for HEV antibodies have greater sensitivity when they employ recombinant antigens that are highly conserved across genotypes, such as the capsid protein of HEV (or synthetic peptides of this protein). Immunoassays that utilize antigens derived from less conserved portions of the HEV genome are less sensitive.

Serum anti-HEV IgM can be detected in up to 96% of patients with hepatitis E 1 to 4 weeks after disease onset. After 6 to 7 weeks, the titer of aHEV IgM will gradually decrease and become undetectable in 50% of patients, 3 months after the onset of disease.[48] Serum aHEV IgG can be detected as late as 14 years after HEV infection.

Monitoring HEV Infection

Serum ALT and bilirubin levels or aHEV IgM can be used to monitor the HEV infection process. Because an HEV infection is usually self-limiting, additional testing is rarely needed.

HEV Assays

The ELISA microtiter plate aHEV IgM assay (Anogen, Ontario, Canada; not FDA approved in 2008) has a sensitivity of approximately 92% and a specificity of 97%. The sensitivity of ELISA microtiter plate aHEV IgG assay (Anogen, Ontario, Canada) is approximately 95%; testing of healthy individuals in low-risk populations yielded a low false-positive rate (≤1%).[49,50]

KEY CONCEPTS BOX 32-2

- Acute infections by a hepatitis virus can be determined by measurement of IgM produced against specific viral proteins or the detection of specific viral proteins. HBV infection is detected by IgM antibody against core antigen and detecting the surface antigen.
- All acute hepatitis infections are noted by increase in amino transaminases and by hyperbilirubinemia.
- Past viral infections can be determined by measuring IgG antibodies against specific viral proteins and noting the absence of specific viral proteins; past HBV infection is noted by the absence of surface antigen and the presence of aHBV for surface, core or e antigens.
- Individuals vaccinated against HBV will have negative results for aHBcT but will have positive results for aHBs. Natural HBV infections are noted by having positive results for both aHBcT and aHBs.
- The reproducibility about cutoff values separating negative and positive results can result in false positive and false negative results. Clinically, there can be false negative results for HBe Ag because of mutants that prevent synthesis of the HBV eAg. The low specificity of the aHCV assays requires confirmation tests by either RIBA testing or by measurement of HCV RNA.

REFERENCES

1. Lemon SM, Jasen RW, Brown EA: Genetic, antigenic and biological differences between strains of hepatitis A virus, Vaccine 10(suppl 1):S40, 1992.
2. Centers for Disease Control and Prevention: Update: Prevention of hepatitis A after exposure to hepatitis A virus and in international travelers. Updated recommendations of the Advisory Committee on Immunization Practices, MMWR 56:1080, 2007.
3. Cuthbert JA: Hepatitis A: Old and new, Clin Microbiol Rev 14:38, 2001.
4. Bower WA, Nainan OV, Han X, et al: Duration of viremia in hepatitis A virus infection, J Infect Dis 182:12, 2000.
5. Centers for Disease Control and Prevention: A comprehensive immunization strategy to eliminate transmission of hepatitis B virus infection in the United States, MMWR 54:RR-16, 2005.
6. Koziel MJ, Siddiqui A: Hepatitis B virus and hepatitis delta virus. In Mandell GL, editor: *Principles and Practice of Infectious Diseases*, 6th ed, Philadelphia, 2005, Elsevier Churchill Livingstone, pp. 1864-1885.
7. Arauz-Ruiz P, Norder H, Robertson BH, et al: Genotype H: a new American genotype of hepatitis B virus revealed in Central America, J Gen Virol 83:2059, 2002.
8. Westland C, Delaney W, Yang H, et al: Hepatitis B genotypes and virologic response in 694 patients in phase III studies of adefovir dipivoxil 1, Gastroenterology 125:107, 2003.
9. Ramvis AK, Kew M, Francois G: Hepatitis B virus genotypes, Vaccine 23:2409, 2005.
10. Kao JH, Chen PJ, Lai MY, et al: Hepatitis B genotypes correlate with clinical outcomes in patients with chronic hepatitis B, Gastroenterology 118:554, 2000.
11. Erhardt A, Blondin D, Hauck K, et al: Response to interferon alpha is hepatitis B virus genotype dependent: genotype A is more sensitive than genotype D, Gut 54:1009, 2005.
12. Chien RN, Yeh CT, Tsai SL, et al: Determinants for sustained HBeAg response to lamivudine therapy, Hepatology 38:1267, 2003.
13. Wai CT, Chu CJ, Hussain M, et al: HBV genotype B is associated with better response to interferon therapy in HBeAg(+) chronic hepatitis than genotype C. Hepatology 36:1425, 2002.
14. Liang TJ, Hasegawa K, Rimon N, et al: A hepatitis B virus mutant associated with an epidemic of fulminant hepatitis, N Engl J Med 324:1705, 1991.
15. Hussain M, Chu CJ, Sablon E, et al: Rapid and sensitive assays for determination of hepatitis B virus genotypes and detection of HBV precore and core promoter variants, J Clin Microbiol 41:3699, 2003.
16. Weber B: Genetic variability of the S gene of hepatitis B virus: clinical and diagnostic impact, J Clin Virol 32:102, 2005.
17. Carmen WF, Zanetti AR, Karayiannis P, et al: Vaccine-induced escape mutant of hepatitis B virus, Lancet 336:325, 1990.
18. Carman WF, Trautwein C, van Deursen FJ, et al: Hepatitis B virus envelope variation after transplantation with and without hepatitis B IG prophylaxis, Hepatology 24:489, 1996.
19. Van Helden J, Denoyel G, Karwowska S, et al: Performance of hepatitis B assays on the Bayer ADVIA Centaur immunoassay system, Clin Lab 50:63, 2004.
20. Siemens Healthcare: ADVIA Centaur HBsAg product insert: Detection of hepatitis B surface antigen in serum, plasma on the ADVIA Centaur system, revision B, Tarrytown, NY, 2007, Siemens Medical Solutions Diagnostics.
21. Baumert TF, Liang TJ: Precore mutants revisited, Hepatology 23:184, 1996.
22. Farrell G: Hepatitis B serocoversion: effects of lamivudine alone or in combination with interferon alpha, J Med Virol 61:374, 2000.
23. Wchiff ER: Lamivudine for hepatitis B in clinical practice, J Med Virol 61:386, 2000.
24. Rokuhara A, Tanaka E, Matsumoto A, et al: Clinical evaluation of a new enzyme immunoassay for hepatitis B virus core-related antigen: a marker distinct from viral DNA for monitoring lamivudine treatment, J Viral Hepat 10:324, 2003.
25. Kimura T, Rokuhara A, Sakamoto Y, et al: Sensitive enzyme immunoassay for hepatitis B virus core-related antigens and their correlation to virus load, J Clin Microbiol 40:439, 2002.
26. Chen D, Kaplan LA, Liu Q: Evaluation of two chemiluminescent immunoassays of ADVIA Centaur for hepatitis B serology marker, Clin Chim Acta 355:41, 2005.
27. Chen D, Kaplan LA: Performance of a new-generation chemiluminescent assay for hepatitis B surface antigen, Clin Chem 52:1592, 2006.
28. Hochberger S, Althof D, Gallegos de Schrott R, et al: Fully automated quantitation of hepatitis B virus DNA in human plasma by the COBAS AmpliPrep/COBAS TaqMan system, J Clin Virol 35:373, 2006.
29. Siowy CO, Giles E: Evaluation of the INNO-LiPA HBV genotyping assay for determination of hepatitis B virus genotype, J Clin Microbiol 12:5473, 2003.

30. Payungporn S, Tangkijvanich P, Jantaradsamee P, et al: Simutaneous quantitation and genotyping of hepatitis B virus by real-time PCR and melting curve analysis, J Virol Methods 120:131, 2004.
31. Farci P, Roskams T, Chessa L, et al: Long term benefit of interferon alpha therapy of chronic hepatitis D: regression of advanced hepatic fibrons, Gastroenterology 126:1740, 2004.
32. Gerin JL, Casey JL, Purcell RH: Hepatitis delta virus. In Knipe DM, Howley PM, editors: *Fields Virology*, 4th ed, Philadelphia, PA, 2001, Lippincott Williams & Wilkins, pp. 3037-3048.
33. Modahi LE, Lai M: Hepatitis delta virus: the molecular basis of laboratory diagnosis, Crit Rev Clin Lab Sci 37:45, 2000.
34. HDV Ag enzyme immunoassay for the determination of HDVAg to hepatitis delta virus in human serum and plasma, product insert, Foster City, CA, 2005, International Immuno-Diagnostics.
35. HDV Ab competitive enzyme immunoassay for the determination of antibodies to hepatitis delta virus in human serum and plasma, product insert, Foster City, CA, 2005, International Immuno-Diagnostics.
36. HDV IgM enzyme immunoassay for the determination of IgM antibody to hepatitis delta virus in human serum and plasma, product insert, Foster City, CA, 2005, International Immuno-Diagnostics.
37. Zanetti AR, Romano L, Bianchi L: Primary prevention of hepatitis C infection, Vaccine 21:692, 2003.
38. Hnatyszyn HJ: Chronic hepatitis C and genotyping: the clinical significance of determining HCV genotypes, Antivir Ther 10:1, 2005.
39. Guidelines for laboratory testing and result reporting of antibody to hepatitis C virus, MMWR 52:RR-3, 2003.
40. Thomas DL, Ray SC, Lemon SM: In Mandell GL, Bennett JE, Dolin R, editors: *Principles and Practice of Infectious Diseases*, 6th ed Chapter 150: *Hepatitis C: Principles and Practice of Infectious Diseases*, 6th ed, Philadelphia, 2005, Elsevier, pp. 1950-1973.
41. Strader DB, Wright T, Thomas DL, et al: American Association for the study of liver diseases: diagnosis, management, and treatment of hepatitis C, Hepatology 39:1147, 2004.
42. Dufour DR, Talastas M, Fernandez M, et al: Chemiluminescence assay improves specificity of hepatitis C antibody detection, Clin Chem 49:940, 2003.
43. Denoyel G, Van Helden J, Bauer R, et al: Performance of a new hepatitis C assay on the Bayer ADVIA Centaur immunoassay system, Clin Lab 50:75, 2004.
44. Bouchardeau F, Cantaloube JF, Chevaliez S, et al: Improvement of hepatitis C virus genotype determination with the new version of the INNO-LiPA HCV assay, J Clin Microbiol 45:1140, 2007.
45. Khuroo MS, Kamili S, Jameel S: Vertical transmission of hepatitis E virus, Lancet 345:1025, 1995.
46. Hamid SS, Jafri MW, Khan H, et al: Fulminant hepatic failure in pregnant women: acute fatty liver or acute virus hepatitis? J Hepatol 25:20, 1996.
47. Mushahwar IK, Dawson GJ, Bile KM, et al: Serological studies of an enterically transmitted non-A, non-B hepatitis in Somalia, J Med Virol 40:218, 1993.
48. Purcell RH, Emerson SU: Hepatitis E virus. In Mandell GL, Bennett JE, Dolin R, editors: *Principles and Practice of Infectious Diseases*, 6th ed, Philadelphia, 2005, Elsevier, pp. 2207-2217.
49. HEV IgM antibody ELISA Kit insert from Anogen: Anogen Mississauga, Ontario Canada.
50. HEV IgG antibody ELISA Kit insert from Anogen: Anogen Mississauga, Ontario Canada.

BIBLIOGRAPHY

Liang T, Hoofnagel J, editors: *Hepatitis C: Biomedical Research Reports*, St. Louis, MO, 2002, Academic Press.

Mandell GL, Bennett JE, Dolin R, editors: *Principles and Practice of Infectious Diseases*, 6th ed, Philadelphia, 2005, Elsevier.

Thomas HC, Lemon S, Zuckerman AJ, editors: *Viral Hepatitis*, 3rd ed, Malden, MA, 2005, Wiley-Blackwell.

INTERNET SITES

http://www.who.int/topics/hepatitis/en/—WHO site

http://digestive.niddk.nih.gov/ddiseases/pubs/viralhepatitis/—NIH site

http://emedicine.medscape.com/article/185463overview—Hepatitis, viral, by Wolf DC (updated 3/21/07)

http://www.aasld.org/practiceguidelines/Pages/ViralHepatitis.aspx—Practice guidelines

http://www.cdc.gov/hepatitis/HepatitisA.htm—CDC site on hepatitis A

http://www.cdc.gov/hepatitis/HepatitisB.htm—CDC site on hepatitis B

http://www.cdc.gov/hepatitis/HepatitisC.htm—CDC site on hepatitis C

http://www.emedicinehealth.com/hepatitis_c/article_em.htm—EMed site

http://www.medicinenet.com/hepatitis_c/article.htm—Hepatitis C

Bone Disease

33

Chapter

Oussama Itani and Reginald C. Tsang

Chapter Outline

Key Terms

bone density Expressed as grams of mineral per area or volume of bone.

bone mass The total amount of bone material, including calcium and phosphorus.

bone quality The architecture, turnover, damage accumulation, and mineralization of bone.

bone remodeling The coupling of bone formation and bone resorption.

bone resorption Breakdown of the bone matrix.

bone sialoprotein Part of the noncollagen bone matrix.

calcidiol 25-Hydroxyvitamin D (25-OHD) is produced when cholecalciferol is hydroxylated at the carbon-25 position in the liver.

calcitonin A hormone of 32 amino acids involved in calcium regulation.

calcitriol 1,25-Dihydroxyvitamin D (1,25-$[OH]_2$D), the active vitamin D metabolite, is produced when cholecalciferol is hydroxylated at both the carbon-1 and carbon-25 positions.

cholecalciferol The parent vitamin D compound.

cortical bone Dense compact bone that provides structural support.

diaphysis Shaft of a long bone.

epiphysis End of a long bone.

ionized calcium The unbound divalent calcium ion that is biologically active.

metaphysis Region in which the diaphysis and epiphysis converge.

N-telopeptides Peptide fragments of the protein that link collagen fragments in bone.

osteoblasts Cells that synthesize bone matrix.

osteocalcin The major component of bone's noncollagen proteins.

osteoclasts Cells that resorb bone.

osteocytes Mature bone cells that have limited function and are encased in bone matrix, the composition of which they help to maintain.

osteoid Bone matrix.

osteolysis Process of being able to resorb bone.

osteomalacia Disorder in which bone contains normal amounts of osteoid but deficient amounts of mineral.

osteopenia The roentgenographic appearance of subnormally mineralized bone.

osteoporosis A generalized reduction in bone mass involving both mineral and osteoid.

parathyroid hormone An 84 amino acid polypeptide hormone that regulates calcium levels in blood.

peak bone mass Maximum bone material during the life of an individual.

phosphatonins Class of phosphate-regulating peptides that increase renal phosphorous excretion and inhibit 25-hydroxyvitamin D 1α-hydroxylase activity, reducing 1α,25$(OH)_2$D synthesis and, thus, intestinal phosphorous absorption.

RANKL Receptor Activator for Nuclear Factor κ B Ligand, also known as TNF-related activation-induced cytokine (TRANCE), osteoprotegerin ligand (OPGL), and ODF (osteoclast differentiation factor). RANKL activates osteoclasts.

rickets Osteomalacia in childhood.

trabecular bone Interlacing delicate spicules of bone that are predominantly involved in mineral homeostasis.

vitamin D Major hormone that controls calcium and phosphorous homeostasis and bone mineralization.

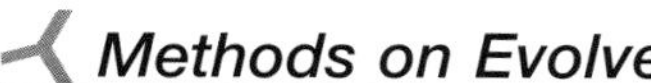

Methods on Evolve

Alkaline phosphatase, total
Calcium
Ionized calcium
Magnesium
Parathyroid hormone
Phosphorus
Vitamin D, 25 hydroxy

SECTION OBJECTIVES BOX 33-1

- Describe the structure and function of normal bone.
- List the primary structural proteins of bone.
- Name and describe the functions of the three types of bone cells.
- List some of the endocrine and autocrine factors that affect osteoblasts.
- List the factors that determine adult bone mass.

BONE STRUCTURE AND FUNCTION

More than 90% of the cells in bone are encased in calcified tissue and are separated by great distances from a vascular supply. This gives the cells the appearance of inactivity. However, the skeletal system is a dynamic organ, with bone having two interdependent roles: provision of support and maintenance of mineral homeostasis. Both functions are successfully achieved by continuous **bone remodeling.** Disturbances in the balance and nature of bone formation and resorption produce the common bone diseases.

Bone Structure

This section provides a basic overview of the complex function of bone. Excellent, recent references provide more advanced knowledge of this field.[1-8]

Macroscopically, the major bones are classified as long bones or flat bones. Long bones are confined to the limbs and consist of a shaft **(diaphysis),** two ends **(epiphyses),** and a region in which the two converge **(metaphysis)** (Fig. 33-1, *A*). Seen in cross section, the diaphysis is lined by dense, compact (cortical) bone, whereas the metaphysis contains interlacing bony spicules that resemble the structure of a sponge (trabecular or cancellous bone) (Fig. 33-1, *B*). Flat bones, typified by the bones of the skull, consist of two thin layers of **cortical bone** that enclose a layer of **trabecular bone.** Trabecular bone is an important contributor to mechanical support, particularly in the vertebrae. It is also more metabolically active than cortical bone and provides initial supplies of mineral in acute deficiency states. Dense cortical bone, which accounts for 80% of the skeleton, provides the strength needed for structural support, and the spicules of trabecular bone provide a large surface area for bone synthesis and resorption and provide a reservoir of minerals for the maintenance of mineral homeostasis.

Bone contains three major types of mature cells—**osteoblasts, osteocytes,** and **osteoclasts.**[9,10] Osteoblasts, which are found along surfaces of both cortical and trabecular bone, are specialized fibroblasts derived from precursor cells that are partially differentiated and ordinarily can further differentiate only into osteoblasts. Osteoclasts secrete and calcify a specific bone matrix that consists of collagen and noncollagen proteins. The plasma membrane of the osteoblast is very rich in alkaline phosphatase (ALP), the activity of which is an index of bone formation. Osteoblasts have receptors for a large number of hormones, both endocrine and autocrine factors produced by the osteoblasts (Box 33-1; see Chapter 48). Stimulation by parathyroid hormone (PTH), 1,25$(OH)_2$D, growth hormone, and estrogen causes osteoblasts to produce insulin-like growth factor I (IGF-I), which has a significant role in local bone regulation and modeling. As osteoblasts become embedded in bone matrix, they differentiate into mature osteocytes. Osteocytes synthesize small amounts of matrix continuously to maintain bone integrity, and they are able to resorb bone (osteocytic **osteolysis**) in exceptional circumstances when normal mineral homeostasis is altered.[11,12] They also are part of the system that senses mechanical force on the bone from weight loads. In response, they produce nitric oxide

Box 33-1

Endocrine and Autocrine Factors Affecting Osteoblasts and Osteoclasts

Calcitriol (1,25-dihydroxyvitamin D)
Glucocorticoids
Growth hormone (GH)
Parathyroid hormone (PTH)
Sex hormones
Serotonin
Thyroid hormone
Growth factors (insulin-like growth factors, interleukin [IL]-1, tumor necrosis factor-alpha, prostaglandins, transforming growth factor beta, bone morphogenetic proteins, fibroblast growth factors, and platelet-derived growth factor)

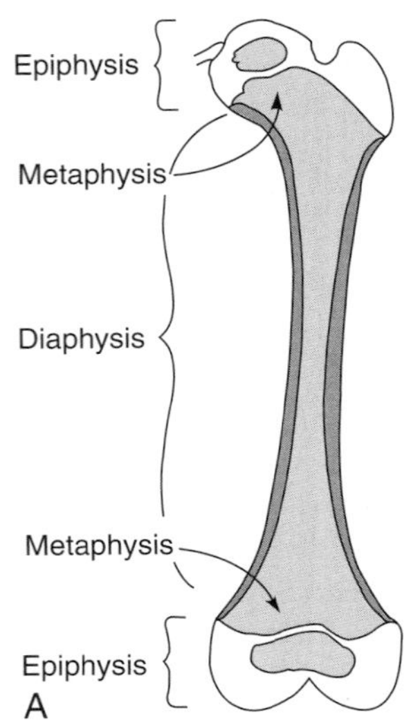

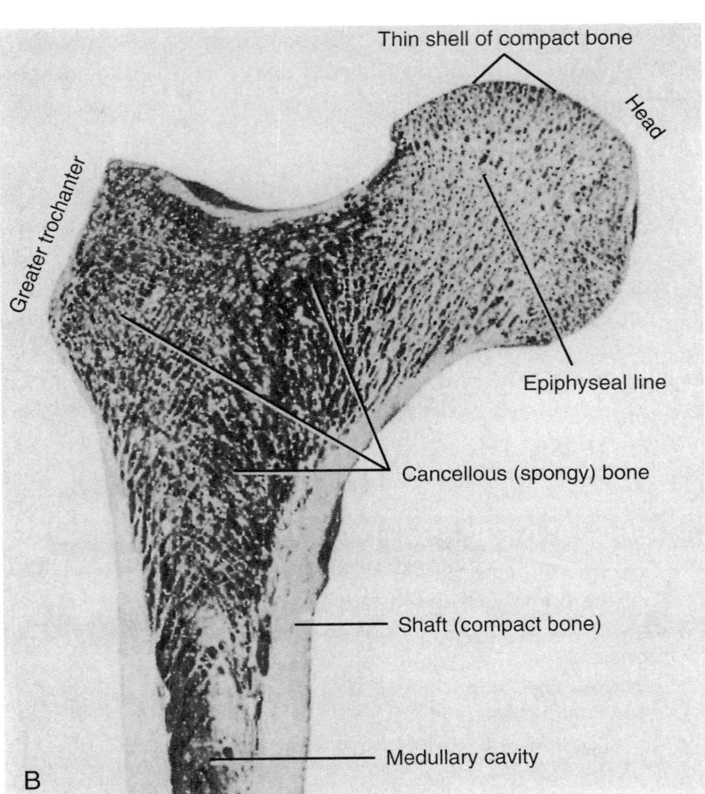

Fig. 33-1 **A,** Parts of a long bone. **B,** Long bone in cross section: note the predominance of trabecular, cancellous bone in the diaphysis. (From Copenhaver WM, Kelly DE, Wood RL, editors: *Bailey's Textbook of Histology,* ed 17, Baltimore, 1978, Williams & Wilkins.)

and prostaglandins that mediate the bone's response to the load.

Osteoclasts resorb bone by dissolving mineral and degrading matrix.[13] The locally acidic pH (≈4.5) decalcifies the tissue, exposing the organic matrix to degradation by lysosomally derived proteases, particularly cathepsin K. Excessive osteoclastic resorption occurs in **osteoporosis,** Paget's disease, hyperparathyroidism, and inflammatory bone loss. On the other hand, osteoclastic resorption is deficient in osteopetrosis. Osteoclasts are related to monocyte/macrophage cells, and macrophage colony-stimulating factor (MCSF) is required to initiate osteoclast differentiation. Osteoclast formation requires an interaction with cells of the osteoblastic lineage.[14] Many hormones and local factors also can act on osteoblasts to promote (**calcitriol,** PTH, tumor necrosis factor [TNF]-alpha, prostaglandin E2, and interleukin [IL]-1, IL-11, and IL-6) or inhibit (IL-4, -12, -13, and -18 and interferon gamma) osteoclastogenesis.[14] Serotonin produced by cells in the gastrointestinal tract also can regulate bone formation.[15] The presence of excess serotonin depresses bone formation while low serotonin levels produce strong, dense bones. Although **bone resorption** is primarily affected by the osteoclast, other cells influenced by bone-resorbing hormones can direct the osteoclasts. The moth-eaten appearance of bone that indicates bone resorption is evident in histological sections of areas in which osteoclasts are numerous.

Only a small portion of bone is cellular; calcified matrix predominates. This matrix is primarily composed of collagen fibers (mostly type I), a glycosaminoglycan-containing ground substance, and noncollagenous proteins. Type I collagen is the major collagen produced by osteoblasts; it represents more than 90% by weight of the nonmineral component of bone. Noncollagen, calcium-binding proteins are critical for regulating mineralization and strengthening the collagen backbone. These include **osteocalcin** (bone Gla protein, the major component of non-collagen proteins) and matrix Gla protein; both contain gamma-carboxyglutamic acid, whose synthesis is vitamin K dependent. These proteins delay mineralization and allow bone matrix to mature. **Bone sialoprotein** and osteopontin bind both calcium and collagen and may play a role in the adherence of osteoclasts to the bone surface. Spindle-shaped hydroxyapatite, $Ca_{10}(PO_4)_6(OH)_2$, crystals are present in the ground substance and are aligned on and within collagen fibers.

Collagen is deposited in a lamellar fashion and is strengthened by multiple cross-links, both within and between the triple-helical collagen molecules. These cross-links are pyridinolines that are resistant to degradation and are released during bone resorption as free or peptide-bound forms that can be measured in serum and urine. Glycosaminoglycans are highly anionic complexes that play a major role in the calcification process and the fixation of hydroxyapatite crystals to collagen fibers. Approximately one-fourth of the amino acids present in collagen consist of proline or hydroxyproline, neither of which is present to any great extent in other tissues. When collagen is metabolized, hydroxyproline-containing oligopeptides are excreted in the urine, and the amount present correlates with the amount of bone turnover. The mineral elements of bone consist mostly of crystals of calcium and phosphate arranged amorphously or as hydroxyapatite. A wide range of other elements, including sodium, magnesium, copper, zinc, lead, and fluoride, may be present.

Skeletal Development[16]

The processes of cellular differentiation that give rise to the skeleton are regulated by genes[17,18] that first establish the pattern of skeletal structure in the form of cartilage and mesenchyme and then replace them with bone through the differentiation of osteoblasts. Replacement of cartilage by more rigid bone begins early in fetal life. As the skeleton grows, not only in fetal life but during childhood and adolescence, modeling (the formation of new bone at sites where none previously existed and the removal of old bone at other sites) is critical for the formation of normal skeletal structures. However, even during fetal life, much of the cellular activity is devoted to remodeling (removing and replacing skeletal structures already present). This becomes the dominant form of bone cell activity after puberty. The first bone formed from mesenchyme in early development as well as bone formed during rapid repair may have a relatively disorganized pattern of collagen fibers in the matrix and is termed "woven" bone. However, all other bone is laid down in an orderly fashion with successive layers of well-organized collagen; this is termed *lamellar bone.*

Bone Mass

About 45% of the adult skeleton is built and enlarged during adolescence.[19-23] The concept of **peak bone mass** has become crucial to an understanding of osteoporosis, especially postmenopausal osteoporosis. Peak bone mass is determined by several factors, including genetics, nutrition, mechanics, and environment.[24,25] The genetic effect on adult female bone mass may be mediated largely through effects on bone formation that occur premenopausally and postmenopausally, rather than through effects on resorption. A strong positive relationship exists between current and past calcium intake and the peak bone mass achieved. Higher calcium intake during adolescence theoretically may optimize, within genetic limits, peak bone mass. Physical activity, use of estrogenic oral contraceptives, and dietary calcium intake exert a positive effect on bone gain in young adult women. Androgens and estrogen are important determinants of peak **bone density** in young women. The optimal dietary calcium intake for bone growth is a debatable issue. The daily calcium intake recommended by the Institute of Medicine[26] is less than the higher calcium intakes suggested by recent studies as needed to meet calcium retention requirements for growth. These higher requirements are as follows: an average of 180 mg/day (dietary calcium intake of 700 mg/day) must be retained during childhood,[27] 220 to 280 mg/day during adolescence (dietary calcium intake of 1300 to 1500 mg/day with an upper limit of 2500 mg/day),[28] and probably 20 to 30 mg/day during early adulthood from 20 to 30 years of age.[29]

Bone strength is determined by bone density and bone quality. Bone density is expressed as grams of mineral per area or volume, and in any given individual is determined by peak bone mass and amount of bone loss. Bone mineral density (BMD) accounts for approximately 70% of bone strength. **Bone quality** refers to architecture, turnover, damage accumulation (e.g., microfractures) and mineralization. A fracture occurs when a failure-inducing force (e.g., trauma) is applied to osteoporotic bone.

Bone Function

The large surface area and excellent blood supply of trabecular bone permit a quick response to perturbations in plasma mineral concentrations. In contrast, the abundant calcified matrix of cortical bone provides the strength to support body weight. Despite this segregation of structure and function, disturbances in both often coexist. Examples include **vitamin D** deficiency, which causes both hypocalcemia and easily fractured bone, and immobilization, which causes bone resorption, osteoporosis, and hypercalcemia. Under normal circumstances, such disturbances do not occur because, in bone remodeling that occurs throughout the body, bone formation and bone resorption are "coupled," resulting in equal amounts of bone formation and resorption.[30] Most bone diseases result from alterations in coupling that are new or that occur secondary to hormonal imbalance, which produces excessive bone formation or excessive resorption.

KEY CONCEPTS BOX 33-1

- The most important functions of bone are to provide physical strength and support for the body and to control calcium (Ca) homeostasis.
- Bone formation is maintained through the actions of the osteoclasts, osteocytes, and osteoblasts; the latter lay down the protein and hydroxyapatite, the mineral matrix of bone.
- The important bone protein is collogen, which contains large amounts of the amino acids proline and hydroxyproline.
- Peak bone mass, the mass of bone attained by adulthood, affects bone strength in later life. It is highly dependent on dietary intake of Ca, general health, and exercise.

SECTION OBJECTIVES BOX 33-2

- Define "bone modeling" and "bone remodeling"; differentiate between the two terms, and explain how the two processes combine to maintain bone.
- List the hormones that affect bone remodeling.
- List the biochemical markers of bone turnover.

BONE CHANGES[16]

Bone Modeling

Growth of the skeleton and changes in bone shape are produced by *modeling.* Linear growth of bones during childhood and adolescence occurs by growth of cartilage at the end plates, followed by endochondral bone formation. The width of the bones increases during childhood; this is accompanied by resorption of the inner bone surface with concomitant enlargement of the marrow cavity. During puberty and early adult life, endosteal apposition and trabecular thickening provide maximum skeletal mass and strength (peak bone mass). These processes are influenced by locally and systemically produced factors and mechanical forces.

Bone Remodeling

Inherent to bone physiology is the physiological "coupling" of the processes of bone formation and resorption, called *remodeling.* Although bone remodeling begins early in skeletal development, it continues throughout life and requires a balance between bone formation and resorption. At any time, approximately 10% of bone mass participates in bone remodeling. Growth during infancy and adolescence is associated with a predominance of bone formation over bone resorption, resulting in increased bone mass and bone deposition. In young adults, the processes of bone resorption and formation are equal. With aging, bone resorption exceeds bone formation, thereby predisposing the older individual to net bone loss and osteoporosis. In bone disease states, this balance is altered. For instance, in osteoporosis, the volume of bone resorbed outweighs the volume of bone formed, resulting in a net loss of bone at each remodeling site. The fact that most of the skeleton consists of remodeled bone led to the concept of bone structural units (BSU), also called bone multicellular or remodeling units. A bone remodeling cycle begins with activation of bone formation mediated by cells of the osteoblast lineage. Activation may involve the osteocytes, the "lining cells" (resting osteoblasts on the bone surface), and pre-osteoblasts in the marrow. These cells undergo shape changes and secrete collagenase and other enzymes that digest proteins on the bone surface; they also express a cell differentiating factor[16] that causes the activation, migration, differentiation, and fusion of hematopoietic cells of the osteoclast lineage to begin the process of resorption. Osteoblasts and other marrow cells produce osteoprotegerin (OPG; osteoclastogenesis inhibitory factor).[14] OPG appears to have important regulatory functions; women with osteoporosis and increased biochemical markers of bone turnover have higher serum osteoprotegerin concentrations than do nonosteoporotic controls. Administration of osteoprotegerin to postmenopausal women results in rapid reduction of biochemical markers of bone turnover. This may occur as a compensatory mechanism in response to increased **RANKL** production. The subsequent remodeling cycle consists of three phases: resorption, reversal, and formation.

Resorption

Osteoclastic resorption begins with the migration of partially differentiated mononuclear pre-osteoblasts to the bone surface; these then coalesce to form the large, multinucleated osteoclasts that are required for bone resorption. Osteoclasts remove mineral and matrix to a limited depth on the trabecular surface or within cortical bone. It is unclear what stops this process, but high local concentrations of calcium or substances released from the matrix may be involved.

Reversal

After osteoclastic resorption is completed, a reversal phase occurs, in which mononuclear cells, possibly of monocyte/macrophage lineage, appear on the bone surface. These cells prepare the surface for new osteoblasts to begin bone formation. A layer of glycoprotein-rich material is laid down on the resorbed surface, the so-called cement line, to which the new osteoblasts can adhere. Osteopontin may be a key protein in this process. The cells at the reversal site may also provide signals for osteoblast differentiation[31] and migration.

Formation

The formation phase follows, with successive waves of osteoblasts laying down bone until the resorbed bone is completely replaced and a new bone structural unit is fully formed. When this phase is complete, the surface is covered with flattened lining cells, and there is a prolonged resting period with little cellular activity on the bone surface until a new remodeling cycle begins. The stages of the remodeling cycle have different lengths. Resorption probably continues for about 2 weeks. The reversal phase may last up to 4 or 5 weeks, and formation can continue for 4 months, until the new bone structural unit is fully formed.

Normal and Abnormal Coupling of Modeling and Remodeling

In healthy adults, bone resorption and bone formation are tightly coupled, so that the amount of bone formed in new BSUs equals the amount of bone resorbed. The size and shape of cortical BSUs, the *osteons,* are relatively uniform. Pathological remodeling can result in bone loss in several ways. One important mechanism is excessive resorption depth, which can result in complete loss of trabecular structures. Second, bone thinning can occur when the extent of resorption or the number of resorbing sites (activation frequency) is increased. Osteoblasts normally completely fill the resorption cavity; if this does not occur, the BSU is incomplete, which results in decreased "wall thickness" in trabecular bone. Last, a progressive decrease in wall thickness occurs with aging, along with a marked decrease in wall thickness, in patients treated with glucocorticoids. These decreases are attributed to defective osteoblast renewal or shortened osteoblast lifespan. Remodeling imbalance can also occur because of failure of the resorptive process. This can result in dense bones (osteopetrosis or osteosclerosis) and impaired hematopoiesis. As described below, macrophage colony-stimulating factor (M-CSF) is required to initiate osteoclast differentiation. In humans, the most common mutation linked to osteopetrosis is a defect in the osteoclast-specific proton-pump subunit *(TCIRG1);* 60 percent of patients with severe autosomal recessive osteopetrosis have this mutation. Other clinically significant mutations have been identified in *CLCN7,* a gene that encodes an osteoclast-specific chloride channel, and in CAII, the carbonic anhydrase II gene. All of these mutations cause defects in the acidification of bone.

Hormonal Regulation of Bone Remodeling[18,32]

Both systemic and local regulators control the dynamic balance between bone formation and resorption. Systematic and local (autocrine and paracrine) regulators of bone homeostasis are listed in Box 33-1. PTH and 1,25$(OH)_2$D (calcitriol) play an important role in activating bone remodeling. PTH has a biphasic effect on bone homeostasis: on the one hand, intermittent administration of PTH stimulates bone formation, possibly through production of local growth factors IGF-I and IGF-II; on the other hand, continuous PTH administration has a catabolic effect on bone and favors bone resorption. Prostaglandins, particularly of the E series, are potent local bone resorbing agents. 1,25$(OH)_2$D and thyroid hormones also have a biphasic effect on bone homeostasis. Bone turnover is increased in hyperthyroidism, and thyrotoxicosis is a significant risk factor for bone loss and osteoporosis. Calcitriol increases intestinal absorption of calcium and phosphorus, thereby promoting bone mineralization. At high concentrations, under conditions of calcium and phosphate deficiency, calcitriol also stimulates bone resorption, thereby helping to maintain the supply of these ions to other tissues. Gastrointestinal-derived serotonin is also a potent inhibitor of bone-forming cells and increases net bone loss.

Growth hormone also has an anabolic effect on bone metabolism; it increases bone formation by increasing local concentrations of IGF-I, which is important for skeletal growth.[33] Increases in IGF-I occur during childhood, with peak levels noted during pubertal development; IGF-I correlates better with Tanner stage of physical development than with chronological age. Glucocorticoids have both stimulatory and inhibitory effects on bone cells. They are essential for differentiation of osteoblasts, and they sensitize bone cells to regulators of bone remodeling, including IGF-I and PTH. Inhibition of bone formation is the major cause of glucocorticoid-induced osteoporosis.

Sex Hormones

Androgens may stimulate bone formation, either directly or through their effects on adjacent muscle tissue.[34] Both androgens and estrogens, via their respective cell receptors (ERs), maintain cancellous bone mass and integrity, regardless of age or sex. Androgen action on cancellous bone depends on local aromatization of androgens into estrogens. Androgens increase cortical bone size via stimulation of both longitudinal and radial growth. Both sex hormones have a biphasic effect on endochondral bone formation: at the start of puberty, sex steroids stimulate endochondral bone formation, whereas they induce epiphyseal closure at the end of puberty. Androgen action on the growth plate is, however, clearly mediated via aromatization to estrogens and subsequent interaction with estrogen receptors. Androgens increase radial growth, whereas estrogens decrease outer bone formation. This effect of androgens may be important because bone strength in males seems to be determined by relatively higher outer bone formation and, therefore, greater bone dimensions, relative to muscle mass at older age. The action of androgens on bone via both sex hormone receptors may protect men against osteoporosis via maintenance of cancellous bone mass and expansion of cortical bone.[35] Estradiol and progesterone stimulate osteoblastic activity to increase bone formation. Estrogen increases production of both IGF-I and IGF-II and affects the production of local factors, including cytokines and prostaglandins.

Estrogens regulate bone turnover and are critical for epiphyseal closure in puberty in both sexes. In fact, estrogen has a greater effect than androgen in inhibiting bone resorption in men, although androgen may still play a role. Estrogen may also be important in the acquisition of peak bone mass in men. In late puberty, estrogens decrease bone turnover by inhibiting bone resorption. Moreover, osteoporosis in older men is more closely associated with low estrogen than with low androgen levels.

Effects of Estrogen on Growth, Modeling, and Remodeling[36-38]

Estrogen has a biphasic effect on growth. In low doses, it stimulates growth hormone production, resulting in accelerated growth, whereas high doses slowed growth and accelerated fusion of the epiphyses. Arrested growth and delayed closure of the growth plate resulting in delayed bone age and osteoporosis have been reported in men with estrogen receptor deficiency[39] or aromatase deficiency.[40] Estrogen mediates the sexual dimorphism of bone and accounts for lesser linear growth and smaller bones relative to size in women compared with men. Estrogen decreases bone remodeling and bone turnover markers in girls during puberty[36] by decreasing the numbers of osteoclasts and osteoblasts. The effects of estrogen on the osteoclast probably are mainly indirect and are mediated by factors secreted by the osteoblast, which regulate the differentiation of osteoclast precursors to osteoclasts and then modulate the activity of the mature osteoclast and regulate its rate of apoptosis.[36] Estrogen binds to receptors on the osteoblasts; it increases the production of osteoprotegerin and decreases the production of colony stimulating factor (CSF)-1. Estrogen decreases secretion of the proinflammatory cytokines interleukin-1 and tumor necrosis factor-alpha by marrow monocytes, resulting in decreased production of osteoclasts and a reduction in their activity and their survival. In the growth plate, estrogen induces apoptosis (programmed death) of chondrocytes, resulting in arrest of linear growth. The effects of biomechanical forces[41] and the remodeling effects of estrogen, as well as growth plate effects, are mediated mainly by the estrogen receptor-α, but the effects on outer bone may be mediated by the β-receptor.[42]

Interaction of Estrogen with GH and IGF-I

Estrogen increases GH secretion by the pituitary gland at puberty, and this has direct and indirect effects (by increasing IGF-I) on bone growth, modeling, and remodeling.[43] Estrogen antagonizes the effects of GH and of IGF-I on the growth plate by stimulating fusion of the epiphysis.[44] It opposes their effects at the periosteum and on bone remodeling.

Prostaglandins have biphasic effects on bone resorption and formation, but their dominant effects in vivo are stimulatory.[45] Prostaglandin production can be increased by impact loading and by inflammatory cytokines, such as nitric oxide and leukotrienes. Nitric oxide inhibits osteoclastic bone resorption and increases bone density, perhaps by increasing OPG production. Leukotrienes, the products of lipoxygenase, stimulate osteoclastic bone resorption and inhibit bone formation. Polymorphisms in the human gene for lipoxygenase, *ALOX15*, are associated with differences in peak bone density in postmenopausal women. Bone morphogenetic proteins (BMPs) increase osteoblast differentiation and bone formation. Polymorphisms of the *BMP2* gene are linked to low bone mineral density and increased fracture risk.[16]

Osteoclasts carry receptors for **calcitonin.** In pharmacologic doses, calcitonin directly inhibits bone resorption by binding to specific receptors on osteoclasts to inhibit osteoclast formation, motility, and activity.[3] However, its physiological role is minimal in the adult skeleton, and it is only transiently effective in treating hypercalcemia caused by excessive bone resorption. Fibroblast growth factors (FGFs) are another family of proteins involved in skeletal development. Mutations in the receptors for these factors result in abnormal skeletal phenotypes, such as achondroplasia.[46] Other growth factors such as vascular endothelial growth factor (VEGF) are produced in bone and may play a role in bone remodeling.[47]

Biochemical Markers of Bone Turnover[48-50]

The processes of bone formation and resorption are accompanied by production of a plethora of proteins. Measurement of several of these molecules in serum and urine provides a valuable indicator of ongoing homeostatic bone processes (Box 33-2). These markers serve as noninvasive indicators of osteoblastic or osteoclastic activities. However, interpretation of their results is difficult because the concentrations depend on age, pubertal stage, growth velocity, mineral accrual, hormonal regulation, nutritional status, circadian variation, method of expression of results of urinary markers, specificity for bone tissue, and the sensitivity and specificity of different assays. In addition, studies have shown that the accuracy of these markers for osteoporosis diagnosis and monitoring is inferior to bone mineral density measurements. Furthermore, no pediatric reference ranges are available for many of the newer markers. However, measurement of these markers in conjunction with clinical evaluation and radiological findings may aid in the initial investigation of osteoporosis and may facilitate monitoring of therapy. Because of their multiple limitations, bone metabolism markers should not be relied on exclusively for important clinical decision making. Measurement of several indices at once, as well as serial measurements, may help to overcome some of these limitations.

Box 33-2
Biochemical Markers of Bone Turnover

Bone Formation
- Serum osteocalcin
- Serum alkaline phosphatase (ALP), bone-specific ALP
- Serum procollagen I extension peptides

Bone Resorption Markers
- Urine hydroxyproline
- Urine deoxypyridinoline
- Urine pyridinoline
- Type I collagen telopeptides (peptides that contain cross-links)
  - N-terminal telopeptide to helix in urine (NTX-I)
  - C-terminal telopeptide-1 to helix in serum (ICTP)
  - C-terminal telopeptide-2 in urine and serum (CTX)
- Serum tartrate–resistant acid phosphatase, hydroxylysine, and its glycosides

KEY CONCEPTS BOX 33-2

- The thickening and lenghtening of bone with new bone protein and mineral matrix is called *bone modeling.* Bone modeling stops at puberty, but thereafter, bones are constantly resorbing bone and laying down new bone, a process called *bone remodeling.*
- Growth hormone and male and female sex hormones affect both bone modeling and remodeling. Parathyroid hormone (PTH) and vitamin D are important in ensuring the supply of Ca for the mineral matrix.
- Markers of bone remodeling (turnover) include the urinary telopeptides and pyridinoline, which are breakdown products of collagen.

SECTION OBJECTIVES BOX 33-3

- List the primary determinant of healthy bone.
- List the primary mineral components of bone.
- Outline the metabolism of calcium.
- Describe the effects of vitamin D metabolites, parathyroid hormone (PTH), magnesium, and phosphorus on calcium metabolism and regulation.

BIOCHEMISTRY AND PHYSIOLOGY

Determinants of Bone Health[19,20,51,52]

Although most growth in bone size and strength occurs during childhood, bone accumulation is not completed until the third decade of life, after the cessation of linear growth. The bone mass attained early in life is perhaps the most important determinant of lifelong skeletal health. Individuals with the highest peak bone mass after adolescence have the greatest protective advantage when declines in bone density associated with increasing age, illness, and diminished sex steroid production take their toll. Peak bone mass is influenced by genetic, physiological, environmental, and lifestyle factors. Among these are adequate nutrition and body weight, exposure to sex hormones at puberty, and physical activity.[24,25] Therefore, maximizing bone mass early in life presents a critical opportunity to reduce the impact of bone loss related to aging. Childhood is also a critical time for the development of lifestyle habits conducive to maintaining good bone health throughout life. Cigarette smoking, which usually starts in adolescence, may have a deleterious effect on achieving bone mass.

Nutrition (see Chapter 41)

Good nutrition is essential for normal bone growth and health.[29] Supplementation of calcium and vitamin D may be necessary. Proper calcium intake is most important for attaining peak bone mass and for preventing and treating osteoporosis. Although the IOM recommends calcium intakes of 800 mg/day for children ages 3 to 8 and 1300 mg/day for children and adolescents ages 9 to 17 years, only about 25% of boys and 10% of girls ages 9 to 17 are estimated to meet these recommendations. For older adults, calcium intake should be maintained at 1000 to 1500 mg/day, yet only about 50% to 60% of this population meets this recommendation.[53]

Vitamin D Requirements for Optimal Calcium Absorption and Bone Health[54] (see later discussion)

Most infants and young children in the United States have some vitamin D intake because of supplementation and fortification of milk. During adolescence, when consumption of dairy products decreases, vitamin D intake is less likely to be adequate, and this may adversely affect calcium absorption. Suboptimal intake of vitamin D in children and adolescents, and the persistence of clinical vitamin D deficiency contributing to bone disease in late adulthood and in the elderly, have necessitated a recommendation of higher vitamin D intake of 2000-4000 IU/day.[55-57] The actual dietary requirement during pregnancy and lactation may actually be as high as 6000 IU/day.[57] The primary function of vitamin D—optimizing intestinal calcium absorption—is fully expressed at a serum 25-hydroxyvitamin D concentration of approximately 80 nmol/L. At this level, elevated parathyroid activity, typical of aging populations, is minimized, and osteoporotic fractures are reduced. Achieving a level at least this high may require a daily oral intake of at least 2200 IU (55 μg) of vitamin D. Actual vitamin D toxicity is not seen at continuing oral intakes of 10,000 IU (250 μg)/day.[58,59]

In preterm infants, a calcium retention level ranging from 60 to 90 mg/kg/day ensures appropriate mineralization; it decreases the risk of fracture and diminishes the clinical symptoms of **osteopenia** of prematurity. Therefore, an intake of 100 to 160 mg/kg/day of highly bioavailable calcium salts, 60 to 90 mg/kg/day of phosphorus, and 800 to 1000 IU/day of vitamin D is recommended.[60]

High dietary protein, caffeine, phosphorus, and sodium can adversely affect calcium balance, but their effects appear not to be important in individuals with adequate calcium intake. Recent studies have underlined the importance of optimal dietary protein intake in increased bone mineral mass and a reduced incidence of osteoporotic fractures.[61] Dietary proteins enhance IGF-I, a factor that exerts positive activity on skeletal development and bone formation.

Exercise

Physical activity early in life contributes to higher peak bone mass, with resistance and high-impact exercise providing the greatest benefit.[24,25] It is clear that exercise later in life, even beyond 90 years of age, can increase muscle mass and strength twofold or more in frail individuals, and can have a modest effect on slowing the decline in bone mass and density (BMD).

Gonadal Steroids (see Chapter 50)

Sex steroids secreted during puberty increase BMD and peak bone mass in both women and men. In adolescent girls and women, sustained production of estrogens is essential for the maintenance of bone mass.[62] Reduction in estrogen production with menopause is the major cause of loss of BMD during later life. Timing of menarche, absent or infrequent menstrual cycles, and the timing of menopause influence both the attainment of peak bone mass and the preservation of BMD. Testosterone production is important for achieving and maintaining maximal bone mass in adolescent boys and men; estrogens have also been implicated in the growth and maturation of the male skeleton. Delayed onset of puberty is a risk factor for diminished bone mass in men, and hypogonadism in adult men results in osteoporosis.

Growth Hormone and Body Composition

Growth hormone and IGF-I, which are secreted maximally during puberty, play a role in the acquisition and maintenance of bone mass and the determination of body composition into adulthood. Growth hormone deficiency is associated with a decrease in BMD. Children and youth with low body mass index (BMI) are likely to attain lower than average peak bone mass. Although a direct association between BMI and bone mass has been noted throughout the adult years, it is not known whether the association between body composition and bone mass is due to hormones, nutritional factors, higher impact during weight-bearing activities, or other factors.

Mineral Physiology

Calcium and mineral metabolism represents a delicate and complex biological process composed of many intricate and interrelated components. Normal homeostatic metabolism depends on the availability of mineral substrates and the interactions of tissues such as bone, kidney, and the gastrointestinal tract with the calcitropic hormones PTH, calcitonin (CT), and $1,25(OH)_2D$.

Calcium and Phosphorus

Calcium is the fifth most abundant inorganic element in the human body. The human body contains about 1200 g of calcium in the adult and approximately 28 g in a full-term newborn. Almost all the body's calcium (99%) resides in bone. The remainder resides in body fluids and serves a crucial role in a multitude of physiological processes, including muscular contraction, neurotransmission, membrane transport, enzyme reactions, hormone secretion, and blood coagulation. In the circulation, calcium exists in three forms: 45% of total serum calcium is the biologically active **ionized calcium,** 45% is protein bound, mainly to albumin, and 10% is complexed to anions (phosphate, lactate, citrate).

Bone contains 80% to 85% of total body phosphorus; approximately 9% is found in muscle, and the remainder is present in the viscera and extracellular fluid. The intracellular concentration of phosphorus (phosphates and organic phosphorus) is greater than the extracellular levels. Inorganic phosphate (PI) is required for energy metabolism, nucleic acid synthesis, bone mineralization, and cell signaling. The activity of cell-surface sodium-phosphate (Na^+-PI) co-transporters, regulated by PTH and 1α,25-dihydroxyvitamin D, mediates the uptake of PI from the extracellular environment.

Metabolism

In the adult, dietary calcium is absorbed by specific calcium-binding proteins in the gut. This process is under the active control of vitamin D (see the following text for details). Most absorbed calcium is deposited in bone. The major route for excretion of body calcium is through the kidneys. Both processes—deposition and renal excretion—, which together maintain serum calcium homeostasis, are under the control of PTH, as is described later.

By an active energy-dependent process, the placenta transfers calcium ions from mother to fetus against a concentration gradient. This leads to relative fetal hypercalcemia and a calcium concentration that is higher in cord blood than in maternal blood. An intrinsic placental calcium-binding protein (CaBP; calbindin) is present only in the presence of specific receptors for $1,25(OH)_2D$, which have been demonstrated in the human placenta and the human fetal gut. It is likely that calbindin may play a significant role in the active transplacental transport of calcium to the fetus.

Magnesium

Magnesium (Mg) is the fourth most abundant cation and the second most abundant intracellular cation within the body.[63] Most of the total body Mg content (50% to 60%) is concentrated in bone tissue as an integral component of the hydroxyapatite lattice (30% to 40%) and as an exchangeable fraction (15% to 20%) adsorbed to apatite and in equilibrium with the extracellular fluid compartment. About 20% of total body Mg is concentrated in muscle, and another 20% is found in the intracellular compartment of blood cells and other body tissues. Changes in total body Mg content are reflected largely by changes in skeletal Mg and to a lesser extent in serum Mg concentrations. Only 1% of the body's magnesium is present in plasma. Magnesium serves as a co-factor for a multitude of enzymatic reactions involved in storage, transfer, and production of energy and the synthesis of nucleic acid. Further, Mg plays a significant role in calcium and bone homeostasis.

Metabolism

Magnesium is absorbed through the intestinal tract, with absorption rates ranging from 44% on an ordinary diet to 76% on a low-magnesium diet. Conservation of magnesium in the kidney is efficient, so that in magnesium deficiency, extremely low magnesium excretion rates occur. PTH appears to cause increased serum magnesium concentrations, possibly the result of mobilizing magnesium from bone. In acute conditions, an increase in the serum magnesium concentration results in suppression of the parathyroids, thus theoretically preventing further PTH increase and completing a "feedback" loop for magnesium-parathyroid interrelationships. This feedback mechanism is thus similar to that for calcium-parathyroid interrelationships (see p. 626).

Although acute lowering of serum magnesium appears to increase serum PTH concentrations, chronic magnesium deficiency results in decreased release of PTH. In addition to this impairment in parathyroid function, magnesium deficiency can decrease the response of target organs to PTH. Thus magnesium deficiency leads to hypoparathyroidism and, secondarily, hypocalcemia, because of the concomitant decrease in calcium release from bone. Under normal circumstances, magnesium and calcium undergo an exchange in bone related to their release into the circulation. Lowered magnesium content in bone results in lowered interchange with calcium and lowered release of calcium from bone.[64]

Hormone Physiology

Vitamin D[54-56,65]

Attention has been focused on vitamin D since its discovery in 1925 led to the elimination of the widespread problem of nutritional **rickets.** Initially considered a vitamin because rachitic patients were cured with oral supplementation of vitamin D, vitamin D now is regarded as a hormone.[55,56] The major source of vitamin D is not the diet, but its production in skin after exposure to sunlight.[55,56] Dietary vitamin D includes vitamins D_2 (derived from plant sterols) and D_3 (from animal or synthetic origin). Normally, in adults, at least 90% of vitamin D requirements are provided by endogenous photosynthesis in the skin, which may amount to 1.5 to 10 mg/day (100 to 400 IU/day). Vitamin D then is transported in the bloodstream to the liver and kidneys for activation. It subsequently localizes at sites of activity in intestine and bone because of the presence of specific cellular receptors in these organs. Finally, as in other hormone systems, the plasma level of activated vitamin D is rigidly controlled by feedback regulation. Vitamin D is regarded as one of the three major hormones that control homeostasis of calcium and phosphorus and bone mineralization.[55,56]

Biochemistry and Metabolism

Under the effect of small intestinal mucosal dehydrogenase, dietary cholesterol is converted into 7-dehydrocholesterol,

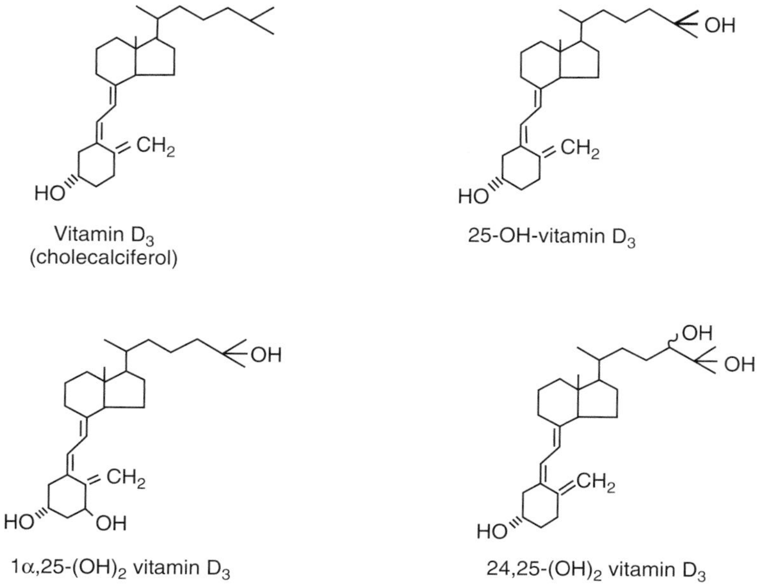

Vitamin D_3 (cholecalciferol)

25-OH-vitamin D_3

1α,25-$(OH)_2$ vitamin D_3

24,25-$(OH)_2$ vitamin D_3

Fig. 33-2 Some common metabolites of cholecalciferol.

which then is transported to the malpighian layer of the skin (see Color Plate 8). Ultraviolet (UV) radiation (of wavelengths 290 to 320 nm) penetrates the skin to break the C9-C10 bond of 7-dehydrocholesterol (provitamin D_3) to form previtamin D_3. Previtamin D_3 undergoes several reactions: it may be photoisomerized to lumisterol and tachysterol or converted by a temperature-dependent isomerization to **cholecalciferol** (vitamin D_3). Cholecalciferol then is released in the circulation, where it is bound to vitamin D–binding protein and transported to the liver.

Bioactivation of vitamin D involves the sequential actions of two 25-hydroxylase enzymes (cytochrome P450, family 27A [CYP27A] and CYP2R1) in the liver and a 1-hydroxylase enzyme (CYP27B) in the kidney, leading to the synthesis of hormonally active 1,25$(OH)_2D_3$. In the liver, cholecalciferol undergoes 25-hydroxylation to yield 25-hydroxyvitamin D, or 25$(OH)D_3$ **(calcidiol)** (see Color Plate 8 and Fig. 33-2), which is released into the circulation before reaching the kidney. In the kidney mitochondrion, 25$(OH)D_3$ undergoes 1-α-hydroxylation to produce 1,25-dihydroxyvitamin D_3 (calcitriol), or 24-hydroxylation to form 24,25-dihydroxyvitamin D_3 (24,25-$[OH]_2D_3$) (see Color Plate 8 and Fig. 33-2).

Plasma calcitriol concentrations are relatively low (approximately 30 pg/mL). Although normal plasma concentrations vary with age, they are probably under strict feedback control. The details of this control are discussed later. If plasma calcitriol concentrations are sufficient, calcidiol is hydroxylated in the kidney at the C-24 position to yield 24,25-dihydroxycholecalciferol (see Color Plate 8 and Fig. 33-2). Most investigators currently regard this metabolite as a waste product of vitamin D metabolism.

Although the human newborn has undetectable plasma vitamin D concentration, vitamin D metabolites are necessary for optimal human fetal and maternal bone mineralization. The fetus is totally dependent on maternal vitamin D.

Mechanisms of Action[54,66]

Cholecalciferol and its metabolites pass through the circulation attached to vitamin D–binding protein.[55,56,65,67] The cytosol of the kidney, intestine, bone, and selected other tissues contains an intracellular protein, the vitamin D receptor (VDR),[68,69] which serves as a specific receptor for calcitriol. After the binding of 1,25$(OH)_2D_3$ or other VDR ligands, VDR forms a heterodimer with the retinoid X receptor (RXR) and associates with vitamin D–response elements (VDREs) on target genes, where it then can positively or negatively affect the expression of these target genes.[70] 1,25$(OH)_2D_3$ is catabolized by 25-hydroxyvitamin D (24-hydroxylase) in the kidney; this is followed by sequential metabolism, yielding the terminal product calcitroic acid. It also undergoes additional 23- and 24-hydroxylations in the liver and small intestine.

The balance between bioactivation and degradation of 1,25$(OH)_2D_3$ is critical for ensuring appropriate biological effects and is tightly controlled in vivo. Elevated levels of **parathyroid hormone** associated with low-calcium states function to upregulate CYP27B (stimulate activation) and downregulate degradative CYP24 enzymes. This increases plasma and cellular levels of 1,25$(OH)_2D_3$ to correct for calcium deficiency. In turn, 1,25$(OH)_2D_3$ shows feedback regulation of its own synthesis by suppressing CYP27B and upregulating CYP24 expression via activation of VDR. CYP24-mediated 24-hydroxylation of 1,25$(OH)_2D_3$ is a critical step in the catabolism of 1,25$(OH)_2D_3$ and appears to be responsible for controlling intrarenal and systemic 1,25$(OH)_2D_3$ levels. CYP24 is directly regulated by VDR, and it is expressed mainly in the kidney, where VDR is also abundant.

Box 33-3

Target Organs for Calcitriol

Intestine—Increased absorption of calcium and phosphorus
Bone—Enhanced parathyroid hormone (PTH)-induced bone resorption
Kidney—Increased resorption of Ca and phosphorus-negative endocrine regulator of the renin-angiotensin system
Skin—Induced keratinocyte differentiation
Pancreas—May have a role in the regulation of insulin secretion and the pathogenesis of diabetes mellitus
Parathyroid gland—Regulatory effect through vit D receptor to suppress the proliferation of parathyroid gland cells and to suppress PTH secretion
Bone marrow and immune system—Immunomodulatory role stimulates cellular differentiation of the roles of promyelocytes, monocyte-macrophages, antigen-presenting cells, dendritic cells (DC), and lymphocytes in the maintenance of B-cell homeostasis; B-cell–mediated autoimmune disorders influence the production of cytokines and transforming growth factor (TGF) through vitamin D receptors (VDRs) on white blood cells. Stimulate Th-2 T-helper cells to produce TGF-1 and interleukin (IL)-4 that might serve to suppress tumor necrosis factor and interferon production by Th-1 cells that mediate autoimmune disorders; inhibit proinflammatory processes by suppressing the enhanced activity of immune cells that take part in the autoimmune reaction.

From Dusso, 2005; Cantorna, 2004; Napgal, 2005.

Box 33-4

Primary Stimuli for Calcitriol Synthesis

Decreased serum calcium concentration
Increased parathyroid hormone secretion
Decreased intracellular phosphorous concentration

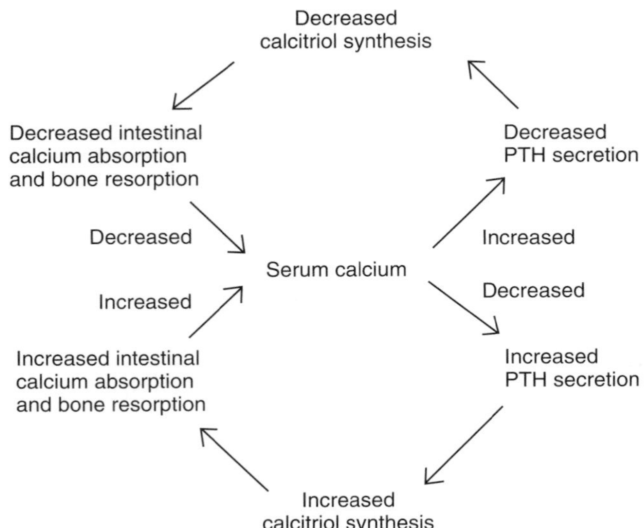

Fig. 33-3 Interrelationships of serum calcium concentrations and parathyroid hormone (PTH) and calcitriol.

The three major target organs of calcitriol are intestine, bone, and kidney (Box 33-3). Calcitriol facilitates both calcium and phosphate absorption in the intestine and induces a specific calcium-binding protein in the intestines, calbindin D. Phosphate transport accompanies calcium transport, but it is also increased by an unknown, calcium-independent mechanism. Calcitriol works cooperatively with PTH to increase bone resorption by increasing osteoclast activity. This may be considered paradoxical because vitamin D is believed to enhance bone mineralization. However, the net effect of the action of calcitriol at bone and intestine is to increase available blood concentrations of calcium and phosphorus, which subsequently facilitates mineralization of newly formed bone matrix. Calcitriol increases the renal reabsorption of both calcium and phosphorus, but because 99% of filtered calcium is normally reabsorbed, the overall effect of alterations in plasma calcitriol concentrations on renal calcium reabsorption is small.

Calcitriol has a regulatory effect on PTH and CT gene transcription. In humans with secondary hyperparathyroidism, intravenous $1,25(OH)_2D$ administration leads to a sharp reduction in serum PTH concentration. Oral administration of calcitriol to children with hypophosphatemic rickets and secondary hyperparathyroidism also has an inhibitory effect on PTH secretion. Calcitriol upregulates its own receptor in the parathyroid glands; $1,25(OH)_2D$ administration increases the concentration of vitamin D receptor mRNA in the parathyroid gland.

Regulation of Vitamin D Metabolism

The regulation of vitamin D metabolism is easily understood once calcitriol function is known (Box 33-4). Although plasma calcidiol levels are poorly controlled, control of plasma calcitriol concentrations appears to be relatively strict. The activity of renal 1-α-hydroxylase is stimulated by IGF-I, PTH, and hypophosphatemia and by periods of high calcium demand such as growth, pregnancy, or low calcium intake. Activity may be inhibited by $1,25(OH)_2D_3$ and other vitamin D metabolites.

PTH is the major stimulus for calcitriol formation. PTH administration is used as a clinical tool to assess the ability of the kidney to produce calcitriol.[71] PTH may indirectly stimulate renal 1-α-hydroxylase, the enzyme that hydroxylates calcidiol at the C-1 position, by lowering intracellular concentrations of phosphorus. Because phosphorous depletion increases calcitriol synthesis in normal or parathyroidectomized animals, decreased intracellular phosphorous levels may be the ultimate common stimulus for calcitriol synthesis.

Understanding the metabolic control of vitamin D allows comprehension of the control of serum calcium and phosphorous concentrations (Fig. 33-3). When serum calcium concentration falls, PTH is secreted and acutely restores normal serum calcium concentrations by stimulating osteoclasts to resorb bone and release calcium. Within hours, calcitriol production is increased, which causes enhanced intestinal calcium absorption; this subsequently restores the serum calcium concentration and indirectly the PTH concentration to normal. Elevations in serum calcium concentration produce the opposite effect, that is, a reduction in both serum PTH concentrations and calcitriol synthesis.

Plasma calcitriol concentrations are altered by aging and pregnancy; they are elevated during adolescence and decline in old age.[72] Pregnancy and subsequent lactation are associated with elevated serum estrogen or prolactin concentrations; both hormones increase calcitriol synthesis.[73] It should be noted that the adolescent growth spurt, pregnancy, and lactation all increase requirements for calcium. Thus, elevated serum calcitriol concentrations represent an appropriate response to a physiological need.

Parathyroid Hormone[74,75]

Biochemistry and Metabolism

PTH is an 84 amino acid polypeptide (at 9500 D) that is synthesized in the parathyroid glands. The precursor protein for PTH is preproparathyroid hormone. This precursor is sequentially converted in the gland, first to proparathyroid and then to PTH, which is released into the circulation. Full biological activity resides in the amino-terminal 1-34 peptide; the middle and carboxy-terminal sequences (35 to 84 amino acids) are biologically inert although immunologically highly reactive. Thus fragments of PTH that bear the amino terminal generally are active, whereas those that bear the carboxy terminal are inactive.

Mechanisms of Action

PTH acts on two major target organs—bone and kidney—to produce three major effects: increase in serum calcium concentrations, decrease in serum phosphorous concentrations, and increase in the active hormonal form of vitamin D_3 (calcitriol). In bone, PTH predominantly mobilizes calcium and phosphorus to the extracellular fluid, thus raising serum calcium and phosphorus concentrations. PTH has a synergistic effect with $1,25(OH)_2D$ in stimulating bone resorption.

At the other target organ, the kidney, PTH causes increased calcium retention, increased phosphorous excretion, stimulation of renal 1-α-hydroxylase activity (see earlier discussion), and increased conversion of 25-hydroxycholecalciferol (calcidiol) to 1,25-dihydroxycholecalciferol (calcitriol). Calcitriol, in turn, as described earlier, predominantly causes increased intestinal calcium and phosphorous absorption. The effects of PTH on the kidney are mediated through the formation of cyclic adenosine monophosphate (cAMP), and urinary levels of this substance rise when PTH production is increased. The resultant effect of PTH on the bone, the kidney, and indirectly, the intestine is to increase calcium concentrations in the blood. Although phosphorous concentrations may be elevated through parathyroid actions on bone and indirectly on the intestine, the effect on increased renal phosphorous excretion overwhelms the other effects and, overall, results in decreased serum phosphorous concentrations (Fig. 33-4).

Serum ionized calcium (iCa) (the unbound divalent calcium ion) concentration is the main determinant of PTH secretion: a drop in serum iCa concentration stimulates PTH secretion, whereas a rise in serum iCa concentration suppresses it. A calcium-sensing receptor is located on the surface of the parathyroid glands and is the main regulator of PTH secretion. Other ions and hormones also influence PTH secretion by the parathyroid glands, for instance, a rise in serum $1,25(OH)_2D_3$ decreases PTH secretion. An acute drop in serum Mg concentration stimulates PTH secretion but to a much smaller extent (tenfold less on a molar basis) compared with the effect of acute hypocalcemia.[76] Chronic hypomagnesemia impairs PTH secretion and causes blunting of PTH action at target organs.[63] Magnesium ions are essential for adenylate cyclase–mediated secretion of secretory granules and subsequent release of PTH from the parathyroid chief cells. Therefore, magnesium deficiency may cause secondary hypocalcemia. Hypermagnesemia also suppresses PTH secretion.

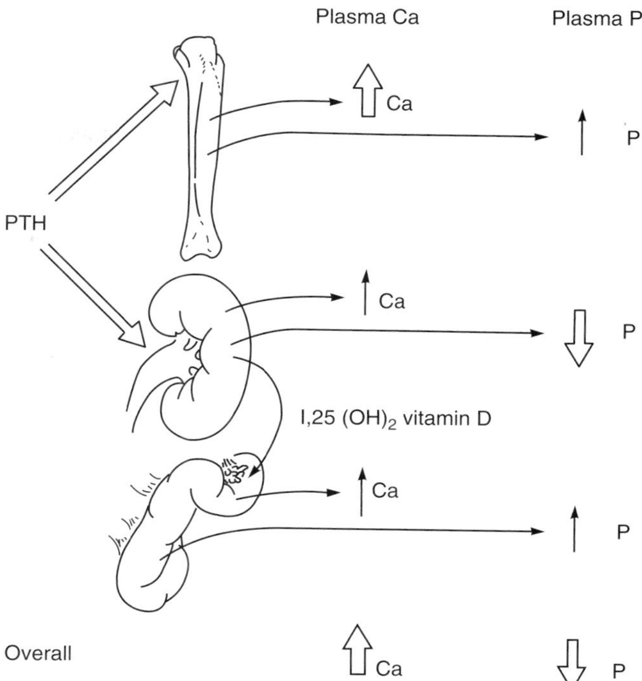

Fig. 33-4 Normal parathyroid hormone (PTH) physiology. PTH action increases serum calcium concentrations predominantly through its bone and kidney effects but reduces plasma phosphorous concentrations (P) by increasing excretion of renal phosphorus. (From Tsang RC, Noguchi A, Steichen JJ: Pediatric parathyroid disorders, Pediatr Clin North Am 26:223, 1979.)

Perinatal PTH Homeostasis

Theoretically, because PTH does not cross the placenta, the relative fetal hypercalcemia should suppress the fetal parathyroid glands. Paradoxically, fetal PTH secretion is not suppressed. A possible explanation for the nonsuppression of PTH secretion, despite relative fetal hypercalcemia, is that the negative-feedback system regulating PTH secretion by calcium concentration operates with a higher "set point" in the fetus, so that suppression of PTH secretion in the fetus requires higher serum calcium concentrations than are required after birth. Both PTH and PTH-related peptide (PTHRP) may have a significant role in the placental transport of calcium, and PTHRP may contribute significantly to PTH bioactivity in fetal serum.

PTH-Related Peptide[77,78]

Biochemistry and Metabolism

PTHRP and PTH genes are members of the same gene family; the amino terminal of PTHRP has a sequence homology in eight amino acids with the PTH amino terminal and PTHRP is also found to be equipotent to PTH. PTH synthesis is restricted to the parathyroid glands in normal individuals, but PTHRP messenger RNA is widely distributed in normal tissues, including the skin, thyroid, bone marrow, hypothalamus, pituitary, parathyroid, adrenal cortex, adrenal medulla, and stomach. Several studies suggest that PTHRP may have a significant physiological role. One of the major production sites of this peptide is lactating breast tissue, and PTHRP is present in large quantities in milk.

Mechanisms of Action

In healthy adults, plasma PTHRP concentrations range from less than 2 to 5 pmol/L. Infusion of PTHRP causes an elevation in serum 1,25-dihydroxy vitamin D concentration and an increase in bone formation parameters. PTHRP may play a causal role in the hypercalcemia of malignancies. It is possible that PTH and PTHRP act on the same bone receptor to cause increased bone resorption and formation and hypercalcemia and hypophosphatemia. PTHRP, produced in the fetal parathyroid glands, may be responsible for the stimulation of placental calcium transport.

Calcitonin (CT)

Calcitonin,[79,80] which was discovered in 1962, is generally regarded as one of three hormones (along with vitamin D and PTH) responsible for the control of calcium and phosphorous homeostasis. Despite great research efforts, a definitive role for CT in calcium homeostasis has not yet been clarified. Neither CT deficiency nor CT excess is clearly associated with bone disease or alteration of serum calcium homeostasis.

Localization, Biochemistry, and Metabolism

CT is produced by the parafollicular C-cells of the thyroid gland, although the pituitary gland, gastrointestinal tract, and liver also may produce the hormone. CT is secreted in a precursor form, with a molecular weight of 15,000 D, and is cleaved into the active 32 amino acid CT polypeptide, which has a molecular weight of 3500 D. Normal serum CT concentrations are less than 100 pg/mL. CT is rapidly excreted, with a half-life of 10 minutes after intravenous administration.[81] Excretion occurs predominantly through the kidney, and serum CT concentrations are increased in patients with renal failure.[82]

Biological Effects

The best recognized physiological effect of CT is counteraction of the action of PTH at several organ sites in the human body. The biological effects of CT may be divided into those related to calcium and phosphorous homeostasis and those related to gastrointestinal function. Intravenous CT administration causes a prompt decline in serum calcium and phosphorous concentrations. This occurs because of the effects of CT on both bone and kidney. CT alters cell function by increasing intracellular cAMP production.[83] Receptors specific for CT have been demonstrated on bone osteoclasts, and CT antagonizes PTH-mediated bone resorption by suppressing osteoclastic activity. Consequently, CT decreases the flux of calcium and phosphorus from bone into the circulation, with urinary hydroxyproline excretion decreasing in parallel with the inhibition of bone resorption. CT also decreases the renal reabsorption of calcium, phosphorus, sodium, potassium, and magnesium.[83] CT also acts on vitamin D metabolism and enhances $1,25(OH)_2D$ production by proximal renal tubules. These described effects on both bone and kidney have been produced with pharmacological CT concentrations.

In the human fetus, the thyroid C-cells appear to be well developed by 14 weeks of gestation. However, the role of CT in fetal mineral and bone homeostasis is not very well understood. CT does not cross the placenta, and, as with PTH, fetal CT function may be autonomous from that of the mother and may play a role in fetal bone mineralization.

Regulation of CT Secretion[79,80]

CT secretion is influenced by serum calcium concentrations; the gastrointestinal hormones gastrin, cholecystokinin, and glucagon; and sex steroids. CT release is affected primarily by the concentration of serum iCa and is stimulated by hypercalcemia and inhibited by hypocalcemia. Vitamin D has a direct inhibitory effect on CT gene expression and CT secretion; receptors for $1,25(OH)_2D_3$ have been demonstrated on parafollicular C-cells. Serum CT concentrations may be higher in pregnant and lactating women than in controls. Men have higher circulating CT concentrations when compared with women.

KEY CONCEPTS BOX 33-3

- Good general nutrition, especially intake of Ca and vitamin D, is needed for proper bone mass. Exercise, especially weight bearing, is very important for the development of good bone mass.
- The mineral mass of bone consists primarily of Ca and phosphate; most of the body's stores of these minerals reside in bone. Magnesium is also an important part of the mineral matrix.
- Under the influence of vitamin D_3, Ca is absorbed in the small intestines and is deposited in bone.
- Total serum Ca is ≈50% bound to proteins (mostly albumin), and ≈40% is found in the unbound, ionized state. It is only the latter that is biologically active.
- Parathyroid hormone (PTH) controls the removal of Ca from bone and its renal excretion.
- When serum Ca is decreased, PTH increases the renal synthesis of active vitamin D_3, calcitriol, which increases intestinal absorption of dietary Ca. PTH also increases the release of Ca from bone and the renal reabsorption of urinary Ca.

SECTION OBJECTIVES BOX 33-4

- Describe the changes on bone associated with *osteoporosis, osteomalacia, rickets, osteitis fibrosa,* and *Paget's disease.*
- List the primary and secondary causes of osteoporosis, osteomalacia, and rickets.
- State the expected levels of calcidiol, parathyroid hormone (PTH), calcium, phosphorus, magnesium, and alkaline phosphatase in the disease states listed above.

Box 33-5

A Partial Differential Diagnosis of Osteopenia

Osteoporosis
Primary
Premature and low birth weight infants
Aging (senile)
Postmenopausal
Juvenile

Secondary
Malnutrition and malabsorption syndromes
Immobilization
Cushing's syndrome
Hyperthyroidism
Multiple myeloma
Rheumatoid arthritis
Leukemia
Turner's syndrome
Alcoholism
Chronic liver disease
Irradiation
Drug-induced
Glucocorticoid therapy
Anticonvulsant therapy
Immunosuppressive therapy (e.g., cyclosporine)

Osteomalacia
Vitamin D deficiency
Chronic gastrointestinal disease
Anticonvulsant medication induced
Vitamin D dependency
Vitamin D resistance (hypophosphatemia)
Chronic acidosis
Fanconi's syndrome
Chronic renal failure
Phosphorous and calcium deficiency

Osteitis Fibrosa
Primary hyperparathyroidism
Chronic renal failure

BONE DISORDERS

Disorders of calcium, phosphorous, vitamin D, or PTH homeostasis frequently produce osteopenia, a general term for the x-ray appearance of a subnormal amount of mineralized bone. Many illnesses are associated with osteopenia[84] (Box 33-5). The bone histopathological condition of osteopenia can reveal decreased **osteoid** (bone matrix) formation, decreased osteoid mineralization, or increased bone resorption.[85] These histological categories correlate with the clinical diagnosis of osteoporosis, **osteomalacia,** or osteitis fibrosa, respectively. Osteopenia can result in the crush-fracture syndrome in adults and in fractures or growth failure in children. Trabecular bone is affected more frequently than cortical bone, and so fractures most often occur in vertebrae, the femoral neck, and the distal ends of the long bones, where trabecular bone is abundant. Whereas specific diagnoses of osteopenic bone are best made histologically, occasionally, characteristic laboratory abnormalities will permit differentiation among osteoporosis, osteomalacia, and osteitis fibrosa (Table 33-1).

Osteoporosis[22,86-90]

The National Institutes of Health (NIH) has declared osteoporosis to be a major health threat to Americans.[19,51] The NIH believes that at least 10 million individuals have osteoporosis, and 18 million more have low bone mass, placing these individuals at increased risk for this disorder. Osteoporosis is no longer considered a disease of postmenopausal women only, and it is by no means entirely age or gender dependent. Prevention of osteoporosis necessitates optimizing the factors that influence bone health (see earlier discussion) throughout the life span in both men and women.[20]

Osteoporosis is characterized by a disturbed balance between bone resorption and bone formation, which results in a progressive decrease in bone mass and a decrease in the amount of normally mineralized bone; the mineral-to-collagen ratio is normal. Major sequelae include fragility of bone and predisposition to fracture, particularly spine-vertebral crush fracture, hip–femoral neck fracture, and fracture of the distal radius, which may occur spontaneously or in response to minor trauma. The World Health Organization (WHO) associates osteoporosis with bone density 2.5 standard deviations below the mean for young white adult women. It is not clear how this diagnostic criterion should be applied to men and children, and across ethnic groups. Because of the difficulty associated with accurate measurement and standardization between instruments and sites, controversy exists among experts regarding the continued use of this diagnostic criterion.

Osteoporosis can be characterized further as primary or secondary.

Primary Osteoporosis

Primary osteoporosis can occur in both genders at all ages but often follows menopause in women and occurs later in life in men and women (senile osteoporosis). However, osteoporosis is not always the result of bone loss, and individuals who do not reach optimal bone mass during childhood and adolescence may also develop osteoporosis without occurrence of accelerated bone loss. Hence suboptimal bone growth in childhood and adolescence is as important as bone loss to the development of osteoporosis. It occurs only rarely in childhood as an idiopathic illness and can also accompany certain systemic diseases.

Table 33-1 Common Serum Abnormalities Associated with Metabolic Bone Disease

Disease	Ca	P	PTH	Alk PO_4	Calcidiol	Calcitriol
Osteoporosis	NL	NL	NL	NL	NL	LO
Osteomalacia	LO	LO	HI	HI	NL or LO	NL or LO
Osteitis fibrosa	HI or NL	LO or NL	HI	HI	NL	HI or NL

Alk PO_4, Alkaline phosphatase; *HI,* increased; *LO,* decreased; *NL,* normal; *PTH,* parathyroid hormone.

Table 33-2 Treatments That Increase the Risk of Secondary Osteoporosis

Treatments	Comments
Irradiation	Direct effects on bone; decreased osteoblastic activity
	Pituitary hormone deficiencies from cranial irradiation
Long-term glucocorticoid use	Definitely with oral use and possibly with high-dose inhaled steroids
Chemotherapy	Methotrexate
	Cyclosporin A
	FK-506
Long-term anticonvulsant therapy	Vitamin D deficiency

Table 33-3 Disorders That Increase the Risk of Secondary Osteoporosis

Disorder	Pathophysiology
Celiac disease	Malabsorption of calcium and vitamin D
Inflammatory bowel disease	Glucocorticoid use
Cholestatic liver disease	Decreased vitamin D production and calcium absorption
Solid organ and bone marrow transplants	Glucocorticoid use
	Immunosuppressive use
Collagen-vascular disease	Glucocorticoid use
Hypogonadism/amenorrhea	Secondary amenorrhea in female athletes
Chronic renal disease	Secondary hyperparathyroidism
	Impaired vitamin D hydroxylation
Growth hormone deficiency	Decreased osteoblastic activity
Cushing's syndrome	Increased bone resorption caused by excess adrenal hormones
Spina bifida	Lack of weight bearing
Neuromuscular disorders	Hypotonia and decreased weight bearing
Severe cerebral palsy	Effect of anticonvulsants on vitamin D synthesis and action
Cystic fibrosis	Malabsorption of calcium and vitamin D
	Glucocorticoid use
"Steroid-dependent" asthma	Long-term oral glucocorticoids
	High doses of inhaled glucocorticoids
Anorexia nervosa	Malnutrition
	Secondary amenorrhea
Osteogenesis imperfecta	
Hyperthyroidism	Increased bone resorption
Hyperparathyroidism	Increased bone resorption

Secondary Osteoporosis

Secondary osteoporosis can result from medications, medical conditions (see Box 33-5 and Table 33-2), and environmental factors. Medical disorders (Table 33-3) associated with osteoporosis can be organized into several categories: genetic disorders, hypogonadal states, other endocrine disorders, gastrointestinal diseases, hematological disorders, connective tissue disease, nutritional deficiencies, drugs, and a variety of chronic systemic disorders, such as congestive heart failure, end-stage renal disease, and alcoholism. Among men, 30% to 60% of osteoporosis is associated with secondary causes, with hypogonadism, glucocorticoids, and alcoholism among the most common. In perimenopausal women, more than 50% of osteoporosis is most commonly associated with secondary causes; the most common of these are hypoestrogenemia, glucocorticoid therapy, thyroid hormone excess,[91] and anti-convulsant therapy.[92]

Environmental factors that predispose to bone loss and osteoporosis include medications (see Table 33-2), cigarette smoking, chronic low dietary calcium intake, a sedentary life-style, a high-acid animal protein diet, and alcohol intake. The incidence of osteoporotic fracture is increased by various risk factors (Box 33-6), in addition to decreased bone strength and density.

Senile Osteoporosis

Progressive bone loss normally occurs during aging. This process begins at 50 years of age in women and at 65 to 70 years of age in men and results in a loss of 0.5% of total bone mass per year and approximately 20% in a lifetime.[86,87] Patients with senile osteoporosis experience accelerated losses of 1% to 2% per year, with symptoms of osteoporosis beginning when 30% of bone mass is lost. It has been suggested that osteoporosis is a natural part of the aging process that manifests earlier in those persons who have accrued less skeletal mass during early adult life. The causes of senile osteoporosis are largely unknown. Hormonal alterations that occur during senescence undoubtedly potentiate bone loss (Box 33-7). Decreased serum calcitriol concentrations found in elderly persons[72] probably result from a blunted synthetic response to PTH. In addition, serum PTH concentrations increase[93,94] and

Box 33-6

Risk Factors Associated with Low Bone Density and Fracture

Female gender
Estrogen deficiency
Late menarche
Early menopause
Low endogenous estrogen
Increased age (both genders)
White race
Hypogonadism (males)
Low weight and body mass index (BMI)
Family history of osteoporosis
Smoking and alcohol use
Excessive caffeine-containing beverages
Chronic low dietary calcium intake
Sedentary lifestyle
High-acid animal protein diet
History of prior fracture

Box 33-7

Calcium-Regulating Hormone Abnormalities Associated with Aging

Decreased serum calcitriol concentration and calcitriol secretory reserve
Increased serum parathyroid hormone (PTH) concentration
Decreased serum calcitriol (CT) concentration

serum CT concentrations decrease[95] with aging. The net effect of these hormonal alterations is diminished intestinal calcium absorption and increased bone resorption.

Residents of long-term care facilities, such as nursing homes, are at particularly high risk of fracture. Most have low BMD and a high prevalence of many of the risk factors associated with fracture, including advanced age, poor physical function, low muscle strength, decreased cognition and high rates of dementia, poor nutrition, and, often, use of multiple medications. There also appears to be a significant role for vitamin D deficiency in the cause of senile osteoporosis. Up to 60% of elderly persons living in nursing homes develop vitamin D deficiency by the end of the winter season; also, a significant number of elderly subjects with hip fractures (40% of males and 30% of females) are vitamin D deficient. Evidence supports defective renal 1-α-hydroxylase activity with aging and secondary hyperparathyroidism as a cause of vitamin D deficiency in elderly people and of secondary osteoporosis.

Postmenopausal Osteoporosis

Postmenopausal osteoporosis, which occurs in females at a younger age than senile osteoporosis does, is caused by estrogen deficiency.[96] Affected women have diminished intestinal calcium absorption and lower serum calcitriol concentrations

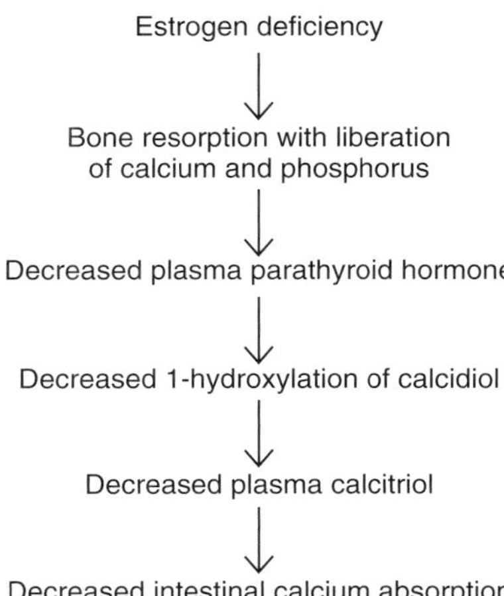

Fig. 33-5 Hypothesized pathogenesis of postmenopausal osteoporosis.

compared with their normal age-matched peers.[97] Although serum PTH concentrations are normal when compared with those of controls with normal serum calcitriol concentrations, they are low when viewed in the context of calcitriol deficiency. Estrogen supplementation increases intestinal calcium absorption and serum calcitriol and PTH concentrations.[93,94] These data have been interpreted to indicate that estrogen deficiency produces postmenopausal osteoporosis by causing bone resorption, which releases calcium into the extracellular space and which, in turn, suppresses PTH secretion, calcitriol synthesis, and intestinal absorption of calcium (Fig. 33-5). It has been suggested that magnesium deficiency may play a role in postmenopausal osteoporosis.

Approximately 30% of postmenopausal white women sustain at least one osteoporotic fracture. However, the true incidence of these fractures is difficult to assess because a large number of vertebral fractures remain asymptomatic. Osteoporotic hip fractures occur in the third and fourth decades after menopause; they are twice as common in women as in men. By 90 years of age, about 33% of women and at least 17% of men sustain a hip fracture.

Idiopathic Juvenile Osteoporosis

Idiopathic juvenile osteoporosis is a rare form of bone demineralization that affects prepubertal children. Clinical features manifest as fractures of long bones and vertebrae, in addition to bone pain. It is characterized by spontaneous recovery after puberty. In severe cases, characteristic metaphyseal compression fractures of the lower extremities occur because of compaction of osteoporotic newly formed bone, a pathognomonic feature of this disease. The origin of this disease is unknown to date. Some patients have transient calcitriol deficiency, which correlates with the clinical course of the disease. Treatment of these patients with calcitriol reduces the bone fracture rate and increases bone mineralization within a year. Other patients may have a negative calcium balance, low $25(OH)D_3$ and high $1,25(OH)_2D_3$, or possible CT deficiency.

Corticosteroid-Induced Osteoporosis[98,99]

Diseases that are treated with glucocorticoid therapy may affect more than 30 million Americans. It is estimated that up to 50% of patients on long-term glucocorticoid therapy will experience loss of bone substance and osteoporotic fractures. The mechanism of steroid-induced bone resorption is complex. Corticosteroids do exert direct inhibitory effects on osteoblast function, thus decreasing bone formation. Serum osteocalcin concentration, an indicator of bone formation, is significantly reduced in steroid-treated patients. Corticosteroid therapy reduces intestinal calcium and phosphorous absorption. Fractures appear early after initiation of treatment, and effective treatment requires primary prevention in those at high risk of fracture. Bisphosphonates are the treatment of choice, and calcium and vitamin D supplements are indicated in most individuals.[98]

Hyperthyroidism[91]

The major role of thyroid hormone in bone metabolism is to increase the number of bone-remodeling units, thereby increasing bone remodeling activity. Thyrotoxicosis causes increased bone resorption and a decrease in bone mineral density.

Hypogonadal States

Hypogonadism, characterized by delayed menarche, oligomenorrhea, or amenorrhea, is relatively common in adolescent girls and young women. Settings in which these occur include strenuous athletic training, emotional stress, and low body weight. Failure to achieve peak bone mass, bone loss, and increased fracture rates have been reported in this group. Anorexia nervosa, a hypogonadic state, is complicated further by associated profound undernutrition and nutrition-related bone demineralization. This latter point is evidenced, in part, by the failure of estrogen replacement to correct the bone loss.

Drugs

Patients with impaired renal function are not able to excrete aluminum contained in antacids, dialysis fluids, foods, and nutritional supplements. Accumulation of aluminum in bone can increase the risk for fracture. Immunosuppressant drugs, such as cyclosporine, predispose to osteoporosis by stimulating bone resorption. Lithium stimulates the production of PTH and increases the rate of bone resorption; long-term lithium therapy therefore can increase the risk for osteoporosis. Cytotoxic medications inhibit bone turnover and predispose to osteoporosis. An excessive amount of vitamin D increases the rate of bone resorption and can increase the risk for osteoporosis.

Diagnosis of Osteoporosis[20,22,86-88]

The diagnosis of osteoporosis should (1) confirm the presence of osteoporosis, (2) rule out secondary causes of osteoporosis, and (3) establish a baseline against which the patient's progress can be monitored. The most commonly used measurement to diagnose osteoporosis and predict fracture risk is assessment of BMD by bone densitometry, which is principally a measure of the mineral content of bone.[100-102] BMD measurements correlate strongly with the load-bearing capacity of the hip and spine and with the risk of fracture. Bone density measurements are performed by dual energy x-ray densitometry (DEXA) and are scored by criteria developed by WHO. Patients with evidence of osteoporosis are started on medications (alendronate 10 mg, hormonal replacement therapy, or CT), whereas patients with osteopenia (see later discussion) need medication to prevent osteoporosis (alendronate 5 mg, hormonal replacement therapy, or raloxifene).[103]

The National Osteoporosis Foundation (NOF) recommends that women be given a bone density test if they meet the following criteria[51]:

- Older than 65 years old
- Postmenopausal with at least one risk factor besides menopause or with a fracture
- Considering osteoporosis therapy
- On prolonged hormone replacement therapy

Other patients who are candidates for a bone density measurement include individuals who meet the following criteria:

- On long-term (longer than 2 months) corticosteroid therapy
- With parathyroid gland disorders
- With x-ray films that are suggestive of osteoporosis

Repeat DEXA scans at annual or biennial intervals allow clinicians to determine whether the patient is responding to the prescribed medication to correct a condition of low bone density.

Laboratory Tests to Rule Out Secondary Causes of Osteoporosis

The main purposes of laboratory investigations are (1) to rule out secondary causes of osteoporosis and (2) to monitor the patient's response to therapy. As yet, no laboratory tests can be used to diagnose osteoporosis. The most frequently ordered tests are listed in Box 33-8 and are discussed in greater detail in the Change of Analyte with Disease section.

Box 33-8

Serum Tests to Rule Out Secondary Osteoporosis

Calcium
Alkaline phosphatase
Inorganic phosphate
Total protein
Creatinine and urea (renal function)
Aspartate aminotransferase (AST), alanine aminotransferase (ALT), total bilirubin (liver function)
Testosterone

Treatment for Osteoporosis[53,62,104-108]

Therapies available for treating osteoporosis are listed in Box 33-9.

Box 33-9

Current and Emerging Therapies for Osteoporosis

Inhibitors of osteoclastic bone resorption:
- Estrogenic compounds
- Bisphosphonates
- Monoclonal antibody (inhibitor) to receptor activator of nuclear factor–kappa B ligand signaling (RANKL)
- Cathepsin K inhibitors
- C-src kinase inhibitors
- Integrin inhibitors
- Chloride channel inhibitors

Osteoblast-targeted (anabolic) agents:
- Intermittent parathyroid hormone (PTH) therapy
- Oral PTH analogs
- Calcium-sensing receptor antagonists
- PTH-related peptide analogs

Induction of osteoblast anabolism by means of pathways involving molecular targets:
- With low-density lipoprotein receptor–related protein 5 signaling
- Sclerostin
- Matrix extracellular phosphoglycoprotein

Adapted from Grey A: Emerging pharmacologic therapies for osteoporosis, Expert Opin Emerg Drugs 12:493, 2007.

Adequate calcium and vitamin D intake modulates age-related increases in PTH levels and bone resorption, thereby increasing spine BMD and reducing fractures.[109] The maximal effective dose of vitamin D is thought to be 400 to 1000 IU/day. Optimal treatment of osteoporosis with any drug therapy also requires that calcium and vitamin D intake must meet recommended levels. The consensus opinion of the North American Menopause Society (NAMS) on the role of calcium in the prevention and treatment of osteoporosis in postmenopausal women include the following[110-112]:

1. Daily calcium intake should not exceed 2500 mg because excessive intake increases the risk of hypercalcemia.
2. The NIH recommends the following calcium intake:
   a. 1000 mg/day for women aged 25 to 50 years and for postmenopausal women younger than 65 years who are taking hormone replacement therapy (HRT)
   b. 1500 mg/day for menopausal women who are not using HRT and for all women 65 years and older

Bisphosphonates[103]

Bisphosphonates are the drugs of choice for preventing and treating postmenopausal osteoporosis. These compounds inhibit osteclastic bone resorption and thus promote a higher bone density.

Hormone Replacement Therapy (HRT)[105,106]

Estrogen increases bone mass and BMD by (1) reducing bone resorption directly by preventing osteoclast differentiation, activity, and survival, and indirectly by stimulating the secretion of CT; (2) increasing collagen synthesis and osteoid formation, probably by stimulating the activity of osteoblasts; and (3) enhancing the absorption of calcium across the intestines. Numerous trials have demonstrated the positive effect that estrogen has on the improvement in bone mineral density, and lower doses have proved efficacious with fewer side effects. Both observational and randomized clinical trials have demonstrated the ability of estrogen treatment to prevent fractures. The appropriate length of estrogen treatment for postmenopausal women remains controversial.[106]

Calcitonin

Although it is preferable to treat osteoporosis with a more potent agent than calcitonin,[105] CT remains an effective alternative for osteoporotic women more than 5 years postmenopausal who refuse estrogens, or for whom estrogens are contraindicated. The role of calcitonin in corticosteroid-induced osteoporosis remains controversial; hence, it can be considered only as a second-line agent for the treatment of patients with low bone mineral density who are receiving long-term corticosteroid therapy.

Parathyroid Hormone (PTH)[75,104,113]

Intermittent administration of recombinant human PTH (1-84) stimulates the formation of new bone by increasing osteoblast number and reverses bone loss in most osteoporotic individuals regardless of the underlying pathophysiology. PTH has reduced the overall risk for new or worsened vertebral fracture in postmenopausal women with osteoporosis, providing an alternative therapeutic option for fracture prevention.[104] PTH can build bone in men with osteoporosis and in women who take glucocorticoid medications increasing the number of osteoblast beyond that needed to replace the bone removed by osteoclasts during bone remodeling.[75] The U.S. Food and Drug Administration (FDA) recommends the use of parathyroid hormone for the treatment of osteoporosis for a maximum of 2 years because of concern regarding the development of osteosarcoma.[105]

Monitoring Osteoporosis and Treatment

Patients with osteoporosis have not only decreased bone mass but also increased rates of bone remodeling (see p. 619). Monitoring of patients' responses to therapy for osteoporosis can be achieved by the measurement of a baseline DEXA, with repeat measurements taken every 1 to 3 years, depending on the expected rate of loss and the clinical situation. Alternatively, surrogate markers of bone turnover in the blood or urine (N-telopeptides) assayed at baseline and then 8 to 12 weeks after specific therapy has been initiated are useful. These markers are discussed on pp. 621 and 639. The level of these markers may identify changes in bone remodeling within a relatively short time interval of several days to months before changes in BMD can be detected. However, marker levels do not predict bone mass or fracture risk, are only weakly associated with changes in bone mass, and thus are of limited utility in the clinical evaluation of individual patients. Despite these limitations, these markers have been shown in research studies to correlate with changes in indices of bone remodeling and may provide insights into mechanisms of bone loss.[51,110-112]

Table 33-4 Biochemical Abnormalities Associated with Rickets

	Serum Calcium	Serum Phosphorus	Parathyroid Hormone	Calcidiol	Calcitriol
Vitamin D deficiency	LO	LO	HI	LO	LO, NL, or HI
Vitamin D dependency					
I	LO	LO	HI	HI	LO
II	LO	LO	HI	HI	HI
Vitamin D resistance	NL	LO	NL	NL	NL or LO
Dietary phosphorous deficiency	NL	LO	NL	LO	HI

HI, Increased; *LO,* decreased; *NL,* normal.

Osteomalacia

Osteomalacia is diagnosed when bone contains normal quantities of osteoid that fail to mineralize. When seen in the growing child, osteomalacia is termed *rickets.* The terms *rickets* and *osteomalacia* are used interchangeably in this chapter. The major causes of osteomalacia are listed in Box 33-5, and their associated biochemical abnormalities are summarized in Table 33-4.

Clinically, the earliest rachitic features in infancy may be hypocalcemic tetany or seizures, particularly in vitamin D–unsupplemented, exclusively human milk–fed infants, and in infants with congenital rickets born to vitamin D–deficient osteomalacic mothers. Acute infection may precipitate hypocalcemic tetany, possibly by mobilizing bone phosphate into the circulation and thereby decreasing serum calcium concentration. In the first 6 months of life, abnormal bones will be seen on x-ray film. The wrist and the knee are most useful in demonstrating even the earliest signs of rickets. "Rachitic lungs" indicate ribcage weakening, with secondary defective pulmonary ventilation. This feature occurs in the very young child, particularly among preterm infants. Beyond infancy, increased weight bearing aggravates rachitic changes, particularly in vertebral, pelvic, and lower limb bones, resulting in spinal and pelvic deformities that cause a waddling gait and bowed legs, or "knock knees." Muscular weakness and hypotonia frequently involve proximal muscle groups in rickets and contribute to waddling gait, protuberance of the abdomen, and inefficient lung ventilation in rachitic children. The muscular weakness is believed to be caused by decreased calcium uptake by myocytes.

Vitamin D–Deficient Osteomalacia[55,56,114]

Historically, the most common cause of osteomalacia was vitamin D deficiency caused by a combination of insufficient sunlight exposure and inadequate dietary intake of vitamin D–containing foods. Serum calcidiol concentrations, which reflect the adequacy of vitamin D in the body, are low in osteomalacia. Supplementation of foods with vitamin D has virtually eliminated the problem in industrialized countries, but it still may be seen in underdeveloped nations, particularly among dark-skinned individuals, because skin pigment decreases the production of cholecalciferol, which normally occurs after UV radiation exposure. It is also encountered in exclusively human milk–fed infants and in strict vegetarian adults, even in developed countries. These individuals have limited exposure to sunshine and do not ingest vitamin D–fortified milk.

Alterations in vitamin D metabolism that can lead to rickets range from conditions of insufficient intake or production of cholecalciferol to disturbances in its activation by the liver and kidneys. Generally, the biochemical response to a deficiency of calcitriol can be predicted (see Fig. 33-3). The absorption of intestinal calcium will decrease and produce hypocalcemia. This will stimulate PTH release (secondary hyperparathyroidism), which will mobilize calcium from bone and increase phosphorous excretion by the kidney. Initially, serum calcium concentrations will be maintained at the expense of bone resorption, but as minerals are depleted, hypocalcemia occurs. Hypophosphatemia occurs because of increased urinary phosphorous losses. Thus the characteristic serum abnormalities associated with calcitriol deficiency are hypocalcemia, hypophosphatemia, and hyperparathyroidism (see Table 33-4). In addition, hyperphosphaturia, aminoaciduria, rachitic bone disease, and elevated serum alkaline phosphatase concentration will be observed.

Osteomalacia also results from phosphorous deficiency. In this situation, low intracellular phosphorous concentrations should stimulate calcitriol synthesis, which will increase both intestinal and renal phosphate absorption. Serum calcium and PTH concentrations should be unaffected (see Table 33-4).

Osteomalacia Secondary to Gastrointestinal Disorders

Patients with gastrointestinal disease, particularly those with hepatobiliary disease, often develop osteomalacia. Vitamin D is fat soluble and requires bile acids for absorption (see Chapter 35). Patients with hepatobiliary disease have low serum calcidiol levels that appear to be caused in part by defective intestinal cholecalciferol or ergosterol absorption, impaired calcidiol production by the liver, and enhanced calcitriol metabolism. Osteopenia also may be seen after gastric surgery, although the pathogenesis is not understood.

Hepatic Rickets[115]

Hepatobiliary disease predisposes to rickets, presumably because of decreased 25-hydroxylase activity, vitamin D malabsorption, and decreased enterohepatic circulation of $25(OH)D_3$. Malabsorption of vitamin D is probably a major factor in the pathogenesis of hepatic rickets. Biochemically, serum $25(OH)D_3$ and $1,25(OH)_2D_3$ concentrations are low.

Clinically, signs of rickets are superimposed on the primary hepatic disease. Infants with hepatitis and infants who require prolonged parenteral hyperalimentation may develop varying degrees of hepatic dysfunction and secondary rickets.

Osteomalacia Secondary to Anticonvulsant Medication[92]

Rickets may occur in up to 30% of children receiving anticonvulsant medications such as phenytoin (Dilantin) and phenobarbital, which induce the hepatic microsomal mixed-oxidase enzyme system. This enzyme system, when stimulated, converts calcidiol to polar inactive metabolites, which results in calcidiol deficiency. Other biochemical effects of therapy may include hypocalcemia, hypophosphatemia, hypocalciuria, and elevated serum concentrations of alkaline phosphatase and PTH. In addition, anticonvulsants inhibit calcitriol-dependent intestinal calcium uptake.

Vitamin D–Dependent Osteomalacia (Types I and II)[116]

After foods were fortified with vitamin D, it became apparent that normal antirachitic doses of analogs of vitamin D failed to heal the rickets of a small subpopulation of rachitic patients. One group of such patients had the classical signs and symptoms of vitamin D deficiency, including early infantile hypocalcemia, hypophosphatemia, and tetany, but these patients, who required up to 100 times the normal intake of vitamin D to heal their rickets, are included in the two types of vitamin D–dependent hereditary *rickets* (VDDR) caused by mutations in the renal 1-α-hydroxylase enzyme [1-α(OH)ase] and VDR genes. The defective 1-α(OH)ase gene is responsible for VDDR type I and defective VDR genes for VDDR type II. Both diseases are inherited as an autosomal recessive trait, but their clinical features and response to administered calcitriol are distinct.

Patients with vitamin D–dependent rickets type I have the classical biochemical abnormalities of vitamin D–deficient rickets, but their serum calcidiol concentrations are normal and they lack circulating calcitriol. Clinically, the disease occurs before 2 years of age, most often in the first 6 months of life. A sporadic form of the disease has been described less often, and its onset occurs in late childhood and adolescence. The osteomalacia of these patients heals when physiological doses of calcitriol are administered.

Patients with vitamin D–dependent rickets type II have low serum calcium and phosphorous concentrations, normal serum calcidiol concentration, and elevated serum $1{,}25(OH)_2D_3$ and PTH concentrations. The disease is an end-organ resistance to the effect of $1{,}25(OH)_2D_3$ caused by a defective VDR and patients are resistant to physiological doses of calcitriol. Mechanistically, this disease should be called *calcitriol (1,25[OH]$_2$D$_3$)–resistant rickets.* Clinically, the disease manifests as rickets and osteomalacia, most commonly before 2 years of life, rarely later in life.

Five classes of defective calcitriol receptors are known: (1) defect in the hormone-binding domain. Calcitriol concentration is elevated, but this does not evoke a biochemical response; this is the most common defect; (2) hormone-binding affinity is normal, accompanied by reductions in the numbers of receptors and hormone-binding sites (10% of normal); (3) hormone-binding affinity is reduced 20-fold to 30-fold, although the number of binding sites is normal; (4) defective nuclear localization; in this form, calcitriol does not localize to the cell nucleus; and (5) decreased affinity of the hormone-receptor complex to DNA. Intracellular defect categories 1, 2, and 5 do not respond to therapy with high vitamin D doses. In contrast, intracellular defects types 3 and 4 can be cured with high vitamin D doses. Prenatal diagnosis of this disease is now feasible and is indicated in high-risk families.

Vitamin D–Resistant Osteomalacia

Patients with vitamin D–resistant osteomalacia lack most of the usual biochemical markers associated with rachitic patients.[117] Serum phosphorus is severely decreased, whereas serum calcium concentrations may be normal or decreased. Serum PTH concentration is normal or increased, and serum $1{,}25(OH)_2D_3$ concentration is normal or low. This disorder is caused by a congenital defect in phosphate resorption in the proximal renal tubules, resulting in massive phosphaturia and hypophosphatemia. The defective gene responsible for this disease has been mapped to the short arm of the human X chromosome. Because low intracellular phosphorous concentrations are a major stimulus for calcitriol synthesis, serum calcitriol concentrations should be elevated in this disorder; however, when measured, serum calcitriol concentrations have been found to be low or low-normal. This finding is suggestive of a potential second defect in this condition, that is, dysfunction of the renal 1-α-hydroxylase enzyme. Vitamin D–resistant rickets may be inherited in a sex-linked recessive or an autosomal dominant pattern. The most frequent type, the X-linked dominant pattern, affects males. Traditionally, patients with vitamin D–resistant rickets have been treated with cholecalciferol and phosphate supplements. Phosphate-wasting peptides, **phosphatonins** such as FGF-23, play a major role in the pathogenesis of renal phosphate wasting disorders with bone disease, including X-linked hypophosphatemic rickets (XLH), autosomal dominant hypophosphatemic rickets (ADHR), and tumor-induced osteomalacia (TIO). XLH results from a mutation in the *PHEX* gene (phosphate-regulating gene with endopeptidase activity) located on the X chromosome. Patients with X-linked hypophosphatemia have hypophosphatemia caused by renal phosphate loss and low or inappropriately normal levels of 1,25-dihydroxyvitamin D_3. The renal phosphate loss and suppressed calcitriol are likely the results of an increase in phosphatonins.[118-120]

Calcium Deficiency Rickets[121]

Also termed *calcipenic rickets,* this form of osteomalacia occurs when the diet is low in calcium, or when the bioavailability of calcium is reduced. Children who follow strict vegetarian or high cereal diets are at risk of developing rickets. Some of these children have clinical and biochemical features of vitamin D deficiency, attributed to vitamin D binding by dietary phytates within the intestinal lumen.

Clinically, affected children have rachitic features with "knock" knees, bow legs, or "wind-swept" deformities, but no muscular weakness. Radiological features correspond to clinical findings of rachitic changes (see earlier discussion). The bone histological pattern reveals features of osteomalacia and secondary hyperparathyroidism. Biochemical features of calcipenic rickets include hypocalcemia and hypocalciuria, normal serum 25(OH)D, elevated serum alkaline phosphatase, and elevated serum calcitriol and PTH concentrations.

Hyperalimentation-Induced Osteopenia

Long-term parenteral alimentation (TPN) has been associated with osteopenia and bone demineralization. The main feature seen in this metabolic bone disease is hypercalciuria. Several factors have been implicated as the causes of hypercalciuria, including cyclic infusion of TPN solutions, sulfur-containing acidic amino acids, and hypertonic dextrose infusions, which results in hyperinsulinemia and decreased tubular resorption of calcium, acidosis, and low phosphate in infused solutions. Hypercalciuria may be ameliorated by phosphate supplementation.

Aluminum-containing parenteral hyperalimentation solutions are responsible for causing a peculiar metabolic bone disease characterized by reduced bone formation. The degree of aluminum accumulation in bone correlates with decreased bone formation.

Other Causes of Osteomalacia

Chronic acidosis causes osteomalacia, hypercalciuria, and hyperphosphaturia as the result of neutralization of acids by bone with subsequent release of bone mineral. Patients with renal Fanconi's syndrome have diminished proximal tubule reabsorption of bicarbonate (resulting in chronic acidosis), phosphorus, glucose, and amino acids. Osteomalacia may be severe because of the chronic acidosis and severe hypophosphatemia. In addition, as part of the proximal tubulopathy, activity of the renal 1-α-hydroxylase enzyme may be subnormal.

Sufficient substrate must be supplied in the diet for proper bone mineralization. Delayed bone mineralization commonly occurs in very low birth weight, premature infants who are fed normal infant formulas or breast milk,[122] both of which contain insufficient quantities of calcium and phosphorus to accommodate the rapid bone mineralization of premature infants.

Drug-Induced Osteomalacia[123,124]

Prolonged administration of heparin has been associated with osteoporosis and decreased bone density. The incidence of heparin-induced osteopenia is unknown. It appears that an individual has to receive a dose of at least 15,000 U/day for 6 months before osteopenia can occur. The symptoms, which are nonspecific, basically manifest as back pain and vertebral fractures; these are reversible after withdrawal of heparin. Methotrexate is a commonly used antineoplastic agent, particularly in childhood leukemias. It has been shown to decrease osteoblastic activity in animals and to increase bone resorption in humans. Consequently, prolonged use of this agent may induce osteopenia.

Osteitis Fibrosa

Osteitis fibrosa is the histopathological bone lesion produced by excessive PTH secretion. It is primarily seen in two conditions, primary hyperparathyroidism and chronic renal failure. Bone disease is of lesser significance in primary hyperparathyroidism because surgical removal of the involved parathyroid glands cures the disease. The pathophysiological condition of secondary hyperparathyroidism associated with chronic renal failure is more complex and less amenable to treatment. Thus uremic patients frequently suffer from severe bone disease.

The complex bone abnormality associated with chronic renal failure is termed *renal osteodystrophy (ROD)*.[125] ROD develops as the early stages of chronic renal failure (CRF) and covers a spectrum of bone changes observed in the uremic patient, which extend from osteitis fibrosa to more mild disease. Between these two extremes are cases of bone mineralization compromised to variable degrees, as in "mixed bone disease" and osteomalacia. The dynamic process of bone remodeling is compromised in CRF, and a positive or negative *bone* balance can be observed in uremic patients. In addition to the classic modulators of bone remodeling, such as parathyroid hormone, calcitriol and calcitonin, and cytokines and growth factors (see Box 33-1) that act at an autocrine or paracrine level, significant modulators of osteoblast and osteoclast activation are present in uremic patients.

Two distinct histopathological forms of renal osteodystrophy, osteomalacia and osteitis fibrosa (Box 33-10), frequently coexist in the same patient. Osteomalacia is probably caused by decreased synthesis of calcitriol secondary to renal parenchymal disease. Serum concentrations of calcitriol and 24,25-dihydroxyvitamin D_3 are decreased in both children and adults with chronic renal failure, and calcidiol concentrations are normal. Factors that contribute to secondary hyperparathyroidism of renal disease include (1) decreased phosphorous excretion and hyperphosphatemia, which directly decreases renal calcitriol synthesis (Figs. 33-6 and 33-7); (2) decreased renal hydroxylase activity caused by renal damage; (3) a higher set point for PTH secretion in uremia possibly caused by a decrease in the number of vitamin D receptors in parathyroid cells; (4) hypocalcemia; and (5) skeletal resistance to PTH.

Box 33-10

Pathological Forms of Renal Osteodystrophy

Predominant osteitis fibrosa
- Normal serum calcium level—Calcitriol responsive
- Pretreatment hypercalcemia—Exacerbated by calcitriol

Predominant osteomalacia
- Small amount of fibrosis present—Calcitriol responsive
- Pure osteomalacia—Hypercalcemia with calcitriol treatment

Mixed osteitis fibrosa and osteomalacia—Calcitriol responsive

Mild—Calcitriol responsive

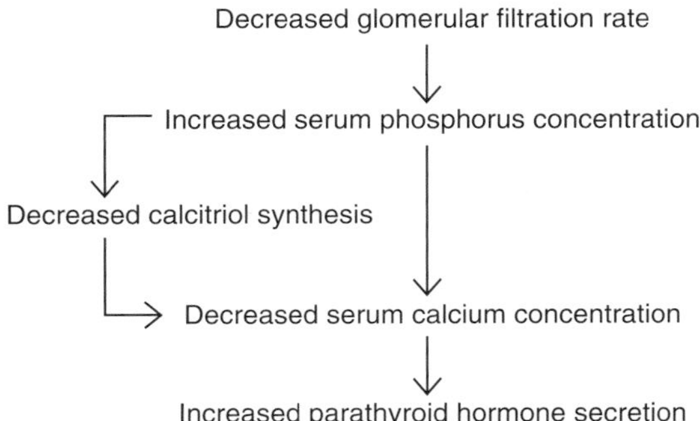

Fig. 33-6 Pathogenetic mechanism of secondary hyperparathyroidism in renal failure according to phosphate theory.

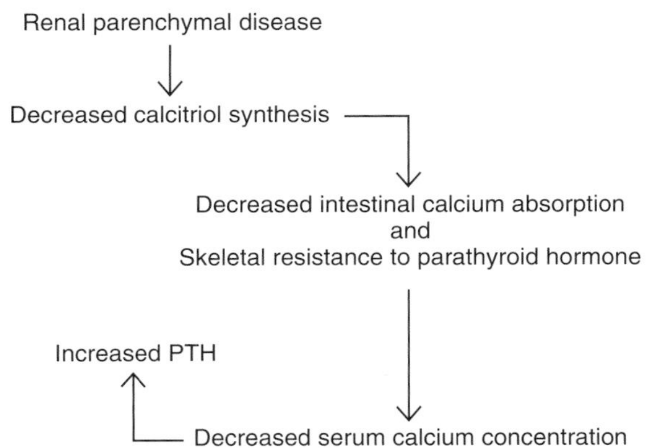

Fig. 33-7 Pathogenetic mechanism of secondary hyperparathyroidism in renal failure according to vitamin D theory.

Paget's Disease[126-128]

Paget's disease of bone (PDB) is a disorder of bone metabolism characterized by increased osteoclastic bone resorption followed by disordered, excessive bone formation. This results in weakened, deformed bones of increased mass in which collagen fibers assume a haphazard irregular mosaic pattern instead of the normal parallel symmetry. The incidence of this disease is difficult to determine because most affected patients are asymptomatic. The incidence of Paget's disease varies with age. PDB rarely occurs before middle age, and its prevalence increases steadily with age. It is more common among elderly than among middle-aged people. In an autopsy series of persons older than 40 years of age, 3% of this group was affected. The overall prevalence in whites is approximately 3%, although it appears to be declining. Family history is positive in 14% of cases. Males are more prone to have the disease than females (3:2). A geographic variation in prevalence has been noted, with highest rates found in the United Kingdom. The disease occurs more frequently among people of European ancestry. It is uncommon among Scandinavians, Asians, and black Africans. The cause of the disease is unknown. Although its origin remains elusive, genetic factors and environmental influences have been implicated.

The histological pattern of patients with Paget's disease proceeds through three stages. In the early phase of the illness, resorption predominates and the bone marrow is replaced by a highly vascular fibrous connective tissue. In the second phase of the disease, bone formation predominates. Pagetic bone is coarse fibered, dense trabecular bone. In the final phase, the rate of bone resorption declines, and continued bone formation produces hard, dense bone. The largest amount of bone resorption that initially occurs produces greatly elevated urinary hydroxyproline concentrations, and the subsequent rapid rate of bone formation results in dramatically elevated serum alkaline phosphatase concentrations. Serum calcium and phosphorous concentrations are normal. However, pathological fractures occur and are treated by immobilization of the patient. In general, diagnosis may be confirmed both by x-ray and by the biochemical marker serum alkaline phosphatase, which is elevated in 85% of individuals with untreated active PDB. Hypercalcemia frequently occurs because immobilization increases the rate of bone resorption. Treatment is indicated for all patients with symptoms and for asymptomatic patients with active PDB in areas of the skeleton with the potential to produce complications of clinical importance. Paget's disease is treated successfully with CT and with bisphosphonates.

Heritable Bone Disease (Table 33-5)

Hypophosphatasia[129]

Hypophosphatasia is a rare heritable bone disease characterized by generalized reduction in alkaline phosphatase activity in liver, bone, and kidney tissues. Placental and intestinal alkaline phosphatase isoenzyme activities remain normal. The disease occurs in all races but is especially common among Mennonites in Canada, among whom the incidence is up to 1 per 100,000 live births. Clinically, the disease affects bone and dentition and ranges from a severe, lethal in utero form to an asymptomatic adult disease. Four clinical forms of the disease are known: (1) the perinatal (lethal) form, commonly associated with stillbirth and polyhydramnios; (2) the infantile form, usually seen during the first 6 months of life; (3) the childhood form; and (4) the adult form, which usually appears in middle age.

Osteogenesis Imperfecta[130]

Osteogenesis imperfecta is a heritable disorder of bone formation that results in low bone mass and a propensity to fracture. It exhibits a broad range of clinical severity, ranging from multiple fracturing in utero and perinatal death to normal adult stature and a low incidence of fracture. The disorder is currently classified into seven types based on differences in clinical presentation and bone architecture. Osteogenesis imperfecta types I through IV are characterized by abnormal synthesis of type I collagen fibers, the most abundant protein in bone matrix. Mutation in one of the type I collagen genes (*COL1A1* or *COL1A2*) is commonly associated with osteogenesis imperfecta, but is not a prerequisite for the diagnosis. The pathogenesis of the disease involves defective mutations

Table 33-5 Common Genetic Diseases Associated with Bone and Mineral Disorders

Disease	OMIM	Gene Involved	Lab Tests	Comment
Achondroplasia	100800	*FGFR3* >95% of patients have point mutation in the gene for fibroblast growth factor receptor 3 (FGFR3) on chromosome 4p >80% are new mutations		Most common form of short limb dwarfism. The mutation most often affects the cartilaginous growth plate in growing *skeleton*.
Hypochondroplasia	146000	*FGFR3*		Milder form
Thanatophoric dysplasia	187600 187601	*FGFR3*		Severe dysplasia
Osteogenesis imperfecta	166200 166210 166220 259440	*COL1A1* *COL1A2*		
Achondrogenesis type II	200610	*COL2A1*		Very short limbs, flat midface, micrognathia
Hypochondrogenesis	200610	*COL2A1*		Less severe changes
Spondylo-epiphyseal dysplasia congenita (SEDC)	183900	*COL2A1*		Milder form
Stickler dysplasia	120140	*COL11A1* *COL11A2*		
Campomelic dysplasia	114290	*SOX9*		
Cleidoclanial dysplasia	119600	*CBFA1/RUNX2*		
Autosomal dominant hypophosphatemic rickets	605380	*FGF* mutation		
X-linked hypophosphatemic rickets		*PHEX*		
Multiple Epiphyseal Dysplasias (EDM)				
EDM1	132400	*COMP*		Severe form
Pseudoachondroplasia	177170	*COMP*		Short limb dwarfism
EDM2	600204	*COL9A2*		
EDM3	600969	*COL9A3*		
EDM 5	607078	Matrillin 3 *MATN 3*		
EDM 4	226900	*DTDST*		Clubfoot, scoliosis, double-layered patella
Genetic Conditions of Abnormal Bone Mineralization				
Hypophosphatasia	146300 171760 241500	*TNAP*	Low serum alkaline phosphatase	
Craniometaphyseal dysplasia	123000	*ANKH*		Hyperostosis
Genetic Conditions of Osteoblast Dysfunction				
Osteopetrosis type 1	166600	*LRP5* gene Chromosome 11q13		Endosteal hyperostosis, autosomal dominant osteosclerosis
Osteoporosis		ER beta aromatase		Accelerated osteoporosis due to estrogen loss
Genetic Conditions of Osteoblast-Osteoclast Signaling Dysfunction				
Paget's disease		*SQSTM1* on chromosome 5q31		Excessive bone formation
Idiopatic osteolysis	605156	MMP-2		Recessive, osteolyses resulting in ankylosis
Genetic Conditions of Osteoclast Dysfunction				
Infantile malignant osteopetrosis	259700	*TCIRG1*		Autosomal recessive, dense bones, usually lethal
Osteopetrosis with RTA	259730	Carbonic anhydrase II		
Osteopetrosis type 2	166600	*CLCN7*		
Pycnodysostosis	265800	Cathepsin k		Short stature, bone fragility, skull deformity

Adapted from Kornak U, Mundlos S: Genetic disorders of the skeleton: a developmental approach, Am J Hum Genet 73:447, 2003.
Aromatase, Enzyme that converts androgens into estrogen; *CLCN7,* chloride channel gene; *COMP,* cartilage oligometric matrix protein; *DTDST,* diastrophic dysplasia sulfate transporter; *ER beta,* estrogen receptor beta; *LRP5,* low-density lipoprotein receptor protein 5; *MMP-2,* matrix metalloproteinase-2; *RTA,* renal tubular acidosis; *TNAP,* tissue-nonspecific alkaline phosphatase.

in the genes that code for pro-α 1 and pro-α 2 chains of type I collagen, resulting in bone fragility.

Newer forms of osteogenesis imperfecta (types V, VI, and VII) are not associated with type I collagen gene defects. The prime clinical manifestations of this disease include pronounced bone fragility, generalized osteopenia, and recurrent fractures in response to mild trauma. Hearing loss occurs in about 50% of patients younger than 30 years of age. Treatment of osteogenesis imperfecta by bisphosphonate therapy can improve bone mass in all types of the disorder.

Achondroplasia[131,132]

Achondroplasia is the most common form of short limb dwarfism. More than 95% of patients have the same point mutation in the gene for fibroblast growth factor receptor 3 (FGFR3), and more than 80% of these are new (spontaneous) mutations. The mutation affects many tissues, most strikingly the cartilaginous growth plate in the growing skeleton, leading to a variety of manifestations and complications.

Osteopetrosis[133]

Osteopetrosis encompasses a group of diseases characterized by failure of osteoclast-mediated bone resorption. The disease is classified into eight types according to clinical and genetic factors. The main two forms of osteopetrosis include a more common benign type, which often is asymptomatic and is inherited as an autosomal dominant mode, and the rare malignant form, which typically occurs in infancy and childhood and is inherited in an autosomal recessive mode. Rare forms of osteopetrosis may be associated with renal tubular acidosis, carbonic anhydrase deficiency, or neuronal storage disease.

Albright Hereditary Osteodystrophy (AHO)[134,135]

AHO, also known as pseudohypoparathyroidism or pseudopseudohypoparathyroidism, has a wide range of clinical features, including short stature, obesity, rounded face, low nasal bridge, short neck, dental defects, osteoporosis, cataracts, subcutaneous ossifications, and characteristic shortening and widening of long bones in the hands and feet, as well as syndactyly between the second and third toes. Mental retardation is present in some, but not all, patients. AHO is caused by heterozygous inactivating mutations of the G protein alpha-subunit (Gs alpha) of the *GNAS* gene. Gs alpha is activated in a tissue-specific manner, in renal proximal tubules, thyroid, pituitary, and ovaries, and is expressed only from the maternal allele. Patients who have Gs alpha mutations that are inherited maternally likely show resistance to PTH, thyroid-stimulating hormone (TSH), and gonadotropins, in addition to the clinical findings of AHO. When this occurs, the resulting syndrome is also known as *pseudohypoparathyroidism*. Paternally inherited mutations of the same gene result only in clinical AHO without parathyroid resistance, also known as *pseudopseudohypoparathyroidism*.

KEY CONCEPTS BOX 33-4

- Bone disease can involve an imbalance of minerals in the collagenous part of the matrix. In osteomalacia, the bone contains normal amounts of collagen base but deficient amounts of mineral. In osteopenia, mineralized bone is decreased.
- Osteoporosis, a significant disease of older people, is noted by decreases in bone mass involving both mineral and osteoid. Loss of estradiol increases the risk of osteoporosis among postmenopausal women.
- Rickets, caused by poor Ca nutrition or lack of vitamin D during the prepubertal years, is associated with decreased bone mineralization and bowed legs. The lack of vitamin D can result from a dietary, genetic defect in synthesis, or from receptor deficits.
- Increases in serum parathyroid hormone (PTH) and alkaline phosphatase are associated with these diseases.

SECTION OBJECTIVES BOX 33-5

- Describe the effects on bone and serum Ca levels of elevated or low serum concentrations of the following:
  - Vitamin D
  - Parathyroid hormone (PTH) (primary and secondary)
- List the disease states associated with elevated and decreased levels of serum calcium.
- Describe the conditions that might require measurement of ionized calcium.
- List the disease states associated with elevated and decreased levels of serum magnesium.
- Describe how serum levels of phosphate change with serum Ca levels.

CHANGE OF ANALYTE IN DISEASE

Biochemical Measurements of Bone Turnover

Biochemical measurements of bone turnover are helpful in the study of the pathophysiology of skeletal metabolism and growth. However, interpretation of their results is difficult because it depends on a number of physiological variables, including age, pubertal stage, growth velocity, mineral accrual, hormonal regulation, nutritional status, and circadian variation. Methodological considerations, including expression of the results of urinary markers, specificity of the markers for bone tissue, and the sensitivity and specificity of assays, also affect interpretation. These limitations have minimized the widespread use of these markers.[136-138]

Urine Collagen Pyridinoline Cross-Linking Amino Acids

These are among the best available specific biomarkers of bone resorption. These compounds, which include hydroxylysylpyridinoline and lysylpyridinoline, are released upon degradation of mature collagen from skeletal tissues. The hydroxypyridinium collagen cross-links, pyridinoline and deoxypyridinoline, are also released upon degradation of mature collagen. These compounds are present in urine in the free, non–peptide-bound (40%) or peptide-bound state (60%).

Urinary Telopeptides

Urinary **N-telopeptides** are the peptide fragments of the protein that links the collagen bundles in bones. These fragments are liberated into the circulation as a result of the breakdown of collagen within the bones, and they are excreted unchanged in the urine. Urine levels of N-telopeptides therefore reflect the degree of bone resorption. Because of diurnal variations in the degree of bone resorption, with highest levels occurring during the night, the N-telopeptides are best measured either in a 24-hour urine sample or in the early morning sample. A single urine N-telopeptide level on its own is not of much use because the normal range is so wide. On the other hand, a reduction of 40% to 50% in these levels over a period of 8 to 12 weeks suggests that the increased rate of bone resorption has been suppressed, and that the patient probably is responding well to the prescribed therapy.

Pyridinoline cross-links and collagen telopeptides are the best indices of bone resorption.

Vitamin D

Serum concentrations of vitamin D metabolites may be altered in a variety of disease states (Box 33-11). Decreased concentrations result from deficient intake, defective metabolic regulation, or increased excretion. Serum calcidiol concentrations are low in patients who have both an insufficient exposure to sunlight and a low intake of foods that contain vitamin D. Patients who receive anticonvulsant drugs convert calcidiol into biologically inactive polar metabolites. Production of calcidiol is impaired in patients with liver disease. Inactive or absent renal 1-α-hydroxylase activity and secondary low serum calcitriol concentrations are associated with vitamin D–dependent rickets type I, postmenopausal and senile osteoporosis,[72,93,94] hypoparathyroidism, pseudohypoparathyroidism, vitamin D–resistant rickets,[116,139] and chronic renal failure. Patients with nephrotic syndrome have low serum concentrations of both calcidiol and calcitriol caused by urinary losses of both metabolites, as well as the serum protein (vitamin D–binding protein) to which they are attached.

High serum calcidiol concentrations result from increased exogenous intake or increased endogenous production following an unusually large sunlight exposure. High serum calcitriol concentrations occur in physiological states of increased calcium requirements such as growth and pregnancy and lactation.[73] High serum calcitriol concentrations are also seen in sarcoidosis, in which an extrarenal source of calcitriol production has been implicated, and in hyperparathyroidism, in which the serum concentrations of PTH, a major stimulus for calcitriol production, are elevated.

Box 33-11

Diseases and Conditions Associated With Changes in Serum Concentrations of Vitamin D Metabolites

- Calcidiol (25-hydroxycholecalciferol) deficiency
  - Nutritional osteomalacia
  - Anticonvulsant-induced osteomalacia
  - Liver disease
  - Nephrotic syndrome
- Calcitriol (1,25-dihydroxycholecalciferol) deficiency
  - Vitamin D–dependent rickets type I
  - Postmenopausal and senile osteoporosis
  - Hypoparathyroidism
  - Pseudohypoparathyroidism
  - Vitamin D–resistant rickets
  - Nephrotic syndrome
- Calcidiol (25-hydroxycholecalciferol) excess
  - Vitamin D intoxication
  - Excessive sunlight exposure
- Calcitriol (1,25-hydroxycholecalciferol) excess
  - Childhood
  - Pregnancy and lactation
  - Sarcoidosis
  - Hyperparathyroidism

Parathyroid Hormone

Hypoparathyroidism

Primary Idiopathic Hypoparathyroidism

Idiopathic hypoparathyroidism describes the condition of decreased production of PTH whose cause is not known. In pseudohypoparathyroidism, production of PTH is intact, but there is target organ resistance to PTH, in other words, PTH, although present, does not exert its physiological actions because the target organs are not responsive. In current terminology, there may be a "receptor defect" for PTH. Another way of describing idiopathic hypoparathyroidism is *hormone-deficient hypoparathyroidism,* and pseudohypoparathyroidism can be described as *hormone-sufficient, receptor-deficient hypoparathyroidism* (Fig. 33-8). Hypoparathyroidism classically manifests with hypocalcemia and hyperphosphatemia, usually in childhood.

Secondary Hypoparathyroidism

Hypoparathyroidism may result from other disorders. Inadvertent surgical removal of the parathyroids may occur during thyroidectomy. Because magnesium is important for PTH secretion, magnesium deficiency may result in hypoparathyroidism. An interesting physiological hypoparathyroidism occurs in infants. In utero, calcium is transferred actively across the placenta, and serum calcium concentrations in the fetus are extremely high. These high serum calcium concentrations appear to inhibit fetal parathyroid function. Inhibited parathyroid function persists for a short interval after birth and appears to be a cause of hypocalcemia in the first 3 days of life, especially in the premature infant.[140,141]

The diagnosis of hypoparathyroidism is made from the clinical presentation of lowered serum calcium and elevated serum phosphorous concentrations. PTH concentrations will be low in hypoparathyroidism but elevated in pseudohypoparathyroidism. To further distinguish idiopathic hypoparathyroidism from pseudohypoparathyroidism, PTH infusion is

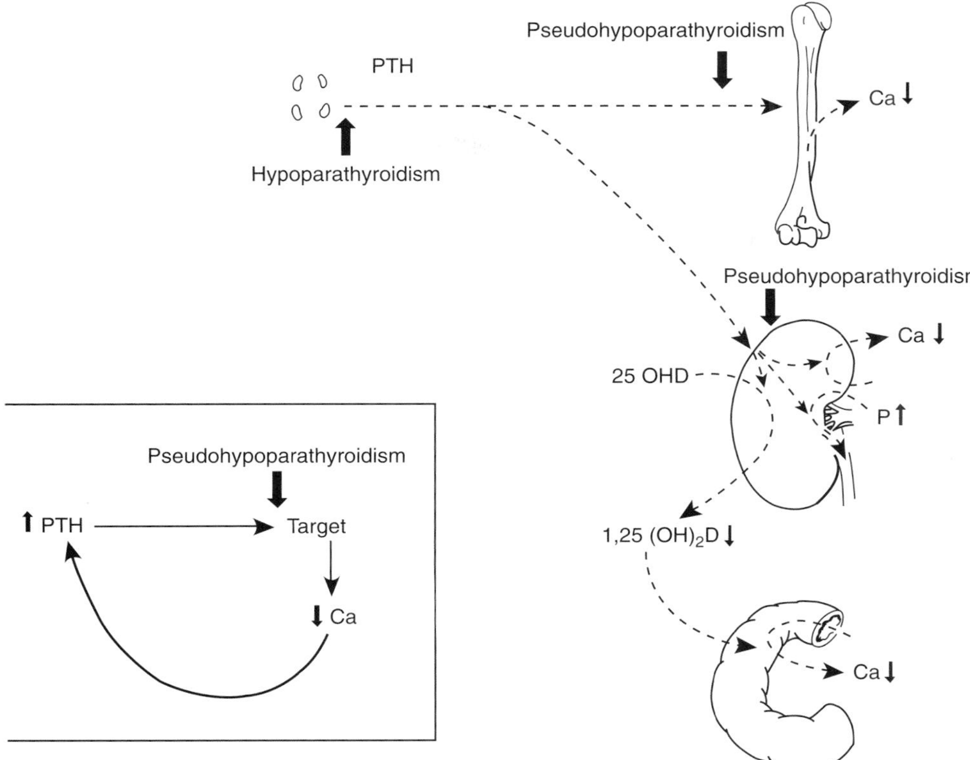

Fig. 33-8 In idiopathic hypoparathyroidism, decreased parathyroid hormone (PTH) results in decreased serum calcium, increased serum phosphorus, and decreased production of 1,25-dihydroxyvitamin D. In pseudohypoparathyroidism, although sufficient hormone is present, target organs are unresponsive and the biochemical result is similar. *Inset,* In pseudohypoparathyroidism, resultant low serum calcium concentrations serve as a stimulus to PTH production. Because parathyroid glands are intact, in contrast to idiopathic hypoparathyroidism, serum PTH concentrations will be elevated in an attempt to overcome target organ resistance and rectify hypocalcemia.

administered. After the infusion has been given, serum calcium and urinary phosphorus and cAMP concentrations are measured. Patients with pseudohypoparathyroidism may have varying "degrees of block" in response to PTH, at the bone site or at various "levels" in the kidney. Patients with hypoparathyroidism are treated with supplements of calcium salts and calcitriol.

Hyperparathyroidism

Primary Hyperparathyroidism (PHPT)[142]

Primary hyperparathyroidism is often described as related to hyperplasia or adenoma of the parathyroids. In contrast to hypoparathyroidism, which usually begins in childhood, hyperparathyroidism is usually discovered in adulthood, predominantly in postmenopausal women. As expected from the physiological action of PTH, excess concentrations of the hormone result in increased serum calcium concentrations and decreased serum phosphorous concentrations. Demineralization occurs as a consequence of the bone-lytic action of PTH and is associated with areas of extensive resorption. Many clinical problems are associated with the high serum calcium concentrations. Major organ systems adversely affected by hypercalcemia are the nervous system and the kidney.

The diagnosis of primary hyperparathyroidism is based on the findings of high serum calcium, low serum phosphorus, and high serum PTH concentrations. However, not all hyperparathyroid patients will have increased serum calcium concentrations or increased serum PTH concentrations. Ionized calcium measurements in blood may provide additional diagnostic help because the ionized calcium fraction is the physiologically active calcium.

Inherited syndromes (Table 33-6), most of which are associated with multiglandular disease, can be found in a minority of patients. These syndromes include multiple endocrine neoplasia (MEN) type 1 and type 2a, familial hypocalciuric hypercalcemia, and neonatal severe primary hyperparathyroidism (HPT), as well as hyperparathyroidism–jaw tumor syndrome. In sporadic parathyroid adenomas, two specific genetic defects have been further characterized: inactivating mutations of the *MEN1* gene (in >25% of parathyroid adenomas), and activation of the *PRAD1/cyclinD1* oncogene.

Two autosomal disorders—familial hypocalciuric hypercalcemia (FHH) and neonatal severe primary hyperparathyroidism (NSHPT)—result from loss of parathyroid calcium-sensing receptor (CASR) function.[144,145] FHH is characterized by moderate elevations in serum calcium concentration (hypercalcemia), lower urinary calcium excretion (hypocalciuria), and inappropriately normal PTH levels. NSHPT represents the most severe expression of familial hypocalciuric hypercalcemia. In most patients with CASR mutations, the two gene copies are mutated. Neonatal severe hyperparathyroidism causes a marked elevation in serum calcium and PTH levels. It appears very early, in the first days of life, and the baby presents with hypotonia, poor feeding, failure to thrive, and respiratory distress associated with ribcage deformities. PTH concentrations are very high and are associated with calcium levels that are life threatening.

Table 33-6 Genetic Disorders of the Parathyroid Gland

Disease	Gene Involved	Comment
Pseudohypoparathyroidism type 1	*GPCR*	Hormone resistance (pseudohypoparathyroidism caused by *loss-of-function mutations*)
	Mutations in the gene encoding the α-subunit of the G protein–coupling receptors	– Inherited Gsα mutations from the mother – Develop resistance to various hormones (PTH, TSH, LH, and FSH) – AHO phenotype
Pseudohypoparathyroidism type 1b		Renal PTH resistance in absence of AHO or resistance to other hormones; PTH resistance occurs only when the disease is inherited maternally
Pseudopseudohypoparathyroidism (PPHP)		– Inherited Gsα mutations from the father: • AHO phenotype • No hormone resistance
Albright hereditary osteodystrophy (AHO)		Inactivating Gsα heterozygous mutations AHO phenotype: Short stature, brachydactyly, subcutaneous ossifications, centripetal obesity, depressed nasal bridge, hypertelorism, and mental or developmental deficits
McCune-Albright syndrome		Hormone hypersecretion (McCune-Albright syndrome caused by *gain-of-function mutations*). Triad of polyostotic fibrous dysplasia, cafe-au-lait skin lesions, and gonadotropin-independent sexual precocity
Neonatal hyperparathyroidism	*GPCR* Loss-of-function mutation Ca-sensing receptor	Autosomal recessive loss-of-function mutation of two copies of the gene encoding the Ca-sensing receptor that controls PTH secretion
Familial hypocalciuric hypercalcemia	*GPCR* Loss-of-function mutation Ca-sensing receptor	Autosomal dominant relative resistance to extracellular Ca action caused by loss-of-function mutation of one copy of the gene encoding the Ca-sensing receptor that controls PTH secretion from the parathyroid and resorption of Ca by the kidney
Blomstrand chondrodysplasia	*GPCR* Loss-of-function mutation PTH/PTHRP	Autosomal recessive Defects in breast and tooth formation
Jansen metaphyseal chondrodysplasia	*GPCR* Gain-of-function mutation PTH/PTHRP	Autosomal dominant Hypercalcemia, hypophosphatemia mimicking PTH hypersecretion Defective endochondral bone formation and short-limb dwarfism
Familial hypocalcemia	*GPCR* Gain-of-function mutation Ca-sensing receptor	Autosomal dominant PTH deficiency, hypocalcemia, and hyperphosphatemia

Adapted from Spiegel AM, Weinstein LS: Inherited diseases involving G proteins and G protein-coupled receptors, Annu Rev Med 55:27, 2004.
AHO, Albright hereditary osteodystrophy; *FSH,* follicle-stimulating hormone; *LH,* luteinizing hormone; *PTH,* parathyroid hormone; *PTHRP,* PTH-related peptide; *TSH,* thyroid-stimulating hormone.

Secondary Hyperparathyroidism

Conditions that are associated with chronic hypocalcemia will result in chronic stimulation of the parathyroids and secondary hyperparathyroidism. Two major factors that result in chronic hypocalcemia of nonparathyroid cause are vitamin D–metabolite deficiencies and high phosphorous loads. Any deficiency of vitamin D or its major metabolites will result in decreased intestinal absorption of calcium and hypocalcemia. The initial response to this hypocalcemia will be secondary hyperparathyroidism, which helps maintain serum calcium concentrations in the normal range. High phosphorous loads occur with infusion of phosphorus-containing fluids, ingestion of high phosphorous content milk (such as cow milk given to newborn infants), or retention of phosphorus by failing kidneys.[143] High serum phosphorous concentrations result in a secondary decrease in serum calcium concentrations. With decreased serum calcium concentrations, compensatory secondary hyperparathyroidism occurs.[141]

In secondary hyperparathyroidism, serum calcium concentrations are low or normal because parathyroid overactivity results from an initial decline in serum calcium. Serum phosphorous concentrations are low except in situations of phosphorous overload, when they are high. Serum PTH concentrations should be elevated in secondary hyperparathyroidism.

Calcium (see Methods on Evolve)

Hypercalcemia

Hypercalcemia resulting from primary hyperparathyroidism has been described earlier. Other causes of hypercalcemia are listed in Box 33-12.

Box 33-12

Causes of Hypercalcemia

- Primary hyperparathyroidism
- Thyrotoxicosis
- Addison's disease
- Withdrawal of steroids
- Tumors
- Vitamin D and vitamin A intoxication
- Sarcoidosis
- Idiopathic hypercalcemia of infancy
- Immobilization
- Subcutaneous fat necrosis in infants
- Thiazide diuretics
- Milk-alkali syndrome
- Benign familial hypercalcemia

Endocrine and Tumor-Related Hypercalcemia

Hypercalcemia may occur with disorders of endocrine organs other than the parathyroids. Overproduction of thyroid hormone (thyrotoxicosis) and underproduction of corticosteroids (Addison's disease or abrupt withdrawal of steroid hormones) are associated with hypercalcemia. A wide variety of tumors appear to produce PTH-like substances with osteoclast stimulatory activity, which results in hypercalcemia. Hypercalcemia and hyperparathyroidism sometimes are associated with pheochromocytoma or MEN type 2 syndrome. Pancreatic VIPoma tumors secrete vasoactive intestinal peptide (VIP), which causes severe diarrhea. About 50% of these patients have hypercalcemia, possibly caused by VIP-induced bone resorption. The mechanism of hypercalcemia in malignancy may, in part, be the result of tumor production of PTH-related proteins (PTHRP) or other substances that cause bone resorption.

Vitamin D–Related Disorders

Excessive intake of vitamin D may result in hypercalcemia. Hypercalcemia may be a feature of granulomatous diseases such as tuberculosis and sarcoidosis, which are associated with abnormal vitamin D metabolism and increased serum levels of $1,25(OH)_2D_3$. In sarcoidosis, elevated calcitriol concentrations appear to be the cause of the hypercalcemia. Therapy for vitamin D–resistant rickets or hypoparathyroidism with high doses of vitamin D is a common cause of hypercalcemia. Idiopathic hypercalcemia of infants is believed to be related to disordered vitamin D metabolism, possibly with increased sensitivity to vitamin D.

Iatrogenic Causes

Immobilization of patients, especially male adolescents, results in rapid mobilization of calcium from bone and resultant hypercalcemia. Lactation causes a transient increase in bone resorption and secondary hypercalcemia, reversed by weaning. In infants born after traumatic deliveries, a curious condition of hypercalcemia can occur that is related to subcutaneous fat necrosis. Use of thiazide diuretics is classically associated with hypercalcemia. Thiazides act directly to increase calcium release from the skeleton and to promote renal tubular reabsorption of calcium. Chronic lithium intake may cause hyperparathyroidism and mild hypercalcemia and hypermagnesemia. Excessive ingestion of milk and alkali in the treatment of peptic ulcer (the milk-alkali syndrome) also results in hypercalcemia.

Neonatal hypercalcemia (total serum calcium concentration higher than 11 mg/dL or serum ionized calcium concentration higher than 5.8 mg/dL) can be the result of prolonged maternal hypocalcemia produced by a multitude of causes. Consequently, a variable degree of congenital, transient hyperparathyroidism may result. Neonatal hypercalcemia in the phosphorous deficiency syndrome has been reported in preterm infants fed human milk.

Familial Form

A benign form of familial hypercalcemia is inherited as a dominant trait. Mild hypercalcemia (less than 13 mg/dL) occurs, apparently without adverse effects.

Box 33-13

Causes of Hypocalcemia

Vitamin D
- Decreased solar exposure and endogenous synthesis
- Decreased intestinal intake (malabsorption, dietary deficiency)
- Altered hepatic metabolism of vitamin D (hepatic disease, anticonvulsant therapy)
- Decreased renal synthesis of calcitriol (vitamin D dependency, renal failure)

Parathyroid
- Hypoparathyroidism (primary and secondary)
- Pseudohypoparathyroidism

Calcitonin
- Calcitonin or mithramycin infusion

Calcium
- Intestinal malabsorption
- Acute pancreatitis
- Infusion of agents complexing calcium
- Alkalosis decreasing ionized calcium

Magnesium
- Magnesium deficiency (see Box 33-15)

Phosphorus
- Renal failure
- Phosphate infusion
- Cow milk formulas

Hypocalcemia

The causes of hypocalcemia are currently classified in relation to the major hormone or biochemical involved as vitamin D, PTH, CT, calcium, magnesium, and phosphate (Box 33-13).

Vitamin D deficiency,[55,56] which was discussed earlier, occurs as a result of reduced synthesis or intake of the parent vitamin D, altered hepatic metabolism of vitamin D, and decreased renal synthesis of calcitriol, the final active metabolite of vitamin D.

Hypoparathyroidism (primary and secondary) and pseudohypoparathyroidism have been discussed previously. CT or mithramycin infusions decrease calcium transport from bone to extracellular space, which results in hypocalcemia. Intestinal malabsorption of calcium may lead to hypocalcemia. Acute pancreatitis is associated with fatty acid–calcium complex precipitates in the pancreas and hypocalcemia. Decreased blood ionized calcium occurs with infusion of agents that complex calcium (citrate and acid-citrated blood for transfusion, or ethylenediaminetetraacetic acid [EDTA]), or with alkalosis, which shifts the fraction of calcium that is ionized to that which is protein bound.

Conditions in which phosphorous concentrations in blood are elevated, such as renal failure (see earlier discussion), phosphate infusion, or infants receiving cow milk formulas with their high phosphate content, will result in decreased serum calcium concentrations because calcium is shifted from the extracellular space into bone and soft tissues, probably as the result of a blunted bone response to the effects of PTH.[146]

Neonatal hypocalcemia is defined as a total serum calcium concentration of less than 7 mg/dL for preterm infants or 8 mg/dL for term infants (serum ionized calcium concentration less than 4.4 mg/dL). Neonatal hypocalcemia is the direct result of the relatively high PTH set point (see p. 626) established in the fetus. After birth, this PTH set point is lowered, with a commensurate lowering of serum calcium. At birth, termination of the high transplacental calcium influx to the fetus can result in a transient hypocalcemia. Prematurity is the major cause of neonatal hypocalcemia, which may develop in a large proportion (30% to 90%) of preterm infants. The incidence of hypocalcemia correlates inversely with gestational age and birth weight. Its cause is uncertain. About 30% of infants with birth asphyxia may develop hypocalcemia in the neonatal period.

Parathyroid gland adenoma is the most common cause of maternal hyperparathyroidism and hypercalcemia. Maternal hypercalcemia suppresses the fetal parathyroid glands, resulting in transient neonatal, or congenital, hypoparathyroidism. At least 50% of infants born to hyperparathyroid mothers have hypocalcemic tetany.

Mothers with insulin-dependent diabetes mellitus have excessive urinary magnesium losses, especially if euglycemia is not maintained. Consequently, these mothers, and theoretically their fetuses, may be magnesium depleted. Hypomagnesemia impairs PTH secretion, which may explain the transient neonatal hypoparathyroidism and hypocalcemia that may develop in about 50% of infants of diabetic mothers.

Hypocalcemia in infants born to mothers with gestational exposure to anticonvulsant therapy may be related to the effect of phenobarbital or phenytoin in enhancing accelerated hepatic metabolism of 25(OH)D. Hypocalcemia has also been described in a few infants born to hypercalcemic women with familial hypocalciuric hypercalcemia.

Changes in PTH include vitamin D–axis analytes in hypercalcemia and hypocalcemia. Changes in the serum concentrations of phosphorus, in the PTH–vitamin D axis, and in vitamin D status are helpful in evaluating the causes of hypercalcemia and hypocalcemia. If the PTH–vitamin D axis is intact, two effects are seen: (1) cAMP production by the kidney is active; renal cAMP is best determined as "nephrogenous" cAMP, which takes into account the cAMP not produced in the kidney, and (2) 1,25-dihydroxycholecalciferol (calcitriol) production is also active (Tables 33-7 and 33-8).

Of the hypercalcemic disorders listed in Table 33-7, serum phosphorous concentrations are decreased in hyperparathyroidism because of the phosphaturic effects of PTH; in the remaining hypercalcemic disorders, little effect on serum phosphorus is evident. In hyperparathyroidism, serum PTH concentrations and PTH–vitamin D axis analytes are increased. In hypercalcemia from other causes, serum PTH is suppressed. In turn, the PTH–vitamin D axis may be suppressed, except in sarcoidosis, in which elevation of serum calcitriol concentrations appears to be a primary problem.

Vitamin D status is best assessed through measurement of serum 25-hydroxycholecalciferol (calcidiol) concentrations. Thus serum 25-hydroxycholecalciferol concentrations are elevated in vitamin D intoxication, with or without elevations in serum 1,25-dihydroxycholecalciferol (calcitriol) concentrations.

In hypocalcemia (see Table 33-8) related to parathyroid disorders, hypoparathyroidism, or pseudohypoparathyroidism, serum phosphorus is elevated because of decreased urinary phosphorous excretion. The PTH–vitamin D axis generally is hypofunctioning, except in pseudohypoparathyroidism, in which serum PTH concentrations are elevated because of target organ resistance to the hormone.

In the vitamin D disorders, serum phosphorous concentrations are generally low because one of the major actions of vitamin D is to raise serum phosphorous concentrations. However, in renal osteodystrophy (renal failure), serum phosphorous concentrations are elevated because of decreased renal phosphorous excretion. The PTH-cAMP axis in this circumstance may be increased because of hyperparathyroidism that follows hypocalcemia; however, serum 1,25-dihydroxycholecalciferol concentrations will remain decreased because of deficiency of vitamin D or blocks in vitamin D metabolism. In the condition of increased resistance to 1,25-dihydroxycholecalciferol, high serum concentrations of the metabolite are found, analogous to elevated PTH concentrations in pseudohypoparathyroidism. Serum 25-hydroxycholecalciferol measurements will be low in vitamin D deficiency or when there is a block in 25-hydroxylation of vitamin D but normal in vitamin D disorders caused by metabolic blocks beyond the liver step of hydroxylation.

In mineral disorders that cause hypocalcemia, little effect on the PTH–vitamin D axis has been reported. Secondary hyperparathyroidism can be a consequence of hypocalcemia. In hypomagnesemia, however, hypoparathyroidism can occur following magnesium deficiency.

Hypomagnesemia

Hypocalcemia can result from hypomagnesemia because of the adverse effect of hypomagnesemia on parathyroid function.

Table 33-7 Parathyroid Hormone–Vitamin D Axis Analytes in Hypercalcemia

			PARATHYROID HORMONE–VITAMIN D AXIS		*VITAMIN D STATUS*
Disorder	Serum Phosphorus	Parathyroid Hormone (PTH)	Nephrogenous Cyclic AMP	Calcitriol (1,25-Dihydroxycholecalciferol)	Calcidiol (25-Hydroxycholecalciferol)
Hyperparathyroidism	LO	HI	HI	HI	NL
Vitamin D disorders					
Vitamin D intoxication	NL	LO	LO	HI or NL	HI
High calcitriol in sarcoidosis	NL	LO	LO	HI	NL
Sensitivity to vitamin D:	NL	LO	LO	NL	NL
Idiopathic					
Hypercalcemia of infancy					
Non–parathyroid hormone, non–vitamin D disorders					
Malignancy	NL	LO	HI/LO	LO or HI	NL
Immobilization	NL	LO	LO	LO	NL
Thyrotoxicosis	NL	LO	NL	LO	NL

HI, Increased; *LO,* decreased; *NL,* normal.

Table 33-8 Parathyroid Hormone–Vitamin D Axis Analytes in Hypocalcemia

			PARATHYROID HORMONE–VITAMIN D AXIS		*VITAMIN D STATUS*
Disorder	Serum Phosphorus	Parathyroid Hormone (PTH)	Nephrogenous Cyclic AMP	Calcitriol (1,25-Dihydroxycholecalciferol)	Calcidiol (25-Hydroxycholecalciferol)
Parathyroid disorders					
Hypoparathyroidism	HI	LO	LO	LO	NL
Pseudohypoparathyroidism	HI	HI	LO	LO	NL
Vitamin D disorders					
Vitamin D deficiency	LO	HI	HI	HI,* NL, or LO	LO
Hepatic disease and anticonvulsant therapy	LO	HI	HI	NL or LO	LO
Renal					
Vitamin D–dependent rickets	LO	HI	HI	LO	NL
Osteodystrophy	HI	HI	—	LO	NL
Resistance to 1,25-dihydroxycholecalciferol	LO	HI	HI	HI	NL
Mineral disorders					
Calcium malabsorption	NL	NL or HI	—	—	—
Hypomagnesemia	NL	LO, NL, or HI	—	—	NL
High phosphate load	NI	NL or HI	—	—	NL

HI, Increased; *LO,* decreased; *NL,* normal.
*Especially in childhood.

Box 33-14

Causes of Hypermagnesemia

Magnesium sulfate therapy
Magnesium-containing antacids and purgatives
Renal failure

Magnesium (see Methods on Evolve)

Hypermagnesemia

An excess of magnesium is usually a consequence of increased medicinal intake of magnesium. Magnesium ($MgSO_4$) is used in the treatment of hypertension induced by pregnancy (preeclampsia). The mother will become hypermagnesemic (up to 11 mg/dL), as will her infant. Recent clinical studies have demonstrated the apparent benefits of maternal magnesium supplementation in reducing the incidence of preterm labor and allowing greater fetal growth. Reduced magnesium excretion may occur in severe renal failure, and the use of medicines that contain magnesium (antacids, purgatives) in this situation may result in hypermagnesemia (Box 33-14).

Hypomagnesemia and Magnesium Deficiency

Severe magnesium deficiency in humans is uncommon, possibly because of the body's highly developed ability to conserve magnesium. Decreased uptake of magnesium caused by gastrointestinal disorders (steatorrhea, malabsorption syndromes, gut resections) can cause magnesium deficiency. Specific intestinal malabsorption of magnesium also occurs and can cause hypomagnesemia in infancy. Protein-calorie malnutrition is often associated with magnesium depletion. Increased urinary magnesium losses may result from generalized renal disease or a specific renal defect in the reabsorption of magnesium. Dialysis of patients may result in magnesium depletion if a low magnesium–content dialysate is used. High rates of production of aldosterone (hyperaldosteronism), hyperparathyroidism, and diabetes mellitus may increase urinary magnesium losses. Alcoholism, intensive diuretic therapy, and treatment with the antibiotic gentamicin also may lead to increased urinary magnesium losses (Box 33-15).

Magnesium deficiency is often associated with hypocalcemia, and the signs and symptoms of magnesium deficiency normally are the signs of hypocalcemia. Although serum magnesium concentrations can be low, serum measurements may not reflect intracellular concentrations because magnesium is predominantly an intracellular mineral. Red blood cell magnesium concentrations have been advocated as a measure of intracellular magnesium status.

Phosphate (see Methods on Evolve)

Hyperphosphatemia

Hyperphosphatemia is most often the result of decreased renal excretion of phosphate anions as encountered in acute or chronic renal failure, particularly when the glomerular filtration rate is reduced to less than 25% of normal. Hyperphosphatemia can also be caused by an increased body phosphate load, which, in turn, can be caused by phosphate-containing laxatives and enemas, blood transfusions, or hyperalimentation, or by massive cell destruction after cell lysis by cytotoxic therapy (the tumor lysis syndrome) or tissue injury (hyperthermia, hypoxia, or crush injuries), which may result in rhabdomyolysis (muscle breakdown) and hemolysis. Increased renal tubular reabsorption of phosphate is responsible for the hyperphosphatemia seen in hypoparathyroidism, hyperthyroidism, hypogonadism, and growth hormone excess.

Box 33-15

Causes of Hypomagnesemia

- Decreased intake of magnesium
  - Steatorrhea
  - Malabsorption syndromes
  - Gut resections
  - Specific intestinal malabsorption of magnesium
  - Protein-calorie malnutrition
- Increased loss of magnesium
  - Renal tubular loss
  - Dialysis with low magnesium dialysate
  - Hyperaldosteronism
  - Hyperparathyroidism
  - Diabetes mellitus
  - Alcoholism
  - Diuretic therapy
  - Aminoglycoside therapy

Hypophosphatemia

Moderate hypophosphatemia, which is defined as a serum phosphorous concentration between 1.0 and 2.5 mg/dL in adults, is usually asymptomatic. In children, serum phosphorous concentrations below 4.0 mg/dL are often considered abnormal. Hypophosphatemia may be caused by decreased intestinal absorption of phosphate or by increased urine losses of phosphate and an endogenous shift of inorganic phosphorus from extracellular to intracellular fluid compartments.

Calcitonin (CT)

Abnormal serum CT concentrations are rarely found (Box 33-16). Serum measurements are most useful in patients suspected of having medullary thyroid carcinoma, a malignancy of the thyroid C-cells. This cancer is frequently seen in different members within families and is often associated with a tendency for other malignancies (such as the MEN syndrome type 2).[147] Serum CT measurements are useful both in the screening of family members who are potentially at risk of developing the disease and in the follow-up examination of previously treated patients suspected of recurrent metastatic disease. Serum CT elevations are produced by a wide variety of other neoplasias, the most frequent being bronchogenic carcinoma. Because gastrin is a potent stimulus for CT secretion, serum CT concentrations are elevated in Zollinger-Ellison syndrome, a pancreatic tumor of gastrin-secreting cells. Finally, CT excretion is decreased in patients with renal

Box 33-16

Diseases Associated with Abnormal Serum Calcitonin Concentrations

Deficiency
- Thyroid agenesis
- Thyroidectomy
- Osteoporosis

Excess
- Medullary thyroid carcinoma
- Bronchogenic carcinoma
- Zollinger-Ellison syndrome
- Renal failure

failure, and this decrease results in secondary elevation of serum concentrations of CT.

Because the thyroid gland is usually the sole source of CT production, athyroid patients lack circulating CT. CT levels are also decreased in some patients with osteoporosis. This may be caused by altered regulation of CT synthesis or release.[148]

Alkaline Phosphatase (ALP) (see Methods on Evolve)

In clinical practice, ALP determinations measure a group of enzymes that catalyze the hydrolysis of phosphate esters in an alkaline medium. Alkaline phosphatase is produced by many tissues (Box 33-17), but only the portion produced by bone and liver is usually detected in serum from healthy persons. Box 33-18 lists bone diseases associated with abnormal serum bone alkaline phosphatase concentrations. Note that ALP lacks sensitivity and specificity for bone disease, particularly in patients with osteoporosis, when serum ALP is usually within reference ranges. Alkaline phosphatase is produced by osteoblasts and lowers bone pyrophosphate levels; this probably facilitates mineralization. Alkaline phosphatase synthesis is deficient in hypophosphatasia, a rare hereditary illness associated with undermineralized bones and pathological fractures, and in achondroplasia, an inherited disorder of endochondral bone growth. Production is also decreased with generalized malnutrition or scurvy.

Far more common than decreased concentrations are diseases associated with elevated bone serum alkaline phosphatase concentrations. Such elevations signify increased osteoblastic activity, as may be seen in osteoblastic sarcoma, rickets, Paget's disease, and acromegaly. The elevated levels associated with hyperparathyroidism result from secondary bone mineralization rather than from PTH-induced osteoclastic activity. Caution should be exercised when the pathological significance of alkaline phosphatase increases in childhood is considered, because growth is an important physiological cause of such elevations. Liver alkaline phosphatase elevations reflect biliary obstruction and do not occur to any great extent with pure hepatocellular disease (see p. 596).

Box 33-17

Sources of Alkaline Phosphatase

- Osteoblasts
- Bile canalicular cells
- Placenta
- Leukocytes
- Proximal renal tubule cells
- Active mammary gland

Box 33-18

Bone Diseases Associated with Abnormal Serum Alkaline Phosphatase Concentrations

Deficiency
- Hypophosphatasia
- Achondroplasia
- Severe malnutrition
- Scurvy

Excess
- Osteoblastic sarcoma
- Osteomalacia
- Paget's disease
- Hyperparathyroidism
- Growing children

Osteocalcin

Clinically, serum osteocalcin concentration is elevated in bone diseases characterized by increased osteoblastic activity such as Paget's disease, osteomalacia, osteitis fibrosa, and renal osteodystrophy. Serum osteocalcin levels in these diseases correlate with other markers of bone formation, such as serum alkaline phosphatase and bone histomorphometry. Decreased serum concentrations of PTH, thyroid hormone, or growth hormone are associated with a decrease in the serum osteocalcin concentration, whereas the reverse is true; hyperparathyroidism, thyrotoxicosis, and acromegaly are associated with elevated serum osteocalcin concentrations. Puberty is associated with a rise in serum osteocalcin concentration, consistent with the increase in osteoblastic activity that accompanies the pubertal growth spurt and gonadal hormone surges. Circadian variations in serum osteocalcin concentration (peak levels at 4 AM and nadir at 5 PM) and in other serum markers of bone formation and resorption have been reported, but the origin and physiological implications of these observations remain unknown.[149]

Hydroxyproline (HP)[150]

Collagen, which is present predominantly in bone and skin, is the sole source of the amino acid hydroxyproline, which, together with proline, makes up approximately one third of the total amino acid content of collagen. Collagen digestion, which is associated with bone or skin breakdown, results in elevated urinary hydroxyproline (UHP) concentrations (Box 33-19). However, the determination of UHP concentration is

Box 33-19

Conditions Associated with Elevated Urinary Hydroxyproline Concentrations

Paget's disease
Acromegaly
Osteomalacia
Rheumatoid arthritis
Neoplastic bone disease
Osteoporosis
Hyperthyroidism
Aseptic bone necrosis
Osteomyelitis
Chronic renal failure
Burns

not a specific test because sources of hydroxyproline include bone, diet, connective tissue, serum protein, and degradation of propeptides from collagen biosynthesis. UHP correlates poorly with bone resorption as assessed by bone histomorphometric and calcium kinetic studies.

KEY CONCEPTS BOX 33-5

- Low levels of vitamin D, or vit D, activity will result in low levels of serum Ca and increased serum parathyroid hormone (PTH). Elevated levels of vitamin D will result in decreased serum PTH and increased serum Ca.
- Primary hyperparathyroidism will result in increased serum Ca and vitamin D levels. Primary hypothyroidism will result in decreased serum Ca and vitamin D levels. Serum PTH levels will be increased by low serum Ca levels and decreased by chronically elevated levels of serum Ca.
- Serum phosphate tends to increase or decrease opposite to changes in serum Ca. Low levels of plasma phosphate will increase renal synthesis of vitamin D and increase serum Ca.
- Ionized calcium may have to be measured when serum levels of protein, especially albumin, are abnormal. Abnormal levels of serum protein may result in low levels of total Ca, but normal levels of ionized Ca.

REFERENCES

1. Cohen M: The new bone biology: pathologic, molecular, and clinical correlates, Am J Med Genet A 140:2646, 2006.
2. Seeman E: Bone quality: the material and structural basis of bone strength, J Bone Miner Metab 26:1, 2008.
3. Shipman P, Walker A, Bichell D, editors: *The Human Skeleton,* Cambridge, MA, 1985, Harvard University Press.
4. Herrero MA, López JM: Bone formation: biological aspects and modelling problems, J Theoret Med 6:41, 2005.
5. Olsen BR, Reginato AM, Wang W: Bone development, Ann Rev Cell Devel Biol 16:191, 2000.
6. Duplomb L, Dagouassat M, Jourdon P, et al: Concise review: embryonic stem cells: a new tool to study osteoblast and osteoclast differentiation, Stem Cells 25:544, 2007.
7. Kogianni G, Noble BS: The biology of osteocytes, Curr Osteoporos Rep 5:81, 2007.
8. Bonewald LF: Osteocytes as dynamic multifunctional cells, Ann N Y Acad Sci 1116:281, 2007.
9. Downey PA, Siegel MI: Bone biology and the clinical implications for osteoporosis, Phys Ther 86:77, 2006.
10. Rauner M, Sipos W, Pietschmann P: Osteoimmunology, Int Arch Allergy Immunol 143:31, 2007.
11. Tanaka Y, Nakayamada S, Okada Y: Osteoblasts and osteoclasts in bone remodeling and inflammation, Curr Drug Targets Inflamm Allergy 4:325, 2005.
12. Klein-Nulend J, Nijweide PJ, Burger EH: Osteocyte and bone structure, Curr Osteoporos Rep 1:5-10, 2003.
13. Asagiri M, Takayanagi H: The molecular understanding of osteoclast differentiation, Bone 40:251, 2007.
14. Boyce BF, Xing L: Biology of RANK, RANKL, and osteoprotegerin, Arthritis Res Ther 9(suppl 1):S1, 2007.
15. Yadav VK, Ryu J-H, Suda N, et al: Lrp5 controls bone formation by inhibiting serotonin synthesis in the duodenum cell. Cell 135: 825-837, 2008.
16. Raisz LG: Pathogenesis of osteoporosis: concepts, conflicts, and prospects, J Clin Invest 115:3318, 2005.
17. Krane SM: Identifying genes that regulate bone remodeling as potential therapeutic targets, J Exp Med 201:841, 2005.
18. Stains JP, Civitelli R: Cell-to-cell interactions in bone, Biochem Biophys Res Commun 18:721, 2005.
19. NIH: Consensus statement: osteoporosis prevention, diagnosis, and therapy, NIH Consens Statement 17:1, 2000.
20. Simmons J, Zeitler P, Steelman J: Advances in the diagnosis and treatment of osteoporosis, Adv Pediatr 54:85, 2007.
21. Bianchi ML: Osteoporosis in children and adolescents, Bone 41:486, 2007.
22. Shaw NJ: Osteoporosis in paediatrics, Arch Dis Child Educ Pract Ed 92:169, 2007.
23. Davies JH, Evans BA, Gregory JW: Bone mass acquisition in healthy children, Arch Dis Child 90:373, 2005.
24. Daly RM: The effect of exercise on bone mass and structural geometry during growth, Med Sport Sci 51:33, 2007. Review.
25. Ondrak KS, Morgan DW: Physical activity, calcium intake and bone health in children and adolescents, Sports Med 37:587, 2000. Review.
26. Institute of Medicine, Food and Nutrition Board: *Dietary Reference Intakes: Calcium, Phosphorus, Magnesium, Vitamin D and Fluoride,* Washington, DC, 1997, National Academy Press.
27. Lynch MF, Griffin IJ, Hawthorne KM, et al: Calcium balance in 1-4-y-old children, Am J Clin Nutr 85:750, 2007.
28. Whiting SJ, Vatanparast H, Baxter-Jones A, et al: Factors that affect bone mineral accrual in the adolescent growth spurt, J Nutr 134:696S, 2004.
29. Anderson JJ: Calcium requirements during adolescence to maximize bone health, J Am Coll Nutr 20(2 suppl):186S, 2001.
30. Phan TC, Xu J, Zheng MH: Interaction between osteoblast and osteoclast: impact in bone disease, Histol Histopathol 19:1325, 2004.
31. Nakashima K, Zhou X, Kunkel G, et al: The novel zinc finger–containing transcription factor osterix is required for osteoblast differentiation and bone formation, Cell 108:17, 2002.
32. Robling AG, Castillo AB, Turner CH: Biomechanical and molecular regulation of bone remodeling, Annu Rev Biomed Eng 8:455, 2006.
33. Kasukawa Y, Miyakoshi N, Mohan S: The anabolic effects of GH/IGF system on bone, Curr Pharm Des 10:2577, 2004. Review.
34. Vanderschueren D, Vandenput L, Boonen S, et al: Androgens and bone, Endocr Rev 25:389, 2004.

35. Cauley JA: Osteoporosis in men: prevalence and investigation, Clin Cornerstone 8(suppl 3):S20, 2006. Review.
36. Eastell R, Hannon RA: Biomarkers of bone health and osteoporosis risk, Proc Nutr Soc 67:157, 2008.
37. Lindberg MK, Vandenput L, Movèrare Skrtic S, et al: Androgens and the skeleton, Minerva Endocrinol 30:15, 2005.
38. Weitzmann MN, Pacifici R: Estrogen deficiency and bone loss: an inflammatory tale, J Clin Invest 116:1186, 2006.
39. Zhao C, Dahlman-Wright K, Gustafsson JA: Estrogen receptor beta: an overview and update, Nucl Recept Signal 6:e003, 2008.
40. Gennari L, Nuti R, Bilezikian JP: Aromatase activity and bone homeostasis in men, J Clin Endocrinol Metab 89:5898, 2004.
41. Lanyon L, Armstrong V, Ong D, et al: Is estrogen receptor alpha key to controlling bones' resistance to fracture? J Endocrinol 182:183, 2004.
42. Riggs BL, Khosla S, Melton LJ 3rd: Sex steroids and the construction and conservation of the adult skeleton, Endocr Rev 23:279, 2002.
43. Veldhuis JD, Anderson SM, Patrie JT, et al: Estradiol supplementation in postmenopausal women doubles rebound-like release of growth hormone (GH) triggered by sequential infusion and withdrawal of somatostatin: evidence that estrogen facilitates endogenous GH-releasing hormone drive, J Clin Endocrinol Metab 89:121, 2004.
44. Caufriez A: The pubertal spurt: effects of sex steroids on growth hormone and insulin-like growth factor I, Eur J Obstet Gynecol Reprod Biol 71:215, 1997.
45. Hadjidakis DJ, Androulakis II: Bone remodeling, Ann NY Acad Sci 1092:385, 2006.
46. Chen L, Li C, Qiao W, et al: A Ser(365)→Cys mutation of fibroblast growth factor receptor 3 in mouse downregulates Ihh/PTHrP signals and causes severe achondroplasia, Hum Mol Genet 10:457, 2001.
47. Zelzer E, McLean W, Ng YS, et al: Skeletal defects in VEGF (120/120) mice reveal multiple roles for VEGF in skeletogenesis, Development 129:1893, 2002.
48. Pagani F, Francucci CM, Moro L: Markers of bone turnover: biochemical and clinical perspectives, J Endocrinol Invest 28(10 suppl):8, 2005.
49. Lello S, Paoletti AM, Migliaccio S, et al: Bone markers: biochemical and clinical significance, Aging Clin Exp Res 16(suppl 3):33, 2004.
50. Löfman O, Magnusson P, Toss G, et al: Common biochemical markers of bone turnover predict future bone loss: a 5-year follow-up study, Clin Chim Acta 356:67, 2005.
51. National Osteoporosis Foundation: *Physicians' Guide to Prevention and Treatment of Osteoporosis,* Belle Mead, NJ, 1999, Excerpta Medica.
52. Heaney RP: Bone health, Am J Clin Nutr 85:300S, 2007.
53. Straub DA: Calcium supplementation in clinical practice: a review of forms, doses, and indications, Nutr Clin Pract 22:286, 2007.
54. DeLuca HF: Overview of general physiologic features and functions of vitamin D, Am J Clin Nutr 80(6 suppl):1689S, 2004. Review.
55. Holick MF, Chen TC, Lu Z, et al: Vitamin D and skin physiology: a D-lightful story, J Bone Miner Res 22(suppl 2):V28, 2007.
56. Holick MF: Vitamin D deficiency, N Engl J Med 357:266, 2007.
57. Hollis B: Vitamin D requirement during pregnancy and lactation, J Bone Miner Res 22(suppl 2):V39, 2007.
58. Heaney RP: The vitamin D requirement in health and disease, J Steroid Biochem Mol Biol 97:13, 2005.
59. Hathcock JN, Shao A, Vieth R, et al: Risk assessment for vitamin D, Am J Clin Nutr 85:6, 2007.
60. Rigo J, Pieltain C, Salle B, et al: Enteral calcium, phosphate and vitamin D requirements and bone mineralization in preterm infants, Acta Paediatr 96:969, 2007.
61. Bonjour JP: Dietary protein: an essential nutrient for bone health, J Am Coll Nutr 24(6 suppl):526S, 2005. Review.
62. Shelly W, Draper MW, Krishnan V, et al: Selective estrogen receptor modulators: an update on recent clinical findings, Obstet Gynecol Surv 63:163, 2008.
63. Aikawa JK: *Magnesium: Its Biologic Significance, CRC Series on Cations of Biological Significance,* Boca Raton, FL, 1981, CRC Press.
64. Tsang RC: Neonatal magnesium disturbances, Am J Dis Child 124:282, 1972.
65. Lips P: Vitamin D physiology, Prog Biophys Mol Biol 92:4, 2006.
66. Nagpal S, Na S, Rathnachalam R: Noncalcemic actions of vitamin D receptor ligands, Endocr Rev 26:662, 2005.
67. Christakos S, Dhawan P, Benn B, et al: Vitamin D: molecular mechanism of action, Ann N Y Acad Sci 1116:340, 2007.
68. Pike JW, Shevde NK: The vitamin D receptor. In Feldman D, Glorieux FH, Pike JW, editors: *Vitamin D,* ed 2, Boston, MA, 2005, Elsevier Academic Press, p. 167.
69. Zhou C, Assem M, Tay JC, et al: Steroid and xenobiotic receptor and vitamin D receptor crosstalk mediates CYP24 expression and drug-induced osteomalacia, J Clin Invest 116:1703, 2006.
70. Dusso AS, Brown AJ, Slatopolsky E: Vitamin D, Am J Physiol Renal Physiol 289:F8, 2005.
71. Eisman JA, Wark JD, Prince RL, et al: Modulation of plasma 1,25-dihydroxyvitamin D in man by stimulation and suppression tests, Lancet 2:931, 1979.
72. Gallagher JC, Riggs BL, Eisman J, et al: Intestinal calcium absorption and serum vitamin D metabolites in normal subjects and osteoporotic patients: effect of age and dietary calcium, J Clin Invest 64:729, 1979.
73. Hsu SC, Levine MA: Perinatal calcium metabolism: physiology and pathophysiology, Semin Neonatol 9:23, 2004.
74. Potts JT: Parathyroid hormone: past and present, J Endocrinol 187:311, 2005.
75. Jilka RL: Molecular and cellular mechanisms of the anabolic effect of intermittent PTH, Bone 40:1434, 2007.
76. Martin KJ, Olgaard K, Coburn JW, et al: Bone Turnover Work Group: Diagnosis, assessment, and treatment of bone turnover abnormalities in renal osteodystrophy, Am J Kidney Dis 43:558, 2004.
77. Strewler GJ: Mechanisms of disease: the physiology of parathyroid hormone-related protein, N Engl J Med 342:177, 2000.
78. Broadus AE, Macica C, Chen X: The PTHrP functional domain is at the gates of endochondral bones, Ann N Y Acad Sci 1116:65, 2007.
79. Huang CL, Sun L, Moonga BS, et al: Molecular physiology and pharmacology of calcitonin, Cell Mol Biol 52:33, 2006.
80. Inzerillo AM, Zaidi M, Huang CL: Calcitonin: physiological actions and clinical applications, J Pediatr Endocrinol Metab 17:931, 2004.
81. Huwyler R, Born W, Ohnhaus EE: Plasma kinetics and urinary excretion of exogenous human and salmon calcitonin in man, Am J Physiol 236:15, 1979.
82. Ardaillou R: Kidney and calcitonin, Nephron 15:250, 1975.
83. Heersche JNM, Marcus R, Aurbach GD: Calcitonin and the formation of 3′,5′-AMP in bone and kidney, Endocrinology 94:241, 1974.
84. Khosla S, Melton LJ III: Osteopenia, N Engl J Med 356:2293, 2007.
85. Parfitt AM: Renal bone disease: a new conceptual framework for the interpretation of bone histomorphometry, Curr Opin Nephrol Hypertens 12:387, 2003.
86. Simon LS: Osteoporosis, Rheum Dis Clin North Am 33:149, 2007.

87. MacLaughlin EJ, Raehl CL: ASHP therapeutic position statement on the prevention and treatment of osteoporosis in adults, Am J Health Syst Pharm 65:343, 2008.
88. MacLean C, Newberry S, Maglione M, et al: Systematic review: comparative effectiveness of treatments to prevent fractures in men and women with low bone density or osteoporosis, Ann Intern Med 148:197, 2008.
89. Canalis E, Giustina A, Bilezikian JP: Mechanisms of anabolic therapies for osteoporosis, N Engl J Med 30:905, 2007. Review.
90. Ralston SH: Genetics of osteoporosis, Proc Nutr Soc 66:158, 2007. Review.
91. Wexler JA, Sharretts J: Thyroid and bone, Endocrinol Metab Clin North Am 36:673, 2007.
92. Gissel T, Poulsen CS, Vestergaard P: Adverse effects of antiepileptic drugs on bone mineral density in children, Expert Opin Drug Saf 6:267, 2007. Review.
93. Gallagher JC, Riggs BL, Jerpbak CM, et al: The effect of age on serum immunoreactive parathyroid hormone in normal and osteoporotic women, J Lab Clin Med 95:373, 1980.
94. Gallagher JC, Riggs BL, DeLuca HF: Effect of estrogen on calcium absorption and serum vitamin D metabolites in postmenopausal osteoporosis, J Clin Endocrinol Metab 51:1359, 1980.
95. Shamonki IM, Frumar AM, Tataryn IV, et al: Age-related changes of calcitonin secretion in females, J Clin Endocrinol Metab 50:437, 1980.
96. Ivey JL, Baylink DJ: Postmenopausal osteoporosis: proposed roles of defective coupling and estrogen deficiency, Metab Bone Dis Rel Res 3:3, 1981.
97. Avioli LV: Postmenopausal osteoporosis: prevention versus cure, Fed Proc 40:2418, 1981.
98. Compston JE: Emerging consensus on prevention and treatment of glucocorticoid-induced osteoporosis, Curr Rheumatol Rep 9:78, 2007.
99. Woolf AD: An update on glucocorticoid-induced osteoporosis, Curr Opin Rheumatol 19:370, 2007.
100. Blake GM, Fogelman I: The role of DXA bone density scans in the diagnosis and treatment of osteoporosis, Postgrad Med J 83:509, 2007.
101. Lewiecki EM, Borges JL: Bone density testing in clinical practice, Arq Bras Endocrinol Metabol 50:586, 2006.
102. Lewiecki EM, Richmond B, Miller PD: Uses and misuses of quantitative ultrasonography in managing osteoporosis, Cleve Clin J Med 73:742, 2006.
103. Boonen S, Haentjens P, Vandenput L, et al: Preventing osteoporotic fractures with antiresorptive therapy—implications of microarchitectural changes, J Intern Med 255:1, 2004.
104. Greenspan SL, Bone HG, Ettinger MP, et al: Treatment of Osteoporosis with Parathyroid Hormone Study Group: Effect of recombinant human parathyroid hormone (1-84) on vertebral fracture and bone mineral density in postmenopausal women with osteoporosis: a randomized trial, Ann Intern Med 146:326, 2007.
105. Gupta G, Aronow WS: Treatment of postmenopausal osteoporosis, Compr Ther 33:114, 2007.
106. Fitzpatrick LA: Estrogen therapy for postmenopausal osteoporosis, Arq Bras Endocrinol Metabol 50:705, 2006.
107. Gennari L, Merlotti D, Valleggi F, et al: Selective estrogen receptor modulators for postmenopausal osteoporosis: current state of development, Drugs Aging 24:361, 2007.
108. Grey A: Emerging pharmacologic therapies for osteoporosis, Expert Opin Emerg Drugs 12:493, 2007.
109. Francis RM, Anderson FH, Patel S, et al: Calcium and vitamin D in the prevention of osteoporotic fractures, QJM 99:355, 2006.
110. North American Menopause Society: The role of calcium in peri- and postmenopausal women: 2006 position statement of the North American Menopause Society, Menopause 13:862, 2006.
111. North American Menopause Society: Management of osteoporosis in postmenopausal women: 2006 position statement of The North American Menopause Society, Menopause 13:340, 2006.
112. North American Menopause Society: Estrogen and progestogen use in peri- and postmenopausal women: March 2007 position statement of The North American Menopause Society, Menopause 14:168, 2007.
113. Stroup J, Kane MP, Abu-Baker AM: Teriparatide in the treatment of osteoporosis, Am J Health Syst Pharm 65:532, 2008.
114. Schwalfenberg G: Not enough vitamin D: health consequences for Canadians, Can Fam Physician 53:841, 2007.
115. Klein GL, Soriano H, Shulman RJ, et al: Hepatic osteodystrophy in chronic cholestasis: evidence for a multifactorial etiology, Pediatr Transplant 6:136, 2002.
116. Kato S, Yoshizawa T, Kitanaka S, et al: Molecular genetics of vitamin D–dependent hereditary rickets, Hormone Res 57:73, 2004.
117. Bouillon R, Verstuyf A, Mathieu C, et al: Vitamin D resistance, Best Pract Res Clin Endocrinol Metab 20:627, 2006. Review.
118. Garabedian M: Regulation of phosphate homeostasis in infants, children, and adolescents, and the role of phosphatonins in this process, Curr Opin Pediatr 19:488, 2007.
119. Berndt T, Kumar R: Phosphatonins and the regulation of phosphate homeostasis, Ann Rev Physiol 69:341, 2007.
120. Stubbs J, Liu S, Quarles LD: Role of fibroblast growth factor 23 in phosphate homeostasis and pathogenesis of disordered mineral metabolism in chronic kidney disease, Semin Dial 20:302, 2007. Review.
121. Thacher TD, Fischer PR, Strand MA, et al: Nutritional rickets around the world: causes and future directions, Ann Trop Paediatr 26:1, 2006.
122. Steichen JJ, Tsang RC, Greer FR, et al: Elevated serum 1,25-dihydroxyvitamin D concentrations in rickets of very low-birth-weight infants, J Pediatr 99:293, 1981.
123. Bannwarth B: Drug-induced musculoskeletal disorders, Drug Saf 30:27, 2007.
124. Goodman SB, Jiranek W, Petrow E, et al: The effects of medications on bone, J Am Acad Orthop Surg 15:450, 2007.
125. Schwarz C, Sulzbacher I, Oberbauer R: Diagnosis of renal osteodystrophy, Eur J Clin Invest 36(suppl 2):13, 2006.
126. Whyte MP: Clinical practice: Paget's disease of bone, N Engl J Med 355:593, 2006.
127. Whyte MP: Paget's disease of bone and genetic disorders of RANKL/OPG/RANK/NF-kappaB signaling, Ann N Y Acad Sci 1068:143, 2006. Review.
128. Josse RG, Hanley DA, Kendler D, et al: Diagnosis and treatment of Paget's disease of bone, Clin Invest Med 30:E210, 2007.
129. Mornet E: Hypophosphatasia, Orphanet J Rare Dis 2:40, 2007.
130. Roughley PJ, Rauch F, Glorieux FH: Osteogenesis imperfecta—clinical and molecular diversity, Eur Cell Mater 30:41, 2003.
131. Carter EM, Davis JG, Raggio CL: Advances in understanding etiology of achondroplasia and review of management, Curr Opin Pediatr 19:32, 2007. Review.
132. Horton WA, Hall JG, Hecht JT: Achondroplasia, Lancet 370:162, 2007.
133. Tolar J, Teitelbaum SL, Orchard PJ: Osteopetrosis, N Engl J Med 351:2839, 2004.
134. Spiegel AM, Weinstein LS: Inherited diseases involving G proteins and G protein-coupled receptors, Annu Rev Med 55:27, 2004.
135. Weinstein LS, Liu J, Sakamoto A, et al: Minireview: GNAS: normal and abnormal functions, Endocrinology 145:5459, 2004.
136. Seibel MJ: Biochemical markers of bone turnover, Part I: biochemistry and variability, Clin Biochem Rev 26:97, 2005.

137. Seibel MJ: Biochemical markers of bone turnover, Part II: clinical applications in the management of osteoporosis, Clin Biochem Rev 27:123, 2006.
138. Seibel MJ: Clinical application of biochemical markers of bone turnover, Arq Bras Endocrinol Metabol 50:603, 2006.
139. Tosiano D, Weisman Y, Hochberg Z: The role of the vitamin D receptor in regulating vitamin D metabolism: a study of vitamin D-dependent rickets, type II, J Clin Endocrinol Metab 86: 1908-2002, 2001.
140. Tsang RC, Brown DR: The parathyroids. In Kelley V, editor: *Practice of Pediatrics,* vol 1, New York, 1979, Harper & Row.
141. Tsang RC, Venkataraman P: Pediatric parathyroid and vitamin D-related disorders. In Kaplan LA, editor: *Clinical Pediatric and Adolescent Endocrinology,* Philadelphia, 1982, Saunders.
142. Miedlich S, Krohn K, Paschke R: Update on genetic and clinical aspects of primary hyperparathyroidism, Clin Endocrinol (Oxf) 59:539, 2003.
143. Rodriguez M, Cañadillas S, Lopez I, et al: Regulation of parathyroid function in chronic renal failure, J Bone Miner Metab 24:164, 2006. Review.
144. D'Souza-Li L: The calcium-sensing receptor and related diseases, Arq Bras Endocrinol Metabol 50:628, 2006.
145. Brown EM: The calcium-sensing receptor: physiology, pathophysiology and CaR-based therapeutics, Subcell Biochem 45:139, 2007. Review.
146. Carmeliet G, Van Cromphaut S, Daci E, et al: Disorders of calcium homeostasis, Best Pract Res Clin Endocrinol Metab 17:529, 2003. Review.
147. Massoll N, Mazzaferri EL: Diagnosis and management of medullary thyroid carcinoma, Clin Lab Med 24:49, 2004.
148. Muñoz-Torres M, Alonso G, Raya MP: Calcitonin therapy in osteoporosis, Treat Endocrinol 3:117, 2004.
149. Szulc P, Seeman E, Delmas PD: Biochemical measurement of bone turnover in children and adolescents, Osteoporos Int 11: 281, 2000.
150. Simsek B, Karacaer O, Karaca I: Urine products of bone breakdown as markers of bone resorption and clinical usefulness of urinary hydroxyproline: an overview, Chin Med J (Engl) 117:291, 2004.

BIBLIOGRAPHY

AAP Committee on Nutrition: Calcium requirements of infants, children, and adolescents, Pediatrics 104:1152, 1999.

Bachrach LK: Consensus and controversy regarding osteoporosis in the pediatric population, Endocr Pract 13:513, 2007.

Braun M, Martin BR, Kern M, et al: Calcium retention in adolescent boys on a range of controlled calcium intakes, Am J Clin Nutr 84:414, 2006.

Broadus AE: Nephrogenous cyclic AMP, Recent Prog Horm Res 37:665, 1981.

Caetano-Lopes J, Canhão H, Fonseca JE: Osteoblasts and bone formation, Acta Reumatol Port 32:103, 2007.

Cantorna MT, Zhu Y, Froicu M: Vitamin D status, 1,25-dihydroxyvitamin D3, and the immune system, Am J Clin Nutr 80(6 suppl):1717S, 2004.

Chan GM: Calcium needs during childhood, Pediatr Ann 30:666, 2001.

Chan GM, McElligott K, McNaught T, et al: Effects of dietary calcium intervention on adolescent mothers and newborns: a randomized controlled trial, Obstet Gynecol 108:565, 2006.

DeLuca HF: The kidney as an endocrine organ for production of 1,25-dihydroxyvitamin D_3, a calcium-mobilizing hormone, N Engl J Med 289:359, 1973.

DeLuca HF: The vitamin D system in the regulation of calcium and phosphorus metabolism, Nutr Rev 37:161, 1979.

Goldstein DA, Haldimann B, Sherman D, et al: Vitamin D metabolites and calcium metabolism in patients with nephrotic syndrome and normal renal function, J Clin Endocrinol Metab 52:116, 1981.

Gomez BJ, Ardakani S, Ju J, et al: Monoclonal antibody assay for measuring bone-specific alkaline phosphatase activity in serum, Clin Chem 41:1560, 1995.

Ham AW, Cormack DH: *Histology,* ed 8, Philadelphia, 1979, Lippincott.

Heikkinen S, Auwerx J, Argmann CA: PPARgamma in human and mouse physiology, Biochim Biophys Acta 1771:999, 2007.

Itani O, Niedbala B, Tsang RC: The small for gestational age infant and problems of prematurity. In Ekvall S, Ekvall V, editors: *Pediatric Nutrition in Chronic Diseases and Developmental Disorders,* New York, 2005, Oxford University Press.

Itani O, Tsang RC: Calcium, bone metabolism in the newborn: pathophysiology and management. In Thureen PJ, Hay WW, editor: *Neonatal Nutrition and Metabolism,* ed 2, New York, 2006, Cambridge University Press.

Itani O, Tsang RC: Calcium, phosphorus, magnesium, vitamin D and bone metabolism in the newborn: pathophysiology and management. In Hay W, editor: *Neonatal Nutrition and Metabolism,* ed 2, New York, 2006, Cambridge University Press.

Juttmann JR, Buurman CJ, De Kam E, et al: Serum concentrations of metabolites of vitamin D in patients with chronic renal failure: consequences for the treatment with 1-alpha-hydroxy derivatives, Clin Endocrinol 14:225, 1981.

Karsenty G: The genetic transformation of bone biology, Genes Dev 13:3037, 1999.

Komori T, Yagi H, Nomura S, et al: Targeted disruption of Cbfa1 results in a complete lack of bone formation owing to maturational arrest of osteoblasts, Cell 89:755, 1997.

Kornak U, Mundlos S: Genetic disorders of the skeleton: a developmental approach, Am J Hum Genet 73:447, 2003. Review.

Kronenberg HM: PTH regulates the hematopoietic stem cell niche in bone, Adv Exp Med Biol 602:57, 2007.

Lacativa PG, de Farias ML: Office practice of osteoporosis evaluation, Arq Bras Endocrinol Metabol 50:674, 2006.

Lane NE: Epidemiology, etiology, and diagnosis of osteoporosis, Am J Obstet Gynecol 194(2 suppl):S3, 2006.

Lee B, Thirunavukkarasu K, Zhou L, et al: Missense mutations abolishing DNA binding of the osteoblast-specific transcription factor OSF2/CBFA1 in cleidocranial dysplasia, Nat Genet 16:307, 1997.

Levis S, Altman R: Bone densitometry: clinical considerations, Arthritis Rheum 41:577, 1998.

Mundlos S, Otto F, Mundlos C, et al: Mutations involving the transcription factor CBFA1 cause cleidocranial dysplasia, Cell 89:773, 1997.

Murphy NM, Carroll P: The effect of physical activity and its interaction with nutrition on bone health, Proc Nutr Soc 62:829, 2004. Review.

Ornitz DM: Regulation of chondrocyte growth and differentiation by fibroblast growth factor receptor 3, Novartis Found Symp 232:63, 2001; discussion 76, 272.

Otto F, Thornell AP, Crompton T, et al: *Cbfa1,* a candidate gene for cleidocranial dysplasia syndrome, is essential for osteoblast differentiation and bone development, Cell 89:765, 1997.

Prins SH, Jørgensen HL, Jørgensen LV, et al: The role of quantitative ultrasound in the assessment of bone: a review, Clin Physiol 18:3, 1998.

Prostko M: Meta-analysis of prevention of nonvertebral fractures by alendronate, JAMA 278:631, 1997.

Ross FP, Christiano AM: Nothing but skin and bone, J Clin Invest 116:1140, 2006.

Samaniego EA, Sheth RD: Bone consequences of epilepsy and antiepileptic medications, Semin Pediatr Neurol 14:196, 2007.

INTERNET SITES

www.meddean.luc.edu—Loyola University Medical Education Network

Osteoporosis

www.nof.org—National Osteoporosis Foundation
www.osteo.org—NIH Osteoporosis and Bone Related Disease
www.nos.org.uk—National Osteoporosis Society

Osteomalacia

http://uwcme.org—University of Washington CME credits for a fee

Osteitis Fibrosa

www.nlm.nih.gov—NIH MEDLINE plus Medical Encyclopedia

The Pancreas: Function and Chemical Pathology

D. Robert Dufour

34 Chapter

Chapter Outline

Key Terms

acinar From the Latin word *acinus*, meaning "berry" or "grape." In anatomy, the term refers to a small saclike dilation.

adenocarcinoma A malignant growth that begins in the epithelial cells; for the pancreas, it affects the cells that line the pancreatic ductules and duct. Nearly all pancreatic cancers are adenocarcinomas.

ampulla of Vater A flasklike dilation at the point where the biliary and pancreatic ducts join. The ampulla joins the duodenal papilla (a nipple-shaped structure), and its orifice is encircled by a ring of smooth muscles called the "sphincter of Oddi." Note that the ampulla and the sphincter are two distinct structures.

cachexia A state of progressive weakness, loss of appetite, malnutrition, and weight loss that is observed in some chronic disorders, such as advanced cancer.

cholecystitis Inflammation of the gallbladder.

cholecystokinin (CCK) A gastrointestinal hormone that is released when the duodenum is distended after ingestion of food or alcohol. CCK is a powerful stimulant for the pancreas, causing it to produce a high-volume secretion that is high in bicarbonate concentration but low in proteins and enzymes. CCK and secretin potentiate each other's actions.

endoscopic retrograde cholangiopancreatography (ERCP) An invasive diagnostic technique whereby the pancreatic duct is cannulated and an x-ray contrast medium is injected into the duct to visualize the biliary and pancreatic ducts.

enterokinase An enzyme produced by the mucosa of the small intestine that converts the inactive, digestive proenzymes from the pancreas into their active forms.

gastrin A hormone produced primarily by the G-cells of the stomach that stimulates the secretion of HCl by parietal cells in the stomach. Plasma gastrin is increased greatly in Zollinger-Ellison syndrome, usually as a pancreatic or duodenal neoplasm, but gastrin is not normally produced by the pancreas.

glucagon An islet cell hormone that has multiple actions to raise plasma glucose.

hypoglycemia A low blood glucose concentration, generally <2.8 mmol/L (<50 mg/dL), which causes some individuals to become symptomatic.

immunoreactive trypsin (IRT) A form of the digestive enzyme found in blood. Because of the presence of potent antiproteases in blood, the enzyme must be measured in serum as a protein. It has little or no enzymatic activity in blood.

insulin An islet cell, anabolic hormone that controls cellular glucose uptake, fat synthesis, and synthesis of proteins.

islets of Langerhans Clusters of cells in the pancreas that produce the endocrine secretions of the gland. They constitute about 1% of the pancreatic mass.

laparoscopy A technique used to view the pancreas or any other abdominal organ. A small incision is made in the abdomen to allow insertion of the viewing instrument. It is probably the most objective and reliable method for diagnosing pancreatitis.

multiple endocrine neoplasia (MEN) An autosomal dominant inherited disorder that has many different clinical presentations. Type I MEN disorder often involves the pancreatic islets and other endocrine organs, particularly the pituitary and parathyroid glands.

pancreatic duct A conduit that passes through the pancreas, collects the pancreatic exocrine secretions of enzymes, water, and electrolytes, and carries them to the ampulla of Vater.

pancreatic polypeptide An islet cell hormone (PP) that slows the absorption of food, stimulates gastric and intestinal secretions, and inhibits intestinal mobility.

proteolytic Having the ability to break down proteins to peptides and amino acids.

secretin A gastrointestinal hormone that is released when the duodenum is distended after ingestion of food or alcohol. It is a powerful stimulant for the pancreas, causing it to produce a secretion high in protein and enzymes but low in volume.

somatostatin An islet cell hormone that has largely inhibitory effects on insulin and glucagon secretion, gastric secretions, and exocrine pancreatic secretions.

trypsin A potent proteolytic enzyme that is produced in the pancreas but is stored there in zymogen granules as the enzymatically inactive protrypsin form.

trypsinogen The enzymatically inactive or zymogen form of trypsin; also called protrypsin.

vasoactive intestinal peptide (VIP) A hormone that can be produced by pancreatic islet cell tumors. When present in excess, it stimulates production of profuse diarrhea and is associated with hypokalemia and non–anion gap metabolic acidosis.

Zollinger-Ellison syndrome The clinical picture of a patient with a gastrinoma (frequently malignant) in the pancreas, duodenum, or both. It causes excessive acid production in the stomach, typically resulting in multiple peptic ulcers and diarrhea.

zymogen granules The storage form of digestive enzymes in the pancreatic acinar cells. Some of these enzymes, especially the proteolytic and lipolytic forms, are present as their zymogens or inactive precursors.

Methods on Evolve

Amylase
Chloride
Fecal fat and fat absorption
Insulin and C-peptide
Lipase
Sweat electrolytes: the sweat test

SECTION OBJECTIVES BOX 34-1

- Describe the location of the pancreas in relation to the stomach, bile duct, and small intestine.
- For each of the pancreatic enzymes (amylase, lipase, trypsin, phospholipase), describe its major function, and indicate whether it is produced in an active or inactive state.
- List the major components of pancreatic secretions and their functions.
- Describe the functions and regulation of the secretion of insulin, glucagon, and somatostatin, as well as their relationships.

ANATOMY

The pancreas is an elongated, flattened pyramidal organ that is located mostly behind the stomach; the tail points to the spleen, and the head is nestled in the duodenal loop (see Color Plate 9). This soft, easily traumatized gland lies behind the peritoneum, the serous membrane lining the abdominal cavity. Blood from the pancreas drains into the portal vein allowing pancreatic islet cell hormones (such as **insulin** and **glucagon**) to be both active in and metabolized by the liver. The exocrine acini (Fig. 34-1) are drained by ductules that combine into a single **pancreatic duct.** In most individuals, this duct joins the common bile duct at the **ampulla of Vater;** however, a variety of other arrangements of drainage of the liver and pancreas are found in some individuals. The ampulla of Vater opens through the duodenal papilla, the orifice of which is encircled by the sphincter of Oddi, so that pancreatic exocrine secretions can flow into the gastrointestinal tract. Except when pancreatic fluid is secreted, the sphincter is tightly closed, preventing stomach and duodenal contents from reaching the pancreas. Exocrine **acinar** cells and their associated structures account for more than 98% of the pancreatic mass.

About 1% of the pancreas consists of unique cell clusters, the **islets of Langerhans,** that produce endocrine hormones. A normal pancreas contains about 1 million islets (Fig. 34-2). Nerve fibers in pancreatic tissue stimulate production of

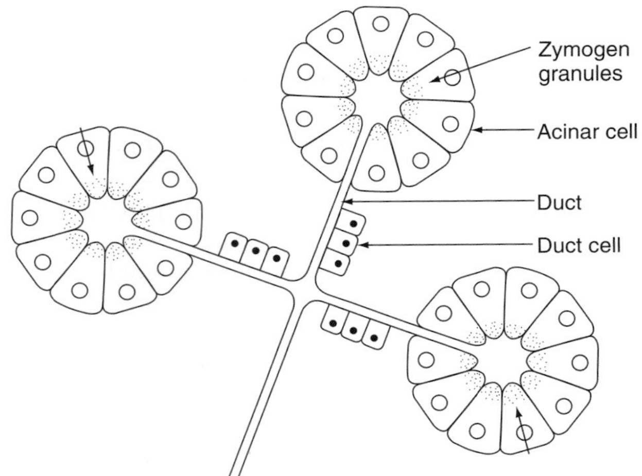

Fig. 34-1 Diagram of acinar cells and associated ductules. The exocrine acini terminate with a collection of acinar cells that contain zymogen granules; the latter contain the proenzymes and other digestive enzymes described in Fig. 34-3. Special cells line the ductules that secrete fluid and electrolytes, especially bicarbonate.

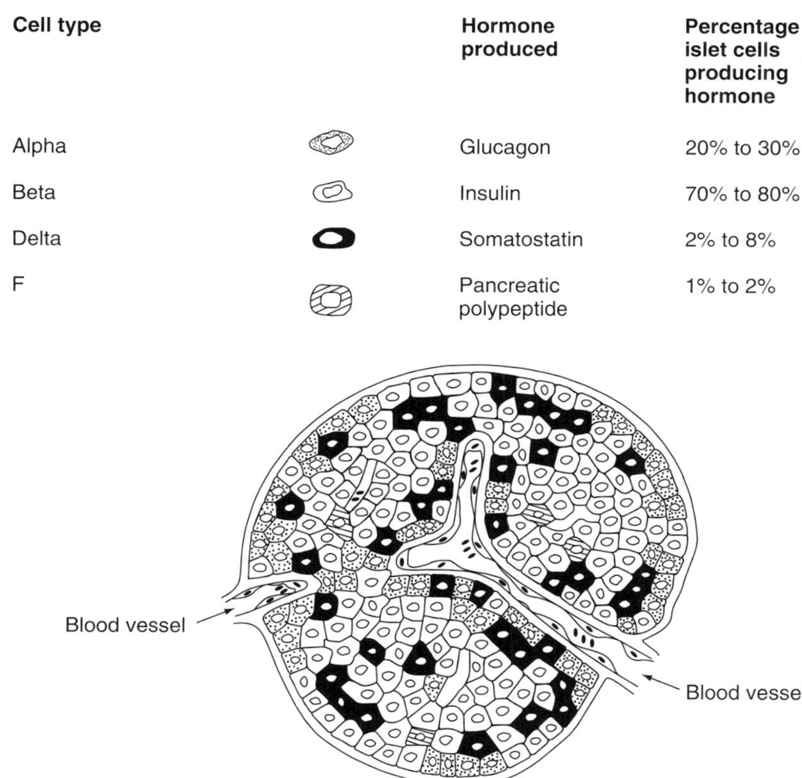

Cell type
Hormone produced
Percentage of islet cells producing hormone
Alpha
Glucagon
20% to 30%
Beta
Insulin
70% to 80%
Delta
Somatostatin
2% to 8%
F
Pancreatic polypeptide
1% to 2%
Blood vessel
Blood vessel

Fig. 34-2 Diagram of an islet of Langerhans. At least four types of cells secrete hormones into the blood. Most of these cells (beta-cells) produce insulin; only a small fraction are F-cells, which produce pancreatic polypeptide. (Adapted from Unger RH, Orci L: Glucagon and the A cell: physiology and pathophysiology (first of two parts), N Engl J Med 304:1518, 1981. Copyright 1981, Massachusetts Medical Society. All rights reserved.)

vasoactive intestinal peptide (VIP), substance P, **somatostatin,** enkephalin-related peptides, and bombesin-like peptides (see also p. 668).

ENDOCRINE PHYSIOLOGY

Pancreatic endocrine secretion from the islets of Langerhans includes the hormones glucagon from the alpha-cells, insulin from the beta-cells, somatostatin from the delta-cells, and **pancreatic polypeptide** from the F-cells. The action and control of these hormones are summarized in Table 34-1. **Gastrin** was once believed to be present in the normal pancreas; however, normally, gastrin originates only from G-cells in the stomach and duodenum.

Alpha-cells, which constitute 20% to 30% of the islet cells, produce glucagon, a hormone that increases plasma glucose concentrations (see Chapter 38); it has a half-life in blood of 5 to 10 minutes. Beta-cells (70% to 80% of islet cells) produce proinsulin, which consists of A and B chains and the C-peptide (see Chapter 38). Proinsulin is stored in secretory granules; when plasma glucose is high, their contents are released by exocytosis. Proinsulin is normally converted to insulin and C-peptide before release by the islet cell, although a small amount is normally found in plasma. Insulin has a half-life of about 10 to 25 minutes. C-peptide has no insulin-like action but can be measured in plasma for evaluation of beta-cell function, even in persons receiving insulin (which does not contain the C-peptide). Production of insulin in response to glucose is markedly increased by the intestinal hormones glucagon-like peptide 1 (GLP-1) and glucose-dependent insulinotropic polypeptide (GIP, formerly called gastric inhibitory polypeptide), which collectively are termed *incretins*[1]; these are discussed in greater detail in Chapter 35.

Delta-cells, which constitute about 2% to 8% of islet cells, produce somatostatin, a hormone that inhibits the production of insulin, glucagon, and gastrin (among other hormones), inhibits the secretion of exocrine pancreatic enzymes, and decreases the flow of bile. Somatostatin is also produced in other sites, notably the hypothalamus, and is important in inhibiting growth hormone production. The F-cells produce pancreatic polypeptide (PP), a hormone that stimulates gastric and intestinal enzyme secretion and inhibits intestinal motility.

EXOCRINE PHYSIOLOGY

Normal Pancreatic Exocrine Secretions

The pancreas produces at least 22 digestive enzymes, 15 of which are proteases, which act on three major dietary sources of energy: proteins, digested by the enzymes **trypsin,** chymotrypsin, and elastase; lipids, digested by the enzymes lipase, phospholipase A_2, and cholesterol esterase; and complex carbohydrates, digested by α-amylase. The functional units of the exocrine pancreas consist of clusters of acini that store most of the digestive enzymes in inactive forms (zymogens, in **zymogen granules**); free enzymes are not normally present in the acinar cell cytoplasm (see Fig. 34-1). Granules are released from the acinar cells by exocytosis into the collecting ductules

Table 34-1 Normal Pancreatic Islet Cell Hormones

Cell of Origin	Hormone	Release Stimulated by	Release Inhibited by	Hormone Causes
Alpha	Glucagon (3500*)	Low plasma glucose, sympathetic nervous system, epinephrine, any factors that lower plasma glucose	Somatostatin, glucose, secretin, insulin	Increased plasma glucose by stimulating hepatic glycogenolysis, gluconeogenesis; adipose tissue lipolysis; mobilizes amino acids
Beta	Proinsulin (11,500*) Insulin (5734*) C-peptide (3000*)	Plasma glucose above 100 mg/dL, keto acids, arginine, leucine, sympathetic and parasympathetic nervous system stimulation, gastric inhibitory polypeptide, gastrin, secretin, cholecystokinin (CCK), glucagon, cortisol, growth hormone, thyroxine, progesterone, sex hormones, sulfonylureas	Alpha-adrenergic agonists, somatostatin, insulin, thiazide diuretics, phenytoin	Glucose uptake by liver, muscle, adipose tissue; inhibition of gluconeogenesis; glycogen formation; fat synthesis and storage; inhibition of mobilization and oxidation of fats; conversion of glucose to fatty acids or cholesterol; production of acetyl CoA; synthesis of proteins; inhibition of protein breakdown; increased RNA synthesis; entry of K, phosphate, Mg into muscle and liver cells
Delta	Somatostatin (1640*)	Food intake, increased plasma glucose, arginine, leucine, CCK	Unknown	Inhibition of insulin and glucagon release, inhibition of gastric and exocrine pancreatic secretions
F	Pancreatic polypeptide (2400*)	Food intake, especially protein; fasting; exercise; hypoglycemia	Hyperglycemia	Decreased rate of food absorption, stimulation of gastric and intestinal enzyme secretion, inhibition of intestinal mobility

*Molecular weight in daltons.

and finally reach the pancreatic duct. Ribonuclease, deoxyribonuclease, cholesterol esterase, amylase, lipase, and co-lipase are the only digestive enzymes produced in their active forms.

Fig. 34-3 illustrates the modification of exocrine digestive enzymes from zymogen granules in the acinar cells to their active forms after entry into the duodenal lumen. The potent **proteolytic** enzymes trypsin, chymotrypsin, carboxypeptidase A and B, and elastase constitute more than 75% of the mass of digestive enzymes secreted. The proenzyme forms of the proteolytic enzymes contain a small amino acid chain that blocks their proteolytic site. This prevents autodigestion of the zymogen granules, the acinar cells, and of course the pancreas itself. The pancreas also secretes protease inhibitors to neutralize any prematurely activated enzymes. Congenital deficiency of one of the major **trypsinogen** inhibitors (*serine protease inhibitor Kazal type 1* [produced by the *SPINK1* gene]), or mutations in the cationic trypsinogen (trypsinogen-1) gene interfering with its inactivation, have been both linked to inherited predisposition to acute pancreatitis.[2] Upon entering the duodenum, **enterokinase** (also called *enteropeptidase*), a duodenal peptidase that is active at acid pH, converts trypsinogen to active trypsin. Free trypsin activates the other proenzymes in a cascade or chain reaction–like fashion and, to a small degree, trypsinogen itself (see Fig. 34-3).

Normal Pancreatic Fluid Secretions

A normal adult weighing 75 kg produces about 2 to 3 liters of water-clear, colorless pancreatic juice per day, which contains the proenzymes and enzymes described above and 120 to 300 mmol/day of bicarbonate. Amylase and lipase, for example, are present in pancreatic juice in activities of about 500,000 to 1 million U/L, with an approximately 10,000:1 gradient in enzyme activities between pancreatic fluid and plasma.[3] Damage to the pancreas thus can produce considerable increases in plasma activities of amylase, lipase, trypsin, and other digestive enzymes. The principal cations in pancreatic fluid, totaling about 150 mmol/L, are Na^+, K^+, Ca^{++}, and Mg^{++}. The principal anions are bicarbonate (120 mmol/L) and Cl^- (30 mmol/L).

Water and electrolytes in pancreatic fluid are secreted by the ductal and acinar cells. The healthy pancreas can secrete bicarbonate into the pancreatic juice and hydrogen ions into blood. Normally, more than enough pancreatic bicarbonate is present to neutralize the acid coming from the stomach; this is critical, because the activity of pancreatic enzymes is inhibited at acid pH.

Control of Exocrine Pancreatic Secretions

Exocrine secretions from the pancreas have both neural and hormonal controls, as is summarized in Table 34-2. Three upper gastrointestinal tract hormones—**cholecystokinin (CCK), secretin,** and gastrin—affect pancreatic juice secretion; these are discussed more fully in Chapter 35. Ingestion of ethanol or distension of the duodenum by food leads to the release of all three hormones. Fat and ethanol are particularly active stimulators of secretin production. A negative-feedback loop exists; trypsin released as a consequence of CCK

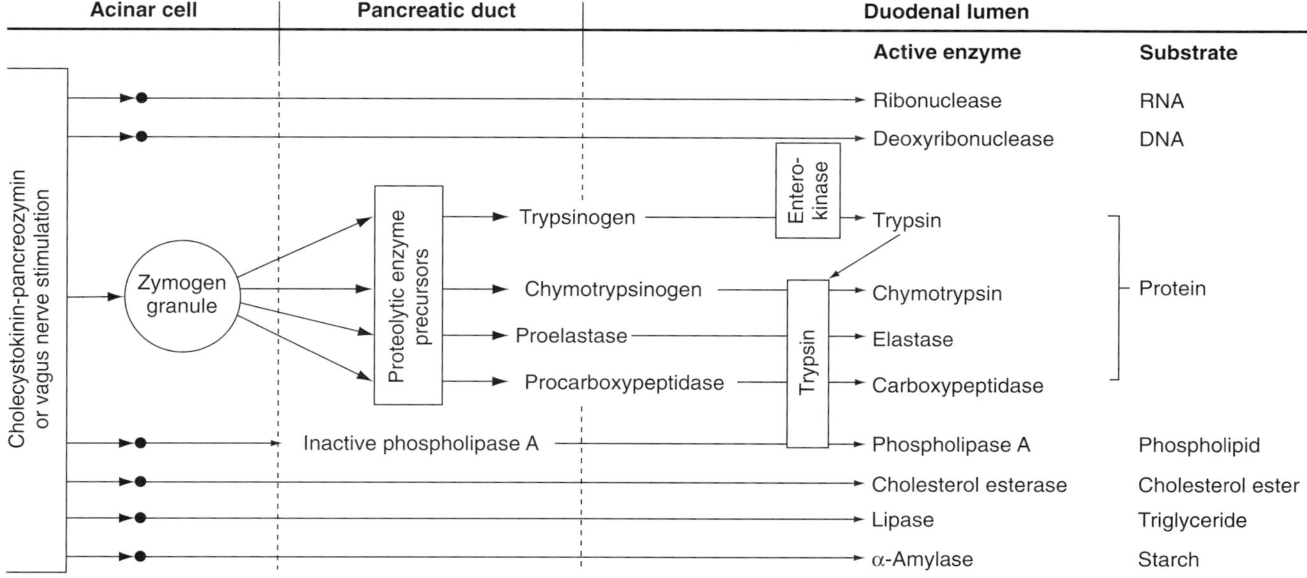

Fig. 34-3 The pancreatic enzymes and their conversion to active forms in the duodenum. Enzymes are stored in zymogen granules that reach the pancreatic duct by exocytosis. Upon reaching the duodenum, proenzymes are converted to their active form by enterokinase and by active trypsin.

Table 34-2 Factors That Control Normal Exocrine Pancreatic Secretions

Event or Release of Factor	Result
Vagal nerve stimulation of pancreas	Secretion of fluid high in protein and enzymes (such as trypsin), low in bicarbonate, low in volume; release of pancreatic polypeptide
Distension of duodenum by food; alcohol ingestion	Cholecystokinin (CCK) and gastrin secretion by duodenum
CCK or gastrin release	Release of zymogen granules from acinar cells; secretion of fluid high in protein and enzymes, low in bicarbonate, low in volume; release of pancreatic polypeptide
Secretin release	Secretion of fluid high in bicarbonate and volume but low in enzymes
Fatty acids or acid food ingestion	CCK release
Amino acids or Ca^{++} ingestion	CCK, gastrin release
Vasoinhibitory polypeptide (VIP) release	Secretin-like effect on gland
Somatostatin release	Inhibition of basal pancreatic secretions, increased fecal fat, decreased intestinal mobility
Trypsin in duodenum	Inhibition of CCK release
Thyroid hormone release	Maintenance of normal pancreatic function and response to stimuli

activity has an inhibitory action on further CCK secretion. VIP is structurally similar to secretin and glucagon; this probably explains the similar action of VIP on the pancreas. All pancreatic exocrine secretions and other gastrointestinal functions are inhibited by somatostatin.

KEY CONCEPTS BOX 34-1

- The pancreas is located deep in the abdomen, but close to the stomach, duodenum, and common bile duct.
- The major pancreatic hormone is insulin, which is needed to maintain normal blood glucose levels.
- Pancreatic exocrine secretions include bicarbonate (to neutralize gastric acid) and digestive enzymes; many of these are released initially as inactive proenzymes that need activation for their digestive functions.

SECTION OBJECTIVES BOX 34-2

- For the following pancreatic diseases, describe their common mode of presentation: acute pancreatitis, chronic pancreatitis, cystic fibrosis, pancreatic cancer.
- List at least three hormones produced by islet cell tumors of the pancreas; for each, describe the clinical picture that should lead to laboratory testing to evaluate for its presence.

PATHOLOGICAL CONDITIONS

Diseases of the pancreas can be grouped broadly into islet cell disorders such as diabetes mellitus (insulin deficiency) and glucagon excess; exocrine insufficiency, producing pancreatic insufficiency and associated malabsorption; inflammatory disorders such as acute or chronic pancreatitis; and neoplastic disorders such as **adenocarcinomas** and islet cell tumors, which may lead to bile duct obstruction if the mass occurs in the head of the pancreas. The emphasis here is on those disorders associated with chemical changes in body fluids or abnormal chemical responses to certain stimuli. Interpretation of laboratory tests is one of the major tools used in defining pancreatic diseases. A carefully obtained history and physical examination may suggest pancreatic disease; imaging techniques such as **endoscopic retrograde cholangiopancreatography (ERCP),** ultrasonography, computerized tomography, and magnetic resonance imaging are also of great importance. Estimating pancreatic size with the use of imaging methods is important in suspected acute pancreatitis, because an inflamed, edematous gland is generally larger than normal. Mass lesions usually can be diagnosed only by imaging, and chronic pancreatitis typically is associated with calcification in the region of the pancreas. Laparotomy or **laparoscopy** with visual observation and palpation are useful in defining pancreatic anatomy.

Endocrine Pancreatic Disorders

Diabetes Mellitus

The major endocrine disorder is diabetes mellitus (DM), which is discussed more fully in Chapter 38. Diabetes mellitus is characterized by inadequate insulin action, which can be caused by autoimmune islet cell destruction (type 1 diabetes) and a state of insulin absence, or insulin resistance (most type 2 diabetes). Chronic inflammation of the pancreas (as in chronic pancreatitis), pancreatic resection, or drugs toxic to the islets (such as pentamidine) are rare causes of DM. Laboratory findings in DM are discussed fully in Chapter 38. An abnormal serum amylase in the absence of pancreatitis is common in uncontrolled DM, especially in the presence of diabetic ketoacidosis. Typically, the increase is the result of high levels of salivary amylase. Transplantation of the pancreas (often along with renal transplantation) is currently being used with excellent success for patients with DM and end-stage renal disease (see Chapter 54). With whole organ transplantation, exocrine pancreatic function is unnecessary and can cause destruction of normal tissue if the enzymes are not eliminated from the body. For many years, the main approach to diversion of exocrine secretions was attachment of the pancreatic duct in a transplanted gland to the bladder. Measurement of urinary amylase is a good test of graft function and can be used to monitor evidence of graft rejection (which causes decreased urine amylase excretion).[4] However, bladder drainage is associated with urinary tract infections, and reflux from the bladder can cause pancreatic injury. Moreover, pancreatic enzymes can degrade urine protein, making it difficult to monitor diabetic patients for renal injury.[4] Intestinal loop drainage is now preferred; amylase can be measured in the intestinal loop as a monitor of graft function.[5]

Pancreatic islet cell tumors often are associated with overproduction of hormones; different tumors thus can produce distinct clinical syndromes, as is discussed below. In some cases, however, symptoms are absent and the tumor is detected as a mass lesion. A neuroendocrine cause may be suspected by markedly elevated levels of chromogranin A in plasma, because chromogranin is present in the secretory granules of most neuroendocrine cells.[6] Specific syndromes of hormone overproduction are discussed later in the chapter under Pancreatic Neoplasms.

Exocrine Pancreatic Disorders

Inflammatory or Necrotic Pancreatic Injury

Acute Pancreatitis

Acute pancreatitis is an inflammatory disorder that is associated with activation of local pancreatic enzymes, which causes destruction of pancreatic tissue. Severe acute pancreatitis can be a life-threatening emergency. Acute pancreatitis is most commonly the result of alcohol abuse (the most common cause in males) or to biliary tract obstruction by gallstones (the most common cause in females); together, these two conditions are responsible for about 75% of cases of acute pancreatitis. Other important causes of acute pancreatitis are listed in Box 34-1. Acute pancreatitis is a relatively uncommon disorder, with an estimated 10 to 20 cases reported per 100,000 population per year.

The pathogenesis of acute pancreatitis is thought to be caused by factors that lead to inappropriate activation of pancreatic enzymes within the gland itself, typically starting with conversion of trypsinogen to trypsin. Alcohol, for example, stimulates pancreatic secretions and can lead to proteinaceous plugs that obstruct small ductules in the pancreas. Gallstones are thought to cause inflammation that activates pancreatic enzymes, which cannot reach the duodenum because of the obstruction. A proposed mechanism for the evolution of pancreatitis is shown in Table 34-3, although the precise factors leading to pancreatitis are unknown. The mechanism by which other causes of pancreatitis cause injury is even less clear. Routine laboratory tests often suggest that gallstones are the cause; alanine aminotransferase (ALT) over 150 U/L has a positive predictive value of 95% for gallstone pancreatitis, but sensitivity is only 50%.[7]

Acute pancreatitis typically presents as sharp upper abdominal pain, often radiating to the back, associated with nausea and vomiting; however, physical examination typically is not diagnostic, and pancreatitis must be distinguished from other disorders with a similar presentation. Box 34-2 lists several of the leading differential diagnoses of patients with abdominal pain, many of which may also cause increased levels of one or more pancreatic enzyme.

In most cases, pancreatitis leads to complete recovery; however, in severe pancreatitis, mortality is 10% to 20%.[8] Interest in trying to predict disease severity and, therefore, risk of mortality is long-standing. Serum and urine enzymes (with the possible exception of urine trypsinogen-2) are not helpful in predicting disease severity. The most commonly used severity scores include a pancreatitis-specific scoring system developed by Ranson and the Acute Physiology and Chronic Health Evaluation (APACHE) II system, which is a general

Table 34-3 Proposed Events in the Development of Acute Pancreatitis

Event	Likely Causes
Injury to acinar cell membranes	Reflux of bile or pancreatic juice into pancreas, alcoholic irritation of duodenum or precipitation of protein plugs in gland, infection or inflammation in gallbladder spreading to pancreas, viral and other microbiological infections of pancreas, ischemia, circulatory failure, trauma, surgery
Biochemical changes in gland	Activation of proenzymes such as protrypsin, proelastase, prophospholipase A_2 to their biochemically active forms; occlusion of pancreatic ductules or duct; conversion of kallikreinogen to kallikrein
Edema, swelling of pancreatic capsule	Inflammation of gland, disturbance of gland's afferent or efferent blood flow
Tetany and cardiac arrhythmias, respiratory distress	Peripancreatic fat necrosis, Ca^{++} sequestration by fatty acids, refractory hypocalcemia, unknown toxic substance(s) (phospholipase A_2?) acting on lung and other organs
Hemorrhagic necrosis of gland, shock, circulatory collapse, profound reduction in plasma volume	Autolysis and digestion of gland with bleeding into retroperitoneal space, release of hypotensive kinins, cytotoxic effects of lysolecithin (from bile)
Death	Acute circulatory and respiratory failure, refractory hypotension

Box 34-1

Causes of Acute Pancreatitis

Causes include alcoholism, biliary tract diseases, surgery to the pancreas or nearby organs, atherosclerotic plaques in the pancreatic arteries, abdominal trauma, post endoscopic retrograde cholangiopancreatography (ERCP), hypertriglyceridemia (especially with triglyceride concentrations above 1000 mg/dL), and infections.

Drugs associated with or possibly causing pancreatitis include azathioprine, cimetidine, cytarabine, didanosine, estrogens, furosemide, 6-mercaptopurine, methyldopa, metronidazole, nitrofurantoin, pentamidine, sulfonamides, sulindac, tetracycline, and valproic acid.

Box 34-2

Diseases Associated With Secondary Pancreatitis

These include all types of biliary tract disorders, any inflammatory process or abscess in the abdomen, renal failure, burns, shock, sepsis, diabetic ketoacidosis, post abdominal surgery, volvulus, gastrointestinal perforation of any kind, and pancreas and kidney transplantation.

disease severity scoring system that is used widely in intensive care. The Ranson criteria are summarized in Table 34-4; the presence of three or more of these findings indicates severe disease. Although their positive predictive value for determining a poor prognosis is less than 50%, their negative predictive value in ruling out severe disease is about 90%.[8] In Europe, C-reactive protein (CRP) has been used to evaluate prognosis; CRP levels >150 mg/L at 48 hours after onset of symptoms are associated with a positive predictive value of about 67% for severe disease, and a negative predictive value of 86% for severe disease. The American Gastroenterology Association technical review recommends wider use of CRP measurement to assess prognosis in persons with acute pancreatitis.[9]

Table 34-4 Ranson's Laboratory Indicators of Severity in Acute Pancreatitis*

On Admission	Within 48 Hours
Glucose > 200 mg/dL (11.1 mmol/L) [220 mg/dL (12.2 mmol/L)]	Hematocrit decrease > 10%
	BUN increase > 5 mg/dL (1.8 mmol/L) [>2 mg/dL (0.7 mmol/L)]
LDH > 350 IU/L [400 IU/L]	Calcium < 8 mg/dL (2 mmol/L)
AST > 250 IU/L	Po_2 < 60 mm Hg [not used]
WBC > 16,000/mm^3 [18,000/mm^3]	Base deficit > 4 mmol/L [>6 mmol/L]

Modified from Ranson JH, Rifkind KM, Turner JW: Prognostic signs and nonoperative peritoneal lavage in acute pancreatitis, Surg Gynecol Obstet 143:109, 1976.

AST, Aspartate aminotransferase; *BUN*, blood urea nitrogen; *LDH*, lactate dehydrogenase; *WBC*, white blood cell count.

*Initial numbers represent values used in pancreatitis not caused by gallstones; numbers in brackets indicate values used in pancreatitis due to gallstones.

Chronic Pancreatitis

Chronic pancreatitis is often a consequence of repeated bouts of acute pancreatitis and extensive destruction of the gland; usually, much of the pancreas has been replaced with scar (fibrotic) tissue. Chronic pancreatitis is an uncommon disorder, with a prevalence estimated to be 0.04% to 0.05% of the adult population.[3] Chronic pancreatitis usually has the same risk factors detailed above for acute pancreatitis. Atherosclerosis of the pancreatic artery causing recurrent pancreatic ischemia is an uncommon cause of chronic pancreatitis. The genetic disorders discussed earlier, involving cationic trypsinogen and *SPINK1*, as well as mutations in the cystic fibrosis transmembrane conductance regulator *(CFTR)* gene, may be responsible for up to 25% of cases of chronic pancreatitis.[10] Although cystic fibrosis commonly causes pancreatic destruction, individuals who are simple heterozygotes or compound heterozygotes for two different mutations in the *CFTR* gene may develop chronic pancreatitis without exhibiting other clinical manifestations of cystic fibrosis.[11] Chronic pancreatitis also may be caused by autoimmune processes, often recognized by the presence of polyclonal gammopathy (particularly involving immune globulin [Ig]G4), other autoimmune organ injury, and autoantibodies against pancreatic acinar tissue.[12]

Chronic pancreatitis typically presents as intermittent episodes of abdominal pain, typically associated with calcification of the pancreas on imaging studies. Often, in later stages, chronic pancreatitis is associated with pancreatic dysfunction that leads to malabsorption; in some cases, destruction of pancreatic islets results in diabetes mellitus. During episodes of acute exacerbation, serum activities of amylase and lipase usually are increased, but between episodes, they may be below the lower limit of normal in up to 60% of cases.[13]

Cystic Fibrosis

Exocrine pancreatic malfunction is a hallmark of cystic fibrosis (CF), an autosomal, recessively inherited disease that is diagnosed primarily in infants and children (see also Chapters 45 and 52). CF is caused by a number of different mutations in the chloride transporter gene that lead to a missing or nonfunctional CFTR protein, which plays a role in the selective cellular uptake of ions. In CF, pancreatic secretions (as well as those of the lungs and other organs) are viscous and of low volume. In the pancreas, this leads to greatly reduced pancreatic flow, in many cases resulting in pancreatic duct obstruction and atrophy.

Newborn screening for cystic fibrosis in the United States now is based on initial screening with serum **immunoreactive trypsin (IRT);** genetic testing is done on infants whose results are above the cutoff value. By 2009, 48 states had mandated neonatal screening for cystic fibrosis, The exact cutoff used varies from state to state, and the methods used produce different absolute values. In some states, cutoffs are based on specific values, although others use particular percentile values (90th or 95th) as the decision point. A few states use a second measurement at 2 weeks of age and then only do genetic testing if results are high on both measurements.[14] If genetic tests (which typically identify only the 25 to 30 most common mutations) are negative, and IRT values are markedly elevated (typically above the 99.9th percentile), additional testing with sweat chloride measurement is recommended.

Pancreatic Insufficiency

Reduction or loss of pancreatic exocrine (digestive) function leads, in its late stages, to severe gastrointestinal disturbances, such as diarrhea, constipation, and malabsorption (see Chapter 35). With advanced disease, a catabolic state leading to weight loss and **cachexia** appears. The exocrine pancreas has extensive reserve capacity; symptoms generally appear only after about 85% to 90% of the acinar tissue has been lost. The most common causes of pancreatic insufficiency differ in children and adults; in children, it is almost always due to cystic fibrosis, and in adults it is usually due to chronic pancreatitis. The causes of acinar cell loss are listed in Box 34-3.

Box 34-3

Causes of Acinar Cell Loss

- Repeated bouts of pancreatitis, especially that caused by chronic alcoholism
- Cystic fibrosis (CF)
- Atherosclerosis and subsequent pancreatic atrophy
- Any obstruction of the pancreatic ductules or duct as caused by a stone or stones or calcification of the gland, a benign or malignant tumor pressing on the pancreas, or other types of mechanical blockage

Pancreatic Neoplasms

Adenocarcinoma

Most pancreatic cancers are adenocarcinomas that arise from the ductal epithelial cells and carry an ominous prognosis. Only about 1% of pancreatic cancers originate in the acinar cells. Pancreatic cancer is the fifth most lethal malignancy in the developed world after colorectal, breast, lung, and prostate cancer. The death rate from pancreatic cancer in the United States is about 12 per 100,000 and is increasing. Predisposing factors include smoking, diabetes mellitus, a diet high in fat, and exposure to certain carcinogens such as coal tar, coke, benzidine, and β-naphthylamine.[3] Most pancreatic cancers are invasive and inoperable when clinically apparent. Death within 1 year of diagnosis is common, and the 5-year survival rate is a dismal 1%. Jaundice develops early in 60% to 70% of patients with cancer in the head of the pancreas because of tumor-caused occlusion of the bile duct. If jaundice does occur with carcinoma of the body or tail of the pancreas, it usually manifests late in the disease. Malabsorption of fats and proteins with weight loss is common.

Islet Cell Tumors

Islet tumors account for only about 1% of pancreatic neoplasms. They often are identified by hormone overproduction, causing distinct clinical pictures based on the hormone produced in excess (see below). Islet cell tumors may occur as part of the type I **multiple endocrine neoplasia** syndrome (see Chapter 35).

Insulinoma

One of the less common causes of **hypoglycemia** is overproduction of insulin by a tumor of the pancreatic islets, termed an *insulinoma*. Although insulinoma is the most common islet cell tumor, it is still a rare disease; only about four cases develop per million population per year.[15] Insulinomas typically are small, benign tumors that can be difficult to locate with the use of imaging procedures. Hypoglycemia is most commonly the result of an imbalance between glucose ingestion or production and medications in patients with diabetes. Among adult patients who do not have diabetes, hypoglycemia often occurs in ill patients because of shock, renal failure, liver failure, and endocrine diseases such as adrenal insufficiency and hypopituitarism.[16] In otherwise healthy individuals, excess insulin production or ingestion is usually the cause of hypoglycemia and requires careful evaluation of the patient. The initial workup of hypoglycemia in such persons involves a period of fasting (24 to 72 hours), with frequent determinations of blood glucose. If the person becomes hypoglycemic (plasma glucose <40 mg/dL [2.2 mmol/L]), samples should be collected for insulin and C-peptide measurement.

Glucagonoma

Tumors that produce glucagon almost always arise in the pancreas and present with a distinctive combination of hyperglycemia, weight loss, and a peculiar skin rash that often calls attention to the presence of the tumor. Most cases occur in adults older than 40.

Somatostatinoma

Tumors of the pancreas (or, less frequently, the intestine) can produce excess somatostatin. These tumors usually occur in older adults (average age of onset is about 50), and they are somewhat more common in women. The most common clinical features are nonspecific and include glucose intolerance or diabetes, gallbladder disease, and diarrhea (often with steatorrhea). However, these symptoms are much more likely to be present with intestinal tumors than with pancreatic tumors, in which these symptoms occur in a minority of cases; an endocrine tumor usually is not suspected until the tumor is removed and is examined histologically. Within the pancreas, the tumors are often large and malignant and predominantly arise in the head of the pancreas (in contrast to most other endocrine tumors), where they may cause bile duct obstruction.[15] Because these tumors are usually malignant, plasma somatostatin levels typically are elevated even after surgery. Excess production of other hormones (such as insulin, calcitonin, and gastrin) is common.

PPoma

Tumors producing pancreatic polypeptide (PP) are uncommon and usually asymptomatic. Similar to somatostatinomas, they are usually large, malignant tumors found in the head of the pancreas, often presenting as a mass or with obstructive jaundice, with diagnosis becoming apparent only at the time of resection. Elevations of PP levels and levels of other hormones such as chromogranins usually are present even after surgery; these can be used as tumor markers to monitor the success of therapy.[15]

Gastrinoma, VIPoma

Tumors that produce gastrin and VIP often arise in the pancreas. Excess production of gastrin produces **Zollinger-Ellison syndrome,** whereas excess production of VIP produces the syndrome of watery diarrhea, hypokalemia, and achlorhydria (WDHA). Because the manifestations of these tumors are primarily intestinal, they are discussed in Chapter 35.

KEY CONCEPTS BOX 34-2

- Acute pancreatitis is the most common pancreatic disease in adults, presenting as upper abdominal pain; it usually is recognized by elevated pancreatic enzyme levels. Laboratory tests may be helpful in predicting prognosis.
- Cystic fibrosis is the most common pancreatic disease in infants and children; it is screened for by serum immunoreactive trypsin.
- Pancreatic tumors are derived most commonly from acinar cells and often are not detected until they are far advanced, but islet cell tumors are detected often by their hormone products.

EXOCRINE PANCREATIC TESTS

Tests performed to evaluate exocrine pancreas function can be divided into two groups: those that evaluate pancreatic function directly, and those that detect pancreatic injury.

Pancreatic function tests measure the ability of the pancreas to produce enzymes, proteins, and bicarbonate and to secrete an adequate volume of fluid into the duodenum. In a review of chronic pancreatitis, the limitations of all pancreatic function tests were emphasized.[13] Evaluation of response of the pancreas to secretin stimulation, although considered the gold standard function test, requires lengthy endoscopy and is not practical. Various other simpler tests (such as stool elastase or trypsin activity, and the bentiromide test) have good sensitivity only in cases of severe pancreatic dysfunction, when the diagnosis can be made clinically based on symptoms, imaging studies, and response to oral administration of pancreatic enzymes. In mild to moderate dysfunction, these simpler tests have sensitivities of <75% at most; with mild dysfunction, sensitivity is usually below 50%. In the author's institution, such pancreatic function tests are never used. Nonetheless, some physicians still order tests to evaluate pancreatic function. The different categories of function tests can be summarized as follows:

1. Tests that directly sample pancreatic fluid
2. Tests on feces that measure pancreatic enzymes or undigested dietary contents
3. Indirect tests that measure the ability of pancreatic enzymes to digest exogenous substances

Direct sampling of pancreatic fluid has been the gold standard test of pancreatic function for many years. A double-lumen tube is inserted through the esophagus and stomach to a point in the duodenum below the ampulla; pancreatic secretion then is stimulated, typically by intravenous administration of secretin. Bicarbonate, fluid volume, and/or pancreatic enzymes (especially amylase, trypsin, or chymotrypsin) are measured in duodenal fluid. Bicarbonate production and fluid volume are reasonably insensitive tests of adequate pancreatic function, and patients with significant losses of pancreatic function may show a normal bicarbonate and volume because of the large reserve capacity. Although duodenal fluid enzyme levels are the first to become decreased, reference values are not widely available for fluid enzyme content. Recently, a newer approach has been developed that does not use laboratory tests, but rather relies on magnetic resonance imaging (MRI) to evaluate pancreatic secretion following administration of secretin, and has similar accuracy to secretin testing in those with clinical evidence of pancreatic dysfunction.[17] However, testing in persons with mild to moderate pancreatic dysfunction has not yet been evaluated.

Tests on Feces

An abnormal fecal fat test on a 72-hour collection has been the standard, noninvasive test for pancreatic insufficiency; however, fat excretion becomes abnormal only after 85% to 90% of pancreatic acinar tissue is lost. In general, the percentage of stool weight composed of fat is higher in pancreatic insufficiency than in intestinal disease, but overlap is seen in the results. Tests for trypsin and chymotrypsin in feces are unreliable (sensitivity 30% or less) in early pancreatic insufficiency, although chymotrypsin as measured by immunoassay typically is decreased when steatorrhea results from pancreatic insufficiency. Probably the most sensitive enzyme measurement is that of elastase-1 in stool; assays for its measurement are commercially available. Although early data suggested that measurement of stool elastase-1 was reliable in evaluating pancreatic function,[18] newer data indicate that it is also insensitive (sensitivity <50% compared with secretin test) in early pancreatic insufficiency.[19] (See Chapter 35 for additional information on fecal fat measurement.)

Indirect Tests of Pancreatic Function

A variety of substances have been developed to indirectly measure the activity of pancreatic enzymes within the intestine. These involve administration of a substance that contains a compound that is further metabolized after absorption; this metabolite then is measured as an indicator of pancreatic enzymatic digestion. The N-benzoyl tryrosyl para-aminobenzoic acid (NBT-PABA) (bentiromide) test is used in a few laboratories to estimate pancreatic digestive function, but it is not commercially available in the United States or Canada. NBT-PABA is *p*-aminobenzoic acid linked to a short chain of synthetic amino acids; after digestion by chymotrypsin to release PABA, PABA is absorbed by the small intestine and is metabolized in the liver to hippurate, which is excreted in urine. Urine hippurate excretion is quantified to determine PABA release and absorption. Unfortunately, this test has poor sensitivity for early pancreatic damage and is affected not only by pancreatic enzyme secretion but also by intestinal absorption, liver function (conjugation), and renal excretion. Fats and peptides labeled with radioactive isotopes also have been used; radioactivity can be measured in breath or urine (depending on the element labeled) to detect absorption.

Pancreatic enzyme tests measure the levels of pancreatic enzymes in the blood as markers of cellular injury to the pancreas. The three most widely used tests are amylase, lipase, and various forms of trypsin and its precursor, trypsinogen. Because the cell-to-plasma gradient is very high for pancreatic enzymes, such tests are sensitive indicators of pancreatic injury; however, specificity of several of the tests is less than optimal, because of other factors that are discussed later.

Historically, amylase has been the most widely used test for the diagnosis of pancreatitis; however, amylase is not specific to the pancreas. The major groupings of amylase isoenzymes are salivary and pancreatic. Salivary isoenzymes are increased in a number of conditions, including salivary gland inflammation or injury, ectopic pregnancy, and serous ovarian carcinoma, as well as after open heart surgery. Lipase can be used to differentiate pancreatic and salivary types as the main source of elevation of serum amylase.

Autoantibodies to amylase are relatively common, producing macroamylase; up to 5% of those with elevated amylase levels are found to have macroamylasemia.[20] In most cases, no cause is found for the autoantibodies, although an association with certain immune disorders such as celiac disease[21] and HIV[22] has been noted. Macroamylase can be suspected in a person with persistent stable increases in amylase, particularly with low urinary amylase excretion. Macrolipase has been reported, but much less frequently than macroamylase; rarely, the two can coexist.[23]

Amylase and lipase levels are affected by other conditions.[7] Both are small enzymes, and their clearance is at least partially due to renal filtration; however, measurement of urine amylase is no longer believed to be useful for the diagnosis of acute pancreatitis. Serum amylase and, to a lesser extent, lipase therefore are increased in renal disease. Intestinal disease leads commonly to increased amylase, and less commonly to increased lipase. Some clinicians prefer amylase as an initial test for evaluation of those with abdominal pain, because a normal result makes significant abdominal pathology unlikely; with such uses, lipase then is used to confirm pancreatitis in a person with elevated amylase.

CHANGE IN ANALYTES WITH DISEASE

Amylase and Lipase

Although imaging studies often are used to identify pancreatitis, diagnosis typically is based on increased serum or plasma levels of pancreatic enzymes, notably amylase, lipase, and immunoreactive trypsin. The gradient of amylase between the pancreas and the plasma is high, making amylase a sensitive test of pancreatic injury. Because of the nonspecificity of amylase, several studies have suggested a threshold of three to five times the upper reference limits for diagnosis of pancreatitis.[8] Lipase is much more specific for pancreatitis than is amylase; studies have found that values above the reference limit can be used as the threshold for diagnosis of pancreatitis. Both serum amylase and lipase are elevated within a few hours of occurrence of pancreatic injury; amylase remains increased an average of 3 to 5 days, and lipase typically remains increased for 5 to 7 days after injury. Guidelines put forth by the American Gastroenterological Association suggest that use of only one of the enzymes is needed to diagnose pancreatitis.[9] UK guidelines state that lipase is the preferred test for diagnosis of acute pancreatitis.[24]

Although not currently commercially available in the United States, assays for measurement of trypsinogen-2 and trypsinogen activation peptide may prove more sensitive and specific than those for amylase or lipase. Urine dipsticks to detect increased trypsinogen-2 have a 99% negative predictive value for acute pancreatitis in several studies.[25] A peptide cleaved during conversion to active trypsin, termed *trypsinogen activation peptide*, also may be measured in urine and has improved specificity for pancreatitis. Some of the data suggest that trypsinogen-2 may be able to predict the severity of pancreatitis.

Cancer Markers

A number of genetic markers and hereditary genetic traits have been linked to pancreatic carcinoma. Mutations in the cationic trypsinogen gene, discussed earlier as a cause of pancreatitis, also are associated with a markedly increased risk of pancreatic carcinoma. Peutz-Jegher syndrome, usually associated with GI tract malignancy, and mutations in the *BRCA* gene, usually associated with breast and ovarian cancer, also increase the risk of pancreatic carcinoma.

A number of tumor markers are increased in pancreatic cancer but are not recommended for screening of high-risk individuals or for diagnosis in persons with suspicious lesions on imaging study because of poor specificity and low sensitivity in small tumors.[26] The most widely used tumor marker is CA 19-9, a sialylated form of the Lewis A blood group antigen. An additional problem is that marked elevations of CA 19-9 can occur with benign obstruction of the biliary tract,[27] as well as in cirrhosis.[28]

Endocrine Tumor Markers

About 20% of islet cell tumors are biochemically silent and do not secrete active hormones. Islet cell tumors have been found that secrete one or more of the following hormones: insulin, glucagon, somatostatin, pancreatic polypeptide, gastrin, vasoactive intestinal peptide (VIP), adrenocorticotropic hormone (ACTH), β-chorionic gonadotropin, calcitonin, prostaglandins, secretin, and serotonin.

Insulin

Insulin levels are best reported as a ratio of insulin to glucose, with glucose reported in mg/dL and insulin in U/L; a ratio above 0.3 indicates inappropriate insulin production. In insulinoma, the ratio is increased along with elevated C-peptide, whereas exogenous insulin administration causes a high ratio but undetectable C-peptide. Ingestion of oral insulin secretagogues, which can produce a pattern similar to that of insulinoma, can be detected by screening for their presence in urine or serum. Proinsulin, which sometimes is the dominant peptide produced in insulinoma, is almost never present with oral insulin secretagogues.

Glucagon

Diagnosis of glucagonomas depends on measurement of plasma glucagon; the upper reference limit is 200 pg/mL, but 70% to 90% of such cases have glucagon levels greater than 1000 pg/mL. Although increased glucagon also occurs in renal failure, starvation, pancreatitis, and other endocrine diseases, glucagon levels are rarely above 500 pg/mL in these disorders (although they may be over 1000 pg/mL in cirrhosis). Most glucagon-producing tumors are very large at the time of diagnosis, and most behave in a malignant fashion.[15]

KEY CONCEPTS BOX 34-3

- Tests of exocrine pancreatic function typically are insensitive for early pancreatic insufficiency and (except for secretin test) are not highly reliable in detecting pancreatic damage.
- Serum lipase is more specific for acute pancreatitis and is of similar sensitivity; amylase still is used often as the primary test although it is also elevated in many other significant abdominal disorders; lipase is the better test for diagnosing pancreatitis.
- In persons with hypoglycemia, serum insulin, C-peptide, and proinsulin typically all are elevated with insulin-producing tumors; those who inject insulin, in contrast, would have only elevated insulin.

REFERENCES

1. Baggio L, Drucker D: Biology of incretins: GLP-1 and GIP, Gastroenterology 132:2131, 2007.
2. Whitcomb D: Hereditary pancreatitis: new insights into acute and chronic pancreatitis, Gut 45:317, 1999.
3. Hruban R, Wilentz R: The pancreas. In Fausto N, editor: *Robbins and Cotran Pathologic Basis of Disease*, Philadelphia, 2005, Elsevier Saunders.
4. Bernard D, Delanghe J, Langlois M: Difficulties in evaluating urinalysis following combined pancreas-kidney transplantation, Ann Clin Biochem 34:664, 1997.
5. Zibari G, Boykin K, Sawaya D, et al: Pancreatic transplantation and subsequent graft surveillance by pancreatic portal-enteric anastamosis and temporary venting jejunostomy, Ann Surg 233:639, 2001.
6. Giovanella L, La Rosa S, Ceriani L, et al: Chromogranin-A as a serum marker for neuroendocrine tumors: comparison with neuron-specific enolase and correlation with immunohistochemical findings, Int J Biol Markers 14:160, 1999.
7. Matull W, Pereira S, O'Donohue J: Biochemical markers of acute pancreatitis, J Clin Pathol 59:340, 2006.
8. Whitcomb D: Clinical practice: acute pancreatitis, N Engl J Med 354:2142, 2006.
9. Forsmark C, Baillie J: AGA Institute technical review on acute pancreatitis, Gastroenterology 132:2022, 2007.
10. Witt H: Chronic pancreatitis and cystic fibrosis, Gut 52:ii31, 2003.
11. Bishop M, Freedman S, Zielenski J, et al: The cystic fibrosis transmembrane conductance regulator gene and ion channel function in patients with idiopathic pancreatitis, Hum Genet 118:372, 2005.
12. Kim M, Kwon S: Diagnostic criteria for autoimmune chronic pancreatitis, J Gastroenterol 42(suppl 18):42, 2007.
13. Witt H, Apte M, Keim V, et al: Chronic pancreatitis: challenges and advances in pathogenesis, genetics, diagnosis, and therapy, Gastroenterology 132:1557, 2007.
14. Grosse S, Boyle C, Botkin J, et al: Newborn screening for cystic fibrosis: evaluation of benefits and risks and recommendations for state newborn screening programs, MMWR 53(RR-13):1, 2004.
15. Mittendorf E, Shifrin A, Inabnet W, et al: Islet cell tumors, Curr Probl Surg 43:685, 2006.

16. Service F: Hypoglycemia, Endocrinol Metab Clin North Am 26:937, 1997.
17. Merkle E, Baillie J: Exocrine pancreatic function: evaluation with MR imaging before and after secretin stimulation, Am J Gastroenterol 101:137, 2006.
18. Elphick D, Kapur K: Comparing the urinary pancreolauryl ratio and faecal elastase-1 as indicators of pancreatic insufficiency in clinical practice, Pancreatology 5:196, 2005.
19. DiMagno M, Dimagno E: Chronic pancreatitis, Curr Opin Gastroenterol 22:487, 2006.
20. Lawson G: Prevalence of macroamylasemia using polyethylene glycol precipitation as a screening method, Ann Clin Biochem 38:37, 2001.
21. Rabsztyn A, Green P, Berti I, et al: Macroamylasemia in patients with celiac disease, Am J Gastroenterol 96:1096, 2001.
22. Foo Y, Konecny P: Hyperamylasaemia in asymptomatic HIV patients, Ann Clin Biochem 34:259, 1997.
23. Zaman Z, Van Orshoven A, Marien G, et al: Simultaneous macroamylasemia and macrolipasemia, Clin Chem 40:939, 1994.
24. Werner J, Feuerbach S, Uhl W, et al: Management of acute pancreatitis: from surgery to interventional intensive care, Gut 54:426, 2005.
25. Al-Bahrani A, Ammori B: Clinical laboratory assessment of acute pancreatitis, Clin Chim Acta 362:26, 2005.
26. Dimagno E, Reber H, Tempero M: AGA technical review on the epidemiology, diagnosis, and treatment of pancreatic ductal adenocarcinoma, Gastroenterology 117:1464, 1999.
27. Akdogan M, Sasmaz N, Kayhan B, et al: Extraordinarily elevated CA 19-9 in benign conditions: a case report and review of the literature, Tumori 87:337-339; 2001.
28. Fabris C, Basso D, Leandro G, et al: Serum CA 19-9 and alpha-fetoprotein levels in primary hepatocellular carcinoma and liver cirrhosis, Cancer 68:1795, 1991.

INTERNET SITES

http://www.pancreas.org/index.html

http://www.vivo.colostate.edu/hbooks/pathphys/digestion/pancreas/index.html

http://www.pancreasfoundation.org/index.shtml

http://www.emedicine.com/MED/topic1720.htm—live as of 4/09/08

http://www.emedicine.com/med/TOPIC1721.htm—live as of 4/09/08

http://www.aafp.org/afp/20000701/164.html—live as of 4/09/08

http://pathology.jhu.edu/pancreas/BasicOverview3.php?area=ba—live as of 4/09/08

Gastrointestinal Function and Digestive Disease

35 Chapter

D. Robert Dufour

Chapter Outline

Key Terms

achlorhydria Literally "without hydrochloric acid." Refers to lack of acid production by the stomach.

brain-gut axis The connections between the central nervous system and the intestinal tract, which include neural control of intestinal function, input from the intestinal tract to the brain to control hunger, and the production of similar hormones both within the central nervous system and the intestine.

carcinoid A tumor of the endocrine cells of the intestinal tract, usually slowly growing (compared with carcinomas) but capable of metastasis. The tumor typically produces hormones such as serotonin, which can produce flushing, diarrhea, and heart valve damage; this spectrum of symptoms is known as *the carcinoid syndrome.*

chyme The semisolid end product of gastric action on food. Chyme consists of mucus, gastric secretions, and broken-down food.

gliadin The major antigen in the protein gluten, the major trigger for the immune reaction found in celiac sprue.

gluten A protein found in wheat and wheat products.

micelle A tiny droplet of fat molecules, arranged in such a way as to allow it to be soluble in water.

microvilli Innumerable, microscopic fingerlike projections on the surfaces of cells that increase the surface area of intestinal cells, facilitating absorption of nutrients.

mucosa The layer of cells that covers the inside of a hollow organ such as the mouth or intestine.

pancreatic exocrine enzymes Enzymes required for digestion. Often released in a precursor form. These enzymes include trypsinogen, chymotrypsinogen, proelastase, procarboxypeptidase, ribonuclease, deoxyribonuclease, amylase, lipase, phospholipase A, and cholesterol esterase.

pancreatic hormones Endocrine hormones mainly concerned with carbohydrate intermediary metabolism and including glucagon, insulin, and gastrin.

portal vein A vein that carries blood from one organ to another, without modification; specifically refers to a vein that carries blood from the intestinal tract to the liver, allowing nutrients and hormones to reach that vital organ.

tissue transglutaminase An enzyme found on the surfaces of lymphoid cells; it is involved in processing foreign substances (such as gliadin).

Methods on Evolve

Carbohydrate antigen 19-9 (CA 19-9)
Carcinoembryonic antigens (CEA)
D-Xylose
Fecal fat absorption
Fecal electrolytes and osmolality
Fecal occult blood
Gastric fluid analysis

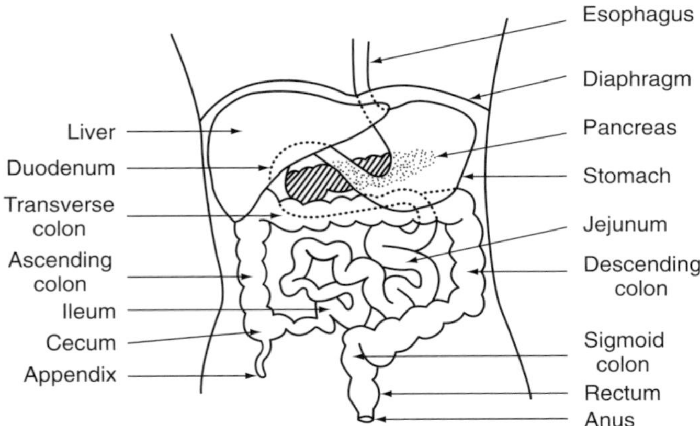

Fig. 35-1 Diagram of gastrointestinal tract.

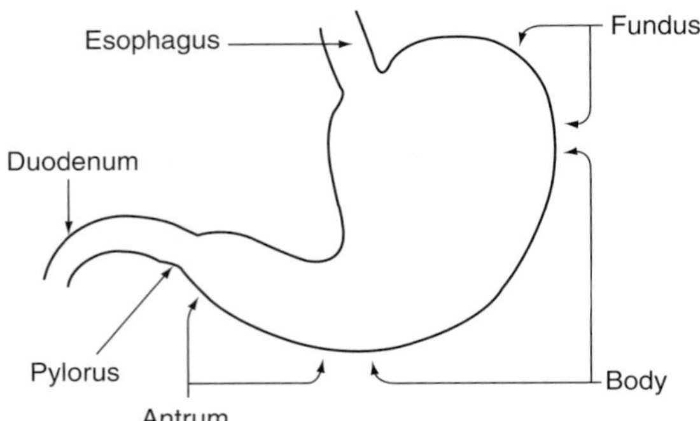

Fig. 35-2 Diagram of stomach.

The gastrointestinal tract is a muscular tube that is lined with epithelial cells and extends 10 m from the mouth to the anus. Along its course, its structure is modified to suit particular requirements for the digestion and absorption of food.

The gastrointestinal tract is an extremely elaborate organ with several structural and functional regions; it serves as both a digestive and an absorptive organ. In addition, the gastrointestinal tract is controlled by an elaborate hormonal and neural regulatory network, and it produces a number of hormones that largely act locally to affect the function of the intestine and other organs (particularly the pancreas and gallbladder) involved in the digestive process. The lower digestive tract contains a large number of microorganisms that coexist with the body without causing disease; in some cases, they serve a symbiotic role in providing nutrients (such as vitamin K) to the body. Changes in the microbial flora or the introduction of unusual microorganisms can lead to disease of the intestinal tract.

SECTION OBJECTIVES BOX 35-1

- Identify the major regions of the intestinal tract.
- For each region, list its major functions.
- Summarize the roles taken by the stomach, pancreas, small intestine, and large intestine in the digestion and absorption of fat, carbohydrate, and protein.

ANATOMY AND FUNCTION

The gastrointestinal tract has seven distinct regions: mouth, esophagus, stomach, duodenum, jejunum, ileum, and large bowel (Fig. 35-1).

The mouth contains teeth, tongue, salivary glands, and an elaborate swallowing mechanism. Ingestion of food stimulates the production of saliva from three pairs of salivary glands: parotid, mandibular, and sublingual. These glands produce viscid, water-based, mucin-containing secretions that act as a lubricant. They also secrete salivary amylase to initiate the digestion of starch and lingual lipase to initiate metabolism of complex lipids. Chewing breaks up food into smaller pieces, increasing the surface area to enhance the action of digestive enzymes. The swallowing mechanism propels food down the esophagus, through the chest cavity, and into the stomach.

The stomach is a rough-surfaced, muscular bag that is coated with a protective mucous layer; it consists of four functional areas (Fig. 35-2). The very top part is known as the *fundus*, and the main portion is known as the *body*. The outlet of the stomach, known as the *antrum*, is segregated from the duodenum by the *pylorus*, which contains a strong, muscular sphincter. The gastric **mucosa** is arranged in numerous coarse folds known as *rugae*. The rugae assist in mixing and breaking down food particles during the churning action of the stomach.

The gastric mucosa contains a number of types of cells with specific functions. Mucous cells, found throughout the stomach, secrete a layer of mucus to protect the mucosa from attack by acid and enzymes. Parietal cells produce hydrochloric acid (HCl) and intrinsic factor. Chief cells produce the proenzyme pepsinogen. These last two cell types are found mainly in the body of the stomach. G-cells in the antrum produce the hormone gastrin.

The sight and smell of food trigger messages from the brain through the vagus nerve to stimulate the production of HCl, both directly and through production of gastrin, which further stimulates HCl production. Distension of the gastric antrum stimulates the production of additional gastrin (Fig. 35-3). Chief cells contain receptors that respond to the acid environment by secreting pepsinogen, which is rapidly converted into its active form (pepsin) at pH 3. These actions convert food into **chyme.**

Chyme enters the duodenum, into which bile and **pancreatic exocrine enzymes** (see Chapter 34) are secreted. Further enzymatic degradation of the basic food materials takes place in the duodenum and continues as food material enters the rest of the small intestine. Through this process, complex macromolecules in food are broken down to amino acids, simple sugars, free fatty acids, and glycerol to allow their absorption by the intestines and ultimate entry into the bloodstream.

The small intestine is 4 m long. Its microvillous substructure increases its absorptive surface area. Along with the duodenum, the small intestine consists of two additional segments (see Fig. 35-1)—the jejunum proximally and the ileum distally, the sites of final digestion and absorption. The nondigestible residual matter enters the large intestine, where

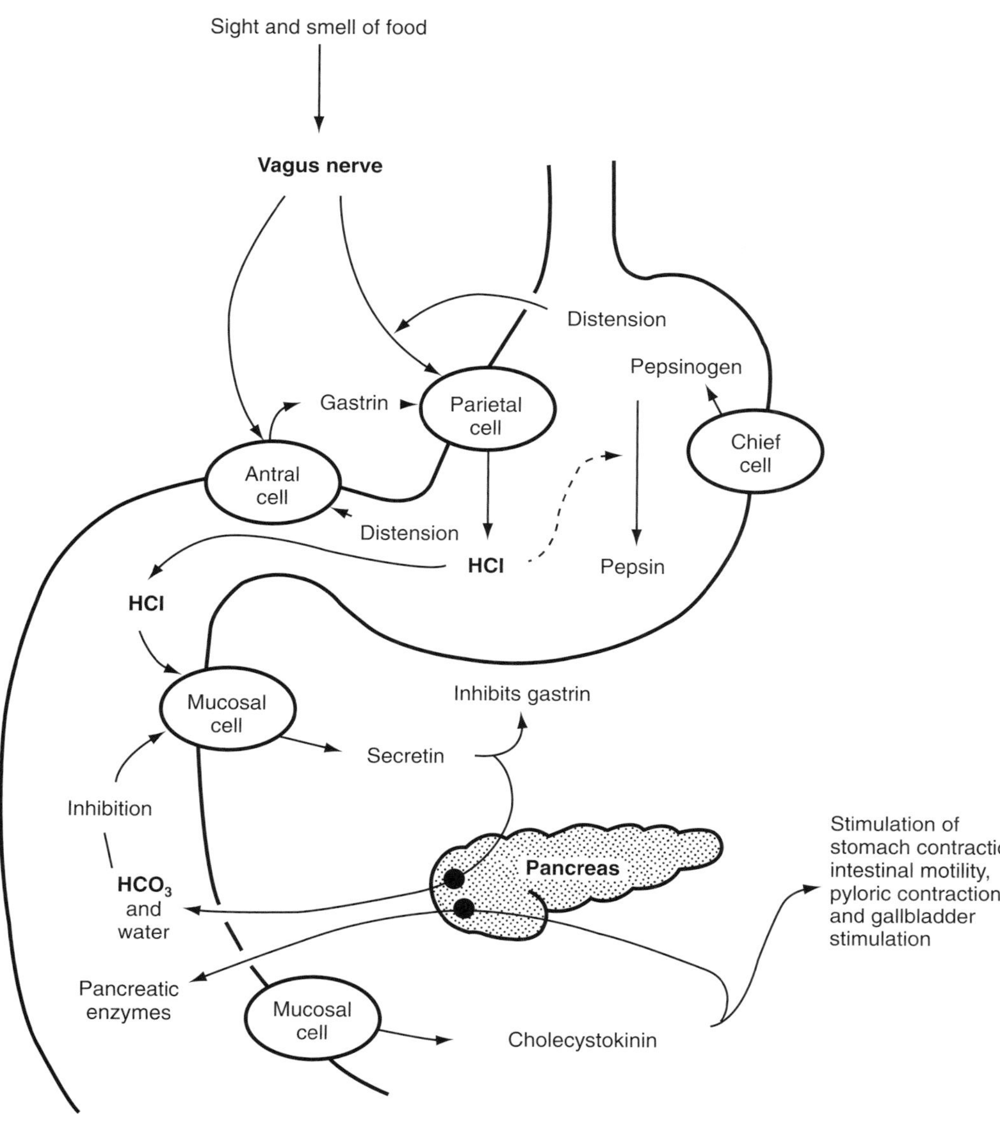

Fig. 35-3 Schema demonstrating various stimuli of stomach and duodenum.

a process of selective water and electrolyte absorption occurs. The digestive process terminates with the formation of feces.

The entire absorptive surface of the gastrointestinal tract is drained by branches of the **portal vein.** These convey the newly absorbed materials directly to the liver so that they may be used immediately. The intestinal tract, from the stomach to the small bowel, also contains many endocrine cells. The peptide hormones produced by these cells are involved in the regulation of gastrointestinal function. In addition, receptors for a significant number of these peptides are present in the central nervous system, while neural impulses control the secretion of many intestinal hormones; these relationships are often termed the **brain-gut axis.**

DIGESTION

Digestion is the chemical process of rendering food into a form that can be absorbed by the body. The digestive process begins in the mouth and generally is completed in the proximal portion of the small intestine. The digestive process for various nutrients is summarized in Table 35-1.

Carbohydrate Digestion

Carbohydrates are present in the diet primarily as complex polysaccharides (starches), but also as monosaccharides and disaccharides (especially sucrose and lactose). Only the polysaccharides and the disaccharides require digestion before their carbohydrate constituents can be absorbed.

Starch is the most common complex polysaccharide. It has a branching structure that is based on 1,4-carbohydrate or 1,6-carbohydrate linkages. Amylase is capable of hydrolyzing the 1,4 linkages in starch into oligosaccharides and ultimately into disaccharides. The dominant disaccharide produced from starch is maltose. Thus, as chyme leaves the duodenum, monosaccharides and disaccharides from the diet and disaccharides produced by the action of amylase are passed to the jejunum and the ileum, where hydrolysis of disaccharides and absorption of monosaccharides take place.

Protein Digestion

Dietary protein is partially degraded in the stomach by hydrochloric acid and pepsin. In the duodenum, trypsin, chymotrypsin, and carboxypeptidase secreted by the pancreas (see Chapter 34) act on the partially degraded protein to yield polypeptides, dipeptides, and amino acids. These tiny molecules then pass into the ileum and jejunum for assimilation.

Fat Digestion

Fat digestion is more complex than digestion of other basic food substances. Most dietary fats are long-chain triglycerides (palmitic, stearic, oleic, and linoleic acids). The stomach decreases the particle size of fatty substances through its churning action. In the duodenum, fats are emulsified by the detergent action of bile salts (synthesized in the liver; see Chapter 31). Emulsification allows the pancreatic enzyme, lipase, in the presence of co-lipase, to attack the otherwise water-insoluble lipids. Lipase causes stepwise hydrolysis, which forms first diglycerides, then monoglycerides, and finally free fatty acids and glycerol.

Table 35-1 Chemical Processes for Digestion of Food

Food Material	Digestive Action	End Product
Starch	Pancreatic amylase	Disaccharides (mainly maltose)
Disaccharides	Mucosal disaccharidases	Monosaccharides
Monosaccharides	None	
Protein	Gastric hydrochloric acid and pepsin	Partial degradation into large polypeptides
	Pancreatic trypsin, chymotrypsin, and carboxypeptidase	Polypeptides, dipeptides, and amino acids
Long-chain triglycerides	Emulsification with bile, hydrolysis by lipase	Fatty acids and glycerol

ABSORPTION

Absorption is the process whereby digested food substances enter the body. The intestinal mucosa is thrown into many fingerlike projections known as *villi* (Fig. 35-4 and see Color Plate 10). Each villus increases the absorptive surface many times. Each surface epithelial cell in the villus is covered by hairlike projections known as **microvilli;** 200 million microvilli are found per centimeter of epithelium. The villous and microvillous structures give the small intestine a massive absorptive surface area of 500 m^2.

Rather than being a purely passive sieve through which food substances are permitted to pass, the intestinal mucosa contains a highly selective mechanism for the absorption of each nutrient. Although there are regional differences in the ability of the intestine to absorb different food substances, these details are not considered here.

Carbohydrate Absorption

The monosaccharides (glucose, galactose, and fructose) are absorbed by specific active-transport mechanisms. Disaccharides are split into monosaccharides by the enzymatic activity of disaccharidases located on the microvilli. For example, the milk sugar, lactose, is split by lactase into glucose and galactose, whereas sucrose (table sugar) is cleaved by sucrase into glucose and fructose. Maltose, the common product of starch hydrolysis, is split by a surface maltase into two molecules of glucose. Lactase deficiency is discussed later in the text.

Protein Absorption

The digested products of protein are small polypeptides, dipeptides, and amino acids. Dipeptides are absorbed more rapidly than amino acids because of special transport mechanisms. Proteins are not absorbed directly. A very large number

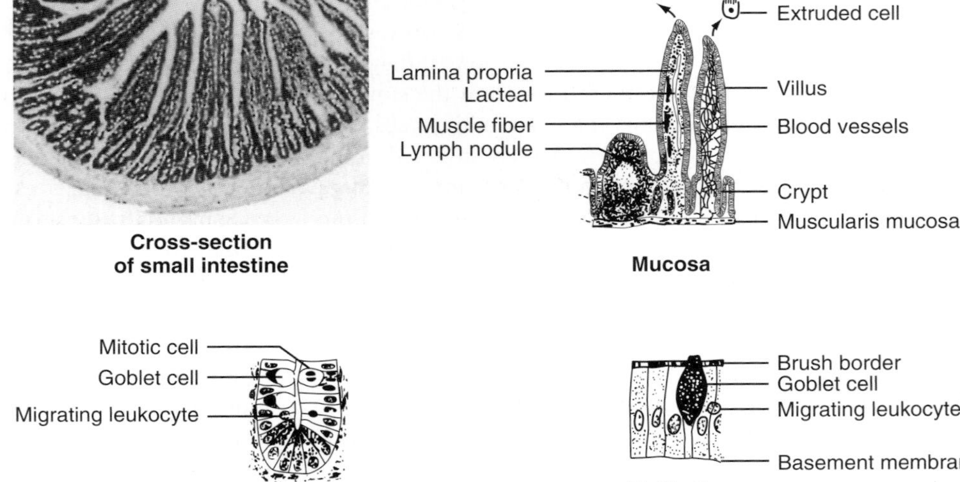

Fig. 35-4 Structures of functional components of small intestine. (From Arey LB: *Human histology: a textbook in outline form*, ed 4, Philadelphia, 1974, Saunders.)

of specific absorptive mechanisms designed for various types of amino acids are located on the mucosal surface.

Fat Absorption (see also Chapter 37)

Successfully digested fat enters the intestine as a **micelle.** By diffusion, fatty acids and monoglycerides enter the intestinal epithelial cells, where they then interact with a binding protein. Long-chain fatty acids of 16 to 18 carbons are reesterified to form triglycerides and then are bound to apolipoprotein B-48 to form chylomicrons, which are released into the lymphatic system before entry into the bloodstream. Medium-chain fatty acids (8 to 10 carbons) are not reesterified and rapidly enter the portal bloodstream bound to albumin. Vitamins D, E, A, and K (see also Chapter 43) are not water soluble and therefore must be absorbed and transported with lipids.

Water and Sodium Absorption

Control over water absorption is not fully understood, but it is believed that bulk flow with sodium absorption is the mode of water transport in the small intestine. Sodium is absorbed by an active-transport mechanism that is linked to the absorption of amino acids, bicarbonate, and glucose. Additional water is absorbed in the large intestine.

Calcium and Iron Absorption

Calcium absorption and iron absorption in the small intestines are highly regulated processes. These processes are described in full detail in Chapters 33 and 39, respectively.

KEY CONCEPTS BOX 35-1

- The mouth breaks up food into small pieces and begins digestion of carbohydrates with amylase. The stomach continues to degrade food and HCL (parietal cells) and pepsin (chief cells) begin to digest proteins.
- Stomach chyme enters the duodenum where pancreatic HCO_3 neutralizes stomach acid and pancreatic enzymes and hepatic bile salt digest proteins and fats to amino acids/dipeptides and fatty acids/glycerol, respectively. Carbohydrates are degraded to monosaccharides and disaccharides.
- Microvilli in the small intestines absorb digested food, usually by specific transport mechanisms. Fatty acids are reesterified and released as chylomicrons.
- Water and electrolytes are absorbed in the large intestines.

SECTION OBJECTIVES BOX 35-2

- List at least four different intestinal tract hormones.
- For each hormone, list its major functions and at least one factor that regulates its production.

HORMONE PHYSIOLOGY

Gut Hormone Structure and Functions

The two main families of gut hormones are the gastrin and secretin families. The gastrin family consists primarily of gastrin and cholecystokinin; in addition, motilin and enkephalin share several structural similarities. The secretin group includes secretin, glucose-dependent insulinotropic polypeptide (GIP), vasoactive intestinal polypeptide (VIP), glucagon, glucagon-like peptide 1 (GLP-1), and bombesin. Many of these hormones are present in multiple forms of varying molecular size.

Gut hormones regulate digestion and absorption; they are released in response to nutrients in the lumen of the gastrointestinal tract and stimulate the release of acid, bicarbonate, and enzymes for the digestion of food. Once nutrients enter the blood, **pancreatic hormones** are released from the islets of Langerhans. Various steps of digestion, absorption, and storage are stimulated and inhibited by different gastroenteropancreatic peptides.

Each gastrointestinal function involves several agonists and antagonists. Final control thus depends on a fine balance of numerous influences. In the case of gastric acid secretion, at least 21 different factors appear important in its normal control. Motilin, gastrin, VIP, and glucagon are the major hormones involved in the control of digestive function in the stomach and intestine. Secretin, cholecystokinin (CCK), VIP, and pancreatic polypeptide (PP) control exocrine pancreatic function; GLP-1 and GIP are involved in regulating insulin and glucagon production. Insulin, glucagon, and somatostatin are primarily involved in the metabolism of carbohydrate, fats, and protein. Substance P, VIP, and the enkephalins have major neurotransmitter involvement in the central, peripheral, and autonomic nervous systems. In addition, a number of other gut hormones have effects on the central nervous system to control nutrient ingestion; GLP-1 inhibits appetite, and ghrelin (a hormone produced by the stomach) stimulates appetite. Only the most important of these hormones are discussed in detail; they are summarized in Table 35-2.

Gastrin

Gastrin exists in multiple molecular forms that contain from 14 to 34 amino acids. The normal cellular origin of gastrin is the gastric G-cell. The main function of gastrin is to stimulate gastric acid secretion; gastrin also stimulates gastric motility and the growth of small bowel mucosa. The secretion of gastrin is mediated by stimuli from the brain, with histamine used as a signal, as well by the presence of various factors in the stomach (gastric distension, amino acids, calcium, and a more alkaline pH than normal). Excess acid inhibits gastrin release, as do a number of hormones, including secretin, glucagon, calcitonin, and somatostatin.

Cholecystokinin (CCK)

CCK is a basic peptide of 33 amino acid residues. CCK is found in the brain and in the K-cells of the upper small intestinal mucosa.

The main physiological role of CCK is the regulation of gallbladder and intestinal motility and pancreatic secretion. Physiological actions of CCK in the pancreas include release of enzymes, potentiation of the action of secretin, and stimulation of growth of the pancreas. A mixture of polypeptides and amino acids is a strong stimulus for the release of CCK.

Table 35-2 Major Intestinal Hormones

Hormone	Number of Amino Acids	Source	Stimulating Factor	Function
Cholecystokinin	33	Mucosa of upper small intestine	Amino acids, fatty acids, hydrochloric acid, and food in duodenum	Stimulates pancreatic enzyme secretion, gallbladder contraction, contraction of stomach and pylorus, intestinal motility
Gastrin	14 to 34	Stomach, gut lumen	Protein digestion products, food in duodenum	Stimulates stomach acid secretion, gastric mobility, gastric mucosal growth
Secretin	27	Throughout gut mucosa but concentrated in duodenum	Acid in duodenum	Stimulates pancreatic secretion of water and bicarbonate, gastric pepsin secretion; relaxes pyloric sphincter
Motilin	22	Upper small intestine	High-fat meal, duodenal acidification	Stimulates motility of small intestines and duodenum
Glucagon	29	Pancreatic and intestinal mucosa	Arginine, alanine, stress	Stimulates gluconeogenesis; raises blood glucose
Gastric inhibitory polypeptide (GIP)	43	Duodenal mucosa	Glucose and fat	Cholecystokinin-like activity
Vasoactive intestinal polypeptide (VIP)	28	Wide distribution throughout gut	Glucose and fat	Vasodilation and hypotensive effects; inhibits histamine, pentagastrin acid release, and pepsin secretion; stimulates electrolyte and water secretion from pancreas; stimulates bile flow
Enteroglucagon (glucagon-like peptides)	29	Lower small intestine	Meal	Inhibits intestinal transit; enhances mucosal growth; stimulates pancreatic secretion and gastrin release

Fatty acids with chains longer than nine carbons also stimulate CCK release.

Secretin

Secretin, the first intestinal hormone to be recognized, is a basic peptide of 27 amino acid residues with strong similarities in sequence to glucagon. Secretin is located predominantly in the S-cells of the mucosa of the duodenum and jejunum. Secretin inhibits smooth muscle contraction, decreases gastric acid secretion, lowers lower esophageal sphincter pressure, and stimulates pancreatic growth. In addition to these effects, it stimulates water and bicarbonate secretion from the pancreas and Brunner's glands. It works together with CCK to stimulate gallbladder contraction and pancreatic enzyme secretion. The primary physiological role of secretin appears to be the modulation of pancreatic bicarbonate secretion.

A principal stimulus for duodenal secretin release is the presence of stomach acid, but in the adult jejunum, there is seldom if ever likely to be sufficient acid to liberate secretin. Fatty acids with 10 or more carbons weakly stimulate duodenal secretin release.

Vasoactive Intestinal Polypeptide

VIP has 28 amino acids and has been shown to be present in both endocrine cells and nerves of the gut and central nervous system. VIP exhibits a wide range of gastrointestinal activities, including inhibition of gastric acid secretion, stimulation of insulin release, stimulation of pancreatic water and bicarbonate secretion, and stimulation of intestinal fluid and electrolyte secretion. Recently, increasing attention has been paid to the role of VIP in immune function.

Glucagon-Like Peptides

Several molecular forms of this family of hormones, which includes pancreatic glucagon, have been identified. The most important of these is glucagon-like peptide 1 (GLP-1), which is produced by L-cells in the intestine and also in the central nervous system. GLP-1 is the most important of the incretins, which are hormones synthesized by the intestinal tract that increase the production of insulin in response to glucose; GLP-1 also decreases appetite. Analogs of GLP-1 now are being used to treat patients with diabetes.

KEY CONCEPTS BOX 35-2

- Most of digestion processes are under the control of hormones produced through out the intestinal tract.
- Gastrin (stomach G-cells) stimulates parietal cell release of HCl while intestinal secretin stimulates pancreatic and gallbladder secretions and inhibits gastrin release.
- Intestinal cholecystokinin stimulates pancreatic release of digestive enzymes and controls intestinal motility. Vasoactive intestinal polypeptide inhibits gastric secretions and stimulates pancreatic electrolyte secretion.
- Many of the intestinal hormones are also produced in the brain.

Box 35-1

Factors Contributing to Ulcers

- Excess acid production (stomach, duodenum)
- Genetic factors (blood group O)
- Decreased mucosal prostaglandin production (caused by nonsteroidal antiinflammatory agents)
- *Helicobacter pylori*
- Stress

SECTION OBJECTIVES BOX 35-3

- Name the factor most commonly involved in causation of ulcers, as well as other stomach conditions that can be caused by this same factor.
- Identify the most common disorders of the intestinal tract by region, and name the laboratory tests that may be helpful in detecting their presence.
- List at least three consequences of malabsorption.

PATHOLOGICAL CONDITIONS

Stomach Diseases

Ulcers

An ulcer results from loss of the normal internal or external surface of the body caused by a variety of factors; in the intestinal tract, mucosal ulcers occur most commonly in the stomach and duodenum, where excess acid action (peptic ulcers) is responsible for most cases. Although a number of conditions can contribute to ulcer development (Box 35-1), *Helicobacter pylori (H. pylori)* infection now is considered to be the direct cause of most cases of chronic gastritis and peptic ulcer; it also increases the risk of development of gastric cancer and primary gastric lymphoma. Ulcers often are suspected in a patient with pain in the upper abdomen, termed *dyspepsia*, that may be improved transiently by eating a meal. Unfortunately, a number of other conditions also can cause dyspepsia. Although definitive diagnosis of an ulcer generally is based on morphological grounds, with roentgenographic and endoscopic examinations of prime importance, an increasing emphasis now is placed on identifying patients with dyspepsia who are infected with *H. pylori* and treating the infection, rather than performing more expensive and invasive imaging procedures.[1] *H. pylori* can survive in the acid environment of the stomach; it attaches to gastric mucosal cells (most strongly in those of blood group O) and causes damage through production of cytotoxins, as well as activation of the host inflammatory response. Eradication of *H. pylori* is associated with reduced symptoms of gastric pain and cure of ulcers. It is interesting to note that only a minority (10% to 20%) of those infected with *H. pylori* actually develop ulcers,[2] suggesting that other factors within individuals determine the likelihood of ulcer development.[3]

Stomach Cancer

The incidence of stomach cancer is declining in the United States, but it remains high in the Soviet Union and in Japan (54% of all cancers). It appears most often in the seventh and eighth decades of life, and 5-year survival remains at 15%. More than half of all gastric cancers are found in the pylorus or the antrum. *H. pylori* infections of the stomach are associated with an approximately sixfold increase in the incidence of gastric cancer, and most cases of gastric cancer are associated with *H. pylori* infection. Although tumor markers are of no use in initial diagnosis, many gastric carcinomas produce carcinoembryonic antigen (CEA) and CA 19-9, which may be useful for monitoring response to treatment.

Zollinger-Ellison Syndrome

The Zollinger-Ellison syndrome is an extreme form of peptic ulcer disease that is caused most commonly by a gastrin-secreting tumor of the pancreas or duodenum (most, a gastrinoma) or rarely by G-cell hyperplasia. The unrelenting gastrin release stimulates hypersecretion of hydrochloric acid by the stomach. The typical clinical presentation (not seen in all patients) is recurrent peptic ulceration, often accompanied by diarrhea. Seventy-five percent of patients with this syndrome have ulcers in the duodenal bulb or in the immediate postbulbar area.

Gastrin-secreting tumors are often very small and can be difficult to identify. Sixty percent of pancreatic (but only 10% of duodenal) tumors metastasize, and multiple tumors are common. The excess secretion of hydrochloric acid accounts for most of the clinical manifestations of the syndrome. The large amount of gastric acid that enters the duodenum interferes with fat digestion and leads to steatorrhea. Because gastrin also inhibits salt and water absorption by the intestine, diarrhea occurs in 50% of patients. The very large volumes of gastric contents that are presented to the intestine enhance the diarrhea. Prolonged secretion of gastrin causes hypertrophy of the stomach, with parietal cell hyperplasia. Often, more distal parts of the intestine also become ulcerated. The Zollinger-Ellison syndrome is associated with hyperparathyroidism in 20% of patients. Other endocrine abnormalities that appear less commonly include pituitary, adrenal, ovarian, and thyroid tumors. This cluster of endocrine adenomas and carcinomas is known as the multiple endocrine neoplasia (MEN) syndrome I. It may occur with autosomal dominant inheritance, as was described originally by Werner, or it may occur sporadically. This syndrome, whch results from mutations in the MEN 1 tumor suppressor gene, located on the long arm of chromosome 11, manifests from the second decade to old age with an equal sex distribution. The areas involved in order of frequency are parathyroids (88%), pancreatic islets (81%), anterior pituitary (65%), adrenal cortex (38%), and thyroid follicular cells (19%).[4]

A fasting serum gastrin concentration four times the upper limit of normal in the absence of **achlorhydria** or renal failure is strongly suggestive of the Zollinger-Ellison syndrome. This criterion is not met in 40% of cases. Because marked elevation of gastrin also can occur with achlorhydria (as occurs with atrophic gastritis), it is important before proceeding further to document that a patient actually is producing excess gastric acid.

Provocative testing has been used for diagnosis of the Zollinger-Ellison syndrome. Serum gastrin can be measured after administration of (1) intravenous secretin, 1 to 2 U/kg (as an intravenous bolus); (2) intravenous calcium gluconate; or (3) a standard meal. When secretin is administered, serum gastrin is collected at 2, 5, 10, 15, 30, and 60 minutes. A post-secretin increase of gastrin of ≥110 pg/mL is the most reliable criterion for Zollinger-Ellison syndrome, because secretin responses of this magnitude typically do not occur with antral G-cell hyperplasia or other causes of hypergastrinemia. The sensitivity of the test is 95%, and the specificity is virtually 100%.

Pernicious Anemia and other Causes of Vitamin B_{12} Malabsorption

Vitamin B_{12}, which is an essential nutrient that is required for normal synthesis of myelin and nucleic acids (see Chapter 43), is absorbed in a complex series of steps. After liberation from food in the stomach, vitamin B_{12} becomes bound nonspecifically to proteins termed *R-binders*. In the duodenum, pancreatic proteases degrade R-binders but cannot digest the specific vitamin B_{12} binding protein, intrinsic factor (produced by gastric parietal cells). In the terminal ileum, receptors bind the intrinsic factor–vitamin B_{12} complex, leading to absorption of vitamin B_{12}.

Pernicious anemia is a disease that consists of gastric achlorhydria, gastric atrophy, and failure to secrete intrinsic factor. It is caused by autoimmune destruction of gastric mucosa (particularly parietal cells), often associated with antibodies to parietal cells (a nonspecific finding) and intrinsic factor–blocking antibodies (specific, but seen in only 50% to 70% of cases). The intrinsic factor deficiency prevents absorption of vitamin B_{12}. This leads to damage to the posterior columns of the spinal cord (causing a sensory neuropathy) and, in many cases, megaloblastic anemia. Pernicious anemia is covered in greater detail in Chapter 43.

Small Intestine Diseases

Malabsorption Syndromes

Malnutrition is caused by an inadequate supply of nutrients to the body; the clinical consequences and laboratory manifestations of malnutrition are covered in Chapter 41. Malabsorption results from diseases of the gastrointestinal tract that, by affecting digestion or absorption of nutrients, cause malnutrition. Clinical features of malabsorption syndromes commonly include loose stools, typically containing fat that gives a greasy appearance and a foul odor to the stools (steatorrhea); loss of weight or failure to gain weight (in children); and features caused by deficiencies of fat-soluble vitamins (bone disease, prolonged clotting times, poor night vision, neuropathy). It is important to distinguish steatorrhea (which indicates malabsorption) from other causes of diarrhea.

In true malabsorption, the gastrointestinal tract is impaired so that it cannot absorb a variety of nutrients; this generally is the result of a disorder that causes damage to the intestinal mucosa. Common causes of intestinal injury are celiac disease and Crohn's disease, both of which are discussed in detail later, along with extensive removal of the small bowel for disease. The other category of malabsorption syndrome in fact should be called *maldigestion*, in which the digestive process is in some way impaired. This is caused most commonly by pancreatic insufficiency (see Chapter 34) but also may occur with inadequate pancreatic enzyme activation in severe achlorhydria or with excessive acid production (see ulcers and Zollinger-Ellison syndrome described earlier) or inadequate bile acid production or secretion with cholestatic disorders (see Chapter 31).

A variety of serum tests may be abnormal in patients with malabsorption syndromes, including anemia, increased prothrombin time, and decreases in serum iron, vitamin B_{12}, albumin, calcium, and phosphorus. Immunoglobulin determinations can be useful for ruling out immune globulin (Ig)A deficiency, a condition that is associated with overgrowth of certain parasites (such as *Giardia*) and celiac disease (discussed later). In persons suspected of malabsorption syndromes, laboratory tests can be useful in confirming its presence and in distinguishing true malabsorption from maldigestion.

Celiac Disease (Celiac Sprue)

Celiac disease is one of the most common intestinal disorders and a common cause of malabsorption in children; most estimate its prevalence as 1% of adults in much of the world, although many are not aware that they have the disease.[5] This autoimmune condition involves an abnormal immunological response to the proteins in **gluten,** which is found principally in wheat, but also in barley and rye in the diet. Ingestion of **gliadin,** an alcohol-soluble protein in gluten, leads to inflammation of the intestine and loss of both villi and microvilli, drastically reducing the absorptive surface area and causing malabsorption. **Tissue transglutaminase,** which removes amide linkages from gliadin, increasing their propensity to cause damage, is also a target of immune attack. The incidence of intestinal lymphoma also is increased in individuals affected by celiac disease, as is the incidence of other autoimmune disorders, particularly those involving the endocrine system. Celiac disease may manifest in very subtle ways such as iron deficiency anemia or osteoporosis; it may be diagnosed definitively in such cases only by the response to a gluten-free diet.

The diagnosis of celiac disease has been based classically on intestinal biopsy that shows the loss of villi, followed by improvement in symptoms when a gluten-free diet is introduced. Close to 100% of those with active celiac disease diagnosed in this fashion have serum antibodies (usually of the IgA type) to gliadin, especially deamidated gliadin,[6] and/or antibodies to tissue transglutaminase.[7] One complicating factor is that up to 3% of those with celiac disease have IgA deficiency, a condition otherwise found in less than 0.5% of the population; those with both celiac disease and IgA deficiency will not have IgA antibodies to tissue transglutaminase or gliadin, only the less specific IgG antibodies. With removal of gluten from the diet, antibody titers typically decline and may fall below the limits of detection; antibodies may not be detectable in mild forms of the disease. A fall in antibody titer can be used to evaluate compliance with a gluten-free diet, which is the treatment for the disease.[7]

Lactose Intolerance and Other Carbohydrate Malabsorption Disorders

The most common isolated carbohydrate malabsorption disorder is lactose intolerance. All infants have the intestinal enzyme lactase, which is necessary to break the milk disaccharide, lactose, into glucose and galactose, thereby allowing their absorption. In those population groups who continue to ingest milk throughout life, mainly those of European ancestry, intestinal lactase persists into adulthood. However, in about 70% of the world's population, lactase production in the intestine diminishes markedly after the first few years of life.[8] If persons who lack lactase ingest milk or milk products, they may fail to split the lactose. The unabsorbed sugar creates an osmotic force that pulls fluid into the intestinal lumen, causing cramping, bloating sensations, and diarrhea. Moreover, large bowel bacteria can metabolize the sugar to produce gas. It is interesting to note, however, that not all who have lactase deficiency have symptoms of lactose intolerance. Although most people with lactose intolerance are aware of their problem and avoid milk products, persons with milder forms experience discomfort in much more subtle ways. In infants, transient lactase deficiency can occur after episodes of gastroenteritis, producing similar symptoms; lactase activity typically becomes normal in less than 2 weeks. The diagnosis of lactose malabsorption can be made by using the lactose tolerance procedures discussed later in the chapter, but this step is usually unnecessary, and the sensitivity of the test for lactase deficiency is low.[8] Malabsorption syndromes of other disaccharides have been reported but are extremely rare. Malabsorption of monosaccharides is seen only in extreme impairment of the mucosal surface.

Carcinoid Syndrome

A syndrome that manifests as vascular flushing, diarrhea, occasional tricuspid valve insufficiency, and, rarely, pellagra associated with an intestinal **carcinoid** tumor is called the *carcinoid syndrome*. Carcinoid tumors are growths of endocrine cells, usually arising in the intestinal tract but sometimes in the lungs or gonads, that are slowly growing tumors capable of metastasis to other parts of the body.[9] In the intestine, these are most common in the distal ileum or appendix. These tumors metastasize most commonly to the regional lymph nodes, liver, and skeleton. Primary carcinoid tumors of the appendix are common but rarely metastasize, whereas those that arise from other parts of the gastrointestinal tract are less common but do metastasize. Carcinoid tumors of the small bowel produce serotonin and kinins in vast excess; these are responsible for the characteristic clinical syndrome. Chromogranin, a marker of neuroendocrine cells, is elevated in a high percentage of persons with carcinoid syndrome and a number of other neuroendocrine tumors.[10]

The presence of the disorder can be detected by measuring serotonin or its metabolite 5-hydroxy-indoleacetic acid (5-HIAA). Serotonin is formed by the conversion of tryptophan to 5-hydroxytryptamine (serotonin), which ultimately is converted to 5-HIAA. The amount of 5-HIAA found in the urine is highly method dependent. Many screening procedures are very nonspecific and therefore should not be used to make diagnoses. An appropriate approach is the use of a screening procedure for all requests for 5-HIAA values; those that exhibit an elevated value should be subjected to a more specific test.

In healthy adults, up to 6 mg (31.2 mmol) of 5-HIAA is excreted per 24 hours. In the carcinoid syndrome, results are usually between 25 and 1000 mg (130 and 5200 mmol) per day. False-negative and false-positive results are produced by many drugs and food substances, as summarized in a recent review article.[11] Reduced urinary excretion of 5-HIAA is seen in renal disease and in phenylketonuria. False-positive results have been reported in celiac disease, intestinal obstruction, pregnancy, and sleep deprivation.

Large Intestine Diseases

Diarrhea

Diarrhea is defined as the excessive production of feces, usually as a result of overabundance of water in the stool. Severe diarrhea causes sodium and water depletion and loss of potassium and bicarbonate. Three main mechanisms for diarrhea are known: solute malabsorption, secretion of fluid into the intestine, and motility disturbance.

Solute malabsorption is caused most commonly by the ingestion of poorly absorbed substances, such as some laxatives and magnesium compounds, or by intestinal malabsorption (see above). Secretion of fluid occurs in many conditions. Passive secretion occurs if obstruction or inflammation increases epithelial permeability. Secretion of ions (with water) occurs through the activity of 3′,5′-cyclic adenosine monophosphate, as stimulated by cholera toxin, endotoxin, prostaglandins, bile acids, and certain hormones, such as VIP. Laxatives and irritable bowel syndrome can cause motility disturbances. These will increase motility and decrease transit time, as well as absorptive efficiency.

At high serum levels, VIP causes vasodilation with facial flushing and increased intestinal blood flow, inducing watery diarrhea and inhibiting gastric secretion. The diarrhea, which is explosive and consists of up to 30 stools per day, causes profound hypokalemia (1 to 3 mmol/L). Diarrhea caused by VIP is called the *Verner-Morrison syndrome*,[12] but it also is sometimes called the *WDHA syndrome* after the initial letters of its main characteristics: *w*atery *d*iarrhea, *h*ypokalemia, and *h*ypochlorhydria or *a*chlorhydria. The syndrome is rare, about one-tenth as common as Zollinger-Ellison syndrome. It sometimes occurs as part of the multiple endocrine neoplasia syndromes (see p. 670).[1] In patients with Verner-Morrison syndrome, a non-β islet cell tumor (VIPoma) of the pancreas is usually present; about half of these tumors are malignant. VIP-secreting tumors such as small cell carcinoma or retroperitoneal neuroblastoma may occur elsewhere. The diagnosis is suspected by elimination of common causes of watery diarrhea and hypokalemia, and is confirmed by elevated blood levels of VIP.

Colorectal Cancer

Malignancies of the colon and rectum account for more than half the cancers of the entire gastrointestinal system; they are the third most common cause of cancer death in both men and women. Early detection through screening is the most effective approach to curing this often fatal disorder. Many organizations have recommended routine screening for colorectal cancer through one of two major approaches.[13] Direct imaging of the entire large bowel by colonoscopy is considered the "gold standard" and needs to be done only once every 10 years if no premalignant polyps of the colon are found. Annual screening of stool for the presence of occult blood, along with performance of colonoscopy if a positive result is found, is another approved alternative. Screening stool for the presence of DNA mutations,[14] has recently been endorsed in screening guidelines.[13]

Inflammatory Bowel Disease

Two idiopathic, probably autoimmune, inflammatory disorders of the intestinal tract—ulcerative colitis and Crohn's disease—may present with signs and symptoms such as abdominal pain, diarrhea, and (in the case of Crohn's disease) malabsorption. The exact pathogenesis of these disorders is unknown, but evidence of familial predisposition and autoimmune phenomena has been found in many cases. Characteristically, Crohn's disease affects the small intestine (although it may involve the colon as well as other parts of the intestinal tract), and ulcerative colitis is limited to the large intestine, but in some cases, it is not possible to distinguish these two disorders clinically or through pathologic examination of samples. Autoantibodies can be found in about half of patients with each disorder.[15] In ulcerative colitis, atypical perinuclear antineutrophil cytoplasmic antibodies are present, whereas in Crohn's disease, antibodies to *Saccharomyces cerevisiae* are found. The specificity of these autoantibodies is about 90% to 95% for each disorder.

KEY CONCEPTS BOX 35-3

- Ulcers, caused by over-production of stomach HCl, are most commonly caused by the presence of *H. pylori* in the stomach mucosa. Uncontrolled production of gastrin (Zollinger-Ellison syndrome) also will cause ulcers.
- Inability to properly digest food (maldigestion) or absorb digested material (malabsorption) can both be seen in malabsorption syndromes. Maldigestion is usually caused by pancreatic dysfunction or overproduction of stomach acid. Malabsorption is usually caused by pathological changes to the intestinal mucosa (celiac disease, Crohn's disease; both autoimmune disorders).
- Malabsorption syndromes can affect the ability of the large intestines to reabsorb water, leading to diarrhea. Diarrhea can also be caused by hypersecretion into the large intestines (excess VIP).

SECTION OBJECTIVES BOX 35-4

- Describe the advantages and disadvantages of commonly used tests for *Helicobacter pylori.*
- List the function tests commonly used to evaluate malabsorption and diarrhea, and explain how their use helps in the differential diagnosis of causes of these conditions.

GASTROINTESTINAL FUNCTION TESTS

Helicobacter pylori Diagnostic Tests

A number of tests are available for determination of exposure to or infection by *H. pylori.*[16] The most widely employed have been serological tests that detect antibodies to *H. pylori;* these are relatively sensitive but nonspecific, and cannot be used to evaluate the effectiveness of treatment because they remain positive for years. Because *H. pylori* produces the enzyme urease, a number of tests have been developed to detect the presence of urease activity in the stomach. The most widely used is the urea breath test, in which the individual ingests a test meal that contains carbon-13– or carbon-14–labeled urea. Urease releases CO_2, and the amount of labeled CO_2 in breath is directly related to urease activity. The sensitivity and specificity of urea breath tests are around 99% in untreated patients; treatment with proton pump inhibitors such as lansoprazole markedly reduces test sensitivity. Recently, a stool test for an *H. pylori* antigen has become available for the detection of *H. pylori;* its sensitivity and specificity are similar to those of urea breath tests. With successful eradication of *H. pylori*, the antigen test remains positive for a short period but becomes negative within 4 to 6 weeks.

If endoscopy is performed, a number of additional methods are available to detect *H. pylori*. Urease activity can be detected through gastric biopsy; the most widely used method is the *Campylobacter*-like organism (CLO) test, in which a small fragment of gastric tissue is incubated with urea and a pH indicator. Direct examination of histological sections is also available. Culture and nucleic acid amplification techniques can be used; culture is becoming more important in detecting antibiotic resistance in those individuals who do not respond to therapy. In patients who have actively bleeding ulcers, tests done on biopsy tissue become less sensitive, as do stool antigen tests; however, urea breath tests seem to remain accurate.[17]

Fat Absorption Tests (see Evolve)

The definitive test of fat absorption is the quantitative measurement of fat in timed collections of feces obtained while the patient is maintained on a diet that contains an approximately known amount of fat. Because collection is extremely difficult for the patient, a variety of alternative approaches have been promoted. Unfortunately, none of these entirely replaces the diagnostic ability of quantitative fecal fat measurement.

Fat Screening

Fat screening is carried out first by evaluation of the weight and appearance of the stool. A pale, frothy appearance is virtually diagnostic of excessive fat. More reliable than this is the application of a small amount of fecal material onto a standard microscopic slide, followed by staining with a fat-specific stain. Trained observers are able to identify excessive fat in 80% to 90% of persons with fat malabsorption. Using quantitative microscopy (including grading size and number of fat droplets) improves the sensitivity and specificity of fecal fat stains.[18] Another screening procedure is the steatocrit, in which the percentage of fat is quantified in a random stool sample; this correlates reasonably well with quantitative fecal fat determination.

Quantitative fecal fat estimation is performed after collection of feces for 3 consecutive days. In the 2 days preceding the collection and during the period of collection, patients must include approximately 100 g of medium-chain triglycerides in their diet. The actual amount of fat in the diet can be difficult to determine, even for a dietitian; however, within the range of fat intakes from about 60 to 200 g, normal fecal fat excretion is less than 7 g per day. Quantitative fecal fat measurements are unreliable in patients without diarrhea (defined as stool output >200 g per day). The nonabsorbable fat substitute Olestra is also measured as fat in quantitative measurements[19]; individuals who collect stool fat specimens should be instructed to discontinue use of products that contain this compound for 72 hours before they start a fecal fat collection.

Feces can be collected in plastic bags, which then may be closed with a tin tie and held in a preweighed, 5-gallon paint can. On arrival in the laboratory, the can and contents are weighed, and the weight of the collection is determined. Chemical analysis then is carried out on a thoroughly mixed aliquot of this 3-day collection. Persons who consume a 100 g fat diet will excrete no more than 5 g of fecal fat per day. Excretion of more than 10 g per day is certain evidence of fat malabsorption. Failure to adhere to the diet may invalidate the results; low fat intake will mask minimum fat malabsorption, whereas grossly excessive fat intake will raise the fecal fat content to above 5 g.

D-Xylose Absorption Test (see Methods on Evolve)

D-Xylose is an aldopentose that is absorbed passively in the small intestine; its successful absorption is a reflection of the integrity of the surface area of the small intestine. Once D-xylose is absorbed, at least 50% is excreted in the urine within the next 24 hours. The amount excreted over a 5-hour period is closely correlated with the amount absorbed in the gastrointestinal tract.

The patient is instructed to fast overnight but is encouraged to drink an ample amount of water during this time. Two doses have been advocated; most authors suggest that 25 g of D-xylose dissolved in approximately 300 to 500 mL of water is a suitable dose for adults, but a 5 g dose appears adequate and is less likely to cause abdominal cramps. Smaller subjects are given 1 g/kg of body weight to a maximum of 25 g. After administration, urine is collected over a 5-hour period. At least 25% of the administered dose will appear in the urine over a 5-hour period if renal function is within the reference interval. For children who cannot be relied on to collect a urinary sample, or for subjects with severe renal insufficiency, blood collections at 1 and 2 hours may be substituted. Most persons demonstrate plasma levels greater than 300 mg/L in one of the samples. In children, values above 100 mg/L should be considered within the reference interval.

Low levels of urine or plasma xylose are suggestive of an absorptive defect in the jejunum. Low levels are also seen in ascites, vomiting, delayed gastric emptying, improper urine collection, and high-dose aspirin therapy, and with neomycin, colchicine, indomethacin, atropine, and impaired renal function. Values within the reference interval are seen in persons who have absorptive defects that occur in a skip pattern (such as Crohn's disease). Such a disease distribution allows a sufficient amount of healthy mucosa to remain and absorb an amount of D-xylose within the usual interval.

Lactose Tolerance Test

In this test, 50 g of lactose dissolved in water is administered orally to the patient, who is observed carefully for the onset of symptoms. The standard protocol includes the collection of a baseline specimen and 5-, 10-, 30-, 60-, 90-, and 120-minute specimens for plasma glucose measurements. Glucose levels will be increased if lactose has been cleaved successfully and its components absorbed. The galactose moiety of the lactose is converted quickly into glucose by the liver. Healthy persons will demonstrate a glucose rise to greater than 200 mg/dL (11.1 mmol/L) over the baseline sample. Those with lactase deficiency will exhibit notable abdominal discomfort and will have a peak plasma glucose of less than 100 mg/dL (5.5 mmol/L).

An alternate method of determining lactose absorption involves measuring the amount of hydrogen that appears in exhaled breath after oral administration of lactose. Lactase-deficient persons will not absorb lactose, and it will find its way into the large bowel, where bacteria will metabolize it. Hydrogen, one of the by-products of this bacterial action, passes quickly into the bloodstream and is removed in the exhaled breath. Special-purpose gas chromatographs can detect the presence of post-lactose hydrogen. A healthy person allows no lactose to enter the colon and therefore has less than 10 parts per million (ppm) of hydrogen in the exhaled breath. Persons with lactase deficiency demonstrate at least 50 ppm of hydrogen. Intermediate amounts of hydrogen in the breath can be caused by large doses of lactose and are of questionable significance. The definitive diagnosis is made by tissue enzyme assays that are carried out on biopsy samples of the intestinal mucosa.

KEY CONCEPTS BOX 35-4

- Measurement of antibodies to *H. pylori* for evaluation ulcers is sensitive but nonspecific and cannot be used to evaluate effectiveness of treatment. The urea breath tests have 99% sensitivity and specificity in untreated patients but treatment reduces test sensitivity. A stool test for an *H. pylori* antigen also has ~99% sensitivity and specificity
- Fecal fat excretion, an important test to evaluate malabsorption, can be performed as a screening test by counting stained fecal fat droplets or as a quantitative test on a 72-hour stool collection.
- The urine or plasma D-xylose test can differentiate between malabsorption and diarrhea caused by pancreatic (normal results) or intestinal (abnormal result) disease.
- The lactose intolerance test diagnoses suspected lactase deficiency. An abnormal increase in serum glucose following a lactose challenge is evidence of a lactase deficiency. Alternatively, the hydrogen breath test can be used, but is technically more difficult to perform and less available.

SECTION OBJECTIVES BOX 35-5

- List the tests used to test for malabsorption syndrome and diarrhea.
- Describe how occult blood in stool is measured, and explain the pitfalls of such testing.

CHANGE OF ANALYTE IN DISEASE (Table 35-3)

Malabsorption Testing

Screening Approach

Screening for malabsorption syndromes is best done by using clinical signs and symptoms associated with malabsorption and by investigating populations at high risk. For example, elderly persons are at greatest risk for occult malabsorption. Laboratory screening for malabsorption is not very sensitive; however, measurement of serum albumin, calcium, and vitamin B_{12}, combined with a peripheral smear to look for evidence of macrocytosis and iron deficiency anemia, constitutes a reasonable general laboratory screen for malabsorption. If necessary, more specific tests for iron deficiency can be carried out. Persons believed to have specific malabsorption syndromes should be tested accordingly. Those with steatorrhea and suspected fat malabsorption first should have their feces examined visually. Next, a rapid slide evaluation of a stool sample should be carried out, to look for meat fibers and excessive fat. A D-xylose absorption test (see earlier discussion) will indicate whether significant absorptive problems are present. Protein malabsorption is difficult to assess biochemically, and only when amino acid malabsorption is serious will serum albumin be depressed. Measurements to evaluate for pancreatic insufficiency as a cause of maldigestion and malabsorption are discussed in Chapter 34.

Evaluation of Diarrhea

In persons with acute onset of diarrhea, laboratory tests (other than culture and gram stain for fecal leukocytes) usually are not required or indicated, because most acute diarrhea will resolve with or without treatment. With persistent diarrhea, infectious and inflammatory causes are still common; examination of the stool for ova and parasites (especially *Giardia*), examination of the stool for leukocytes (for infectious and inflammatory processes), and testing for blood (often present in inflammatory bowel disease and some infections) are helpful initial tests. In those without positive findings on these tests, laboratory tests can be helpful in distinguishing secretory diarrhea from that resulting from the presence of osmotically active substances (as also occurs in those who have malabsorption). Normally, most of the stool solute is composed of electrolytes, and normal stool osmolality is approximately 290 mOsm/kg. Measurement of stool electrolytes in liquid stools (after centrifugation) can be used to calculate an osmotic gap, defined as the difference between normal stool osmolality (290) and stool electrolytes (two times the sum of Na^+ and K^+ concentrations in mmol/L). Measurement of actual stool osmolality, although theoretically more accurate in calculating osmotic gap, is limited by the rise in stool osmolality that occurs because of bacterial metabolism of undigested solutes after sample collection. A normal stool osmotic gap (<50 mmol/L) indicates the presence of increased water and electrolytes in normal balance, caused by secretory diarrhea or abnormal motility. An increased osmotic gap indicates the presence of unabsorbed solutes, as can be found with malabsorption and with ingestion of nonabsorbable solutes such as magnesium salts. Alkalinization of a stool sample and inspection for the pink color of phenolphthalein can be used to detect occult ingestion of this laxative.

Occult Blood in Stool

A number of methods are available to detect trace amounts of hemoglobin in feces. Most rely on the ability of hemoglobin and its derivatives to act as peroxidases and catalyze the reaction between hydrogen peroxide and a chromogenic, organic compound. Benzidine has been used but is carcinogenic and therefore is not currently available; most commercial assays employ guaiac. A number of immunochemical tests to detect hemoglobin directly are also available; these are more specific and sensitive than guaiac-based tests.[20] Immunochemical tests produce false-negative results if stool is exposed to toilet bowl sanitizers. With peroxidase-based tests, a number of dietary substances, including iron and peroxidases found in red meat and various plants, are capable of producing false-positive results. Most kit manufacturers and practice guidelines suggest putting the patient on a diet in which red meat is withheld for several days before the time

Table 35-3 Change of Analyte and Function Tests in Disease

Condition	Fecal Fat	B_{12} Folate	D-Xylose Absorption	Stool Occult Blood	CEA	5-HIAA	Stool Examination
Pancreatic insufficiency	↑↑	N, ↓ B_{12} N folate	N	Neg	N	N	Foul smelling, greasy
Celiac disease	N, ↑	N B_{12} N, ↓ folate	AB	Neg	N	N	Variable
Carcinoid syndrome	N	N	N	Neg, pos	N	↑↑	Loose, in association with cutaneous flushing
Functional diarrhea	N	N	N	Neg	N	N	Loose
Bowel carcinoma	N	N	N	Neg, pos	N, ↑	N	Change in bowel habits
Inflammatory bowel disease	N, may be ↑ with Crohn's	N, may be ↑ with Crohn's	N	Neg, pos	N, ↑	N	Loose, bloody

AB, Abnormal; *N*, normal (within reference interval); *Neg*, negative; *pos*, positive; *S*, serum; ↑, increased; ↓, decreased.

of collection, but this may not be necessary to prevent false-positive results. Allowing samples to stand for 2 to 3 days (as occurs with mailing of completed collection cards to the laboratory) reduces the rate of false-positives derived from plant peroxidases and may reduce interference from other food peroxidases as well. Rehydration of dried stool samples before testing reduces the rate of false-negative results but increases the rate of false-positive results as well, and is not currently recommended.

Carcinoembryonic Antigen

Carcinoembryonic antigen (CEA), which also is discussed in Chapter 53, is a glycoprotein that is abundant in fetal entodermally derived tissues (gastrointestinal mucosa, pancreas, lung). CEA is not a single chemical compound; numerous glycoproteins, including fetal sulfoglycoprotein, normal colonic antigen, and normal glycoprotein, cross-react in CEA assays. CEA is produced in a variety of tumors, including most tumors of the GI tract, but especially in colon cancer. Serum CEA levels are related to tumor mass; CEA is elevated in less than one fourth of localized tumors, preventing its use in screening for colon cancer. CEA is most useful in monitoring the course of disease in persons who have been treated for colon cancer. CEA should be measured at the time of surgery for establishment of a baseline level, and it should be checked again starting at least 1 month after surgery. Persistent elevations and increases after surgery indicate residual and metastatic disease, respectively. The reference interval for CEA is typically 0 to 5 ng/mL. Higher values occur in liver disease, inflammatory bowel disease, heavy smoking, and chronic renal failure, but levels above 10 to 15 ng/mL are rare in these conditions. Immunoassays for CEA are not interchangeable; patients who are being followed for colon cancer should have levels checked by old and new assays in parallel (re-baselining) before the laboratory switches to a new CEA method.

KEY CONCEPTS BOX 35-5

- Initial testing for malabsorption syndromes should include routine tests for malnutrition such as serum albumin, calcium, and vitamin B_{12}, combined with a peripheral smear to look for evidence of macrocytosis and iron deficiency anemia. Follow-up tests can include fecal fat analysis, and the D-xylose absorption test to differentiate between pancreatic and intestinal disease.
- Investigation of persistent diarrhea should include examination of the stool for ova and parasites, examination of the stool for leukocytes (for infectious and inflammatory processes), and testing for blood. Measuring the fecal osmolar gap can help differentiate secretory diarrhea from the presence of osmotically active substances.
- Measuring hemoglobin by its enzymatic activity is the most common method for detecting fecal blood. False positives can result form the presence of food-derived iron and peroxidases.

REFERENCES

1. Talley N, Vakil N, Practice Parameters Committee of the American College of Gastroenterology: Guidelines for the management of dyspepsia, Am J Gastroenterol 100:2324, 2005.
2. Makola D, Peura D, Crowe S: *Helicobacter pylori* infection and related gastrointestinal diseases, J Clin Gastroenterol 41:548, 2007.
3. Amieva M, El-Omar E: Host-bacterial interactions in *Helicobacter pylori* infection, Gastroenterology 134:306, 2008.
4. Gibril F, Schumann M, Pace A, et al: Multiple endocrine neoplasia type 1 and Zollinger-Ellison syndrome: a prospective study of 107 cases and comparison with 1009 cases from the literature, Medicine (Baltimore) 83:43, 2004.
5. Green P, Cellier C: Celiac disease, N Engl J Med 357:1731, 2007.
6. Niveloni S, Sugai E, Cabanne A, et al: Antibodies against synthetic deamidated gliadin peptides as predictors of celiac disease: prospective assessment in an adult population with a high pretest probability of disease, Clin Chem 53:2186, 2007.

7. Agardh D: Antibodies against synthetic deamidated gliadin peptides and tissue transglutaminase for the identification of childhood celiac disease, Clin Gastroenterol Hepatol 5:1276, 2007.
8. Lomer M, Parkes G, Sanderson J: Review article: lactose intolerance in clinical practice—myths and realities, Aliment Pharmacol Ther 27:93, 2008.
9. Raut C, Kulke M, Glickman J, et al: Carcinoid tumors, Curr Probl Surg 43:383, 2006.
10. Syversen U, Ramstad H, Gamme K, et al: Clinical significance of elevated serum chromogranin A levels, Scand J Gastroenterol 39:969, 2004.
11. de Herder W: Biochemistry of neuroendocrine tumours, Best Pract Res Clin Endocrinol Metab 21:33, 2007.
12. Nikou G, Toubanakis C, Nikolaou P, et al: VIPomas: an update and management in a series of 11 patients, Hepatogastroenterology 52:1259, 2005.
13. Levin B, Lieberman DA, McFarland B, Smith RA, Brooks D, Andrews KS, et al.: Screening and Surveillance for the Early Detection of Colorectal Cancer and Adenomatous Polyps, 2008: A Joint Guideline from the American Cancer Society, the US Multi-Society Task Force on Colorectal Cancer, and the American College of Radiology. Ca Cancer J Clin 58:161-179, 2008.
14. Itzkowitz S, Jandorf L, Brand R, et al: Improved fecal DNA test for colorectal cancer screening, Clin Gastroenterol Hepatol 5:111, 2007.
15. Bossuyt X: Serologic markers in inflammatory bowel disease, Clin Chem 52:171, 2006.
16. Ricci C, Holton J, Vaira D: Diagnosis of *Helicobacter pylori:* invasive and non-invasive tests, Best Pract Res Clin Gastroenterol 21:299, 2007.
17. Gisbert J, Abraira V: Accuracy of *Helicobacter pylori* diagnostic tests in patients with bleeding peptic ulcer: a systematic review and meta-analysis, Am J Gastroenterol 101:848, 2006.
18. Fine K, Ogunji F: A new method of quantitative fecal fat microscopy and its correlation with chemically measured fecal fat output, Am J Clin Pathol 113:528, 2000.
19. Balasekaran R, Porter J, Santa Ana C, et al: Positive results on tests for steatorrhea in persons consuming Olestra potato chips, Ann Intern Med 132:279, 2000.
20. Young G, Cole S: New stool screening tests for colorectal cancer, Digestion 76:26, 2007.

INTERNET SITES

http://www.iffgd.org/site/gi-disorders

MEN 1

http://endocrine.niddk.nih.gov/pubs/men1/men1.htm

Ulcers

http://digestive.niddk.nih.gov/ddiseases/pubs/pepticulcers_ez/
http://digestive.niddk.nih.gov/ddiseases/pubs/hpylori/
http://www.corecharity.org.uk/Peptic-ulcers.html
http://opa.faseb.org/pdf/pylori.pdf

Malabsorption

http://www.worldgastroenterology.org/assets/downloads/en/pdf/guidelines/13_malabsorption_en.pdf

Celiac Disease

http://celiac.nih.gov/Materials.aspx
http://www.celiac.org/cd-main.php

Lactose Intolerance

http://digestive.niddk.nih.gov/ddiseases/pubs/lactoseintolerance/

Carcinoid Disease

www.carcinoid.com
http://www.mayoclinic.com/health/carcinoid-syndrome/DS00690

Cardiac and Muscle Disease

Chapter 36

Wendy R. Sanhai, Benjamin C. Eloff, and Robert H. Christenson

Chapter Outline

Key Terms

actin One of the two contractile, fibrous proteins involved in muscle contraction, in myocardial, skeletal, and arterial smooth muscles. Chains of actin proteins form "thin" filaments that transmit the force generated by myosin to the ends of the muscle.

action potential An electrical event produced by the ion flux across a membrane when its permeability is changed upon stimulation.

acute coronary syndromes The continuum of ischemic heart disease from unstable angina (reversible injury) through myocardial infarction (irreversible injury), in which the unstable coronary plaque is a common physiological feature.

adenosine-5′-triphosphate (ATP) The high-energy compound that can be hydrolyzed to adenosine-5′-diphosphate (ADP) or adenosine-5′-monophosphate (AMP), while releasing energy that can be used to drive metabolic reactions.

atherosclerosis A process that results in gradual deposition of lipid, fibrin, and calcium in the walls of arteries. Often called "hardening of the arteries," this condition is one of the most common causes of death.

atria The chambers of the heart that collect blood from the veins and contract to expel the blood into their respective ventricles. There are two atria: the right atrium collects blood from systemic veins and fills the right ventricle; the left atrium collects blood from the pulmonary vein and expels it into the left ventricle.

cardiac failure Inability of the heart to maintain blood circulation through efficient contraction, which leads to inadequate perfusion of essential organs, usually resulting in accumulation of salt and water.

cardiomyopathy A heterogeneous group of disorders that may be caused by a genetic component and/or a physiological pathology, which may affect contracting myocardial cells directly.

creatine phosphate (CP) Also known as phosphocreatine, this phosphorylated creatine molecule is an important energy store in skeletal muscle.

Embden-Meyerhof pathway The pathway of anaerobic glycolysis that converts glucose or glycogen to lactate.

glycoside A generic term for a group of drugs originally obtained from the foxglove plant. These drugs improve the contractility of the failing heart and slow the rate of ventricular contraction in atrial fibrillation. Digoxin is a member of this family of drugs.

infarction A process of cell death caused by an inadequate blood supply (ischemia).

ischemia A reduction in blood supply to tissue that is sufficient to prevent the tissue from functioning normally.

Krebs citric acid cycle The pathway of intermediary metabolism that will accept metabolic products from the Embden-Meyerhof pathway and oxidize, decarboxylate, and reduce them, with production of a relatively large amount of ATP.

myocardial infarction, or **MI** (also known as a heart attack or a coronary thrombosis) Occurs when part of the heart muscle suddenly loses its blood supply. This results in injury to the heart muscle, which can lead to severe chest pain and pressure.

myofibril Small fibers that run through each muscle cell and have alternate "light" (actin) and "dark" (myosin) bands; responsible for muscle contraction.

myocardiocyte (cardiac muscle cell, cardiomyocyte) A type of involuntary striated muscle cell that is found in the walls of the heart. As it contracts with other myocardiocytes, the heart propels blood through the blood vessels of the circulatory system.

myosin A contractile, fibrous protein that is part of a super family of motor proteins that that contains ATP- and actin-binding sites and is involved in skeletal, cardiac, and smooth muscle contraction.

sarcolemma The plasma membrane of muscle cells.

sarcomere Basic unit of a muscle's cross-striated myofibril. Sarcomeres are multi-protein complexes that are composed of two different filament systems: thick filaments and thin filaments. Other muscle proteins, such as **titan** and nebulin, stabilize the filaments.

sarcoplasm The cytoplasm of muscle cells.

sarcoplasmic reticulum The endoplasmic reticulum of muscle cells.

syncytium A group of cells that maintain cytoplasmic continuity and contain many nuclei.

technetium 99m (**^{99m}Tc**) An isotope that is injected intravenously to measure left ventricular output (m = metastable).

thallium 201 An isotope that is injected intravenously to delineate the ischemic part of the ventricular muscle mass or a scar caused by an old infarction.

titin A giant (3 mDa) protein that is a major constituent of the sarcomere in vertebrate skeletal muscle. It spans half the length of the sarcomere, joining the Z-line to the M-band. Functions include thick-filament assembly, muscle elasticity, and tension generation. Also called *connectin.*

tropomyosin A rigid, rod-shaped protein made up of two identical α-helical proteins that wind around each other in a coiled fashion. It binds along the length of the actin filaments, making them more rigid and altering their affinity for other proteins, such as myosin.

troponins Three distinct polypeptides: troponin T, responsible for tropomyosin-binding activity; troponin I, which binds to actin and inhibits the activity of actomyosin ATPase; and troponin C, responsible for calcium-binding activity of muscle contraction. Together with tropomyosin, the troponins (T, I, and C) form a complex that regulates actin and myosin interactions and muscle contraction.

ventricles The main right and left pumping chambers of the heart that expel blood. The right ventricle pumps blood into the pulmonary artery, and the left ventricle pumps blood to the aorta. The left ventricle is more massive and powerful than the right ventricle because the pressure in the systemic circulation, against which it must expel blood, is greater than that in the pulmonary circulation.

Methods on Evolve

B-Type natriuretic peptide
C-Reactive protein
Creatine kinase
Creatine kinase isoenzymes
Digoxin and digitoxin
Lactate dehydrogenase and lactate dehydrogenase isoenzymes
Myoglobin
Procainamide and *N*-acetylprocainamide
Troponin

SECTION OBJECTIVES BOX 36-1

- List the proteins involved in muscle contraction, and describe how they function in contraction.
- List the major types of muscles and their functions.
- Describe the differences between fast- and slow-twitch skeletal muscles.

MUSCLE ANATOMY AND FUNCTION

Types of Muscle

There are three distinct groups of muscle: skeletal, cardiac, and smooth. Skeletal muscle consists of unbranched, cylindrical muscle cells that are multinucleated (a **syncytium**) and arranged in parallel bundles (see Color Plate 11) as a result of the fusion of many individual progenitor cells (myoblasts) during myogenesis. The nuclei are located just under the plasma membrane (**sarcolemma**), and the fibers run the whole length of the muscle. They have well-defined nerve end plates and are under voluntary control. Contractions are initiated by nerve impulses and are termed *neurogenic.* Nerve endings are attached to the outer surface of the sarcolemma through the motor end plate of an axon. Within the sarcolemma-enclosed space, the fibrils are bathed by the intracellular fluid of muscle, the **sarcoplasm.**

Each muscle cell contains bundles of cylindrical *myofibrils,* which make up about two thirds of the dry mass of the cytoplasm (see Color Plate 11). Myofibrils, the contractile elements of muscle cells, are surrounded by an extensive network of tubular channels known as the **sarcoplasmic reticulum,** which is analogous to a "net stocking" around the muscle fibers (see Color Plate 11). Myofibrils, which have a diameter of 1 to 2 mm and run parallel to the long axis of the muscle fiber, consist of an end-to-end chainlike arrangement of repeating **sarcomeres.** The parallel arrangement of the filaments within each sarcomere gives muscle its characteristic cross-striation, a pattern of light and dark bands visible at high magnification. The darker bands are called A bands (anisotropic, containing both thick and thin filaments); the light bands are called I bands (isotropic, containing only thin filaments). In the electron microscope, each I band is bisected by a dense transverse band called the *Z line,* or *Z disc,* which

Table **36-1** Characteristics of Myofibrillar Proteins

Proteins	Location	Protein (as a Percentage of Total Cellular Protein)	Molecular Weight (kD)
Myosin II	A band	60	2 ∞ 260 (2 heavy and 4 light chains)
Actin	I band	20.0	42
Tropomyosin	I band	3	2 ∞ 35
Troponin (TIC- triple complex)	I band	4.5	T-component = 31
			T-component = 21
C-protein	A band	<1	128
α-Actinin	Z line, I band	<1	2 ∞ 100 (dimer)
Titin (also called connection)	Z line	<1	3 MDa
Desmin	Z line	<1	55

Data from Politou AS, Thomas DJ, Pastore A: The folding and stability of titin immunoglobulin-like modules with implications for the mechanism of elasticity, Biophys J 69:2601, 1995; Squire JM: Architecture and function in the muscle sarcomere, Curr Opin Struct Biol 7:247, 1997; Trinick J, Tskhovrebova L: Titin: a molecular control freak, Trends Cell Biol 9:377, 1999.

separates one sarcomere from the next. Each sarcomere contains a precisely arranged assembly of partially overlapping thick and thin filaments. The thick filaments are polymers of specific isoforms of **myosin** II. Thin filaments composed of **actin** and associated proteins are attached to the Z discs at either end of the sarcomere. They extend toward the middle of the sarcomere, where they overlap with the thick filaments (see Color Plate 11).

Skeletal muscles can also be divided into two types, "fast-twitch" and "slow-twitch," which differ in their biochemical nature (see p. 684) and their motor nerve endings (see p. 682).

Cardiac muscle is found exclusively in the heart and, like skeletal muscle, it contains actin and myosin filaments arranged in a similar banding pattern. However, cardiac muscle cells bifurcate, or branch, and contain only 1 or 2 nuclei per cell. Cardiac muscle consists of tightly knit bundles of interwoven cells, or cardiomyocytes, that form a quasi-syncytium, which contributes to the characteristic wave of contractions that leads to the "pumping" of blood from **atria** and **ventricles.** Cardiac muscle control is involuntary, that is, no conscious effort is required to initiate and maintain contraction of cardiac muscle; it therefore is termed *myogenic.*

Smooth muscle is composed of elongated, nonstriated cells with a single, centrally located nucleus. The smooth muscle cell does not have a structurally defined end plate and is not under voluntary control; therefore, it is also called *involuntary muscle.* Found in the walls of tubes or sacs such as blood vessels, the wall of the uterus, the urinary bladder, the intestines, and the bronchioles, smooth muscle is characterized by slow contraction and can maintain tension or a given length without fatigue at low energy cost.

Proteins Involved in Muscle Contraction (Table 36-1)

Many proteins, including myosin II (consisting of heavy and light chains), actin, **troponins,** and **tropomyosin,** are required for muscle contraction. Muscle myosin belongs to the myosin II subfamily, and myosin I is present in nonmuscle cells. Myosin II is a large filamentous molecule (540 kD) that is made up of six peptide chains—two heavy chains (230 kD) and four light chains (myosin light chains [MLCs]; 26 kD). The heavy chains contain two head domains and a long rodlike tail composed of two α-helical peptide chains arranged in a coiled motif, as is shown in Fig. 36-1. When stimulated by the binding to actin filaments in skeletal muscle, the globular head, or motor domain, of myosin II hydrolyzes **adenosine-5′-triphosphate (ATP)** to adenosine-5′-diphosphate (ADP) and inorganic phosphate (Pi), using the energy released to contract the muscle.

Two types of MLCs bind to the head domains of the myosin heavy chains: cardiac and noncardiac. Phosphorylation of one of the two light chains by myosin light chain kinase (MLCK) causes a change in the conformation of the myosin head, exposing its actin-binding site. MLCs from cardiac and noncardiac sources can be differentiated by using antibodies specific for cardiac MLCs.

Actin, a critical component of a wide range of structures in eukaryotic cells, has the same fundamental structure in all cells, and consists of long filamentous (F-actin) polymers made up of two strands of globular (G-actin) monomers. However, the length of the filaments, their stability, and the number and geometry of attachments vary, depending on the actin-binding proteins, such as α-actinin and desmin. α-Actinin, a major component of the Z line, is thought to anchor the actin filaments. Specialized accessory proteins, tropomyosin and troponins, also associate with polymerized actin filaments and mediate the Ca^{2+} regulation of muscle contraction. Sarcomere shortening is caused by sliding of the myosin filaments past the actin filaments with no change in the length of either filament.

The troponin complex is a set of three proteins that, together with Ca^{++} ions and tropomyosin, regulate muscle contraction (seen as the spherical triple complex in Fig. 36-1). Localized primarily in the myofibrils (94% to 97%) with a smaller soluble, cytoplasmic fraction (3% to 6%), the troponin complex consists of three proteins: troponin C (the calcium-binding component), troponin T (the tropomyosin-binding component), and troponin I (the inhibitory component). The subunits exist in a number of different isoforms,

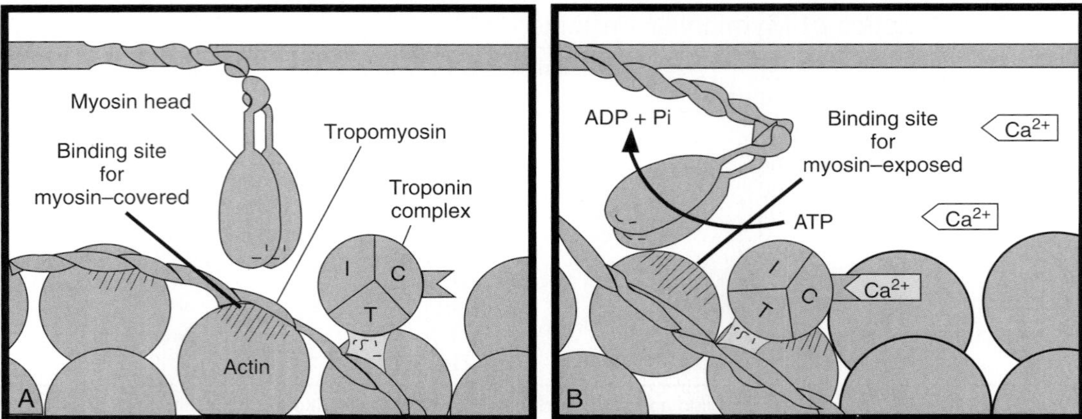

Fig. 36-1 Schematic representation of the spatial configuration of myosin, actin, tropomyosin, and the troponin complex in the presence and absence of calcium ions. **A**, In the absence of calcium ions, the long tropomyosin molecule is bound to the myosin-binding site on the actin filament (large spheres representing actin monomers polymerize to form the actin filament). **B**, Calcium ions (Ca^{2+}), upon their release from the sarcoplasmic reticulum, bind to the troponin C subunit of the troponin complex (total ion current [TIC] spherical complex with Ca^{2+}-binding site on the C subunit); subsequent conformational changes increase the affinity of the troponin T subunit for the tropomyosin molecule. The troponin-tropomyosin-Ca^{2+} complex triggers movement of the tropomyosin molecule away from the myosin-binding site on the actin filament. Adenosine-5′-triphosphate (ATP) binds to a site on the myosin head domain and, upon hydrolysis to adenosine-5′-diphosphate (ADP) and inorganic phosphate (Pi), triggers a conformational change that allows the myosin head to move along the actin filament in the direction of the Z line (not shown). (Drawing adapted with permission from Wu A: *Cardiac Markers*, Totowa, NJ, 1998, Humana Press.)

whose distributions vary between cardiac muscle and slow- and fast-twitch skeletal muscle. Troponin C is found in human heart and skeletal muscle. However, cardiac-specific troponin T (cTnT) and cardiac-specific troponin I (cTnI) isoforms have been isolated. cTnI and cTnT have different amino acid sequences compared with skeletal muscle isoforms and are encoded by different genes. Only one form of cTnI has been identified, and it has never been shown to be expressed in normal, regenerating, or diseased skeletal muscle.

Tropomyosin is a rod-shaped molecule that contains two polypeptide chains that bind within the grooves of the actin filaments (see Fig. 36-1). Troponin T is bound to tropomyosin and positions the complex on the actin filament. The troponin T–tropomyosin complex, together with troponin I, which binds to actin filaments, inhibits interactions between actin filaments and the head domain of myosin II. However, when **action potentials** (produced by an ion flux across membranes, resulting in increased permeability) stimulate Ca^{2+} ion release from the sarcoplasmic reticulum, troponin C binds up to four Ca^{2+} ions. This binding changes the conformation of the tropomyosin-troponin complex and removes the inhibition of myosin binding to actin produced by the other two troponin components. With the myosin-binding site on the actin filament now exposed, the myosin head domain is free to bind to actin filaments, and in the presence of ATP, muscle contraction can occur.

The above machinery is applicable to single cells and holds true for all types of muscle cells. However, a collection of individual cells that interact in a coordinated manner is needed to create a working muscle or heart. At the ends of cardiac myocytes, actin and the intermediate filaments that make up the cytoskeleton bind with members of the cadherin family of proteins to link with adjacent cells. The cadherin proteins are transmembrane proteins with a cytoplasmic C-terminus that bind to actin and an extracellular N-terminus that binds to another cadherin protein, thereby mechanically linking the cells together.

Gap junctions are plaques of transmembrane pores that link to adjacent cells to provide a pathway for transmitting ions and molecules up to approximately 1 kDa in size. Each complete pore consists of two hemi-channels, one in each cell membrane, consisting of a hexameric complex of proteins from the connexin (Cx) family. Gap junctions are throught to play a vital role in organizing electrical communication in the heart to promote orderly contraction of the myocardium.

The Neuromuscular Connection

The force-generating molecular interactions just described take place only when a signal passes to the muscle from its motor nerve. At the site of muscle innervation, motor nerves have no myelin sheath, and the exposed end sits within a trough on the muscle cell surface. This structure is called the *motor end plate*, or *myoneural junction*. Within the nerve axon terminal are numerous mitochondria and synaptic vesicles, the latter containing the neurotransmitter acetylcholine. When an action potential is transmitted from the neuron to the muscle through the neuromuscular junction, acetylcholine is liberated from the axon terminal, diffuses through the synaptic cleft, and binds with receptors in the sarcolemma of the adjacent muscle cell. Binding of the transmitter makes the sarcolemma more permeable to sodium, which results in membrane depolarization. This depolarization is propagated along the length of the muscle cells and triggers the release of Ca^{2+} ions, which are stored in the sarcoplasmic reticulum, into the vicinity of the myofibrils. Ca^{2+} ions initiate the contraction by acting as second messengers, activating the ATPase in the troponin complex and triggering the interaction between myosin and actin (see Fig. 36-1). When depolarization ceases, the Ca^{2+} ions are actively transported back into the sarcoplasmic reticulum, and the muscle relaxes.

Motor nerve endings differ, depending on the main fiber type. A single nerve fiber (axon) can innervate one muscle fiber/cell, or it may branch and innervate more than 160 muscle fibers. Slow-twitch fibers, which respond to nerve stimuli with prolonged contractions, generally are innervated by multiple nerve endings. Fast-twitch fibers usually are innervated by individual end plates. Acetylcholine, which serves as a neurotransmitter (see Chapter 47, p. 910), is synthesized and stored in vesicles of both types of neurons.

Mechanism of Contraction

The general function of the muscles is to respond mechanically to stimulation, producing fiber shortening and force development, both of which usually occur together. Skeletal muscle function is modified by leverage, as a result of attachment to the skeleton. In cardiac muscle, force development is manifested by the development of pressure within the chambers of the heart during cardiac muscle shortening, which results in reduced chamber size and the characteristic pumping action of the heart. Smooth muscle shortening is seen when smooth muscle sacs or cavities are emptied, as in the expulsion of urine from the bladder or of a child from the uterus during the birthing process.

Muscle contraction is driven by the interaction between myosin II heads and adjacent actin filaments. The sequence of events in a reaction cycle during muscle contraction is summarized as follows:

- Myosin heads interact with actin filaments
- ATP binds to the head of the myosin filaments and causes a conformational change that causes myosin to be released from the actin
- ATP is hydrolyzed, which results in a second conformational change causing myosin to weakly bind to a different actin binding site; this *ratcheting* movement moves the myosin head along the actin filament
- A phosphate molecule is released and another conformational change results, which leads to stronger myosin binding, and the power stroke.
- ADP dissociates from the myosin head and leaves the myosin head tightly bound to actin. In the absence of further binding of ATP, this state results in muscle rigidity called rigor.

The energy for muscle contraction is generated by the hydrolysis of ATP by myosin's motor domain *(heads)*. The amount of ATP hydrolyzed in contraction is not constant but depends on the duration of the contraction and on the amount of work done by the muscle. With each cycle of ATP hydrolysis, the myosin molecule alters its affinity for the actin filaments and moves or "walks" along the actin filament in the direction of the Z line (i.e., toward the positive end of the actin filament), sliding the myosin and actin filaments past one another at rates up to 15 mm/sec. This sliding filament mechanism of contraction can shorten the sarcomere by as much as one-third its original length.

Relaxation of the muscle is a passive process. Interdigitated filaments slide back to a less overlapped position, thereby increasing the length of the muscle. The same basic mechanism of contraction/relaxation applies to all muscle types. In the absence of ATP, the myosin-actin complex becomes stable; this accounts for the extreme muscular rigidity (rigor mortis) that occurs after death.

KEY CONCEPTS BOX 36-1

- The three muscle types are cardiac, skeletal, and smooth muscle: all work by contracting the myofibrils to produce force.
- The heart is a multi-chambered organ that is designed to pump blood into the circulatory system with little rest.
- Smooth muscles line sacs or cavities and are designed to produce a steady force to move material from that sac.
- Skeletal muscles are designed to move rapidly to produce the force to move limbs, but they tend to tire rapidly.
- The important contraction proteins are the actins, myosins, and troponins.
- The contraction proteins combine with Ca^{++} to contract the muscle fibers and create force.
- Slow- and fast-twitch muscles differ in terms of their neuromuscular connections, their numbers of mitochondria, and their myoglobin content.

ANATOMY AND FUNCTION OF THE HEART

The pumping action of the heart is the prime factor in the maintenance of the body's circulation. The heart is a muscular organ that is composed of four chambers—two atria and two ventricles. The right atrium collects blood from the systemic circulation and pumps it into the right ventricle. The right ventricle pumps blood to the lungs for reoxygenation; the blood then is collected by the left atrium, which pumps blood to the left ventricle. The left ventricle pumps blood to the rest of the body, including the heart itself. Synchronization of the pumping function of the heart is performed through the specialized conduction system, which consists of the sinoatrial (SA) node, followed by the atrioventricular (AV) node and the His-Purkinje system. The SA node acts as a pacemaker and creates electrical impulses that initiate contractions within the atria. These impulses travel to the AV node, then are distributed through the His-Purkinje system to the ventricles to begin contraction there. Cardiac output is determined primarily by the volume of blood pumped, heart rate, by the systemic blood pressure, and by the contractile force developed in the wall of the left ventricle. Cardiac muscle, which is extremely active, requires large quantities of energy (as ATP) and oxygen for metabolism. Delivery of the oxygen needed to fuel the heart requires a rich capillary bed.

ENERGY METABOLISM

Various substrates are used by muscle cells for energy production. Energy is liberated from these fuels by several pathways, including the Embden-Meyerhof glycolytic pathway, the pentose phosphate shunt, fatty acid oxidation, and the **Krebs citric acid cycle** (see Chapter 38). Energy produced by the breakdown of substrates then is transported through the electron-transport system of the mitochondria to produce ATP, the chemical form of stored energy that is used by muscle tissue to perform work. To perform their functions, muscle cells must maintain a high [ATP]/[ADP] ratio, and all muscles require an effective storage method to maintain a reserve of ATP. This is achieved through the synthesis of **creatine phosphate (CP),** which functions as an energy reservoir source that can be used for rapid regeneration of ATP when levels fall as a result of increased demand.

This high-energy reservoir uses the enzymes creatine kinase (CK) and myokinase (MK) to maintain an equilibrium concentration of ATP, ADP, and creatine phosphate (CP). The immediate effect of increased ADP concentrations caused by the hydrolysis of ATP during contraction is a disturbance of the equilibrium of the creatine kinase–catalyzed reaction:

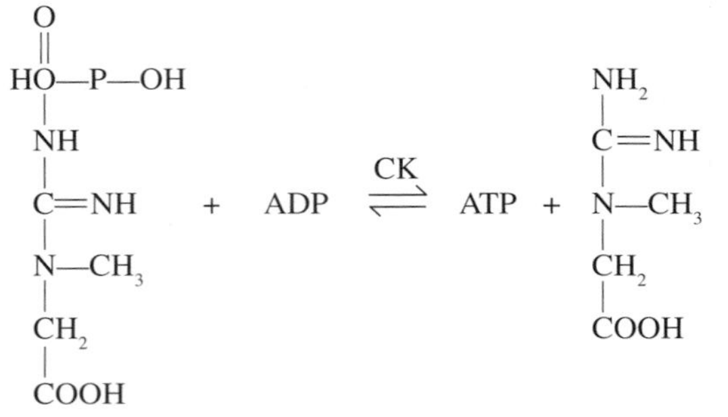

$$\underset{\textbf{Creatine phosphate}}{HO{-}P(=O)(OH){-}NH{-}C({=}NH){-}N(CH_3){-}CH_2{-}COOH} + ADP \underset{}{\overset{CK}{\rightleftharpoons}} ATP + \underset{\textbf{Creatine}}{NH_2{-}C({=}NH){-}N(CH_3){-}CH_2{-}COOH}$$

The equilibrium is reestablished by the phosphorylation of ADP to ATP by this reaction, thus preserving a high [ATP]/[ADP] ratio. Another enzyme, myokinase, catalyzes the reaction:

$$2\ ADP \xleftrightarrow{MK} ATP + AMP$$

This reaction also ensures the reestablishment of the original high [ATP]/[ADP] ratio.

A third enzyme present in the muscle, adenosine deaminase (AD), prevents the accumulation of AMP produced by the myokinase reaction through deamination of the AMP:

$$AMP \xleftrightarrow{AD} IMP + NH_3^+$$

Inosine monophosphate (IMP) then either returns to the nucleoside pool as inosine or is degraded further to uric acid. For a single contraction (twitch) or for short periods of muscle activity, the only measurable change in the intracellular high-energy phosphate pool is a small change in CP concentration.

ENERGY DEMANDS OF DIFFERENT MUSCLE TYPES

Skeletal Muscle

Human skeletal muscle contains both red and white fibers, which differ in their metabolic properties. Red or slow fibers are rich in myoglobin and mitochondria. In these fibers, the main metabolic pathway is oxidative phosphorylation. White or fast fibers contain little myoglobin and mitochondria, and the main route for energy metabolism is glycolysis. Rested, well-nourished muscle synthesizes and stores glycogen, which serves as a ready source of fuel that can be converted to glucose-6-phosphate for entry into the glycolytic pathway. Skeletal muscle at rest uses about 30% of the oxygen consumed by the human body. At maximum activity, skeletal muscle can increase its oxygen uptake 20-fold or more during the transition from rest to full activity to supply the oxygen needed for the oxidative process. However, its rate of ATP hydrolysis can increase by a much greater amount. Therefore, at maximum activity, the skeletal muscles still are relatively oxygen poor (anoxic), and lactate, the end product of anaerobic glucose metabolism, is increased in blood.

Acidosis occurs when either metabolic or other abnormal processes result in a lower than normal pH of the arterial blood. Lactic acidosis, which results from excessive production of lactic acid, can occur in normal skeletal muscles after excessive exercise. Localized imbalance of sodium and potassium ions along with a metabolic acidosis in skeletal muscle contributes to fatigue and can result in muscle cramps and pain.

Cardiac Muscle

The highly aerobic metabolism of the heart allows it to use as fuel many substrates normally present in plasma; cardiac uptake of most of these substances is proportional to their arterial concentration once certain levels are exceeded. In general terms, the heart uses free fatty acids as its predominant fuel. It also consumes significant quantities of glucose and lactate, as well as lesser amounts of pyruvate, ketone bodies, and amino acids. Most of the energy for cardiac function is obtained from the breakdown of metabolites through the citric acid cycle and oxidative phosphorylation. These enzyme pathways are found principally in the mitochondria, which make up some 35% of the total volume of cardiac muscle. Although free fatty acids are the resting heart's fuel of choice, upon the imposition of a heavy workload the heart greatly increases its rate of glucose consumption, derived mainly from its relatively limited glycogen supply.

Smooth Muscle

Compared with skeletal and cardiac muscle, the energy needs of smooth muscle contraction are very modest. An influx of Ca^{2+} ions is involved in the initiation of contraction in smooth muscle cells. Ca^{2+} complexes with the binding protein calmodulin, and the Ca^{2+}-calmodulin complex activates MLCK, the enzyme responsible for the ATP-dependent phosphorylation of myosin. The myosin of smooth muscle interacts with actin only when its light chain is phosphorylated. For this reason, and because troponin is absent, the contraction mechanism of smooth muscle differs from that of skeletal and cardiac muscle. Smooth muscle contraction is slow and concerted, is not subjected to voluntary control, and does not demand the high aerobic metabolism of skeletal and cardiac muscle.

KEY CONCEPTS BOX 36-2

- Energy demands of all muscle cells are met with the production of adenosine triphosphate (ATP) via the Embden-Meyerhof and Kreb cycle pathways.
- Because energy needs can vary greatly, all muscle cells store high-energy phosphate bonds in the form of creatine-phosphate, formed by the reaction of creatine and ATP.
- Skeletal muscles depend almost entirely on glucose metabolism to create ATP. When levels of oxygen, which is required for the Krebs cycle and is stored in muscle cells bound to myoglobin, are low, muscle cells depend only on the Embden-Meyerhof pathway, which soon leaves them depleted of ATP.
- Red (slow-twitch) fibers contain higher levels of myoglobin and mitochondria than do white (fast-twitch) fibers and depend more on the Krebs cycle for energy.
- Cardiac muscle does not depend solely on glucose for energy needs, but can use organic acids such as lactic and fatty acids as fuel.

SECTION OBJECTIVES BOX 36-2

- Define MI.
- Describe the clinical spectrum of ACS.
- Define CHF, and explain the use of BNP in CHF.
- Define and list the types of arrhythmias.

PATHOLOGICAL CONDITIONS

Cardiac Disorders

Ischemic Heart Disease

Ischemia is a condition in which an organ has an inadequate blood supply for maintaining its essential functions. Although myocardial ischemia has many causes, including vascular contraction and spasm, the most common cause by far is coronary **atherosclerosis,** which is believed by many to be an inflammatory condition of arterial vessels that generally progresses over many years, often beginning at an early age. Atherosclerosis causes the arteries that supply blood to the heart to gradually narrow (occlude) because of deposition of cholesterol and other substances in the arterial wall. The most common cause of ischemia is related to unstable lipid-filled deposits, termed *plaques* (see p. 720, Chapter 37). Unstable plaques are the common physiological feature of acute coronary syndrome, a continuum of ischemic disease ranging from unstable angina, associated with reversible myocardial cell injury, to frank **myocardial infarction (MI)** with large areas of necrosis. Another condition that can cause ischemia and cell death is coronary vasospasm, in which the arterial wall constricts in an abnormal and prolonged fashion because of hypersensitivity to normal vasoconstrictor signals. Other less common causes of myocardial ischemia are severe anemia and hypotension.

Effects of Occlusion on Myocardium

Cessation of blood flow produces a complex series of metabolic consequences for the cells deprived of blood flow. Severe hypoxia occurs because tissue oxygen concentration drops drastically; also contributing to this condition are delayed clearance of toxic cellular metabolites from ischemic tissue and the production of free radicals after reperfusion of damaged tissues. Hypoxia prevents aerobic metabolism, and oxygen supplies remaining in the microvasculature are readily consumed. Instead of the aerobic Krebs cycle, myocardial metabolism switches to the use of glycogen or glucose in the anaerobic **Embden-Meyerhof pathway.** The end product of anaerobic glucose metabolism, pyruvate, is reduced to lactate, which accumulates and is one of the earliest and most dramatic signs of myocardial ischemia.

As ischemia continues, accumulation of lactate and other acidic intermediates of glycolysis occurs. CP reserves are depleted, and ATP levels fall. Generally, if tissue is reperfused, it will recover in 15 to 20 minutes after an ischemic incident. However, after 15 to 20 minutes of occlusion, more than 60% of the cellular ATP is depleted, and the amount of lactate in myocardial tissue is 12-fold higher than its normal aerobic level. In addition, all cellular glycogen is exhausted. With glycogen and CP reserves depleted, dramatic ultrastructural changes occur, indicating irreversible cell damage. At this point, even if the obstruction is relieved and the myocardial tissue is reperfused, the myocardial tissue is unable to tolerate the arrival of oxygenated blood, resulting in cell lysis, necrosis, loss of muscle tone, and fibrosis.

During ischemia, three major factors—elevated $[K^+]$, acidosis, and anoxia—all contribute to abnormalities in the action potential conduction in the heart. These abnormalities can lead to ventricular fibrillation. Ventricular fibrillation (VF), if not treated immediately, results in cessation of blood pumping to the brain and other vital organs, leading to death.

At the point at which reversible ischemic injury becomes irreversible, the cell is no longer able to maintain membrane integrity, and the intracellular contents are released into the extracellular environment. The rate of release of intracellular proteins into the circulation depends on the clearance mechanism, the rate and extent of reperfusion of the damaged myocardium, and the size of the protein molecule. The greater the reperfusion and the smaller the size, the sooner the molecule will be seen in peripheral blood. For example, myoglobin with a molecular weight of 17,800 daltons will be observed in peripheral blood before CK and the cardiac troponins T and I, which have molecular weights in the range of 85,000 daltons. Release of these proteins can be used as biomarkers for the evaluation and confirmation of irreversible ischemic injury. Release of biomarkers (cTnT, cTnI, or CK-MB) that reflect death to myocytes indicates that the patient has had an MI rather than a transient ischemic episode. Mitochondrial enzymes are also released, but there is usually some delay before they appear in plasma.

Acute Coronary Syndromes (ACS)

The **acute coronary syndromes** represent the following continuum of events:

angina

↓

reversible tissue injury

↓

unstable angina, frequently associated with minor myocardial damage

↓

myocardial infarction

↓

extensive tissue necrosis

Based on World Health Organization (WHO) criteria for ischemic symptoms, assessment of coronary artery disease has focused mainly on electrocardiogram changes and a rise and fall in biochemical markers. From the 1980s to the mid-1990s, CK-MB was the benchmark for markers; however, CK-MB is not specific for myocardium. The cardiac-specific proteins cTnT and cTnI have emerged as sensitive and specific biomarkers of myocardial infarction and, more important, for risk stratification of patients with acute coronary syndrome (see below). In addition to these markers of necrosis, other indicators are of potential use, for example, markers for inflammation (C-reactive protein and serum amyloid A), "angry" platelets (P-selectin), and the procoagulant state and thrombosis (soluble fibrin). Also, CK-MB and myoglobin have been combined with clinical indicators to monitor reperfusion after thrombolytic therapy.

Each year, millions of patients with chest pain are evaluated in hospital emergency departments in the United States and are given the diagnosis of MI. The cost of caring for patients with suspected and confirmed MI is estimated to be in the billions per year. A system of patient triage based on the results of cardiospecific biomarkers obtained within 12 hours after onset of symptoms could reduce the number of patients admitted to coronary care units by as much as 70%. This system would operate under the assumption that all patients with negative results, even those with unstable angina (chest pain but without ischemic injury), could be adequately cared for in a regular hospital unit. The use of biomarkers, therefore, will continue to be a cost-effective and important clinical adjunct for MI diagnosis, risk assessment, patient stratification, and reperfusion monitoring in the future. Rapid testing is crucial because the faster ACS is diagnosed and treated, the less heart muscle will be affected, thereby decreasing the severity of the event (see National Academy of Clinical Biochemistry [NACB] updated guidelines in Bibliography). When blood vessels are occluded, revascularization is performed by opening the blood vessel with an angioplasty balloon and placing bare metal or drug-eluting stents (DES) in blood vessels to prevent reocclusion.

Congestive Heart Failure (CHF)

Congestive heart failure (CHF) is a disease that is related to the decreased capability of the heart to pump blood. The prevalence of CHF in the United States is rising, and the projection is that this trend will continue. It is now recognized that CHF represents a spectrum of diseases that can progress from left ventricular dysfunction (LVD), in which at least half of subjects are asymptomatic, to end-stage overt CHF, with markedly high morbidity and mortality. Contributing factors to CHF include increased age, hypertension, and coronary atherosclerosis. Regardless of its origin, CHF is divided into four classes according to symptoms delineated by the New York Heart Association (NYHA) classification index. Class I represents ventricular dysfunction in the absence of symptoms. Class II represents minimal symptoms that may occur with exercise. Class III is classified as moderate symptoms associated with mild exercise, and Class IV represents symptoms that may occur at rest. The symptom-based diagnosis of CHF is difficult because the symptoms may occur with pulmonary disease, syndromes associated with edema, and syndromes associated with fatigue.

An important therapy for CHF is treatment with angiotensin-converting enzyme (ACE) inhibitors, which usually is provided throughout the spectrum of CHF from Class I through Class IV. An increasing role for beta-adrenergic blockers has emerged, particularly in symptomatic heart failure. Diuretics are indicated for patients with sodium retention, and digitalis is recommended for those with symptomatic heart failure, to reduce the progression of disease and hospitalization. The laboratory may be used to monitor these therapeutic agents.

Brain natriuretic peptide (BNP), a protein released from the heart in response to cardiac stretch receptors, may help to differentiate between CHF and other conditions that have similar clinical presentations, and to guide therapy for CHF. However, it is unclear to what extent other conditions (such as renal disease) or medications (such as beta-blockers) might interfere with the use of BNP as a biomarker in the diagnosis of heart failure.

Cardiomyopathy

Cardiomyopathy represents a diverse group of disorders, which generally fall into two categories: disease originating in heart tissue, and disease that is related to other, nonmyocardial disorders. Cardiomyopathy is characterized by inadequate muscle contraction caused by direct damage to myocardial cells and typically results in hemodynamic overload and heart failure. Although some specific forms of cardiomyopathy are known, most clinical cases are idiopathic, that is, the causes are unclear. Cardiomyopathy usually manifests as an enlargement of all four chambers of the heart and as **cardiac failure.** Biochemical findings in most cases of cardiomyopathy are nonspecific and reflect cardiac failure, the major clinical presentation. At least two forms of this disease, familial hypertrophic cardiomyopathy and viral myocarditis, now can be diagnosed with the use of molecular genetic techniques.

Arrhythmias

A complex neuroregulatory system controls and coordinates the pattern of contraction for the four chambers of the heart and regulates cardiac function in relation to the changing needs of body organs. Arrhythmias can be structural in nature or may be related to an acute or progressive cardiac disease process. Damage to the neuroregulatory system, which can occur during and after cardiac injury (such as MI), is relatively nonspecific and frequently is related to the disease process that affects the heart muscle. Whatever the cause, distortion of the transmission of cardiac nerve impulses, which produces abnormal, irregular, and self-sustaining contractile activity of the heart, is termed *arrhythmia*.

In functional terms, arrhythmias are classified as bradycardias (resulting in heartbeat rates less than 60 beats/min) or as tachycardias (producing heartbeat rates faster than 100 beats/min). The arrhythmia can affect atrial or ventricular contractions and can be acute or chronic. VF, a chaotic contraction of the ventricular muscle, is a common and fatal arrhythmia that often requires a defibrillation shock. Atrial fibrillation is a fairly common rhythm abnormality in which the atria beat in an irregular and abnormally rapid fashion. Chronic arrhythmias can be controlled by medications, the serum levels of which should be monitored routinely during the initial period to determine optimal therapeutic dosing levels.

Congenital and Valvular Heart Disease

Many congenital heart abnormalities have been described, but these are beyond the scope of this chapter. In general terms, all components of the heart can be affected by maldevelopment or infectious disease. In many cases, the causes of these defects are unknown. One important exception is rubella infection of the mother during the first trimester of pregnancy, which is associated with a very high risk for fetal cardiac malformation. Of acquired valvular diseases of the heart, one large group is caused by rheumatic carditis. In susceptible patients affected by hemolytic streptococcus, the body develops an immune reaction against all myocardial tissue, but particularly the valves, which become damaged and deformed.

Skeletal Muscle Disorders

Diseases of muscle are characterized by motor dysfunction such as muscular weakness. The three major categories of muscle disorders, according to the part of the motor unit affected, are (1) neurogenic muscular atrophies, (2) muscle fiber disorders (myopathies), and (3) disturbances of the neuromuscular junction. Within each major class, further distinctions are made based on the loci, or known origins, of the defects. These categories are listed below.

The muscular atrophies are caused by loss of efferent innervation as a result of degeneration of an anterior horn cell or an axon at the level of an anterior efferent root or peripheral nerve cell. The myopathies are characterized by major defects at the level of the muscle fiber. Certain hereditary progressive myopathies are called, by convention, muscular dystrophies. Nonhereditary myopathies can result from inflammation or from an endocrine or metabolic abnormality.

Anterior Root and Peripheral Nerve Involvement

Acute polyneuropathy, or Guillain-Barré syndrome, is a parainfectious and postinfectious disease presumed to be caused by an immunological reaction with peripheral nerves. Metabolic neuropathies include damage to nerves that results from metabolic diseases such as diabetes mellitus or malnutrition.

Disorders of Muscle Fibers: Muscular Dystrophies

Muscular dystrophy is a general name for a group of chronic diseases of muscle. General characteristics include progressive weakness and degeneration of skeletal muscle with no evidence of neural degeneration. These genetic diseases have different inheritance patterns. The age of onset, the course of the disease, and its effects on different fiber types differ among the individual diseases.

Pseudohypertrophic muscular dystrophy, or Duchenne's muscular dystrophy (DMD), is the most common of the muscular dystrophies. DMD is an X-linked recessive disease that causes progressive muscle weakness and muscle wasting starting at 1 or 2 years of age and progressing to heart failure or weakness of the respiratory muscles; most patients are confined to wheelchairs by 10 to 12 years of age, and death typically occurs in early adulthood. Most patients with DMD have deletions that eliminate large portions of the dystrophin gene, one of the largest known genes in the human genome. This gene codes for the protein dystrophin, which is thought to stabilize the sarcolemma during muscle contraction.

Serum enzymes are greatly elevated in the disease even before symptoms develop; especially noted is the rise in CK. CK values in heterozygous females and in normal individuals overlap, so the enzyme is elevated in only about 50% to 70% of heterozygous females. Diagnosis of this disease by DNA analysis and genetic counseling has significantly decreased DMD occurrence in the past 10 years. No effective treatment is available for DMD, but the disease is a prime candidate for gene therapy.

Disturbances of the Neuromuscular Junction

Myasthenia gravis is an autoimmune disorder that is characterized by progressive muscular weakness caused by a reduction in the number of functionally active acetylcholine receptors in the sarcolemma of the myoneural junction. Circulating antibodies bind to acetylcholine receptors in the junctional folds and inhibit normal nerve-muscle communication. As the body attempts to correct the condition, membrane segments with affected receptors are internalized, digested by lysosomes, and replaced by newly formed receptors. These receptors, however, are rapidly rendered unresponsive to acetylcholine by the same antibodies, and the disease follows in its progressive course.

KEY CONCEPTS BOX 36-3

- Myocardial infarction (MI) occurs when an area of the heart dies following cessation of blood flow to that area because of occlusive disease of the myocardial blood vessels.
- As the degree of blockage varies, so do the clinical symptoms; symptoms can range from increasing pain that occurs with less stress on the heart, to frank MI.
- The clinically important proteins used to diagnose acute coronary syndrome (ACS) are myoglobin, creatine kinase (CK)-MB, and the troponins I and T. The troponins are the most sensitive biomarker for ACS and MI.
- Congestive heart failure (CHF) is the result of weakening of cardiac tissue and the inability of the heart to perform its pumping function.
- As a result of excess fluid that accumulates in CHF, the atria release brain natriuretic peptide (BNP), which is used as a biomarker for CHF.
- An arrhythmia is any abnormality of the conductive system of the heart that resuts in an abnormal beating pattern of the heart. Bradycardia is a decreased heart rate (<60 beats/min), and tachycardia is an increased heart rate (>100 beats/min).
- Atrial and ventricular fibrillations are uneven rhythms of the atria and ventricles; the latter fibrillation can be deadly.

SECTION OBJECTIVES BOX 36-3

- List the primary function tests used to assess myocardial function.
- List cardioactive drugs whose serum levels might need monitoring.
- List the expected time frame for cardiac biomarkers to become elevated following myocardial infarction and then return to normal.
- Compare the use of the troponins, CK-MB, and myoglobin in the diagnosis of MI.
- Compare the diagnostic use of cardiac troponins T and I in assessing cardiac injury.

FUNCTION TESTS

The most important tests for assessment of cardiac function are the electrocardiogram (ECG) and myocardial imaging techniques. The ECG, which involves noninvasive recording of electrical impulses through the heart, is an effective but not perfect means of assessing cardiac rhythm abnormalities and diagnosing an MI. Although relatively specific for MI, the diagnostic sensitivity of the ECG is believed to range from 43% to 65%. Data suggest that the diagnostic reliability of the initial ECG in the emergency department setting found the sensitivity and specificity for acute MI to be 79% and 83%, respectively. Myocardial imaging techniques (**technetium 99m** [^{99m}Tc] pyrophosphate, and **thallium 201**) are used to assess cardiac output and wall motion abnormalities, and to detect nonfunctioning regions of the myocardium caused by infarction. The diagnostic sensitivity of the technetium 99m pyrophosphate scan may be as high as 84% in transmural infarctions; however, the sensitivity may be as low as 32% in patients with nontransmural infarctions. The thallium 201 scan is not typically used for initial diagnosis of infarction.

DRUG THERAPY

Two groups of drugs have a direct effect on cardiac tissue and therefore are monitored by the clinical chemistry laboratory. These include the cardiac **glycosides** and antiarrhythmic drugs.

Glycosides

The glycosides increase contractility in the heart and are particularly useful in treating heart failure. The problem with glycosides is that the therapeutic-to-toxic ratio is very low. At toxic dosage levels, the glycosides can upset the electrical activity of the heart and induce fatal arrhythmias. Because they have long half-lives in the body, they tend to have cumulative effects, necessitating careful monitoring of blood levels to reduce the possibility of toxic side effects. Testing for the most commonly used cardiac glycoside, digoxin, is often needed on a stat. basis.

Antiarrhythmic Drugs

Lidocaine is an anesthetic compound that is given intravenously as a bolus or infusion to suppress ventricular irregularities and to prevent the induction of life-threatening arrhythmias, such as ventricular tachycardia. Lidocaine is a particularly attractive drug because it has few side effects, and because it has little or no effect on myocardial function and cardiac conduction. Rare requests for serum lidocaine measurements most often are associated with cardiac surgery patients.

Many antiarrhythmic drugs have a major side effect of inducing severe arrhythmias; for this reason, drug blood levels usually are monitored, so that one may use antiarrhythmic drugs as safely as possible. Infrequently monitored antiarrhythmic drugs are quinidine and procainamide and its metabolite, N-acetyl procainamide (NAPA).

CHANGE OF ANALYTE IN DISEASE

Myocardiocyte Biomarkers

When cardiac myocytes become necrotic, they lose membrane integrity, and intracellular macromolecules diffuse into the cardiac interstitium and ultimately into the cardiac microvasculature and lymphatics. Eventually, these biomarkers are detectable in the peripheral circulation. The term currently used to collectively describe these macromolecules is *cardiac biomarkers*. The ideal cardiac marker of MI should be abundant in myocytes and low in blood, released early after injury, and absent from nonmyocardial tissue. It should be rapidly released into the blood at the time of myocardial injury, and there should be a direct relation between the plasma level of the cardiac marker and the extent of myocardial injury. The marker should persist in blood for a sufficient length of time

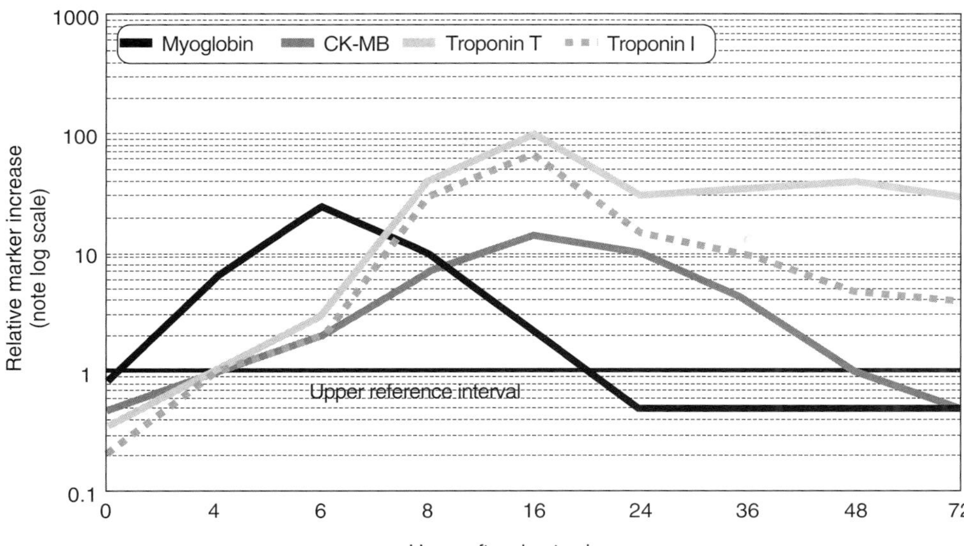

Fig. 36-2 Relative marker increase after myocardial infarction. Markers are expressed as multiples of the upper limit of the reference interval. Therefore, the relative increase varies, depending on the normal reference interval used. The time scale above (*x*-axis) is not linear. (Drawing adapted with permission from Wu A: *Cardiac Markers*, Totowa, NJ, 1998, Humana Press.)

to allow a high rate of diagnosis. Finally, measurement of the marker should be easy, inexpensive, and rapid.

Definition of Myocardial Infarction (MI)

MI represents the end of the acute coronary syndrome continuum, in which ischemic injury is irreversible, leading to cell death and necrosis. Diagnosis of acute myocardial infarction relies upon the clinical history of the patient, interpretation of the electrocardiograms, and measurement of serum levels of cardiac-specific biomarkers. Based on the ECG, two classifications of MI are possible: ST elevation MI, which tends to be larger and tends to affect the anterior location of the heart, and non-ST elevation (NSTE) MI, which tends to involve less myocardial tissue. In the past, a general consensus existed for the clinical entity designated as MI. In studies of disease prevalence conducted by the WHO, MI was defined by a combination of at least two of three characteristics: typical symptoms (such as chest discomfort), a rise in biochemical marker levels, and a typical ECG pattern involving the development of Q waves. However, current clinical practice, health care delivery systems, epidemiologic studies, and clinical trials all require a more precise definition of MI.

In response to increased evidence gained by new cardiac biomarkers such as troponin and the development of other technologies for assessment of the acute coronary syndromes, including MI, the European Society of Cardiology (ESC) and the American College of Cardiology (ACC) held a consensus conference in July 1999 to reexamine the definition of MI. As a result of these activities, cTnT and cTnI now represent the cornerstone for the definition and detection of MI. It became apparent from these deliberations that the term *MI* required further qualifications. Such qualifications should refer to the amount of myocardial cell loss (infarct size), the circumstances leading to the infarct (spontaneous or in a setting of a coronary artery diagnostic or therapeutic procedure), and the timing of the myocardial necrosis relative to the time of the observation (evolving, healing, or healed MI).

Also necessitating reevaluation of established definitions of MI is the advent of sensitive and specific serological biomarkers capable of detecting small infarcts (as little as 1.0 g of dead tissue) that may not have been considered an MI in an earlier era. If it is accepted that any amount of myocardial necrosis caused by ischemia should be labeled as an infarct (as proposed by the ESC/ACC), then individuals formally diagnosed with severe, stable, or unstable angina might be diagnosed today as having had MI. According to the ESC/ACC document, the cutoff for cardiac biomarkers used to diagnose MI is the 99th percentile of a reference control population. The increased sensitivity criterion for MI means that more cases will be identified. In contrast, increased specificity of the troponins would lessen the number of false-positive MI results.

Cardiac Biomarkers in MI

After the onset of symptoms in MI is a "time window," during which elevated values for the cardiac markers released from myocardial tissue become elevated in blood. This temporal relationship is unique for each cardiac marker and varies somewhat among individuals, although a typical pattern is defined for each marker (Fig. 36-2). Usually, 4 to 6 hours is required after the onset of chest pain before CK-MB or the troponins become elevated in the serum of patients with MI. These biomarkers have high diagnostic sensitivity and specificity within 8 to 12 hours after presentation. This time course represents the classic temporal sequence of CK-MB changes and often is helpful in distinguishing uncomplicated MI from extension or reinfarction.

Clinical interpretation of cardiac biomarker data for the diagnosis of MI requires that samples be collected and analyzed at appropriate intervals. Because the temporal sequence of events is critical in the assessment of biochemical changes, the diagnosis of an MI with cardiac markers should not be made on the basis of a single isolated specimen, particularly if the result is negative. Some studies have recommended a sampling sequence that includes samples collected on admission and at 2 to 4 hours, 6 to 8 hours, and 12 hours after an MI is suspected. The ESC/ACC consensus report stressed the importance of serial sampling for cardiac markers, recommending sampling upon presentation, at 6 to 9 hours, and again at 12 to 24 hours if earlier samples were negative and the clinical index of suspicion was high.

Results of cardiac marker measurement should be available 24 hours a day, within 30 to 60 minutes of sample collection. Numerous cases in which elevated CK-MB levels were accompanied by normal total CK levels during the initial course of an MI have been documented.[22] In most of these cases, however, a distinct rise and fall of the total CK values occurs, although no value ever exceeds the upper limit of normal.

Recommendations for the Use of Cardiac Biomarkers in Coronary Disease

The assays for cardiac troponins T and I have revolutionized clinical assessment of cardiac disease and patient care. Troponin elevations are substantially more sensitive and specific for cardiac injury than CK-MB, essentially indicating only cardiac disease. High quality assays for the cardiac troponins have significantly decreased the incidence of analytical false positives caused by fibrin interferences and/or cross-reacting antibodies. Thus, the troponins have been generally accepted by the scientific community as the preferred biomarker for clinical investigation of cardiac disease.

Diagnostic Use of Cardiac Troponin T (cTnT) and Cardiac Troponin I (cTnI)

Troponin plays a vital role in the diagnosis and risk stratification of ACS. Several general impressions can be made regarding cTnT and cTnI. First, the release kinetics of cTnT and of cTnI are similar to those of CK-MB after MI. Second, troponin remains elevated in blood for 4 to 10 days after MI. Third, very low troponin values in patients without cardiac disease permit the use of lower discriminator values for determination of MI based on cutoff at the 99th percentile of a reference control population. Finally, troponin's cardiac specificity helps eliminate the diagnostic uncertainty caused by increased CK-MB following skeletal muscle injury.

It must be emphasized that the use of troponins for MI diagnosis requires a setting of cardiac ischemia. Clinical interpretation of elevated cardiac troponin levels that are common in heart failure, end-stage renal disease, and other conditions is uncertain at this time. However, as a biomarker of adverse events, the presence of cardiac troponins suggests that these patients are at greater risk for adverse cardiac events. It should be noted that even though troponin measurements are based on immunoassays, false-positive results may be associated with a variety of factors unrelated to heart disease (see Toponin Methods review on Evolve).

cTnI

Although cTnI has a lower molecular weight (27 kDa) than cTnT (37 kDa) and CK-MB (85 kDa), its release kinetics and use as an early indicator of MI are similar to those of cTnT and CK-MB. cTnI is similar to cTnT in most clinical applications, and its measurement offers the same advantages over CK-MB. cTnI remains elevated 3 to 7 days after acute MI. Thus cTnI and CK-MB have comparable diagnostic sensitivity for MI during the initial 48 to 72 hours after MI, with improved cTnI sensitivities 72 to 96 hours after MI.

In contrast to CK-MB and total CK, cTnI is not elevated in patients with extreme skeletal muscle injury, including (1) acute skeletal muscle injury following marathon racing, (2) chronic myopathy of Duchenne's muscular dystrophy, or (3) chronic renal failure requiring dialysis.

cTnT

Once an MI has occurred, cTnT increases in serum after 4 hours, achieving an initial peak or plateau at 1 to 6 days. A second cTnT peak is observed in some patients with MI, which is thought to occur because cTnT has both cytosolic and structurally bound cTnT pools. The first peak is believed to result from release of the cytosolic pool; the second peak may reflect slower release of the bound fraction later in the myocardial necrosis process.

According to the traditional WHO definition of MI, the clinical sensitivity of cTnT is similar to that of CK-MB during the first 48 hours after onset of chest pain. Thus cTnT is not an early marker of MI; it shows clinical sensitivity of 50% to 65% from 0 to 6 hours after chest pain onset. Because of the extended lifetime of cTnT in serum, levels may provide important diagnostic information about an MI after serum CK-MB has achieved normal levels. In addition, cTnT may offer substantial information about the recent history of myocardial dysfunction. cTnT is useful for risk stratification of patients with ACS and is advocated in clinical guidelines for coronary intervention and for targeting therapy with low-molecular-weight heparin and platelet inhibitors in high-risk patients.

cTnI Versus cTnT

For practical purposes, no major clinical difference has been noted between cTnT and cTnI assays. As much as a 30-fold difference in values has been observed among the various analytical methods used to measure cTnI. Explanation for this disparity is related not only to calibration but also to the fact that the reagent antibodies used in various assays recognize different epitopes on the troponin molecule. In addition, cTnI may be present in the circulation in three forms: (1) free, (2) bound as a two-unit complex (cTnI-cTnC), and (3) bound as a three-unit complex (cTnT-cTnI-cTnC). Issues involving calibration and antibody targets represent an active area of investigation by American Association for Clinical Chemistry (AACC) and International Federation of Clinical Chemistry (IFCC) committees.

Myoglobin

Myoglobin is present in both cardiac and skeletal muscle, limiting its diagnostic specificity. The value of myoglobin assay in MI is its early appearance in serum after MI. Because the interval between onset of symptoms and clinical presentation is variable, it has been suggested that multiple biomarkers are needed to enable detection of MI in patients who present very early or late after the onset of pain. Currently, myoglobin most effectively fits the role of an early marker. A rise in myoglobin is detectable in blood as early as 1 to 2 hours after symptom onset and is highly sensitive for MI diagnosis and effective for rule-out in the 2- to 6-hour time frame after onset of symptoms (see Fig. 36-2). Myoglobin is not cardiac specific, and patients with renal failure, or injury, trauma, or diseases involving the skeletal muscle, can have abnormal concentrations in the absence of MI. The presence of myoglobinuria can be used to confirm massive muscle cytolysis (trauma or drug induced) and as a diagnostic aid for assessing myoglobin-induced acute renal failure.

CK and CK Isoenzymes in Conditions Other Than MI

Frequently, the pattern of cardiac isoenzyme elevation in conditions other than MI does not follow a rise and fall pattern, but instead is chronically elevated. These potential false-positive situations emphasize the importance of documenting an acute ischemic event in the time frame of testing and measuring multiple samples obtained at appropriate intervals. The pattern of CK isoenzymes that is found in the developing fetus is duplicated in the adult in certain pathological states. This alteration is observed most commonly in skeletal muscle. In the adult, CK is present predominantly in the MM form. Fetal muscle, however, is predominantly BB until the 16th week of gestation, at which time expression of the gene coding for the M subunit is significantly increased. Diseases of skeletal muscle characterized by blood perfusion regeneration often are associated with chronically increased levels of the fetal isomeric forms of CK. Thus Duchenne's muscular dystrophy, polymyositis, and some forms of rhabdomyolysis frequently show increased levels of CK-MB in serum. These increases are proportionate to the degree of muscle fiber regeneration. Because normal skeletal muscle contains CK-MB, serum levels of CK-MB are frequently in the range associated with MI following extensive muscle damage. Because the absolute amount of CK in skeletal muscle is about 5- to 10-fold that observed in cardiac tissue, actual elevations in total CK observed in serum in skeletal muscle abnormalities are frequently dramatically higher than those observed in MI, although the proportion that is CK-MB (CK-MB/total CK) is typically quite low.

Caveats for Diagnostic Performance of Cardiac Biomarkers for MI

Interpretation of cardiac biomarkers for the diagnosis of MI can be obscured by false-positive and false-negative results. A fundamental issue in the use of cardiac biomarkers is that the diagnosis of myocardial ischemia without cell death is extremely difficult because few objective data are available, and ischemia can present clinically with many signs and symptoms. Proper interpretation requires an understanding of the clinical setting of ischemia for which testing will occur. The use of cardiac biomarkers in the setting of a coronary care population, with 50% prevalence of disease assumed, clearly increases the predictive values of cardiac biomarkers. In a low-prevalence population such as the emergency department (3%), the usefulness of positive predictive values of cardiac biomarkers for MI will be diminished. In all cases, laboratory data must be used within the context of other clinical findings, such as history of prior cardiac disease, history of coronary pain, and ECG changes.

B-type Natriuretic Peptide, or Brain Natriuretic Peptide (BNP)

BNP and atrial natriuretic peptide (ANP) act as a dual natriuretic system in regulating blood pressure and fluid balance. See Chapter 28 for additional details on the natriuretic peptides. The heart releases BNP in response to ventricular volume expansion and pressure overload. The underlying rationale for the use of BNP as a diagnostic tool for heart failure is its substantial release from the failing heart into the plasma, making it an appealing target for further development.

KEY CONCEPTS BOX 36-4

- Electrocardiogram (ECG) and myocardial imaging can detect malfunctioning hearts.
- Few cardioactive drugs require monitoring of blood levels. Rarely, there may be requests for quinidine or lidocaine. Blood digoxin levels, because of the drug's high potential for toxicity, must be monitored.
- Following a myocardial infarction (MI), myoglobin can be elevated within 4 to 6 hours, and creatine kinase (CK)-MB and the troponins within 6 to 12 hours. Serum levels of myoglobin tend to normalize within 24 hours after an MI, and CK-MB ≈48 hours after an MI; the troponins may not become normal until 7 to 10 days after an MI.
- The best use of serum myoglobin is for the very early detection of MI. However the "gold standard" biomarker for the diagnosis of MI is either of the troponins. Cardiac-specific troponin T (cTnT) and cardiac-specific troponin I (cTnI) appear to be equally effective. CK-MB is not as effective as the troponins but may have limited use in the diagnosis of reinfarction.

BIBLIOGRAPHY

Abbott BG, Wackers FJ: Use of radionuclide imaging in acute coronary syndromes, Curr Cardiol Rep 5:25, 2003.

Andersen HR, Nielsen TT, Rasmussen K, et al: A comparison of coronary angioplasty with fibrinolytic therapy in acute myocardial infarction, N Engl J Med 349:733, 2003.

Antman EM, Tanasijevic MJ, Thompson B, et al: Cardiac-specific troponin I levels to predict the risk of mortality in patients with acute coronary syndromes, N Engl J Med 335:1342, 1996.

Boersma E, Mercado N, Poldermans D, et al: Acute myocardial infarction, Lancet 361:847, 2003.

Gershlick AH, Stephens-Lloyd A, Hughes S, et al: Rescue angioplasty after failed thrombolytic therapy for acute myocardial infarction, N Engl J Med 353:2758, 2005.

Fesmire FM, Hughes AD, Fody EP, et al: The Erlanger chest pain evaluation protocol: a one-year experience with serial 12-lead ECG monitoring, two-hour delta serum marker measurements, and selective nuclear stress testing to identify and exclude acute coronary syndromes, Ann Emerg Med 40:584, 2002.

Kwong RY, Schussheim AE, Rekhraj S, et al: Detecting acute coronary syndrome in the emergency department with cardiac magnetic resonance imaging, Circulation 107:531, 2003.

Newby LK, Rutsch WR, Califf RM, et al: Time from symptom onset to treatment and outcomes after thrombolytic therapy: GUSTO-1 Investigators, J Am Coll Cardiol 27:1646, 1996.

Ohman EM, Armstrong PW, Christenson RH, et al: Cardiac troponin T levels for risk stratification in acute myocardial ischemia: GUSTO IIA Investigators, N Engl J Med 335:1333, 1996.

Ohman EM, Armstrong PW, White HD, et al: Risk stratification with a point-of-care cardiac troponin T test in acute myocardial infarction: GUSTO III Investigators: global use of strategies to open occluded coronary arteries, Am J Cardiol 84:1281, 1999.

Tsai TN, Yang SP, Tsao TP, et al: Delayed diagnosis of post-traumatic acute myocardial infarction complicated by congestive heart failure, J Emerg Med 29:429, 2005.

Yuichi S, Takako I, Fumio I, et al: Detection of atherosclerotic coronary artery plaques by multislice spiral computed tomography in patients with acute coronary syndrome: report of 2 cases, Circ J 68:263, 2004.

Chen HH, Burnett JC: Natriuretic peptides in the pathophysiology of congestive heart failure, Curr Cardiol Rep 2:198, 2000.

Cheng V, Kazanagra R, Garcia A, et al: A rapid bedside test for B-type peptide predicts treatment outcomes in patients admitted for decompensated heart failure: a pilot study, J Am Coll Cardiol 37:386, 2001.

Effects of metoprolol CR in patients with ischemic and dilated cardiomyopathy: the randomized evaluation of strategies for left ventricular dysfunction pilot study, Circulation 101:378, 2000.

Cody RJ: Hormonal alterations in heart failure. In Hosenpud JB, Greenberg BH, editors: *Congestive Heart Failure: Pathophysiology, Diagnosis and Comprehensive Approach to Management*, Philadelphia, 2000, Lippincott Williams & Wilkins, pp. 199-212.

Dao Q, Krishnaswamy P, Kazanegra R, et al: Utility of B-type natriuretic peptide in the diagnosis of congestive heart failure in an urgent-care setting, J Am Coll Cardiol 37:379, 2001.

Feldman AM, Combes A, Wagner D, et al: The role of tumor necrosis factor in the pathophysiology of heart failure, J Am Coll Cardiol 35:537, 2000.

Fenton DE: Myocardial infarction, 2007. Available at http://www.emedicine.com/emerg/TOPIC327.htm.

Febton DE: Acute coronary syndrome, 2007. Available at http://www.emedicine.com/EMERG/topic31.htm.

Fonarow GC: The treatment targets in acute decompensated heart failure, Rev Cardiovasc Med 2(suppl 2):S7, 2001.

He J, Ogden LG, Bazzano LA, et al: Risk factors for congestive heart failure in US men and women: NHANES I epidemiologic follow-up study, Arch Intern Med 161:996, 2001.

Krumholz HM, Chen YT, Wang Y, et al: Predictors of readmission among elderly survivors of admission with heart failure, Am Heart J 139(1 Pt 1):72, 2001.

Maisel AS, Koon J, Hope J, et al: A rapid bedside test for brain natriuretic peptide accurately predicts cardiac function in patients referred for echocardiography, Am Heart J 141:374, 2001.

NACB Writing Group Members, Apple FS, Jesse RL, Newby LK, et al: National Academy of Clinical Biochemistry and IFCC Committee for Standardization of Markers of Cardiac Damage Laboratory Medicine Practice Guidelines: Analytical Issues for Biochemical Markers of Acute Coronary Syndromes, Clin Chem 53:545, 2007.

Rich MW, McSherry F, Williford WO: Effect of age on mortality, hospitalizations and response to digoxin in patients with heart failure: the DIG study, J Am Coll Cardiol 38:806, 2001.

Saenger and Jaffe: Requiem for a Heavyweight; The Demise of Creatine Kinase-MB. Circulation 118:2200-2206, 2008.

Thygesen K, Alpert JS, Jaffe, AS, et al. Universal definition of myocardial infarction. Circulation 116:2634-2653, 2007.

Zevitz ME: Heart failure, 2006. Available at http://www.emedicine.com/MED/topic3552.htm.

INTERNET SITES

http://health.howstuffworks.com—Animations of heartbeat, descriptions of muscle types, and percutaneous transluminal coronary angioplasty

http://www.blackwellpublishing.com/matthews/myosin.html—Animated illustration from *Neurobiology Molecules, Cells and Systems*, by Gary G. Matthews

http://www.nhlbi.nih.gov/health/dci/Browse/Heart.html—NHLBI website with information and animations for various heart and blood vessel diseases

http://content.onlinejacc.org/cgi/content/full/50/7/e1—ACC/AHA 2007 Guidelines for the management of patients with unstable angina/non-ST-elevation myocardial infarction

http://www.acc.org/qualityandscience/clinical/data_standards/ACS/pdf/ACS_clinicaldata.pdf—American College of Cardiology key data elements and definitions for measuring the clinical management and outcomes of patients with acute coronary syndromes

http://content.onlinejacc.org/cgi/content/full/j.jacc.2007.10.001—2007 Focused update of the ACC/AHA 2004 guidelines for the management of patients with ST-elevation myocardial infarction

http://content.onlinejacc.org/cgi/content/full/j.jacc.2007.09.011—Universal definition of myocardial infarction

http://www.acc.org/qualityandscience/clinical/guidelines/stemi/STEMI%20Full%20Text.pdf—ACC/AHA guidelines for the management of patients with ST-elevation myocardial infarction

http://www.mhhe.com/biosci/esp/2002_general/Esp/folder_structure/tr/m1/s7/trm1s7_3.htm—McGraw-Hill animation of blood clotting cascade

http://www.science-art.com/image.asp?id=3181&search=1—Animation of motor neuron delivering action potential to a muscle cell

http://www.johnkyrk.com/krebs.html—Animation of the Krebs cycle

Guidelines for MI

www.acc.org/qualityandscience/clinical/consensus/mi_redefined/index.cfm—Myocardial infarction redefined: a consensus document

www.escardio.org—European Society of Cardiology

http://medlib.med.utah.edu/WebPath/TUTORIAL/MYOCARD/MYOCARD.html—University of Utah tutorial

www.nlm.nih.gov/medlineplus/ency/article/000158.htm—National Medical Library, *Encyclopedia: Heart Failure*

http://users.rcn.com/jkimball.ma.ultranet/BiologyPages/M/Muscles.html

Coronary Artery Disease: Lipid Metabolism

John R. Burnett

Chapter 37

Chapter Outline

PART 1: LIPIDS
Normal Physiology of Lipids
Lipid Composition of Foods
Fat Digestion, Absorption, and Metabolism of Lipids
Cholesterol Metabolism
Biological Functions
Physiology
Synthesis
Catabolism
Expected Cholesterol Values
Triglyceride Metabolism
Biological Functions
Physiology
Synthesis
Catabolism
Expected Triglyceride Values
PART 2: APOLIPOPROTEINS
Apolipoprotein A
Apolipoprotein B
Apolipoprotein C
Apolipoprotein E
Apolipoproteins as Markers of Cardiovascular Disease Risk
PART 3: LIPOPROTEINS
Classification of Lipoproteins
Chylomicrons
Very-Low-Density Lipoprotein
Low-Density Lipoprotein
High-Density Lipoprotein
Other Lipoproteins
Lipoprotein Metabolism
Chylomicrons
Very-Low-Density Lipoprotein
Intermediate-Density Lipoprotein
Low-Density Lipoprotein
High-Density Lipoprotein
PART 4: PATHOLOGICAL DISORDERS
Hyperlipidemia
Hyperlipoproteinemia
Metabolic Syndrome
Genetic Dyslipoproteinemias
Familial Hyperchylomicronemia
Familial Hypertriglyceridemia
Monogenic Hypercholesterolemia
Monogenic Hypocholesterolemia
Familial Hypoalphalipoproteinemia
Tangier Disease
Transformation of Hyperlipidemia to Hyperlipoproteinemia
From Lipids to Lipoproteins: Laboratory Considerations
Secondary Hyperlipoproteinemia
Clinical Implications of Hyperlipidemia
Coronary Artery Disease
Atherosclerotic Plaque Formation
Change of Analyte in Disease: Therapeutic Guidelines and Treatment

Key Terms

acanthocytosis A cell membrane defect of red cells.

amphipathic From amphi- ("on both sides") and -pathic ("of feeling"); pertaining either to a molecule that has two sides with characteristically different properties, or to a detergent that has both a polar (hydrophilic) end and a nonpolar (hydrophobic) end but is long enough so that each end demonstrates its own solubility characteristics.

apo, apolipoprotein Lipid-binding protein constituents of lipoproteins.

chylomicron Large lipid-protein complexes that are made by the gut and serve an important function in the transport of fats (mainly dietary triglycerides).

corneal arcus A white ring in the corneal margin that can occur in familial hypercholesterolemia.

lipoproteins Lipid-protein complexes consisting of discrete families of macromolecules with known physical, chemical, and physiological properties.

mitogens Cellular factors that induce a cell to commence cell division.

retinitis pigmentosa A disorder in which abnormalities of the retina lead to progressive visual loss.

xanthomas Deposits of yellowish cholesterol-rich material in vasculature and skin, especially around tendons and eyelids.

Abbreviations

ABCA1 ATP-binding cassette transporter A1. A membrane-associated protein that is a major regulator of cellular cholesterol homeostasis.

ABL Abetalipoproteinemia. An extremely rare recessive disorder characterized by an absence of plasma apoB-containing lipoproteins that interferes with the normal absorption of fat and fat-soluble vitamins from food.

ACAT Acyl-coenzyme A:cholesterol acyltransferase. ACAT catalyzes the intracellular formation of cholesteryl esters from cholesterol and fatty acids.

ATP Adenosine triphosphate.

CAD Coronary artery disease.

CETP Cholesteryl ester transfer protein. A plasma protein involved in the transfer of cholesteryl esters and triglycerides between lipoproteins.

CHD Coronary heart disease.

CVD Cardiovascular disease.

CoA Coenzyme A.

EFA Essential fatty acids. Fatty acids that cannot be synthesized by humans and must be obtained from the diet.

ER Endoplasmic reticulum. A cellular organelle responsible for synthesis of lipids and transport of proteins.

FCHL Familial combined hyperlipidemia. A common dominant disorder characterized by mixed hyperlipidemia and premature coronary heart disease (CHD).

FDB Familial defective apoB-100. A rare dominant disorder characterized by very high LDL levels in the blood and early cardiovascular disease (CVD) that runs in families.

FFA Free fatty acids.

FH Familial hypercholesterolemia. A rare dominant disorder characterized by very high LDL levels in the blood and early CVD.

FHA Familial hypoalphalipoproteinemia. An inheritable disorder characterized by low HDL levels in the blood.

FHBL Familial hypobetalipoproteinemia. A rare dominant disorder characterized by very low LDL levels in blood and protection from CVD.

HDL High-density lipoprotein. A lipoprotein complex also called α-lipoprotein, and the most dense of the lipoproteins.

HMG-CoA 3-Hydroxy-3-methylglutaryl CoA.

IDL Intermediate-density lipoprotein. A lipid-protein complex that has a density between VLDL and LDL and a very short half-life. It is present in the blood in very low concentrations in a healthy person. In a person with dysbetalipoproteinemia, the IDL concentration in the blood is elevated.

LCAT Lecithin:cholesterol acyltransferase. An enzyme that converts free cholesterol, which is incorporated into new HDL particles into cholesteryl ester.

LDL Low-density lipoprotein. A lipid-protein complex that is the end product of VLDL catabolism and the major carrier of serum cholesterol. Also called β-lipoprotein.

LPL Lipoprotein lipase. An enzyme that hydrolyzes triglyceride in lipoproteins.

Lp(a) Lipoprotein (a). An LDL-like lipoprotein that consists of apo(a) covalently bound to apoB-100.

Lp-X Lipoprotein X. An abnormal lipoprotein found in cholestasis.

MI Myocardial infarction. More commonly known as a "heart attack," it is a medical condition that occurs when the blood supply to a part of the heart is interrupted, most commonly as the result of rupture of a vulnerable plaque.

MTTP Microsomal triglyceride transfer protein. A chaperone protein that plays a central role in lipoprotein assembly and secretion.

NCEP ATP National Cholesterol Education Program Adult Treatment Panel.

NEFA Non-esterified fatty acids.

NIH National Institutes of Health.

PHLA Post-heparin lipolytic activity.

SR-BI Scavenger receptor B type I. A liver cell membrane protein that facilitates hepatic uptake of cholesteryl esters from HDL.

TD Tangier disease. An extremely rare recessive disorder characterized by a severe reduction or absence of HDL in plasma.

TLC Therapeutic lifestyle change.

TRL Triglyceride-rich lipoproteins. These are primarily chylomicrons and very-low-density lipoproteins (VLDL).

VLDL Very-low-density lipoprotein. A relatively large lipid-protein complex that transports mainly endogenously synthesized triglycerides.

Methods on Evolve

Apolipoproteins A1 and B
Cholesterol
High-density lipoprotein (HDL) cholesterol
Lipoprotein(a)
Triglycerides

SECTION OBJECTIVES BOX 37-1

- Describe the various phases of lipid digestion.
- Describe the processes of absorption and metabolism of cholesterol and triglycerides, including the roles of the intestine, liver, and adipose tissue.

PART 1: Lipids

NORMAL PHYSIOLOGY OF LIPIDS

Lipid Composition of Foods

About 98% to 99% of the fat found in food is composed of triglycerides, of which 92% to 95% are fatty acids and the remainder is glycerol. The remaining 1% to 2% of dietary lipids includes cholesterol, phospholipids, diglycerides, monoglycerides, fat-soluble vitamins, steroids, terpenes, and other fats. Most triglycerides contain four or five major fatty acids, including both saturated and unsaturated fatty acids. Several polyunsaturated acids (linoleic, linolenic, and arachidonic acids) cannot be synthesized in the animal body and must be provided in the diet. These have been termed **essential fatty acids (EFA)** (see Chapter 41).

The small amount of nonhydrolyzable matter in food fats consists of sterols, fatty alcohols, hydrocarbons, pigments, glycerol esters, and various other compounds. Most sterols consist of cholesterol, especially in animal fat, but depending on the diet, other sterols, such as phytosterols, can make up an appreciable percentage of total sterols, particularly in individuals on vegetarian diets. The phytosterols are important because they compete with cholesterol for uptake by the mucosal cell. Thus the more phytosterols consumed, the less dietary cholesterol is absorbed by the mucosal cells of the gut.

Fat Digestion, Absorption, and Metabolism of Lipids

Fat absorption occurs in three phases: the intraluminal phase (or digestive phase), during which dietary fats are modified both physically and chemically before absorption; the cellular phase (or absorptive phase), in which digested material enters the intestinal mucosal cells, where it is reassembled into its preabsorptive form; and the transport phase, during which absorbed lipids are carried from the mucosal cell to other tissues through the lymphatics and blood (Fig. 37-1).[1]

Intraluminal Phase

After ingestion of a meal, fat digestion by salivary and gastric lipases begins in the stomach. The products of this hydrolysis are carried in an emulsion to the small intestine. Most digestion of food fat occurs in the intestine through the action of intestinal and pancreatic enzymes (lipases) and bile acids (see Chapters 35 and 34, respectively). Because of their surface-active properties, the bile salts emulsify dietary triglycerides into very small particles with diameters of about 1 μm. The emulsification process thus forms particles that can be readily acted on by the digestive enzymes. In the intestinal lumen, the action of pancreatic lipase on ingested fat results in the progressive digestion of triglycerides to 1,2-diglycerides, and then to 2-monoglycerides and fatty acids. Only a small percentage of the fat is completely hydrolyzed to **non-esterified fatty acids (NEFA)** and glycerol. Cholesteryl esters (about 10% of total) are hydrolyzed by the enzyme cholesterol esterase to free cholesterol and NEFA.

Absorptive Phase

After monoglycerides and fatty acids enter the endoplasmic reticulum (ER) of the mucosal cell of the brush border membranes, presumably by diffusion, the monoglycerides and

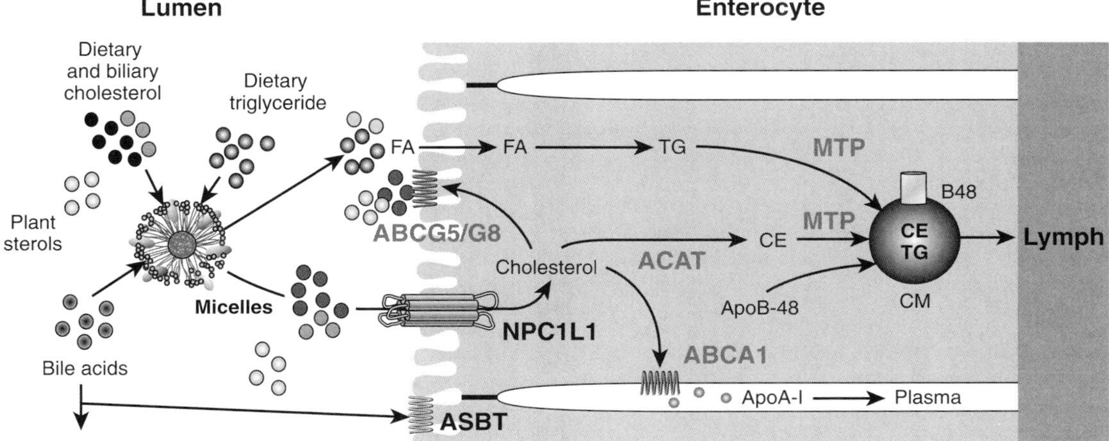

Fig. 37-1 Cholesterol absorption pathway. *ABCA1,* ATP binding cassette transporter A1; *ABCG5/G8,* ATP binding cassette transporter G5/G8; *ACAT,* acyl-coenzyme A:cholesterol acyltransferase; *ApoA-I,* apolipoprotein A-I; *ASBT,* apical sodium-dependent bile acid transportor; *B48,* apolipoprotein B-48; *CE,* cholesteryl ester; *CM,* chylomicron; *FA,* fatty acid; *MTP,* microsomal triglyceride transfer protein; *NPC1L1,* Niemann-Pick C-1–like 1; *TG,* triglyceride; ●, biliary cholesterol; ●, dietary cholesterol; ●, dietary triglyceride; ○, plant sterols; ●, bile acids; ○, fatty acids. (Modified with permission from Burnett JR, Huff MW: Cholesterol absorption inhibitors as a therapeutic option for hypercholesterolemia, Exp Opin Investig Drugs 15:1337, 2006.)

fatty acids are re-esterified into triglycerides by either of two pathways. The monoglyceride pathway is peculiar to the intestinal mucosa and involves the direct acylation of the absorbed monoglyceride from the lumen with activated NEFA. The α-glycerophosphate pathway present in most tissues, including the intestine, involves the formation of a **coenzyme A (CoA)** derivative of the fatty acid (acyl-CoA). This reaction, which requires **adenosine triphosphate (ATP),** is catalyzed by the enzyme fatty acid:CoA ligase, which has a pronounced specificity for longer-chain fatty acids. Thus long-chain fatty acids appear in thoracic duct lymph transported as triglycerides in the **chylomicrons,** whereas short- and medium-chain fatty acids are transported bound to albumin in the portal circulation.

Intraluminal cholesterol includes about 400 mg of dietary cholesterol (in an average Western diet), 200 to 400 mg of non-cholesterol sterols (derived mostly from plants), 800 to 1200 mg of biliary cholesterol, and ≈300 mg derived from intestinal mucosal cell turnover. The transporter protein Niemann-Pick C-1–like 1 (NPC1L1), which is localized to the brush border membrane of jejunal enterocytes, is critical for absorption of intestinal cholesterol and plant sterols.[2,3] Once within the enterocytes, about 75% of absorbed cholesterol is esterified by **acyl-coA:cholesterol acyltransferase (ACAT),** an enzyme thought to be critical for net cholesterol absorption. Cholesterol esterification facilitates chylomicron assembly, which prevents the transport of cholesterol via the ATP binding cassette transporters ABCG5 and ABCG8, back into the lumen of the small intestine. An understanding of the molecular mechanisms of intestinal cholesterol absorption and transport[4] has led to novel therapeutic approaches to inhibiting the cholesterol absorption process.[5]

Transport Phase

Resynthesized triglycerides, along with cholesterol, cholesteryl esters, and phospholipids, are packaged within the intestinal mucosal cell ER, together with the protein apoB-48, into water-soluble macromolecules called *chylomicrons,* facilitated by the **microsomal triglyceride transfer protein (MTTP).**[6] The intestinal **lipoproteins** leave the mucosal cells presumably by reverse pinocytosis. They first appear in the lymphatic vessels of the abdominal region and later enter the systemic circulation via the thoracic duct. The intestinal release of chylomicrons persists for several hours after ingestion of a fat meal. Because the chylomicrons are large enough to scatter light (up to 0.5 μm in diameter), the plasma becomes lactescent (turbid)—the alimentary lipemic response. These chylomicrons are mixtures of triglycerides (82%), some proteins (2%, as apoproteins), small amounts of cholesterol (9%, mainly as ester), and phospholipids (7%). Although the amount of protein is small, a good deal of evidence suggests that its presence is necessary for the release of chylomicrons. For example, in **abetalipoproteinemia** (ABL, a genetically determined disease in which apoB-containing lipoproteins cannot be made in the body), triglycerides are not released from the intestinal cells.

The bloodstream transports chylomicrons to all tissues in the body, including adipose tissue, which is their principal site of uptake. The chylomicrons (Fig. 37-2) are removed rather rapidly (within minutes) and normally are present in only

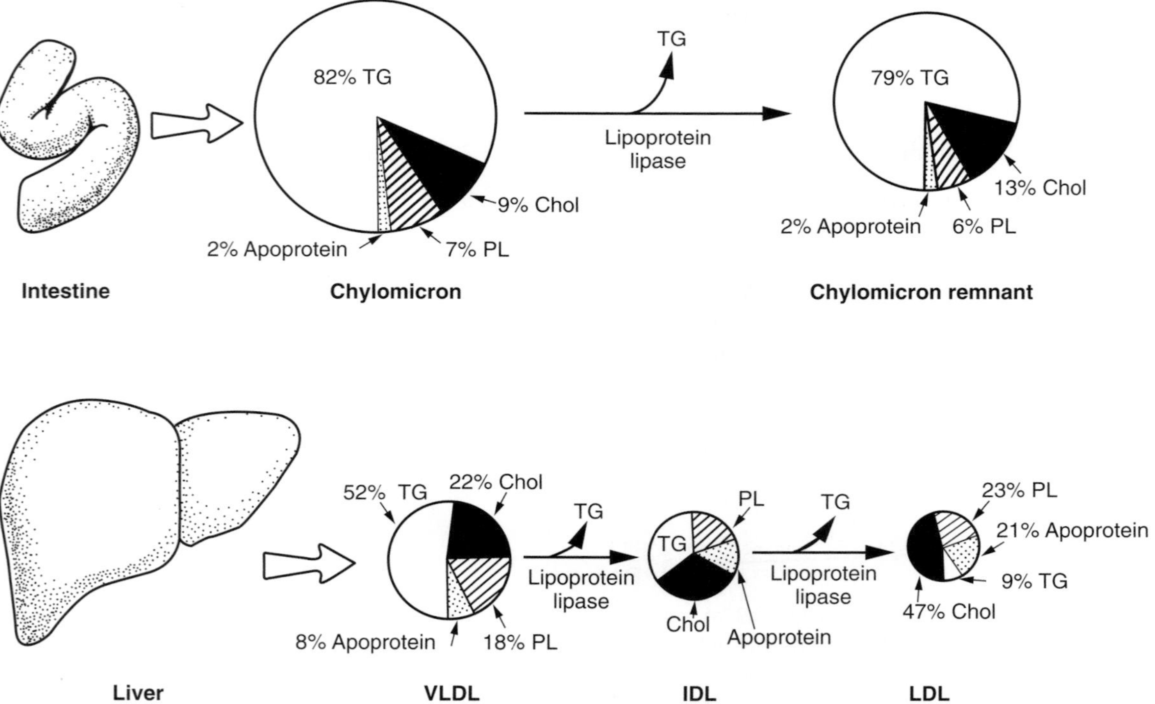

Fig. 37-2 Origin and catabolic pathway of chylomicron and very-low-density lipoprotein (VLDL). End product of chylomicron is chylomicron remnant; end product of VLDL is LDL. *Chol,* Cholesterol; *PL,* phosphatidyl lecithin; *TG,* triglyceride.

trace amounts in blood samples taken from individuals after an overnight fast.

Under normal conditions, chylomicron catabolism proceeds in two known phases. In the first, triglycerides are hydrolyzed at extrahepatic tissue sites under the influence of **lipoprotein lipase (LPL),** the key enzyme for regulating the catabolism of **triglyceride-rich lipoproteins (TRL)** in the circulation. LPL belongs to a family that includes hepatic lipase, pancreatic lipase, and the recently discovered endothelial lipase. The process of removing triglycerides by LPL hydrolysis results in a relatively triglyceride-poor, cholesterol-rich remnant particle. In the second catabolic phase, remnant particles, which are believed to be highly atherogenic, are removed from the circulation by the liver.

Hydrolysis by LPL of TRL takes place at the luminal surface (bloodstream side) of the capillary endothelium. The enzyme is bound to the capillary endothelial cells in muscle and adipose tissue and can be released by intravenous administration of heparin **(post-heparin lipolytic activity [PHLA]).**

As a result of the first phase of chylomicron metabolism, NEFA are released into the bloodstream, and the diglycerides and monoglycerides are taken up in vacuoles and transported across the capillary wall for hydrolysis. Within tissue cells, the NEFA derived from triglycerides in chylomicrons (or **very-low-density lipoproteins [VLDL],** see following) can be stored or used for energy when needed, especially by the heart. NEFA also are used for cellular phospholipid synthesis, including synthesis of prostaglandins, the ubiquitous local hormones.

Role of Liver in Metabolism of Lipids

In addition to the intestine, the liver can synthesize lipoprotein particles from recently absorbed dietary constituents. In fact, the liver is the major organ that synthesizes cholesterol; about 70% of daily cholesterol production comes from the liver. Dietary-derived and newly synthesized hepatic triglycerides are coupled with phospholipid, cholesterol, and proteins to form VLDL. These macromolecules then are released into the circulation and transported to adipose tissue, where they are metabolized as other TRL, to deliver triglycerides to muscle and adipose cells.

Hepatic triglyceride synthesis is accelerated when the diet is rich in excess calories, resulting in VLDL overproduction; this may explain the hypertriglyceridemia observed when diets are particularly rich in simple sugars.

During fasting, metabolic pathways in the liver are reversed. Blood glucose concentration falls, insulin concentrations are diminished, and hepatic VLDL triglyceride synthesis is reduced. NEFA derived from adipose tissue are taken up by the liver; their oxidation to ketone bodies provides energy for gluconeogenesis. NEFA of adipose tissue origin can be esterified to triglycerides, incorporated into hepatic VLDL, and then secreted into the bloodstream. During periods of stress and in certain metabolic conditions, such as uncontrolled diabetes, NEFA are the principal precursors of hepatic VLDL. VLDL remnants, the end products of the first phase of VLDL catabolism, are metabolized further at extracellular sites, resulting in the formation of low-density lipoprotein (LDL), a cholesterol-rich particle.

KEY CONCEPTS BOX 37-1

- Dietary lipids are hydrolyzed in the intestinal tract and reassembled within the intestinal epithelium.
- Reassembled dietary fats are released into the circulation as chylomicrons, which function to deliver triglyceride to peripheral cells (primarily adipose cells).
- Remnant chylomicrons are taken up by the liver, which re-exports fats as VLDL; VLDL also serve to deliver triglyceride to adipose tissue.

SECTION OBJECTIVES BOX 37-2

- Describe the functions and biosynthesis of cholesterol and triglycerides.
- Describe the role of cholesterol esterification and the role of triglycerides in the process of lipoprotein metabolism.
- Describe the variables that affect plasma cholesterol and triglyceride concentrations.

CHOLESTEROL METABOLISM

Biological Functions

Cholesterol is a member of a large class of biological compounds called *steroids* that have a similar four-ring structure, a cyclopentanoperhydrophenanthrene ring (Fig. 37-3).

Because of the well-established positive association between plasma cholesterol concentration and **coronary heart disease (CHD),** we are apt to think of cholesterol as a harmful substance. Contrary to that belief, cholesterol is essential for normal functioning of the organism because it is

1. An essential structural component of the membranes of all animal cells and subcellular particles
2. An obligatory precursor of bile acids
3. A precursor of all steroid hormones, including sex and adrenal hormones

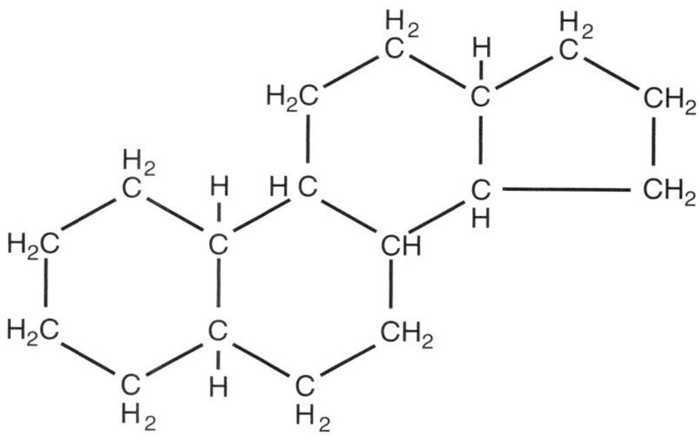

Fig. 37-3 Chemical structure of cyclopentanoperhydrophenanthrene ring. This common four-ring structure is the basic structure of all steroids.

Physiology

Tissue cholesterol is in constant exchange with plasma cholesterol; the turnover rate and the amount of tissue cholesterol that is exchangeable with plasma cholesterol vary from one tissue to another. About 55% of dietary cholesterol is normally absorbed and retained; in contrast, <1% of the non-cholesterol sterols are retained. Although most of the total body pool of cholesterol is derived from de novo cholesterol synthesis, dietary sources play an important role in maintaining total body sterol balance. Dietary cholesterol regulates the amount of de novo synthesis, and the liver is a key organ in maintaining this balance. Excess body cholesterol, derived from endogenous synthesis or from dietary absorption, is excreted exclusively by the liver, either by direct excretion as free cholesterol into bile or by conversion to bile acids, and is excreted as bile acid conjugates into bile.

Because of loss and replacement, about 2% of the body's cholesterol is renewed each day. The main channel for outflow from the pool is the gastrointestinal tract; the absolute rate of turnover as estimated by measurement of daily fecal output is 1 to 2 g/day of cholesterol, with excretion of bile acids accounting for about half the total turnover. Fig. 37-4 illustrates that the concentration of a given cholesterol pool is under the influence of cholesterol input and output, and turnover rates. It should be stressed that because of the continuous cycling of cholesterol into and out of the bloodstream, the plasma cholesterol concentration is not a simple additive function of dietary cholesterol intake and endogenous cholesterol synthesis. Rather, it reflects the rates of synthesis of cholesterol-carrying lipoproteins and the efficiency of the cellular receptor mechanisms that determine their catabolism. A detailed discussion of the dynamics of lipoprotein concentration can be found in the section on lipoprotein metabolism.

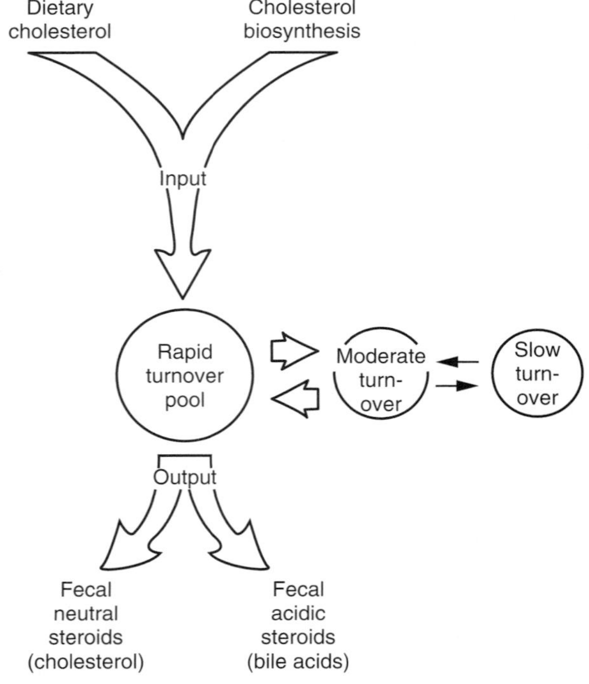

Fig. 37-4 Scheme of dynamics of cholesterol metabolism.

Cholesterol is present in all plasma lipoproteins, but about 60% of the total cholesterol in plasma from a fasting human is carried in the LDL. About two thirds of plasma total cholesterol is esterified with long-chain fatty acids, with linoleic acid being the predominant fatty acid in humans. The cholesteryl esters in the plasma are in a state of constant turnover because of their continual hydrolysis and resynthesis. Hydrolysis of cholesteryl esters takes place in the liver, but synthesis occurs mainly in the plasma through transfer of a fatty acid residue from lecithin to free cholesterol (Fig. 37-5). A plasma enzyme known as **lecithin:cholesterol acyltransferase (LCAT)** catalyzes this reaction. The preferred lipoprotein substrate for human LCAT is **high-density lipoprotein (HDL),** and it seems likely that the bulk of esterified cholesterol in the plasma is formed on HDL. The cholesteryl ester then is transferred from HDL to LDL and VLDL, partly in exchange for triglyceride.

One of the functions of HDL is to transport cholesterol, in esterified form, from the tissues to the liver by the following sequence of events.[7] The liver and intestine synthesize lipid-poor apoA-I to create a lipid-poor pre-HDL (see below). This particle interacts with the **ATP-binding cassette transporter A1 (ABCA1)** located on the arterial macrophages, transferring free cholesterol to extracellular lipid-poor HDL. The HDL cholesterol then is esterified by LCAT, enabling HDL to take up more free cholesterol. The esterified cholesterol formed on HDL is transferred by the **cholesteryl ester transfer protein (CETP)** to LDL and VLDL, where it is incorporated into the nonpolar core of these lipoprotein molecules. LDL, carrying its load of cholesteryl ester to peripheral tissues, reaches the liver, where the cholesteryl esters are hydrolyzed, and subsequently enters the pool of free cholesterol in the hepatocyte. The free cholesterol can leave the hepatic pool by secretion into the bile, directly or after conversion into bile acids, or by reincorporation into VLDL. Hepatic excretion of cholesterol via the biliary pool is one of the major mechanisms for removing cholesterol from the circulation.

Synthesis

Almost all animal tissues synthesize cholesterol from acetyl CoA, which is derived from the partial oxidation of glucose and from breakdown of fatty acids (see Chapter 38). In adults, the liver and the intestinal wall supply >90% of the plasma cholesterol of endogenous origin. Hepatic cholesterogenesis, unlike intestinal cholesterol synthesis, is inhibited by dietary cholesterol. The cholesterol production rate (absorbed cholesterol plus endogenously synthesized cholesterol) amounts to about 1 g/day. In most tissues, the rate of synthesis of cholesterol is determined by the capacity of **3-hydroxy-3-methylglutaryl CoA (HMG-CoA)** reductase, which catalyzes the rate-determining step in the biosynthetic sequence from acetyl CoA to cholesterol. Hepatic HMG-CoA reductase is subject to induction and repression by several hormones, dietary factors, and drugs. Feedback control of hepatic

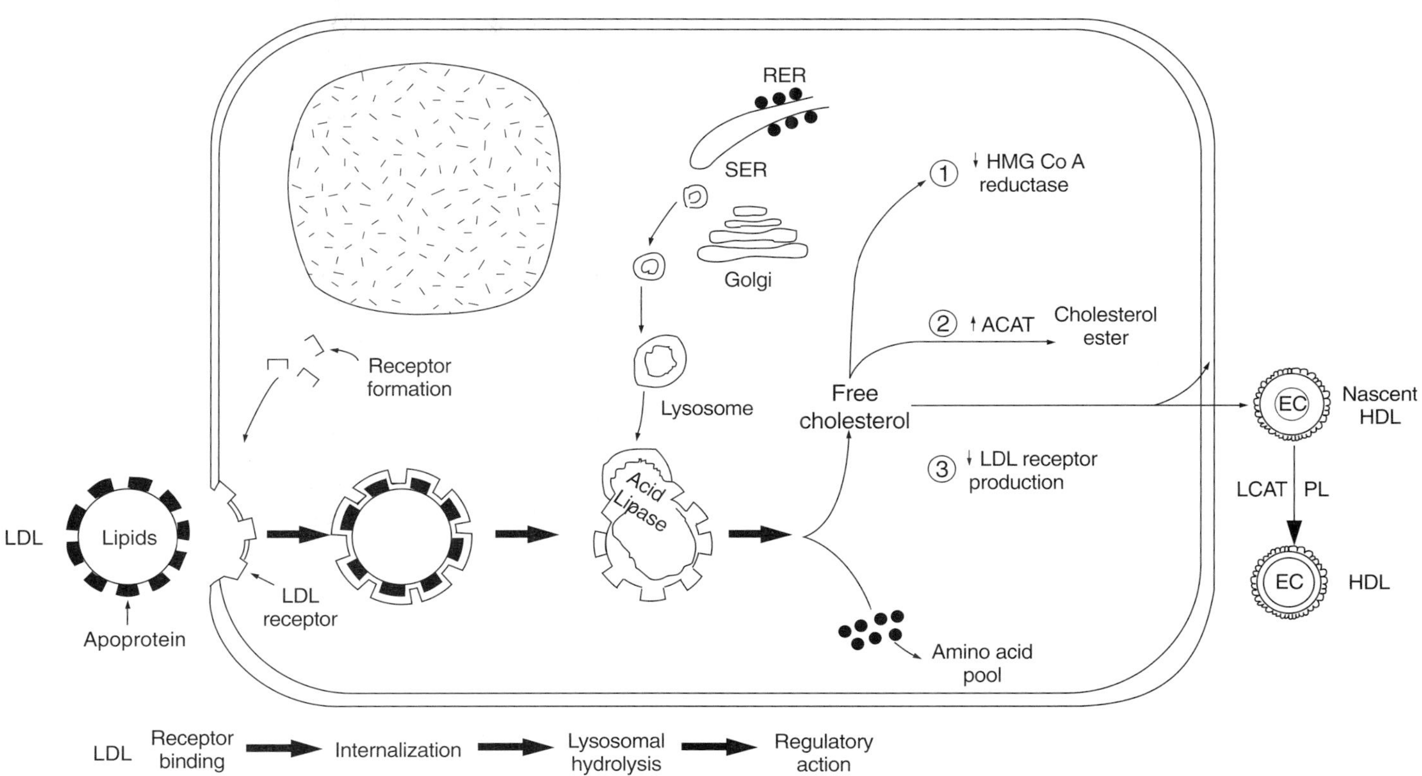

Fig. 37-5 Scheme of low-density lipoprotein (LDL) uptake and catabolism by a cell. Mechanism not only clears LDL from circulation but also aids in regulation of cholesterol synthesis and storage. High-density lipoprotein (HDL) plays an integral role in removing cellular cholesterol, esterifying free cholesterol in blood, and transporting cholesterol to the liver for catabolism. *ACAT,* Acyl-CoA:cholesterol acyltransferase; *EC,* cholesteryl ester; *HMG-CoA reductase,* 3-hydroxy-3-methylglutaryl-coenzyme A reductase; *LCAT,* lecithin:cholesterol acyltransferase; *PL,* phospholipid; *RER,* rough endoplasmic reticulum; *SER,* smooth endoplasmic reticulum.

cholesterogenesis is also mediated by cholesterol itself and by bile acids. A brief scheme of the control of hepatic cholesterogenesis is shown in Fig. 37-6.

Catabolism

In humans, increased absorption of dietary cholesterol is followed by increased excretion of cholesterol from the exchangeable pool. Increased conversion of cholesterol into bile acids can be brought about by interruption of the enterohepatic circulation of bile salts. Bile salts returning to the liver from the intestine repress the formation of an enzyme that would catalyze the rate-limiting step in the conversion of cholesterol into bile acids. When bile salts are prevented from returning to the liver, the activity of this enzyme increases, and degradation of cholesterol to bile acids is stimulated. This effect may be exploited therapeutically in the treatment of hypercholesterolemia by the use of nonabsorbable resins, which bind bile acids in the lumen of the intestine and prevent their return to the liver.

These mechanisms for excretion of cholesterol by means of bile acids or cholesterol in the bile depend on receptor-mediated activity in the hepatocytes. The hepatocytes have receptor sites specific for **apolipoproteins (apo)** B and E. The major function of the liver in lipoprotein clearance is to remove from plasma, lipoproteins that contain apoE (such as chylomicron remnants and VLDL remnants) and apoB (such as LDL). However, apoE-containing lipoproteins are cleared with much greater efficiency than apoB-containing lipoproteins. For this reason, chylomicron remnants and VLDL remnants (**intermediate-density lipoprotein** [**IDL**]) are not normally measurable in healthy individuals (see Fig. 37-2).

The uptake of LDL by peripheral tissues is also receptor site dependent (see Fig. 37-5). The binding of LDL to the receptor site, followed by internalization and hydrolysis of LDL, serves to deliver free cholesterol to the cell. The intracellular free cholesterol then functions (1) as a regulator for the rate of receptor synthesis, (2) as a regulator for cholesterol synthesis by the end-product negative-feedback mechanism, or (3) as a regulator for ACAT activity, which determines how much cholesterol is stored in the cell as cholesteryl oleate, a cholesteryl ester. It is believed that the availability of HDL is one of the determining factors for the efflux of cholesterol from the cell into the blood. By this process, cholesteryl oleate in the cell is hydrolyzed to free cholesterol and fatty acid. The liver and to some extent the gastrointestinal tract and other organs, such as the adrenal glands and gonadal tissues, take up the HDL and catabolize it to its protein and lipid constituents (including cholesterol).

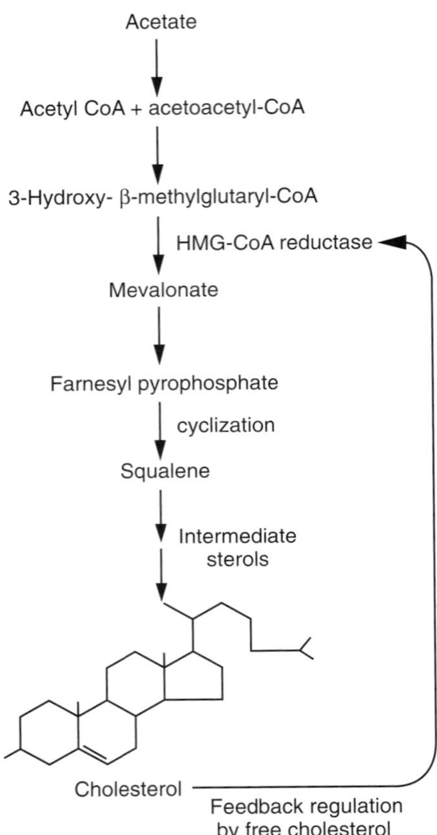

Fig. 37-6 Metabolic pathway of cholesterol synthesis, emphasizing negative feedback end-product inhibition by cholesterol on the rate determining enzyme HMG-CoA reductase.

Box 37-1

National Institutes of Health National Cholesterol Education Program Adult Treatment Panel III[8] Guidelines

Optimal Fasting Levels
Total cholesterol <200 mg/dL
LDL cholesterol <100 mg/dL
HDL cholesterol >40 mg/dL
Triglycerides <150 mg/dL

Near or Above Optimal Fasting Levels
LDL cholesterol 100 to 129 mg/dL

Borderline High Fasting Levels
LDL cholesterol 130 to 159 mg/dL

High Fasting Levels
LDL cholesterol 160 to 189 mg/dL

Very High Fasting Levels
LDL cholesterol >190 mg/dL

Expected Cholesterol Values

Unlike many of the blood analytes that we measure in the laboratory, lipids and lipoproteins require a different approach when reference values are being defined. For example, a cholesterol value of 250 to 280 mg/dL (to convert mg/dL to mmol/L, divide by 38.7) may be within the 95th percentile of the distribution of an apparently healthy male population between 51 and 59 years of age in the United States, but about 40% to 50% of these persons eventually will develop CHD. Critical values for serum lipids and lipoproteins have been established that are better predictors of disease or disease risk (see the discussion of the National Cholesterol Education Program). Because of the positive correlation between blood cholesterol concentration and increased risk for CHD, the average cholesterol concentration for the entire population should be as low as possible.

The latest guidelines of the **National Institutes of Health (NIH) National Cholesterol Education Program Adult Treatment Panel III**[8] **(NCEP ATP III)** suggest that total cholesterol should be <200 mg/dL for the high-risk adult. These guidelines identify LDL cholesterol as critical for assessment of CHD risk, therapeutic goal setting, and the primary target of therapy, and not for total and HDL cholesterol concentrations, as in the past.[9] These guidelines recommend that all adults 20 years or older have a fasting lipoprotein profile (total cholesterol, LDL cholesterol, HDL cholesterol, and triglycerides) every 5 years (Box 37-1).

In addition to LDL cholesterol, risk determinants for CHD include the current presence or absence of CHD, other clinical forms of atherosclerotic disease, and major biochemical risk factors other than LDL cholesterol (Box 37-2). NCEP ATP III guidelines[8] focus attention on intensive treatment of patients with CHD and on primary prevention of CHD in persons with multiple risk factors; the latter have a relatively high risk for CHD and will benefit from more intensive LDL-lowering treatment than is recommended in ATP II.[9]

As people age, they become more susceptible to the atherosclerotic process (**coronary artery disease [CAD]**, peripheral arterial disease, abdominal aortic aneurysm, and carotid artery disease) because of changes in lifestyle and accumulation of CHD risk factors. The more risk factors that are accumulated, the greater the risk for early CHD, including angina pectoris, **myocardial infarction (MI)**, and, for an unfortunate 35% of the population, acute cardiac death. It has been calculated that, for an individual with a total cholesterol concentration of 200 mg/dL and no other risk factors, a critical degree of significant atherosclerosis (>60% stenosis) may be reached by the time the person reaches the age of 70 years. If the same individual had a cholesterol value of 250 or 300 mg/dL, this degree of CAD probably would be attained by 60 or 50 years of age, respectively. This timetable is accelerated when multiple risk factors for CHD are involved (see Box 37-2). With the addition of a single CHD risk factor (smoking), the critical age is reached by 60 years of age; with the addition of a second CHD risk factor (hypertension), this age drops to 50 years. A plasma cholesterol concentration of 250 mg/dL moves the critical age back to 50 years with one risk factor and to 40 years

Box 37-2

Risk Factors Associated With the Development of Coronary Heart Disease

Major

Age (years): Male, >45 years; female, >55 years or premature menopause without estrogen replacement therapy
Family history of premature coronary heart disease
Current cigarette smoking
Hypertension (BP ≥140/90 mm Hg) or on hypertensive medication
Diabetes mellitus
Low HDL cholesterol, <40 mg/dL (1.0 mmol/L)

Other

Obesity
Physical inactivity
Atherogenic diet
Elevated CRP
Elevated Lp(a)
Elevated homocysteine
Elevated triglycerides
Remnant lipoproteins
Metabolic syndrome (high triglycerides, low HDL, abdominal obesity, physical inactivity, insulin resistance, hypertension, high fasting glucose)
Prothrombogenic and proinflammatory factors
Impaired fasting glucose
Subclinical atherosclerotic disease (peripheral arterial disease, abdominal aortic aneurysm, symptomatic carotid artery disease)
Multiple risk factors and 10-year increased risk for CHD

Negative Risk Factors

High HDL cholesterol, >60 mg/dL (1.6 mmol/L)

with two risk factors. More than 20% of the general population can expect to develop CHD or to have a recurrent CHD event within 10 years if they have multiple risk factors (two or more). Thus the number of CHD risk factors is a determinant in deciding how aggressive the patient's treatment protocol should be.

Genetics

Genetic factors are probably the most important influence on a person's cholesterol concentration. It is estimated that about half of the variability in blood cholesterol concentrations has a genetic basis.

Age

Serum cholesterol concentration starts out at around 65 mg/dL at birth and steadily increases with age (about 1.5 mg/dL per year).

Sex

The cholesterol concentration in the blood of males generally is higher than that in premenopausal females. After menopause, however, the cholesterol concentration is higher in females than in males. Serum cholesterol concentrations in males seem to reach a plateau by 50 to 60 years of age.

Diet

Saturated fat in the diet increases serum cholesterol concentrations, whereas polyunsaturated fat decreases cholesterol concentration; monounsaturated fats have some cholesterol-lowering effect. *Trans*-fatty acids are another LDL-raising fat that should be kept at a low intake. Dietary cholesterol elevates serum cholesterol concentrations. Plant sterols and certain types of fiber decrease serum cholesterol concentration. Fish oils lower triglycerides and lipoprotein (a) (**Lp(a)**) more than they lower cholesterol. Current guidelines[8] suggest that saturated fat intake should not exceed 7% of total calories, and total fat intake should not exceed 35% of total calories with cholesterol intake of <200 mg/day. In addition, it is recommended that other therapeutic options for lowering LDL cholesterol can be achieved with greater dietary intake of phytosterols (plant sterols) and viscous fiber (both found in fruits and vegetables).

Obesity

Although obesity commonly is regarded as an important contributor to the development of hypertriglyceridemia, it is well established that as the percentage of individuals with obesity increases with age, so do blood cholesterol concentrations. About 30% of American adults can be considered obese (see Chapter 41). The problem is especially pronounced for Hispanic populations, low socioeconomic Caucasian populations, and African American women. It is estimated that >70 million American adults are obese, and the problem is acute for American children. Weight reduction therapy for overweight or obese patients will enhance lowering of LDL cholesterol concentrations and will provide other health benefits, including modification of other lipid and nonlipid risk factors. Current NCEP ATP III guidelines[8] recommend that diet should be focused on a balanced energy intake and expenditure to maintain desirable body weight and to prevent weight gain. Additional risk reduction can be achieved by simultaneously increasing physical activity.

Physical Activity

Physical activity tends to lower serum total cholesterol. Much of this effect depends on the type, intensity, duration, and frequency of physical activity. Exercise also lowers total and LDL cholesterol, triglycerides, and VLDL cholesterol, and it increases HDL cholesterol concentration. Physical activity can lower blood pressure, reduce insulin resistance, and reduce stress. Physical inactivity further enhances the risk for CHD by impairing cardiovascular fitness and coronary blood flow. More than 60% of American adults have a sedentary lifestyle or perform no regular physical activity. This prevalence is higher in women, minority groups, and older adults. It has been demonstrated that when women with diabetes exercised at least 4 hours per week (moderate to vigorous exercise), they had a 40% reduced risk for cardiovascular disease (CVD).

Hormones

Growth hormone, L-thyroxine, and glucagon decrease serum cholesterol concentrations, whereas anabolic steroids and progestins increase cholesterol concentrations. The loss of estrogen in postmenopausal women is associated with elevated blood concentrations of total cholesterol, Lp(a), and homocysteine in older women.

Primary Disease States

Diabetes mellitus, thyroid dysfunction, obstructive liver disease, acute porphyria, dysgammaglobulinemias, and nephrotic syndrome all have an effect on blood cholesterol concentrations. Current guidelines[8] categorize diabetic patients as high-risk individuals who need aggressive intervention therapy. This is based on the fact that diabetes confers a high risk for new CHD within 10 years from the onset of the disease, in part through its frequent association with multiple risk factors. Furthermore, a more intensive prevention strategy is recommended for diabetic patients because MI in these patients results in an unusually high death rate, either immediately or over the long term. Primary hypothyroidism is relatively common in the geriatric population and is a common cause for secondary hypercholesterolemia. Thus, appropriate screening and treatment for thyroid dysfunction in older adults are warranted (see Chapter 49).

TRIGLYCERIDE METABOLISM

Biological Functions

Triglycerides are the major form of fat found in nature, and their primary function is to provide energy for the cell. One gram of fatty acids liberates about 9 kcal. The human body stores large amounts of fatty acids in ester linkages with glycerol in the adipose tissue. This form of reserve energy storage is highly efficient because of the magnitude of the energy released when fatty acids undergo catabolism. Most of the fatty acids come from our diets, can be synthesized endogenously, and are called *non-EFA*. Three fatty acids (linoleic, linolenic, and arachidonic acids) cannot be made by the human body. These fatty acids, called *EFA*, are important for the proper growth and development of cells, cell membrane integrity, prostaglandin synthesis, and myelinization of the central nervous system. Insufficient intake of EFA will lead to an EFA deficiency.

Physiology

Triglycerides by far make up the most abundant subclass of neutral glycerides in nature. Mammalian tissues also contain diglycerides and monoglycerides, but these occur in trace concentrations when compared with triglycerides. Most triglyceride molecules in mammalian tissues are mixed glycerides, that is, containing mixed types of fatty acids.

Because of their water insolubility, triglycerides are transported in the plasma in combination with other more polar lipids (phospholipids) and proteins, as well as with cholesterol and cholesteryl esters, within complex lipoprotein macromolecules. It appears that the essentially nonpolar triglycerides (and cholesteryl esters) are largely in the center of the lipoprotein, whereas the more polar protein and the phospholipid components are at the surface, with their polar groups directed outward to stabilize the whole structure in the aqueous plasma environment.

Synthesis

The concentration of triglyceride in the plasma at any given time represents a balance between rate of entry into the plasma and rate of removal. A change in concentration therefore may result from a change in either or both of these factors. Moreover, a primary change in one may result in a secondary change in the other. Thus, perhaps the main problem to be considered in any situation in which the plasma triglyceride concentration is abnormally high is whether this is attributable to a rise in rate of entry, or to a fall in rate of removal, of plasma triglycerides.

Plasma triglycerides are derived from two sources—intestine and liver. Intestinal triglycerides are synthesized from dietary fat. The source of fatty acids present in triglycerides that enter the blood from the liver depends greatly on the individual's nutritional state. Thus in the fasting state, fatty acids derived from adipose cell triglycerides are taken up by the liver, and some are re-excreted as VLDL. Following a meal, dietary carbohydrates are taken up by the liver and converted to triglycerides, which are secreted as VLDL. It is important to realize that, except during absorption of dietary fat, the liver is the main contributor of triglyceride to plasma.

The size, triglyceride content, and particle density of the lipoprotein complexes formed by the intestines and by the liver vary according to the amount of triglyceride that is being released. Thus high rates of release result in large complexes with a higher triglyceride load and a correspondingly lower density. In fact, lipoprotein complexes released from the liver under such conditions may reach a size not much smaller than that of the intestinal chylomicrons, even though normally, they may have a lower triglyceride content, and therefore, a higher density.

Catabolism

The action of lipase at the endothelial cell surface not only facilitates the removal of triglyceride fatty acid from the blood, but also determines where it is used, and this has important consequences. For example, in a state of caloric excess, the amount of triglyceride fatty acid in the bloodstream in excess of immediate caloric needs is taken up by adipose tissue. Most fatty acids are reconverted to intracellular triglyceride and stored. In contrast, in a state of caloric deficit (as during "chronic" fasting), the tissues derive their energy primarily from the oxidation of NEFA, which are mobilized from adipose tissue and carried to body tissues in the blood. Triglyceride is still present in the blood in VLDL under these conditions, but instead of being taken up by adipose tissue, it now is directed away from this tissue and toward muscle, to supplement the supply of energy from mobilized fatty acids. This switch in triglyceride fatty acid uptake is achieved through changes in the activity of intracellular lipase in the tissues concerned. Thus fasting results in a decrease in the activity of the enzyme in adipose tissue and an increase in its activity in muscle.

The intracellular adipose triglyceride enzyme is distinct from the plasma enzyme and is called *hormone-sensitive lipase* because it is converted from an inactive to an active form by epinephrine, norepinephrine, adrenocorticotropin, thyroid-stimulating hormone, and glucagon. Moreover, its activity is promoted by growth hormone. On the other hand, insulin inhibits the activity of this lipase. Unlike the LPL of adipose tissue, hormone-sensitive lipase of other tissues exhibits increased activity during fasting, possibly because of falling insulin concentrations.

Expected Triglyceride Values

NCEP ATP III guidelines recommended that the most useful triglyceride value to remember is 500 mg/dL or greater, which represents an increased risk for acute pancreatitis.[8] (To convert triglyceride units from mg/dL to mmol/L, divide by 88.6.) Other clinical presentations may occur when a patient has marked elevations in triglycerides, such as lipemia retinalis, eruptive **xanthomas,** hepatomegaly, and splenomegaly. These guidelines[8] define the upper reference limit for serum triglycerides as <150 mg/dL. Borderline-high triglyceride concentration now is defined as 150 to 199 mg/dL, and high triglyceride concentration is 200 to 499 mg/dL. Very high triglyceride concentration is defined as ≥500 mg/dL. Factors that contribute to elevated serum triglycerides are listed in Box 37-3.

According to the guidelines, the treatment strategy for elevated triglycerides depends on the causes and severity of the elevation. For all persons with borderline-high or high triglyceride concentrations, the primary aim of therapy is to achieve the target goal for LDL cholesterol. Emphasis should be placed on weight reduction and increased physical activity. In many instances, lowering of triglycerides will normalize below-normal HDL cholesterol concentrations (<40 mg/dL), because of the existence of the reverse relationship between triglyceride and HDL cholesterol concentrations. However, NCEP ATP III recommendations do not specify a goal for raising HDL cholesterol. Although many clinical trial results suggest that raising HDL cholesterol will reduce CHD risk, the evidence is insufficient to specify a goal for therapy, unless the patient has documented CHD.

Box 37-3

Factors That Contribute to Elevated Serum Triglycerides

- Excess weight or obesity
- Physical inactivity
- Cigarette smoking
- Excess alcohol intake
- Excessively high carbohydrate diets (>60% of caloric intake)
- Primary disease states
    - Type 2 diabetes
    - Chronic kidney disease
- Drugs (such as corticosteroids, estrogens, retinoids, high doses of β-adrenergic blocking agents)
- Certain genetic metabolic disorders (including familial combined hyperlipidemia, familial hypertriglyceridemia, and familial dysbetalipoproteinemia)

KEY CONCEPTS BOX 37-2

- Cholesterol is a lipid that is synthesized in the body from acetyl CoA, but also has dietary sources.
- Cholesterol is an essential structural component of cell membranes and a precursor of bile acids and steroid hormones that is transported in the circulation within lipoproteins.
- Plasma cholesterol concentrations are determined by the synthetic rate of cholesterol-carrying lipoproteins (revealed by HMG-CoA reductase activity) and the efficiency of receptor mechanisms that determine their catabolism; increased cholesterol levels are associated with CHD.
- Triglycerides are major components of the triglyceride-rich lipoproteins, namely, chylomicrons and VLDL, that play a key role as a source of energy for the cells.
- At the endothelial surface, triglyceride is broken down to glycerol and **free fatty acids (FFA)** by the enzyme lipoprotein lipase; both adipose and liver cells can synthesize and store triglyceride.

SECTION OBJECTIVES BOX 37-3

- Describe the functions of apolipoproteins.
- Describe the roles of the various apolipoproteins in the process of lipoprotein metabolism.
- Describe the usefulness of apolipoproteins as markers of CVD risk.

PART 2: Apolipoproteins

Apolipoproteins are the lipid-binding protein components of plasma lipoproteins. Each lipoprotein class contains a variety of apoproteins in varying proportions, except LDL, which contains only apoB-100 (Table 37-1). The **amphipathic** properties of apoproteins solubilize the hydrophobic lipid constituents of lipoproteins. In addition to their structural role, apoproteins function as enzyme cofactors and receptor ligands (Table 37-2).

Apolipoprotein A

ApoA-I is the primary protein constituent of the antiatherogenic HDL that promotes cholesterol efflux from cells, which is important in maintaining cellular cholesterol homeostasis.[10] ApoA-I is a 243 amino acid protein that contains a globular amino terminal domain and a lipid-binding carboxyl-terminal domain. ApoA-I is secreted by the intestines and liver principally in a lipid-free form, and HDL biosynthesis proceeds with the stepwise formation of nascent pre-β HDL and diskoidal HDL particles through the addition of cell membrane–derived phospholipid and cholesterol. These

Table 37-1 Physical and Chemical Descriptions of Plasma Lipoproteins in Humans

Feature	Chylomicrons	VLDL	IDL	LDL	HDL
Density, g/mL	<1.006	<1.006	1.006 to 1.019	1.019 to 1.063	1.063 to 1.21
Electrophoretic mobility	Origin	Pre-β	β	β	α
Flotation rate, S_f	>400	20 to 400	12 to 20	0 to 10	—
Diameter, nm	80 to 500	40 to 80	24.5	20	7.5 to 12
Lipids, % by weight	98	92	85	79	50
Cholesterol	9	22	35	47	19
Triglyceride	82	52	20	9	3
Phospholipid	7	18	20	23	28
Apoproteins, % of weight	2	8	15	21	50
Major	A-I, A-II B-48 C-I, C-II, C-III	B-100 C-I, C-II, C-III E	B-100 C-I, C-II, C-III E	B-100	A-I, A-II C-I, C-II, C-III
Minor	B-100 D E-II, E-III, E-IV	A-I, A-II B-48	B-48	C-I, C-II, C-III E-II, E-III, E-IV	B-100 D E-II, E-III, E-IV

Table 37-2 Characteristics and Functions of Serum Apolipoproteins

Apoprotein	Molecular Weight, kDa	Lipoprotein Class	Function
ApoA-I	28	Chylomicron, HDL	Structural (HDL), activator of LCAT
ApoA-II	17	Chylomicron, HDL	Structural (HDL), activator of HL, LPL
ApoA-IV	46	Chylomicron, HDL	Activator of LCAT, modulator of LPL
ApoB-48	264	CM	Structural, secretion of chylomicrons
ApoB-100	550	VLDL, IDL, LDL	Structural, secretion of VLDL, LDL receptor ligand
ApoC-I	6.6	Chylomicron, VLDL, IDL, HDL	Activator of LCAT, inhibitor of CETP, LRP, and LDLR
ApoC-II	8.9	Chylomicron, VLDL, IDL, HDL	Activator of LPL
ApoC-III	8.8	Chylomicron, VLDL, IDL, HDL	Inhibitor of LPL, inhibitor of TRL uptake by liver
ApoE	34	Chylomicron, VLDL, IDL, HDL	Ligand for LDL receptor and LRP, reverse cholesterol transport, regulator of cell growth and immune responses

particles then are converted to spherical HDL particles through the action of LCAT and are remodeled further by the action of plasma enzymes and transfer proteins or by exchange of apoA-I. ApoA-I is one of the protein ligands that binds to **scavenger receptor B type I (SR-BI),** a selective receptor that transfers lipids but not apoprotein into cells.

ApoA-II, the second major protein component of HDL, is produced by the liver. Although apoA-II has structural features similar to those of apoA-I, it does not possess athero-protective properties. ApoA-II may displace apoA-I from the surface of HDL. ApoA-IV is present in chylomicrons, but its function is unknown. ApoA-V is a newly discovered member of the *APOA1/C3/A4/A5* gene cluster located on chromosome 11q23 that reduces plasma triglyceride concentrations by inhibiting VLDL production, stimulating LDL-mediated VLDL triglyceride hydrolysis, and accelerating hepatic uptake of VLDL particles.[11]

Apolipoprotein B

ApoB, a large amphipathic glycoprotein, plays a central role in human lipoprotein metabolism.[5] The human *APOB* gene is located on the short arm of chromosome 2 and produces two forms of apoB in circulating lipoproteins, apoB-48 (2152 amino acids) and apoB-100 (4536 amino acids). ApoB-48 is the product of a C-to-U change in apoB mRNA, which creates a UAA stop codon at amino acid 2153 and produces a truncated form of apoB-100, consisting of the N-terminal 48% of full-length apoB-100. ApoB-48 is synthesized in the intestine and is essential for the formation and secretion of chylomicrons. ApoB-100 is synthesized in the liver and is an essential structural component of VLDL and its metabolic products, IDL and LDL; it is also a ligand for the LDL-receptor mediated endocytosis of LDL particles by cells. There is only one apoB molecule per TRL particle and, unlike the other apoproteins, apoB does not participate in inter-lipoprotein exchange. Elevated plasma concentrations of apoB-containing lipoproteins are key risk factors for the development of atherosclerosis and CHD.

Apolipoprotein C

ApoC-I and apoC-III are constituents of HDL and TRL. They slow the clearance of TRL through a variety of mechanisms. ApoC-I is an inhibitor of lipoprotein binding to LDL receptors, LDL receptor–related protein, and the VLDL receptor. It is also the major plasma inhibitor of CETP, and it appears to interfere directly with fatty acid uptake into tissues. ApoC-III interferes with lipoprotein particle clearance, but its principal role is as an inhibitor of LPL activity by interfering with lipoprotein binding to the cell-surface glycosaminoglycan matrix, where lipolytic enzymes and lipoprotein receptors reside.[12] ApoC-III also interferes with remnant lipoprotein clearance. Although most apoC-III is carried on HDL, there is a close correlation between plasma apoC-III concentrations and triglyceride levels. ApoC-II is a necessary co-factor for normal activation of LPL required for the metabolism of chylomicrons and VLDL.

Apolipoprotein E

ApoE is a glycoprotein that plays an essential role in the catabolism of TRL.[13] The *APOE* gene is located on chromosome 19 in a cluster with *APOC1* and *APOC2*. The gene has three major alleles—apoE2, apoE3, and apoE4—which translate into three isoforms, namely, wild-type ε3, ε2, and ε4. These isoforms differ from each other only by single amino acid substitutions at positions 112 and 158. Individuals who carry the ε4 allele have higher serum cholesterol levels, and those who carry the ε2 allele have lower total cholesterol levels than individuals with the commonest ε3/ε3 genotype. Compared with individuals with the ε3/ε3 genotype, ε2 carriers have a 20% lower risk of CHD, and ε4 carriers have a slightly higher risk.[14] Although apoE2 isoforms bind to LDL receptors much more weakly than does apoE3 or apoE4, most ε2 carriers have advantageous lipid profiles and reduced CHD risk, perhaps because of compensatory upregulation of LDL receptors. By contrast, about 5% of ε2/ε2 homozygotes develop familial dysbetalipoproteinemia.

Apolipoproteins as Markers of Cardiovascular Disease Risk

Cardiovascular disease (CVD) risk increases as plasma LDL cholesterol increases, but decreases as HDL cholesterol increases. Based on these relationships, cholesterol ratios such as LDL cholesterol to HDL cholesterol and total cholesterol to HDL cholesterol are used in CVD risk prediction. However, apoB and apoA-I also may serve as CVD risk predictors.[15-17]

There is one molecule of apoB-100 in each VLDL, IDL, LDL and Lp(a) particle, and one molecule of apoB-48 in chylomicrons and chylomicron remnants. Both apoB-100 and apoB-48 are recognized by conventional clinical immunoassays for apoB, and the assays are standardized. Total plasma apoB, therefore, is an estimate of total atherogenic particle number, of which LDL makes up the vast quantity.[16] Because LDL particles differ in composition, LDL cholesterol is not equivalent to LDL particle number. This discordance becomes critical when small dense LDL is the dominant LDL species, as is the case in the atherogenic lipoprotein phenotype. ApoA-I is the major apoprotein in HDL, and, as is the case with HDL cholesterol, higher concentrations of apoA-I, in general, are associated with a reduced risk of CVD.[10] As apoB increases, CVD risk increases, and as apoA-I increases, CVD decreases. The apoB–to–apoA-I ratio integrates the risk due to proatherogenic and antiatherogenic lipoproteins. Thus, the apoB–to–apoA-I ratio may represent a surrogate marker not only for predicting future CVD risk, but also for evaluating the effects of lipid-lowering therapy. However, at this time, guidance documents, such as the NCEP ATP III,[8] still rely on LDL cholesterol measurements to assess risk and guide therapy.[17]

KEY CONCEPTS BOX 37-3

- Apolipoproteins are the lipid-binding protein components of lipoproteins that, in addition to their structural role, may act as co-factors and receptor ligands.
- ApoB-48 is synthesized in the intestine and is essential for the formation and secretion of chylomicrons, whereas apoB-100 is synthesized in the liver and is an essential structural component of VLDL and its metabolic products, and is a ligand for the LDL receptor; apoB and apoA-I may play a role in CVD risk prediction.

SECTION OBJECTIVES BOX 37-4

- Describe the structure and functions of a lipoprotein.
- Describe the physical and chemical properties of the various plasma lipoproteins.
- Describe the various lipoprotein transport systems.
- Describe the synthesis and metabolic fate of the various lipoproteins.

PART 3: Lipoproteins

A lipoprotein can be visualized most simply as a globular structure with an outer coat of protein, phospholipid, and free cholesterol, and an inner hydrophobic, neutral core of triglycerides and cholesteryl esters (Fig. 37-7). The protein and the phospholipid impart solubility to the otherwise insoluble lipids. The binding of the inner lipid to the phospholipid and protein coat is noncovalent, occurring primarily through

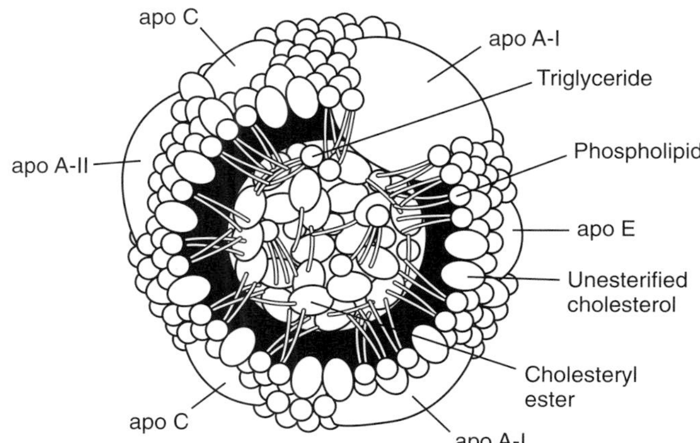

Fig. 37-7 Scheme of HDL (high-density lipoprotein), a lipoprotein complex showing polar outer surface and a core filled with neutral lipids.

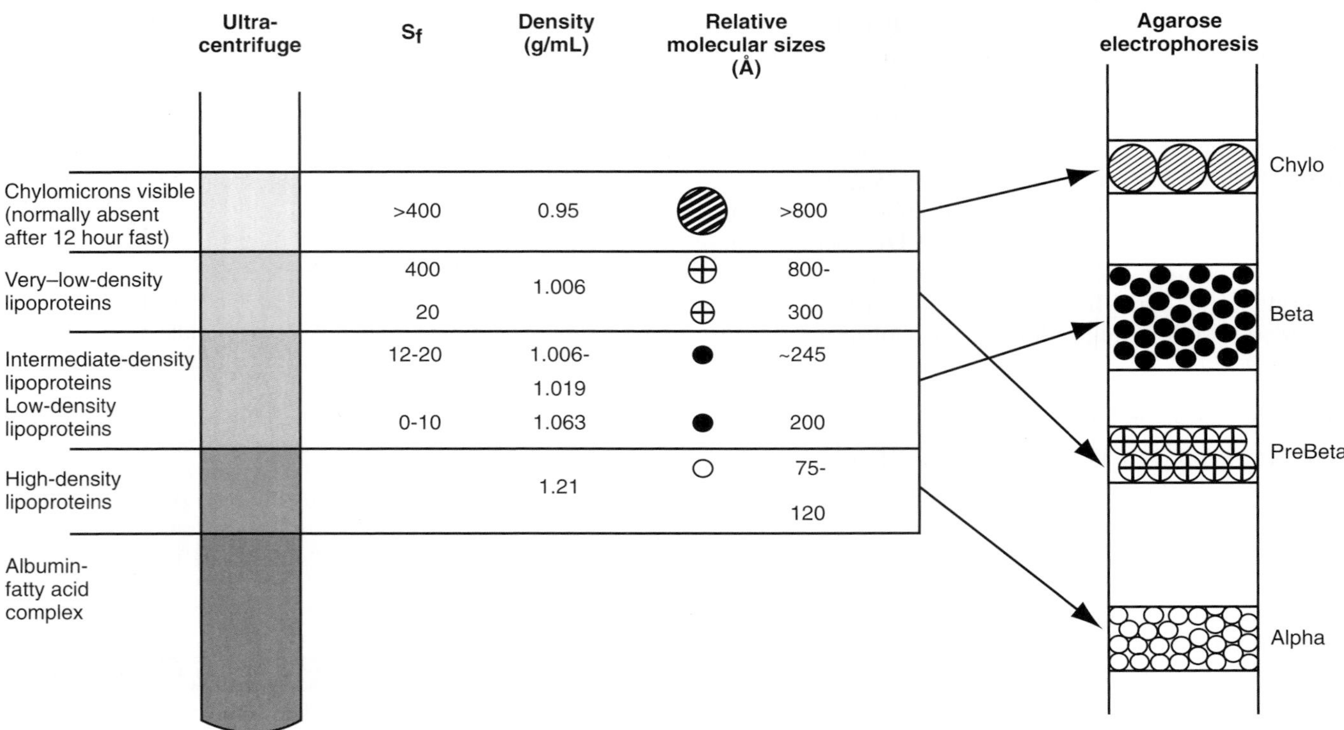

Fig. 37-8 Overview of major types of lipoproteins, showing some basic chemical and physical properties. *alpha,* α-Lipoprotein; *beta,* β-lipoprotein; *chylo,* chylomicrons; *preBeta,* a very-low-density lipoprotein; *Sf,* Svedberg flotation rate.

hydrogen bonding and van der Waals forces. The protein, free of lipid, is called *apoprotein.* Note that the lipids, which are weakly bound to the protein and the phospholipid, are bound loosely enough to allow the ready exchange of lipid between serum lipoproteins, as well as between serum and tissue lipoproteins. On the other hand, the lipids are bound strongly enough to allow the lipid and protein moieties to be separated within the analytical systems used to isolate and classify the lipoproteins.

CLASSIFICATION OF LIPOPROTEINS

The four systems most frequently used to isolate, separate, and characterize lipoproteins are based on analytical ultracentrifugation, preparative ultracentrifugation, electrophoresis, and precipitation techniques. The most frequently used systems are those based on ultracentrifugation and electrophoresis (Fig. 37-8). With a paper or agarose support medium, electrophoretic patterns show that chylomicrons remain at the origin, whereas pre–β-lipoproteins and β-lipoproteins migrate within β1- and β2-globulin areas, respectively, and α-lipoproteins migrate within the α_1-globulin area. High-definition agarose support media can identify Lp(a) as a fast-migrating pre–β-lipoprotein that typically migrates between the α- and pre–β-lipoprotein bands. Using conventional ultracentrifuge methods and taking advantage of the fact that lipoproteins are lighter than the other serum proteins, one can separate the lipoproteins into chylomicrons (the lightest lipoproteins) of a density less than plasma, with VLDL at a density below 1.006 g/mL (after chylomicron removal), LDL of density 1.006 to 1.063 g/mL, and HDL of density 1.019 to 1.210 g/mL. These lipoprotein classes correlate with electrophoretic patterns, for example, pre–β-lipoprotein generally is synonymous with VLDL, β-lipoprotein with LDL, and α-lipoprotein with HDL. Table 37-1 and Fig. 37-8 summarize the physical, chemical, and physiological characteristics of the major plasma lipoproteins.

Chylomicrons

Chylomicrons contain mainly triglyceride combined with cholesterol, small amounts of phospholipid, and specific apoproteins (apoB-48, A-I, A-II, C-I, C-II, and C-III, with small amounts of apoB and E-II, E-III, and E-IV) (see Table 37-1). Most models for chylomicron structure have been made under the assumption that the neutral lipids (triglycerides and cholesteryl ester) are partially surrounded by an outer shell of phospholipid, free cholesterol, and protein. Under fasting conditions (longer than 10 to 12 hours after a meal), no chylomicrons generally are found in the blood of healthy persons. The presence of chylomicrons makes the serum appear turbid or milky.

Very-Low-Density Lipoprotein

An average preparation of VLDL contains 52% triglyceride, 18% phospholipid, 22% cholesterol, and about 8% protein. Cholesterol and cholesteryl esters occur in a ratio of about 1:1 by weight. Sphingomyelin and phosphatidylcholine are the major phospholipids. The larger the size of a VLDL particle, the greater is the proportion of triglycerides and apoC, and the smaller is the proportion of phospholipid, apoB, and other apoproteins. ApoB appears to be present in a constant absolute quantity in all VLDL fractions. ApoB-100 accounts for about 30% to 35%, with apoC-I, C-II, and C-III making up >50%, of the apoprotein content in VLDL. ApoE-II, E-III, and E-IV and varying quantities of other apoproteins (apoA-I, A-II, B-48) also may be present. The relative quantity of each protein varies with the individual and with the degree of hyperlipidemia. Partially degraded VLDL, the remnant lipoprotein, is a triglyceride-poor lipoprotein, known to be highly atherogenic. In clinical practice, remnant lipoproteins are not measured easily. Although VLDL is not known to be atherogenic, it would be prudent to lower VLDL cholesterol only if triglycerides are >200 mg/dL (or VLDL cholesterol >30 mg/dL) and LDL cholesterol values are abnormal.

Low-Density Lipoprotein

LDL contains, by weight, 80% lipid and 20% protein. Consistent with this increased protein content, LDL is smaller (21 to 25 nm) and is of higher hydrated density (1.006 to 1.063 g/mL) than VLDL and chylomicrons. About 50% of LDL lipid is cholesterol. LDL constitutes 40% to 50% of the plasma lipoprotein mass in humans. LDL is the major carrier of cholesterol and is considered an atherogenic lipoprotein. ApoB-100 is the major apoprotein of normal LDL, and LDL apoB represents 90% to 95% of the total plasma apoB-100; LDL apoB is derived almost entirely from VLDL apoB.

LDL can be separated into at least two classes—LDL1 (or IDL) and LDL2—on the basis of flotation density. The lower-density fraction, IDL (1.006 to 1.109 g/mL), is more lipid-rich than LDL2 (1.019 to 1.063 g/mL) and probably represents an intermediate in VLDL catabolism (see Fig. 37-2). Comparison of IDL with LDL2 demonstrates the gradual disappearance of triglyceride and of apoproteins more characteristic of VLDL (apoC and apoE)—an enrichment with apoB-100 and cholesteryl ester. It has been shown that small dense LDL is metabolically more active and is more atherogenic than conventionally sized LDL. Furthermore, patients who have, or who are at risk for, CHD have increases in small and medium-sized LDL fractions. The NCEP ATP III report[8] has acknowledged this as a CHD risk factor.

High-Density Lipoprotein

The HDL macromolecular complex (see Fig. 37-7) contains about 50% protein and 50% lipid. HDL, the smallest of the lipoproteins (9 to 12 nm), floats at the highest density (1.063 to 1.21 g/mL) of any of the lipoprotein molecules. Quantitatively, the most important HDL lipid is phospholipid, although HDL cholesterol is of particular interest. The major phospholipid species is phosphatidylcholine (also known as lecithin), which accounts for 70% to 80% of total phospholipid. Phosphatidylcholine plays an important functional role as a reactant in plasma cholesterol esterification, which is catalyzed by the enzyme LCAT.

The heterogeneity of HDL is demonstrated by the presence of several different classes and as many as 14 subfractions.[18] HDL may be subfractionated by differential ultracentrifugation into HDL2 (with a density of 1.063 to 1.110 g/mL) and HDL3 (1.110 to 1.21 g/mL); the former is present in premenopausal women at about three times its concentration in men. Persons with lower HDL2 concentrations are apparently more susceptible to premature CHD. CHD severity is positively associated with concentrations of the small, dense HDL3 particles and is inversely associated with intermediate-sized HDL particles, independent of standard lipid measurements. Moreover, individuals with exceptional longevity were found to have significantly larger, less dense HDL2 and LDL particle sizes.

Other Lipoproteins

IDL

This lipoprotein fraction is found in increased concentrations in persons with familial dysbetalipoproteinemia, also called "broad-β disease" and type III hyperlipoproteinemia. The term is derived from the broad smear from β- to pre–β-lipoprotein regions frequently present on whole plasma lipoprotein electrophoresis in these subjects. IDL has a density of 1.006 g/mL, which is a VLDL characteristic, but it has a β-lipoprotein migration pattern. The abnormal lipid composition of VLDL in type III hyperlipoproteinemic persons is attributable to a proportionately larger amount of cholesterol in that fraction. This is considered to be a very atherogenic lipoprotein.

Lp(a)

Similarities in lipid composition, concentration, and density (1.05 to 1.10 g/mL) between Lp(a) and LDL prevented clear discrimination of these two lipoproteins until immunological tests demonstrated the uniqueness of their protein moieties. ApoB-100 makes up 65% of Lp(a) protein, but another 15% is albumin, and the remainder is an apoprotein unique to Lp(a), called apo(a). Lp(a) structurally resembles LDL, and the apoB protein is connected to the apo(a) by disulfide bridges. It is polymorphic in size and has several isomers. Despite its high frequency in the population, the functional significance of this lipoprotein still is not entirely clear.[19,20] However, it is known that Lp(a) competes with plasma plasminogen for the latter's binding sites, resulting in decreased synthesis of plasmin and inhibition of fibrinolysis. Thus Lp(a) may have a role in thrombogenesis. It also plays a role in atherogenesis by causing cholesterol deposition in the arterial wall, inducing monocyte-chemotactic activity in the arterial wall subendothelial space, enhancing foam cell formation, and promoting smooth muscle cell proliferation (see below).

From a pathological standpoint, Lp(a) concentrations >30 mg/dL are associated with an elevated risk for CHD. It appears that a person can have normal LDL cholesterol, but an elevated Lp(a) concentration and be at increased risk for CHD. Most prospective studies have demonstrated that Lp(a) is a primary and independent CHD risk factor that aggravates the CHD risk factors listed in Box 37-2. Persons with elevated concentrations of Lp(a) and **familial hypercholesterolemia (FH)** are at very high risk for premature CHD. Although about a third of Americans have Lp(a) concentrations <10 mg/dL, about 50% have elevated levels. The elevation of Lp(a) occurs early in childhood and persists throughout adulthood. Lp(a) increases are seen in postmenopausal women, and especially in African American males. Lp(a) concentrations are not affected by dietary intervention techniques and are not responsive to most lipid-lowering therapies, except for use of nicotinic acid.

Lipoprotein X

Although **lipoprotein X (Lp-X)** has a flotation density similar to that of LDL, the lipid and protein compositions are different, and this abnormal lipoprotein migrates in an electrophoretically different manner from LDL. Lp-X is characterized by an unusually high proportion of plasma phospholipid and unesterified cholesterol and by a low protein content consisting of apoB, apoC, and albumin. Electrophoretically, Lp-X migrates in the opposite direction from conventional lipoproteins on an agar support medium. On new high-definition agar support media, Lp-X migrates as a slow-migrating β-lipoprotein (a lipoprotein cathodal to the β-lipoprotein band) and is found most characteristically in the plasma of patients with biliary obstruction. Lp-X is not found in healthy persons but often is found in patients with a familial deficiency of the enzyme LCAT and in patients with obstructive liver disease. Lp-X has been used in Europe for differentiating cholestasis from hepatic parenchymal disease. However, it is not a useful marker for differentiating extrahepatic from intrahepatic cholestasis.

LIPOPROTEIN METABOLISM

The lipoprotein transport system carries the hydrophobic core lipids, triglyceride and cholesteryl ester. The circulating lipoproteins that contain these lipids are subjected to continuous modeling by enzymes and proteins in the metabolic cascade. The lipoprotein transport system can be separated into three pathways: exogenous, endogenous, and reverse pathways. The exogenous pathway transports dietary fat to peripheral tissues (Fig. 37-9), whereas the endogenous pathway transports hepatically synthesized lipids, primarily VLDL triglyceride, to their sites of utilization in peripheral tissues (Fig. 37-10). In the peripheral circulation, chylomicrons and VLDL share

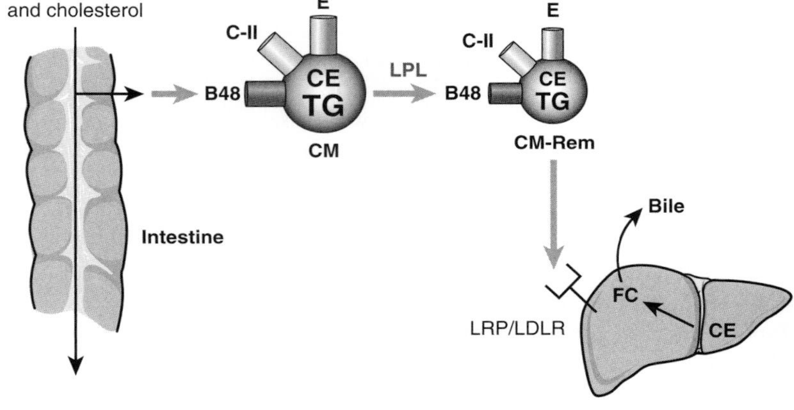

Fig. 37-9 Exogenous lipoprotein transport pathway. B48, Apolipoprotein B-48; *C-II,* apolipoprotein C-II; *CE,* cholesteryl ester; *CM,* chylomicron; *CM-Rem,* chylomicron remnant; *E,* apolipoprotein E; *FC,* free cholesterol; *LPL,* lipoprotein lipase; *LDLR,* LDL receptor; *LRP,* LDL receptor–related protein; *TG,* triglyceride. (Adapted with permission from the Lipids Online Slide Library [www.lipidsonline.org], © Copyright 2000-2008, Baylor College of Medicine.)

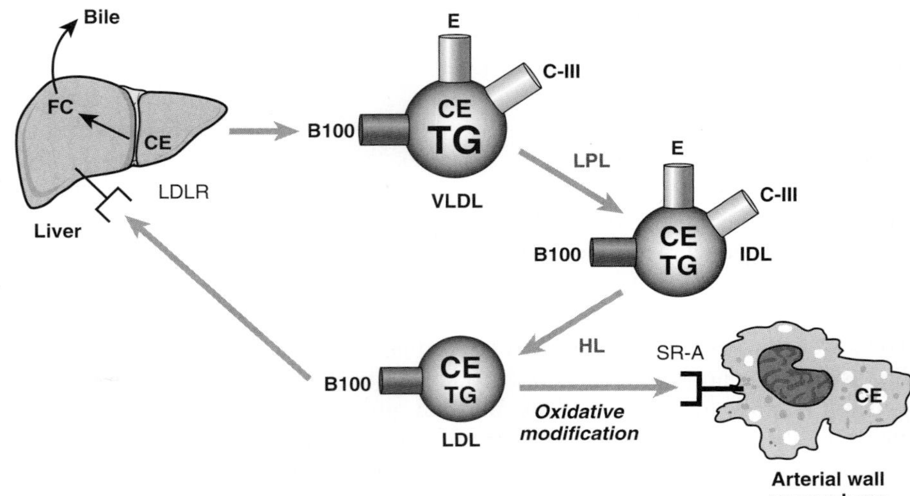

Fig. 37-10 Endogenous lipoprotein transport pathway. *B100,* Apolipoprotein B-100; *C-III,* apolipoprotein C-III; *CE,* cholesteryl ester; E, apolipoprotein E; *FC,* free cholesterol; *HL,* hepatic lipase; *IDL,* intermediate-density lipoprotein; *LDL,* low-density lipoprotein; *LPL,* lipoprotein lipase; *SR-A,* scavenger receptor type A; *VLDL,* very-low-density lipoprotein. (Adapted with permission from the Lipids Online Slide Library [www.lipidsonline.org], © Copyright 2000-2008, Baylor College of Medicine.)

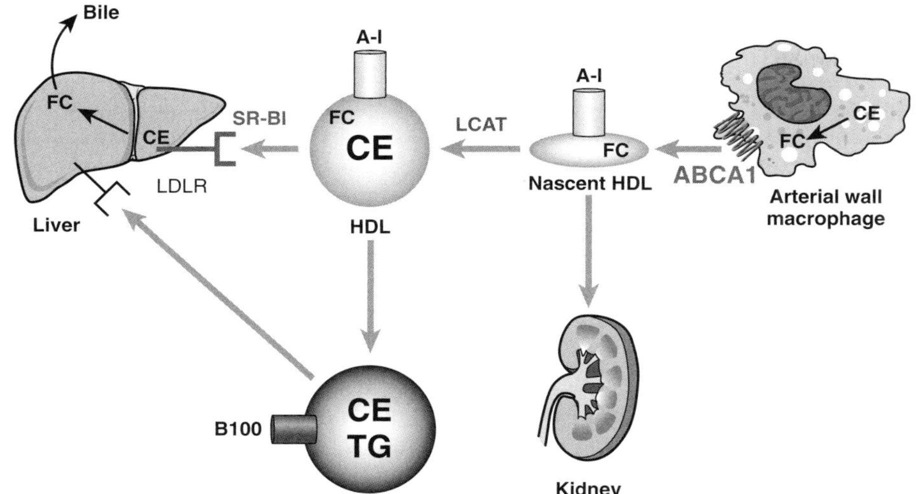

Fig. 37-11 Reverse cholesterol transport pathway. *ABCA1,* ATP binding cassette transporter A1; *A-I,* apolipoprotein A-I; *B100,* apolipoprotein B-100; *CE,* cholesteryl ester; *FC,* free cholesterol; *LCAT,* lecithin:cholesterol acyltransferase; *LDLR,* low-density lipoprotein receptor; *TG,* triglyceride. (Reprinted with permission in a slightly modified form from the Lipids Online Slide Library [www.lipidsonline.org]. © Copyright 2000-2008, Baylor College of Medicine.)

a common metabolic removal pathway catalyzed by LPL. Furthermore, the metabolic end products of the lipolytic process—chylomicron remnants and LDL, respectively—are cleared from the plasma predominantly by hepatic receptor–mediated processes. Reverse cholesterol transport is a process that shuttles cholesterol from peripheral tissues back to the liver directly via HDL and via other endogenously derived lipoproteins (e.g, VLDL, LDL). HDL occupies center stage in reverse cholesterol transport (Fig. 37-11).

Chylomicrons

Chylomicrons are made exclusively in the intestine and traverse the lymphatic system to the thoracic duct, where they then enter the systemic circulation. The major function of the chylomicron is the transport of dietary triglycerides. Newly synthesized and secreted chylomicrons (80 to 500 nm) from the intestinal mucosal cells ultimately pick up apoC-II from HDL, which catalyzes lipoprotein triglyceride hydrolysis by LPL. The hydrolysis results in liberation of NEFA and monoglycerides.

As is shown in Fig. 37-2, endothelial cell LPL-catalyzed hydrolysis results in progressive triglyceride depletion of the chylomicron molecule, resulting in the chylomicron remnant particle. This transformation involves maintenance of the lipoprotein structure by simultaneous removal of phospholipid, unesterified cholesterol, and apoC peptides from the lipoprotein surface to plasma HDL. Reciprocal transfer of cholesteryl ester from HDL may occur, and apoD may aid in this transfer process. The chylomicron remnant particle then is released from the capillary wall and cleared from circulation through the liver, where it is metabolized. This remnant particle, now smaller (30 to 80 nm), retains its cholesteryl ester and apoB and apoE, which play an important role in the uptake of these particles by a high-affinity hepatic receptor uptake mechanism (see Fig. 37-9). When hepatic binding occurs, the remnants are internalized immediately by receptor-mediated endocytosis and are degraded in hepatic lysosomes.

Very-Low-Density Lipoprotein

After the postprandial rise in chylomicron triglyceride, a secondary rise in triglyceride concentration occurs 4 to 6 hours after a meal. This represents predominantly hepatic VLDL triglyceride synthesized from glucose and chylomicron triglyceride not hydrolyzed in the peripheral tissue. The relative contributions of glucose and dietary fat vary with diet composition. Consumption of a high-carbohydrate diet may lead to a phenomenon known as *carbohydrate-induced hypertriglyceridemia.* With high dietary carbohydrate, glucose influx into the hepatocyte is in excess of energy demands and of glycogen-storage capacity. This results in the shunting of acetyl CoA into fatty acid synthesis and dihydroxyacetone phosphate into activated glycerol. This phenomenon may not occur in healthy persons, but others may be unusually susceptible to carbohydrate induction of VLDL synthesis. This serves as the basis for reduction of dietary carbohydrate (simple sugars and alcohol) in the treatment of hypertriglyceridemia, but this approach is not successful if the hypertriglyceridemia results from other causes of VLDL overproduction or from a clearance defect. Normally, VLDLs represent about 10% to 15% of the total circulating lipoproteins in a healthy individual.

VLDL triglycerides undergo the same fate as that of triglycerides from chylomicrons. During catabolism of VLDL, more than 90% of apoC is transferred to HDL, whereas essentially all apoB remains with the original lipoprotein particle. The metabolism of VLDL leads to the formation first of a VLDL remnant particle (IDL, see below) and then of the cholesterol-rich particle LDL. HDL plays an important role by serving as an acceptor macromolecule for apoC and unesterified cholesterol and phospholipids—the excess surface materials from a saturated VLDL. The apoC may recycle from HDL to newly synthesized chylomicrons or VLDL. The half-life of VLDL is 1 to 3 hours.

Intermediate-Density Lipoprotein

IDL is a transient particle (22 to 28 nm) that usually is present in very low concentrations in plasma from fasting persons.

IDL is a remnant lipoprotein derived from VLDL catabolism. HDL particles interact with the plasma enzyme LCAT, which esterifies excess HDL free cholesterol with fatty acids derived from the carbon-2 position of phosphatidylcholine, the major phospholipid of plasma. The newly synthesized cholesteryl ester is transferred back to the IDL particles from HDL, apparently through the action of CETP. The net result of the coupled lipolysis and exchange reactions is replacement of most of the original triglyceride core of VLDL with cholesteryl ester.

After lipolysis, IDL particles are released from the capillary wall into the circulation. They then undergo further conversion in which most remaining triglycerides are removed, and all apoproteins except apoB are lost. The resultant particle, which contains almost pure cholesteryl ester in the core and apoB at the surface, is LDL.

Low-Density Lipoprotein

LDL formation occurs primarily through the catabolism of VLDL. In healthy persons, LDL cholesterol constitutes about two-thirds of total plasma cholesterol; LDL cholesterol concentration in premenopausal women is slightly less than that in men and is similar after menopause. LDL delivers cholesterol to hepatic and extrahepatic tissues, where it is used, deposited, or excreted.

Delivery of LDL particles to peripheral tissue is accomplished when LDL binds to high-affinity receptors located in regions of the cell membrane called *coated pits.* These pits invaginate into the cell, and when LDL binds, they pinch off to form endocytic vesicles that carry LDL to the lysosomes (see Fig. 37-5). Fusion of the vesicle membrane with the lysosomal membrane exposes the latter's LDL hydrolytic enzymes, which degrade apoB to amino acids. The cholesteryl esters are hydrolyzed by an acid lipase, and liberated free cholesterol leaves the lysosomes for use in cellular reactions. As a result of this uptake mechanism, extrahepatic cells have low rates of cholesterol synthesis, relying instead on LDL-derived cholesterol. The free cholesterol thus released is used for membrane synthesis and serves to regulate, that is, depress cellular cholesterol synthesis by HMG-CoA reductase. LDL internalization also regulates synthesis of the LDL receptor itself.

Excess intracellular cholesterol activates the enzyme ACAT, leading to intracellular cholesteryl ester storage. Thus the net result of LDL binding and internalization is the reciprocal inhibition and activation of enzymes that synthesize and store cellular cholesterol and a reduction in the number of receptors available to bind LDL.

It has been recognized that the specificity of the LDL receptor extends to lipoproteins that contain apoE and apoB as well. It appears that although extrahepatic receptors take up LDL readily, hepatic receptors take up chylomicron remnants with greater efficiency (about 20 times greater) and LDL with much less efficiency. This difference is probably attributable to the apoE content of chylomicron remnants and IDL, which has a higher receptor affinity than that of apoB. In addition to its normal degradation mechanism, the high-affinity LDL receptor pathway, plasma LDL can be degraded by less efficient mechanisms that require high plasma concentrations to achieve significant rates of removal. One of these mechanisms occurs in scavenger cells (macrophages) of the reticuloendothelial system. When the plasma concentration of LDL rises, these scavenger cells ingest and degrade increasing amounts of LDL. When macrophages are overloaded with cholesteryl esters, they are converted into foam cells, which are classic components of atherosclerotic plaques (see below). In humans, estimates of the proportion of plasma LDL degraded by the LDL receptor system range from 33% to 66%. The remainder is degraded by the scavenger cell system and perhaps by other mechanisms not yet elucidated.

High-Density Lipoprotein

The liver and the intestine synthesize lipid-poor apoA-I that interacts with ABCA1 located on the arterial macrophages, transporting free cholesterol to extracellular lipid-poor HDL. When this protein is deficient or inactive, as in patients with **Tangier disease (TD),** or familial HDL deficiency, cholesterol accumulates in peripheral tissues. Lipidation of HDL particles generates nascent (pre-β) HDL. Subsequently, LCAT esterifies free cholesterol within nascent HDL to produce mature α-HDL particles (HDL3) and HDL2. Persons with LCAT deficiency have an accumulation of these cholesteryl ester–deficient particles in plasma. The apoprotein profile of newly secreted (nascent) HDL is modified concomitantly by changes in lipid content. ApoE is a major component of nascent HDL, unlike mature HDL, which is characterized by a predominance of apoA with minor contributions by apoC and apoE. The functional significance of this modification is not yet completely understood.

HDL is divided into large, lipid-rich HDL2 and smaller, more dense HDL3, with as many as 14 subfractions, depending on the separation technique used. It appears that HDL2 is more protective in terms of arterial wall damage than is HDL3. HDL also may be subclassified as LpA-I (contains apoA-I alone) and LpA-I:A-II (contains both apoA-I and apoA-II) particles. HDL participates in the regulation of triglyceride catabolism and cholesteryl ester formation by providing the respective cofactors, apoC-II for activation and apoC-III for inhibition of LPL activity. Also, HDL balances LDL transport by mediating cholesterol removal from peripheral sites to degradative and excretory sites. This role of HDL in reverse cholesterol transport may form the basis for the protection afforded by HDL against CVD. In addition to its major role in reverse cholesterol transport, HDL exhibits other biological activities that may contribute to its protective effects against atherosclerosis. These include anti-inflammatory, antioxidant, antimitotic, anticoagulant, anti-aggegatory, and profibrinolytic effects.

Mature HDL has at least two metabolic fates. In the direct pathway, HDL cholesteryl esters undergo selective uptake by hepatocytes and steroid hormone–producing cells via the SR-BI, leaving the HDL-apoprotein complex intact. Cholesterol taken up by hepatocytes is subsequently excreted into bile. In the indirect pathway, cholesteryl esters within HDL are exchanged for triglycerides in apoB-containing lipoproteins through the action of CETP. The subsequent uptake of apoB-containing lipoproteins by hepatic LDL receptors may be responsible for up to 50% of reverse cholesterol transport. Triglyceride-rich HDL then can undergo hydrolysis by hepatic lipase and endothelial lipase to form small HDL for further participation in reverse cholesterol transport.

The plasma half-life of HDL in normal subjects ranges from 3.3 to 5.8 days. HDL catabolism is enhanced in nephrotic patients, but decreased in hypertriglyceridemic individuals, especially those with hyperchylomicronemia. It is also increased in those on high-carbohydrate diets and is greatly enhanced in patients with TD. It appears that changes in HDL catabolism may play a major role in regulating HDL concentrations in plasma.

HDL metabolism represents a major therapeutic target for reduction of risk of atherosclerotic CVD.[21] Advances in our understanding of the molecular regulation of HDL metabolism, macrophage cholesterol efflux, and HDL function will lead to a variety of novel therapeutics.[7]

KEY CONCEPTS BOX 37-4

- Lipoproteins are globular structures with an outer coat of protein, phospholipids, and free cholesterol, and an inner hydrophobic, neutral core of triglycerides and cholesteryl esters.
- The main classes of lipoproteins are, namely, chylomicrons, VLDL, IDL, LDL, and Lp(a), which differ in their physical and chemical properties.
- The lipoprotein transport system carries the hydrophobic core lipids, namely, triglyceride and cholesteryl ester, and can be separated into three pathways.
- The exogenous pathway transports dietary fat to peripheral tissues, whereas the endogenous pathway transports hepatically synthesized lipids, primarily VLDL triglyceride, to their sites of utilization in the peripheral tissues.
- Chylomicrons and VLDL share a common metabolic removal pathway catalyzed by LPL. Furthermore, the metabolic end products of the lipolytic process, chylomicron remnants and LDL, respectively, are cleared from the plasma predominantly by hepatic receptor–mediated processes.
- Reverse cholesterol transport is a process that shuttles cholesterol from peripheral tissues back to the liver directly via HDL and via other endogenously derived lipoproteins (i.e., VLDL and LDL); HDL occupies center stage in reverse cholesterol transport.

SECTION OBJECTIVE BOX 37-5

- Describe the primary and secondary causes of hyperlipidemia.
- Describe the cluster of abnormalities that make up the metabolic syndrome, and explain its importance.
- Describe the clinical, diagnostic, genetic, and biochemical-pathological aspects of the genetic dyslipoproteinemias.

PART 4: Pathological Disorders

HYPERLIPIDEMIA

The major plasma lipids of interest are total cholesterol (free cholesterol + cholesteryl ester) and the triglycerides. When one or more of these major classes of plasma lipids is elevated, a condition referred to as *hyperlipidemia* exists. Cholesterol and triglyceride concentrations can be used to detect hyperlipoproteinemia. More than 90% of persons with hyperlipidemia, as defined previously, have hyperlipoproteinemia. Major exceptions are individuals with excessive amounts of LDL, whose plasma cholesterol is kept within normal limits by a concomitant decrease in HDL.

NCEP ATP III guidelines[8] have lowered the upper cholesterol limit, delineating minimal risk for CHD to <150 mg/dL. Triglyceride concentrations of 150 to 199 mg/dL are considered borderline high, whereas concentrations of 200 to 499 mg/dL are considered high. Values >500 mg/dL are considered undesirable because of the increased risk for acute pancreatitis.

HYPERLIPOPROTEINEMIA

Hyperlipoproteinemia is an elevation of serum lipoprotein concentrations. The classification of hyperlipoproteinemia begins with determination of the type of abnormal lipoprotein profile. However, other differentiation and analyses, such as the following, are necessary:

1. Separation of hyperlipoproteinemia into primary and secondary forms (Table 37-3). The secondary form is caused by another known disease that can result in secondary hyperlipoproteinemia that manifests itself in any of the five major types of lipoprotein profiles.
2. Differentiation of primary hyperlipoproteinemia into heritable and nonheritable forms
3. Determination of the relative concentrations of lipoprotein fractions, that is, VLDL cholesterol, LDL cholesterol, and HDL cholesterol

Numerous types of hyperlipoproteinemias have been identified, but most patients with heritable hyperlipidemia have one of six common abnormal lipoprotein patterns. These patterns are summarized in Fig. 37-12, which illustrates that three of the four lipoprotein families serve as determinants. These three families include (1) chylomicrons, (2) VLDL, and (3) LDL (including IDL). The original Fredrickson phenotyping system, which disregarded the importance of HDL and other lipoproteins discussed in this chapter, has fallen into disuse. For information on our current understanding of the use of lipoprotein profiling for assessment of CHD risk, refer to the NCEP ATP III guidelines[8] discussed in detail in this chapter.

METABOLIC SYNDROME

The NCEP ATP III guidelines[8] describe a disorder called the *metabolic syndrome,*[22] which is a constellation of interrelated

Table 37-3 Causes of Secondary Hyperlipoproteinemia

Pattern	Causes
Hyperchylomicronemia	Type 1 diabetes mellitus
	Dysglobulinemia
	Lupus erythematosus
	Acute pancreatitis
Hyperbetalipoproteinemia	Nephrotic syndrome
	Primary hypothyroidism
	Obstructive liver disease
	Porphyria
	Multiple myeloma
	Portal cirrhosis
	Viral hepatitis, acute phase
	Myxedema
	Stress
	Anorexia nervosa
	Idiopathic hypercalcemia
Dysbetalipoproteinemia	Primary hypothyroidism
	Dysgammaglobulinemia
	Myxedema
	Primary biliary cirrhosis
	Diabetic acidosis
Hyperprebetalipoproteinemia	Diabetes mellitus
	Nephrotic syndrome
	Pregnancy
	Hormone use (oral contraceptives)
	Glycogen storage disease
	Alcoholism
	Gaucher's disease
	Niemann-Pick disease
	Acute pancreatitis
	Primary hypothyroidism
	Dysglobulinemia
Mixed type of hyperlipoproteinemia	Type 1 diabetes mellitus
	Nephrotic syndrome
	Alcoholism
	Myeloma
	Idiopathic hypercalcemia
	Acute pancreatitis
	Macroglobulinemia
	Type 2 diabetes mellitus

risk factors of metabolic origin that appear to directly promote the development of atherosclerotic CVD.[23] This syndrome is linked closely to a generalized metabolic disorder called *insulin resistance,* in which the normal actions of insulin are impaired (see Chapter 38). The most widely recognized of the CHD risk factors associated with metabolic syndrome are atherogenic dyslipidemia, elevated blood pressure, and elevated plasma glucose. Individuals with these characteristics commonly manifest a prothrombotic and proinflammatory state. Atherogenic dyslipidemia consists of an aggregation of lipoprotein abnormalities, including elevated plasma triglyceride and

Box 37-4

Features Characteristic of Metabolic Syndrome

Abdominal obesity
Atherogenic dyslipidemia
Elevated triglycerides, small LDL particles, low HDL cholesterol
Raised blood pressure
Insulin resistance (with or without glucose intolerance)
Prothrombotic and proinflammatory states

apoB concentrations, increased small LDL particles, and reduced HDL cholesterol levels. The predominant underlying risk factors for the metabolic syndrome appear to be abdominal obesity and insulin resistance. Factors characteristic of metabolic syndrome are listed in Box 37-4. The prevalence of metabolic syndrome in the United States varies according to definition, ethnicity, and gender.

GENETIC DYSLIPOPROTEINEMIAS

The classification of genetic dyslipoproteinemias is based on the biochemical phenotype, the concentration of blood lipids, and identification of abnormal lipoprotein patterns, in addition to clinical phenotype (see Fig. 37-12; Table 37-4).[24] With the exception of FH, monogenic disorders of lipid metabolism tend to be infrequent or very rare. Furthermore, these disorders may be difficult to classify unambiguously because of age, gender, disease penetrance, and gene-gene and gene-environment interactions. The genetic dyslipoproteinemias are described with emphasis on distinctive clinical, diagnostic, genetic, biochemical-pathophysiological, and therapeutic aspects.

Familial Hyperchylomicronemia

This lipoprotein disorder is characterized by highly elevated plasma triglyceride concentrations—generally >1000 mg/dL—that result from chylomicronemia.[25] Occasional elevations in cholesterol occur as the result of pronounced elevation in chylomicron concentrations, because these particles also contain cholesterol. LDL and HDL are often low, whereas VLDL may be slightly elevated. The cause of this disorder is reduced clearance of chylomicrons caused by deficiencies in lipase activities, such as post-heparin LPL activity.

Familial Lipoprotein Lipase Deficiency

Familial LPL deficiency is a rare autosomal recessive disorder that is characterized by severe hypertriglyceridemia caused by the accumulation in plasma of TRL, which result from absence of LPL activity. The population frequency is one per million people, with a carrier frequency of about 1 per 500. Patients with familial LPL deficiency often have extremely low or absent LPL activity in post-heparin plasma. This disorder

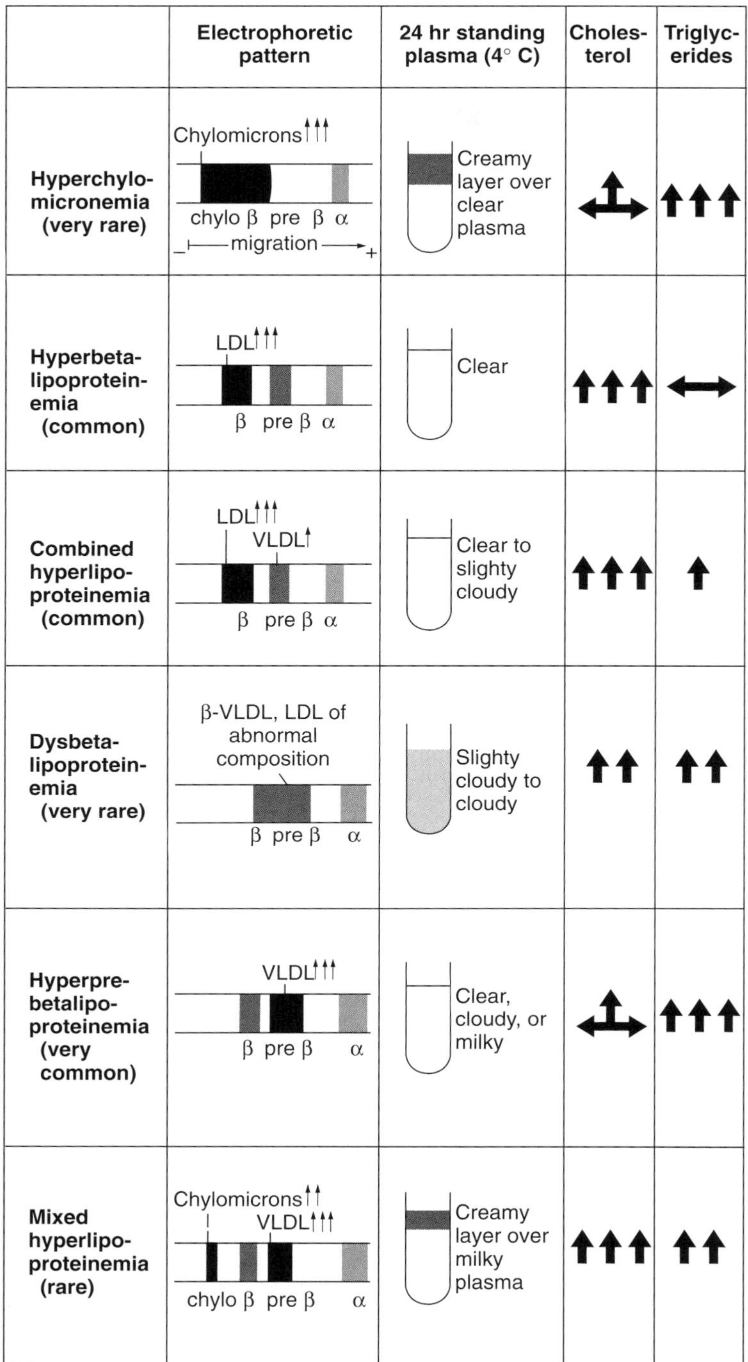

Electrophoretic pattern
24 hr standing plasma (4° C)
Choles-terol
Triglyc-erides
Hyperchylo-micronemia (very rare)
Chylomicrons
chylo β pre β α
migration
Creamy layer over clear plasma
Hyperbeta-lipoprotein-emia (common)
LDL
β pre β α
Clear
Combined hyperlipo-proteinemia (common)
LDL
VLDL
β pre β α
Clear to slighty cloudy
Dysbeta-lipoprotein-emia (very rare)
β-VLDL, LDL of abnormal composition
β pre β α
Slighty cloudy to cloudy
Hyperpre-betalipo-proteinemia (very common)
VLDL
β pre β α
Clear, cloudy, or milky
Mixed hyperlipo-proteinemia (rare)
Chylomicrons
VLDL
chylo β pre β α
Creamy layer over milky plasma

Fig. 37-12 Summary of six types of hyperlipoprotein-emias. Abbreviations as in Fig. 37-8.

usually manifests early in childhood with repeated episodes of abdominal pain, acute pancreatitis, eruptive cutaneous xanthomatosis, and hepatosplenomegaly. The severity of symptoms is proportional to the degree of hyperchylomicro-nemia, which, in turn, is dependent on dietary fat intake. Obligate heterozygotes usually are asymptomatic but can exhibit up to a 50% reduction in post-heparin LPL activity and variable plasma triglyceride concentrations.

The human *LPL* gene, which is located on chromosome 8p22, encodes for a mature protein of 448 amino acids. Numerous structural mutations in the *LPL* gene have been reported to be associated with a catalytically defective LPL protein. Familial LPL–deficient individuals may be homozygous for a single mutation or may be compound heterozygotes. Most of the about 100 *LPL* gene mutations described in humans are missense or nonsense, and they are

Table 37-4 Genetic Dyslipidemias

Disease	Gene	Protein	Gene Locus
Abetalipoproteinemia	*MTTP*	Microsomal triglyceride transfer protein	4q22-q24
Apolipoprotein C-II deficiency	*APOC2*	Apolipoprotein C-II	19q13.2
Cerebrotendinous xanthomatosis	*CYP27A1*	Sterol 27-hydroxylase	2q33-qter
Chylomicron retention disease	*SARA2*	Sar1b	5q31.1
Cholesteryl ester transfer protein deficiency	*CETP*	Cholesteryl ester transfer protein	16q21
Familial hypoalphalipoproteinemia	*ABCA1*	ATP binding cassette transporter AI	9q22-q31
Familial hypoalphalipoproteinemia	*APOA1*	Apolipoprotein A-I	11q23
Familial hypobetalipoproteinemia	*APOB*	Apolipoprotein B	2p24
Familial hypobetalipoproteinemia	*PCSK9*	Proprotein convertase subtilisin/kexin-type 9	1p34.1-p32
Familial dysbetalipoproteinemia	*APOE*	Apolipoprotein E	19q13.2
Fish-eye disease	*LCAT*	Lecithin cholesterol acyl transferase	16q22.1
Hypercholesterolemia, autosomal dominant	*LDLR*	LDL receptor	19p13.2
Hypercholesterolemia, autosomal dominant, type b (familial ligand defective apoB-100)	*APOB*	Apolipoprotein B	2p24
Hypercholesterolemia, autosomal dominant	*PCSK9*	Proprotein convertase subtilisin/kexin-type 9	1p34.1-p32
Hypercholesterolemia, autosomal recessive	*ARH*	Adaptor protein	1p36-p35
Familial lipoprotein lipase deficiency	*LPL*	Lipoprotein lipase	8p22
Sitosterolemia	*ABCG5/G8*	ATP binding cassette transporter G5 and G8	2p21
Tangier disease	*ABCA1*	ATP binding cassette transporter AI	9q22-q31

clustered in the region coded by exons 4, 5, and 6, which forms the proposed catalytic domain of LPL.

ApoC-II Deficiency

Chylomicronemia can result from deficiency or absence of apoC-II, a co-factor necessary for normal activation of LPL. The *APOC2* gene is located on chromosome 19q13.2, and structural mutations in *APOC2* that lead to a defective or absent apoC-II molecule cause the extremely rare autosomal recessive disorder, apoC-II deficiency. Clinical symptoms are identical to those of familial LPL deficiency but are typically milder in nature and occur later in age. Obligate heterozygotes are asymptomatic and have a normal lipid profile because adequate concentrations of apoC-II are present to activate LPL.

Although chylomicronemia is usually primary and familial, the lipoprotein pattern may be produced by several other diseases or metabolic states. Thus secondary forms of this dyslipoproteinemia should be ruled out (see Table 37-3).

Once secondary causes have been ruled out, the primary disorder can be confirmed by (1) the presence of eruptive cutaneous xanthomas, hepatosplenomegaly, lipemia retinalis, abdominal pain, and acute pancreatitis early in life; (2) intake of drugs that can cause secondary hypertriglyceridemia; (3) the presence of reduced post-heparin plasma concentration LPL activities; (4) reduction in triglyceride concentrations and disappearance of chylomicronemia on a fat-free diet; and (5) confirmation by family screening of inheritance as an autosomal recessive trait.

Familial Hypertriglyceridemia

Familial hypertriglyceridemia is defined as an isolated elevation of VLDL. This disorder is common, with a prevalence of 5% to 10%. Its molecular basis still is largely unknown, but it is likely to be polygenic, requiring a secondary factor for expression. Typically, patients with this disorder have moderately elevated plasma triglyceride concentrations (266 to 886 mg/dL), often with low levels of HDL cholesterol. Familial hypertriglyceridemia is associated with increased risk of CVD, obesity, insulin resistance, diabetes, hypertension, and hyperuricemia.

Monogenic Hypercholesterolemia

Monogenic hypercholesterolemia is characterized by marked hypercholesterolemia (increased LDL cholesterol), which results in excessive deposition of cholesterol in tissues, leading to accelerated atherosclerosis and increased risk of premature CHD. Monogenic hypercholesterolemia results from defects in the hepatic uptake and degradation of LDL via the LDL receptor pathway, which commonly is caused by a loss-of-function mutation in the LDL receptor gene *(LDLR)* or by a mutation in the gene that encodes apoB *(APOB)*.[26,27] Monogenic hypercholesterolemia is primarily an autosomal dominant disorder with a gene-dosage effect.

Familial Hypercholesterolemia

FH, one of the most common genetic disorders, affects about 1 per 500 people in the heterozygous and one per million in the homozygous form. FH provides compelling support for the causal role of LDL cholesterol in human atherosclerotic CVD. This disease is characterized by marked hypercholesterolemia from birth, leading to tissue cholesterol deposition such as tendinous and cutaneous xanthomas, **corneal arcus,** and premature CAD. Increased burden of premature CAD and death in FH are delayed by a decade in female patients. Unfortunately, most individuals with FH remain undiagnosed or are diagnosed only after their first coronary event.[28]

FH is an autosomal co-dominant disorder of lipoprotein metabolism caused by mutations in the *LDLR* gene, with homozygotes having a more severe phenotype than heterozygotes.[29] The *LDLR* locus on chromosome 19 (at 19p13.1-p13.3) spans 45 kb, contains 18 exons, and codes for a 96 kDa, 839 amino acid transmembrane receptor protein that binds to both apoB-100 and apoE. To date, about 1000 mutations in the *LDLR* gene have been identified; most are unique, which makes the search for an unknown mutation challenging and expensive. These *LDLR* gene mutations result in a defective or absent LDL receptor and reduced LDL clearance from the circulation, with increased LDL production found in FH homozygotes. Other gene loci cause phenotypes similar to FH, such as *APOB* located on chromosome 2p24, and the recently identified proprotein convertase subtilisin/kexin type 9 *(PCSK9)* on chromosome 1p32.

In heterozygous FH, only 50% of LDL receptors are fully functional, which increases plasma LDL cholesterol concentrations by twofold to threefold over those of the general population. Although heterozygous FH affects about 1 in 500 people, it occurs much more frequently in some populations, such as Afrikaners in South Africa, Christian Lebanese, French Canadians, Finns, and Icelanders, because of founder gene effects. Homozygous subjects have extreme hypercholesterolemia (plasma LDL cholesterol levels fourfold to fivefold normal) and develop coronary atherosclerosis in childhood, typically involving the aortic root and valve, and subsequently involving the coronary ostia, at a rate proportional to the magnitude and duration of plasma LDL cholesterol levels.

The diagnosis of FH currently is based on cholesterol levels, clinical signs, and family history, rather than on identification of disease-causing mutations.[30] The primary clinical diagnostic criteria for FH include marked hypercholesterolemia, the presence of tendon xanthomas (due to tissue cholesterol deposition) in the patient or first-degree relative (characteristically seen in the Achilles tendons and extensor tendons of the hands), and a dominant pattern of inheritance of premature CAD by the third or fourth decade, or of hypercholesterolemia.

Although FH is a monogenic disorder, substantial variation in onset and severity of symptomatic atherosclerotic CVD has been noted. Additional genetic and environmental risk factors probably determine the variable clinical expression in patients with this condition. Given the high prevalence of atherosclerotic CVD in FH, subclinical CAD should be actively sought. Male gender, smoking, hypertension, diabetes mellitus, decreased HDL cholesterol, and increased Lp(a), along with an unhealthy diet, lack of physical exercise, and obesity, compound the risk of CVD in FH.

Before primary hypercholesterolemia can be confirmed, secondary causes of hypercholesterolemia, such as primary hypothyroidism, acute intermittent porphyria nephrotic syndrome, dysgammaglobulinemia, and obstructive liver disease, as well as factors such as obesity, physical inactivity, and highly saturated fat and cholesterol diets, should be ruled out.

Once secondary hypercholesterolemia has been ruled out, the primary disorder can be confirmed by (1) screening of family members, including children; (2) persistent hypercholesterolemia even after 8 weeks on a low-cholesterol (<300 mg/day), high–polyunsaturated fat diet (polyunsaturated fat–to–saturated fat [P/S] ratio of 1:1.2); (3) the presence of tendinous xanthomas, xanthelasma, and corneal arcus; and (4) determination of LDL receptor defect or deficiency or other genetically determined molecular defects.

Familial Defective ApoB-100

Defects in the LDL receptor binding domain of apoB can cause autosomal dominant hypercholesterolemia.[31] **Familial defective apoB-100 (FDB)** is characterized by increased concentrations of LDL cholesterol with normal triglyceride levels, tendon xanthomas, and premature CAD. FDB cannot be distinguished clinically from FH; however, hypercholesterolemia in FDB is less severe and the presence of tendon xanthomas less common, and there appears to be a lower incidence of CAD. Furthermore, it is important to note that plasma LDL cholesterol concentrations are <95th percentile of the population in >25% of FDB heterozygotes. Indeed, FDB homozygotes have plasma LDL cholesterol concentrations that are more comparable with those of heterozygous rather than homozygous FH.

Several mutations in the *APOB* gene that affect the binding affinity for the LDL receptor have been identified. The most common, R3500Q, affects about 1 in 500 individuals of European descent and involves the substitution of a glutamine for arginine at position 3500. Genotyping for the R3500Q mutation is available at many specialist biochemical genetics laboratories. These mutations appear to alter the three-dimensional structure of the binding area, so that LDL particles with mutated apoB have reduced binding affinity to the LDL receptor, resulting in the accumulation of particles that contain the mutant apoB. Stable isotope studies in R3500Q FDB heterozygotes showed a decreased production rate and fractional catabolic rate of LDL-apoB. An increase in clearance of LDL precursors, as well as a decrease in conversion of IDL to LDL, could explain the milder phenotype in FDB compared with FH.

Familial Combined Hyperlipidemia

Familial combined hyperlipidemia (FCHL) is a relatively common, highly atherogenic disorder that affects 1% to 2% of the Western world.[32,33] The characteristic feature of this disorder is the scatter of lipoprotein phenotypes within a family. Most commonly, patients exhibit an elevation in both LDL and VLDL; however, within a family, hyperbetalipoproteinemia and hyperprebetalipoproteinemia also are found, affecting different persons. In contrast to FH, patients with FCHL generally do not manifest their disease until adulthood. Clinically, these patients have an increased incidence of CAD. They also frequently have diabetes, show a tendency for hyperuricemia, and have a low incidence of tendinous and tuberous xanthomas. Although the mode of inheritance of FCHL still is in doubt, it is clear that this lipoprotein pattern is a familial inherited disorder. Genome-wide linkage studies have revealed several linked loci that guide to susceptibility genes. The USF1 transcription factor is the major gene underlying the 1q21-23 linkage. Modifying genes, especially those that influence the high-triglyceride trait, include *APOCA1/C2C3/A4/A5,* the latter representing the downstream target of USF1 and implying a USF1-dependent pathway in the molecular pathogenesis of dyslipidemias.[34]

The typical FCHL lipid profile comprises elevated total cholesterol and/or triglyceride concentrations, elevated apoB levels, and increased numbers of small dense LDL particles. Patients also may have elevated cholesterol-enriched VLDL and/or reduced HDL cholesterol, and this may be associated with enrichment of the HDL2 fraction with triglyceride. It is important to note that in Westernized societies, lipid abnormalities of FCHL may occur as a manifestation of the metabolic syndrome, and the possible effects of dietary carbohydrates should not be overlooked when this lipoprotein disorder is assessed. It has been shown that fasting hypertriglyceridemia in patients with this metabolic lipoprotein profile could be attributable to an acute increase in dietary carbohydrates. It appears that triglyceride values >400 mg/dL are rare in patients with this condition. The few reported cases in the medical literature occurred in postmenopausal women.

Any secondary hypercholesterolemia and hypertriglyceridemia such as obesity and type 2 diabetes should be ruled out before the primary lipoprotein disorder is confirmed. Family screening is mandatory for recognition of this lipid abnormality. Accurate diagnosis of the lipoprotein profile also requires an appreciation of the factors that determine triglyceride concentrations. Studies in free-living populations in the United States have documented increases in triglyceride concentrations with age and have indicated that as many as one-fourth of middle-aged men have triglyceride levels that exceed previously published cutoff values. Thus, although statistically valid, the critical limits for triglyceride concentrations may not represent physiological limits. Therefore, investigators might expect a greater prevalence of FCHL in older age groups.

Familial Dysbetalipoproteinemia

Familial dysbetalipoproteinemia is a very rare genetic disorder that affects about 1 in 10,000 individuals.[35] A hallmark clinical presentation of this disease is palmar xanthoma (also called *xanthoma striatum palmare*). Occasionally, tuberous or tuberoeruptive xanthomas occur on the arms and, less frequently, on the buttocks. In addition to premature CHD, dysbetalipoproteinemia causes cerebral and peripheral vascular disease.

Familial dysbetalipoproteinemia (also called broad-β hyperlipoproteinemia) is characterized by an elevation of plasma cholesterol and triglyceride concentrations (typically in a 1:1 ratio) and specifically marked increases in IDL concentrations. This IDL often merges with the pre-β band on electrophoresis to produce a broad-β band (see Fig. 37-12). For accurate diagnosis of familial dysbetalipoproteinemia, an ultracentrifugal study with measurement of cholesterol and triglyceride in the fractions at a density below 1.006 g/mL is required to document the presence of the IDL. It has been suggested that if the VLDL cholesterol-to-triglyceride ratio is ≥0.30, the subject may have familial dysbetalipoproteinemia. However, when the ratio is between 0.25 and 0.29, a diagnosis of possible familial dysbetalipoproteinemia should be considered. Confirmation of this disorder is made by finding a ε2/2 genotype.

Clinical characteristics of patients with this lipoprotein disorder vary widely as a function of age, sex, degree of adiposity, and the presence of associated disorders such as primary hypothyroidism and alcoholism. The most characteristic xanthoma in subjects with familial dysbetalipoproteinemia is called *xanthoma striatum palmare.* In their most subtle form, these lesions produce an orange or yellowish discoloration of the palmar creases (xanthochromia striata palmaris), a phenomenon most easily detected in patients of fair complexion. When more advanced, these lesions may produce planar elevations and even virtual obliteration of the palmar and digital creases. Raised lesions occasionally can affect the remaining palmar surfaces and in their severe form produce tuberous, incapacitating xanthomas.

Various forms of CHD have been reported in association with familial dysbetalipoproteinemia, which is treated readily by diet and drugs. The form of CVD associated with this form of dyslipoproteinemia differs significantly from that associated with FH in that peripheral disease and even cerebrovascular disease appear to be as common as CHD.

Secondary familial dysbetalipoproteinemia has been associated with primary hypothyroidism, gout, and diabetes mellitus and is found in patients with acute renal failure who are receiving maintenance hemodialysis.

Monogenic Hypocholesterolemia

Many factors such as illness, high-dose statin therapy, or a strict vegan diet can cause hypobetalipoproteinemia. The more common secondary causes in the hospital setting include cachexia, malabsorption, malnutrition, severe liver disease, and hyperthyroidism. Primary causes include FHBL, ABL, and chylomicron retention disease.[27,36]

Familial Hypobetalipoproteinemia

Familial hypobetalipoproteinemia (FHBL) is a rare autosomal co-dominant disorder characterized by low plasma concentrations of total cholesterol, LDL cholesterol, and apoB.[27,31,36] Heterozygotes often are asymptomatic, but have plasma LDL cholesterol and apoB concentrations that are one-quarter to one-third of normal (<5th percentile for age and sex). Clinical and biochemical features of FHBL in homozygous and compound heterozygous form are very similar to those of ABL (see below). Clinical features of homozygous FHBL may include **acanthocytosis,** deficiencies in fat-soluble vitamins following malabsorption, an atypical form of **retinitis pigmentosa,** and neuromuscular abnormalities. Retinitis pigmentosa and other neuropathies primarily result from deficiencies in fat-soluble vitamins, especially vitamins E and A, caused by their impaired absorption and transport. Mild acanthocytosis and fatty liver have been observed in FHBL heterozygotes. FHBL and ABL can be differentiated by inheritance pattern; in contrast to FHBL, ABL is recessive, and obligate heterozygotes for MTTP mutations usually have normal LDL cholesterol concentrations. It has been suggested that FHBL may represent a longevity syndrome that results from low concentrations of LDL cholesterol in affected subjects, along with a presumed decrease in CHD caused by a lower lifetime exposure of LDL and atherogenic apoB-containing lipoproteins.

FHBL is caused primarily by mutations in the *APOB* gene. More than 60 different mutations in *APOB* that interfere with translation of full-length apoB have been described. Most of these mutations in *APOB* cause the production of truncated apoB isoforms of various lengths associated with the missing carboxyl-terminal portion of the molecule. The population frequency of FHBL resulting from truncated forms of apoB has been estimated at 1 in 3000. Recently, two rare missense mutations—R463W and L343V—have been shown to cause FHBL through a mechanism that involves impaired ER exit and enhanced binding to MTTP. Cases of FHBL that are not linked to *APOB* have been identified.

The concentrations of apoB-100 in FHBL heterozygotes are typically about 25% of normal. Possible reasons for these lower than expected concentrations include decreased hepatic secretion of apoB-containing lipoproteins and upregulation of the LDL receptor, which results in an enhanced clearance rate for VLDL and LDL particles produced by the normal *APOB* allele. Decreased production rates and increased clearance rates are responsible for the low plasma concentrations of truncated apoB species.

Abetalipoproteinemia

MTTP is a critical protein involved in the assembly of chylomicrons and VLDL. Individuals with the very rare recessive disorder abetalipoproteinemia (ABL), also known as Bassen-Kornzweig syndrome, carry two defective MTTP alleles and have undetectable plasma concentrations of LDL cholesterol and apoB.[27,36] The plasma cholesterol concentration does not exceed 80 mg/dL and is likely to be no higher than 30 mg/dL. This is accompanied by concentrations of triglycerides lower than those seen in any other disease, usually <20 mg/dL. After a fat load, chylomicrons do not appear in plasma.

Patients often present in childhood with failure to thrive, fat malabsorption (steatorrhea), and low plasma cholesterol and vitamin E concentrations. Vitamin E is essential for neurological function and is transported in plasma in association with apoB-containing lipoproteins. Without high-dose vitamin E and A treatment, progressive spinocerebellar degeneration and an atypical form of retinitis pigmentosa may occur. Liver biopsies have shown marked steatosis, which may or may not be reflected in raised serum transaminase concentrations. Acanthocytosis is found in ABL, with acanthocytes accounting for 50% to 100% of circulating erythrocytes. Acanthocytosis may occur in other diseases in which lipoproteins are not deficient. The acanthocytosis found in ABL may result from vitamin E deficiency or altered membrane lipid composition.

The human MTTP gene, which is located on chromosome 4q22-24, encodes an 894 amino acid protein. MTTP forms a heterodimer with the ubiquitous ER enzyme, protein disulfide isomerase. A variety of mutations in *MTTP* gene have been described, including three missense mutations that affect the protein disulfide isomerase- or apoB-binding ability of MTTP, leading to an increase in degradation of nascent apoB-containing lipoproteins and a corresponding decrease in secretion.

Chylomicron Retention Disease

Chylomicron retention disease, also known as Anderson's disease, is an autosomal recessive form of hypobetalipoproteinemia that is characterized by the selective absence of apoB-48.[27,36] Affected subjects do not have chylomicrons present in plasma after a fat-containing meal. The disorder is accompanied by steatorrhea, growth retardation and malnutrition, and an accumulation of lipid droplets within the enterocyte. Mutations in *SARA2*, a member of the Sar1-ADP-ribosylation factor family of small GTPases that control intracellular trafficking of proteins in coat protein complex (COP)-coated vesicles, are the cause of chylomicron retention disease. Sar1b, the gene product of *SARA2*, initiates the formation of COPII-coated vesicles and seems to be necessary for intracellular trafficking of very large chylomicron particles. Chylomicrons are recruited selectively by the COPII machinery for transport through cellular secretory pathways.

Familial Hypoalphalipoproteinemia

Familial hypoalphalipoproteinemia (FHA) is characterized by normal plasma lipids and LDL cholesterol and reduced HDL cholesterol (<5th percentile for age and sex).[37] The disorder appears to be the result of reduced synthesis or increased catabolism of HDL or apoA-I. Furthermore, mutations in the gene that encodes ATP binding cassette transporter A1 (ABCA1) on chromosome 9q31 have been found in some patients with FHA, a relatively more common disorder than TD. Cellular cholesterol efflux appears to be abnormal in some patients with FHA because of a mutant *ABCA1,* but no tissue deposition of cholesterol esters is evident, and low plasma HDL cholesterol concentrations demonstrate an apparent autosomal co-dominant pattern of expression in *ABCA1* mutation carriers.

Tangier Disease

Tangier disease (TD) is a rare autosomal co-dominant disorder that is characterized by severe deficiency or absence of normal HDL in plasma, caused by increased catabolism and accumulation of cholesteryl esters in many tissues throughout the body.[37] The combination of severe HDL cholesterol deficiency and hyperplastic orange-yellow tonsils and adenoid tissue is pathognomonic of TD. Some persons may exhibit peripheral neuropathy. Small amounts of HDL in TD plasma differ qualitatively and quantitatively from normal HDL, particularly with respect to apoA-I and apoA-II content. Patients with TD appear to be at increased risk for CAD. Mutations in *ABCA1* on chromosome 9q31 have been reported in patients with TD, *ABCA1* has been shown to regulate the apoA-I–mediated lipid removal pathway from cells, and patients with TD exhibit defective transport of lipids from the Golgi to the cell membrane. Heterozygotes in TD families with known homozygotes usually can be identified by low HDL concentrations (about 50% below normal); they do not develop neuropathy and cholesteryl ester accumulation. Plasma total cholesterol concentrations range from about 40 to 125 mg/dL—similar to those observed in ABL and hypobetalipoproteinemia. Individual variation in plasma triglyceride concentration is considerable and is highly contingent on diet. The plasma lipoprotein pattern is distinctive: The α-lipoprotein band is absent, irrespective of the support medium used. Estimation of the cholesterol content of plasma lipoproteins after sequential preparative ultracentrifugation or after ultracentrifugation and selective heparin-manganese precipitation confirms the paucity of HDL.

In addition to HDL absence or deficiency, the following diseases must be excluded:

- Familial deficiency of LCAT. In this case, HDL is very low, but the plasma total cholesterol concentration is normal or high, and most of the cholesterol is unesterified.
- Obstructive liver disease, in which plasma HDL and apoA-I may be reduced to concentrations as low as those seen in TD. In this disorder, the total cholesterol concentration is not low, but high, and most of the cholesterol is unesterified. Appropriate tests of liver function should permit correct diagnosis.
- Severe malnutrition or hepatic parenchymal disease in which HDL is decreased. The reduction in cholesterol will be associated with low triglyceride and LDL concentrations.
- Acquired HDL deficiency attributable to dysglobulinemia, including possible development of antibodies to HDL
- Other storage diseases associated with foam cells and hepatosplenomegaly. In these conditions, HDL concentrations are higher than those seen in TD, and typical tonsillar abnormalities are absent.

TRANSFORMATION OF HYPERLIPIDEMIA TO HYPERLIPOPROTEINEMIA

From Lipids to Lipoproteins: Laboratory Considerations

In the transformation of hyperlipidemia to hyperlipoproteinemia, lipid analyses and the overnight refrigeration test can be used to determine the lipoprotein profile with a fair degree of accuracy. If the plasma is clear, the triglyceride concentration is most likely to be normal or near normal (<200 mg/dL). When triglyceride increases to about 300 mg/dL or higher, the plasma is usually hazy to turbid in appearance and is not translucent enough to allow for clear reading of newsprint through the tube. When plasma triglyceride is >1000 mg/dL, the plasma usually is opaque and milky (lipemic, lactescent). If chylomicrons are present, after overnight incubation at 4°C, a thick homogeneous "cream" layer may be observed floating at the plasma surface. As is summarized in Fig. 37-12, a uniformly opaque plasma sample usually denotes a hyperprebetalipoproteinemia. An opaque plasma sample with a cream layer on top usually is consistent with the mixed form of hyperlipoproteinemia. A thick chylomicron cream layer with generally clear plasma infranate usually is consistent with a hyperchylomicronemic profile.

In patients with hypercholesterolemia without hypertriglyceridemia, most often with raised LDL concentrations, the plasma is clear but may have an orange-yellow tint, because carotene is carried with LDL. After a visual observation that is "simple and free," the diagnosis of the lipid abnormality can be made in as many as 90% of subjects via quantitation of plasma cholesterol and triglyceride alone. It should be noted that the Fredrickson system of hyperlipoproteinemia phenotypes, once widely taught, has fallen into disuse.

The recommended protocol of the NECP ATP III for laboratory analyses required for effective assessment of CHD risk and detection of common lipoprotein abnormalities includes measurement of total cholesterol, triglycerides, and LDL and HDL cholesterol.[8] These measurements can be performed by most clinical laboratories (see Methods on Evolve).[38,39] More demanding analytical techniques, such as analytical ultracentrifugation or apoprotein and lipoprotein subfraction measurements, may be needed to differentiate atypical lipoprotein abnormalities; these usually are available in specialized research laboratories.

Secondary Hyperlipoproteinemia

In general, lipoprotein quantification and typing alone will not distinguish the primary from the secondary form of hyperlipoproteinemia (see Table 37-3). Even the diagnosis of a concurrent disorder that is likely to cause secondary hyperlipoproteinemia does not necessarily establish it as the cause of a patient's hyperlipoproteinemia. Reversal of the lipid abnormality that accompanies treatment for the suspected causative disorder, however, provides compelling evidence of the secondary nature of the hyperlipoproteinemia. Failure of such reversal to occur implies that the hyperlipoproteinemia may be primary and indicates the need for family screening.

Some disorders associated with hyperlipoproteinemia will be obvious from the patient's history and physical examination. Others will require blood or urine tests for diagnosis. If such a screening reveals no abnormalities, it is reasonable to assume that the patient has primary hyperlipoproteinemia. Whether or not the hyperlipoproteinemia is established as familial in origin depends on the results of the family screening.

KEY CONCEPTS BOX 37-5

- Hyperlipoproteinemia is an elevation in serum lipoprotein concentrations that results from primary (genetic) or secondary causes.
- The metabolic syndrome is a constellation of interrelated risk factors (including abdominal obesity, atherogenic dyslipidemia, elevated blood pressure, and elevated plasma glucose) of metabolic origin that appear to directly promote the development of atherosclerotic CVD.
- The classification of genetic dyslipoproteinemias is based on the biochemical phenotype, the concentrations of blood lipids, and identification of abnormal lipoprotein patterns, in addition to clinical phenotype.
- With the exception of FH, monogenic disorders of lipid metabolism tend to be infrequent or very rare.

SECTION OBJECTIVES BOX 37-6

- Explain the basis for using the NCEP ATP III–recommended laboratory protocol to assess CHD risk and detect common lipoprotein abnormalities.
- Describe the risk factors associated with coronary artery disease.
- Describe the process of atherogenesis.

CLINICAL IMPLICATIONS OF HYPERLIPIDEMIA

Hyperlipidemia usually is a symptomless biochemical state that, if present for a sufficiently long time, may be associated with the development of atherosclerosis and CVD. Occasionally, hyperlipidemia may be associated with specific overt symptoms or signs that are directly attributable to the presence of hyperlipidemia. Examples include abdominal pain, acute pancreatitis, and the cutaneous manifestations of hyperlipidemia, such as xanthomas, corneal arcus, and xanthelasmas (yellow plaques on eyelid).

Coronary Artery Disease

Coronary artery disease (CAD) is almost always the result of atherosclerosis, which currently is viewed as an inflammatory disease.[40] Coronary atherosclerosis primarily results from the accumulation of fatty deposits in the walls of coronary arteries, which leads to the formation of fibrous tissue in the vessel wall. CAD is the most common type of heart disease and is a leading cause of death in the United States and many other countries. About 75% of coronary-related mortalities are the result of atherosclerosis. Although death rates from CVD declined 26.4% from 1995 to 2005, CVD accounted for 34.2% of all deaths in the United States in 2005, with CHD making up 52% of this total (i.e., CHD causes about one of every five deaths in the United States).[41] CAD affects middle-aged males; nearly 45% of all heart attacks occur in individuals younger than 65 years of age. CHD develops in men 60 years of age or younger at about twice the rate seen in women, and postmenopausal women have a higher incidence of CHD than do premenopausal women of the same age. For both men and women, the incidence of CVD and the rate of death from atherosclerosis increase with advancing age. In 2009, an estimated 785,000 Americans will have a new MI, and about 470,000 will have a recurrent attack.[40] It is estimated that an additional 195,000 silent first MIs will occur each year.

Box 37-5

Primary and Secondary Risk Factors Associated With Coronary Heart Disease

Primary

Genetic predisposition for CHD
Family history of premature CHD in first-degree relatives (<45 years for males, <55 years for females)
Hypertension
Cigarette smoking
Elevated total cholesterol (LDL cholesterol)
Decreased HDL cholesterol
Elevated triglycerides (VLDL cholesterol, remnant lipoproteins)
Increasing age
Male gender

Secondary

Lack of exercise
Obesity
Stress
Diabetes mellitus
Elevated CRP
Elevated Lp(a)
Elevated homocysteine
Elevated IDL
Patients with chronic kidney disease receiving hemodialysis
Postmenopausal state
Certain thrombogenic disorders

Risk Factors Associated With CAD

Scientists have identified several factors associated with a distinct increase in the likelihood that a person will develop a MI later in life.[42] These primary or secondary risk factors correlate with the presence of CHD (Box 37-5). Some risk factors, such as racial and genetic susceptibility, increased prevalence in males, and increased likelihood of MI as aging occurs, are unavoidable. Many known risk factors, however, are susceptible to behavior modification. Particularly important among these are high blood pressure, cigarette smoking, and elevated serum cholesterol, or, more significantly, elevated LDL cholesterol. About 50% of persons who experience MI have one or more of these three risk factors. The Framingham data reveal a clear gradient of CHD incidence rates in relation to serum HDL cholesterol concentrations. Persons with concentrations <35 mg/dL have eight times the CHD rate of persons with HDL cholesterol concentrations of ≥65 mg/dL.

Important additional risk factors are fibrinogen, oxidized LDL, small lipoprotein particle size (or dense LDL), specific apoproteins (apoA-I, B, E isoforms), and triglyceride-poor remnant lipoproteins.[43] Other possible factors whose relative

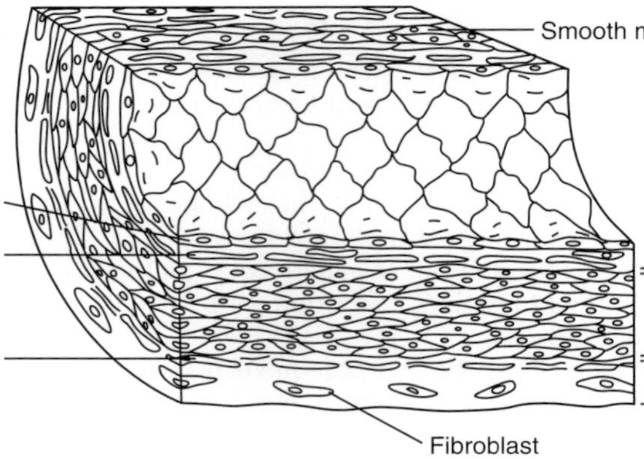

Fig. 37-13 Diagram of a healthy blood vessel (artery) with normal integrity of the intima, media, and adventitia.

importance still is being established include hypertriglyceridemia, level of physical activity, and personality types.

ATHEROSCLEROTIC PLAQUE FORMATION

Normal arteries have a well-developed trilaminar structure. The innermost layer, the tunica intima, is lined by endothelium on the inner, luminal side of the vessel, which is bound by the internal elastic lamina to the tunica media (Fig. 37-13). The outermost layer is the adventitia, which is bound by the external elastic lamina and exterior to the vessel itself. The tunica intima is the site at which atherosclerotic lesions form. The endothelium serves as a barrier to bloodborne materials and as a site where several **mitogens** are synthesized and secreted. The tunica media is the muscular wall of the artery that consists of smooth muscle cells held together by a discontinuous basement membrane and by interspersed collagen fibrils and proteoglycan.[40,44] Smooth muscle cells that proliferate in the arterial intima to form advanced lesions of atherosclerosis originate in the media. This smooth muscle cell proliferation represents the defining condition of the lesions of advanced atherosclerosis. Smooth muscle cells, like the endothelium and fibroblasts, contain receptors for LDL and platelet-derived growth factor (PDGF). One characteristic feature of smooth muscle cells found in the lesions of atherosclerosis is the accumulation of lipids that result in the formation of highly vacuolated cells, or foam cells.

Atherogenesis is the complex interaction of risk factors with cells of the artery wall and the blood, as well as the molecular messages that they exchange.[40,44] The first steps in atherogenesis in humans remain largely speculative, but inflammation plays a major role at all stages of the process. Atherosclerotic plaque formation occurs in three progressive stages: (1) the fatty streaks, which gradually develop into raised lesions, called *fatty plaques;* (2) the fibrous plaque, which has a proliferation of smooth muscle cells and a collagen-rich fibrous cap that covers a lipid core lined by foam cells and surrounding an amorphous extracellular accumulation of cholesteryl esters; and (3) the complicated lesion, which can manifest calcification, hemorrhage, ulceration (rupture), and thrombosis (Fig. 37-14). It is the complicated lesion that frequently underlies the acute clinical event of arterial occlusion that leads to MI.

The formation and accumulation of foam cells in the tunica intima are the hallmark of the early atherosclerotic lesion. Currently, it is believed that most foam cells are derived from bloodborne macrophages, although some may come from smooth muscle cells. A pivotal step in the development of foam cells is the accelerated uptake of modified LDL (see below), followed by proliferation of smooth muscle cells (with and without lipid deposits in their cytoplasm) (Fig. 37-15). Smooth muscle cell proliferation is accompanied by increased synthesis of cellular elastin, collagen, and proteoglycans, which these cells deposit extracellularly in the developing plaque.

When the arterial endothelium encounters certain factors, such as bacteria or dyslipidemia, these cells express adhesion molecules that promote the migration of blood leukocytes to the inner surface of the arterial wall. Macrophage foam cells recruited to the artery wall provide a rich source of proinflammatory cytokines and chemokines and various lipid mediators. These phagocytic cells also can elaborate large quantities of oxidant species such as superoxide anion in the milieu of the atherosclerotic plaque. This collection of inflammatory mediators promotes inflammation in the plaque and thus contributes to the progression of atherosclerotic lesions.[45]

As a major consequence of the inflammatory process under way in the early atheroma, smooth muscle cells migrate from the tunica media into the intima. These cells proliferate and elaborate a rich and complex extracellular matrix. Together with endothelial cells and monocytes, they secrete matrix metalloproteinases in response to various oxidative, hemodynamic, inflammatory, and autoimmune signals. Certain constituents of the extracellular matrix, notably proteoglycans, bind lipoproteins, prolong their residence in the tunica intima, and render them more susceptible to oxidative modification and glycation. The uptake of LDL by macrophages can be enhanced if the LDL lipid is modified by oxidation or there is degradation of apoB by reactive oxygen species (such as free radicals) or via derivatization of apoB through glycosylation or reaction with malonaldehyde (Fig. 37-16). These products of lipoprotein modification sustain and propagate the inflammatory response. As the lesion progresses, calcification can occur. In addition to cell proliferation, cell death commonly occurs in the established atherosclerotic lesion. Extracellular

Fatty streak

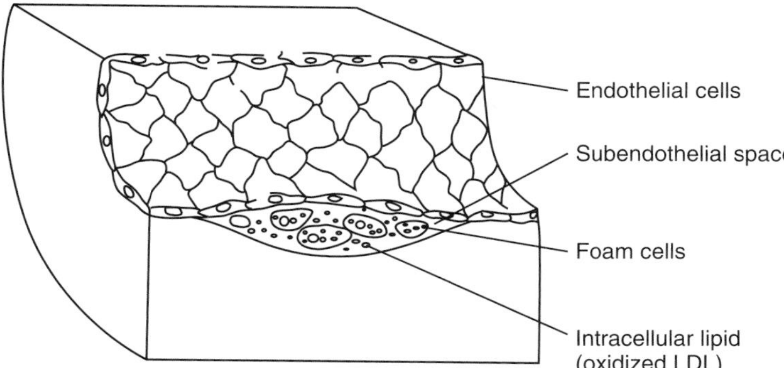

Fibrous plaque

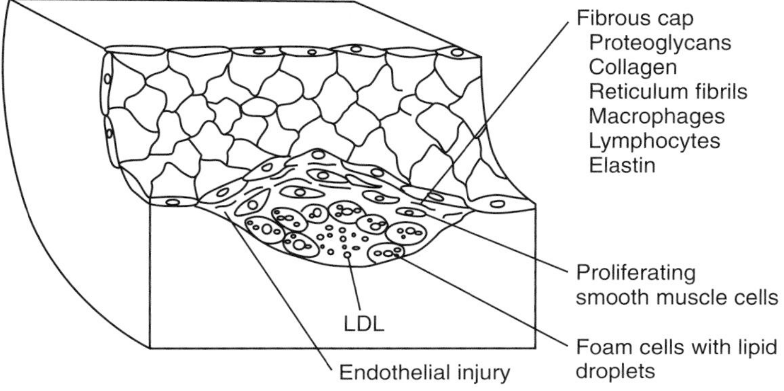

Complicated lesion

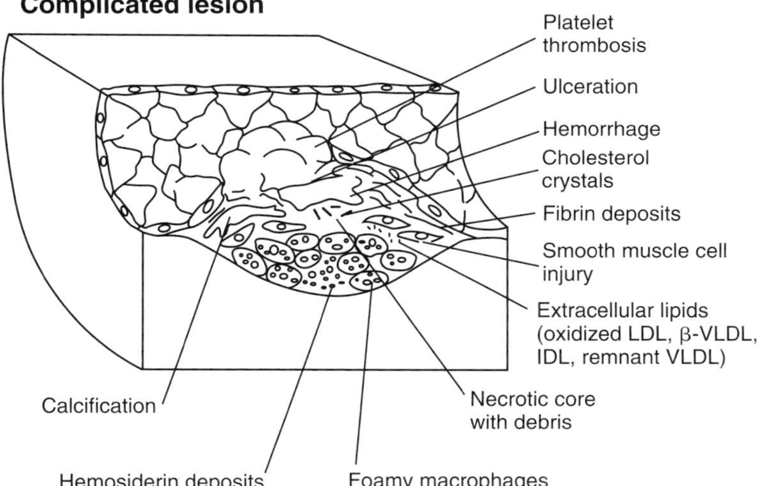

Fig. 37-14 The three stages of atherogenesis: formation of the fatty streak, fibrous plaque, and complicated lesion. Note the development and accumulation of foam cells in the fatty streak, accumulation of smooth muscle cells in the fibrous plaque, and formation of calcification, ulceration, thrombosis, and hemorrhage in the advanced or complicated lesion.

lipid that accumulates in the tunica intima can coalesce to form the classic, lipid-rich necrotic core of the atherosclerotic plaque.

Platelets have a smaller role in some atherosclerotic lesions but play a major role in the formation of thrombi.

It is usually a mural or occlusive thrombus that leads to an MI. Platelets also can produce the same growth factors as activated macrophages. Thus, at sites of injury in which collagen exposure occurs, numerous vasoactive, stimulatory, and proliferative responses can take place and probably play a role in the initiation of atherosclerotic lesions.

Fat-laden macrophages, together with varying numbers of lipid-filled smooth muscle cells, develop into fatty streaks. Most of the lipid in foam cells consists of free cholesterol and cholesteryl ester. Fatty streaks are observed early in childhood, and their transformation into complicated lesions usually takes four to five decades before clinical manifestations of disease, including angina pectoris, MI, or sudden cardiac

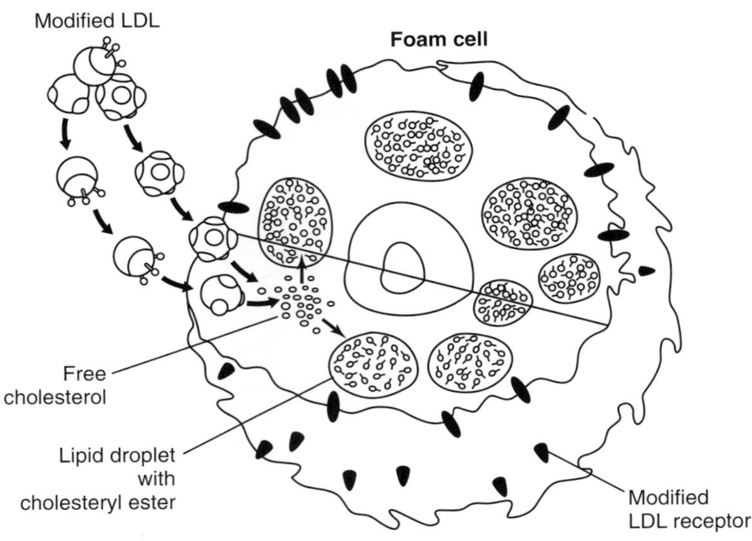

Fig. 37-15 Formation of the foam cell: macrophage uptake (ingestion) of modified low-density lipoprotein (LDL) by the modified LDL receptor pathway, which results in the development of large fat-laden droplets. This process of foam cell formation is the hallmark of fatty streak development in atherogenesis.

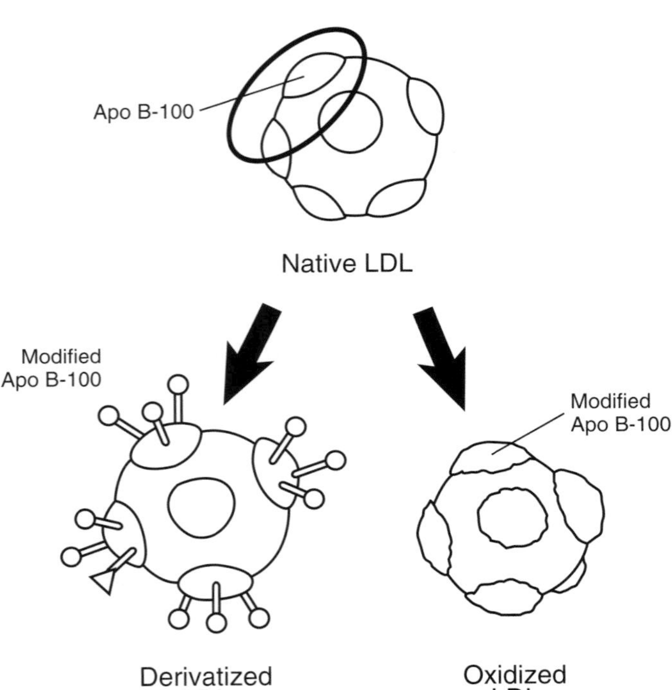

Fig. 37-16 Modification of low-density lipoprotein (LDL). Entrapped native LDL (in the subendothelial space) can undergo two types of modification: derivatization (malondialdehyde attachment to or glycosylation of apoB-100) or oxidation (degradation of apoB-100 by superoxides).

death, appear. In males, the first MI event usually occurs at around 55 years of age, whereas in females, a 10-year delay leads to occurrence at around 65 years of age. This atherosclerotic process can be accelerated by having (1) additional CHD risk factors; (2) endothelial injury, which removes the natural barrier to the entrance of lipoproteins into the arterial wall or causes thrombosis; and (3) a genetic predisposition for FH.

We now recognize that for much of its life history, the atherosclerotic lesion grows outward, away from the arterial wall, rather than inward. Thus, a substantial burden for atherosclerosis can exist without producing stenosis. Pathological studies have established characteristics of rupture-prone plaque, including a thin, fibrous cap and a large lipid core populated by numerous inflammatory cells and relatively lacking in smooth muscle cells. Ruptured plaques are complicit in acute coronary syndromes (Fig. 37-17).

KEY CONCEPTS BOX 37-6

- The NECP ATP III–recommended protocol for the laboratory analyses can assess CHD risk and detect common lipoprotein abnormalities by using measurements of total cholesterol, triglycerides, and LDL and HDL cholesterol.
- Both primary (genetic) and secondary risk factors are associated with CAD.
- Some risk factors, such as racial and genetic susceptibility and male gender, are unavoidable; however, many risk factors are susceptible to behavior modification, for example, high blood pressure, cigarette smoking, and elevated serum LDL cholesterol.

SECTION OBJECTIVES BOX 37-7

- Describe the features of the NCEP ATP III therapeutic guidelines, including implications for treatment.

Change of Analyte in Disease: Therapeutic Guidelines and Treatment

In the late 1980s, health care workers realized that a unified effort was needed to standardize the approach for detection and classification of individuals at high risk for CHD, and to standardize treatment and monitoring of such individuals. This effort required a major educational drive to inform physicians and their patients of CHD risk factors. To fulfill this scientific and educational goal, the federal government and a broad range of professional health care groups worked together to formulate guidelines and recommendations, with the intent

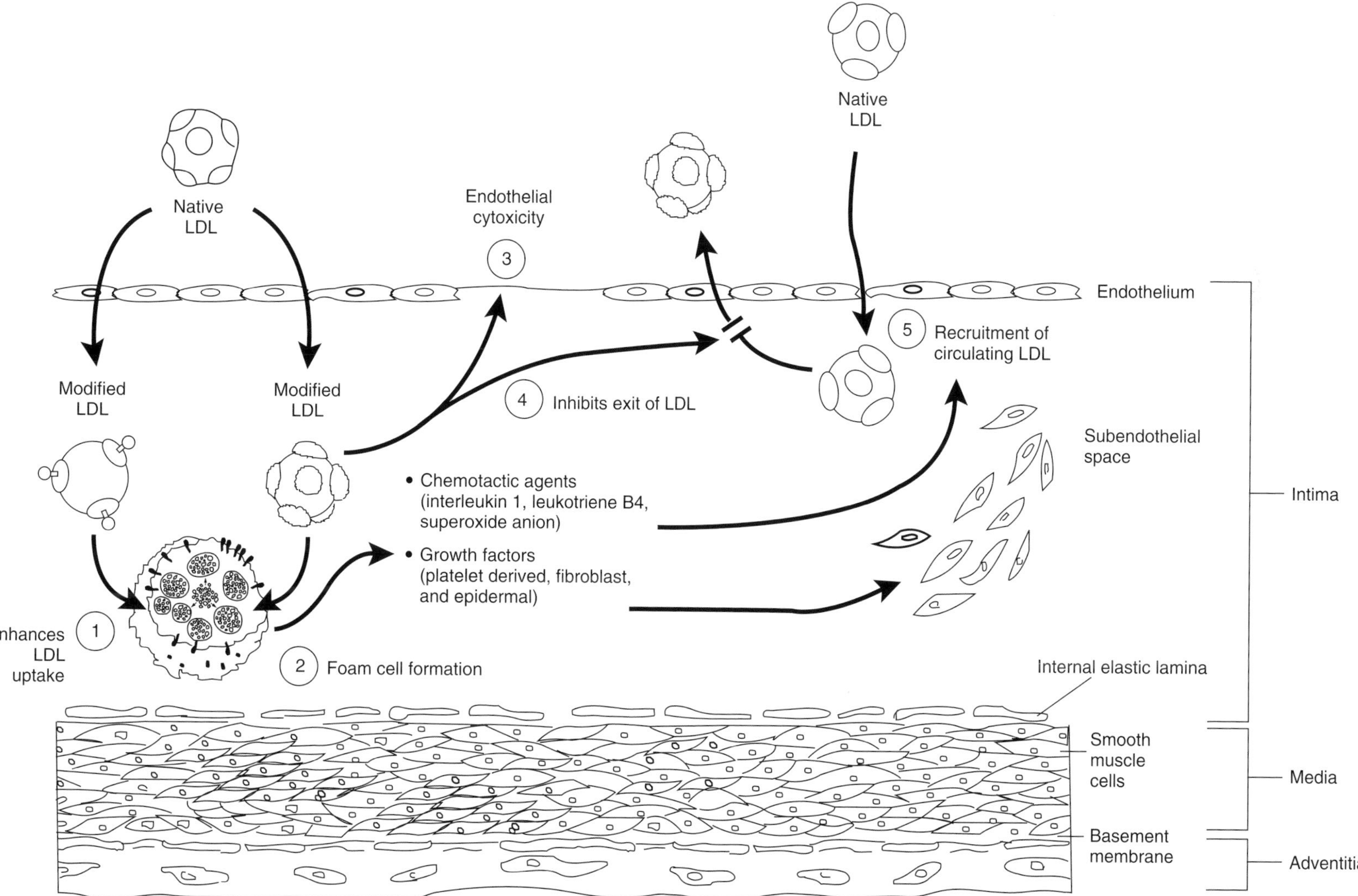

Fig. 37-17 Hypothesis of the multiple roles of oxidized low-density lipoprotein (LDL) in atherogenesis. (Derived from Steinberg D, Parthasarathy S, Carew TE, et al: Beyond cholesterol: modifications of low-density lipoproteins that increase its atherogenicity, N Engl J Med 320:915, 1989.)

of reducing CHD in the United States. This national campaign was called the *NCEP*.

As a result of this effort, the NIH established criteria that defined the high-risk person for medical intervention for CHD and provided clear guidelines on how to detect disease and set goals for treating and monitoring these patients over time. Some of the key features of these landmark reports[8,9,46] on cholesterol are described here.

Features of the most recent NCEP ATP III[8] guidelines are as follows:

- Recommend a complete lipoprotein profile (total, LDL, and HDL cholesterol and triglycerides) as the preferred initial test, rather than screening for total cholesterol and HDL cholesterol alone
- Raise the risk for CHD among individuals with diabetes without CHD, most of whom have multiple risk factors, to the risk level of CHD risk equivalent, that is, a risk for major coronary events equal to that of established CHD
- Identify certain patients with multiple (2+) risk factors as candidates for more intensive treatment
- Identify persons with multiple metabolic risk factors (metabolic syndrome) as candidates for intensified therapeutic lifestyle changes.
- Identify LDL cholesterol <100 mg/dL as optimal
- Raise categorical low HDL cholesterol from <35 mg/dL to <40 mg/dL
- Lower triglyceride classification cutoff point from <200 mg/dL to <150 mg/dL
- Emphasize the use of a sliding scale for LDL cholesterol therapeutic goals: zero or one risk factor, <160 mg/dL; two or more risk factors, <130 mg/dL; and CHD and CHD risk equivalents, <100 mg/dL

All adults 20 years of age or older should have a fasting total cholesterol, triglycerides, and lipoprotein profile done every 5 years. For nonfasting individuals, only the values for total cholesterol and HDL cholesterol should be used. If the total cholesterol (≥200 mg/dL) or HDL cholesterol (<40 mg/dL) value is abnormal, a follow-up fasting lipoprotein profile is required for the development of therapeutic goals.

The more aggressive classification of risk of the NCEP ATP III,[8] which is based on total, LDL, and HDL cholesterol, is defined in Tables 37-5, 37-6, and 37-7. LDL cholesterol, not total cholesterol, will serve as the primary target of CHD risk assessment and therapy.

Along with lipid and lipoprotein testing, all adults should be evaluated for the presence or absence of CHD and of other major CHD risk factors (Box 37-5). The patient is considered to have a high-risk status if he or she has any of the following:

1. Definite CHD (i.e., definite prior MI or myocardial ischemia)
2. The presence of two or more other CHD risk factors
3. A lipid or lipoprotein abnormality with the presence of one other CHD risk factor

Selection of therapeutic LDL cholesterol intervention strategies requires the therapeutic modalities of lifestyle changes and drug intervention (Box 37-6). Increased physical activity

Table 37-5 Classifications of Risk in Adults Based on Low-Density Lipoprotein Cholesterol

LDL Cholesterol, mg/dL*	Classification of Risk
<100	Optimal
100 to 129	Optimal or above optimal
130 to 159	Borderline high
160 to 189	High
>190	Very high

From Adult Treatment Panel III: Executive summary of the third report of the National Cholesterol Education Program (NCEP) expert panel on detection, evaluation, and treatment of high blood cholesterol in adults, JAMA 285:2486, 2001.
*To convert mg/dL of cholesterol to mmol/L, divide by 38.7.

Table 37-6 NCEP ATP III Risk Classification for HDL Cholesterol Levels

Classification of Risk	HDL Cholesterol
High	<40 mg/dL
Low	>60 mg/dL

From Adult Treatment Panel III: Executive summary of the third report of the National Cholesterol Education Program (NCEP) expert panel on detection, evaluation, and treatment of high blood cholesterol in adults, JAMA 285:2486, 2001.

Table 37-7 Recommendations from the NCEP for Children and Adolescents

Total Cholesterol, mg/dL	Classification of Risk	LDL Cholesterol, mg/dL
<170	Acceptable	<110
170 to 199	Borderline high	110 to 129
>200	High	>130

From American Academy of Pediatrics. National Cholesterol Education Program: Report of the Expert Panel on Blood Cholesterol Levels in Children and Adolescents. Pediatrics 89:525, 1992.

Box 37-6
Major Therapeutic Modalities

Therapeutic Lifestyle Changes
Low saturated fat and cholesterol intake diet
Weight reduction
Increased physical activity

Pharmaceuticals
HMG-CoA reductase inhibitors (statins)
Cholesterol absorption inhibitors
Bile acid sequestrants
Nicotinic acid
Fibric acids

is important if the patient has a metabolic syndrome or life habit risk factors such as abdominal obesity, atherogenic dyslipidemia (elevated triglyceride, small LDL particles, low HDL cholesterol), elevated blood pressure, insulin resistance (with or without glucose intolerance), and prothrombotic and proinflammatory states.

The NCEP ATP III[8] report also emphasizes primary prevention of CHD, along with LDL-lowering therapy. Therapeutic lifestyle changes serve as the foundation of clinical primary prevention. Nonetheless, some persons at highest risk for CHD, because of high LDL cholesterol concentrations or multiple risk factors, are candidates for LDL-lowering drugs. Secondary prevention with LDL-lowering therapy is also beneficial, and the goal of therapy should be aggressive (i.e., LDL cholesterol <100 mg/dL). Clinical trials[46] have demonstrated that LDL-lowering therapy reduces total mortality, coronary mortality, major coronary events, coronary artery procedures, and stroke in persons with established CHD. It should be stressed that any person with elevated LDL cholesterol or other forms of hyperlipidemia should undergo clinical or laboratory assessment to rule out secondary dyslipidemia before lipid-lowering therapy is initiated. Major recommendations for modifications to footnote the ATP III treatment algorithm are as follows:

- In high-risk persons, the recommended LDL cholesterol goal is <100 mg/dL, but when risk is very high, an LDL cholesterol goal of 70 mg/dL is a therapeutic option.
- When a high-risk patient has high triglycerides or low HDL cholesterol, consideration can be given to combining a fibrate or nicotinic acid with an LDL-lowering drug.
- For moderately high-risk persons (2+ risk factors and 10-year risk of 10% to 20%), the recommended LDL cholesterol goal is <130 mg/dL; an LDL cholesterol goal <100 mg/dL is a therapeutic option. This option extends to moderately high-risk persons with a baseline LDL cholesterol of 100 to 129 mg/dL.
- Any person at high risk or moderately high risk who has lifestyle-related risk factors (e.g., obesity, physical inactivity, elevated triglycerides, low HDL cholesterol, metabolic syndrome) is a candidate for **therapeutic lifestyle change (TLC)** to modify these risk factors, regardless of LDL cholesterol level.
- When LDL-lowering drug therapy is employed in high-risk or moderately high-risk persons, it is advised that intensity of therapy is sufficient to achieve at least a 30% to 40% reduction in LDL cholesterol levels.
- For individuals in lower-risk categories, recent clinical trials do not modify the goals and cutpoints of therapy.

Additional features of the NCEP ATP III report include the following:

- Age (45 years or older for males and 55 years or older in women) as a major CHD risk factor
- Recommended delay in the use of pharmacological agents for lipid and lipoprotein therapy in most young adult men and premenopausal women with elevated LDL cholesterol levels
- Enhanced recognition that high-risk postmenopausal women and high-risk older adult patients who otherwise are in good health are candidates for cholesterol-lowering therapy
- More attention to HDL cholesterol as a CHD risk factor, which includes the addition of HDL cholesterol measurements to initial cholesterol testing. A high HDL cholesterol level (>60 mg/dL) has been designated as a negative CHD risk factor, whereas low HDL cholesterol (<40 mg/dL) has been designated as a positive CHD risk factor (see Table 37-6). In addition, when a physician is selecting a drug for lowering LDL cholesterol, consideration should be given to the effect of the drug on the patient's HDL cholesterol.
- Increased emphasis on physical activity and weight loss as components of the dietary therapy of high blood LDL cholesterol

The NIH Expert Panel on Blood Cholesterol Levels in Children and Adolescents[47] recommended the following (see Table 37-7):

- Selective screening of high-risk children and adolescents who have a family history of premature CVD or at least one parent with high blood cholesterol (>240 mg/dL) was recommended. Screening also was advocated if the parents or grandparents, at 55 years of age or younger, underwent diagnostic coronary arteriography and were found to have coronary atherosclerosis. These include parents or grandparents who have undergone balloon angioplasty or coronary artery bypass surgery, or who have suffered a documented MI, angina pectoris, peripheral vascular disease, cerebrovascular disease, or sudden cardiac death.
- Universal screening of children and adolescents for high blood cholesterol was not advocated.
- Minimum goals of treatment—for patients with borderline LDL cholesterol, to lower the level to <110 mg/dL; for patients with high LDL cholesterol, to lower the level to <130 mg/dL. Drug therapy should not be used in children who are younger than 10 years of age, or in those who have not been prescribed an adequate cholesterol-lowering diet for at least 6 months to 1 year.

Positive and negative CHD risk factors are used as a guide to the type and intensity of cholesterol-lowering therapy that should be used by the physician (see Box 37-2). For example, a male patient who is >45 years or a female patient who is >55 years is at higher risk for CHD and should be treated more aggressively. Therefore, the goals for lowering serum levels of LDL cholesterol and total cholesterol are more intensive.

It should be stressed that a person with two or more of the positive risk factors listed in Box 37-2, in addition to an elevated LDL cholesterol value, would be classified as a high-risk individual for CHD. Keep in mind that a high amount of HDL cholesterol (>60 mg/dL) represents a negative risk factor.

Treatment strategies still focus on lowering the high blood level of LDL cholesterol to provide primary prevention of CHD.[8] Algorithms of testing and treatment modalities for primary prevention in adults without evidence of CHD are

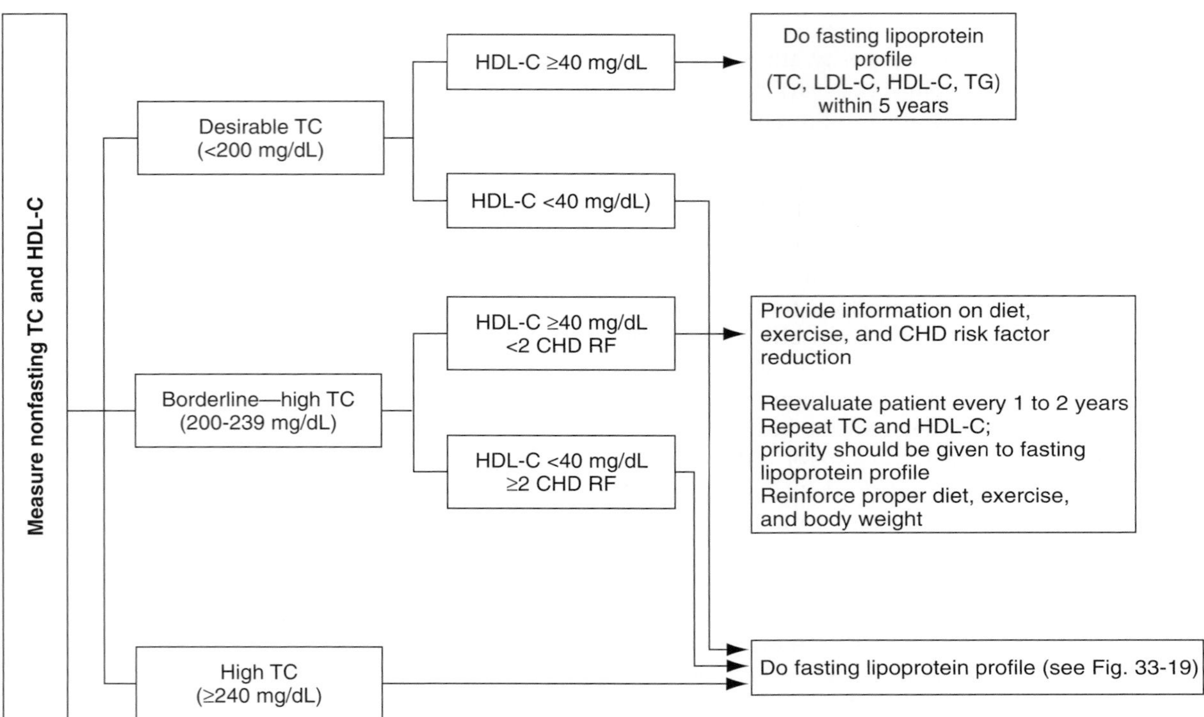

Fig. 37-18 Algorithm of coronary heart disease risk assessment, treatment, and monitoring using the National Cholesterol Education Program (NCEP) Adult Treatment Panel III guidelines[8] for primary prevention in adults with and without evidence of coronary heart disease (CHD). Initial classification of risk is based on nonfasting results of both total cholesterol (TC) and high-density lipoprotein cholesterol (HDL-C) concentrations. *RF,* Risk factor.

shown in Figs. 37-18 and 37-19. For example, for a person with desirable LDL cholesterol (<100 mg/dL), further LDL-lowering therapy is not required. However, emphasis should be placed on controlling other lipid and nonlipid risk factors and on treating the metabolic syndrome, if present. If the patient has CHD (or CHD risk equivalents) and an LDL cholesterol level ≥100 mg/dL, there are three possible approaches:

1. Initiate or intensify TLC—for example, reduction of saturated fat and cholesterol intakes, increased physical activity, weight control—and/or drug therapies specifically designed to lower LDL cholesterol.
2. Emphasize weight reduction and increased physical activity in persons with the metabolic syndrome.
3. Delay the use or intensification of LDL-lowering therapies, and institute treatment for other lipid risk factors (elevated triglycerides; HDL cholesterol <40 mg/dL) or nonlipid risk factors (Tables 37-8 and 37-9).

The therapeutic goal is to lower LDL cholesterol to <100 mg/dL. If the patient has no CHD but has two or more CHD risk factors, intervention should begin if LDL cholesterol is ≥130 mg/dL. The goal for this patient is to lower LDL cholesterol to <130 mg/dL. If the patient has no CHD and has fewer than two risk factors, TLC intervention should not begin until LDL cholesterol is ≥160 mg/dL. The goal for this patient is to lower LDL cholesterol to <160 mg/dL. For secondary prevention of disease in adults with evidence of CHD or other clinical atherosclerotic disease, lipoprotein analyses are required, and LDL cholesterol concentration is the key index for classification of CHD risk and therapy. For secondary prevention, the optimum LDL cholesterol is <100 mg/dL—a far more aggressive goal than that of the primary prevention group. Persons in this category with LDL cholesterol levels >100 mg/dL should undergo appropriate clinical workup and should begin cholesterol-lowering therapy.

It cannot be overemphasized that therapy should always start with dietary intervention to achieve the LDL cholesterol targets described in Tables 37-5 and 37-7. Weight reduction (if appropriate) and physical activity should be part of the intervention process. If elevated LDL cholesterol persists after an appropriate trial of TLC, drug intervention may be considered. The NCEP ATP III report is very specific as to when drug therapy should be used (see Table 37-8). Specifically, with fewer than two risk factors, drug intervention should begin only when LDL cholesterol exceeds 190 mg/dL. If the individual has two or more risk factors, or if the 10-year risk is <10%, drug intervention should be initiated if LDL cholesterol is ≥160 mg/dL; if the 10-year risk is between 10% and 20%, intervention should begin when LDL cholesterol is ≥130 mg/dL. If the person has CHD or a 10-year risk of >20%, drug intervention should begin when LDL cholesterol is ≥130 mg/dL.

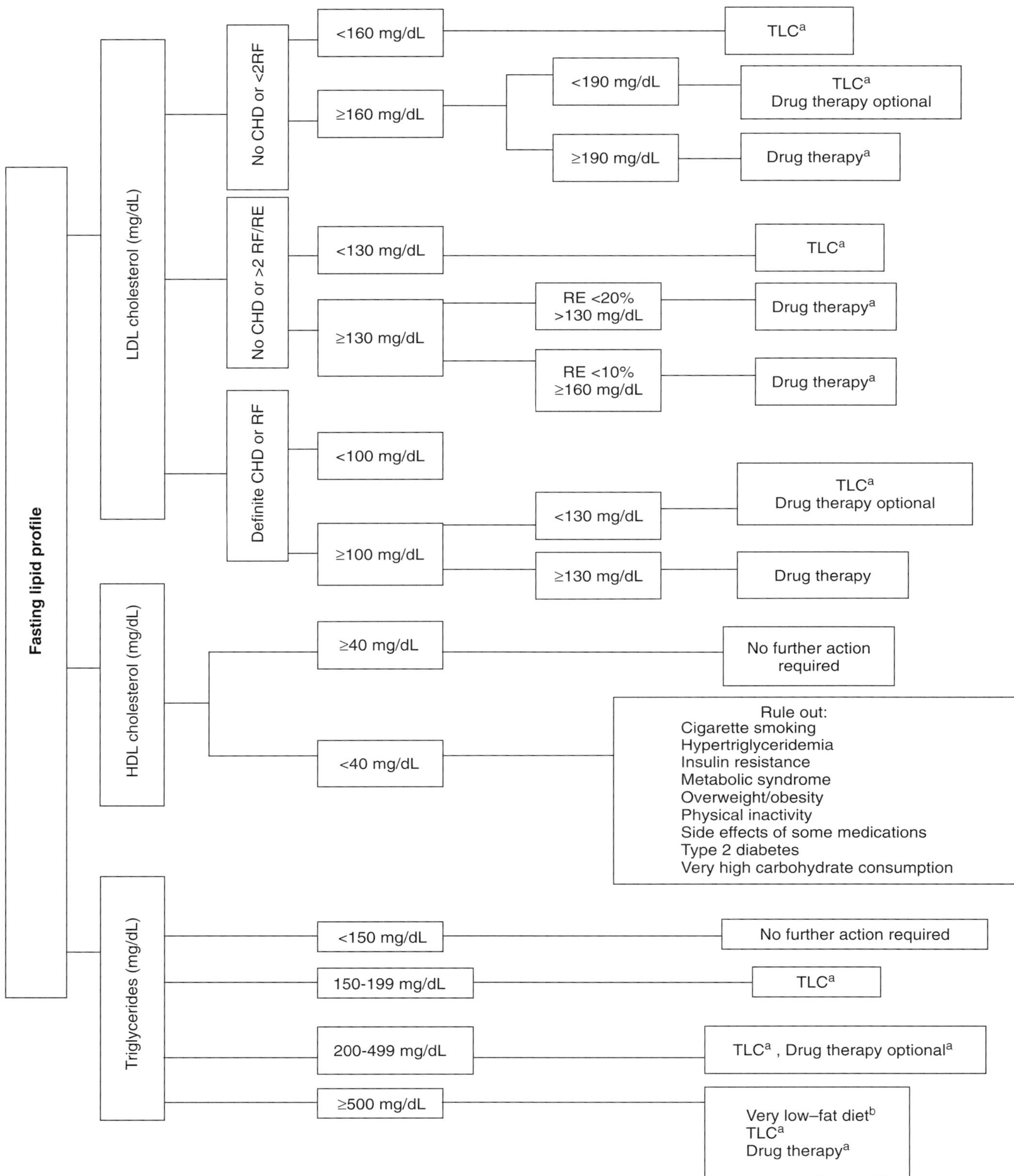

Fig. 37-19 Algorithm of coronary heart disease (CHD) risk assessment, treatment, and monitoring for primary and secondary prevention of CHD in adults with and without evidence of CHD. Classification of risk is based on fasting results on low-density lipoprotein cholesterol (LDL-C), high-density lipoprotein cholesterol (HDL-C), triglyceride (TG) concentrations, and other risk factors. Monitoring of LDL cholesterol response to therapy should be evaluated 6, 12, and 16 to 24 weeks after initiation of therapy. If the initial goal is to reduce the risk for acute pancreatitis, rapid reduction of triglycerides by diet is required; triglyceride monitoring should be done within a few days. *RE,* Risk equivalent; *RF,* risk factor; *TLC,* therapeutic lifestyle changes.

Table 37-8 Three Categories of Risk That Modify LDL Cholesterol Goals

CHD and Risk Factor Status	LDL Cholesterol Decision Level, mg/dL (mmol/L)	Treatment Modality
Without CHD and <2 risk factors	>160 (4.1)	TLC
	>190 (4.9)	Drug optional
Without CHD and >2 risk factors	>130 (3.4)	TLC for 3 months; start drug if LDL is still high
	>160 (4.1)	Drug
With CHD or CHD risk equivalents	>100 (2.6)	TLC
	>130 (3.4)	Drug

From Adult Treatment Panel III: Executive summary of the third report of the National Cholesterol Education Program (NCEP) expert panel on detection, evaluation, and treatment of high blood cholesterol in adults, JAMA 285:2486, 2001.
TLC, Therapeutic lifestyle change.

Table 37-9 Comparison of LDL Cholesterol and Non-HDL Cholesterol Goals for Three Risk Categories

Risk Category	LDL-C Goal, mg/dL	Non–HDL-C Goal, mg/dL
0 to 1 RF	<160	<190
2+ RF and CHD RE ≤20%	<130	<160
CHD and CHD RE >20%	<100	<190

From Adult Treatment Panel III: Executive summary of the third report of the National Cholesterol Education Program (NCEP) expert panel on detection, evaluation, and treatment of high blood cholesterol in adults, JAMA 285:2486, 2001.
RE, Risk equivalent (10-year risk for CHD); *RF,* risk factor.

In young adult men (20 to 35 years old) and premenopausal women (20 to 45 years old) who have LDL cholesterol concentrations ≥130 mg/dL, TLC should be instituted. In contrast to the NCEP ATP II[9] report, which recommended delaying the use of drug therapy, NCEP ATP III[8] guidelines indicate that drugs should be considered when LDL cholesterol reaches or exceeds 190 mg/dL in young men and women. Young men who smoke and have high LDL cholesterol (160 to 189 mg/dL) may be candidates for drug intervention. African Americans have the highest overall CHD mortality rate and the highest out-of-hospital coronary death rates of any ethnic group in the United States, particularly at younger ages. However, the present NCEP ATP III guidelines[8] do not recommend more aggressive strategies for specific racial and ethnic groups.

The NCEP ATP III[8] guidelines consider high triglycerides (or VLDL cholesterol) a risk factor that should be treated. The NCEP ATP III guidelines also regard individuals with the metabolic syndrome as a high-risk group. These persons have a constellation of cardiometabolic risk factors such as abdominal obesity, atherogenic dyslipidemia (elevated triglyceride, small LDL particles, low HDL cholesterol), raised blood pressure, insulin resistance (with or without glucose intolerance), and prothrombotic and proinflammatory states.[48] The absolute CVD risk of the metabolic syndrome, however, is not necessarily higher than that of its individual components. Management of the metabolic syndrome has a twofold objective: (1) to reduce underlying causes (such as obesity and physical inactivity), and (2) to treat associated nonlipid and lipid risk factors.

Table 37-10 National Cholesterol Education Program Recommendations for Triglyceride Classification of Risk

Triglyceride, mg/dL*	Risk
<150	Normal
151 to 199	Borderline high
200 to 499	High
>500	Very high

From Adult Treatment Panel III: Executive summary of the third report of the National Cholesterol Education Program (NCEP) expert panel on detection, evaluation, and treatment of high blood cholesterol in adults, JAMA 285:2486, 2001.
*To convert mg/dL of triglyceride to mmol/L, divide by 88.6.

Changes in the NCEP ATP III guidelines[8] include lowering the normal plasma triglyceride cutoff point from <200 mg/dL to <150 mg/dL (Table 37-10). The treatment strategy for hypertriglyceridemia depends on the cause and severity of the triglyceride elevation.[49] If a patient has borderline-high or high triglycerides, the primary aim is to achieve the target goal for LDL cholesterol. When triglycerides are borderline high (150 to 199 mg/dL), emphasis should be placed on weight reduction and increased physical activity. For high triglycerides (200 to 499 mg/dL), non-HDL cholesterol becomes a secondary target of therapy. The term *non-HDL cholesterol* refers to VLDL, LDL, IDL, and Lp(a) cholesterol. In addition to weight reduction and increased physical activity, lipid-lowering therapy in high-risk persons may be considered, to achieve the non-HDL cholesterol goal.

In rare cases in which triglycerides are very high (>500 mg/dL), treatment may include very-low-fat diets, weight reduction, increased physical activity, and triglyceride-lowering drugs.[49] It should be emphasized that a person's serum or plasma total cholesterol concentration is influenced by many other factors, some of which are controllable and others uncontrollable.

Finally, physicians should remember to differentiate secondary from primary dyslipidemia to avoid misclassifying a patient's CHD risk.[50] Some of the more frequently occurring secondary dyslipidemias are listed in Table 37-3. In these cases, it is imperative that the primary condition leading to secondary hyperlipidemia be treated first.

KEY CONCEPTS BOX 37-7

- Atherosclerosis is a chronic inflammatory process that affects blood vessels.
- Atherosclerotic plaque formation occurs in three progressive stages: (1) the fatty streaks, which gradually develop into raised lesions, called *fatty plaques;* (2) the fibrous plaque, which has a proliferation of smooth muscle cells and a collagen-rich fibrous cap that covers a lipid core lined by foam cells and surrounds an amorphous extracellular accumulation of cholesteryl esters; and (3) the complicated lesion, which can manifest with calcification, hemorrhage, ulceration (rupture), and thrombosis.
- Ruptured plaques are complicit in acute coronary syndromes.
- The goal of the NECP ATP III guidelines is to reduce illness and death from CHD resulting high blood cholesterol in the United States by use of lifestyle changes and drug interventions.

REFERENCES

1. Havel RJ, Kane JP: Introduction: structure and metabolism of plasma lipoproteins. In Scriver CR, Beaudet AL, Sly WS, et al, editors: *The Metabolic and Molecular Bases of Inherited Disease,* ed 8, New York, 2001, McGraw-Hill.
2. Altmann SW, Davis HR Jr, Zhu L, et al: Niemann-Pick C1 like 1 protein is critical for intestinal cholesterol absorption, Science 303:1201, 2004.
3. Huff MW, Pollex RL, Hegele RA: NPC1L1: evolution from pharmacological target to physiological sterol transporter, Arterioscler Thromb Vasc Biol 26:2433, 2006.
4. Lammert F, Wang DQ: New insights into the genetic regulation of intestinal cholesterol absorption, Gastroenterology 129:718, 2005.
5. Burnett JR, Huff MW: Cholesterol absorption inhibitors as a therapeutic option for hypercholesterolaemia, Expert Opin Investig Drugs 15:1337, 2006.
6. Burnett JR, Barrett PHR: Apolipoprotein B metabolism: tracer kinetics, models and metabolic studies, Crit Rev Clin Lab Sci 39:89, 2002.
7. Rader DJ: Molecular regulation of HDL metabolism and function: implications for novel therapies, J Clin Invest 116:3090, 2006.
8. Adult Treatment Panel III: Executive summary of the third report of the National Cholesterol Education Program (NCEP) Expert Panel on Detection, Evaluation, and Treatment of High Blood Cholesterol in Adults, JAMA 285:2486, 2001.
9. Second Expert Panel: Detection, evaluation, and treatment of high blood cholesterol in adults (Adult Treatment Panel II), Circulation 89:1329, 1994.
10. Barter PJ, Rye KA: The rationale for using apoA-I as a clinical marker of cardiovascular risk, J Intern Med 259:447, 2006.
11. Charlton-Menys V, Durrington PN: Apolipoprotein A5 and hypertriglyceridemia, Clin Chem 51:295, 2005.
12. Oii EM, Barrett PHR, Chan DC, et al: Apolipoprotein C-III: understanding an emerging cardiovascular risk factor, Clin Sci (Lond) 114:611, 2008.
13. Mayley RW, Rall SC Jr: Apolipoprotein E: far more than a lipid transport protein, Annu Rev Genomics Hum Med 1:507, 2000.
14. Bennet AM, Di Angelantonio E, Ye Z, et al: Association of apolipoprotein E genotypes with lipid levels and coronary risk, JAMA 298:1300, 2007.
15. Chan DC, Watts GF: Apolipoproteins as markers and managers of coronary risk, QJM 99:277, 2006.
16. Barter PJ, Ballantyne CM, Carmena R, et al: Apo B versus cholesterol in estimating cardiovascular risk and guiding therapy: report of the thirty-person/ten-country panel, J Intern Med 259:247, 2006.
17. Burnett JR, Watts GF: Estimating LDL apoB: informania or clinical advance? Clin Chem 54:782, 2008.
18. Moova R, Rader DJ: Laboratory assessment of HDL heterogeneity and function, Clin Chem 54:788, 2008.
19. Jones GT, van Rij AM, Cole J, et al: Plasma lipoprotein(a) indicates risk for 4 distinct forms of vascular disease, Clin Chem 53:679, 2007.
20. Anuuarad E, Boffa MB, Koschinsky ML, et al: Lipoprotein(a): a unique risk factor for cardiovascular disease, Clin Lab Med 26:751, 2006.
21. Singh IM, Shishehbor MH, Ansell BJ: High-density lipoprotein as a therapeutic target, JAMA 298:786, 2007.
22. Eckel RK, Grundy SM, Zimmet PZ: The metabolic syndrome, Lancet 365:1415, 2005.
23. Grundy SM, Cleeman JI, Daniels SR, et al: Diagnosis and management of the metabolic syndrome: an American Heart Association/National Heart, Lung, and Blood Institute scientific statement, Circulation 112:2735, 2005.
24. Garg A, Simha V: Update on dyslipidemia, J Clin Endocrinol Metab 92:1581, 2007.
25. Merkel M, Eckel RH, Goldberg IJ: Lipoprotein lipase: genetics, lipid uptake, and regulation, J Lipid Res 43:1997, 2002.
26. Rader DJ, Cohen J, Hobbs HH: Monogenic hypercholesterolemia: new insights in pathogenesis and treatment, J Clin Invest 111:1795, 2003.
27. Burnett JR, Hooper AJ: Common and rare gene variants affecting plasma LDL cholesterol, Clin Biochem Rev 29:11, 2008.
28. Watts GF, Lewis B, Sullivan DR: Familial hypercholesterolemia: a missed opportunity in preventive medicine, Nat Clin Pract Cardiovasc Med 4:404, 2007.
29. Soutar AK, Naoumova RP: Mechanisms of disease: genetic causes of familial hypercholesterolemia, Nat Clin Pract Cardiovasc Med 4:214, 2007.
30. Bhatnagar D: Diagnosis and screening for familial hypercholesterolaemia: finding the patients, finding the genes, Ann Clin Biochem 43:441, 2006.
31. Whitfield AJ, Barrett PHR, van Bockxmeer FM, et al: Lipid disorders and mutations in the APOB gene, Clin Chem 50:1725, 2004.
32. Shoulders CC, Jones EL, Naoumova RP: Genetics of familial combined hyperlipidemia and risk of coronary heart disease, Hum Mol Genet 13:R149, 2004.
33. Wierzbicki AS, Graham CA, Young IS, et al: Familial combined hyperlipidemia: under-defined and under-diagnosed? Curr Vasc Pharmacol 6:13, 2008.
34. Naukkarinen J, Ehnholm C, Peltonen L: Genetics of familial combined hyperlipidemia, Curr Opin Lipidol 17:285, 2006.
35. Smelt AH, de Beer F: Apolipoprotein E and familial dysbetalipoproteinemia: clinical, biochemical, and genetic aspects, Semin Vasc Med 4:249, 2004.
36. Hooper AJ, van Bockxmeer FM, Burnett JR: Monogenic hypocholesterolaemic lipid disorders and apolipoprotein B metabolism, Crit Rev Clin Lab Sci 42:515, 2005.
37. Hovingh GK, de Groot E, van der Steeg W, et al: Inherited disorders of HDL metabolism and atherosclerosis, Curr Opin Lipidol 16:139, 2005.
38. Rifai N, Warnick GR, Dominiczak MH, editors: In *Handbook of Lipoprotein Testing,* ed 2, Washington, 2000, AACC Press.
39. McNamara JR, Warnick GR, Cooper GR: A brief history of lipid and lipoprotein measurements and their contribution to clinical chemistry, Clin Chim Acta 369:158, 2006.

40. Libby P, Theroux P: Pathophysiology of coronary artery disease, Circulation 111:3481, 2005.
41. Lloyd-Jones D, Adams R, Carnethon M et al, for the American Heart Association Statistics Committee and Stroke Statistics Subcommittee: Heart disease and stroke statistics—2009 update: a report from the American Heart Association Statistics Committee and Stroke Statistics Subcommittee, Circulation 119:e1, 2009.
42. Libby P: The vascular biology of atherosclerosis. In Zipes DP, Libby P, Bonow RO, et al, editors: *Braunwald's Heart Disease: A Textbook of Cardiovascular Medicine,* ed 7, Philadelphia, 2005, Elsevier Saunders.
43. Ridker PM, Libby P: Risk factors for atherothrombotic disease. In Zipes DP, Libby P, Bonow RO, et al, editors: *Braunwald's Heart Disease: A Textbook of Cardiovascular Medicine,* ed 7, Philadelphia, 2005, Elsevier Saunders.
44. Libby P: Atherosclerosis: disease biology affecting the coronary vasculature, Am J Cardiol 98:3Q, 2007.
45. Packard RR, Libby P: Inflammation in atherosclerosis: from vascular biology to biomarker discovery and risk prediction, Clin Chem 54:24, 2008.
46. Grundy SM, Cleeman JI, Bairey Merz N, et al, for the Coordinating Committee of the National Cholesterol Education Program: Implications of recent clinical trials for the National Cholesterol Education Program Adult Treatment Panel III guidelines, Circulation 110:227, 2004.
47. American Academy of Pediatrics. National Cholesterol Education Program: Report of the Expert Panel on Blood Cholesterol Levels in Children and Adolescents. Pediatrics 89:525, 1992.
48. Qiao Q, Gao W, Zhang L, et al: Metabolic syndrome and cardiovascular disease, Ann Clin Biochem 44:232, 2007.
49. Brunzell JD: Clinical practice: hypertriglyceridemia, N Engl J Med 357:1009, 2007.
50. Durrington PN, editor: In *Hyperlipidaemia: Diagnosis & Management,* ed 3, UK, 2007, Hodder Arnold.

INTERNET SITES

General

www.chestx-ray.com/Coronary/CorCalc.html
www.webmd.com/cholesterol-management/default.htm
www.webmd.com/heart-disease/default.htm
www.familydoctor.org/handouts/239.html
www.lipidsonline.org
www.theheart.org
www.cvspectrum.org
www.ccmdweb.org
www.incirculation.net

Biochemistry of Lipids and Lipoproteins

www.themedicalbiochemistrypage.org/cholesterol.html
www.lipidsonline.org/slides/slide01.cfm?tk=10
www.themedicalbiochemistrypage.org/lipoproteins.html

Diagnosis and Treatment/Adult Treatment Panel/National Institutes of Health Sites

www.nhlbi.nih.gov/guidelines/cholesterol
www.nhlbi.nih.gov/guidelines/cholesterol/atp_iii.htm
www.nhlbi.nih.gov/guidelines/cholesterol/atp3upd04.htm

Atherosclerosis

www.americanheart.org
www.athero.org
www.nhlbi.nih.gov
www.nlm.nih.gov/medlineplus/coronarydisease.html

Diabetes Mellitus

Richard F. Dods

38 Chapter

Chapter Outline

Key Terms

acromegaly Growth hormone excess in adults, characterized by enlargement of features such as the head, hands, and feet.

adenosine 3′,5′-cyclic monophosphate (cAMP) An organic molecule that is obligatory for the action of enzymes such as protein kinases

aerobic glycolysis Glycolysis that is linked to the tricarboxylic acid cycle by the presence of oxygen; aerobic glycolysis produces 36 moles of ATP per mole of glucose.

anaerobic glycolysis Glycolysis that occurs in the absence of oxygen; in this case, glycolysis is not linked to the tricarboxylic acid cycle, and only 2 moles of ATP are produced per mole of glucose.

angiogenesis A complication of diabetes mellitus; abnormal proliferation of blood vessels in a tissue such as the eye lens.

angiopathy A complication of diabetes mellitus that manifests as damage to the basement membranes of blood vessels.

anoxia Lack of oxygen.

atherogenic dyslipidemia Refers to blood fat disorders that promote fatty deposits along arterial walls.

basement membrane A layer of noncellular material that underlies the epithelium.

diabetic ketoacidosis A complication of diabetes mellitus that is characterized by hyperglycemia, hyperosmolarity, low pH, ketonuria and ketonemia, and lethargy or coma.

disaccharide Two monosaccharides linked by a glycosidic bond.

electron transport chain A series of molecules that transfer electrons from NADH and $FADH_2$ to oxygen.

gestational diabetes Glucose intolerance that occurs in some pregnancies.

glucagon A hormone produced by the α-cells of the pancreas; glucagon is involved primarily in energy release.

glucagonoma A tumor that produces excessive serum glucagon levels.

gluconeogenesis Production of glucose from pyruvic acid.

glucose A six-carbon polyhydroxyl aldehyde; primary source of energy in living organisms

glucosuria Excessive quantities of urinary glucose.

glycation Reaction in which a sugar such as glucose binds covalently to protein.

glycogen Highly branched high-molecular-weight polysaccharide composed only of glucose units.

glycogenesis Formation of glycogen from glucose-6-phosphate.

glycolysis Metabolism of glucose-6-phosphate to pyruvic acid or lactic acid.

growth hormone Hormone produced by the anterior part of the pituitary; also called *somatotropin.* Raises blood glucose.

hexose monophosphate shunt Metabolic pathway in which glucose-6-phosphate is metabolized to ribose and carbon dioxide.

histocompatibility antigen (human lymphocyte antigen, HLA) Proteins responsible for rejection of tissue transplanted to an individual from another unrelated individual. Specific HLAs are present at a high frequency in persons who develop certain diseases.

hyperglycemia High blood glucose concentrations.

hyperglycemic hyperosmolar nonketotic coma (HHNC) A complication of diabetes mellitus that is characterized by hyperglycemia, hyperosmolarity, normal keto acid levels, and lethargy or coma.

impaired glucose tolerance (IGT, also called *pre-diabetes*) Abnormal oral glucose tolerance test without elevated fasting blood glucose.

incretins Hormones secreted from the intestinal mucosa upon ingestion of carbohydrates. They result in the release of insulin at a quantity greater than the effect of absorbed glucose alone.

islet cell antibodies (ICA) Antibodies frequently found in patients with type 1 diabetes that are suggestive of an autoimmune cause.

islets of Langerhans Group of cells in the pancreas composed of α-cells, which secrete glucagon; β-cells, which secrete insulin; and δ-cells, which secrete somatostatin.

ketonemia Excess of ketones and derived keto acids in the blood.

ketonuria Excess of ketones and derived keto acids in the urine.

lactic acidosis Acidosis (low blood pH) caused by excess lactic acid.

lipolysis Hydrolysis of triglycerides to free fatty acids and glycerol.

metabolic syndrome A cluster of risk factors found in an individual that increase the likelihood of cardiovascular disease and diabetes.

monosaccharide A polyhydroxyl aldehyde or ketone, such as glucose, fructose, or mannose.

nephropathy A complication of diabetes mellitus characterized by damage to capillaries associated with the glomerulus.

neuropathy The most common complication of diabetes mellitus; refers to reduced motor and sensory nerve conduction velocities caused by axonal degeneration and demyelination.

oral glucose tolerance test (OGTT) Measure of ability to clear glucose from the blood after an oral glucose challenge.

oxidative phosphorylation The process that links the tricarboxylic acid cycle with ATP formation.

polydipsia Excessive thirst; a symptom of diabetes mellitus.

polyphagia Constant hunger; a symptom of diabetes mellitus.

polysaccharide A carbohydrate composed of more than two monosaccharides linked by glycosidic bonds.

polyuria Excessive urinary output; a symptom of diabetes mellitus.

pre-diabetes *See* impaired glucose tolerance.

preproinsulin Precursor to proinsulin.

proinsulin Precursor to insulin.

protein kinases Enzymes that phosphorylate other proteins.

prothrombotic state Refers to elevated fibrinogen and plasminogen activator inhibitor-1.

receptor sites Sites on or in cells where hormones are bound. Hormone binding to the receptor site is the initial step for hormone action.

retinopathy A complication of diabetes mellitus; a disorder of the retina that occurs in diabetes and is characterized by cataract formation or proliferation of small blood vessels (angiogenesis).

somatostatin A hormone produced in the δ-cells of the pancreas; inhibits insulin and glucagon secretion.

somatostatinoma A tumor that produces excessive quantities of somatostatin, resulting in hyperglycemia.

thyroxine A hormone produced by the thyroid gland that increases blood glucose levels.

tricarboxylic acid cycle Metabolic pathway that converts glucose-6-phosphate via pyruvic acid to CO_2 and water. When coupled to oxidative phosphorylation, adenosine triphosphate is formed.

uronic acid pathway Converts glucose-6-phosphate to glucuronic acid.

Methods on Evolve

Albumin in urine
Anion gap
Blood gas analysis and oxygen saturation
Glucose
Glycated hemoglobin
Insulin and C-peptide
Ketones
Lactic acid
Osmolality
Sodium and potassium
Triglycerides
Urea
Urine protein, total

SECTION OBJECTIVES BOX 38-1

- Describe the prevalence and incidence of DM in the American population.
- List its common symptoms.

DIABETES

The prevalence of diabetes has increased from 5.6 million in the 1980s to epidemic numbers of 15.8 million in 2005[1]—an incidence of approximately 7.2%.[2,3] The National Health and Nutrition Examination Survey (NHANES) estimates that in 2005, an additional 6.2 million cases of diabetes remained undiagnosed.[4-6] Persons aged 65 years or older account for 38% of the population with diabetes. Data from 2004 indicate that the number of newly diagnosed diabetes cases among adults aged 18 to 79 years was 1.4 million in that year alone. Before 1999, rates of newly diagnosed diabetes were equal by gender; from 1999, the prevalence for males began to increase at a rate faster than that for females. Race-based differences are significant. Data from 2005 indicate that Hispanic males are 1.3 times, Hispanic females 1.4 times, black males 1.5 times, and black females 1.8 times as likely to have diagnosed diabetes as whites of similar age.[1] American Indians and Alaskan Natives are 2.2 times, Pacific Islanders 2 times, and Californian Asians 1.5 times as likely to have diagnosed diabetes as whites of a similar age. Diabetes was the sixth leading cause of death in the United States according to data compiled in 2005.[6] This figure is likely to be understated because complications of diabetes such as heart disease and stroke often are listed as the primary cause of death. The diabetes epidemic is not limited to the United States. In 2006, the World Health Organization (WHO) estimated that in excess of 180 million people worldwide have diabetes, and that this number will double by 2030. In 2005, WHO estimated that 2.9 million people died from diabetes, including persons who died from diabetic complications such as heart disease or kidney failure. This figure could increase by at least 50% by 2017.[7]

The health implications of diabetes include its direct effects and its long-term complications, including coronary heart disease and cerebrovascular disease (stroke). A person with diabetes has a twofold greater risk of suffering a myocardial infarction than does a nondiabetic person of the same age and sex. Insulin resistance or glucose intolerance is a component of a cluster of metabolic risk factors found in individuals who are prone to cardiovascular disease. This cluster also includes obesity (especially weight gain in the abdominal region), atherogenic dyslipidemia, hypertension, elevated fibrinogen or plasminogen activator inhibitor-1 (the **prothrombotic state**), and an inflammatory state as indicated by elevated C-reactive protein. This widely prevalent condition is called the **metabolic syndrome.** (See also Chapter 37.)[8-10]

Diabetes mellitus (DM) is not a single disease but an array of diseases that exhibit a common symptom—inability of the individual to regulate glucose levels (glucose intolerance). The primary symptoms of DM are abnormally high blood and urine glucose levels (**hyperglycemia and glucosuria,** respectively), **polyuria,** excessive thirst (**polydipsia**), constant hunger (**polyphagia**), sudden weight loss, and, during acute episodes of DM, excessive blood and urinary ketones (**ketonemia** and **ketonuria**, respectively). All these symptoms are the result of an inability to regulate glucose metabolism and are the consequences of high glucose levels.

KEY CONCEPTS BOX 38-1

- DM is a widespread disease that is reaching epidemic proportions in the United States and the world.
- It is found in a cluster of conditions collectively called the *metabolic syndrome.* The metabolic syndrome includes dyslipidemia, hypertension, the prothrombotic state, the inflammatory state, and DM.
- The primary symptoms of DM include abnormally high blood and urine glucose levels, polyuria, excessive thirst, constant hunger, sudden weight loss, and, during acute episodes of DM, excessive blood and urinary ketones.

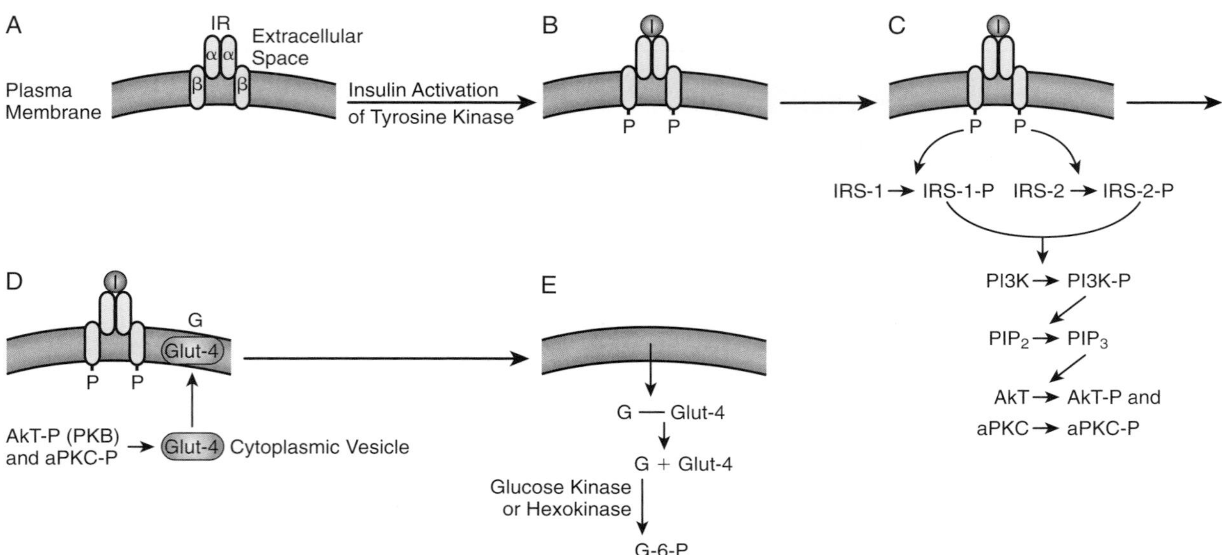

Fig. 38-1 *A* through *E,* The insulin signaling pathway. Insulin binds to the α-unit of the insulin receptor, thus beginning a cascade of phosphorylations that leads to the transport of glucose transporter protein-4 (GLUT-4) from vesicles in the cytoplasm to the plasma membrane. GLUT-4 binds with glucose and transports it to the cytoplasm, where it is phosphorylated to form glucose 6-phosphate. See text for details.

SECTION OBJECTIVES BOX 38-2

- Describe normal glucose homeostasis.
- Describe the role that incretins have in glucose metabolism.
- Describe the effects that hormones other than insulin have on glucose levels.
- Explain the difference between glucose metabolism in a normal individual versus that in a person with diabetes.

GLUCOSE: PROPERTIES AND METABOLISM

Definition

Carbohydrates are defined as polyhydroxyl aldehydes (aldoses) and ketones (ketoses). Simple carbohydrates such as **glucose** are also called **monosaccharides.** Two monosaccharides linked by a bond called a *glycosidic bond* form a **disaccharide.** More than two monosaccharides linked by glycosidic bonds form a **polysaccharide.** Dietary carbohydrates consist of monosaccharides such as glucose, fructose, and galactose; disaccharides such as sucrose, lactose, and maltose; and polysaccharides such as starch. Intestinal enzymes convert disaccharides and polysaccharides to monosaccharides (see pp. 665-666).

Function

The principal biochemical function of glucose is to provide energy for life processes. Adenosine triphosphate (ATP) is the universal energy source for biological reactions. Glucose oxidation by the glycolytic and tricarboxylic acid pathways is the primary source of energy for the biosynthesis of ATP.

Insulin Signaling Pathway

The initial event in glucose metabolism is the transport of glucose across the cell plasma membrane, facilitated by the hormone insulin. As is shown in Fig. 38-1, *A*, insulin receptors are located in the plasma membranes of such cells as **hepatocytes** and **adipocytes.** The insulin receptor (IR) consists of two α-subunits and two β-subunits that are linked by disulfide bonds. When insulin binds to the α-subunit of the IR, a signal is transmitted across the cell membrane, resulting in the activation of tyrosine kinase, which resides on the β-subunit. Tyrosine kinase phosphorylates tyrosine residues on adjacent β-subunits (Fig. 38-1, *B*), initiating a cascade of events that leads to glucose transport across the cell membrane. The following events in the insulin signaling pathway occur in the cytoplasm. As can be seen in Fig. 38-1, *C*, activated IR phosphorylates several tyrosine proteins, including insulin receptor substrates 1 and 2 (IRS-1, IRS-2). Activated IRS-1 phosphorylates type A phosphatidyl inositol 3-kinase (PI3K),[11] which phosphorylates phosphatidyl inositol biphosphate (PIP2) to produce phosphatidyl inositol triphosphate (PIP3). PIP3 activates atypical protein kinase C (aPKC) and protein kinase B (PKB; also called serine/threonine kinase [AkT]; Fig. 38-1, *C* and *D*).[12] Activated aPKC and PKB induce the translocation of glucose transporter 4 (GLUT-4) from vesicles in the cytoplasm to the plasma membrane, where it complexes with glucose. The GLUT-4:glucose complex then travels from the cell membrane into the cytoplasm,[13] where glucose is phosphorylated by glucokinase to glucose 6-phosphate (Fig. 38-1, *E*).

Principal Glucose Metabolic Pathways

Within the cell, glucose is rapidly converted to glucose-6-phosphate (G6P), a major intermediate in glucose metabolism.

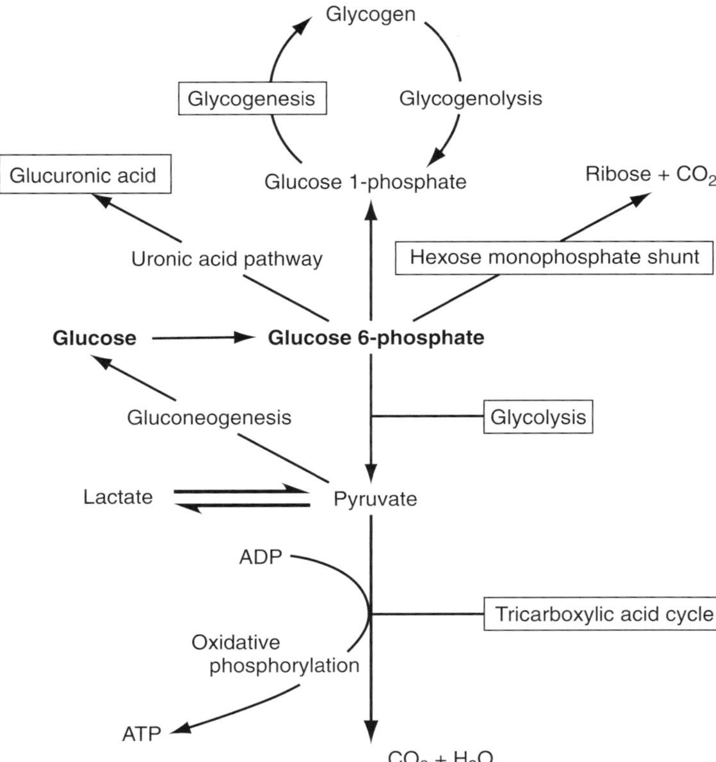

Fig. 38-2 The five principal pathways of glucose metabolism: glycolysis, tricarboxylic acid pathway, glycogenesis, hexose monophosphate shunt, and the uronic acid pathway.

The enzyme that catalyzes the phosphorylation of glucose by ATP is hexokinase (or glucokinase in the liver and β-cells of the pancreas). Glucokinase may play a key role in the regulation of glucose homeostasis by maintaining a gradient for glucose transport in hepatocytes.[14] As is shown in Fig. 38-2, glucose-6-phosphate serves as a starting point for four metabolic pathways. Glucose-6-phosphate is converted by **glycolysis** to pyruvate, a substance that is metabolized further by the tricarboxylic acid pathway to carbon dioxide and water. Glucose-6-phosphate is also oxidized by the **hexose monophosphate shunt** to ribose and carbon dioxide, converted by the **uronic acid pathway** to glucuronic acid, and incorporated into **glycogen** by **glycogenesis.**

Aerobic Glycolysis

Glycolysis

Glucose-6-phosphate metabolism by the glycolytic pathway (also called the Embden-Meyerhof pathway) results in the formation of ATP (Fig. 38-3). Glycolysis converts the six-carbon glucose molecule to two molecules of a three-carbon compound called *pyruvic acid.* This process produces 2 mol of ATP per mole of glucose. An important aspect of glycolysis is the formation of pyruvic acid. In **aerobic glycolysis,** pyruvate is metabolized further by means of the tricarboxylic acid cycle.

Tricarboxylic Acid Cycle

Pyruvic acid enters the **tricarboxylic acid cycle** (citric acid cycle, Krebs cycle), where it is metabolized to carbon dioxide and water. Fig. 38-4 shows the intermediate steps in the tricarboxylic acid cycle and the steps that are used to reduce nicotinamide adenine dinucleotide (NAD) and flavin adenine dinucleotide (FAD) to their corresponding analogs, NADH and FADH2. The tricarboxylic acid cycle does not directly produce ATP, but ATP is produced by the oxidation of NADH and FADH2.

Electron Transport Chain (Oxidative Phosphorylation)

Electron transport is a complex process that takes place in the mitochondria, and that involves electron transfer from NADH and FADH2 to a series of compounds, ending with the reduction of oxygen to yield a water molecule. **Oxidative phosphorylation** involves the phosphorylation of ADP by inorganic phosphate to form ATP; the energy for this reaction is produced by the flow of electrons through the **electron transport chain.** Thus it is the reoxidation of NADH and FADH2—compounds produced by the tricarboxylic acid cycle—that produces ATP. In contrast to glycolysis, which produces 2 mol of ATP per mole of glucose, the tricarboxylic acid cycle linked with oxidative phosphorylation produces 36 mol of ATP per mole of glucose. The oxidative and ATP synthesis processes are tightly coupled because the availability of adenosine diphosphate (ADP) controls the rate of oxidation, and oxygen availability regulates phosphorylation.

Anaerobic Glycolysis

In fatigued muscle, where there is a deficiency of oxygen, or **anoxia,** the above pathways cannot further metabolize glucose converted by glycolysis to pyruvic acid. Instead (see Fig. 38-3), pyruvate is converted by the enzyme lactate dehydrogenase to lactate. This is called **anaerobic glycolysis.** In contrast to aerobic glycolysis, only 2 mol of ATP per mole of glucose is produced by anaerobic glycolysis. Lactic acid produced by anoxic tissue is carried by the circulation to the liver, where it is reconverted to glucose in a process called **gluconeogenesis** (see the following text).

Alternate Energy Sources

As is indicated in Fig. 38-4, amino acids and fatty acids also enter the tricarboxylic acid cycle to produce ATP and therefore are alternative sources of energy.

Glycogenesis, Glycogenolysis, and Gluconeogenesis

Glycogen

Excess glucose is stored in cells as the polymer glycogen for later energy demands. Glycogen (Fig. 38-5) is a high-molecular-weight polysaccharide composed entirely of glucose units in 1,4-glycosidic bonds with 1,6-branches occurring approximately every 10 units. Glycogen is located in the cytoplasm of liver and muscle cells in granules that contain the enzymes involved in the synthesis (glycogenesis) and

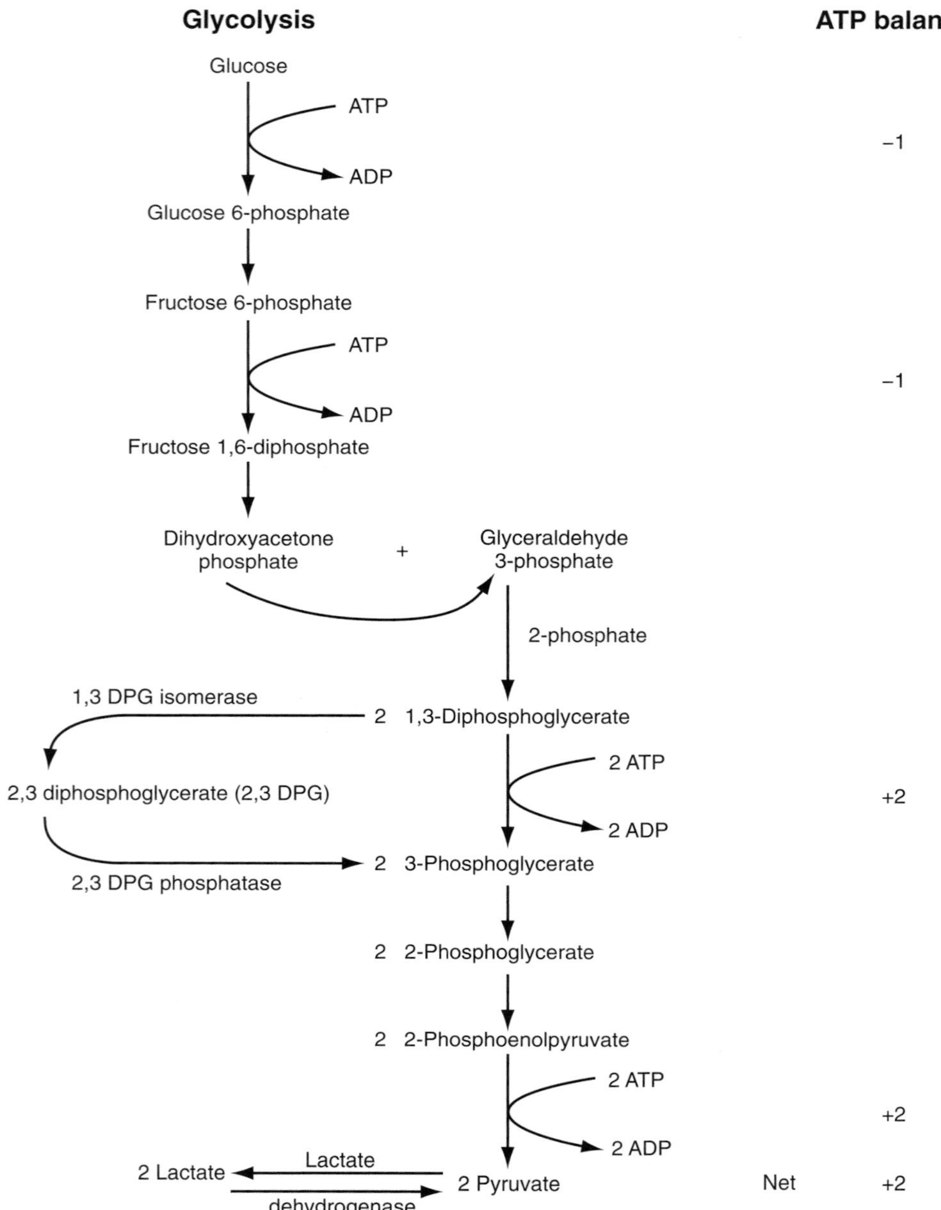

Fig. 38-3 Two stages of glycolysis. First stage proceeds from glucose to formation of 1,3-diphosphoglycerate and consumes 2 mol of adenosine triphosphate (ATP). Second stage proceeds from 1,3-diphosphoglycerate to pyruvate and produces 4 mol of ATP. Glycolysis therefore results in net gain of 2 mol of ATP per mole of glucose. The synthesis of 2,3-DPG by the Rapoport-Luebring cycle is important for the regulation of oxygen transport.

hydrolysis (glycogenolysis) of glycogen. Refer again to Fig. 38-2 to see how glucogenesis and glycogenolysis fit into the overall scheme of glucose metabolism. Fig. 38-6 presents a simplified representation of glycogenesis and glycogenolysis.

Glycogenesis

The first step in glycogenesis is conversion of glucose-6-phosphate to glucose-1-phosphate (see Fig. 38-6). The reaction of glucose-1-phosphate with uridine-5′-triphosphate produces uridine diphosphate glucose, a substance that reacts with a preexisting glycogen molecule to form 1,4-glycosidic linkages. Synthesis of 1,4-glycosidic bonds is catalyzed by the enzyme glycogen synthetase. Glycogen synthetase exists in two forms: the phosphorylated, inactive enzyme form and the dephosphorylated, active enzyme form. Phosphorylation of the active enzyme is accomplished by any of several enzymes of the protein kinase class. **Protein kinases** are activated by low levels of **adenosine 3′,5′-cyclic monophosphate (cAMP).** Thus glycogen synthetase activity—and thereby glycogenesis—is regulated by intracellular cAMP levels. Glycogenesis is enhanced by low cAMP levels and is inhibited by high cAMP

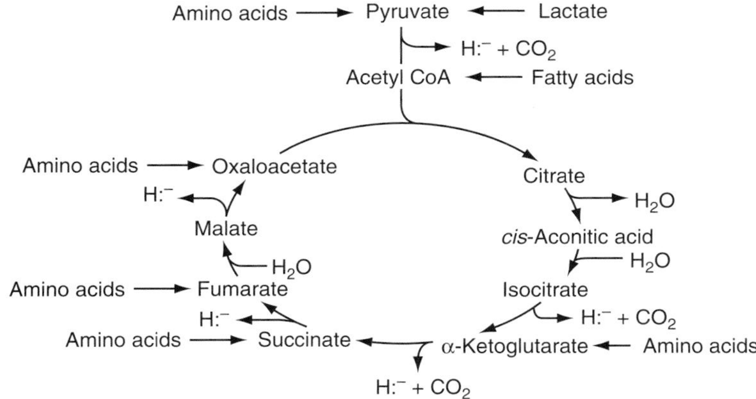

Fig. 38-4 Tricarboxylic acid cycle produces CO_2 and water from pyruvate, fatty acids, and amino acids, which enter the cycle at the points indicated. Hydride ions (H^-) are produced and used in the oxidative phosphorylation process to produce adenosine triphosphate (ATP) from adenosine diphosphate (ADP) and inorganic phosphate.

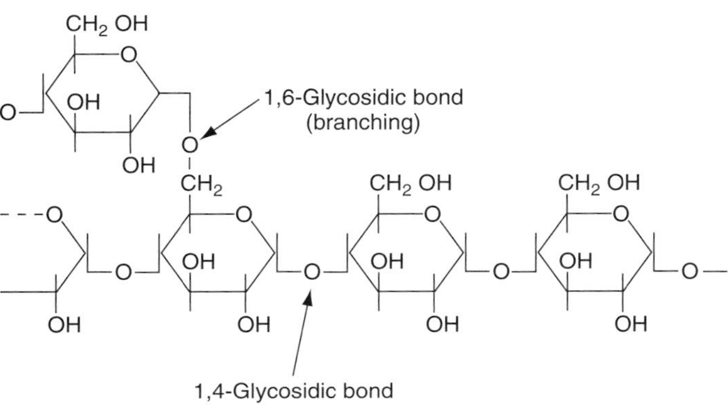

Fig. 38-5 Glycogen is a 1 to 4 million Dalton polysaccharide composed of glucose units in 1,4- and 1,6-glycosidic linkage. The 1,6-bonds produce branches at intervals of approximately 10 glucose units.

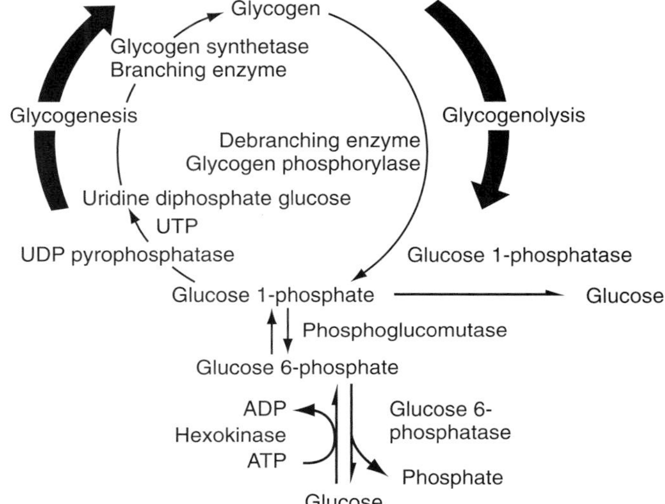

Fig. 38-6 Glycogen, the storage molecule for glucose, is synthesized from glucose-1-phosphate through a process called *glycogenesis (left side).* Glycogenolysis releases glucose units from glycogen. Debranching is the first step in glycogenolysis *(right side).*

levels; cAMP levels in turn are regulated by insulin, which causes decreased cAMP levels.

Branching of glycogen is accomplished by an enzyme called a *branching enzyme.* This branching enzyme hydrolyzes the 1,4-glycosidic bond of glycogen to form five to six glucose unit fragments, which are reattached to the glycogen molecule through 1,6-glycosidic bonds.

Glycogenolysis

Although glycogenolysis (see Fig. 38-6) is the opposite of glycogenesis, it does not occur through a simple reversal of each step of glycogenesis but by a unique enzyme system. The debranching enzyme splits off trisaccharides from branches and reattaches them by 1,4-glycosidic bonds to the ends of the glycogen molecule. Glycogen phosphorylase hydrolyzes the 1,4-glycosidic bond, producing glucose-1-phosphate:

$$\underset{\textbf{(n residues)}}{\text{Glycogen}} + \text{Pi}_1 \rightarrow \underset{\textbf{(n -1 residues)}}{\text{Glycogen}} + \text{Glucose-1-phosphate} \quad \text{Eq. 38-1}$$

Similar to glycogen synthetase, glycogen phosphorylase exists in two forms. The active form, called *phosphorylase a,* is a tetramer. The inactive form, *phosphorylase b,* is a dimer. The active tetramer is formed in three steps: phosphorylation of the dimer by a protein kinase called *phosphorylase kinase,* followed by binding of the phosphorylated dimer with another phosphorylated dimer, then the third and final step in the activation process—the binding of one molecule of pyridoxal phosphate to each subunit of the tetramer. Phosphorylase kinase is activated by cAMP. Note that high cellular cAMP levels favor glycogenolysis over glycogenesis. The activation of glycogen phosphorylase is under hormonal control (see later discussion).

Gluconeogenesis

The steps in gluconeogenesis are shown in Fig. 38-7. Gluconeogenesis produces glucose-6-phosphate from most amino acids (glucogenic amino acids), fatty acids, glycerol, and lactate. Pyruvate is an important intermediary in gluconeogenesis (see Fig. 38-7), because it can be formed directly from lactate oxidation (by lactate dehydrogenase) and from the amino acid alanine (via transamination by alanine transaminase). Glycerol, which is derived from hydrolysis of triglyceride **(lipolysis),** enters the gluconeogenic pathway

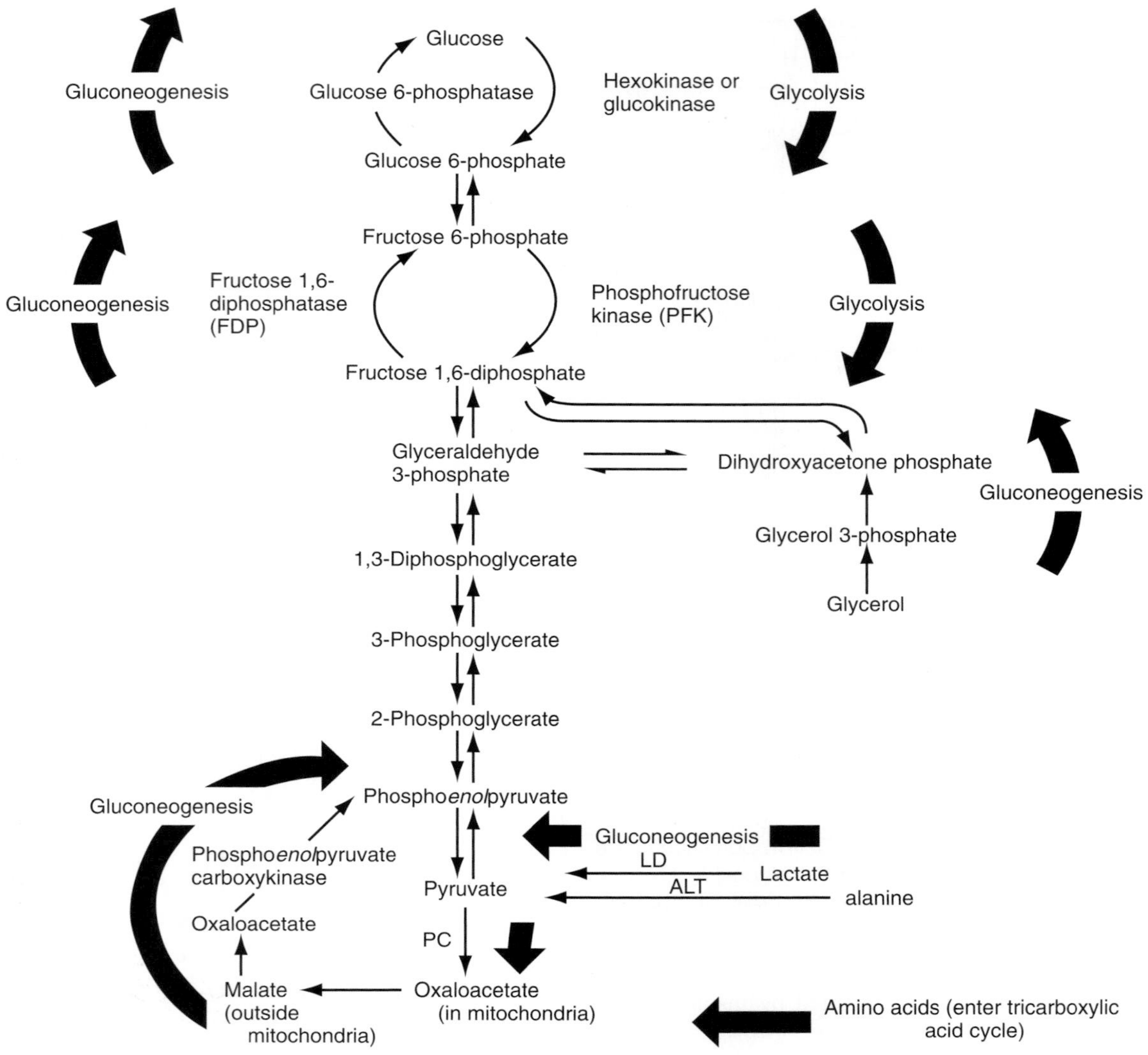

Fig. 38-7 Pathways involved in gluconeogenesis from amino acids, fatty acids, glycerol, and lactate. This pathway shares many of the enzymes of glycolytic and tricarboxylic acid pathways. Gluconeogenesis provides glucose whenever scarcity of glucose occurs, and whenever lactate accumulates. *ALT,* Alanine transaminase; *LD,* lactate dehydrogenase; *PC,* pyruvate carboxylase.

after pyruvate as glycerol-3-phosphate. These three substances—lactate, alanine, and glycerol—are the primary precursors for glucose synthesis. Gluconeogenesis is not a simple reversal of glycolysis, although gluconeogenesis does share some of the enzymes of the glycolytic pathway. Glucose is formed only in liver and kidney, which have the enzyme glucose-6-phosphatase, which hydrolyzes G6P to glucose. In fact, the liver is the major nondietary source of serum glucose and is critical for maintaining blood glucose levels.

Hormone Regulation of Glucose Metabolism

The system for regulating blood glucose levels is designed to achieve two ends. The first is to store glucose in excess of the body's immediate needs in a compact reservoir (glycogen), and the second is to mobilize stored glucose to maintain the blood glucose level. The regulation of blood glucose is essential for keeping the brain, whose primary energy source is glucose, supplied with a constant amount of glucose. The role of insulin is to shift excess extracellular glucose to intracellular storage sites in the form of macromolecules (such as glycogen, fats, and proteins). Thus glucose is stored away in times of plenty for times of need.

In response to low blood glucose, as in periods of fasting, a series of hyperglycemic agents acts on intermediary metabolic pathways to form glucose from storage macromolecules. Thus proteins and glycogen are metabolized to form glucose-6-phosphate (gluconeogenesis), which, in the liver, is hydrolyzed to glucose and released into the blood to maintain blood glucose levels.

The most important hyperglycemic agents are **glucagon,** epinephrine, cortisol, **thyroxine, growth hormone,** and certain intestinal hormones. The behavior of each of these agents in regulating blood glucose is different; whereas insulin promotes anabolic metabolism (synthesis of macromolecules), these hormones in part induce catabolic metabolism to break down large molecules.[15]

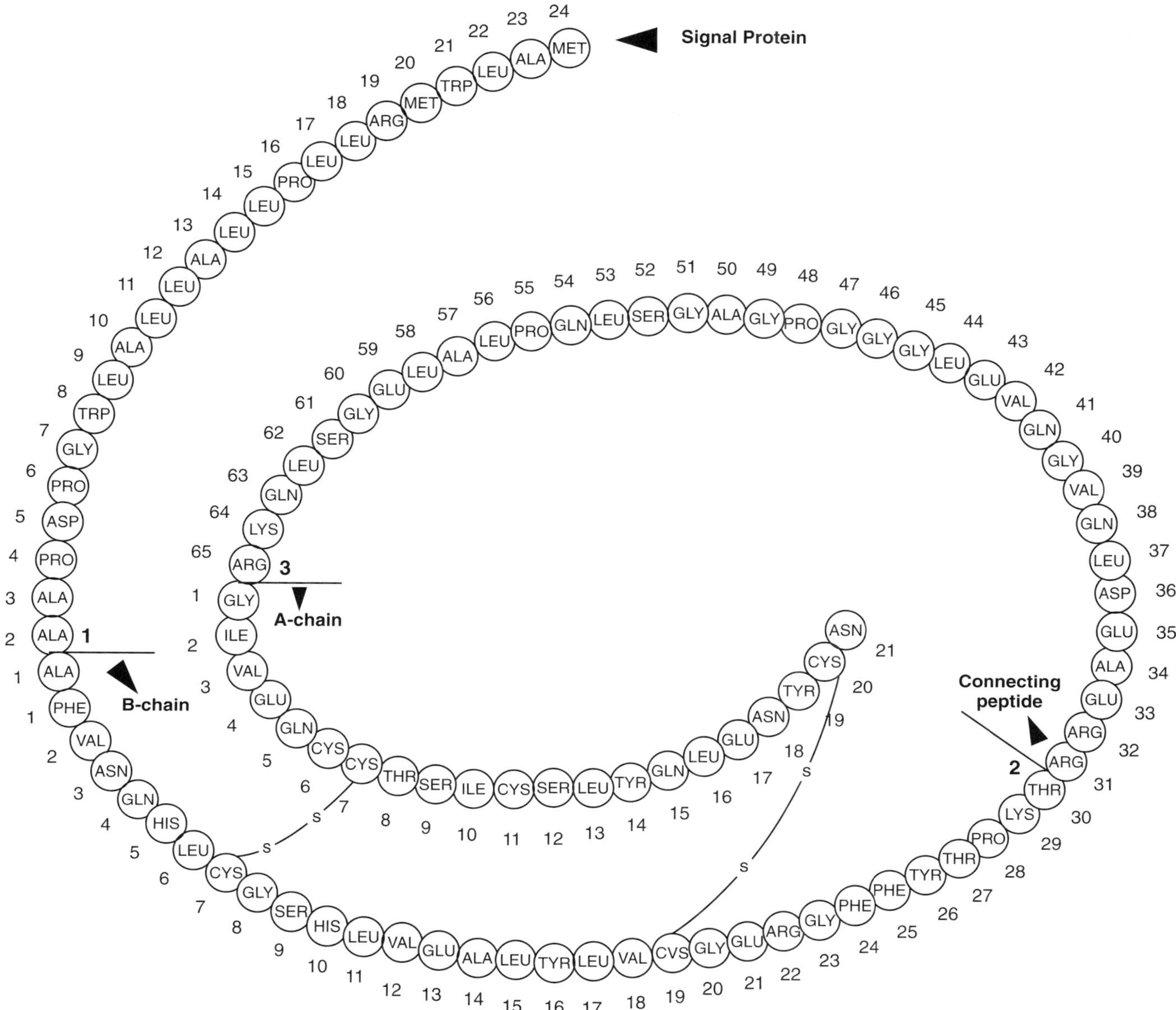

Fig. 38-8 Amino acid sequence of human preproinsulin. The series of enzymatic cleavages of preproinsulin (site 1) to proinsulin and of proinsulin (sites 2 and 3) to insulin are described in text.

Insulin

Insulin is synthesized in the endocrine pancreas by the β-cells of the **islets of Langerhans** as a high-molecular-weight precursor called **preproinsulin** (11,500 D).[16] As can be seen in Fig. 38-8, cleavage at the link marked by the line labeled *1* results in the formation of **proinsulin** (9000 D). Proinsulin has only 5% of the activity of insulin. The proinsulin molecule consists of the A and B chains of insulin connected by disulfide bonds and by a connective peptide called *C-peptide.* During processing, the C-peptide (3000 D) is removed from the molecule by cleavage at the links marked by lines 2 and 3. The resulting insulin molecule (6000 D) consists of chains A and B connected by two disulfide bonds. This entire process occurs within the β-cell. The initial synthesis of preproinsulin occurs at the Golgi apparatus. The molecule is packaged in a vesicle called a *β-granule,* where it is cleaved first to proinsulin and then to insulin. Equal quantities of C-peptide and insulin are released into the circulation when the granule is dissolved at the plasma membrane of the β-cell after neural, dietary, or hormonal stimulation. Only small quantities of proinsulin are found in the circulation.

Glucagon and Cortisol

Glucagon is a 3500 D polypeptide hormone that is synthesized in the α-cells of the pancreas.[17] In DM, because of insulin deficiency, glucagon levels are elevated and are not suppressed by carbohydrate loading. Cortisol[18] and the other adrenal corticosteroids increase the rate of gluconeogenesis from protein and amino acids, especially in the liver. Insulin and glucagon have opposing effects. Insulin inhibits proteolysis, lipolysis, gluconeogenesis, and glycogenolysis and stimulates lipid synthesis and glycogenesis in the liver; increases protein synthesis in muscle; and accelerates triglyceride synthesis in fat cells (Table 38-1). Insulin acts as the body's only hypoglycemic

Table 38-1 Metabolic Action of Insulin

	TISSUE		
	Liver	**Adipose**	**Muscle**
Inhibits	Glycogenolysis Gluconeogenesis Ketogenesis	Lipolysis	Protein breakdown Amino acid release
Stimulates	Glycogen and fatty acid synthesis	Glycerol and fatty acid synthesis	Glucose uptake and metabolism Amino acid uptake Synthesis of protein Glycogenesis

agent. In contrast, glucagon stimulates lipolysis, ketogenesis, gluconeogenesis, and glycogenolysis. A meal rich in carbohydrates induces insulin secretion and suppresses glucagon release. Hypoglycemia stimulates the release of glucagon. Thus, in general, insulin and glucagon act oppositely to each other, with insulin promoting energy storage and glucagon promoting energy release. The net result of the hypoglycemic agent (insulin) and the hyperglycemic agents is glucose homeostasis.

Epinephrine

Epinephrine increases serum glucose levels by stimulating glucagon secretion, glycogenolysis, and gluconeogenesis and by inhibiting insulin secretion.

Incretins

Incretins are hormones that are released from the intestinal mucosa upon ingestion of glucose. Two principal incretins are known—glucose-dependent insulinotropic polypeptide (GIP), also called *gastric inhibitory peptide,* and glucagon-like peptide-1 (GLP-1). These hormones act on islet **β-receptor sites,** resulting in insulin release. In non-diabetic individuals, the incretins are responsible for 50% to 70% of the insulin released when carbohydrates are ingested.[19]

Other Hormones

Growth hormone and thyroxine also act to raise circulating levels of glucose. **Somatostatin** is a polypeptide hormone that is synthesized primarily in the δ-cells of the pancreas. Somatostatin inhibits insulin and glucagon release. Insulin-like growth factors are proteins with structured homology to proinsulin and somatomedin C. These factors may play a role in glucose control.

Glucose Metabolism in Diabetes Mellitus

Metabolic Processes in the Normal Individual

Hormonal regulation of blood glucose levels and metabolic processes is abnormal in persons with diabetes and results in the classic sign of DM: elevated blood glucose levels.

In the postabsorptive (fasting) state of normal individuals, the blood insulin–to–glucagon ratio is low, causing muscle and hepatic glycogen to be degraded as a source of glucose. Again, the liver is the primary source of blood glucose in the fasting state. Additional fasting results in the breakdown of protein to amino acids in skeletal muscle, and the lipolysis of triglycerides to fatty acids in adipose tissue. The amino acid alanine and glycerol are used to synthesize glucose by means of glucagon-stimulated gluconeogenesis. In addition, free fatty acids can be used as fuel by the heart, skeletal muscles, and liver.

Just minutes after ingestion of a meal, blood insulin levels rapidly increase. This is due in part to secretion of the incretins GLP-1 and GIP from the intestinal mucosa. Glucose and amino acids, such as leucine, isoleucine, and lysine, are potent stimulants of the β-cells of the pancreas, causing them to secrete insulin. Most peripheral cells respond to the rise of blood glucose by rapidly increasing glucose transport into cells. Thus following a meal, blood glucose levels increase by only 20% to 40% in nondiabetic individuals. However, approximately 80% of glucose uptake is not insulin dependent, because the brain, red blood cells, liver, and intestines do not require insulin for increased glucose uptake in the presence of elevated blood glucose. Muscle is the most important insulin-dependent tissue. Increased blood insulin and glucose levels do inhibit lipolysis, as well as approximately 60% of the normal hepatic release of glucose.

Metabolic Processes in the Person With Diabetes[15,20]

In the individual with diabetes, both the production and the metabolism of glucose are abnormal. Thus, in the fasting state, hepatic glucose release is greatly elevated, causing the diagnostic, fasting hyperglycemia of persons with diabetes.

In addition, both the release of insulin (type 1 diabetes) and the cellular response to insulin (insulin resistance in type 2 diabetes, see later discussion) are decreased in those with diabetes, especially relative to a given blood glucose level. Decreased insulin control causes the diabetic individual to be in a state of semistarvation, with increased dependence on triglycerides as a source of fuel and on protein as a source of glucose precursors. Thus, in the fasting state, the person with diabetes may have increased blood free fatty acids and ketones (see p. 743).

After a meal, the inhibition of hepatic glucose output is much smaller in the person with diabetes. Combined with diminished insulin output and insulin resistance, this event leads to an abnormal and prolonged rise in blood glucose after a meal in those with diabetes (Fig. 38-9).

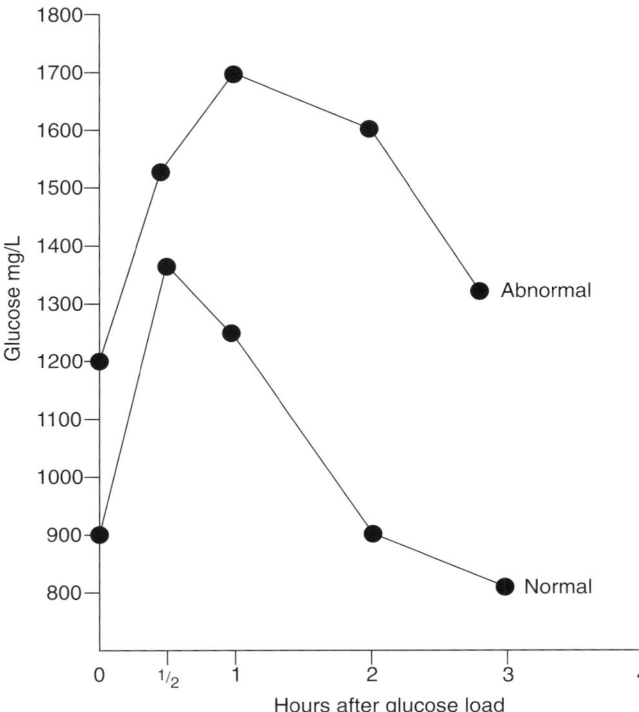

Fig. 38-9 Oral glucose tolerance test (OGTT, see p. 746). Response of person with diabetes to OGTT is compared with normal response. In diabetic individuals, the glucose curve is elevated and delayed. In normal response, a peak is reached after 30 minutes and returns to baseline value after 2 hours. Those with type 1 diabetes produce a nearly flat insulin curve after glucose load. If there is a peak, it occurs late (later than 1 hour). In type 2 diabetes, insulin response often is exaggerated, the peak is late, and the return to baseline value is later than 3 hours.

KEY CONCEPTS BOX 38-2

- The principal biochemical function of glucose is to provide energy for life processes.
- The initial event in glucose metabolism is facilitated transport of glucose across the plasma membrane. This is initiated by the hormone insulin binding to the insulin receptor site found on the plasma membranes of specific cell types. The attachment of insulin results in a cascade of events (the insulin signaling pathway), which leads to transport of glucose across the plasma membrane into the cytoplasm.
- Next, the glucose is metabolized by several pathways, leading to the production of ATP or the storage of glucose as a part of a polymer (glycogen).
- Just after a meal, hormones called *incretins* are secreted from the intestinal wall, acting as a major stimulus for insulin secretion. Glucose that enters the bloodstream accounts for the rest of the stimulus for insulin secretion.
- The metabolism of glucose differs in persons with diabetes as contrasted with normal individuals.
- Glucagon, cortisol, epinephrine, growth hormone, thyroxine, somatostatin, and insulin-like growth factors also play roles in glucose regulation.

SECTION OBJECTIVE BOX 38-3

- Summarize the National Diabetes Group of the NIH classification scheme for diabetes.

CLASSIFICATION OF DIABETES MELLITUS

In 1979, the National Diabetes Data Group of the National Institutes of Health (NIH) developed a classification scheme for DM and other types of glucose intolerance based on current knowledge of the biochemistry of this disease.[21] Table 38-2 summarizes the NIH classification system.

Type 1 Diabetes

Type 1 diabetes accounts for 5% to 10% of the diagnosed cases of diabetes. In 2005, the Centers for Disease Control and Prevention estimated its prevalence to be 1 in 400 to 600 persons younger than 20 years of age—the age at which this disease is usually diagnosed. This represents 0.22% of persons in this age range.[22] This type of diabetes is caused by insufficient insulin secretion (insulinopenia). Insulin injections are necessary to maintain normal glucose metabolism. Individuals with type 1 diabetes are especially prone to ketoacidosis, the excessive formation of keto acids, and low blood pH (acidosis). This condition is discussed on p. 743. Other complications of type 1 diabetes include cataracts, disease of the nerves **(neuropathy),** kidney disease **(nephropathy),** cardiovascular disease, and blood vessel disease **(angiopathy).**

Type 2 Diabetes

Until recently, type 2 diabetes occurred primarily in persons 40 years of age or older. However, regional studies and reports suggest that the appearance of type 2 diabetes has increased significantly among youths 20 years of age or younger. This is particularly true in minorities such as African Americans, American Indians, and Hispanics. The increase in the prevalence of diabetes among youths is considered to have reached epidemic proportions. Coupled with the prevalence of type 2 diabetes among youths is the prevalence of obesity (see the metabolic syndrome on p. 709 and Nutrition chapter, p. 797), which also is increasing at epidemic levels.[22,23] Late-onset diabetes can be divided further by the presence or absence of obesity. The occurrence of type 2 diabetes has no correlation with blood insulin levels. Generally, unlike individuals with type 1 diabetes, those with type 2 diabetes are not dependent on insulin injections, nor are they prone to ketoacidosis.

Secondary Diabetes

DM caused by other conditions and diseases is called *secondary diabetes.* Secondary diabetes can be caused by pancreatic disease, **acromegaly** (growth hormone excess), Cushing's

Table 38-2 Classification of Diabetes and Other Categories of Glucose Intolerance

Class	Description
Type 1 DM	Deficiency of insulin (insulinopenia) Dependence on injected insulin Usually occurs before 40 years of age Prone to ketoacidosis Prone to diabetic complications • Cataracts (six times greater than in nondiabetics) • Neuropathy (60% to 70% show mild to severe symptoms; 10% serious) • Nephropathy (40% to 50% develop renal failure) • Angiopathy (high risk for heart attack and stroke)
Type 2 DM	Variable levels of insulin Not dependent on exogenous insulin for control of hyperglycemia; often obese individuals Usually occurs after 40 years of age Not prone to ketoacidosis Not as prone to diabetic complications
Secondary DM	Diabetes caused by various secondary conditions such as pancreatic disease, acromegaly, Cushing's syndrome, pheochromocytoma, glucagonoma, somatostatinoma, primary aldosteronism, severe liver disease, and certain drugs, chemicals, and hormones Maturity onset–type diabetes of the young (MODY)
Impaired glucose tolerance	Persons who exhibit in their oral glucose tolerance test a 2-hour value between 140 mg/dL and 200 mg/dL[72]
Impaired fasting glucose	Persons who exhibit a fasting plasma glucose level between 100 mg/dL and 126 mg/dL fall into this new category[72]
GDM	Diabetes that occurs during pregnancy
Statistical risk classes; previous abnormality of glucose tolerance	Previous transient hyperglycemia that occurred spontaneously or in response to specific stimuli but presently testing normally
Potential abnormality of glucose tolerance	Persons not presently exhibiting any indications of diabetes but at substantially increased risk to develop diabetes in the future; includes the monozygotic twin of a person with type 2 diabetes; person who has parent, sibling, or offspring who has type 2 diabetes; obese individuals; members of certain racial or ethnic groups with a high prevalence of diabetes

DM, Diabetes mellitus; *GDM,* gestational diabetes mellitus.

syndrome (elevated cortisol), pheochromocytoma (excessive catecholamines), **glucagonoma** (excessive glucagon produced by a tumor), **somatostatinoma** (excessive somatostatin produced by a tumor), primary aldosteronism, severe liver disease, and administration of certain drugs, hormones, and chemicals. Maturity onset–type diabetes (type 2, above) of the young (MODY) occurs in younger individuals (<25 years) who have impaired pancreatic β-cells and still can produce insulin, but demonstrate insulin resistance.[23]

Impaired Glucose Tolerance

Impaired glucose tolerance (IGT) affects persons who have had an abnormal glucose tolerance test but no frank fasting hyperglycemia. The oral glucose tolerance test (OGTT) is discussed later in this chapter (p. 746). It has been established that in adult-onset type 2 diabetes, an intermediate stage of IGT occurs.[24] IGT now is referred to as **pre-diabetes.** A recent study[25] demonstrates that IGT (pre-diabetes) is also the intermediate step in the development of type 2 diabetes among obese youth (ages 8 to 18).

Gestational Diabetes

Gestational diabetes (GD) refers to diabetes that occurs temporarily during pregnancy. GD occurs in 2% to 5% of pregnancies in the United States.[26] Kim et al[27] reviewed articles published between January 1965 and August 2001 in which women were tested for GD and then were tested for type 2 diabetes after delivery. They found that in most women with a diagnosis of GD, the condition progressed to type 2 diabetes. This progression increased significantly over the first 5 years after delivery and leveled off after 10 years. Screening of pregnant women for GD, to prevent perinatal complications associated with maternal hyperglycemia, has become accepted practice (see Chapter 44, p. 875). GD is derived from a woman's inability to secrete sufficient insulin to compensate for the increased nutritional needs of pregnancy, the greater numbers of adipose cells during pregnancy, and the pregnancy-associated secretion of increased quantities of hyperglycemic hormones, including human placental lactogen, cortisol, prolactin, and progesterone. This results in a nearly fourfold increase in the need for insulin secretion. When this need for additional insulin is not totally met, hyperglycemia develops in a pregnant woman.

Table 38-3 Genetic Changes Related to Diabetes Mellitus

Disorder	Symbol(s)	OMIM	Location
DM, gestational, 125851 (3)	GCK, HHF3	138079	7pl5-pl3
DM, insulin-dependent, neonatal (2) (?)	PBCA	600089	Chr.6
DM, insulin-resistant, with acanthosis nigricans and hypertension, 604367 (3)	PPARG.PPARG1, PPARG2	601487	3p25
DM, insulin-resistant, with acanthosis nigricans, 610549 (3)	INSR, HHF5	147670	19pl3.2
DM, neonatal, with congenital hypothyroidism, 610199 (3)	GLIS3, ZNF515	610192	9p24.3-p23
DM, non–insulin-dependent, 125853 (3)	ABCC8, SUR, PHHI, SUR1.HHF1, TNDM2	600509	llpl5.1
DM, non–insulin-dependent, 125853 (3)	TCF2, HNF2, MODY5, FJHN	189907	17cen-q21.3
DM, non–insulin-dependent, 2 (2)	NIDDM2	601407	12q24.2
DM, non–insulin-dependent, late-onset, 125853(3)	GCK, HHF3	138079	7pl5-pl3
DM, permanent neonatal, 606176 (3)	ABCC8, SUR, PHHI, SUR1.HHF1, TNDM2	600509	llpl5.1
DM, permanent neonatal, 606176 (3)	GCK, HHF3	138079	7pl5-pl3
DM, permanent neonatal, with cerebellar agenesis, 609069 (3)	PTF1A	607194	10pl2.3
DM, permanent neonatal, with neurological features, 606176 (3); DM, type 2, susceptibility to, 125853 (3)	KCNJ11,BIR,PHHI, HHF2, TNDM3	600937	llpl5.1
DM, rare form (1)	INS	176730	llpl5.5
DM, transient neonatal type 2, 610374 (3)	ABCC8, SUR, PHHI, SUR1, HHF1, TNDM2	600509	llpl5.1

From http://www.ncbi.nlm.nih.gov/0mim/getmorbid.cgi?start=1095&term=diabetes+mellitus&f . . . , Accessed 9/24/2007.
DM, Diabetes mellitus.

KEY CONCEPTS BOX 38-3

- Type 1 diabetes is caused by insufficient insulin secretion due to the autoimmune destruction of β-islets cells.
- Type 2 diabetes was previously a disease of persons 40 years of age or older. In recent years, it has been occurring in increasing numbers in persons younger than 20 years of age. This is particularly true among youths who have metabolic syndrome.
- Secondary diabetes is caused by other conditions and diseases that affect glucose production and metabolism.
- Impaired glucose tolerance may affect persons who do not exhibit hyperglycemia but who have abnormal oral glucose tolerance tests.
- Gestational diabetes occurs temporarily during pregnancy, although many affected women eventually progress to type 2 diabetes after delivery.

SECTION OBJECTIVES BOX 38-4

- Describe the evidence that suggests that there is a correlation between type 2 diabetes and heredity.
- Describe the evidence that suggests that there is an inherited susceptibility or resistance to type 1 diabetes.
- Describe the evidence that suggests that type 1 diabetes is an autoimmune disease.
- Describe the connection between type 1 diabetes and viruses. What evidence suggests this connection?

PATHOGENESIS OF DIABETES MELLITUS

Introduction

Epidemiologists have studied identical twins and the offspring and siblings of diabetics.[28,29] These studies show clearly that DM develops from a complex interaction between environmental and genetic factors. If the development of diabetes was determined by hereditary factors alone, the disease should always affect both identical twins. Three different studies show that when type 1 diabetes occurs in one twin, it subsequently appears in the other only about 50% of the time. On the other hand, development of type 2 diabetes in one twin presages its appearance in the other nearly 100% of the time. Studies of offspring of type 2 diabetic parents show that diabetes is transmitted to offspring at a frequency of only 6% to 10%. A propensity to diabetes exists in these offspring because 25% to 40% of them have abnormal glucose tolerance test results. Similar results have been obtained in the siblings of diabetic individuals.

Genetic Factors (Type 2 Diabetes)

Recent studies have found clusters of genes that raise the risk of type 2 diabetes (Table 38-3). At least 10 genetic loci now have been linked to type 2 diabetes.[30,31] In fact, individuals with an affected parent or sibling are at 3.5 times greater risk of developing diabetes than are those from diabetes-free families. Clusters of gene variants that increase the risk of type 2 diabetes include three new loci. They are located in a noncoding region of *CDKN2A* and *CDKN2B*, in an intron of *IGF2BP2*, and in an intron of *CDKAL1*. New techniques promise identification of additional gene loci that cause susceptibility to type 2 diabetes.[32,33] However, genetics is not the sole cause of the disease. The development of type 2 diabetes is linked to a combination of genetic and lifestyle factors associated with the development of obesity.[34]

Recently, with elucidation of the insulin signaling pathway, investigators have found associations between type 2 diabetes and genetic defects in the pathway. Models of decreased insulin signaling have as their first step a defect in insulin receptor activation or its subsequent phosphorylation activity.[35,36] Investigators have reported that elevation of plasma fatty acids abolishes insulin activation of PI3K activity.[37] Other investigations have shown that individuals with severe familial insulin resistance carry mutations in their insulin receptor alleles.[11,38]

Genetic Factors (Type 1 Diabetes)

Inherited susceptibility or resistance to type 1 DM is supported by studies that associate the production of specific human lymphocyte antigens (HLAs) with occurrence of the disease.[39] HLAs are dimeric proteins produced by the major histocompatibility complex on chromosome 6. The class II HLA loci so far identified with susceptibility to type 1 diabetes are DP, DQ, and DR. HLA DR3 or DR4 or both types occur in 90% of patients with type 1 diabetes. Resistance to type 1 diabetes is associated with DR2.[40] Susceptibility to type 1 diabetes is greater when DR4 protein was produced in conjunction with a protein produced by the DQ locus, called DQw3.2. The DQw3.2 allele has a gene frequency of 35.7% in those with type 1 diabetes, as contrasted with 10.1% in nondiabetic persons. Individuals who possess the DQw3.1 allele are less likely to acquire type 1 diabetes than are their DQw3.2 counterparts.[41] Susceptibility to type 1 diabetes is increased further when the DQ β-chain lacks aspartic acid at position 57 and has arginine present at position 52 of the DQ α-chain.[42] Table 38-3 lists some of the genetic defects associated with type 1 diabetes.

The autoimmune cause for type 1 DM has been suggested by observations of progressive lymphocytic infiltration of the islet cells of the pancreas with concomitant β-cell destruction and the appearance of **islet cell antibodies (ICA)** before the manifestation of overt diabetes. Markers for autoimmune destruction of the β-cell include autoantibodies to glutamic acid decarboxylase, β-islet cells, insulin, and tyrosine phosphatases. At least one of these autoantibodies is present in 85% to 90% of persons with a diagnosis of diabetes.[43] Assays that lead to the identification of CD4 and CD8 T cells that contain β-islet epitopes could be used to identify individuals likely to exhibit types 1 diabetes, as well as to follow their treatment.[44,45]

Viruses

Viral infections have long been considered to be initiating factors in the autoimmune cause of type 1 diabetes. At present, 14 different viruses have been implicated in β-cell death. Two mechanisms may be involved: β-cell autoimmunity with or without infection of the β-cell by the virus, and cell infection followed by destruction.[46] Evidence for viral infection as a cause of type 1 diabetes comes from studies with coxsackie virus B4.[47] An increase in coxsackie virus B antibodies in Swedish individuals with diabetes has been reported.[48] In addition, mumps virus, B1, and rubella reovirus type 3 have been implicated in the development of type 1 diabetes.[49]

KEY CONCEPTS BOX 38-4

- Evidence demonstrates that type 1 diabetes is an autoimmune disease that may be caused by viruses.
- Substantial evidence reveals gene clusters that make an individual more susceptible or more resistant to the disease.
- Evidence suggests that type 2 diabetes involves defects in the insulin signaling pathway and/or the incretins. Recent studies have found gene clusters that raise the risk of occurrence of type 2 diabetes.

SECTION OBJECTIVES BOX 38-5

- Describe the principal complications of diabetes.
- Explain the effects of hyperglycemia on the fetus.

COMPLICATIONS OF DIABETES MELLITUS

The principal complications of DM are **retinopathy,** neuropathy, angiopathy, nephropathy, susceptibility to infection, hyperlipidemia, ketoacidosis, and **hyperglycemic hyperosmolar nonketotic coma (HHNC).** With the single exception of HHNC, these diabetic complications occur more frequently for individuals with type 1 diabetes than for type 2 diabetic persons.

Retinopathy

Opaque areas in the lens of the eye are called *cataracts.* Cataract formation is the principal retinopathy of diabetes. Retinopathy also is caused by **angiogenesis,** a proliferation of small blood vessels in the lens. Diabetic retinopathy is the primary cause of blindness in persons 20 to 74 years old.

Neuropathy

Neuropathy is the most common complication of DM. It is apparent in about 60% to 70% of diabetic individuals and is recognized by a variety of symptoms that include pain, numbness, tingling or burning sensations in the extremities, dizziness, and double vision. Decreased motor and sensory nerve conduction velocities produced by axonal degeneration and demyelination cause these symptoms. Secondary manifestations of neuropathy include cardiac failure, excessive sweating, and male impotence.

Angiopathy

Angiopathy refers to damage to linings (**basement membranes**) of blood vessels. Angiopathy increases the risk of coronary heart disease and stroke and can lead to retinopathy and nephropathy.

Nephropathy

Nephropathy refers to damage to the capillaries associated with the glomerulus (filtering apparatus of the nephron); this

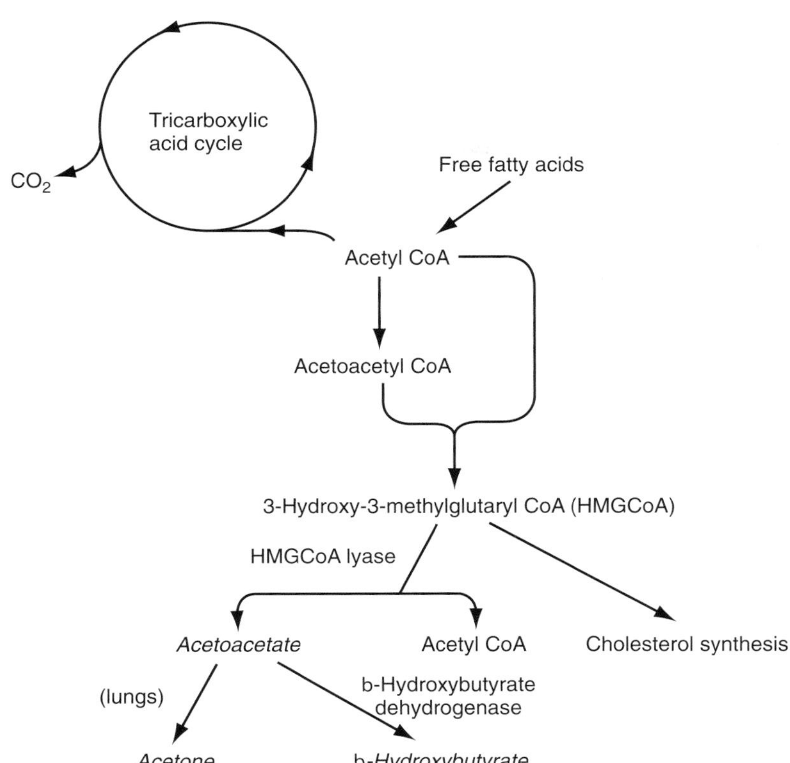

Fig. 38-10 Pathways involved in keto acid metabolism. Accumulation of keto acids, acetoacetate, and β-hydroxybutyrate is a principal feature of diabetic ketoacidosis. The metabolic pathway leading from acetyl-CoA to acetoacetate and β-hydroxybutyrate is accelerated in diabetes because of free fatty acid mobilization.

damage is associated with a reduction in the filtering capability of the kidneys (see Chapter 30). Capillary damage is caused by angiopathy, a common feature of diabetes. Approximately 25% to 30% of individuals treated for end-stage renal failure have diabetes, and approximately 27% of those with diabetes have developed end-stage renal disease. Both the prevalence and the incidence of end-stage renal disease are approximately twice the rates of the early 1990s, and diabetic nephropathy accounted for 44% of new cases in 2002.[50]

Proteinuria is often the first sign of diabetic nephropathy. The Diabetes Control and Complications Trial (DCCT) convincingly demonstrated that maintaining blood glucose levels of a person with diabetes to within or near the healthy range reduced the risk of developing small quantities of protein in the urine by 35%, and the risk of developing substantial quantities of protein in the urine by 56%.[51] Close control of blood glucose levels in combination with new treatment modalities may well make diabetes-associated nephropathy a controllable disease.

Infection

Individuals with diabetes are highly susceptible to infection, ulceration, and gangrene (especially in the extremities). More than 60% of lower limb amputations in the United States occur in diabetic individuals. Skin disorders are also more common in those with diabetes than in nondiabetic individuals.

Hyperlipidemia and Atherosclerosis

Abnormal triglyceride, cholesterol, and very-low-density lipoprotein (VLDL) levels often are associated with type 2 diabetes.[52,53] High-density lipoprotein (HDL) levels have been reported to be significantly lower in diabetic than in nondiabetic persons. These results are consistent with the high incidence and natural history of atherosclerotic coronary heart disease in persons with diabetes, and with the higher death rates from myocardial infarction in diabetic individuals. Heart disease and stroke account for about 65% of deaths in persons with diabetes—an incidence two to four times higher than that in persons without diabetes (see Chapter 37).[54]

Diabetic Ketoacidosis (DKA)

Keto Acid Metabolism

As is shown in Fig. 38-10, acetyl coenzyme A (acetyl CoA) is at the crossroads of glucose, protein, and lipid metabolism. It enters the tricarboxylic acid cycle or is metabolized to 3-hydroxy-3-methylglutaryl coenzyme A (HMG-CoA). HMG-CoA can be metabolized to cholesterol, or it can be converted to acetoacetate. Acetoacetate has two possible fates: spontaneous decarboxylation to acetone (in the lungs), or enzymatic reduction to β-hydroxybutyrate. Acetoacetate, acetone, and β-hydroxybutyrate are commonly called *keto acids,* or *ketone bodies.* Keto acids are normally a source of energy for the brain, kidneys, and cardiac muscle. The kidneys excrete a considerable quantity of acetoacetate and β-hydroxybutyrate, with concomitant loss of sodium and potassium. Kidney excretion of sodium and potassium results in the retention of hydrogen ions.

Keto Acids and Insulin

In nondiabetic individuals, keto acid formation is a minor pathway. In those with type 1 diabetes, insulinopenia causes fat cells to mobilize fatty acids from triglycerides. Fatty acid degradation increases as it becomes the major source of energy for the cell. Increased fatty acid catabolism produces excessive quantities of acetyl CoA. Although a significant portion of the acetyl CoA is able to enter the tricarboxylic acid cycle to produce energy, an excess quantity of acetyl CoA is metabolized to produce abnormal levels of keto acids (ketosis). Increased production of keto acids consumes bicarbonate, thereby lowering blood pH (acidosis). This same metabolic pattern occurs in starvation, except that hypoglycemia is present instead of hyperglycemia.

Diagnosis of Ketoacidosis

Blood gas and blood glucose levels are useful in detecting **diabetic ketoacidosis.** Low pH, normal P_{CO_2}, low bicarbonate, high anion gap, and high glucose are suggestive of uncompensated ketoacidosis. Low pH, low P_{CO_2}, low bicarbonate, high anion gap, and high glucose are suggestive of partially compensated diabetic ketoacidosis. The elevated anion gap is caused by the accumulation of sodium salts of keto acids.

Lactic Acidosis

Lactic acidosis is caused by the accumulation of lactic acid that results from tissue hypoxia (oxygen deficiency). Similar to the accumulation of keto acids, lactate accumulation causes increased blood hydrogen ions and therefore low pH. In the diabetic individual, lactic acidosis often occurs simultaneously with diabetic ketoacidosis, especially if the pH falls to below 7.10, if renal insufficiency occurs, or if certain hypoglycemic agents such as phenformin (DBI) are administered.

Hyperglycemic Hyperosmolar Nonketotic Coma

Hyperglycemic hyperosmolar nonketotic coma (HHNC) has a mortality of 10% to 20%. It is characterized by a blood glucose level above 600 mg/dL, normal or slightly low blood pH, serum osmolality above 350 mOsm/kg, normal keto acid levels, and lethargy or coma. Although diabetic ketoacidosis occurs primarily in persons with type 1 diabetes, HHNC occurs primarily in type 2 diabetic individuals. The absence of keto acids in HHNC probably is caused by the differential sensitivity of lipid and glucose metabolism to insulin. Lipolysis is inhibited by one-tenth the insulin level that is required to enhance glucose metabolism.[55] In persons with type 1 diabetes, insulinopenia enhances lipolysis, with resulting accumulation of keto acids, and glucose utilization is blocked, resulting in hyperglycemia. In type 2 diabetes, although insulin resistance occurs, insulin activity is sufficient to limit lipolysis and thus keto acid production; however, insulin activity is insufficient to avoid hyperglycemia. HHNC often is brought on by stressful events and major illness, especially in older individuals.

Hypoglycemia

Hypoglycemia causes numerous neurogenic problems, ranging from mild to severe coma, seizures, and death. The level of blood glucose when symptoms become obvious varies but tends to be lower than 50 mg/dL for adults and lower than 40 mg/dL for newborns. This potentially life-threatening disorder most often is the result of aggressive use of insulin treatment to maintain normoglycemia. Long-acting insulin derivatives reduce the potential for hypoglycemia (see Treatment, p. 751).

Box 38-1

Causes of Fasting Hypoglycemia

Depressed blood insulin/decreased glucose production
Liver disease
Alcoholism
Renal insufficiency
Galactosemia and glycogen storage disease
Malignancy (increases consumption of glucose or production of insulin-like growth factor)
Infection
Late pregnancy
Malnutrition
Overtreatment with insulin
- Insulinoma
- Factitious (exogenous) treatment with insulin
- Treatment with sulfonylurea drugs
- Antiinsulin antibodies

Several other causes of hypoglycemia[56] are listed in Box 38-1. Many of these are detected in emergency room cases as coma, treatable simply with intravenous glucose. Differential diagnosis may require measurement of blood glucose, insulin, and C-peptide. C-peptide is important in diagnosing surreptitious or overzealous insulin treatment because commercial insulin preparations contain no C-peptide.[57] In these cases, although blood insulin levels are elevated, C-peptide levels are low. Production of autoantibodies against insulin can result in a similar pattern, although these cases often are associated with postprandial hyperglycemia.

The risk for hypoglycemia is increased for some hospitalized patients. This risk often is unrelated to diabetes but is associated with advanced liver disease, renal insufficiency, and malnutrition. Such severely ill patients have an increased likelihood of mortality.

Effects of Diabetes on the Fetus
(see also Chapters 44 and 45)

Poorly controlled diabetes after conception and during the first trimester of pregnancy is associated with an increased number of major birth defects and spontaneous abortions, that is, 5% to 10% and 15% to 20% of pregnancies, respectively. The newborn of a pregnant woman with diabetes is also at increased risk for macrosomia, hypoglycemia, hypocalcemia, polycythemia, and hyperbilirubinemia. The greatest risk for intrauterine death or neonatal mortality occurs when the mother's glucose levels are greater than 110 mg/dL when fasting, or greater than 120 mg/dL after a meal. The risk for perinatal morbidity and mortality is reduced to that seen in the general population when normal fasting and postprandial levels are maintained. A child who has been exposed to hyperglycemia in utero is at greater risk for the development of diabetes later in life.[58] Fetita et al[59] determined that fetuses exposed to maternal GD exhibit a higher incidence of IGT as adolescents. A subsequent study[60] performed on a multiethnic American population suggested that hyperglycemia in pregnancy is associated with an increased risk of childhood obesity.

Increased rates of cesarean section and hypertensive disorder have been reported as maternal complications directly related to the degree of maternal hyperglycemia.

Other Complications of Diabetes

The acutely ill diabetic person, with ketoacidosis or hyperosmolar coma, is at risk for immediately life-threatening complications. The hypovolemia associated with these acute illnesses can result in shock and renal failure. Cerebral edema may arise in patients with ketoacidosis and hyperosmolar coma as a result of insulin and fluid administration. Loss of salts usually occurs in DKA and HHNC. Although patients' serum electrolytes may be elevated, normal, or low, they usually exhibit a deficit of body potassium.

KEY CONCEPTS BOX 38-5

- Diabetes can have immediate and long-term complications. Complications are especially prevalent for type 1 diabetes.
- Complications include retinopathy, neuropathy, angiopathy, nephropathy, infection, hyperlipidemia, ketoacidosis, and hyperglycemic hyperosmolar nonketotic coma.
- Gestational hyperglycemia in association with greater risk for development of diabetes later in life for both the mother and newborn.

SECTION OBJECTIVE BOX 38-6

- Explain the two major theories that have been proposed to explain the causation of diabetic complications.

PATHOGENESIS OF DIABETIC COMPLICATIONS

Protein Glycation

The carbonyl functional groups of glucose and other sugars react with free amino groups of proteins to form intermediates called Schiff bases, or aldimines. The amino group that reacts is an N-terminal amino group or an internal lysine ε-amino group. The aldimine subsequently rearranges to form a ketamine. This rearrangement is called the *Amadori rearrangement.* The aldimine is labile; it can readily hydrolyze to re-form a free amino group and a carbonyl group. The ketamine is relatively stable, and its formation is not reversible. The extent of this nonenzymatic protein **glycation** reaction, which commonly occurs in red blood cells, glomeruli, nerve cells, and other tissues, is directly proportional to extracellular glucose concentrations.[61]

Advanced glycation end products (ketamines) are modified lysine, arginine, cysteine and N-terminal amino groups. Excessive glycation is known to produce significant alterations in a protein's physical and biochemical properties.[62] For example, glycation of α-crystallin, a protein that occurs in the lens of the eye, greatly reduces its solubility.[63] Glycation of basement membranes in kidneys has been shown to be a result and a cause of renal failure.[64] Glycation of proteins and loss of protein function is most likely the biochemical basis of many of the physiological complications of diabetes.

Sorbitol Accumulation

The intracellular accumulation of sorbitol forms the basis for another hypothesis designed to explain diabetic complications. Aldose reductase reduces glucose to sorbitol, which, in turn, is oxidized to fructose by sorbitol dehydrogenase. Sorbitol does not easily cross cell membranes. Removal of sorbitol from the cell depends on its conversion to fructose, which does pass freely through the cell membrane. However, when glucose levels are high, the quantities of sorbitol produced outstrip the ability of the cell to convert sorbitol to fructose, resulting in intracellular accumulation of sorbitol. Intracellular accumulation of ketones, glucose, and sorbitol causes osmotic swelling and injury to cell structures. Only cells that do not depend on insulin for glucose transport across the plasma membrane are affected. These cells include nerve, ocular lens, and glomerulus cells. This osmotic effect is the cause of life-threatening cerebral edema that can occur during treatment for DKA and HHNC.[65] After insulin treatment reduces blood glucose levels, blood osmolality decreases faster than intracellular osmolality in brain cells, causing a shift of extracellular water into brain cells, which can result in brain swelling and death. Supporting this hypothesis are reports of elevations in sorbitol and fructose levels in the nerve and ocular lens cells of diabetic persons and studies in which aldose reductase inhibitors were used.[66]

KEY CONCEPTS BOX 38-6

- Nonenzymatic protein glycation leads to changes in the physical structure of the protein and therefore interferes with protein function.
- The intracellular accumulation of sorbitol and its subsequent metabolism to fructose cause osmotic swelling and injury to cell structures.

SECTION OBJECTIVES BOX 38-7

- Explain in a stepwise manner the protocols for postprandial plasma glucose, oral glucose tolerance, and fasting blood glucose tests.
- Explain the variables that must be controlled for these tests to have validity.
- List the order of the tests that a physician would use to diagnose diabetes.
- Explain how the Carpenter and Coustan test for the detection of gestational diabetes differs from the O'Sullivan-Mahan test.
- Explain under what conditions the intravenous glucose tolerance test is used.
- Explain the disadvantages of the OGTT.
- Explain why the OGTT should be the test of choice.

FUNCTION TESTS

Postprandial Plasma Glucose

Diabetes is detected more readily when carbohydrate metabolic capacity is tested. This can be done by stressing the system with a defined glucose load. Measurement of the rate at which the glucose load is cleared from the blood, as compared with the rate of glucose clearance in healthy persons, detects impairment in glucose metabolism. A meal high in carbohydrates often is used as the carbohydrate load, although a 75 g glucose drink usually is preferred over a meal. This is called the *postprandial test.* Two consecutive postprandial tests are recommended for diagnosis.

Blood is drawn at 2 hours after ingestion of the meal or glucose drink. Two postprandial tests with glucose levels of 200 mg/dL or higher at 2 hours are suggestive of diabetes.[67] The postprandial glucose test, although widely used for detection of diabetes, is highly inaccurate because of several variables that are difficult to control or adjust for. These variables include age, weight, previous diet, activity, illness, medications, time of day that the test is conducted, and actual size of the glucose dose. When a meal is used as the load, the effective glucose load depends on the digestion of disaccharides and polysaccharides and their subsequent absorption from the intestinal tract.

Oral Glucose Tolerance Test

The **oral glucose tolerance test (OGTT)** evaluates glucose clearance from the circulation after glucose loading under defined and controlled conditions. The Committee on Statistics of the American Diabetes Association has standardized the test.[68]

Standard conditions call for a minimum carbohydrate intake of 150 g/day for 3 days before the test. A minimum 8-hour fast is required before testing. The patient must be ambulatory because inactivity decreases glucose tolerance. However, exercise and emotional stress should be avoided.

Factors Affecting Glucose Tolerance

Hormone abnormalities of thyroxine, growth hormone, cortisol, and catecholamines interfere. Drugs and medications such as oral contraceptives, salicylates, nicotinic acid (found in cigarettes, cigars, pipe tobacco, chewing tobacco), diuretics (including caffeine), and hypoglycemic agents (insulin, sulfonylureas) interfere. Testing time affects the test. The best time to conduct the test is between 7 AM and noon. Evaluation criteria should be adjusted for age. If adjustments for age are not made, about 80% of persons over 60 years of age will be judged diabetic.[69]

The glucose load should consist of glucose only. Some commercial preparations labeled "100 grams glucose equivalent" contain disaccharides and polysaccharides. The rate at which these saccharides are hydrolyzed and absorbed from the intestinal tract varies from person to person. Such a preparation obviously is not desirable for individuals with pancreatic or malabsorptive disorders. The size of the load is 40 g of glucose per square meter of body area. For most subjects, 75 g of total glucose is sufficient. The drink can be flavored if caffeine or theophylline is not used.

Table 38-4 Comparison of the Criteria for Evaluation of Oral Glucose Tolerance Test Using 75 G or 100 G Glucose Challenges

Time of Blood Drawing, Hours	*PLASMA GLUCOSE LEVELS, mg/dL*	
	75 g Challenge	100 g Challenge
Fasting	95	95
1	180	180
2	155	155
3		140

Test should be conducted in the morning, with patient seated and nonsmoking. A fast of >8 hours and 3 days of unrestricted diet (greater or equal to 150 g carbohydrate per day) is required. Physical activity is unlimited. Two or more criteria must be met or exceeded for a diagnosis of DM.[72]

In accordance with World Health Organization (WHO) recommendations, a blood glucose measurement should be made 2 hours[70] after a 75 g glucose challenge is given. A glucose value of greater than or equal to 200 mg/dL is suggestive of DM. This value is supported by evidence from several studies (Pima Indians in the United States, Egyptian study, Third National Health and Nutrition Examination Survey in the United States [NHANES III]) that diabetic complications such as retinopathy and nephropathy increase significantly beyond this glucose level. In addition, the Paris Prospective Study showed that the incidence of fatal coronary heart disease increased dramatically as the 2-hour plasma glucose value increased to above 140 mg/dL. The Expert Committee on the Diagnosis and Classification of DM criteria for evaluating the 75 and 100 g glucose challenge OGTT are presented in Table 38-4.[71] The shape of the glucose tolerance curve is useful for evaluating the OGTT (see Fig. 38-9). Healthy subjects peak at $^1/_2$ hour and return to fasting levels at 2 hours. Diabetic individuals peak late (approximately 1 hour) or even show a plateau at 2 to 3 hours and return to baseline value after 3 hours. Insulin determinations performed along with glucose determinations are useful in evaluating the OGTT. Plasma insulin levels after a glucose load differentiate type 1 from type 2 diabetes. In nondiabetic persons, insulin levels peak 1 hour after a glucose load and return to fasting levels at 2 to 3 hours. Persons with type 1 diabetes respond to a glucose load with little or no insulin increase above fasting levels. Those with type 2 diabetes respond to the challenge with an abnormally late and often excessive increase in insulin levels. Type 1 diabetes often is associated with low fasting insulin levels, and type 2 diabetes is characterized by variable fasting insulin levels.

Fasting Blood Glucose

The OGTT has been criticized[72,73] because many of the variables that affect test results are difficult to control, and the reproducibility of the test is poor. In fact, the OGTT is used rather infrequently.[73] The American Diabetes Association recommends a fasting plasma glucose level rather than the OGTT for detection of DM. This has brought criticism from some investigators,[74,75] who have identified a sizable number of patients who test below the 126 mg/dL cutoff for fasting plasma glucose levels, but who are diabetic by OGTT criteria. The consensus opinion is that the OGTT is best used (1) to assess individuals who have borderline fasting glucose levels (see Screening on p. 751) who are at risk for the development of diabetes, (2) to screen pregnant women, and (3) to distinguish (in concert with insulin levels) type 1 from type 2 diabetes.

O'Sullivan-Mahan Glucose Challenge Test and Carpenter-Coustan OGTT for Gestational Diabetes

The O'Sullivan-Mahan glucose challenge test is used frequently to detect gestational diabetes. A 50 g load of glucose is given to a fasting patient, and a blood glucose measurement is made 1 hour after dosage. A plasma glucose level above 140 mg/dL suggests gestational diabetes, and a full oral glucose tolerance test is recommended for such patients.[71,76,77]

In 1982, Carpenter and Coustan proposed a 75 g, 2-hour OGTT for the detection of gestational diabetes.[78] The American Diabetes Association supported this alternative approach for the detection of gestational diabetes in a workshop conducted in March 1997. New criteria[79] for the detection of gestational diabetes as proposed at that workshop are summarized as follows:

1. Women with the following characteristics need not be screened for gestational diabetes: those who are younger than 25 years of age, with normal body weight, no family occurrence of diabetes, no history of abnormal glucose tolerance, no history of poor obstetrical outcome, and not of an ethnic or racial group with a high prevalence of diabetes (Hispanic, Native American, Asian, African, and Pacific Islander).
2. Women who do not fulfill all of the above criteria should be tested as soon as possible after pregnancy has been detected.
3. If glucose tolerance is found to be normal, women should be retested at between 24 and 28 weeks of gestation.
4. The test should consist of a fasting plasma blood glucose or a random plasma blood glucose.
5. A fasting value of greater than 126 mg/dL or a random value of greater than 200 mg/dL suggests gestational diabetes, if subsequently confirmed.
6. If the fasting or random plasma blood glucose is normal, follow-up testing should consist of the O'Sullivan-Mahan glucose challenge or the O'Sullivan-Mahan glucose challenge as modified by Carpenter-Coustan or the Carpenter-Coustan OGTT.
   a. O'Sullivan-Mahan test procedure and criteria are reported earlier.
   b. O'Sullivan-Mahan test (as modified by Carpenter-Coustan) is an OGTT that uses a 100 g glucose load. Cutoff criteria for a normal response to this test include the following: fasting 95 mg/dL, 1-hour 180 mg/dL, 2-hour 155 mg/dL, and 3-hour 140 mg/dL.
   c. Carpenter-Coustan OGTT uses a 75 g glucose load. Criteria for this test include the following: fasting 95 mg/dL, 1-hour 180 mg/dL, and 2-hour 155 mg/dL.
   d. For b and c, two or more plasma glucose values must be equaled or exceeded for a diagnosis of gestational diabetes. The test is done in the morning after a minimum fast of 8 hours and after 3 days of unrestricted diet (greater than 150 g of carbohydrate/day) and unlimited physical activity. During the test, the patient should remain seated and should not smoke.

Two protocols are recommended by the Expert Committee on the Diagnosis and Classification of DM for testing for gestational diabetes.[71] In the one-step approach, an OGTT is the initial action. In the two-step approach, initial screening is performed using the O'Sullivan-Mahan glucose challenge. For those women who test abnormally in the first step, a second step consisting of a diagnostic OGTT (the O'Sullivan-Mahan glucose challenge as modified by Carpenter-Coustan or the Carpenter-Cousin OGTT) is recommended to confirm the diagnosis.

Intravenous Glucose Tolerance Test

The intravenous glucose tolerance test is often used for persons with malabsorptive disorder or previous gastric or intestinal surgery. Glucose is administered intravenously over 30 minutes, using a 20% solution. A glucose load of 0.5 g/kg of body weight is used. Nondiabetic individuals respond with a plasma glucose level of 200 to 250 mg/dL. Discontinuation of glucose loading leads to a decrease in plasma glucose levels, with fasting levels reached at about 90 minutes. Diabetic persons demonstrate plasma glucose levels above 250 mg/dL during administration of the load. On discontinuation of the loading, plasma glucose levels of those with diabetes also return to fasting levels at about 90 minutes. An alternative procedure, called the *Soskin method,* uses 50% glucose delivered intravenously within 3 to 5 minutes. The glucose load used is 0.3 g/kg of body weight. Nondiabetic persons reestablish fasting levels within 60 minutes after discontinuing the glucose infusion. In those with diabetes, fasting levels are reestablished significantly later than 60 minutes.

KEY CONCEPTS BOX 38-7

- Detection of diabetes often requires a glucose challenge test.
- Blood glucose values determined after ingestion of a meal or a defined glucose challenge represent one type of glucose challenge and serve as the rationale for the postprandial plasma glucose test.
- The oral tolerance test evaluates glucose clearance after glucose loading under defined and controlled conditions.
- Fasting blood glucose is a recommended screening test for detecting diabetes.
- Two protocols are used for the detection of gestational diabetes: the O'Sullivan-Mahan glucose challenge test, and the Carpenter-Coustan OGTT.
- The Expert Committee on the Diagnosis and Classification of Diabetes Mellitus suggests two protocols for testing for gestational diabetes: one-step and two-step approaches.
- The intravenous glucose tolerance test is recommended for persons with malabsorptive disorders or previous gastric or intestinal surgery.

SECTION OBJECTIVES BOX 38-8

- Explain how fasting plasma glucose correlates with severity of diabetes and the occurrence of complications.
- Explain why urinary glucose is not a good marker for diabetes.
- What approaches can the person with diabetes use to minimize the acute and long-term complications of the disease?
- Explain how Hb A1c is produced, and how it is used to monitor diabetes.
- Explain how blood plasma insulin levels can be used to determine which type of diabetes an individual possesses.
- Explain the effects of DKA and HHNC on the following factors: keto acids, urinary protein levels, lactic acid, pH, osmolality, body fluid volume, anion gap, BUN, and lipids.
- Describe the effect of insulin on the transport of potassium.
- Explain the effects of DKA and HHNC on plasma sodium.
- Explain the effects of type 1 and type 2 diabetes on plasma potassium.

CHANGE OF ANALYTE IN DISEASE

The following is a summary of analyte changes in DM. For each analyte, levels in controlled diabetes, diabetic ketoacidosis, and HHNC are compared.

Fasting Plasma Glucose

The criteria for diagnosis of DM have been adjusted recently by the Expert Committee.[72] An individual who has symptoms of diabetes (polyuria, polydipsia, unexplained weight loss) and causal plasma glucose levels equal to or greater than 200 mg/dL is a candidate for diabetes. *Causal* is defined as occurring any time of day independent of time since the last meal. If this individual's symptoms are confirmed on a subsequent day, the individual would be diagnosed as having diabetes. Repeated fasting plasma glucose levels greater than 126 mg/dL are strongly suggestive of diabetes, provided that drugs such as glucocorticoids are not being administered, and diseases and conditions such as those listed in Box 38-2 are not present. Values from 100 to 126 mg/dL are suggestive of impaired fasting glucose.

Fasting plasma glucose is directly proportional to the severity of DM. As with the OGTT, results greater than the upper range of normal (99 mg/dL), coincide with a dramatic increase in incidence of retinopathy, nephropathy, and fatal coronary heart disease.[68] Blood glucose levels above 180 mg/dL may produce glucosuria. Ketoacidosis can occur at almost any level above 140 mg/dL but is more common at levels above 180 mg/dL. HHNC is associated with glucose levels above 600 mg/dL.

Persons with diabetes who are under control exhibit wide variation in their plasma glucose concentrations. Plasma glucose levels in those with controlled diabetes range during a typical 24-hour period from as low as 250 mg/dL to as high as 325 mg/dL. These variations are considerably wider than those of nondiabetic individuals.[80] Wide swings in plasma glucose contribute to the development of diabetic complications. Management of insulin therapy remains a significant challenge for the physician. Excessive quantities of insulin cause insulin-induced hypoglycemia, which often leads to coma. On the other hand, inadequate control of glucose levels

Box 38-2

Conditions and Diseases that Often Cause Both Hyperglycemia and Glucosuria or Glycosuria in the Absence of Hyperglycemia

Hyperglycemia and Glucosuria
Septicemia
Hypercortisolism
Pancreatic cancer
Glucagonoma
Acute pancreatitis
Somatostatinoma
Pheochromocytoma
Primary aldosteronism
Hyperthyroidism
Acute myocardial infarction
Acromegaly
Cerebral hemorrhage

Glucosuria and Normal Plasma Glucose
Pregnancy (renal threshold is reduced)
Vitamin D–resistant rickets
Osteomalacia (proximal tubular malfunction)
Hepatolenticular degeneration

causes diabetic complications such as those described earlier. Generally, fasting plasma glucose in diabetics is maintained at normal or slightly above normal concentrations.

Urinary Glucose

Urinary glucose is a poor marker for DM. The normal renal threshold for glucose is 180 mg/dL. Blood glucose levels must exceed this value before excessive glucose is apparent in the urine. Further complicating this picture is the fact that the renal threshold in persons with diabetes often is increased to above 300 mg/dL. Some diseases and conditions that produce both hyperglycemia and glucosuria are listed in Box 38-2. This box also lists conditions that cause glucosuria in the absence of hyperglycemia.

Self-Monitoring and Bedside Monitoring of Blood Glucose[81]

The goal of therapy for patients with diabetes is to maintain normal levels of glucose, so as to minimize acute and long-term complications of the disease. Aggressive therapy to achieve this goal has the primary side effect of an increased risk for hypoglycemia (see earlier discussion). However, close monitoring of blood glucose levels has been aided by the development of increasingly accurate and reliable bedside glucose monitors, for use in hospitals or by the patient (see Chapter 21). Self-monitoring programs now are considered standard treatment for those with diabetes, including pregnant women; patients with unstable diabetes; those with a history of severe ketosis or hypoglycemia, especially those who do not demonstrate warning symptoms of hypoglycemia; patients receiving intensive insulin therapy; and those with abnormal renal thresholds for glucose. Correct use of such devices should minimize the wide variations in blood glucose experienced by persons with diabetes and, as a result, the hypoglycemic events and even long-term complications of diabetes.

Glycated Hemoglobin[82-89]

A minor hemoglobin derivative called *Hb A1c* is produced by glycation, the covalent binding of glucose to hemoglobin. Because this reaction is nonenzymatic, and because the red cell is completely permeable to glucose, the quantity of Hb A1c formed is directly proportional to the average plasma glucose concentration that the red blood cell is exposed to during its 120-day life span, that is, the 4 to 6 weeks before sampling. Thus, in long-term hyperglycemia, Hb A1c constitutes a higher percentage of total hemoglobin than in normoglycemia. Transient elevations in plasma glucose only mildly affect Hb A1c levels.

Total glycated hemoglobin, Hb A1, actually consists of four principal components, called Hb A1a1, Hb A1a2, Hb A1b, and Hb A1c.[82] Each component consists of two parts: a labile component, which is an aldimine, and a stable component, which is a ketamine. For normoglycemic persons, Hb A1a1, Hb A1a2, and Hb A1b constitute 0.4% to 0.8% of total hemoglobin. Hb A1c constitutes 4% to 5% of total hemoglobin. Total Hb A1 is normally 5.0% to 7.0% (see Methods on Evolve). Diabetic persons have total Hb A1 and Hb A1c percentages that are significantly elevated. These elevations are directly proportional to the long-term degree of hyperglycemia.[83]

The DCCT[86] demonstrated that patients with type 1 diabetes reduced their risk of development or progression of retinopathy, nephropathy, and neuropathy by 50% to 70% by maintaining their average Hb A1c at 7.2%, as compared with diabetic individuals, who maintained their values at an average of 9.0%. In addition, the reduction in risk for these complications progressively decreased with decreased levels of Hb A1c, suggesting that if nondiabetic levels Hb A1c were achieved, the risk of complications would approach that of the nondiabetic population, with a reference interval of 4.0% to 6.0%. When Hb A1c levels are kept below 8%, the risk of developing an early sign of diabetic nephropathy, microalbuminuria (see later discussion), is greatly reduced.[87] Although measurements of glycosylated hemoglobins are recommended for the monitoring of diabetes, they are not sufficiently sensitive to effectively detect borderline cases of DM.[88] The American Diabetes Association recommends fasting plasma glucose of <99 mg/dL and Hb A1c of less than 7% as goals for treatment.[89] Hb A1c is currently the measurement of choice in monitoring the treatment of diabetes.[71]

Insulin

Fasting plasma insulin levels in type 1 diabetes are usually low. Those in type 2 diabetes are low only when fasting plasma glucose levels exceed 250 mg/dL. Otherwise, they are normal or even elevated.[90] A glucose challenge with insulin measurement separates type 1 diabetic persons from those with type 2 diabetes. Glucose loading elicits no significant insulin response for type 1 diabetes, and a delayed, often exaggerated response in type 2 diabetes.

Keto Acids

Significant elevations of acetoacetate and β-hydroxybutyrate cause diabetic ketoacidosis. It is important to measure both blood and urinary keto acid levels, because plasma keto acid levels can be normal even though urinary keto acid concentrations are high. This effect is caused by increased urinary keto acid excretion resulting from renal compensation to low pH. Both ketonemia and ketonuria are absent in HHNC. Persons with controlled diabetes should have both normal plasma and normal urinary keto acid levels.

The nitroprusside test (commonly known as Acetest) is useful for the detection of acetoacetic acid (AcAc) in the blood or urine. Nitroprusside does not react with β-hydroxybutyrate (β-HBA) and reacts only weakly (20%) with acetone. In the early stages of diabetic ketoacidosis, acetoacetate levels often are normal (AcAc:β-HBA, 1:3) or only mildly elevated. In later stages of ketoacidosis, β-hydroxybutyrate levels are highly elevated (AcAc:β-HBA, 1:30). Under these conditions, the nitroprusside test can significantly produce an underestimation of the severity of ketoacidosis. As ketoacidosis becomes controlled, the β-hydroxybutyrate is metabolized to acetoacetic acid, and the nitroprusside test can become strongly positive.

Urinary Protein[91-94]

One of the earliest signs of impending glomerular nephropathy is increased excretion of albumin in the urine, also termed *microalbuminuria.* Monitoring patients with diabetes for microalbuminuria is now standard practice, so the glomerular disease complication of diabetes can be treated early and prevented (see Chapter 30). Determination of the urine albumin/creatinine ratio on a random urine sample is an effective screening test.[93] *Microalbuminuria* is defined as an albumin/creatinine ratio equal to or greater than 20 to 30 mg/g.[94]

Lactic Acid

Plasma lactic acid levels frequently are elevated (lactic acidosis) during DKA.

Hydrogen Ion (pH)

High plasma hydrogen ion concentrations (low pH) occur in DKA and ketoacidosis with lactic acidosis. A pH level below 7.00 is associated with a poor prognosis.

Electrolytes

Uncontrolled diabetics can exhibit normal, low, or high plasma sodium levels. Plasma sodium levels in diabetics are influenced by three factors, which are described next.

Hyperglycemia causes an increase in the osmotic pressure of plasma. As a result, water flows from cells to plasma. Plasma substituents are thereby diluted. Thus hyponatremia and hypokalemia are promoted in diabetes. In diabetic ketoacidosis, excessive quantities of sodium are excreted in the urine, further lowering plasma sodium levels. However, complicating matters is the preferential excretion of water relative to sodium. This effect often compensates for sodium loss from high plasma glucose levels and ketosis, thus resulting in normal or even elevated plasma sodium levels.

For potassium, three factors are operative. First, the same urinary losses of potassium are true as in the case of sodium. Second, insulin causes the transport of plasma potassium into cells. Thus hyperkalemia should occur in insulin deficiency (type 1 diabetes). Third, in acidosis, potassium moves out of cells. Thus in DKA, significant quantities of potassium ion are shifted from cells to plasma. For type 1 diabetics, this accentuates the hyperkalemia. On the other hand, type 2 diabetics who have elevated insulin levels normally exhibit hypokalemia or normokalemia. Hypokalemia often occurs in diabetics who are treated with insulin because of the second factor described above. Excessive urinary losses of potassium in diabetics in DKA always require potassium replacement and monitoring during therapy.

Plasma bicarbonate levels are normal in controlled diabetes. Ketoacidosis causes low plasma bicarbonate levels. The body responds to ketoacidosis by kidney retention of bicarbonate and rapid, deep respirations called *Kussmaul breathing,* which remove CO_2. Both of these compensatory mechanisms raise pH. Kussmaul breathing lowers P_{CO_2}. Both plasma bicarbonate and P_{CO_2} are low in DKA.

Osmolality

Serum osmolality is increased in both ketoacidosis and HHNC because of the water loss that accompanies glucose excretion. Serum osmolality in HHNC is usually above 350 mOsm/kg—a hallmark of the condition.

Body Fluid Volume

Renal loss of water in DKA produces severe volume depletion, often as much as 6 to 8 L. Patients with HHNC can have fluid deficits greater than 9 L. Low fluid volume (hypovolemia) often coexists with hyponatremia. Insulin therapy restores both fluid volume and plasma sodium to normal.

Anion Gap

In ketoacidosis, the anion gap is always increased because of excessive formation of sodium salts of keto acids. Lactic acidosis further increases the gap caused by high lactate levels.

Blood Urea Nitrogen (BUN)

BUN levels are increased in both DKA and HHNC because of increased protein catabolism and prerenal azotemia secondary to loss of extracellular fluids. Prerenal azotemia refers to increased BUN caused by decreased renal blood flow. In DKA, prerenal azotemia is also caused by hypovolemia.

Lipids

Elevated plasma triglycerides, cholesterol, and VLDL are commonly found in persons with diabetes. On the other hand, HDL cholesterol levels are usually low.

KEY CONCEPTS BOX 38-8

- Fasting plasma glucose is the principal marker for the diagnosis of diabetes.
- In addition, fasting blood plasma glucose is directly proportional to the severity of diabetes and is a good predictor of complications.
- Urinary glucose is a poor marker for diabetes because of its lack of specificiaty for diabetes.
- Self-monitoring and bedside monitoring of glucose levels have become prevalent as accurate and easy to use portable glucose instruments have become available.
- In DKA and HHNC, the following analytes are usually abnormal:
  - Glucose, lactic acid, osmolality, anion gap, BUN, lipids are elevated.
  - In DKA and HHNC, body fluid volume is low.
  - In DKA ketones and keto acids will be elevated and pH low.
- Several factors affect sodium and potassium levels in persons with diabetes. These include the following:
  - Increased osmotic pressure leading to excessive urinary excretion of sodium and potassium
  - Insulin transports potassium from plasma into cells. In acidosis, potassium is transported from cells to plasma. Insulin treatment results in electrolyte loss from plasma.

SECTION OBJECTIVES BOX 38-9

- Explain why screening for diabetes remains controversial.
- Describe the modalities of diabetes treatment that hold promise for the future.
- Describe how derivatives of the incretins are used for the control of diabetes.

SCREENING

Although screening for gestational diabetes mellitus (GDM) has become routine (see Chapter 44), the best approach to screening for type 1 and 2 DM remains controversial. The American Diabetes Association suggests that all individuals aged 45 years or older be screened every three years. In addition, those identified at risk for diabetes younger than 45 years of age should also be screened every three years.[95] OGTT is the reference standard for diagnosing diabetes but is not cost-effective as a screening tool. Hb A1c and fasting plasma glucose (FPG) are equally effective in screening for type 2 diabetes, but they have low sensitivity (about 50%) for the diagnosis of IGT.[96,97] Early detection of IGT and impaired fasting glycemia (IFG) would reduce the number of individuals who progress to type 2 diabetes but would require the OGTT.[98] A screening system for genetic risk factors of type 1 diabetes appears on the horizon. One method[99] uses dried blood spots from neonates. Early detection of the genetic propensity to type 1 diabetes could lead to new immunotherapies that would be effective in preventing the disease.[100]

TREATMENT

Type 1 Diabetes Mellitus

As was reported earlier, autoimmune destruction of β-islet cells is the usual cause of type 1 diabetes. Thus numerous studies have explored islet cell transplantation,[101] pancreatic transplantation,[102] islet cell regeneration,[103] and insulin gene therapy.[104] Although progress is being observed in each of these modalities, a cure for or the prevention of type 1 diabetes is not imminent.[105] The principal problem with these therapies is the need to turn off the immune response that led to the destruction of β-islet cells in the first place. The treatment of choice remains injectable insulin. Long-acting insulin derivatives such as detemir[106] and glargine[107] have been developed and are presently in use. Inhaled insulin was approved by the U.S. Food and Drug Administration (FDA) in 2006 under the market name, Exubera.[108] Progress continues in insulin pump therapy.[109] Insulin pump therapy reduces the complication of hypoglycemia and avoids the inconvenience of insulin injections.

Type 2 Diabetes Mellitus

Depending on the severity of the type 2 diabetes, therapies vary from lifestyle changes, such as weight loss, to the use of pharmaceutical hypoglycemic agents, to insulin replacement. Individuals with type 2 diabetes start out with normal β-islet cells. As the disease progresses, overworked β-islet cells decrease in number, and the disease becomes more severe and similar to type 1 diabetes. Drugs that augment insulin secretion are presently available for persons with type 2 diabetes.[110] Two types of biopharmacological agents have been approved for use in humans. The first type is GLP-1 itself (see incretin hormones, p. 738) or a derivative that mimics the binding of GLP-1 to its receptor site. The second type is a pharmacological agent that inhibits dipeptidyl peptidase-IV (DPP-IV), the enzyme that destroys incretins.[111] Approved for marketing by the FDA in 2005, Byetta (exenatide) is a compound that was first extracted from Gila monster saliva. It is an analog of GLP-1 that effectively enhances the secretion of insulin by binding to the receptor for GLP-1. Januvia (sitagliptin)[112] is an inhibitor of DPP-IV that increases the concentration of GLP-1, leading to increased insulin secretion. Added benefits resulting from increased GLP-1 levels include inhibition of glucagon secretion, which decreases glucose release from the liver, delayed stomach emptying, which spreads glucose absorption over an increased length of time, and promotion of satiety, which leads to weight loss.[113]

KEY CONCEPTS BOX 38-9

- Screening for gestational diabetes has become routine.
- Screening for type 1 and 2 diabetes remains controversial.
- The objective in curing type 1 diabetes is some means of turning off the immune response.
- Although injectable insulin is used most generally for treatment of type 1 diabetes, long-acting insulin, inhalable insulin, and insulin pumps are also in use.
- For type 2 diabetes, analogs of the incretins are becoming useful.

REFERENCES

1. National Center for Chronic Disease Prevention and Health Promotion: Diabetes public health report, data and trends, prevalence of diabetes, National Diabetes Surveillance System, 2007, Atlanta, GA. Available at www.cdc.gov/diabetes/statistics/prev/national/index.htm. Accessed July 2007.
2. Mainous AG 3rd, Baker AR, Koopman RJ, et al: Impact of the population at risk of diabetes on projections of diabetes burden in the United States: an epidemic on the way, Diabetologia 50:934, 2007.
3. Engelgau MM, Geiss LS, Saaddine JB, et al: The evolving diabetes burden in the United States, Ann Intern Med 140:945, 2004.
4. Mokdad AH, Bowman BA, Ford ES, et al: The continuing epidemics of obesity and diabetes in the United States, JAMA 286:1195, 2001.
5. Centers for Disease Control and Prevention: Prevalence of diabetes and impaired fasting glucose in adults—United States, 1999-2000, MMWR Wkly 52(35):833, 2003. Available at www.cdc.gov/mmwr/preview/mmwrhtml/mm5235a1.htm. Accessed July 2007.
6. National Center for Health Statistics: Deaths: final data for 2005, Table C, compiled in 2008. Available at http://www.cdc.gov/nchs/fastats/lcod.htm. Accessed May 17, 2008.

7. The World Health Organization: Diabetes, fact sheets, 2006, Geneva, Switzerland. Available at www.who.int/mediacentre/factsheets/fs312/en/index.html. Accessed July 10, 2007.
8. Qiao Q, Gao W, Zhang L, et al: Metabolic syndrome and cardiovascular disease, Ann Clin Biochem 44(Pt 3):232, 2007.
9. Gogia A, Agarwal PK: Metabolic syndrome, Indian J Med Sci 60:72, 2006.
10. American Heart Association: Metabolic syndrome. Available at www.americanheart.org/presenter.jhtml?identifer=4756. Accessed July 13, 2007.
11. Pessen JE, Saltiel AR: Signaling pathways in insulin action: molecular targets of insulin resistance, J Clin Invest 106:165, 2000.
12. Farese RV, Sajan MP, Standaert ML: Insulin-sensitive protein kinases (atypical protein kinase C and protein kinase B/Akt): actions and defects in obesity and type II diabetes, Exp Biol Med (Maywood) 230:593, 2005.
13. Schinner S, Scherbaum WA, Bornstein SR, et al: Molecular mechanisms of insulin resistance, Diabet Med 22:674, 2005.
14. Froguel P, Zouali H, Vionnet N, et al: Familial hyperglycemia due to mutations in glucokinase, N Engl J Med 328:697, 1993.
15. Cryer PE, Gerich JE: Glucose counterregulation, hypoglycemia, and intensive insulin therapy in diabetes mellitus, N Engl J Med 131:232, 1985.
16. Chan SJ, Keim P, Steiner DF: Cell-free synthesis of rat preproinsulin: characterization and partial amino acid sequence determination, Proc Natl Acad Sci USA 73:1964, 1976.
17. Unger RH, Orci L: Glucagon and the A cell, N Engl J Med 304:1518, 1981.
18. Hartmann H, Probst I, Jungermann K, et al: Inhibition of glycogenolysis and glycogen phosphorylase by insulin and proinsulin in rat hepatocyte cultures, Diabetes 36:551, 1987.
19. Vilbel T, Holst JJ: Incretins, insulin secretion and type 2 diabetes mellitus, Diabetologia 47:357, 2004.
20. Dinneen S, Gerich J, Rizza R: Carbohydrate metabolism in non–insulin-dependent diabetes mellitus, N Engl J Med 327:707, 1992.
21. National Diabetes Data Group: Classification and diagnosis of diabetes mellitus and other categories of glucose intolerance, Diabetes 28:1039, 1979.
22. Centers for Disease Control and Prevention: Prevalence of diagnosed diabetes in people aged 20 years or younger, National Diabetes Fact Sheet, United States, 2005. Available at www.cdc.gov/diabetes/pubs/estimates05.htm#prev2_on. Accessed August 2007.
23. Zimmet P, Alberti G, Kaufman F, et al: The metabolic syndrome in children and adolescents, The Lancet 369:2059, 2007.
24. Edelstein SL, Knowler WC, Bain RP, et al: Predictors of progression from impaired glucose tolerance to NIDDM: an analysis of six prospective studies, Diabetes 46:701, 1997.
25. Weiss R, Dufour S, Taksali SE, et al: Prediabetes in obese youth: a syndrome of impaired glucose tolerance, severe insulin resistance, and altered myocellular and abdominal fat partitioning, Lancet 362:951, 2003.
26. Engelgau MM, Herman WH, Smith PJ, et al: The epidemiology of diabetes and pregnancy in the U.S., Diabetes Care 18:1029, 1995.
27. Kim C, Newton KM, Knopp RH: Gestational diabetes and the incidence of type 2 diabetes: a systematic review, Diabetes Care 25:1862, 2002.
28. Atkinson MA, Maclaren NK: The pathogenesis of insulin-dependent diabetes mellitus, N Engl J Med 331:1428, 1994.
29. Krolewski AS, Warram JH, Rand LI, et al: Epidemiologic approach to the etiology of type 1 diabetes mellitus and its complications, N Engl J Med 317:1390, 1987.
30. Saxena R, Voight BF, Lyssenko V, et al: Genome-wide association analysis identifies loci for type 2 diabetes and triglyceride levels, Science 316:1331, 2007.
31. Zeggini E, Weedon MN, Lindgren CM, et al: Replication of genome-wide association signals in UK samples reveals risk loci for type 2 diabetes, Science 316:1336, 2007.
32. Diabetes Genetics Initiative of Broad Institute of Harvard and MIT, Lund University, and Novartis Institutes for Biomedical Research: Genome-wide association analysis identifies loci for type 2 diabetes and triglyceride levels, Science 316:1331, 2007.
33. Scott LJ, Mohlke KL, Bonnycastle LL, et al: A genome-wide association study of type 2 diabetes in Finns detects multiple susceptibility variants, Science 316:1341, 2007.
34. Lazar M: How obesity causes diabetes: not a tall tale, Science 307:373, 2005.
35. Youngren JF: Regulation of insulin receptor function, Cell Mol Life Sci 64:873, 2007.
36. Drazin B: Molecular mechanisms of insulin resistance: serine phosphorylation of insulin receptor substrate-1 and increased expression of p85alpha: the two sides of a coin, Diabetes 55: 2392, 2006.
37. Peterson K, Shulman G: Etiology of insulin resistance, Am J Med 119:10S, 2006.
38. Rhodes CJ: Type 2 diabetes—a matter of β-cell life and death, Science 307:380, 2005.
39. Jahromi MM, Eisenbarth GS: Cellular and molecular pathogenesis of type 1A diabetes, Cell Mol Life Sci 64:865, 2007.
40. Baisch JM, Weeks T, Giles R, et al: Analysis of HLA-DQ genotypes and susceptibility in insulin-dependent diabetes mellitus, N Engl J Med 322:1836, 1990.
41. Khalil I, d'Auriol L, Gobet M, et al: A combination of HLA DQ beta Asp 57-negative and HLA DQ alpha Arg 52 confers susceptibility to insulin-dependent diabetes mellitus, J Clin Invest 85:1315, 1990.
42. Hagopian WA, Sanjeevi CB, Kockum I, et al: Glutamate decarboxylase-, insulin- and islet cell-antibodies and HLA typing to detect diabetes in a general population-based study of Swedish children, J Clin Invest 95:1505, 1995.
43. The Expert Committee on the Diagnosis and Classification of Diabetes Mellitus: Report of the Expert Committee on the Diagnosis and Classification of Diabetes Mellitus. In American Diabetes Association: Clinical practice recommendations 2001, Diabetes Care 24(suppl 1):S5, 2001.
44. DiLorenzo TP, Roep BO, Peakman M, et al: Translational mini-review series on type 1 diabetes: systematic analysis of T cell epitopes in autoimmune diabetes, Clin Exp Immunol 148:1, 2007.
45. Mallone R, Martinuzzi E, Blancou P, et al: CD8+ T-cell responses identify beta-cell autoimmunity in human type 1 diabetes, Diabetes 56:613, 2007.
46. McFarlane J: A new look at viruses in type 1 diabetes, Diabetes Metab Res Rev 19:8, 2003.
47. Jones DB, Armstrong NW: Coxsackie virus and diabetes revisited, Nat Med 1:284, 1995.
48. Gupta M, Nikitina-Zake L, Landin-Olsson M, et al: Coxsackie virus B antibodies are increased in HLA DR3-MICA5.1 positive type 1 diabetes patients in the Linkoping region of Sweden, Hum Immunol 64:874, 2003.
49. Craighead JE: Does insulin dependent diabetes mellitus have a viral etiology? Hum Pathol 10:267, 1979.
50. U.S. Renal Data System (USRDS): Annual data report: atlas of end-stage renal disease in the United States, Bethesda, MD, 2001. National Institutes of Diabetes and Digestive and Kidney Disease. Available at http://www. cdc.gov/diabetes/pubs/estimates05.htm.
51. The Diabetes Control and Complications Trial Research Group: The effect of intensive diabetes therapy on the development and progression of nephropathy, Kidney Int 47:1703, 1995.
52. O'Brien T, Nguyen TT, Zimmerman BR: Hyperlipidemia and diabetes mellitus, Mayo Clin Proc 73:969, 1998.

53. Betteridge DJ: Diabetic dyslipidemia, Diabetes Obes Metab 2(suppl 1):S31, 2000.
54. Krolewski AS, Warram JH, Valsania P, et al: Evolving natural history of coronary artery disease in diabetes mellitus, Am J Med 90(suppl 2A):2A, 1991. Available at http://www. cdc.gov/diabetes/pubs/estimates05.htm.
55. Zierler KL, Rabinowitz D: Effect of very small concentrations of insulin on forearm metabolism: persistence of its action on potassium and free fatty acids without its effect on glucose, J Clin Invest 43:950, 1964.
56. Polonsky KS: A practical approach to fasting hypoglycemia, N Engl J Med 326:1020, 1992 (editorial).
57. Fischer KF, Lees JH, Newman JH: Hypoglycemia in hospitalized patients, N Engl J Med 315:1245, 1986.
58. Jovanoic J: The diabetic pregnancy: a clinical challenge. Symposium of the Diabetes and Pregnancy Council, 60th Scientific Sessions of the American Diabetes Association, Day 2, June 11, 2000.
59. Fetita LS, Sobnqwi E, Serradas P, et al: Consequences of fetal exposure to maternal diabetes in offspring, J Clin Endocrinol Metab 91:3718, 2006.
60. Hillier TA, Pedula KL, Schmidt MM, et al: Childhood obesity and metabolic imprinting: the ongoing effects of maternal hyperglycemia, Diabetes Care 30:2287, 2007.
61. Ahmed N, Thornalley PJ: Advanced glycation end products: what is their relevance to diabetic complications? Diabetes Obes Metab 9:233, 2007.
62. Peppa M, Uribarri J, Vlassara H: Glucose, advanced glycation end products, and diabetes complications: what is new and what works, Clin Diabetes 21:186, 2003.
63. Cerami A, Stevens VJ, Montier VM: Role of nonenzymatic glycosylation in the development of the sequelae of diabetes mellitus, Metabolism 28:431, 1979.
64. Bohlender JM, Franke S, Stein G, et al: Advanced glycation end products and the kidney, Am J Physiol Renal Physiol 289:F645, 2005.
65. Chiasson JL, Aris-Jilwan N, Belanger R, et al: Diagnosis and treatment of diabetic ketoacidosis and the hyperglycemic hyperosmolar state, CMAJ 168:859, 2003.
66. Notvest RR, Inserra JJ: Tolrestat, an aldose reductase inhibitor, prevents nerve dysfunction in conscious diabetic rats, Diabetes 36:500, 1987.
67. Report of the Expert Committee on the Diagnosis and Classification of Diabetes Mellitus, Diabetes Care 20:1183, 1997.
68. Report of the Committee on Statistics of the American Diabetes Association: Standardization of the oral glucose tolerance test, Diabetes 18:299, 1969.
69. Davidson MB: The effect of aging on carbohydrate metabolism: a review of the English literature and a practical approach to the diagnosis of diabetes mellitus in the elderly, Metabolism 28:688, 1979
70. Harris MI, Hadden WC, Knowler WC, et al: International criteria for the diagnosis of diabetes and impaired glucose tolerance, Diabetes Care 8:562, 1985.
71. Report of the Expert Committee on the Diagnosis and Classification of Diabetes Mellitus, Diabetes Care 26:S5, 2003.
72. Expert Committee on the Diagnosis and Classification of Diabetes Mellitus: Follow-up report on the diagnosis of diabetes mellitus, Diabetes Care 26:3160, 2003.
73. Meltzer S, Leiter L, Daneman D, et al: Clinical practice guidelines for the management of diabetes in Canada, Canadian Diabetes Association. CMAJ 159(suppl 8):S1, 1998.
74. Stolk RP, Orchard TJ, Grobbee DE: Why use the oral glucose tolerance test? Diabetes Care 18:1045, 1995.
75. The DECODE Study Group on behalf of the European Diabetes Epidemiology Group: Is fasting glucose sufficient to define diabetes? Epidemiological data from 20 European studies, Diabetologia 42:647, 1999.
76. Shaw JE, de Courten M, Boyko EJ, et al: Impact of new diagnostic criteria for diabetes on different populations, Diabetes Care 22:762, 1999.
77. Metzger BE, editor: Proceedings of the Third International Workshop-Conference on Gestational Diabetes Mellitus, Diabetes 40(suppl 2):1, 1991.
78. Carpenter MW, Coustan DR: Criteria for screening tests for gestational diabetes, Am J Obstet Gynecol 144:768, 1982.
79. Metzger BE, Coustan DR: Summary and recommendations of the Fourth International Workshop-Conference on Gestational Diabetes Mellitus, Diabetes Care 21(suppl 2):B161, 1998.
80. Mauer AC: The therapy of diabetes, Am Scientist 67:422, 1979.
81. Consensus Development Panel: Consensus statement on self-monitoring of blood glucose, Diabetes Care 10:95, 1987.
82. Gonen B, Rochman H, Rubenstein AH: Metabolic control in diabetic patients: assessment by hemoglobin A1 values, Metabolism 28:448, 1979.
83. Larsen ML, Horder MN, Mogensen EF: Effect of long-term monitoring of glycosylated hemoglobin levels in insulin diabetes mellitus, N Engl J Med 323:1021, 1990.
84. Bry L, Chen PC, Sachs DB: Effect of hemoglobin variants and chemically modified derivatives on assays for glycohemoglobin, Clin Chem 47:153, 2001.
85. American Diabetes Association: Position statement: Tests of glycemia in diabetes, Diabetes Care 26:S106, 2003.
86. American Diabetes Association: Position statement: Standards of medical care for patients with diabetes mellitus, Diabetes Care 21:S23, 1998.
87. Krolewski AS, Laffel LM, Krolewski M, et al: Glycosylated hemoglobin and the risk of microalbuminuria in patients with insulin-dependent diabetes mellitus, N Engl J Med 332:1251, 1995.
88. Dods RF, Bolmey C: Glycosylated hemoglobin assay and oral glucose tolerance test compared for detection of diabetes mellitus, Clin Chem 25:764, 1979.
89. American Diabetes Association: Position statement: Standards of medical care for patients with diabetes mellitus, Diabetes Care 24(suppl 1):S33, 2001.
90. Ward WK, Beard JC, Halter JB, et al: Pathophysiology of insulin secretion in non–insulin-dependent diabetes mellitus, Diabetes Care 7:491, 1984.
91. Hawthorne V, Herman WH, editors: International symposium on preventing the kidney disease of diabetes mellitus: public health perspectives, Am J Kidney Dis 13:2, 1989.
92. American Diabetes Association: Position statement: Standards of medical care for patients with diabetes mellitus, Diabetes Care 17:616, 1994.
93. Nelson RG, Knowler WC, Pettitt DJ, et al: Assessment of risk of overt nephropathy in diabetic patients from albumin excretion in untimed urines, Arch Intern Med 151:1761, 1991.
94. Emancipator K: Laboratory diagnosis and monitoring of diabetes mellitus, Am J Clin Pathol 112:665, 1999.
95. American Diabetes Association: Position statement: Screening for diabetes, Diabetes Care 24(suppl 1):S21, 2001.
96. Bennett CM, Guo M, Dharmage SC: HbA(1c) as a screening tool for detection of Type 2 diabetes: a systematic review, Diabet Med 24:333, 2007.
97. Simmons D, Thompson CF, Engelgau MM: Controlling the diabetes epidemic: how should we screen for undiagnosed diabetes and dysglycaemia? Diabet Med 22:207, 2005.
98. Waugh N, Scotland G, McNamee P, et al: Screening for type 2 diabetes: literature review and economic modeling, Health Technol Assess 11:iii-iv, ix-xi, 1-125, 2007.
99. Dantonio P, Meredith N, Earley M, et al: A screening system for detecting genetic risk markers of type 1 diabetes in dried blood spots, Diabetes Technol Ther 8:433, 2006.

100. Cernea S, Herold KC: Drug insight: new immunomodulatory therapies in type 1 diabetes, Nat Clin Pract Endocrinol Metab 2:89, 2006.
101. Kaestner KH: Beta cell transplantation and immunosuppression: can't live with it, can't live without it, J Clin Invest 117:2380, 2007.
102. Sutherland DE, Gruessner RW, Dunn DL, et al.: Lessons learned from more than 1,000 pancreas transplants at a single institution, Ann Surg 233:463, 2001.
103. Couri CE, Foss MC, Voltarelli JC: Secondary prevention of type 1 diabetes mellitus: stopping immune destruction and promoting beta cell regeneration, Braz J Med Biol Res 39:1271, 2006.
104. Yoon JW, Jun HS: Recent advances in insulin gene therapy for type 1 diabetes, Trends Mol Med 8:62, 2002.
105. Yoon JW, Jun HS: Approaches for the cure of type 1 diabetes by cellular and gene therapy, Curr Gene Ther 5:249, 2005.
106. Pavlić-Renar I, Prašek M, Djojić M, et al: Insulin detemir—a novel basal insulin, Diabetologia Croatica 32:163, 2003.
107. Barrio Castellanos R: Long-acting insulin analogues (insulin glargine or detemir) and continuous subcutaneous insulin infusion in the treatment of type 1 diabetes mellitus in the paediatric population, JPEM 18:1173, 2005.
108. Pham DQ, Cohen H, Chu V: Inhaled human (rDNA origin) insulin, a novel formulation for diabetes mellitus, J Clin Pharmacol 47:890, 2007.
109. Kapellen TM, Heidtmann B, Bachmann J, et al: Indications for insulin pump therapy in different age groups: an analysis of 1567 children and adolescents, Diabet Med 24:836, 2007.
110. Jeha GS, Heptulla RA: Newer therapeutic options for children with diabetes mellitus: theoretical and practical considerations, Pediatr Diabetes 7:122, 2006.
111. Pratley RE, Salsali A: Inhibition of DPP-4: a new therapeutic approach for the treatment of type 2 diabetes, Curr Med Res Opin 23:919, 2007.
112. Herman GA, Stein PP, Thornberry NA, et al: Dipeptidyl peptidase-4 inhibitors for the treatment of type 2 diabetes: focus on sitagliptin, Clin Pharmacol Ther 81:761, 2007.
113. Baggio LL, Drucker DJ: Biology of incretins: GLP-1 and GIP, Gastroenterology 132:2131, 2007.

INTERNET SITES

http://www.bsc.gwu.edu/bsc/studies/dcct.html—A brief summary of the 10-year Diabetes Control and Complications Trial and links pertaining to it

http://www.aafp.org/afp/981015ap/mayfield.html—Diagnosis and classification of diabetes mellitus: new criteria, by J. Mayfield

http://www.diabetes.org—American Diabetes Association

http://www.cdc.gov—Centers for Disease Control and Prevention

http://www.cdc.gov/diabetes/pubs/pdf/ndfs_2005.pdf

http://www.cdc.gov/diabetes/pubs/estimates05.htm#prev2

http://www.who.int/mediacentre/factsheets/fs312/en/index.html

http://americanheart.org/presenter.jhtml?identifer=4756 http://themedicalbiochemistrypage.org/

http://www.ncbi.nlm.nih.gov/entrez/dispomim.cgi?id=125850

http://www.phlaunt.com/diabetes/14047009.php

http://www.cdc.gov/mmwr/preview/mmwrhtml/mm5443a2.htm

http://www.diabetes.org/diabetes-statistics/kidney-disease.jsp

http://emedicine.medscape.com/article/766804-overview Hyperosmolar Hyperglycemic State, by Sergot, PB and Nelson LS. Updated July 22, 2008

Iron and Porphyrin Metabolism

39 Chapter

William E. Schreiber

Chapter Outline

Key Terms

anemia A reduction in the quantity of hemoglobin or the number of red cells in blood.
chelate A chemical compound in which a metallic ion is bound firmly to a chelating molecule.
cutaneous Related to the skin.
erythropoiesis The production of erythrocytes.
hemolytic anemia Anemia caused by shortened survival of mature red blood cells.
HFE Gene that is defective (usually the C282Y mutation) in most cases of hereditary hemochromatosis.
hypochromic Referring to erythrocytes that are paler than normal because of a decrease in hemoglobin content.
mean corpuscular hemoglobin (MCH) The average amount of hemoglobin per red blood cell.
mean corpuscular hemoglobin concentration (MCHC) The average concentration of hemoglobin per red blood cell.
mean corpuscular volume (MCV) The average red blood cell volume.
microcytic Referring to erythrocytes that are smaller than the reference interval.
parenchyma The functional tissue of an organ (excluding the fibrous framework).
photosensitivity Abnormal reactivity of the skin to sunlight.
reticuloendothelial system A functional system composed of highly phagocytic cells with both endothelial and reticular attributes, located in blood vessels, lymph nodes, liver, spleen, bone marrow, and other tissues.
sideroblastic anemia A heterogeneous group of anemias in which iron stores of the reticuloendothelial tissues are increased, and bone marrow normoblasts contain iron deposits within mitochondria (ringed sideroblasts).
tachycardia Rapid heart rate.
thalassemia A heterogeneous group of hereditary hemolytic anemias that have a decreased rate of synthesis of one or more hemoglobin polypeptide chains.

Methods on Evolve

Ferritin
Iron and total iron-binding capacity
Porphobilinogen screening and quantitation
Porphyrins, urine and fecal
Transferrin and carbohydrate-deficient transferrin

SECTION OBJECTIVES BOX 39-1

- List the physiological functions of iron.
- Describe absorption of iron from the gut and its transport and storage in the body.
- Explain the role of blood cell turnover in the metabolism of iron.

PART 1: Iron Metabolism

DISTRIBUTION AND FUNCTION

Iron is one of the most abundant elements on earth, yet only trace amounts are present in living cells. Most of the iron in humans is located within the porphyrin ring of heme, which is incorporated into proteins such as hemoglobin, myoglobin, catalase, peroxidases, and cytochromes. There are also iron-sulfur proteins, such as NADH dehydrogenase and succinate dehydrogenase, in which iron is present in clusters with inorganic sulfur. In all of these proteins, it is the ability of iron to interact reversibly with oxygen and to function in electron transfer reactions that makes it biologically indispensable.

An average adult male has 4 g of body iron. About 65% to 70% of this total is found in hemoglobin, and about 10% is located in myoglobin and other iron-containing enzymes and proteins. The remaining 20% to 25% consists of a storage pool of iron. By comparison, the average adult woman has only 2 to 3 g of iron in her body. This difference is attributable in part to the much smaller iron reserves in women. Less hemoglobin iron is also present; women have a lower hemoglobin concentration in blood and a smaller vascular volume than men. Iron distribution is summarized in Table 39-1.

METABOLISM

Daily requirements for iron vary depending on the person's age, sex, and physiological status. Although iron is not excreted in the conventional sense, about 1 mg is lost daily through the normal shedding of skin epithelial cells and cells that line the gastrointestinal and urinary tracts. Small numbers of erythrocytes are lost in urine and feces as well. Absorption of 1 mg of iron per day is therefore sufficient for men and postmenopausal women. However, the blood lost in each menstrual cycle drains 20 to 40 mg of iron, so women in their reproductive years need to absorb 2 mg of iron per day. Diversion of iron to the growing fetus during pregnancy, blood loss during delivery, and subsequent breast feeding of the infant account for about 1 g of iron. This increases daily iron demands to 3 or 4 mg in pregnant and lactating women.

Table 39-1 Iron Distribution and Function in a Normal Male Adult

Compound	Function	Iron, mg
Hemoglobin	O_2 transport, blood	2500
Myoglobin	O_2 storage, muscle	500
Enzymes		
Catalase	H_2O_2 decomposition	
Peroxidases	Oxidation	
Cytochromes	Electron transfer	
Iron-sulfur*	Electron transfer	
Transferrin*	Iron transport	3
Ferritin* and hemosiderin*	Iron storage	600 to 1000

*Nonheme iron compounds.

Absorption

A healthy North American diet contains between 10 and 20 mg of iron per day. Only 5% to 10% of this amount is absorbed, mainly in the duodenum and the upper small intestine. Most dietary iron is in the ferric (Fe^{3+}) state, but it must be converted to the ferrous (Fe^{2+}) state before it can enter the intestinal cell. A ferric reductase on the brush border of the enterocyte reduces Fe^{3+} to Fe^{2+}, which then is transported into the cell by a divalent metal transporter (DMT1), as is shown

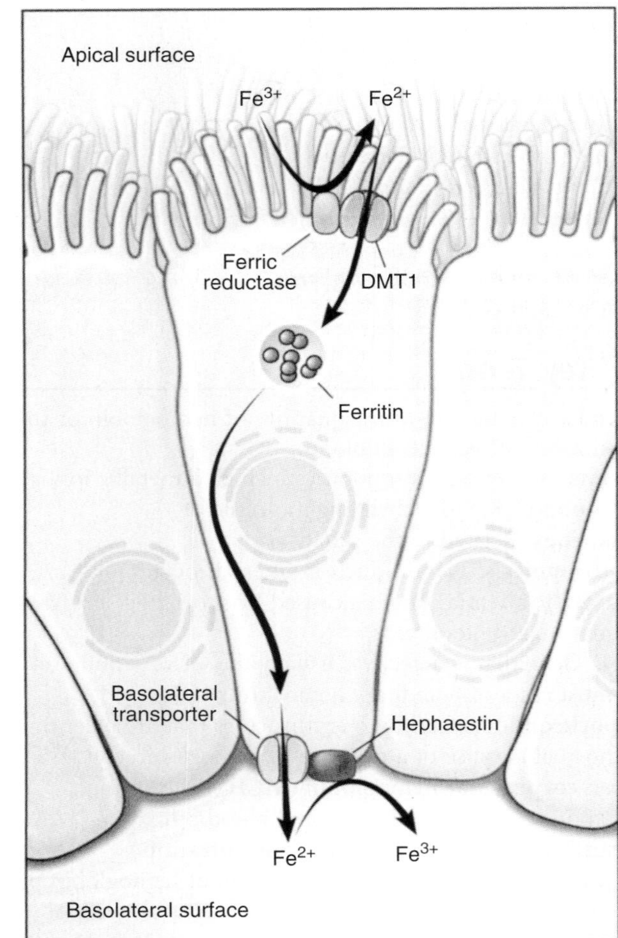

Fig. 39-1 Iron absorption. Dietary iron is reduced from Fe^{3+} to Fe^{2+} at the apical surface of intestinal epithelial cells by a ferric reductase enzyme (known as duodenal cytochrome b, or DcytB). Ferrous iron then is taken into cells by a divalent metal transporter (DMT1). Within the cell, iron may be stored as ferritin, or it may be transported through the basolateral surface to enter the circulation. The basolateral transporter, called *ferroportin,* works in combination with hephaestin, a copper-containing protein that oxidizes Fe^{2+} back to Fe^{3+}. (From Andrews NC: Disorders of iron metabolism, N Engl J Med 341(26):1986, 1999. Copyright © 1999 Massachusetts Medical Society. All rights reserved.)

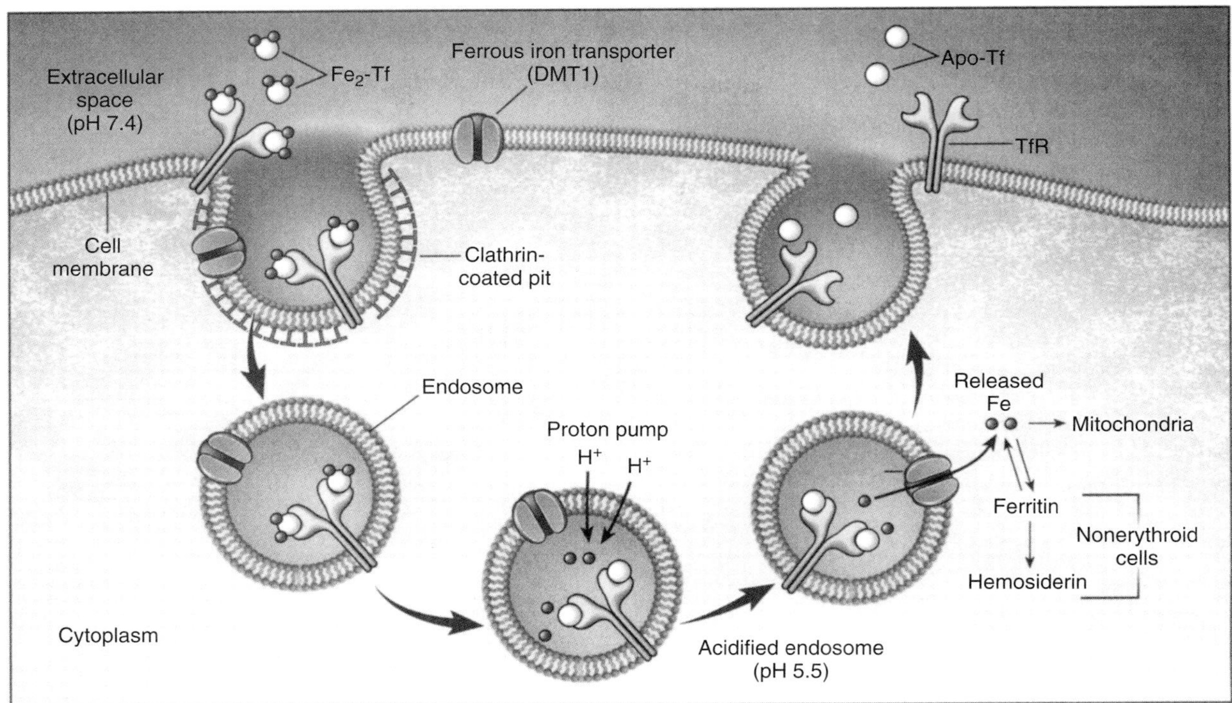

Fig. 39-2 Delivery of iron to cells. Iron-loaded transferrin (Fe_2-Tf) binds to transferrin receptors (TfR) on the cell surface. A portion of the cell membrane then is pinched off to form an endosome, a self-enclosed fragment of the membrane with the Fe_2-Tf-TfR complex inside. Protons (H^+) are pumped into the endosome, releasing iron from transferrin. Iron is transported out of the acidified endosome and into the cytoplasm, where it can enter the mitochondria for heme synthesis or can be stored as ferritin. The endosome then fuses with the cell membrane, and iron-free apotransferrin (Apo-Tf) is released into the extracellular space. (From Andrews NC: Disorders of iron metabolism, N Engl J Med 341(26):1986, 1999. Copyright © 1999 Massachusetts Medical Society. All rights reserved.)

in Fig. 39-1. Gastric acid and dietary components that form soluble iron **chelates** (such as ascorbic acid, sugars, and amino acids) keep ingested iron in solution and increase its absorption. Substances that form insoluble complexes with iron, such as phosphates (in eggs, cheese, and milk), oxalates and phytates (in vegetables), and tannates (in tea), decrease iron absorption. Heme iron, which is derived mainly from meat and fish, is processed differently. After it is released from the surrounding polypeptide chain, heme is absorbed intact by the intestinal cell, where the porphyrin ring is split and iron is liberated. This process is more efficient than the absorption of nonheme iron and is not affected by dietary factors.

Intestinal cells take in considerably more iron than the amount that eventually will enter the circulation. Once inside the intestinal cell, iron is transferred across its basolateral surface into plasma (as reoxidized Fe^{3+}) by the transport protein ferroportin, or it is incorporated into ferritin for storage. Stored intestinal iron subsequently can be mobilized as necessary, but most of this iron is lost when the mucosal cells are shed. New cells take their place, and the cycle of iron buildup starts again.

Red Blood Cell Turnover

Absorbed iron represents only a fraction of the iron required for heme synthesis. Most of the iron, 20 to 25 mg/day, comes from the destruction of old erythrocytes by tissue macrophages, primarily in the spleen. Within these cells, heme oxygenase breaks open the porphyrin ring to release iron. Macrophages transfer most of the iron to plasma transferrin, which then carries it to the bone marrow for hemoglobin synthesis. In this manner, the **reticuloendothelial system** continuously recycles iron from old red cells into new ones.

Macrophages also maintain a storage pool of iron. When red cell destruction exceeds the rate of production, iron accumulates within macrophages, and the storage pool expands. When the balance shifts toward red cell production, macrophages release additional iron from their stores. Infection, inflammation, and malignancy interfere with the release of iron from macrophages and may cause a drop in red cell production, despite the presence of adequate iron reserves.

Transport and Cell Uptake

Free iron is toxic to cells and biomolecules. For this reason, iron is bound to specific proteins during its transport through the body and storage within cells. Transferrin, a single-chain glycoprotein with a molecular weight of 79,500 daltons, is the transport protein for iron in blood. Each transferrin molecule has two binding sites for Fe^{3+} that normally are 20% to 50% saturated. Iron transport is a dynamic process. The circulating iron pool turns over 10 to 20 times per day, so a typical iron atom spends no longer than 2 hours in plasma.

Transferrin delivers iron to cells with specific surface receptors for this protein (Fig. 39-2). After binding to the transferrin receptor, the complex is taken into the cell by endocytosis

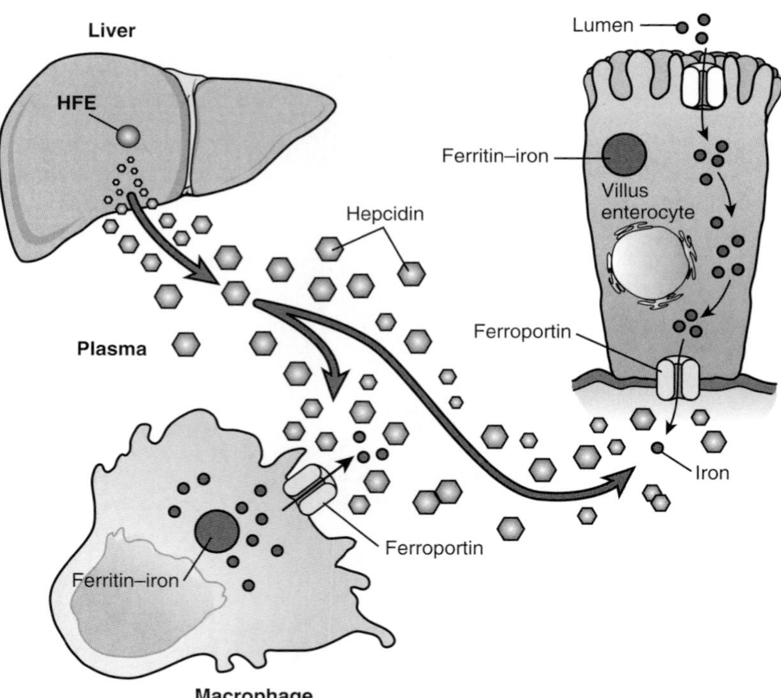

Fig. 39-3 Regulation of iron. Iron may enter the circulation from intestinal cells (absorbed iron) or from macrophages (turnover of red blood cells). Hepcidin, a small polypeptide hormone that regulates the flow of iron from these cells into plasma, is produced in the liver. Several proteins involved in iron metabolism, including HFE, are thought to modulate hepcidin production and release. (From Andrews NC: *Medical Progress: Disorders of Iron Metabolism*. N Engl J Med 350:1986-1995, 1999.)

and is formed into a vesicle. At the acidic pH of the vesicle, iron is released from transferrin. The receptor-transferrin complex then is returned to the cell surface, where both transferrin and the receptor become available for additional rounds of iron transport and uptake. Inside the cell, iron is used for heme synthesis within the mitochondria, or is stored as ferritin.

Storage

Iron is stored in tissue in one of two forms: ferritin or hemosiderin. Ferritin consists of a multi-subunit protein shell, known as *apoferritin,* which surrounds a core of up to 4500 iron atoms. The iron in ferritin is deposited within its core as a ferric hydroxyphosphate complex. Ferritin is present in most cells and is a readily mobilized form of storage iron. It serves to package and isolate iron atoms from the intracellular environment, thus preventing any toxic action on cell constituents. Hemosiderin is an insoluble complex derived from ferritin that has lost some of its surface protein and has become aggregated. It is present in granules 1 to 2 μm in diameter and is visible by light microscopy after tissue sections are stained with Prussian blue dye. Hemosiderin has a higher iron concentration than ferritin, but it releases iron more slowly. About one-third of the body's iron reserve is stored in the liver, one-third in the bone marrow, and the remainder in the spleen and other tissues.

Control of Iron Balance

Because iron loss is a continuous and largely unregulated process, iron balance is controlled by changes in absorption. The major factors that affect iron absorption are body iron stores and the rate of red blood cell production. When necessary, the efficiency of absorption can be increased by threefold or more. Iron deficiency, pregnancy, and the accelerated **erythropoiesis** that occurs in some **anemias** all stimulate increased iron absorption. Absorption is reduced after unusually large amounts of iron are consumed (e.g., dietary supplementation, iron poisoning).

At the molecular level, the central player in this process is a small polypeptide hormone called *hepcidin.* Hepcidin is produced by the liver in response to perceived iron demands. It controls the flow of iron out of intestinal cells by binding to ferroportin and inhibiting iron release (Fig. 39-3). Thus, low levels of hepcidin promote release of iron into the circulation, and high levels restrict the flow of iron from intestinal cells into blood. The mechanisms that govern hepcidin production have not yet been identified.

KEY CONCEPTS BOX 39-1

- The iron-heme-porphyrin complex in proteins such as hemoglobin (≈70%), myoglobin (10%), catalase, peroxidases, and cytochromes is required for oxygen metabolism. Iron-sulfur proteins, such as NADH dehydrogenase and succinate dehydrogenase, function in electron transfer reactions.
- Men have more body Fe than do premenopausal females; serum Fe reference intervals reflect gender.
- Absorption of dietary Fe, 5% to 10% of total, changes with body Fe needs.
- Iron (Fe^{+3}) is transported in serum bound to *transferrin* (Tr), which is taken up by cells with specific Tr receptors.
- Fe is stored primarily in liver (30%) complexed to *ferritin* and in bone (30%).

Table **39-2** Laboratory Measurements of Iron Status

	Serum Iron, µg/dL	TIBC, µg/dL	Transferrin Saturation, %	Serum Ferritin, µg/L	Free Erythrocyte Protoporphyrin, µg/L
Reference interval	65 to 175 (men) 50 to 170 (women)	250 to 450	20 to 50 (men) 15 to 50 (women)	20 to 250 (men) 10 to 120 (women)	170 to 770
Iron deficiency anemia	↓	↑	↓	↓	↑
Anemia of chronic disease	↓	↓	↓	N or ↑	↑
Thalassemia trait	N	N	N	N	N
Sideroblastic anemia	↑	N	↑	↑	N or ↑
Hemochromatosis	↑	↓	↑	↑	N

N, Normal; ↓, decreased; ↑, increased; *TIBC,* total iron binding capacity.

SECTION OBJECTIVES BOX 39-2

- Describe the populations at risk for Fe deficiency, and explain how stages of Fe deficiency are reflected in the body.
- Define *anemia,* and list the laboratory tests that can be used to diagnose and distinguish the causes of anemia.
- Describe two types of iron overload, their causes, and the laboratory tests that can diagnosis them.

PATHOLOGICAL CONDITIONS

Iron Deficiency

When iron intake falls below the amount required for red blood cell production, iron reserves become depleted, and, in time, anemia develops. Iron deficiency, the most common nutritional disorder in humans, is the most frequent cause of anemia. In the United States, about 2% of adult men and more than 10% of women in their reproductive years are deficient in iron. The figures are much higher in pregnant women and among people of low socioeconomic status.

The high prevalence of iron deficiency among women is the result of the blood loss that occurs during each menstrual cycle. Bleeding from the gastrointestinal tract is the usual cause of iron deficiency in men. The increased demand for iron in infants and young children, adolescents, and pregnant women may lead to iron deficiency, especially if these individuals have diets that are low in iron. Impaired absorption of iron after gastrointestinal surgery and in patients with chronic diarrhea or malabsorption also causes depletion of iron reserves.

Iron deficiency develops in stages, the first of which is depletion of storage iron in response to a prolonged negative iron balance. Once iron reserves have been exhausted, biochemical tests of iron metabolism become abnormal, even though anemia may not be present. Next, a drop in the hemoglobin concentration of blood is seen, and over time, red blood cells become smaller (**microcytic**) and paler (**hypochromic**) than normal. In fully developed iron deficiency anemia, a complete blood count reveals a decrease in hemoglobin and in all red blood cell indices: **mean corpuscular volume** (**MCV**), **mean corpuscular hemoglobin** (**MCH**), and **mean corpuscular hemoglobin concentration** (**MCHC**). Examination of a peripheral blood smear shows hypochromic, microcytic erythrocytes with abnormal variations in size and shape (anisocytosis). No stainable iron is visible in the bone marrow.

Laboratory tests of iron status can distinguish iron deficiency from other causes of hypochromic, microcytic anemia (Table 39-2). The concentration of serum iron decreases, and the total iron binding capacity (TIBC), which measures the capacity of transferrin for iron, increases. The transferrin saturation, calculated as iron concentration divided by TIBC, is well below its reference interval. A decrease in serum ferritin, which is a reflection of body iron stores, is the single most reliable indicator of iron deficiency. Free erythrocyte protoporphyrin is increased, but this increase is not specific for iron deficiency.

Iron Overload

Hereditary Hemochromatosis

Hereditary hemochromatosis is a genetic disorder characterized by a progressive increase in iron stores, leading to organ impairment and damage. Inheritance is autosomal recessive. Among populations of northern European descent, about 10% carry the gene, and 0.3% are homozygotes. For reasons that are not clearly understood, only a small fraction of homozygotes develop the full-blown disease. Men are affected five to ten times more frequently than women because of the protective effects of menstrual blood loss and pregnancy. Symptoms of the disease usually are not apparent before 40 years of age.

The molecular defect responsible for most cases of hemochromatosis is a cysteine→tyrosine mutation (C282Y) in the **HFE** protein. This protein is similar in structure to proteins of human leukocyte antigen (HLA) system, the major histocompatibility complex, and plays a role in regulating the amount of iron absorbed by cells. Several other mutations in the HFE gene have been identified, but their relationship to disease expression is more tenuous. Mutations in four other genes related to iron metabolism cause rare forms of hemochromatosis. Characteristics of each genetic type of iron overload are given in Table 39-3.

Table 39-3 Hereditary Disorders Causing Iron Overload

	Classic Hemochromatosis	Juvenile Hemochromatosis		Transferrin Receptor 2 Deficiency	Ferroportin Deficiency
Affected protein	HFE	Hemojuvelin	Hepcidin	Transferrin receptor 2	Ferroportin
Gene symbol	*HFE*	*HJV*	*HAMP*	*TfR2*	*SLC40A1*
Chromosomal location	6p21.3	1q21	19q13	7q22	2q32
Inheritance	Autosomal recessive	Autosomal recessive	Autosomal recessive	Autosomal recessive	Autosomal dominant
Age of onset of clinical disease	Adult	Childhood	Childhood	Adult	Adult
OMIM type	1	2a	2b	3	4

Patients with hereditary hemochromatosis may absorb 4 mg of iron or more per day, even on a usual diet. Iron is deposited directly into **parenchymal** cells of the liver, pancreas, heart, and other organs. After accumulating for years, excessive amounts of intracellular iron lead to tissue injury and ultimately organ failure. At this stage, the amount of storage iron may exceed 20 g.

Several organ systems are affected by hemochromatosis. The liver is nearly always enlarged and in time may become cirrhotic, predisposing patients to an unusually high risk of hepatocellular carcinoma. Damage to the islet cells of the pancreas causes diabetes mellitus in about two-thirds of patients. Most patients show an increase in skin pigmentation as a result of increased melanin production and iron deposition within the skin. Cardiac damage may be expressed as congestive heart failure or arrhythmias. Testicular atrophy in men is caused by a drop in production of gonadotropins by the pituitary gland—another site of iron deposition. Arthritis also occurs in up to half of patients.

In hemochromatosis, serum iron concentration increases and TIBC decreases—the opposite of the changes seen in iron deficiency. Transferrin saturation is much higher than the reference interval and is a particularly sensitive index of iron overload. Serum ferritin concentration is increased early in the course of disease, before signs and symptoms become apparent. Until recently, measurement of iron content in a liver biopsy specimen was considered the definitive test for hemochromatosis. Now that DNA testing for the C282Y mutation is available, most homozygotes can be diagnosed without the need for liver biopsy.

Acquired Hemochromatosis

Iron overload also can be an acquired disorder. At first, excess iron is deposited in reticuloendothelial cells of the liver, spleen, and bone marrow. As the iron load increases, its distribution pattern changes, and iron is deposited in the parenchymal cells of the liver, pancreas, heart, and other organs. The clinical picture then resembles the hereditary form of hemochromatosis.

Acquired hemochromatosis may be a complication of anemias in which erythropoiesis is ineffective, such as β-thalassemia major (see p. 784). Not only is iron absorption increased in this disorder, but patients are treated with multiple blood transfusions, which further increases their iron load. Alcoholics with chronic liver disease may develop an increase in tissue iron stores, but those with massive iron overload probably have the genetic form of hemochromatosis. Medicinal iron supplements do not, on their own, cause hemochromatosis.

KEY CONCEPTS BOX 39-2

- Iron is needed for RBC formation; Fe deficiency caused by increased loss (GI disease, bleeding), increased demands (pregnancy, lactation, growth), or dietary insufficiency leads to decreased RBC formation and *anemia,* usually hypochromic and microcytic.
- Chronic Fe deficiency is noted by changes in serum Fe, TIBC, and ferritin (all low); then decreased Hb levels; and finally frank anemia, usually microcytic and hypochromic with anisocytosis.
- Two types of iron overload are hereditary (HH) and acquired (AH) hemochromatosis; both are associated with decreased TIBC, increased serum Fe and ferritin levels, as well as excess Fe deposited in liver, heart, and spleen.
- HH is an autosomal recessive disorder (in gene coding for HFE protein) common in Europeans.
- AH can be caused by poor RBC production (β-thalassemia) or excessive, chronic transfusions.

SECTION OBJECTIVES BOX 39-3

- List the two major pools of body Fe and the laboratory tests that reflect those pools.
- Describe the components of a CBC, and explain how these indices reflect iron disorders.
- Explain how **free erythrocyte protoporphyrin** is used.
- Explain the role of genetic testing in cases of suspected iron overload.

CHANGE OF ANALYTE IN DISEASE

The clinical laboratory can measure three iron compartments, which account for 90% of total body iron. The largest of these pools is the iron contained in hemoglobin, which is measured as part of a complete blood count. Next largest is the tissue storage compartment, and the serum ferritin concentration is proportional to the size of this pool. Finally, circulating iron is evaluated by measurement of serum concentrations of iron and its transport protein, transferrin. This combination of hematological and biochemical studies enables one to identify disorders of iron metabolism (see Table 39-2).

Complete Blood Count (CBC)

A complete blood count gives the number of erythrocytes per liter, hemoglobin concentration, hematocrit, and red blood cell indices. The World Health Organization defines anemia as a hemoglobin concentration below 13 g/dL in men, 12 g/dL in women, and 11 g/dL in pregnant women. Iron deficiency causes a hypochromic, microcytic anemia in which cell size (MCV), hemoglobin content (MCH), and concentration of hemoglobin per cell (MCHC) all are reduced. The peripheral blood smear shows a wide variation in the size, shape, and hemoglobin content of erythrocytes; a large proportion of cells are smaller and paler than normal. This clear-cut picture will not be present at the early stages of iron depletion, when both hemoglobin concentration and red cell indices remain normal. Hypochromic, microcytic anemia is characteristic of **thalassemia** trait, **sideroblastic anemia,** and anemia of chronic disease, as well as iron deficiency. Red blood cell parameters thus define the presence or absence of anemia and its morphological character, but other tests are required to identify the cause of anemia. Erythrocyte studies do not contribute to the diagnosis of hemochromatosis.

Serum Iron, TIBC, and Transferrin Saturation

The serum iron concentration can fluctuate markedly, even in healthy people, because of momentary imbalances in iron inflow and outflow. Diurnal variation occurs, with a fall in iron concentration in the evening, as well as significant day-to-day variations. These factors limit the diagnostic usefulness of a single iron measurement. Serum iron should always be measured and interpreted in combination with total iron binding capacity (TIBC).

TIBC measures the maximum amount of iron that serum proteins can bind and therefore is an indirect way of assessing transferrin levels. Transferrin also can be measured directly by immunoassay and converted to TIBC by application of a formula. The serum iron concentration divided by TIBC yields the transferrin saturation. Clinical laboratories should report all three values together.

The low serum iron and high TIBC in iron deficiency produce low transferrin saturation; low values also may be seen in pregnancy and chronic disease. High transferrin saturation is characteristic of iron overload and is a sensitive test for hemochromatosis. Thalassemia major, sideroblastic anemia, and acute iron poisoning also cause transferrin saturation to increase.

Serum Ferritin

A small amount of ferritin circulates in plasma, most of it as iron-free apoferritin. Circulating ferritin is in equilibrium with tissue iron stores and, under most circumstances, accurately reflects the amount of storage iron present. A low serum ferritin concentration is diagnostic of iron deficiency. Ferritin levels drop early in the development of iron deficiency, before serum iron and transferrin saturation become abnormally low. An increase in serum ferritin may be the first indication of iron overload, possibly occurring long before signs and symptoms of hemochromatosis appear. However, the release of ferritin from damaged tissues in hepatitis, acute inflammatory conditions, and a variety of tumors also dramatically increases the serum ferritin level. In these situations, normal ferritin values occasionally can mask the presence of iron deficiency.

Free Erythrocyte Protoporphyrin

In the course of heme synthesis, small numbers of protoporphyrin molecules bind Zn^{2+} instead of Fe^{2+} to produce zinc protoporphyrin, which then circulates in the mature erythrocyte (see below). A decrease in the iron available to developing red cells increases the formation of zinc protoporphyrin. Measurement of zinc protoporphyrin as free erythrocyte protoporphyrin (FEP) provides an assessment of the iron available for hemoglobin production. A related assay, the zinc protoporphyrin : heme (ZnPP/H) ratio, yields the same clinical information and can be run on a dedicated instrument (hematofluorometer) that requires only a drop of blood.

Both iron deficiency (absolute lack of iron) and chronic disease (impaired utilization of iron) will increase FEP. Lead interferes with the final step in heme synthesis, and chronic lead poisoning may produce large increases in FEP. Protoporphyria, a hereditary deficiency of ferrochelatase, is associated with very high FEP values. Neither FEP nor the ZnPP/H ratio is a specific test of iron status, but they still are used as screening tests for iron deficiency, particularly in children.

Molecular Genetics

DNA-based testing has become the gold standard for identifying most cases of hereditary hemochromatosis. About 80% of patients with this disease are homozygous for the C282Y mutation in the *HFE* gene. Gene carriers with one mutated allele also can be detected, although they do not develop symptomatic iron overload. Compound heterozygotes for both C282Y and another mutation in the *HFE* gene, H63D, are at increased risk for iron overload compared with C282Y heterozygotes. Genetic testing is indicated in patients with consistently high transferrin saturation and in first-degree relatives of patients with a known mutation. Some patients with clinical and laboratory evidence of hemochromatosis are heterozygous or negative for the C282Y mutation and are presumed to have a different genetic defect.

KEY CONCEPTS BOX 39-3

- Changes in iron status will be reflected by changes in the major iron pools: RBCs and organ storage.
- Complete blood count (CBC) indices reflect chronic hypochromic, microcytic anemia of Fe deficiency by decreased Hb, MCV, MCH, and MHCH.
- The major serum indices that reflect lowered body stores of Fe are increased TIBC and decreased serum ferritin, Fe, and transferrin saturation.
- A decrease in free erythrocyte protoporphyrin (FEP) reflects decreased RBC synthesis caused by Fe deficiency, chronic disease, or lead poisoning.
- Detection of the C282Y mutation in the *HFE* gene can occur in ≈80% of patients with homogenous hereditary hemochromatosis.

SECTION OBJECTIVES BOX 39-4

- List the three major porphyrins, and describe their structure, important physical properties, and function.
- Explain the critical steps in the synthesis of porphyrins leading up to Hb, especially the roles of ALA and PBG, and the distribution of these steps within the cell.

PART 2: Heme Synthesis and the Porphyrias

STRUCTURE AND FUNCTION

The porphyrins are a class of molecules that have a central, macrocyclic ring structure consisting of four pyrrole units joined by methenyl (=CH–) bridges (Fig. 39-4). The cyclic network of alternating single and double bonds causes porphyrins to absorb visible light, and it is this group that imparts a red color to hemoglobin. Porphyrins also fluoresce a reddish-pink color under long-wavelength ultraviolet light—a property that is very useful when porphyrins are detected and measured in body fluids. The arrangement of four nitrogen atoms at the center of the ring enables porphyrin molecules to chelate metal atoms. In biological systems, iron is the most important metal that complexes with porphyrins.

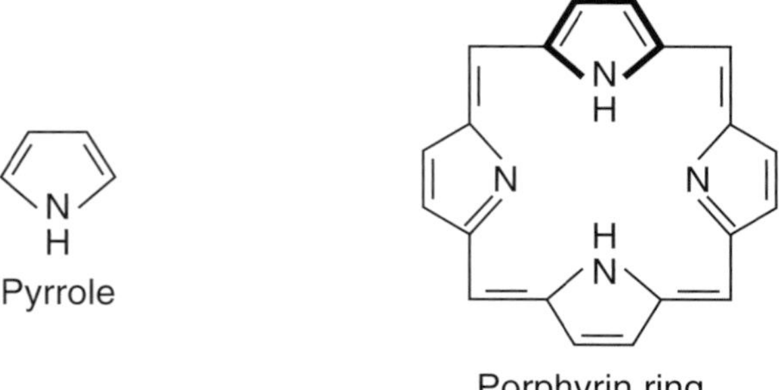

Fig. 39-4 Chemical structures of pyrrole and the porphyrin ring. One of the pyrrole units within the porphyrin ring appears in boldface.

Differences in porphyrin structure depend on the types and positions of side chains located at the corners of the pyrrole rings. In humans, three major porphyrins—uroporphyrin (URO), coproporphyrin (COPRO), and protoporphyrin (PROTO)—are present. URO has four propionate and four acetate side chains, and COPRO has four propionate and four methyl side chains. These groups may be arranged in four different structural configurations, of which the type III isomer is normally produced. PROTO has two propionate, two vinyl, and four methyl groups that can be arranged in 15 different configurations. Only the type IX isomer is produced by the body.

Free porphyrins are by-products of the heme synthetic pathway and have no biological functions of their own. Heme, the iron chelate of protoporphyrin IX, is the prosthetic group for many proteins and enzymes involved in oxygen metabolism and electron transfer reactions (see Table 39-1). Trace amounts of zinc protoporphyrin also occur naturally, although no physiological role has been assigned to this compound.

METABOLISM

Heme synthesis takes place in all cells but occurs to the greatest extent in the bone marrow (red cell precursors) and liver. The process consists of eight steps, each of which is catalyzed by a different enzyme. It is helpful to consider the pathway in two halves: formation of the ring structure by repeated condensations of precursors (Fig. 39-5), and modification of the side chains and insertion of iron (Fig. 39-6).

Synthetic Pathway

The synthetic pathway begins with the condensation of succinyl CoA and glycine to form delta-aminolevulinic acid (ALA). This reaction, catalyzed by ALA synthase, is the rate-limiting step in heme synthesis. Two ALA molecules then condense to form porphobilinogen (PBG), a pyrrole with acetate and propionate side chains at its corners. Next, four PBG molecules are joined in head-to-tail fashion to form a linear tetrapyrrole, hydroxymethylbilane. This unstable intermediate cyclizes spontaneously to form uroporphyrinogen I. To produce the physiological type III isomer of uroporphyrinogen, a specific enzyme, uroporphyrinogen III synthase, rearranges the orientation of propionate and acetate side chains on one of the pyrrole units.

At this point, the basic ring structure is in place. Modification of side chains begins with decarboxylation of the four acetate groups to form coproporphyrinogen III. Two propionate groups then are decarboxylated and dehydrogenated to vinyl groups, producing protoporphyrinogen IX. The bridging carbon atoms are oxidized from methylene ($-CH_2-$) to methenyl (=CH–), to yield protoporphyrin IX. In the final step, Fe^{2+} is inserted into the protoporphyrin ring to produce heme.

Three of the intermediates in this pathway are porphyrinogens. They differ from porphyrins in that the bridging carbon

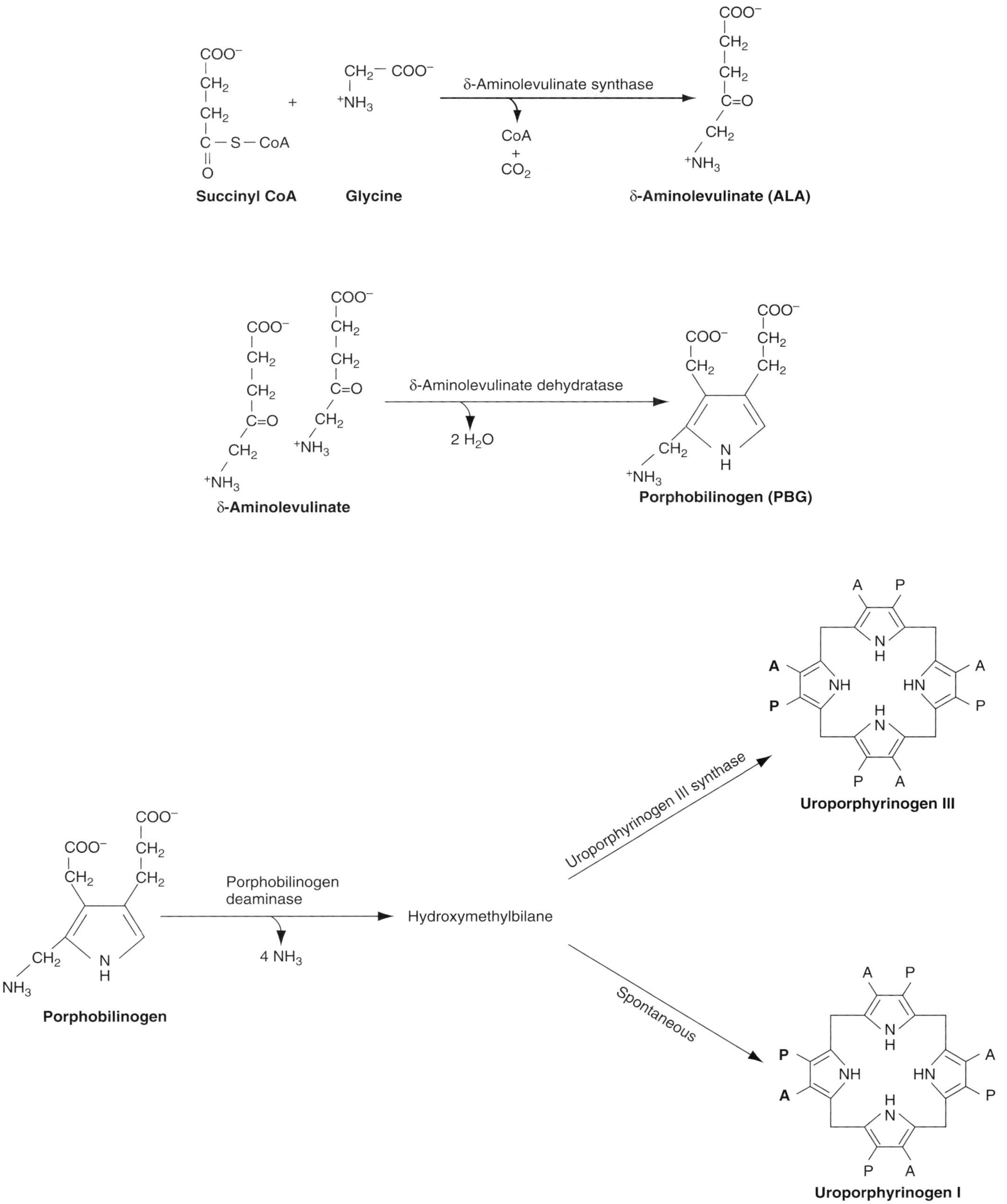

COO^- – CH_2 – CH_2 – C(=O) – S – CoA
Succinyl CoA
+
CH_2 – COO^- / $^+NH_3$
Glycine
δ-Aminolevulinate synthase → (CoA + CO_2)
COO^- – CH_2 – CH_2 – C=O – CH_2 – $^+NH_3$
δ-Aminolevulinate (ALA)

2 × **δ-Aminolevulinate**
δ-Aminolevulinate dehydratase → (2 H_2O)
Porphobilinogen (PBG)

Porphobilinogen
Porphobilinogen deaminase → (4 NH_3)
Hydroxymethylbilane
Uroporphyrinogen III synthase → **Uroporphyrinogen III**
Spontaneous → **Uroporphyrinogen I**

Fig. 39-5 Initial steps in porphyrin synthesis. The difference between the type I and type III isomers of uroporphyrinogen is indicated by the bolded side chains. Only the type III isomer is a precursor of heme. *A,* Acetate; *P,* propionate.

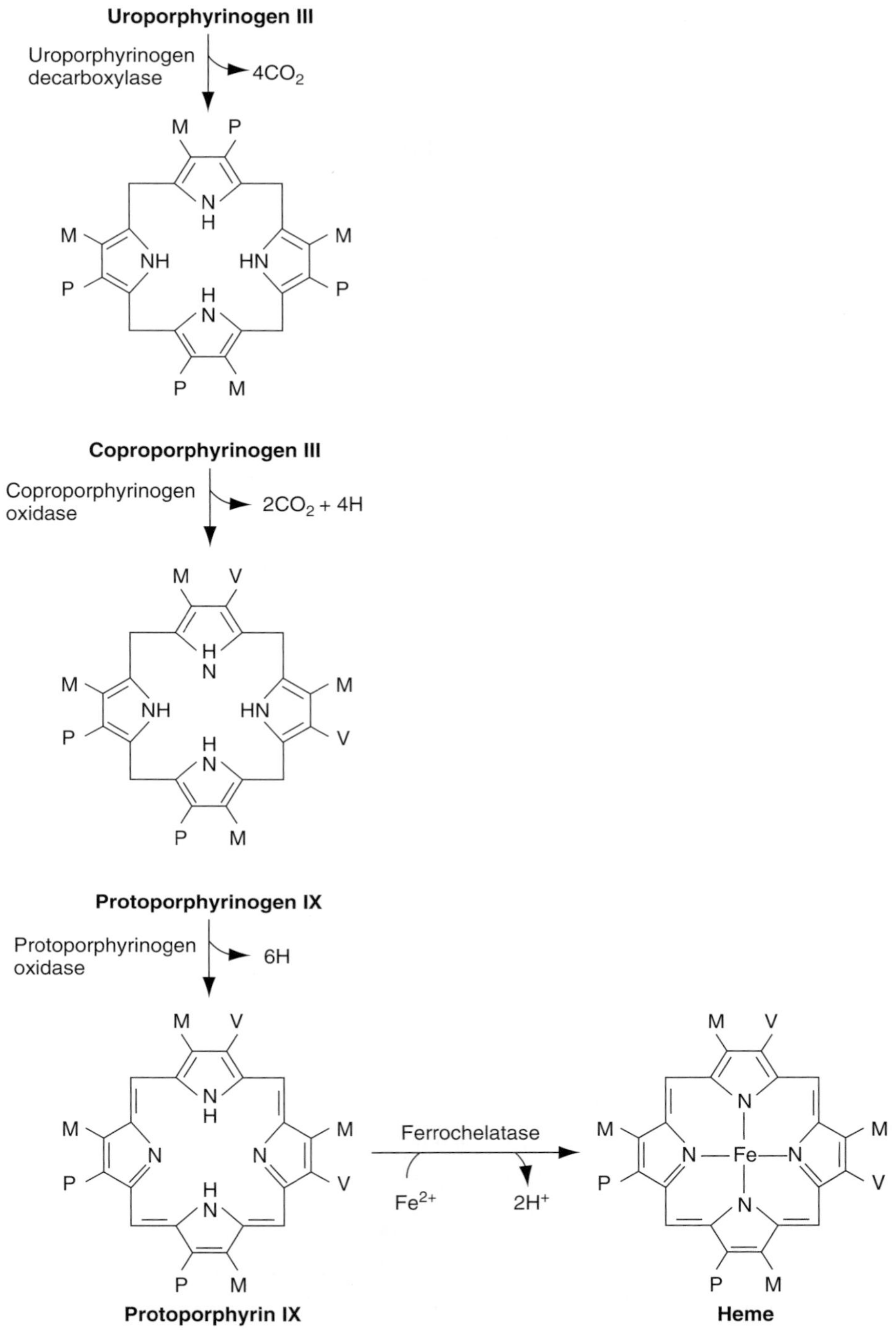

Uroporphyrinogen III

Uroporphyrinogen decarboxylase → $4CO_2$

Coproporphyrinogen III

Coproporphyrinogen oxidase → $2CO_2 + 4H$

Protoporphyrinogen IX

Protoporphyrinogen oxidase → 6H

Protoporphyrin IX

Ferrochelatase (Fe^{2+} → $2H^+$)

Heme

Fig. 39-6 Latter half of the heme biosynthetic pathway. Note the difference in structure between a porphyrinogen and a porphyrin (compare protoporphyrinogen IX to protoporphyrin IX). *M,* Methyl; *P,* propionate; *V,* vinyl.

atoms are fully reduced, and all four nitrogen atoms are protonated. There is no network of alternating single and double bonds, so these compounds are colorless and nonfluorescent. Most of the porphyrinogens that are not used in the regular pathway spontaneously and irreversibly oxidize to the corresponding porphyrins. For this reason, URO, COPRO, and PROTO, and not the porphyrinogens, are the major excretion forms.

The synthetic pathway for heme begins and ends in mitochondria, but four of the intervening steps take place in the cytosol. The intracellular distribution of enzymes is shown in Fig. 39-7. Because developing erythrocytes lose their mitochondria as they mature, only half of these enzymes can be assayed in circulating red blood cells.

Regulation

Heme synthesis in the liver is controlled primarily by changes in the activity of ALA synthase, the first and rate-limiting enzyme. Small amounts of free heme are present within liver cells. An increase in this cellular pool inhibits the activity of ALA synthase, whereas a decrease stimulates the enzyme. Heme synthesis in red cell precursors is regulated in a different manner and is related to the availability of iron.

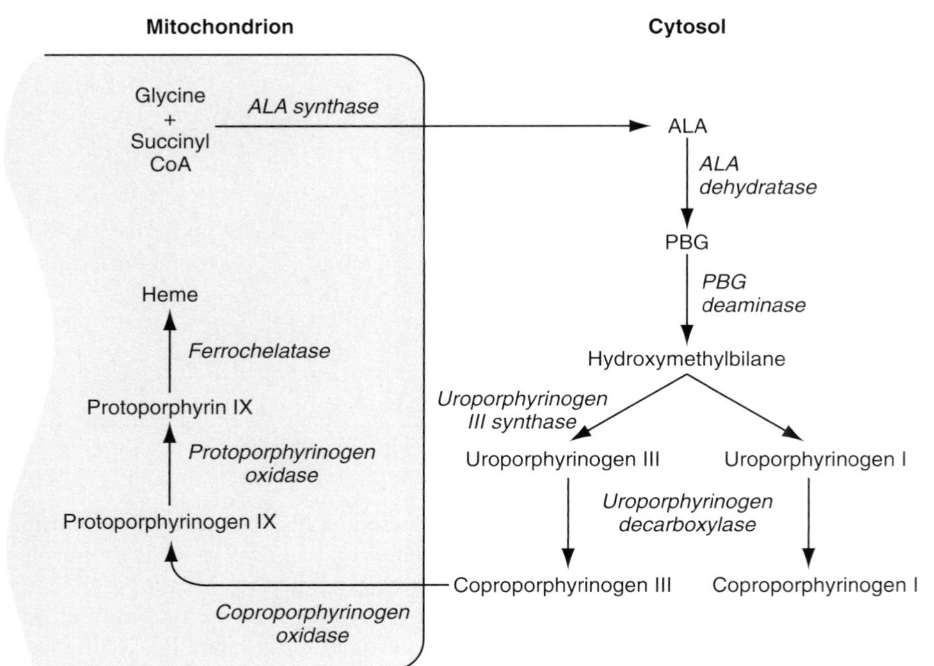

Fig. 39-7 Distribution of the porphyrin pathway between mitochondria and cytosol.

KEY CONCEPTS BOX 39-4

- The porphyrin central, macrocyclic ring structure of four pyrrole units joined by methenyl (=CH–) bridges (see Fig. 39-4), with their cyclic network of alternating single and double bonds, causes porphyrins to absorb visible light.
- The four nitrogen atoms at the center of the ring allow porphyrin molecules to chelate iron and form heme.
- The three major porphyrins are uroporphyrin (URO), coproporphyrin (COPRO), and protoporphyrin (PROTO).
- Heme synthesis occurs primarily in liver and bone, with eight synthetic enzymes distributed between the cytoplasm and the mitochondria.
- ALA and PBG are important synthetic intermediaries to be measured in detecting porphyrias.

SECTION OBJECTIVES BOX 39-5

- List the two major classes of porphyrias and the individual diseases.
- List the enzyme deficiency associated with each porphyria and the metabolic product that can be used to diagnose the porphyria.
- List the causes of the secondary porphyrias.

PATHOLOGICAL CONDITIONS

What would happen if the enzymes involved in heme synthesis did not function properly? The answer to that question can be found in the study of the porphyrias, a group of genetically determined disorders of heme synthesis. Deficiencies in seven of the eight enzymes involved in heme synthesis, each leading to a distinct form of porphyria, have been described. Most of the porphyrias are inherited as an autosomal dominant trait. Because the heterozygote patient has only one gene that produces a functional enzyme, about 50% of normal enzyme activity is observed. This partial defect does not cause a deficiency of heme in red blood cells, so patients do not develop anemia. However, porphyrins and their precursors build up behind the deficient enzyme and accumulate in body tissues and fluids. The photosensitizing properties of porphyrins are responsible for the **cutaneous** signs and symptoms seen in patients with these disorders.

The excretion of excess porphyrins and their precursors serves as the basis for diagnosing the porphyrias. The route of excretion is a function of solubility. URO, with eight carboxyl groups, is the most water soluble and is excreted almost entirely in urine. PROTO, with only two carboxyl groups, is excreted exclusively in feces. COPRO, which has four carboxyl groups, is excreted by either route. The porphyrin precursors ALA and PBG are both water soluble and are eliminated in urine.

Traditionally, the porphyrias have been classified as erythropoietic or hepatic, based on the site of overproduction of the porphyrins and their precursors. A more useful approach is to classify these disorders by signs and symptoms (neurological vs. cutaneous), because this allows one to think in terms of clinical presentation.

Neurological Porphyrias

Four porphyrias are characterized by acute attacks of abdominal pain, neurological signs and symptoms, and/or psychiatric disturbances. Acute attacks, which may last from days to weeks, are accompanied by an increase in the excretion of ALA and PBG in urine. The biochemical basis for the attacks

Table 39-4 Biochemical and Clinical Features of the Neurological Porphyrias

	Acute Intermittent Porphyria	Variegate Porphyria	Hereditary Coproporphyria	ALA Dehydratase Deficiency
Enzyme defect	Porphobilinogen deaminase*	Protoporphyrinogen oxidase	Coproporphyrinogen oxidase	ALA dehydratase
Gene symbol	*HMBS*	*PPOX*	*CPOX*	*ALAD*
Chromosomal location	11q23.3	1q22	3q12	9q34
Inheritance	Autosomal dominant	Autosomal dominant	Autosomal dominant	Autosomal recessive
Abdominal pain, neurological dysfunction	Yes	Yes	Yes	Yes
Photosensitivity, cutaneous lesions	No	Yes	Yes	No
Tissue expression	Liver	Liver	Liver	Liver

*Also known as hydroxymethylbilane synthase.

remains a mystery, although several theories to explain them have been proposed. Three of the four enzyme defects are inherited as autosomal dominant traits.

Signs and symptoms of the neurological porphyrias usually begin during adolescence or early adulthood and affect women more often than men. Abdominal pain, the most constant finding, is accompanied frequently by constipation, nausea, and vomiting. Sensory and motor dysfunction of the peripheral nervous system may be expressed as pain in the extremities, chest, back, head or neck, areas of reduced or altered sensation, muscle weakness, and paralysis. **Tachycardia** and hypertension are common findings, and seizures may occur in a minority of cases. Some patients have a history of nervousness, mood disorders, or delusional thinking, suggestive of a primary psychiatric illness.

Acute attacks can be precipitated by a variety of drugs. Lists of drugs considered to be safe and unsafe for use in patients with a neurological porphyria have been developed to assist in preventing attacks. Fasting, alcohol consumption, infection, and other factors can also precipitate an attack. Between attacks, the signs and symptoms of porphyria are usually absent. Most gene carriers for one of these porphyrias never have an attack, and their disease remains clinically latent. The unique features of each neurological porphyria are reviewed below and in Table 39-4.

Acute Intermittent Porphyria

Acute intermittent porphyria is the most common of the neurological porphyrias, with an estimated prevalence of 1 to 10 per 100,000. Patients with this disease have a 50% deficiency of porphobilinogen deaminase, the enzyme that joins four PBG molecules to form uroporphyrinogen. The defect causes ALA and PBG to accumulate, and partial interruption of the pathway induces the activity of ALA synthase. Consequently, ALA and PBG are excreted in the largest amounts in this porphyria. Because the defect does not involve the porphyrinogen portion of the pathway, porphyrins are not produced in excess, and **photosensitivity** does not occur.

The major laboratory finding is an increase in urine ALA and PBG concentrations during acute attacks. However, between attacks, these values may be only slightly elevated or normal. When PBG is present in high concentrations in urine, it spontaneously condenses and cyclizes to form uroporphyrinogen (type I isomer), which then oxidizes to URO. Large increases in URO may be present in acute intermittent porphyria, as well as other porphyrias in which PBG accumulates. Porphobilinogen deaminase can be assayed in erythrocytes and usually is decreased to about 50% of normal, whether the patient is acutely ill or has the unexpressed latent form.

Variegate Porphyria

Patients with variegate porphyria may suffer from acute neurological attacks, sensitivity of the skin to sunlight and mechanical trauma, or both. The enzymatic defect is a partial deficiency of protoporphyrinogen oxidase. PROTO and COPRO accumulate, giving rise to photosensitivity and cutaneous lesions. The disease is most common among South African whites and has been traced to a couple who emigrated from Holland in 1688. In an interesting but unproved historical footnote, several authors have speculated that King George III of England suffered from variegate porphyria.

The finding of increased ALA and PBG in urine during acute attacks establishes the presence of a neurological porphyria. Variegate porphyria is distinguished from the other neurological porphyrias by the increased excretion of PROTO and COPRO in feces.

Hereditary Coproporphyria

A partial deficiency of coproporphyrinogen oxidase in this disease causes COPRO to accumulate. In addition to the acute attacks, photosensitivity and skin lesions may occur, although less often than in variegate porphyria. Urinary levels of ALA and PBG are increased during acute attacks. The key diagnostic finding is an increase in the fecal excretion of COPRO.

ALA Dehydratase Deficiency

Several patients with a nearly complete deficiency of ALA dehydratase have been described. Homozygotes have neurological symptoms but no photosensitivity; heterozygotes are asymptomatic. Increased excretion of ALA and COPRO in urine is the main laboratory finding.

Table **39-5** Biochemical and Clinical Features of the Cutaneous Porphyrias

	Porphyria Cutanea Tarda	Protoporphyria	Congenital Erythropoietic Porphyria
Enzyme defect	Uroporphyrinogen decarboxylase	Ferrochelatase	Uroporphyrinogen III synthase
Gene symbol	*UROD*	*FECH*	*UROS*
Chromosomal location	1p34	18q21.3	10q25.2-q26.3
Inheritance	Autosomal dominant	Autosomal dominant	Autosomal recessive
Abdominal pain, neurological dysfunction	No	No	No
Photosensitivity, cutaneous lesions	Yes	Yes	Yes
Tissue expression	Liver	Erythroid cells	Erythroid cells

Cutaneous Porphyrias

The three cutaneous porphyrias have in common an excess of porphyrins in body tissues, including skin. Porphyrin molecules absorb light near 400 nm, which raises electrons to a higher energy state. As electrons return to their ground state, some of the energy that they release may be transferred to molecular oxygen, producing activated oxygen species that can react with membranes and other cellular constituents. Leakage of proteolytic enzymes from damaged lysosomes, activation of complement, and release of inflammatory mediators are possible mechanisms for the photosensitivity and skin lesions seen in these disorders. Each of the cutaneous porphyrias is discussed briefly below and is reviewed in Table 39-5.

Porphyria Cutanea Tarda

Porphyria cutanea tarda is a skin disease that usually does not appear until adulthood. It is the most common type of porphyria and is caused by a partial deficiency of uroporphyrinogen decarboxylase. The estimated prevalence of this disease is 1 to 2 per 25,000 population. Some cases of the disease are clearly familial and are inherited as an autosomal dominant trait, but most cases are sporadic and probably represent an acquired deficiency of the hepatic enzyme. Patients may exhibit fragile skin, blister formation, thickening and scarring of sun-exposed skin, and areas of hyperpigmentation. The disease remains dormant until some form of liver dysfunction, such as an overload of hepatic iron or alcoholic liver disease, develops. Estrogen therapy also may activate skin lesions. The rare, homozygous form of this disease, called hepatoerythropoietic porphyria, produces severe photosensitivity.

The deficiency of uroporphyrinogen decarboxylase causes URO as well as porphyrins with 7, 6, and 5 carboxyl groups to accumulate, and their concentrations in urine are greatly increased. Fecal porphyrins are only mildly elevated, but the presence of isocoproporphyrin, which is an isomer of COPRO, is distinctive for this porphyria.

Protoporphyria

Patients with protoporphyria (formally known as erythropoietic protoporphyria) have a partial deficiency of ferrochelatase, the last enzyme in the synthetic pathway for heme. The resulting accumulation of PROTO causes photosensitivity that begins in childhood or adolescence. When exposed to sunlight, patients develop burning, itching, swelling, and redness of the skin. Sun-exposed areas such as the hands and face are affected, but skin changes are mild and scarring uncommon. A minority of patients develop liver disease or protoporphyrin-containing gallstones, because the liver must excrete excess amounts of PROTO.

A large increase in the concentration of free erythrocyte protoporphyrin is the key diagnostic finding. Fecal PROTO usually is increased as well, although the size of the increase is variable.

Congenital Erythropoietic Porphyria

Congenital erythropoietic porphyria is a rare autosomal recessive disorder caused by deficiency of uroporphyrinogen III synthase. The enzyme defect is not complete, and enough uroporphyrinogen III is synthesized to meet metabolic needs. However, large amounts of the type I isomer series also are produced and are eventually oxidized to form URO I and COPRO I. The disease usually presents in early childhood with extreme photosensitivity. Light-exposed areas of the skin become scarred, and, as patients grow older, extensive scarring and mutilation of the fingers, nose, and ears may occur. A unique finding is erythrodontia, the reddish-brown staining of teeth caused by porphyrin deposition. Patients also develop **hemolytic anemia** and enlargement of the spleen. Of all the porphyrias, this one has the worst prognosis.

Patients excrete urine that is pink or red because of the massive amounts of URO and COPRO that are present. Red blood cells contain large quantities of URO and COPRO and fluoresce when examined microscopically under ultraviolet light. Fecal porphyrins also are increased.

Secondary Disorders of Porphyrin Metabolism

Alterations in porphyrin metabolism and excretion can occur in situations other than the porphyrias. Several common examples are described below.

Lead Poisoning

Lead poisoning may occur through ingestion of paint chips that contain lead; consumption of foods, beverages, or folk remedies that contain lead; and exposure to lead compounds in an industrial setting. Signs and symptoms include abdominal pain and neurological abnormalities that may mimic an acute attack of porphyria. Lead inhibits two enzymes in the porphyrin pathway: ALA dehydratase and ferrochelatase.

Table **39-6** Laboratory Diagnosis of the Porphyrias

	Urine ALA and PBG,* mg/day	Urine Porphyrins, µg/day	Fecal Porphyrins, µg/g dry weight	Red Blood Cell Porphyrins, µg/L
Reference interval	ALA: 1.5-7.5 PBG: <2	URO: <50 COPRO: <230	COPRO: <30 PROTO: <60	170-770
Acute intermittent porphyria	↑	↑ URO*	N	N
Variegate porphyria	↑	↑ COPRO	↑ PROTO, COPRO	N
Hereditary coproporphyria	↑	↑ COPRO	↑ COPRO	N
ALA dehydratase deficiency	↑ (ALA only)	↑ COPRO		↑ PROTO
Porphyria cutanea tarda	N	↑ URO, 7-carboxyl	↑ Isocoproporphyrin	N
Protoporphyria	N	N	↑ PROTO	↑ PROTO
Congenital erythropoietic porphyria	N	↑ URO, COPRO	↑ COPRO	↑ URO, COPRO

N, Normal; ↑, increased.
*May be increased only during an acute attack.

Consequently, there is an increase in urine ALA (but not PBG) and in the erythrocyte concentration of zinc protoporphyrin; urine COPRO also is increased. Although these findings are typical of lead poisoning, the diagnosis is based on increased concentrations of lead in whole blood.

Iron Deficiency

Patients with iron deficiency have an imbalance between protoporphyrin, which is produced in normal amounts, and iron, which is not readily available for heme synthesis. Zinc protoporphyrin accumulates in red blood cells to above normal levels. Because it is such a widespread condition, iron deficiency is the most common cause of increased red blood cell porphyrins. Physiological states that decrease the availability of iron, such as acute or chronic inflammation, also increase red cell porphyrins. Measurement of zinc protoporphyrin is a useful screening test for iron deficiency, but the diagnosis must be confirmed by studies of serum iron, TIBC, and ferritin.

Coproporphyrinuria

An increase in COPRO is the most common abnormal result when urine is screened for porphyrins. Although this may indicate a porphyria, it is much more often caused by problems unrelated to heme synthesis, such as liver disease, acute illness, or exposure to toxic compounds. A small (less than twofold), isolated increase in urinary COPRO is usually a nonspecific finding.

KEY CONCEPTS BOX 39-5

- Increases in urinary ALA and PBG are associated with the neurological porphyrias, especially acute intermittent porphyria, the most common of the neurological porphyrias.
- The cutaneous porphyrias usually have urine ALA and PBG in the reference interval, but they have elevated levels of urine and fecal proto-, copro-, and uroporphyrinogens.
- Secondary disorders of porphyrin metabolism include lead poisoning and iron deficiency. Lead poisoning is associated with increased urinary ALA and FEP.

SECTION OBJECTIVES BOX 39-6

- List the diseases associated with increased urinary ALA and PBG.
- List the diseases associated with increases in urinary porphyrins.
- Describe the use of FEP measurements.

CHANGE OF ANALYTE IN DISEASE

The laboratory workup of a suspected porphyria depends on the clinical presentation. For a patient with neurological signs and symptoms, a random urine specimen should be collected during an attack and tested for PBG and porphyrins. When cutaneous symptoms are present, a screening test for urine porphyrins is performed on a random specimen, or, if protoporphyria is suspected, free erythrocyte protoporphyrin is measured. Negative screening tests require no further analysis. Positive screening tests are confirmed by quantitative measurements on a 24-hour urine sample, as well as by identification of which porphyrins are elevated. Analysis of urine ALA, fecal porphyrins, and red cell porphobilinogen deaminase is most helpful in distinguishing among the neurological porphyrias, but these are second-line tests.

Interpretation of results is complicated by the variable excretion of porphyrins and their precursors in health and disease. Urine, fecal, and red blood cell porphyrins typically are increased by fivefold or more in patients with porphyria. The same is true for ALA and PBG in the acute phase of a neurological porphyria. However, some analytes are affected by current disease activity, and the range of values seen in any of the porphyrias can vary greatly. An isolated increase of porphyrins in urine (less than twofold), feces (less than threefold), and red blood cells (less than fivefold) also may occur in individuals who do not have a porphyria. For this reason, diagnosis must be based on a combination of clinical information and careful interpretation of test results. Key laboratory findings in the porphyrias are summarized in Table 39-6.

Porphobilinogen (PBG)

Urine PBG is elevated in acute intermittent porphyria, variegate porphyria, and hereditary coproporphyria. The screening test for PBG is positive during acute attacks but may be negative or weakly positive between attacks. A negative test on a properly collected specimen effectively rules out a neurological porphyria. A positive screening test is confirmed by quantitative PBG analysis performed on a 24-hour urine collection.

Delta-Aminolevulinic Acid (ALA)

Urine ALA values are increased in all four of the neurological porphyrias. ALA excretion is also increased in lead poisoning and hereditary tyrosinemia and therefore is a less specific indicator of these porphyrias than PBG. The exception is ALA dehydratase deficiency, an exceedingly rare condition in which urine ALA, but not PBG, is elevated. Measurements are performed on a 24-hour urine collection.

Urine Porphyrins

Screening tests for urine porphyrins are usually positive in all of the porphyrias except protoporphyria and the latent phase of acute intermittent porphyria. Positive screening tests are followed by quantitative measurement of total porphyrins in a 24-hour urine sample and identification of which porphyrins are elevated. A slight to moderate increase in urinary COPRO concentration is seen in liver disease, lead poisoning, alcohol ingestion, and acute illness. Larger increases in COPRO or URO are more likely to indicate a porphyria.

The most common disorder associated with a large increase in urine porphyrins is porphyria cutanea tarda. The pattern of excretion, which shows large amounts of URO and a distinctive 7-carboxyl porphyrin, is diagnostic for this disease.

Fecal Porphyrins

Fecal porphyrins consist of COPRO, PROTO, and several other dicarboxylic porphyrins (meso-, deutero-, and pemptoporphyrin). The quantity of porphyrins excreted by this route is a function of diet and the anaerobic flora of the colon. Increases in fecal porphyrin excretion up to threefold the upper reference limit may be seen in healthy individuals.

Fecal porphyrins usually are increased in all of the porphyrias except acute intermittent porphyria. The most important application of this test is to distinguish variegate porphyria (PROTO and COPRO both elevated) from hereditary coproporphyria (only COPRO elevated).

Red Blood Cell Porphyrins

Red blood cell porphyrins other than heme are measured as free erythrocyte protoporphyrin (FEP). Under normal conditions, FEP reflects the concentration of zinc protoporphyrin.

The concentration of red blood cell porphyrins is greatly increased in protoporphyria (PROTO) and congenital erythropoietic porphyria (URO and COPRO) but is normal in other porphyrias. Fractionation of red blood cell porphyrins is not necessary, because these two disorders can be differentiated by urine porphyrin assays and clinical presentation. As was mentioned previously, FEP is also increased in iron deficiency and lead poisoning.

Enzyme Assays

Only one enzyme in the synthetic pathway for heme, porphobilinogen deaminase, is routinely measured by clinical laboratories. Its activity is decreased to about 50% of normal in the red blood cells of most individuals with acute intermittent porphyria, whether the disease is latent or in an acute phase. The usefulness of this assay is diminished by two factors. First, an overlap of values is seen between patients and healthy individuals at the lower end of the reference interval. Second, a small subset of patients with the disease have normal PBG deaminase activity in erythrocytes, caused by mutations in the gene that do not affect expression of the enzyme in red cells. Despite these shortcomings, PBG deaminase frequently is the only test that can identify asymptomatic patients who carry the gene for acute intermittent porphyria.

Molecular Genetics

All of the genes that encode enzymes of the heme synthetic pathway have been identified and sequenced. Analysis of these genes has led to the discovery of numerous disease-causing mutations for each of the porphyrias. The most intensively studied disease is acute intermittent porphyria, in which more than 200 mutations have been reported. No single mutation accounts for more than a fraction of cases.

DNA-based testing for a known mutation can be offered to all members of a patient's family. Such testing is more definitive in identifying gene carriers than are conventional biochemical tests, especially in relatives with no signs or symptoms of porphyria. However, a positive test does not predict whether the course of the disease will be asymptomatic, mild, or severe. If the causative mutation is not known, it may be necessary to analyze the entire coding sequence of the gene to identify the molecular defect. A limited number of research and specialty laboratories offer this service.

KEY CONCEPTS BOX 39-6

- Increases in urinary ALA and PBG are associated with the neurological pophyrias, especially acute intermittent porphyria, the most common of the neurological porphyrias.
- The cutaneous porphyrias usually have urine ALA and PBG in the reference interval, but they have elevated levels of urine and fecal proto-, copro- and uroporphyrinogens.
- Red blood cell porphyrins are increased in protoporphyria and congenital erythropoietic porphyria.

BIBLIOGRAPHY

Iron Metabolism

Beutler E: Disorders of iron metabolism. In Lichtman MA, Beutler E, Kipps TJ, editors: *Williams Hematology,* ed 7, New York, 2006, McGraw-Hill, pp. 511-553.

Beutler E: Hemochromatosis: genetics and pathophysiology, Annu Rev Med 57:331, 2006.

Fleming RE, Bacon BR: Orchestration of iron homeostasis, N Engl J Med 352:1741, 2005.

Labbe RF, Dewanji A: Iron assessment tests: transferrin receptor vis-à-vis zinc protoporphyrin, Clin Biochem 37:165, 2004.
Pietrangelo A: Hereditary hemochromatosis—a new look at an old disease, N Engl J Med 350:2383, 2004.
Qaseem A, Aronson M, Fitterman N, et al: Screening for hereditary hemochromatosis: a clinical practice guideline from the American College of Physicians, Ann Intern Med 143:517, 2005.
Swinkels DW, Janssen MCH, Bergmans J, et al: Hereditary hemochromatosis: genetic complexity and new diagnostic approaches, Clin Chem 52:950, 2006.
Zimmermann MB, Hurrell RF: Nutritional iron deficiency, Lancet 370:511, 2007.

Heme Synthesis and the Porphyrias

Anderson KE, Bloomer JR, Bonkovsky HL, et al: Recommendations for the diagnosis and treatment of the acute porphyrias, Ann Intern Med 142:439, 2005.
Badminton MN, Elder GH: Molecular mechanisms of dominant expression in porphyria, J Inherit Metab Dis 28:277, 2005.
Bloomer JR, Brenner DA. Porphyrias. In Schiff ER, Sorrell MF, Maddrey WC, editors: *Schiff's Diseases of the Liver,* ed 10, Philadelphia, 2007, Lippincott Williams & Wilkins, pp. 1085-1116.
Chemmanur AT, Bonkovsky HL: Hepatic porphyrias: diagnosis and management, Clin Liver Dis 8:807, 2004.
Kauppinen R: Porphyrias, Lancet 365:241, 2005.
Nordmann Y, Puy H: Human hereditary hepatic porphyrias, Clin Chim Acta 325:17, 2002.
Sassa S: Modern diagnosis and management of the porphyrias, Br J Haematol 135:281, 2006.
Sassa S: The hematologic aspects of porphyria. In Lichtman MA, Beutler E, Kipps TJ, editors: *Williams Hematology,* ed 7, New York, 2006, McGraw-Hill, pp. 803-822.

INTERNET SITES

Porphyria

http://ghr.nlm.nih.gov/condition=porphyria
http://www.emedicine.com/DERM/topic344.htm
www.porphyriafoundation.com
http://www.ncbi.nlm.nih.gov/entrez/dispomim.cgi?id=176000
http://www.cpf-inc.ca—website of the Canadian Porphyria Foundation—Good resource

Iron Metabolism

http://sickle.bwh.harvard.edu/menu_iron.html
http://themedicalbiochemistrypage.org/heme-porphyrin.html
http://library.med.utah.edu/WebPath/TUTORIAL/IRON/IRON.html

Hemochromatosis

http://digestive.niddk.nih.gov/ddiseases/pubs/hemochromatosis/index.htm
http://www.hemochromatosis.org/
http://www.emedicine.com/MED/topic975.htm
www.cdnhemochromatosis.ca—Website of the Canadian Hemochromatosis Society; good resource

Hemoglobin

Fermina M. Mazzella and Harold R. Schumacher

40

Chapter

Chapter Outline

Key Terms

2,3-biphosphoglycerate A glycolytic intermediate in the red cell that changes the affinity of hemoglobin for oxygen; also known as 2,3-diphosphoglycerate or 2,3- DPG (see Chapter 38).

anemia A disorder that results from low concentrations of hemoglobin in blood.

Bohr effect The change of oxygen affinity of hemoglobin with pH.

carboxyhemoglobin Hemoglobin combined with carbon monoxide.

erythropoietin A renal hormone that stimulates the production of hemoglobin and red blood cells.

fetal hemoglobin The form of hemoglobin that is present during most of fetal development, also in certain hemoglobinopathies. This form has two α-chains and two γ-chains.

globins The polypeptide chains without heme of hemoglobin. The term is used also to describe a class of protein molecules.

heme An iron-containing porphyrin derivative that gives hemoglobin its red color.

heme-heme interaction or **subunit cooperativity** In general, this describes the effect that the binding of one ligand to a protein has on the binding of other ligands at other sites on that protein. With hemoglobin, the binding of oxygen to one heme group increases the affinity of other heme groups for oxygen, resulting in the sigmoidal curve of oxygen uptake by hemoglobin.

hemichromes Greenish ferric compounds formed by the oxidation of the heme group and its subsequent covalent binding to the protein.

hemoglobin A red oxygen-carrying protein found in red blood cells.

hemoglobin A_1 A series of hemoglobin derivatives formed by the postsynthetic, nonenzymatic reaction of various sugars with amino groups of the globin chains of hemoglobin. Hemoglobin A1c (Hb + glucose) is the derivative found in the highest concentration.

hemoglobinopathies Genetic disorders involving the structure and synthesis of one or more of the globin polypeptide chains.

hemogram A formula used to differentiate iron deficiency from milder forms of thalassemia.

hereditary persistence of fetal hemoglobin (HPFH) β-Thalassemia, a condition in which synthesis of the β-chains of hemoglobin is diminished while synthesis of γ-chain is increased.

hypoxia Low Po_2 in tissues.

methemoglobin A form of hemoglobin in which the ferrous ion Fe^{2+} of hemoglobin has been oxidized to the ferric state Fe^{3+}.

sickle cell anemia A chronic, moderate to severe hemolytic anemia in persons homozygous for hemoglobin S.

sickle cell disorders Formation of a morphological, abnormal sickle cell type caused by the presence of a hemoglobin variant.

sickle hemoglobin A genetically altered globin gene in which valine is substituted for glutamine in the β-chain of the hemoglobin, causing reduction in solubility of the hemoglobin molecule.

sulfhemoglobin A stable compound resulting from the linkage of sulfur to hemoglobin.

thalassemias A group of disorders in which there is a quantitative defect in the production of globin chains.

α-thalassemia A group of genetic disorders that result in defective α-chain synthesis.

β-thalassemia A group of genetic disorders that result in defective β-chain synthesis.

Methods on Evolve

Blood gas analysis and oxygen saturation
Haptoglobin
Hemoglobin F
Hemoglobin separation and quantitation
Oximetry

Hemoglobin and myoglobin, respectively, serve to transport and to store oxygen. Erythrocyte hemoglobin, which accounts for up to 95% of the total soluble protein content of blood transports oxygen from the lung to peripheral tissues for cell use. Hemoglobin is a tetramer of two pairs of different globin chains, in association with an iron-containing porphyrin derivative called "heme." Myoglobin, a single-chain globular protein, stores oxygen in skeletal and cardiac muscle, but not smooth muscle.

More than 700 different inherited variants of **hemoglobins** have been described in humans. Most of these are of no clinical consequence. However, some significantly alter hemoglobin stability or function, resulting in **anemia** or other disease manifestations. Most clinical abnormalities are explainable in terms of the structural abnormality. Mutations continue to occur, often resulting in disease states called **hemoglobinopathies.**

SECTION OBJECTIVES BOX 40-1

- Describe the tertiary and quaternary structures of HbA.
- Name alternative Hb molecules and explain when in life they are produced.
- List factors that stimulate Hb and RBC synthesis.
- List factors that affect O_2 binding to Hb, and explain how these factors affect Hb O_2 saturation.
- Discuss the relationship between blood PO_2 and Hb O_2 saturation.
- List five derivatives of HbA, and explain their relationship to disease.

STRUCTURE AND FUNCTION OF HEMOGLOBIN

Genetics

In human genetics, there are two copies of each gene contained within the genome, one inherited from each parent. The different variants of a specific gene are known as alleles. Frequently, the phenotype is determined completely by one of the alleles, which is said to be "dominant". The other allele, which is in effect silent, is said to be recessive. In the case of hemoglobin, though, the globin genes are co-dominant, meaning that both alleles are transcribed. In other words, the hemoglobin of any adult is derived from both chromosomes.

The α-globin genes are found on the short arm of each chromosome 16, between band p13.33 and the terminus. The human α-globin gene cluster located on chromosome 16 spans about 30 kb and includes seven loci: ζ, φζ, $\varphi\alpha_2$, $\varphi\alpha_1$, α_2, α_1, and θ (going from the 5′ to the 3′ direction on the DNA). Both α_1 and α_2 genes are transcribed in adults. The 3′ untranslated regions of these genes differ significantly. This difference leads to the α_2-globin gene being expressed at 2-3-fold higher levels than the α_1-globin gene at both mRNA and protein levels.

The φζ, $\varphi\alpha_2$, and $\varphi\alpha_1$-globin genes are "pseudo-genes" and have no known function. The θ-globin gene appears to exhibit an erythroid-tissue specificity and is primarily active during the fetal stages of development and maintains its activity during adult life, although at low levels.

The human β-globin locus is composed of six genes; ε, G_γ, A_γ, φβ, δ, and β (going from the 5′ to 3′ direction); located on the terminal portion of the short arm of each chromosome 11, at 11p15.5. Expression of all of these genes is controlled by a single locus control region (LCR).

Structure

Hemoglobin (Hb) is a red, oxygen-carrying protein found in red blood cells. It is a tetramer of two pairs of different globin chains with a molecular weight of 64,000 D. Each chain carries an iron-containing porphyrin derivative called *heme,* a ferriprotoporphyrin IX in which one iron atom is bound in the center of the porphyrin ring (see Fig. 39-6). The polypeptide chains (without heme) are collectively called the *globin* moiety of hemoglobin. Each polypeptide chain is designated by a Greek letter: α (alpha), β (beta), γ (gamma), δ (delta), ε (epsilon), and ζ (zeta). Normal mammalian hemoglobin contains two pairs of chains: two α- and two non–α- (β-, γ-, or δ-) chains. The α-chains bind with β-chains to produce normal adult Hb (HbA = $\alpha_2\beta_2$), they bind with the γ-chain to produce fetal Hb (HbF = $\alpha_2\gamma_2$), and they bind with the δ-chain to produce HbA_2 ($HbA_2 = \alpha_2\delta_2$). The latter accounts for only 2.5% of normal adult Hb. The two early embryonic Hb, termed Hb Gower 1 and Hb Gower 2, consist of α-like ζ-chains and β-like ε-chains.

The primary, secondary, tertiary, and quaternary structures of all the hemoglobins have been determined. The β-, γ-, δ-, and ε-chains have similar amino acid sequences, as do the

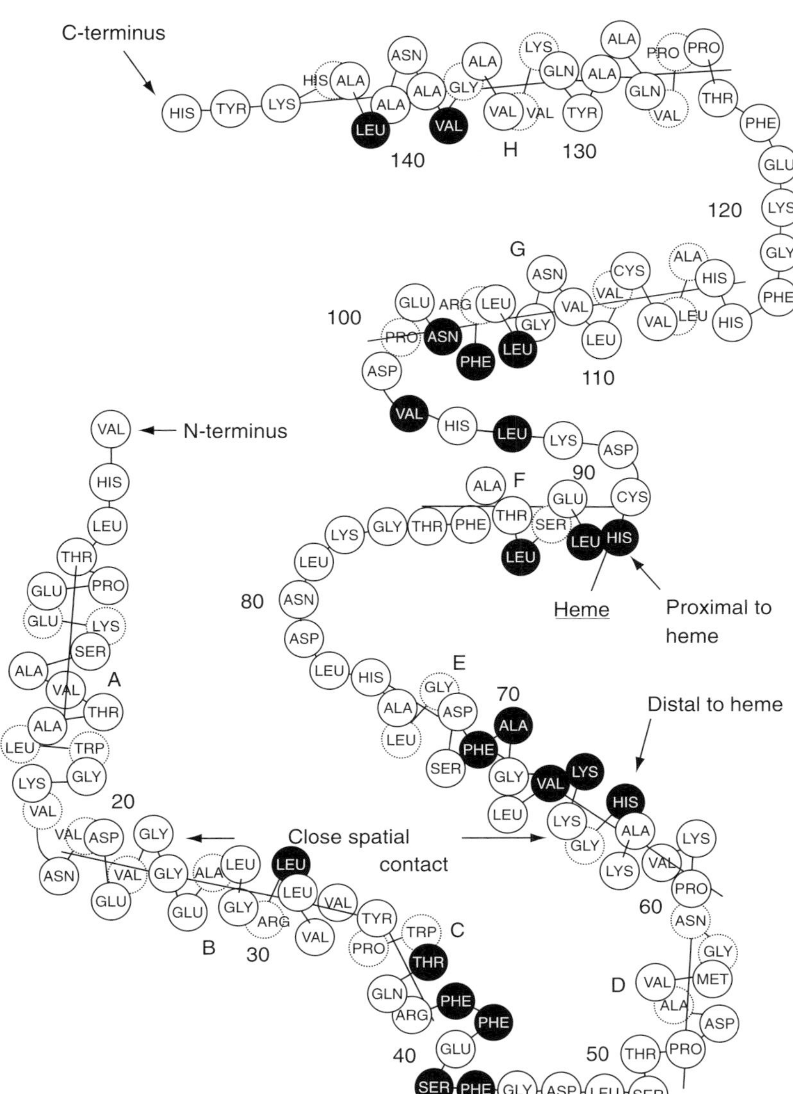

Fig. 40-1 The β-globin chain showing helical and nonhelical segments. The helical segments are labeled *A* through *H,* whereas nonhelical segments are designated *NA* for those residues between the N terminus and the A helix, *CD* for residues between the C and D helices, and so forth. (From Huisman THJ, Schroeder WA: *New Aspects of the Structure, Function and Synthesis of Hemoglobin,* Boca Raton, FL, 1971, CRC Press.)

α- and ζ-chains. The α-chain contains 141 amino acid residues, and each of the β-, δ-, and ε-chains contains 146.

In all hemoglobin and myoglobin chains, approximately 75% of the amino acids are arranged in an α-helix with three to six amino acids per turn (Fig. 40-1). The tertiary structure of hemoglobin is depicted in Fig. 40-2. The folding pattern places polar amino acid residues on the outside of the molecule and provides a pocket with a deep hydrophobic niche for the heme ring between the E and F helices in each protein subunit. Many noncovalent bonds are formed between the heme moiety and surrounding amino acids. An iron atom in the ferrous (Fe^{2+}) state, in the center of the ferriprotoporphyrin IX ring, forms an important bond with the F8, or proximal, histidine and via the bound oxygen with the E7, or distal, histidine. This heme iron is critical because oxygenation and deoxygenation occur at this site.

The complete hemoglobin tetramer composed of two α-globin and two non–α-globin chains fits together to form a quaternary structure (Fig. 40-3). The central cavity is filled with water and allows the entrance of small molecules such as **2,3-biphosphoglycerate** (2,3-BPG) and salts. The motion of individual globin chains, including the movement of globin chains relative to one another during oxygenation and deoxygenation, gives hemoglobin its unique ability to serve as a carrier of oxygen. The substitution of a single amino acid can change the secondary, tertiary, and quaternary structures of hemoglobin, causing severe and even fatal pathophysiological changes.

Ontogeny

The hemoglobin composition of a red blood cell (RBC) varies widely, depending on when, during gestation or postnatal development, the RBC is produced. The first globin chains formed in embryonic red cells are ε-chains, which resemble β-chains in their primary structure.[1] Almost immediately, the synthesis of ζ-, α-, and γ-chains begins. Sequential activation and inactivation, or switching, among genes within the α- and

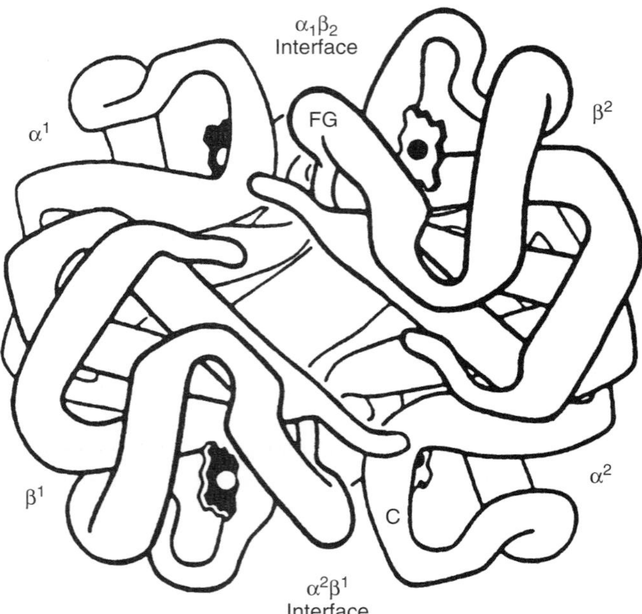

Fig. 40-2 Diagrammatic representation of the tertiary structure of the hemoglobin molecule, showing the location of variant hemoglobins that impart physical instability to the molecule. Each chain carries an iron-containing porphyrin derivative called *heme,* a ferriprotoporphyrin IX in which one iron atom is bound in the center of the porphyrin ring. The FG corner is shown and represents an important area of the molecule that regulates oxygen binding and release. 2,3-Biphosphoglycerate (2,3-BPG), an important oxygen-regulating enzyme, is located in the central clear area of the molecule. (From Irving Geis. Rights owned by Howard Hughes Medical Institute. Not to be used without permission.)

non–α-globin gene clusters results in the formation of four commonly encountered embryonic hemoglobins. These are Gower 1, $\zeta_2\varepsilon_2$, Gower 2, $\alpha_2\varepsilon_2$, Portland, $\zeta_2\gamma_2$, and fetal hemoglobin, $\alpha_2\gamma_2$. Gower 1 and Gower 2 hemoglobins constitute 42% and 24% of total hemoglobin, respectively, at 5 weeks of gestation. The rest is **fetal hemoglobin.** The α-globin genes undergo a switch in expression, from co-expression of the

KEY CONCEPTS BOX 40-1

- Hb is composed of 2 α-like and 2 β-like chains. The quarterary structure allows a heme molecule to bind to each chain.
- During embryonic and fetal life, different α- and β-like chains are expressed to allow the fetal Hbs to be synthesized.
- Low blood PO_2 stimulates renal production of EPO, which directly stimulates Hb and RBC production.
- DPG, an intermediary metabolite of glucose metabolism, binds to N-terminal valine on the β-chain to decrease O_2 binding to Hb. Decreased pH stimulates the release of O_2 from Hb, while the H^+ is bound to, and buffered by, Hb.
- A nonlinear relationship exists between blood PO_2 and Hb O_2 saturation. When one O_2 molecule binds to Hb, this makes it easier for the second and third O_2 molecules to bind as well.
- Derivatized HbA include HbA_1, which includes covalently bound sugars (increased in diabetes); MetHb, which has Fe^{3+} (acquired or genetic, reduced capacity to oxygenate tissues); and HbS, which has covalently bound sulfur from drugs (also reduced capacity to oxygenate tissues).

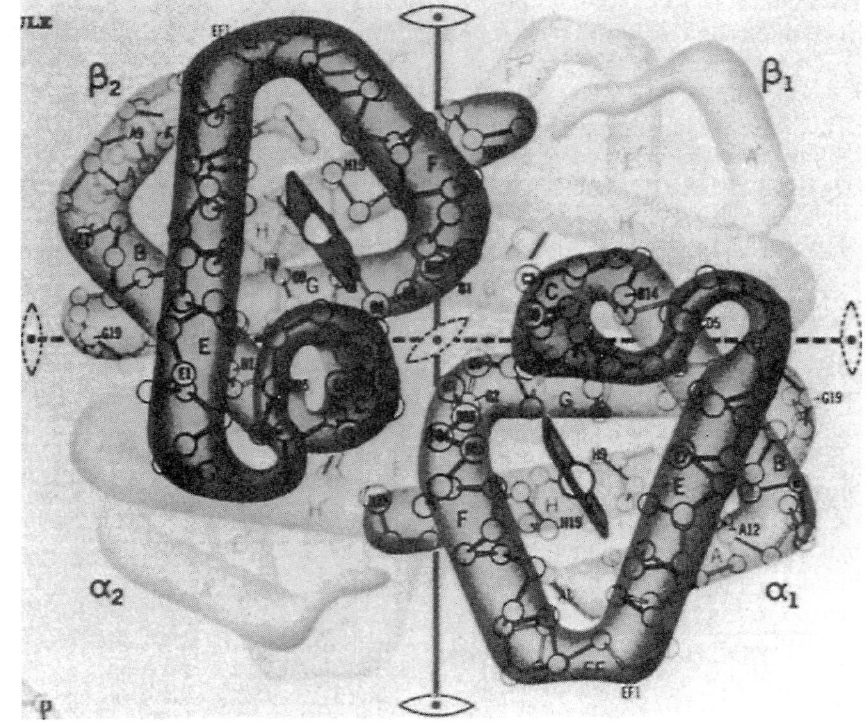

Fig. 40-3 Quaternary structure of hemoglobin. The α_1- and β_2-chains are in the foreground, and $\alpha_1\beta_2$ contact is at the center. (From Dickerson and Geis. *The Structure and Action of Proteins,* Benjamin/Cummings, 1969. From Irving Geis. Rights owned by Howard Hughes Medical Institute. Not to be used without permission.)

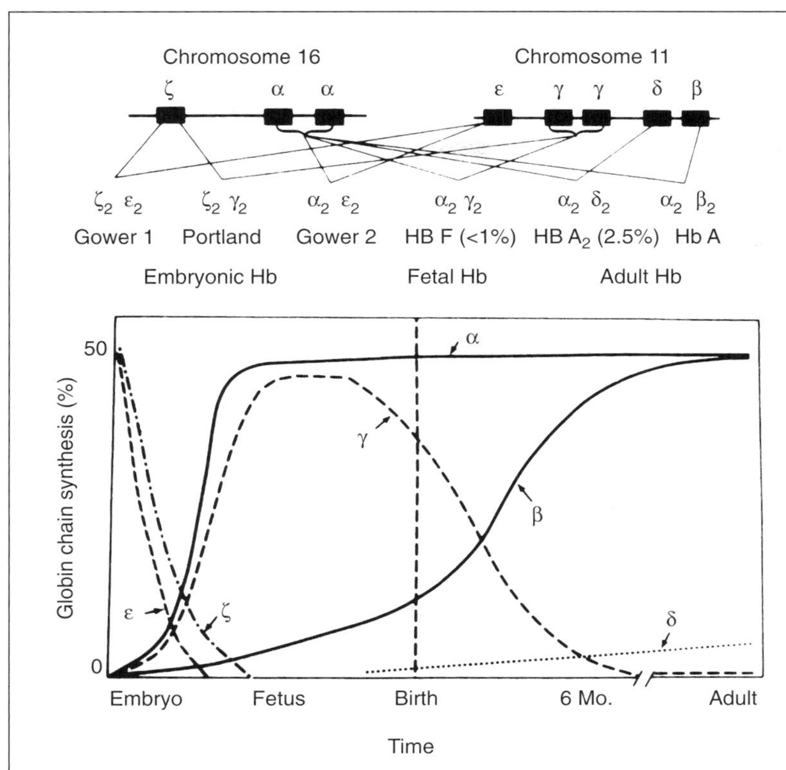

Fig. 40-4 Developmental switching of globin synthesis and the globin chain composition of human hemoglobins. Switching of gene expression within the β-like and α-like gene clusters leads to the synthesis of different hemoglobins within the embryo, fetus, infant, and adult. *Top,* The globin gene–containing chromosomes and their contributions to the hemoglobin molecules of the embryo, fetus, and adult. *Bottom,* Embryonic ε- and ζ-chains rapidly disappear and are replaced by fetal γ-and adult α-chains. γ-Chain synthesis peaks at mid gestation and reaches its adult level at 6 months of age. A progressive rise in β-chain synthesis is seen from the first trimester to its peak at 6 to 12 months of age. Small amounts of synthesized δ-chain peak at about 12 months. (From Steinberg MH: Hemoglobinopathies and thalassemias. In Stein JH, editor: *Internal Medicine,* ed 5, St Louis, 1998, Mosby.)

α and ζ-globin genes in the embryo to exclusive expression of the two α-globin genes in the fetal stage of development. In addition, a switch from an equal proportion of α_1 and α_2 globin transcripts to a predominance of α_2 also occurs at about the eighth week of gestation. The spatial orientation of the individual β-globin genes in relation to the LCR is essential to their proper regulation. In the early embryonic stage the gene located closest to the LCR, the ε-globin locus, is expressed, while the gene expressed at the highest levels in the adult, β-globin, is situated the farthest away. Hemoglobin switching during embryonic, fetal, and adult development is shown in Fig. 40-4.

NORMAL HEMOGLOBIN BIOCHEMISTRY

Assembly of Hemoglobin

The four α-like globin genes of man are located on the short arm of chromosome 16, between band P 13.2 and the terminus, whereas the two β-like genes are located on the terminal portion of the short arm of chromosome 11 (P15).[2] The α- and β-polypeptide chains of an adult hemoglobin are synthesized in equal amounts, although an excess of α-chains may be found in the cytoplasm of young red cells. The assembly process starts with the release of α- and β-chains from the ribosomes in the cytoplasm. They immediately incorporate heme (see Chapter 39 for discussion on the synthesis of heme) and form monomer combinations and dimer aggregates followed by the synthesis of tetramers. In the hemoglobinopathies, the concentrations of two like chains, such as βA and βS; βA and βC; and βA and βE, may differ, even though their rates of synthesis are the same. Evidence suggests that the relative rates of assembly in relation to synthesis of hemoglobins A and S may differ because of differences in affinities of βA and βS for α-chains. The α-chains, if in short supply, prefer to combine with normal β-chains, rather than with variant chains,[3] and excess variant chains then are removed by proteolysis.

The synthesis of hemoglobin is stimulated normally by tissue **hypoxia** (low Po_2 in tissues). Hypoxia causes the kidneys to produce increased amounts of **erythropoietin** (see p. 573), which, in turn, stimulate the production of hemoglobin and RBCs.

Functional and Structural Interrelationships

Hemoglobin and Oxygen: The Oxygen Dissociation Curve

Each of the four subunits of hemoglobin contains a heme moiety deep in the pocket of the globin chains, leaving one edge of the heme exposed to receive the oxygen. Each of the four heme iron atoms can bind reversibly one oxygen molecule. Because iron remains in the ferrous form, the reaction is an oxygenation, not an oxidation.

To fulfill its function as a respiratory pigment, hemoglobin must specifically bind oxygen molecules with high affinity, transport them, and release them at the oxygen tension of tissues. Each gram of hemoglobin binds approximately 1.34 mL of oxygen. The tetrameric structure of hemoglobin, which is responsible for its unique oxygen-binding capacity, renders it physiologically superior to single hemoglobin subunits or to myoglobin. Heme iron has six valence bonds, four

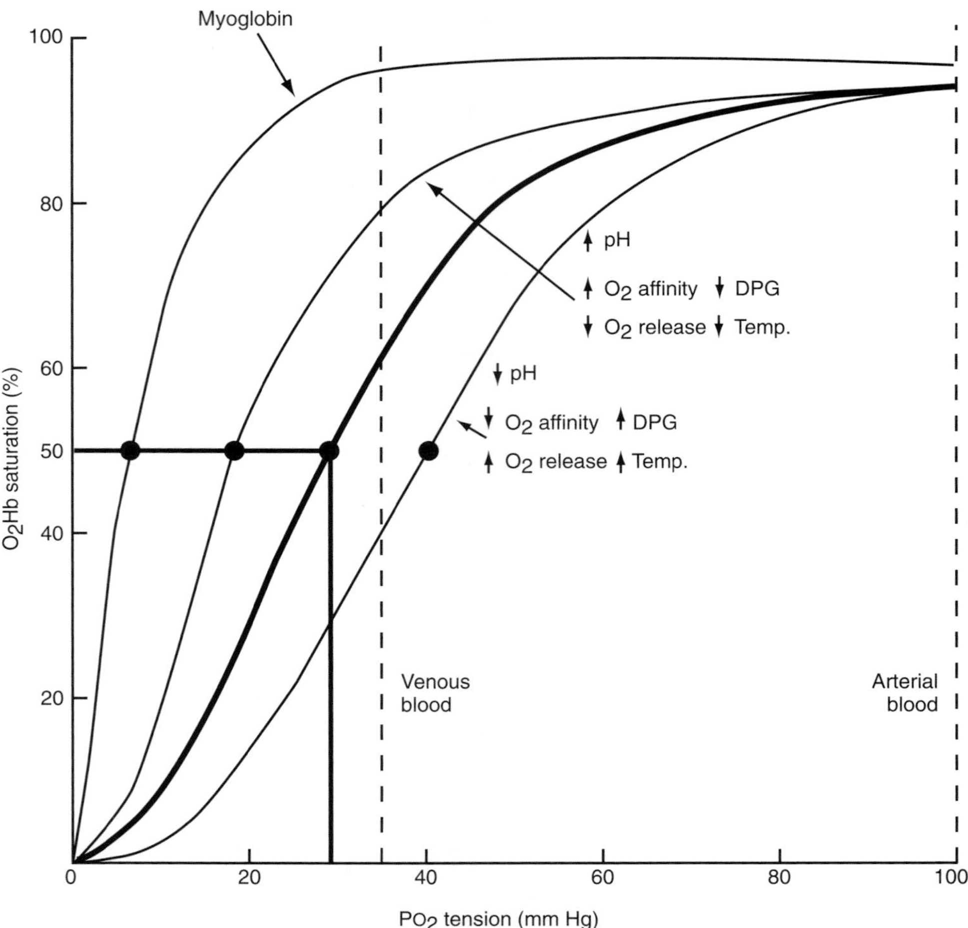

Fig. 40-5 Oxygen dissociation curves of normal human hemoglobin. *Heavy middle line,* Dissociation curve of normal adult blood (temperature 37°C, pH 7.4, P_{CO_2} 35 mm Hg). *Dots,* P_{50} values, partial pressure of oxygen (27 mm Hg) at which hemoglobin solution is 50% oxyhemoglobin and 50% deoxyhemoglobin. If temperature increases, pH decreases, or carbon dioxide tension (P_{CO_2}) increases, the curve shifts to the right. This shift increases the release of oxygen from hemoglobin at given oxygen tension by decreasing its oxygen affinity. If temperature decreases, pH rises, or carbon dioxide tension decreases, the oxygen dissociation curve moves to the left. This shift increases the oxygen-binding capacity of hemoglobin at given oxygen tension, resulting in a decrease in oxygen release. (From Bauer JD: *Clinical Laboratory Methods,* ed 9, St Louis, 1982, Mosby.)

of which are occupied by the four pyrrole rings of heme. The fifth iron valency bond attaches heme to globin, leaving the sixth iron valency bond available for a reversible combination with oxygen or other ligands.

The affinity of hemoglobin for oxygen depends on the partial pressure of oxygen (P_{O_2}). A plot of the oxygen content (percentage of molecule saturated with oxygen) against P_{O_2} for myoglobin subunits results in a hyperbolic oxygen dissociation curve, but a similar plot using hemoglobin gives a sigmoid curve (Fig. 40-5). The hyperbolic curve indicates appreciable release of oxygen at very low partial pressures only, whereas the sigmoid curve indicates much earlier release of oxygen, even at relatively high oxygen tensions, allowing adequate oxygenation of tissues. The curve has a sigmoid shape because oxygenation of one heme group increases the oxygen affinity of the others, a phenomenon called **heme-heme interaction** (or **subunit cooperativity**), which is responsible for the physiologically efficient uptake and release of oxygen. A progressive change in oxygen affinity is seen as each heme molecule becomes oxygenated; the affinity for oxygen is low at first but increases as each heme molecule takes up oxygen. In myoglobin, the hyperbolic dissociation curve indicates that each molecule is oxygenated independently. In the lung, at a P_{O_2} of about 95 mm Hg, arterial blood becomes 97% saturated with oxygen and carries 200 mL of oxygen per 1000 mL of blood. In the capillary bed, venous blood at a P_{O_2} tension of about 40 mm Hg is still about 75% saturated with oxygen but nevertheless is able to give up 46 mL of oxygen per 1000 mL of blood. The 75% of hemoglobin returned to the lung in an oxygenated form establishes a large reservoir for improved oxygen delivery to tissues.

The position of the oxygen dissociation curve is determined by several factors that affect the affinity of hemoglobin for oxygen. The oxygen dissociation curve is conventionally indexed by the P_{50} value, the P_{O_2} at which the hemoglobin is 50% saturated with O_2; this normally occurs at a P_{O_2} of 27 mm Hg. The higher the P_{50}, the lower is the affinity of hemoglobin for oxygen. A decreased P_{50} indicates a shift to the left of the oxygen dissociation curve, an increased oxygen affinity of hemoglobin, and an impaired oxygen release to tissues. P_{50} is decreased in the presence of (1) a high concentration of hemoglobin (Hb)F, the γ-chain of which binds 2,3-BPG poorly; (2) a modified hemoglobin, such as **methemoglobin** and **carboxyhemoglobin;** (3) certain hemoglobin variants, such as Hb Rainier; and (4) 2,3-BPG–depleted blood found after massive transfusions (see Fig. 40-5). Obviously, 2,3-BPG binding to hemoglobin decreases the affinity of hemoglobin for oxygen (see later discussion). A *shift to the right* indicates a decreased oxygen affinity, which causes the delivery of oxygen to tissues. This is seen in various types of hypoxia, such as that occurring at high altitudes, along with severe anemia and heart and lung disease.[2]

Oxygen Affinity and Transport

Oxygen affinity and transport depend not only on Po_2 (see earlier discussion) but also on temperature, pH (Bohr effect), and 2,3-BPG concentration.

Bohr Effect

The **Bohr effect** expresses the fact that the oxygen affinity of hemoglobin varies with the pH. Protons lower the affinity of hemoglobin for oxygen mass; conversely, oxygen lowers the affinity of hemoglobin for protons.

$$Hb(O_2)_4 + 2H^+ \rightleftharpoons Hb \bullet 2H^+ + 4O_2$$

At physiological pH in the tissues, about two protons are taken up for every four molecules of oxygen released, whereas in the lungs, two protons are liberated again when four molecules of oxygen are bound to hemoglobin. This reciprocal action is known as the Bohr effect and is essential to the mechanism of oxygen transport and the buffering of carbon dioxide (see Chapter 29).

In the physiological pH range, the affinity of hemoglobin for oxygen decreases in the tissues as acidity increases and the dissociation curve shifts to the right (see Fig. 40-5). The Bohr effect aids in the transport of oxygen and the buffering of carbon dioxide in the acid milieu of tissues in which carbon dioxide and acid metabolites accumulate and in the more alkaline milieu of the lungs, where carbon dioxide is released and oxygen is picked up. Both 2,3-BPG and chloride enhance the Bohr effect.

2,3-Biphosphoglycerate

Other molecules influence the structure and function of hemoglobin. Of the factors that affect oxygen release from hemoglobin (temperature, pH, Po_2, Pco_2, and 2,3-BPG), 2,3-BPG is the most important. It is the most abundant glycolytic intermediate in red blood cells and is present at a concentration equimolar with that of deoxyhemoglobin. In oxyhemoglobin, the helices of the β-chains are not open enough to permit firm stereospecific binding of 2,3-BPG within the central cavity of the hemoglobin tetramer to the N-terminal valine, the H21 histidine (position 143), and the EF6 lysine (position 82) of the β-chain. Thus 2,3-BPG binding stabilizes the deoxygenated form at the expense of the oxyhemoglobin form. This, along with other conformational changes in the oxygenated molecule, favors binding of 2,3-BPG to the deoxygenated rather than the oxygenated form, reducing the affinity of hemoglobin for oxygen and shifting the oxygen dissociation curve to the right.

$$HbO_2 + BPG \rightleftharpoons Hb \bullet BPG + O_2$$

During anaerobic metabolism, red cells increase the production of 2,3-BPG, thereby facilitating oxygen release.

The controlling factor of the 2,3-BPG-Bohr effect is the rate of glycolysis, which is stimulated by alkalosis and suppressed by acidosis, because the former stimulates phosphofructokinase activity (converting fructose 6-phosphate to fructose 1,6-diphosphate) and the latter suppresses it. 2,3-BPG is formed from 1,3-BPG, an intermediary of the Embden-Meyerhof pathway (Rappaport-Leubering cycle; see Fig. 38-3). When the pH drops, as in acidosis, the oxygen dissociation curve moves to the right, but the resulting reduction of 2,3-BPG production corrects the shift through an equal change to the left. An elevated red blood cell pH shifts the dissociation curve to the left, but the rising RBC 2,3-BPG concentration shifts it to the right, returning it to base position (see Fig. 40-5).

Other Chemical Derivatives of Hemoglobin

Besides oxyhemoglobin and deoxyhemoglobin (see earlier discussion and Chapter 29), other chemically modified forms of hemoglobin exist.

Hemoglobin A1

Hemoglobin A1 is formed by the postsynthetic, nonenzymatic reaction of various sugars with amino groups of the globin chains. HbA1 actually consists of four principal components, called HbA1a1, HbA1a2, HbA1b, and HbA1c. Hemoglobin A1c, the major sugar derivative, is produced by the reaction of glucose with the terminal amino group (valine) of the β-chain. The glycosylated hemoglobins are useful for the monitoring of diabetes; other hemoglobins are the adducts of glucose-6-phosphate or fructose-1,6-diphosphate and the β-chain. See Chapter 38 for further discussion of glycosylated hemoglobins.

Carbaminohemoglobin

Approximately 20% of the CO_2 carried in blood is covalently bound to the globin portion of hemoglobin. This CO_2-Hb complex is termed carbaminohemoglobin (see Chapter 29). Carbaminohemoglobin has a blue tinge, rendering venous blood darker than arterial blood.

Carboxyhemoglobin

Carbon monoxide (CO) is a ligand that, similar to oxygen, binds reversibly to the ferrous ion of hemoglobin. However, it forms a toxic compound, carboxyhemoglobin (CO-Hb). It also binds to other heme-containing proteins, such as myoglobin, cytochrome P-450, and cytochrome oxidase.[4] CO combines with hemoglobin more slowly than oxygen, but because the union is much firmer, the release of CO is 10,000 times slower than the release of oxygen from oxyhemoglobin. Also, the affinity of hemoglobin for CO is 218 times greater than that for oxygen. Because CO and O_2 compete for the same binding sites on heme, the presence of CO reduces the concentration of oxyhemoglobin. At a CO concentration of 0.1% in inhaled air, more than 50% of hemoglobin is unavailable for O_2 transport. In the presence of CO, oxyhemoglobin dissociates more slowly, because the iron atoms not bound to CO have a higher affinity for O_2, causing the oxygen dissociation curve to shift to the left. CO-Hb can be identified in blood by spectroscopic, spectrophotometric, chemical, or gas chromatographic techniques.[5] The presence of CO-Hb in blood does not cause substantial error in pulse oximetry[6]—a determination that has great clinical importance.

Methemoglobin

Methemoglobin (Met-Hb) is a form of hemoglobin (with oxy- or deoxy- forms) in which the ferrous ion (Fe^{2+}) of hemoglobin has been oxidized to the ferric state (Fe^{3+}) to form ferrihemoglobin. Met-Hb cannot bind oxygen reversibly and is unable to act as an effective oxygen transporter. If Met-Hb is present in high enough concentrations (over 30% of total hemoglobin), hypoxia and cyanosis (methemoglobinemia) will result. Normally, a small amount of methemoglobin forms continuously in RBCs; however, this usually does not exceed 1% of total hemoglobin because the methemoglobin is reduced back to Hb (see p. 785).

After prolonged exposure to air, the oxyhemoglobin in normal blood is autooxidized and the blood turns brown as methemoglobin is formed. This process is also responsible for the brown color of blood in acid urine.

Hemichromes

Hemichromes are greenish ferric compounds with characteristic absorption spectral profiles. During the oxidation of hemoglobin to Met-Hb, superoxide anions are formed, and hydrogen peroxide is produced. As a result, more Met-Hb is formed, and oxidative changes occur in the globin protein. These changes in the heme group and in the protein alter the stereochemical binding of heme to protein, and heme iron may form ligands with various side chains in the proteins (hemichromes), rather than with proximal histidine or with oxygen. The heme group can be displaced physically from the protein and can precipitate as free ferriheme (or hematin) onto the interior of the RBC membrane. Polypeptide chains also precipitate when they are denatured. These hemoglobin breakdown products form inclusions on the interior of the RBC membrane, called *Heinz bodies,* which are responsible for lysis of affected red cells.[7] The steps that lead to cell lysis occur as follows:

Oxyhemoglobin
↓
Methemoglobin
↓
Hemichrome 1, reversible
↓
Hemichrome 2, irreversible
↓
Heinz bodies
↓
Lysis

Hematologists use supravital stains to identify Heinz bodies, which are found in a group of anemias known as *Heinz body anemias.*

Sulfhemoglobin

Sulfhemoglobin (S-Hb) is a stable compound that results from linkage of sulfur to hemoglobin. The toxic effects of certain drugs on hemoglobin lead not only to the formation of methemoglobin, but also to concomitant S-Hb production.[5]

Sulfhemoglobinemia occurs in some persons after exposure to sulfonamides, phenacetin, acetanilid, and trinitrotoluene. It is not clear why Met-Hb is found in the blood of some individuals, whereas S-Hb is reported in the blood of others after exposure to these drugs. The structure of S-Hb is unknown, but sulfur probably is linked to heme. The S-Hb complex is stable and irreversible (thus differing from Met-Hb) and does not disappear from the circulation until affected RBCs complete their life cycle. Sulfhemoglobin produces anoxia and cyanosis, which clinically are indistinguishable from the anoxia and cyanosis of Met-Hb. Sulfhemoglobin shows a characteristic absorption of light at 620 nm that does not shift when cyanide is added. Rarely, sulfhemoglobin causes Heinz body formation.

This form of hemoglobin is unable to transport oxygen, however, in contrast to methemoglobin, a high concentration of sulfhemoglobin can be tolerated despite the resulting physiological anemia. Sulfhemoglobinemia does not respond to methylene blue, a reducing agent effective in methemoglobinemia, since S-Hb is an irreversible state and thus not amenable to reduction. The treatment is supportive, with removal of the suspected causative agent.

SECTION OBJECTIVES BOX 40-2

- Describe the Hb forms found in healthy adults.
- Define the term *hemoglobin variants,* and describe how they may be formed.
- Describe the types of hemoglobinopathies.
- List the clinical outcomes that may be associated with an Hb variant.
- List four clinical manifestations of HbSS.
- Name and describe two other common hemoglobinopathies.
- Differentiate between α- and β-thalassemias.

NORMAL HUMAN HEMOGLOBINS (Table 40-1)

Hemoglobin A ($\alpha_2\beta_2$)

Hemoglobin A makes up the major portion (95% to 98%) of the adult hemolysate. Small amounts of HbA are produced in the last 6 weeks of fetal life (see Chapter 44), along with the predominant fetal hemoglobin. Over 6 to 12 months postpartum, the shift to the adult form of hemoglobin is completed (see later discussion).

Hemoglobin A_2 ($\alpha_2\delta_2$)

Hemoglobin A_2 is a minor component of hemoglobin that makes its first appearance before the completion of intrauterine development (0.2% of cord blood hemolysate) and

Table 40-1 Normal Human Hemoglobins

		HEMOLYSATE (%)	
Designation	Tetrameric Structure	Adult	Newborn
Adult			
HbA	$\alpha_2\beta_2$	95 to 98	20 to 30
HbA_2	$\alpha_2\delta_2$	2 to 3	0.2
Fetal			
HbF	$\alpha_2\gamma_2$	<1	80
Embryonic			
Gower 1	$\zeta_2\varepsilon_2$	0	0
Gower 2	$\alpha_2\varepsilon_2$	0	0
Hb Portland	$\zeta_2\gamma_2$	0	0

remains at low concentration (2.5%) throughout adult life. Its exact function is unknown but is probably similar to that of HbA.

Fetal Hemoglobin ($\alpha_2\gamma_2$)

Hemoglobin F is the major hemoglobin of fetal life and is preceded by the embryonic hemoglobins Gower 1, Gower 2, and Portland. HbF is a mixture of two molecular species in which the γ-chains have glycine (Gγ) or alanine (Aγ) at position 136. At birth, the HbF Gγ/Aγ ratio is about 3:1, whereas in the normal adult, the Gγ/Aγ ratio of the small amount of HbF (less than 1%) is 2:3. In the first months of fetal life, small amounts of HbF are produced along with the Gower hemoglobins, which are replaced by HbF at the end of the second month. From this time to just before birth, the percentage of fetal hemoglobin is about 90%. At birth, the RBCs contain about 70% to 90% HbF, although higher concentrations have been reported. After birth, HbF normally decreases rapidly to about 50% to 70% at the end of the first month, 25% to 60% at the end of the second month, and 10% to 30% at the end of the third month. Between 6 months and 12 months, the HbF concentration falls from 8% to 2%; in the second year, it falls to 1.8%; and in the third year, it falls to 1%. It finally levels off to the adult level of less than <1%, a level not detectable by routine laboratory methods. It normally is slightly increased (up to 3%) during pregnancy.

The functions and molecular characteristics of HbF are as follows:

1. Electrophoretically, it is slower than HbA.
2. It resists alkali denaturation—a feature that forms the basis of the Singer test for HbF.[7]
3. It is twice as resistant to acid elution as HbA—a characteristic that forms the basis of the Kleihauer elution technique.[8]
4. HbF is oxidized to Met-Hb twice as quickly as HbA, predisposing the newborn to cyanosis.
5. It has a higher oxygen affinity than HbA has, because it binds 2,3-BPG to a lesser degree than adult hemoglobin because of its γ-chain. This characteristic allows oxygen transport across the placental villi, despite their low oxygen concentration (80%).[9]

The molecular properties of HbF allow HbF to function as the primary oxygen carrier for the fetus. The other embryonic hemoglobins have similar properties and are able to combine with oxygen at the low oxygen tension and low pH of interstitial fluid, facilitating fetal growth and development. Embryonic hemoglobins are detectable in red cells through modification of the Kleihauer method for HbF.

PATHOLOGICAL CONDITIONS

Hemoglobinopathies

The inherited disorders of hemoglobin, the hemoglobinopathies, are genetic disorders involving the structure and synthesis of one or more of the globin polypeptide chains. Hemoglobinopathies may be divided into several overlapping groups[10]: (1) structural hemoglobin variants that involve substitution, addition, or deletion of one or more amino acids of the globin chain; (2) **thalassemias,** a group of disorders in which a quantitative defect in globin chain production is present; (3) combinations of types 1 and 2 that result in complex hemoglobinopathies; and (4) **hereditary persistence of fetal hemoglobin (HPFH),** an asymptomatic disorder.

Structural Hemoglobin Variants (see Chapter 5)

Nomenclature

Hemoglobins A, F, and S were the first hemoglobins to be discovered and were assigned letters. As additional variants were discovered, they were assigned successive letters of the alphabet, beginning with HbC. Subsequently, hemoglobins were discovered so rapidly that the letters of the alphabet were depleted. Therefore, hemoglobins with similar electrophoretic mobility, but with different structures, were distinguished by adding (properly as a subscript) the place of discovery of the new hemoglobin, such as $HbC_{Georgetown}$, HbD_{Punjab}. Finally, some hemoglobins are called by the names of the families in which they were first discovered, such as Hb_{Lepore}. When the exact amino acid substitution of the new variant and the spatial structure of hemoglobin were determined, the expression became more complex. For instance, HbS evolved into the scientific designation: HbS B6 (A3) Glu → Val. This designation reveals that the substitution is located at the sixth position of the amino acid sequence, in the A3 position of the β-chain. It also shows that glutamine (Glu) has been replaced by a valine (Val). More than 700 variant hemoglobins have been identified in humans up to the present. Some of the more important ones demonstrating clinical disorders are shown in Table 5-2. Excellent tables on nomenclature, molecular structure, clinical manifestations, and electrophoretic mobility of hemoglobin variants are found in reference 11.

Classification

Hemoglobin variants are classified according to (1) molecular mechanism, (2) clinical and functional manifestations, and (3) electrophoretic behavior.

Molecular Mechanisms Responsible for Structural Hemoglobin Variants

Five basic molecular mechanisms are responsible for the structural changes found in most hemoglobin variants: (1) amino acid substitution, (2) amino acid deletions and insertions, (3) unequal crossing over (fusion genes), (4) chain elongation, and (5) frame shift variance.[11]

Clinical Consequences of Structural Alterations of Hemoglobin Molecules

Structural alterations of the hemoglobin molecule are responsible for a wide range of clinical manifestations. Most mutations are asymptomatic because they do not interfere with hemoglobin function. Others produce disease, because they affect the stability, shape, or function of the hemoglobin molecule. A person homozygous for abnormal hemoglobin may have striking clinical manifestations such as **sickle cell anemia,** whereas a person heterozygous for abnormal hemoglobin (HbA-HbS) usually is asymptomatic. Some hemoglobins (HbC, HbD, HbE) even in the homozygous state produce only mild symptoms, whereas others are responsible for almost specific pathophysiological changes, such as cyanosis and erythrocytosis. Some combinations, such as HbS with HbO_{Arab}, are actually more aggressive disease states than either alone. Conversely, other combinations, such as HbS and HbC generate milder symptoms than either Hb alone.

The clinical disorders can be grouped as follows.

Hemolytic Anemias

Intraerythrocytic crystals of HbS and HbC may form and cause deformity of the RBCs. Such deformities, such as the sickle-shaped cells of sickle cell anemia, are recognized easily by light microscopy. Unstable hemoglobins and enzyme abnormalities of the hexose-monophosphate shunt are also responsible for intraerythrocytic Heinz body inclusions. Affected cells are destroyed prematurely in the spleen, resulting in a greatly shortened red cell life span. HbS adults are functionally asplenic, because of the continuous splenic damage induced by the malformed erythrocytes.

Cyanosis

Amino acid substitution near the heme pocket produces *M-hemoglobins,* which result in methemoglobinemia and cyanosis. Cyanosis also may occur because of hemoglobin mutants such as Hb_{Kansas}, and $Hb_{BethIsrael}$ that result in increased deoxyhemoglobin. Both types of hemoglobin show decreased oxygen affinity.

Erythrocytosis

Some amino acid substitutions result in high oxygen affinity and tissue hypoxia. Because of the hypoxia, erythropoietin synthesis is stimulated, resulting in an increased production of RBCs *(erythrocytosis)* and peripheral blood nucleated erythrocytes. Examples are $Hb_{Rainier}$, $Hb_{Chesapeake}$, and $Hb_{Ypsilanti}$.

Hypochromic Anemias

Some mutations reduce hemoglobin output. Examples are Hb_{Lepore} and $Hb_{ConstantSpring}$.

Electrophoretic and Chromatographic Behavior of Hemoglobins

Hemoglobin electrophoresis and cation-exchange high performance liquid chromatography (HPLC) are the most important laboratory procedures used to diagnose and classify a hemoglobin abnormality (see p. 119). However, no single hemoglobin test can accurately distinguish an abnormal hemoglobin from a thalassemic disorder.

Sickle Cell Disorders: Sickle Hemoglobin

Sickling disorders are caused by the homozygous form of the sickle cell gene (sickle cell anemia), the heterozygous form of the sickle cell gene (sickle cell trait), and the combination of either with other structural hemoglobin variants or thalassemias.

Sickle hemoglobin (HbS) results when valine is substituted for the normally occurring glutamine residue, and intracellular crystals of deoxygenated HbS form, causing the RBC to sickle.

HbS is not the only hemoglobin that causes RBCs to sickle, because RBCs that contain $HbC_{Georgetown}$, HbI, and $Hb_{Bart's}$ also sickle. Nevertheless, in America and Africa, HbS is the most common hemoglobin variant, with an incidence of the heterozygous form of approximately 8% in American blacks and 30% in African blacks. HbS also can be found among nonblack inhabitants in the areas bordering Africa. In Africa, the high frequency of the sickle cell gene has persisted because heterozygotes for HbS are somewhat protected from malaria because *Plasmodium* organisms fail to grow in HbS-containing RBCs.[12] Even more marked protection may be conferred by Hgb SS.

Table 40-2 Varying Clinical Severity of the Different Sickle Syndromes

Genotype	% of Hemoglobin S	% of Non-S Hemoglobin	Clinical Severity
SA	30 to 40	60 to 70 (A)	0
SF*	70	30 (F)	0
SS	80 to 90	5 to 15 (F)	++/++++
S-thalassemia	80	20 (A + F)	+/+++
SC	50	50 (C)	+/+++
SO.SD	30 to 40	60 to 70	++/++++

From Bunn HF: Sickle cell anemia and other hemoglobinopathies. In Beck WS, editor: *Hematology,* Cambridge, Mass 1981, MIT Press.
*Double heterozygous state for hemoglobin S and hereditary persistence of fetal hemoglobin.

Molecular Mechanism of Sickling

The substitution of valine for normal glutamic acid at position 6 in the β-chain results in a hemoglobin whose deoxy form (deoxy-HbS) polymerizes within the RBCs and forms long fibers that are readily visible on electron microscopy of red cells from patients homozygous for the β^S mutation. Oxyhemoglobin S does *not* form such fibers.

Several facts about the polymerization are relevant to the pathogenesis of the sickle configuration and to possible therapeutic intervention. The polymerization occurs in two phases. The first of these, the slow nucleation (or *delay*) phase, reflects the initial association of a few molecules of deoxy-HbS. This phase varies in duration from milliseconds to a few minutes, depending on several factors, including temperature and the presence of hemoglobins other than HbS.

The duration also depends, exponentially, on the concentration of HbS. Thus a prolonged delay time, resulting from a decreased concentration of HbS within the RBC, might permit the deoxygenated cell to traverse the microcirculation without sickling. Factors that favor increasing polymerization of HbS within red cells and thus the severity of the disease have their effect by increasing the relative abundance of deoxy-HbS. Such factors include a decrease in Po_2, increased organic phosphates, increased hydrogen ion concentrations, and increased temperature.[13] The varying clinical severity of the different sickle syndromes is depicted in Table 40-2.

Pathophysiology of Sickle Cell Disease

HbS is inherited as an autosomal co-dominant trait. The sickle-shaped cells temporarily or permanently block microcirculation, and the resulting stasis leads to hypoxia and ischemic infarcts of various organs, including liver, kidneys, spleen, lungs, heart, bones, and nervous system. Such infarcts lead to increased morbidity and, if located in a vital area, may cause death.[14] Based on studies from numerous laboratories, the emerging consensus is that a key contributor to vasoocclusion may be the increased tendency of sickle red cells to adhere to vascular endothelium.[15,16] Vasoocclusion can occur when the transit time of red cells through the capillaries is longer than the delay time for deoxyhemoglobin-induced hemoglobin polymerization of sickle hemoglobin. Consequently, adherence of the sickle red cells to vascular endothelium impedes blood flow and thereby increases capillary transit time. Therefore, it has been suggested that increased cell adherence can initiate and propagate vasoocclusion. Factors such as inflammatory mediators that activate endothelial cells and thereby enhance the endothelial adversity of sickle red cells thus have the potential to trigger vasoocclusive episodes. A partial list of agonists of the endothelium includes tumor necrosis factor (TNF)-α/β, interferon γ, 1L-1B, vascular endothelial growth factor (VEGF), thrombin, histamine, and the effects of hypoxia and reperfusion.

Sickle red cells exhibit increased adherence to endothelial cells in vitro, and the extent of in vitro sickle adherence correlates with vasoocclusive severity.[17] Adhesive ligands identified for sickle red cells include CD36, α4 B1 integrin, sulfated glycolipid, and the Lutheran blood group antigen. On the endothelial side, cytokine-induced vascular cell adhesion molecule-1 (VCAM-1), a ligand for $\alpha_4 B$, and $\alpha_v B_3$ subunits of integrin that binds von Willebrand factor and thrombospondin, has been shown to mediate sickle cell adherence. Bridging molecules connect adhesive receptors on sickle cells and endothelial cells.

In addition to adherence, viscosity plays an important role in affecting the rate of blood flow (hypoxia) and the production of thrombosis. Studies indicate that membrane viscosity and deformability in sickle cell disease are altered markedly, even when the red cell is fully oxygenated.[18-20] Although internal viscosity of red cells is of great importance in determining the flow characteristics of blood, the hematocrit is a major determinant of whole blood viscosity. Effects on the circulation caused by increased viscosity are seen in larger blood vessels compared with the effects of adherence and occlusion. Thrombosis can be seen on the arterial or venous side of the circulation and has been known for many years in the pathophysiology of polycythemia and macroglobulinemia.[21]

Sickled cells have a greatly shortened life span. The ensuing hemolytic anemia is exacerbated by the inability of the bone marrow to respond adequately to the anemia because of ineffective erythropoiesis. Increased RBC destruction is responsible for hyperbilirubinemia, reticulocytosis, bone marrow erythroid hyperplasia, gallbladder pigment stones, and osteoporosis as a result of the expanding bone marrow.

Sickle cells exhibit oxygen transport abnormalities.[22] In sickled cells, the oxygen dissociation curve is shifted to the right. The resulting decreased oxygen affinity favors the release of oxygen at higher oxygen tensions but also supports the formation of deoxyhemoglobin and sickling. The shift to the right of the oxygen equilibrium is caused by an elevated 2,3-BPG concentration and by HbS polymerization. In vitro studies have shown that the oxygen affinity of HbS depends upon the severity of its polymerization, and that in the absence of polymer formation, sickle hemoglobin (HbS) has normal oxygen affinity.

Sickle Cell Trait (HbAS)

Persons with sickle cell trait are usually asymptomatic and have a normal **hemogram** (RBC profile; including RBC count, mean corpuscular volume [MCV], and mean corpuscular hemoglobin [MCH]); and normal RBC survival. The demonstration of HbS is usually of no clinical significance, because a normal HbA gene has been inherited along with the HbS gene, but it should indicate the need for genetic counseling. Sickling complications have been reported rarely in HbAS patients. These include (1) spontaneous hematuria in about 3% of patients and more frequently hyposthenuria (urine of low specific gravity) caused by impairment of the concentrating power of the kidneys, both signs pointing to sickling within the blood vessels of the medulla; (2) rupture of the infarcted spleen; (3) sickling crisis at elevated altitudes; and (4) rarely, proliferative retinopathy.

Sickle Cell Anemia (HbSS)

Sickle cell anemia is a chronic, moderate to severe, hemolytic anemia in a person homozygous for HbS who has inherited the HbS gene from both parents. The finding of HbSS is useful for differentiating sickle cell anemia from sickle cell–β-thalassemia or HbS hereditary persistence of HbF. The disease is not evident at birth and does not manifest until the γ-chains of the newborn are replaced by β^S-chains after 3 to 6 months of life.

The clinical severity of HbSS disease varies from patient to patient. Such variation has been clarified further by the investigation of haplotypes (Fig. 40-6). These genetic variations are of hematological, genetic, and anthropological interest, because they offer new insights into sickling disorders. Each haplotype has a different combination of 14 cleavage sites for 10 DNA restriction endonucleases in the vicinity of the β-globin locus. Each haplotype, plus genetic modifiers on the X-chromosome, contributes additively to the proportion of HbF, with the Senegal and Indian haplotypes contributing more than those from Benin, Bantu, and Cameroon poulations. Clinical manifestations may be divided into acute and chronic episodes. Acute problems result from vasoocclusive crises involving several areas, as well as acute hematological crises (Box 40-1).

Box 40-1

Acute Clinical Manifestations of HbSS

Hematological
Accelerated hemolytic anemia
Megaloblastic anemia
Aplastic crisis

Vasoocclusive
Bone and joints
Abdomen, spleen
Lungs
Central nervous system
Back

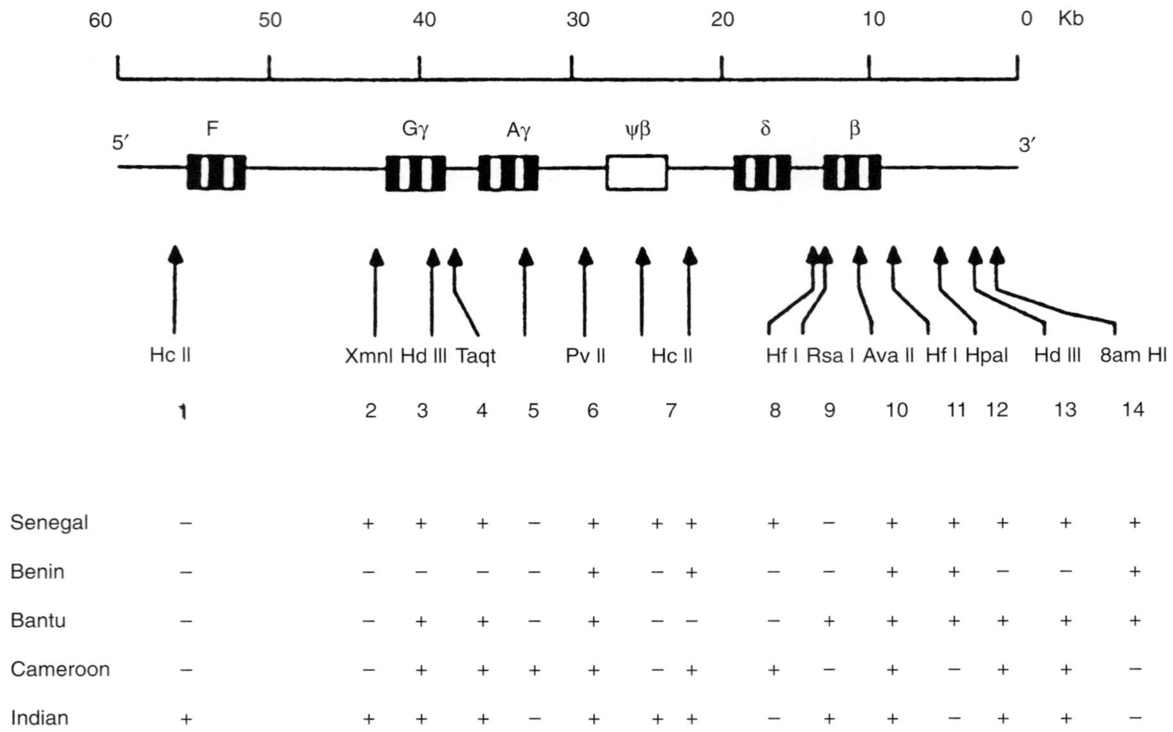

Fig. 40-6 Restriction endonuclease polymorphisms in the β-globin cluster. *Top,* Arrows point to the cleavage sites for each of the enzymes. *Bottom,* Haplotypes defined by patterns of cleavage typical of the regions in which each haplotype is most prevalent. (From Nagel RL: Origins and dispersions of the sickle gene. In Embury SH, Hebbel RP, Mohandas N, et al: *Sickle Cell Disease: Basic Principles and Clinical Practice,* New York, 1994, Raven Press.)

Splenic crisis may result from sudden trapping of blood in the spleen. Chronic manifestations of sickle cell disease usually appear after mid-childhood. These include disturbances in growth and development, bone and joint disease, and organ damage involving cardiovascular, pulmonary, hepatobiliary, genitourinary, ocular, and dermatological systems. Renal failure may occur in many patients with sickle cell anemia, probably as the result of glomerular capillary disease.

Hemoglobin values hover around 7 to 8 g/dL and are accompanied by a greatly elevated reticulocytosis (10%). The hemoglobin electrophoretogram shows absence of HbA (no β^A-chains), 80% to 95% HbS, 2% to 4% HbA_2, and 2% to 20% HbF. Outstanding biochemical findings include (1) hyperuricemia in patients with altered tubular function; (2) reduced zinc levels in plasma, red cells, and hair; and (3) high serum lactate dehydrogenase levels in patients in crisis.

Treatment of HbSS is designed to (1) inhibit HbS polymerization, (2) decrease intracellular levels of total Hb, and (3) increase the concentration of HbF. Many drugs have been used to increase HbF, which early on was recognized to interfere with HbS polymerization. The first "hemoglobin switching" agent, a nucleoside analog 5-azacytidine, was postulated to increase HbF by inducing gene expression. Hydroxyurea promotes HbF production indirectly, perturbing the maturation of erythroid precursors. Butyrates appear to directly modulate globin gene expression by binding to transcriptionally active elements.[23] Hydroxyurea is the cornerstone of treatment for sickle cell disease. Bone marrow transplant has also been introduced for young children with severe symptomatology from both sickle cell disease and β-thalassemia.

Sickle Cell–HbC Disease

Sickle cell–HbC disease has a relatively high incidence (1 in 833 births among blacks in the United States) because HbS and HbC are common hemoglobin variants. The patient inherits one abnormal gene from each parent, and the resulting disease is a mild to moderate hemolytic anemia associated with the same vasoocclusive complications that are seen in sickle cell disease. However, these complications usually occur at a lower frequency. Because genes in this disease are allelic β-chain mutations, no normal β-chains are formed, and HbA is absent.

Peripheral blood smear reveals many target cells, rare sickle cells, and red cells with straight, curved, or misshapen crystals. Erythrocytes containing Hb SC exhibit unusual morphologic features, particularly the tendency for membrane "folding", crystals, and cells containing round Hb aggregates, called "billiard-ball cells." Hemoglobin values range from 10 to 13 g/dL, with only HbC and HbS bands seen on electrophoresis. The reticulocyte count varies from 3% to 10%.

HbC Trait (Hgb AC)

Hgb C results from an amino acid substitution of Lys for Glu at the β6 position. HbC trait (HbAC) is a clinically benign condition that affects about 2.3% of American blacks. It is asymptomatic, and the peripheral blood smear is normal except for a few target cells. Hemoglobin analysis show about 30% to 40% HbC, 50% to 60% HbA, 3% to 4% HbA_2, and 7% HbF.

Hemoglobin C Disease (HbCC)

The homozygous form is uncommon, with a prevalence of about 0.017% in American blacks, and is asymptomatic. Upon examination, the patient has features of mild to moderate anemia, some degree of splenomegaly, numerous target cells, and HbC crystals.

Hemoglobin E Trait (HbAE) and Disease (HbEE)

The variant HbE, or B26 Glu → Lys, is the second most common hemoglobin abnormality worldwide. Because of the large influx of immigrants from Southeast Asia, an increasing number of patients with HbE are encountered in the United States. HbE trait (HbAE), although clinically silent, exhibits moderately severe microcytosis and no anemia. The amount of HbE in HbE trait is 30% to 35%. This is lower than expected for a heterozygous condition, for example, 45% HbS is observed in patients with sickle cell trait. This discrepancy is attributable to the thalassemia-like defect of the HbE gene.

HbE results in a heterogeneous group of disorders whose phenotype range from asymptomatic to severe. Patients with HbE disease exhibit mild microcytic, normochromic anemia with many target cells, conferring a thalassemic phenotype.

Because many Southeast Asians have α- and β-thalassemic gene abnormalities, combinations of HbE with these genes become much more clinically significant. For example, patients with HbE-β^0 thalassemia have significant anemia and require transfusions—a clinical situation similar to that seen with thalassemia intermedia.

Unstable Hemoglobin Disorder

The unstable hemoglobins are structural variants of HbA, in which the mutant hemoglobin is less stable than normal hemoglobin. Approximately 150 variants of HbA have been shown to be unstable in in vitro tests. However, only 70 have been shown to have significant clinical manifestation, usually hemolysis. The molecular distortion responsible for unstable hemoglobin produces a series of pathophysiological effects that can be evaluated by laboratory methods, although they are not expressed equally by all unstable hemoglobins. These include (1) hemolytic anemia, (2) increased methemoglobin and sulfhemoglobin production, (3) hemichrome formation, (4) inclusion (Heinz) body formation, (5) altered oxygen dissociation, (6) drug sensitivity, (7) altered electrophoretic mobility (rare), (8) altered response to hemoglobin stability tests, and (9) passage of dark urine. The deeply pigmented urine is caused by mesobilifuscin, a dipyrrole derived from the catabolism of Heinz bodies or free heme.

THALASSEMIAS[24-28]

Definitions

Thalassemias are inherited hemoglobinopathies that result from a decreased rate of production of one or more globin chains of hemoglobin.[10,26] They are quantitative hemoglobinopathies that differ from qualitative hemoglobinopathies in that the structure of the affected globin chain (or chains) is normal, but its synthesis is reduced or absent. The thalassemias are classified according to which chain of the hemoglobin molecule is affected. In α-thalassemias decreased production of the α globin chain is seen, while in β-thalassemia, production of the β globin chain is affected. The decreased hemoglobin synthesis results in decreased RBC hemoglobin, hypochromia, microcytosis, and a variable degree of hemolysis. Generally, thalassemias are prevalent in populations where malaria was endemic. The thalassemias are particularly associated with people of Mediterranean origin (especially in Greece and southern Italy), Arabs, and Asians, but are found in all races. Deletion of one of the α loci has a high prevalence in people of African-American or Asian descent, making them more likely to develop an α-thalassemia. β-thalassemias are common in African-Americans, but also in Greeks and Italians. Defective synthesis of one set of globin chains results in excessive production of the unaffected pair[10] (imbalanced globin chain synthesis), which precipitates in the RBCs in the form of inclusion bodies that cause hemolysis.

Classification

The most common phenotypic classification of thalassemias as *thalassemia major, intermedia, minor,* and *minima* describes the clinical severity of the disorder and disregards the genetic makeup. The preferred genetic classification is based on the particular deficient polypeptide chain. In **α-thalassemia,** the synthesis of α-chains is diminished; in **β-thalassemia,** the synthesis of β-chains is diminished. The major forms of thalassemia are depicted in Table 40-3.

Thalassemias involving γ-, ε-, or ζ-genes may lead to fetal or embryonic death.[26] A thalassemia-like condition that is asymptomatic is HPFH. The inheritance of thalassemia is autosomal and is similar to that of HbS. From the clinical viewpoint, it is recessive because the heterozygous form is asymptomatic. Similar to the HbS(β^S) gene, the thalassemia gene may express itself in homozygous, heterozygous, and doubly heterozygous states.

The clinical range varies from normal to a severe, life-threatening condition and can include growth retardation, hepatomegaly, bone overgrowth, bone pain, and jaundice.

α-Thalassemias

The α-thalassemias are a group of genetic disorders that result in defective α-chain synthesis. The α-thalassemias are inherited in an autosomal recessive fashion; they may also be secondary to a deletion of the short arm of chromosome 16.

The α-thalassemias are more difficult to diagnose because characteristic elevations in HbA_2 or HbF seen in the β-thalassemias are not observed. Diminished α-chain synthesis depresses the production of HbA, HbF, and HbA_2 because they contain α-chains, and this leads to excess β- and γ-chains, which polymerize to the tetrameric forms γ_4 ($Hb_{Bart's}$) and β_4 (HbH, which demonstrate an abnormal oxygen dissociation

Table 40-3 Laboratory Findings in α-Thalassemias

Genotype	Anemia (Hypochromic)	Hb Types	α-Chain Deletions
α-Thalassemia 1 trait	±	Birth: $Hb_{Bart's}$ 5% to 10% HbCS 1% to 2% Adult: HbA, A_2, F	2
α-Thalassemia 1/α-thalassemia 1 (hydrops fetalis)	+++	Birth: $Hb_{Bart's}$ 80% Traces of HbH and Portland Adult: Not compatible with life	4
α-Thalassemia 2 trait	±	Birth: $Hb_{Bart's}$ 1% to 2% HbCS 1% to 2% Adult: HbA, A_2, F	1
α-Thalassemia 1/α-thalassemia 2 (HbH disease)	± (Inclusions)	Birth: $Hb_{Bart's}$ 1% to 15% HbB 4% to 30% Adult: HbA, A_2, F HbH 8% to 10%	3
α-Thalassemia 1/HbCS (Hb H/CS)	++ (Inclusions)	Birth: $Hb_{Bart's}$ HbH, HbCS Adult: HbH HbA, A_2, F, CS	2 plus α-chain termination mutation
α-Thalassemia 2/HbCS	+	Birth: $Hb_{Bart's}$ Adult: HbA, CS	1 plus α-chain termination mutation
HbCS/HbCS	+	Birth: $Hb_{Bart's}$ Adult: HbA, A_2, F, CS	α-chain termination mutation

curve). The presence of these hemoglobins is the hallmark of α-thalassemia. Four classical α-thalassemias include α-thalassemia-2 trait (silent carrier), in which one of the four α-globin gene loci fails to function; α-thalassemia-1 trait (mild hypochromic anemia) with two dysfunctional loci; HbH (moderate severe hemolytic anemia) with three loci affected; and $Hb_{Bart's}$ (hydrops fetalis incompatible with life), in which all four loci are affected. α-Thalassemia also may result from the production of $Hb_{ConstantSpring}$ (HbCS). This hemoglobin is the result of a mutation in the terminal codon of the 3′ portion of DNA that normally stops α-chain production. Therefore, HbCS contains 172 amino acids in the α-chain rather than 141. Production of this elongated α-chain causes an inadequacy of α-chains relative to non–α-chains, with a resultant thalassemic condition (see Table 40-3).

β-Thalassemias[25,26]

The β-thalassemias are a group of genetic disorders that result in diminished (β^+ and β^{++} thalassemias) or absent (β^0-thalassemia) β-chain synthesis. They are inherited in a multitude of genetic combinations responsible for a heterogeneous group of clinical syndromes. Similar to α-thalassemia, β-thalassemia is transmitted as a Mendelian autosomal recessive characteristic. The output of β-chains is reduced or absent because of a defect in transcription of the β-thalassemia genes. Currently, point mutations that result in the various β-thalassemias number approximately 200. β-Thalassemia major, also known as *Cooley's anemia,* or *homozygous β-thalassemia,* is a clinically severe disorder caused by the inheritance of two β-thalassemia alleles, one on each copy of chromosome 11. The hypochromic anemia of thalassemia major is so severe that lifetime blood transfusions usually are required.

β-Thalassemias are distributed widely throughout the world but occur most frequently in the Mediterranean population; they also occur in Southeast Asia, the Middle East, India, and Pakistan. In Greeks and in American blacks, the β^+-thalassemia is most common, whereas in Italy, the β^0 is predominant.

The severity of the disease depends on the nature of the mutation. Structural mutations within the coding region of the globin gene allele may result in nonsense or truncation mutations of the corresponding globin chain, leading to complete loss of globin synthesis from that allele (β^0 thalassemia). Alternatively, abnormalities of transcriptional regulation or mutations that alter splicing may cause markedly decreased, but not absent, globin gene synthesis (β^+ thalassemia).

β-Thalassemia minima, also called β^{++} thalassemia, is known as the silent form of the disorder. There are no major hematologic abnormalities. The only noted abnormality is a decrease in β globin production.[61]

If only one β globin allele bears a mutation, the disease is called **β-thalassemia minor** (or **β-thalassemia trait**).

Heterozygous β-thalassemia, whether β^+ or β^0, is an asymptomatic disorder that may or may not be associated with a mild degree of anemia.[27] It is the most commonly found thalassemia in North America.[10,27] Characteristically, slight to moderate erythrocytosis of poorly hemoglobinized RBCs is seen. The MCH and the MCV are always strikingly decreased. The mean corpuscular hemoglobin content (MCHC) is variable.

The designation **thalassemia intermedia** describes clinical manifestations of a form of β-thalassemia more severe than thalassemia trait, but milder than the homozygous form. It is usually seen in patients who are double heterozygotes for thalassemic alleles, at least one of which is β^+. Affected individuals can often manage a normal life but may need occasional transfusions at times of illness, pregnancy, or surgery, depending on the severity of their anemia. Most patients have splenomegaly and prominent bony expansion.

β-thalassemia major, also known as *Cooley's anemia*, or β^0 *thalassemia*, is a clinically severe disorder caused by the inheritance of 2 abnormal β-thalassemia alleles, leading to a severe deficiency in β chain synthesis. Symptoms are usually evident within the first 6 months of life, as the levels of Hgb F begin to decline. This is a severe microcytic, hypochromic anemia associated with marked bone marrow hypertrophy. The ineffective erythropoiesis leads to skeletal changes, growth retardation, progressive hepatosplenomegaly, gallstone formation and heart disease. Untreated, this progresses to death before age twenty. Treatment consists of periodic blood transfusion; splenectomy if splenomegaly is present, and treatment of transfusion-caused iron overload. Cure is possible by bone marrow transplantation.

Homozygous β^0-thalassemia leads to complete suppression of β-chain synthesis and to complete absence of HbA. It is the cause of a severe lethal transfusion-dependent hemolytic anemia accompanied by characteristic clinical and hematological findings. Homozygous β^+ thalassemia is a heterogeneous disorder that, on the basis of the amount of HbA synthesized, is best divided into three main types. Type 1, in which 5% to 15% HbA is synthesized, is the Mediterranean and Oriental form, characterized by a severe transfusion-dependent anemia. Type 2, of African background, has 20% to 30% HbA and is responsible for a milder disease. Type 3 leads to a mild form of thalassemia intermedia.[27]

Pregnancy may lead to severe anemia in patients with thalassemia trait.[28] The hemoglobin electrophoretogram shows a slightly elevated HbF (1% to 7%) in 50% of cases and a diagnostic elevation of A_2 (3.5% to 7.5%).[22] Distribution of HbF within the RBCs demonstrated by acid elution technique reveals a heterogeneous pattern.

Thalassemias and Hemoglobinopathies

Thalassemia can co-exist with other hemoglobinopathies. The most common of these are:

- Hb E/thalassemia: common in Cambodia, Thailand, and parts of India; clinically similar to β thalassemia major or thalassemia intermedia.
- Hb S/thalassemia, common in African and Mediterranean populations; clinically similar to sickle cell anemia, with the additional feature of splenomegaly
- Hb C/thalassemia: common in Mediterranean and African populations, hemoglobin C/β^0 thalassemia causes a moderately severe hemolytic anemia with splenomegaly; hemoglobin C/β^+ thalassemia produces a milder disease.

Hereditary Persistence of Fetal Hemoglobin (HPFH)

HPFH consists of a group of rare conditions characterized by continued synthesis of high levels of HbF in adult life. No deleterious effects on patients are observed, and such an absence supports the concept that prevention or reversal of the switch from fetal hemoglobin to adult hemoglobin would benefit patients with sickle cell anemia and β-thalassemia. It is considered to be a form of δβ-thalassemia[29] because the persistence of γ-chain synthesis compensates for the deficient δ- and β-chain production.

Two major types of HPFH exist: pancellular and heterocellular. The pancellular type has very high levels of fetal hemoglobin synthesis and uniform distribution of HbF among all RBCs. It can be divided further by mutation type into deletional and nondeletional forms. HPFH shows ethnic differences in that blacks with heterozygous pancellular deletional disease have HbF ranges between 15% and 35% and contain γ^{Gly} and γ^{Ala} chains in a ratio of 2:3. On the other hand, Greeks with pancellular nondeletional HPFH demonstrate lower HbF levels (10% to 20%) and contain 90% γ^{Ala}.

A few black patients may have homozygous HPFH. All the Hb within red cells is HbF. These patients demonstrate mild microcytic hypochromic erythrocytes but no anemia.

HPFH–β-thalassemia is similar to the β-thalassemia trait except for a greater proportion and regular distribution of HbF in the RBCs.[30] Some patients with HPFH–δβ-thalassemia may have a more severe clinical condition similar to thalassemia intermedia.

Heterocellular HPFH seems to result from mutations outside the globin gene cluster and results in a variable increase in the number of F-cells. HbF levels are usually lower than those in the pancellular forms.

Methemoglobinemia[31,32]

Methemoglobinemia is classified into acquired and hereditary forms.[5] Four metabolic pathways are available for the reduction of methemoglobin to hemoglobin: (1) the NADH methemoglobin reductase pathway, (2) the reverse (NADPH) methemoglobin reductase pathway, (3) reduction by ascorbic acid, and (4) reduction by reduced glutathione. Methemoglobinemia caused by an inherited deficiency of NADH methemoglobin reductase is transmitted as an autosomal recessive trait.

Acquired Methemoglobinemia[32]

Normal individuals develop methemoglobinemia after exposure to agents that increase methemoglobin production beyond the capacity of the methemoglobin-reducing pathways. Most agents capable of producing methemoglobinemia are aromatic compounds that contain amino, hydroxy, or nitro functional groups. Some of the agents responsible for methemoglobinemia include nitrites, nitrates, sulfonamides, aniline dyes (laundry markings), acetanilid, phenacetin, and phenazopyridine HCl (Pyridium). The nitrites and nitrates account for most occurrences. The blood may be chocolate-brown. Symptoms vary in intensity, depending on the level of methemoglobin.

Hereditary Methemoglobinemia

Hereditary methemoglobinemia can be subdivided into two forms: one resulting from mutations leading to NADH methemoglobin reductase deficiency, and the other resulting from methemoglobin accumulation caused by an amino acid substitution in the globin chain that stabilizes methemoglobin, rendering it poorly susceptible to subsequent reduction. These hemoglobins are termed *M-hemoglobins.*

M-hemoglobins show a recessive inheritance pattern and, unlike many hemoglobinopathies, do not produce hemolytic anemias. The mutation causes the formation of an abnormally stable methemoglobin. This stability is attributable to amino acid substitution in or near the heme pocket, resulting in direct heme-globin bonding. Tyrosine is substituted for histidine at or across from the heme-binding site in many of the M-hemoglobins. HbM_{Iwate} and M_{Boston} have this substitution in the α-chain, whereas HbS $M_{Hyde\ Park}$ and $M_{Saskatoon}$ have it in the β-chain. Methemoglobin rarely exceeds 25% to 30% in these individuals. If α-chains are involved, cyanosis may be present at birth, whereas β-chain substitutions are responsible for cyanosis in later months because of the later appearance of these chains.

Clinically, patients with hereditary methemoglobinemia have erythrocytosis and slate gray cyanosis from birth, which is not associated with cardiopulmonary disease. Methemoglobin concentrations of 10% to 20% of the total hemoglobin produce cyanosis but no other ill effects. Methemoglobin concentrations of 30% may be responsible for headache and dyspnea, and concentrations of 70% and greater may be fatal. A low incidence of mental retardation and early death can be observed in cases of methemoglobinemia caused by NADH methemoglobin reductase deficiency, a disease that lends itself to prenatal diagnosis.[32]

KEY CONCEPTS BOX 40-2

- HbA, HbA_2 ($\alpha_2\delta_2$), and HbF ($\alpha_2\gamma_2$) are found in healthy adults.
- An HbA variant is one in which the amino acid sequence of the α- or β-chains is different from the usual sequences. This can occur by deletion or substitution of an amino acid, by genetic recombinations of globin genes, or by improper transcription of the globin gene. Variants may be benign or may cause disease, such as anemia, RBC changes, or cyanosis.
- Hemoglobinopathies are diseases caused by either an Hb variant, defective production of α- or β-chains, or a combination of the two. HPFH, a benign disorder, is a hereditary persistence of large amounts of HbF into adult life.
- Homozygous HbSS disease consists of severe megaloblastic anemia with sickled RBCs, bone pain, CNS disorders, and abnormal spleen.
- HbC is an asymptomatic disease (found most often in American blacks). Homozygous HbC disease (HbCC) is accompanied by mild anemia.
- α-Thalassemia results from insufficient production of α-chains, decreasing α-containing HbA, HbF, and HbA_2. Excess β-chains polymerize to produce characteristic HbBarts (γ_4) and HbH (β_4). The degree of sickness of the α-thalassemia depends on how many of the four α-genes are defective.
- β-Thalassemias result from reduced or absent production of β-chains, which decreases β-containing HbA. In response, levels of HbF and HbA_2 are increased. Clinical manifestations, usually anemia, are dependent on the severity of the reduction in β-chain production.

SECTION OBJECTIVE BOX 40-3

- List the laboratory results associated with thalassemias and sickle cell anemia.

Table 40-4 Reference Intervals for Hemoglobin in Grams per Deciliter in "Apparently Healthy" Subjects, White and Black

Subjects	Mean (Reference Interval)
Adult men	15.1 (13.6 to 16.3)
Adult women	13.5 (12.0 to 15.0)
Boys	
Birth	20.0 (18.5 to 21.5)
1 mo	17.0 (15.5 to 18.5)
3 mo	15.0 (13.5 to 16.5)
6 mo	14.0 (13.0 to 16.0)
9 mo	13.0 (12.0 to 14.0)
1 yr	12.1 (10.0 to 14.0)
2 yr	12.3 (10.5 to 14.2)
4 yr	12.6 (11.2 to 14.3)
8 yr	13.4 (12.0 to 14.8)
14 yr	14.0 (12.5 to 15.0)
Girls	
Birth	19.5 (18.0 to 21.0)
1 mo	17.0 (15.8 to 18.9)
3 mo	14.8 (13.3 to 16.4)
6 mo	13.8 (12.8 to 14.8)
9 mo	12.8 (11.7 to 13.9)
1 yr	12.2 (10.0 to 14.0)
2 yr	12.2 (10.5 to 14.2)
4 yr	12.7 (11.3 to 14.2)
8 yr	13.0 (11.5 to 14.5)
14 yr	13.2 (11.6 to 14.8)

From Miale JB: *Laboratory medicine: hematology,* ed 6, St Louis, 1982, Mosby.

CHANGE OF ANALYTE IN DISEASE

Interpretation of Hemoglobin Values

Mean and reference intervals for hemoglobin in healthy adults are 15.1 (13.6 to 16.3) g/dL for men and 13.5 (12.0 to 15.0) g/dL for women. Values of hemoglobin vary greatly for newborns, infants, children up to puberty, and adults (Table 40-4).

Physiological variations and pathological processes influence hemoglobin concentrations. The physiological variations include age, sex, physical exercise, posture, dehydration, and altitude. The influence exerted by age is readily apparent in Table 40-4. During puberty, the male hemoglobin level increases over the female value as a result of the influence of testosterone. Strong exercise raises the hemoglobin level probably through fluid loss, and a transient increase is experienced after a change from the recumbent to the standing position. Dehydration is responsible for a rise in hemoglobin concentration of such magnitude that it can mask a significant anemia. High altitude is responsible for increased hemoglobin levels because of the erythropoietin-stimulating effect of hypoxia.

Three main causes of anemia have been identified: impaired production, increased destruction, and excessive blood loss. Impaired production occurs with aplastic anemias; increased destruction occurs with hemolytic anemia; and excessive blood loss usually results in iron deficiency anemia. The reticulocyte count usually is depressed in chronic iron deficiency, reflecting the effect of lack of iron on erythropoiesis.

Increased hemoglobin values are encountered in polycythemia vera, erythrocytosis, dehydration, newborn chronic heart and lung disease, high altitude, renal cysts, and numerous erythropoietin-producing tumors, as well as in cigarette smoking and chronic lung disease.

HbF

In normal adults, the concentration of F-cells is fairly constant at 0.2% to 0.7%, but in some genetic and acquired hematological conditions, the concentration is increased. Genetic disorders include thalassemias (β and δβ), hereditary persistence of HbF, sickle cell anemia, and unstable β-chain variants. Acquired conditions include pregnancy at about midterm, recovery from bone marrow depression,[33] leukemias (highest values in Philadelphia chromosome–negative juvenile chronic myelocytic leukemia), thyrotoxicosis, and hepatoma.[9,34,35]

Hb A1c

Hb A1c levels depend on the time-integrated blood levels of glucose (see Chapter 38 for a more detailed discussion). Hb A1c levels are decreased in hemolytic anemia because the RBC life span is shortened by lysis,[36] and in hemoglobinopathies in which HbA is decreased (although the percentage of Hb A1c in relation to total HbA may be normal).

Carboxyhemoglobin (CO-Hb)

Some carboxyhemoglobin produced endogenously as 1 mol of CO is generated by the degradation of 1 mol of heme to bilirubin (see Chapter 31). Although this endogenous production of carboxyhemoglobin can present a hazard when exhaled air is concentrated in poorly ventilated, small spaces, the exogenous generation of CO from combustion of organic material in confined spaces causes intoxication. Exogenous CO is derived from the exhaust of automobiles, from industrial pollutants such as coal gas and charcoal burning, and from tobacco smoke. In the absence of exogenous CO, the endogenous CO-Hb concentration is 0.2% to 0.8%. Co-Hb levels can be elevated in hemolytic anemias,[37] and in smokers the Co-Hb may range from 4% to 20%. In smokers, who have a greater exposure to CO, the average level may be 10%.[5]

Because of the firm binding of CO to hemoglobin, long exposure to even low CO concentrations can lead to toxic accumulations to which the most oxygen-dependent organs, such as brain and heart, are most susceptible. Mild symptoms such as slight headache and slight dyspnea on exertion can occur at levels of 10% to 15% saturation. At levels of 20% to 30%, the headaches are more severe and are accompanied by impaired vision and judgment. Levels greater than 50% cause increasingly severe symptoms, coma, and convulsions, and levels of 60% and greater are usually fatal, although death has occurred at levels as low as 20%. The half-life of elimination of CO is about 4 hours for a person breathing atmospheric air, but in smokers the level may remain high.[38] Chronic exposure to CO may be responsible for a relative polycythemia.[39]

Carboxyhemoglobin produces a cherry-red color of the blood and skin. Sometimes the blood may have a violet tinge, because of the simultaneous presence of moderate quantities of reduced hemoglobin. Exposure to toxic levels of CO is treated with oxygen, often at elevated pressures (hyperbaric treatment), to displace CO from hemoglobin. Both exposure and therapy are followed closely by blood-gas analysis for CO-Hb.

Oxygen Saturation

Clinically, oxygen saturation is used as an indicator of tissue hypoxia or hyperoxia. Tissue hypoxia is produced by decreased oxygen content of inspired air, as in high altitude, or by decreased alveolar capillary oxygen exchange in the lungs, as in pulmonary fibrosis, emphysema, and chronic heart disease with a left-to-right shunt. Tissue hypoxia also is produced (1) by a defect in erythrocytic oxygen transport as occurs in severe anemia; (2) when hemoglobin ligands are present that prevent oxygen binding, such as carboxyhemoglobin, sulfhemoglobin, and methemoglobin; (3) in hemoglobinopathies; (4) in inappropriate concentrations of erythrocytic 2,3-BPG; and (5) in intraerythrocytic enzyme deficiencies. Therapeutic oxygen treatment must be monitored carefully because of the danger of oxygen toxicity. In newborns, it can be responsible for retrolental fibroplasia, and in adults, for hyaline membrane disease of the lungs (adult respiratory distress syndrome).

2,3-Biphosphoglycerate

2,3-BPG and hemoglobin interaction in hypoxia is related to the increased intraerythrocytic levels of deoxyhemoglobin, which binds large amounts of BPG. This binding sequesters the 2,3-DPB, which results in a feedback mechanism that stimulates glycolysis and additional BPG synthesis. Increased deoxyhemoglobin concentrations raise the pH, which, in turn, stimulates the synthesis of BPG. It has been emphasized that a reciprocal relationship exists between hemoglobin and BPG concentrations. Pyruvate kinase deficiency leads to a buildup of BPG and decreased oxygen affinity. Hexokinase deficiency leads to a decrease in BPG and to a compensatory erythropoietic response with increased hemoglobin values. Many hemoglobin mutations result in an increased oxygen affinity by the abnormal hemoglobin; some, such as $HbS_{ShepherdsBush}$, HbS_{Ohio}, and $HbS_{LittleRock}$, increase this affinity further by impairing BPG binding.

Other Hemoglobins

The HbF concentration can vary from 10% to 90%, and HbF distribution within the RBCs as determined by the Kleihauer technique can be heterogeneous. Possible abnormal cellular distribution patterns are as follows:

1. *Separate cell patterns.* RBCs that contain HbA or HbF are observed in cases of fetal-maternal hemorrhage if the mother's blood is examined, or in cases of maternal-fetal hemorrhage if the infant's blood is examined.
2. *Even distribution.* HbA and HbF are distributed equally in all red blood cells. This distribution is observed in hereditary persistence of HbF (HPFH).

3. *Uneven distribution.* Red blood cells have varying amounts of HbA and HbF. This pattern is seen in thalassemia, sickle cell disease, Fanconi's anemia, and hereditary spherocytosis.

The HbA_2 concentration may range from 1.4% to 20%, including low, normal, elevated, and very high values. The concentration of HbA_2 is increased in β-thalassemia, β-chain unstable hemoglobinemias, sickle cell trait, megaloblastic anemias, and hyperthyroidism. Normal or decreased values are seen in α-thalassemias, δβ-thalassemias (Lepore heterozygotes), δ-thalassemia, and HPFH. In Hb_{Lepore} homozygotes, HbA_2 is absent because no δ-chain synthesis occurs. HbA_2 is decreased in acquired disorders such as iron deficiency, sideroblastic anemias, and lead poisoning.

In homozygous β-thalassemia, the HbA_2 value, even if it is low or normal in the patient, will be high in both parents. If the HbA_2 level in the patient is expressed as a percentage of the total hemoglobin, it spans the previously mentioned range from low to high, but if it is expressed in relation to the HbA value only, the ratio is decreased in all cases of β-thalassemia, that is, the A/A_2 ratio is about 10:1 as compared with the normal A/A_2 ratio of about 40:1. If the HbA_2 level is greatly increased, HbF is normal or only slightly elevated and vice versa. In β^0-thalassemia, a total absence of HbA is seen, and so the patient's hemoglobin consists only of HbF and HbA_2, whereas in β^+-thalassemia, diminished amounts of HbA are found (5% to 20%). In both these β-thalassemias, free α-chains may be seen close to the application point of the electrophoretogram at alkaline pH. The severe reduction in β-globin chains leads to a β/α ratio of less than 0.25 to 0.3. Some of the more common hemoglobinopathies as evaluated by cation-exchange HPLC are depicted in Figs. 5-5 to 5-10.

Other Related Biochemical Findings

Because of the hemolytic components of anemia in most hemoglobinopathies, serum unconjugated bilirubin levels are elevated, and haptoglobin is decreased or absent. Serum aspartate aminotransferase, lactate dehydrogenase, and erythropoietin concentrations also are raised. Erythropoietin elevation is responsible for the 20% to 30% increase in erythropoietic marrow and is a result of the anemia and high oxygen affinity of HbF, which further increases the tissue anoxia. Liver involvement (transfusion hemosiderosis) can lead to a bleeding tendency. Gross examination of the urine may show the brown color of dipyrroles caused by excessive hemolysis.

Use of Hemogram Results to Differentiate Iron Deficiency from Thalassemias

Various formulas may be used to differentiate iron deficiency from milder forms of thalassemia. One such formula is the discriminant function (DF):

$$DF = MCV - RBC - (5 \times Hb) - 3.4$$

in which MCV is in fL (femtoliters), RBC is in millions/mm^3, and Hb is in g% (g/dL). The 3.4 is an instrument constant and varies with the instrument. A positive DF result is suggestive of iron deficiency, whereas a negative DF result is suggestive of a thalassemia. For example, in a patient with MCV of 65 fL, Hb of 13 g/dL, and RBC of 6 million/mm^3, the following is true: $DF = 65 - 6 - (5 \times 13) - 3.4 = -9.4$. The example indicates a diagnosis of thalassemia minor. A simpler formula is the ratio MCV/RBC. Values of this ratio greater than 13 are associated with iron deficiency anemia; values less than 13 are associated with thalassemias. In the above example, the ratio would be 10.8.

KEY CONCEPTS BOX 40-3

- α-Thalassemias are associated with decreased HbA and the presence of Hb Bart's and HbH.
- β-Thalassemias are associated with increased HbA2 and HbF.
- Sickle cell anemia is associated with HbAS or HbSS, hemolytic anemia, and in seed HbF.

REFERENCES

1. Bunn HF, Forget BG: *Hemoglobin: Molecular, Genetic and Clinical Aspects,* Philadelphia, 1986, Saunders.
2. Hardison R: Hemoglobins from bacteria to man: evolution of different patterns of gene expression, J Exp Biol 201:1099, 1998.
3. Shaeffer JR: Evidence for a difference in affinities of human hemoglobin β^A and β^S chains for α chains, J Biol Chem 255:2322, 1980.
4. Hawkins M: Carbon monoxide poisoning, Eur J Anaesthesiol 16:585, 1999.
5. Gorman D, Drewry A, Huang YL: The clinical toxicology of carbon monoxide, Toxicology 187:25, 2003.
6. Bozeman WP, Hampson NB: Pulse oximetry in CO poisoning—additional data, Chest 117:295, 2000.
7. Sepulveda W, Be C, Youlton R, et al: Accuracy of the haemoglobin alkaline denaturation test for detecting maternal blood contamination of fetal blood samples for prenatal karyotyping, Prenat Diagn 19:927, 1999.
8. Nelson M, Zarkos K, Popp H, et al: A flow-cytometric equivalent of the Kleihauer test, Vox Sang 75:234, 1998.
9. Weatherall DJ, Pembrey ME, Pritchard J: Fetal hemoglobin, Clin Hematol 3:467, 1974.
10. Clarke GM, Higgins TN: Laboratory investigation of hemoglobinopathies and thalassemias: review and update, Clin Chem 46:1284, 2000.
11. Fairbanks VF: Nomenclature and taxonomy of hemoglobin variants. In Fairbanks VF, editor: *Hemoglobinopathies and Thalassemias,* New York, 1988, Brian Decker.
12. Destro Bisol G: Genetic resistance to malaria, oxidative stress and hemoglobin oxidation, Parassitologia 41:203, 1999.
13. Buihl RW: The rheology of sickle cell hemoglobin, Ann NY Acad Sci 565:279, 1989.
14. Bunn HF: Hemoglobin II, sickle cell anemia and other hemoglobinopathies. In Beck WS, editor: *Hematology,* Cambridge, MA, 1981, MIT Press.
15. Hebbel RP, Mohandas N: Sickle cell adherence. In Embury SH, et al, editors: *Sickle Cell Disease: Basic Principles and Clinical Practice,* New York, 1994, Raven.
16. Embury SH, et al: Pathogenesis of vasoocclusion. In Embury SH, Hebbel RP, Mohandas N, et al, editors: *Sickle Cell Disease: Basic Principles and Clinical Practice,* New York, 1994, Raven.
17. Hebbel RP, Boogaerts MA, Eaton JW, et al: Erythrocyte adherence to endothelium in sickle cell anemia: a possible determinant of disease severity, N Engl J Med 302:992, 1980.
18. Chien S, Usami S, Bertles JF: Abnormal rheology of oxygenated blood in sickle cell anemia, J Clin Invest 49:623, 1970.

19. Nash GB, Johnson CS, Meiselman HJ: Mechanical properties of oxygenated red blood cells in sickle cell (HbSS) disease, Blood 63:73, 1984.
20. Clark MFR, Mohandas N, Shohet SB: Deformability of oxygenated irreversibly sickled cells, J Clin Invest 65:189, 1980.
21. Rosse W: *New Views of Sickle Cell Disease: Pathology and Treatment,* Washington, DC, 2001, American Society of Hematology.
22. Nagel RL, Bookchin RM: Oxygen transport and the sickle cell. In Wallach DFH, editor: *The Function of Red Blood Cells: Erythrocyte Pathobiology,* New York, 1981, Alan Liss.
23. Provan D, Gribben J: *Molecular Hematology,* ed 2, Oxford, UK, 2005, Wiley-Blackwell.
24. Schrier SL, Angelucci E: New strategies in the treatment of the thalassemias, Annu Rev Med 56:157, 2005.
25. Thein SL: Pathophysiology of β thalassemia—a guide to molecular therapies, Hematology Am Soc Hematol Educ Program 31-37, 2005.
26. Rund D, Rachmilewitz E: Beta-thalassemia, N Engl J Med 353:1135, 2005.
27. Higgs DR: Gene regulation in hematopoiesis: new lessons from thalassemia, Hematology Am Soc Hematol Educ Program 1-13, 2004.
28. Steensma DP, Gibbons RJ, Higgs DR: Acquired alpha-thalassemia in association with myelodysplastic syndrome and other hematologic malignancies, Blood 105:443, 2005.
29. Forget BG: Molecular basis of hereditary persistence of fetal hemoglobin, Ann NY Acad Sci 850:38, 1998.
30. Weatherall DJ, Clegg JB: Hereditary persistence of fetal haemoglobin, Br J Haematol 29:191, 1975.
31. Price D: Methemoglobin inducers. In Flomenbaum NE, Goldfrank LR, Hoffman RS, et al: *Goldfrank's Toxicologic Emergencies,* ed 8, New York, 2006, McGraw-Hill Professional, pp. 1734-1745.
32. Ash-Bernal R, Wise R, Wright SM: Acquired methemoglobinemia: a retrospective series of 138 cases at 2 teaching hospitals, Medicine 83:265, 2004.
33. Dover GJ, Boyer SH, Zinkhorn WH: Production of erythrocytes that contain fetal hemoglobin in anemia, J Clin Invest 63:173, 1979.
34. Honig GR, Suarez CR, Vida LN, et al: Juvenile myelomonocytic leukemia (JMML) with the hematologic phenotype of severe beta thalassemia, Am J Hematol 58:67, 1998.
35. Rochette J, Craig JE, Thein SL: Fetal hemoglobin levels in adults, Blood Rev 8:213, 1994.
36. Bunn HF, Haney DN, Kamin S, et al: The biosynthesis of human hemoglobin A_{1c}, J Clin Invest 57:1652, 1976.
37. Landau SA, Winchell HS: Endogenous production of ^{14}CO: a method for calculation of RBC life-span in vivo, Blood 36:642, 1970.
38. Astrup P: Carbon monoxide inhalation—time for clearance from blood in reversible coma, JAMA 230:1064, 1974.
39. Smith JR, Landau SA: Smoker's polycythemia, N Engl J Med 298:6, 1978.

BIBLIOGRAPHY

Bick RL, editor: *Hematology: Clinical and Laboratory Practice,* St Louis, 1993, Mosby.

Brenner MK, Hoffbrand AV: *Recent Advances in Haematology,* vol 8, New York, 1996, Churchill Livingstone.

Brown JM, Leach J, Reittie JE, et al. Coregulated human globin genes are frequently in spatial proximity when active. *J Cell Bio,* 2006, 172:2; 177-187.

Bunn HF, Forget BG: *Hemoglobin: Molecular, Genetic and Clinical Aspects,* Philadelphia, 1986, Saunders.

Forget BG: Thalassemia syndromes. In Hoffman R, Silberstein L, Benz EJ (Editors): *Hematology: Basic Principles and Practice,* ed 3, New York, 2000, Churchill Livingstone, pp 485-509.

Greer JP, Foerster J, Lukens JN, editors: *Wintrobe's Clinical Hematology,* ed 11, Baltimore, 2003, Lippincott Williams & Wilkins.

Hoffman R, Benz E, Shattil S, et al: *Hematology: Basic Principles and Practice,* ed 4, New York, 2004, Churchill Livingstone.

Jandl JH: *Blood: Textbook of Hematology,* Boston, 1996, Little, Brown.

Kutlar F. Diagnostic approach to hemoglobinopathies. *Hemoglobin,* 2007, 31: 243-250.

Lichtman MA, Beutler E, Kaushansky K, et al: *Williams Hematology,* ed 7, New York, 2005, McGraw-Hill Professional.

McKenzie S: *Clinical Laboratory Hematology,* Upper Saddle River, NJ, 2003, Prentice Hall.

Old JM, "Screening and genetic diagnosis of haemoglobinopathies", *Scan J Clin Lab Invest,* 2007, 67:1; 71-86.

Rappaport SI: *Introduction to Hematology,* ed 3, Philadelphia, 1997, Lippincott, Raven.

Rucknagel DL: Hemoglobinopathies and thalassemias. In Schumacher H, Rock W, Stasse S, editors: *Handbook of Hematologic Pathology,* New York, 2000, Marcel Dekker.

Schumacher HR, Garvin DF, Triplett DA: *Introduction to Laboratory Hematology and Hematopathology,* New York, 1984, Alan Liss.

Schumacher HR, Rock WA, Stass SA: *Handbook of Hematologic Pathology,* New York, 2000, Marcel Dekker.

Stamatoyannopoulos G, Majerus P, Perlmutter R, et al, editors: *The Molecular Basis of Blood Diseases,* ed 3, Philadelphia, 2001, Saunders.

Steinberg M: *Disorders of Hemoglobin: Genetics, Pathophysiology and Clinical Management,* London, 2001, Cambridge University Press.

Weatherall DJ, Clegg JB, editors: *The Thalassaemia Syndromes,* ed 4, Oxford, 2004, Blackwell Science.

Williams W: *Hematology,* ed 6, New York, 2000, McGraw-Hill.

INTERNET SITES

http://www.emedicine.com/med/topic2259.htm—Thalassemia alpha, by Bleibel SA, et al

http://www.emedicine.com/med/TOPIC2260.htm—Thalassemia beta, by Takeshita K

http://www.emedicine.com/emerg/TOPIC313.htm—Methemoglobinemia, by Lee DC, Ferguson KL

http://www.emedicine.com/ped/topic1432.htm—Methemoglobinemia, by Verive M, Kumar M

http://www.emedicine.com/EMERG/topic817.htm—Toxicity, Carbon monoxide, by Shochat G, Lucchesi M

http://www.nhlbi.nih.gov/health/dci/Diseases/Sca/SCA_SignsAndSymptoms.html

http://www.scinfo.org/

http://www.emedicine.com/med/TOPIC976.htm—Hemoglobin C disease, by Carter SM, Gross SJ

http://www.hematology.org/—American Society of Hematology

http://www.cooleysanemia.org/—Cooley's Anemia Foundation, for patients with thalassemia

http://sickle.bwh.harvard.edu/—Joint Center for Sickle Cell and Thalassemic Disorders

http://omlc.ogi.edu/spectra/hemoglobin/index.html

http://www.slh.wisc.edu/newborn/guide/hemoglobinopathies.dot—*The Wisconsin State Laboratory of Hygiene Health Professionals' Guide to Newborn Screening for Hemoglobinopathies*

http://en.wikipedia.org/wiki/Pyruvate_kinase_deficiency-Pyruvate kinase deficiency, by Frye RF and DeLoughery TG

Human Nutrition

Nancy W. Alcock

Chapter 41

Chapter Outline

Key Terms

anabolic Biochemical pathways that synthesize macromolecules such as proteins and nucleic acids.

anthropometric Study of human body measurements, such as body and upper arm circumference; to assess nutritional status.

basal metabolic rate (BMR) The energy expended to maintain basic physiological functions.

bioavailability Amount quantity (usually expressed as a percentage) of dietary components that can be absorbed from the gastrointestinal tract, either intact or after degradation.

cachexia Physical wasting caused by starvation and malnutrition.

catabolic Metabolic degradation or breakdown of macromolecules.

diet The food that is ingested orally.

Dietary Reference Intakes (DRI) Recommended intakes of various dietary components (see Box 42-1, p. 805).

dysphagia Difficulty in swallowing.

enteral feeding Provision of synthetic nutrients to the gastrointestinal tract through a tube.

essential nutrients Nutrients required for normal growth and development and for maintaining the adult body in equilibrium; these nutrients cannot be synthesized at all or cannot be synthesized in sufficient amounts. They include vitamins, minerals, trace elements, certain amino acids, and at least two fatty acids.

kilocalorie (kcal) The amount of energy-producing food equivalent to the energy required to raise the temperature of 1 kg of water from 15°C to 16°C.

kilojoule (kJ) A unit of heat; 1 kJ is equivalent to approximately 0.24 kcal.

kwashiorkor Malnutrition caused by a diet deficient in protein; "the disease of the displaced child" in Western African Ga language.

malnutrition Suboptimal nutrition arising from inadequate or unbalanced intake, bioavailability, or utilization of nutrients.

marasmus A protein-calorie malnutrition arising from inadequate food intake as the result of partial or complete starvation.

nitrogen balance The difference between total nitrogen intake and the sum of fecal and urinary nitrogen excretion; an estimate of net synthesis of body proteins.

nutrient A dietary component used by the body in any metabolic pathway.

nutrition The branch of science that studies the processes of requirement, intake, bioavailability, absorption, utilization, and excretion of nutrients.

parenteral nutrition Nutrition administered by a route other than the gastrointestinal tract.

peripheral parenteral nutrition (PPN) Parenteral nutrition introduced through a peripheral vein.

Recommended Dietary Allowance (RDA) Suggested daily requirements of some essential nutrients for healthy subjects of various ages as published by the Food and Nutrition Board of the National Research Council; now referred to as Dietary Reference Intakes (see above).

resting energy expenditure (REE) Energy expended at resting state, that is, at a basal metabolic rate (BMR).

total parenteral nutrition (TPN) Parenteral nutrition administered as the sole source of nutrition.

undernutrition Without the wasted look of marasmus, undernourished individuals are underweight for one's age, too short for one's age, thin, and deficient in vitamins and minerals.

Methods on Evolve

Albumin
Iron and iron binding capacity
Transferrin
Transthyretin (prealbumin)
Triglycerides
Urea
Vitamin B_{12}
Zinc

SECTION OBJECTIVES BOX 41-1

- Describe the various estimates of allowable nutrition, including RDA, DRI, AI, and UL.
- Discuss the contributions of individual nutrient classes to human metabolism, with specific reference to energy, protein, fats, and carbohydrates.
- Describe the hypermetabolic state and its medical consequences.

NUTRIENT CLASSES

The science of **nutrition** is concerned with the qualitative and quantitative aspects of the **diet** and utilization of dietary components required to sustain health. The major component groups required for human nutrition—carbohydrates, proteins, lipids, minerals, trace elements, vitamins, and fiber—are biochemically well defined. Some biochemicals can be synthesized via endogenous metabolic processes, but others cannot be synthesized and therefore must be specifically provided in the diet as **nutrients.** These nutrients are termed *essential* and include the essential amino acids and fatty acids (see below). All water-soluble vitamins, as well as the fat-soluble vitamins A, E, and K, are essential (see Chapter 43). Vitamin D, the fourth fat-soluble vitamin, is required for growing children, but adequate supplies usually are formed in the adult from its endogenous precursor, 7-dehydrocholesterol (see Chapter 33). Dietary fat and its absorption are prerequisites for absorption of the fat-soluble vitamins (see Chapter 35).

Variation in the requirement of nutrients depends on the age and sex of the individual, on reproductive status, and on the altered nutritional demands associated with disease, injury, and therapeutic interventions. The Food and Nutrition Board of the Commission on Life Sciences, National Research Council, estimates the levels of dietary **essential nutrients** that should be adequate to meet the known nutrient needs of practically all healthy persons. These estimates, initially reported as **Recommended Dietary Allowances (RDA)** were updated as **Dietary Reference Intakes (DRI)** in 2004 and 2005.[1,2] The DRI contains at least four nutrient-based reference values that are useful for planning and assessment of diets. The RDA remains as the first requirement. The second is the adequate intake (AI) guideline, which is to be used when an RDA is unobtainable. The AI is based on the recommended intake value for groups of healthy individuals and is derived from experimental or observational sources. The tolerable upper limit, or UL, is the highest level of a nutrient that can be tolerated in one day without experiencing adverse effects. The fourth value in the DRI is the estimated average requirement (EAR), the daily nutrition value that is estimated to suffice for half of a group of healthy individuals.

Table 41-1 Basic Classes of Nutrients

Nutrient	Chapter Discussed
Carbohydrate	Diabetes, 38
Lipids	Lipid, 37
Proteins	Liver, 31
Inorganic Elements	**Chapter Discussed**
Na, K, Cl	Electrolytes and water balance, 28
Ca, Mg, inorganic phosphorus	Bone, 33
Fe^{++} (Fe^{+++})	Iron and porphyrins, 39
Trace minerals	Trace elements, 42
Vitamins	Vitamins, 43
Water	Renal, 30 Electrolytes and water balance, 28

Various estimates indicate that at least 50% of hospitalized patients are malnourished (see below). The Joint Commission (formally the Joint Commission on Accreditation for Healthcare Organizations [JCAHO]) has stressed the importance of a nutrition care plan for institutionalized individuals that addresses detection of malnutrition, establishment of a nutrition intervention plan for patients at nutritional risk, and monitoring of the response to that plan. Although **anthropometric** measurements (see below) are first-tier indicators of suboptimal nutrition, nutritional assessment using biochemical parameters can help to alert the physician to deficiencies.

Biochemical and clinical aspects of the essential minerals, electrolytes, trace metals, and vitamins and their functions are discussed in detail in relevant chapters (Table 41-1).

Energy Requirements[3-6]

The World Health Organization defines the energy requirement of an individual as follows: "The level of energy intake that will balance energy expenditure when the individual has a body size and composition, and a level of physical activity, consistent with long-term good health. The energy requirement should also allow the maintenance of economically necessary and socially desirable physical activity. In children and pregnant or lactating women, the energy requirement includes the energy requirements associated with the deposition of tissues or the secretion of milk at rates consistent with good health."[7]

The body is in energy balance when the metabolizable energy intake is equal to the sum of energy expenditure and changes in stored energy. Resting energy expenditure, an individual's **basal metabolic rate,** can be determined by direct calorimetry (generation of heat), by indirect calorimetry (from measurement of oxygen consumption and carbon dioxide production), and by isotope dilution methods with the use of doubly labeled water. An estimate of the expenditure of endogenous energy stores can be quantitated from measurement of the **nitrogen balance** (see below). A positive nitrogen balance is essential for growth (children and fetus), pregnancy, and lactation, and during physiologically stressful pathological states. Excess nutrients are stored as fat and protein, and an extreme state of overnutrition can lead to obesity. When insufficient nutrients are available, stored protein and fat are mobilized to supply energy and glucose; extreme lack of nutrients can lead to starvation.

Hormones and cytokines, such as tumor necrosis factor, may initiate a heightened metabolic response to injury and infection. The increased metabolism associated with physiological stress is termed the *hypermetabolic state.*[8] Observations associated with the hypermetabolic state are listed in Box 41-1. It is important to note the difference between starvation, when both muscle and fat stores are used up for fuel, and the hypermetabolic state, characterized by a primary dependence on muscle protein as a source of amino acids for gluconeogenesis.

Patients suffering from trauma, burns, and sepsis often are in a hypermetabolic state within 1 to 2 weeks after acute injury. Individuals with major burns experience a 180% to 200% increase in the body's normal basal metabolic rate (MR) for as long as 50 days after the burn. In contrast, peritonitis is associated with an increased MR of 140% or greater for 10 to 20 days, and fractures lead to a peak in MR at 120% within 7 days. Individuals who are hypometabolic will experience a 60% to 70% decrease in MR. The increased metabolic rate, which is proportionate to the severity of the condition, results in insulin insensitivity and hyperglycemia. Although stored triglycerides are mobilized and oxidized, the body turns to muscle protein as its primary energy source. If the patient is not fed, stores of fat and especially protein may be depleted. Loss of adipose tissue (fat) and muscle tissue (protein) may result in a wasted appearance resembling that of individuals suffering from extreme protein-calorie malnutrition. To meet the increased nutritional needs in these cases, health care providers should give minimal nutritional support at first and then increase this support gradually to maintain body cell mass. Biochemical parameters useful in monitoring such patients are discussed below.

Energy intake at birth is approximately 120 **kilocalories (kcal)**/kg/day (30 **kilojoules**) for both males and females. During the first 2 years of life, there is a gradual drop to 90 to 100 kcal/kg/day. From 2 to 14 years of age, energy requirements decrease gradually to approximately 40 kcal/kg/day, with males requiring 5 kcal/kg/day more than females.

Box 41-1

Observations Associated With the Hypermetabolic State

- Increased basal metabolic rate (BMR)
- Increased nutritional needs
- Fever
- Increased heart rate and cardiac output
- Altered immune system activity
- Increased levels of catabolic hormones, including glucagon, catecholamine, and cortisol; decreased insulin levels
- Negative nitrogen balance
- Breakdown of muscle protein
- Use of amino acids rather than fat to produce glucose; no ketosis
- Increased hepatic gluconeogenesis
- Synthesis of acute-phase proteins

Carbohydrates (see Chapter 38)

Carbohydrates are the principal source of energy for the body, contributing 50% to 60% of total calories. Complex carbohydrates, such as starches and sugars found in fruits and vegetables, are a better source of energy than simple refined sugars and may lower the incidences of hypertension, metabolic syndrome and maturity-onset diabetes, hyperlipidemia, and cardiovascular disease. Excessive carbohydrate intake leads to an increase in body weight, whereas insufficient intake stimulates mobilization of lipid stores with associated ketosis, loss of electrolytes, and dehydration. In a healthy adult, carbohydrate is stored as glycogen, principally in muscle (about 150 g) and in the liver (about 90 g). One gram of carbohydrate provides 4 kcal (1 kJ) of energy.

Proteins

Requirements

Dietary proteins are the source of amino acids, the building blocks for synthesis and maintenance of tissue proteins. Some amino acids cannot be synthesized by the body at all or cannot be synthesized in sufficient amounts to satisfy requirements; these "essential" amino acids must be obtained in the diet. The essential amino acids are listed in Box 41-2. The quality of

Box 41-2

Essential Amino Acids

Isoleucine	Phenylalanine	Histidine*
Leucine	Threonine	Arginine*
Lysine	Tryptophan	Taurine†
Methionine	Valine	

*Indicated to be unnecessary for maintenance of nitrogen equilibrium in adults in short-term studies but probably necessary for normal growth of children.

†Required in infants.

Table 41-2 Daily Recommended Dietary Allowance for Protein and for Some Minerals and Trace Elements for Various Ages

Category	Age (Years) or Condition	Ca, mg	P, mg	Mg, mg	Fe, mg	Zn, mg	I, μg	Se, μg	Protein, g
Infants	0.0 to 0.5	210*	100*	30*	0.27*	2*	100*	10	9.1*
	0.5 to 1.0	270*	75*	75*	11	3	130*	15	11
Children	1 to 3	500*	460	80	7	3	90	20	13
	4 to 8	800*	500	130	10	5	90	20	19
Males	9 to 13	1300*	1250	240	8	8	120	40	32
	14 to 18	1300*	1250	410	11	11	150	50	54
	19 to 30	1000*	700	400	8	11	150	70	56
	31 to 50	1000*	700	420	8	11	150	70	56
	51+	1200*	700	420	8	11	150	70	56
Females	9 to 13	1300*	1250	240	8	8	120	45	44
	14 to 18	1300*	1250	360	15	8	150	50	46
	19 to 30	1000*	700	310	18	8	150	55	46
	31 to 50	1000*	700	320	18	8	150	55	46
	51+	1200*	700	320	8	8	150	55	46
Pregnant		1100-1300*	700-1250	354-400	27	11-12	220	65	71
Lactating		1100-1300*	700-1250	310-360	9-10	12-13	220	75	71

From United States Department of Agriculture, National Agricultural Library: http://fnic.nal.usda.gov/nal_display/index.php?info_center=4&tax_level=2&tax_subject=256&topic_id=1342.
*Adequate intakes.

dietary protein is determined by its content of all essential amino acids. For infants, children 10 to 12 years of age, and adults, essential amino acids should make up 43%, 36%, and 10%, respectively, of the total amino acid intake. Good-quality protein is required to replace losses during the acute phase of physiological (hypermetabolic) stress associated with fevers, burns, surgical trauma, fractures, and other pathological states. On the other hand, protein restriction is required to manage acute liver failure and end-stage renal disease.

Nitrogen Balance

Nitrogen balance studies are used to assess utilization of dietary amino acids for protein synthesis and to determine the balance between **anabolic** and **catabolic** processes. An accurate diet record is used to calculate dietary intake of protein nitrogen. Accurate assessment of nitrogen output requires the measurement of fecal and urinary nitrogen and a correction for nitrogen losses through sweat, hair, nails, and sloughed cells from the skin. The most accurate quantitative assessment of nitrogen excretion measures total nitrogen excretion in urine or feces by chemiluminescence analysis after pyrolysis of the sample. Because this technique is not in widespread use, an approximate estimate of nitrogen excretion can be obtained through measurement of urine urea nitrogen (UUN). The UUN must be adjusted by a factor that is intended to account for other nitrogen losses. In an adult, a positive nitrogen balance is associated with general good health. A positive nitrogen balance (protein intake >protein loss) is necessary during periods of growth and development and during pregnancy. A negative nitrogen balance during periods of starvation, in **cachexia,** and in many hypermetabolic disease states should alert the physician to consider corrective nutritional support. The frequency of quantitative measurements is dictated by the patient's response to therapy, but it has been suggested that several assessments per week may be needed during the most catabolic state of an acute illness.[9]

The RDA for protein among various ages and conditions is shown in Table 41-2. One gram of protein provides 4 kcal of energy.

Lipids

Lipids are the most energy-dense of the macronutrients, providing 9 kcal/g of fat. Although a typical American diet contains 35% to 45% of calories as fat, the American Heart Association and the Food and Nutrition Board of the National Research Council recommend that fat consumption be reduced to less than 30% of total calorie intake (see Chapter 37).

In view of the association of saturated fats from animal sources with heart disease, it is recommended that at least 10% of ingested fat be polyunsaturated. Some fatty acids found in the structural lipids of cells and the mitochondrial membranes cannot be synthesized in sufficient quantity, and their supply is thus essential. The essential fatty acids are linoleic acid, linolenic acid, and arachidonic acid. Arachidonic acid accounts for 5% to 10% of the fatty acids in phospholipids of the cell membrane. Approximately 2.7 g/day of the essential fatty acids—linoleic, linolenic, and arachidonic acids—is required for normal health. Lipids are stored as triglycerides, mainly in adipose tissue. Lipid metabolism and associated diseases are discussed in Chapter 37.

Minerals[1-3]

The DRI for the major inorganic components, the macrominerals, of the diet are shown in Table 41-2. The role of each of the macrominerals is discussed in detail in the relevant chapters, as listed in Table 41-1. Important aspects of the biological roles and symptoms of deficiency or excess of the

Table 41-3 Major Role of Macrominerals and Associated Abnormalities

Element	Major Role	Associated Abnormality	Comments
Calcium	Major component with phosphorus of skeletal and dental tissues	Deficiency: rickets in children; osteomalacia in adults; contributes to osteoporosis	Hormonal regulation: parathyroid hormone, vitamin D, calcitonin
Chloride	Important in fluid and electrolyte balance; major extracellular fluid anion; contributes to osmolality	Deficiency may occur as the result of vomiting, diarrhea, diuretics, renal disease	
Magnesium	Major pools intracellular, bone; cofactor for many enzymes	Deficiency may occur because of malabsorption, diarrhea, alcoholism	Symptoms of deficiency; muscle weakness
Phosphorus	Major component with calcium in skeletal and dental tissue; energy source from ATP; phosphorylated intermediate in metabolic pathways; component of nucleic acids	Deficiency: in children, rickets: in adults, osteomalacia	Parathyroid hormone and vitamin D regulatory mechanisms
Potassium	Major intracellular cation; important in muscle and nerve functions Na^+, K^+-ATPase	Muscle weakness, confusion, paralysis	Hormonal regulation of potassium excretion by aldosterone; urine loss increased by diuretics
Sodium	Major extracellular fluid cation; contributes to osmolality; important in acid-base balance, Na^+, K^+-ATPase	Excess may cause hypertension in some individuals	Hormonal regulation of sodium reabsorption by aldosterone

individual minerals are shown in Table 41-3. A discussion of the biological role of trace elements, microminerals, is found in Chapter 42.

Fiber

Fiber, an important component of the diet, comprises plant cell components that cannot be digested by enzymes found in the gut. The more insoluble fibers, such as cellulose and lignin found in wheat bran, are beneficial to colonic function, whereas the more soluble gums and pectins found in fruits and vegetables have been associated with lowering of blood cholesterol. High-fiber diets and their phytate content provide binding sites for the divalent metals calcium, iron, and zinc, lowering these metals' **bioavailablity.** Hence, a requirement for increased intake of these metals should be addressed when high-fiber diets are consumed.

KEY CONCEPTS BOX 41-1

- Maintenance of good health requires sufficient supply dietary nutrients to meet body needs; neither an undersupply or an oversupply is associated with good health.
- The hypermetabolic state is associated with an injury response in which the metabolic rate increases and protein becomes the primary source of glucose to meet body energy needs.
- If physicians do not meet the additional nutrition demands of a patient with the hypermetabolic state, the patient is at increased risk for poor medical outcomes.

SECTION OBJECTIVES BOX 41-2

- Describe the different types of malnutrition.
- Discuss the prevalence of various types of malnutrition states in the following populations: worldwide, in the United States, and in institutionalized populations.
- Discuss the problem of drug-nutrient interactions.

MALNUTRITION[1-5]

The world's general population can be divided into those at risk for **malnutrition** (likely to become malnourished) and those who are at low risk for becoming malnourished (likely to remain well nourished). Among the former group are those who become at risk for malnutrition because of changing nutritional needs, such as illness or change in socioeconomic status.

Types of Malnutrition[10]

This chapter considers several basic types of malnutrition. The first is protein-energy malnutrition (PEM), caused by the lack of sufficient protein and food (energy, measured in calories) to meet physiological needs. PEM is what is referred to when world hunger or starvation is discussed. The second type of malnutrition is a micronutrient (vitamin and mineral) deficiency. This type of malnutrition is important because of its impact on the occurrence of other diseases. A variation of PEM and micronutrition deficiency is **undernutrition,** in which the signs and symtoms of PEM are lacking, yet individuals are at risk for developing PEM.

The third type of malnutrition, obesity, is caused by eating calories in excess of body needs; this results in accumulation

Box 41-3

Characteristics of Kwashiorkor

Edema ("swollen belly")
Rashes and skin lesions ("flaky paint" dermatosis)
Diarrhea
Thinning and discoloration of the hair
Enlarged, fatty liver
Apathy, lethargy
Retarded physical and cognitive growth
Immunodeficiency

Box 41-4

Consequences of Malnutrition and Undernutrition

Decreased capacity for physical or school work
Decreased ability of women to nourish fetus or breast-feed child
Delayed wound healing
Impaired immune function
Increased risk for infectious diseases (diarrhea, pneumonia, malaria, and HIV/AIDS)
Increased risk for marasmus or kwashiorkor
Increased death rates

Table 41-4 WHO Classification of Marasmus

Evidence of Malnutrition	Moderate	Severe (Type)
Symmetrical edema	No	Yes (edema PEM)*
Weight for height	SD[†] score −3 SD score <−2 (70%-90%)[‡]	SD score <−3 (i.e., severe wasting) (<70%)
Height for age	SD score −3 SD score <−2 (85%-89%)	SD score <−3 (i.e., severe stunting) (<85%)

Modified from http://www.emedicine.com/ped/TOPIC164.HTM.
*Includes kwashiorkor-like symptoms (presence of edema always indicates serious protein-energy malnutrition [PEM]).
†Below the median National Center for Health Statistics/WHO reference: SD score = (observed value − median reference value) ÷ standard deviation of reference population.
‡Percentage of the median NCHS/WHO reference.

of high levels of body fat. Obesity is a matter of concern because of the severe health problems associated with it, primarily cardiovascular disease and diabetes. The incidences of these types of malnutrition in various populations are discussed below.

Protein Malnutrition—Kwashiorkor

Conditions of severe protein deficiency, termed **kwashiorkor,** occur in underdeveloped countries when breast-fed infants are transferred to a high-carbohydrate diet. The major characteristics of kwashiorkor, which primarily affects children younger than age 5, are listed in Box 41-3.

Protein-Energy Malnutrition—Marasmus

Severe overall nutritional deficiency in both calories and protein occurs in **marasmus** (wasting away) and appears with classic signs of starvation, including the loss of subcutaneous adipose mass and muscle mass, which produces a wasted appearance. Muscle protein is catabolized in order to synthesize glucose from glucogenic amino acids (see Chapter 38). The World Health Organization (WHO) classification of marasmus is shown in Table 41-4.

Overlap may occur between the conditions of kwashiorkor and marasmus (marasmic kwashiorkor malnutrition), and the two are often difficult to distinguish. Patients with marasmus may not have the severe edema present in kwashiorkor and usually retain their mental alertness. PEM can occur primarily because of the lack of available dietary nutrition, or secondarily, as a result of physical or mental illness that prevents proper intake of available foods.

Undernutrition

Individuals who have marasmic or kwashiorkor malnutrition are aften easy to observe and therefore treat. More difficult to identify are those individuals who are receiving insufficient nutrients to meet their needs, but who do not have severe PEM. Such individuals may appear thin, not wasted, and may be able to function to a limited degree. Yet the social and medical consequences of undernutrition are as severe as for frank PEM (Box 41-4).

Approximately 50% of child deaths in developing countries can be attributed to undernutrition.[11]

Micronutrient Deficiency[12]

Micronutrient deficiency results from a deficiency in one or more vitamins or minerals. It usually is caused by a diet lacking these nutrients and results in a disease associated with such a deficiency. Micronutrient deficiencies can result in blindness, impaired immune function, and increased severity of common infections (e.g., measles, diarrhea). They also may decrease intellectual potential, physical growth, and adult productivity.

Obesity[13-15]

Obesity is defined by a body mass index (BMI) greater than or equal to 30.0. Although protein-calorie malnutrition remains a major problem in developing countries, obesity is a growing problem in affluent societies in all countries. The medical consequences of obesity are shown in Box 41-5. Individuals who are obese have a 10% to 50% increased risk of death from all causes, compared with individuals with a normal BMI (18.5 to 24.9). Most of this increased risk is the result of cardiovascular causes.[16]

General Populations

World Population[17-19]

More than 900 million people, most of them in the developing world, cannot meet basic needs for energy and protein, and

Box 41-5

Medical Consequences of Obesity

Hypertension (high blood pressure)
Osteoarthritis (degeneration of cartilage and its underlying bone within a joint)
Metabolic syndrome
Dyslipidemia (e.g., high total cholesterol, high levels of triglycerides)
Type 2 diabetes
Coronary heart disease
Sleep apnea
Stroke
Gallbladder disease
Sleep apnea and respiratory problems

Box 41-6

Conditions Associated With Undernutrition or Malnutrition

Aging
Alcoholism
Cancer
Coronary heart disease
Diabetes
Growth
Hyperlipidemia
Injury, severe (e.g., burns, trauma)
Immunoincompetence
Lactation
Low birth weight infant
Malabsorption
Marasmus
Obesity
Poverty
Pregnancy
Sepsis

more than billions lack essential micronutrients. The malnutrition in these poverty-stricken countries disproportionately affects children; 174 million children younger than 5 years of age in the developing world are malnourished, and 230 million have stunted growth. Associated with malnutrition and undernutrition are poor physical and mental development, lower resistance to infectious disease, and a high mortality rate. In developing countries, approximately half of the deaths of children younger than 5 years of age—about 10 million each year—are associated with malnutrition.

PEM

Marasmus and kwashiorkor represent a serious worldwide problem that involves more than 50 million children younger than 5 years. WHO estimates that 49% of the 10.4 million deaths occurring in children younger than 5 years in developing countries are associated with PEM, marasmus, or kwashiorkor. In 2006, more than half of young children in South Asia were estimated to have PEM; in sub-Saharan Africa, 30% of children had PEM. Almost 60% of the total worldwide mortality in 2006, approximately 62 million people, resulted from malnutrition.

Undernutrition

The United Nations Food and Agriculture Organization (FAO) estimates that in 2006, 12% of the world's population—854 million people—were undernourished, and more than 36 million died of hunger or diseases caused by deficiencies in micronutrients. More than 96% of the undernourished were living in developing countries. UNICEF estimates that in 2004, one of every four children in the developing world (primarily in South Asia [46%] and sub-Saharan Africa [28%]) younger than 5 years old was undernourished. These figures parallel those for PEM prevalence and emphasize the connection between undernutrition and frank PEM.

Micronutrient Deficiency

Worldwide, 2 billion people are deficient in a specific micronutrient, such as vitamin A, iron, or iodine. Deficiency in vitamin A, a major cause of blindness, affects up to 250 children younger than 5 years of age. Iron deficiency affects approximately one-third of the world's women and children, with resulting anemia. Globally, 20% of maternal mortality, 22% of perinatal mortality, and 18% of mental retardation can be attributed to iron deficiency. Iodine deficiency is still the leading cause of preventable mental retardation, with as many as 50 million infants born annually at risk for iodine deficiency.

Obesity[20]

WHO estimates that worldwide in 2005, 20 million children younger than 5 years of age and 1.6 billion adults (age 15+) were overweight, and at least 400 million adults were obese; WHO projects that by 2015, the latter number will rise to 700 million adults. It has been estimated that there are now more overweight individuals worldwide than there are undernourished or malnourished ones.

American Population

The American population generally reflects the developed counties in the world in terms of nutritional issues. These countries have emphasized a good diet as a path to good health and to prolonged life. The increased consumption of fruits and vegetables, especially citrus fruits, leafy vegetables, tomatoes, and orange-colored vegetables, is recommended because these foods are good sources of vitamins. A reduction in caloric intake has been demonstrated to be beneficial; excessive caloric intake leads to obesity and its accompanying health problems (see below).

Malnutrition

Nevertheless, undernutrition and malnutrition do exist, albeit at much lower levels than in the developing world. Much of the world's malnutrition is experienced by at-risk populations with the conditions listed in Box 41-6. Less than 1% of all children in the United States have chronic malnutrition, and the incidence of malnutrition is less than 10%, even in the highest-risk group (children in shelters for the homeless). Up to 10% of children of nonurban populations may have poor growth resulting from inadequate nutrition.[10]

It is important to note that the malnourished adult population includes ambulatory individuals who are not acutely ill and may even be completely healthy (such as pregnant women). Undernutrition occurs frequently in older people. About 1 of 7 older individuals consumes fewer than 1000 calories a day—not enough for adequate nutrition. Many at-risk populations may become acutely protein-calorie malnourished as the result of illness or trauma. This is a particular problem for developed countries with aging populations, whether free living or institutionalized (see later).

Obesity[20,21]

The trend for increasing obesity in the United States has been rising since 1985. The National Health and Nutrition Examination Survey (NHANES) data for 2003-2004 show that among individuals 20 years and older, 66% are overweight (BMI >25) and 32% of these are obese (BMI >30). Among American children in 2003-2004 aged 2 to 5, 6 to 11, and 12 to 19 years, the prevalences of overweight individuals are 14%, 19%, and 15%, respectively. Adult Americans show a similar trend of steadily increasing weight, with the percentage of overweight individuals almost doubling since the late 1980s. American black and Hispanic women have greater percentages of overweight and obese individuals than do non-Hispanic whites. The problem is equally serious in other Western, developed countries. Obesity data for Europe suggest that 10% to 28% of European men and up to 38% of women are obese. European children also are manifesting rising rates of overweightness and obesity.

Institutionalized Populations

Malnutrition in chronic and acute care institutions can be a major problem.[22-24] It is estimated now that about 20% to 50% of hospitalized patients show signs of malnutrition or undernutrition; the rates for elderly patients are even higher. Studies of hospitalized individuals suggest that as many as one-fourth of patients have some form of acute PEM, and 27% have chronic PEM. These include individuals who enter the hospital with preexisting chronic conditions (such as individuals with acquired immunodeficiency syndrome [AIDS] or cancer), as well as those who may become acutely ill as the result of their hospital stay (such as trauma patients, surgery and burn patients, and very low birth weight babies). Individuals in chronic care facilities (such as nursing homes) may not eat properly and may become chronically malnourished.[25] Rates of undernutrition and PEM among institutionalized elderly are estimated to range from 23% to 85%. The problem of pressure ulcers among inactive elderly in long-term care is a nutritional problem with medical consequences.

PEM can have both medical (Box 41-7) and economic consequences in institutionalized patients.[26,27] The medical complications resulting from PEM are associated with greatly increased costs to hospitals and nursing homes. These costs result from the increased length of stay (LOS) in intensive care units (ICUs) or regular hospital beds, as well as from increased use of medical resources. It now is required that hospital and long-term care institutions must establish policies that will enable early detection of PEM, early and effective treatment of PEM, and careful monitoring of that treatment.

Box 41-7

Medical Consequences of Protein-Calorie Malnutrition in Institutionalized Individuals

Delayed wound healing
- Bed sores (pressure ulcers)

Increased risk for postoperative complications
- Pneumonia
- Wound site infection

Impaired immune function
Increased length of stay in hospital
Increased death rate

Drug-Nutrient Interactions

Comprehensive reviews of the nature of interactions between drugs and nutrients and their consequences are available.[28-30] Physicochemical interaction may occur in the gastrointestinal tract and may impair absorption of drug or nutrient, or both. Factors involved may include solubility properties, pH of the milieu, adsorptivity, chelation, gel formation, and ion exchange. Physiological interactions in which gastrointestinal function is altered may alter transit time of intestinal contents and hence absorption rate of dietary nutrients, may produce electrolyte imbalance or vasodilation, or may have a modifying effect on appetite, resulting in excessive or inadequate food intake.

The intestinal absorption of specific drugs may be reduced or retarded by food or food supplements, and the intestinal absorption of other drugs may be increased by food or by enteral formulas.[30] Although drug-nutrient interactions can occur in any individual, some populations are especially susceptible (Box 41-8). Older populations are among the most highly vunerable to diet-drug interactions because they frequently are given multiple drug prescriptions and are at high risk for poor nutrition (see above).

Low-protein diets reduce renal plasma flow, creatinine clearance, and renal clearance of drugs such as the antiuricemic drug allopurinol, which inhibits xanthine oxidase. Basic drugs such as gentamicin are altered by the alkalinizing effect of low-protein diets, thus presenting a less ionized form of the drug to the kidney and resulting in increased reabsorption. Amphetamines are known to decrease appetite. Likewise, digitalis given at high levels for long periods may cause nausea and cachexia. Many cancer chemotherapeutic drugs also decrease appetite; in some cases, this may be attributable to gastrointestinal ulceration.

Many drugs appear to act as vitamin antagonists. Although evidence of this has been provided by in vitro studies and observed in animal experiments for many drugs, confirmation in vivo in humans often is lacking. Table 41-5 lists some drugs that are vitamin antagonists. The effects of drugs on retention or loss of major minerals in humans are well established and are summarized in Table 41-6.

Table 41-5 Examples of Drugs That Are Vitamin Antagonists*

Drug	Use/Effect	Vitamin Affected
Adriamycin	Cancer chemotherapy; dose-dependent cardiomyopathy, if accumulation >500 mg/m^2; histological pattern resembles that of vitamin E deficiency	Incidence, severity of damage reduced by vitamin E supplementation in animals, not in humans
Alcohol	Impaired utilization of B vitamins	Thiamine administration improves, as in Wernicke-Korsakoff syndrome
Coumarin drugs Warfarin Dicumerol	Anticoagulants	Vitamin K antagonists; high vitamin K intake decreases anticoagulant effects
Hydralazine	Antihypertensive drug	B_6 antagonist; inhibits nicotinamide synthesis
Isoniazid	Antituberculosis drug	B_6 antagonist; inhibits nicotinamide sythesis
Methotrexate	Cancer chemotherapeutic drug	Folate antagonist
Moxalactam	Antibiotic	Decreases vitamin K–dependent clotting factors
Nitrous oxide	Anesthetic; important in cardiac bypass surgery	B_{12} antagonist
Pentamidine	*Pneumocystis carinii* pneumonia therapy	Folate antagonist
Pyrimethamine	Antimalarial agent	Folate antagonist
Sulfasalazine	Antiinflammatory drug	Folate antagonist
Triamterine	Diuretic	Folate antagonist
Trimethroprim	Antibiotic	Folate antagonist

It should be noted that demonstration of vitamin antagonism by a drug in vitro in animal models often lacks confirmation in humans.
*From Roe DA: Diet, nutrition, and drug interactions. In Shils ME, Olson JA, Shike M, editors: *Modern Nutrition in Health and Disease,* ed 8, Philadelphia, 1993, Lea & Febinger, with extensive bibliography.

Table 41-6 Some Classes or Individual Drugs That Influence Mineral Status

	MINERAL STATUS	
Mineral	Overload	Depletion
Potassium	Succinylcholine increases serum potassium; potassium-sparing diuretics	Laxatives; potassium-losing diuretics; nephrotoxic antibiotics
Sodium	Antacids containing $NaHCO_3$; diazoxide, an antihypertensive, may increase serum sodium	Sodium-losing diuretics
Calcium	Thiazide diuretics, calcium retention; etidronate, a biphosphonate, increases bone mass; pharmacological doses of vitamin D and metabolites—potential hypercalcemia and soft tissue calcification	Aluminum-containing antacids or parenteral fluids—osteomalacia may occur; corticosteroids, phenobarbital, phenytoin
Magnesium	Magnesium-containing antacids	Nephrotic antibiotics; diuretics; cisplatin
Iron		Aspirin; indomethacin
Zinc		Penicillamine; nephrotic antibiotics

Box 41-8 Populations at High Risk for Drug-Nutrient Interactions

Persons who have a poor diet
Persons who have health problems that affect the liver or kidney
Growing children
Pregnant women
Older adults
Persons who are taking two or more medications at the same time
Persons who are using prescription and over-the-counter medications together
Persons who are not following medication directions
Persons who are taking medications for a long period of time
Persons who drink alcohol or smoke excessively

KEY CONCEPTS BOX 41-2

- The basic types of malnutrition are marasmus, kwashiorkor, and obesity. These result from protein-calorie insufficiency, protein insufficency, and overnutrition, respectively.
- Variations of kwashiorkor/marasmus include undernutrition and micronutrient deficiency.
- Kwashiorkor is found most often in children; marasmus is found in both children and adults. Both conditions are associated with increased illness and death.
- Obesity is increasing in all parts of the world and is associated with illness and death.
- Drug and nutrients can interact to adversely affect a drug's effect as well as a person's ability to be nourished properly.

SECTION OBJECTIVES BOX 41-3

- Discuss therapeutic nutrition support by enteral and parenteral routes.
- Discuss the role of the laboratory in supporting nutrition programs and in supporting patients with inborn errors of metabolism.
- List the biochemical parameters used to monitor nutritional status.

Box 41-9

Conditions for Which Enteral Nutrition Is Indicated

Severe dysphagia
Persistent anorexia
Coma
Short bowel syndrome
Inflammatory bowel disease
Partial obstruction of stomach or small bowel
Nausea, vomiting (except with intestinal obstruction)
Need for excessive nutritional requirements, as in burn patients
Fistula of small bowel or colon
Requirement for specific nutrient(s)
Persistent aspiration via jejunostomy

From Shike M: Enteral feeding. In Shils ME, et al, editors: *Modern Nutrition in Health and Disease,* ed 9, Philadelphia, 1999, Lea & Febiger.

THERAPEUTIC NUTRITION SUPPORT[1-3,31]

In all cases of PEM, undernourishment, or specific nutrient deficiencies, appropriate nutritional intervention is needed to treat the malnourished patient. The nutritional therapy must be tailored to the needs of the individual patient. The route of nutritional administration depends on the ability of the gut to function effectively; for patients who are unable to receive nutritional care orally, enteral feeding or parenteral feeding may be necessary.

Enteral Feeding

Enteral feeding refers to the introduction of nutrients into the stomach through a tube. This method is necessary when patients are unable to consume sufficient food normally. Box 41-9 provides a brief list of conditions in which enteral feeding may be indicated. The availability of a variety of commercial enteral formulas tailored to meet specific circumstances has made this an increasingly practical route for maintaining adequate nutrition. A nasogastric tube, used for short-term feeding, is inserted through the nose, down the esophagus, and into the stomach. For long-term enteral feeding, percutaneous endoscopic gastrostomy (PEG) is used to place gastric tubes into the stomach through an incision in the abdominal wall and stomach.

Enteral nutrition is used for burn patients who require increased nutritional support, coma patients, patients with partial obstruction of the stomach or small bowel or fistulas of the small bowel or colon; and individuals with persistent anorexia. It also is useful for disorders with specific requirements that can be met by the introduction of tailored solutions. Whenever possible, enteral feeding is preferred to **total parenteral nutrition (TPN),** because enteral nutrition enables the patient to maintain a functioning gut, with its contribution to normal metabolic processes. In addition, enteral formulas are simpler to manage and preferable to parenteral nutrition. However, when enteral feeding is not possible, nutrients must be administered intravenously.

Box 41-10

Clinical States of Patients Likely to Benefit from Parenteral Nutrition

Inability to digest food
Persistent vomiting (such as that related to obstruction, increased intracranial pressure, or medications given intracranially)
Intestinal motility disorders (such as severe pseudointestinal obstruction)
Massive bowel resection
Severe inflammatory bowel disease
Small bowel fistula unable to be bypassed by tube feedings
Immune disease with intestinal villous atrophy
Support for the underweight premature infant
Persistent hypermetabolic states wherein enteral feeding is contraindicated or is inadequate (such as severe burns with trauma or sepsis)

From Shils ME: Parenteral nutrition. In Shils ME, et al, editors: *Modern Nutrition in Health and Disease,* ed 9, Philadelphia, 1999, Lea & Febiger.

Parenteral Nutrition (PN)

Parenteral nutrition aims to maintain or improve the nutritional status of patients who are unable to obtain the necessary nutrients from normal feeding or from enteral formulas. Parenteral nutrient solutions are intravenously administered by peripheral vein, that is, by **peripheral parenteral nutrition (PPN),** or through a central vein in which a central catheter has been maintained (TPN). Isotonic lipid emulsions containing 5% or 10% glucose, 5% amino acids, electrolytes, and micronutrients supplying up to 2500 kcal in 3 L can be administered peripherally.[28] When a critically ill patient is unstable, continued access to a vein is required; hence a central catheter is essential and must be readily available. Total parenteral nutrition allows larger volumes and therefore more nutrients to be administered than can be delivered by the PPN route. Conditions in which patients may benefit from TPN are summarized in Box 41-10.

Dietary Therapy

Dietary regimens for the treatment of individuals with obesity, hyperlipidemia, or coronary heart disease include restrictions on calories, total fat, saturated fat, and animal protein, and increased consumption of complex carbohydrates, fiber, and vegetable proteins, as well as an increase in the proportions of polyunsaturated and monounsaturated fats. The intake of cholesterol should be less than 100 mg/1000 kcal.

Nutrition plans for patients with diabetes who are at risk for development of atherosclerosis recommend that carbohydrates supply at least 55% to 60% of calories. Complex carbohydrates should provide at least two-thirds of the total. Protein intake should provide 12% to 16% of calories. Fat intake should be reduced to 20% to 25% of calories, no more than 10% of which should be saturated fats. A high-fiber intake that includes as much as 30 to 50 g/day usually is well tolerated and beneficial. Additional details can be found in Chapter 37. Dietary intervention usually is required for populations with other medical conditions, including obesity, cancer, end-stage renal disease, pregnancy and lactation, and inborn errors of metabolism. Often, dietary therapy will require supplemental pharmaceutical intervention.

NUTRITION AND INBORN ERRORS OF METABOLISM[1,32-34]

Inherited metabolic diseases are the result of "inborn errors" in genes that result in alterations in the structure and function of enzymes or protein molecules (see Chapter 52). Intervention during the first few weeks of life is mandatory for phenylketonuria, galactosemia, isovaleric acidemia, homocystinuria, maple syrup urine disease, argininosuccinic aciduria, and citrullinemia. The metabolic diseases associated with inborn errors of amino acid, sugar, and glycogen metabolism are those most readily treatable by diet. Diet must be established specifically for each metabolic disease with the goals of (1) restricting intake of the particular nutrient that cannot be broken down properly, (2) reducing the risk of brain or other organ damage, and (3) promoting proper physical and mental development. Such diets may require specific dietary supplements to attain these goals.

BIOCHEMICAL PARAMETERS USED TO MONITOR NUTRITIONAL STATUS

Early detection and treatment of PEM in hospitals and chronic care facilities has become a required standard of care of the Joint Commission. Institutions are required to have plans to screen for malnutrition within 24 hours after admission of a patient to an institution, to effectively treat the condition, and to monitor the success of that intervention. A recent U.S. government report revealed continuing problems with malnutrition and bed sores in nursing home patients, and highlighted the difficulties involved in detecting and responding to the nutritional needs of institutionalized patients.[35]

General Detection and Monitoring of PEM[9,36]

Assessment of the nutritional status of institutionalized patients and monitoring of nutritional therapies involve both anthropometric and laboratory measurements. Because taking anthropometric measurements (Box 41-11) is a difficult task for nonspecialized health care workers to perform, laboratory tests serve increasingly as more precise surrogate markers for PEM.

Box 41-11

Anthropometric Measurements

Body mass index (BMI) (weight [kg]/[height {m^2}]; http://www.nhlbisupport.com/bmi/)
Mid upper arm circumference (MUAC)
Skinfold thicknesses
Weight-for-height index
Weight-for-age index
Height-for-age index

Box 41-12

Properties of an Ideal Nutritional Marker

Is specific for analyte to be measured
Has a high degree of sensitivity
Is indicative of status of a particular analyte
Has very short biological half-life
Responds rapidly to supplementation
Indicates onset and degree of deficiency early

The properties of an ideal laboratory marker in biological fluids for detecting and monitoring nutritional status are summarized in Box 41-12. Although these properties cannot all be met for every clinical situation, when used in conjunction with consideration of a patient's medical history, they enable interpretation of the patient's nutritional status. Routine biochemical testing can provide data on the patient's basic nutritional status (see Table 41-1).

Although classic cases of micronutrient deficiency (trace minerals and vitamins) are rarely seen in developed countries, they can be found in war-ravaged, poverty-stricken populations. In developed countries, individuals who chronically receive parenteral nutrition may be at high risk for developing a deficiency in micronutrients and may need monitoring of specific nutrients (e.g., zinc, selenium).[9] In most other at-risk populations (see Box 41-6), routine measurement of a micronutrient is rarely needed; monitoring patients for specific signs of a nutrient deficiency (see Chapters 42 and 43) will suffice.

Refeeding Syndrome[37,38]

The refeeding syndrome describes the negative sequelae that can result when patients who have been chronically starved and severely malnourished receive aggressive nutritional support. This syndrome may begin when the starved individual receives more glucose than can be processed physiologically. Under normal conditions, the maximum rate at which glucose can be metabolized is 2 to 4 mg/kg/min. Under stress, this metabolic rate can increase to 3 to 5 mg/kg/min. If these rates are exceeded, an exaggerated insulin response may occur. In addition to its hypoglycemic effect (see Chapter 38), insulin has strong antidiuretic properties. Thus in an exaggerated insulin response, which can occur if a malnourished patient is treated with excessive glucose, water and salt retention may occur, increasing the vascular space and leading to fluid overload and stress to the heart.

Other biochemical sequelae to elevated insulin levels include profound decreases in serum phosphate, magnesium, and potassium as the insulin drives these analytes into peripheral cells, primarily muscle cells. In a body that might already be deficient in these nutrients, hypophosphatemia, hypokalemia, and hypomagnesemia may result.

- Deficiency in serum magnesium may reduce the activity of key enzymes in other tissue, especially cardiac tissue.
- Hypophosphatemia can lead to decreased cellular levels of adenosine triphosphate (ATP) and, in red blood cells, of 2,3-diphosphoglycerate (2,3-DPG). Decreased 2,3-DPG alters the shape of red blood cells, decreases the half-life of red blood cells, and alters the binding of oxygen to hemoglobin (see Chapters 29 and 40). This results in diminished delivery of oxygen to peripheral cells and tissue hypoxia.
- Hypokalemia results in increased irritability of cardiac tissue and reduced ability of cells to take up glucose.

In a severely protein-malnourished individual, muscles already have been weakened because muscle proteins have been catabolized to amino acids that are consumed in the gluconeogenic pathway to increase the availability of blood glucose for the brain. In this weakened condition, the biochemical stresses listed above act to further reduce the capability of muscles to function, leading to respiratory failure and tissue hypoxia, which, in turn, lead to congestive heart failure and cardiac arrest. These sequelae of aggressive nutrition therapy can be avoided by careful monitoring of the serum levels of these analytes and a cooperative relationship among the dietician, physician, laboratory, and pharmacist.

Nitrogen Balance

Tests that may be used to monitor nitrogen balance and provide some estimate of the liver's protein synthesis capabilities are shown in Table 41-7. Nitrogen balance may be estimated from calculated dietary intake and determination of 24-hour excretion of urine urea. An adjustment factor for estimated fecal and other nitrogen losses, such as creatinine, uric acid, ammonia, and losses to hair, nails, and sweat, is determined from an individual patient's condition. This method has limitations, particularly when the factor urine urea × 1.25 grams is used to estimate total nitrogen in the critically ill patient. A more accurate measure of nitrogen excretion can be made through direct analysis of total nitrogen (see earlier and reference 9).

Protein Synthesis

Interpretation of results of plasma albumin and of specific proteins must take into account the individual patient's condition. Alterations in fluid volume status and fluid shifts into or out of the vascular system produce changes in the concentrations of plasma albumin and transferrin. Conditions that initiate the acute-phase response, including trauma, infection, malignancy, and myocardial infarction, can affect the levels of specific hepatic proteins. Of the commonly measured specific proteins, ceruloplasmin is a positive acute-phase reactant, and serum levels are increased because of increased synthesis at the site of injury. At the same time, the serum levels of negative-phase reactants are decreased, because of enhanced catabolism and decreased synthesis. Hence, a decrease in plasma transthyretin (prealbumin), transferrin, retinol binding protein, and albumin may result, at least in part, in conditions other than malnutrition. Nevertheless, analyses of specific proteins with short biological half-lives are useful in monitoring the response to nutritional supplementation. Half-lives of some of the specific proteins, as well as suggested levels at which supplementation is indicated, are shown in Table 41-8. Response to protein supplementation is reflected most rapidly by an increase in retinol binding protein, but prealbumin has been found to be more predictive of improved status. Because prealbumin can be readily measured with the use of routine laboratory equipment, its use as a rapid marker to screen for PEM and to monitor treatment has been recommended,[9] and it is being used increasingly for this purpose.

Table 41-7 Laboratory Tests to Monitor Response to Nutrient Supplements

Parameter	Rationale/Comments
Urine urea nitrogen	Approximate nitrogen balance in anabolic and catabolic states
Total urine nitrogen	Direct measure of excreted nitrogen
Plasma albumin	Low in malnutrition, affected by redistribution with fluid shifts or retention
Plasma transthyretin* (prealbumin)	Low in malnutrition; half-life of 2 days; reflects hepatic protein synthesis
Plasma transferrin*	Low in malnutrition; half-life of 8 days
Plasma retinol-binding protein*	Low in malnutrition; half-life of 10 hours
Plasma zinc	Low levels (500 μg/L) with skin lesions indicate immunoincompetence
Plasma triglycerides	Essential to monitor hypertriglyceridemia in peripheral parenteral nutrition

*Acute-phase reactants, see text.

Table 41-8 Proteins Used in Nutrition Assessment

Protein	Half-life	Normal Values	Suggested Medical Decision Point
Albumin	21 days	3.5 to 5.5 g/dL	3.0 g/dL
Transferrin	8 days	2000 to 4000 mg/L	1500 mg/L
Prealbumin	2 days	160 to 350 mg/L	110 mg/L
Retinol-binding protein	10 hours	26 to 76 mg/L	16 mg/L

KEY CONCEPTS BOX 41-3

- Patients who are unable to consume sufficent nutrients can receive them by tube directly in the stomach (enteral feed) or via a vein (parenteral nutrition).
- Diets can be specialized to meet specific needs.
- Treatment of neonates with inborn errors of glycogen, amino acid, or fat metabolism with specialized diets must occur early to prevent disease and maintain proper mental and physical development.
- Several laboratory tests can be used to detect malnutrition and to monitor dietary response.

REFERENCES

1. http://fnic.nal.usda.gov/nal_display/index.php?info_center=4&tax_level=3&tax_subject=256&topic_id=1342&level3_id=5141
2. Otten JJ, Hellwig JP, Meyers DL: *Dietary Reference Intakes: The Essential Guide to Nutrient Requirements,* Washington, DC, 2006, The National Academies Press.
3. Shils ME, Shike M, Ross AC, et al, editors: *Modern Nutrition in Health and Disease,* ed 10, New York, 2006, Lippincott Williams & Wilkins.
4. Gibney MJ, Elia M, Ljungqvist O, et al, editors: *Clinical Nutrition,* Oxford, 2005, Blackwell Publishing.
5. Whitney EN, Rolfes SR: *Understanding Nutrition,* ed 10, Belmont, CA, 2005, Thomson/Wadsworth Publishing Co.
6. World Health Organization: *Energy and Protein Requirements: A Joint FAO/WHO/UNU Expert Consultation Technical Report,* series 724, Geneva, Switzerland, 1985, WHO.
7. Scrimshaw NS, Waterlow JC, Schürch B, supplement editors: Proceedings of an IDECG workshop, held at the London School of Hygiene and Tropical Medicine, UK (October 31 to November 1994), Eur J Clin Nutr 50(suppl 1):S1, 1996 (see also www.unu.edu/unupress/food2/UID01E/UID01E00.htm).
8. http://www.medscape.com/viewarticle/432384_4
9. National Academy of Clinical Biochemistry: Laboratory support in assessing and monitoring nutritional status. In Kaplan LA, general editor: *Standards of Laboratory Practice Series,* Washington, DC, 1994, National Academy of Clinical Biochemistry.
10. Scheinfeld NS, Mokashi A, Lin A: Protein-energy malnutrition, updated February 18, 2008. Available at http://www.emedicine.com/derm/topic797.htm.
11. Black RE, Allen LH, Bhutta ZA, et al, for the Maternal and Child Undernutrition Study Group: Maternal and child undernutrition: global and regional exposures and health consequences, Lancet 371:243, 2008.
12. Caulfield LE, de Onis M, Blossner M: Undernutrition as an underlying cause of child deaths associated with diarrhea, pneumonia, malaria, and measles, Am J Clin Nutr 80:193, 2004.
13. Centers for Disease Control and Prevention: State-specific prevalence of obesity among adults—United States, 2005, MMWR 55:985, 2006.
14. Dietz WH: Overweight in childhood and adolescence, N Engl J Med 350:855, 2004.
15. Bray GA: Obesity is a chronic, relapsing neurochemical disease, Int J Obes Relat Metab Disord 28:34, 2004.
16. Flegal KM, Graubard BI, Williamson DF, et al: Excess deaths associated with underweight, overweight, and obesity, JAMA 293:1861, 2005.
17. World Health Organization: Global database on child growth and malnutrition. Available at http://www.who.int/nutgrowthdb/en/.
18. http://www.who.int/child_adolescent_health/documents/pdfs/cah_01_10_tsslides_malnutrition.pdf
19. Blecker U, Mehta DI, Davis R, et al: Nutritional problems in patients who have chronic disease, Pediatr Rev 21:29, 2000.
20. Ogden CL, Carroll MD, Curtin LR, et al: Prevalence of overweight and obesity in the United States, 1999-2004, JAMA 295:1549, 2006. Available at http://www.euro.who.int/obesity; http://www.who.int/mediacentre/factsheets/fs311/en/index.html.
21. Ogden CL, Flegal KM, Carroll MD, et al: Prevalence and trends in overweight among US children and adolescents, 1999-2000, JAMA 288:1728, 2002.
22. Demling RH: The incidence and impact of pre-existing protein energy malnutrition on outcome in the elderly burn patient population, J Burn Care Rehabil 26:94, 2005.
23. Harris CL, Fraser C: Malnutrition in the institutionalized elderly: the effects on wound healing, Ostomy Wound Manage 50:54, 2004.
24. Thomas D: Undernutrition in the elderly, Clin Geriatr Med 18: XIII, 2002.
25. Suominen M, Muurinen S, Routasalo P, et al: Malnutrition and associated factors among aged residents in all nursing homes in Helsinki, Eur J Clin Nutr 59:578, 2005.
26. Correia MITD, Waitzberg DL: The impact of malnutrition on morbidity, mortality, length of hospital stay and costs evaluated through a multivariate model analysis, Am J Clin Nutr 22:235, 2003.
27. Horn SD, Bender SA, Ferguson ML, et al: The national pressure ulcer long-term care study: pressure ulcer development in long-term care residents, J Am Geriatr Soc 52:359, 2004.
28. Boullata JI, Armenti VT, editors: Handbook of Drug-Nutrient Interactions, Totowa, NY, 2004, Humana Press.
29. Pronsky ZM: Food-medication interactions. In Gibney MJ, Elia M, Ljungqvist O, et al, editors: *Clinical Nutrition,* ed 15, Oxford, 2008, Blackwell Publishing.
30. Chan L-N: Drug-nutrient interactions. In Shils ME, Shike M, Ross AC, et al, editors: *Modern Nutrition in Health and Disease,* New York, 2006, Lippincott Williams & Wilkins.
31. Gibney MJ, Elia M, Ljungqvist O, et al, editors: *Clinical Nutrition,* Oxford, 2005, Blackwell Publishing.
32. Fernandes J, Saudubray JM, van den Berghe G, et al: *Inborn Metabolic Diseases: Diagnosis and Treatment,* ed 4, Berlin, 2006, Springer.
33. Blau N, Hoffmann GF, Leonard J, et al: *Physicians' Guide to the Treatment and Follow-up of Metabolic Diseases,* Berlin, 2006, Springer.
34. Saudubray JM, Sedel F, Walter JH: Clinical approach to treatable inborn metabolic diseases: an introduction, J Inherit Metab Dis 29:261, 2006.
35. U.S. Government Accountability Office: Report on nursing homes, May 2008. Available at http://www.gao.gov/new.items/d08517.pdf.
36. Teo YK, Wynne HA: Malnutrition of the elderly patient in hospital: risk factors, detection and management, Rev Clin Gerontol 11:229, 2001.
37. Kraft M, Btaiche I, Sacks G: Review of the refeeding syndrome, Nutr Clin Pract 20:625, 2005.
38. Lauts N: Management of the patient with refeeding syndrome, J Infus Nurs 28:337, 2005.

INTERNET SITES

General

www.nutrition.org.uk—British Nutrition Foundation

www.who.int/nut/topics/nutrition/en/—World Health Organization: Nutrition

http://whqlibdoc.who.int/hq/2000/WHO_NHD_00.7.pdf or

http://cms.unescobkk.org/fileadmin/user_upload/appeal/ECCE/Advocacy_letters/NUTRITION.pdf—
http://www.css.cornell.edu/FoodSystems/nutr%26health.html
http://www.nps.ars.usda.gov/programs/programs.htm?NPNUMBER=107—Dade Behring nutrition articles
http://www.ars.usda.gov/—U.S. Department of Agriculture: Agriculture Research Service (Click on Search, type in Nutrition)
http://emedicine.medscape.com/article/985140-overview
http://www.eatright.org/cps/rde/xchg/ada/hs.xsl/index.html—American Dietetic Assn
http://fnic.nal.usda.gov/nal_display/index.php?info_center=4&tax_level=2&tax_subject=256&topic_id=1342
http://emedicine.medscape.com/article/1104623-overview—Protein-energy malnutrition

World Malnutrition

http://www.who.int/en
http://www.doctorswithoutborders.org/images/news/malnutrition/map_hotspots_large.jpg
http://www.unicef.org/progressforchildren/2006n4/index_howmany.html
http://www.usaid.gov/our_work/global_health/nut/techareas/micro.html
http://www.who.int/child_adolescent_health/documents/pdfs/cah_01_10_tsslides_malnutrition.pdf
http://www.who.int/mediacentre/factsheets/fs311/en/index.html
http://www.who.int/nutgrowthdb/en/—WHO Global Database on Child Growth and Malnutrition
http://www.childinfo.org/nutrition.html

Obesity

http://www.euro.who.int/obesity
http://www.euro.who.int/document/RC57/epres_nut.pdf
http://www.cdc.gov/nchs/products/pubs/pubd/hestats/overweight/overwght_adult_03.htm#Table%201—Adult obesity data
http://www.cdc.gov/nccdphp/dnpa/obesity/trend/maps/obesity_trends_2006.ppt#485,1—Citations: Obesity data with time
http://www.cdc.gov/nchs/products/pubs/pubd/hestats/overweight/overwght_child_03.htm—Childhood obesity data
http://www.cdc.gov/nchs/data/nhanes/databriefs/overwght.pdf
www.iotf.org/—WHO International Obesity Task Force
www.cdc.gov/nccdphp/dnpa/obesity/—National Center for Chronic Disease Prevention and Health Promotion: Obesity and Overweight
www.nhlbi.nih.gov/guidelines/obesity/ob_home.htm—National Heart, Lung, and Blood Institute Clinical Guidelines on the Identification, Evaluation, and Treatment of Overweight and Obesity in Adults
www.cdc.gov/brfss—National Center for Chronic Disease Prevention and Health Promotion Behavioral Risk Factor Surveillance System

Drug-Nutrient Interactions

http://www.cc.nih.gov/ccc/patient_education/drug_nutrient/
http://www.ext.colostate.edu/PUBS/foodnut/09361.html
http://www.merck.com/mmhe/sec02/ch013/ch013c.html

Enteral Feeding

http://www.rxkinetics.com/tpntutorial/2_2.html
http://ahca.myflorida.com/Medicaid/dme/category_lists_for_hcpcs_codes_042508.pdf

Genetic Disease

http://rarediseases.info.nih.gov/—Web pages for rare diseases
http://www.ncbi.nlm.nih.gov/sites/entrez?db=omim—National Center for Biotechnology Information for known gene defects and their metabolic consequences
http://ghr.nlm.nih.gov/

Refeeding Syndrome

http://www.ccmtutorials.com/misc/phosphate/page_07.htm

42

Chapter

Trace Elements

Nancy W. Alcock

Chapter Outline

Classification

Essential Trace Elements

Chromium (Cr)

Method

Reference Intervals

Copper (Cu)

Fluorine (F)

Iodine (I)

Manganese (Mn)

Molybdenum (Mo)

Selenium (Se)

Zinc (Zn)

Toxic Trace Metals

Aluminum (Al)

Cadmium (Cd)

Lead (Pb)

Mercury (Hg)

Considerations in Assessing Trace Element Status in Humans

Key Terms

adequate intake (AI) Recommended daily intake value of a micronutrient that is assumed to be adequate; used when an RDA cannot be determined.

deficiency Status of a nutrient in which an abnormal symptom or biochemical function is reversed by supplementation with the nutrient.

dental caries A condition in which the calcified dentin or enamel, or both, of a tooth is destroyed by the action of microorganisms on carbohydrates.

essential trace element An element that, if removed from the diet, produces a biochemical abnormality that is reversed by supplementation with the element.

metallothionein A 6200 D protein, with approximately 30% of its amino acid residue content composed of cysteine, which firmly binds Cd>Cu>Zn ions. Metallothionein plays an important role in zinc-copper interactions, and its synthesis is readily induced by zinc.

micronutrients Essential food components that are required or present in the body in very small amounts. Include vitamins and some metals.

RDA Recommended daily allowance of a micronutrient; covers the needs of 97% to 98% of the population.

tolerable upper intake level (UL) The highest level of daily nutrient intake that is likely to pose no risk of adverse health effects for almost all individuals in the general population. The potential risk of adverse effects increases at dietary intakes above the UL.

toxic trace elements Those elements found in the environment that are antagonistic to biochemical processes. When present in tissues in elevated levels, they can be toxic and eventually may be fatal.

trace elements Elements present in the body in very low amounts (micrograms/gram or less). Some are essential; others may be toxic, even at relatively low levels. Most trace elements are metals; the halogens iodine and fluorine are the exceptions.

zinc fingers Specific zinc binding (by histidine and cysteine residues) regions that occur at defined intervals of regulatory proteins. These proteins bind to deoxyribonucleic acid (DNA) and regulate gene expression by controlling DNA transcription.

Methods on Evolve

Aluminum

Ceruloplasmin

Copper

Iron and iron binding capacity

Lead

Thyroxine (total)

Thyroxine, free and free triiodothyronine

Vitamin B_{12}

Zinc

SECTION OBJECTIVES BOX 42-1

- Review and be able to describe the definitions for dietary reference intakes.
- Review the various classifications of trace metals.

CLASSIFICATION[1]

In 1997, the Food and Nutrition Board of the National Academy of Sciences created a new set of criteria for dietary assessment—the Dietary Reference Intakes (DRIs). There are four types of DRI reference values: the Estimated Average Requirement (EAR), the Recommended Dietary Allowance (RDA), the Adequate Intake (AI), and the **Tolerable Upper Intake Level (UL).** The definitions of these new categories are provided in Box 42-1.

Trace elements are present in the body in very low amounts, usually less than 1 microgram per gram of tissue. They are part of the **micronutrients** of the body and can be subdivided into four major groupings based on their physiological function:

1. Essential trace elements for which a **recommended daily allowance (RDA)** has been established. These elements have been shown to be essential for normal growth, development, and maintenance, and a specific biological role has been identified. The elements in this group that are considered in this chapter are zinc, iodine, and selenium. The RDAs for these elements are listed in Table 42-1. Iron, the most abundant of the essential trace metals, is discussed in Chapter 39. Iron and zinc are transition elements in Mendeleev's original classification of the elements, whereas selenium and iodine are members of the "normal" series in group VI and group VII, respectively.
2. Trace elements for which there is definite evidence of an essential role in human metabolism but for which an RDA has not yet been established. These include the transition metals copper, manganese, chromium, cobalt, and molybdenum and the group VII halogen fluorine. The estimated RDAs and **adequate intakes (AIs)** for these elements also are listed in Table 42-1. The only known requirement for cobalt in humans is as a component of the B_{12} molecule, which is discussed in Chapter 43.

Box 42-1

Dietary Reference Intakes (DRI) Definitions

Recommended Dietary Allowance (RDA): The average daily dietary intake level that is sufficient to meet the nutrient requirements of nearly all (97% to 98%) healthy individuals in a particular life stage and gender group.

Adequate Intake (AI): A recommended intake value based on observed or experimentally determined approximations or estimates of nutrient intake by a group (or groups) of healthy individuals, which is assumed to be adequate; it is used when an RDA cannot be determined.

Tolerable Upper Intake Level (UL): The highest level of daily nutrient intake that is likely to pose no risk of adverse health effects for almost all individuals in the general population. As intake increases above the UL, the potential risk of adverse effects increases.

Estimated Average Requirement (EAR): A daily nutrient intake value that is estimated to meet the requirement of half of healthy individuals in a life stage and gender group; used to assess dietary adequacy and serves as the basis for the RDA.

Source: http://ific.org/publications/other/driupdateom.cfm?renderforprint=1

Table 42-1 Recommended Daily Dietary Allowances Established for Zinc, Iodine, and Selenium (the RDA for Iron is Included for Comparison)

Category	Age (Years) or Condition	Iron, mg	Zinc, mg	Iodine, µg	Selenium, µg	Copper, µg	Manganese,* µg	Fluoride,* µg	Chromium,* µg	Molybdenum µg
Infants	0.1 to 0.5	0.27*	2*	110*	15*	200*	0.003	0.01	0.2	2*
	0.51 to 1.0	11	3	130*	20*	220*	0.6	0.5	5.5	3*
Children	1 to 3	7	3	90	20	340	1.2	0.7	11	17
	4 to 8	10	5	90	30	440	1.5	1	15	22
Males	9 to 13	8	8	120	40	700	1.9	2	25	34
	14 to 18	11	11	150	55	890	2.2	3	35	43
	19 to 30	8	11	150	55	900	2.3	4	35	45
	31 to 50	8	11	150	55	900	2.3	4	35	45
	51+	8	11	150	55	900	2.3	4	30	45
Females	9 to 13	8	8	120	40	700	1.6	2	21	34
	14 to 18	15	8	150	55	890	1.6	3	24	43
	19 to 30	18	8	150	55	900	1.8	3	25	45
	31 to 50	18	8	150	55	900	1.8	3	25	45
	51+	8	8	150	55	900	1.8	3	20	45
Pregnant		27	11 to 12	220	60	1000	2.0	3	29 to 30	50
Lactating	14 to 50	9 to 10	12 to 13	290	70	1300	2.6	3	44 to 45	50

Modified from *Dietary Reference Intakes (DRIs): Recommended Intakes for Individuals, Elements,* Washington, DC, 2006, Institute of Medicine, Food and Nutrition Board, National Academies. Available at: http://www.iom.edu/Object.File/Master/21/372/0.pdf

Recommended dietary allowances (RDAs) are listed unless marked with an asterisk (*), which indicates Adequate Intakes (AIs).

Table 42-2 Biological Roles of Essential Trace Elements and Associated Abnormalities

Element	Biological Role	Comments	Deficiency/Abnormality/Toxicity
Chromium	Metabolism of glucose	Potentiates insulin action	Glucose intolerance in deficiency
Cobalt	Component of vitamin B_{12}	No other function known in man	Vitamin B_{12} deficiency; anemia
Copper	Co-factor for oxidase enzymes	90% to 95% plasma copper bound to ceruloplasmin	Inherited diseases: Wilson's, Menkes'
Fluorine	Inhibits dental caries; therapeutically improves quality of hydroxyapatite crystals in bone	Usually supplied as supplement to drinking water	Excessive intake causes fluorosis
Iodine	Component of T_3 and T_4	Concentrated in the thyroid; supplementation by addition to salt is common	Iodine deficiency still occurs in various geographic areas
Iron	Component of heme enzymes; hemoglobin, cytochromes	In plasma, bound to transferrin; stored as ferritin	Deficiency: Hypochromic, microcytic anemia
Manganese	Required for glycoprotein and proteoglycan synthesis	Component of mitochondrial peroxide dismutase	Deficiency not known in man
Molybdenum	Component of sulfite and xanthine oxidases	Essential for production of uric acid	Deficiency reported in TPN patient; inability to metabolize methionine
Selenium	Component of glutathione peroxidase and iodinothyronine-5′-deiodinase	Antioxidant properties; selenium and vitamin E act synergistically	Deficiency may occur where soil Se is low and in long-term TPN patients with inadequate supplements
Silicon	Involved in calcification in bone	Role in bone, cartilage, and connective tissue is poorly understood	Deficiency: Impairment of normal growth in animals; silicosis may occur from industrial exposure
Zinc	Co-factor or component of more than 200 metalloenzymes	Involved in many metabolic processes: Protein synthesis; immunological function; growth and development	Deficiency: Growth failure, hypogonadism, impaired wound healing; genetic disease: acrodermatitis enteropathica–impaired absorption; toxicity: vomiting, gastrointestinal irritation

TPN, Total parenteral nutrition.

3. Trace elements that are consistently found in tissues or biological fluids in "ultratrace" amounts but that have not yet been shown to be either essential or detrimental at these levels of concentration. These include lithium, nickel, tin, silicon, and vanadium. They are not discussed in this chapter.
4. Trace metals that have no known biological function in humans but that, if present at relatively low levels, cause pathological changes. These **toxic trace elements** include aluminum, beryllium, cadmium, mercury, lead, and arsenic. They are discussed in this chapter. Cadmium, arsenic, and mercury are transition elements, whereas aluminum and lead are members of the normal series in group III and group IV, respectively.

KEY CONCEPTS BOX 42-1

- There are 4 definitions of recommended dietary intake of trace, these are the RDA, the AI, UL, and EAR (see Box 42-1). This hierarchy is based on the levels of knowledge of the amount of trace element needed or tolerated in the diet.
- The trace elements can be divided into those known to be necessary for life when present in sufficient amounts (the essential trace elements, Tables 42-1 and -2.) and those with no known biological function and that are harmful when present above a certain level in the body (Table 42-4).

SECTION OBJECTIVES BOX 42-2

- Explain the biochemical mechanisms by which the essential trace elements perform their functions.
- Describe the primary methods used for measuring each trace metal.

ESSENTIAL TRACE ELEMENTS

The biological role of **essential trace elements** and some abnormalities arising from a **deficiency** or excess of the respective elements are shown in Table 42-2. Reference intervals, taken from the literature, for essential trace elements are listed in Table 42-3, and those for toxic metals are given in Table 42-4.

Chromium (Cr)[2-8]

Chromium is a transition element in period 4 of the periodic table of the elements, with an atomic weight of 52.

Biochemistry

Chromium exists in several oxidation states; the most prevalent are hexavalent chromium (Cr VI, which is associated with industrial exposure and toxicity) and trivalent chromium (Cr III, which is stable and the biologically active form). Cr (III) binds to transferrin in plasma, and Cr (VI) is rapidly taken up

Table 42-3 Suggested Reference Intervals for Essential Trace Elements

Element	Specimen Type or Source	REFERENCE INTERVAL Concentration	IU
Cr	S	<0.5 μg/L	<9.6 nmol/L
	RBC	20 to 36 μg/L	384 to 692 nmol/L
	U	<0.5 μg/L	<9.6 nmol/L
Co	S	0.11 to 0.45 μg/L	1.9 to 7.6 nmol/L
	RBC	16 to 46 μg/L	272 to 781 nmol/kg
	U	1 to 2 μg/L	17 to 34 nmol/L
Vitamin B_{12}	S	180 to 960 pg/mL	133 to 708 pmol/L
Cu	S	μg/dL	μmol/L
	Birth to 6 mo	20 to 70	3.14 to 10.99
	6 years	90 to 190	14.13 to 29.83
	12 years	80 to 160	12.56 to 25.12
	Adult (male)	70 to 140	10.99 to 21.98
	Adult (female)	80 to 155	12.56 to 24.34
	Term pregnancy	118 to 302	18.53 to 47.41
	U	3 to 35 μg/day	0.047 to 0.55 μmol/day
F	P	0.01 to 0.2 μg/mL	0.5 to 10.5 μmol/L
	U	0.2 to 1.1 μg/mL	10.5 to 57.9 μmol/L
I	P	0.8 to 6.0 μg/L	102 to 761 μmol/L
T_4 free	Newborn	2.6 to 6.3 ng/dL	33.5 to 81.3 pmol/L
	Adult	0.8 to 2.3 ng/dL	10.3 to 31.0 pmol/L
T_4 total	S adult	5 to 12 μg/dL	65 to 155 μmg/L
T_3 free (equilibrium dialysis)	S cord blood	15 to 391 pg/dL	0.2 to 6.0 pmol/L
	Children and adults	260 to 380 pg/dL	4.0 to 7.4 pmol/L
	Adult	208 to 674 pg/dL	3.2 to 104 pmol/L
T_3 total	Adult	100 to 200 ng/dL	1.54 to 3.08 nmol/L
Mn	S	0.5 to 1.5 μg/L	9 to 27 nmol/L
	B	≈11 μg/L	≈200 nmol/L
	U	0.2 to 0.5 μg/L	3.6 to 9.0 nmol/L
Mo	S	0.1 to 3.0 μg/L	1.0 to 31.3 nmol/L
Se	S (Mean ± SEM)		
	Adult males	86.7 ± 7.9 μg/L	1.10 (±0.10) μmol/L
	Adult females	94.4 ± 7.9 μg/L	1.20 (±0.10) μmol/L
	Toxicity	>400 μg/L	>5.06 μmol/L
	U	7 to 60 μg/L	0.09 to 0.78 μg/L
Zn	S	70 to 120 μg/dL	10.7 to 18.3 μmol/L
	U	300 to 500 μg/day	4.58 to 7.64 μmol/day

B, Whole blood; *IU,* standard international units; *P,* plasma; *RBC,* red blood cell; *S,* serum; *U,* urine.

by erythrocytes after absorption and is reduced to Cr (III) within the cell.

Clinical Significance

Trivalent chromium is a potentiator of insulin action,[3] either directly by increasing receptor number or affinity, or by activating other mediators, such as the insulin receptor kinase.[4] In humans, signs and symptoms indicative of chromium deficiency include impaired glucose tolerance, elevated circulating insulin, glucosuria, elevated fasting blood glucose, elevated serum triglycerides and cholesterol, encephalopathy, and neuropathy. Patients who are receiving long-term total parenteral nutrition (TPN) are at risk for chromium deficiency if their TPN fluids are not supplemented. In a case of chromium deficiency,[5] a nondiabetic patient developed hyperglycemia, glucose intolerance, and glucosuria after he was on TPN therapy for several months. The patient's low serum chromium levels and glucose metabolism returned to normal after chromium supplementation.

Although the physiological role of chromium is accepted, its role in the development and treatment of diabetes remains controversial.[6] Chromium picolinate has been advocated as part of the treatment for diabetes, but again, this remains controversial.

The adequate intake level of chromium intake is shown in Table 42-1. It is estimated that less than 2% of dietary trivalent chromium is absorbed from the gastrointestinal tract.

Table **42-4** Acceptable and Toxic Reference Ranges for Toxic Trace Metals

Element	Specimen Type	REFERENCE RANGE Concentration	SIU
Al	S	<4 µg/L	<148 nmol/L
	U	<10 µg/day	<0.4 µmol/day
	S toxic	See text	
As	B	2 to 62 µg/L	26 to 826 µmol/L
	U	5 to 50 µg/day	66 to 660 nmol/day
	B chronic toxicity	600 to 9300 µg/L	8 to 125 µmol/L
Cd	B	<5 µg/L	<44.6 nmol/L
	U	<3 µg/day	<26 nmol/L
	Toxic	>50 µg/L	>446 nmol/L
Hg	B	<7 µg/L	<35 nmol/L
	U (dentists)	7 to 15 µg/L	35 to 74.7 nmol/L
	U	<20 µg/day	<99.5 nmol/L
	B toxicity	>150 µg/L	>750 nmol/L
	Hair	<1 µg/g	<4.9 nmol/g
Pb	B (children)	<10 µg/dL	<480 nmol/L

B, Whole blood; *SIU,* standard international units; *S,* serum; *U,* urine.

Toxicity

Cr VI is 1000 times as toxic as Cr III, and toxicity from trivalent sources of chromium has not been reported in humans. Hexavalent chromium toxicity from industrial exposure through inhalation and skin contact has been associated with an increased incidence of lung cancer.[7]

Food Sources

Chromium is found in brewer's yeast, mushrooms, molasses, nuts, wine, beer, asparagus, prunes, meats, cheeses, and whole grains. It is difficult to assess accurately the chromium content of foods, because preparation for analysis usually involves homogenization in equipment with stainless steel parts, and some contamination usually occurs.

Method[8]

Graphite furnace flameless atomic absorption spectrometry is the preferred method of analysis. Although a tungsten halogen lamp provides adequate background correction, graphite furnace atomic absorption spectrophotometry with the use of Zeeman background correction is the preferred instrumentation.

Reference Intervals

Normal, nonsupplemented human adults excrete approximately 0.5 µg of chromium/L of urine and have serum levels <0.5 µg/L (see Table 42-3).[8] Erythrocytes have a concentration of 20 to 36 µg/L.

Copper (Cu)[9-16]

Biochemistry

Copper is a transition element in period 4 of the periodic table of the elements, with an atomic weight of 64.

Divalent copper forms complexes with proteins, many of which are copper metalloenzymes with oxidase activity. These take part in a large number of physiological activities (see Table 42-3), including energy production (cytochrome C oxidase), iron metabolism (ceruloplasmin and ferroxidase II), antioxidant functions (superoxidase dismutase), connective tissue formation (lysly oxidase), neurotransmitter metabolism (dopamine β-hydroxylase and monoamine oxidase), spermine oxidase, melanin formation (tyrosinase), and intermediate metabolism (uricase, benzylamine oxidase, diamine oxidase, and tryptophan 3,3-di-oxygenase). In biological systems, copper has the ability to induce the synthesis of **metallothionein,** which is involved in the uptake, transport, and regulation of zinc. Approximately 50% of dietary copper is absorbed, and the process is facilitated by the complexing of copper with amino acids. In plasma, approximately 95% of copper is bound to ceruloplasmin, an α_2-globulin with ferroxidase activity. Copper also is transported in the plasma bound loosely to albumin. A small fraction of plasma copper is complexed with amino acids.

Although the RDA for dietary copper for adults is 0.9 mg/day (see Table 42-1), it is estimated that 35% of diets in the United States provide <1 mg/day. Excretion of copper occurs mainly in the bile, with urinary excretion normally measured at <40 µg/day.

Clinical Significance

A relatively high carbohydrate intake in the American diet accompanied by marginal intake of copper possibly potentiates subclinical copper deficiency.[11] Evidence suggests that marginal copper deficiency is associated with heart disease, bone and joint osteoarthritis, and osteoporosis. Microcytic hypochromic anemia, as well as neutropenia, hypothermia, and demineralization, has been associated with copper deficiency. Copper deficiency, which is rare among healthy, well-nourished individuals, is more frequent among severely undernourished, premature infants, patients receiving

Table 42-5 Genetic Changes Associated With Disease

Disease	Gene	Protein	Gene Locus
Menkes' syndrome, kinky hair disease, steely hair disease, copper transport disease	*ATP7A*	Cu(2+)-transporting ATPase, alpha peptide	Xq12-q13
Wilson's disease	*ATP7B*	ATPase, Cu(2+)-transporting, beta polypeptide	13q14.3-q21.1
Aceruloplasminemia	*CP* gene	Copper/iron binding protein	3q23-q24
Copper deficiency, familial benign	Not known	Not known	X-linked or autosomal dominant
Sulfite oxidase deficiency	*SUOX*	Enzyme, sulfite oxidase (EC 1.8.3.1)	Chromosome 12
Molybdenum co-factor deficiency*	*MOCOD*	Mo-containing co-factor, essential to the function of sulfite oxidase, xanthine dehydrogenase, and aldehyde oxidase	14q24, 6p21.3, 5q11
Glutathione peroxidase deficiency	*GPX1*	Red cell glutathione peroxidase (EC 1.11.1.9)	3p21.3
Glutathione peroxidase deficiency	*GPX3*	Plasma glutathione peroxidase (EC 1.11.1.9)	5q32-q33.1

*Disease has more than one associated genetic focus.

long-term intravenous total parenteral nutrition (TPN), and individuals with severe, chronic malabsorption syndromes, such as celiac disease, Crohn's disease, cystic fibrosis, or tropical sprue.

In Menkes' kinky hair syndrome, an X-linked genetic defect (Table 42-5) seen in 1 in 35,000 to 50,000 infants by 2 to 3 months,[12] absorption of copper from the gastrointestinal tract is impaired. The resulting copper deficiency is manifested by severe cerebellar and cerebral degeneration, subdural hematoma and/or thrombosis of arteries in the brain, osteoporosis, motor delay, and failure to thrive.[13] Many infants with Menkes' syndrome die within the first decade of life, usually by the age of three. A number of similar X-linked genetic defects that may be allelic variants of Menkes' syndrome have been investigated because they are associated with abnormal copper metabolism, including Haas Chir Robinson syndrome and familial benign copper deficiency.

Wilson's disease is an inherited autosomal recessive error (see Table 42-5) in copper metabolism that results in excessive accumulation of copper in liver, brain, cornea, and kidneys.[14] With 10 to 30 million cases worldwide, the estimated gene frequency of this defect is 0.3% to 0.7%, and the disease presents more often in females than in males (4:1). In this disease, the liver has an impaired ability to excrete excess copper, leading to deposition in the liver, nerves, and cornea. This leads to the symptoms (neuropsychiatric, severe brain damage, and liver failure) associated with Wilson's disease, and the best diagnotic sign, the green-gold Kayser-Fleischer rings in the cornea, formed by the deposition of copper. Ceruloplasmin levels are low, and levels of non–ceruloplasmin-bound copper are elevated. Tissue copper deposits may be diminished and then excreted by the intravenous administration of a chelating agent.[14]

Marginal copper deficiency, especially in adults, so far has proved difficult to detect biochemically. Milne and Johnson[15] have concluded that diminished cytochrome oxidase activity in leukocytes or diminished superoxide dismutase activity in erythrocytes is likely to be the most reliable laboratory index of reduced levels of metabolically active copper.

Plasma copper is not a reliable indicator of copper status. Although long-term copper deprivation, as occurs in treatment by TPN, results in low plasma levels, long-term therapy with corticosteroids and adrenocorticotropic hormone (ACTH) also reduces copper levels. The primary criterion used to estimate the Estimated Average Requirement (EAR) for copper consists of a combination of indicators, including plasma copper and ceruloplasmin concentrations, erythrocyte superoxide dismutase activity, and platelet copper concentration in controlled human depletion/repletion studies.

Food Sources of Copper

Most foods contain appreciable quantities of copper. Those rich in copper include shellfish, liver, kidney, egg yolk, and some legumes.

Methods[16]

Flame atomic absorption spectrophotometry for serum or plasma and graphite furnace flameless atomic absorption spectrophotometry for urine, wherein concentration usually is <40 μg/L, are the preferred methods of analysis.

Reference Intervals

Serum or plasma levels vary with age and are higher in adult women than in men (see Table 42-3). Most copper is excreted through the bile, and urine levels usually are <40 μg/day.

Fluorine (F)[17-21]

Fluorine, atomic weight 19, is the first member of period 2 of the group VII halogens of the periodic table of elements.

Biochemistry

The fluoride anion may substitute for the hydroxyl ion in the hydroxyapatite crystal structure in calcified tissues, bone, and teeth.[17] The production of a "harder" crystal is believed to account for the protective effect of fluoride against **dental caries.**[18] Fluoride also has been used therapeutically, alone or in combination with vitamin D, in the treatment of osteoporosis.

Clinical Significance

A direct, inverse association between the incidence of dental caries and the fluoride concentration in drinking water of ≤1 mg/L has long been recognized. Less convincing is a reported beneficial effect of sodium fluoride as a therapy for osteoporosis.[19]

Requirement

The daily requirement is 2 to 4 mg/day. Usually, a fluoridated water supply with 1 mg/L of fluoride provides the daily requirement.

Food Sources

Traces of fluoride are present in most foods. Fluoride can be present in drinking water, either naturally or because of artificial supplementation.

Toxicity

High intake of fluoride causes dental fluorosis characterized by discolored and mottled teeth.[17,18] Increased bone density and calcification of muscle evident by radiography occur in areas where 10 to 45 mg/L of fluoride is present in water. Exposure to hydrofluoric acid solutions, through contact of exposed skin or by oral ingestion, is associated with high morbidity.[20] The hydrofluoric acid molecule rapidly burns through the skin, and once it enters the circulation, it will react with, and precipitate, calcium and magnesium. This results in a profound hypocalcemia and hypomagnesemia, which can cause cardiac arrhythmias and cardiac arrest.

Method

An ion-selective electrode[21] method is the preferred method of analysis.

Reference Intervals[21]

Reference intervals in plasma are 0.01 to 0.2 µg/mL; 0.5 to 10.5 µmol/L. Reference intervals in urine are 0.2 to 1.1 µg/mL; 10.5 to 57.9 µmol/L.

Iodine (I)[22-24]

Iodine, atomic weight 127, is in period 5 of the group VII halogens of the periodic table of elements.

Biochemistry

Although iodine is widely distributed throughout the earth's surface, the sea is the major source of iodine. Iodides, oxidized by sunlight to the volatile elemental iodine, are estimated to provide annually some 400,000 tons of iodine to the atmosphere from seawater. The iodide concentration in seawater, approximately 50 µg/L, is similar to that in human serum.

Iodine is of significance in human biology as a constituent of the thyroid gland hormones thyroxine (3,5,3′,5′-tetraiodothyronine; T_4) and 3,5,3′-triiodothyronine (T_3), which are synthesized by the iodination of tyrosine (see Chapter 49 for details). These hormones are essential for healthy growth, cell differentiation, and development. Iodine deficiency occurs in areas where soil is depleted of iodide. Uptake by crops is directly proportional to soil content. Iodine-deficiency disease is still a frequent occurrence in various underdeveloped countries.

Clinical Significance[22,24]

Both maternal and fetal thyroid hormones contribute to fetal development. Iodine deficiency during pregnancy may result in spontaneous abortions, stillbirths, an increase in infant or perinatal mortality, congenital abnormalities or neurological cretinism, fetal hypothyroidism, and psychomotor defects. Most areas in the United States screen for neonatal hypothyroidism, which is readily treatable. In the child and adolescent, goiter, mental retardation, and retarded development are prominent signs of hypothyroidism. Myxedematous, or neurological, cretinism also is seen. Approximately 2.2 billion of the population of the world live in areas of iodine-deficient soil, and ≈11% of the population in the United States have low urinary iodine; these indiviuals are at risk for endemic goiter. Iodine status may be determined by measurement of serum thyroid hormone levels or urine iodine excretion.

Requirements

Iodine requirements vary with age (see Table 42-1).

Food Sources

Marine fish and seaweed are rich in iodine.

Toxicity

Prolonged excessive iodine intake (>2 mg/day) results in iodide goiter and myxedema.

Methods

Immunoassay for thyroid hormones and ion-selective electrode methods for iodide are the recommended methods of analysis (see reference 24 and Methods section on Elsevier Evolve Website).

Reference Intervals[23]

See Chapter 49 for levels of iodine-containing hormones. Reference intervals for plasma inorganic iodide are 0.8 to 6.0 µg/L. Urine inorganic iodide correlates with plasma level. The lower limit of the reference interval is age dependent: 5 to 10 years, 32.5 µg/g creatinine; adolescents, 50 µg/g creatinine; adults, 75 µg/g creatinine.

Manganese (Mn)[25-29]

Manganese is a transition element in period 4 of the periodic table of the elements with an atomic weight of 55.

Biochemistry

Manganese forms divalent and trivalent salts. It is important for proper metabolism in connective tissue, physical growth and development of reproductive functions, and proper carbohydrate and lipid metabolism.[25] It functions as an enzyme activator; however, other divalent cations, in particular magnesium, may substitute for manganese. Enzymes that may have high specificity for manganese include the glycosyl transferases and mitochondrial pyruvate carboxylase and superoxide dismutase; the latter is the principal antioxidant in mitochondria.[26] The total manganese content in adult humans is 12 to 20 mg, of which 25% is in the skeleton. Usual intake ranges from 1.7 to 8.3 mg/day, of which 2% to 15% is absorbed. Absorption occurs in the small intestine and is inhibited by the presence of other divalent cations, including Fe, Ca, and Mg, and by phosphate, fiber, and phytate. Excess manganese is excreted through bile and pancreatic secretions; only a small amount is excreted in the urine.

Clinical Significance

Manganese deficiency in humans has not been unambiguously demonstrated. Manganese deficiency has been suspected in hip abnormalities, joint disease, congenital skeletal deformities, and childhood epilepsy. Industrial poisoning, especially among welders, produces schizophrenia-like psychiatric effects and neurological disorders similar to those of Parkinson's disease.[27,28]

Requirement

The estimated safe and adequate dietary intake for various ages is shown in Table 42-1.

Food Sources

Bran flakes and wheat are rich in manganese. Refined grains and meat contain little manganese.

Toxicity

Manganese toxicity from prolonged industrial exposure results in neurological changes that resemble those of Parkinson's disease.[28]

Method

Zeeman graphite furnace atomic absorption spectrophotometry is the preferred analytical procedure. Magnesium nitrate is recommended as a matrix modifier.[29]

Reference Intervals

Reference intervals in whole blood are approximately 11 μg/L, or approximately 200 nmol/L. Intervals in serum are 0.5 to 1.5 μg/L and 9 to 27 nmol/L; and in urine are 0.2 to 0.5 μg/L; 3.6 to 9.0 nmol/L.

Molybdenum (Mo)[30-34]

Molybdenum is a transition element in period 5 of the periodic table of the elements, with an atomic weight of 96.

Biochemistry

Molybdenum is a co-factor of the metalloenzymes xanthine oxidase, sulfite oxidase, and aldehyde oxidase, and thus plays a role in the metabolism of purines to uric acid, the final stages of oxidation of sulfur-containing amino acids, and the oxidation of aldehydes, respectively.[30,31] In these enzymes, the molybdenum atom is complexed by the dithiolene moiety of tricyclic pyranopterin structures, the simplest of which is known as molybdopterin. Although absorption of molybdenum from the gastrointestinal tract may be inhibited by competition from elevated dietary copper, increased molybdenum intake can cause a physiological copper deficiency.

Clinical Significance

Most of the available evidence on the metabolism of molybdenum has been derived from animal studies. Increased intake of molybdenum inhibits copper utilization; this effect is potentiated by increased sulfate intake. Molybdenum retention is decreased in the presence of excess copper or sulfate.[31] An increase in molybdenum intake is accompanied by increased serum levels of uric acid and the development of gout.

Mild cases of molybdenosis or deficiency are identified most easily by biochemical changes, for example, by changes in uric acid or methionine levels, reflecting the activity of molybdenum-containing enzymes. A case of molybdenum deficiency was reported in a patient maintained on TPN.[32] Elevated levels of the amino acid methionine and decreased uric acid excretion and sulfate excretion were corrected by administration of molybdenum, indicating reduced activity of molybdenum-containing metalloenzymes in the molybdenum-deficient patient. Excessive molybdenum intake is accompanied by increased serum levels of uric acid and the development of gout.

Requirement

An estimate of the adequate daily intake of molybdenum ranges from 2 to 3 μg in infancy, and the RDA is 34 to 45 μg in adults.

Food Sources

Milk, milk products, organ meats, and dried legumes and cereals contain molybdenum, primarily in an organic form.

Toxicity

The toxicity of molybdenum from dietary sources has been documented.[33,34] Symptoms of gout were reported, as were others that indicated possible involvement of the liver, gastrointestinal tract, and kidney.

Method

Graphite furnace atomic absorption spectrophotometry is the recommended method of analysis for molybdenum.

Reference Interval

The reference interval for serum molybdenum is 0.1 to 3.0 μg/L.

Selenium (Se)[35-44]

Selenium is in period 4, group VI, of the periodic table of the elements and has an atomic weight of 79.

Biochemistry[35-38]

Selenium is a member of the same group of elements as oxygen and sulfur. In animals, selenium is found primarily as selenocysteine, in which an atom of selenium has replaced the usual sulfur atom of cysteine. From one to four selenocysteine residues are incorporated into glutathione peroxidases (4 residues), tetraiodothyronine 5′ deiodinases, thioredoxin reductases, formate dehydrogenases, glycine reductases, and some hydrogenases. Glutathione peroxidase, which is present in the cytoplasm and the mitochondria of tissues, has strong antioxidant properties. Thioredoxin reductases facilitate the reduction of other proteins, thereby regenerating several antioxidant systems.[38] The thioredoxins are kept in the reduced state by the flavoenzyme thioredoxin reductase, in a NADPH-dependent reaction. The selenium-metalloenzyme iodothyronine deiodinases play a role in the conversion of T_4 to T_3.

Clinical Significance

Low selenium status has been recognized when intake is below the RDA shown in Table 42-1; chronic ingestion of levels above the RDA produces clinical symptoms.

Selenium deficiency has been demonstrated in Keshan (pronounced *kuh-shahn*), a city in Manchuria, China, where soil selenium content is very low.[39] Although Keshan disease, which often is associated with cardiomyopathy in children and young females, responded to supplementation by selenium, the selenium deficiency is not considered to be the sole cause of this condition, and the implication of a virus or other agent has been considered. In other areas such as New Zealand, Finland, and Sweden, where low selenium status has been demonstrated, serious detrimental effects of the low soil selenium have not been observed. A second disease associated with low selenium intake in China is Kashin-Bek disease, which causes cartilage degeneration and osteoarthritis in adolescents and preadolescents.[40] Patients maintained on long-term TPN are at risk of developing selenium deficiency if fluids are not supplemented.[41,42] Numerous such cases have been reported, and several deaths associated with cardiomyopathy have occurred.

Requirement

The RDA and the AI for selenium for various ages are shown in Table 42-1.

Food Sources

Selenium enters the food chain via plants. Because of wide variability in the concentration range of selenium in various areas throughout the world, the availability of selenium may be low in some areas, whereas in seleniferous areas, excessive selenium is taken up by plants.[35] However, the form in which selenium occurs in foods remains unknown. In decreasing order of magnitude, organ meats and seafood, cereals and grains, dairy products, and fruits and vegetables are sources of dietary selenium.

Toxicity

Selenium toxicity is rare in the United States, where the tolerable upper intake level (UL) for selenium is 400 μg. Selenium toxicity is characterized by dermatitis, loose hair, and diseased nails. Selenium poisoning caused by excessive intake of supplements results in acute toxicity. Symptoms include a metallic taste, odor of garlic, mucosal irritation, gastroenteritis, paronychia (infection of soft tissue around fingernail), and reddening of nails, hair, and teeth.[43] Evidence indicates that chronic ingestion of moderately elevated levels of selenium may be carcinogenic.

Method[44]

Zeeman graphite furnace atomic absorption analysis with nickel nitrate or reduced palladium as the matrix modifier is the recommended analysis method.

Reference Intervals

Although no single marker for selenium status has been identified, plasma selenium is an indication of recent ingestion. Erythrocyte and platelet glutathione peroxidase activity correlates well with selenium supplementation in patients maintained on TPN.[41,42] Urine selenium varies with intake, and at very high levels of intake, volatile forms of selenium are exhaled. Nails and hair, which can include a large number of sulfur- or selenium-containing proteins, both have been assessed for measurement of selenium status. In the United States, the use of selenium-containing shampoos precludes the use of hair for such measurement.

Reference intervals in serum vary from region to region, depending on the selenium content of the soil of food sources. The mean serum levels (±1 SEM) for adults in the United States are 1.10 (±0.10) μmol/L for men and 1.20 (±0.18) μmol/L for women.

Zinc (Zn)[45-52]

Zinc is a transition element in period 4 of the periodic table of the elements and has an atomic weight of 65.

Biochemistry

Zinc forms stable complexes, called **zinc fingers,** with the histidine and cysteine amino acid residues of proteins. These proteins bind to, and control, regulatory regions of DNA.[45] More than 1600 zinc metalloenzymes have been identified,[46] including those involved in nucleic acid replication, (i.e., DNA and RNA polymerases, and reverse transcriptase), protein synthesis, and intermediary metabolism (i.e., carbonic anhydrase, sorbitol dehydrogenase, and carboxypeptidase A).

Zinc induces the synthesis of metallothionein, which serves an important regulatory function for zinc and copper metabolism. The protein binds copper more firmly than zinc and forms an unabsorbable complex in the gastrointestinal tract, hence reducing copper absorption. In the liver, induction of metallothionein synthesis is significant in cases of stress and infection when this organ sequesters zinc.

Zinc is an intracellular cation that is present in all body tissues and fluids and, next to iron, is the second most abundant of the trace metals in humans. Muscle contains 50% to 60% of the 2 g of total body zinc, bone contains 28% of body zinc stores, and 0.5% is found in blood. Erythrocytes contain 75% to 88% of blood zinc. In the plasma, approximately 8% of zinc (reference range, 700 to 1200 μg/L) is tightly bound to an α_2-macroglobulin, 90% is loosely bound to albumin, 2% is bound to transferrin, ceruloplasmin, or the amino acids histidine and cysteine, and a small fraction is present as free zinc.

The RDA of 11 mg of zinc for adult males and 8 mg for females is not likely to be provided by many diets consumed in the United States. Red meat is a prime source of bioavailable zinc. Hence, vegetarians are at risk for zinc insufficiency. In addition, the high fiber content of a vegetarian diet binds zinc and hence diminishes its bioavailability. From a usual nonvegetarian diet, approximately 20% of zinc is absorbed. Meats, liver, eggs, and seafood enhance absorption, whereas vegetables, whole grain foods, fiber, phytate, calcium, and iron inhibit absorption.

Clinical Significance[47,48]

Because zinc is required for the activity of enzymes that are critical for nucleic acid replication and protein synthesis, it is a necessary component of cell replication. Adequate supplies of zinc are imperative for healthy development of the fetus, and in early pregnancy, plasma zinc falls despite increased intake. During pregnancy, an increase is noted in the plasma zinc fraction bound to α_2-macroglobulin, as is a decrease in the zinc bound to albumin. Plasma zinc is elevated during lactation. Zinc deficiency was first described by Prasad[49] in Iran and Egypt. Male adolescents showed retarded development and hypogonadism. Acute zinc deficiency in humans is apparent from skin lesions (especially on body extremities or around orifices), diarrhea, irritability, hair loss, growth retardation, and increased susceptibility to infection.[50,51] Individuals at risk for zinc deficiency include infants and children; pregnant and lactating women; patients receiving total parenteral nutrition; individuals with severe or persistent diarrhea or with malabsorption syndromes, such as celiac disease or short bowel syndrome; and individuals with inflammatory bowel disease, such as Crohn's disease and ulcerative colitis.

Impaired immunological function is associated with zinc insufficiency. In vitro, stimulation of lymphocytes by phytohemagglutinin and concavalin A is enhanced by zinc. In vivo, a delayed hypersensitive response to skin allergens occurs that is consistent with the degree of zinc deficiency.

A reliable marker for assessment of zinc status has yet to be identified. Although abnormal plasma zinc levels are associated with many pathological conditions, plasma zinc concentrations are a poor indicator of the body status of zinc. Plasma levels of zinc may be lowered in response to stress and trauma, but they do not reflect intracellular status. Leukocyte zinc has been suggested as a reliable marker, but consistent findings have yet to be reported. Urinary excretion of zinc in response to a zinc challenge has been explored as a marker of zinc nutriture, as has the level of zinc in the hair. Further investigation is required before any of these markers can be recommended.

Requirement

The RDAs for zinc is shown in Table 42-1. An increase in intake to 11 mg/day is recommended during pregnancy.

Food Sources

Seafoods, meat, milk, and eggs are good sources of zinc. Although vegetables contain appreciable amounts of zinc, the presence of high concentrations of fiber and phytate account for the low bioavailability of zinc in these food sources.

Toxicity[52]

Epigastric pain, diarrhea, and vomiting have been observed as the result of high zinc intake from food stored in galvanized containers. Supplements of as little as 25 mg of zinc have resulted in diminished absorption of copper, presumably caused by competition.

Method

The preferred method for zinc analysis is flame atomic absorption spectrophotometry for serum or plasma, for erythrocytes, and for urine.

Reference Intervals

Reference intervals in serum are 700 to 1200 μg/L and 10.7 to 18.3 μmol/L, and in urine are 300 to 500 μg/day and 4.58 to 7.64 μmol/day.

KEY CONCEPTS BOX 42-2

- The common mechanism by which most of the essential trace metals function is as a cofactor for metabolic enzymes (Cr, Cu, Mn, Mo, Se, and Zn). F works by forming stronger hydroxyapatite crystal in teeth while I modifies the amino acid tyrosine to form active thyroid hormones.
- A direct relationship between blood concentration of an essential trace metal and symptoms is not always present. Deficiencies often must be detected based on clinical symptomology.
- Flame or flameless atomic absorption spectroscopy is the method used most commonly for measuring most of the essential trace metals. F and I (in urine) are best measured by ion selective electrodes; the best measure of I nutriture is measurement of thyroid hormones.

SECTION OBJECTIVES BOX 42-3

- Discuss the known mechanisms of the biological toxicity of trace levels of the toxic metals.
- Review the most important symptoms of critical concentrations of toxic trace metals.
- List the critical levels of toxic trace metals, such as lead and mercury.
- Discuss considerations involved in assessing the status of trace metals in humans.
- Explain the primary methods used for measuring each trace metal.

TOXIC TRACE METALS

Many toxic trace metals have no or little known biological function. We shall limit our discussion to the ones that are monitored more commonly.

Aluminum (Al)[53-59]

Aluminum is classified as a period 3 element with an atomic weight of 27.

Basis for Toxicity

Aluminum, the third most common element in the earth's crust, is present in plants and water. Ingested aluminum, which is 90% bound to serum transferrin,[53] is readily excreted by the kidneys, and individuals with normal renal function are at low risk for aluminum toxicity. Aluminum toxicity can result from exposure to industrial sources of aluminum, but most commonly the cause is iatrogenic.[54] Populations at highest risk for aluminum toxicity include patients with chronic renal failure, infants, and those given long-term parenteral nutrition.[55-58]

Patients who have chronic renal failure are at high risk for aluminum toxicity.[55] Previous sources of aluminum contamination for dialysis patients now are controlled; aluminum-containing antacids to decrease phosphate absorption are no longer used and aluminium-free water is used in dialysate fluid; and it has been suggested that routine monitoring of the plasma aluminum of dialysis patients is no longer necessary.[56] Monitoring of patients and dialysate fluids for aluminum levels is still routine practice.

Many of the components of parenteral fluids can be contaminated with aluminum.[57] Premature infants who receive parenteral nutrition or artificial food supplements are particularly at risk for aluminum toxicity because of their reduced renal clearance.[58]

In all cases of aluminum toxicity, the skeleton, brain, and muscle are the primary target organs.[59] Although the biochemical basis for the neurotoxic effects of aluminum is uncertain, an association was found between high brain-aluminum concentrations at autopsy and dialysis dementia or dialysis encephalopathy in a large number of patients with renal failure who were undergoing chronic dialysis.

Deposition of aluminum along the calcification front in bone has long been recognized. The development of bone pain in dialysis patients can indicate an excessive accumulation of aluminum. Bone morphology in these cases is consistent with osteomalacia (see p. 633, Chapter 33). Another major sign of aluminum toxicity is microcytic anemia.

Monitoring the aluminum content of dialysate fluid and of components of artificially prepared nutrients used for enteral and parenteral nutritional supplements is necessary to ensure minimal exposure to aluminum.

Serum Levels and Indications for Treatment

Reference intervals for serum aluminum vary among laboratories because of the ease of contamination. An upper limit of 4 μg/L (0.15 μmol/L) is considered to be within the reference interval. Serum aluminum levels do not necessarily reflect the amount of metal deposited in bone, liver, and brain. Bone pain is a useful clinical indicator of the degree of aluminum toxicity. The effectiveness of chelation therapy with desferrioxamine during dialysis can be monitored by measurement of serum aluminum.

Method

Zeeman graphite furnace atomic absorption spectrophotometry with magnesium nitrate used as the matrix modifier is the recommended method of analysis.

Arsenic (As)[60-66]

Arsenic is a period 4 element with an atomic weight of 75.

Basis for Toxicity

Arsenic in food and in drinking water is the most common mechanism for chronic exposure.[60-62] A fatal acute dose is estimated to be 10.2 to 26 nmol (0.76 to 1.95 μg) of arsenic per kilogram of body weight.[62] Trivalent arsen*ite* is more rapidly absorbed from the gastrointestinal tract than is pentavalent arsen*ate*, and it is considered the more toxic form. Once absorbed, arsenite can form methylated compounds, which may be important toxic forms.[63]

Arsenic usually is found in all tissues, with skin, hair, and nails showing the highest concentrations. The mechanism for the toxicity of arsenic involves its binding to the sulfhydryl (—SH) groups of compounds, which greatly deminishes their biological activity. For example, when arsenic binds to dihydrolipoic acid, a pyruvate dehydrogenase co-factor, the conversion of pyruvate to acetyl coenzyme A is blocked, thereby inhibiting citric acid cycle activity, production of cellular ATP, and gluconeogenesis. Arsenic also competes with phosphates for adenosine triphosphate, forming adenosine diphosphate monoarsine and causing the loss of high-energy bonds. The reaction of arsenite with sulfhydryl groups in enzymes destroys enzymatic activity.

In the United States, where the limit of arsenic in drinking water is set at 10 parts per billion, approximately 1000 cases of arsenic poisoning occur per year, about one-third of which are derived from pesticide exposure. Worldwide, approximately 100 million people are exposed to excessive arsenic in drinking water.[64] Symptoms of acute toxicity in humans from oral intake of arsenic include nausea, vomiting, diarrhea, burning of the mouth and throat, and severe abdominal pain. Chronic exposure to smaller toxic doses causes weakness, prostration, muscle aches, and, in children, loss of hearing at low frequencies. Headaches, drowsiness, and confusion occur in both acute and chronic toxicity. An association between industrial exposure to arsenic and the increased prevalence of lung and skin cancer has been noted.

The absorption of organic forms of arsenic from the gastrointestinal tract and its excretion in the urine are highly efficient. Urine excretion is an effective mode of monitoring body status; hair and toenail analysis also has been used to determine past exposure.[65]

Treatment[66]

Treatment of acute poisoning with D-penicillamine, 2,3-dimercapto-1-propanesulfonate, 2,3-dimercaptosuccinic acid, or 2,3-dimercaptopropanol (BAL) has been successful in humans.

Method

The recommended method of total arsenic analysis is flameless atomic absorption. High-performance liquid chromatography can characterize the form in which arsenic is excreted.

Cadmium (Cd)[67-73]

Cadmium is a period 5 element with an atomic weight of 112.4.

Basis for Toxicity

The primary organs affected by cadmium toxicity are liver and kidney.[67,68] The exact mechanism of cadmium toxicity, as well as the role that cadmium-metallothionein may play, is not known.[69,70]

Clinical Significance

Only small amounts of cadmium (<5%) are absorbed from the gut, but Cd is absorbed readily by the lungs.[68] Absorbed cadmium is stored in the liver and preferentially in the renal cortex, where the metal accumulates rapidly within the first 3 years of life and continues to accumulate up to approximately 50 years of age. It is estimated that the biological half-life of cadmium is approximately 30 years. Sources of cadmium include food and water, industrial activity (especially CdNi battery manufacture and the air and water in proximity to Cd-use industry), the burning of coal and Cd-containing municipal wastes, and cigarette smoking. The level in blood, which usually is <5 μg/L, is increased about 50% in smokers.[67,68] Urinary excretion is normally approximately 1 μg/L, and it is higher in smokers. Children exposed to idustrial pollution are also at high risk for elevated blood Cd.[71]

Inhalation of cadmium results in renal damage even before impaired lung function is detected, causing a low-molecular-weight proteinuria and a reduced glomerular filtration rate. Osteomalacia (itai-itai disease) in Japanese women has been ascribed to cadmium exposure.[72,73]

Testing for acute Cd exposure can be accomplished by measuring serum Cd levels. The best screen for chronic exposure is a 24-hour urinary cadmium measurement. Measurement of Cd in the hair has not proved useful for estimating exposure.

Treatment

Standard chelation therapy with ethylenediaminetetraacetic acid (EDTA), British anti-Lewisite (BAL or dimercaprol), or dimercaptosuccinic acid (DMSA) generally has not proved effective, probably because of an inability to chelate the less accessible intracellular cadmium.[68]

Method

The recommended method of analysis is flameless atomic absorption.

Lead (Pb)[74-82]

Lead is considered to be a heavy metal and lies in period 6 of the periodic table of elements. Its atomic weight is 207.

Basis for Toxicity

Worldwide, a major source of lead in the environment is industrial waste in the water and air; an estimated 120 million individuals are at risk for the adverse effects of ingested lead.[74] In the United States, the primary source is lead-based paint in the interior and exterior of pre-1978 wooden houses. A significant number (≈25%) of children in the United States still live in such houses.[75] Subsequent removal or decay of the paint leads to environmental contamination and exposure of children to lead contamination. Immigrant populations are at risk for lead exposure from home medicines and cosmetics.[76] Lead absorption by the intestines is increased when a deficiency of iron, calcium, magnesium, zinc, phosphate, or vitamin D is present.

Lead toxicity most likely is based on its ability to substitute for calcium and zinc in proteins, especially those with sulfhydryl groups; lead binding to proteins renders them dysfunctional.[77] For example, inhibition by lead of the enzymes ferrochelatase and δ-aminolevulinic acid dehydratase (see also p. 769) results in anemia when the blood-lead level exceeds 40 μg/dL (1.92 μmol/L). In both iron deficiency and lead poisoning, incorporation of ferrous iron into protoporphyrin IX is decreased—a step needed for the synthesis of heme—and iron is replaced by zinc to form zinc protoporphyrin. Erythrocyte protoporphyrin begins to rise at a blood-lead level of 20 μg/dL.

Clinical Significance of Lead Toxicity

Lead toxicity produces neurological, gastrointestinal, renal, immunological, endocrinological, and hematopoietic changes in humans. Children 6 months to 6 years of age are affected the most, because they are growing rapidly and lead crosses the blood-brain barrier at an age when brain development is critical. Lead also can cross the placenta,[78] placing the fetus at risk for lead toxicity.[79] It is now believed that these neurological effects occur at lower blood-lead concentrations than was previously believed; there may be no threshold for the toxic effects of lead.[80,81] Lead decreases children's measured intelligence (IQ),[78-81] but it also can adversely affect sociological development.[82]

Because of the magnitude of the problem, which affects millions of children, well-recognized, widespread efforts have been undertaken to prevent or minimize the possibility of lead exposure. Testing of children's blood-lead levels is required routinely by many states and countries.[83]

Blood-Lead Levels

Although the level of blood lead considered to be safe is currently <10 μg/dL, evidence suggests that even lower blood-lead concentrations may be detrimental in growing children.[80,81] Although no specific action level has been suggested, the Centers for Disease Control and Prevention (CDC) has recommended diagnostic evaluation and medical management of children at lead levels >20 μg/dL. Adults are less vulnerable than children to the neurological damage caused by lead, but a blood-lead level of 30 μg/dL or higher in an adult requires evaluation. In New York State, all blood-lead values in children must be reported to the State Department of Health; values >20 μg/dL in children and >40 μg/dL in adults are considered critical, and immediate treatment is required (see New York State website, http://www.health.state.ny.us/environmental/lead/).

Treatment

Treatment for lead toxicity with chelating agents has included the use of penicillamine, calcium-ethylenediaminetetraacetic acid (Ca-EDTA), 2,3 dimercaptopropane-1-sulfonic acid sodium salt (DMPS), and 2,3-dimercaptopropanol (BAL, British anti-Lewisite). Dimercaptosuccinic acid (Succimer), which may be administered orally, appears to have the fewest side effects, but its clinical efficacy has been questioned.[84] Effectiveness of treatment may be monitored by measurement of both blood lead levels and urine excretion.

Method

Zeeman graphite furnace atomic absorption spectrophotometry is the recommended method of analysis. Matrix modifiers of ammonium dihydrogen phosphate and magnesium nitrate together are effective. To facilitate blood-lead screening of children, the U.S. Food and Drug Administration has expanded the availability of a portable lead testing system.[85]

Mercury (Hg)[86-92]

Mercury is a transition element that also appears in period 6 of the periodic table of elements, with an atomic weight of 201.

Basis for Toxicity[86,87]

In addition to natural sources of mercury, mercury is added to the environment by human activity, such as manufacturing (e.g., batteries), gold and silver mining, and coal and waste combustion. Worldwide, human activities have increased the atmospheric burden of mercury by two- to threefold, currently increasing the atmospheric mercury by about 1.5% a year. In the United States, power plants and other industrial facilities emit as much as 150 tons of mercury into the air. Much of the environmental mercury enters fresh water and seawater, where microorganisms in sediments convert elemental and inorganic salts to alkyl derivatives, especially methyl mercury. These organic forms of mercury then enter seafood, which is consumed by humans. The most common food source of mercury is fish, in which the element is present as methyl mercury.[86,88] In the United States and in other countries, limits have been established for the safe consumption of fish; by 2006, 35 states had issued advisories that limit fish consumption.

Exposure to inorganic mercury, as to lead (see above), can occur by use of unregulated medicinals[89] and beauty products.[90] However, dental amalgam is *not* considered a significant health threat.[91,92]

Inorganic mercury is poorly absorbed, alkyl derivatives of mercury are >90% absorbed, and mercury vapor is approximately 80% absorbed by inhalation. Mercury usually is present at from 0.1 to 0.5 μg/g in all human body tissues, even in the absence of any identified exposure from dental amalgams. The highest levels occur in skin, nails, and hair. In populations exposed to industrial mercury, the pituitary and the thyroid concentrate mercury to a greater degree than other organs. Red blood cells readily take up methyl mercury, at a blood cell-to-plasma ratio of approximately 20:1. Methyl mercury crosses the placenta, and the level in cord blood correlates well with that in the mother. Preganant women are asked to carefully limit their consumption of mercury-contaminated fish.[93] Organic mercury is excreted into bile, and intestinal flora convert it to inorganic mercury, which is excreted in feces.[94] The biological half-life of mercury in human tissue is estimated to be 70 days; blood mercury has a half-life of about 44 days.

In the United States, a national effort has reduced the presence of mercury in hospitals and laboratories (see p. 27, Chapter 1), and the exposure of newborns to mercury has been reduced by the removal from vaccines of a common preservative—Thimerosal, which contains ≈50% mercury by weight.[95]

Clinical Significance

Mercury has a high affinity for sulfhydryl groups; as with lead, the biochemical basis for the toxicity of mercury is believed to be its binding to these groups in proteins, rendering the proteins dysfunctional. Mercury poisoning affects the central nervous system (CNS). Acute mercury vapor toxicity ("metal fume fever") is manifested by fatigue, weakness, fever, chills, dizziness, headache, abdominal cramping, and dyspnea. Acute, cutaneous inorganic mercury poisoning in children is seen as acrodynia, a pink peeling rash, along with generalized pain.[96] Signs of chronic toxicity, which include irritability, excitability, anxiety, insomnia, and social withdrawal, may be described as erethism, which also is known as "Mad Hatter's Disease." These signs were noted in the felt hat makers of 19th century London.

The passage of methyl mercury across the placenta is associated with increases in congenital abnormalities, mental retardation, cerebral palsy, and fetal mortality. All these symptoms were present after an incident termed the Minamata Bay incident, in which industrial wastes containing mercury were dumped into Minamata Bay, Japan. In Minamata disease, increased levels of methyl mercury were found in fetal tissue, most particularly within the brain.[97]

In spite of its widespread presence, acute clinical exposure to mercury is rare. In 2003, only 3362 exposures to mercury were recorded, and no patients died as a result.[98]

Mercury concentration in the hair has been shown to correlate well with blood levels of mercury. The concentration in hair is approximately tenfold higher than levels seen in the blood. Clinical manifestations of mercury intoxication appear at whole blood levels of 200 to 300 μg/L; it can result from exposure to about 0.3 mg of mercury per day as methyl mercury; this dosage is equivalent to approximately 4 mg of mercury per kilogram of body weight in an adult. For workers chronically exposed to mercury compounds, urinary mercury levels higher than 50 μg/L are associated with an increased frequency of tremor.

Treatment

Dimercaprol (BAL), penicillamine, and 2,3-dimercaptosuccinic acid (Succimer) all are used for the treatment of acute mercury toxicity; the latter is considered superior because it binds both inorganic and organic forms.[99] Urinary mercury is a good indicator of inorganic and elemental mercury exposure but is unreliable for organic mercury (methyl mercury) because elimination occurs most often in the feces. Elimination of mercury by chelation therapy can be monitored by following urine excretion.

Method[100]

Cold vapor atomic absorption spectrophotometry is the preferred method for analysis of inorganic mercury. Predigestion is required to convert methyl mercury to inorganic mercury.

Levels in Biological Samples

Because mercury levels are so high in red blood cells, blood mercury is a good indicator of acute exposure. Usual levels (95% population, NHANES data[101]) in blood are <7.1 μg/L and 0.035 μmol/L, in red blood cells <40 μg/L and 0.20 μmol/L, and in urine (mostly inorganic mercury) <5 μg/L and 0.025 μmol/L. Long-term exposures can be determined by measurement of mercury in hair (high sulfur content; 90% population, 1.2 μg/g); however, ease of environmental contamination can result in a high rate of false positives. Mercury levels in toetail clippings (population mean, 0.25 to 0.45 μg/g) have been shown to correlate well with seafood consumption and can serve as a reasonable alternative.[102]

CONSIDERATIONS IN ASSESSING TRACE ELEMENT STATUS IN HUMANS

The roles of essential trace elements in biology are summarized in Table 42-2. The status of most of the essential trace elements cannot be assessed from their concentrations in whole blood or plasma, the most easily accessible body component, and this remains a problem in patient care. Because it is not possible to assign a threshold for plasma or serum zinc, copper, selenium, chromium, or manganese below which supplementation of the respective element is indicated, other biochemical and clinical parameters should be considered concomitantly for assessment of trace metal nutriture. These include dietary availability, existing conditions that may involve re-distribution within the body, genetic disorders, hormonal regulation in the case of iodine, and the functional state of excretory organs. Most important, the presence of clinical signs and symptoms that usually are associated with a deficiency of a trace metal is an important diagnostic finding. Hence, a plasma zinc amount less than 500 μg/L in association with dermatological lesions, especially in a rapidly growing child, is suggestive of severe acute zinc deficiency. Investigation would be necessary to determine whether the deficiency resulted from an insufficient dietary intake of zinc or from malabsorption of zinc, as occurs in the genetic disorder acrodermatitis enteropathica. In cases of trauma such as burns, a similarly low plasma zinc level indicates re-distribution of zinc, and the necessity for zinc supplementation is equivocal. Usually, the main route of excretion of endogenous zinc is the gastrointestinal tract, with contributions from pancreatic secretions and bile. Intestinal absorption of trace metals can be reduced as a result of the competition between zinc, iron, copper, manganese, and other divalent minerals in the diet. Trace metal absorption also may be decreased in high-fiber diets because of binding of the metals to phytates.

Although very low levels of plasma copper, such as 300 μg/L, and ceruloplasmin (which binds 60% to 95% of the copper) are indicative of frank copper deficiency, plasma level generally is not a good indicator of copper status. Hence, functional tests, such as response to antigenic challenge for zinc and measurement of a copper-requiring enzyme such as superoxide dismutase or cytochrome oxidase, are considered to be useful in assessing the status of these metals. Serum selenium is an acceptable indicator of recent selenium absorption.

Deficiencies of trace elements in patients maintained on TPN or enteral feeding now are rare, but consideration must be given to ensure adequate supplementation in these groups of patients, especially when therapy is provided over a long term. If periodic estimations of zinc, copper, selenium, or manganese reveal a decrease in plasma levels of a trace metal when the patient's condition is stable, the possibility of a deficiency should be explored further.

Individuals who consume over-the-counter nutritional supplements may have an intake of trace elements that greatly exceeds suggested limits (see Tables 42-1 and 42-2). Very often, claims of improved health with supplements are not validated by proper studies, and these supplements may cause health problems, rather than improved health.

An emerging problem is the potential and actual exposure of individuals to toxic levels of trace metals that rarely were present in the environment. For example, an increasing number of persons receive metal implants that contain significant levels of trace metals. The long-range effects of such implants are not known. In addition, beryllium is being used with increasing frequency in computers, cellular telephones, and dental work. Workers who manufacture these materials are at risk for berylliosis, an often fatal lung disease.

Identification of the biochemical parameters that can be measured to indicate the status of trace elements in the body remains a challenge. Appropriate function tests or tests that measure the activity of an enzyme that has a specific requirement for a particular trace metal that are suitable for routine use in a clinical chemistry laboratory have yet to be determined.

KEY CONCEPTS BOX 42-3

- The mechanism by which most toxic trace metals produce symptoms involves binding to small molecules (As) or proteins (particularly enzymes; e.g., Hg, Pb), and inhibiting their biological activity.
- The exception is aluminium, which inserts into bone structure and diminishes bone strength.
- The most common mechanism of exposure to toxic trace elements is industrial and environmental contamination.
- The most common symptom of many of the toxic trace metals is neurological, including diminished intelligence caused by lead (>20 μg/dL) and mercury (>7 μg/L).
- A direct relationship between blood concentration of a toxic trace metal and symptoms is not always present.
- Atomic absorption spectroscopy, with flame or flameless, is the method used most commonly for measuring trace metals.

REFERENCES

Classification of Trace Elements

1. Otten JJ, Hellwig JP, Meyers LD, editors, National Academy of Sciences: *The Dietary Reference Intakes: The Essential Guide to Nutrient Requirements,* Washington, DC, 2006, Institute of Medicine, Food and Nutrition Board.

Essential Trace Elements

Chromium

2. Anderson RA: Chromium. In Mertz W, editor: *Trace Elements in Human and Animal Nutrition,* vol 1, ed 5, New York, 1987, Academic Press.
3. Cefalu WT, Hu FB: Role of chromium in human health and in diabetes, Diabetes Care 27:2741, 2004.
4. Wang H, Allison Kruszewski A, Brautigan DL: Cellular chromium enhances activation of insulin receptor kinase, Biochemistry 44:61679, 2005.
5. Brown RO, Forloines-Lynn S, Cross RE, et al: Chromium deficiency after long-term total parenteral nutrition, Dig Dis Sci 31:661, 1986.
6. Althuis MD, Jordan NE, Ludington EA, et al: Glucose and insulin responses to dietary chromium supplements: a meta-analysis, Am J Clin Nutr 76:148, 2002.
7. Kornhauser C, Wrobel K, Wrobel K, et al: Possible adverse effect of chromium in occupational exposure of tannery workers, Industrial Health 40:207, 2002.
8. Chakraborty R, Das AK, Cervera ML, et al: Determination of chromium by electrothermal atomic absorption spectrometry after rapid microwave-assisted digestion of sediment and botanical samples, J Anal At Spectrom 10:353, 1995.

Copper

9. Genetic and environmental determinants of copper metabolism. In Proceedings of an International Conference, Bethesda, MD, March 18-20, 1996; Am J Clin Nutr 67:951, 1998.
10. Manuel O, Magdalena A, Ricardo U: Copper homeostasis in infant nutrition: deficit and excess, J Pediatr Gastroenterol Nutr 31:102, 2000.
11. Turnlund JR: Human whole-body copper metabolism, Am J Clin Nut 67:960S, 1998.
12. Tonnesen T, Kleijer WJ, Horn N: Incidence of Menkes disease, Hum Genet 86:408, 1991.
13. Barbagallo JS, Kolodzieh MS, Silverberg NB, et al: Neurocutaneous disorders, Dermatol Clin 20:3, 2002.
14. Schilsky ML: Wilson disease: new insights into pathogenesis, diagnosis, and future therapy, Curr Gastroenterol Rep 7:26, 2005.
15. Milne DB, Johnson PE: Assessment of copper status: effect of age and gender on reference ranges in healthy adults, Clin Chem 39:883, 1993.
16. Alcock NW: Copper. In Pesce AJ, Kaplan LA, editors: *Laboratory Medicine: A Scientific and Management Infobase,* version 5.0, Cincinnati, 2002, Pesce Kaplan.

Fluorine

17. Krishnamachari KAVR: Fluorine. In Mertz W, editor: *Trace Elements in Human and Animal Nutrition,* vol 1, ed 5, New York, 1987, Academic Press.
18. Aoba T, Fejerskov O: Dental fluorosis: chemistry and biology, Crit Rev Oral Biol Med 13:155, 2002.
19. Riggs BL, Hodson SF, O'Fallon WM, et al: Effect of fluoride treatment on the fracture rate in postmenopausal women with osteoporosis, N Engl J Med 322:802, 1994.
20. Kao WF, Deng JF, Chiang SC: A simple, safe, and efficient way to treat severe fluoride poisoning—oral calcium or magnesium, J Toxicol Clin Toxicol 42:33, 2004.
21. Blancke RV, Decker WJ: Analysis of toxic substances: determination of fluoride in plasma and urine by ion specific potentiometry. In Tietz NW, editor: *Textbook of Clinical Chemistry,* New York, 1986, Saunders.

Iodine

22. Hetzel BS, Maberly GF: Iodine. In Mertz W, editor: *Trace Elements in Human and Animal Nutrition,* vol 2, ed 5, New York, 1986, Academic Press.
23. Clugston GA, Hetzel BS: Iodine. In Shils ME, Olsen JA, Shike M, editors: *Modern Nutrition in Health and Disease,* ed 10, Philadelphia, 2005, Lippincott Williams & Wilkins.
24. Demers LM, Spencer CA: Laboratory medicine practice guidelines: laboratory support for the diagnosis and monitoring of thyroid disease, Thyroid 13:1, 2003.

Manganese

25. Yocum CF, Pecoraro VL: Recent advances in the understanding of the biological chemistry of manganese, Curr Opin Chem Biol 3:182, 1999.
26. Nielsen FH: Ultratrace minerals. In Shils M, Olson JA, Shike M, et al, editors: *Nutrition in Health and Disease,* ed 9, Baltimore, MD, 1999, Williams & Wilkins, p. 283.
27. Pal PK, Samii A, Calne DB: Manganese neurotoxicity: a review of clinical features, imaging and pathology, Neurotoxicology 20:227, 1999.
28. Racette B, McGee-Minnich L, Moerlein SM, et al: Welding-related parkinsonism: clinical features, treatment, and pathophysiology, Neurology 56:8, 2001.
29. Garnrick GR, Slavin W: *Techniques for Graphite Furnace Atomic Absorption Spectrophotometry,* Norwalk, CT, 1985, Perkin-Elmer Corp.

Molybdenum

30. Nielsen FH: Ultratrace minerals. In Shils ME, Olson JA, Shike M, et al, editors: *Modern Nutrition in Health and Disease,* ed 9, Baltimore, MD, 1999, Williams and Wilkins, p. 283.
31. Kisker C, Schindelin H, Rees DC: Molybdenum-cofactor–containing enzymes: structure and mechanism, Ann Rev Biochem 66:233, 1997.
32. Abumrad NN, Schneider AJ, Steel D, et al: Amino acid intolerance during prolonged TPN reversed by molybdate therapy, Am J Clin Nutr 34:2551, 1981.
33. Momcilovic B: A case of acute human molybdenum toxicity from a dietary molybdenum supplement—a new member of the "Lucor metallicum" family, Arh Hig Rada Toksikol 50:289, 1999.
34. Vyskocil A, Viau C: Assessment of molybdenum toxicity in humans, J Appl Toxicol 19:185, 1999.

Selenium

35. Lavender OA, Burke RF: Selenium. In Shils ME, Olsen JA, Shike M, editors: *Modern Nutrition in Health and Disease,* ed 9, Baltimore, MD, 1999, Williams & Wilkins.
36. Foster LH, Sumar S: Selenium in health and disease: a review, Crit Rev Food Sci Nutr 37:211, 1997.
37. Holben DH, Smith AM: The diverse role of selenium within selenoproteins: a review, J Am Diet Assoc 99:836, 1999.
38. Arnér E, Holmgren A: Physiological functions of thioredoxin and thioredoxin reductase, Eur J Biochem 267:6102, 2000.
39. Keshan Disease Research Group: Epidemiologic studies on etiologic relationship of selenium and Keshan disease, Chin Med J 92:477, 1979.
40. Iodine, selenium, and joints: Kashin-Beck disease, Arch Dis Child 80:261, 1999.
41. Gramm HJ, Kopf A, Bratter P: The necessity of selenium substitution in total parenteral nutrition and artificial alimentation, J Trace Elem Med Biol 9:1, 1995.
42. Kuroki F, Matsumoto T, Lida M: Selenium is depleted in Crohn's disease on enteral nutrition, Dig Dis 21:266, 2003.
43. McLaren CS: Clinical manifestations of human vitamin and mineral disorders. In Shils ME, Olsen JA, Shike M, editors: *Modern Nutrition in Health and Disease,* ed 8, Philadelphia, 1993, Lea & Febiger.
44. Jacobson BE, Lockitch G: Direct determination of selenium in serum by graphite furnace atomic absorption spectrometry with deuterium background correction and a reduced palladium modifier: age specific reference ranges, Clin Chem 34:709, 1988.

Zinc

45. Laity JH, Lee BM, Wright PE: Zinc finger proteins: new insights into structural and functional diversity, Curr Opin Struct Biol 11:39, 2001.
46. Andreini C, Banci L, Bertini I, et al: Counting the zinc-proteins encoded in the human genome, J Proteome Res 5:196, 2006.
47. Wolfgang M: Zinc biochemistry, physiology, and homeostasis—recent insights and current trends, BioMetals 14:187, 2001.
48. Prasad AS: Zinc: an overview, Nutrition 11:93, 1995.
49. Prasad AS: Zinc deficiency in humans: a neglected problem, J Am Coll Nutr 17:542, 1998.
50. Hambidge M: Human zinc deficiency, J Nutr 130(5 suppl):1344S, 2000.
51. Wapnir RA: Zinc deficiency, malnutrition and the gastrointestinal tract, J Nutr 130(5 suppl):1388S, 2000.
52. Fosmire GJ: Zinc toxicity, Am J Clin Nutr 51:225, 1990.

Toxic Trace Metals

Aluminum

53. Soldado AB, Gonzales EB, Sanz-Medel A: Quantitative studies of aluminium binding species in human uremic serum by fast protein liquid chromatography coupled with electrothermal absorption spectrometry, Analyst 122:573, 1997.
54. Becaria A, Campbell A, Bondy SC: Aluminum as a toxicant, Toxicology and Industrial Health 18:309, 2002.
55. Cannata-Andia JB, Fernandez-Martin JL: The clinical impact of aluminum overload in renal failure, Nephrol Dial Transplant 17(suppl 2):9, 2002.
56. Gault PM, Allen KR, Newton KE: Plasma aluminium: a redundant test for patients on dialysis? Ann Clin Biochem 42:51, 2005
57. Popińska K, Kierkuś J, Lyszkowska M, et al: Aluminum contamination of parenteral nutrition additives, amino acid solutions, and lipid emulsions, Nutrition 15:683, 1999.
58. Advenier E, Landry C, Colomb V, et al: Aluminum contamination of parenteral nutrition and aluminum loading in children on long-term parenteral nutrition, J Pediatr Gastroenterol Nutr 36:448, 2003.
59. Yokel RA, McNamara PJ: Aluminum toxicokinetics: an updated minireview, Pharmacol Toxicol 88:159, 2001.

Arsenic

60. Florea A-M, Büsselberg D: Occurrence, use and potential toxic effects of metals and metal compounds, BioMetals 19:419, 2006.
61. Duenas-Laita A, Perez-Miranda M, Gonzalez-Lopez MA, et al: Acute arsenic poisoning, Lancet 365:1982, 2005.
62. Klaassen CD: *Casarett and Doull's Toxicology, The Basic Science of Poisons,* ed 6, New York, NY, 2001, McGraw-Hill.
63. Stýblo M, Drobná Z, Jaspers I, et al: The role of biomethylation in toxicity and carcinogenicity of arsenic: a research update, Environ Health Perspect 110(suppl 5):767, 2003.
64. Bhattacharjee Y: Toxicology: a sluggish response to humanity's biggest mass poisoning, Science 315:1659, 2007.
65. Slotnick MJ, Meliker JR, AvRuskin GA, et al: Toenails as a biomarker of inorganic arsenic intake from drinking water and foods, J Toxicol Environ Health A 70:148, 2007.
66. Kalia K, Flora SJ: Strategies for safe and effective therapeutic measures for chronic arsenic and lead poisoning, J Occup Health 47:1, 2005.

Cadmium

67. Aitio A, Tritscher A: Effects on health of cadmium—WHO approaches and conclusions, BioMetals 17:491, 2004.
68. Pope AM, Rall DP, editors: *Environmental Medicine: Integrating a Missing Element Into Medical Education,* Washington, DC, 1995, Institute of Medicine, National Academy Press.
69. Klaassen CD, Liu J, Choudhuri S: Metallothionein: an intracellular protein to protect against cadmium toxicity, Ann Rev Pharm Tox 39:267, 1999.
70. Liu J, Liu Y, Goyer RA, et al: Metallothionein-I/II null mice are more sensitive than wild-type mice to the hepatotoxic and nephrotoxic effects of chronic oral or injected inorganic arsenicals, Toxicol Sci 55:460, 2000.
71. Yapici G: Lead and cadmium exposure in children living around a coal-mining area in Yataan, Turkey Tox Ind Health 22:357, 2006.
72. Nogowa K, Kobayashi E, Okubo Y, et al: Environmental cadmium exposure, adverse effects, and preventative measures in Japan, Y Biometals 17:581, 2004.
73. Nakagawa H, Tabata M, Morikawa Y, et al: High mortality and shortened life-span in patients with itai-itai disease and subjects with suspected disease, Arch Environ Health 45:283, 1990.

Lead

74. Rodgers A, Murray CJL, Lopez AD, et al: *Comparative Quantification of Health Risks: Global and Regional Burden of Disease Attributable to Selected Major Risk Factors,* Geneva, Switzerland, 2004, World Health Organization.
75. Committee on Environmental Health: Lead exposure in children: prevention, detection, and management, Pediatrics 116:1036, 2005.
76. Handley MA, Hall C, Sanford E, et al: Globalization, binational communities, and imported food risks: results of an outbreak investigation of lead poisoning in Monterey County, California, Am J Public Health 97:900, 2007.
77. Garza A, Vega R, Soto E: Cellular mechanisms of lead neurotoxicity, Med Sci Monit 12:57, 2006.
78. Lead exposure among females of childbearing age—United States, 2004, Morb Mortal Wkly Rep 56:397, 2007.
79. Schnaas L, Rothenberg SJ, Flores M-J, et al: Reduced intellectual development in children with prenatal lead exposure, Environ Health Perspect 114:791, 2006.
80. Lanphear BP, Hornung R, Khoury J, et al: Low-level environmental lead exposure and children's intellectual function: an

international pooled analysis, Environ Health Perspect 113:894, 2005.

81. Canfield RL, Henderson CR, Cory-Slechta DA, et al: Intellectual impairment in children with blood lead concentrations below 10 micrograms per deciliter, N Engl J Med 348:1517, 2003.
82. Needleman HL, McFarland C, Ness RB, et al: Bone lead levels in adjudicated delinquents: a case control study, Neurotoxicol Teratol 24:711, 2002.
83. Hu H, Shih R, Rothenberg S, et al: The epidemiology of lead toxicity in adults: measuring dose and consideration of other methodologic issues, Environ Health Perspect 115:455, 2007.
84. Rogan WJ, Dietrich KN, Ware JH, et al: The effect of chelation therapy with succimer on neuropsychological development of children exposed to lead, N Engl J Med 344:1421, 2001.
85. The FDA Broadens Access to Lead Screening Test, FDA Consumer 40:24, 2006,US Department of Health and Human Services. (see also http://www.fda.gov/fdac/features/2006/606_lead.html)

Mercury

86. Clarkson TW, Magos L, Myers GJ: The toxicology of mercury—current exposures and clinical manifestations, N Engl J Med 349:1731, 2003.
87. Graeme KA, Pollack CV Jr: Heavy metal toxicity, Part I: arsenic and mercury, J Emerg Med 16:45, 1998.
88. Ruedy J: Methylmercury poisoning, CMAJ 165:1193, 2001.
89. Sallon S, Namdul T, Dolma S, et al: Mercury in traditional Tibetan medicine—panacea or problem? Hum Exp Toxicol 25:405, 2006.
90. Tang HL, Chu KH, Mak YF, et al: Minimal change disease following exposure to mercury-containing skin lightening cream, Hong Kong Med J 12:316, 2006.
91. Bellinger DC, Trachtenberg F, Barregard L, et al: Neuropsychological and renal effects of dental amalgam in children: a randomized clinical trial, JAMA 295:1775, 2006.
92. DeRouen TA, Martin MD, Leroux BG, et al: Neurobehavioral effects of dental amalgam in children: a randomized clinical trial, JAMA 295:1784, 2006.
93. Stern AH, Jacobson JL, Ryan L: Do recent data from the Seychelles Islands alter the conclusions of the NRC report on the toxicological effects of methylmercury? Environ Health 3:2, 2004.
94. Ballatori N, Clarkson TW: Biliary transport of glutathione and methylmercury, Am J Physiol 244:435, 1983.
95. Bigham M, Copes R: Thiomersal in vaccines: balancing the risk of adverse effects with the risk of vaccine-preventable disease, Drug Saf 28:89, 2005.
96. Jao-Tan C, Pope E: Cutaneous poisoning syndromes in children: a review, Curr Opin Pediatr 18:410, 2006.
97. Eto K: Pathology of Minamata disease, Toxicol Pathol 25:614, 1997.
98. Watson WA, Litovitz TL, Klein-Schwartz W, et al: 2003 Annual Report of the American Association of Poison Control Centers Toxic Exposure Surveillance System, Am J Emerg Med 22:335, 2004.
99. Risher JF, Amler SN: Mercury exposure: evaluation and intervention—the inappropriate use of chelating agents in the diagnosis and treatment of putative mercury poisoning, Neurotoxicology 26:691, 2005.
100. Magos L, Clarkson TW: Atomic absorption determination total, inorganic and organic mercury in blood, J Assoc Office Anal Chem 55:966, 1972.
101. http://www.cdc.gov/nchs/nhanes.htm, National Health and Nutrition Examination Survey, Centers for Disease Control.
102. Rees JR, Sturup S, Chen C, et al: Toe nail mercury and dietary fish consumption, J Expos Sci Environ Epidemiol 17:25, 2007.

INTERNET SITES

General

http://www.nal.usda.gov/—National Agriculture Library Recommended Dietary Allowances (RDA)—McMaster University nutrition health care information links

http://www.lhsc.on.ca/cgibin/view_labtest.pl?lab=Trace+Elements&action=browse_dept&Browse=Browse&.cgifields=lab—London Health Sciences Center of Canada trace elements laboratory—Type in "Trace Metals"

http://water.usgs.gov/nawqa/trace/—USGS, for general information about trace metal in US waters

Arsenic

http://www.epa.gov/safewater/arsenic/basicinformation.html—United States EPA

http://www.atsdr.cdc.gov/HEC/CSEM/arsenic/index.html—DHHS Agency for Toxic Substances and Disease Registry

http://www.atsdr.cdc.gov/tfacts2.pdf—DHHS Agency for Toxic Substances and Disease Registry

http://www.bt.cdc.gov/agent/arsenic/index.asp—DHHS CDC

http://www.who.int/mediacentre/factsheets/fs210/en/index.html—World Health Organization

http://www.osha.gov/SLTC/arsenic/index.html—OSHA

http://phys4.harvard.edu/~wilson/arsenic/arsenic_project_introduction.html—Harvard University

http://emedicine.medscape.com/article/812953-overview—Marcus S: Toxicity, arsenic (last updated: August 21, 2006)

http://emedicine.medscape.com/article/165429-overview—Graziano C, Hamilton RJ: Toxicity, arsenic (Last updated: August 21, 2006)

Cadmium

http://www.atsdr.cdc.gov/tfacts5.html—CDC

http://www.osha.gov/SLTC/cadmium/—OSHA

http://www.osha.gov/doc/outreachtraining/htmlfiles/cadmium.html—OSHA

Chromium

http://www.nap.edu/books/030906354X/html/index.html—National Academy Press, Division of the National Academy of Sciences: *The Role of Chromium in Animal Nutrition,* 1997, online book

Copper

www.nutrition.org—American Society for Nutritional Sciences: To find information, type name of element into the search engine

http://lpi.oregonstate.edu/infocenter/minerals/copper/—Oregon State University

Wilson's Disease

http://www.wilsonsdisease.org/—Wilson's Disease Association International

http://www.niddk.nih.gov/—National Institutes of Diabetes & Digestive & Kidney Diseases: To find information, type Wilson's disease into the search engine

http://www.ninds.nih.gov/—National Institute of Neurological Disorders and Stroke: To find information, type Wilson's disease into the search engine

http://emedicine.medscape.com/article/183456-overview—Shah R, Piper MH: Wilson disease (last updated: December 8, 2006)

Menkes' Syndrome

http://www.ncbi.nlm.nih.gov/—National Center for Biotechnology Information: Click on OMIM (Online Mendelian Inheritance in Man), and type Menkes' syndrome into the search engine http://dmoz.org—Open Directory Project, type Menkes' syndrome into the search engine for website links

http://emedicine.medscape.com/article/1153622-overview—Chang CH: Menkes disease (last updated: May 18, 2006)

http://www.ninds.nih.gov/health_and_medical/disorders/menkes.htm—National Institute of Neurological Disorders and Strokes

Fluoride

http://emedicine.medscape.com/article/814774-overview—Nochimson G: Toxicity, fluoride (last updated: January 8, 2007)

Iodine

http://emedicine.medscape.com/article/122714-overview—Lee SK: Iodine deficiency (last updated: July 27, 2006)

http://indorgs.virginia.edu/iccidd/aboutidd.htm—International Council for the Control of Iodine Deficiency Disorders (ICCIDD) (last updated: August 18, 2005)

http://whqlibdoc.who.int/publications/2004/9241592001.pdf—Iodine status worldwide, 2004 WHO report

Manganese

http://www.digitalnaturopath.com/cond/C686313.html

Lead

http://www.who.int/water_sanitation_health/diseases/lead/en/—WHO

http://www.iehmsp.com/online/sscba/leadResources.pdf Listing of lead resources

http://www.cdc.gov/nceh/lead/—CDC

http://www.haz-map.com/—Brown JA: NIH review of workplace health issues, Haz-Map: Information on hazardous chemicals and occupational diseases

http://www.epa.gov/lead/—EPA

http://www.nlm.nih.gov/medlineplus/leadpoisoning.html—NIH, general

http://www.niehs.nih.gov/kids/lead.htm—NIH, children

http://emedicine.medscape.com/article/815399-overview—Marcus S: Toxicity, lead (last updated: October 25, 2005)

http://emedicine.medscape.com/article/167157-overview—Habel R: Toxicity, lead (last updated: January 12, 2006)

http://pediatrics.aappublications.org/cgi/content/full/116/4/1036

http://www.health.state.ny.us/environmental/lead/ NY State

http://www.slh.wisc.edu/—Wisconsin State Laboratory of Hygiene, lead proficiency testing program: Type lead into the search engine

Mercury

http://www.aap.org/—American Academy of Pediatrics: Type mercury into the search engine

http://www.epa.gov/mercury/—Environmental Protection Agency: Type mercury into the search engine

http://www.usgs.gov/mercury/—USGS search engine

http://www.unido.org/doc/44254—United Nations project to reduce mercury in gold mining

http://mercurypolicy.org/—Advocacy group

http://rais.ornl.gov/tox/profiles/methyl_mercury_f_V1.shtml—U.S. government site, prepared 1992

http://emedicine.medscape.com/article/819872-overview—Diner B: Toxicity, mercury (last updated: October 18, 2005)

http://emedicine.medscape.com/article/1175560-overview—Olson DA: Mercury (last updated: September 19, 2006)

Selenium

www.cc.nih.gov—NIH Clinical Center: Type selenium into the search engine

www.cce.cornell.edu—Cornell Cooperative Extension: Type selenium into the search engine

http://ods.od.nih.gov/factsheets/selenium.asp—Office of Dietary Supplements, NIH

http://en.wikipedia.org/wiki/Selenocysteine—Wikipedia

Zinc

http://www.tamu.edu/—Texas A & M University: Type zinc into the search engine

http://en.wikipedia.org/wiki/Zinc_finger—Last modified, 7 April 2007

http://ods.od.nih.gov/factsheets/cc/zinc.html#issues—NIH Office of Dietary Supplements

http://lpi.oregonstate.edu/infocenter/minerals/zinc/—Linus Pauling Instit, Oregon State University

http://www.intox.org/databank/documents/chemical/zincsalt/ukpid89.htm

Vitamins

Hans G. Schneider

Chapter 43

Chapter Outline

Key Terms

avidin A glycoprotein in raw egg white with strong affinity for biotin.

carotenoids Compounds structurally similar to β-carotene (provitamin A) that occur naturally in vegetables and fruits.

chylomicrons Large lipoprotein particles formed in the small bowel that carry dietary lipids into the circulation.

dry beriberi A degenerative neurological disease that affects motor neurons.

endocytosis A process whereby cells take up molecules from the outside. Cells make tubular intrusions into the cell that then separate from the cell membrane and form intra-cellular vesicles.

flavins A group of yellow water-soluble pigments that include riboflavin, flavin adenine dinucleotide (FAD), and flavin mononucleotide (FMN).

osteomalacia Bone disease in adults caused by vitamin D deficiency and characterized by decreased calcification of the newly formed bone matrix.

pellagra Niacin deficiency resulting in the 3 "D's": diarrhea, dementia, and dermatitis.

pyridine nucleotides A group of nucleotides that bear a pyridine structure and are involved in electron transfer reactions: NAD, NADH, NADP, NADPH.

rickets Skeletal deformities caused by bone softening due to vitamin D deficiency.

scurvy Severe ascorbic acid deficiency characterized by spongy gums with loosening of teeth, weakened capillary beds, and defective cartilage synthesis.

Wernicke-Korsakoff syndrome Neurological pathology that occurs in alcoholic individuals with severe nutritional deficiencies, particularly thiamine deficiencies.

wet beriberi Similar to dry beriberi, but also includes left ventricular failure and concomitant edema.

Methods on Evolve

Folic acid
Holotranscobalamin
Vitamin B_{12}
Vitamin 25-OH D_3

SECTION OBJECTIVES BOX 43-1

- Define the term *vitamin.*
- Define the terms *RDA, DRI,* and *UL* with respect to recommended dietary requirements for vitamins.
- List ways of assessing vitamin status.

Vitamins (from Latin *vita* for "life," and *amine,* meaning "amines necessary for life") are a group of chemically unrelated low-molecular-weight compounds that must be provided in the diet because they are either not synthesized or they are synthesized in inadequate quantities to meet metabolic demands. They function as cofactors to certain enzymes. In addition, some vitamins have been shown to function as hormones or transcriptional regulators. Classical deficiency states of individual vitamins are rare but well described; however, low blood levels of vitamins, which might not always be associated with disease, are found much more frequently. Good evidence recommends dietary supplementation with specific vitamins in specific situations (e.g., folate in pregnancy, vitamin D in osteoporosis).

GENERAL CONSIDERATIONS

In the clinical setting, the investigation of possible vitamin deficiencies is often the primary focus, although a shift toward preventing disease by maintaining adequate intake has occurred. Both of these efforts require knowledge of the causes of deficiencies beyond inadequacies of diet. Deficiencies can be absolute or may result from an inability to utilize a vitamin optimally. Absolute vitamin deficiencies can be the result of a nutritional deficit, an inability to properly absorb a vitamin, increased metabolism and clearance, or markedly increased utilization. The inability to make use of a vitamin is typically the result of an inherited genotype that results in the synthesis of a defective enzyme or reduced enzyme quantities. These inherited defects often present with symptoms that can be quite different from those seen with an absolute deficiency of the vitamin (Table 43-1), and normal vitamin levels may be observed on measurement.

Historically, vitamin deficiencies were defined by overt clinical signs that often presented only after a prolonged and gross insufficiency of the vitamin. However, the clinical appearance of vitamin deficiencies constitutes a continuum that is dependent on the duration of deficiency and metabolic demand, as well as on the cellular concentration and form of the vitamin. Different physiological conditions and certain individual genetic differences in a vitamin's associated apoenzyme or receptor can influence an individual's nutritional requirement for a vitamin. This confounds the use of population-based reference intervals that do not account for these genetic differences.

Insufficient nutritional intake resulting in the deficiency of a vitamin often does not occur in isolation. One must consider the presence of other nutritive deficits, including other vitamins or other essential nutrients (see Chapter 41). Metabolic demand is another important consideration. Periods of marked growth or repair of tissues such as pregnancy, recovery from surgery, or recovery from a major infection will affect vitamin intake requirements.

Clinical symptoms of vitamin deficiencies can be nonspecific and vague, often delaying a definitive diagnosis. In many cases, clinical and dietary history, as well as physical examination, can be more informative than biochemical measurements when a vitamin deficiency is diagnosed. Vitamin functions and the usual symptoms seen in deficient and toxic states are listed in Table 43-2.

Recommended Dietary Allowances and Intakes

Suspicion of dietary deficiency of a vitamin arises primarily from knowledge of dietary sources and dietary practices likely to provide inadequate intake or absorption, resulting in deficiency states.[1] Recommended Dietary Allowances (RDA) for vitamins have been replaced by dietary reference intakes, or DRI (see Box 42-1, p. 805 and Chapter 41).[2,3]

An estimated 35% to 50% of American adults regularly consume vitamin mineral supplements purchased as "dietary supplements" sold at nutritional outlets. The health benefits of these supplements have not been substantiated. Evidence in the literature suggests that certain diets (like the so-called Mediterranean diet), rather than the intake of multivitamin supplements, are associated with health benefits. A health-conscious population lacking clear direction from scientific bodies[4] is susceptible to the influence of vendors who promote unsubstantiated nutritional value for these compounds. This problem is not limited to Western countries; in many non-Western countries, specific food supplements and "medications" are touted as maintaining or restoring health and potency. The tolerable upper intake level (UL) designated as part of the DRI has become a necessary guideline because food fortification and the use of supplements have increased the risk that a person may reach or exceed the critical level of a vitamin or mineral, which may result in toxic side effects.[5] The tolerable level is derived for the most part through human data, and each vitamin or nutrient is set at a level that is thought to pose no risk to humans. The European Food Safety Authority has published values for tolerable upper limits for minerals and vitamins.[6] It is important to consider that most humans have no need to achieve the UL in their diet, and that this maximum allowable limit is not intended to be a target value.

Vitamin Deficiencies

Vitamin deficiencies are relatively common, and identification of patients at risk for decreased intake, malabsorption, or impaired utilization should be considered for many patient settings. For patients at risk for vitamin deficiencies, the use of supplements on a prophylactic basis is generally accepted.

Vitamin deficiency is more common among individuals living in lower socioeconomic groups, among whom the condition is usually part of a general malnourished state (see p. 797-798, Chapter 41), as well as among older adults, alcoholics, and persons consuming unconventional diets. This last group is represented in all age groups and races and can include patients with psychiatric disorders. Patients with end-stage renal disease (ESRD) also present a special challenge for clinicians because dialysis adversely affects their ability to maintain adequate levels of vitamins.

Biochemical indices of vitamin status sometimes can become abnormal before obvious clinical changes are observed, thus allowing some vitamin deficiencies to be detected indirectly. Chemical determination of human vitamin status has been approached in the following ways:

1. Measurement of the vitamin, the active cofactor(s) or precursor(s) in biological fluids or blood cells
2. Measurement of urinary metabolite(s) of the vitamin
3. Measurement of a biochemical function that requires the vitamin (such as enzymatic activity) with and without in vitro addition of the cofactor form

Table 43-1 Genetic Changes Associated With Disease

Disease	Phenotype	Gene	Protein	Gene Locus	Relative Vitamin Deficiency
Thiamine-responsive megaloblastic anemia syndrome (TRMA)	Megaloblastic anemia, diabetes mellitus, sensorineural deafness	*SLC19A2*	Thiamine transporter 1	1q23.3	Thiamine
Imerslund-Grasbeck syndrome, recessive hereditary megaloblastic anemia 1	Megaloblastic anemia, proteinuria, later neurological defects	*CUBN, AMN*	Cubilin and amnionless form the Cbl-IF receptor in the small bowel	10p12.1, 14q32	Cobalamin
Homocystinuria due to methylenetetrahydrofolate reductase deficiency	Developmental delay, severe mental retardation, perinatal death, psychiatric disturbances, and later-onset neurodegenerative disorders	*MTHFR*	Methylenetetrahydrofolate reductase	1p36.3	Folate
Carnitine-O-palmitoyltransferase I deficiency		*CPT1B*	Carnitine-O-palmitoyltransferase I, muscle isoform	22q13.33	Carnitine
Retinol binding protein deficiency	Disturbed night vision, atrophy of the retinal pigment epithelium	*RBP4*	Retinol binding protein	10q24	Vitamin A
Vitamin D–dependent rickets, Type I	Rickets, inability to walk, bone deformities, or seizures	*CYP27B1*	25-Hydroxyvitamin D_3-1-alpha-hydroxylase (CYP27B1)	12q13.1-q13.3	Vitamin D
Vitamin E, familial isolated deficiency (VED)	Progressive ataxia, areflexia, and loss of proprioception	*TTPA*	α-Tocopherol transfer protein and TTP1	8q13.1-q13.3	Vitamin E
Combined deficiency of vitamin K–dependent clotting factors	Increased bleeding tendency, intracranial hemorrhage in the first weeks of life	*GGCX*	γ-Glutamyl carboxylase	2p12	Vitamin K
Epilepsy, pyridoxine-dependent (EPD)	Various seizures in the first hours of life unresponsive to anticonvulsants, but improved with pyridoxine	*ALDH7A1*	Aldehyde dehydrogenase 7, family member A1	5q31	Pyridoxine (vitamin B_6)
Multiple carboxylase deficiency, late-onset	Seizures, hypotonia, ataxia, hearing loss, optic atrophy, skin rash, alopecia, ketolactic acidosis, and organic aciduria	*BTD*	Biotinidase	3p25	Biotin (vitamin H)
Pantothenate kinase–associated neurodegeneration (PKAN)	Dystonia, parkinsonism, and iron accumulation in the brain	*PANK2*	Pantothenate kinase 2	20p13-p12.3	Pantothenic acid (vitamin B_5)

4. Measurement of urinary excretion of vitamin(s) or metabolite(s) after a test load of the vitamin
5. Measurement of urinary metabolites of a substance, the metabolism of which requires the vitamin, after administration of a test load of the substance
6. Measurement of accumulated metabolic substances that are increased because of vitamin deficiencies

Reduced serum concentrations of a vitamin do not always indicate a deficiency that interrupts cellular function, just as values within a reference interval as defined by population

Table 43-2 Vitamin Functions and Symptoms of Deficiency or Toxicity

Vitamin	Function	Clinical Deficiency	Toxicity
Fat-Soluble			
A	Vision, growth, reproduction, mucous secretion, immune responses	Night blindness, growth reduction, appetite loss, reduced taste, recurrent infection, dermatitis, dry mucous membranes *Late:* Bone growth failure, aspermatogenesis, xerophthalmia (dry, thickened, lusterless eyeballs), blindness	*Acute:* Raised intracranial pressure and skin desquamation; teratogen *Chronic:* Liver damage, skin changes and exostoses, osteoporosis, hypercalcemia
D	Bone calcification	*Children:* Rickets *Adults:* Osteomalacia	Anorexia, vomiting, headache, drowsiness, diarrhea, hypercalcemia
E	Antioxidant (membrane stability), neurological function	Mild hemolytic anemia, ataxia, loss of tendon reflexes, pigmentary retinopathy	Creatinuria, decreased platelet aggregation, impaired wound healing, anti-inflammatory activity, hepatomegaly, impaired fibrinolysis, potentiation of vitamin K deficiency, coagulopathy
K	Coagulation (γ-carboxylation of inactive clotting factors—prothrombin, factors II, IX, and X)	Hemorrhage (ranging from easy bruising to massive ecchymoses, mucous membrane hemorrhage, or posttraumatic bleeding)	*Adults:* Cardiac and pulmonary signs *Newborns:* Hemolytic anemia
Water-Soluble			
B_{12}	Myelin formation, methionine synthesis, folate interconversions, and DNA synthesis	Cognitive impairment, dementia, megaloblastic anemias, neurological abnormalities (paresthesias progressing to spastic paraparesis) (subacute combined degeneration)	Infrequent adverse reactions are most often allergic (possibly related to contaminants or preservatives)
Biotin	Coenzyme for CO_2 carboxylation relations and for carboxyl group exchange	Dermatitis progressing to mental and neurological changes, nausea, anorexia, peripheral vasoconstriction, or coronary ischemia in some cases	None described
C	Collagen formation, catecholamine synthesis, cholesterol catabolism, antioxidant	*Early:* Weakness, lassitude, irritability, vague aches and pains *Late:* Scurvy (hemorrhages into skin, alimentary and urinary tracts, other tissues; osteoporotic bones, defective tooth formation, anemia, pyrexia, delayed wound healing)	Increased excretion of oxalate and urate, diarrhea, dyspepsia
Carnitine	Energy metabolism and acyl group transport	Muscle weakness, fatigue	None known
Folate	One-carbon transfers	Megaloblastic anemia	Few reports—most often allergic reactions
Niacin	Oxidation-reduction (as pyridine nucleotides NAD and NADP)	*Early:* Lassitude, anorexia, weakness, digestive disturbances, anxiety, irritability, and depression *Late:* Pellagra (dermatitis, mucous membrane inflammation weight loss, disorientation, delirium, dementia)	Cutaneous flushing, gastric irritation, mild liver dysfunction, jaundice, hyperuricemia, impaired glucose tolerance
Pantothenate	Acyl group transfer reactions (as part of coenzyme A and acyl carrier protein)	Never spontaneously seen; with chemical agonist: Apathy, depression, increased infection, paresthesias (burning sensations), muscle weakness	None described
Pyridoxine	Enzyme systems involving amino acid transaminases, phosphorylases, racemases, decarboxylases, deaminases	*Infants:* Irritability, seizures, anemia, vomiting, weakness, ataxia, abdominal pain *Adults:* Facial seborrhea	Usually low systemic toxicity. Reduced milk production? Sensory neuropathy?

Continued

Table 43-2 Vitamin Functions and Symptoms of Deficiency or Toxicity—cont'd

Vitamin	Function	Clinical Deficiency	Toxicity
Water-Soluble—cont'd			
Riboflavin	Oxidative enzymatic reactions	Angular stomatitis (mouth lesions), glossitis (smooth tongue), photophobia, blepharospasm (eyelid spasm), conjunctival congestion and other ocular changes, dermatological changes, neurological alterations (behavior changes, decreased hand grip strength, burning feet in adults, retarded intellectual development and EEG changes in children), and hematological dyscrasias (anemia and reticulocytopenia)	Low toxicity
Thiamine	Decarboxylations, ketol formation	*Infants:* Dyspnea and cyanosis, diarrhea, vomiting, wasting, aphonia *Adults:* "Dry beriberi" (poor appetite, fatigue, peripheral neuritis) or "wet beriberi" (edema and cardiac failure), Wernicke-Korsakoff syndrome (apathy, ataxia, double vision, nystagmus, drooping eyelids, loss of short-term memory)	Anxiety, headache, convulsions, weakness, trembling, neuromuscular collapse

studies do not always reflect adequate supply. Typically, classical vitamin deficiencies are associated with lower levels of metabolites than are borderline or preclinical deficiencies. The absolute values will depend on the individual compound and the method used for its measurement. Table 43-3 lists biochemical data that are usually associated with classical deficiency symptoms. These values are, however, affected by age and laboratory method used. Some method references are included with the description of individual vitamins.[7,8]

Vitamins historically have been classed as fat or water soluble. This classification was adopted, in part, because the absorption of so-called fat-soluble vitamins depends on normal fat absorptive processes in the bowel (see Chapter 35 and below).

KEY CONCEPTS BOX 43-1

- Vitamins include a group of compounds that are necessary for a number of biological processes and that the body cannot make, totally or in part.
- Several ways are available to estimate the dietary intakes needed for a healthy body. These include the following:
  - RDA, Recommended Dietary Allowance
  - DRI, Dietary Reference Intakes
  - UL, Upper Limit of Normal Intake
- Laboratory assessment of vitamin status can be accomplished by measuring the vitamin or its metabolites in serum or urine, or by measuring a functional aspect of the vitamin (such as enzyme activity). However, the best way to identify vitamin deficiency is to look for signs and symptoms.

SECTION OBJECTIVES BOX 43-2

- List the fat-soluble vitamins and their functions, and conditions that result from their deficiency.
- List water-soluble vitamins and their functions, and conditions that result from their deficiency.
- Explain the functions of vitamin B_{12} and folic acid, and describe disease conditions that may result from deficiencies of these vitamins.
- Explain the roles of absorption, metabolism, and genetics in the development of relative or absolute vitamin deficiencies.
- Describe the role of vitamin deficiencies in the development of disease.
- Discuss toxicities that can develop as a consequence of oversupply of vitamins.
- Describe the main ways used to measure vitamins and their shortfalls.
- Explain the differences between measured levels of vitamins, determination of metabolites to identify vitamin deficiency, and clinically developed vitamin deficiency.
- Discuss areas of controversy involving vitamin deficiency states.

FAT-SOLUBLE VITAMINS

Because the fat-soluble vitamins (A, E, K, and D) are absorbed as part of the chylomicron complex (see Chapter 37), their absorption depends on the presence of adequate bile and pancreatic secretions, as well as healthy bowel mucosa. Therefore, chronic malabsorptive states often are associated with a deficiency of one or more of these vitamins (see Chapters 34 and 35). Malabsorptive states include chronic bowel inflammatory conditions, impaired bile flow, pancreatic insufficiency, and alcoholic liver disease (see Chapter 31). A new acquired form

Table 43-3 Concentration or Excretion Rates Associated With Classical Vitamin Deficiency Symptoms*†

Vitamin	Chemical Value
Fat-Soluble	
A	<0.2 mg/L of plasma retinol
	>20% relative dose response (RDR) in plasma
D	See Chapter 33
E	<5.0 mg/L of plasma α-tocopherol
K	Plasma prothrombin time greater than normal
Water-Soluble	
Ascorbic acid (C)	<2.4 mg/L of serum ascorbate
	<3 mg/L of whole blood ascorbate
	<80 mg/L of leukocyte ascorbate
B_{12}	<150 ng/L of serum vitamin B_{12}
	≥24 mg of urinary methylmalonic acid per day
	>0.44 nM serum methylmalonic acid
	>4 mmol methylmalonic acid/mole of creatinine in urine
	>15 nM serum total homocysteine
Biotin‡	<0.7 μg/L of whole blood?
Carnitine	<30 nM plasma total carnitine
	15 μg of urinary biotin per day?
Folate	<140 μg/L of erythrocyte folate
	<3.0 μg/L of serum folate
	≥30 mg of urinary N^5-formiminoglutamic acid (FIGLU) per 8 hours
	>15 nM serum homocysteine
Niacin	≥1 urinary ratio (α-pyridone/N′-methyl-nicotinamide)
Pantothenic acid‡	<1.0 mg/L of whole blood pantothenate
	<1.0 mg of urinary pantothenate per day
Pyridoxine (B_6)	≥1.5 AC of erythrocytic AST
	≥1.25 AC of erythrocytic ALT
	<0.8 mg of urinary 4-pyridoxic acid per day
	>25 mg of urinary xanthurenic acid per day
	<30 nM plasma pyridoxal phosphate
Riboflavin (B_2)	>1.4 AC of erythrocytic glutathione reductase
	<0.1 mg of riboflavin per liter of erythrocytes
	<0.12 mg of urinary riboflavin per day
	≥0.08 mg of urinary riboflavin per gram of creatinine
Thiamine	>1.25 AC of erythrocyte transketolase
	<0.1 mg of urinary thiamine per day

AC, Activity coefficient; ratio of activities with and without added cofactor.
*These are general guidelines with reference intervals that are dependent on age and method used.
†Compiled from references 3, 4, and 42.
‡Deficient values for biotin and pantothenate are not well established.

of lipid-soluble vitamin deficiency can occur with the use of gastrointestinal lipase inhibitors, such as Xenical, or the ingestion of non-bioavailable fat substitutes, such as Olestra. Deficiency of fat-soluble vitamins has been described to occur in more than 60% of patients after biliopancreatic diversion for obesity.[9] Deficiency of this class of vitamins generally develops slowly as stored supplies of vitamins are depleted. Vitamin A can be stored in liver parenchymal cells for a year or longer, and vitamin E can be stored in body fat for several months. Paradoxically, although they are fat soluble, vitamins K and D appear to be stored for only days or weeks.

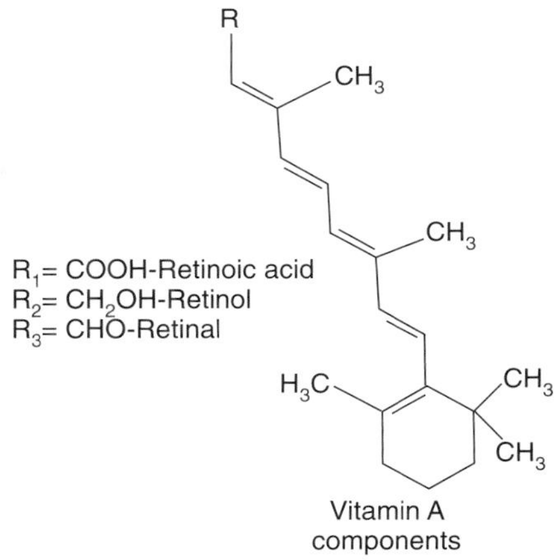

R
CH_3
CH_3
R_1= COOH-Retinoic acid
R_2= CH_2OH-Retinol
R_3= CHO-Retinal
H_3C
CH_3
CH_3
Vitamin A components

Fig. 43-1 Structures of vitamin A compounds.

Vitamin A and Carotenoids

First described in 1909 and found to prevent night blindness in 1925, vitamin A now is known to be made up of three biologically active forms: retinol, retinal, and retinoic acid. These major vitamin A compounds all contain a trimethylcyclohexenyl group and an all-*trans* polyene chain with four double bonds (Fig. 43-1). These compounds are derived directly from dietary sources, primarily as retinyl esters, or from metabolism of dietary carotenoids, primarily β-carotene (provitamin A). **Carotenoids** have been proposed to have additional functions such as scavenging of free radicals and protection of low-density lipoproteins (LDLs) from oxidation.[10]

Major dietary sources of these compounds include animal products, mainly liver for vitamin A and pigmented fruits and vegetables for carotenoids. β-Carotene (provitamin A) is the major plant source of vitamin A and supplies two-thirds of vitamin A. Each of these compounds is soluble in organic solvents, with retinoic acid being more polar than the others. Oxidation of retinol or retinal by peripheral cells is irreversible; thus neither retinoic acid nor retinal is converted metabolically to retinol.

Vitamin A has a very important role as a hormone that binds to nuclear hormone receptor proteins. The natural ligand for the receptors is the 9-*cis*-retinoic acid form of vitamin A, which appears to play a role in cellular differentiation, growth, and apoptosis (cell death). Although retinoic acid administration is beneficial in clearly defined instances, the broader application of vitamin A in cancer prevention and treatment has been unsuccessful.[11]

The recommended intake of vitamin A is dependent on age and starts from 300 μg/d in infants to 770 μg/d in adults, rising up to 1200 to 1300 μg/d in pregnancy. The tolerable upper intake level is 600 μg/d in children and rises to 3000 μg/d in adults. This shows the relatively small therapeutic window for vitamin A. The European Food Safety Authority recommends that β-carotene as a supplement is contraindicated in smokers at doses of 20 mg/d, about 3 to 4 times the normal intake.

Metabolism

Enzymes of the small intestinal mucosa convert dietary β-carotene and retinyl esters to the predominant form of vitamin A, retinol. The retinyl esters of dietary animal products are cleaved to retinol by pancreatic and mucosal hydrolases (vitamin A esterases). Uptake into the mucosal cells probably occurs through a facilitated process. Once in the mucosal cell, retinol is reesterified, forming retinyl esters (primarily retinyl palmitate) that are transported in lymph **chylomicrons** to the systemic circulation. After the chylomicrons release their triglycerides, the retinyl esters are transported to the liver, where they are stored bound to intracellular retinol binding proteins within the liver.[12] The retinoids are biologically inactive when bound to these proteins; this may serve as a protective mechanism to prevent unwanted or inappropriate retinoid transcriptional activity. This is supported by the observation that increased exposure to retinoids can lead to dramatic increases in retinoid binding protein.[12] The more polar retinoic acid does not require this lipoprotein transport route but is directly absorbed into the portal circulation. However, this form is not stored in the liver but is excreted through bile as a glucuronide conjugate. The exact role of these water-soluble glucuronide derivatives is unknown.

When body demands require mobilization of hepatic vitamin A, the stored retinyl palmitate is hydrolyzed and the free retinol combines with retinol binding protein (RBP). RBP-retinol then is secreted into the circulation, where it complexes with prealbumin. Cellular uptake from the vitamin A–RBP complex is mediated by STRA6, a multitransmembrane domain protein, which acts as a specific membrane receptor for RBP.[13] STRA6 is widely expressed in embryonic development and in adult organ systems. Retinol is transferred intracellularly to another specific binding protein termed cytosol-retinol binding protein (CRBP). CRBP-retinol presumably transports the retinol to its functional site within the cell.

Function (see Table 43-2)

A physiological role for retinol in vision is clearly defined. Retinol is oxidized in the rods of the eye to retinal, which, when complexed with opsin, forms rhodopsin, allowing dim-light vision. In the visual cycle, rhodopsin is reversibly bleached by a photon of light. During this process, 11-*cis*-retinal is converted to all-*trans*-retinal, forcing the dissociation of opsin. Activated rhodopsin stimulates transducin, a G-protein, which ultimately decreases the cellular content of cyclic guanosine 3′,5′-monophosphate (cyclic GMP) via the activation of a cyclic-GMP phosphodiesterase. This effect culminates in nervous conduction in the optic nerve to the brain. All-*trans*-retinal then isomerizes to 11-*cis*-retinal, which then associates with opsin to reform rhodopsin, completing the visual cycle. When retinal is depleted in the retina, opsin becomes destabilized and is catabolized. This eventually results in the permanent destruction of the rod cells. A similar reaction uses iodopsin in the cone cells of the retina, and visual pigments absorb light at different wavelengths in different types of cone cells. Apart from this role in retinal physiology, vitamin A has been shown to be important in immunity and mucosal physiology. Vitamin A deficiency reduces the functional efficiency of neutrophils, natural killer cells, and macrophages.[14]

In the gut, retinoic acid (RA) has an important role in maintaining immunity. After exposure to picomolar concentrations of RA (but not retinol), activated T cells express subunits α4β7 of the cell surface receptor integrin and the chemokine receptor CCR9, markers that help T cells migrate to the gut. Dendritic cells from gut-associated lymphoid tissue (GALT) can convert retinol to retinoic acid, in contrast to dendritic cells from the spleen.[15] Removing vitamin A from the diet in an animal model reduced the number of α4β7-positive T cells in lymphoid organs, as well as depletion of CD4+ T-cells specifically from the small intestinal mucosa. Gut-homing immunoglobulin (Ig)A-producing B-memory cells also required RA to induce expression of the gut-homing molecules integrin α4β7 and CCR9. To stimulate IgA production, additional interleukin (IL)-5 or IL-6 was needed.[16] An additional role of RA was identified recently in the balance of proinflammatory and anti-inflammatory immunity.[17] RA might promote differentiation of activated T cells to regulatory T cells, which can prevent autoimmunity.

In vitamin A deficiency, epithelial cells (cells in the outer skin layers and cells in the lining of the gastrointestinal, respiratory, and urogenital tracts) become dry and keratinized. Thus vitamin A may help to maintain epithelial cells, which provide protection against infectious organisms. Retinoic acid and retinol play a significant role in epithelial differentiation in mucus and keratinizing tissues. Retinoic acid induces production of mucus in basal epithelial cells and inhibits keratinization of epithelium, whereas goblet cell formation occurs in the presence of retinoids. The end result is the formation of a healthy, non-stratified, non-keratinizing epithelial layer. Because the mucous secretions of the goblet cells are part of the natural immune system, retinoid compounds function to bolster the immune system.

The role that retinoids play in cellular differentiation and regulation occurs at the level of nuclear transcription. Two superfamilies of retinoid nuclear receptors have been described. The retinoic acid receptor (RAR) and the retinoid X receptor (RXR; because more than one retinoid may naturally bind to the receptor) groups each consist of alpha, beta, and gamma subtypes. In general, the role of these receptors is to activate the transcriptional machinery of cells, activating specific genes in a concerted manner.

Clinical and Chemical Deficiency Signs

Vitamin A deficiency is a serious nutritional problem in a large part of the world, especially in Africa, South America, and Southeast Asia. In infants younger than 5 years, vitamin A deficiency can be fatal. A recent review estimated that vitamin A deficiency is responsible for 600,000 deaths and about 5.4% of global disability-adjusted life-years (DALYs) for children younger than 5 years.[18]

Clinical signs of vitamin A deficiency can be separated into early and late signs (see Table 43-2). Although night blindness frequently is seen in vitamin A deficiency, keratomalacia is seen in children who have a severe deficiency. Keratinization of the respiratory tract with subsequent reduction in mucous secretion can result in respiratory infection, a significant cause for mortality in developing countries. Other symptoms include increased mortality from diarrheal illness in children with vitamin A deficiency and increased mortality after measles. In transplant patients, the retinol level is associated with future mortality, underlining the importance of a sufficient vitamin A supply in the immunosuppressed patient.[19]

The chemical sign of deficiency is reduction in plasma vitamin A. Generally, retinol values below 0.1 mg/L are associated with clinical symptoms, and values above 0.2 mg/L are not.[7,20] However, values below 0.29 mg/L may be inadequate for post-adolescent persons. Vitamin A itself is not excreted in human urine. Although several metabolites are excreted, they do not seem to reflect the tissue status of vitamin A. One method for assessment of vitamin A status is the relative dose response (RDR) test and a modified version of it (MRDR); these tests measure the increase in plasma retinol after administration of retinyl palmitate (RDR) or dehydroretinol (MRDR) and are meant to better reflect the vitamin A stores in the liver than serum retinol. However, some have questioned the value of the RDR and MRDR[21] as indicators of vitamin A stores in liver. Another functional measure of vitamin A status involves evaluation of the morphology of conjunctival epithelial cells, referred to as conjunctival impression cytology (CIC).[22-24]

Pathophysiology

Because retinol and RBP are secreted from the liver as a 1:1 complex, low plasma concentrations of both are seen in vitamin A deficiency. An adequate concentration of plasma retinol usually indicates dietary and tissue adequacy, but low concentrations do not always indicate dietary deficiency. Factors that reduce hepatic synthesis of RBP or secretion of the RBP-retinol complex also lower plasma concentrations of retinol and RBP, even though dietary intake and the hepatic retinol store are adequate. These states, which are recognized primarily by the absence of an increase in plasma retinol after oral therapy with vitamin A, include protein-calorie malnutrition, liver disease, zinc deficiency, and cystic fibrosis.

Pathophysiological conditions that can result in increased retinol and RBP include chronic renal disease and use of oral contraceptives.

Therapeutic Uses and Toxicity

In countries with endemic vitamin A deficiency in pregnancy and childhood, small doses of vitamin A have been shown to reduce death rates from diarrheal illness and measles in small children. Premature infants are born with lower serum retinol and RBP levels, as well as low hepatic stores of retinol. Newborns thus are treated with vitamin A as a preventative measure. In addition, retinoids have been used therapeutically to treat a variety of skin disorders, including acne (isotretinoin and tretinoin) and psoriasis (etretinate). Retinoids in higher doses are known to result in congenital malformations, and women who use high-dose retinoid therapy should practice contraception for up to 2 years after discontinuation of the drug.

Clinically, all-*trans* retinoic acid (ATRA) plays an important role in acute promyelocytic leukemia (APL), a form of leukemia in which the differentiation of white cell precursors to neutrophils is blocked at the level of the promyelocyte. In APL, a chromosomal translocation produces a chimeric protein between RARα and a protein called promyelocyte leukemia protein (PML). PML-RARα works as a dominant negative receptor in leukemic cells, interfering with the normal function of RARα and/or PML, which, in turn results in the arrest of cell maturation at the stage of promyelocytes. Oral administration of ATRA induces differentiation of promyelocytic leukemic cells to mature neutrophils and leads to a high rates (>90%) of complete remission. ATRA therapy has become standard in the treatment of APL; however, because of toxicity and only short-term effectiveness, it must be combined with standard chemotherapy.

Vitamin A toxicity, one of the more common hypervitaminosis states, can occur in adults or children. Typically, it is the result of overmedication with vitamin supplements, but it can also result from the use of topical retinoids for acne. Infants are more susceptible to retinoid toxicity than are adults. A well-known, albeit rare, cause of hypervitaminosis A that can be fatal occurs with the ingestion of polar bear liver, which contains up to 1.2% vitamin A by weight. Signs of vitamin A toxicity include dry, itchy skin; dermatitis; fissures of the lips; bone pain; edema; fatigue; renal disorders; intracranial hypertension; and hemorrhage. Further increased vitamin A intake increases bone resorption, can cause hypercalcemia,[25] and may increase the risk of hip fracture.[26]

Hypervitaminosis A can also result in the development of numerous congenital malformations in the fetus. Indeed, the dose required to cause defects in the fetus can be reached with dietary supplements.[27] As was mentioned earlier, retinoid therapy can result in significant stores of retinoids in fat, which extend the length of time that women of childbearing years should wait before discontinuing contraceptive use.

Vitamin E

A factor in cereal oils that prevented infertility in deficient rats was isolated in the early 1920s as vitamin E; later, it was given the generic name tocopherol and was shown to include several biologically active isomers. α-Tocopherol, which is the predominant isomer in plasma, is the most potent isomer by current biological assays (Fig. 43-2). Other isomers include β-, γ-, and δ-tocopherol and β-, γ-, and δ-tocotrienol. The actively maintained form of α-tocopherol in plasma is the RRR form (for explanation of stereochemistry, see reference 28). However, synthetic α-tocopherol contains a mixture of all eight isomers (all racemic) and exhibits only about half the activity of naturally occurring vitamin E.

Dietary sources of tocopherols include vegetable oils, fresh leafy vegetables, egg yolk, legumes, peanuts, and margarine. Diets suspect for vitamin E deficiency are those low in

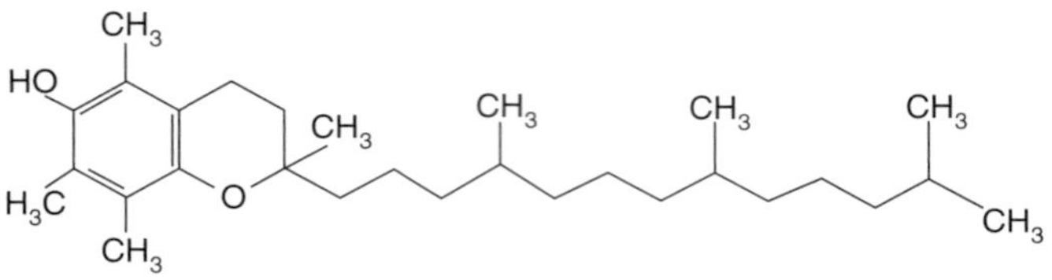

Fig. 43-2 Vitamin E α-tocopherol.

vegetable oils or fresh green vegetables, or those high in unsaturated fats.

Metabolism

Absorption of vitamin E is associated with intestinal fat absorption, and bile acids are required for solubilization. Although previously believed to be a passive process, active uptake in enterocytes with a scavenger receptor has been described.[29] Approximately 40% of ingested tocopherol is absorbed and integrated into chylomicrons.

Chylomicron remnants are taken up by the liver, and α-tocopherol is re-secreted as a component of liver-derived very low-density lipoproteins (VLDLs) (and perhaps high-density lipoproteins [HDLs]).[30] A specific α-tocopherol transfer protein (α-TTP) is crucial in this process, and deficiency of this protein causes a neuropathy secondary to vitamin E deficiency.[31] This α-TPP preferentially transports RRR α-tocopherol and is responsible for the fact that most circulating vitamin A is present in this form.[32]

Vitamin E is stored predominantly in adipose tissue, although increased dietary α-tocopherol acetate is reflected by increased concentrations in all animal tissues, including plasma, erythrocytes, and platelets.

Function

The main recognized function of vitamin E in humans is as an antioxidant. It functions as a free radical scavenger and protects oxidative modification of polyunsaturated fatty acids, which make up a significant percentage of the cell membrane. A number of biological effects, such as inhibition of platelet or monocyte adhesion, are observed, which are not related to the antioxidant function.[33] Recently, the preservation of neurological function has begun to be recognized as an important function of vitamin E.

Clinical Deficiency Signs (see Table 43-2)

Vitamin E deficiency is rare because the vitamin is distributed so widely in different food sources. Patients with conditions that result in fat malabsorption, such as cholestasis, chronic pancreatitis, cystic fibrosis, or abetalipoproteinemia, are suspect for vitamin E deficiency, but they may be deficient in all fat-soluble vitamins. A relationship has been noted between vitamin E deficiency and progressive loss of neurological function in infants and children with chronic cholestasis.[34]

Neuronal signs of vitamin E deficiency include ataxia and peripheral neuropathy, although myopathies have also been seen. Vitamin E deficiency can occur without lipid malabsorption.[35]

The nervous system is particularly sensitive to vitamin E deficiency. In humans, a macrocytic megaloblastic anemia is associated with α-tocopherol deficiency. It is important to understand that this anemia is related to severe protein–calorie deficiency and may not be totally attributable to vitamin E. Premature infants may be susceptible to a hemolytic anemia that results from oxidative damage to their cell membranes. Premature newborns often are supplemented with multivitamins, including vitamin E, to stabilize their red blood cells and prevent hemolytic anemia. In addition, a rare genetic disorder that results in a beta-lipoprotein deficiency with concomitant vitamin E deficiency produces acanthocytosis. This disorder also appears to be associated with a malabsorptive state for vitamin E. Steatorrhea affects α-tocopherol absorption; subsequent premature erythrocyte destruction occurs.

Chemical Deficiency Signs

Plasma concentrations of α-tocopherol below 5 mg/L are associated with increased erythrocyte hemolysis in the presence of hydrogen peroxide and thus are designated "deficient." A strong correlation has been observed between plasma α-tocopherol and plasma lipids, indicating that plasma concentrations should be interpreted relative to plasma lipid levels; 0.8 mg of α-tocopherol per gram of total plasma lipids appears to indicate adequate levels of vitamin E in infants. Others have suggested that vitamin E should be corrected for total cholesterol.[36]

Pathophysiology

At the present time, assessment of vitamin E status is indicated primarily in persons with fat-malabsorption states and in those receiving synthetic diets. Dietary insufficiency rarely causes vitamin E deficiency.

Toxicity

Toxicity may result from chronic voluntary overdoses. Premature infants receiving vitamin E sufficient to sustain serum levels above 30 mg/L have an increased incidence of sepsis and necrotizing enterocolitis. Patients who are receiving synthetic diets should be monitored to avoid vitamin E toxicity (see Table 43-1). In a meta-analysis, high-dose supplementation of vitamin E has been linked to increased mortality.[37]

Vitamin K

Experiments in the mid-1930s led to the discovery of the antihemorrhagic factor that later was called vitamin K. Purification efforts revealed that several quinone-containing compounds possess this antihemorrhagic activity, and the term *vitamin K* now is used as a generic descriptor for substances containing a 2-methyl-1,4-napthoquinone nucleus with a lipophilic side chain. A large number of these compounds are related to those shown in Fig. 43-3 by number and substituents of polyisoprenoid side chains and degree of saturation.

The two major forms of vitamin K are phylloquinone (vitamin K_1) and the menaquinones (vitamin K_2). The phylloquinone derivatives of vitamin K are found in plants and constitute the dietary source of vitamin K. Menaquinone forms of vitamin K are produced in gram-positive bacteria and represent the bowel-derived source of vitamin K in humans. Major dietary sources of phylloquinones include cabbage, cauliflower,

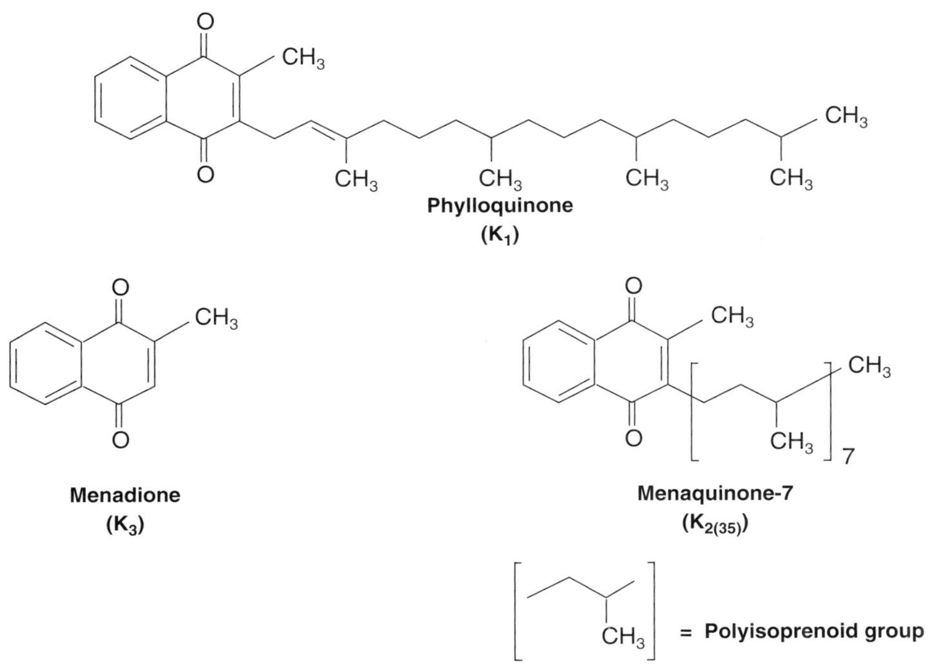

Phylloquinone (K_1)

Menadione (K_3)

Menaquinone-7 ($K_{2(35)}$)

= Polyisoprenoid group

Fig. 43-3 Structures of vitamin K forms.

spinach, and other leafy vegetables, as well as pork, liver, soybeans, and vegetable oils. Uncomplicated dietary deficiency is considered rare in healthy children and adults.

Metabolism

Absorption of vitamin K in the intestine requires pancreatic enzymes to release phylloquinone from binding proteins and bile for solubilization in micelles. After absorption, vitamin K is incorporated into chylomicrons. Bacterial production in the intestine provides for menaquinone. Vitamin K malabsorption states include cystic fibrosis, biliary atresia, cholelithiasis, and obstructive jaundice, as well as other disorders leading to dysfunction of the upper small intestine. Tissue stores of the vitamin diminish through normal metabolism. As tissue stores become saturated, vitamin K is excreted in urine. Depletion of body stores sufficient to manifest deficiency usually requires 3 weeks.

Function

The phylloquinone and menaquinone forms of vitamin K are largely inactive. Vitamin K must be reduced to the hydroquinone form to act as a cofactor. First shown to be involved in prothrombin synthesis, vitamin K also has been found to be required for the synthesis of the active form of clotting factors VII, IX, and X, as well as for the γ-carboxylation of the clotting inhibitor proteins C and S. Vitamin K–dependent γ-carboxylation of glutamic acid residues of inactive precursor proteins occurs in the liver. The conversion of glutamic acid (glu) to a γ-carboxyglutamic acid (gla) permits the coagulation proteins to bind calcium, which then can serve as an ionic bridge to bind with phospholipids. This is essential to the coagulation pathway. γ-Carboxylation occurs in the presence of oxygen and carbon dioxide. A microsomal carboxylase enzyme facilitates the conversion of the hydroquinone form to a 2,3-epoxide. The hydroquinone form of vitamin K is regenerated from the 2,3-expoxide via the action of epoxide reductase, which is inhibited by coumarin (for further explanation and formulas, see reference 38).

Other proteins that contain gla include osteocalcin, which is secreted from osteoblasts, and matrix gla-protein. Osteocalcin may be involved in bone matrix calcification (see Chapter 33). Epidemiological studies have shown an association between higher intake of vitamin K and reduced hip fracture rate.[39] Data are inconclusive regarding an effect of vitamin K supplementation on fracture prevention.[40,41]

Clinical Deficiency Signs (see Table 43-2)

The primary clinical manifestation of a vitamin K deficiency is an increased tendency to hemorrhage as a result of decreased hemostatic function, primarily from a reduction in active prothrombin, as well as other clotting factors. Major signs of hemorrhage include ecchymosis (bleeding under the skin), nosebleeds (epistaxis), and intestinal bleeding.

Vitamin K supplies in the newborn are frequently insufficient, and without supplementation, vitamin K deficiency bleeding in infancy (previously known as hemorrhagic disease of the newborn) has been described. This is caused by a low amount of vitamin K in the breast milk and a lack of bacterial production of vitamin K_2 in the immature gut. Vitamin K administration at birth reduces this condition.[42]

Administration of oral anticoagulants during the first trimester of pregnancy results in fetal bone growth retardation deformities known as fetal warfarin syndrome. This congenital syndrome may result from decreased γ-carboxylation of osteocalcin and matrix protein, although this has not yet been proven. The defects are the result of premature calcification of cartilage, which can be associated with breathing problems caused by nasal hypoplasia.

Chemical Deficiency Signs

Direct measurement of vitamin K in blood usually is not performed for adults. Prothrombin time (PT) is an excellent index of prothrombin adequacy. PT is prolonged in deficiency of vitamin K and in liver diseases characterized by decreased synthesis of prothrombin. Deficiency of vitamin K also results in prolongation of partial thromboplastin time, but the thrombin time is within the reference interval. Immunological measurement of acarboxyprothrombin (protein induced by vitamin K absence; PIVKA-II) is useful in the detection of vitamin K deficiency in neonates and appears to have greater sensitivity than the coagulation tests.[43] Vitamin K status can be directly assessed by high-performance liquid chromatography (HPLC) measurement of phylloquinone, and a relationship to plasma triglycerides has been described.[44] The reporting of vitamin K levels as a ratio to triglyceride levels may be beneficial. Subclinical deficiency has been described recently in patients with terminal malignancies[45] and in patients on hemodialysis.[46]

Pathophysiology

The vitamin K malabsorptive states are described above. The prothrombin reduction seen in patients with chronic liver disease is corrected by administration of vitamin K only if there is associated malnutrition or malabsorption. Vitamin K action is antagonized by coumarin or indanedione anticoagulants. Oral contraceptive use increases the levels of prothrombin and factors VII, IX, and X and apparently reduces the requirement for vitamin K.

Vitamin D (see Chapter 33)

The naturally occurring vitamin D in humans is cholecalciferol (vitamin D_3) that is produced in the skin from ultraviolet conversion of 7-dehydrocholesterol (for formulas, see reference 47). Vitamin D_3 is a prohormone that is converted in the liver to 25-hydroxycholecalciferol (calcidiol), which is hydroxylated further in the kidney to form the active hormone 1,25-dihydroxycholecalciferol (calcitriol). Ergocalciferol (vitamin D_2) is obtained through the diet (mainly plants) and with food fortification and makes up a portion of the total vitamin D level.

Major dietary sources include irradiated foods and commercially prepared milk in the United States. Small amounts are found in butter, egg yolk, liver, salmon, sardines, and tuna. Calcidiol is the form that usually is measured in the clinical laboratory.

Evidence of insufficient vitamin D levels has been found in a significant percentage of the adult population in countries with reduced sunlight exposure. Studies have shown annual variability of vitamin D levels, with reduced levels at the end of winter and increased levels at the end of summer. This is physiologically important in that parathyroid hormone levels increase with reduction in vitamin D, and bone resorption is also increased. Increases in PTH and bone absorption are associated with increased fracture incidence.[48] Vitamin D deficiency is especially frequent in elderly patients in nursing homes and supported accommodation. Because of the high frequency of vitamin D deficiency, elderly institutionalized individuals should be supplemented with additional vitamin D.

Physiological actions, regulation, and assessment of the hormone forms of vitamin D are discussed in Chapter 33. The concentration of 25-hydroxycholecalciferol in serum reflects overall vitamin D status, because it represents an average of dietary and sunlight-induced vitamin D. Measurement of vitamin D is performed by immunological assays, by HPLC with ultraviolet (UV) detection, or by liquid chromatography–mass spectrometry (LC-MSMS). The different immunological assays for vitamin D do not all recognize vitamin D_3 and vitamin D_2 to the same extent. Some evidence indicates that vitamin D_2 is less biologically active than vitamin D_3, and its half-life is shorter; however, other studies have disputed this.[49] No general agreement has been reached on the reference interval for vitamin D levels, with one group of physicians setting the lower reference limit at 50 nmol/L, the level below which PTH levels start to increase.[50] Others suggest higher levels of 70 to 80 nmol/L, based on epidemiological studies.[51]

The concentration of 1,25-dihydroxycholecalciferol in serum in general is not useful in the evaluation of disorders of calcium and bone metabolism. One exception is seen in the setting of unexplained hypercalcemia with suppressed parathormone (PTH) levels, where an inappropriately elevated 1,25-dihydroxycholecalciferol level indicates a likely granulomatous process (like sarcoidosis), which causes unregulated 1,25-dihydroxycholecalciferol production.

Deficiency results in **rickets** (in children) or **osteomalacia** (in adults) in its full-blown form, both of which are forms of abnormal bone synthesis. Osteoporosis might be associated with low vitamin D levels, and vitamin D supplementation has been shown to reduce fracture rates in elderly institutionalized patients, but not in the remaining population.[52] Excess dietary intake is uncommon, especially when only small amounts of vitamin D are available for dietary supplementation. Excessive supplementation with vitamin D can cause hypercalcemia that takes weeks to months to resolve. Patients with a tendency toward hypercalcemia, such as those with primary hyperparathyroidism or with sarcoidosis, are particularly at risk.

KEY CONCEPTS BOX 43-2

- Fat soluble vitamins (FSV) include vitamins A, D, E, and K.
- FSV are absorbed as part of the chylomicron complex and require adequate bile and pancreatic secretion as well as healthy bowel mucosa for absorption.
- In addition to malabsorption, treatment with weight loss agents or gastrointestinal surgery for obesity can lead to FSV deficiency.
- Vitamin A stores last a year, vitamin E lasts for months, while vitamin D lasts for weeks and vitamin K for days.
- HPLC assays are useful for vitamins A and E, vitamin D is most commonly assayed by immunoassay, the prothrombin time is used to assay the biological effect of vitamin K.
- Vitamin A deficiency is common in the developing world and leads to excess mortality in children (mainly through diarrhea). The therapeutic window is small and toxicity is well described.
- Vitamin E is transported in plasma lipid particles and should be reported as a ratio to lipids.

SECTION OBJECTIVES BOX 43-3

- List water-soluble vitamins (WSV) and their functions, and describe conditions that may result from their deficiency.
- Describe the functions of vitamin B_{12} and folic acid, and discuss disease conditions that may result from deficiencies of these vitamins.
- Describe the roles of absorption, metabolism, and genetics in the development of relative and absolute vitamin deficiencies.
- Describe the role of vitamin deficiency in the development of disease.
- List toxicities that can occur as a consequence of oversupply of WSV.
- List the primary ways used to measure WSV, and discuss their shortfalls.
- Describe the differences between measured levels of WSV, determination of metabolites to identify vitamin deficiency, and clinically developed vitamin deficiency.

WATER-SOLUBLE VITAMINS

The water-soluble vitamins include the B vitamin group and ascorbic acid. The B vitamin group is large and varied (Box 43-1).

Although choline and inositol historically have been considered part of the B vitamin complex, a detailed description of these two nutrients is not included in this chapter because their status as vitamins is debatable.

Choline (trimethylethanolamine), a constituent of the phospholipid lecithin, is lipotropic (removes lipid from the liver), functions as a methyl donor in hepatocytes, and is required for acetylcholine synthesis. Recently, choline levels have attained interest as a possible prognostic marker of unstable angina.[53] Inositol is an isomeric form of glucose. Similar to choline, inositol is a constituent of phospholipids in cell membranes. Phosphatidylinositol is also found in lipoproteins in serum. Phosphorylated inositol functions as an intracellular second messenger in response to hormones, neurotransmitters, and autocoids (local and often self-acting hormones).

Box 43-1
B Vitamin Group

Folic acid
Cobalamin
Thiamine
Pyridoxine
Pantothenic acid
Nicotinic acid
Thiamine
Riboflavin
Choline
Inositol

All water-soluble vitamins are absorbed without the involvement of fat absorption, and excess vitamin is excreted almost immediately in the urine. Thiamine is stored for only a few weeks, and most other B-complex vitamins and ascorbic acid are stored for less than 2 months. Development of deficiency therefore can be rapid. The exception is vitamin B_{12}, which, although it is a water-soluble vitamin, is stored in the liver for several years. The water-soluble vitamins function as coenzymes, and all except ascorbic acid and biotin must be converted metabolically to active forms.

Ascorbic Acid (Vitamin C)

The symptom cluster known as **scurvy** (Box 43-2) was clearly described during the time of the Crusades and became commonplace when long sea voyages began. In 1747, a naval surgeon who was experimenting with diets to cure scurvy identified the efficacy of citrus fruits. The antiscurvy agent, vitamin C, was isolated in 1932 and later was given the name *ascorbic acid* because of its antiscorbutic effect. The structures of this water-soluble vitamin and its oxidized form, dehydroascorbate (DHAA), are shown in Fig. 43-4. By virtue of its ene-diol group, ascorbate is a very strong reducing compound. Together with DHAA, from which it can be recycled, it forms an important redox system. Although plants and most animals can synthesize this vitamin, primates cannot; thus dietary ingestion is essential.

Major dietary sources include fruits (especially citrus) and vegetables (tomatoes, green peppers, cabbage, leafy greens, and potatoes). Because ascorbate is labile to heat and oxygen, fresh and uncooked foods are highest in ascorbate content.

Box 43-2
Symptoms of Scurvy

Bruising
Ecchymosis
Swollen gums with loss of teeth
Skin lesions
Weakness in the lower extremities

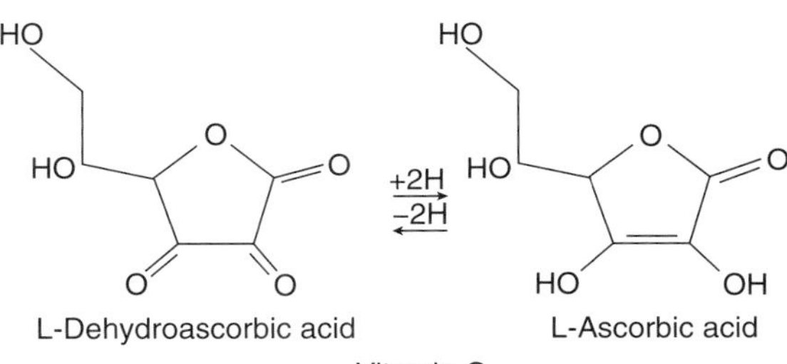

Fig. 43-4 Structures of ascorbic acid and dehydroascorbate.

Metabolism

Ascorbate is absorbed along the whole small intestine by a sodium ascorbate cotransporter. DHAA is also absorbed via facilitated diffusion but with a different sodium-independent transporter. Two isoforms of sodium-ascorbate cotransporters—SVCT1 and SVCT2—have been cloned. They mediate ascorbate uptake from the small intestine, nephron reuptake of ascorbate filtered by the glomerulus, and cellular uptake. Cellular uptake of DHAA is mediated by glucose transporters of the GLUT-family.[54]

Vitamin C is distributed widely in tissues (most concentrated in the adrenal cortex and pituitary) and passes the placenta readily. The normal body store requires several months to deplete before symptoms of scurvy appear. Cerebrospinal fluid (CSF) concentrations are higher than those in plasma. Excess ascorbate and a metabolite, oxalate, are eliminated readily in the urine. Generally, ascorbate metabolism accounts for about half the urinary oxalate.

Function

Ascorbic acid functions as an antioxidant and an electron donor for enzymes that are involved in selected reductive processes. This is essential for the conversion of proline and lysine in procollagen to hydroxyproline and hydroxylysine, respectively. Thus ascorbic acid is important in the formation and stabilization of collagen by hydroxylation of proline and lysine, which are required to allow the formation of the triple helix and cross-linking of the collagen chains. This effect may be demonstrated clinically because scurvy is a disease of impaired collagen synthesis. Formation of small skin hemorrhages (petechiae) and subsequent bruising in scurvy are thought to reflect decreased fibrous tissue support for capillary beds, which results in their bursting when stressed. Tyrosine conversion to catecholamines via dopamine β-hydroxylase also requires ascorbic acid, and the adrenals have much higher ascorbate concentrations than do other tissues. In addition, ascorbic acid is involved in the synthesis of carnitine and the amidation of peptide hormones. Uptake of the nonheme form of iron in the gut is facilitated by ascorbic acid through the nonenzymatic reduction of ferric iron to the ferrous state.

Clinical and Chemical Deficiency Signs

Clinical signs of ascorbic acid deficiency are listed in Table 43-2. Fatigue, an early sign, is followed by small areas of hemorrhage (petechiae, ecchymoses, bleeding gums) and follicular hyperkeratosis. In children, gum bleeding can be associated with a pseudoparalysis (caused by pain) and irritability.

Serum vitamin C levels are highly specific for scurvy but not very sensitive and may be normal even in cases of severe vitamin C depletion. A level of 11 μmol/L or less supports the diagnosis of scurvy. Leukocyte and lymphocyte vitamin C levels offer a more accurate assessment of the true status of vitamin C stores because they are not affected by circadian rhythm or dietary changes.[55]

Reference levels of serum vitamin C measure around 23 to 85 μmol/L, with maximally achieved levels at about 200 μmol/L, as downregulation of SVCT1 in the gut and increased renal clearance limit the concentration of vitamin C in plasma. Leukocyte ascorbate is considered to reflect tissue stores more closely but is technically more difficult to assay. Although plasma vitamin C is predominantly found in the ascorbic acid form, leukocyte cell types also contain considerable dehydroascorbic acid. The different vitamin C stores in each leukocyte cell type, the possibility of artifactual interconversion of vitamin C forms, and the numerous assay methods used have led to widely divergent reference intervals for leukocytes. Measurement of urinary ascorbate is not recommended for status assessment because the value reflects recent intake and is subject to numerous analytical difficulties. Drugs known to increase the urinary excretion of ascorbate include aspirin, aminopyrine, barbiturates, hydantoins, and paraldehyde.

Lower plasma concentrations of ascorbic acid are seen frequently in patients on dialysis and are associated with increased cardiovascular mortality.[56] No reliable functional assessment of vitamin C status has yet been described.

Pathophysiology

Ascorbic acid requirements appear to be increased in chronic illness, as well as during pregnancy.

Toxicity and Therapeutic Uses

Although earlier reports of trials in which vitamin C supplementation was used to alter the outcome of malignant disease have not been confirmed, it was argued that sufficiently high blood concentrations have not been achieved. Although a high dose of oral vitamin C achieves plasma levels of only about 220 μmol/L, 5- to 100-fold higher concentrations are required to achieve a pro-oxidant effect that leads to selective killing of cancer cells.[57]

Although little toxicity is associated with this ascorbate, excess intake may interfere with metabolism of vitamin B_{12} and with drug actions (aminosalicylic acid, tricyclic antidepressants, and anticoagulants) and could lead to increased hydroxyl formation, which itself is a contributor to free radicals. A sudden discontinuation of megadose intake can result in rebound scurvy, which likely is the result of the induction of clearance mechanisms of vitamin C.

Intravenous vitamin C might prove helpful in mobilizing iron in patients on dialysis, because low vitamin C levels are common in dialysis patients[58]; several small trials have shown that patients supplemented with vitamin C exhibited better hemoglobin responses to erythropoietin, despite requiring smaller doses.[59]

Riboflavin (Vitamin B_2)

This highly pigmented yellow compound consists of flavin attached to D-ribitol. Its structure and that of its two cofactor-active forms, riboflavin 5′-phosphate (flavin mononucleotide [FMN]) and flavin adenine dinucleotide (FAD), are shown in Fig. 43-5. FAD, the most water-soluble of these three **flavins,** exhibits orange fluorescence, whereas the other two fluoresce greenish yellow. Aqueous solutions of flavins are stable to heat and oxidizing agents, but the riboflavin in milk is reduced dramatically on exposure to sunlight.

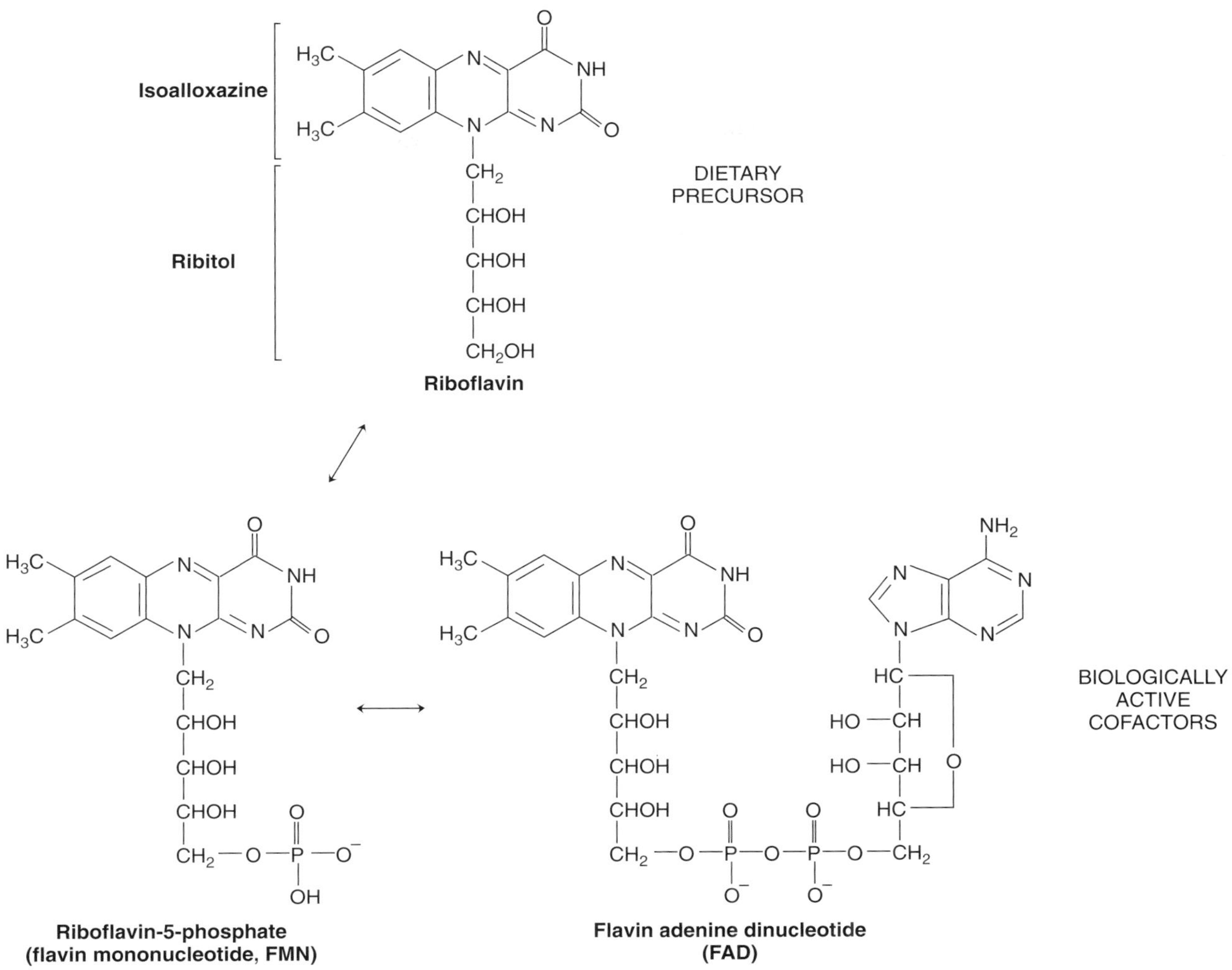

Fig. 43-5 Riboflavin and its active cofactor forms.

Foods high in riboflavin include milk, liver, eggs, meat, and some green leafy vegetables. Intestinal organisms also synthesize riboflavin.

Metabolism

Dietary protein complexes of FAD and FMN release these flavins on gastric acidification and proteolysis. After dephosphorylation, riboflavin is absorbed via sodium-independent carrier-mediated transport in the proximal small intestine and is rephosphorylated. A similar mechanism of uptake seems to be active in the colon.[60] Endocytic uptake into cells with the use of clathrin-coated pits has also been described and may contribute. Flavins then appear in the circulation weakly bound to albumin and other plasma proteins, including specific riboflavin-binding proteins. The liver and the kidneys quickly take up most flavins, although measurable amounts are found in most tissues. The liver is the main storage organ for riboflavin. The three flavin forms can be interconverted enzymatically. FAD is the predominant tissue form. Small amounts of flavin are excreted in bile, feces, sweat, and breast milk; urinary flavin excretion is greater. Flavin is excreted in urine, most often in free riboflavin form; the amount excreted depends on tissue stores and on the amount ingested. The body metabolizes only a small amount of ingested riboflavin. Riboflavin, but not FMN or FAD, is the moiety that is transferred from plasma into the brain. The flavins in blood are present primarily in the erythrocytes and function in the two FAD enzymes, glutathione reductase and methemoglobin reductase. The fetus obtains free riboflavin derived from maternal erythrocytic FAD through the placenta, which uses an endocytic mechanism.[61]

Function

The active vitamin B_2 compounds function as important cofactors for the large group of flavoproteins.[62] There are hundreds of flavoproteins; 1% to 3% of the genes of procariotes and eucariotes code for flavoproteins. These are used mainly in redox reactions that cover a large variety of functions. Riboflavin has key roles in respiratory enzymes such as D-amino acid oxidase, pyruvate dehydrogenase, xanthine oxidase, glutathione reductase, and NADH dehydrogenase. In addition, flavins are involved in the metabolism of iron, pyridoxine, and folate, and they play a role in protection against peroxidation, in metabolism of xenobiotics, and in

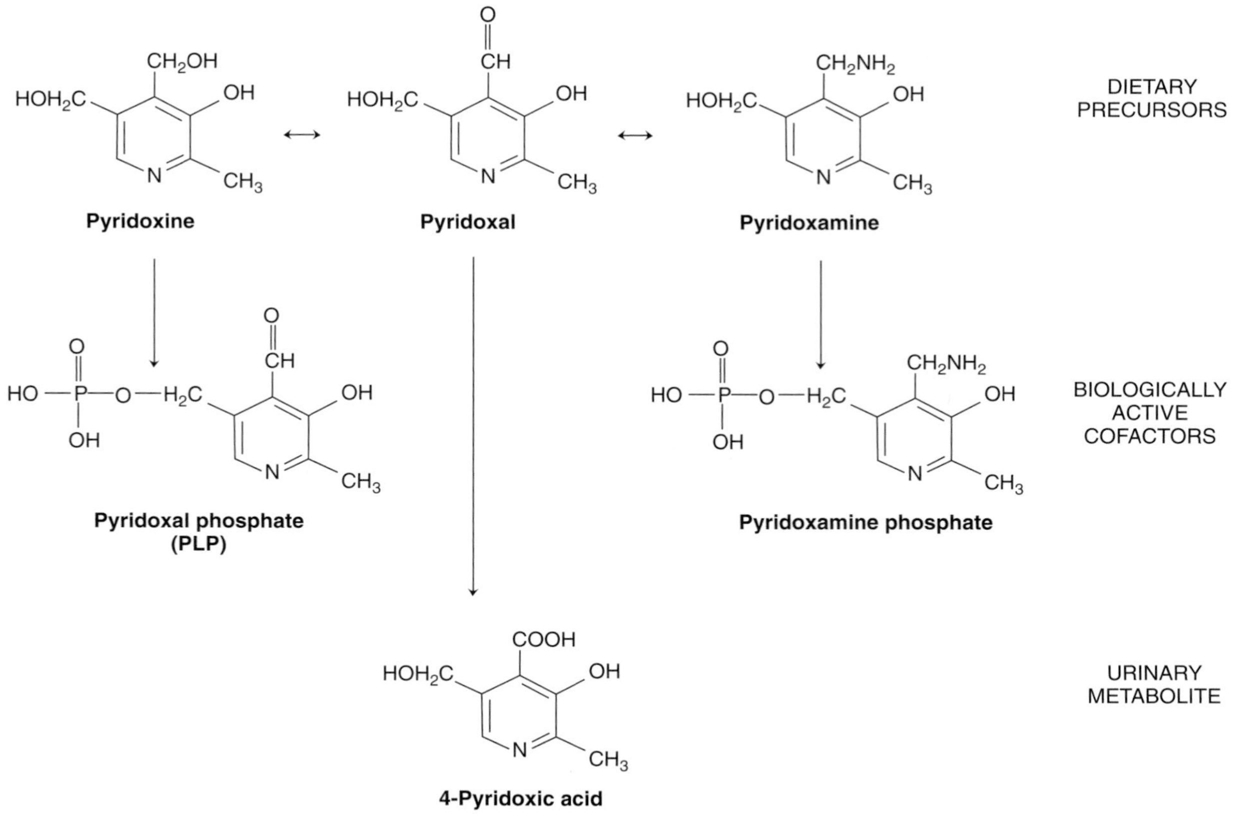

DIETARY PRECURSORS

Pyridoxine ⟷ **Pyridoxal** ⟷ **Pyridoxamine**

BIOLOGICALLY ACTIVE COFACTORS

Pyridoxal phosphate (PLP) **Pyridoxamine phosphate**

URINARY METABOLITE

4-Pyridoxic acid

Fig. 43-6 Vitamin B_6 forms and major metabolites.

superoxide generation by granulocytes. New flavoenzymes are implicated in biological processes such as nucleotide biosynthesis, protein folding, apoptosis, axon guidance, and chromatin remodeling.

Clinical and Chemical Deficiency Signs

Clinical signs of riboflavin deficiency are listed in Table 43-2. Erythrocytic concentrations of riboflavin, FMN, and FAD are more sensitive indices of riboflavin status than are flavin measurements in urine or plasma, but these blood indices are altered only late in the progression of deficiency. A functional approach to assessment of riboflavin status involves measurement of the increase in erythrocytic glutathione reductase (EGR) activity after in vitro addition of FAD (EGR index). This EGR index plateaus rapidly and does not continue to increase as deficiency progresses. In subjects deficient in glucose-6-phosphate dehydrogenase (G6PD), the EGR index is misleading because EGR does not lose its coenzyme even in severe riboflavin deficiency.[63]

Pathophysiology

A riboflavinosis is encountered most commonly when intake is inadequate as a result of poverty. American surveys have indicated inadequate riboflavin nutrition in up to 10% of children, up to 47% of teenagers, and up to 32% of geriatric subjects. Riboflavin deficiency can occur as a result of disease states that cause malnutrition (such as anorexia nervosa) or malabsorption (such as celiac disease or short bowel syndrome). Riboflavin and other nutrients are decreased in alcoholics. Riboflavin decomposition is accelerated by phototherapy for neonatal jaundice, but the induced deficiency does not appear to limit riboflavin-dependent fatty acid oxidation. Negative nitrogen balance, seen in all catabolic states (including stress, physical exertion, fasting, and prolonged bed rest), results in increased urinary riboflavin excretion. Riboflavin deficiency often occurs concomitantly with deficiencies of other B vitamins. Additionally, riboflavin interacts in metabolic processes involving other vitamins. These interactions therefore can result in a mixed clinical picture and may explain how therapy with one vitamin may improve symptoms of another vitamin deficiency. Treatment with riboflavin might help in some rare mitochondrial β-oxidation defects and in patients with HIV who are treated with zidovudine and develop lactic acidosis.[64]

Pyridoxine (Vitamin B_6)

Vitamin B_6 is known chemically as pyridoxine. Pyridoxal and pyridoxamine are metabolites that were first identified through vitamin activity; then their phosphorylated forms were recognized as active cofactors. The structure is shown as pyridoxal phosphate (PLP) in Fig. 43-6. Pyridoxine occurs mainly in plants, whereas pyridoxal and pyridoxamine are present primarily in animal products. These three pyridine derivatives are interconverted metabolically.

Major dietary sources of vitamin B_6 include meat, poultry, fish, potatoes, and vegetables; dairy products and grains contribute lesser amounts. The predominant food form is PLP, which is readily lost in food processing.

Metabolism

Pyridoxine does not bind to plasma proteins; pyridoxal and PLP bind mainly to albumin. Erythrocytes rapidly take up pyridoxine, convert it to PLP and pyridoxal, and then release pyridoxal into plasma. Metabolism of pyridoxal appears to occur primarily in the liver with formation of 4-pyridoxic acid, which is excreted in urine (see Fig. 43-6). PLP synthesis depends on a flavin enzyme, which coordinates riboflavin and pyridoxine nutrition. Vitamin B_6 concentration is high in the brain and in the CSF; the nonphosphorylated forms enter the CSF, choroid plexus, and brain.

Function

PLP is the active metabolite that interacts as a cofactor with a variety of enzyme-catalyzed reactions involving transformations of amino acids; the major exception is seen in the phosphorylases. Decarboxylation, transamination, and racemization reactions depend on pyridoxine. Pyridoxine cofactor forms act in more than 60 different enzyme systems, catalyzing a variety of reaction types, including the clinically relevant transaminases aspartate aminotransferase (AST) and alanine aminotransferase (ALT). The best known functions of the pyridoxine cofactors are their roles in the conversion of tryptophan to 5-hydroxytryptamine (serotonin) and in the separate pathway of tryptophan to nicotinic acid ribonucleotide (the "niacin pathway"), both of which are shown in Fig. 43-7.

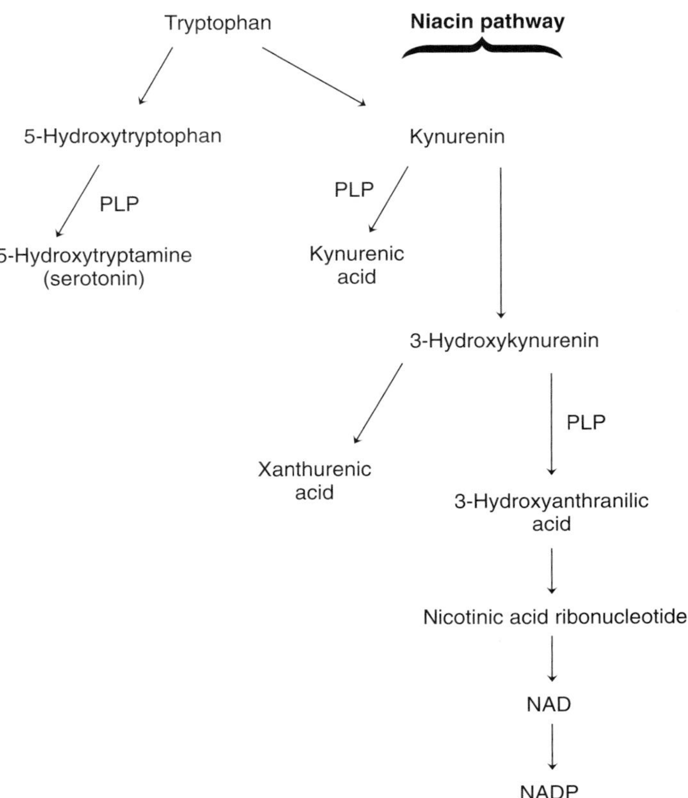

Fig. 43-7 Role of vitamin B_6 in tryptophan metabolism. *NAD,* Nicotinamide adenine dinucleotide; *NADP,* nicotinamide adenine dinucleotide phosphate; *PLP,* pyridoxal phosphate.

Clinical and Chemical Deficiency Signs

Clinical signs of pyridoxine deficiency for infants and adults are listed in Table 43-2. Chemical indices of pyridoxine depletion include reduction in plasma and erythrocyte concentrations of pyridoxine or pyridoxal phosphate. Urinary pyridoxine (usually representing less than 10% of the pyridoxine intake) and pyridoxic acid, the major urinary metabolite, are also reduced. An oral tryptophan load given to persons suspected of being deficient in pyridoxine results in excretion of several tryptophan metabolites in higher amounts than usual; xanthurenic acid is the one that is measured most commonly (see Fig. 43-7). The involvement of other metabolic and hormonal factors in this pathway necessitates cautious interpretation of the tryptophan challenge test.

The tissue status of pyridoxal phosphate can be assessed by measurement of the increase in erythrocytic aspartate (or alanine) aminotransferase activity (AST or ALT, respectively) after in vitro addition of the pyridoxal phosphate cofactor. Elevation in the ratio of activity plus or minus pyridoxal phosphate (the EAST index) is suggestive of inadequate tissue stores. Plasmas from healthy subjects primarily contain pyridoxal phosphate and 4-pyridoxic acid with lesser amounts of pyridoxal. All the known B_6 vitamins can be measured simultaneously by HPLC. Of the direct measures of B_6 status, plasma pyridoxal phosphate currently is considered most reflective of tissue status. Measurement of plasma pyridoxal phosphate and urinary 4-pyridoxic acid and an indirect measure (the EAST index or urinary xanthurenic acid) are all recommended for evaluation of B_6 status.

Pathophysiology

Conditions that may affect pyridoxine concentrations in the body include celiac disease, ulcerative colitis, lactation, and alcoholism. Certain mental illnesses such as psychoses and schizophrenia in the past have been associated with pyridoxine deficiency; however, to what extent this is simply an associated finding of individuals who have marginal or deficient nutritional intake is uncertain. Pyridoxine requirements increase during pregnancy as a result of fetal demand and hormonal induction of maternal enzymes, which increases maternal requirements. Pyridoxine inadequacy during pregnancy has been linked to suboptimal birth outcomes (infants with low Apgar scores and low birth weight); however, evidence is insufficient to suggest that pyridoxine supplementation should be recommended in normal pregnancies.[65]

Drugs known to antagonize pyridoxine include isonicotinic acid hydrazide (isoniazid, INH), steroids, and penicillamine. Isoniazid combines with pyridoxine to form a hydrazone, which is not available for enzymatic reactions. Because hepatic enzymes dependent on pyridoxine as a cofactor can be inactivated, liver function is monitored during isoniazid therapy. The vitamin B_6 compounds are considered to be of low systemic toxicity, although toxicity has been reported with high dosages. Pyridoxine now is regarded as a first-line treatment to control hyperemesis gravidarum; no evidence of any teratogenic effect has been found.[66] However, pyridoxine deficiency in pregnancy does confer teratogenic risk. In rare forms of early childhood seizures, pyridoxine supplementation is required to control the epilepsy. These disorders are due to disturbed neurotransmitter formation and breakdown.[67]

Niacin (Vitamin B_3)

Pellagra (from the Italian, meaning "rough skin") is associated with diarrhea, dementia, and dermatitis (the "three D's") and has been attributed to poor diet for more than two centuries. In 1912, nicotinic acid was extracted from rice polishings and was claimed to have vitamin-like effects, but it was not until 1935 that nicotinic acid (also called niacin) was shown to cure black tongue in dogs (a disease similar to pellagra in humans).

Niacin is a simple derivative of pyridine and is extremely stable. The active cofactor forms of NAD and NADP (Fig. 43-8) derived from niacin can also be synthesized in situ from tryptophan (see Fig. 43-7), and so sufficient dietary tryptophan can abolish the requirement for niacin. This makes niacin relatively unique with respect to the other vitamins in that we are only partially dependent on diet for a direct source. Sources of niacin include meats and grains, as well as many food products that are supplemented with this vitamin. Corn is especially poor in tryptophan, and part of the niacin in corn is not bioavailable. Pellagra continues to be prevalent in areas with high reliance on maize products.[68]

It has been noted that high levels of dietary leucine somehow interfere with niacin pathways. The niacin equivalent of tryptophan is approximately 60 mg of tryptophan, which equals 1 mg of niacin. The typical diet consists of approximately 600 mg of tryptophan, which is not sufficient to meet the nutritional needs for niacin in all adults.

Metabolism

Both niacin and nicotinamide are readily absorbed in the gut. Niacin is transported in blood, mainly in erythrocytes. Little storage of niacin occurs in the body, and urine contains nicotinamide and other metabolites of niacin (see Fig. 43-8). Plasma nicotinamide readily enters the CSF, whereas niacin does not. Brain tissue does not express the niacin pathway of tryptophan and so must use plasma nicotinamide from the diet or dephosphorylated forms of the cofactors.

Function

NAD and NADP are involved in a large number of oxidation-reduction reactions catalyzed by dehydrogenases, including alcohol, glutamate, glucose-6-phosphate, and glycerol-3-phosphate dehydrogenases. Reduction yields dihydronicotinamide (NADH or NADPH), which has a strong absorption at 340 nm—a feature widely used in assays of **pyridine nucleotide**–dependent enzymes (see Chapter 15). Apart from the reactions where NAD/NADP are recycled from NADH/NADPH, a number of reactions use up the cofactors. Examples include reactions that break the bond between the nicotinamide and the ADPribose.

Clinical and Chemical Deficiency Signs

Clinical signs of niacin deficiency are listed in Table 43-2. Diagnosis of niacin deficiency is usually made with a careful evaluation of the patient's socioeconomic and behavioral status in addition to the clinical picture. Niacin deficiency usually does not occur in isolation, and other nutritional deficits also will be present. One exception is carcinoid tumors, in which tryptophan is metabolized preferentially to serotonin and is not available for NAD formation. In carcinoid, the frequency of pellagra has been found to be increased.[69] The diagnosis of niacin deficiency usually can be confirmed with treatment. Biochemical detection of niacin deficiency usually is not necessary, although niacin and several metabolites can be detected in biological fluids. Chemical measures of niacin status primarily involve the two major urinary metabolites N′-methylnicotinamide and N′-methyl-2-pyridone-5-carboxylamide. The ratio of the 2-pyridone compound to N′-methylnicotinamide is reduced in niacin deficiency; reduction in the individual metabolites is also seen. In contrast to earlier reports, low NAD and NADP concentrations are not helpful.[70]

For some time, pharmacological doses of niacin have been recognized as an efficacious means of reducing mixed dyslipidemias while increasing HDLs. Increased lipoprotein a, or Lp(a), is also treatable with niacin. The effect of niacin is mediated via the nicotinic acid receptor. This has been identified as an orphan receptor called GPR109A, which is linked through G_i to inhibition of the adenylate cyclase. It is expressed in fat cells and in various immune cells.[71]

Large doses of niacin are associated with gastrointestinal discomfort and flushing; however, it is hoped that newer drug combinations and sustained-release niacin preparations that can be taken at bedtime will reduce these side effects and enhance compliance.

Thiamine (Vitamin B_1)

Thiamine consists of a pyrimidine linked by a methylene group to a substituted thiazole (Fig. 43-9). Thus the name reflects its components of amine and sulfur (thia-) groups. Highly water-soluble, thiamine is easily leached out of foodstuffs when they are being washed or boiled.

Sources of thiamine include yeast, wheat, whole grain and enriched breads and cereals, nuts, peas, potatoes, and most vegetables. In Western society, alcoholics experience thiamine deficiency most often, although the elderly and individuals with psychiatric disorders also may be at risk. Outbreaks of thiamine deficiency in prison and detention populations with poor dietary intake continue to be reported.[72]

Metabolism

Dietary thiamine is absorbed in the intestine by a pH-dependent, carrier-mediated process that is saturated at an

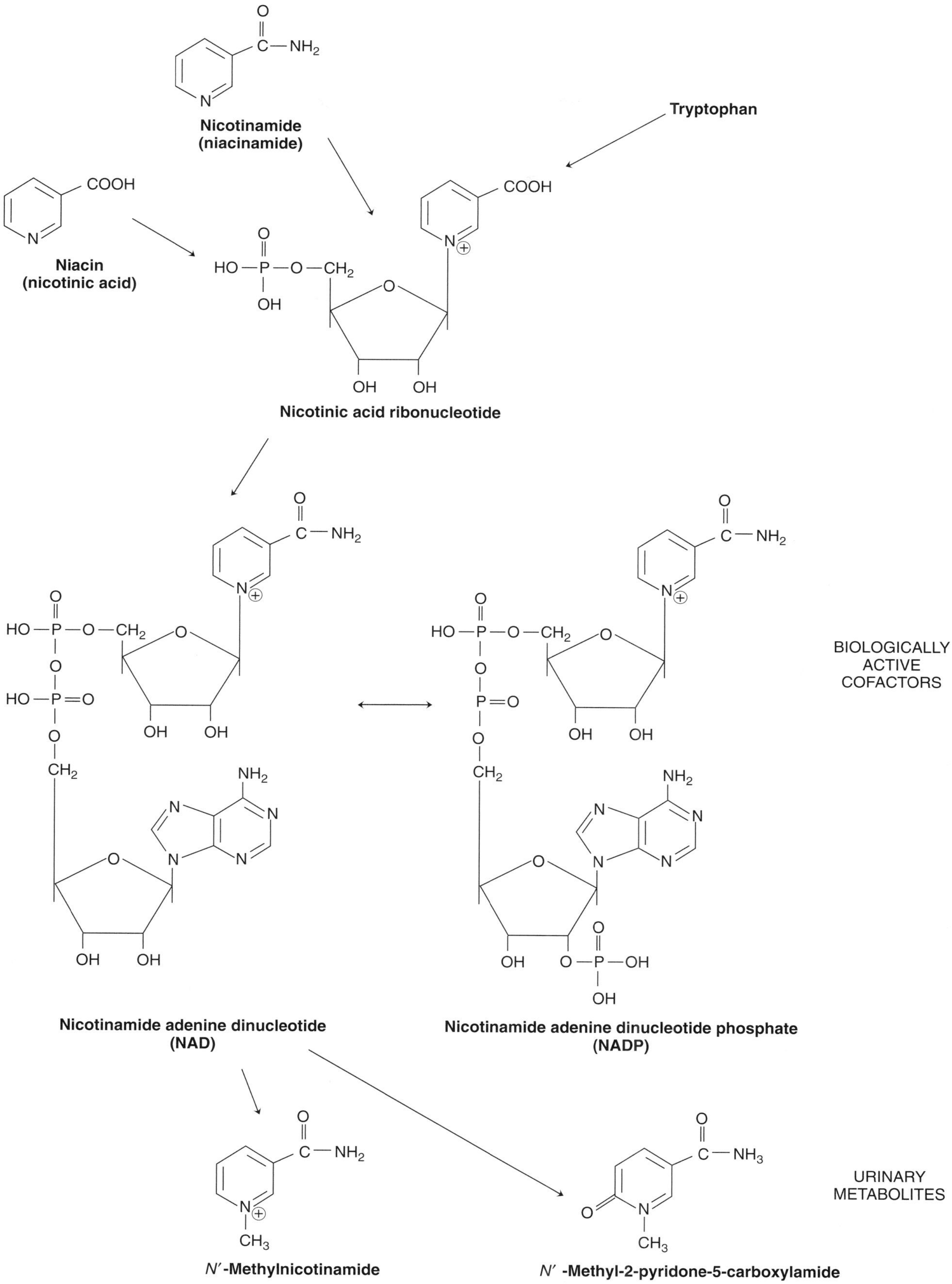

Fig. 43-8 Cofactor forms and metabolites derived from niacin or tryptophan.

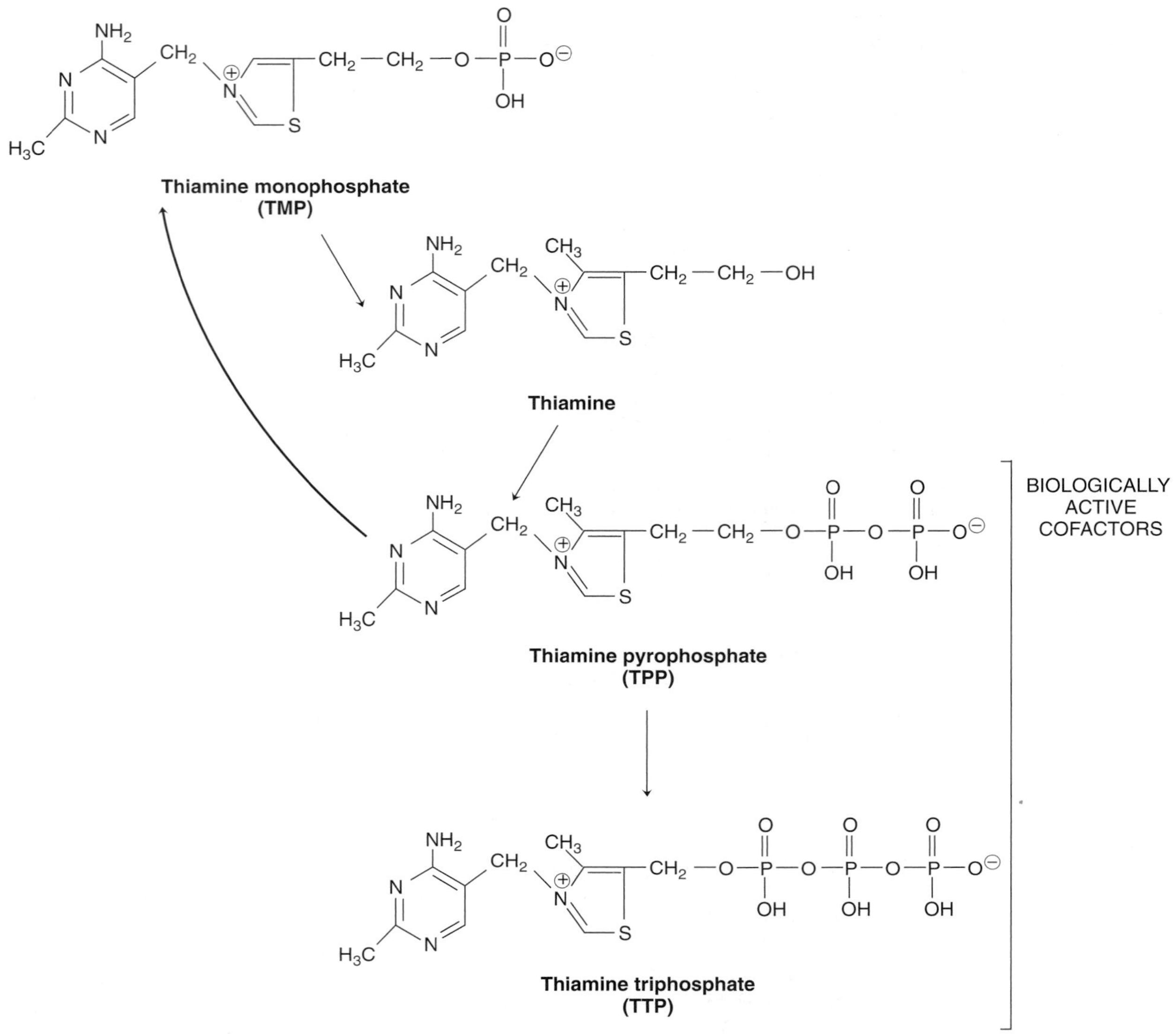

Thiamine monophosphate (TMP)

Thiamine

Thiamine pyrophosphate (TPP)

Thiamine triphosphate (TTP)

BIOLOGICALLY ACTIVE COFACTORS

Fig. 43-9 Thiamine and its cofactor forms.

oral intake of about 10 mg. In plasma, it is bound to albumin. Phosphorylation in the tissues generates thiamine monophosphate (TMP), thiamine diphosphate (also called thiamine pyrophosphate-TPP), and thiamine triphosphate (TTP). TPP is the predominant moiety in tissues, whereas the major form in plasma is thiamine. The mechanism of thiamine transport has been clarified with the cloning of transporters SLC 19A1, -2, and -3 and SLC 25A19.[73] SLC 19A2 and SLC 19A3 are involved in absorption of thiamine from the gut and reabsorption from the kidney. Absence of SLC 19A2 in humans leads to a thiamine-responsive megaloblastic anemia without the CNS complications of thiamine deficiency.[74] SLC 19A1 is a reduced folate carrier that also transports TMP, although with lower affinity than the other carriers. Concentrations of thiamine in the CNS are similar to those in plasma, and thiamine crosses the blood-brain barrier through facilitated diffusion and the choroid plexus, likely with the use of active transport, possibly involving SLC 19A3. In addition, mitochondrial uptake is mediated by SLC 25A19.[75]

Sequestration of thiamine occurs at saturable levels as TPP in tissue is reflected in the differential between erythrocyte and plasma concentrations of this vitamin. Tissues such as liver, heart, and brain have higher concentrations than muscle and other organs.

Function

In its TPP cofactor form, thiamine catalyzes the decarboxylation of α-keto acids (pyruvate and α-ketoglutarate), the oxidative decarboxylation by α-keto acid dehydrogenases, and the formation of ketols. TPP functions in major carbohydrate pathways and in the metabolism of branched chain amino acids. Thiamine triphosphate (TTP) is involved in nerve membrane conduction (Na^+ gating).

Clinical Deficiency Signs

Table 43-2 lists the major clinical signs of thiamine deficiency. The **Wernicke-Korsakoff syndrome** responds to thiamine therapy, and evidence of an abnormality of neurotransmitter metabolism, perhaps involving TTP, has been found. These patients typically accumulate excessive amounts of pyruvate and lactate in physiological fluids.

Genetic variations in TPP-dependent enzymes modify the effects of dietary thiamine deficiency. Although most patients with thiamine deficiency do not develop Wernicke-Korsakoff syndrome, mild deficiency leads to impairment in higher integrative functions (including memory). More severe deficiency leads to **dry beriberi** or **wet beriberi** (see Table 43-1).

Chemical Deficiency Signs

Chemical indices of thiamine deficiency that are commonly used include reduction in urinary thiamine, reduction in erythrocyte transketolase (ETK) activity, and stimulation of ETK by in vitro TPP. Prolonged deficiency results in decreased synthesis of the ETK apoenzyme, and so the ETK stimulation test may underestimate the magnitude of deficiency. Evidence of reduction in ETK has been found in undernutrition, diabetes, and liver disease, without a TPP stimulation effect. As is possible with all proteins, the genetic heterogeneity of ETK has been demonstrated in humans. Correlation between ETK stimulation and dietary thiamine or clinical signs is not always seen. HPLC can be used to measure thiamine and its metabolites and has been shown to correlate with the ETK assay.[76] Recently, a rapid whole blood assay that uses HPLC has been described that allows separation of thiamine and its metabolites.[77]

Pathophysiology

The clinical manifestations of thiamine deficiency depend on the degree of depletion. Mild thiamine deficiency is common among elderly persons and alcoholics. Cardiovascular disease associated with thiamine deficiency is relatively common in the elderly and chronic alcoholics. Less commonly, pregnant women are susceptible to a form of cardiac failure that typically presents with high cardiac output, which is corrected readily with the administration of thiamine. Paradoxically, thiamine deficiency can be precipitated by furosemide therapy for edema.[78] Cardiac failure precipitated or exacerbated by furosemide therapy should be treated empirically with thiamine. Magnesium deficiency, which is commonly encountered in alcoholics, impairs thiamine activation. This can exacerbate Wernicke's encephalopathy in the already thiamine-depleted alcoholic. Wernicke's encephalopathy is also common in patients with AIDS, those with cancer, and patients who have undergone gastric bypass. It has also been described after bariatric surgery to affect weight loss. Wernicke's encephalopathy is recognized in only about 15% of cases premortem and is characterized by confusion, ataxia, and ophthalmoplegia.[79]

This disorder is so common among alcoholics that preventative treatment with intravenous thiamine often is given at hospital admission without clear clinical signs of the disorder. In four cases of Wernicke's encephalopathy, a primary respiratory alkalosis together with primary lactic acidosis has been described and might prove helpful in the diagnosis.[80] After acute presentation with Wernicke's encephalopathy, up to 80% of these patients will develop the Korsakoff syndrome. This psychiatric disorder is characterized by short-term memory loss and learning deficits. Confabulation (misleading statements) occurs to compensate for the memory loss. Leigh disease, a necrotizing encephalopathy of childhood, is associated with decreased brain TTP. Leigh disease is a congenital disorder of oxidative phosphorylation that results in lesions in numerous areas of the brain, including the brain stem, optic nerve, and thalamic region. The disease may present early in childhood, with gait problems progressing to severe neurological deterioration. Defects in at least three enzymes—pyruvate dehydrogenase, pyruvate carboxylase, and cytochrome c oxidase—are associated with Leigh disease. The common feature is that thiamine-dependent oxidative pathways are affected. Treatment can include high-dose thiamine, lipoic acid, and creatine.

The time course to thiamine deficiency with a thiamine-deficient diet is relatively short, although the development of deficiency could be predicted only under controlled experimental conditions. Groups susceptible to unrecognized thiamine deficiency include chronically ill children (those receiving nasogastric feeding or intensive chemotherapy or receiving intensive care for a period of weeks) and individuals who are experiencing chronic vomiting or a behaviorally based eating disorder. Patients who are administered carbohydrates or who are treated for hyperglycemia are at risk for thiamine deficiency (as a result of thiamine consumption that occurs in normal carbohydrate metabolism). Those most at risk are patients who are already nutritionally compromised.

Biotin (Vitamin H)

The water-soluble coenzyme, biotin (structure shown in Fig. 43-10), was discovered through administration to rats of experimental diets that consisted of raw egg whites. The cause of biotin deficiency in this diet was **avidin,** a heat-labile component of egg white that binds with biotin in one of the

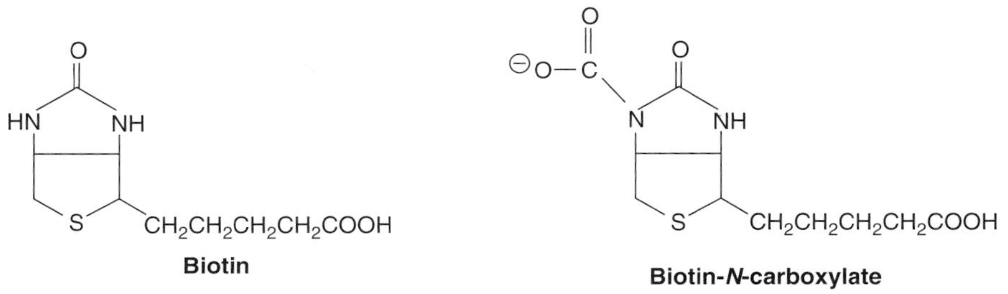

O
HN NH
S $CH_2CH_2CH_2CH_2COOH$
Biotin

O
⊖O—C
O
N NH
S $CH_2CH_2CH_2CH_2COOH$
Biotin-*N*-carboxylate

Fig. 43-10 Biotin and its active form.

highest noncovalent associations known. The presence of avidin prevents biotin from being absorbed. Numerous foods contain biotin, although no one food is especially rich (up to 2 mg/100 g).

Metabolism

Dietary protein–bound biotin is released during degradation of ingested food by the enzyme biotininase. Biotin then is absorbed via the sodium-dependent multivitamin transporter (SMVT), which it shares with the vitamin pantothenic acid and the metabolic substrate lipoate. Uptake occurs primarily in the proximal half of the small intestine. Bacteria in the colon generate a significant amount of free biotin, and a similar uptake exists in the colon.[81] Biotin circulates in blood largely bound to plasma proteins. Forms of excreted biotin in urine include bisnorbiotin, bisnorbiotin methyl ketone, biotin sulfoxide, and biotin sulfone. Little else is known about the catabolic pathways of this cofactor. Uptake into lymphocytes occurs with 100-fold higher concentrations that involve the monocarboxylate transporter 1 (MCT1).

Function

Biotin acts as a coenzyme, participating in the metabolic pathways of gluconeogenesis, fatty acid synthesis, and amino acid catabolism. D-Biotin is the only active isomer. Biotin functions as a prosthetic group for carboxylation and carboxyl exchange reactions. Important enzymes include acetyl CoA, propionyl CoA, and the pyruvate carboxylases, as well as methylmalonyl-oxaloacetic transcarboxylase. In addition, biotin affects the expression of a large number of genes, many of them associated with cell signaling. The enzyme biotinidase has been shown to have biotin transferase activity, in addition to its hydrolase activity. Biotin, which has been observed covalently attached to the nuclear histone proteins, downregulates protein transcription of specific genes.

Clinical and Clinical Deficiency Signs

Pure biotin deficiency is extremely rare. Table 43-2 lists the major signs of biotin deficiency. In recent years, interest in mild and borderline biotin deficiency has been increasing.

Dietary deficiency is accompanied by decreased urinary and plasma biotin and increased urinary organic acids, indicating functional deficiency of β-methylcrotonyl CoA carboxylase and propionyl CoA carboxylase. A lymphocyte assay that measures propionyl-CoA carboxylase has been described as very sensitive in experimentally induced biotin deficiency.[82]

Genetic alterations in these carboxylases may result in biotin-dependent states that cause a high anion gap metabolic acidosis and require pharmacological biotin doses; these enzyme deficiencies are confirmed in leukocytes. Genetic deficiency of biotinidase, which can be detected by a blood spot assay, is treated with biotin.

Pathophysiology

With proper modern nutrition, biotin deficiencies are extremely rare. However, biotin deficiency might be suspected in newborns on special diets, in patients receiving long-term total parenteral nutrition, and occasionally in individuals who practice unusual eating habits, such as the ingestion of raw eggs. Apparent biotin deficiency also occurs with inherited metabolic disorders of biotin metabolism. Biotinidase deficiency and holocarboxylase synthetase deficiency are autosomal recessive disorders that prevent the completion of biotin-dependent pathways.

Pantothenic Acid (Vitamin B_5)

Pantothenic acid is the precursor to 4′-phosphopantothenine, a cofactor that is indispensable in fatty acid metabolism. The vitamin is widely distributed in foods including liver and other organ meats, milk, eggs, peanuts, legumes, mushrooms, salmon, and whole grains. Although many organisms are capable of synthesizing pantothenic acid, no evidence suggests that intestinal microorganisms are responsible for part of the human daily requirement of this cofactor.

Metabolism

As shown in Fig. 43-11, pantothenate is metabolically converted to 4′-phosphopantothenine, which becomes covalently bound to either serum acyl carrier protein (ACP) or to coenzyme A. Little is known about pantothenate metabolism. Urinary excretion of pantothenate decreases with experimental deficiencies. Free pantothenate is the major form in both urine and serum, whereas coenzyme A is the major erythrocytic form.

Function

Coenzyme A is an important acyl group transfer coenzyme that is involved in a large number of reactions of a great variety of reaction types. Acyl derivatives of coenzyme A are formed first (by thioester linkage), followed by transfer of the acyl group to an acceptor molecule.

Clinical and Chemical Deficiency Signs

No clear-cut case of a pantothenate deficiency has been reported; Table 43-2 lists clinical signs observed in experimentally induced deficiencies. Cellular levels of coenzyme A remain unchanged in pantothenate deficiency, indicating a pantothenate-conserving process that minimizes the effects of reduced nutritional intake.

Pathophysiology

Low urinary excretion and reduced blood levels of pantothenate have been reported in patients with chronic malnutrition and alcoholism. Pantothene deficiency has been seen in severe malnutrition and famine. The clinical significance of pure pantothenate deficiency is unclear. No toxicity from increased intake is known.

Cobalamin (Vitamin B_{12})

Vitamin B_{12}, as an isolate from liver extracts, was shown to reverse some forms of pernicious anemia. Another compound isolated from leafy vegetables was shown to reverse other types of macrocytic anemia. Purification of this substance led to its identification as pteroylglutamic acid, more commonly known

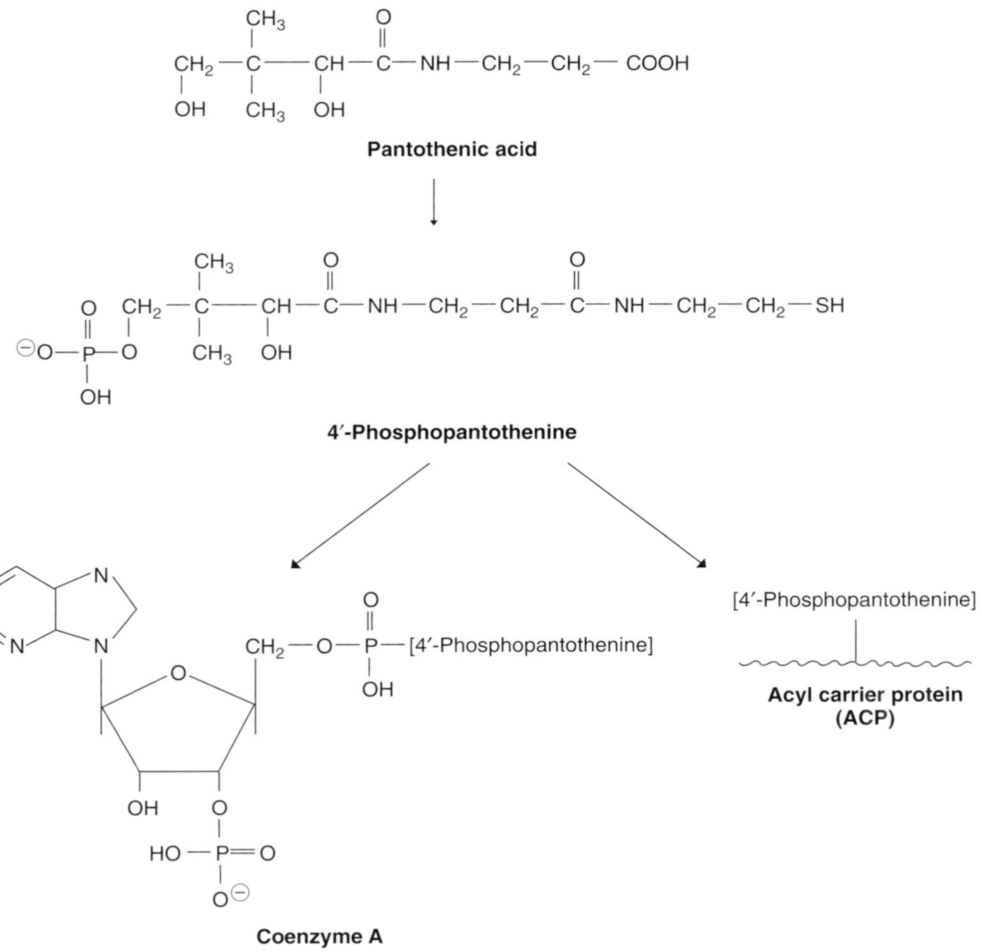

Fig. 43-11 Pantothenic acid and its active cofactors.

as folic acid. Thus similar clinical symptoms were found to result from deficiencies of two totally different structures (Figs. 43-12 and 43-13), neither of which could replace the other. The clinical similarities of deficiency and the metabolic interactions of vitamin B_{12} and folic acid usually dictate their simultaneous assessment. This is of particular importance when one or the other vitamin is administered because methyl trapping, that is, sequestration of folate, can occur when cobalamin (vitamin B_{12}) is administered. Conversely, symptoms of cobalamin deficiency can be masked by folate administration.

Vitamin B_{12} (see Fig. 43-12), which has the most complex structure of all the vitamins, is characterized by a central cobalt ion with a surrounding corrin ring (containing pyrroles similar to porphyrin). Different cobalamins are distinguished by different substituents in the R-position linked to the central cobalt. In humans, methylcobalamin and 5′-deoxyadenosylcobalamin are the only two coenzyme forms.

Humans are not able to synthesize vitamin B_{12} and require dietary intake. Sources of vitamin B_{12} are primarily of animal origin (meat, dairy products, eggs). Total vegetarian diets therefore are likely settings for deficiency. The average daily diet contains 3 to 30 μg of vitamin B_{12}, of which 1 to 5 μg is absorbed in normal individuals. The frequency of vitamin B_{12} deficiency increases with age, and because of significant body stores (1 to 5 mg) and an efficient enterohepatic recycling mechanism, it might take many years for an individual to develop B_{12} deficiency. Although strictly defined, pernicious anemia is present in about 2% to 4% of the elderly population,[83] decreased cobalamin levels are seen in up to a quarter of this group.[84] In these studies of vitamin B_{12} deficiency, decreased levels of vitamin B_{12} and elevated metabolites as a consequence of vitamin B_{12} deficiency were used as indicators of B_{12} deficiency, rather than the development of clinical complications.

Absorption

Vitamin B_{12} absorption involves three related proteins with very high affinity for cobalamin: haptocorrin, intrinsic factor (IF), and transcobalamin.[85] Haptocorrin (previously called R-binder) is present in saliva and binds available cobalamin (Fig. 43-14). Acidification of the stomach content is required to release cobalamin from exogenous binding proteins and allow it to bind to haptocorrin, which is produced along with intrinsic factor by the gastric parietal cells. A significant amount of B_{12} bound to haptocorrin is also secreted in bile. In the duodenum, pancreatic proteases digest haptocorrin and make B_{12} available for binding to IF, which is not degraded. The IF-B_{12} complex is transported further through the ileum and is bound to specific receptors (a complex of the two

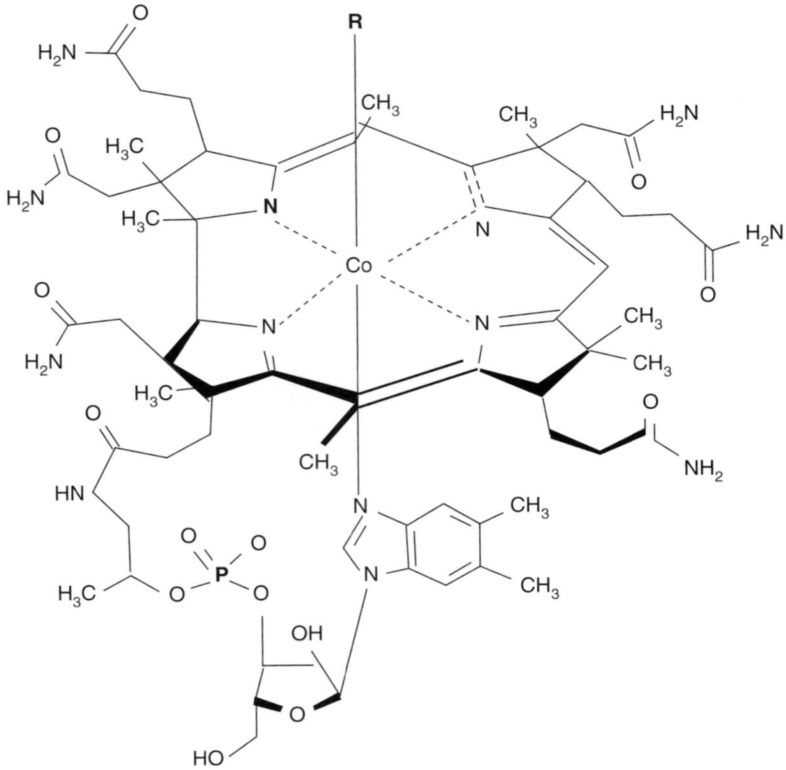

Fig. 43-12 Active vitamin B_{12} forms in humans: R = CH_3 (methylcobalamin) and R = 5′-Deoxyadenosine (deoxyadenosylcobalamine).

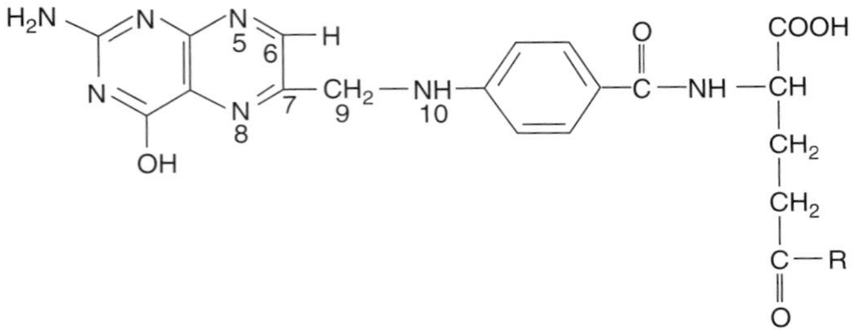

Fig. 43-13 Structure of folic acid.

proteins, cubilin and amnionless) present on intestinal cells in the final 80 cm of the ileum.[86] After **endocytosis,** the IF is degraded and cobalamin is bound to transcobalamin for transport in serum. IF antibodies are present in classical pernicious anemia; they prevent binding of vitamin B_{12} to IF and absorption through the ileal receptor. Parietal cell antibodies have also been identified as a cause of pernicious anemia.

About 75% of circulating vitamin B_{12} is bound to haptocorrin. Haptocorrin seems to bind cobalamin that becomes available upon cell death. However, haptocorrin-bound vitamin B_{12} is only taken up in the liver and is not available to tissues such as bone marrow and other cells. The physiologically important fraction of vitamin B_{12} seems to be bound to transcobalamin, and this complex (holotranscobalamin) is taken up by a receptor-mediated mechanism.[87] The structure of the transcobalamin-cobalamin complex has recently been resolved.[88]

Functions

In contrast to bacteria, in mammals only two distinct roles for cobalamin are known. The deoxyadenosylcobalamin form (AdoCbl) is a cofactor for the mitochondrial enzyme methylmalonyl CoA mutase, which is responsible for the conversion of methylmalonyl CoA to succinyl CoA. This enzyme is required for metabolism of odd numbered and branched fatty acids (β-oxidation metabolizes two C-groups at each cycle) and for conversion of the three-carbon-group (methylmalonic acid) to succinyl-CoA for further metabolism in the Krebs cycle. An absolute deficiency of cobalamin or a congenital lack of the enzyme results in accumulation of the intermediate methylmalonyl-CoA and subsequent hydrolysis to methylmalonic acid (MMA). MMA elevation is thought to be specific for vitamin B_{12} deficiency, although renal failure also increases the levels. The second important reaction involves methylcobalamin (MeCbl) and occurs in the cytoplasm. MeCbl functions as a methyl donor for methionine synthase. A deficiency of MeCbl leads to accumulation of homocysteine, the precursor to methionine (see also Fig. 43-15). A lack of functional methionine synthase or methionine synthase reductase causes an accumulation of homocysteine. Folate deficiency also causes accumulation of homocysteine in that methyltetrahydrofolate is responsible for the de novo methylation of cobalamin to sustain the reaction. Methionine, obtained from remethylated homocysteine, is necessary for the generation of adenosylmethionine, which bears a high-energy methyl group and participates in more than 100 intracellular reactions. Notably, intact DNA synthesis requires adequate methylation activity to ensure the incorporation of thymidine and not uridine. Insertion of uridine into the DNA double strand increases the need for DNA repair, placing the organism at increased risk for flawed DNA replication. Dietary deficiency of the precursor of these two coenzyme forms results in deficiencies of both active cobalamins. Genetic deficiencies of

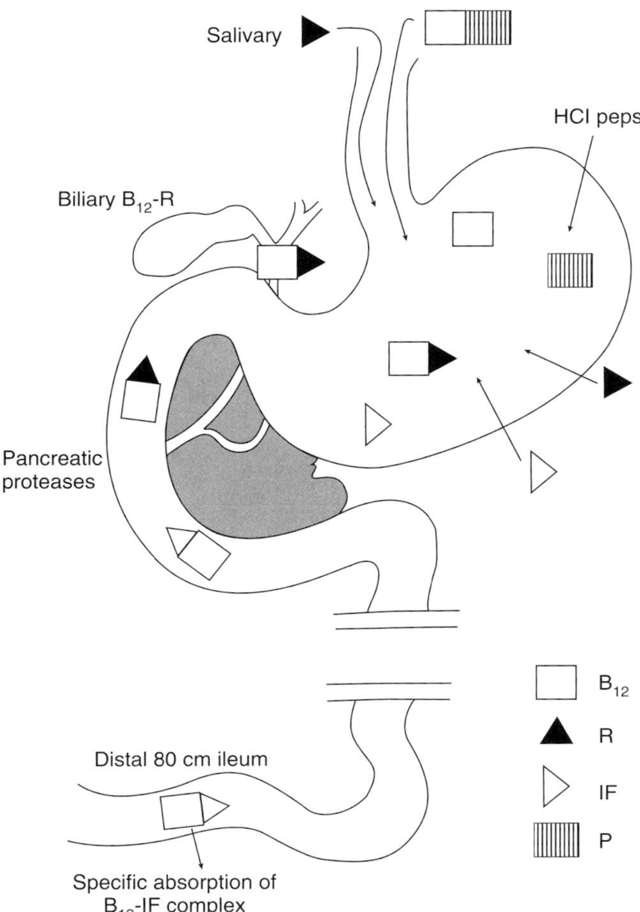

Fig. 43-14 Absorption of dietary vitamin B_{12}: *R,* Haptocorrin; *IF,* intrinsic factor; *P,* exogenous binding proteins.

enzymes in either pathway are known. In the few case reports of inherited deficiency of transcobalamin, symptoms of pancytopenia and failure to thrive developed within a few months of birth.

Diagnostic Testing and Deficiency

Table 43-2 lists signs of vitamin B_{12} deficiency. Diagnostic tests for vitamin B_{12} deficiency today mainly include immunoassays on automated platforms; microbiological or radioligand assay methods are no longer used. In addition, measurement of urinary or serum methylmalonic acid or total homocysteine, as well as the Schilling test, may be helpful, as may be the measurement of intrinsic factor antibodies or parietal cell antibodies. In many countries, the Schilling test, which uses radioactively labeled vitamin B_{12}, is no longer available. Measurement of holotranscobalamin, the biologically available fraction of vitamin B_{12}, has been claimed to be superior to vitamin B_{12} measurement.[89]

Early serum B_{12} competitive-binding methods used B_{12} binders with variable purity and binding specificity, yielding unreliable results; numerous reports have described cobalamin deficiency in patients with normal serum cobalamin concentrations. However, even with the use of modern vitamin B_{12} assays, patients can have levels in the low part of the reference interval and still have pernicious anemia.[90] In addition, patients with a clinical response to vitamin B_{12} therapy (in their neuropathy) may have normal vitamin B_{12} levels.[91] Analysis of serum methylmalonic acid concentration by gas chromatography-mass spectrometry (GC-MS) appears to be a more sensitive and specific indicator of cobalamin deficiency than are direct measures of serum cobalamin, even though response to vitamin B_{12} has been shown in the absence of ele-

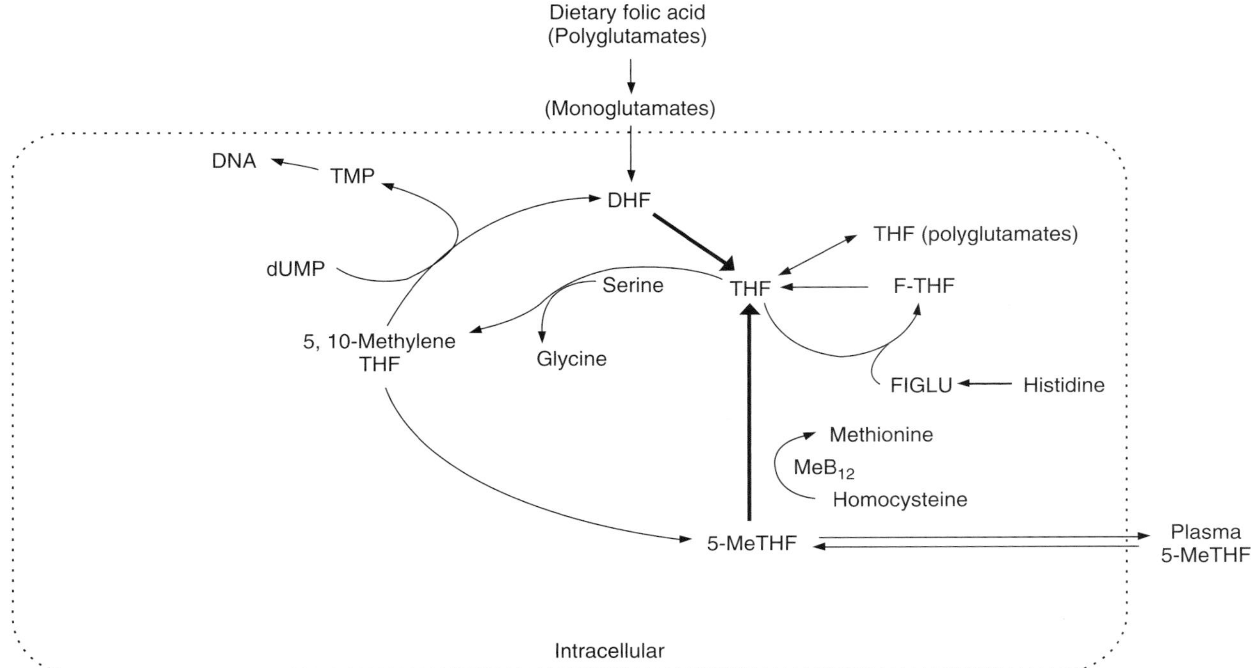

Fig. 43-15 One-carbon transfer with the use of folic acid forms as cofactors. *DHF,* Dihydrofolate; *DNA,* deoxyribonucleic acid; *dUMP,* deoxyuridine monophosphate; *FIGLU,* formimino-L-glutaric acid; *F-THF,* folinic acid; MeB_{12}, methylcobalamin; *5-MeTH,* N^5-methyltetrahydrofolate; *THF,* tetrahydrofolate; *TMP,* thymidine monophosphate.

vated MMA. In addition, the treatment with B_{12} injections of patients identified only by elevation of MMA has not resulted in hematological response or a convincing improvement in quality of life[92]; the cost and complexity of the MMA assay (using isotope dilution GC-MS or LC-MSMS) prohibit its use as a first-line test in the assessment of cobalamin deficiency. Urinary methylmalonic acid excretion has been recommended as a sensitive screening test for undetected cobalamin deficiency among the elderly and the newborn. Uremic patients show elevated serum methylmalonic acid, apparently unrelated to cobalamin status. This may be a function of the form and location of cobalamin, or it may reflect decreased methylmalonyl CoA mutase activity. Hyperhomocysteinemia is seen in deficiency of B_{12}, folate, or vitamin B_6. It likely is not an early indicator of B_6 status and does not appear to be superior to serum methylmalonic acid as an index of B_{12} deficiency.

Pathophysiology

A variety of disorders of the gastrointestinal tract can lead to reduced absorption of cobalamin (see Fig. 43-14). Inadequate acid production can result from gastric atrophy or gastrectomy, or frequently may result from proton pump inhibitor therapy. This seems to be the most frequent cause of B_{12} deficiency in the elderly.[93] Inadequate secretion of intrinsic factor may accompany lesions of the gastric mucosa, iron deficiency, and some endocrine disorders. The IF-B_{12} complex may be formed inadequately in pancreatic insufficiency because pancreatic protease activity is insufficient to split the dietary vitamin B_{12} from haptocorrin within the duodenum. The IF-B_{12} complex may be absorbed inadequately in ileal malfunction (sprue, enteritis, ileal resection, neoplasias, and granulomas). The term *pernicious anemia* is applied most commonly to vitamin B_{12} deficiency resulting from lack of IF. Antibodies to IF and to parietal cells are common in patients with pernicious anemia, in their healthy relatives, and in patients with other autoimmune disorders. In addition to deficiencies of cobalamin, congenital defects of the enzymes directly and indirectly involved with cobalamin transport and metabolism of the IF-B_{12} receptor can present in childhood with a wide range of clinical signs, including megaloblastic anemia, developmental delay, and failure to thrive.

Treatment

Treatment is given most often as intramuscular injections of cyanocobalamin or hydroxocobalamin. Newer studies indicate that in most patients (probably not in IF antibody–positive patients), oral B_{12} supplementation will suffice. However, guaranteed compliance and the relative infrequency of the intramuscular injections make them attractive to patients and health care providers.

Folic Acid (Vitamin B_{11})

Folates (from *folium*—Latin for "leaf") are structural relatives of pteroylglutamic acid (folic acid) (see Fig. 43-13). Up to eight glutamate residues may be found in these naturally occurring compounds. Glutamate residue number may function as a "handle" for the channeling of folate from enzyme to enzyme. Channeling is the movement of cofactor or substrate from enzyme to enzyme within a biochemical complex without equilibration to the external environment. This serves to conserve a rare cofactor or substrate and to prevent degradation if it is unstable. Also, it is thought that the various enzymes that use folate as a cofactor preferentially have affinity to a specific number of glutamate residues attached to the folate molecule. Therefore, if cells control the number of glutamate residues added to the folate cofactor, efficient and coordinated use of the species can be facilitated.[94]

Food folates are found primarily in green and leafy vegetables, fruits, and organ meats. Excessive heating of foods and use of large quantities of water when boiling vegetables may result in folate destruction. Absorption of food folate occurs at a rate that is only about 50% that of synthetic folic acid absorption.

Metabolism

The naturally occurring folate polyglutamates are hydrolyzed to monoglutamate forms before absorption. These are absorbed in the duodenum and the upper small intestine and are transported to the liver. The rare disease of hereditary folate malabsorption, which probably is autosomal recessive, provides evidence for a specific intestinal folate transporter. This has been identified recently as the protein HCP1, which previously was thought to be a heme carrier protein.[95] The folate transporter is pH dependent, exhibits high affinity for folate, and is located primarily in the apical brush border of the duodenum, where most of the folate is absorbed. It also is expressed in the choroid plexus and might contribute to higher CSF concentrations of folate. A second transporter is the reduced folate carrier, which exhibits lower affinity.

Although the liver converts some folate monoglutamates to polyglutamates for its own use, folate that is excreted into bile as N^5-methyltetrahydrofolate (MeTHF) is the primary source of folate available to tissues. The enzyme responsible for the synthesis of methyltetrahydrofolate is methylenetetrahydrofolate reductase (MTHFR). MeTHF is reabsorbed from the gut but is not taken up by the liver and therefore becomes the major circulating form of folate. MeTHF, in the monoglutamate form, readily enters the choroid plexus and the CSF. Folic acid, on the other hand, is readily transported from CSF to plasma. The CSF form is mainly MeTHF; brain folates are predominantly polyglutamate forms of dihydrofolate (DHF). Folate catabolism involves cleavage of the pterin ring, followed by acetylation to form the excreted product, p-acetamidobenzoylglutamic acid.

Function

Folate (MeTHF) is a cofactor for enzymatic reactions involving one-carbon transfers. After cellular uptake, the MeTHF is converted to THF during transfer of a carbon to homocysteine to yield methionine. As was mentioned previously, this reaction requires vitamin B_{12}. In the absence of vitamin B_{12}, the folate is essentially trapped in the MeTHF form, making it unavailable for other reactions, including the synthesis of thymidine for DNA (see Fig. 43-15).

Clinical and Chemical Deficiency Signs

The major clinical symptom of frank and prolonged folate deficiency is megaloblastic anemia. Although moderate hyperhomocysteinemia is an early marker of insufficient folate, it also can result from B_6 and B_{12} deficiency.

Serum folate reflects the very recent intake of folate; one meal can normalize values in a folate-deficient person. Low erythrocyte folate better reflects the levels of folate stores.[96]

The urinary formiminoglutamic acid test (FIGLU; a histidine metabolite accumulating in absence of folate) requires ingestion of an oral load of histidine, followed by a timed urine collection, and can be abnormally high in deficiencies of folate or vitamin B_{12}. Because most folate storage occurs after the vitamin B_{12}–dependent step, erythrocyte folate also can be reduced in deficiency of B_{12} or folate. As was indicated in the discussion of vitamin B_{12}, homocysteine elevation in serum or urine occurs in folate deficiency. Generally total homocysteine is measured, which is the sum of all homocysteine species (both free and protein-bound forms). Homocysteine measurements should be interpreted in conjunction with the determination of folate and cobalamin status.[97]

Changes in blood cell morphology, similar to hypersegmentation of neutrophils, are late signs of folate deficiency, as are macro-ovalocytosis, megaloblastic marrow, and finally anemia.

Pathophysiology

Folate requirement increases during pregnancy and lactation. This increase is the result of elevated demand in the rapidly growing tissues of the placenta and fetus and the newborn. The increased need during lactation results in part from the presence in milk of high-affinity folate binders, which likely serve to concentrate folate in milk for the infant. Other conditions that may result in an increased need for folate include hemolytic anemias, iron deficiency, prematurity, and malignant neoplasia, particularly neoplasia in which bone marrow infiltration is present. Patients with end-stage renal disease who are receiving dialysis treatment rapidly lose folate and pyridoxine. Folate deficiency as a result of malabsorption can occur in sprue, celiac disease, and inflammatory bowel disease. Intestinal transport of folate is pH sensitive at the microenvironmental level. Conditions that may interfere with intestinal transport include inflammatory bowel disease, but some of the drugs used to treat it, notably sulfasalazine, may have this effect as well.

Genetic alterations in most of the folate-interconverting enzymes have been reported. The best described genetic defect occurs in the gene for MTHFR and consists of a *C677T* transition, resulting in a thermolabile phenotype in the expressed enzyme. Approximately 12% of Caucasians are homozygous for this defect. A second defect is found at allele 1298 on the gene, *A1298C*. This mutation has nearly the same allele frequency as the *C677T* mutation in Caucasians, and some cases of combined *677/1298* mutations have been reported.[98]

Both mutations result in reduced MTHFR activity, which, in turn, decreases the quantity of folate delivered to bile and subsequently to the systemic circulation. These and other mutations of folate metabolizing enzymes have been shown to be associated with an increased risk of neural tube defects.[99] An increased risk for Down syndrome also has been associated with the presence of the MTHFR point mutation *C677T* and with methionine synthase mutations in the mother.[100] Although it seems compelling that lower levels of bioavailable folate might be causing some cases of Down syndrome, the introduction of folate food fortification has not reduced the incidence of Down syndrome in Canada.[101]

Several rare cases of folate transport defects involving children who are unable to transfer folates from the lumen of the gut to blood and, in some cases, into CSF have been described. Mutations of the intestinal folate transporter that cause this disease have been identified. Failure to thrive and mental retardation are common among these children. Mothers of children with neural tube defects have been found to have specific antibodies to the folate receptor.[102]

Folate deficiency of dietary origin commonly occurs in the elderly. Phenytoin (Dilantin) therapy accelerates folate metabolism. Alcohol interferes with the enterohepatic circulation folate, whereas the chemotherapeutic agent methotrexate inhibits the enzyme dihydrofolate reductase.

Therapeutic Uses

Inadequate maternal intake of folate is associated with fetal neural tube defects—mainly spina bifida and anencephaly—and it has been clearly demonstrated that folate supplementation lowers these rates.[103] Because it is the periconceptual folate that prevents neural tube defects, several countries, among them the United States, Canada, and Chile, have introduced mandatory food fortification with folate (in cereal and grain foods, as well as flours). Other countries like Australia and a number of EU members have introduced voluntary folate fortification. Still others do not allow fortification with folic acid for fear that it could mask symptoms of vitamin B_{12} deficiency and precipitate neurological complications, and because of concerns regarding a possible detrimental effect on cancer.[104]

The therapeutic form of folate is 5-formyl-THF (also known as leucovorin, citrovorum factor, or folinic acid). This form of folate can bypass MeTHF and enter the cycles of one-carbon transfer reactions of folate (see Fig. 43-15). This feature is useful in the "leucovorin rescue" of cancer patients who are given high-dose methotrexate therapy with toxic levels of methotrexate. The use of folate supplements prior to conception and early pregnancy is recommended to reduce the occurrence of neural tube defects. Although the introduction of mandatory folate fortification has reduced the incidence of neural tube defects, it also has reduced the incidence of other birth defects (transposition of great arteries, cleft palate, renal agenesis, and others).[105]

Carnitine

Carnitine, including L-carnitine and its fatty acid esters (acylcarnitines) (Fig. 43-16), is described as a "conditionally essential" nutrient.

Major dietary sources include meat, poultry, fish, and dairy products. Foods of plant origin generally contain very little carnitine (exceptions being peanut butter, asparagus, and avocados). Average diets provide more than half the human requirement; strict vegetarian diets provide only 10% of the total available carnitine. Most dietary carnitine is absorbed.

Metabolism

De novo synthesis involves N-tri-methyllysine residues of proteins; the biosynthetic rate is determined by the available supply of these N-tri-methyllysine residues. Synthesis occurs in liver, brain, and kidney, with storage primarily in muscle. Uptake from the gut occurs via a specific carnitine transport protein, which is mutated in primary systemic carnitine deficiency.[106] Carnitine is not degraded but is excreted mainly in the urine in both free and esterified forms.

Function

L-Carnitine facilitates entry of long-chain fatty acids into mitochondria for oxidation and energy production. As is shown in Fig. 43-17, coenzyme A esters of the long-chain fatty acids (acyl-S-CoA) are transesterified to L-carnitine by means of catalysis by an enzyme of the mitochondrial outer membrane, CPT I (carnitine palmitoyltransferase I). Once inside the inner membrane, the long-chain fatty acid once again is transesterified (by CPT II), yielding the CoA ester, which can enter the beta-oxidation pathway for energy production. The carnitine "transporter" then can leave the mitochondria to be reused, or it can serve its other known role and carry out from the mitochondria short- and medium-chain fatty acids that accumulate during normal or abnormal metabolism. The carnitine esters may be excreted in urine or distributed in tissues; some may be used for specific purposes.

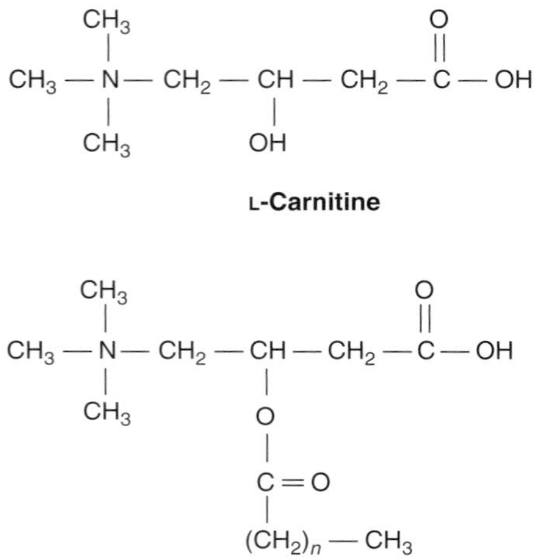

$$CH_3-N(CH_3)_2-CH_2-CH(OH)-CH_2-C(=O)-OH$$

L-Carnitine

$$CH_3-N(CH_3)_2-CH_2-CH(O-C(=O)-(CH_2)_n-CH_3)-CH_2-C(=O)-OH$$

Acylcarnitine

Fig. 43-16 L-Carnitine and fatty acid esters.

Clinical and Chemical Deficiency Signs

The major signs of carnitine deficiency are muscle weakness and fatigue. Chemical indices of deficiency include decreased total or free carnitine in serum, urine, or tissues. Total carnitine is measured after hydrolysis of ester forms to free carnitine; acylcarnitines represent the difference between these two measures. Short- and long-chain esters can be distinguished by their differing solubility. Characterization of individual esters is helpful in identification of disorders of fatty acid metabolism; techniques include gas chromatography-mass spectrometry and liquid chromatography electrospray tandem mass spectrometry.[107] The first applications on routine analyzers are being published now.[108] Abnormally high ratios of acylcarnitines to free carnitine can be seen in disorders of fatty acid oxidation, in ketosis, and in chronic renal failure.

Pathophysiology

Primary systemic carnitine deficiency is very rare. In this autosomal recessive disorder, affected children have cardiomyopathy, hypoglycemia, elevated ammonia, and muscle weakness. Administration of large doses of carnitine reverses the disorder, which is to the result of a mutation of the organic cation transporter *OCNTN2*.[109] Other causes of primary carnitine

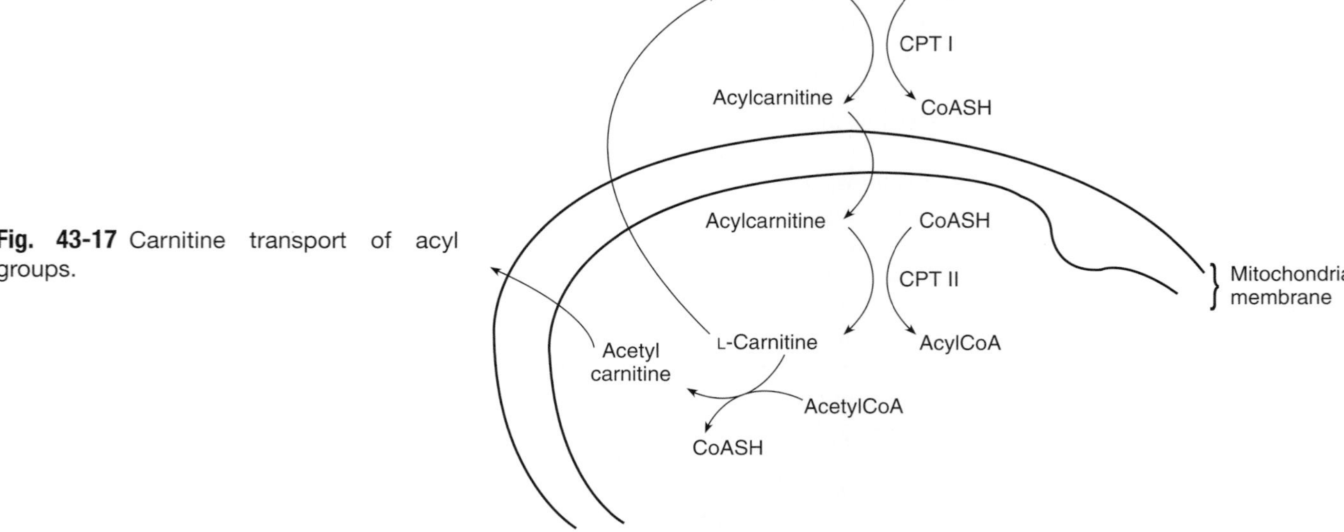

Fig. 43-17 Carnitine transport of acyl groups.

deficiency without cardiomyopathy are not as clearly understood and do not always respond to carnitine supplementation.

Acquired deficiency can be caused by inadequate intake, increased requirement (pregnancy and breast feeding), or increased urinary loss. Infants, patients following a course of long-term parenteral nutrition, and perhaps children constitute the groups most vulnerable to deficiency, as judged by decreased circulating levels and altered indicators of energy metabolism. Patients who are receiving hemodialysis may lose carnitine in the dialysis fluid. However, evidence from controlled trials is not sufficient to recommend carnitine supplementation in patients on dialysis.[110] Secondary deficiencies may result in muscular dysfunction. Carnitine therapies are being evaluated for these circumstances and also for use in patients with disorders of ammonia metabolism. Valproate, which is used for the treatment of epilepsy, is associated with liver toxicity, and carnitine may prove helpful in the management of liver injury caused by valproate. The three-carbon ester propionyl-L-carnitine has been shown to protect the ischemic heart from reperfusion injury. Propionyl-L-carnitine also seems to help in cases of intermittent claudication, but additional studies are needed.[111] Studies in patients with Alzheimer's disease show a small benefit of treatment with acetyl-carnitine.[112]

L-Acetyl carnitine has been described to be beneficial in various trials for HIV-associated neuropathy that is thought to be caused by the nucleoside analog reverse transcriptase inhibitors—drugs that disrupt mitochondrial energy generation.[113] In diabetic nephropathy, early studies indicate a beneficial effect of high doses of acetyl-carnitine.[114]

KEY CONCEPTS BOX 43-3

- Vitamins with high water solubility—the "water-soluble vitamins" (WSV)—include vitamin C and the large group of B vitamins and their derivatives.
- WSV are absorbed in the intestines during normal food absorption. Specific protein binders may be needed to absorb the WSV. WSV are carried in the water portion of blood.
- Vitamin C acts as an antioxidant, and the B vitamins are used to synthesize cofactors (e.g., FAD, NAD) for a whole host of biological reactions. Serum levels of WSV do not reflect well body (tissue) levels of the vitamins.
- Because WSV are not stored in the body, no toxic levels are associated with excessive WSV.
- WSV are best measured by HPLC, although the best indications of WSV deficiency are clinical signs and symptoms associated with a deficiency, such as symptoms of scurvy with vitamin C deficiency.
- Functional enzyme assays have been used for some of the cofactors, such as FAD, vitamin B_2, and NAD (vitamin B_6).

SECTION OBJECTIVES BOX 43-4

- Discuss the arguments for and against taking supplemental vitamins in the absence of disease or high risk for disease.
- Review the use of vitamin therapy for the prevention or treatment of cancer or cardiovascular disease.

VITAMIN SUPPLEMENTATION IN DISEASE PREVENTION: THE BUSINESS OF MULTIVITAMIN SUPPLEMENTATION

Free radicals are highly reactant molecules that are generated during ordinary metabolism and from certain drugs or xenobiotics (foreign chemicals). Exposure to ultraviolet radiation, cigarette smoke, and other environmental pollutants increases the body's burden of free radicals. These short-lived free radicals can damage membranes, enzymes, and DNA. An array of antioxidant defenses exists in cells and tissues to prevent formation or limit the effects of free radicals. Free radicals have been implicated as a possible cause of cancer and cardiovascular disease. Vitamins C and E and β-carotene theoretically should protect against cancer of the lung and other epithelial tissues through a variety of mechanisms.

The other argument for the use of multivitamins is the fact that some members of the population have marginal stores of vitamins. This is especially true for the elderly and marginalized groups. Numerous observational studies have shown that higher vitamin levels are associated with better outcomes for malignancy and for cardiovascular disease.

In the meantime, the use of multivitamin supplements has become a major business, with public expenditures worth many millions of dollars.

Prospective, randomized, controlled studies have not demonstrated a cancer protective role for vitamins when taken as supplements. Indeed, the role of vitamin supplements in the prevention of disease most likely is limited to individuals with marginal nutritional intake. For example, supplementation with multivitamins decreased the incidence of low birth weight and small for gestational age births and improved maternal hemoglobin in women in Tanzania.[115]

The data from randomized, controlled trials of the antioxidant vitamins A, C, and E in general have been negative for prevention of cardiovascular disease and prevention of cancer.[116]

Some studies even resulted in excessive mortality, as with vitamin E in the VITAL (VITamins And Lifestyle) study and vitamin A in the ATBC (Alpha-Tocopherol Beta-Carotene Cancer Prevention) study. It is interesting to note that higher baseline values of vitamin E in the ATBC study were associated with lower mortality, but a reduction in mortality was not seen after additional supplementation. Similarly, most studies that planned to reduce cardiovascular mortality with vitamin supplementation have been unsuccessful. Most recently, no reduction in cardiovascular or total mortality was reported among high-risk women who were supplemented with folate and B_6 and B_{12} vitamins.[117]

Current trials may have not been planned well enough in terms of length of treatment, frequency of events, and statistical power, or perhaps the lack of reported effect reflects reality. It is possible that measured vitamin levels reflect other parameters that currently are not appropriately assessed, such as other compounds present in the nutrition of participants that might cause a lower risk. At this stage, multivitamin supplementation in healthy participants cannot be recommended to reduce cancer or cardiovascular disease.

KEY CONCEPTS BOX 43-4

- The RDA, UL, and DRI estimate dietary intakes of vitamins needed for health. NO evidence suggests that intakes in excess of what is needed for general health are useful.
- When the utility of "megadoses" of vitamins has been studied, whether vitamin C to prevent the common cold or vitamins A and E to prevent cancer or heart disease, the data thus far have been negative.
- Large commerce has resulted from selling such megadoses, and concerns have arisen that aside from the money that is being spent without proof of improved health, these megadoses actually may be causing increased risks for disease and toxicity.

REFERENCES

1. *Vitamin and Mineral Requirements in Human Nutrition,* Geneva, Switzerland, 2004, World Health Organization, Food and Agriculture Organization of the United Nations.
2. Food and Nutrition Board of the Institute of Medicine: Dietary Reference Intakes: The Essential Guide to Nutrient Requirements Released On: September 15, 2006.
3. Otten JJ, Hellwig JP, Meyers DL: *Dietary Reference Intakes: The Essential Guide to Nutrient Requirements,* Washington, DC, 2006, The National Academies Press.
4. Position of the American Dietetic Association: Fortification and Nutritional Supplements, J Am Diet Assoc 105:1300, 2005.
5. Walter P: Towards ensuring the safety of vitamins and minerals, Toxicol Lett 120:83, 2001.
6. European Food Safety Authority: Tolerable Upper Intake Levels for Vitamins and Minerals by the Scientific Panel on Dietetic products, nutrition and allergies (NDA) and Scientific Committee on Food (SCF) December 2006. http://www.efsa.europa.eu/en/publications/scientific.html
7. Pesce AJ, Kaplan LA, editors: *Methods in Clinical Chemistry,* electronic version 4.3, St Louis, 1996, Mosby.
8. Berdanier CD, Dwyer J, Felman EB: *Handbook of Nutrition and Food,* ed 2, Boca Raton, 2007, CRC Press.
9. Slater GH, Ren CJ, Siegel N, et al: Serum fat-soluble vitamin deficiency and abnormal calcium metabolism after malabsorptive bariatric surgery, J Gastrointest Surg 8:48, 2004; discussion, 54.
10. Voutilainen S, Nurmi T, Mursu J, et al: Carotenoids and cardiovascular health, Am J Clin Nutr 83:1265, 2006.
11. Krinsky NI, Johnson EJ: Carotenoid actions and their relation to health and disease, Mol Aspects Med 26:459, 2005. Epub 23 Nov, 2005.
12. Jessen KA, Satre MA: Mouse retinol binding protein gene: cloning, expression, and regulation by retinoic acid, Mol Cell Biochem 211:85, 2000.
13. Kawaguchi R, Yu J, Honda J, et al: A membrane receptor for retinol binding protein mediates cellular uptake of vitamin A, Science 315:820, 2007.
14. Stephensen CB: Vitamin A, infection, and immune function, Ann Rev Nutr 21:167, 2001.
15. Iwata M, Hirakiyama A, Eshima Y, et al: Retinoic acid imprints gut-homing specificity on T cells, Immunity 21:527, 2004.
16. Mora JR, Iwata M, Eksteen B, et al: Generation of gut-homing IgA-secreting B cells by intestinal dendritic cells, Science 314:1157, 2006.
17. Mucida D, Park Y, Kim G, et al: Reciprocal TH17 and regulatory T cell differentiation mediated by retinoic acid, Science 317:256, 2007.
18. Black RE, Allen LH, Bhutta ZA, et al, for the Maternal and Child Undernutrition Study Group: Maternal and child undernutrition: global and regional exposures and health consequences, Lancet 371:243, 2008.
19. Connolly GM, Cunningham R, Maxwell AP, et al: Decreased serum retinol is associated with increased mortality in renal transplant recipients, Clin Chem 53:1841, 2007.
20. Garry PJ: Vitamin A. In Labbe RF, editor: *Clinics in Laboratory Medicine: Laboratory Assessment of Nutritional Status,* vol 1, Philadelphia, 1981, WB Saunders.
21. Verhoef H, West CE: Validity of the relative-dose-response test and the modified-relative-dose-response test as indicators of vitamin A stores in liver. Am J Clin Nutr. 2005 Apr;81(4):835-839.
22. Shamberger RJ: Vitamin A alterations in disease. In Brewster MA, Naito HK, editors: *Nutritional Elements and Clinical Biochemistry,* New York, 1980, Plenum Publishing.
23. Sklan D: Vitamin A in human nutrition, Prog Food Nutr Sci 11:39, 1987.
24. Underwood BA: Methods for assessment of vitamin A status, J Nutr 120(suppl 11):1459, 1990.
25. Bhalla K, Ennis DM, Ennis ED: Hypercalcemia caused by iatrogenic hypervitaminosis A, J Am Diet Assoc 105:119, 2005.
26. Feskanich D, Singh V, Willett WC, et al: Vitamin A intake and hip fractures among postmenopausal women, JAMA 287:47, 2002.
27. Dolk HM, Nau H, Hummler H, et al: Dietary vitamin A and teratogenic risk, Eur J Obstet Gynecol Reprod Biol 83:31, 1999.
28. Dinan FJ, and Yee GT, National Center for Case Study Teaching in Science, University at Buffalo, State University of New York An Adventure in Stereochemistry: Alice in Mirror Image Land www.sciencecases.org/alice/alice.asp
29. Reboul E, Klein F, Bietrix B, et al: Scavenger receptor class B type I (SR-BI) is involved in vitamin E transport across the enterocyte, J Biol Chem 281:4739, 2006. Epub 27 December, 2005.
30. Traber G, Arai H: Molecular mechanisms of vitamin E transport, Ann Rev Nutr 19:343, 1999.
31. Ouahchi K, Arita M, Kayden H, et al: Ataxia with isolated vitamin E deficiency is caused by mutations in the alpha-tocopherol transfer protein, Nat Genet 9:141, 1995.
32. Traber MG, Burton GW, Hamilton RL: Vitamin E trafficking, Ann NY Acad Sci 1031:1, 2004.
33. Zingg JM, Azzi A: Non-antioxidant activities of vitamin E, Curr Med Chem 11:1113, 2004.
34. Sokol RJ, Guggenheim MA, Heubi JE, et al: Frequency and clinical progression of the vitamin E deficiency neurologic disorder in children with prolonged neonatal cholestasis, Am J Dis Child 139:1211, 1985.
35. Sokol RJ: Vitamin E and neurological deficits, Adv Pediatr 37:119, 1990.
36. Cham BE, Smith JL, Colquhoun DM: Correlations between cholesterol, vitamin E, and vitamin K1 in serum: paradoxical relationships to established epidemiological risk factors for cardiovascular disease, Clin Chem 44:1753, 1998.

37. Miller ER III, Pastor-Barriuso R, Dalal D, et al: Meta-analysis: high-dosage vitamin E supplementation may increase all-cause mortality, Ann Intern Med 142:37, 2005.
38. Desai UR: Virginia Commonwealth University School of Pharmacy - Dept of Medicinal Chemistry January 5, 2000, http://www.people.vcu.edu/~urdesai/cou.htm
39. Booth SL, Tucker KL, Chen H, et al: Dietary vitamin K intakes are associated with hip fracture but not with bone mineral density in elderly men and women, Am J Clin Nutr 71:1201, 2000.
40. Cockayne S, Adamson J, Lanham-New S, et al: Vitamin K and the prevention of fractures: systematic review and meta-analysis of randomized controlled trials, Arch Intern Med 166:1256, 2006.
41. Tamura T, Morgan SL, Takimoto H: Vitamin K and the prevention of fractures, Arch Intern Med 167:93, 2007; author reply, 94.
42. Puckett RM, Offringa M: Prophylactic vitamin K for vitamin K deficiency bleeding in neonates, Cochrane Database Syst Rev (4):CD002776. 2000.
43. Motohara K, Endo F, Matsuda I: Screening for late neonatal vitamin K deficiency by acarboxyprothrombin in dried blood spots, Arch Dis Child 62:370, 1987.
44. Azharuddin MK, O'Reilly DS, Gray A, et al: HPLC method for plasma vitamin K1: effect of plasma triglyceride and acute-phase response on circulating concentrations, Clin Chem 53:1706, 2007.
45. Harrington DJ, Western H, Seton-Jones C, et al: A study of the prevalence of vitamin K deficiency in patients with cancer referred to a hospital palliative care team and its association with abnormal haemostasis, J Clin Pathol 61:537, 2008. Epub 8 Oct, 2007.
46. Pilkey RM, Morton AR, Boffa MB, et al: Subclinical vitamin K deficiency in hemodialysis patients, Am J Kidney Dis 49:432, 2007.
47. University of California, Riverside Vitamin D Home Page http://vitamind.ucr.edu/chem.html
48. Pasco JA, Henry MJ, Kotowicz MA, et al: Seasonal periodicity of serum vitamin D and parathyroid hormone, bone resorption, and fractures: the Geelong osteoporosis study, J Bone Miner Res 19:752, 2004. Epub 19 January, 2004.
49. Holick MF, Biancuzzo RM, Chen TC, et al: Vitamin D2 is as effective as vitamin D3 in maintaining circulating concentrations of 25-hydroxyvitamin D, J Clin Endocrinol Metab 93:677, 2008. Epub 18 December, 2007.
50. Working Group of the Australian and New Zealand Bone and Mineral Society, Endocrine Society of Australia, Osteoporosis Australia: Vitamin D and adult bone health in Australia and New Zealand: a position statement, Med J Aust 182:281, 2005.
51. Bischoff-Ferrari HA: Optimal serum 25-hydroxyvitamin D levels for multiple health outcomes, Adv Exp Med Biol 624:55, 2008.
52. Holick MF: Vitamin D deficiency, N Engl J Med 357:266, 2007.
53. Danne O, Möckel M, Lueders C, et al: Prognostic implications of elevated whole blood choline levels in acute coronary syndromes, Am J Cardiol 91:1060, 2003.
54. Wilson JX: Regulation of vitamin C transport, Annu Rev Nutr 25:105, 2005.
55. Emadi-Konjin P, Verjee Z, Levin AV, et al: Measurement of intracellular vitamin C levels in human lymphocytes by reverse phase high performance liquid chromatography (HPLC), Clin Biochem 38:450, 2005.
56. Deicher R, Ziai F, Bieglmayer C, et al: Low total vitamin C plasma level is a risk factor for cardiovascular morbidity and mortality in hemodialysis patients, J Am Soc Nephrol 16:1811, 2005.
57. Li Y, Schellhorn HE: New developments and novel therapeutic perspectives for vitamin C, J Nutr 137: 2171, 2007.
58. Singer R, Rhodes HC, Chin G, et al: High prevalence of ascorbate deficiency in an Australian peritoneal dialysis population, Nephrology 13:17, 2008.
59. Attallah N, Osman-Malik Y, Frinak S, et al: Effect of intravenous ascorbic acid in hemodialysis patients with EPO-hyporesponsive anemia and hyperferritinemia, Am J Kidney Dis 47:644, 2006.
60. Said HM, Ortiz A, Moyer MP, et al: Riboflavin uptake by human derived colonic epithelial NCM460 cells, Am J Physiol Cell Physiol 278:C270, 2000.
61. Foraker AB, Ray A, Da Silva TC, et al: Links dynamin 2 regulates riboflavin endocytosis in human placental trophoblasts, Mol Pharmacol 72:553. Epub 12 June, 2007.
62. De Colibus L, Mattevi A: New frontiers in structural flavoenzymology, Curr Opin Struct Biol 16:722, 2006.
63. Bates CJ: Human riboflavin requirements and metabolic consequences of deficiency in men and animals, World Rev Nutr Diet 50:215, 1987.
64. Fouty B, Frerman F, Reves R: Riboflavin to treat nucleoside analogue–induced lactic acidosis, Lancet 352:291, 1998.
65. Thaver D, Saeed MA, Bhutta ZA: Update of Cochrane Database Syst Rev (2):CD000179, 2000: Pyridoxine (vitamin B6) supplementation in pregnancy, Cochrane Database Syst Rev (2): CD000179. 2006.
66. Sheehan P: Genetic defects of the hyperemesis gravidarum—assessment and management, Aust Fam Physician 36:698, 2007.
67. Pearl PL, Taylor JL, Trzcinski S, et al: The pediatric neurotransmitter disorders, J Child Neurol 22:606, 2007.
68. Seal AJ, Creeke PI, Dibari F, et al: Low and deficient niacin status and pellagra are endemic in postwar Angola, Am J Clin Nutr 85:218, 2007.
69. Shah GM, Shah RG, Veillette H, et al: Biochemical assessment of niacin deficiency among carcinoid cancer patients, Am J Gastroenterol 100:2307, 2005.
70. Creeke PI, Dibari F, Cheung E, et al: Whole blood NAD and NADP concentrations are not depressed in subjects with clinical pellagra, J Nutr 137:2013, 2007.
71. Bodor ET, Offermanns S: Nicotinic acid: an old drug with a promising future, Br J Pharmacol 153(suppl 1):S68, 2008. Epub 26 November, 2007.
72. Ahoua L, Etienne W, Fermon F, et al: Outbreak of beriberi in a prison in Côte d'Ivoire, Food Nutr Bull 28:283, 2007.
73. Spector R, Johanson CE: Vitamin transport and homeostasis in mammalian brain: focus on vitamins B and E, J Neurochem 103:425, 2007.
74. Subramanian VS, Marchant JS, Said HM: Targeting and trafficking of the human thiamine transporter-2 in epithelial cells, J Biol Chem 281:5233, 2006.
75. Lindhurst MJ, Fiermonte G, Song S, et al: Knockout of Slc25a19 causes mitochondrial thiamine pyrophosphate depletion, embryonic lethality, CSF malformations, and anemia, Proc Natl Acad Sci 103:15927, 2006.
76. Talwar D, Davidson H, Cooney J, et al: Vitamin B1 status assessed by direct measurement of thiamin pyrophosphate in erythrocytes or whole blood by HPLC: comparison with erythrocyte transketolase activation assay, Clin Chem 46:704, 2000.
77. Lu J, Frank EL: Rapid HPLC measurement of thiamine and its phosphate esters in whole blood, Clin Chem 54:901, 2008.
78. Tsujino T, Nakao S, Wakabayashi K, et al: Loop diuretic precipitated beriberi in a patient after pancreaticoduodenectomy: a case report, Am J Med Sci 334:407, 2007.
79. Donnino MW, Vega J, Miller J, et al: Myths and misconceptions of Wernicke's encephalopathy: what every emergency physician should know, Ann Emerg Med 50:715, 2007.

80. Donnino MW, Miller J, Garcia AJ, et al: Distinctive acid-base pattern in Wernicke's encephalopathy, Ann Emerg Med 50:722, 2007.
81. Said HM: Recent advances in carrier-mediated intestinal absorption of water-soluble vitamins, Annu Rev Physiol 66:419, 2004.
82. Stratton SL, Bogusiewicz A, Mock MM, et al: Lymphocyte propionyl-CoA carboxylase and its activation by biotin are sensitive indicators of marginal biotin deficiency in humans, Am J Clin Nutr 84:384, 2006.
83. Carmel R: Prevalence of undiagnosed pernicious anemia in the elderly, Arch Intern Med 156:1097, 1996.
84. Flood VM, Smith WT, Webb KL, et al: Clinical prevalence of low serum folate and vitamin B12 in an older Australian population, Aust N Z J Public Health 30:38, 2006.
85. Wuerges J, Geremia S, Randaccio L: Structural study on ligand specificity of human vitamin B_{12} transporters, Biochem J 403:431, 2007.
86. Moestrup SK: New insights into carrier binding and epithelial uptake of the erythropoietic nutrients cobalamin and folate, Curr Opin Hematol 13:119, 2006.
87. Quadros EV, Nakayama Y, Sequeira JM: The binding properties of the human receptor for the cellular uptake of vitamin B12, Biochem Biophys Res Commun 327:1006, 2005.
88. Wuerges J, Garau G, Geremia S, et al: Structural basis for mammalian vitamin B12 transport by transcobalamin, Proc Natl Acad Sci USA 103:4386, 2006. Epub 14 Mar, 2006.
89. Clarke R, Sherliker P, Hin H, et al: Detection of vitamin B_{12} deficiency in older people by measuring vitamin B_{12} or the active fraction of vitamin B_{12}, holotranscobalamin, Clin Chem 53:963, 2007. Epub 15 Mar, 2007.
90. Devalia V: Diagnosing vitamin B-12 deficiency on the basis of serum B-12 assay, BMJ 333:385, 2006.
91. Solomon LR: Cobalamin-responsive disorders in the ambulatory care setting: unreliability of cobalamin, methylmalonic acid, and homocysteine testing, Blood 105:978, 2005.
92. Hvas AM, Juul S, Nexø E, et al: Vitamin B-12 treatment has limited effect on health-related quality of life among individuals with elevated plasma methylmalonic acid: a randomized placebo-controlled study, J Intern Med 253:146, 2003.
93. Andrès E, Loukili NH, Noel E, et al: Vitamin B_{12} (cobalamin) deficiency in elderly patients, CMAJ 171:251, 2004.
94. Donnelly JG: Folic acid, Crit Rev Clin Lab Sci 38:183, 2001.
95. Qiu A, Jansen M, Sakaris A, et al: Identification of an intestinal folate transporter and the molecular basis for hereditary folate malabsorption, Cell 127:917, 2006.
96. Clifford AJ, Noceti EM, Block-Joy A, et al: Erythrocyte folate and its response to folic acid supplementation is assay dependent in women, J Nutr 135:137, 2005.
97. Donnelly JG, Isotalo PA: Occurrence of hyperhomocysteinemia in cardiovascular, hematology and nephrology patients: contribution of folate deficiency, Ann Clin Biochem 37:304, 2000.
98. Isotalo PA, Wells GA, Donnelly JG: Neonatal and fetal methylenetetrahydrofolate reductase genetic polymorphisms: an examination of C677T and A1298C mutations, Am J Hum Genet 67:986, 2000.
99. Tamura T, Picciano MF: Folate and human reproduction, Am J Clin Nutr 83:993, 2006.
100. Eskes TK: Abnormal folate metabolism in mothers with Down syndrome offspring: review of the literature, Eur J Obstet Gynecol Reprod Biol 124:130, 2006.
101. Ray JG, Meier C, Vermeulen MJ, et al: Prevalence of trisomy 21 following folic acid food fortification, Am J Med Genet A 120A:309, 2003.
102. Rothenberg SP, da Costa MP, Sequeira JM, et al: Autoantibodies against folate receptors in women with a pregnancy complicated by a neural-tube defect, N Engl J Med 350:134, 2004.
103. Eichholzer M, Tönz O, Zimmermann R: Folic acid: a public-health challenge, Lancet 367:1352, 2006.
104. van Guelpen B: Folate in colorectal cancer, prostate cancer and cardiovascular disease, Scand J Clin Lab Invest 67:459, 2007.
105. Canfield MA, Collins JS, Botto LD, et al, for the National Birth Defects Prevention Network: Changes in the birth prevalence of selected birth defects after grain fortification with folic acid in the United States: findings from a multi-state population-based study (Birth Defects Research), Clin Molec Teratol 73:679, 2005.
106. Nezu J, Tamai I, Oku A, et al: Primary systemic carnitine deficiency is caused by mutations in a gene encoding sodium ion-dependent carnitine transporter, Nat Genet 21:91, 1999.
107. Chace DH, Kalas TA: A biochemical perspective on the use of tandem mass spectrometry for newborn screening and clinical testing, Clin Biochem 38:296, 2005.
108. Kerspern H, Carré JL: Adaptation of free and total plasma carnitine determination on the Dimension HM, X-Pand model (Dade Behring), Ann Biol Clin (Paris) 66:207, 2008.
109. Melegh B, Bene J, Mogyorósy G, et al: Phenotypic manifestations of the OCTN2 V295X mutation: sudden infant death and carnitine-responsive cardiomyopathy in Roma families, Am J Med Genet A 131:121, 2004.
110. Eknoyan G, Latos DL, Lindberg J: Practice recommendations for the use of L-carnitine in dialysis-related carnitine disorder: National Kidney Foundation Carnitine Consensus Conference, Am J Kidney Dis 41:868, 2003.
111. Hiatt WR, Regensteiner JG, Creager MA, et al: Propionyl-L-carnitine improves exercise performance and functional status in patients with claudication, Am J Med 110:616, 2001.
112. Hudson S, Tabet N: Acetyl-L-carnitine for dementia, Cochrane Database Syst Rev (2):CD003158, 2003.
113. Youle M: Acetyl-L-carnitine in HIV-associated antiretroviral toxic neuropathy, CNS Drugs 21(suppl 1):25, 2007; discussion, 45.
114. Sima AA, Calvani M, Mehra M, et al: Acetyl-L-carnitine improves pain, nerve regeneration, and vibratory perception in patients with chronic diabetic neuropathy: an analysis of two randomized placebo-controlled trials, Diabetes Care 28:89, 2005.
115. Fawzi WW, Msamanga GI, Urassa W, et al: Vitamins and perinatal outcomes among HIV-negative women in Tanzania, N Engl J Med 356:1423, 2007.
116. Bjelakovic G, Nikolova D, Gluud LL, et al: Antioxidant supplements for prevention of mortality in healthy participants and patients with various diseases, Cochrane Database Syst Rev (2)CD007176, 2008.
117. Albert CM, Cook NR, Gaziano JM, et al: Effect of folic acid and B vitamins on risk of cardiovascular events and total mortality among women at high risk for cardiovascular disease: a randomized trial, JAMA 299:2027, 2008.

INTERNET WEBSITES

http://www.efsa.europa.eu/en/publications/scientific.html—European food safety authority with a publication on tolerable upper limit of vitamin intake

http://www.dentistry.leeds.ac.uk/biochem/lecture/nutritio/nutritio.htm—Helpful lecture notes from the Leeds Dental Institute

http://www.iom.edu/?id=2138—Institute of Medicine dietary reference intake tables

www.asns.org/—American Society for Nutrition

http://www.nutritioncare.org/—American Society for Parenteral and Enteral Nutrition

http://vm.cfsan.fda.gov/list.html—United States Food and Drug Administration Center for Food Safety and Applied Nutrition

www.nalusda.gov/fnic/—Food and Nutrition Information Center of the National Agriculture Library

http://books.nap.edu/books/—Dietary reference intakes report. This site takes you to the Crawler List of all NAP searchable open books. Search for dietary reference intake for vitamins

http://www.iom.edu/Object.File/Master/7/296/webtablevitamins.pdf—This site takes you to the National Agriculture Library Dietary Reference Intakes for Vitamins

http://themedicalbiochemistrypage.org/vitamins.html—Indiana State University Terre Haute Center for Medical Education: Introduction to vitamins

Chapter 44 Pregnancy and Fetal Development

John F. Chapman, Jr., Catherine A. Hammett-Stabler, and David G. Grenache

Chapter Outline

Key Terms

anencephaly A defective development of the brain wherein the cerebral and cerebellar hemispheres are absent.

blastocyst An early stage in embryonic development characterized by a fluid-filled cavity within the cell mass covered by the trophoblast.

corpus luteum A yellow glandular mass in the ovary formed by an ovarian follicle that has matured and discharged its ovum.

eclampsia Convulsions and coma occurring during pregnancy associated with prior development of hypertension, proteinuria, and edema (see preeclampsia).

ectopic pregnancy Pregnancy that occurs outside the uterine cavity, most commonly in the fallopian tubes.

endometrium The mucous membrane that lines the uterus.

hematopoietic Related to the process of formation and development of various types of blood cells.

hydatidiform A structure that resembles a hydatid cyst.

isoantibodies Antibodies produced by an individual that reacts with isoantigens of other individuals of the same species.

isoantigen Antigens that are found in many alternative forms in a species. These multiple forms (alleles) may ellicit an immune response when introduced into individuals who do not possess that specific allele.

keratinization The process of skin development and differentiation wherein keratin, a proteinaceous substance, is produced.

lamellar bodies The physical form of pulmonary surfactant that is extruded from type II pneumocytes.

meningomyelocele A protrusion of the membranes and spinal cord that results from a defect in the vertebral column.

neural tube defect A developmental abnormality characterized by defective closure of the spinal cord.

oligohydramnios The presence of less amniotic fluid than is usual for a given gestational age.

polyhydramnios The accumulation of an excessive amount of amniotic fluid.
preeclampsia The presence of hypertension, proteinuria, and edema during pregnancy.
tocolytic agents Chemicals used to supress contractions of pre-term labor.
transudation The passage of a substance through a membrane as a result of a difference in hydrostatic pressure.
trophoblast The cell layer covering of the blastocyst, which erodes the inner lining of the uterus during the process of implantation. Trophoblastic cells do not become part of the embryo itself but contribute to formation of the placenta.
ultrasonography The visualization of internal body structures by evaluation of the reflection of ultrasonic waves directed at tissues.

Methods on Evolve

α-Fetoprotein
β-Human chorionic gonadotropin (β-hCG)
Bilirubin
Creatinine
Fetal lung maturity (amniotic fluid phospholipids [AFPL] LS ratio and PG)
Glucose
Magnesium
Maternal fetal screening
Uric acid
Urine protein, total

SECTION OBJECTIVES BOX 44-1

- Describe the process of implantation of fertilized ovum within the uterus.
- Explain the maternal and fetal changes that occur after implantation of an ovum.
- List the maternal hormonal changes that allow the uterus to provide a suitable environment for the implanted ovum.
- Describe the role of the placenta in the exchange of nutrients, water, and gases between the mother and the fetus.
- Describe the formation and list the functions of amniotic fluid.

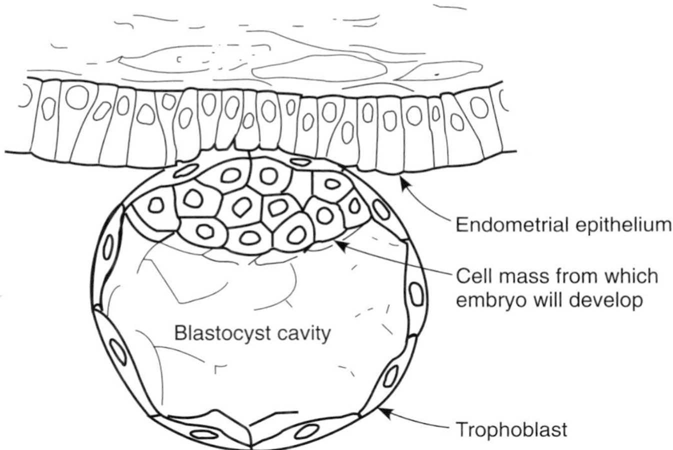

Fig. 44-1 Attachment of blastocyst to endometrial wall.

ANATOMICAL AND PHYSIOLOGICAL INTERACTION OF MOTHER AND FETUS

Fertilization and Implantation of the Ovum

Chapter 50 reviews the biochemical changes required for the successful development and release of an ovum. After ovulation, the ovum is expelled into the peritoneal cavity, where it is moved into either of the two fallopian tubes by the action of ciliated epithelial cells of the fimbriated tentacles. Fertilization normally occurs before the ovum enters the tube or shortly thereafter. Approximately 3 days is required for transport of the fertilized ovum through the tube and into the cavity of the uterus. An additional 2 to 5 days is required for implantation of the ovum in the **endometrium** of the uterus. Thus, implantation of the developing ovum, the **blastocyst,** typically occurs 5 to 8 days after fertilization. Implantation results from the proteolytic digestion of the endometrium by the **trophoblasts** covering the surface of the blastocyst (Fig. 44-1). Once implantation is complete, both trophoblastic and endometrial cells proliferate rapidly in a coordinated fashion, forming the placenta and its membranes. The placenta serves to separate the foreign body, the fetus, from the maternal host, and to provide an interface between the fetal and maternal circulatory systems. Through this interface, nutrients from maternal blood are delivered to the fetus, and fetal wastes are delivered to the mother for eventual disposal.[1]

As the demands for nourishment and oxygen for the rapidly growing embryo increase, the trophoblast increases its surface area by forming villi. The surface area of these villi is enormous, and from the villi, the fetal circulation of the placenta is established. The innermost membrane, the amnion, immediately surrounds the embryo and is filled with fluid. This fluid, referred to as the liquor amnii, or amniotic fluid, bathes the fetus, thereby preventing desiccation, and buffers the fetus against physical shocks. The blood in the placenta is derived from the fetal circulation.

Fetal Growth and Nutrition

Fetal growth is dependent on the availability of essential nutrients, which are delivered to the fetus from the maternal/uterine circulation via the placenta. Placental transfer of nutrients is a dynamic process that is controlled by hormonal signals from maternal and fetal somatotropic axes. Growth hormone (GH) and insulin-like growth factor (IGF-I) produced from maternal and fetal sources are pivotal regulators in this process. Placental size and architecture, developmental and pathological processes, and interaction of maternal and fetal somatotropic mechanisms act in concert to regulate placental-fetal nutrient exchange.[2,3]

Unlike the infant, whose diet includes a complex mixture of carbohydrates, fats, and proteins, the fetus has a diet that consists largely of glucose and sufficient quantities of amino acids to satisfy the nitrogen requirements of protein synthesis. Also included are small amounts of essential fatty acids, ketones, vitamins, and minerals. Although glucose provides most of the energy needed for the formation of tissues, amino acids can serve as an alternative source of oxidizable fuel. Ketones also may serve as alternative fetal energy sources and as precursors for proteins and lipids during periods of maternal fasting.

The amount of glucose available to the fetus depends on the concentration of glucose in maternal blood, which is regulated by the action of numerous hormones, including insulin and the placental hormone, human chorionic somatomammotropin (also called human placental lactogen, or hPL). hPL increases the breakdown of maternal fat and counters the action of insulin; both factors in raising maternal blood glucose.

Glucose passes readily from the maternal to the fetal circulation by means of "facilitated diffusion," crossing the placenta at a faster rate than would be expected on physiological grounds alone. A rise in the glucose concentration in maternal blood is followed rapidly by a comparable increase in its concentration in fetal blood. The two levels do not become equal, however, and a concentration gradient from mother to fetus is always present. In addition, the placenta consumes a significant quantity of glucose to meet its own energy requirements.

Because glucose levels in the fetus mirror those in the mother, there usually is little need for the fetus to regulate its own blood glucose concentrations. Mechanisms for doing so are developed during the fetal period, but, except in infants of hyperglycemic diabetic mothers, these mechanisms are largely dormant until birth, when the supply of glucose through the placenta ends abruptly. Nevertheless, two important processes are active from an early stage. The first is the storage of glucose as glycogen or fat to provide for the metabolic needs of the newborn until feeding begins. The second involves control of the rate at which glucose is used by the growing tissues; this is attributable primarily to the action of insulin as secreted by the fetal pancreas beginning at 8 to 9 weeks of gestational age.

Role of Placenta in Gas Exchange

To meet its metabolic needs, the fetus is completely dependent on continuous delivery of oxygen across the placenta. Transplacental exchanges, including those of gases, depend on both perfusion and permeability. Placental perfusion is a composite of uterine and umbilical blood flows, whereas permeability is a characteristic of the placental membrane. Under healthy conditions with well-oxygenated maternal blood, oxygen transport across the placenta is regulated primarily by blood flow. However, maternal placental or fetal blood flows and O_2 capacities may be altered by as much as 50% without significant effect on fetal uptake of oxygen. To meet the increasing demands of the growing fetus, uterine blood flow and placental membrane permeability increase during gestation. In the presence of maternal hypoxia, oxygen transport across the placenta becomes limited primarily by the permeability of the placental membrane.[4]

Carbon dioxide rapidly diffuses across the placenta in either direction. This allows the fetus to maintain a normal P_{CO_2} and the mother to eliminate fetal carbon dioxide. The placenta has limited permeability to bicarbonate ions. The placenta therefore allows the fetus to dispose of carbon dioxide while protecting it from maternal metabolic acidosis.

Formation of Amniotic Fluid

The volume of fluid in the amniotic sac, which surrounds the developing embryo, increases throughout pregnancy until it reaches a maximum volume at about 36 weeks of gestation (Table 44-1). Many maternal and fetal abnormalities can produce **oligohydramnios** or **polyhydramnios** states. Amniotic fluid volume and composition at any point in time are the result of a dynamic balance between production and removal. Amniotic fluid originates from multiple sources, including the placenta, fetal kidneys, skin, membranes, lungs,

Table 44-1 Amniotic Fluid Volume in Normal Pregnancy

Gestational Age, Weeks	Volume of Fluid, mL
12	5 to 200
14	50 to 200
16	150 to 300
18	200 to 400
20	225 to 775
22	300 to 500
24	500 to 675
26	500 to 700
28	500 to 875
30	400 to 1300
32	400 to 1375
34	500 to 1350
36	525 to 1500
38	300 to 1525
40	325 to 1450
42	600

and intestine. The relative contribution of each source depends on the stage of fetal development. In the first half of pregnancy, amniotic fluid forms as a transudate (see Chapter 46) from the skin surface of the fetus. The composition of amniotic fluid is similar to that of extracellular fluid, and amniotic fluid should be considered as an extension of the fetal extracellular fluid space. Later in pregnancy, fetal kidneys and lungs assume a major role in the formation of amniotic fluid, and its volume now depends on a balance between fetal urination and volume of amniotic fluid that is swallowed.[1]

Fluid that moves from the trachea and pharynx into the esophagus can enter the amniotic cavity. This provides an explanation for the appearance of pulmonary surfactant in amniotic fluid. Respiratory movements (pseudo-breathing) by the fetus readily mix amniotic fluid with lung surfactant because these movements produce a tidal volume exchange (into and out) of about 600 to 800 mL/day[2] through the fetal lungs throughout the third trimester.

Amniotic fluid disappearance is affected in part by fetal swallowing. It is estimated that between 200 and 450 mL of amniotic fluid per day flows out from the amniotic cavity by this route, accounting for about half of the daily urine production of the fetus. Because the amniotic cavity gains a fluid volume of no more than 10 mL/day in the third trimester (the total solute concentration always remains in the normal range), a sizable quantity of urine must be reabsorbed by other pathways.[3,5]

KEY CONCEPTS BOX 44-1

- Implantation of a fertilized ovum that occurs 5 to 8 days after fertilization initiates a series of physiological processes that result in a uterine environment suitable for fetal development, especially the establishment of a suitable placental blood supply.
- Placental delivery of glucose to the fetus is controlled largely by maternal glucose levels.
- Placenta allows diffusion of maternal O_2 to the fetus and removal of CO_2 and other wastes.
- Amniotic fluid is formed initially as a transudate from fetal skin, and later in development, from fetal urine and fluids originating from the lungs. It serves to hold and protect the fetus.

SECTION OBJECTIVES BOX 44-2

- Describe the biochemical and biophysical changes that occur in amniotic fluid as pregnancy progresses.
- Describe the origin of amniotic fluid proteins.
- Explain the diagnostic significance of specific amniotic fluid proteins.

BIOCHEMISTRY OF AMNIOTIC FLUID[6]

Water, Electrolytes, and Nitrogenous Products

Because of the shift in the source of amniotic fluid that occurs about midway through pregnancy, constituents of amniotic fluid also change during gestation. Before **keratinization** of the skin, amniotic fluid can result as a **transudation** from the surface of the fetus. After keratinization and with progressive development of the renal system, fetal urine makes a more prominent contribution to the amniotic fluid compartment. The biochemical composition of amniotic fluid therefore reflects the routes of formation of the fluid and is related to the developmental stage of the fetus.

Amniotic fluid is isotonic during early pregnancy but by term becomes moderately hypotonic (mean total solute concentration, 255 mOsm/kg of water) compared with fetal and maternal plasma. This changing concentration of amniotic fluid reflects the maturation of fetal renal function. Osmotic and oncotic pressures in fetal and maternal tissues cause the transfer of water from mother to fetus to amniotic fluid, then back to the mother. It has been calculated that the net transfer of water from mother to fetus reaches 20 to 25 mL/day in late pregnancy.[6]

Amniotic fluid concentrations of nitrogenous products of metabolism, creatinine, urea, and uric acid increase toward the end of the term (see later discussion) but many times are lower than concentrations found in maternal urine. The composition difference between amniotic fluid and maternal urine is readily measurable and can be used to determine whether a sample obtained from vaginal leakage or from an errant amniocentesis is amniotic fluid.

Proteins

Proteins derived from many sources have been identified in amniotic fluid. Under healthy conditions, amniotic fluid proteins of fetal origin come from the skin, the urinary and gastrointestinal tracts (urine and meconium, respectively), and the respiratory tract. Proteins from the respiratory tract are part of the proteolipid product secreted by type II epithelial cells of the fetal lung. These products function as components of the lung surfactant system[7] (see later discussion). At least four surfactant protein (SP) species have been described: SP-A, SP-B, SP-C, and SP-D. These differ in molecular weight and charge and possibly function.

Proteins of maternal origin can enter amniotic fluid by transudation across the amnion. Under abnormal circumstances, unusual avenues for protein exchange can occur, such as neural tube developmental defects, which increase the α-fetoprotein levels in amniotic fluid (see later discussion).

More than 50 enzymes have been identified in amniotic fluid,[4,5] but the origin of many of these enzymes and their significance in the fluid are not understood. Enzymes fall into two categories: those that exhibit greatest activity early in pregnancy (12 to 20 weeks), and those that are active at a later stage of pregnancy (35 to 40 weeks). Acetylcholinesterase, an enzyme of fetal origin, is used in the diagnosis of neural tube defects.

Hormones

Examples of the hormones that have been identified in amniotic fluid are listed in Box 44-1. This list includes hormones derived from steroids, peptides, and amino acids. Although many of these hormones are products of urinary or biliary excretion from the fetus, a few have clinical usefulness and are discussed later. A more extensive list is available.[4,5]

Box 44-1

Hormones Identified in Amniotic Fluid

Proteins and Polypeptides
Adrenocorticotropic hormone
Angiotensin
Endorphin
Follicle-stimulating hormone
Growth hormone
Human chorionic gonadotropin
Human placental lactogen
Insulin
Luteinizing hormone
Oxytocin
Prolactin
Relaxin
Renin
Somatomedin
Somatostatin
Thyrotropin
Thyroxine

Steroids
Estradiol
Estriol
Estrone

Prostaglandins
E2
F2α

KEY CONCEPTS BOX 44-2

- Amniotic fluid (AF) composition begins to reflect fetal kidney maturation, with decreasing fluid tonicity and increasing blood urea nitrogen (BUN) and creatinine as pregnancy progresses.
- AF levels of creatinine become higher than serum levels, but never as high as in adult urine.
- AF proteins can originate from fetal skin and from the urinary, GI, and respiratory tracts.
- AF AFP levels can be useful for the diagnosis of neural tube disorders, and lung surfactant found in AF can be used to assess fetal lung maturity.

SECTION OBJECTIVES BOX 44-3

- Describe the structure of hCG and its function during pregnancy.
- Describe the synthesis of estriol by the fetoplacental unit and the function of estriol in pregnancy.
- Explain the changes in maternal thyroid hormone levels that occur during early pregnancy, and discuss the importance of thyroid hormones to the fetus.
- Describe the changes in maternal serum proteins and urinary protein and glucose that occur during pregnancy.

MATERNAL BIOCHEMICAL CHANGES DURING PREGNANCY

Human Chorionic Gonadotropin

Human chorionic gonadotropin (hCG) is one of a family of closely related glycoprotein hormones that regulate reproductive and metabolic functions. This family includes follicle-stimulating hormone (FSH), luteinizing hormone (LH), and thyroid-stimulating hormone (TSH). All four are composed of two dissimilar polypeptide subunits, α and β, which are noncovalently combined. The α-subunit is identical among these hormones while the β-subunit differs in both amino acid sequence and carbohydrate structure; the β-subunit thereby confers physiological and immunological specificity on the dimeric hormone.[8] The β-subunits of hCG and LH are 80% homologous, and the two hormones share a common cell-surface receptor (the LH-hCG receptor). hCG is the most extensively glycosylated human hormone, with 30% of its weight from carbohydrate. The α-subunit contains 2 N-linked oligosaccharide side chains, and the β-subunit has 2 N-linked and 4 O-linked side chains. The carbohydrate moieties stabilize the half-life of hCG in the plasma to ≈36 hours. In contrast, the half-life of LH is ≈60 minutes. These differences in metabolic clearance correlate well with our understanding of the functions of these hormones, with LH regulating the complicated process of ovulation and subsequent formation of the **corpus luteum,** and hCG providing continued stimulation of the corpus luteum to ensure uninterrupted progesterone production until the placenta can provide sufficient progesterone to maintain the pregnancy (see Chapter 50 for details).

Placental production of hCG begins upon implantation of the blastocyst into the uterus and is first detected in maternal serum 6 to 9 days following conception.[9] Plasma hCG concentrations increase exponentially during the first trimester and peak at between 8 and 10 weeks (Fig. 44-2). Afterward, concentrations decline to one-tenth of peak concentration, at

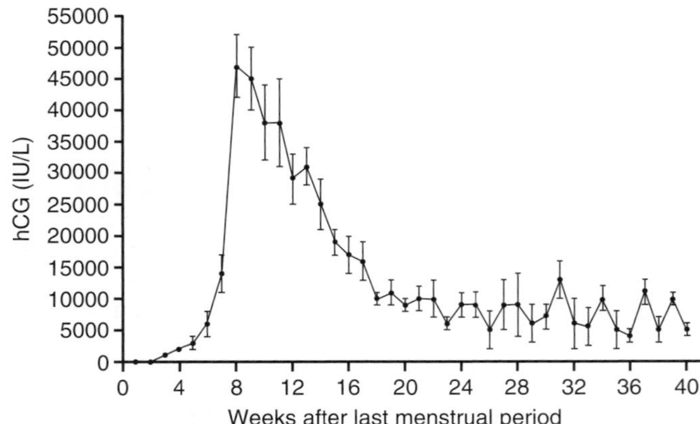

Fig. 44-2 Mean (±SE) maternal serum human chorionic gonadotropin (hCG) concentrations throughout normal pregnancy. (Adapted from Braunstein GD, Rasor J, Danzer H, et al: Serum human chorionic gonadotropin levels throughout normal pregnancy, Am J Obstet Gynecol 126:678, 1976; used with permission from Elsevier.)

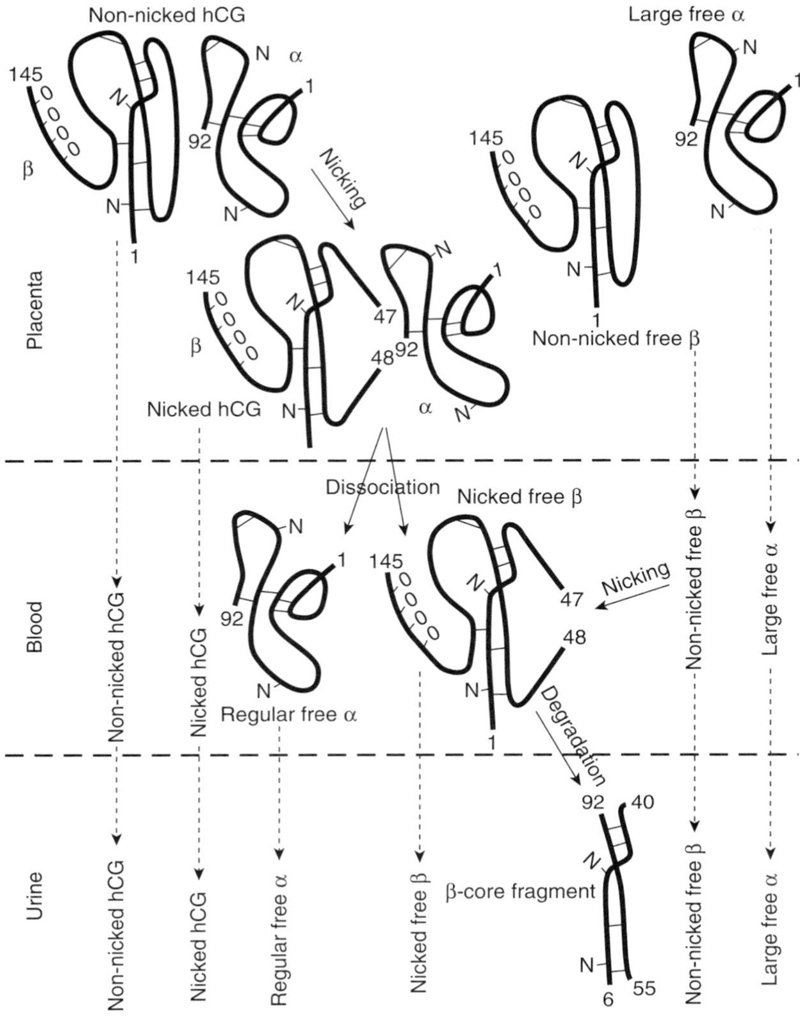

Fig. 44-3 Representation of the structures of human chorionic gonadotropin (hCG) and related molecules in the placenta, blood, and urine. (From Cole LA: Immunoassay of human chorionic gonadotropin, its free subunits, and metabolites, Clin Chem 43:2233, 1997; reprinted with permission from the American Association for Clinical Chemistry.)

Fig. 44-4 Structures of the three clinically relevant estrogens.

between weeks 18 and 20, where they remain until delivery. The appearance of hCG in urine closely parallels that in serum.

hCG demonstrates considerable molecular heterogeneity (Fig. 44-3). In addition to intact hCG, distinct isoforms present in the serum and urine include hyperglycosylated hCG, nicked hCG, free β-subunit, and nicked free β-subunit. The terminal degradation product of hCG, the β-core fragment, is detected only in maternal urine.[10]

Estrogens

The estrogens constitute a group of steroid hormones that function as the primary female sex hormone (see Chapter 50). Although more than 20 estrogens have been identified, only estrone, estradiol, and estriol are clinically relevant (Fig. 44-4). In non-pregnant women, the major estrogen is estradiol produced by the ovaries. During pregnancy, the predominant estrogen is estriol produced by the placenta in quantities that are 1000-fold greater than those of ovarian estradiol. This quantitative and qualitative change results from the combined effects of the fetal adrenal gland and the placenta, also referred to as the *fetoplacental unit*[11] (Fig. 44-5).

Placental trophoblast cells lack 17α-hydroxylase and therefore are unable to directly convert pregnenolone to estradiol. Placental pregnenolone enters the fetal circulation and is taken up by the fetal adrenal gland, itself a source of pregnenolone,

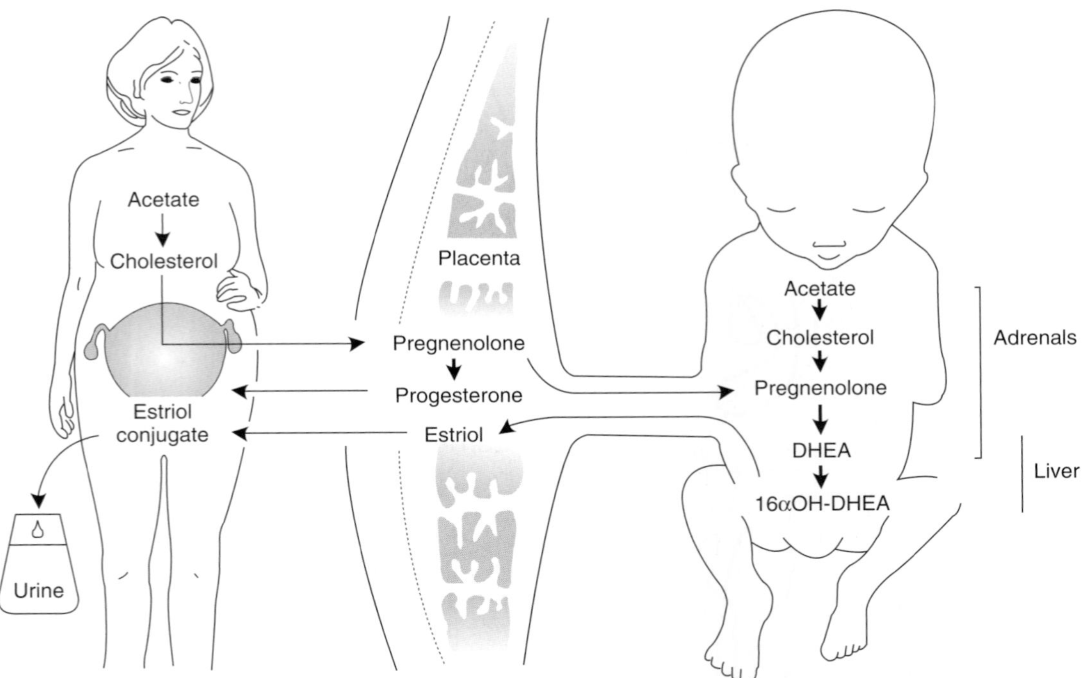

Fig. 44-5 Schema of fetoplacental unit. *DHEA,* Dehydroepiandrosterone; *16α-OH-DHEA,* 16α-hydroxydehydroepiandrosterone.

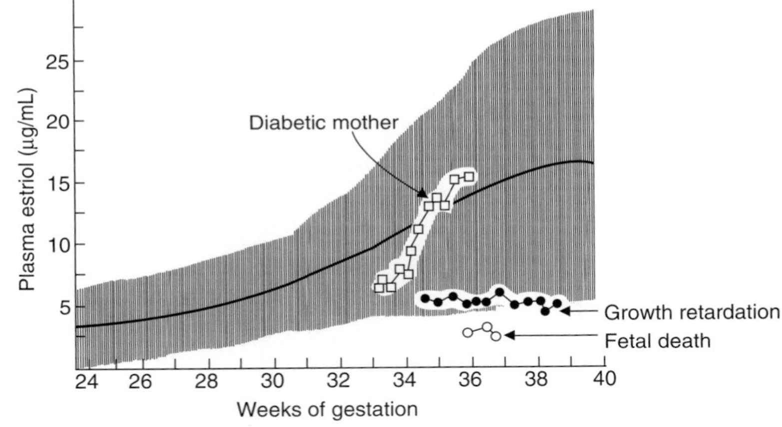

Fig. 44-6 Mean *(solid line)* and estimated 5th and 95th percentiles *(shaded areas)* for plasma unconjugated estriol during normal pregnancy. Estriol patterns from three actual pregnancy conditions are shown.

which is deficient in 3β-hydroxysteroid dehydrogenase and Δ4 isomerase activities. This limits the fetal adrenal conversion of pregnenolone to progesterone and favors the production of dehydroepiandrosterone sulfate (DHEAS), which is converted by the fetal liver to 16α-hydroxy-DHEAS. The 16α-hydroxy-DHEAS is transported to the placenta, where it is used to synthesize estriol via sequential desulfurylation and aromatization. Through this complex synthetic pathway, 90% of estriol present in the maternal serum has its origin in the fetus, and so maternal estriol concentrations can serve as an indicator of fetal well-being.[12]

Estriol is metabolized by maternal liver to both sulfate and glucuronide conjugated forms. These conjugates are the primary excretory forms of estriol. Concentrations in maternal serum increase with advancing gestation and reach nearly 40 ng/mL at the end of the term. In Fig. 44-6, the patterns of a normal increase in plasma estriol and the patterns seen in a diabetic patient, along with fetal death and with growth retardation, are shown.

The functional role of estriol in pregnancy has prompted much speculation. In many biological test systems, estriol is a weak estrogen, which demonstrates only a hundredth of the potency of estradiol and one-tenth of the potency of estrone per unit weight. However, estriol can be demonstrated to be equipotent to estradiol in its ability to promote uteroplacental blood flow. For this reason, its role in pregnancy may be to ensure optimum blood flow in the gravid uterus. Estriol also functions to enhance the cellular uptake of low-density lipoprotein (LDL) cholesterol necessary for the increased steroidogenesis of pregnancy, to simulate the hepatic synthesis of many proteins, and to prepare the breasts for lactation.[13] It is interesting to note that conditions associated with low concentrations of estriol do not appear to impair progesterone synthesis or fetal development.

Measurements of serum estriol are used as part of biochemical screening programs for Down syndrome (see below).

Thyroid

Although maternal thyroid disease can occur in pregnancy (see Chapter 49), the changes that occur in the maternal serum levels of thyroid hormones are a normal response related to the changing physiology of the mother and needs of the developing fetus.[14] Three factors contribute to the changes observed in thyroid function during this time: increases in hCG, increases in estriol, and increases in urinary iodide excretion. The increase in maternal thyroid hormone requirements is such that pregnant women who are hypothyroid need 25% to 50% more thyroxine (T_4) to maintain normal thyrotropin (TSH) concentrations than do non-pregnant women. In areas of iodine sufficiency, the maternal thyroid increases in volume by 10% to 20% during pregnancy.[15,16] During the first 1 to 2 months of pregnancy, the mother serves as the primary source of thyroid hormones for the fetus.[17] Studies of children who have congential hypothyroidism or who are conceived under conditions of severe iodine deficiency have demonstrated that thyroid hormones are essential for normal brain development, and that insufficient exposure during fetal development results in permanent neurological consequences. Furthermore, growing evidence suggests a relationship between the type and severity of cognitive and neurological deficits and the timing and severity of hormone insufficiency.[18,19]

The thyroid is the first fetal gland to develop, with the earliest evidence of formation noted at between 3 and 4 weeks. By week 8, the structures that evolve into thyroid follicles become apparent, but the cells may not be functional until about the third month. Until this time, the fetus relies on thyroid hormones and iodide received exclusively from the mother. These are acquired by placental transfer or by placental deiodination. Even after the fetal thyroid becomes functional, during the second and into the third trimester, the fetus continues to need maternal hormones to supplement its own.

Although many of the initiating mechanisms remain unknown, hCG and estriol contribute to changes in maternal thyroid hormone production. TSH concentrations decrease as hCG concentrations begin to rise and remain suppressed into midpregnancy. Although not as potent, hCG exhibits TSH-like activity (about 1/4000 the thyrotropic activity of pituitary TSH), and the large amounts of hCG produced by the placenta stimulate TSH receptors on the maternal thyroid gland. This leads to an increase in production of T_4 and T_3. At the same time, increased estriol stimulates the maternal liver to synthesize more thyroid-binding globulin (TBG) and to increase the number of carbohydrate residues of the protein (sialylation), to reduce its renal clearance. By the end of the first trimester, maternal serum TBG levels have almost doubled, and they remain elevated throughout pregnancy. The net result of these events is that although the amount of total T_4 and T_3 in maternal serum increases, the free hormone concentrations usually remain within reference intervals, and the pregnant woman is euthyroid. In the second and third trimesters, the maternal pituitary releases additional TSH in response to decreasing hCG levels.

The incidence of hypothyroidism in the pregnant population is between 2% and 5%. In addition to its deleterious effects on neurological development, the disease is associated with an increased incidence of miscarriage, preterm delivery, preeclampsia, and placental abruption. Except in high-risk populations, however, screening for the disease is not recommended currently.

Serum Lipids

Hyperlipidemia develops during a healthy pregnancy, most likely as the result of alterations in hormone levels. Total serum lipid concentrations are increased progressively throughout pregnancy, with highest levels observed in the second and third trimesters.[20,21] After delivery, these levels return to the levels seen before, thus lending support for the role of pregnancy-related hormones in regulating serum lipid levels. All components of serum lipids are increased, but the triacylglyceride fraction shows the largest proportionate rise. High-density lipoprotein/low-density lipoprotein (HDL/LDL) ratios decrease with increasing duration of pregnancy, and HDL levels remain decreased at 1 year after pregnancy.

Serum Proteins and Liver Function

The total concentration of serum proteins decreases by about 0.1 g/dL during pregnancy. Most of this decrease occurs during the first trimester and is related to increased excretion and utilization. The decrease is seen mainly in serum albumin. Levels of α_1-, α_2-, and β-globulins rise slowly and progressively during pregnancy. The maternal antibody (immunoglobulin [Ig]G) component, which is transferred to the fetus, declines progressively. Throughout pregnancy, fibrinogen increases progressively, and values at term are 30% to 50% above non-pregnant levels. Clotting factors VII, VIII, IX, and X also increase, whereas prothrombin and factors V and XII are reduced. Alterations in the levels of clotting factors and plasminogen probably are brought about by the action of estriol on the liver.

Under the influence of increased estriol, the maternal liver enhances the synthesis of transcortin (corticoid-binding globulin). This results in increased total cortisol levels during pregnancy, and these levels are almost doubled by late pregnancy. However, the levels of free, active cortisol are normal.

Nonspecific alkaline phosphatase activity in serum nearly doubles during pregnancy with a healthy mother and fetus, and can reach levels that would be considered abnormal in the non-pregnant woman. Much of this increase is attributable to isoenzymes that originate from the placenta.[22]

Proteinuria

Proteinuria, which is a common occurrence during pregnancy, results from changes in the glomerular filtration rate. Studies of healthy pregnant women have found 10% to 40% will have at least one episode of proteinuria, defined as >30 mg/dL.[23] For this reason, the test no longer is considered a hallmark of impending preeclampsia in uncomplicated pregnancy.[24]

Glucosuria

Glucosuria occurs during pregnancy in up to 50% of nondiabetic women as the result of an increase in the glomerular filtration rate.[25] The cardinal feature of the glucosuria of pregnancy is a conspicuous variability both during the course of the day and from day to day. For these reasons, urinary glucose measurements should not be used to screen for gestational diabetes, or to monitor women known to be diabetic. (See later discussion and Chapter 38 for additional information on gestational diabetes.)

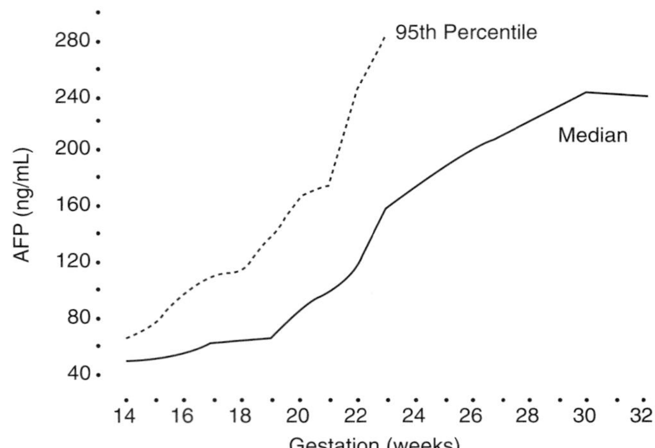

Fig. 44-7 Median and 95th percentile of α-fetoprotein (AFP) in maternal serum. (From Crandall BF: In Kirkpatrick AM, Nakamura RM, editors: *Alpha-Fetoprotein: Laboratory Procedures and Clinical Applications,* New York, 1981, Masson.)

KEY CONCEPTS BOX 44-3

- hCG is a highly glycosylated protein hormone produced by the placenta that is required to maintain progesterone production by the corpus luteum in early pregnancy.
- Although present in many molecular forms, hCG is the earliest biochemical marker of pregnancy.
- Estriol, produced by the fetoplacental unit, exhibits the least biological activity of the estrogens; it may function to maintain placental blood supply. It also increases protein synthesis in the liver. Low maternal serum estriol is associated with Down syndrome.
- TSH-like activity of hCG, increased hepatic TBG production, and fetal demand for thyroid hormones result in many changes to maternal thyroid hormones.
- Thyroxine (T_4) is needed for proper development of fetal brain.
- Estriol increases synthesis of many hepatic proteins (e.g., TBG), and an increase in synthesis of clotting factors, including factors VII, VIII, IX, and X and fibrinogen, is seen.
- Loss of protein and glucose in maternal urine is increased as pregnancy progresses.

SECTION OBJECTIVES BOX 44-4

- Describe the functional changes that occur to the liver and kidneys during the fetal and neonatal period.
- Describe the composition of pulmonary surfactant, and explain its synthesis and function.
- Discuss the hepatic processing of bilirubin, and explain why neonates develop hyperbilirubinemia.
- Define RDS, and describe its cause.
- Describe the changes in hemoglobin synthesis that occur during the fetal gestational period.

FETAL BIOCHEMICAL CHANGES DURING PRENATAL DEVELOPMENT

Liver Function

The liver begins to develop from the embryonic foregut during the first few weeks of life and continues to develop after birth. Initially, it serves as the primary source of hematopoiesis, until the bone marrow assumes this responsibility at around 22 to 24 weeks of gestation. Although not fully functional, the fetal hepatocytes nevertheless produce many necessary enzymes and proteins and are involved in a variety of metabolic processes. Ongoing development and maturation produce circulating concentrations and activity patterns for most enzymes and proteins that often are different from those observed in adults.

α-Fetoprotein (AFP) is a major protein produced by the fetal liver. After its release into the fetal circulation, AFP is excreted by the fetal kidneys into amniotic fluid. AFP appears in maternal serum throughout gestation (Fig. 44-7), where it can be measured easily to screen for neural tube defects.

The need of the fetus for increased quantities of amino acids for protein synthesis is satisfied by placental transport. This is an active process against a concentration gradient that depends on placental blood flow and, to a lesser degree, on the concentration of amino acids in maternal plasma.

Because maturation of the fetal liver is not complete by the time of birth, the liver may not be able to fully clear bilirubin from the blood; as a result, some jaundice may occur during the first week of life, particularly if the birth is preterm. Known as physiological jaundice, the yellow pigmentation, or jaundice, is caused by bilirubin that is produced by the normal destruction of red blood cells (see p. 885 for details). This condition should be mild, should resolve rapidly, and should not be confiused with more serious causes of hyperbilirubinemia in a newborn (see Chapter 45).

Renal Function

The primary function of the mammalian kidney is to maintain water and electrolyte homeostasis. These tasks are accomplished by selective excretion or retention of water and solutes as conditions dictate. In the fetus, however, the placenta is the

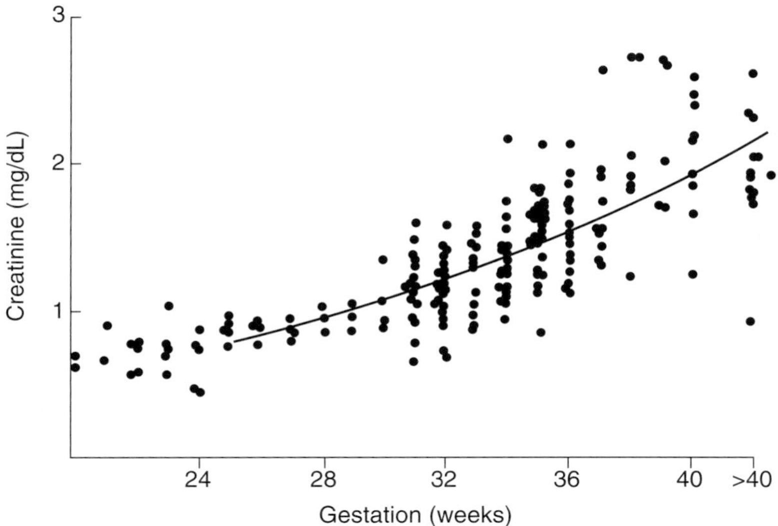

Fig. 44-8 Distribution and regression curve of amniotic fluid creatinine concentration in milligrams per deciliter. (From Lind T: In Fairweather DVI, Eskes TKAB, editors: *Amniotic Fluid: Research and Clinical Application,* ed 2, Amsterdam, 1978, Excerpta Medica.)

primary organ responsible for body water and electrolyte balance. For this reason, a fetus with nonfunctioning kidneys often shows no water or electrolyte abnormalities. As with the liver, the fetal kidneys continue to mature after birth.

Organic nitrogenous compounds such as urea, uric acid, and creatinine (Fig. 44-8) gradually increase in amniotic fluid as the renal system of the fetus matures. In early pregnancy, these compounds are present in amniotic fluid in concentrations similar to those found in maternal and fetal blood. Concentrations increase gradually to become significantly higher than levels in maternal or fetal blood. A sharp rise in creatinine at about the 37th week of gestation elevates the amniotic fluid concentrations of urea and creatinine to levels two to three times higher than those of the reference interval of serum in healthy persons.[26]

Lung Development

At birth, an abrupt physiological transition requires the newborn infant to assume vital functions that previously were handled by the maternal circulation. The lung is shifted from a fluid-filled organ to a gas exchange system within a few brief minutes. This functional transition is possible only if sufficient maturation of the fetal lung has occurred during development. The fetal lung maturation process appears to consist of two distinct components: (1) morphological development of the fetal lungs; and (2) synthesis, storage, and release of pulmonary surfactant. In the latter process, the control mechanisms for synthesis and storage of pulmonary surfactant appear to be distinct from those responsible for surfactant release.[27] Thus, functional lungs should have developed alveoli with adequate surface area and vascularization for gas exchange, and sufficient surfactant must be available to sustain the ventilatory movements needed for pulmonary function. These processes are highly organized and are coordinated by the timing of anatomical and biochemical events.

Surfactant facilitates pulmonary function in at least two ways: It maintains alveolar stability by preventing collapse of the terminal respiratory tree, and it reduces the pressure that is needed to distend the lungs in the initial phase of inspiration. Infants who develop the respiratory distress syndrome (RDS) have higher surface tension at the alveolar air-liquid interface as a result of a pulmonary surfactant deficiency.

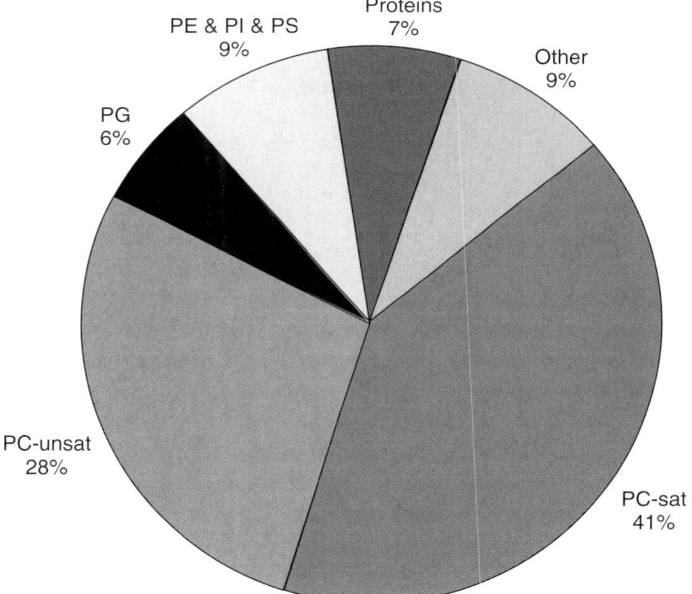

Fig. 44-9 Composition (by weight percent) of human surfactant. *PC-sat,* Saturated phosphatidylcholine; *PC-unsat,* unsaturated phosphatidylinositol; *PE,* phosphatidylethanolamine; *PG,* phosphatidylglycerol; *PI,* phosphatidylinositol; *PS,* phosphatidylserine. Proteins include 3.8% surfactant protein (SP)-A (SP-B and SP-C detected but not quantified). (From Hallman M: Rev Perinatal Med 6:197, 1989.)

Human surfactant is composed principally of phospholipid that contains highly saturated fatty acid moieties.[28] The major constituents and their relative concentrations are shown in Figs. 44-9 and 44-10. In addition to the highly unusual satu-

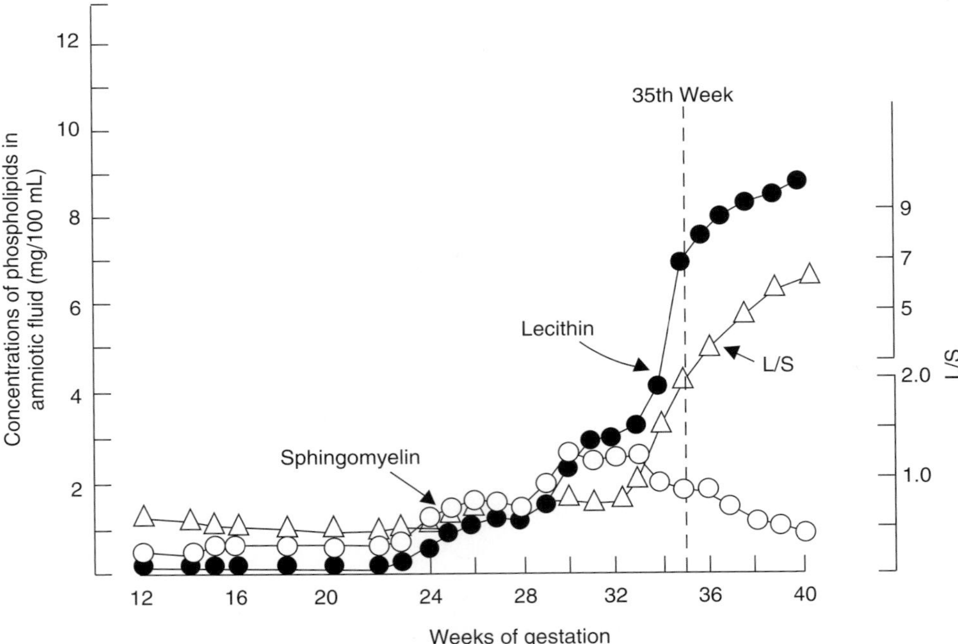

Fig. 44-10 Lecithin, sphingomyelin, and lecithin/sphingomyelin ratios in amniotic fluid during normal pregnancy. (Modified from Gluck L, Kulovich MV: Lecithin-sphingomyelin ratios in amniotic fluid in normal and abnormal pregnancy, Am J Obstet Gynecol 115:539, 1973.)

rated lecithins, other important constituents of the surface-active system include phosphatidylglycerol and the surfactant proteins (SPs) mentioned previously. These proteins may play a key role in enabling surfactant function by enhancing the rapidity with which surfactant can spread to form a monolayer along the air-water interface of the alveolus. Although functional differences between the individual SPs are described incompletely, surfactant protein B (SP-B) may be the most important of the proteins in pulmonary surfactant.[29] This is believed to be the result of the unique interaction of this protein with phospholipid moieties in surfactant. This interaction adds stability to the surfactant monolayer, thus enhancing the ability of this layer to lower surface tension and prevent alveolar collapse. Detailed accounts of the function and biochemical composition of pulmonary surfactant have been published.[30-32]

Surfactant is formed in the large alveolar epithelial cells known as type II pneumocytes, which make up about 10% of the cells of the lung. Although biosynthetic pathways for the individual phospholipids have been well described, much remains to be learned about the factors responsible for their regulation. Synthesis and storage begin at between 24 and 28 weeks of gestational age. At about 32 weeks, this material begins to be released from type II pneumocytes in the form of specialized unique structures called **lamellar bodies** (LBs). This term describes the concentrically wound, or "onionlike," structure of these particles when viewed with the electron microscope. Once in the alveolar air space, LBs unravel to form tubular myelin. Tubular myelin then remains in the alveolar space, where it eventually spreads into a surfactant monolayer at the air-liquid interface with the alveoli. During normal respiration, up to 50% of the surface-active material is reabsorbed and subsequently re-released by the type II pneumocytes. The complex synthesis and degradation of pulmonary surfactant are shown in Fig. 44-11.

Hemoglobin

Embryos have a hemoglobin that is unique to the embryonic stage of development. This is replaced during fetal life by fetal hemoglobin (HbF) and finally by adult hemoglobin (HbA).[33] The pattern of hemoglobins formed during development is presented in Fig. 44-12. Fetal hemoglobin has been found to constitute 34% of the total hemoglobin in an embryo just younger than 7 weeks.[34] By approximately 10 weeks of gestation, the embryonic hemoglobins decrease to 10% of the total hemoglobin present. Before the end of the first trimester (within the first 12 weeks), the HbF has increased to approximately 90% of the total, with the remaining percentage consisting of HbA. From this point, the percentage of HbF remains constant until about the 36th week of gestation, when a decline is evident. This decline is caused primarily by an increase in HbA synthesis, rather than by a decrease in HbF synthesis. Sharp increases in HbA are seen in reticulocytes and erythrocytes by the time of birth. Developmental changes in **hematopoietic** sites, the red cell morphology, and the hemoglobin types are shown in Fig. 44-13.

The physiological differences between the hemoglobins are summarized by Kleihauer[33] and include differences in affinity for oxygen; resistance to acid, base, and heat denaturation; and electrophoretic and chromatographic properties. The higher affinity that fetal hemoglobin has for oxygen is reflected in the fetal oxyhemoglobin saturation curve, which lies to the left of the maternal oxyhemoglobin curves under standard conditions. In fact, when oxygen is diffusing from maternal blood

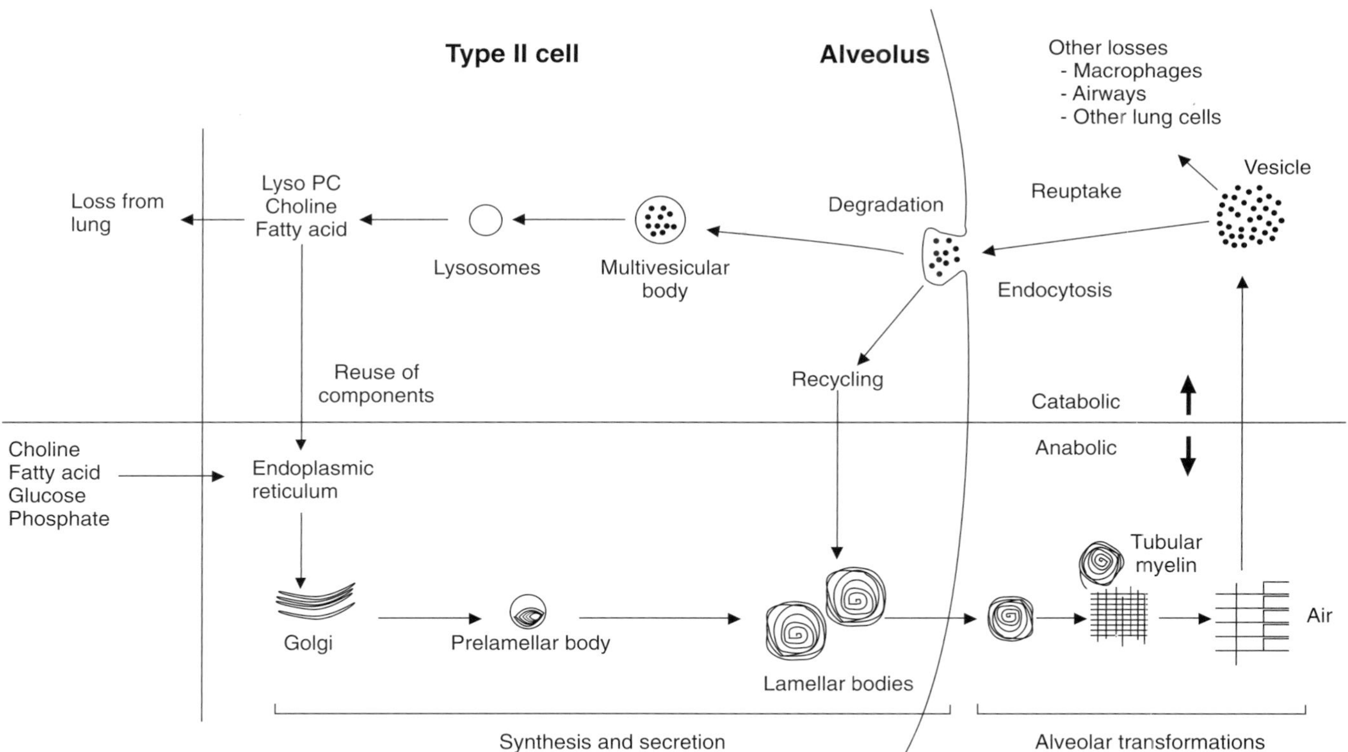

Fig. 44-11 Illustration of surfactant metabolism. The anabolic synthetic and secretory pathways link with the alveolar transformation of lamellar bodies to tubular myelin that forms the functional surfactant monolayer. During the newborn period, most surfactant is taken up by type II pneumocytes and is recycled. (From Jobe AH, Ikegami M: Surfactant metabolism, Clin Perinatol 20:687, 1993; with permission.)

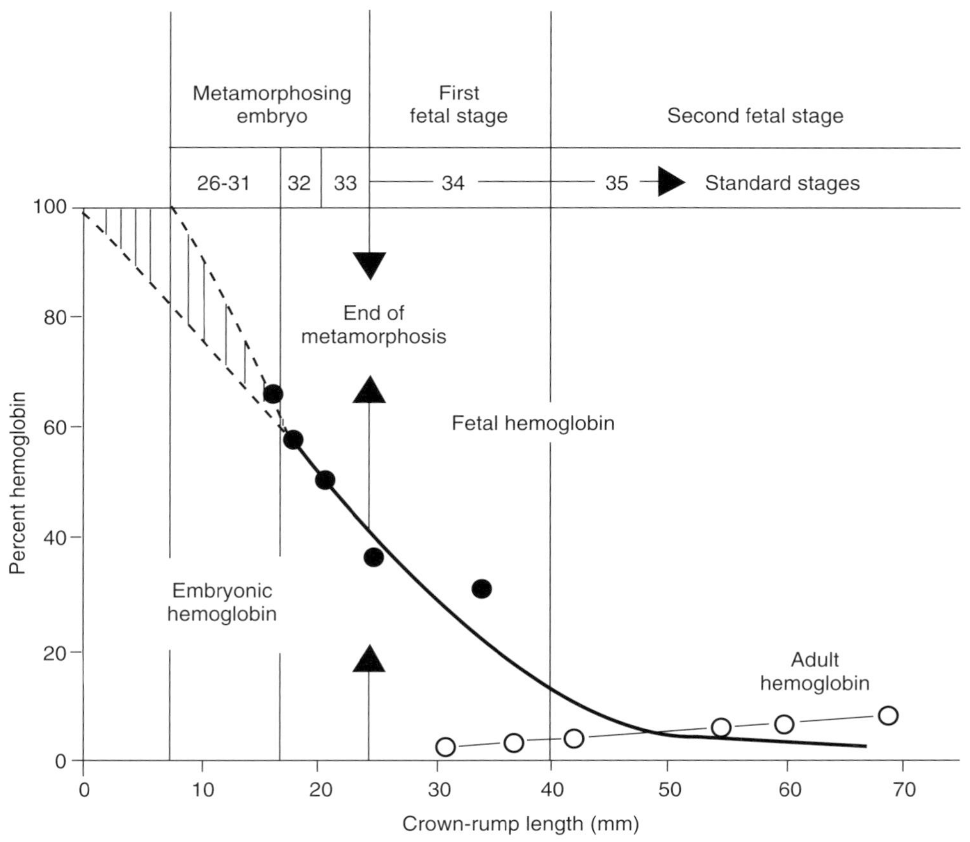

Fig. 44-12 Relationship between hemoglobin types and developmental stages in early human life. *Dashed lines and hatched area,* Expected development. (From Kleihauer E: In Stave U, editor: *Perinatal Physiology,* New York, 1978, Plenum.)

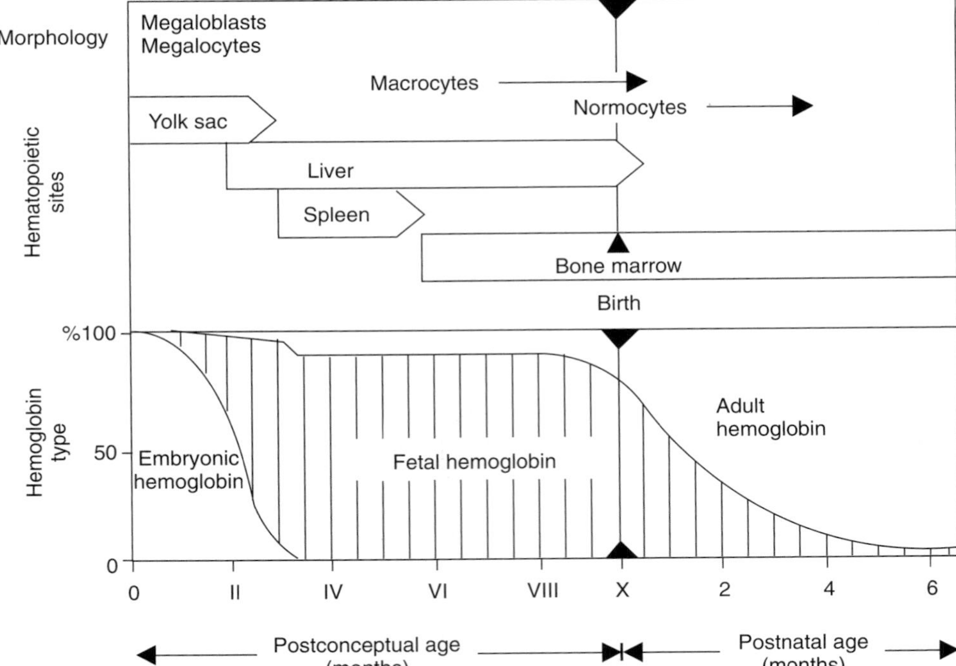

Fig. 44-13 Developmental changes in hematopoietic sites, red blood cell morphology, and hemoglobin types. (From Kleihauer E: In Stave U, editor: *Perinatal Physiology,* New York, 1978, Plenum.)

with a Pco_2 of about 34 mm Hg to fetal blood with a Pco_2 of about 30 mm Hg, the oxygen is actually moving against a concentration gradient.

Bilirubin

Erythrocyte destruction precedes the formation of bilirubin. Biliverdin is the principal and initial degradation product of hemoglobin and is an important intermediate pigment in the formation of bilirubin (see Chapter 31 for details). These relationships are presented in simplified terms as follows:

$$\text{Hemoglobin} \rightarrow \text{Biliverdin} \xrightarrow{\text{Biliverdin reductase}} \text{Bilirubin}$$
$$\searrow \text{Globin}$$

Plasma concentrations of bilirubin in the fetal circulation usually are low, except in unusual circumstances, as in severe erythroblastosis fetalis (see p. 871). Even in circumstances in which the rapid breakdown of erythrocytes leads to accelerated bilirubin production, as in severe maternal-fetal blood group incompatibility, cord blood bilirubin rarely exceeds 5 mg/dL. This fact attests to the rapid, efficient transfer of this pigment across the placenta and the equally efficient disposal of fetal bilirubin by the mother.

After birth, the newborn loses the placental mechanism for bilirubin removal. As a result, a modest accumulation of unconjugated bilirubin occurs in the plasma. The jaundice that results from this change in physiological circumstance is related to the limited uptake, conjugation, and excretion of bilirubin by the immature liver. The degree of neonatal jaundice that occurs at birth depends on the maturity and health of the fetal liver at birth (see Chapter 45). A discussion of the transport and liver metabolism of bilirubin can be found in Chapter 31.

KEY CONCEPTS BOX 44-4

- Many fetal organs are not fully mature until near or after birth.
- Liver produces AFP as the primary serum protein until late in gestation, and the ability of the liver to process and excrete bilirubin does not reach full maturity until after birth.
- Immature hepatic function often leads to hyperunconjugated bilirubinemia (jaundice, icterus).
- Mature, functional lungs require surfactant (phospholipids, proteins) to maintain alveoli stability.
- Immature pulmonary function at birth can result in respiratory distress syndrome (RDS); prebirth testing can detect a fetus at risk for RDS.
- Hemoglobin synthesis changes throughout fetal and newborn life, with the production of embryonic hemoglobin chains gradually switching to the production of adult hemoglobin A.

SECTION OBJECTIVES BOX 44-5

- Define ectopic pregnancy, and list its causes and effects on the mother.
- Define preterm labor, list its causes, and describe the problems associated with it.
- Explain the causes of preeclampsia and risks to the mother and fetus.
- Explain the causes of maternal diabetes and its effects on the mother and the fetus.
- Explain the causes of fetal hemolytic disorders, and describe how the laboratory can monitor.
- Discuss the major liver disease of pregnancy and its effects on mother and fetus.
- Describe the primary congenital diseases that are screened by laboratory testing.

PATHOLOGICAL CONDITIONS ASSOCIATED WITH PREGNANCY AND PERINATAL PERIOD

Placental Disorders

Adequate exchange across the placenta between the maternal and fetal circulations is essential for normal fetal growth and metabolism. Less than optimum quantities of nutrients result in small-for-gestational-age fetuses, whereas excessive quantities of nutrients, as in maternal diabetes, result in large-for-gestational-age infants.

Monitoring of chemicals by the laboratory is useful in only a few pathological conditions involving the placenta. One such example is the **hydatidiform** mole. Molar tissue is a developmental anomaly of the placenta that has the potential for malignant growth. It is the most common lesion antecedent to choriocarcinoma. Because the mole is made up of trophoblastic tissue, hCG is produced, leading to a positive pregnancy test result. If serum or urinary hCG levels exceed values typical of specific times in pregnancy, a mole may be suspected. However, because of variations in gonadotropin values possible for normal pregnancy, no single value can be established as the borderline between normal and abnormal. Because highly sensitive and specific methods are available for monitoring serum hCG, this hormone is useful in monitoring the response of hydatidiform moles to therapy. Recent studies indicate that structural variants of hCG, with distinct oligosaccharide glycosylation patterns, may be found in a variety of pregnancy-related disorders, including choriocarcinoma and hydatidiform mole.[35,36]

Ectopic Pregnancy

Following fertilization, the fertilized egg migrates down the fallopian tube and enters and implants in the uterus. An **ectopic pregnancy** occurs when implantation takes place outside the uterus. In 99% of such cases, implantation occurs in the fallopian tube itself (a tubal pregnancy). An ectopic pregnancy can be caused by endocrine imbalances, residual effects stemming from tubal infection, especially recurring salpingitis, or retrograde movement of the embryo from the uterus to the fallopian tube.[37] The prevalence of ectopic pregnancy is approximately 20 per 1000 pregnancies.[38] Risk factors include a previous occurrence of pelvic inflammatory disease (infection with *Chlamydia trachomatis* or *Neisseria gonorrhoeae* is most common), tubal surgery, previous ectopic pregnancy, and infertility treatment.

Clinical symptoms include lower abdominal pain and vaginal bleeding, although the former is highly variable in intensity and perceived location. Amenorrhea is not a characteristic feature. Before rupture of the fallopian tube occurs, tubal pregnancies usually yield a positive pregnancy test result. However, because compromised placentas (i.e., those in the process of abruption, degeneration, or penetration of the tubal wall) cannot produce chorionic gonadotropin in usual quantities, these tests may have low diagnostic sensitivity and/or may be misleading. Ectopic pregnancy is the leading cause of pregnancy-related, first-trimester death, so early diagnosis is important for reducing morbidity and mortality from hemorrhage and preserving fertility (see later discussion).

Preterm Delivery

Preterm labor, defined as labor that occurs before 37 weeks of gestation, is the leading cause of perinatal morbidity and mortality in the United States. Its incidence has increased by 13% since the early 1990s, and currently, it affects approximately 12.5% of births.[39] A higher rate of multiple gestation is likely the major reason for the increased incidence. Babies born before 37 completed weeks are at higher risk for pulmonary immaturity with resultant RDS and intraventricular hemorrhage. In addition, premature rupture of membranes (PROM) can increase the risk of fetal infection.

Symptoms of preterm labor include vaginal bleeding and spotting, increased vaginal discharge, abdominal cramping, and back pain. Because clinical findings are relatively nonspecific, this condition is difficult to diagnose with absolute certainty. Patients usually are hospitalized for observation, and many times, the symptoms subside. If preterm labor advances, **tocolytic agents** (such as magnesium sulfate), which can slow or halt uterine contractions, may be used over the course of several days to delay labor. This allows time in which the physician can administer corticosteroids in an attempt to induce fetal lung maturity. In some cases, the patient is not in labor, but the placental membranes have ruptured; this can cause preterm delivery. Causes of premature labor and PROM are listed in Box 44-2 and can be grouped as maternal, fetal, and

Box 44-2

Risk Factors Associated With Preterm Birth

Maternal
History of preterm birth (most significant risk factor)
Maternal age, younger than 18 and older than 35 years
Maternal weight, less than 100 lb
Nonwhite race
Maternal behaviors, including smoking and cocaine, amphetamine, or alcohol use
Multiple gestation
No prenatal care
Cervical incompetence
Exposure to DES (diethylstilbestrol)
Placenta previa
Retained intrauterine device

Fetal
Chromosomal abnormalities
Intrauterine fetal death
Intrauterine growth restriction

Infectious
Acute pyelonephritis
Bacterial vaginosis
Gonorrhea
Group B streptococcus
Chorioamnionitis
Chlamydia
Periodontal disease

infectious. Although these risk factors can guide the physician in deciding which patients to monitor closely, their value in assessing the risk of premature labor has proved to be limited. Currently, two tests with a proven high positive predictive value for preterm labor are used in the clinic: The first is **ultrasonography,** which is performed to measure cervical length. Pregnant women with a cervical dimension of 1.5 cm or less display an increased risk of premature birth.[40,41]

The second test measures fetal fibronectin (fFN), a large, extracellular glycoprotein that is produced by the chorion and is found in fetal membranes, decidua, and amniotic fluid, but not in blood or urine. The detection of fFN in vaginal fluids can indicate the loss of membrane integrity. This protein is discussed further under Change of Analyte in Disease.

Preeclampsia

Preeclampsia refers to the new onset of hypertension along with proteinuria after week 20 of the pregnancy. The condition complicates 2% to 10% of all pregnancies and is a major cause of obstetrical morbidity and mortality for both mother and fetus. One of the more serious complications of preeclamsia is the development of grand mal seizures, also known in this setting as **eclampsia.**

It was recognized even as early as 1939 that the placenta, not the fetus, is central to the pathogenesis of preeclampsia. Numerous genetic, immunological, and environmental mechanisms can result in abnormalities within the developing placenta that may lead to hypertension and preeclampsia. The role of placental tissue in the development of the disorder is emphasized further by the fact that the condition occurs in molar pregnancies. Preeclampsia develops in two stages.[42] In stage 1, the placental vasculature fails to develop properly, resulting in placental ischemia. Whether this is a cause or a result of abnormal placental development is unclear, but oxidative stress, lipid peroxidation, increased endothelial cell permeability, and activation of the coagulation cascade within placental tissues may occur in response. The vessels that develop tend to be narrow and fail to deliver needed nutrients and oxygen. In response to these stresses, placental endothelial cells release numerous cytokines, tissue factors, vasoactive mediators, and so forth, into the maternal circulation. Stage 2 begins with the onset of clinical signs and symptoms that include hypertension, edema, renal impairment, proteinuria, consumptive coagulopathy, sodium retention, and hyperreflexia. Life-threatening complications of eclampsia, including seizures and coma, also can occur. Preeclampsia occurs twice as often in primagravidas (those having first pregnancies), and about half of these women will have a recurrence in subsequent pregnancies.[43] Other risk factors include chronic hypertension, gestational diabetes, pregestational diabetes, obesity, and maternal age greater than 35 years.[44] Management includes bed rest, dietary restriction of salt, and administration of antithrombotic drugs.[45] Unfortunately, no tests currently allow for risk screening or early detection. Urinary glucose and protein have been used, but given the high rates of glucosuria and proteinuria that are seen during a healthy pregnancy, routine use of either of these is no longer recommended.[44] Once the condition has been diagnosed, laboratory tests for monitoring the patient include uric acid, aspartate aminotransferase (AST), alanine aminotransferase (ALT), creatinine, and urine protein.

Maternal Diabetes (also see Chapter 38)

The metabolic changes within a normal pregnancy first promote maternal fat deposition; they then increase insulin resistance and lipolysis. As the placenta increases in size, it produces increasing amounts of human placental lactogen (hPL), human placental growth hormone (hPGH), and numerous proinflammatory cytokines that modify or oppose the action of insulin within the maternal circulation.[46] hPL increases by as much as 30-fold during pregnancy raising maternal blood glucose; maternal pancreatic β-cells respond accordingly by increasing insulin secretion to control glucose. Complicating glucose homeostasis for the nondiabetic pregnant woman is the fact that severe insulin resistance develops within her skeletal muscle and adipose tissue during the latter half of pregnancy through mechanisms that are as yet unclear. For the diabetic woman (type 1 or type 2) and for the woman who develops gestational diabetes, hyperglycemia is a serious concern, because a clear relationship has been established between poor glycemic control and increased risk of intrauterine death, congenital malformation, and perinatal mortality and morbidity, as well as subsequent health risks for both mother and child. Not only should the diabetic woman be monitored closely throughout the course of her pregnancy, but considerable evidence suggests that it is also important to maintain a euglycemic state during the period around and immediately after (first 7 weeks of gestation) conception, to minimize congenital malformations that may result from the teratogenic effects of glucose.[47] Although maternal glucose readily crosses the placenta, insulin does not, which means that insulin produced by the fetus has no impact on the mother's glycemic control.[48] Exogenous insulin therapy and diet therefore are necessary for management of the diabetic mother's insulin-deficient state.

When insufficient insulin is available to maintain normal glucose homeostasis, maternal hyperglycemia results; this, in turn, increases blood glucose and insulin within the fetus, resulting in unusually large babies (macrosomia), who are at increased risk for becoming diabetic in later life. At delivery, when the fetus is deprived of the maternal glucose source, excess insulin in the newborn rapidly decreases blood glucose levels, so that the newborn becomes hypoglycemic. Life-threatening hypoglycemic crises frequently are encountered in untreated infants of diabetic mothers. When this happens, glucose must be administered to the newborn until a proper glucose-insulin balance can be achieved.

In pregnancies complicated by diabetes, a significant increase in the incidence of RDS has been noted, although this is by no means a universal finding. These apparent contradictions may relate to glycemic control and the number of episodes of hypoglycemia encountered by the mother.

Intrahepatic Cholestasis of Pregnancy

Intrahepatic cholestasis of pregnancy (ICP) is the most frequent liver disorder of pregnancy, with an incidence of between 1 : 1000 and 1 : 10,000 pregnancies. Mild to severe itching that begins during the third trimester is the major clinical complaint of the mother. This itching is caused by an increase in serum bile acids, which is the key diagnostic finding for the disease. ICP is associated with increased risks of premature birth and stillbirth (perinatal mortality can be as high as 1%). If ICP is diagnosed, it is best treated by early delivery of the fetus. Diagnosis can be made when an increase in hepatic enzymes associated with complaints of itching is reported and most important, when an increase in serum bile acids is found.

Fetal Lung Immaturity

The last of the organ systems to mature sufficiently to support extrauterine life are the lungs. Fetal lung immaturity, or RDS, occurs most often when insufficient lung surfactant is present.[49] Infants with RDS require increased respiratory effort. The tremendous effort needed to inflate uncooperative lungs often results in the grunting, nasal flaring, and substernal retractions that are characteristic physical signs in these infants. The greater expenditure of energy that is required for breathing can result in the death of weak, premature newborns.

In 2003, infant mortality from RDS in the United States was 20 per 100,000 live births which is considerably lower than it was in previous decades.[50] Therapy for newborns with RDS is basically supportive, and clinical therapy is aimed at effective management of pulmonary exchange of oxygen and carbon dioxide, acidosis, and circulatory insufficiency. The effect of administration of pulmonary surfactant from exogenous sources (human, mammalian, and artificially synthesized) has been investigated in infants with RDS. Several recent studies have established clear benefits from surfactant replacement therapy in reducing the severity of pulmonary damage and mortality caused by RDS.[51,52]

Glucocorticoids stimulate the process of pulmonary maturation, and it is well established that prenatal administration of maternal dexamethasone or betamethasone at between 30 and 33 weeks of gestational age can promote lung development and reduce the risk and/or severity of RDS,[53,54] although only about 15% of eligible pregnant patients actually receive hormonal therapy.[55] Intrauterine infection, diabetes, and severe preeclampsia represent contraindications to antenatal steroid administration. The potential risks of glucocorticoid administration and the short window of therapeutic response (24 hours to 7 days before birth) are probably largely responsible for its limited use.

Although the therapies discussed have demonstrated significant reductions in RDS morbidity and mortality, no ideal preventative therapy has yet been developed for infants who are at risk for developing RDS. Thus obstetrical management efforts continue to be directed toward prevention of the syndrome in premature infants through delivery management based, in part, on antenatal assessment of lung maturation. Because the status of fetal surfactant synthesis and release correlates so well with the probability of lung maturity at delivery, amniotic fluid tests that assess the quantity or quality of pulmonary surfactant present before delivery are used widely for obstetrical management. These tests are discussed in detail in a later section.

Fetal Hemolytic Disorders (Rh Isoimmunization)

Hepatic capacity to conjugate bilirubin does not become fully mature until nearly 4 weeks post partum in full-term human infants. Hepatic processing of unconjugated bilirubin therefore insufficient to clear bilirubin before that time. When bilirubin production exceeds the capacity of the liver to excrete the quantity formed, as in infants with severe hemolytic disease, unconjugated bilirubin accumulates in tissues and serum.

Hemolytic disease of the newborn (HDN) results from the destruction of fetal red blood cells (RBCs) by maternal IgG antibodies directed against paternally inherited RBC antigens. Most often, these **isoantibodies** have specificity toward **isoantigens** of the Rhesus (Rh) blood group system, but other blood group antigens such as ABO, Kell, Duffy, Kidd, and MNS may be involved. Anti-D is the most common cause of HDN. Maternal sensitization can develop from antepartum or intrapartum fetomaternal hemorrhage during the first pregnancy with a fetus that expresses RBC antigens not expressed by the mother. Although this fetus is unlikely to develop HDN, subsequent antigen-positive fetuses are at considerable risk for developing the disease. The passage of IgG antibodies across the placenta typically induces fetal RBC hemolysis that can vary from subclinical, to mild anemia, to the life-threatening condition of erythroblastosis fetalis.[56]

The healthy fetus generates approximately 35 mg of bilirubin from the catabolism of 1 g of hemoglobin. The high maternal-to-fetal plasma protein gradient facilitates rapid transplacental extraction of unconjugated fetal bilirubin and at the same time suppresses glucuronide conjugation by the fetal liver. The transferred bilirubin is so efficiently conjugated and excreted by the mother that it is uncommon for the neonate to have an elevated cord blood bilirubin level. However, in severe erythroblastosis, particularly when coupled with placental deterioration, unconjugated bilirubin levels can run as high as 8 mg/dL. Fetuses who receive intrauterine transfusions often are born with high levels of conjugated bilirubin, probably arising from stimulation of fetal glucuronide formation coupled with decreased placental permeability to the bilirubin glucuronide.

Also unique to the newborn and related to developmental immaturity is the tissue toxicity of unconjugated bilirubin, especially to the brain. In the adult, serum bilirubin elevations are viewed as an important clinical or laboratory sign of disease or altered physiological state. In the newborn, hyperbilirubinemia has dual significance as a clinical sign and as a toxin.

Bilirubin glucuronide is highly water soluble, while unconjugated bilirubin is insoluble in aqueous solution but highly soluble in lipids (see Chapter 31). Usually, unconjugated bilirubin is bound to plasma albumin, which prevents the entrance of unconjugated bilirubin into the lipid-rich central nervous system. When the bilirubin-binding capacity of albumin is exceeded, unbound, unconjugated bilirubin readily passes into the cells of the central nervous system. Unconjugated bilirubin is toxic to the central nervous system and causes necrosis, a pathological process referred to as kernicterus. Surviving infants may have mental retardation, hearing deficits, or cerebral palsy. Many affected infants, particularly those of low birth weight, may have no neonatal symptoms, but later in childhood can develop hearing deficits, perceptual handicaps, and hyperkinesis.

Usually, no bilirubin is detected in amniotic fluid when the fetus and the mother are healthy.[57] However, a newborn who demonstrates significant elevations of unconjugated bilirubin in serum, as in HDN, frequently also passes bilirubin into the amniotic fluid as a fetus. The route by which bilirubin is transferred into amniotic fluid from the fetus is unclear. Measurements of the concentration of amniotic bilirubin (the ΔA_{450} test; see later discussion) are used to assess the risk for fetal complications resulting from HDN.

Newborns with severe HDN are clearly at risk for life-threatening anemia or hyperbilirubinemia. Following delivery and stabilization, cord blood hematological and biochemical tests should be performed. These generally include conjugated and total bilirubin, direct Coombs', blood type, hemoglobin, reticulocyte count, and nucleated RBCs. Results of these tests are used to determine the need for continued close monitoring versus immediate exchange transfusion.

Neural Tube Defects

Neural tube defects (NTDs) are congenital anomalies that result from failure of the neural tube to close during early embryogenesis. In the United States, the overall incidence is <0.5 per 1000 births, but this varies with ethnic and geographic factors.[58] Caucasian and Hispanic populations demonstrate a higher incidence, as do infants born in the eastern and southern parts of the United States.

NTDs can affect the spine or the cranium and are classified as open (neural tissue exposed) or closed (neural tissue not exposed). Spina bifida, which refers to a cleft in the spinal column, ranges in severity from spina bifida occulta, a closed defect in which the dorsal portions of some vertebrae fail to fuse with one another, to **meningomyelocele,** in which both the meninges and the spinal cord herniate through the vertebral defect. Cranial defects are more severe and include **anencephaly,** the congenital absence of a major portion of the brain, skull, and scalp, and encephalocele, in which herniation of cranial contents occurs through a defect in the skull.

It is possible, by measuring serum α-fetoprotein (AFP) in maternal serum, to identify women who are at increased risk of carrying fetuses with NTDs.[59] AFP has physicochemical properties similar to those of albumin (see Evolve). It is synthesized by the fetal yolk sac and liver and reaches its peak concentration in fetal serum at ≈9 weeks of gestation. It is excreted by the fetal kidney into the amniotic fluid and ultimately reaches the maternal circulation through transplacental passage, albeit at a concentration that is thousands of times lower than in the fetal blood.

Screening tests for NTD are based on the fact that maternal serum AFP (MSAFP) concentrations are greater when the fetus has an *open* NTD. Closed defects cannot be readily detected by biochemical screening. Approximately 80% of fetuses with open spina bifida and 95% of anencephalic fetuses are detectable by MSAFP at 16 to 18 weeks of gestation.[60]

Diagnostic testing, which includes ultrasound to visualize the defect and amniocentesis for biochemical analysis of amniotic fluid AFP and fetal acetylcholinesterase (AChE), an enzyme present in fetal blood cells, muscle, and nerves, is offered to all women with a positive screening test. Increased amounts of both amniotic fluid AFP and AChE are virtually diagnostic of an open NTD.

Down Syndrome

Down syndrome (DS), or trisomy 21, is the most common genetic cause of mental retardation. The birth prevalance increases dramatically with increasing maternal age, but is approximately 1:700 in the general population. Infants with DS demonstrate characteristic dysmorphic features such as abnormal epicanthic folds (upper eyelid), a flat nasal bridge, an open mouth, and a short neck. In addition to defects in mental development, patients with DS are at increased risk for heart defects, gastrointestinal (GI) anomalies, and childhood leukemias. Trisomy 21 is the most common autosomal trisomy; 95% of cases result from meiotic nondisjunction (most often of matenal origin). Other causes include translocations involving chromosome 21 and mosaicism (see Chapter 52).

Biochemical screening for Down syndrome has become a standard of care. Risk for Down syndrome is estimated on the basis of maternal age plus maternal serum AFP, unconjugated estriol, and hCG measurements ("triple screen"), and, with the addition of inhibin A measurement, the "quad screen." When used at 16 to 18 weeks of gestation, triple and quad screens provide DS detection rates of ≈65% and 80%, respectively, with a 5% false-positive rate.[61]

Screening for DS is also performed in the first trimester (11 to 14 weeks of gestation). First-trimester screening combines biochemical measurements of maternal serum hCG, total or free β chains, and pregnancy-associated plasma protein A (PAPP-A) with ultrasound measurement of fetal nuchal translucency (NT), that is, the width of space between the fetal skin and the cervical spine. Together, these markers produce a detection rate for DS that is higher than that associated with the quad screen performed during the second trimester.[62]

Recurrent Pregnancy Loss

Recurrent pregnancy loss (RPL), defined as three or more consecutive losses of intrauterine pregnancy before 28 weeks of gestation, occurs in approximately 2% to 5% of women.[63] Major causes of RPL can be categorized into problems associated with the fetus (e.g., chromosomal anomaly) and problems with the fetal environment (e.g., hormonal, immunological, anatomic). Because chromosomal anomalies are responsible for the majority of first-trimester spontaneous abortions, it is likely that some cases of RPL are the result of repeated genetic aberrations. Emerging evidence points to immunological mechanisms that lead to interference with blood supply to the fetus as the major cause of RPL among karyotypically normal fetuses.[64] This interference can be caused by the production of cytokines by uterine immune cells, antiphospholipid antibodies produced by systemic B cells, or an inherited predisposition to thrombotic events.

Antiphospholipid antibodies (APLAs) are autoantibody-directed phospholipid binding proteins. They can be categorized broadly into those antibodies that prolong phospholipid-dependent coagulation assays, known as lupus anticoagulants, and anticardiolipin antibodies. The presence of these antibodies in patients with arterial or venous thrombosis or RPL is known as the antiphospholipid antibody syndrome (APS). Approximately 18% of women with RPL have detectable APLAs in their blood. Although the association of APLAs with RPL is clear, no agreement has been reached on their mechanisms of action in women with RPL. Numerous hypotheses have been proposed, including (1) that the antibodies act on coagulation factors or placental endothelial cells to promote thrombosis of placental vessels; (2) that they act directly on trophoblast cells and inhibit implantation; and (3) that they are only markers of other immunological processes that are harmful to the pregnancy.

Laboratory testing for APS includes the lupus anticoagulant test (LA) and enzyme immunoassays for anticardiolipin antibodies (aCL). As named, the LA test is a misnomer because most patients with LA do not have systemic lupus erythematosus, and the antibodies are procoagulant, not anticoagulant.

The presence of LA causes prolongation of the phospholipid-dependent, activated partial thromboplastin time (aPTT). To identify the presence of LA, two additional tests must be performed. First, a mixing study is done to demonstrate the presence of an inhibitor rather than a clotting factor deficiency. If aPTT remains prolonged, then the second test, dilute Russell's viper venom time, is used to confirm the presence of the phospholipid-neutralizing LA. It is recommended that these tests be performed on a minimum of two occasions at least 12 weeks apart and that they be positive on each occasion before the diagnosis of APS is established.[65]

KEY CONCEPTS BOX 44-5

- Ectopic pregnancy, the implantation of a fertilized egg outside of the uterus, can be a life-threatening event that requires rapid laboratory testing for diagnosis and monitoring.
- Preterm delivery, that is, delivery of an infant before 37 weeks of gestation, is associated with PROM and the birth of immature babies with RDS, infection, and intraventricular hemorrhage. The fetal fibronectin test can rule out PROM.
- Preeclampsia associated with maternal hypertension and proteinuria can be life threatening and may result in premature birth.

KEY CONCEPTS BOX 44-5—cont'd

- Hemolytic disease of the newborn results from the destruction of fetal RBCs caused by maternal IgG antibodies directed against paternally inherited RBC antigens.
- Maternal antibodies against fetal RBC antigens cause destruction of the RBC and possible loss of the fetus. Levels of amniotic fluid bilirubin are used to monitor risk to the fetus.
- Neural tube defects result from failure of the neural tube to close completely during early embryogenesis. Down syndrome is caused by the third copy of chromosome 21 and is the most common genetic cause of mental retardation. Both are screened for by laboratory tests performed in the first and second trimesters of pregnancy.
- Recurrent pregnancy loss is defined as three or more consecutive losses of intrauterine pregnancy before 28 weeks of gestation. Lupus anticoagulants (anticardiolipin antibodies) may be the cause of recurrent loss of pregnancy.
- Glucose levels of newborns of diabetic mothers should be monitored to determine proper glucose control and to detect life-threatening hypoglycemia.

SECTION OBJECTIVES BOX 44-6

- Describe the use of the following laboratory tests: hCG, fetal fibronectin, AFP, unconjugated estriol, magnesium, ΔA_{450}, and bile acids.
- Describe the laboratory tests used to assess fetal lung maturity.
- Explain the use of laboratory tests for the detection of isoimmune antibodies.
- Describe the tests and procedures used to diagnose and monitor maternal diabetes.

CHANGE OF ANALYTE IN DISEASE

The development and application of improved analytical techniques and the improved safety of amniocentesis through ultrasound visualization have dramatically altered the course of management of problem or "high-risk" pregnancies. Amniocentesis is performed most commonly to obtain amniotic fluid for prenatal genetic studies and assessment of fetal lung maturity. It also may be performed to determine the degree of fetal hemolytic anemia, to determine fetal blood type, to identify hemoglobinopathies, and to detect the presence of a neural tube defect. Genetic disorders are discussed in Chapter 52.

Human Chorionic Gonadotropin

Human chorionic gonadotropin (hCG) is used to identify and follow both gestational trophoblastic disease and the course of normal pregnancy, including screening for Down syndrome. In a healthy pregnancy, hCG levels become detectable in maternal serum within a week following conception and reach their peak near the end of the first trimester; they then decline to approximately one-tenth the peak concentration, where they remain until delivery. The urine concentration parallels that of serum, and hCG can be detected as early as the day of the missed menses in 90% of women.[66] After delivery, hCG rapidly decreases and eventually becomes undetectable.

Patients with gestational trophoblastic disease such as a molar pregnancy usually have marked elevations of hCG, frequently exceeding 100,000 IU/L.[67] The amount of hCG correlates well with tumor mass and is used to monitor the patient's response to therapy. Successful treatment is indicated by decreasing concentrations of the hormone; stable or increasing concentrations are indicative of persistent or recurrent disease. Currently, the American College of Obstetricians and Gynecologists (ACOG) recommends that patients who have been treated successfully for trophoblastic disease should continue to be monitored for possible relapse by hCG testing for at least 6 months after the end of treatment.

The concentration of serum hCG is often low for gestational age in patients with ectopic pregnancy, and serum hCG is used in conjunction with ultrasound for evaluation of a suspected ectopic pregnancy. Serial hCG tests can be used to examine the rate at which hCG increases. In a uterine pregnancy, hCG concentrations should double every 48 hours, but in an ectopic pregnancy, this doubling time often is prolonged. It is not a particularly sensitive test, however, in that prolonged doubling is observed in only ≈85% of ectopic pregnancies.[68] Although ultrasound can be used to help visualize a fetal sac, it is largely insensitive for detecting ectopic pregnancy or an early intrauterine pregnancy. The two tests can be combined to improve the detection rate. One common approach is to use serum hCG as a screening tool when selecting patients for ultrasound. A concentration >1500 IU/L has been shown to be a reliable threshold for identifying an intrauterine pregnancy; therefore, patients with this threshold and no uterine pregnancy observed by ultrasound are diagnosed as having an ectopic pregnancy. Patients with hCG <1500 are monitored by serial hCG testing. An abnormal increase identifies an ectopic pregnancy; a normal increase is followed until the cutoff is reached, at which point the patient undergoes ultrasound and is managed accordingly.[69] It should be noted that this test cannot distinguish a failing intrauterine pregnancy from an ectopic pregnancy.

Progesterone concentrations are lower than expected in ectopic pregnancy. Unlike hCG, however, no single progesterone concentration can be recommended as a cutoff, and so the progesterone concentration merely confirms the diagnostic impressions already obtained by hCG and ultrasonography.

Estriol

Estriol has been investigated as a biochemical test of the fetoplacental unit in an effort to identify high-risk pregnancies and predict adverse fetal outcomes. Although some studies have suggested that low serum or urinary estriol levels or, more important, declining estriol levels carry an unfavorable prognostic significance,[70] most available evidence does not support its use for this purpose.

As a predictor of preterm delivery, salivary estriol has been shown to have a high negative predictive value. However, its reduced effectiveness in identifying patients at risk for early preterm delivery (<30 weeks) and the long analytical time required present significant limitations. Serum unconjugated estriol levels are used to screen for Down syndrome and trisomy 18.

Fetal Fibronectin

Fetal fibronectin (fFN) is a member of the fibronectin family of proteins that are present in the extracellular matrix and plasma. During gestation, the location of fFNs at the choriodecidual interface suggests a role for this protein as a "trophoblast glue" that anchors the fetal trophoblast within the uterus. Although fFN is detectable in cervicovaginal secretions during the first 24 weeks of pregnancy, it typically declines to undetectable concentrations between weeks 24 and 34. The release of fFNs into cervicovaginal secretions when the chorionic-decidual interface is disrupted underlies the rationale for measurement of fFN as a predictor of preterm delivery. Although the presence of fFN in symptomatic women during weeks 24 through 34 of gestation indicates an increased risk of preterm delivery, the absence of fFN is a much more reliable predictor, because it indicates that the pregnancy is likely to continue for at least another 2 weeks.

Currently, only one qualitative test for fFN has received U.S. Food and Drug Administration (FDA) approval. The chromatographic immunoassay produces a positive (>50 ng/mL) or a negative result. In a meta-analysis of 40 studies, fFN exhibited sensitivities of 77%, 74%, and 70% for predicting delivery in symptomatic women within 7, 14, and 21 days of testing, respectively.[71] Unfortunately, the positive predictive value of fFN is consistently low (<30%), and many women with positive results go on to deliver term infants. The real value of the assay appears to lie in its high negative predictive value (≈95%), which helps women with a negative result to avoid potentially dangerous or expensive interventions. The high negative predictive value of the fFN test also has been demonstrated to decrease health care costs in women who undergo evaluation for possible preterm delivery.[72]

Tests of Fetal Lung Maturation

Antenatal laboratory tests for fetal lung maturity (FLM) are used by the obstetrician to predict the likelihood of RDS subsequent to preterm delivery. Typically, these tests include biochemical or biophysical evaluations of amniotic fluid for the presence of surfactant components derived from maturing fetal lungs. These tests have been designed either to quantify specific surfactant-associated phospholipids (biochemical approach) or to measure the surface-active effects of these pulmonary surfactant components within the amniotic fluid sample (biophysical approach).

Biochemical Assays

Before 34 weeks of gestation, lecithin and sphingomyelin are present in amniotic fluid in approximately equal amounts, but at about 34 weeks, the concentration of lecithin begins to rise rapidly compared with that of sphingomyelin. Gluck and Kulovich[73] used the relative concentrations of lecithin and sphingomyelin in amniotic fluid to estimate the functional status of the fetal lung. Rather than quantifying lecithin and sphingomyelin, the test used the ratio of these compounds, that is, the lecithin/sphingomyelin ratio (LSR), after separation by thin-layer chromatography (TLC). When the TLC methods of the type originally proposed by Gluck are used, LSR values of 2 or greater have been found to correlate with fetal lung maturity and a low likelihood of respiratory distress after delivery.

Because early reports suggested that a greater risk for RDS is associated with the diabetic pregnancy, values of 2.5 or greater often have been used for these pregnancies. More recent reports indicate that fetal lung maturity testing is no more necessary for diabetic mothers with good glycemic control and accurate gestational dating than it is for mothers without diabetes.[74]

The clinical predictability of the LSR, similar to most FLM tests, varies widely. Reported sensitivities and specificities for this test range between 80% and 85%.[75] This variability is likely to result from poor analytical standardization, differences in study populations, inherent lack of consistency in the diagnosis of RDS, and the use of different reference values.

Contamination of samples with blood that has an LSR of ≈1.4 tends to produce falsely elevated values for very immature samples and falsely lowered values for very mature samples; however, a mature result obtained from a bloody specimen remains clinically useful. Meconium, vaginal secretion, and maternal urine contamination also can produce false results. RDS can develop in an asphyxiated neonate, despite a mature LSR.

Because phosphatidylglycerol (PG) contributes to the functional properties of the surfactant, tests for this phospholipid came to be popular as an adjunct to the LSR. Functional lung maturity is clearly associated with measurable quantities of PG[76]; however, the absence of PG does not necessarily mean that RDS is inevitable. Collective experience with the PG test indicates that, whereas the predictive value of the presence of PG is nearly 100% for lung maturity, the predictive value of the absence of PG in predicting RDS may be so low as to be virtually uninformative. Because PG appears to be a very small constituent of blood, the measurement of PG is especially valuable at times when fetal lung status must be predicted from blood- or meconium-contaminated amniotic fluid samples. When amniotic fluid obtained from leakage into the vagina is the most readily accessible sample, PG is the only phospholipid that should be measured. If a proper vaginal pool sample is obtained, false-positive results are rare. Creatinine or urea values should be obtained on vaginal pool samples suspected of being heavily contaminated with maternal urine, to help determine the nature of the sample.

Biophysical Assays

The methods in this group were designed to measure some specific biophysical property of pulmonary surfactant in the amniotic fluid sample.[77,78] They generally are easier, faster, and cheaper to perform than traditional TLC techniques.

The ability of surfactant to maintain a stable foam is a function of surface tension at the air-solvent interface; this property was exploited by foam-stability assays, the shake test, and foam stability index (FSI) tests.

Measurement of the surfactant/albumin ratio by fluorescence polarization is now the most common quantitative method for assessing fetal lung maturity.[75] This method is based on binding of a fluorescent probe to albumin and to pulmonary surfactant in amniotic fluid. Polarization of fluorescent light is high when the probe is bound to albumin and low when bound to surfactant. The degree of net polarization is correlated with fetal lung maturity. Results greater than the high cutoff are associated with lung maturity, and results below the lower cutoff are associated with lung immaturity. Results between these two values are reported as indeterminate.

Lamellar bodies represent the structural form of pulmonary surfactant extruded by type II pneumocytes. Their similarity in size to blood platelets permits the use of a standard automated hematological cell counter to quantify the number of lamellar bodies in amniotic fluid. Known as the lamellar body count (LBC), the result is used to estimate surfactant production in utero and thus predict the degree of fetal lung maturity.[75]

Tests for FLM can provide important clinical information; however, the low prevalence of RDS causes a high proportion of false-positive predictions of immaturity throughout gestation for all FLM tests. Testing strategies have been developed for the purpose of enhancing the predictive value of test results that are positive for respiratory immaturity.[79-82] Such strategies rely heavily on the availability of rapid methods for FLM that can be performed in a sequential, or cascade, fashion without substantially lengthening the total turnaround time for results. Typically, the easiest and fastest tests are performed first, followed by additional tests until the first mature result is obtained, or until all tests in the cascade indicate immaturity.

Traditionally, cutoffs for fetal lung maturity testing have been selected so as to maximize sensitivity and the predictive value of a mature result in order to reduce the risk of delivering infants with immature lungs. A limitation of this approach is that the same cutoff is applied to all gestational ages despite the fact that the risk of RDS decreases with increasing gestational age. The alternative is to report the probability of RDS based on gestational age and test results[75] with the use of published risk tables. This approach produces consistent sensitivities and specificities across the gestational age range and can help physicians to individualize risk-benefit decisions according to gestational age and results from the surfactant/albumin ratio by fluorescence polarization.[83,84]

Tests for Hemolytic Disease (Isoimmunization)

Maternal sensitization to paternally inherited RBC antigens places the fetus at risk for developing hemolytic disease of the newborn (HDN). In conjunction with ABO and RhD typing of maternal red blood cells as part of the initial tests performed on an obstetrical patient at her first prenatal visit, the indirect antiglobulin test (IAT), also known as the indirect Coombs' test, is performed to identify antibodies, such as anti-D, that have the potential to cause HDN. When isoantibodies are detected, semi-quantitative assessment is accomplished by titration of the serum, which then is tested by the IAT for antibody activity. The titer is recorded as the reciprocal of the highest dilution that gives a 1+ agglutination reaction. A "critical titer," the titer below which fetal hydrops is not anticipated and additional fetal monitoring is unnecessary, is employed. Patients with rising or elevated titers require subsequent monitoring, such as measuring absorbance at 450 nm (ΔA_{450}) in amniotic fluid (see below).

During normal pregnancy, amniotic fluid bilirubin peaks at ≈19 to 22 weeks at concentrations of 0.16 to 0.18 mg/dL.[56] Intrauterine hemolysis severe enough to cause erythroblastosis fetalis can dramatically increase the bilirubin concentration of amniotic fluid. Because the concentration of amniotic fluid bilirubin is usually too low to be measured by standard chemical techniques, an alternative method that uses scanning spectrophotometry has been devised. The principle of this approach is based on the fact that amniotic fluid light absorbance at 450 nm results primarily from the presence of bilirubin. Because bilirubin absorbs light maximally at 450 nm, the extent to which the absorbance curve deviates from a base line (drawn between absorbance readings at 350 and 550 nm) at this wavelength is proportionate to the concentration of bilirubin in the amniotic fluid; it is this change in absorbance that is known as the ΔA_{450} test (Fig. 44-14).

Liley[85] developed a graph that reasonably allows the prediction of the severity of hemolytic disease and the recommendation of clinical management (Fig. 44-15). The higher the ΔA_{450}, the more severe is the hemolytic disease relative to the gestational age of the pregnancy. In general, a decreasing amniotic fluid bilirubin trend is a good prognostic indicator that a fetus will survive, whereas a horizontal or rising bilirubin level indicates more severe HDN. The main source of error is the fetus with polyhydramnios, because this can cause a falsely low bilirubin determination. In addition, maternal hyperconjugated bilirubinemia may result in elevation of bilirubin in amniotic fluid in the absence of fetal hemolytic disease. In recent years, this invasive test has been replaced largely by the more sensitive and specific Doppler ultrasonography, to measure blood flow through the fetus' middle cerebral artery as an assessment of fetal anemia.

Cord Blood/Venous Bilirubin

Most newborn infants develop a hyperunconjugated bilirubinemia >1.0 mg/dL and jaundice (see Chapter 31), usually caused by excess neonatal production (increased RBC destruction) combined with an immature hepatic bilirubin conjugation system. In infants born at ≥35 weeks of gestation, hyperbilirubinemia is defined as a total serum bilirubin concentration that exceeds the 95th percentile for hours-of-age reference limits (see Chapter 45).[86] In infants born at term, hyperbilirubinemia is transient and usually resolves within 1 to 2 weeks after birth. Box 44-3 lists bilirubin concentrations for which pathological causes should be sought.[87] Infants with significant bilirubin elevations may be treated with phototherapy or exchange transfusion. Specific recommendations

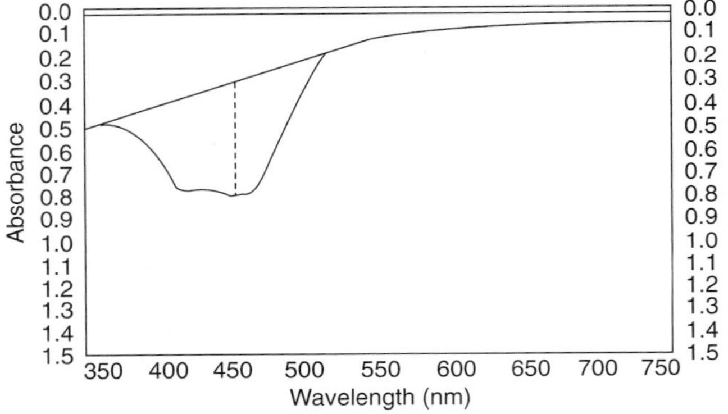

Fig. 44-14 Spectrum of bilirubin in amniotic fluid. *Dashed line,* Absorbance at 450 nm. (From Queenan JT: Amniotic fluid analysis, Clin Obstet Gynecol 14:505, 1971.)

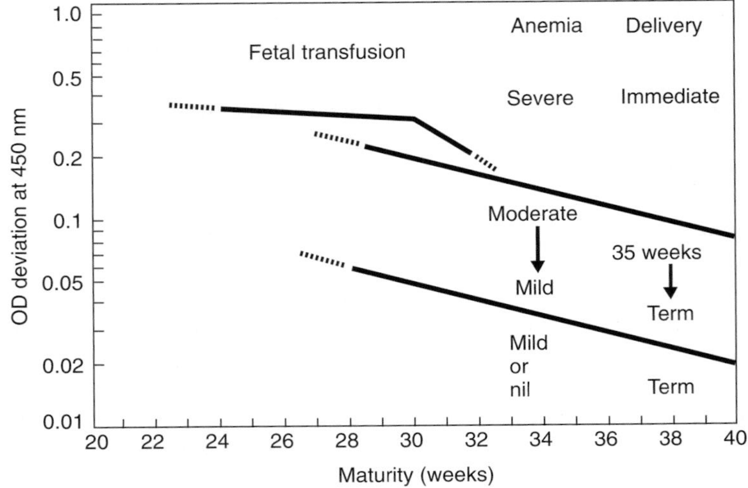

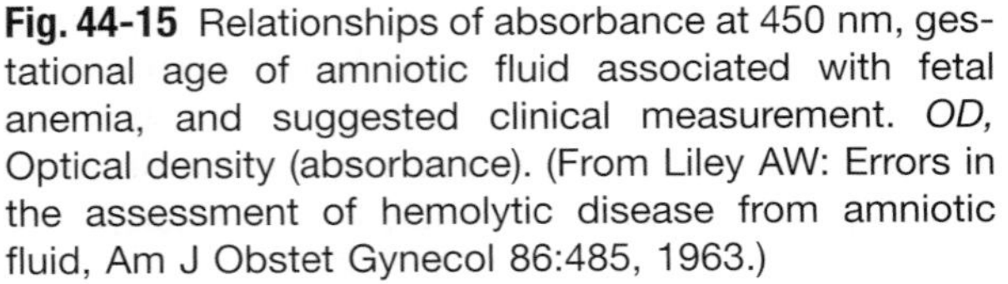

Fig. 44-15 Relationships of absorbance at 450 nm, gestational age of amniotic fluid associated with fetal anemia, and suggested clinical measurement. *OD,* Optical density (absorbance). (From Liley AW: Errors in the assessment of hemolytic disease from amniotic fluid, Am J Obstet Gynecol 86:485, 1963.)

Box 44-3

Bilirubin Values Typically Associated With Pathological Causes

Serum bilirubin >5 mg/dL during first 24 hours of life
Serum bilirubin levels rising to more than 5 mg/dL/day
Term infants with serum bilirubin (unconjugated) values >12 to 13 mg/dL
Preterm infants with serum bilirubin (unconjugated) values >15 mg/dL

for treatment are somewhat controversial and typically differ according to premature versus mature infants, breast-feeding status (which promotes an increase in bilirubin levels), birth weight, and possibly race. Detailed treatment guidelines for management of hyperbilirubinemia in healthy term infants have been published.[88]

Glucose Screening and Monitoring (see also pp. 746 and 747)

Two issues have arisen with respect to pregnancy and diabetes. The first deals with the identification of gestational diabetes.[89] Not only are a significant number of pregnancies affected by gestational diabetes, but many of these women may go on to develop diabetes while not pregnant. At risk are women who develop glycosuria, have a positive family history of diabetes, have a history of large-for-gestational-age infants, have had a stillbirth, and have a parity of five or more, as well as those who are obese or are older than 35 years. Because of the adverse effects of diabetes on the fetus, ACOG recommends that all women undergo diabetes screening by 24 to 28 weeks of gestation.[90] The American Diabetes Association recommends screening unless the woman is considered at low risk (i.e., maternal age <25 years and ethnicity other than African American, Hispanic, or Native American).[89] (See p. 747, Chapter 38, for details on the recommended screening procedure.)

The second issue involves careful monitoring and control of the pregnant diabetic woman. High maternal glucose, high fetal glucose and insulin, or a combination of these delays the biochemical and morphological development of the fetal lung. The exact mechanisms involved remain to be determined, but it has been suggested that high glucose concentrations block the movement of lipids from fibroblasts to type II cells,[91] or that fetal hyperinsulinemia inhibits the synthesis of SP-A.[92]

When diabetic mothers are in good or strict metabolic control, little difference is seen in the lung development of their fetuses compared with those of nondiabetic mothers. It is interesting to note that the fetuses of mothers who are poorly controlled but who have more than five episodes of hypoglycemia per week often are found to have accelerated lung maturation, possibly caused by stress on the fetus.[93]

The pregnant diabetic woman is at risk for other complications as well, including hypertension, infection, acidosis, and nephropathy, and should be monitored carefully so these conditions can be detected early.[94] Frequent self-monitoring of blood glucose is considered an important part of managment. Not only is elevated glucose a concern, but as indicated above, recognition of episodes of hypoglycemia may be useful in identifying fetal stress. Blood glucose goals in the pregnant diabetic woman as recommended by ACOG include fasting glucose concentrations of <95 mg/dL and 1- and 2-hour postprandial glucose concentrations no higher than 140 mg/dL and 120 mg/dL, respectively.[95] Although some recommend that hemoglobin A_{1c} (HbA_{1c}) should be monitored at frequent intervals, it is important to realize that levels of glycated hemoglobin reflect both changes in glucose tolerance and changes in red cell mass and survival time during pregnancy. These changes result in an initial decrease in HbA_{1c}, followed by a rise during the third trimester.[96] Thus it should be remembered that the HbA_{1c} level may be lower than when the patient is not pregnant. Miller found an increased risk of congenital anomalies (e.g., ventricular septal defects, anencephaly) when the HbA_{1c} was greater than 8.5% in early pregnancy.[97]

Because diabetic nephropathy in association with hypertension presents a risk of fetal death, urinary microalbumin and creatinine clearance should be monitored. Creatinine clearance below 50 mL/min has been associated with fetal demise. Because the risk of hypothyroidism is increased in these patients, early screening is recommended.

Renal Function Tests (see also p. 580)

During pregnancy, the glomerular filtration rate increases by 40% to 65% and renal plasma flow by 50% to 85%.[98] Many women experience a transient decline in renal function during pregnancy, and so an initial assessment of renal function should include protein excretion, serum creatinine, and creatinine clearance, particularly in women with diabetes.

In patients with preeclampsia, renal perfusion and glomerular filtration are reduced, yet creatinine or urea concentration in plasma usually is not appreciably elevated. Excretion of glucose and protein usually is increased, but these are no longer considered diagnostic. The plasma uric acid concentration is much more commonly elevated, especially in women with more severe renal disease. This elevation results primarily from decreased renal clearance of uric acid by the kidney, a decrease that exceeds the reduction in glomerular filtration rate and creatinine clearance. However, uric acid is not helpful in differentiating preeclampsia from the transient hypertension of pregnancy.

α-Fetoprotein

In contrast to other analytes, elevations or decreases in serum AFP levels do not directly confirm a pathological process. However, this analyte is unique as an identifier of patients at risk for having fetuses with a variety of birth defects, as well as of malignant disease in men and nonpregnant women.

Elevated maternal serum AFP levels are associated with an increased risk for NTD, whereas decreased levels are associated with an increased risk for Down syndrome. However, because maternal AFP levels are dependent on numerous factors, including gestational age, maternal weight and age, race, insulin-dependent diabetes, multiple pregnancies, and drug ingestion, the results are not diagnostic. Thus maternal serum

AFP levels are most useful in identifying (screening) those pregnant women who require additional testing (such as ultrasonography and amniocentesis) to exclude the possibility of an affected fetus.

Maternal serum α-fetoprotein results are reported routinely as a multiple of the normal median (MoM) for the gestational week, once the value has been normalized for the factors mentioned earlier. Spina bifida, anencephaly, gastroschisis, and omphalocele are among the differential diagnoses at 15 to 20 weeks of gestation, when both maternal serum and amniotic fluid AFP levels are above 2.0 MoM, and amniotic fluid acetylcholinesterase levels are increased. Increased maternal age and decreased maternal serum AFP levels are associated with increased risk for Down syndrome.

Screening for Down Syndrome in the First and Second Trimesters

Screening for Down syndrome is performed by combining the risks associated with maternal age and those related to abnormal levels of specific biochemicals. At maternal age 20 to 24, the risk for Down syndrome is 1/1490; at age 40, the risk is 1/60; and at age 49, the risk is 1/11.[99] Despite this, most Down babies are born to younger mothers because far more pregnancies occur in the third and fourth decades of life. Screening tests are not diagnostic for DS, but they do identify which patients should undergo more definitive tests. Diagnostic tests for the presence of trisomy 21 include amniocentesis and chorionic villous sampling, both of which isolate fetal cells for karyotypic analysis (see p. 1044, Chapter 52).

Multiple screening strategies for DS are currently available, and revised recommendations from ACOG state that all women, regardless of age, should be offered Down syndrome screening. Screening for DS can be performed during the second (weeks 16 to 18) or the first trimester (weeks 11 to 14). With a DS detection rate that is higher than that of the second trimester quadruple screen, first-trimester biochemical screening offers the benefits of earlier detection and safer methods of pregnancy termination, if needed. First-trimester screening also may include ultrasound inspection of the fetus for other developmental abnormalities associated with Down syndrome, such as increased nuchal translucency and nasal septal bone abnormalities.

Combinations of first- and second-trimester screening protocols have been described. This "integrated" screening test is accomplished by measuring maternal serum hCG and PAPP-A concentrations and by nuchal translucency testing in the first trimester, followed by the quadruple screen in the second trimester. When all tests have been completed, a final DS risk is calculated on the basis of test results and patient age. Data from two large, prospective studies have confirmed that this approach provides the highest rates of DS detection.[100,101]

Magnesium

Women with toxemia of pregnancy, preeclampsia, or premature labor often are treated with high levels of magnesium sulfate ($MgSO_4$). These women, usually under hospital care, must be closely monitored for excessive hypermagnesemia (>8 mg/dL).

Bile Acids

Liver function tests are not performed routinely during a normal pregnancy. However, if a pregnant woman shows signs suggestive of intrahepatic cholestasis of pregnancy (ICP), the measurement of serum bile acids is a sensitive yet nonspecific marker of hepatic and biliary disease. Measurement of total bile acid is sufficient for this purpose.

KEY CONCEPTS BOX 44-6

- hCG can detect early pregnancy, and prolonged doubling time for hCG is one indicator of ectopic pregnancy.
- The clinical utility of fetal fibronectin lies in its high negative predictive value for ruling out increased risk for preterm delivery.
- Tests of fetal lung maturity have high sensitivity for detecting lung immaturity but suffer from low specificity.
- Amniotic fluid concentrations of bilirubin are assessed indirectly by the ΔA_{450} and are used to assess fetal hemolytic disease.
- Screening the pregnant mother for gestational diabetes is common, and diabetes mellitus in the pregnant patient requires careful monitoring and control to prevent adverse effects to the fetus.
- Multiple screening strategies for detecting Down syndrome are now available and should be recommended to all women, regardless of age.
- Serum bile acids can be used to diagnose cholestasis of pregnancy.
- Serum magnesium is used to monitor tocolytic therapy for treating eclampsia.

REFERENCES

1. Heikinheimo O, Gibbons WE: The molecular mechanisms of oocyte maturation and early embryonic development are unveiling new insights into reproductive medicine, Mol Human Reprod 4:745, 1998.
2. Bauer MK, et al: Fetal growth and placental function, Mol Cell Endocrinol 140:115, 1998.
3. Hay WW: Placental transport of nutrients to the fetus, Hormone Res 42:215, 1994.
4. Carter AM: Factors affecting gas transfer across the placenta and the oxygen supply to the fetus, J Dev Physiol 12:305, 1989.
5. Gilbert WM, Brace RA: Amniotic fluid volume and normal flows to and from the amniotic cavity, Semin Perinatol 17:150, 1993.
6. Sandler M, editor: *Amniotic Fluid and Its Clinical Significance,* New York, 1981, Marcel Dekker.
7. Weaver TE: Pulmonary surfactant-associated proteins, Gen Pharmacol 18:1, 1987.
8. Pierce JG, Parsons TF: Glycoprotein hormones: structure and function, Annu Rev Biochem 50:465, 1980.
9. Lenton EA, Neal LM, Sulaiman R: Plasma concentrations of human chorionic gonadotropin from the time of implantation until the second week of pregnancy, Fertil Steril 37:773, 1982.

10. Cole LA: Immunoassay of human chorionic gonadotropin, its free subunits, and metabolites, Clin Chem 43:2233, 1997.
11. Vinson GP: *The Adrenal Cortex,* Englewood Cliffs, NJ, 1992, Prentice Hall.
12. Miller WL: Steroid hormone biosynthesis and actions in the materno-feto-placental unit, Clin Perinatol 25:799, 1998.
13. Pepe GJ, Albrecht ED: Actions of placental and fetal adrenal steroid hormones in primate pregnancy, Endocr Rev 16:608, 1995.
14. Burrow GN, Fisher DA, Larsen PR: Mechanisms of disease: maternal and fetal thyroid function, N Engl J Med 331:1072, 1994.
15. Glinoer D, de Nayer P, Bordoux P, et al: Regulation of maternal thyroid during pregnancy, J Clin Endocrinol Metab 71:276, 1990.
16. Lowe TW, Cunningham FG: Pregnancy and thyroid disease, Clin Obstet Gynecol 34:72, 1991.
17. Calvo RM, Jauniaux E, Gulbis B, et al: Fetal tissues are exposed to biologically relevant free thyroixine concentrations during early phases of development, J Clin Endocrinol Metab 87:1767, 2002.
18. Zoeller RT, Rovet J: Timing of thyroid hormone action in the developing brain: clinical observations and experimental findings, J Neuroendocrinol 16:809, 2004.
19. Chan S, Rovet J: Thyroid hormones in the fetal central nervous system development, Fetal Maternal Med Rev 14:177, 2003.
20. van Stiphout WAHJ, Hofman A, de Bruijn AM: Serum lipids in young women before, during, and after pregnancy, Am J Epidemiol 126:922, 1987.
21. Herrera E: Lipid metabolism in pregnancy and its consequences in the fetus and newborn, Endocrine 19:43, 2002.
22. Studd JW, Wood S: Serum and urinary proteins in pregnancy. In Wynn RM, editor: *Obstetrics and Gynecology Annual,* New York, 1976, Appleton-Century-Crofts.
23. Murray N, Homer CSE, Davis GK, et al: The clinical utility of routine urinalysis in pregnancy: a prospective study, Med J Aust 177:477, 2002.
24. American College of Obstetricians and Gynecologists: ACOG Practice Bulletin 33, *Diagnosis and Management of Preeclampsia and Eclampsia,* Washington, DC, 2002, ACOG, p. 312.
25. Davison JM: The urinary system. In Hytten F, Chamberlain G, editors: *Clinical Physiology in Obstetrics,* Oxford, UK, 1980, Blackwell Scientific.
26. van Geuns HJ, van Kessel H: Creatinine in amniotic fluid and fetal renal function. In Fairweather DVI, Eskes TKAB, editors: *Amniotic Fluid: Research and Clinical Application,* ed 2, Amsterdam, 1978, Excerpta Medica.
27. Spillman T, Cotton DB: Current perspectives in the assessment of fetal pulmonary surfactant status with amniotic fluid, CRC Rev Clin Lab Sci 27:341, 1989.
28. Hallman M: Recycling surfactant: a review of human amniotic fluid as a source of surfactant for treatment of respiratory distress syndrome, Rev Perinatal Med 6:197, 1989.
29. Cochrane CG, Revak SD: Pulmonary surfactant protein B (SP-B): structure-function relationships, Science 254:566, 1991.
30. Martin RJ, Fanaroff AA, Skalina MEL: The respiratory system. In Fanaroff AA, Martin RJ, editors: *Behrman's Neonatal/Perinatal Medicine,* St. Louis, 1987, Mosby.
31. Reynolds MS, Wallander KA: Use of surfactant in the prevention and treatment of neonatal respiratory distress syndrome, Clin Pharmacol 8:559, 1989.
32. Gibson AT: Surfactant and the neonatal lung, Br J Hosp Med 58:381, 1997.
33. Kleihauer E: The hemoglobins. In Stave U, editor: *Perinatal Physiology,* New York, 1978, Plenum.
34. Hecht F, Jones RT, Koler RD: Newborn infants with Hb Portland 1, an indicator of α-chain deficiency, Ann Hum Genet 31:215, 1967.
35. Lustbader JW, Lobel L, Wu H: Structural and molecular studies of human chorionic gonadotropin and its receptor, Recent Prog Hormone Res 53:395, 1998.
36. Kobata A, Takeuchi M: Structure, pathology and function of the N-linked sugar chains of human chorionic gonadotropin, Biochim Biophys Rev 1445:315, 1999.
37. Lehner R, Kucera E, Jiracek CE, et al: Ectopic pregnancy, Arch Gynecol Obstet 263:87, 2000.
38. Centers for Disease Control and Prevention: Ectopic pregnancy—United States, 1990-1992, MMWR Morb Mortal Wkly Rep 44:46, 1995.
39. Hoyert DL, Mathews TJ, Menacker F, et al: Annual summary of vital statistics: 2004, Pediatrics 117:168, 2006.
40. Iams JD, Goldenberg RL, Meis PJ, et al: The length of the cervix and the risk of spontaneous premature delivery, N Engl J Med 334:567, 1996.
41. Hartmann K, Thorp JM Jr, McDonald TL, et al: Cervical dimensions and risk of preterm birth: a prospective cohort study, Obstet Gynecol 93:504, 1999.
42. Hladunewich M, Karumanchi SA, Lafayette R: Pathophysiology of the clinical manifestations of preeclampsia, Clin J Am Soc Nephrol 2:543, 2007.
43. Dildy GA, Belfort MA, Smulian JC: Preeclampsia recurrence and prevention, Semin Perinatol 31:135, 2007.
44. American College of Obstetrics and Gynecology: ACOG Practice Bulletin 33, *Diagnosis and Management of Preeclampsia and Eclampsia,* Washington, DC, 2002, ACOG.
45. Redman CRG, Roberts JM: Management of pre-eclampsia, Lancet 341:1451, 1993.
46. Barbour LA, McCurdy CE, Hernandez TL: Cellular mechanisms for insulin resistance in normal pregnancy and gestational diabetes, Diabetes Care 30(suppl 2):S112, 2007.
47. Taylor R, Davison JM: Type 1 diabetes and pregnancy, BMJ 334:742, 2007.
48. Posner BI: Insulin metabolizing enzyme activities in human placental tissue, Diabetes 22:552, 1973.
49. Cotran RS, Kumar VK, Collins T, editors: *Robbins Pathologic Basis of Disease,* Philadelphia, 1999, Saunders.
50. Hoyert DL, Kung H, Smith BL. Deaths: preliminary data for 2003. Natl Vital Stat Rep 53(15):1-48, 2005.
51. Dekowski SA, Holtzman RB: Surfactant replacement therapy: an update on applications, Pediatr Clin North Am 45:549, 1998.
52. Hudak ML, Martin DJ, Egan EA, et al: A multicenter randomized masked comparison trial of synthetic surfactant versus calf lung surfactant extract in the prevention of neonatal respiratory distress syndrome, Pediatrics 100:39, 1997.
53. Moya FR, Gross I: Combined hormonal therapy for the prevention of respiratory distress syndrome and its consequences, Semin Perinatol 17:267, 1993.
54. Robertson B: Corticosteroids and surfactant for prevention of neonatal RDS, Ann Med 25:285, 1993.
55. Taeusch HW, Ballard RA: *Avery's Diseases of the Newborn,* Baltimore, 1998, Williams & Wilkins.
56. Grenache DG: Hemolytic disease of the newborn. In Gronowski AM, ed: *Handbook of Clinical Laboratory Testing During Pregnancy,* Totowa, NJ, 2004, Humana Press.
57. Liley AW: The administration of blood transfusions to the foetus in utero, Triangle 7:184, 1966.
58. Centers for Disease Control and Prevention: Spina bifida and anencephaly before and after folic acid mandate—United States, 1995-1996 and 1999-2000, MMWR Morb Mortal Wkly Rep 53:362, 2004.
59. Sundaram SG, Goldstein PJ, Manimekalai S, et al: Alpha-fetoprotein and screening markers of congenital disease, Reprod Med 12:481, 1992.

60. Milunsky A, Jick SS, Bruell CL, et al: Predictive values, relative risks, and overall benefits of high and low maternal serum alpha-fetoprotein screening in singleton pregnancies: new epidemiologic data, Am J Obstet Gynecol 161:291, 1989.
61. Ashwood ER, Knight GJ: Clinical chemistry of pregnancy. In Burtis CA, Ashwood ER, Bruns DE, editor: *Tietz Textbook of Clinical Chemistry and Molecular Diagnostics,* ed 4, St. Louis, 2006, Elsevier Saunders.
62. Malone FD, Canick JA, Ball RH, et al, for the First- and Second-Trimester Evaluation of Risk (FASTER) Research Consortium: First-trimester or second-trimester screening, or both, for Down's syndrome, N Engl J Med 353:2001, 2005.
63. Christiansen OB, Andersen AN, Bosch E, et al: Evidence-based investigations and treatments of recurrent pregnancy loss, Fertil Steril 83:821, 2005.
64. Coulam CB: Recurrent pregnany loss. In Gronowski AM, editor: *Handbook of Clinical Laboratory Testing During Pregnancy,* Totowa, NJ, 2004, Humana Press.
65. Miyakis S, Lockshin MD, Atsumi T, et al: International consensus statement on an update of the classification criteria for definite antiphospholipid syndrome (APS), J Thromb Haemost 4:295, 2006.
66. Wilcox AJ, Baird DD, Dunson D, et al: Natural limits of pregnancy testing in relation to the expected menstrual period, JAMA 286:1759, 2001.
67. Berkowitz RS, Goldstein DP: Chorionic tumors, N Engl J Med 335:1740, 1996.
68. Silva C, Sammel MD, Zhou L, et al: Human chorionic gonadotropin profile for women with ectopic pregnancy, Obstet Gynecol 107:605, 2006.
69. Barnhart K, Mennuti MT, Benjamin I, et al: Prompt diagnosis of ectopic pregnancy in an emergency department setting, Obstet Gynecol 84:1010, 1994.
70. Little B, Billar RB: Endocrine disorders. In Romney SL, et al, editors: *Gynecology and Obstetrics: The Health Care of Women,* New York, 1980, McGraw-Hill.
71. Leitich H, Kaider A: Fetal fibronectin—how useful is it in the prediction of preterm birth? BJOG 110(suppl 20):66, 2003.
72. Joffe GM, Jacques D, Bemis-Heys R, et al: Impact of the fetal fibronectin assay on admissions for preterm labor, Am J Obstet Gynecol 180:581, 1999.
73. Gluck L, Kulovich MV: Lecithin/sphingomyelin ratios in amniotic fluid in normal and abnormal pregnancies, Am J Obstet Gynecol 115:539, 1973.
74. Langer O: The controversy surrounding fetal lung maturity in diabetes in pregnancy: a re-evaluation, J Matern Fetal Neonatal Med 12:428, 2002.
75. Grenache DG, Gronowski AM: Fetal lung maturity, Clin Biochem 39:1, 2006.
76. Bent AE, Gray JH, Luther ER, et al: Assessment of fetal lung maturity: relationship of gestational age and pregnancy complications to phosphatidylglycerol levels, Am J Obstet Gynecol 139:664, 1981.
77. Dubin SB: The laboratory assessment of fetal lung maturity, Am J Clin Pathol 97:836, 1992.
78. Haymond S, Luzzi VI, Parvin CA, et al: A direct comparison between lamellar body counts and fluorescent polarization methods for predicting respiratory distress syndrome, Am J Clin Pathol 126:894, 2006.
79. Herbert WNP, Chapman JF, Schnoor MM: Role of the TDx FLM assay in fetal lung maturity, Am J Obstet Gynecol 168:808, 1993.
80. Garite TJ, Freeman RK, Nageotte MP: Fetal maturity cascade: a rapid and cost effective method for fetal maturity testing, Obstet Gynecol 67:619, 1986.
81. Herbert WNP, Chapman JF: Clinical and economic considerations associated with testing for fetal lung maturity, Am J Obstet Gynecol 155:820, 1986.
82. American College of Obstetricians and Gynecologists: ACOG Educational Bulletin: assessment of fetal lung maturity, Int J Gynecol Obstet 56:191, 1996.
83. Kaplan LA, Chapman JF, Bock JL, et al: Prediction of respiratory distress syndrome using the Abbott FLM II amniotic fluid assay, Clin Chim Acta 326:61, 2002.
84. Parvin CA, Kaplan LA, Chapman JF, et al: Predicting respiratory distress syndrome using gestational age and fetal lung maturity by fluorescent polarization, Am J Obstet Gynecol 192:199, 2005.
85. Liley AW: Liquor amnii analysis in the management of the pregnancy compicated by rhesus sensitization, Am J Obstet Gynecol 82:1359, 1963.
86. Bhutani VK, Johnson L, Sivieri EM: Predictive ability of a predischarge hour-specific serum bilirubin for subsequent significant hyperbilirubinemia in healthy term and near-term newborns, Pediatrics 103:6, 1999.
87. Kaplan LA, Tange SM, editors: *Guidelines for the Evaluation and Management of the Newborn Infant,* Washington, DC, 1998, National Academy of Clinical Biochemistry.
88. American Academy of Pediatrics Subcommittee on Hyperbilirubinemia: Management of hyperbilirubinemia in the newborn infant 35 or more weeks of gestation, Pediatrics 114:297, 2004.
89. Report of the Expert Committee on the Diagnosis and Classification of Diabetes Mellitus, Diabetes Care 23(suppl 1): S4, 2000.
90. ACOG Practice Bulletin, Gestational diabetes, Obstet Gynecol 98:525, 2001.
91. Gewolb IH, Torday HS: High glucose inhibits maturation of the fetal lung in vitro: morphometric analysis of lamellar bodies and fibroblast lipid inclusions, Lab Invest 73:59, 1995.
92. Mendelson CR: Role of transcription factors in fetal lung development and surfactant protein gene expression, Annu Rev Physiol 62:875, 2000.
93. Zapata A, Grande C, Hernandez-Garcia JM: Influence of metabolic control of pregnant diabetics on fetal lung maturity, Scand J Clin Lab Invest 54:431, 1994.
94. Javanovic L: Medical emergencies in the patient with diabetes during pregnancy, Endocrinol Metab Clin North Am 29:771, 2000.
95. ACOG Practice Bulletin 60: Pregestational diabetes mellitus, Obstet Gynecol 105:675, 2005.
96. Worth R: Glycosylated hemoglobin in normal pregnancy: a longitudinal study with two independent methods, Diabetologia 28:76, 1985.
97. Miller E: Elevated maternal hemoglobin A_{1c} in early pregnancy and major congenital anomalies in infants of diabetic mothers, N Engl J Med 304:1331, 1981.
98. Jeyabalan A, Conrad KP: Renal function during normal pregnancy and preeclampsia, Front Biosci 12:2425, 2007.
99. Centers for Disease Control and Prevention: Improved national prevalence estimates for 18 selected major birth defects—United States, 1999-2001, Morb Mortal Wkly Rep 54:1301, 2006.
100. Malone FD, Canick JA, Ball RH, et al: First-trimester or second-trimester screening, or both, for Down's syndrome, N Engl J Med 353:2001, 2005.
101. Wald NJ, Rodeck C, Hackshaw AK, et al: First and second trimester antenatal screening for Down's syndrome: the results of the Serum, Urine and Ultrasound Screening Study (SURUSS), J Med Screen 10:56, 2003.

INTERNET SITES

http://www.babycenter.com/pregnancy/fetaldevelopment/
http://www.pregnancy.about.com/
http://www.fpnotebook.com/ – Family Practice Notebook

http://www.atlanta-mfm.com/body.cfm?id=25 – Atlanta Fetal-Medicine PC Clinical Discussion

http://www.docboard.org/me/rules/allch078.htm – Maine Board of Licensure in Medicine: Medical Board Rules 2. Procedure: Assessment of fetal maturity prior to repeat cesarean delivery or elective induction of labor

http://www.acog.org/ – The American College of Obstetricians and Gynecologists: Type "diabetes" into the website's search engine

http://video.google.com/videoplay?docid=-2745043160590391764&q=fertilization&total=626&start=0&num=10&so=0&type=search&plindex=0

http://video.google.com/videoplay?docid=-5556029667786989666&q=Down+syndrome+screening&total=30&start=0&num=10&so=0&type=search&plindex=0

The Newborn

Chapter 45

Andre Mattman, Anne Catherine Halstead, and Gillian Lockitch

Chapter Outline

Key Terms

apnea Temporary cessation of respiration.

Apt test Test to differentiate maternal from newborn/fetal blood. Test is based on the principle that hemoglobin F resists alkaline denaturation. Thus, a maternal blood sample changes from red to yellow after addition of NaOH whereas newborn/fetal blood does not.

enteral feeding Feeding via the gastrointestinal tract.

extremely low birth weight Birth weight less than 1500 g.

ex utero Outside the uterus (i.e., after birth).

gastroschisis A congenital defect in the abdominal wall usually accompanied by protrusion of viscera.

gestational age Fetal age of a newborn, calculated from the number of completed weeks since the first day of the mother's last menstrual period to the date of birth.

LGA Large for gestational age.

low birth weight Birth weight less than 2500 g.

meconium Sterile stools passed by an infant within the first few days of life, containing materials ingested during the time the infant spent in the uterus.

necrotizing enterocolitis A gastrointestinal disorder primarily of premature infants, in which portions of the bowel undergo tissue necrosis.

neonatal period Birth to four weeks (28 days).

nephrocalcinosis A form of renal stone disease wherein numerous deposits of calcium phosphate and calcium oxalate are found in tissues of the kidney.

nephrolithiasis The presence of calculi in the kidney or collecting system.

parenteral nutrition Providing nutrients intravenously.

phototherapy Treatment of a newborn with jaundice with light.

polycythemia Too many red blood cells; hemoglobin, red blood cell count, and total RBC volume all above normal.

premature Born before 37 weeks of gestation.

term newborn Born between 37 and 42 weeks of gestation.

Methods on Evolve

aHBs
aHBcIgM
Alanine aminotransferase
Albumin
Albumin in urine
Alkaline phosphatase, total
α-Fetoprotein
Alpha_1-antitrypsin
Ammonia
Anion gap

Aspartate aminotransferase
β-human chorionic gonadotropin (β-hCG)
Bilirubin
Blood gas analysis
Blood gas analysis and oxygen saturation
Carbon dioxide and bicarbonate
Chloride
Creatinine
Creatinine clearance algorithm
Electrolytes (sodium, potassium, calcium, magnesium, phosphate)—serum and urine
Fetal lung maturity (amniotic fluid phospholipids [AFPL] LS ratio and PG)
Gamma-glutamyl transferase
Glucose
Glycated hemoglobin
HBsAg
Henderson-Hasselbalch calculating algorithm
Insulin and C-peptide
Ketones
Lactate dehydrogenase and lactate dehydrogenase enzymes
Lactic acid
Magnesium
Maternal fetal screening
Osmolality
Oximetry
Pyruvic acid
Sodium and potassium
Triglycerides
Urea
Uric acid
Urine protein, total

THE NEWBORN

During birth and the immediate postpartum period, major physiological changes occur as the fetus transitions from a dependent, intrauterine state to postnatal existence as an independent entity, the newborn. These transitions may be exacerbated by **premature** birth, abnormal intrauterine growth, or maternal disease or drug use. Among the challenges to providing timely, accurate, and clinically useful diagnostic services for newborns and infants are restrictions on blood volume, difficulties in blood sampling, lack of appropriate reference values, and disorders unique to the newborn.

SECTION OBJECTIVES BOX 45-1

- Summarize routine chemistry tests whose reference ranges differ significantly between neonates and adults.
- Contrast mechanisms employed in utero and in the neonatal period with adult mechanisms for the maintenance of water, electrolyte, and mineral balance.
- Contrast the hematological, coagulation, and immune systems in neonates and adults.
- Discuss the maturity of the systems that control release of TRH, TSH, CRH, ACTH, and growth hormone in the neonate.

PHYSIOLOGICAL CHANGES ASSOCIATED WITH TRANSITION FROM INTRAUTERINE TO EXTRAUTERINE STATE

In utero, the fetus depends on the placenta for gas exchange and metabolic functions, including nutrition and removal of toxic waste products (see Chapter 44). At birth, fetal systems must adapt immediately to independent existence. The reorganization of body systems and tissues for extrauterine life is associated with changing blood levels of hormones, metabolites, plasma proteins, and tissue enzyme levels. Thus, neonatal reference intervals in many cases are significantly different from those in older children or adults. In general, reference intervals for tests that reflect trace element, vitamin, protein, carbohydrate, and lipid nutritional status are lower than those for adults, and markers of tissue turnover or inflammation are higher. Transplacental transfer of maternal estrogens results in relative elevations in the neonate; however, androgen levels are much lower than in adults. Chemistry tests that differ significantly (normal median >±25%) between adults and neonates are listed in Table 45-1.[2,21,29,35,36]

Cardiorespiratory Adaptation

To facilitate in utero oxygen transport, the fetus is relatively polycythemic, and fetal erythrocytes contain for the most part

Table 45-1 Chemistry Testing in Neonates: Expected Reference Intervals (Normal Values) Relative to Adults

Test	Similar Median Adult & Neonatal Normal values	Neonatal Values Higher than Adults	Neonatal Values Lower than Adults
Electrolytes	Na, K, Cl, Total CO2, Ca, Mg, Osmolality, pCO2, pH	Phosphate	Base excess
Metabolites	Ammonia, lactate, uric acid	Bilirubin (total and unconjugated)	Carnitine, creatinine, glucose, urea
Plasma proteins	Alpha 1 antitrypsin, Apolipoprotein A and Apolipoprotein B, Immunoglobulin G	AFP, cystatin C, CRP	Albumin, ceruloplasmin, complement (C3, C4), haptoglobin, IgA, IgM, prealbumin, RBP, total protein, transferrin
Enzymes & markers of tissue turnover	ALT, lipase	Alkaline phosphatase, AST, CPK, GGT, LD, cardiac troponins	Amylase
Nutrients	Fe, Zn		Cholesterol, Cu, Se, triglycerides, vitamins (A, E, 25-OH Vitamin D)
Hormones	DHEA, DHEA-S, 11-Deoxycortisol, Gastrin	Aldosterone, estradiol, 17-OH progesterone, prolactin, renin, TSH, free T4	Cortisol, IGF-1, PTH, androgens

Where higher and lower refer to differences in the expected normal median value for neonates that deviate by more than 25% from the corresponding adult median.

Table 45-2 Fetal and Neonatal Body Composition

	FETAL			*ADULT*	
Stage of Development	**24-25 Weeks**	**28 Weeks**	**40 Weeks (Term Neonate)**	**Male**	**Female**
Mean weight	650-750 g	1500 g	3500 g	70 kg	55 kg
Subcutaneous fat	Minimal	3.5% TBW	12%		
Total body water (% of TBW)		84%	78%	60%	55%
Extracellular fluid (% of TBW)		65%	40%	20%-25%	20%

TBW, Total body weight.

higher oxygen affinity fetal hemoglobin (HbF). A normal **term newborn** has a hematocrit of around 60%. At 36 weeks, HbF accounts for about 90% of total hemoglobin; when term is approached, the percent of HbF decreases to 70%. Maturation of the pulmonary surfactant system occurs during the last 4 to 6 weeks of gestation. Neonatal respiratory distress syndrome resulting from insufficient production of surfactant is the most common disorder diagnosed in the neonatal intensive care unit (NICU). At birth, with separation of the placenta, systemic vascular resistance increases, fluid is cleared from the lungs, pulmonary vascular resistance drops, and blood flow to the lungs is enhanced. Closures of the ductus venosus, ductus arteriosus, and foramen ovale separate the pulmonary and systemic circulations. If healthy, the newborn cries, becomes pink, and has good muscle tone. Such predictors of health along with heart rate and reflex irritability are assessed at 1 and 5 minutes by the Apgar score. Low Apgar scores (<3) identify neonates in need of immediate resuscitation (5% to 10% of newborns).

Fluid, Electrolyte, and Mineral Homeostasis (see Chapters 28, 30, and 33)

The neonate's capacity to maintain fluid and electrolyte homeostasis is dependent on the degree of in utero maturation. Extreme changes in body composition occur between 24 weeks of gestation and term (Table 45-2). Extracellular fluid, which approximates 20% to 25% of body weight in adults, decreases from 60% of body weight in the second trimester fetus to about 45% at term. Relative to total body weight, the term newborn has three times more interstitial water content than an adult, and body water content is inversely proportionate to the maturity of the infant. A term neonate may lose 5% to 10% of body weight owing to a combination of renal and insensible losses of extracellular fluid. Neonatal growth replaces this weight loss in a healthy neonate within 7 to 10 days. A premature neonate may lose 10% to 15% of body weight during the first week of life.[37] Transdermal fluid loss is particularly high in premature neonates who have a fragile permeable epidermis with a disproportionately large surface area for body mass, and are cared for in warm ambient temperatures. **Phototherapy** is used more frequently in this population, which increases transdermal fluid losses. Because of all these factors, extremes of fluid volumes and fluid electrolyte composition are common in the premature infant.[37]

Neonatal fluid and electrolyte homeostasis improves with maturation of the renal system. In utero, fetal cardiac output to the kidneys is only about 5% (compared with 25% in the adult) because 40% to 60% of cardiac output goes to the placenta. Maturation of the renal system occurs during the third trimester. Urine production by the fetus increases from 10 mL/hr around 30 weeks to 27 mL/hr at term.

Despite increased production of urine **ex utero,** the neonatal kidney is still immature. Although nephrogenesis is complete by 34 weeks of gestation, the proximal tubular and collecting duct epithelial cells of the newborn incompletely express the transporters necessary for uptake of sodium and secretion of potassium. Consequently, hormonal regulation of sodium and water by antidiuretic hormone (ADH) and the renin-angiotensin-aldosterone (RAA) system is limited. These effects are magnified as the degree of premature delivery increases.

All neonates experience a postnatal surge of ADH, but blood levels normalize within 24 hours. The amplitude of the surge reflects birth-related factors such as vaginal vs non-vaginal delivery, degree of hypoxia, and increased intracranial pressure (ICP). As in adults, ADH is regulated primarily by plasma osmolality and secondarily by plasma volume. However, lack of a well-developed renal medullary concentration gradient blunts the ADH effect, leading to a maximum urine osmolality of 350 to 500 mOsm/kg. Similarly, although plasma renin activity, angiotensin-converting enzyme (ACE), angiotensin I, angiotensin II, and aldosterone all are relatively high in the neonate, tubular sodium reabsorption is poor, because the immature cells of the renal collecting duct respond only partially to aldosterone stimulation. In addition, atrial natriuretic peptide and brain natriuretic peptide surge postnatally. Together, these hormonal changes produce an early natriuresis that facilitates volume contraction in the **neonatal period.** However, with limited capacity for sodium conservation and renal concentrating capacity, either hyponatremia or hypernatremia may develop, especially in the premature infant.[25]

Calcium, phosphate, and essential trace elements such as iron, copper, and zinc are acquired primarily during the third trimester. Sixty-six percent of these minerals are accumulated at between 28 and 40 weeks of gestation. Premature infants who need prolonged parenteral nutrition or who have diuretic-induced phosphate loss are at risk for metabolic bone disease.

Calcium homeostasis is regulated tightly from birth. Calcium exists in free (ionized) and bound (albumin-bound, anion conjugate) forms. The free form, which constitutes about 50% of the total, is the bioavailable functional fraction. The concentration of ionized calcium is regulated by parathyroid hormone and vitamin D activity. Although parathyroid hormone is present from birth, newborn vitamin D levels reflect maternal vitamin D status. Calcium and phosphate levels tend to be lower in prematurely born infants. Alkaline phosphatase activity is relatively high compared with adult levels.

Gastrointestinal Functions
(see Chapters 31, 34, and 35)

All organs needed for the digestion, absorption, and metabolism of nutrients are immature in the preterm newborn, and parenteral nutrition often is needed. However, protein and carbohydrate digestive enzymes are present in sufficient quantities to permit **enteral feeding** in newborns older than 28 weeks of gestation.[42]

The premature infant has higher protein requirements, and inadequate intake results in poor growth in weight and length, hypoalbuminemia, and low total serum protein. **Meconium** begins to form after 3 months of gestation and accumulates in the GI tract until birth. After birth, meconium is passed for the first 1 to 3 days; then stools evolve through a transitional greenish-brown coloration with some milk curds to yellow-brown milk stools, which may be passed up to seven times a day in a breast-fed infant. Failure to pass meconium (meconium ileus) is a strong predictor of cystic fibrosis. Testing for cystic fibrosis involves collection of an ample amount of sweat. After 2 weeks of age, this amount of sweat may be collected without difficulty in 95% of cases; however, before 2 weeks of age, the frequency of inadequate sweat collection increases. If possible, testing should not be attempted before a neonate has reached 7 days of age and weighs a minimum of 3 kg. The earliest that sweat testing can be attempted is after 48 hours of age.[23,41] Molecular testing for cystic fibrosis transmembrane conductance regulator (CFTR) gene mutations may obviate the need for neonatal sweat testing in some cases.

Hematological and Immune Systems
(see Chapter 40)

Blood erythrocyte counts and hemoglobin levels rise in the first 2 hours of life, drop by 10% to 20% during the first 6 to 10 weeks of life, and then rise again. The transient physiological anemia results from a combination of shorter fetal red blood cell life ($t_{1/2}$ = 60 to 80 days) and blunted renal erythropoietin production. In term neonates, this anemia is asymptomatic, but it may be important in preterm neonates (see Anemia of Prematurity). The reduced half-life of fetal erythrocytes and the hemoglobin gene switch from gamma- to β-chain production result in a gradual postnatal decline in fetal hemoglobin from about 55% to 65% of total hemoglobin at birth, to about 5% by 4 to 5 months of age. Degraded fetal hemoglobin is converted into unconjugated bilirubin by reticuloendothelial cells, contributing to the physiological jaundice of newborns (see Neonatal Jaundice).

Neonatal and adult coagulation systems are similar, aside from transiently reduced levels of vitamin K–dependent cofactors in the first week of life. Classic hemorrhagic disease of the newborn affects 2% of neonates and is prevented effectively with routine administration of 1 mg of intramuscular vitamin K_1 to all neonates. Exclusively breast-fed neonates receive almost no vitamin K and may be at risk for a late-onset form (>2 months) of vitamin K–deficient bleeding, despite receiving the neonatal vitamin K_1 injection.[48]

Neonatal T cells and B cells are relatively immature. T cells are shifted toward CD4+ cells, producing adult levels of the proinflammatory cytokines interleukin (IL)-1, IL-6, and tumor necrosis factor (TNF)-alpha. Thus, cell-mediated immunity is functional. However, adaptive immunity cytokines such as IL-5 and IL-10 are present in much lower levels as compared with those in adults, indicating a decreased ability to stimulate B-cell proliferation. Although B cells are present at adult levels, they are functionally immature and have a reduced ability to generate an antibody response to many antigens. Antibody production involves mainly immunoglobulin (Ig) M, with B cells demonstrating delayed isotype switching. Term infants have IgG levels that are greater than adult levels because of placental transfer of IgG antibodies during the third trimester. As maternally derived antibodies are cleared, the neonatal IgG level (typically 10 g/L) decreases over the first 3 months of life to a nadir of 3.0 to 5.0 g/L, before increasing after 3 to 5 months because of accelerated intrinsic antibody production.[30]

Endocrine Functions (see Chapters 48 and 49)

Several quiescent fetal endocrine axes are stimulated immediately after birth. Thus, an underlying inborn deficiency in endocrine system function may present during the neonatal period.

Production of thyrotropin-releasing hormone (TRH), thyroid-stimulating hormone (TSH), and thyroid hormones is active from birth. A postnatal rise in TRH induces an increase in blood TSH and T_4 levels as the fetus makes the transition from the in utero environment (37°C) to the postnatal delivery room environment (25°C). Peak levels correlate with **gestational age.** Adult thyroid hormone levels are achieved by 4 weeks of age.[20]

Corticotropin-releasing hormone is active at birth and regulates adrenocorticotropic hormone (ACTH), as in adults. ACTH stimulates adrenal cortex cortisol release at adult levels by 1 week of age. The ACTH stimulation test gives comparable results by day 3 of life. Increases in serum cortisol and catecholamines represent the primary counterregulatory response to low blood glucose and are used to maintain euglycemia in newborns.[20,26,27]

Growth hormone–releasing hormone is released in an adult, pulsatile fashion, starting at 4 weeks of age. Before 4 weeks, growth hormone production increases in response to hypoglycemia and physical stress. Insulin-like growth factor (IGF)-I and IGFBP3 levels remain low for the first year of life.

Glucose levels tend to be low in the first 24 hours after birth and increase modestly to a new equilibrium state, which lasts until adult levels are reached at 2 years of life.[14] Fetal pancreatic insulin production is mature at midgestation, and several problems can arise from overactive pancreatic insulin secretion (see Disorders of Glucose Regulation). Newborn diabetes mellitus is extremely rare. Oxytocin, prolactin, gonadotropin-releasing hormone, follicle-stimulating hormone (FSH), and luteinizing hormone (LH) have no known role in normal neonatal physiology; consequently, blood levels are low or undetectable.

Blood-Brain Barrier (see Chapter 47)

Neonatal cerebrospinal fluid (CSF) has a relatively high protein concentration. The integrity of the neonatal blood-brain barrier is intact, and very-high-molecular-weight proteins such as plasma immunoglobulins do not readily cross into the CSF. CSF immunoglobulin concentrations and cell counts are similar to those found in adults and can be used to check the integrity of the blood-brain barrier. CSF glucose, lactate, and bilirubin levels parallel serum concentrations, as they do in adults.[50]

KEY CONCEPTS BOX 45-1

- At birth, the newborn suddenly makes the transition from dependency on maternal function to an independent state for nutritional, respiratory, and waste removal functions.
- Organ systems mature at different periods of gestation, so the degree of prematurity affects the physiological capacity to adapt to extrauterine life.
- A number of routinely available laboratory tests can be used to determine the degree of maturity of an organ, but they must be interpreted with an understanding of healthy neonatal physiology.

SECTION OBJECTIVES BOX 45-2

- Summarize pathological causes of, typical laboratory results for, and treatment for hyperunconjugated and hyperconjugated bilirubinemia.
- Discuss the primary causes of disorders of fluid and electrolyte homeostasis, disorders of glucose regulation, and calcium and phosphate disorders.
- Discuss the primary hematological disorders in the neonate.
- Discuss neonatal screening tests for hypothyroidism, hyperthyroidism, and congenital adrenal hyperplasia.
- List common pathogens that cause neonatal infections and typical laboratory tests used to diagnose those infections.

PATHOLOGICAL CONDITIONS IN NEONATAL MEDICINE

Premature or inappropriately small or large neonates are susceptible to a wide range of medical problems, but appropriately grown, term neonates are also at risk. Three percent to 5% of neonates are born with a congenital anomaly. In addition, neonatal problems may result from fetal exposure to an abnormal intrauterine environment, from limitations in physiological adaptations needed by all newborns for normal birth transition, or from problems arising during the birth process or in the early neonatal period (Table 45-3).

Laboratory management of the newborn requires the ability to rapidly provide information on blood gases, hematocrit, and glucose from small blood samples available from newborns. Cord blood gas parameters, pH, and base excess are used in combination with clinical findings as a retrospective indication of possible intrapartum asphyxia. Although respiratory complications (e.g., transient tachypnea of the newborn, meconium aspiration syndrome, persistent pulmonary hypertension, congenital diaphragmatic hernia) may arise in term neonates, the most common respiratory problems—respiratory distress syndrome and apnea of prematurity—occur in premature neonates.

Table 45-3 Major Concerns in Neonatal Medicine

Neonatal Maturation	Intrauterine Environment	Intrapartum/Early Neonate
—Preterm delivery (respiratory distress syndrome)	**Maternal Disease**	**Intrapartum**
—Congenital anomalies	—Gestational diabetes	—Chorioamnionitis
—Inborn error of metabolism	—ITP	—Hypoxia/asphyxia
—Endocrine deficiency	—Graves disease	—Meconium aspiration
—Physiological jaundice	—SSA/SSB	—Hemorrhage
	—Phenylketonuria	—Trauma
	—Maternal infection (e.g., HIV, hepatitis, TORCH)	**Early Neonatal Period**
	—Hemolytic disease of the newborn	—Neonatal sepsis
	—Maternal medication/illicit drug use, teratogens	
	Placental Insufficiency	

ITP, Idiopathic thrombocytopenic purpura.

Box 45-1

Pathological Causes of Hyper-unconjugated Bilirubinemia

Deficient hepatic uridine diphosphoglucuronyl transferase activity
- Genetic (Gilbert or Crigler-Najjar syndrome)
- Hypothyroidism

Genetic defects affecting the following:
- Hemoglobin structure (e.g., sickle cell anemia)
- Red blood cell enzyme activity (e.g., glucose-6-phosphate dehydrogenase deficiency)
- RBC membrane characteristics (e.g., hereditary spherocytosis)

Increased deconjugation and re-uptake of enteral bilirubin:
- Limited enteral feeding
- Breast feeding

Hemolytic disease of the newborn; blood group incompatibility
High rate of RBC (hemoglobin) catabolism
Neonatal hemorrhage
Polycythemia
Sepsis
Trauma

Neonatal Jaundice (see p. 591, Chapter 31)

The high rate of red blood cell breakdown (see earlier) and consequent bilirubin synthesis, along with an immature liver, cause a transient (physiological) neonatal unconjugated hyperbilirubinemia. Total bilirubin measurements remain below the 75th percentile for age of life (in hours), peak within 2 to 3 days, and show substantial decline by days 4 and 5 in physiological jaundice. If bilirubin parameters exceed these limits, pathological causes of hyperbilirubinemia must be investigated.[16] Pathological causes of unconjugated and conjugated hyperbilirubinemia are listed in Boxes 45-1 and 45-2, respectively.

Extrahepatic biliary atresia (EHBA) caused by an absent or blocked common bile duct leads to conjugated hyperbilirubinemia. EHBA affects 1 in 10,000 neonates and can be diagnosed when jaundice presents in the second to third week of life in association with acholic (pale-colored) stools, reflecting lack of biliary pigments. A conjugated bilirubin level greater than 20% of the total bilirubin must be followed up with appropriate radiological imaging and hepatic biopsy as necessary to confirm or rule out the diagnosis.[52]

Box 45-2

Pathological Causes of Cholestasis and Hyper-conjugated Bilirubinemia

Biliary tree obstruction
Extrahepatic biliary atresia
Impaired hepatic excretion of conjugated bilirubin from nonspecific or infectious hepatitis
Metabolic derangements of bilirubin excretion or bile synthesis
Other neonatal metabolic syndromes

Neonatal hyperbilirubinemia is defined as a total serum bilirubin that is above the 95th percentile for hour-of-age on a bilirubin nomogram.[10] The unconjugated fraction of bilirubin that exceeds the binding capacity of albumin is able to pass the blood-brain barrier and cause bilirubin-induced neurological damage (BIND). The American Academy of Pediatrics has detailed guidelines for the identification of at-risk neonates and the prevention of BIND (Pediatrics 114:297, 2004; http://pediatrics.aappublications.org/cgi/content/full/115/3/824). In general, phototherapy must be considered when the bilirubin concentration exceeds the 95th percentile for age (in hours), with decision limits dependent on the gestational age and weight of the neonate. For infants who have risk factors (Box 45-3), the threshold for BIND is lower; thus, therapy may be initiated at lower bilirubin levels in these neonates as compared with others. Neonates who do not respond to phototherapy may undergo exchange transfusion to keep bilirubin levels below BIND thresholds (428 to 513 μmol/L; 25 to 30 mg/dL). The guidelines recommend screening for hyperbilirubinemia by plasma bilirubin measurement or by an approved transcutaneous photometric bilirubinometer.

Disorders of Fluid and Electrolyte Homeostasis

Disorders of fluid, electrolyte, and glucose homeostasis are common even in term neonates. Hyponatremia is frequent in

Box 45-3

Risk Factors That May Affect Phototherapy Intervention

Acidosis
Asphyxia
Glucose-6-phosphate dehydrogenase (G6PD) deficiency
Hemolytic disease of the newborn
Hypoalbuminemia (<3 g/dL)
Lethargy
Prematurity
Sepsis
Temperature instability

From http://newborns.stanford.edu/BiliSummary.html#PhototxGuide

Box 45-4

Causes of Neonatal Hypoglycemia

Increased Glucose Utilization
- Catabolic stress
- Cold-induced thermogenesis
- Shock (sepsis)

Decreased glucose supply
- Low glycogen stores (preterm or small for gestational age [SGA])
- Insufficient supply of calories

Endocrine disorders
- Growth hormone deficiency
- Adrenal insufficiency

Genetic disorders
- Unregulated insulin production
- Fatty acid oxidation disorder

Hypoxia
Maternal diabetes

the first week of life because of prenatal transfer of free water from the maternal to the fetal circulation. Later in the neonatal period, hyponatremia may arise from impaired sodium transport and sodium loss in the proximal tubules (immature epithelial cells) and collecting ducts (mineralocorticoid deficiency). Pseudohyponatremia associated with elevated serum lipids (especially parenterally administered) or protein can cause an apparent hyponatremia.

Hypernatremia is common in neonates who suffer from excessive insensible free water loss, particularly if associated with a specific anomaly such as **gastroschisis.** Neonatal hypernatremic dehydration associated with impaired breast feeding may result from delayed maturation of breast milk secretion. Excessive urine free water loss also results from impaired nephron-concentrating ability.

Hypokalemia resulting from the use of diuretics and nasogastric tubes is common, as is hyperkalemia resulting from impaired renal excretion (low glomerular filtration rate [GFR] or mineralocorticoid deficiency), cellular damage (hemolysis, necrosis), or iatrogenic causes. Therapy is aimed at preventing cell membrane instability (calcium), stabilizing plasma K levels (insulin and glucose), and removing excess body stores (diuretics).

Disorders of Glucose Regulation

Neonatal hypoglycemia is common (10% of neonates) and may result in short- or long-term neurological deficits. Asymptomatic hypoglycemia is more common and is identified by screening of high-risk infants. Symptomatic hypoglycemia is more likely to be associated with adverse neurological outcomes. Neonatal hypoglycemia most commonly results from increased glucose utilization (Box 45-4) but also may result from impaired glucose production. Persistent hypoglycemia requiring high rates of intravenous glucose administration suggests an underlying hormonal or metabolic abnormality. When such hypoglycemia is present, the neonate should be investigated for plasma glucose, lactate, ketone, insulin, cortisol, and growth hormone levels. Other tests such as TSH, amino acids, acyl carnitine profile, and urine organic acids may prove useful.

The diagnosis of hypoglycemia is based on plasma glucose levels relative to gestational age, postnatal age, and fasting status. Thresholds for intervention have been established at 40 mg/dL (2.2 mmol/L) and 50 mg/dL (2.2 to 2.8 mmol/L) for neonates younger than 24 hours and older than 24 hours, respectively. Neonates at risk for hypoglycemia should be tested for plasma glucose at 1 to 2 hours (before feeding). If glucose is less than 40 mg/dL, the infant should be fed and retested after feeding. Glucose testing may be done by bedside glucometers, but low results should be confirmed by a backup assay. Treatment should take place while one is waiting for confirmatory testing.[13]

Neonatal hyperglycemia is a rare finding in a term neonate. Its presence suggests hypercortisolemia (i.e., stress response) or the very rare congenital diabetes syndrome (1:500,000). Iatrogenic hyperglycemia from intravenous glucose therapy also must be considered, particularly in preterm infants, in whom the ability to regulate hepatic gluconeogenesis and pancreatic B-cell insulin production is immature. Blood glucose concentrations greater than 180 mg/dL (10 mmol/L) should be treated by decreasing glucose infusion or providing insulin, depending on the caloric needs of the neonate. Plasma glucose levels must be monitored for all neonates on intravenous glucose until the glucose level stabilizes.

Calcium and Phosphate Disorders

Nephrolithiasis and **nephrocalcinosis** are common concerns. Nephrocalcinosis affects up to 60% of at-risk neonates (low birth weight, preterm delivery, and treatment with loop diuretics) and is associated with long-term relative impairment in tubular and glomerular function.[31]

Early (24 to 72 hours) neonatal hypocalcemia and associated hyperphosphatemia are common in preterm neonates and infants of diabetic mothers. Preterm and small-for-gestational-age (SGA) neonates may have hypocalcemia as the result of hypoalbuminemia, insufficient acquisition of calcium stores in utero, a blunted response to parathyroid hormone, renal tubular calcium losses associated with high sodium passage, and high calcitonin production. Between 10% and 50% of infants of diabetic mothers have hypocalcemia caused by hypoparathyroidism of unknown pathogenesis. Neonatal asphyxia also predisposes to hypocalcemia and hyperphosphatemia.

Late (>72 hours) neonatal hypocalcemia arises from neonatal hypoparathyroidism, high phosphate intake, phototherapy, and disorders of vitamin D metabolism. Hypoparathyroidism may be caused by Di George syndrome, maternal hyperparathyroidism, and hypomagnesemia (transient decrease to 0.80 to 1.41 mg/dL [0.33 to 0.58 mmol/L]; normal, >1.60 mg/dL [0.66 mmol/L]). High phosphate intake occurs rarely now because current infant formulas are lower in phosphate.

Hypocalcemic neonates present with jitteriness, neuromuscular irritability, and seizures. Most commonly, hypocalcemia is asymptomatic, so high-risk infants should be assessed by ionized calcium measurements at 12, 24, and 48 hours. Treatment with calcium and magnesium repletion should be monitored.

Thyroid Disorders

Congenital hypothyroidism, a rare but treatable condition that affects 1 in 4000 neonates, is usually the result of a developmental thyroid migration abnormality (i.e., sublingual thyroid). Rarer causes include thyroid aplasia, a genetic disorder of thyroid hormone synthesis, and hypopituitarism. Recognition that cognitive impairment correlates with length of treatment delay led to the establishment of newborn screening for this disorder in all developed countries. Primary hypothyroidism is readily detectable by neonatal TSH screening (follow-up if TSH >20 mU/L), whereas neonatal free T4 screening will identify both primary and secondary hypothyroidism. TSH screening is prone to false positives in the first 24 hours because of the high TSH levels associated with the neonatal transition from in utero to ex utero life. Premature infants tend to have low free T_4 levels with normal TSH values.

Neonatal hyperthyroidism is a rare but very serious condition that is caused primarily by transfer of maternal TSH receptor–stimulating antibodies, which results in neonatal Graves' disease. The mother may have subclinical, treated, or untreated Graves' disease. A minority of such women (2% to 17%) will have fetuses or neonates with hyperthyroidism; the level of maternal antibodies in the third trimester of pregnancy is the strongest predictor of neonatal Graves' disease. Neonatal Graves' disease is characterized by preterm delivery, microcephaly, warm body, tachycardia with bounding pulses, irritability, restlessness, poor weight gain, and Graves' ophthalmopathy. Symptoms are suppressed by maternal antithyroid medications and worsen as maternally derived medication is cleared. Conversely, the syndrome lessens over 3 to 12 weeks of life as maternal antibodies are cleared from the infant's circulation. In the interim, neonates require treatment with antithyroid therapy. Diagnosis and monitoring of neonatal Graves' disease requires measurement of free T_4 levels, which must be compared against appropriate, age-adjusted norms.[47]

Adrenal Disorders

Classical congenital adrenal hyperplasia (CAH) affects between 1:10,000 and 1:20,000 neonates. In 90% of cases, the defect is an autosomal recessive (CYP2A2) deficiency of 21-hydroxylase activity. Deficiency of this enzyme leads to impaired conversion of steroid precursors (17-hydroxyprogesterone and 17-hydroxypregnenelone) into the respective glucocorticoid (cortisol) and mineralocorticoid (aldosterone) derivatives. Instead, progesterone steroids are converted into androgen steroids (dehydroepiandrosterone [DHEA], DHEA-sulfate, and androstenedione). Infants present with signs of virilization (ambiguous genitalia in females) and, depending on the severity of the enzyme deficiency, a hypotensive salt-wasting syndrome characterized by high renin, low aldosterone, hyponatremia, hyperkalemia, and low plasma-free metanephrines produced by deficient stimulation of activity in the adrenal medulla. Many health regions in North America screen all neonates for this treatable and potentially fatal condition by testing neonatal blood 17-hydroxyprogesterone levels (levels typically >95 nmol/L). When the diagnosis is in doubt, an ACTH (250 μg) stimulation test reveals marked post-stimulation elevations in 17-hydroxyprogesterone.

Neonatal Infections

Neonates, because of their immune compromised status (immature humoral immune system), are prone to infection caused by peripartum bacterial (e.g., group B streptococcus, *Escherichia coli, Chlamydia trachomatis, Neisseria gonorrhoeae*) and viral (herpes simplex, enterovirus, varicella, HIV, hepatitis B) exposures. Late-onset infection (greater than 72 hours) usually is nosocomially acquired (*Staphylococcus aureus*, gram-negative rods, *Candida*). In the setting of a neonatal fever or other signs of sepsis, neonatal meningitis, urinary tract infection, and gastroenteritis must be considered.[54]

Body fluids for bacterial or fungal culture are necessary to confirm a presumptive diagnosis before antibiotic therapy is provided. Empirical antibiotic therapy typically is started while culture results are awaited. Additional laboratory tests may provide assistance in guiding the decision to initiate empirical antibiotic therapy. High-sensitivity C-reactive protein has been recognized as a sensitive but late marker of sepsis. Procalcitonin is a more sensitive marker of bacterial infection but is less specific in the neonatal population. Serum amyloid A protein is an early, sensitive, and specific marker of sepsis. This latter test has sufficient accuracy to guide initial use of antibiotic therapy in neonates.[7] A combination of these markers may provide a more accurate assessment of those at risk for neonatal sepsis.[43]

Although bacteriuria is present in 1:1000 newborns, urinary tract infection (UTI) is unusual before 3 days of age. Most UTIs occur during the second week of life. UTI can be assessed by urinalysis, particularly if the sample is taken by suprapubic aspiration or catheterization. Urine dipstick leukocyte esterase and nitrite tests are 95% sensitive for detection of a significant UTI. A urine culture test is required if clinical suspicion for UTI is high.[5,22,38,56]

Neurological Disorders

Neonatal encephalopathy affects 2 to 9 in 1000 newborns. The cause is largely unknown, although hypoxia and ischemia are risk factors. Predictors of neonatal encephalopathy include a 5-minute Apgar score <5, umbilical artery pH <7.0, and base deficit ≥12 mmol/L.[3,33] Radiological and electroencephalographic (EEG) studies also provide prognostic information.

About 1:1000 newborns have seizures, with the risk increasing in preterm neonates. Many factors, including intraventricular hemorrhage, neonatal (hypoxic ischemic) encephalopathy, metabolic abnormalities (hypoglycemia, hypocalcemia, hypomagnesemia), or specific genetic syndromes associated with a seizure disorder, may predispose neonates to seizure. Treatment for neonatal seizures requires specific treatment of the cause, such as correction of metabolic problems or provision of pyridoxine. Prolonged, frequent seizures may require anticonvulsant medications. Phenobarbital has a longer half-life in premature infants, especially in those with renal or hepatic insufficiency. Plasma levels must be monitored because clearance changes as the child matures. Phenytoin also exhibits variable clearance in preterm neonates and requires an individualized dosing schedule.

Hematological Disorders

Neonatal thrombocytopenia may result from a disorder of platelet survival (e.g., alloimmune thrombocytopenia), platelet consumption (e.g., disseminated intravascular coagulation [DIC]), or platelet production (thrombocytopenia-absent radii syndrome). Laboratory tests to differentiate these categories of disease include complete cell counts of neonate and parents, parental antiplatelet antibodies, prothrombin time (PT) and activated partial thromboplastin time (aPTT), and D-dimer tests for possible DIC. Neonatal bleeding in gastric aspirates or stool should be investigated with occult blood tests and, if maternal or fetal origin of stool blood is unclear, **Apt tests.**[34]

Neonatal **polycythemia** (peripheral vein hematocrit >0.68) is associated with thrombocytopenia (unknown cause), hypoglycemia (increased red blood cell glycolysis), and hyperbilirubinemia (increased red blood cell turnover). Clinical signs of neonatal polycythemia include decreased cardiac output secondary to increased peripheral vascular resistance, as well as impaired perfusion of brain, kidneys, and intestines. Acrocyanosis occurs when reduced hemoglobin levels exceed 1 g/dL (unlikely with oxygen saturation >90%).

Blood group incompatibility with the D or an alternate antigen can cause hemolytic disease of the newborn (see pp. 873-874, Chapter 44), an important cause of neonatal anemia and pathological jaundice.[39] Infants with atrioventricular heart block should be given serum tests for anti-Ro/SSA and anti-La/SSB antibodies. If present, the mother should be tested as well, so neonatal lupus syndrome can be diagnosed.

Cardiovascular Disorders

Neonatal hypertension affects 3% of infants in an NICU. The most common cause is renovascular thrombosis secondary to umbilical venous catheterization. Other renal, pulmonary, and iatrogenic causes need consideration, as do endocrine causes (e.g., hyperthyroidism, congenital adrenal hyperplasia). Laboratory testing in the form of urinalysis for hematuria and proteinuria, serum electrolytes, calcium, urea, and creatinine may assist the clinician in making the diagnosis. Plasma renin and aldosterone levels also may be helpful.

Distinct Problems of Small-for-Gestational-Age (SGA) and Large-for-Gestational-Age (LGA) Infants

Multiple medical conditions are more common in **LGA** and SGA neonates than in infants of normal birth weight. These medical conditions arise as a consequence of the pathophysiology that underlies abnormal fetal growth rates.

The most common factor that results in an LGA baby is gestational diabetes. Factors that cause an SGA baby differ, depending on whether a general or a specific decrease in growth parameters occurs. General SGA may result from maternal drug use (e.g., narcotics, alcohol) or intrauterine infection (e.g., cytomegalovirus [CMV], toxoplasmosis, syphilis, rubella). In contrast, specific growth retardation suggests impaired oxygen supply to the fetus rather than toxic exposure. When faced with relatively impaired delivery of oxygenated blood, the fetus will direct a disproportionate amount of oxygenated blood to the largest and most critical organ, the brain. Thus, head size may be relatively preserved despite the undersupply of oxygenated blood that led to the stunted growth of other tissues. Impairment of the total fetal oxygenated blood supply may result from maternal smoking or placental insufficiency.

LGA neonates of gestational diabetic mothers are at risk for hypoglycemia and anemia, particularly if the maternal glucose level is poorly controlled in pregnancy. SGA neonates are at increased risk for hypoglycemia and hyperviscosity. Hypoglycemia arises from decreased glycogen reserves caused by compromised placental supply of nutrients. Polycythemia-induced hyperviscosity represents a physiological response to compromised placental oxygen supply to the fetal circulation.

Distinct Problems of Preterm Neonates

Preterm neonates are at risk for many minor and potentially severe complications. **Low birth weight** (LBW; <2500 g) and very low birth weight (<1500 g) neonates account for approximately 7% and 1% of births, but are responsible for 50% to

60% of infant mortality. Preterm birth, with or without SGA, accounts for the majority of low birth weight neonates in developed countries (SGA is the major cause of LBW neonates in countries with increased poverty). Their care requires significant resources from laboratories that serve NICUs.

Electrolyte Disorders

As was noted previously, fluid, electrolyte and glucose homeostasis is suboptimal in a preterm neonate. Frequent monitoring of sodium, potassium, and glucose is required to guide supplementation. Non-oliguric hyperkalemia is particularly common in preterm babies, because low activity of cell membrane sodium-potassium-triphosphatase (Na^+, K^+-ATPase) activity in the first 2 days of life shifts potassium from intracellular to extracellular fluid. Potassium is omitted from maintenance IV fluids for the first 2 days, to prevent exacerbation of this tendency.[40,55]

Nutritional Disorders

Premature neonates are at risk for nutritional deficiencies because their nutritional requirements are greater than at any other stage of life, and their ability to obtain nutrients is limited. The premature infant has not been able to accumulate the massive nutrient stores (e.g., fat, calcium, iron, other minerals) that would have been provided in utero in the third trimester of pregnancy. Clinical goals in treating the premature infant include trying to restore these nutrients ex utero. Inability to achieve this goal leads to nutritional and metabolic problems. The best indicator of success in meeting the neonate's nutrient requirements is the infant's growth rate.[24] Monitoring of blood tests is a secondary but helpful indicator. Weekly measurements of plasma Ca, Mg, phosphate, albumin, and hemoglobin levels provide useful information to guide nutritional supplementation.

Respiratory Disorders

Respiratory distress syndrome (RDS) is a syndrome of respiratory insufficiency that arises from insufficient pulmonary surfactant production (see p. 869, Chapter 44). The incidence of this disorder increases with increasing degree of prematurity. Severe RDS leads to multi-organ failure and severe bronchopulmonary dysplasia among those who survive. However, these severe manifestations of RDS have become much less frequent because of current interventions, including accelerated fetal lung maturation via antenatal corticosteroid therapy given to women in threatened preterm labor, postnatal administration of surfactant, and more conservative mechanical ventilation.[53] Nevertheless, ventilation often is required, and the overall prevalence of chronic lung disease resulting from a milder form of bronchopulmonary dysplasia remains high in preterm neonate survivors.[8] Therefore, prevention of unnecessary delivery of a fetus with insufficient surfactant production remains important. Prenatal testing of amniotic fluid is done to assess the risk for respiratory distress syndrome, as discussed in Chapter 44 (see p. 872). Monitoring of neonates at risk for RDS consists of measuring blood oxygen saturation, P_{CO_2}, and pH.

Apnea of prematurity is characterized by apneic episodes lasting longer than 20 seconds and associated with low oxygen saturation or bradycardia. Apneic episodes are more likely with greater prematurity and typically do not occur after the neonate has reached the equivalent of 36 weeks of gestation. This idiopathic disorder must be differentiated from more deadly causes of prolonged apnea, including disease of the central nervous system, lungs, heart, and gastrointestinal system, or metabolic abnormalities. Prolonged or frequent apneic episodes are treated routinely with caffeine to stimulate respiration. This treatment is effective in reducing the incidence of bronchopulmonary dysplasia and the severity of retinopathy of prematurity.[51] These benefits are achievable when a standard dosing protocol is used and adjustments are made according to clinical signs of toxicity (i.e., tachycardia, feeding intolerance) or lack of effect (i.e., persistent prolonged apnea).[46]

Necrotizing Enterocolitis (NEC)

The origin of this serious complication of prematurity is unknown, but preventative measures involve early exposure of the bowel to breast milk and normal gut flora (commensal bacteria).[17] Bell's criteria for diagnosis and staging include clinical and radiographic factors. DIC, respiratory and metabolic acidosis, and neutropenia are laboratory indicators of advanced NEC. Fecal occult blood monitoring is a very nonspecific indicator of NEC, because almost two-thirds of preterm neonates have occult blood–positive stools resulting from swallowing of maternal blood, anal stricture, polyps, or inflammation.

Anemia of Prematurity

Anemia of prematurity occurs as an acceleration and amplification of the physiological anemia seen during the first 6 to 10 weeks of life in term neonates.[12] The exaggerated response results from a shorter half-life of HbF-containing red blood cells combined with a greater deficit of erythropoietin production. Both factors correlate with greater immaturity. Iatrogenic blood loss compounds the anemia. Very sick infants have greater blood loss. In **extremely low birth weight** neonates, 20% to 40% of their blood volume may be taken for laboratory testing over the course of an NICU stay. Iron deficiency can delay recovery from anemia and must be prevented. Blood transfusions correct symptoms of anemia (e.g., increased cardiac output, poor weight gain, lactic acidosis) but may further blunt erythropoietin production.[19] The preterm infant is able to respond to erythropoietin, but the role of erythropoietin in the management of anemia of prematurity has not been well defined. Early treatment with erythropoietin may increase the risk for retinopathy of prematurity.[44]

Neonatal Jaundice

Physiological jaundice has a more protracted, severe course in premature newborns with a relatively delayed onset of peak bilirubin levels (4 to 7 days). Preterm neonates also are at increased risk for kernicterus. Thus, phototherapy decisions are based on lower thresholds for interventions.

KEY CONCEPTS BOX 45-2

- Physiological jaundice is a common neonatal problem that requires measurement of total bilirubin to diagnose and monitor the disease.
- Pathological jaundice may be caused by disease states, such as hepatitis B, and may require measurement of conjugated and total bilirubin to diagnose and monitor the disease.
- Hypoglycemia is a common life-threatening disorder that requires close laboratory monitoring of blood glucose.
- Medical problems can arise from fetal exposure to an abnormal intrauterine environment (drugs, infectious diseases) or from limitation in physiological adaptations, which can affect the intrauterine growth of the fetus. These abnormally sized newborns require special attention during the early neonatal period.
- Prematurely born newborns also have a large number of medical problems, most often associated with immature organs, that can result in life-threatening disease, especially jaundice and respiratory problems.

SECTION OBJECTIVES BOX 45-3

- Explain the reasons for special neonatal specimen collection protocols.
- Contrast the benefits and problems associated with using serum whole blood, or plasma for laboratory investigations in neonates.

LABORATORY REQUIREMENTS FOR NEWBORN CARE

Laboratories that test neonatal samples must actively collaborate with clinical care providers in setting standards for quality and volume of sample collection (Box 45-5). The laboratory should take an active role in educating clinical staff regarding minimum blood volumes needed for individual tests, and in developing laboratory protocols that will allow the laboratory to efficiently use the sample that is available, which, in turn, will minimize blood loss and sample collection trauma.

Sample Volume and Sample Collection

Sample volume is a major consideration in neonatal care. A 10 mL blood sample represents about 0.2% of an adult's blood volume, whereas it represents 3% to 4% of the blood volume of a term newborn and 8% to 10% of the blood volume of a 1000 g newborn born at 26 to 28 weeks of gestation. High hematocrit in neonates further compromises the amount of plasma available (Fig. 45-1). In the 1000 g neonate, a 10 mL blood loss at one time, or over 1 week, could be an indication for transfusion. No common standard is used for maximum blood collection in infants, but typical institutional guidelines for infants with body weight <7 kg advise that single collections should consist of <1 mL/kg body weight, or approximately 1% of total blood volume.

Laboratories that do neonatal testing may be responsible for capillary and venous blood sample collection or training, because any sample loss or compromise of the sample may have a significant adverse effect on the quality of neonatal care.

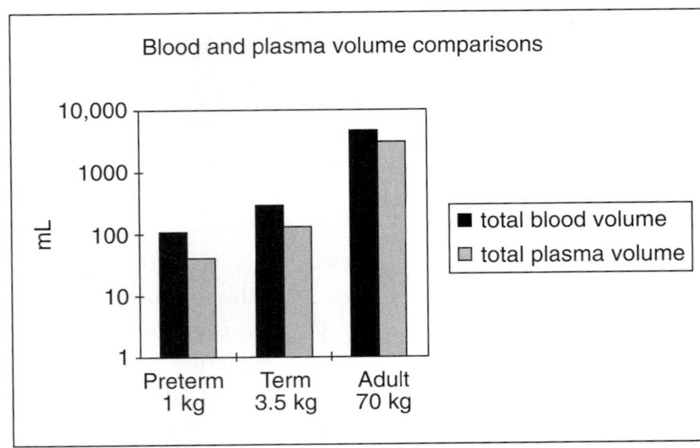

Fig. 45-1 Expected blood and plasma volumes for preterm neonates, term neonates, and adults, respectively.

Box 45-5

Neonatal Sample Considerations

Collection Consideration

General:
Blood loss
Pain (stress response, feeding during sample collection)
Trauma (line sampling, transcutaneous monitoring, no second attempt)
Risk of infection
Crying (affects blood gases, glucose, lactate)

Line Samples: Infection Control
Line patency (heparin solutions)
Clearing of line to prevent sample contamination with IV fluids

Heelstick Capillary Samples
Capillary-venous differences in analyte concentrations (thyroid-stimulating hormone [TSH], thyroid-binding globulin [TBG], thyroxine [T_4], glucose, lactate, ammonia, hemoglobin)
Peripheral perfusion
Site selection (reuse of site, bruising, edema-affected results)
Warming of site (for blood flow, arterialization of sample)
Antiseptic (analytical interferences with isopropanol, betadine)
Lancet usage (affects flow, trauma to site)
Blood flow (tissue contamination, coagulation activation, hemolysis)
Appropriate sample
Appropriate sample containers

Laboratory Considerations
Processing of samples
Prioritization of testing
Preanalytical decisions to match available sample volume with tests ordered: control of dead volume, predilutions

Current recommendations related to sample collection may be found in recent references.*

Laboratory personnel responsible for testing samples from newborns should match the available sample volume with the volume needed for the tests ordered. The calculation must include the analytical instrument's dead volume, which for

*References 1, 4, 6, 9, 15, 18, 28.

Box 45-6

Alternative Laboratory Monitoring Techniques for Neonates in Critical Care

Transcutaneous
Po_2, Pco_2, and oxygen saturation
Bilirubin (at >28 to 30 weeks of gestation)

Blood Gases: Whole blood analysis
Blood gases, cooximetry, electrolytes, hemoglobin, ionized calcium, glucose, lactate, and total bilirubin

Point-of-Care Testing
Glucose, electrolytes, etc. (see Chapter 21 for expanded list of available tests)

many automated analyzers is often much greater than the total sample volume required for the testing. Prioritization of tests can be based on protocols developed with the clinical staff or by telephone consultation with a neonatologist. In some cases, manual dilution may be appropriate to expand the available volume, provided that (1) the sample is sufficient for an accurate dilution, and (2) results on the diluted sample are expected to be within the analytical range. Instruments that employ whole blood analysis may serve as a suitable alternative to those that use serum or plasma, given the low yield of serum from neonatal blood.

Blood testing in neonates often is integrated with other monitoring techniques. For critical care, transcutaneous monitoring, point-of-care testing, and whole blood analysis offer rapid turnaround time with minimum sample collection and handling (Box 45-6).[11,45,49] Instruments used for such alternative testing should be validated in neonates, because factors such as skin characteristics, oxygen exposure in incubators, binding of unconjugated bilirubin, and the unique metabolic activity of neonatal blood cells may not be replicated accurately in vitro with the use of adult blood. If method performance in neonates has never been documented adequately, whole blood and point-of-care analyzers can be validated with the use of plasma left over from other tests requested at the same time. In settings where this is not feasible, consultation with a laboratory that has experience with the test in newborns is advisable, to review other strategies for method validation such as in vitro modification of adult or cord blood samples.

Some of the challenges associated with whole blood methods and whole blood versus plasma comparisons for neonates are outlined in Box 45-7.

For more complex testing in neonates, lithium heparin plasma is preferred to serum because of more rapid processing times, reduced hemolysis and microclots, and higher yield. Selection of laboratory analyzers for testing neonatal plasma samples requires close attention to sample handling (Box 45-8).

Therapeutic drug monitoring for the sick neonate can be difficult because of the many problems that can occur with administration of low amounts of drug, as well as the physiological differences between neonates and adults in terms of

Box 45-7

Factors Affecting Whole Blood Tests in Neonates

Blood gases and cooximetry
- Fetal hemoglobin

Potassium
- Undetected hemolysis in whole blood

Ionized calcium
- Heparin contamination (false decrease)

Glucose
- In vitro glycolysis (falsely low plasma glucose)
- Sequential sampling during or soon after feeding

Box 45-8

Instrumentation Considerations for Testing of Neonatal Plasma/Serum Samples

Adaptability to capillary tubes and microsamples
Small labels/bar codes
Low dead volume sample cup (40 to 50 μL)
Minimum on-board evaporation
Preservation of residual sample with minimum evaporation
Operator notification and option to triage tests with the following:
- Inadequate sample
- Clots, air bubbles
- Interferences such as hemolysis, lipemia, and icterus

Quantitative information on effects of interference
Adequate analytical range for typical neonate results
Low sample volume for common neonatal tests
Off-line dilution capability
User-defined test options

drug absorption, distribution, and administration.[32] The main drugs of interest for the neonate include aminoglycosides and other antibiotics (e.g., vancomycin, amikacin, chloramphenicol), digoxin, phenobarbital, and phenytoin. Before the introduction of caffeine for neonatal apnea, theophylline monitoring was required, but caffeine can be titrated by clinical response, and caffeine levels are rarely required. Digoxin methods must be assessed for reactivity with digoxin-like immunoreactive substances (DLIS) present in newborn blood in the first 1 to 4 weeks of life, and clinicians must be advised of any interferences. Testing of digoxin in blood from neonates not receiving the drug demonstrates the potential amount of interference.

Although the majority of neonatal laboratory testing is done on venous, line, or capillary samples, a laboratory that serves neonates encounters requests for analysis of a variety of other sample types. An overview is presented in Table 45-4.

Metabolic Diseases (see Chapter 52)

One in 600 infants has an inborn error of metabolism, and newborn screening (NBS) will pick up the most common and the most treatable of these conditions. However, newborn screening panels vary regionally in North America, and physicians must be familiar with the panel of disorders detected by

Table 45-4 Special Samples for Neonatal Assessment

Sample Type	Collection	Clinical Use	Interpretation	Notes
Umbilical cord blood	Umbilical artery (blood from fetus) and umbilical vein (blood from placenta)	Assess possibility of intrapartum asphyxia	pH Base excess Lactate: may indicate prolonged acidosis	Medicolegal use Methods described for delayed analysis if laboratory not open 24 hr/d Umbilical vein results differentiate respiratory from metabolic acidosis that suggests hypoxia
	Cord arterial or venous blood	Postnatal investigation for possible hemolytic disease of newborn	Includes newborn ABO group, Rh type, direct antiglobulin test	
		Risk of developing hyperbilirubinemia	Risk correlated with cord blood bilirubin	Not routine Neonatal results more predictive
Arterial blood	Arterial line in aorta (through umbilical or other artery) Arterial puncture (radial or other)	Validate transcutaneous monitoring	Discrepancies when Pa_{O_2} >100 torr, hypoperfusion, vasoactive drugs, edema, thick skin, poor transcutaneous electrode application	Arterial puncture rare. Crying affects results If no arterial line, arterialized capillary blood gas is adequate for most monitoring
Urine	Suprapubic aspirate (gold standard for UTI but invasive) Catheter Clean catch (not very practical at this age) Bag Diaper pad	Investigate urinary tract infection Investigate nephropathy Document intrauterine drug exposure	Culture is diagnostic, especially at <3 months. Test strip positive for nitrites/leukocytes or white blood cells (WBC)/bacteria is a good screen in older infants Catheterize for reliable collection Bag specimens may be pooled until enough volume, in first day of life	Too few studies to evaluate bags or diaper pad specimens Negative dipstick likely excludes infection, but samples are too contaminated to culture False-negative drug screens common (dilute urine, delayed collection, low drug concentration)
GI Samples				
Meconium	From diaper at 1 to 2 days of life	Document intrauterine drug exposure	Detects drugs from last two trimesters of gestation	Not routine Specialized labs only Urine contamination or transition to stool may cause false negatives Clinical need for test should be justified
Gastric, vomitus	Gastric aspirate, clothing	Differentiate maternal (ingested) from fetal blood (Apt test)	Fetal blood is more resistant to alkali denaturation than is maternal blood	Use visual screen for low-volume fresh samples (e.g., clothing) Spectrophotometric method more reliable but needs additional sample
Stool	From diaper	Blood Bilirubin color pH Reducing substance Fat globules	Abnormal: Distinguish maternal from fetal Absence of color is abnormal Lower if breast-fed >2% is normal 50 to 100/low-power field is normal	Stool culture if diarrhea with blood/mucus
Sweat	Pilocarpine iontophoresis	Diagnosis of cystic fibrosis (CF)	Sweat Cl >60 mmol/L is diagnostic	Sweat Cl not accurate before 48 hours of age. Inadequate collection more common in first 2 weeks of life Low birth weight or preterm infants must be big enough for electrodes not to touch
Hair	Instructions from referral laboratory	Document intrauterine drug exposure up to 3 months of age	Drugs incorporated in last trimester of gestation	Not routine Specialized labs only Clinical need for test should be justified
Maternal Samples				
Breast milk	Expressed breast milk (fat increases toward end of feed: Collect one side through a complete feed to simulate infant's intake)	Na, in neonatal hypernatremia Therapeutic drugs or drugs of abuse, to estimate dose to neonate	High Na in colostrum, lower in mature milk Drug concentration varies with time of dose and through each feed	Not routine Delayed transition to mature milk is secondary, not causative Analysis not routine. Consult reference on drugs in lactation (Briggs) instead

Table **45-4** Special Samples for Neonatal Assessment—cont'd

Sample Type	Collection	Clinical Use	Interpretation	Notes
Maternal Samples—cont'd				
Urine	Random urine	Document drug use in pregnancy	Detects drug use in few days before delivery	Easier collection and higher drug levels than newborn urine Intrapartum drugs may cause positive screens
Blood	Maternal blood testing sometimes may be an adjunct to neonatal testing	Confirm presence of a maternal disease that affects the newborn Confirm or investigate an inherited condition that affects the neonate		

the local NBS program. Each NBS laboratory must have the testing capacity to diagnose quickly and guide treatment for potentially life-threatening genetic illnesses that may present in the neonatal period.

Common laboratory presentations of inborn errors of metabolism include neonatal hypoglycemia, jaundice, metabolic acidosis, lactic acidosis, and hyperammonemia. Severe neonatal hyperammonemia (>150 μmol/L) may be caused by a urea cycle disorder, other inborn errors of metabolism, or the rare but severe transient hyperammonemia of the newborn. In each of these conditions, neonatal encephalopathy may arise if prompt treatment is not initiated. Asymptomatic hyperammonemia (40 to 150 μmol/L) is common in preterm neonates and does not require treatment.

KEY CONCEPTS BOX 45-3

- The small blood volume available from the sick newborn and the need for laboratory testing make anemia of prematurity a major concern for the laboratory.
- Practical steps must be taken to minimize collection errors to reduce unnecessary blood loss and harm to the newborn.
- The laboratory must ensure efficient use of precious samples by matching available sample volume with required test volume, prioritizing tests, and prediluting samples to extend the available volume.
- Alternative, rapid-testing modes that require smaller sample volumes include transcutaneous, whole blood, and point-of-care-testing.
- Instruments should be chosen with specifications that allow efficient neonatal testing.
- Neonatologists may require the laboratory to handle a wide variety of nonroutine sample types.

REFERENCES

1. NCCLS. Procedures and Devices for the Collection of Diagnostic Capillary Blood Specimens; Approved Standard-Fifth Edition. NCCLS document H4-A5 [ISBN 1-56238-538-0], 2004.
2. Pediatric reference intervals, ed 5th, Washington, DC, 2005, AACC Press.
3. ACOG Committee Opinion No. 348, November 2006: Umbilical cord blood gas and acid-base analysis, Obstet Gynecol 108:1319, 2006.
4. National Academy of Clinical Biochemistry. Laboratory medicine Practice Guidelines. Maternal-Fetal Risk Assessment and Reference Values in Pregnancy (2006) Section VII. Current Practices and Guidelines for Evaluation of the Newborn Infant, 2006.
5. Al Orifi F, McGillivray D, Tange S, Kramer MS: Urine culture from bag specimens in young children: are the risks too high? J Pediatr 137:221, 2000.
6. Arena J, Emparanza JI, Nogues A, Burls A: Skin to calcaneus distance in the neonate, Arch Dis Child Fetal Neonatal Ed 90: F328, 2005.
7. Arnon S, Litmanovitz I, Regev RH, Bauer S, Shainkin-Kestenbaum R et al: Serum amyloid A: an early and accurate marker of neonatal early-onset sepsis, J Perinatol 27:297, 2007.
8. Baraldi E, Filippone M: Chronic lung disease after premature birth, N Engl J Med 357:1946, 2007.
9. Batton DG, Barrington KJ, Wallman C: Prevention and management of pain in the neonate: an update, Pediatrics 118:2231, 2006.
10. Bhutani VK, Johnson L, Sivieri EM: Predictive ability of a predischarge hour-specific serum bilirubin for subsequent significant hyperbilirubinemia in healthy term and near-term newborns, Pediatrics 103:6, 1999.
11. Borgard JP, Szymanowicz A, Pellae I, Szmidt-Adjide V, Rota M: Determination of total bilirubin in whole blood from neonates: results from a French multicenter study, Clin Chem Lab Med 44:1103, 2006.
12. Brugnara C. , POS: The Neonatal Erythrocyte and its Disorders. In Nathan DG, Orkin SH, Ginsburg D, and Look AT, editors: *Hematology of Infancy and Childhood*, 2003, pp. 38-39.
13. Cornblath M, Ichord R: Hypoglycemia in the neonate, Semin Perinatol 24:136, 2000.
14. Cowett RM, Farrag HM: Selected principles of perinatal-neonatal glucose metabolism, Semin Neonatol 9:37, 2004.
15. Davies MW, Mehr S, Morley CJ: The effect of draw-up volume on the accuracy of electrolyte measurements from neonatal arterial lines, J Paediatr Child Health 36:122, 2000.
16. Dennery PA, Seidman DS, Stevenson DK: Neonatal hyperbilirubinemia, N Engl J Med 344:581, 2001.
17. Flidel-Rimon O, Branski D, Shinwell ES: The fear of necrotizing enterocolitis versus achieving optimal growth in preterm infants–an opinion, Acta Paediatr 95:1341, 2006.

18. Folk LA: Guide to capillary heelstick blood sampling in infants, Adv Neonatal Care 7:171, 2007.
19. Gibson BE, Todd A, Roberts I, Pamphilon D, Rodeck C et al: Transfusion guidelines for neonates and older children, Br J Haematol 124:433, 2004.
20. Gluckman PD, Sizonenko SV, Bassett NS: The transition from fetus to neonate–an endocrine perspective, Acta Paediatr Suppl 88:7, 1999.
21. Gomez P, Coca C, Vargas C, Acebillo J, Martinez A: Normal reference-intervals for 20 biochemical variables in healthy infants, children, and adolescents, Clin Chem 30:407, 1984.
22. Gorelick MH, Shaw KN: Screening tests for urinary tract infection in children: A meta-analysis, Pediatrics 104:e54, 1999.
23. Green A, Kirk J: Guidelines for the performance of the sweat test for the diagnosis of cystic fibrosis, Ann Clin Biochem 44:25, 2007.
24. Hawthorne KM, Griffin IJ, Abrams SA: Current issues in nutritional management of very low birth weight infants, Minerva Pediatr 56:359, 2004.
25. Holtback U, Aperia AC: Molecular determinants of sodium and water balance during early human development, Semin Neonatol 8:291, 2003.
26. Hume R, Burchell A, Williams FL, Koh DK: Glucose homeostasis in the newborn, Early Hum Dev 81:95, 2005.
27. Jackson L, Williams FL, Burchell A, Coughtrie MW, Hume R: Plasma catecholamines and the counterregulatory responses to hypoglycemia in infants: a critical role for epinephrine and cortisol, J Clin Endocrinol Metab 89:6251, 2004.
28. Janes M, Pinelli J, Landry S, Downey S, Paes B: Comparison of capillary blood sampling using an automated incision device with and without warming the heel, J Perinatol 22:154, 2002.
29. Kanakoudi F, Drossou V, Tzimouli V, Diamanti E, Konstantinidis T et al: Serum concentrations of 10 acute-phase proteins in healthy term and preterm infants from birth to age 6 months, Clin Chem 41:605, 1995.
30. Kapur R, Yoder MC, Polin RA: The Immune System: Part 1 Developmental Immunology. In Martine RJ, Fanaroff AA, and Walsh MC, editors: *Neonatal-Perinatal Medicine: Diseases of the Fetus and Infant*, Philadelphia, PA, 2006, Mosby, Elsevier, pp. 761-791.
31. Kist-van Holthe JE, van Zwieten PH, Schell-Feith EA, Zonderland HM, Holscher HC et al: Is nephrocalcinosis in preterm neonates harmful for long-term blood pressure and renal function? Pediatrics 119:468, 2007.
32. Koren G: Therapeutic drug monitoring principles in the neonate. National Academy of CLinical Biochemistry, Clin Chem 43:222, 1997.
33. Liston R, Sawchuck D, Young D: Fetal health surveillance: antepartum and intrapartum consensus guideline, J Obstet Gynaecol Can 29:S3, 2007.
34. Liu N, Wu AH, Wong SS: Improved quantitative Apt test for detecting fetal hemoglobin in bloody stools of newborns, Clin Chem 39:2326, 1993.
35. Lockitch G, Halstead AC, Albersheim S, MacCallum C, Quigley G: Age- and sex-specific pediatric reference intervals for biochemistry analytes as measured with the Ektachem-700 analyzer, Clin Chem 34:1622, 1988.
36. Lockitch G, Halstead AC, Wadsworth L, Quigley G, Reston L et al: Age- and sex-specific pediatric reference intervals and correlations for zinc, copper, selenium, iron, vitamins A and E, and related proteins, Clin Chem 34:1625, 1988.
37. Modi N: Clinical implications of postnatal alterations in body water distribution, Semin Neonatol 8:301, 2003.
38. Mori R, Lakhanpaul M, Verrier-Jones K: Diagnosis and management of urinary tract infection in children: summary of NICE guidance, BMJ 335:395, 25-8-2007.
39. Murray NA, Roberts IA: Haemolytic disease of the newborn, Arch Dis Child Fetal Neonatal Ed 92:F83, 2007.
40. Nash PL: Potassum and sodium homeostasis in the neonate, Neonatal Netw 26:125, 2007.
41. NCCLS, NCCLS et al: Sweat Testing: Sample Collection and Quantitative Analysis; Approved Guideline, C34-A2, Vol. 20 No. 14:2000.
42. Neu J: Gastrointestinal maturation and implications for infant feeding, Early Hum Dev 83:767, 2007.
43. Ng PC, Lam HS: Diagnostic markers for neonatal sepsis, Curr Opin Pediatr 18:125, 2006.
44. Ohlsson A, Aher SM: Early erythropoietin for preventing red blood cell transfusion in preterm and/or low birth weight infants. Cochrane. Database, Syst Rev 3:CD004863, 2006.
45. Peake M, Mazzachi B, Fudge A, Bais R: Bilirubin measured on a blood gas analyser: a suitable alternative for near-patient assessment of neonatal jaundice? Ann Clin Biochem 38:533, 2001.
46. Pesce AJ, Rashkin M, Kotagal U: Standards of laboratory practice: theophylline and caffeine monitoring. National Academy of Clinical Biochemistry, Clin Chem 44:1124, 1998.
47. Peters CJ, Hindmarsh PC: Management of neonatal endocrinopathies–best practice guidelines, Early Hum Dev 83:553, 2007.
48. Puckett RM, Offringa M: Prophylactic vitamin K for vitamin K deficiency bleeding in neonates. Cochrane Database Syst Rev CD002776, 2000.
49. Rolinski B, Okorodudu AO, Kost G: Evaluation of total bilirubin determination in neonatal whole-blood samples by multiwavelength photometry on the Roche OMNI S Point-of-care analyzer. Point of Care: the Journal of Near Patient Testing and Technology 4:3, 2005.
50. Saunders NR, Habgood MD, Dziegielewska KM: Barrier mechanisms in the brain, II. Immature brain, Clin Exp Pharmacol Physiol 26:85, 1999.
51. Schmidt B, Roberts RS, Davis P, Doyle LW, Barrington KJ et al: Long-term effects of caffeine therapy for apnea of prematurity, N Engl J Med 357:1893, 2007.
52. Schreiber RA, Barker CC, Roberts EA, Martin SR, Alvarez F et al: Biliary atresia: the Canadian experience, J Pediatr 151:659, 2007.
53. Smith VC, Zupancic JA, McCormick MC, Croen LA, Greene J et al: Trends in severe bronchopulmonary dysplasia rates between 1994 and 2002, J Pediatr 146:469, 2005.
54. Stoll BJ: The Fetus and the Neonatal Infant;Infections of the Newborn Infant. In Kliegman R, Behrman R, Jenson H, and Stanton, B. , editors: *Nelson Textbook of Pediatrics*, St Louis, MO, 2004, WB Saunders, Elsevier, pp. 623-640.
55. Vemgal P, Ohlsson A: Interventions for non-oliguric hyperkalaemia in preterm neonates. Cochrane Database Syst Rev CD005257, 2007.
56. Whiting P, Westwood M, Watt I, Cooper J, Kleijnen J: Rapid tests and urine sampling techniques for the diagnosis of urinary tract infection (UTI) in children under five years: a systematic review, BMC Pediatr 5:4, 2005.

INTERNET SI10TE

http://bilitool.org

Extravascular Biological Fluids

Lewis Glasser

Chapter 46

Chapter Outline

Serous Fluids
Formation
Change of Analyte in Disease
Synovial Fluid (Synovia)
Normal Synovial Fluid
Change of Analyte in Disease
Other Body Fluids

Key Terms

arthritis Inflammation of a joint.
ascites Pathological accumulation of serous fluid within the peritoneal cavity.
chyle Fatty lymph fluid that originates from the intestinal lymphatics. Chyle is milky white in appearance.
colloid osmotic pressure The difference in osmotic pressure between plasma and interstitial fluid that drives water into the bloodstream from the interstitial spaces.
effusion Pathological accumulation of fluid within a body cavity.
empyema The presence of pus in a body cavity, usually the pleural cavity.
epicardium The visceral layer of pericardium.
exudate A fluid with a high concentration of protein that accumulates within a body cavity when capillary permeability is increased.
gout An inflammatory arthritis of the joint secondary to crystallization of monosodium urate in the joint.
hemothorax Blood in the pleural cavity secondary to rupture of the blood vessels.
hyaluronic acid A high-molecular-weight polymer made up of repeating units of the disaccharide N-acetylglucosamine and glucuronic acid.
hydrostatic pressure The lateral pressure of water within a blood vessel that tends to drive fluid out of the capillaries into the interstitial space.
joint An articulation between bones.
neuroarthropathy Disease of a joint secondary to a disease of the nervous system.
osmotic pressure The force with which a solvent passes through a semipermeable membrane.
osteoarthritis A degenerative form of arthritis that is primarily a disease of the bones with joint involvement.
osteochondromatosis A joint disease characterized by the development of cartilaginous nodules within the synovial tissues.
paracentesis Aspiration of fluid from a body space.
parietal membrane The lining covering the wall of a cavity.
pericardium The sac that encloses the heart.
peritoneum The serous membrane that lines the abdominal cavity and the organs of the abdominal cavity.
peritonitis An inflammation of the peritoneum.
permeability Condition that allows the passage of fluid through a membrane.
pigmented villonodular synovitis A disease of the joints of unknown cause; it is characterized by fingerlike proliferative growths of the synovial tissue with hemosiderin deposition within the synovial tissue.
pleura The serous membrane that lines the inner surface of the thorax, the diaphragm, and the outer surface of the lungs.
pseudogout An inflammatory arthritis of the joint secondary to crystals of calcium pyrophosphate.
psoriatic arthritis A chronic destructive joint disease that occurs in some patients with skin disease psoriasis.
Reiter's syndrome A syndrome of unknown cause that is characterized by inflammation of the joints, urethra, skin, and conjunctivae.
rheumatoid arthritis A chronic progressive inflammatory disease of unknown cause that involves multiple joints.
serous fluid Fluid that has the characteristics of serum.
synovial fluid Joint fluid.
systemic lupus erythematosus (SLE) A multisystem disease that is caused by an autoimmune reaction and most often involves the skin, kidneys, joints, and serosal membranes.
thoracentesis Removal of fluid from the pleural cavity.
transudate Fluid with a low concentration of protein that has accumulated within a body cavity.
visceral membrane The outer wall of an organ.

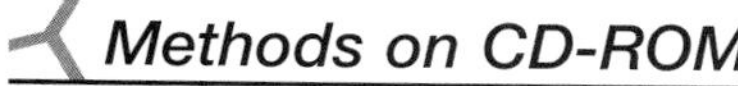

Methods on CD-ROM

Albumin
Alkaline phosphatase

Amylase
C-reactive protein (CRP)
Carcinoembryonic antigen (CEA)
Complement (C_3 and C_4)
Creatinine
Glucose
Lactate dehydrogenase and lactate dehydrogenase enzymes
Osmolality
Total serum protein
Triglycerides
Urea

SECTION OBJECTIVES BOX 46-1

- Define serous fluid and name some serous fluids.
- Describe the formation of serous fluids.

SEROUS FLUIDS

In this chapter, use of the term *serous fluids* is restricted to pleural, pericardial, or peritoneal fluid. The word *serous,* which is derived from serum, accurately expresses the derivation of body fluids from plasma. Body fluids are designated by a variety of medical terms. Pleural fluid (thoracic or chest fluid) is obtained by surgical puncture of the chest wall (**thoracentesis.**) **Empyema** refers to pus in the pleural cavity. Peritoneal fluid frequently is designated by the nonanatomical term "ascitic fluid." **Ascites** is derived from the Greek word *askos* (which means "wineskin, belly") and describes the bloated abdomen of the patient afflicted with a massive accumulation of peritoneal fluid. **Paracentesis** is aspiration of fluid from a cavity, and abdominal paracentesis fluid is synonymous with peritoneal fluid. Whole blood in the body cavities is designated with the prefix hemo-, as in **hemothorax.** A chylous effusion refers to the accumulation of lymph (chyle) within the body cavity.

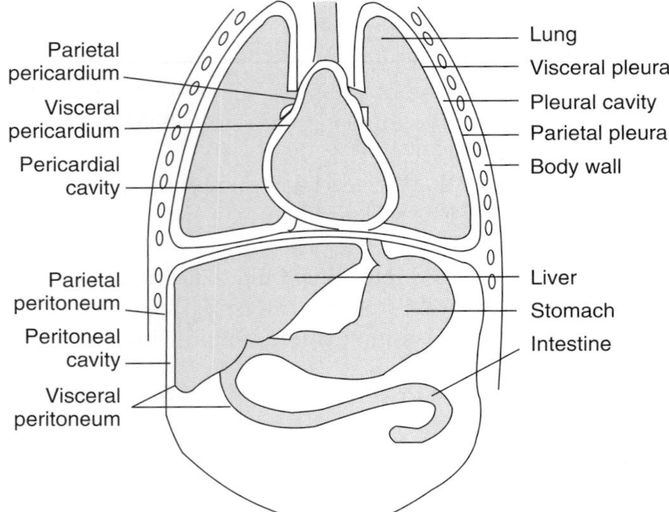

Fig. 46-1 Relationships of serous membranes, body cavities, and viscera. The heart is enclosed within the pericardial sac. The outer layer of **pericardium** is called the *parietal pericardium.* Lining the exterior surface of the heart is the visceral pericardium, which also is called the **epicardium.** Parietal peritoneum lines the wall of the abdominal cavity. Visceral peritoneum invests stomach, liver, and intestines. The peritoneal cavity is the space between the two layers of peritoneum.

Formation

Normal Formation

Each body cavity is lined by a thin serosal membrane. The lining of the body wall is the **parietal membrane,** and the outer lining of the organs is the **visceral membrane.** The two membranes, which together form the serosal membrane, are continuous, and the space between them is the body cavity (Fig. 46-1). The serosal membrane is composed of a thin layer of connective tissue that contains numerous capillaries and lymphatics and a superficial layer of flattened mesothelial cells.

Serous fluid is an ultrafiltrate of plasma derived from the rich capillary network in the serosal membrane. Its formation is similar to the production of extravascular interstitial fluid anywhere in the body. Three factors are important: hydrostatic pressure, colloid **osmotic pressure,** and capillary **permeability. Hydrostatic pressure** (HP) drives a protein-free filtrate out of the capillaries and into the body cavities. Impermeable protein molecules remaining in the plasma exert a force that counteracts the hydrostatic pressure and causes fluid to flow back into the capillaries. This force is called the *colloid osmotic pressure* (COP) and is proportional to the molar concentration of protein. Lymphatics also play an important role in the absorption of water, protein, and particulate matter from the extravascular space.

In the thoracic (chest) cavity, fluid is formed at the parietal **pleura** because the high hydrostatic pressure of the systemic circulation exceeds the colloid osmotic pressure. This fluid is reabsorbed at the visceral pleura because the capillary colloid osmotic pressure exceeds the low hydrostatic pressure of the pulmonary circulation (Fig. 46-2). Normally, less than 15 mL of fluid is found in each pleural cavity, 10 to 50 mL in the pericardial sac, and less than 50 mL in the peritoneal cavity.[1]

Abnormal Formation

Effusions, abnormal accumulations of serosal fluid, will form when the normal physiological mechanisms responsible for

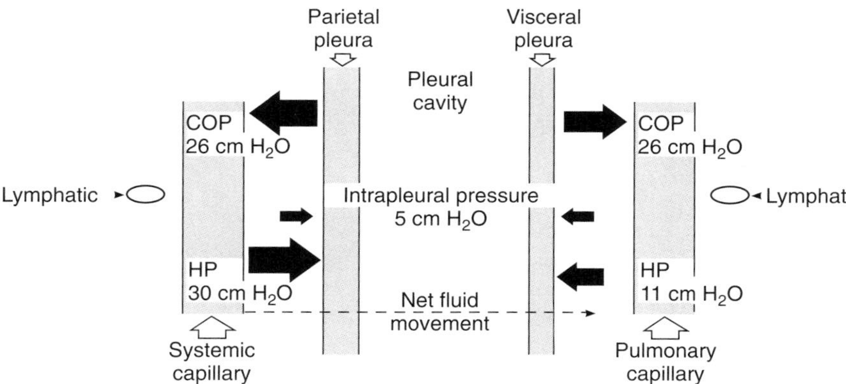

Fig. 46-2 Pleural fluid is formed at the parietal pleura because net forces for flow of fluid out of the systemic capillaries exceed net colloid osmotic pressures. Fluid moves toward the visceral pleura, where net colloid osmotic pressure exceeds outward forces because of low hydrostatic pressure in pulmonary capillaries. Lymphatics play a role in absorption of water, protein, and particulate matter. *COP,* Colloid osmotic pressure; *HP,* hydrostatic pressure.

the formation or absorption of serosal fluid are impaired. Thus, fluid will accumulate if capillary permeability increases, hydrostatic pressure increases, colloid osmotic pressure decreases, or lymphatic drainage is obstructed; in each case, the normal balance between fluid accumulation (HP) and fluid removal (COP and lymphatic drainage) is disrupted. Hydrostatic pressure is increased in congestive heart failure, a frequent cause of effusions. Hypoproteinemia decreases the colloid osmotic pressure. Decreased plasma protein can occur secondary to decreased synthesis or increased loss of protein. Albumin, which is synthesized in the liver, is the most important protein in the maintenance of colloid osmotic pressure. Diseases of the liver or severe malnutrition may result in decreased albumin synthesis; the liver disease most frequently associated with hypoproteinemia and effusions is cirrhosis. Hypoalbuminemia also is caused by an increased loss of serum protein, which occurs in the nephrotic syndrome. Capillary permeability increases if the pleural surfaces are inflamed. Increased capillary permeability also results in loss of protein from the vascular space, so the physical forces that lead to excessive fluid formation are accentuated. Conditions that cause an increase in capillary permeability include inflammatory disease, infection, and metastatic tumor. If the lymphatics are obstructed, a protein-rich fluid will accumulate. Neoplasms of the lymph nodes frequently produce pleural effusions. The causes of effusions and their underlying pathogeneses are listed in Table 46-1.

KEY CONCEPTS BOX 46-1

- **Serous fluids** are serum-derived fluids that accumulate in body cavities.
- **Pleural fluid** is found in the chest cavity, peritoneal fluid is formed in the abdomen, and synovial fluid is formed in joints.
- **Serous fluids** form when HP forces protein-free fluid out of capillaries. The amount is kept small by COP, causing fluid to return to the capillaries and to the lymphatic system, which drains excess fluid.
- **Abnormal** formation of serous fluids, *effusions,* results with one or more of the following forces: increased HP, decreased COP, increased capillary permeability, or a blocked lymphatic system.

Table 46-1 Causes of Effusions

Cause	Finding	Pathogenesis
Transudates		
Congestive heart failure	↑ HP	Systemic and pulmonary venous hypertension
Hepatic cirrhosis	↑ HP	Portal and inferior vena cava hypertension
	↓ COP	Hypoalbuminemia
Nephrotic syndrome	↓ COP	Hypoalbuminemia
Exudates		
Pancreatitis	↑ CP	Inflammation caused by chemical injury
Bile peritonitis	↑ CP	Inflammation caused by chemical injury
Rheumatoid disease	↑ CP	Inflammation of serosa
Systemic lupus erythematosus	↑ CP	Inflammation of serosa
Infection (bacterial, tuberculosis, fungal, viral)	↑ CP	Inflammation caused by microorganisms
Infarction (myocardial, pulmonary)	↑ CP	Inflammation caused by extension of the process to the serosal surface
Neoplasms	↑ CP	Increased permeability of capillaries that supply tumor implants; pleuritis related to obstructive pneumonitis
	↓ LyD	Lymphatic obstruction secondary to lymph node infiltration
Chyle		
Trauma Surgery Neoplasms Idiopathic	↓ LyD	Disruption of lymphatic ducts

COP, Colloid osmotic pressure; *CP,* capillary permeability; *HP,* hydrostatic pressure; *LyD,* lymphatic drainage.

SECTION OBJECTIVES BOX 46-2

- Differentiate transudate and exudate on the basis of the following:
  - Mode of formation
  - Protein, enzyme, and glucose levels
- List analytes of transudate and exudate that may be markers of disease conditions.
- List analytes found in serous fluids that can serve as markers for diseases of organs.

Change of Analyte in Disease

Transudates and Exudates

Serous effusions are designated as **transudates** or **exudates,** depending on the protein content of the fluid. This distinction is important because transudates are not caused by inflammation, but by disturbances in hydrostatic or colloid osmotic pressure, whereas exudates are caused by increased capillary permeability related to diseases that directly involve inflammation of the surfaces of body cavities.

Distinguishing between transudates and exudates involves the use of arbitrary medical decision levels that have been determined empirically. The higher the protein content, the more likely it is that the fluid is caused by a process that alters capillary permeability and involves disturbances to surfaces of the body cavity. Measuring the specific gravity will indirectly measure the protein concentration. Pleural fluids are classified as exudates if the specific gravity is greater than 1.015 g/mL, or the total protein is 3 g/dL or greater. Measurement of total protein is preferable to measurement of specific gravity. The distinction between exudates and transudates in pleural fluids is even more precise if the fluid protein is compared with the serum total protein. A ratio is calculated by dividing the concentration of the protein in the fluid by the concentration of the protein in serum; a ratio of 0.5 or greater is indicative of an exudate.[2] This distinction is improved if a large protein molecule such as lactate dehydrogenase (LD) is used as a marker of capillary permeability. Pleural fluid-to-serum LD ratios of 0.6 or greater are diagnostic of exudates.[2] The differences between transudates and exudates in pleural effusions are summarized in Table 46-2.

Different cutoff values are used for abdominal (peritoneal) fluid. Protein levels greater than 2.5 g/dL classify the fluid as an exudate.[1] Determining the difference between serum and peritoneal fluid albumin concentrations allows significantly better discrimination between transudative and exudative ascites than does use of total protein levels; differences less than 1.1 g/dL correlate with malignant effusions.[3,4]

Table 46-2 Diagnostic Criteria for Transudates and Exudates in Pleural Fluid

Test	Transudate	Exudate
Appearance	Clear	Cloudy
Fibrinogen	No clot	Clots
Specific gravity	<1.015	≥1.015
Total protein	<3 g/dL	≥3 g/dL
Total protein (fluid/serum)	<0.5	≥0.5
Lactate dehydrogenase (fluid/serum)	<0.6	≥0.6
Glucose	≈Serum	Often <60 mg/dL

Glucose

Pleural fluid glucose concentrations are similar to plasma glucose levels in normal fluids and transudates. Glucose is decreased in exudates, and a pleural fluid glucose concentration of less than 60 mg/dL, or a difference between plasma and fluid glucose concentrations of greater than 30 mg/dL, is clinically significant. Low fluid glucose levels are seen with bacterial infection, tuberculosis, neoplasia, and rheumatoid disease.[5,6] Only low glucose levels are diagnostically useful, and the various diseases associated with low glucose levels are also associated with normal values. Any etiological diagnosis that is based on a low glucose level alone is unreliable. Two mechanisms are operative in producing low values. One is increased glucose consumption by microorganisms or cells in the fluid, and the second is a relative block in the transport of glucose from blood to the fluid. The latter occurs with rheumatoid effusions.[7] Interpretation of low glucose concentrations in peritoneal and pericardial fluid is similar to that in pleural fluid.

pH

Measurement of pleural fluid pH is clinically useful in the management of patients with pneumonia who develop pleural effusions, because the infectious process extends to the visceral pleura, causing an exudate to form in the pleural space. Complications of these exudates include formation of pus in the pleural cavity. Fluids are divided into potentially benign and complicated exudates on the basis of pH. Fluids with a pH greater than 7.30 resolve spontaneously, whereas a pH lower than 7.20 indicates the need for tube drainage.[8] A cautionary note: The specimen must be collected anaerobically in a heparinized syringe, stored on ice, and measured at 37°C. A significant relationship exists between pleural fluid pH and glucose concentration.[9]

Lipid

Chyle is a milky white emulsion of fatty lymph fluid that originates from the intestinal lymphatics. The accumulation of chyle in the pleural space is rare. Even less frequent is chyle accumulation in the peritoneal or pericardial cavity. Chylous fluid accumulates as the result of blockage of the thoracic duct. Chylomicrons found on lipoprotein analysis provide the best evidence for a chylous effusion. Triglyceride values above 110 mg/dL for a milky fluid are highly suggestive of chylous effusion.[10] Cholesterol values do not distinguish between chylous and nonchylous effusions.

Box 46-1

Laboratory Analysis of a Pleural Fluid

- Cell count with differential
- Total protein level
- Glucose level
- Lactate dehydrogenase (LD) level
- Amylase level
- pH
- Cytological analysis (especially for patients with history of undiagnosed exudative effusions, suspected malignancy, or *Pneumocystis carinii* infection, or exudative effusions with normal fluid glucose and amylase levels)
- In the appropriate clinical setting, the following may be helpful: gram staining, acid-fast bacilli staining, fungal (KOH) staining, and culture and sensitivity testing for aerobic and anaerobic organisms and fungi
- Blood culturing (two tests, preferably from different sites and one-half hour apart)
- Determination of serum total protein, glucose, LDH, and amylase levels; determination of arterial pH (especially if acidemia is suspected)

From Abrahemian FM: Pleural Effusion. Available at http://www.emedicine.com/emerg/topic462.htm. Accessed June 2005.

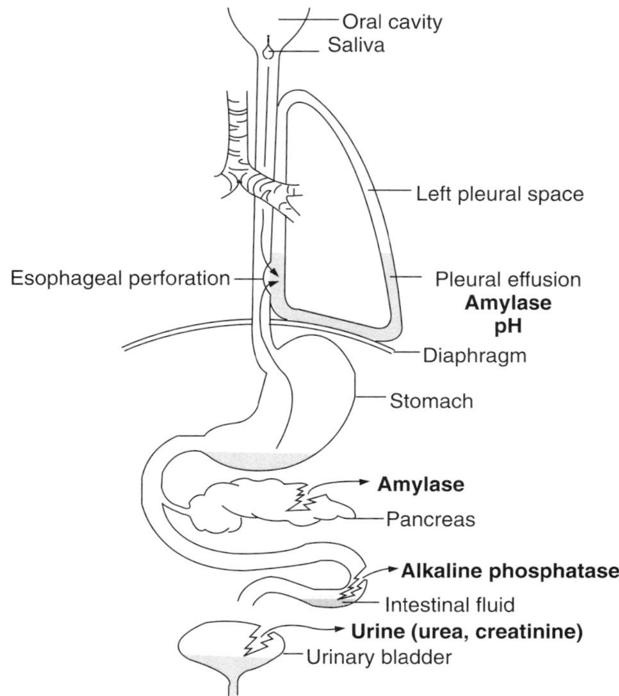

Fig. 46-3 Chemical determinations of body fluids as markers for specific organ involvement.

A complete laboratory workup suggested for pleural effusions is listed in Box 46-1.

Analytes as Markers for Organs and Disease

Chemical substances can serve as markers for the specific organ involved in the pathogenesis of the effusion. The rationale for these tests is easily understood when one considers the anatomical location of the viscera and normal biochemistry (Fig. 46-3). Analytes that have been used as markers include amylase, lipase, pH, alkaline phosphatase, urea nitrogen, and creatinine. Pleural effusions accompany most cases of esophageal rupture. The perforation allows secretions from both the oral cavity and the stomach to contaminate the effusion fluid. Pleural fluid amylase levels can be elevated to higher than the serum amylase, and electrophoretic studies indicate that amylase is derived from the saliva.[11] Another indicator of esophageal perforation is the pH of the pleural fluid. Normal gastric juice has a pH below 3.5. Leakage of gastric contents through the esophageal tear acidifies the pleural fluid.[12,13] A pH below 6.0 is clinically significant. This measurement may be taken at the bedside with the use of pH reagent paper.

Amylase and lipase are well-accepted markers of pancreatic disease. In acute pancreatitis, amylase and lipase-rich fluid seep into the tissue surrounding the pancreas, causing a chemical **peritonitis** and, in most cases, the formation of small amounts of peritoneal fluid. One study reports fluid amylase levels of 27,800 ± 7560 U/L.[14] Fluid amylase levels are higher and persist longer than corresponding blood amylase levels.[15] Pancreatic *ascites* is the chronic accumulation of massive amounts of fluid in association with pancreatitis. It is not certain whether this fluid represents leakage of pancreatic secretions from ruptured ducts or exudation of fluid from serosal surfaces secondary to chemical irritation.[16] In pancreatic ascites, peritoneal fluid amylase concentrations range from 680 to 129,500 U/L.[17] Pleural effusions are present in 15% of cases of pancreatitis. Increased amylase levels in pleural effusions are caused by transdiaphragmatic lymphatic drainage or seepage of the enzyme across the diaphragm.[17] In rare cases, pleural fluid is present as the result of direct communication between the pleural and peritoneal cavities.[18] Elevated lipase and amylase levels in the peritoneal dialysis fluid of patients undergoing peritoneal dialysis have been shown to be useful in differentiating between acute pancreatitis and pancreatic infection.[19,20]

Alkaline phosphatase has been shown to be a marker enzyme for pathological processes of the small intestine. The source of this enzyme can be leakage of alkaline phosphatase–rich fluid from the intestinal contents or from the wall of the intestine.[21] The enzyme is elevated in peritoneal serous effusions in association with intestinal perforation and infarction of the small bowel, and in peritoneal blood in patients with physically induced injury of the small intestine.[22] These values are higher than corresponding peripheral blood levels.

Both urea nitrogen and creatinine are helpful in the differential diagnosis of a ruptured urinary bladder after abdominal trauma. Leaked urine will have high levels of both urea nitrogen and creatinine. The former is freely diffusible and will elevate the blood urea nitrogen; however, the **peritoneum** is relatively impermeable to creatinine, and blood levels of creatinine will not increase. In uncomplicated serous effusions, the fluid urea nitrogen and creatinine are low. If the physician inadvertently aspirates urine from the bladder, both urea nitrogen and creatinine will be high, but their concentrations in the blood will be within the reference interval. Urinothorax, defined as urine in the pleural space, has been described in patients with urinary tract obstruction and acute pyelonephritis.[23] Pleural effusions in these cases exhibited elevated creatinine.

KEY CONCEPTS BOX 46-2

- **Transudates** are caused by increased leakage *(increased hydrostatic pressure)* or decreased fluid return into capillaries *(decreased colloid osmotic pressure).*
- **Exudates** are caused by *increased capillary permeability*, which results from inflammatory processes that allow plasma to leak out of capillaries.
- **Appearance,** fibrinogen, specific gravity, total protein, total protein ratio (fluid/serum), lactate dehydrogenase ratio (fluid/serum), and glucose are useful measures for differentiating between exudates and transudates (see Table 46-2).
- **Analytes** that have been used as markers for organ disease include amylase and lipase (slivary glands and pancreas), pH (stomach), alkaline phosphatase (intestines), and urea nitrogen and creatinine (kidney and bladder).

SECTION OBJECTIVES BOX 46-3

- Briefly describe the structure of joints.
- List the major proteins and carbohydrates that constitute normal synovial fluid.
- List the most useful analytes of synovial fluid when assessing the disease state of joints.

SYNOVIAL FLUID (SYNOVIA)

Joints are articulations between bones. Freely movable joints are composed of hyaline articular cartilage and a fibrous capsule that is lined on its inner surface by a membrane (Fig. 46-4). **Synovial fluid** fills the joint cavity and acts as a lubricant, to minimize the friction between bones during movement or weight bearing. This fluid also provides the sole nutrition for cartilage. Synovial fluid enters the cartilage by diffusion and through a spongelike effect when the cartilage is compressed and relaxed. The term *synovia,* coined by Paracelsus, is derived from the Greek *syn* ("with"), along with *oon* (from the Latin *ovum,* meaning "egg") and *-ia* (probably "condition"), suggesting the fluid's resemblance to raw egg white.

Synovial fluid is a dialysate of plasma that is mixed with **hyaluronic acid.** Ultrafiltration by the rich vascular network in the synovial tissue produces this fluid, whereas hyaluronic acid, a mucoprotein, is secreted into the dialysate by synovial cells.

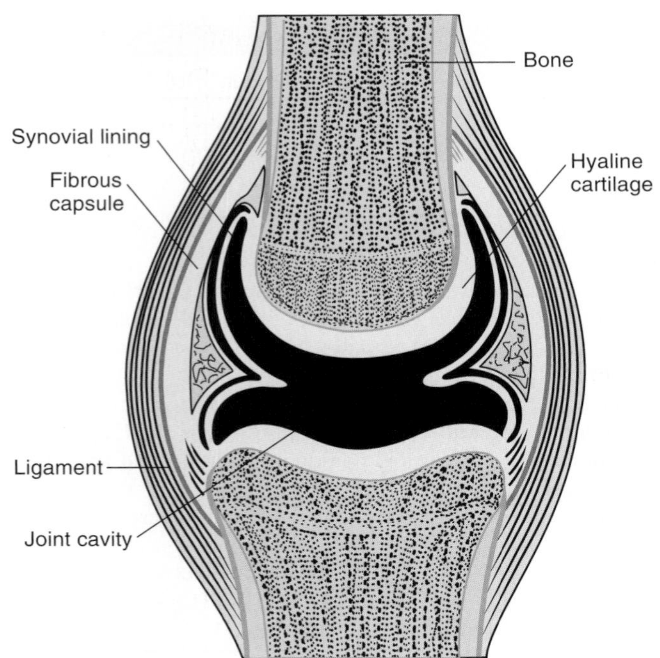

Fig. 46-4 Diagram of normal synovial joint. (From Beck EW: *Mosby's Atlas of Functional Human Anatomy,* St Louis, 1982, Mosby. Courtesy of Ernest Beck.)

Normal Synovial Fluid

The fluid volume in the normal joint depends on the size of the structure. The knee joint usually contains 0.1 to 3.5 mL of fluid.[24] Normal synovial fluid is clear or pale yellow with a specific gravity close to that of plasma. The viscosity is high relative to that of water because of protein complexes with the polysaccharide, hyaluronic acid; these complexes constitute 99% of the mucoproteins present in the fluid. *Hyaluronic acid,* a long-chain, high-molecular-weight polymer made up of repeating units of acetylglucosamine and glucuronic acid, is destroyed in inflammatory states by hyaluronidase, an enzyme that is contained in neutrophils. When this occurs, fluid viscosity decreases significantly, giving the clinician a bedside test for the presence of inflammatory fluid.

Synovial protein concentrations are related to the molecular weight of each protein because of the molecular sieving effect in the synovia. Thus, albumin is present in relatively higher concentrations than are the higher-molecular-weight globulins. Fibrinogen is not present because of its high molecular weight, so normal synovium does not coagulate. Glucose and uric acid diffuse freely into the synovia, and in the fasting state are as concentrated in synovia as in plasma.

The characteristics of normal synovia are summarized in Table 46-3.[25-28]

Change of Analyte in Disease

Physical and chemical changes that occur in the synovia during disease reflect basic pathological processes that occur in the joint. A pathological classification of synovial fluids and the diseases associated with each category are summarized in Table 46-4. The laboratory tests discussed in this section include viscosity, fibrinogen, total protein, complement, glucose, uric acid, and the number and composition of white blood cells, as well as the percentage of neutrophils. In addition, crystal indentification and microbiological tests (gram stain and culture) are needed to complete examination of the fluid.

Clinically, there is no need for a sophisticated measurement of viscosity. Instead, this may be measured at the time of aspiration by placing a finger at the tip of the syringe and stringing out the fluid. Noninflammatory fluids will "string out" longer than 4 cm. An alternative method is to drip fluid off the needle and syringe and observe it. Generally, if the fluid strings, it is a noninflammatory fluid; if it drips similar to water, the fluid is the result of inflammation. The depolymerization of hyaluronic acid by neutrophil hyaluronidase decreases the viscosity in inflammatory disease.

Table 46-3 Physical and Chemical Characteristics of Normal Synovia

	Mean	Range
Volume, mL*	1.1	0.13 to 3.5
Relative viscosity at 38°C	235	5.7 to 1160
Hyaluronic acid, g/L	3600	1700 to 4050
Total protein, g/dL	1.7	1.0 to 2.1
Immunoglobulins, mg/dL		
IgG	453	33 to 850
IgA	74	27 to 177
IgM	37	0 to 84
Fibrinogen, mg/L	0	0
Complement, CH_{50} U/mL	20†	16 to 25
Glucose, mg/dL	‡	65 to 120
Uric acid, mg/dL	‡	2.5 to 7.2

Ig, Immunoglobulin. *CH_{50},* total (hemolytic) complement.
*Knee.
†Values are approximately 10% of plasma values.
‡Fasting values are similar to plasma values.

Normal synovia contain no fibrinogen, but because inflammatory synovitis permits the passage of high-molecular-weight proteins into the fluid, fibrinogen can be present, and spontaneous clotting can occur; clot size is roughly proportionate to the degree of inflammation. Thus anticoagulants are necessary when specimens are collected for microscopic and bacteriological examination.

In synovia, unlike in serous fluids, total protein concentration is *not* used to distinguish noninflammatory from inflammatory fluids, because the leukocyte count is used to make that distinction. Thus, total protein is not included in the routine examination of synovial fluids; however, its measurement can be helpful for interpreting complement levels.[29]

Complement proteins usually are present at lower concentrations in synovial fluid than in serum. In systemic inflammatory conditions, complement behaves as an acute-phase reactant, and hypercomplementemia occurs. In some conditions, such as Reiter's disease, the joint fluid complement concentration has been reported to be even higher than that of serum.

In systemic immune complex diseases such as **systemic lupus erythematosus (SLE),** complement is consumed widely and can be low in both serum and synovial fluid. In other diseases, such as rheumatoid **arthritis** and viral synovitis, complement is consumed locally in the synovia, whereas serum levels are usually normal or high. In rheumatoid arthritis, synovial fluid complement levels generally are low, and many types of immunoglobulins are present.[30] The proper approach to interpreting complement levels in synovia is controversial. For practical purposes, compare synovia versus serum complement levels, and consider synovium complement low if it is less than 30% of serum levels. However, in SLE and other severe immune complex diseases, both levels may be low. In such a situation, one can compare synovium and serum complement levels versus total protein in each fluid.

Interpretation of synovial glucose levels requires knowledge of the patient's simultaneous serum glucose. This is done

Table 46-4 Pathological Classification of Synovial Fluids

Test	Noninflammatory	Inflammatory	Septic	Hemorrhagic
Volume, mL	>3.5	>3.5	>3.5	>3.5
Color	Yellow	Yellow-white	Yellow-green	Red-brown
Viscosity	High	Low	Low	Low
Leukocytes, cells/μL	200 to 2000	2000 to 100,000	10,000 to >100,000	>500
Neutrophils, %	<25	>50	>75	>25
Glucose, mg/dL	≈Serum	>25 mg/dL lower than serum	>40 mg/dL lower than serum	≈Serum
Culture	Negative	Negative	Positive	Negative
Diseases	Osteoarthritis	Gout	Bacterial infection	Hemophilia
	Osteochondritis dissecans	Pseudogout	Fungal infection	Trauma
	Osteochondromatosis	Psoriatic arthritis	Tuberculous infection	Pigmented villonodular synovitis
	Traumatic arthritis	Reiter's syndrome		
	Neuroarthropathy	Rheumatoid arthritis		
		Systemic lupus erythematosus		

Table 46-5 Genetic Changes With Disease

Disease	Gene	Protein	Gene Locus
Gout, HPRT-related	HPRT	Enzyme	Xq26-q27.2
Rheumatoid arthritis; RA*	Multiple		multiple, see 21q22.3
Rheumatoid arthritis, systemic juvenile*	Macrophage migration inhibitory factor	Cytokine	22q11.2
Psoriatic arthritis, susceptibility*	Multiple		16q12
Reiter's syndrome	HLA B27	Surface protein	6p21.3

*Disease has more than one associated genetic foci.

best in the fasting state, but such preparation is not always clinically feasible. In the ideal situation, after an 8-hour fast, the difference between serum and synovia is less than 10 mg/dL; levels 25 mg/dL or more below the serum level are suggestive of inflammation, and differences greater than 40 mg/dL are suggestive of sepsis. In the nonfasting state, synovial glucose levels that are less than half of serum levels should definitely arouse suspicion of a septic process. Rarely, such findings are noted in rheumatoid arthritis effusions.

Serum uric acid levels are important in the diagnosis of **gout.** The synovial fluid uric acid concentration is similar to that of serum, and measurement of uric acid in synovial fluid is of no diagnostic value[31]; however, formation of monosodium urate crystals and their identification by polarized light microscopy in synovia are central to the diagnosis of gouty arthritis.

Rheumatoid arthritis (RA) is a chronic disorder that affects approximately 2.1 million Americans. Several laboratory tests on serum, including erythrocyte sedimentation rate (ESR), C-reactive protein (CRP), rheumatoid factor (RF), and antinuclear antibodies (ANA), may be used to make a diagnosis of RA. Although most of these serum tests are nonspecific for rheumatoid arthritis, the RF assay is positive in about 70% to 90% of patients with this disease; RF can be positive in patients with other types of autoantibody disease, such as Sjögren's syndrome. A genetic susceptibility to this disease and to other diseases of joints has been noted; these are listed in Table 46-5.

KEY CONCEPTS BOX 46-3

- **Synovial** fluid fills the space between two bones and serves to "cushion" bone contact.
- Synovial fluid is an ultrafiltrate of serum that contains large amounts of *hyaluronic acid,* a long-chain, high-molecular-weight polymer.
- **Fibrinogen,** viscosity, complement, glucose, uric acid, the number and composition of white blood cells, and rheumatoid factor are useful laboratory tests for investigating abnormal synovial fluid.
- **Decreased viscosity,** the presence of clots, and an increased number of neutrophils are associated with inflammatory joint disease.
- **RF** increases in serum are associated with *rheumatoid arthritis.*
- **Gout** is best diagnosed by the presence of uric acid crystals in joint fluid.

OTHER BODY FLUIDS

The laboratory may be called on to examine a number of other body fluids, including cerebrospinal fluid (CSF; see Chapter 47), amniotic fluid (see Chapter 44), ocular fluid,[32] tears,[33] and cystic fluid.[34] The examination may be ordered for a current or postmortem diagnostic problem, and it may require extending the analytical boundary beyond that defined by current analytical procedures. For example, pancreatic cysts can indicate a large number of possible diseases, including inflammatory pseudocysts, benign serous tumors, and mucinous neoplasms; some of these are relatively benign, and others are malignant. The tumor marker carcinoembryonic antigen (CEA; see Chapter 53), normally performed only in serum, has been shown to be useful in helping to differentiate between malignant and non-malignant cysts.[34]

REFERENCES

1. Smith GP, Kjeldsberg CR: Cerebrospinal fluid, synovial and serous body fluids. In McPherson RA, Pincus MR, editors: *Henry's Clinical Diagnosis and Management by Laboratory Methods,* ed 21, Philadelphia, 2006, Saunders.
2. Light RW: Clinical practice: pleural effusion, N Engl J Med 346:1971, 2002.
3. Pare P, Talbot J, Hoefs JC: Serum-ascites albumin concentration gradient: a physiologic approach to the differential diagnosis of ascites, Gastroenterology 85:240, 1983.
4. Rector WG Jr, Reynolds TB: Superiority of the serum-ascites albumin difference over the ascites total protein concentration in the separation of "transudative" and "exudative" ascites, Am J Med 77:83, 1984.
5. Light RW, Ball WC Jr: Glucose and amylase in pleural effusions, JAMA 225:257, 1973.
6. Carr DT, Mayne JG: Pleurisy with effusion in rheumatoid arthritis, with reference to the low concentration of glucose in pleural fluid, Am Rev Respir Dis 85:345, 1962.
7. Dodson WH, Hollingsworth JW: Pleural effusion in rheumatoid arthritis: impaired transport of glucose, N Engl J Med 275:1337, 1966.
8. Sokolowski JW Jr, et al: Guidelines for thoracentesis and needle biopsy of the pleura, Am Rev Respir Dis 140:257, 1989.
9. Sahn SA, Good JT: Pleural fluid pH in malignant effusions, Ann Intern Med 108:345, 1988.
10. Staats BA, et al: The lipoprotein profile of chylous and nonchylous pleural effusions, Mayo Clin Proc 55:700, 1980.
11. Sherr HP, et al: Origin of pleural fluid amylase in esophageal rupture, Ann Intern Med 76:985, 1972.
12. Dye RA, Lafaret EG: Esophageal rupture: diagnosis by pleural fluid pH, Chest 66:454, 1974.
13. Abbott OA, Mansor KA, Logan WD: Atraumatic so-called spontaneous rupture of the esophagus, J Thorac Cardiovasc Surg 59:67, 1970.

14. Geokas MC, et al: Studies on the ascites and pleural effusion in acute pancreatitis, Gastroenterology 58:950, 1970.
15. Keith LM, Zollinger RM, McCleery RS: Peritoneal fluid amylase determinations as an aid in diagnosis of acute pancreatitis, Arch Surg 61:930, 1950.
16. Donowitz M, Kerstein MD, Spiro HM: Pancreatic ascites, Medicine 53:183, 1974.
17. Salt WB, Schenker S: Amylase—its clinical significance: a review of the literature, Medicine 55:269, 1976.
18. Goldman M, Goldman G, Fleischner FG: Pleural fluid amylase in acute pancreatitis, N Engl J Med 266:715, 1962.
19. Burkart J, Hagler S, et al: Usefulness of peritoneal fluid amylase levels in the differential diagnosis of peritonitis in peritoneal dialysis patients, J Am Soc Nephrol 1:1186, 1991.
20. Bruno MJ, van Westerloo DJ, van Dorp WT, et al: Acute pancreatitis in peritoneal dialysis and haemodialysis: risk, clinical course, outcome, and possible aetiology, Gut 46:385, 2000.
21. Lee YN: Alkaline phosphatase in intestinal perforation, JAMA 208:361, 1969.
22. Delany HM, Moss CM, Carnevale N: The use of enzyme analysis of peritoneal blood in the clinical assessment of abdominal organ injury, Surg Gynecol Obstet 42:161, 1976.
23. Looi LM, Lee P: An unusual case of unilateral transudative pleural effusion, Chest 130:328S, 2006.
24. Ropes MW, Rossmeisl EC, Bauer W: The origin and nature of normal human synovial fluid, J Clin Invest 19:795, 1940.
25. Shmerling RH, et al: Synovial fluid tests: what should be ordered? JAMA 264:1009, 1990.
26. Shmerling RH: Synovial fluid analysis: a critical reappraisal, Rheum Dis Clin North Am 20:503, 1994.
27. Pekin TJ, Zvaifler NJ: Hemolytic complement in synovial fluid, J Clin Invest 43:1372, 1964.
28. Pruzanski W, et al: Serum and synovial fluid proteins in rheumatoid arthritis and degenerative joint diseases, Am J Med Sci 265:483, 1973.
29. McCarty DJ: Synovial fluid. In McCarty DJ, Koopman WJ, editors: *Arthritis and Allied Conditions: A Textbook of Rheumatology,* ed 14, Philadelphia, 2001, Lea & Febiger.
30. Agarwal V, Misra R, Aggarwal A: Immune complexes contain immunoglobulin A rheumatoid factor in serum and synovial fluid of patients with polyarticular juvenile rheumatoid arthritis, Rheumatology 41:466, 2002.
31. Baker DG: Chemistry, serology, and immunology. In Gatter RA, Schumacher HR, editors: *A Practical Handbook of Joint Fluid Analysis,* ed 2, Philadelphia, 1991, Lea & Febiger.
32. de Groot-Mijnes JDF, Rothova A: Diagnostic testing of vitrectomy specimens, Am J Ophthalmol 141:982, 2006.
33. Tear fluid analysis, Acta Ophthalmol Scand 78:26, 2000.
34. van der Waaij LA, van Dullemen HM, Porte RJ: Cyst fluid analysis in the differential diagnosis of pancreatic cystic lesions: a pooled analysis, Gastrointest Endosc 62:383, 2005.

INTERNET SITES

www.arthritis.org—Arthritis Foundation

www.niams.nih.gov/—National Institute of Arthritis and Musculoskeletal and Skin Diseases

www.arthritis-research.com—Arthritis Research

www.aafp.org/afp/20000415/2391.html—American Academy of Family Physicians: Knee Effusions: A Systematic Approach to Diagnosis

www.postgradmed.com/index.php?art-pgm_O5.1_1999?article-736—Postgraduate Medicine: Evaluating Pleural Effusions

www.nlm.nih.gov/medlineplus/ency/article/003629.htm—National Library of Medicine: Synovial Fluid Analysis

http://www.geocities.com/soho/gallery/6412/diagnostic1.htm

http://emedicine.medscape.com/article/299959-overview

http://emedicine.medscape.com/article/807375-overview

http://www.clevelandclinicmeded.com/medicalpubs/diseasemanagement/rheumatology/septicarthritis/septicarthritis.htm—Rheumatoid arthritis

http://www.labtestsonline.org/understanding/analytes/rheumatoid/test.html—Rheumatoid arthritis

Nervous System

Michael D. Privitera, Tarek Zakaria, and Rakesh Khatri

47 Chapter

Chapter Outline

Key Terms

affective disorder A disorder of mood regulation that is manifested clinically by episodes or sustained periods of depression or mania or both.

antiepileptic drugs Medications given therapeutically to prevent seizures of various types. Many of these drugs are used widely for various nervous system disorders such as pain, headache, or bipolar disorder.

antipsychotic drugs Drugs that are used for the reversal or attenuation of psychotic symptoms (e.g., hallucinations, delusions, disorders of cognition).

anxiety disorder Chronic disorder characterized by inappropriate, pervasive, continuous, or paroxysmal feelings of worry or fear.

bipolar affective disorder Affective disorder in which episodes of depression and mania are present episodically in the same patient.

blood-brain barrier The barrier between the brain and the blood that allows the brain to maintain a cerebrospinal fluid composition different from that of blood.

cerebrospinal fluid (CSF) Clear, colorless fluid contained within the four ventricles of the brain, the subarachnoid space, and the spinal cord.

coma A state of unconsciousness from which patients cannot be aroused, even by the strongest stimuli.

depression A mood disturbance often described as being sad, blue, hopeless, low, "down in the dumps," or irritable, accompanied by pervasive loss of interest or pleasure in almost all usual activities or pastimes.

epilepsy A disorder characterized by a tendency to have seizures.

IgG index The ratio (CSF IgG × Serum albumin)/(Serum IgG × CSF albumin) used as an indicator of the source of elevated cerebrospinal fluid protein.

mania A periodic disturbance of mood in which the mood is elevated, expansive, or irritable, accompanied by hyperactivity, pressure of speech, flight of ideas, inflated self-esteem, and a decreased need for sleep.

meninges The three membranes that cover the brain and the spinal cord: the dura, arachnoid, and pia.

meningitis Inflammation of the meninges, often caused by viral or bacterial infection.

neurotransmitter A chemical substance released by one neuron onto a specific receptor on an adjacent cell; it alters the physiological functioning of the cell.

receptor A protein complex embedded in the cell membrane that binds to a particular neurotransmitter and initiates a series of events that alter the physiological functioning of the membrane.

reuptake A process by which neurons conserve their own neurotransmitter by recovering it from the synaptic cleft for storage and subsequent re-release.

schizophrenia A chronic psychotic illness with delusions, hallucinations, and disorders of cognition that has lasted longer than 6 months, and from which full recovery is not expected.

seizure A sudden and transient disturbance of mental function or body movement that results from an excessive electrical discharge of a group of brain cells.

stroke Sudden onset of symptoms caused by acute ischemia in the brain resulting from hemorrhage, embolism, or thrombosis; it is evidenced by loss of neurological function.

subarachnoid space The space between the arachnoid and the pia membranes.

synapse The structural junction of two neurons, where chemical messages are carried from the presynaptic neuron to the postsynaptic receptor by neurotransmitters.

unipolar affective disease Affective disorder in which episodes of depression occur alone without episodes of mania.

ventricles Four cavities within the brain filled with cerebrospinal fluid and lined by the pia and the choroid plexus.

xanthochromia A yellow coloring to the cerebrospinal fluid caused by the presence of breakdown products of hemoglobin.

Methods in Evolve

Anticonvulsive drugs
Barbiturates
Carbamazepine
Catecholamines—Plasma, urine
CSF proteins
Drug screen
Glucose
Lithium
Opiates
Phenytoin
Serum protein electrophoresis
Thyroid tests
Lithium
Tricyclic antidepressants

BASIC NEUROANATOMY

The central nervous system (CNS) consists of the brain and the spinal cord. The brain includes the two cerebral hemispheres, which roughly are mirror images of one another; the cerebellum, a rounded structure about the size of a baseball that helps control movement and balance; and the brain stem, a narrow structure through which all the pathways entering and leaving the two hemispheres must pass (Fig. 47-1). The brain stem contains the centers that control breathing, heart rate, eye movements, and many other critical functions. The lower brainstem flows into the spinal cord. The spinal cord is the point of exit for nerves on their way out to the muscles they control and the point of entry for sensory fibers returning from the body's sensory organs. All nerves outside the CNS are collectively called the peripheral nervous system.

The two cerebral hemispheres are built around a connecting system of hollow spaces called the ventricular system. The **ventricles** are filled with **cerebrospinal fluid (CSF)** (Fig. 47-2).

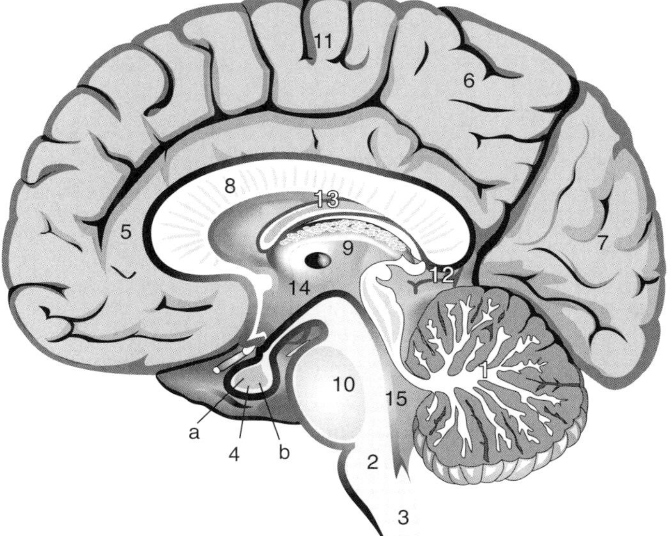

Fig. 47-1 Scheme of functional or motor control areas of the brain (right hemisphere, medial view). *1,* Cerebellum; *2,* medulla oblongata; *3,* spinal cord; *4,* pituitary gland: *a,* anterior lobe; *b,* posterior lobe; *5,* frontal lobe; *6,* parietal lobe; *7,* occipital lobe; *8,* corpus callosum; *9,* thalamus; *10,* pons; *11,* cerebrum; *12,* pineal body; *13,* fornix; *14,* third ventricle; and *15,* fourth ventricle. (From Beck EW: *Mosby's Atlas of Functional Human Anatomy,* St. Louis, 1982, Mosby.)

The brain and spinal cord both are covered by a double membrane called the **meninges** (Fig. 47-3). Its inner membrane, the arachnoid, lies next to the outermost covering of the brain and spinal cord, the dura. The dura is a tough, nonelastic membrane that essentially wraps the brain and spinal cord in a nondistensible sac. The brain, blood, and CSF thus are sealed within a space, the volume of which is fixed. The space between the pia and the arachnoid, called the **subarachnoid space,** communicates directly with the ventricular system.

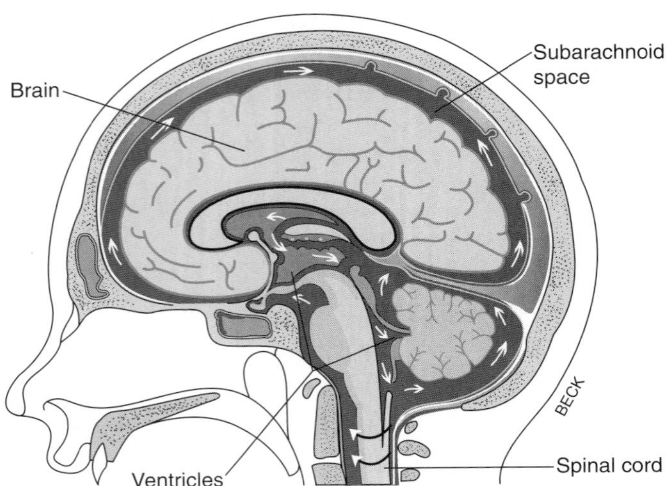

Fig. 47-2 Scheme of brain showing relationships of ventricles and subarachnoid space with rest of brain. (From Beck EW: *Mosby's Atlas of Functional Human Anatomy,* St. Louis, 1982, Mosby.)

SECTION OBJECTIVES BOX 47-1

- Describe the normal formation and reabsorption of cerebrospinal fluid (CSF).
- Explain the physiological function of the blood-brain barrier, including factors that influence access to the brain and the effects of inflammation, neovascularity, presence of toxins, and age have on its permeability.
- List four functions of CSF.
- Describe the normal composition of CSF.
- Describe the composition of CSF and the relationship of CSF protein and glucose levels to their serum levels.
- Explain the neurotransmitter systems in the CNS, including the functions of norepinephrine, dopamine, acetylcholine, serotonin, GABA, and glutamate.

PHYSIOLOGY AND BIOCHEMISTRY

Formation of Cerebrospinal Fluid

The ventricular system and the subarachnoid space are filled with CSF. The total volume of CSF in adults is about 150 mL. CSF is constantly produced and reabsorbed at a rate of approximately 500 mL/day (0.35 mL/min). This means that the total amount of CSF is replaced every 6 to 8 hours. CSF is produced in the ventricles by a specialized, spongelike structure called the *choroid plexus.* Beginning in the lateral ventricles, where it is formed, CSF circulates into the third ventricle and then into the fourth ventricle. It leaves the fourth ventricle through three small openings, or foramina, to circulate through the intracranial and spinal subarachnoid spaces. Circulation may be blocked in any of the ventricles or at the foramina between them, leading to an obstructive hydrocephalus (accumulation of fluid within the brain).

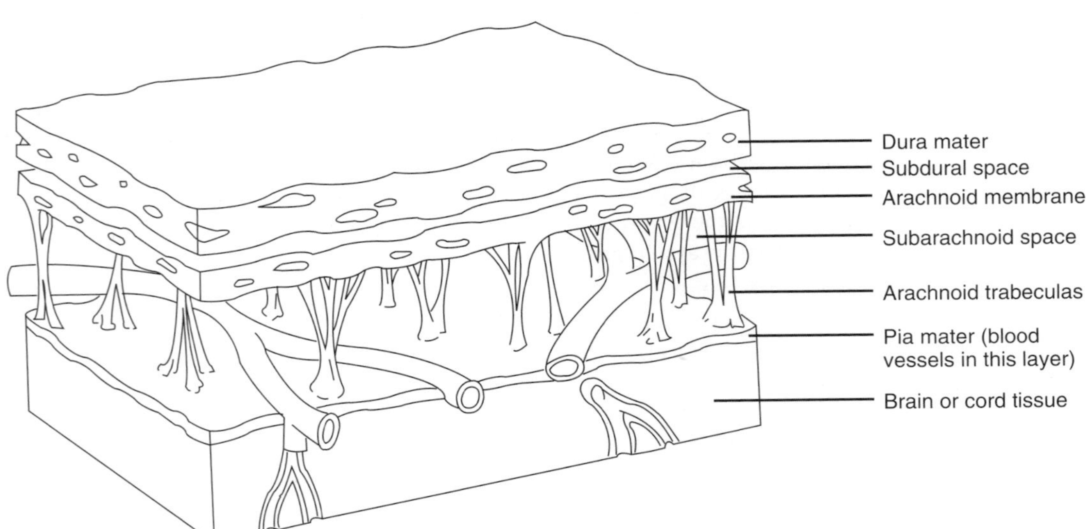

Fig. 47-3 Scheme of meninges. Arrangement may be compared with that of an underground parking garage. Dura and arachnoid form the roof with pia membrane as the floor. Cerebrospinal fluid (CSF) flows in the subarachnoid space. (From Prezbindowski KS: *Guide to Learning Anatomy and Physiology,* St. Louis, 1982, Mosby.)

New CSF is constantly produced and absorbed at the arachnoid villi and granulations to keep volume constant. These arachnoid villi and granulations are scattered along the entire inner table of the skull and down the spinal canal to the points at which the spinal nerves exit the dura. Thus CSF reabsorption can occur along the entire neuraxis. If absorption is impaired (as after meningeal inflammation, bacterial **meningitis,** or subarachnoid hemorrhage), CNS pressure and CSF volume both rise; this is called a *communicating hydrocephalus.*

Factors that determine the rate at which CSF is formed and absorbed are complex and are not completely understood. Any increase in the size of one component (i.e., brain, CSF, or blood) leads to a sharp increase in pressure within the system, unless a corresponding decrease occurs in the volume of one of the other two components. With increased CSF pressure, the brain may suffer from direct effects of the abnormally high pressure, or from having its blood flow decreased.

Blood-Brain Barrier

The term **blood-brain barrier** refers to a physiological barrier that separates the brain and CSF from substances borne in the blood. The blood-brain barrier allows brain and CSF composition to be maintained at levels quite different from those of blood with respect to proteins, ions, and other molecular elements. The blood-brain barrier is extremely important in clinical practice. It determines the access of antibiotics to the brain and meninges and contributes to exquisite control exercised over the brain's chemical milieu despite simultaneous changes that occur in the peripheral blood.

The extracellular fluid (ECF) compartment of the brain is in relatively free communication with the CSF, whereas a barrier exists between capillary blood and the ECF compartment–CSF combination.

Factors that significantly influence the access of substances to brain and CSF include molecular weight, protein binding, and lipid solubility. With molecular weight, entry is inversely related to size, hence the 1 : 200 CSF-to-plasma ratio of albumin (molecular weight, 69,000 daltons). Drugs that are highly protein bound enter the CSF much less readily than unbound smaller-molecular-weight substances. For example, phenytoin is 90% protein bound and 10% free in blood; only free phenytoin is easily able to enter the CNS. Calcium, magnesium, and metabolites such as bilirubin are also highly protein bound and thus are relatively restricted from CSF. Highly lipid-soluble substances such as carbon monoxide, neuroactive drugs, and alcohol readily enter the CNS. Substances that are highly ionized at physiological pH are relatively excluded. Highly polar substances, such as some amino acids, enter slowly and require an active transport mechanism.

The blood-brain barrier is readily permeable to water but not to electrolytes. The cations sodium and potassium require hours to reach equilibrium with CSF after changes occur in peripheral blood. Changes in blood osmolality are followed by parallel CSF changes after a lag time of a few hours.

In the case of drugs, their pK_a, or ionic dissociation constant, is important in determining how readily they cross the blood-brain barrier. pK_a refers to the pH at which 50% of a compound is ionized. A nonionized drug is relatively lipid soluble and so more freely enters the CNS. The polar ionized fraction is relatively excluded.

Finally, characteristics of the blood-brain barrier can be altered dramatically by disease states. Penicillin, an acidic substance, normally is excluded from the CNS after parenteral injection, and yet it is an effective agent for treating meningitis. The reason is that meningeal inflammation alters (damages) the blood-brain barrier, allowing greater access to drugs, such as penicillin, that normally would not reach infected tissue.

Specific factors that alter permeability of the blood-brain barrier include the following:

- Inflammation can increase the ease of entry into the nervous system of macromolecules such as albumin and penicillin.
- Neovascularity, in association, for example, with tumor, trauma, or ischemia, alters the blood-brain barrier. This may result from defects in the new vessels or may be caused by their immaturity.
- Toxins can change blood-brain barrier characteristics, and some agents used in radiographic studies increase the permeability of the barrier through direct toxic effects. When they are injected in hyperosmolar concentrations, the effect is greater.
- Finally, the blood-brain barrier of the immature nervous system is more permeable to a variety of substances. For infants below 6 months of age, CSF protein is normally as high as 100 mg/dL.

Functions of Cerebrospinal Fluid

Why should the brain be suspended in and bathed by this distinctive fluid? First, CSF provides mechanical support to the brain. Second, CSF probably functions to help remove metabolic products from the brain—a function that is poorly understood but probably important in both healthy and diseased states. Third, evidence suggests that CSF transports biologically active compounds that may function as chemical messengers. Finally, it plays an important role in maintaining the chemical environment of the brain. Although its communication with the plasma compartment is tightly regulated, CSF seems to be in relatively free communication with the extracellular fluid compartment of the brain, which aids brain cells themselves. The following section examines the composition of CSF more closely.

Composition of Cerebrospinal Fluid

The ionic and molecular composition of CSF differs from that of plasma for some components and is the same for others (Box 47-1). Changes in serum sodium are followed by corresponding changes in CSF sodium, so that after a lag time of about 1 hour, sodium values are nearly the same. However, CSF potassium is lower than plasma potassium and is maintained within a very narrow concentration range despite wide fluctuations in plasma values. Active transport into and out of the CSF space appears to be largely responsible for maintaining these differences. Chloride and magnesium are somewhat

Box 47-1

Characteristics of Normal Spinal Fluid

Total volume: 150 mL
Color: Colorless, like water
Transparency: Clear, like water
Osmolarity at 37°C: 281 mOsm/L
Specific gravity: 1.006 to 1.008
Acid-base balance:

pH	7.31
P_{CO_2}	47.9 mm Hg
HCO_3^-	22.9 mEq/L

Sodium: 138 to 150 mmol/L
Potassium: 2.7 to 3.9 mmol/L
Chloride: 116 to 127 mmol/L
Calcium: 2.0 to 2.5 mEq/L (4.0 to 5.0 mg/dL)
Magnesium: 2.0 to 2.5 mEq/L (2.4 to 3.1 mg/dL)
Lactic acid: 1.1 to 2.8 mmol/L
Lactate dehydrogenase: Absolute activity depends on method; approximately 10% of serum value
Glucose: 45 to 80 mg/dL
Proteins: 20 to 40 mg/dL

At different levels of spinal tap:

Lumbar	20 to 40 mg/dL
Cisternal	15 to 25 mg/dL
Ventricular	15 to 10 mg/dL

Normal values in children:

Up to 6 days of age	70 mg/dL
Up to 4 years of age	24 mg/dL

Electrophoretic separation of spinal fluid proteins (% of total protein concentration):

Prealbumin	2% to 7%
Albumin	56% to 76%
α_1-Globulin	2% to 7%
α_2-Globulin	3.5% to 12%
β- and γ-globulin	8% to 18%
γ-Globulin	7% to 12%
Immunoglobulin (Ig)G	10 to 40 mg/L
IgA	0 to 0.2 mg/L
IgM	0 to 0.6 mg/L
κ/λ ratio	1

Erythrocyte count:

Newborn	0 to 675/mm^3
Adult	0 to 10/mm^3

Leukocyte count:

<1 year of age	0 to 30/mm^3
1 to 4 years of age	0 to 20/mm^3
5 years of age to puberty	0 to 10/mm^3
Adult	0 to 5/mm^3

higher in CSF than in plasma, and bicarbonate is somewhat lower.

CSF glucose normally ranges from 45 to 80 mg/dL (2.5 to 4.44 mmol/L), that is, between 60% and 80% of the blood glucose concentration after equilibration. Blood and CSF glucose equilibrate only after a lag period of about 4 hours, and so CSF glucose at any given time reflects blood glucose levels during the past 4 hours. When a lumbar spinal puncture (LP) is performed and CSF glucose is to be determined, a simultaneous sample of peripheral blood must also be drawn. CSF glucose is altered by certain disease processes, as is discussed later. Equilibrated CSF glucose is definitely abnormal when it is less than 40% of the simultaneous blood glucose value; values less than 40 to 45 mg/dL are almost always abnormal.

One should also be aware that the expected percentage of CSF glucose to blood glucose (60% to 80%) falls as blood glucose rises, that is, one would expect a CSF-to-blood ratio of 0.5 when blood glucose values reach 500 mg/dL, and a ratio of 0.4 when blood glucose reaches 700 mg/dL.

Proteins found in the CSF ordinarily originate from serum and reach the CSF space by pinocytosis across the capillary endothelium. The normal ratio of serum to CSF protein is 200:1 (with serum equal to 7 g/dL, and CSF equal to 35 mg/dL).

Brain Metabolism

The metabolic rate of the brain is one of the highest of any of the body's organs, whether one is awake or asleep. However, unlike most other organs, which store and reserve some supplies of energy to sustain themselves, the brain has almost no energy reserve. It depends entirely on an uninterrupted supply of glucose and oxygen delivered by peripheral blood. The brain uses glucose almost exclusively to supply its energy needs (see Chapter 38). To get an idea of just how hungry the brain is and how dependent it is on a constant, swift flow of blood, consider that under resting conditions, total cerebral blood flow equals 15% to 20% of cardiac output (or about 500 mL per 100 g of brain per minute). Although total cerebral blood flow remains remarkably constant, discrete areas within the brain show striking variability; gray matter receives three to four times the blood flow compared with white matter. Moreover, regional blood flow is known to vary during performance of certain tasks, with regional flow increasing in appropriate areas during tasks such as hand movement, speaking, or mental problem solving. Blood flow also is altered in response to disease states, as in stroke.

Neurotransmitter Systems

Neurons (nerve cells) within the central nervous system process information arriving from multiple internal and external sources. To maintain physiological and psychobiological homeostasis, CNS neurons communicate both with one another and eventually with effectors outside the central nervous system by means of neurotransmitters released by each neuron onto specific **receptors** (Fig. 47-4).

The function of the **neurotransmitter** is to propagate an electrical impulse from one neuron to another. The electrical

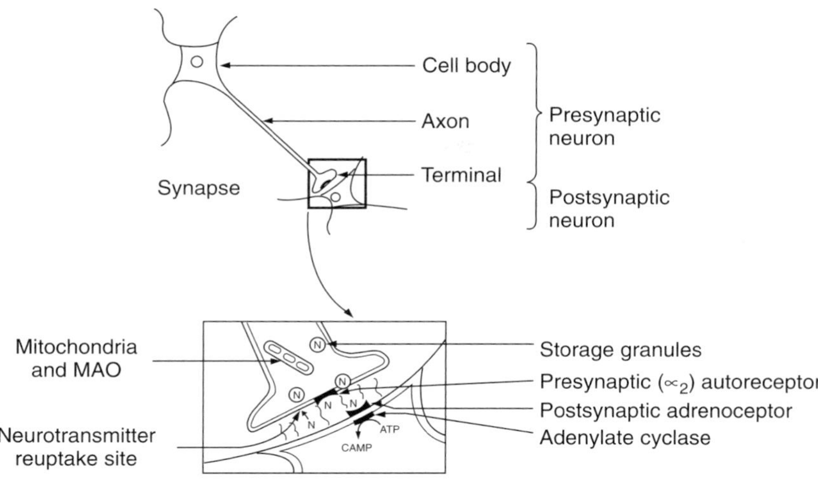

Fig. 47-4 Norepinephrine (N) neuron, synapse, and postsynaptic connections. *MAO,* Monoamine oxidase.

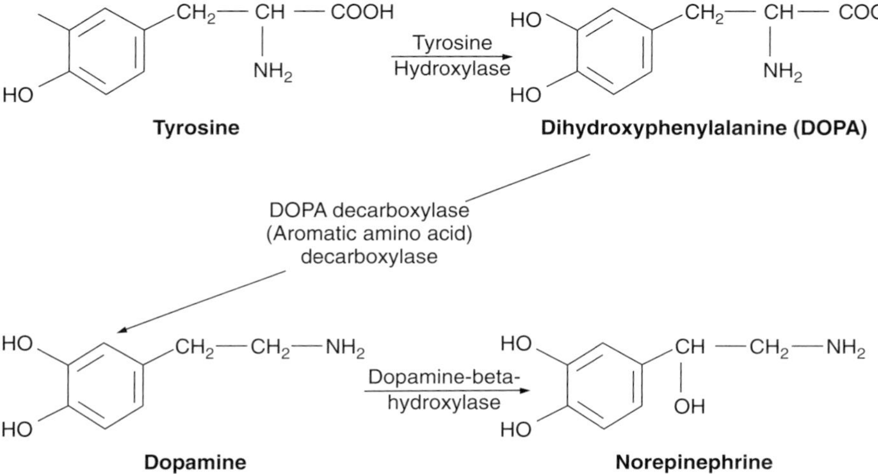

Fig. 47-5 Enzymatic pathway for synthesis of dopamine and norepinephrine. (From Kaplan H, Sadock B: *Clinical Psychiatry,* Baltimore, 1988, Williams & Wilkins.)

impulse travels down a neuron, causing the release of a neurotransmitter from presynaptic vesicles in which the neurotransmitter is synthesized and stored. Subsequently, several thousand molecules of neurotransmitter are released into the synaptic cleft, the space between the presynaptic and postsynaptic neurons. There they bind to transmitter-specific receptors of the postsynaptic neurons and produce an excitatory or inhibitory impulse. Neurotransmitters are broken down by enzymes in the synaptic cleft. Both the metabolites and the parent compounds bind to receptors on the presynaptic membrane, where they are again taken back into the presynaptic neuron (**reuptake**) for formation of a new neurotransmitter.

Norepinephrine

Norepinephrine is formed in presynaptic noradrenergic neurons from the substrate tyrosine by means of the intermediary products of dopa and dopamine (Fig. 47-5). Norepinephrine produces an excitatory response at postsynaptic receptors. It is either broken down in the cleft to 3-methoxy-4-hydroxyphenylglycol (MHPG) by a cytoplasmic enzyme called monoamine oxidase, or it is taken up into the presynaptic neuron. This reuptake is inhibited by cocaine and tricyclic antidepressants. MHPG crosses the blood-brain barrier, enters the circulatory system, and is excreted into urine; approximately 50% of urinary MHPG is derived from the CNS.

Dopamine

Dopamine is formed by the same metabolic pathway as is shown in Fig. 47-5 in dopaminergic neurons that lack the enzymes for further metabolism of dopamine into norepinephrine. These neurons project from the brain stem to the limbic system and frontal cortex. Dopamine appears to be mainly inhibitory in action. There now appear to be five to seven different types of dopamine receptors; these subtypes may have significance in pharmacological treatment of mental disorders. Typical neuroleptics (phenothiazines and thioxanthenes) primarily block D2 receptors and are associated with extrapyramidal adverse effects, including Parkinson's disease and tardive dyskinesias; atypical neuroleptics (clozapine and olanzapine) that have additional D3-D4 blocking effects are less likely to have these side effects. Dopamine is metabolized to homovanillic acid and is excreted into urine.

Acetylcholine

Acetylcholine, the first demonstrated neurotransmitter, is formed in presynaptic cholinergic neurons from acetyl CoA, a ubiquitous metabolite, and choline, which is derived from lipid metabolism. The essential enzyme for this reaction is choline acetyltransferase.

Once released from presynaptic vesicles into the synaptic cleft, acetylcholine binds to postsynaptic receptors and acts as an excitatory neurotransmitter. The **synapses** are located in all neuromuscular junctions, in the major portion of the autonomic nervous system, and in brain areas such as motor pathways, the hippocampus, which is part of the limbic system, and the basal ganglia.

It is broken down in the synaptic cleft by the enzyme acetylcholinesterase. Drugs that inhibit this enzyme (rivastigmine, pyridostigmine, etc.) are used for the treatment of Alzheimer's disease and myasthenia gravis, an autoimmune disease with antibodies directed against acetylcholine receptors.

Serotonin (5-Hydroxytryptamine, 5-HT)

Serotonin is formed in presynaptic serotoninergic neurons from the amino acid tryptophan, by means of hydroxytryptophan. Most serotoninergic neurons originate in the raphe nuclei in the pons, from where projections run diffusely throughout the brain and spinal cord. The raphe nuclei are part of the reticular formation, which regulates general arousal. Serotonin binds to the postsynaptic hydroxytryptamine receptor, where it produces an excitatory response. Both serotonin and its metabolite 5-hydroxyindoleacetic acid (5-HIAA) are taken up into the presynaptic neuron. Most antidepressants (fluoxetine) inhibit serotonin reuptake transporters, causing an increase in serotonin levels within the synaptic clefts.

GABA (γ-Aminobutyric Acid)

GABA is formed from the amino acid glutamic acid through decarboxylation. GABA is used as a neurotransmitter by 30% to 40% of all synapses in the brain and is located diffusely throughout the brain, brain stem, and spinal cord. It acts as an inhibitory neurotransmitter. Postsynaptic GABA receptor complexes also bind drugs like phenobarbital, valproate, and the benzodiazepines. Tiagabine, one of the new **antiepileptic drugs,** is believed to enhance the activity of the GABA system by binding to recognition sites associated with the GABA uptake carrier. This results in reduced GABA reuptake, thereby increasing the GABA concentration available to the receptor.

Glutamate

Glutamate, a major excitatory neurotransmitter, is synthesized by astrocytes either from glutamine or α-ketoglutarate by glutamate dehydrogenase. Three different ionic receptors (AMPA, NMDA, and Kainate receptors) mediate the function of glutamate, which is cleared from synaptic clefts by the high-affinity Na- and K-coupled glutamate carriers, called *excitatory amino acid transmitters (EAATs).* Increased glutamate excitotoxicity has been implicated in a wide range of neurological diseases, including stroke, **epilepsy,** and chronic CNS degenerative disorders (e.g., amyotrophic lateral sclerosis [ALS], Parkinson's disease).

Other Neurotransmitters

A variety of other substances make up the majority of neurotransmitters in the central nervous system, but their clinical significance is poorly understood at the present time. Such substances include glycine, another amino acid that has inhibitory function in the spinal cord; endogenous opioids, such as endorphin and enkephalin; and substance P, which is found in neuronal pathways that transmit pain. Two gases—nitric oxide and carbon monoxide—have been shown to act as neurotransmitters.

KEY CONCEPTS BOX 47-1

- Through charge, lipid solubility, and molecular weight, the blood-brain barrier prevents substances in blood from entering the CSF.
- Inflammation of meninges, altered vascularity, and toxins can alter the blood-brain barrier.
- CSF functions as a mechanical support to the brain; it removes metabolic wastes and delivers nutrients to brain tissue.
- CSF is in slow equilibrium with blood components and has lower K, glucose (60% to 80%), and protein than are seen in serum.
- The high metabolic rate of the brain is dependent upon a constant supply of glucose.
- Neurotransmitters are chemical messengers; when released from one nerve cell, they stimulate the next nerve cell to transmit an electrical signal. Reuptake of neurotransmitters is an important part of their metabolic clearance.
- The primary neurotransmitters include norepinephrine, dopamine, acetylcholine, serotonin, GABA, and glutamate.

SECTION OBJECTIVES BOX 47-2

- List the major causes of coma or altered mental status.
- List characteristic laboratory findings in multiple sclerosis.
- Describe changes in CSF white blood cell count and differential, glucose, protein, and microbiological findings that are associated with the following disorders:
  - Infectious diseases
  - Intracranial bleeding
  - Neuromuscular diseases
- List endocrine disorders that occur with mood-changing symptoms.

PATHOLOGICAL CONDITIONS: NEUROLOGICAL

Loss of neural function with resultant disease states is caused by abnormalities of the neurotransmitter biochemical pathways. For example, in the early stages of Alzheimer's disease, a large decrease in choline acetyltransferase activity occurs, along with degeneration of neurons that use acetylcholine. Loss of acetylcholine activity in the hippocampus may explain the hallmark symptom of early memory loss in Alzheimer's disease, because the hippocampus is involved in acquisition of memory. In Huntington's disease, degeneration of cholinergic neurons occurs in the basal ganglia, contributing to the movement disorder and dementia seen in Huntington's disease. Dysfunction of GABA-ergic systems is postulated in idiopathic generalized epilepsy, Huntington's disease, and anxiety disorders. Clinical disease states attributable to dopaminergic neuron dysfunction vary according to the anatomical locations of the dysfunctional neurons. Dopaminergic neuron dysfunction in pathways from the brain stem to the frontal cortex and limbic system may contribute to clinical symptoms of schizophrenia, whereas dysfunction of dopaminergic neurons that project from the brain stem to the corpus striatum is important in movement disorders such as Parkinson's disease.

Damage to discrete (focal) areas of the brain or spinal cord produces predictable circumscribed signs and symptoms, such as paralysis of an arm, leg, or side of the body, loss of ability to speak or comprehend spoken language, incoordination, and visual or sensory loss. Diffuse impairment of cerebral tissue, on the other hand, leads to a different characteristic clinical picture. Failure of various intellectual functions such as attention, concentration, judgment, memory, problem-solving ability, and insight is an early finding with mild diffuse disease. Other symptoms include changes in alertness, beginning with clouding of consciousness and proceeding to drowsiness, stupor, and coma. Excessive synchronized nerve transmission can cause sudden transient abnormalities of mental function or body movement, called **seizures.** Seizures can accompany both diffuse and focal brain damage.

Various disease states tend to produce either focal or diffuse brain damage, and so the pattern of deficits described above is often helpful to the clinician in working backward toward a specific diagnosis. Examples of conditions that cause focal damage include stroke caused by arterial occlusion or hemorrhage; trauma; cerebral abscess; and tumors. Many of these conditions also cause changes in the CSF by damaging the blood-brain barrier (elevating CSF protein) and stimulating inflammatory changes (with leukocytosis), tissue necrosis (elevating CSF protein and cell count), or shedding of tumor cells (observed in cytological specimens).

Examples of conditions associated with diffuse cerebral dysfunction (encephalopathic states) include anoxia, generalized ischemia, hypoglycemia, sepsis, thyroid abnormalities, disseminated intravascular coagulation, and the entire group of toxic and metabolic derangements. Diagnosis of these states often rests on laboratory findings.

Some of the clinical and pathological changes commonly found in many conditions are briefly discussed here.

Coma

Coma is a state of unconsciousness from which the patient cannot be aroused. A coma is but one aspect of altered states of consciousness that can be present in patients. With confusion, which is the least altered state, there is disorientation with respect to time, along with associated drowsiness and altered attention span. Stupor is a state in which the patient is unresponsive but can be aroused back to a near-normal state with appropriate stimuli.

A patient with an altered mental state, as may be seen in an emergency department, first must be given any life support, such as ventilation, necessary to maintain vital functions. The next step is to determine the underlying cause of the altered mental status. Readily treatable causes can be corrected by procedures, such as administration of dextrose to relieve coma caused by severe hypoglycemia. Table 47-1 lists the most important causes of coma and altered mental states; these

Table 47-1 Some Causes of Coma and Altered Mental States

Type	Cause	Laboratory Findings
Metabolic	Alcoholism	Increased blood ethanol, metabolic acidosis, and ketosis
	Hyperosmolar coma	Blood glucose >500 mg/dL, no ketosis, dehydration
	Diabetic ketoacidosis	Increased blood glucose, ketosis, acidosis, dehydration
	Metabolic acidosis of other origin	Decreased pH, increased lactic acid
	Hypoglycemia	Decreased blood glucose (<50 mg/dL)
	Hypercalcemia or hypocalcemia	Changes in calcium levels; hypomagnesemia can be found with hypocalcemia
	Drugs	Presence of any of many drugs on serum or urine toxicology screen, often at very high levels
Systemic metabolic diseases	Hepatic coma	Increase in blood ammonia, increased liver function tests
	Uremic coma	Increased serum urea and creatinine; with metabolic acidosis
	Ischemia: cardiac, pulmonary	Lactic acidosis
	Hypothyroidism or hyperthyroidism	Abnormal thyroid function tests
Encephalopathy	Intracranial hemorrhage	Blood in CSF
Trauma	—	None, or blood in CSF if traumatic hemorrhage is present
Infectious	Bacterial, viral	Decreased CSF glucose, increased protein
Psychiatric	—	None

include metabolic, structural, and infectious causes. Many of these causes are described in detail in the following sections.

Intracranial Bleeding

Bleeding from a vessel on the surface of the brain, such as an arterial aneurysm, pours blood between the surface of the brain and the pia and arachnoid layers; this is called a subarachnoid hemorrhage. Blood thus mingles with CSF, and red blood cells appear on examination of the CSF. Furthermore, because blood is an extremely irritating substance when it escapes from its usual vascular channels, it may provoke an inflammatory response in the meninges, called chemical meningitis, and leukocytes may be shed into the CSF by the irritated meninges. Because meninges are pain sensitive, a subarachnoid hemorrhage typically causes acute, severe headache.

Inflammatory Diseases

Multiple sclerosis (MS) and sarcoidosis are inflammatory CNS diseases of unknown cause. MS, which usually affects young adults, produces numerous areas of demyelination in the CNS and is characterized by waxing and waning of symptoms, but usually with a progressive course. The diagnosis of MS is best made clinically on the basis of the presence of two different events that affect two separate areas of the CNS on two different occasions; clinicians often refer to this as "two lesions separated in time and space." Magnetic resonance imaging (MRI) of brain and spinal cord is helpful in detecting white matter lesions. Examination of CSF can help in supporting the diagnosis, especially in patients who do not meet all the clinical criteria for MS. Five major CSF abnormalities are seen in MS (Box 47-2). However, none of these CSF abnormalities is specific for multiple sclerosis. Devic's disease is a newly recognized demyelinating disease that affects the spinal cord and the optic nerves. The major difference between Devic's disease and MS is the absence or very small number of brain lesions on MRI, negative oligoclonal bands, and prominent neutrophils in the CSF in patient with Devic's disease.

Box 47-2

CSF Abnormalities Associated With MS

Elevation of up to 40 cells/mm^3 of white blood cells
Elevation in protein up to 100 mg/dL
Elevation in immunoglobulin (Ig)G
Presence of oligoclonal bands
Elevation in myelin basic protein

Sarcoidosis is a generalized disease of unknown cause that may affect the nervous system. Serum angiotensin-converting enzyme (ACE) usually is elevated, and CSF shows similar findings to those seen with MS.

Infectious Diseases

CNS infections may be limited to meninges, causing meningitis, or brain parenchyma, causing encephalitis. Both the type of invading bacterial or viral organism and the intracranial structures that they invade help to determine CSF changes seen in the infectious process. CSF parameters that reflect CNS invasion by an infectious agent include white blood cell (WBC) count and differential, glucose, and, to a lesser extent, protein concentration (Table 47-2).

Bacterial, or purulent, meningitis is associated with a CSF polymorphonuclear (PMN) leukocytosis, with cell counts ranging from very few to many thousands of PMNs. CSF glucose levels may be depressed to strikingly low values, and CSF protein concentrations may be elevated. Later in the course of illness, lymphocytes can become prominent or dominant, especially if the infection has been treated in part with

Table 47-2 CSF Findings in CNS Infections

Meningitis	Pressure, mm H_2O	WBC (per mm^3)	Protein (mg/dL)	Glucose (mg/dL)
Acute bacterial	Usually elevated	100s to >60,000, usually a few thousand, PMNs	Usually 100-500, occasionally >1000	5-40 in most cases
Tuberculous	Usually elevated, but can be low with spinal block	25-100, rarely >500, lymphs (except early in some with PMN)	Usually 100-200, can be higher with block	Usually low, <45 in 75% of cases
Cryptococcal	Usually elevated	0-800, average 50, lymphs	20-500, usually 100	Reduced, average 30 May be normal
Viral	Normal to moderately elevated	5-few hundred, maybe up to 1000, lymphs except early	Normal or slightly elevated, <100	Normal (except mumps, HSV, or CMV, which is low in 25%)
Acute syphilis	Usually elevated	Average 500, usually lymphs	Average 100	Normal
Cysticercosis	Often increased but can be low with block	Increased, with eosinophils in 50%	50-200	Reduced in 20%
Sarcoid	Normal to considerably low	0-100, mononuclear	Slight to moderate elevation	Reduced in 50%
Carcinomatosis	Normal to increased	0-several hundred, mono + malignant	Elevated, often very high	Normal to low in 75%

CMV, Cytomegalovirus; *HSV,* herpes simplex virus; *PMN,* polymorphonuclear leukocyte; *WBC,* white blood cell count; *lymphs,* lymphocytes.

antibiotics. Partial treatment of bacterial meningitis that fails to eradicate the infection can produce confusing findings and may make diagnosis difficult.

Viral meningitis causes a predominantly or exclusively lymphocytic leukocytosis. Rarely, PMN leukocytes may predominate within the first few hours of viral meningitis, especially in patients with West Nile virus (WNV), mumps, Eastern equine virus, or echovirus-9. Red blood cells may be seen with herpes simplex encephalitis. CSF glucose levels usually remain within the healthy reference interval but may be decreased in mumps, herpes simplex, or herpes zoster encephalitis. Protein usually is present within the healthy reference interval or may be slightly elevated in these diseases.

Fungi also invade the CNS and may cause no change in CSF other than a lymphocytosis and increased protein concentration. Glucose levels usually remain within the healthy reference interval.

Viral encephalitis, a viral infection of the brain parenchyma, is characterized by acute fever, headache, altered mentation, and evidence of parenchymal involvement such as seizures, focal cerebral symptoms or signs, stupor or coma, and signs of increased intracranial pressure. In the United States, common pathogens include herpes simplex virus-1 (HSV-1), arbovirus, enterovirus, measles, and mumps. HSV-1 encephalitis is the most common viral encephalitis; it manifests with fever, headache, focal or generalized seizures, behavioral changes, amnestic syndrome (short-term memory loss), and aphasia (loss of language use). CSF is under normal or elevated pressure, with lymphocytic pleocytosis and a cell count of 10 to 1000 WBCs/μL; red blood cells (RBCs) and **xanthochromia** also may be present. Protein is elevated, and glucose is normal or decreased. Culture and serology are important diagnostic tools for identifying specific viral agents. Herpes viral (human cytomegalovirus [CMV], HSV, varicella zoster virus [VZV], Epstein-Barr virus [EBV]), enteroviral, Jacob-Creutzfeldt (JC) viral, and measles viral nucleic acid can be detected by polymerase chain reaction (PCR) in CSF specimens. WNV has emerged recently as one of the most common causes of epidemic meningoencephalitis in North America. Neuroinvasive cases may have variable presentations, including meningitis, meningoencephalitis, and acute flaccid paralysis syndrome (poliomyelitis-like picture).

The presence of bacteria should be determined by gram stain and culture of CSF. Gram stain is positive in identifying the organism in 60% to 90% of cases of bacterial meningitis. CSF culture is positive in about 80% of untreated patients. Latex agglutination testing against some bacterial antigens can provide diagnostic confirmation. The PCR test can detect small numbers of viable and nonviable bacterial organisms in CSF.

Viruses can be detected with appropriate serological tests or culture, and fungi can be found by means of culture or immunological procedures and with appropriate staining. For example, carefully performed India ink staining may reveal *Cryptococcus* species.

CSF findings in syphilis depend on the stage of illness, disease activity, and whether previous treatment was given in adequate amounts. Pleocytosis may be lymphatic or mononuclear in character, with white cell counts in the range of 100 to 1000/μL. CSF protein levels may be elevated. CSF Venereal Disease Research Laboratory (VDRL) and serum fluorescent treponemal antibody (FTA) tests usually are positive, and oligoclonal bands may be present.

Organisms can invade the brain substance, in which case the term *encephalitis* is used. CSF findings are comparable with those in meningitis or may be minimal.

Abscess formation within the brain may produce no CSF changes, even though a potentially deadly infection may be present. Finally, any of the above conditions can and frequently will lead to increased CSF pressure. This is especially true of meningitis, which obstructs the usual flow of CSF, causing an obstructive hydrocephalus. Meningitis can also impair CSF absorption, causing a communicating hydrocephalus.

A variety of organisms that do not usually cause serious infection in healthy individuals may produce life-threatening infection in patients whose immune system is compromised. Patients at risk for these "opportunistic" infections include those with acquired immunodeficiency syndrome (AIDS) or cancer, and those taking immunosuppressant drugs for other reasons (e.g., steroids, chemotherapeutic drugs for cancer).

AIDS is caused by the human immunodeficiency virus (HIV). Direct HIV invasion of the nervous system may produce neurological manifestations, but AIDS also predisposes affected individuals to opportunistic infections and unusual malignant tumors that can involve the nervous system. Opportunistic infections, AIDS-related neoplasms, or HIV can affect the brain, spinal cord, or peripheral nerves; usually, multiple sites are affected by multiple causes. With direct HIV infection of the CNS, oligoclonal bands and elevated protein concentrations usually are present in the CSF. The most common CNS tumors include lymphoma and metastatic Kaposi's sarcoma. Common infections include toxoplasmosis, progressive multifocal leukoencephalopathy (PML), fungal and mycobacterial granulomas, and herpes simplex virus (HSV) encephalitis.

Lyme disease is caused by a spirochete *(Borrelia burgdorferi)* and is spread through tick bites. Clinical symptoms include arthritis, meningitis, radiculitis, neuropathy, and, in late stages, concentration, memory, and sleep disorders. The diagnosis is made by organism-specific immunoglobulin (Ig)G or IgM in the serum, but CSF typically shows elevated WBCs and protein levels, and the presence of oligoclonal bands.

Parasitic infections are rare except for neurocysticercosis, which is common in Mexico and Central and South America. Most cases are reported in individuals who have emigrated from these countries. It develops through the consumption of *Taenia solium* ova shed in stools from hosts infected with a mature tapeworm.

Prion diseases are a group of transmissible neurological degenerative diseases that exhibit characteristic pathological changes that led to the early designation of spongiform encephalopathy. They result from the accumulation of an abnormal amyloid form of a host-encoded protein-resistant protein (PrP, or prion), specified by a gene on chromosome 20. The most common prion disease in humans is Creutzfeldt-Jacob disease (CJD). Clinical features include progressive dementia, behavior changes, and abnormal movements. The average time of survival is approximately 7 months. Routine examination of CSF usually is normal. An immunoassay that detects a class of 14-3-3 proteinase released into the CSF from damaged neurons has proved useful in the diagnosis. One series showed a sensitivity of 85% for 14-3-3 in sporadic CJD. Other new emerging tests include detection of abnormal prion protein isoforms within the spinal fluid.

Ischemia

Although immensely dependent on glucose for its energy source, the brain's own glucose reserves are small. Because oxygen is available, and because the metabolic needs of the brain are met by respiration in which only glucose stored within the brain is used, those stores could supply the needs of the brain for only 2 to 3 minutes. If both glucose and oxygen are cut off (as in ischemia), glycolysis becomes the dominant source of energy, and glucose stores in the brain can support its energy metabolism for only about 14 seconds. When energy metabolism ceases, the integrity of cellular membranes fails, potassium begins to leak from the cells, osmotic balance is lost, fluid rushes into the damaged cells, and within seconds cells begin to die.

The term *ischemia* can be defined as inadequate blood flow to a tissue. In the brain, ischemia can be present for many reasons. For example, if the heart stops, total cerebral blood flow ceases; if the blood pressure drops low enough, the flow of blood becomes inadequate; and if a single large vessel such as the carotid artery becomes narrowed, too little blood passes through. If a cerebral blood vessel becomes occluded by an embolus or an atherosclerotic plaque, the tissue that it irrigates becomes ischemic. Other blood vessels usually try to supply the area and make up the difference, but if the area of brain supplied by an occluded vessel cannot be supplied with blood from surrounding vessels, the cells in that area die. This is called a *cerebral infarction,* or a *stroke.*

Stroke

The symptoms of brain ischemia may be transient, lasting seconds to minutes, or may persist for longer periods, causing cerebral infarction, or **stroke.** When a stroke occurs, the functions served by the infarcted region are compromised. For example, if the area that controls strength and movement in one extremity or on one side of the body is infarcted, that extremity or side becomes weak or paralyzed. If the area that serves speech is damaged, the patient may lose the ability to talk or to comprehend what is heard (aphasia). The dying or dead area of brain may release protein into the CSF. Because blood vessels in the area are damaged by ischemia, some bleeding may occur. Only a few cells may appear in the CSF, if only a little blood has escaped from the area, or the CSF may become frankly bloody, if an actual hemorrhage has occurred within the damaged area. Finally, as the brain begins to clear away damaged tissue, some WBCs may appear in the CSF.

Diffuse Cerebral Ischemia and Hypoxia

If total cerebral circulation stops, as in cardiac arrest, consciousness is lost within 6 to 8 seconds. On the other hand, if oxygen supply becomes inadequate but circulation continues, the clinical result is usually a feeling of light-headedness followed by mental confusion in mild cases, and proceeding to loss of consciousness, seizures, and coma with moderate to severe hypoxia. Precipitating events include pulmonary edema, carbon monoxide poisoning, pulmonary embolism, strangulation, respiratory failure during mechanical ventilation, and exposure to ambient air at high altitudes. Failure to restore cerebral circulation and oxygenation within 4 to 5 minutes after their total cessation may result in cell death and irreversible damage.

Neuromuscular Diseases (see also Chapter 36)

The term *neuromuscular disease* refers to disorders that affect peripheral nerves, neuromuscular junctions, or muscle cells, typically causing weakness, sensory loss, or loss of autonomic function. A detailed discussion of these disorders is beyond the scope of this chapter, but laboratory aids in their diagnosis will be discussed.

Peripheral nerve disorders may be hereditary or acquired. The diagnosis of hereditary neuropathy usually requires nerve biopsy for histological evaluation of the nerve; however, neuropathy resulting from porphyria frequently is associated with elevated levels of δ-aminolevulinic acid and porphobilinogen in urine (see Chapter 39). Guillain-Barré syndrome (acute idiopathic demyelinating polyneuropathy) and its chronic form cause weakness and loss of reflexes, with a characteristic CSF finding of elevated protein levels without elevated cell counts. Other causes of neuropathy in which laboratory diagnosis is essential include diabetes (see Chapter 38), hypothyroidism (see below), vasculitis, uremia (see Chapter 30), hepatic dysfunction (see Chapter 31), and heavy metal (arsenic, lead, mercury, and thallium) poisoning (see Chapter 42). Infectious causes of neuropathy include AIDS, Lyme disease, herpes zoster, diphtheria, and leprosy. Amyloidosis causing neuropathy can occur as the result of a plasma cell dyscrasia or hereditary amyloidosis.

Myasthenia gravis is a disorder of the neuromuscular junction in which antibodies are directed against the acetylcholine receptor. Patients have fluctuating weakness that typically affects the face and limbs, as well as eye movements. Approximately 85% of patients with active myasthenia show elevated acetylcholine receptor antibody titers.

Muscular disorders may be hereditary or acquired. Hereditary forms include genetic myopathies, which usually are caused by an abnormal structural protein. Duchenne's muscular dystrophy and Becker's muscular dystrophy are caused by absence or deficiency of dystrophin, which causes progressive destruction of muscle. The serum concentration of creatine kinase (CK) is markedly elevated in these illnesses; levels greater than 10,000 U/L are common. The dystrophin gene is located on the X chromosome. The diagnosis is confirmed by performing DNA studies that reveal a deletion within the dystrophin gene or muscular biopsy that proves absence or reduced dystrophin.

Several familial muscular illnesses, including hyperkalemic and hypokalemic periodic paralysis and myotonia congenita, are caused by abnormalities in ion channels (particularly of sodium and chloride). This group of diseases is characterized by attacks of generalized weakness, dystonia, and elevated or decreased serum potassium concentrations. Myoglobinuria occurs when necrosis of the muscle is acute and myoglobin from muscle escapes into the blood and then into the urine.

Mitochondrial disorders are inherited diseases caused by disturbances in mitochondrial function that produce CNS neurological damage and abnormalities within the muscle. They are characterized clinically by muscle weakness, exercise intolerance, seizures, myoclonus, and stroke. Blood lactate levels are elevated. Muscle biopsy shows "ragged-red fibers," and abnormalities in the mitochondria may be seen under the electron microscope.

Polymyositis and dermatomyositis, termed *inflammatory myopathies,* are believed to be abnormalities of the autoimmune system. Dermatomyositis is an illness in which weakness is associated with a characteristic skin rash. It is the most common form of myositis in childhood. Serum CK concentrations usually are elevated at the range of several hundred to a thousand U/L. Blood tests also provide evidence of an altered immune state with development of unusual antibodies, including Jo-1 antibody and anti-Mi-2 antibody. Muscle biopsy reveals perifascicular atrophy that may be diagnostic. Polymyositis may occur at any age, producing widespread weakness, often more proximally than distally. CK levels may be markedly elevated, and anti-Jo-1 antibodies are found in one-fifth of patients. Muscle biopsy shows muscle fibrosis associated with inflammatory reactions.

Neoplastic and Paraneoplastic Syndromes

Neoplasms that affect the CNS can be present in neural tissue (brain, cranial nerves, spinal cord, or peripheral nerves) or related structures (skull, meninges, blood vessels, pituitary or pineal glands). *Carcinomatous meningitis* refers to invasion of the CSF and meninges by neoplastic cells. If the neoplasm arises directly from these structures, it is termed *primary;* it is termed *metastatic* if it has spread from a neoplasm elsewhere in the body. Symptoms that develop with various types of nervous system tumors are related to the nature of the tumor, its size, and its location. Approximately one-third of patients with cerebral tumors develop seizures.

Paraneoplastic syndromes are neurological disorders associated with cancer, but not caused by direct effects of the tumor mass or its metastases. The presence of antibodies in many patients suggests that immune mechanisms participate in these disorders. The antibodies found in neoplastic syndromes are different from each other but share some common characteristics. Most consist of polyclonal immunoglobulin G (IgG) that fix complement. They react predominantly or exclusively with both target neurological tissue and underlying tumor. Antibodies often are found in a subset of patients with a specific clinical syndrome and a specific tumor. The anti-Yo antibody is found in patients with paraneoplastic cerebellar degeneration and gynecological tumors; the anti-Hu antibody is found in patients with limbic encephalitis, sensory neuropathy, and small cell lung cancer. Anti-Ri antibody is found in patients with opsoclonus-myoclonus syndrome or breast and gynecological cancer. Anti–voltage-gated calcium channel antibody is found in Lambert-Eaton myasthenic syndrome and in small cell lung cancer. These antibodies have proved useful in identifying the presence of a paraneoplastic syndrome, but their sensitivity and specificity for a paraneoplastic syndrome and the accuracy of specific antibodies in identifying a specific syndrome or a specific tumor have not been determined.

Modern imaging techniques such as MRI and computerized tomography (CT) can identify nervous system neoplasms with extraordinary accuracy. Laboratory diagnosis, however, still can prove useful for certain neoplasms. Diagnosis of carcinomatous meningitis is made through examination of the CSF for neoplastic cells. Elevations in CSF β-glucuronidase and carcinoembryonic antigen (CEA) also are found in some cases.

Epilepsy

A seizure is a sudden and transient disturbance of mental function or body movement that results from an excessive electrical discharge by a group of brain cells. Two main types of seizures are known: focal onset and generalized onset. Focal-onset seizures begin in a discrete region of the brain and exhibit varying degrees and patterns of spread. Generalized-onset seizures begin throughout the brain all at once. The clinical manifestations of the seizure depend on the areas of the brain involved. For example, a focal-onset seizure involving the motor cortex may manifest as twitching of one hand, whereas a seizure involving the temporal lobe may result in alteration in consciousness with staring and memory loss (known as a complex partial seizure). Staring spells of generalized onset are known as absence or petit mal seizures. Focal-onset or generalized-onset seizures may spread to involve the entire brain and may cause a generalized tonic-clonic seizure with generalized motor activity, sometimes called a *convulsion,* or a *grand mal seizure.*

Focal-onset seizures usually are caused by some localized abnormality of the brain that may be identified through the use of brain-imaging procedures such as CT or MRI. Frequent causes of focal-onset seizures include stroke, brain tumors, birth injury, and severe head injury. Generalized seizures may be idiopathic (no obvious cause) or symptomatic, resulting from a generalized insult to the brain such as drug overdose, renal failure, encephalitis, or use of illicit drugs. The type and duration of treatment are determined by the seizure type and presumed cause. Each person who has seizures must undergo careful evaluation by a physician who is searching for an underlying cause that can be corrected.

Persons with seizures usually are placed on antiepileptic drugs (AEDs) for months or even for the rest of their lives, in an attempt to stop or at least reduce the frequency of seizures. Once treated, most persons with seizures obtain excellent control and can live normal lives; often, their medication can be stopped after a period of time. However, about 30% to 40% of persons with seizures will obtain inadequate seizure control or will have unacceptable side effects caused by the AEDs.

Intoxication With Drugs and Poisons

Many drugs and poisons affect the nervous system directly, producing confusion, drowsiness, stupor, coma, seizures, or psychotic states (see Chapter 55). Drugs also may cause respiratory depression, may alter the systemic metabolic balance, or otherwise may indirectly damage the nervous system, causing neuropathy or movement disorder. In many cases, the differential diagnosis of these states requires laboratory confirmation of the presence of an offending drug or toxin. When specific drugs are known or suspected to be available to the patient, the search is simplified.

Physical findings may raise suspicion of a certain class of drugs, for example, small pupils are suggestive of the presence of opiates, and widely dilated pupils are suggestive of drugs with atropine-like effects such as tricyclic antidepressants or amphetamines with adrenergic actions. Unfortunately, many cases of intoxication involve multiple substances, whether "street" drugs or medications. In these cases, or when the circumstances surrounding an ingestion are unclear, a toxic screen for common substances is necessary.

Metabolic Diseases

Neurometabolic diseases include (1) acquired or hereditary inborn errors of metabolism related to metabolism of sugar, fat, protein, and nucleic acids; and (2) acquired metabolic disorders related to nutritional deficiency of electrolytes, glucose, and other metabolites. These conditions usually present with episodic confusion, stupor, or coma. Hypercapnia (elevated pressure of CO_2 in the blood) can produce alterations in the level of consciousness. Hypoglycemia can cause CNS symptoms when plasma glucose falls to below 25 to 30 mg/dL (1.4 to 1.7 mmol/L), as may occur with insulin overdose, acute severe alcohol intoxication, and various conditions in children and neonates. Hyperglycemia may cause stupor or coma when severe ketoacidosis or hyperosmolar nonketotic hyperglycemia occurs (see Chapter 38). Hepatic failure can result in impaired consciousness resulting from elevated serum ammonia. Altered consciousness in patients with renal insufficiency may be attributable to uremia or to a disequilibrium syndrome associated with dialysis. Altered consciousness sometimes accompanied by seizures may result from a variety of electrolyte disturbances, including (but not limited to) metabolic acidosis, hypernatremia and hyponatremia, hypokalemia, and hypocalcemia. Deficiencies in nutrients such as thiamine can cause memory dysfunction and eye movement and gait problems; vitamin B_{12} deficiency may cause nerve and spinal cord damage.

Endocrine Diseases

Adrenal Disease

Inadequate release of cortisol affects the brain in ways that are complex and are not well understood. In chronic untreated hypoadrenalism, apathy, **depression,** fatigue, and even mild delirium are common. Stupor and coma usually occur only when there is an abrupt severe worsening of chronic illness, the so-called Addisonian crisis. Other metabolic derangements related to the hypoadrenalism such as hyponatremia, hyperkalemia, hypoglycemia, and hypotension may occur and may produce additional CNS dysfunction.

Excessive glucocorticoid products and administration of steroid medications are associated in some patients with disturbances in mood (e.g., depression, elevation, hypomania), mild confusion, delusions, hallucinations, impaired insight, and grossly inappropriate behavior.

Hypothyroidism

In the fetus and during infancy, hypothyroidism can cause irreversible brain damage and profound mental retardation (cretinism), unless the condition is corrected without delay. Chronic hypothyroidism is associated with depression or lability of mood, listlessness, confusion, and sometimes delusions and hallucinations (see Chapter 49). Peripheral neuropathy and unsteady gait related to impaired cerebellar function also occur together with abnormal deep tendon reflexes. Elevated CSF protein is a common finding in hypothyroidism. Severe hypothyroidism (myxedema coma) may cause decreased body temperature, slowed respiration, and hypometabolism, usually occurring in a setting of chronic hypothyroidism on which some acute event, such as infection, surgery, trauma, or congestive heart failure, is superimposed. Because myxedema coma is rapidly fatal, correct diagnosis and prompt treatment are essential.

Signs of thyroid hypermetabolism (thyrotoxicosis) distinguish the state of thyroid excess that is associated with disturbances in thinking and emotion. Because the clinical appearance of thyroid disease can mimic psychiatric disease or CNS dysfunction, thyroid function tests are frequently ordered from psychiatric and emergency areas of the hospital.

Neuropathic Pain

Neuropathic pain results from damage to, or dysfunction of, the peripheral or central nervous system, rather than from stimulation of pain receptors. Diagnosis is suggested by pain out of proportion to tissue injury, dysesthesia (burning, tingling), and signs of nerve injury detected during neurological examination. Multiple neuropathic pain syndromes have been identified, and the interested reader is referred to resources on the Internet site for the International Association for the Study of Pain (in the bibliography).

Several classes of drugs are moderately effective in treating pain, but complete or near-complete relief is unlikely. Antide-

Table 47-3 Drugs for Neuropathic Pain

Class/Drug	Dose	Comments
Anticonvulsants		
Carbamazepine	200-800 mg daily	Monitor WBCs when starting treatment
Gabapentin	300-3600 mg daily	Preferred drug in this class; starting dose usually 300 mg once/day
Phenytoin (Dilantin)		Limited data; second-line drug
Pregabalin	50-600 mg daily	Mechanism similar to gabapentin
Valproate	250-2000 mg daily	Limited data, but data support use in treatment of headache
Antidepressants		
Amitriptyline	10-25 mg at bedtime	May increase dose to 75-150 mg over 1-2 wk, particularly if significant depression is present; may not need high doses; not recommended for the elderly or patients with a heart disorder because it has strong anticholinergic effects
Desipramine	10-25 mg at bedtime	Usually better tolerated than amitriptyline
Duloxetine	30 mg bid	Usually better tolerated than tricyclic antidepressants
Central α_2-Adrenergic Agonists		
Clonidine	0.1 mg once/day	Also can be used transdermally or intrathecally
Tizanidine	2-20 mg bid	Less likely than clonidine to cause hypotension
Corticosteroids		
Dexamethasone	0.5-4 mg qid	Used only for pain with an inflammatory component
NMDA-Receptor Antagonists		
Memantine	10-30 mg once/day	Limited evidence of efficacy
Dextromethorphan	30-120 mg qid	Usually considered second-line
Oral Na Channel Blockers		
Mexiletine	150 mg once/day to 300 mg q8h	Used only for neuropathic pain For patients with a significant heart disorder, consider cardiac evaluation before the drug is started
Topical		
Capsaicin 0.025%-0.075%	tid	Some evidence of efficacy in neuropathic pain and arthritis
EMLA	tid, under occlusive dressing if possible	Usually considered for a trial if lidocaine patch is ineffective; expensive
Lidocaine	Daily	Available as patch
Other		
Baclofen	20-60 mg bid	May act via GABA receptor Helpful in trigeminal neuralgia; used in other types of neuropathic pain

EMLA, Eutectic mixture of local anesthetics; *GABA,* γ-aminobutyric acid; *NMDA,* *N*-methyl-D-aspartate; *WBC,* white blood cell count.

pressants and anticonvulsants are used most commonly (Table 47-3). Psychological factors must be constantly considered from the start of treatment. Anxiety and depression must be treated appropriately. When dysfunction is severe, patients may benefit from the comprehensive approach provided by a pain clinic.

Opioid analgesics can provide some relief but are less effective for neuropathic-type pain than for acute pain resulting from tissue irritation, impending injury, or actual injury (nociceptives). Adverse effects from these analgesics may prevent adequate pain relief (Table 47-4). Topical drugs and a lidocaine patch may be effective for peripheral syndromes.

Neurogenetics

A neurogenetic disorder is a clinical disease that is caused by a defect in one or more genes that affect the differentiation and function of the neuroectoderm and its derivatives. Genetic findings in various neurogenetic disorders are summarized in Table 47-5. The molecular basis of genetic disorders is discussed more fully in Chapter 52. In many neurogenetic disorders, such as hereditary forms of dystonia, the disease gene has not yet been identified. In these situations, molecular diagnosis relies on indirect approaches based on methods such as analysis of linkage and of allelic association (see Chapter 13).

Table **47-4** Opioid Analgesics Used in Treating Pain

Drug (Trade Name)	Route of Administration	Onset of Action, min	Time to Peak Effect, min
Strong Agonists			
Fentanyl (Sublimaze)	IM	7-15	20-30
	IV	1-2	3-5
Hydromorphone (Dilaudid)	Oral	30	90-120
	IM	15	—
	IV	10-15	30-60
	Sub-Q	30	—
Levorphanol (Levo-Dromoran)	Oral	10-60	90-120
	IM	—	—
	IV	—	60
	Sub-Q	10-60	Within 20
Meperidine (Demerol)	Oral	15	60-90
	IM	10-15	—
	IV	—	30-50
	Sub-Q	1	—
Methadone (Dolophine)	Oral	30-60	90-120
	IM	—	—
	IV	10-20	60-120
Morphine (many trade names)	Oral	—	60-120
	IM	10-30	—
	IV	—	30-60
	Sub-Q	—	—
	Epidural	10-30	20
Oxymorphone (Numorphan)	IM	10-15	30-90
	IV	—	—
	Sub-Q	5-10	15-30
	Rectal	—	—
Mild to Moderate Agonists			
Codeine (many trade names)	Oral	30-40	60-120
	IM	10-30	30-60
	Sub-Q	10-30	—
Hydrocodone (Hycodan)	Oral	10-30	30-60
Oxycodone (Percodan)	Oral	—	60
Propoxyphene (Darvon, Dolene)	Oral	15-60	120
Butorphanol (Stadol)	IM	10-30	30-60
	IV	2-3	30
Nalbuphine (Nubian)	IM	Within 15	60
	IV	2-3	30
	Sub-Q	Within 15	—
Pentazocine (Talwin)	Oral	15-30	60-90
	IM	15-20	30-60
	IV	2-3	15-30
	Sub-Q	15-20	30-60

KEY CONCEPTS BOX 47-2

- Altered metal status can be caused by intracranial bleeding, infectious and inflammatory diseases, reduction in blood flow (ischemia, stroke), neoplasms, and epilepsy (seizures).
- In addition, drugs and toxins and metabolic disorders such as hypoglycemia or hyperglycemia, thyroid disease, and hypoadrenalism can result in altered mental acuity and function.
- Intracranial bleeding or disruption of the meninges can be seen in the presence of RBCs or xanthochromia in CSF.
- Infection can be noted by the presence of WBCs, bacteria, and fungi, as well as by decreased CSF glucose and increased CSF protein.
- Epileptic patients receive antiepileptic drugs that require monitoring of blood levels.

Table 47-5 Genetic Bases of Some Important Neurological Diseases

Syndrome/ Localization	Disease	Locus	Protein	Inheritance	Implication/Mechanism	Chromosome
Dementia	Familial Alzheimer's disease	AD1	Amyloid precursor protein	AD	Proteolysis yields neurotoxic β-amyloid	21
	Creutzfeldt-Jakob disease (prion disease)		Prion protein	AD	Conformational change, protein aggregation	20
Movement disorder	Familial Parkinson's disease	PARK1	α-Synuclein	AD	Major component of Lewy body	4
		PARK5	Ubiquitin carboxyterminal hydrolase L1	AD	Dysfunction of ubiquitin-protease system	4
	Huntington's disease		Huntington's	AD	Expanded CAG repeat, protein aggregation	4
Epilepsy	Juvenile myoclonic epilepsy		GABA A receptor, α_1-polypeptide	AD	Altered function of GABA receptor	5
	Progressive myoclonus epilepsy		Cystatin B	AR	Reduced activity of a protease inhibitor	21
Myelopathy	Hereditary spastic paraplegia	SPG4	Spastin	AD	Putative regulator of microtubule disassembly	2
Anterior horn cell	Familial amyotrophic lateral sclerosis	ALS1	Superoxide dismutase-1	AD	First of seven or more loci for familial ALS	21
Peripheral nerve	Charcot-Marie-Tooth disease (Schwann cell)	CMT1A	Peripheral myelin protein-22	AD	Gene duplication leads to overexpression of pmp-22	17
Neuromuscular junction	Congenital myasthenic syndrome		Acetylcholine receptor, α-subunit	AD	Altered synaptic response to acetylcholine	2
Muscle	Duchenne's muscular dystrophy		Dystrophin	X-LR	Loss of essential membrane-associated protein	X
	Myotonic dystrophy		Myotonic dystrophy protein kinase	AD	Expanded CTG repeat, production of toxic RNA	19

AD, Autosomal dominant; *ALS,* amyotrophic lateral sclerosis; *AR,* autosomal recessive; *X-LR,* X-linked recessive.

SECTION OBJECTIVES BOX 47-3

- Differentiate between the following: schizophrenia, affective disorders, and anxiety disorders.
- Describe the two types of affective disorders, and list two classes of drugs used for treatment.
- Describe two types of anxiety disorders and several drugs used for treatment.

PATHOLOGICAL CONDITIONS: PSYCHIATRIC

Schizophrenia

Description

Approximately 1% of the population is afflicted with the mixed group of chronic psychotic disorders termed **schizophrenia;** these usually start in young adulthood and persist throughout life. Schizophrenia disease patterns include active phases in which illogical thinking, delusions (fixed false beliefs), auditory hallucinations (often with threatening content), and bizarre behavior may be prominent. Because of the chronic nature of the disorder and the frequent gradual decline in the ability of the schizophrenic patient to function appropriately and independently, the cost of care to society is tremendous. In the current classification of psychiatric disorders (*Diagnostic and Statistical Manual of Mental Disorders, Fourth Edition* [DSM-IV]), several subtypes, including disorganized, paranoid, undifferentiated, catatonic, and residual, are described.

Pathophysiology

The cause of this disorder remains unknown; theories involve developmental abnormalities and aberrant neurotransmitter function. In contrast to some forms of psychiatric illness that seem to result from childhood experience and stressful life circumstances, schizophrenia runs in families and has a genetic and a biological basis. Increased production of neurotransmitters in the mesolimbic dopaminergic pathway appears to be correlated with hallucinations and delusions (referred to as positive symptoms), whereas decreased production in the mesocortical dopaminergic pathway is postulated to be associated with withdrawn, asocial behavior (referred to as negative symptoms) and a gradual decline in function in patients with chronic schizophrenia. Supporting this concept is the observation that at postmortem examination, the neurons of substantial numbers of patients with chronic schizophrenia have an increased number of dopamine-related postsynaptic receptors.

Treatment

Antipsychotic drugs ameliorate and stabilize schizophrenic disorder; however, these medications do not cure the disease and typically must be taken on a lifelong basis. The mechanism by which these medications act on schizophrenic symptoms is poorly understood, but all share the blockade and antagonism of dopamine receptors to a variable extent. The antipsychotics (also known as neuroleptics) available for the past 50 years are now known as conventional antipsychotics. Conventional agents probably are effective because of blockade of dopamine receptors, but they also may cause adrenergic and cholinergic blockade that leads to sedation, orthostatic hypotension, dry mouth, urinary retention, and constipation.

The conventional agents primarily block dopamine D1 receptors, which produce unwanted muscular side effects and probably cause tardive dyskinesia, a chronic movement disorder that begins after some period of use of the antipsychotics. These side effects include muscle stiffness and rigidity, often in the jaw. Patients who take these medications may appear to have Parkinson's symptoms such as difficulty initiating movement and a masklike face. Tardive dyskinesia often involves dystonic movements of the mouth and tongue. Another dangerous side effect is the neuroleptic malignant syndrome, which if untreated can be lethal; it is characterized by mental status changes, fever, muscle rigidity, elevated white blood cell count, and elevated CK levels. Some of the typical antipsychotics (haloperidol and fluphenazine) are available in injectable depot forms that are effective for up to 4 weeks after a single injection.

The neuroleptic agents known as atypical antipsychotics, are designed to block dopamine D2, D3, and D4 receptors. By avoiding D1 blockade, these atypical agents rarely cause side effects and seem much less likely to cause tardive dyskinesia. The atypical antipsychotics affect serotonin receptors, which confer effectiveness in treating depressive and anxiety symptoms. They also block histamine receptors, which may cause weight gain and sedation.

Affective Disorders

Description

The **affective disorders** are diseases of mood regulation. Clinical symptoms may include depression, **mania** (abnormally elevated mood), or **bipolar affective disorder** (mood alternating between depression and mania). Depression may be seen in **unipolar affective disorder** or bipolar affective disorder and is accompanied by changes in neurovegetative functions such as sleep, appetite, motivation, psychomotor regulation, and energy, as well as distinct cognitive effects with loss of concentration and capacity to make decisions. Major depression causes loss of enjoyment of one's usual activities, feelings of worthlessness, and severe hopelessness that may lead to suicidal thoughts or actions. Major depression or bipolar depression may be accompanied by psychotic symptoms such as hallucinations and delusions, often of a persecutory nature. Dysthymic disorder is a milder form of depression that is chronic, lasting at least 2 years; cyclothymia refers to a milder form of bipolar mood swings that are not as severe as those seen in bipolar affective disorder.

Major depression and bipolar affective disorder tend to run in families and have a genetic and biological basis, whereas dysthymia and cyclothymia may result from stressful life events and from maladaptive behavior. Evidence from epidemiological studies in which identical twins were compared with fraternal twins suggests a substantial genetic background for many psychiatric illnesses.

Pathophysiology

The monoamine theory of depression states that depression results from deficits in norepinephrine, serotonin, or dopamine, or all three. The first available treatments for depression were the tricyclic antidepressants, compounds that enhance synaptic activity of both serotonin and norepinephrine within the central nervous system. Norepinephrine affects mood, cognition, sexual function, sleep, and attention via projections from an area of norepinephrine neurons in the brain stem to the frontal cortex. Depressed patients have been shown to have abnormally low levels of CSF norepinephrine and urinary MHPG, half of which has its origin from central nervous system norepinephrine metabolism. Patients with decreased urinary MHPG excretion often respond to antidepressants that selectively inhibit the reuptake of norepinephrine into the presynaptic neuron. As a consequence of this reuptake inhibition, more norepinephrine is available in the synaptic cleft to act on the postsynaptic receptor, thereby correcting the central norepinephrine deficiency.

Evidence for the role of serotonin in depression comes from numerous reports of diminished quantities of its metabolite, 5-HIAA, in the cerebrospinal fluid of depressed patients; furthermore, 5-hydroxytryptophan (5-HT), a precursor of serotonin, is an effective antidepressant only in depressed patients with decreased cerebrospinal fluid 5-HIAA.

Treatment

Although tricyclic antidepressants and monoamine oxidase inhibitors are very effective, these medications cause significant unwanted side effects such as dizziness, constipation, dry mouth, increased sweating, and tachycardia. Tricyclics can be dangerous in patients with coronary artery disease because they can cause arrhythmias and are fatal in overdose. First-line treatment of depression now is provided with the selective serotonin reuptake inhibitors (SSRIs), which include fluoxetine (Prozac), sertraline, paroxetine, fluvoxamine, and citalopram. These medications work by blocking reuptake of serotonin on the presynaptic side of the synapse, leading to

Table 47-6 Site of Action of Some Antidepressants

	REUPTAKE BLOCKADE		*RECEPTOR BLOCKADE*		
	NE	**5-HT**	**Muscarinic ACh**	**H1**	**H2**
Imipramine	+	+	++	±	±
Desipramine	+++	±	±	–	–
Trimipramine	±	±	++	++	?
Amitriptyline	±	++	+++	++	++
Nortriptyline	++	±	+	±	±
Protriptyline	+++	±	+	+++	–
Amoxapine	++	±	+	±	?
Doxepin	+	±	++	+++	+
Maprotiline	+++	–	+	±	?

From Kaplan H, Sadock B: *Clinical Psychiatry,* Baltimore, 1988, Williams & Wilkins.
ACh, Acetylcholine; *H,* histamine; *5-HT,* 5-hydroxytryptophan; *NE,* norepinephrine.

increased available serotonin in the synaptic cleft. The subsequent generation of antidepressants includes the serotonin and norepinephrine reuptake inhibitors, or SNRIs, agents that affect reuptake of both monoamines. These include venlafaxine, nefazodone, and mirtazapine. Bupropion is the only agent currently used that seems to affect dopamine transmission, as well as that of norepinephrine (Table 47-6).

The tricyclics include amitriptyline, nortriptyline, imipramine, desipramine, protriptyline, and clomipramine. These agents variably bind to presynaptic and postsynaptic noradrenergic and serotoninergic receptors within the synaptic cleft. The mechanism of action of these medications appears to involve competitive blockade of these receptors, which become unavailable for binding to norepinephrine and serotonin, resulting in increased availability of neurotransmitter. Antidepressant drugs that are relatively selective in terms of inhibition of neuronal reuptake of norepinephrine include desipramine, protriptyline, and the tetracyclic maprotiline. Pharmacological agents such as amitriptyline, trazodone, and clomipramine, which are effective in the treatment of depression, have been shown to inhibit selectively the neuronal reuptake of 5-HT from the synapse.

The monoamine oxidase inhibiters work by irreversibly inhibiting cytoplasmic monoamine oxidase A and B in the presynaptic neuron, thus inhibiting the breakdown of norepinephrine, serotonin, and dopamine. This inhibition takes place within 5 to 10 days after medication is started and makes additional neurotransmitter available for neuronal transmission (see later discussion).

Lithium, which has nonspecific membrane-stabilizing properties, remains the first-line treatment for bipolar disorder that includes episodes of euphoric mania, called bipolar type I. Psychiatrists increasingly recognize the existence of other forms of bipolar illness, including bipolar type II, which is characterized by episodes of severe depression alternating with mild mania or hypomania and spells of irritability and anger. Valproate (Depakote), an antiepileptic medication with mood-stabilizing properties, is now the first-line treatment for this form of bipolar disorder and for bipolar disorder that primarily manifests as depression. Carbamazepine (Tegretol and others) is another antiepileptic drug that is effective in mania.

Anxiety Disorders

Description

Anxiety disorders are defined as pervasive chronic or paroxysmal feelings of apprehension that often are accompanied by physical signs such as dizziness, sweating, shortness of breath, increased heart rate, tingling or numbness of the mouth or extremities, and agitation or restlessness.

The spectrum of anxiety disorders includes generalized anxiety disorder, which is chronic rather than experienced as spells. Generalized anxiety disorder frequently disrupts the individual's capacity to fall asleep, because it involves excessive worrying and tension. Panic disorder is defined as circumscribed anxiety attacks that may occur at any time, including on awakening from sleep. Patients with panic disorder often have such fear that another attack will occur that they may have difficulty leaving their homes, or agoraphobia. Obsessive-compulsive disorder is characterized by obsessions, pervasive ruminative worries, often quite implausible (such as fearing that one's environment is somehow contaminated by blood), and compulsions, or repetitive acts meant to undo the obsessive fear (such as repeatedly washing one's hands to overcome the imagined contamination). The obsessions and compulsions are beyond the person's ability to control, but both are responsive to behavioral desensitization treatment. Phobias are irrational fears of specific places, objects, or activities, such as heights, elevators, snakes, insects, or driving on highways. Some phobias involve social activities such as speaking, eating, writing, or using the bathroom in public.

Pathophysiology

The pathophysiological characteristics of anxiety disorders are poorly understood at the present time, and a variety of biological, genetic, and behavioral theories have been put forth.

Research into neurotransmitter systems is focused on the noradrenergic, serotonergic, and GABA-ergic systems.

Treatment

As with depression, first-line pharmacological treatment for the anxiety disorders now consists of the SSRIs, because these are effective and safe. Serotonergic medications are uniquely effective for obsessive-compulsive disorder, which does not respond to noradrenergic antidepressants like the tricyclics, with the exception of clomipramine, which has prominent serotonergic activity.

Generalized anxiety disorder and panic disorder also respond to drugs that affect the noradrenergic system and downregulate its activity. Such drugs consist of beta-adrenergic receptor blockers, tricyclic antidepressants, monoamine oxidase inhibitors, and benzodiazepines, in addition to the SSRIs. Benzodiazepines bind to specific receptor sites throughout the brain and spinal cord. These binding sites are coupled with a GABA-benzodiazepine receptor complex that mediates the anxiolytic, sedative, and antiepileptic actions of these agents. Because of the potential for tolerance and addiction, the benzodiazepines should not be considered first-line treatment for the anxiety disorders.

KEY CONCEPTS BOX 47-3

- Schizophrenia is associated with delusional, often hallucinogenic, behavior. Haloperidol and fluphenazine are used in treatment.
- Depression, mania, and bipolar disorder are the primary affective disorders. The tricyclic antidepressants and serotonin reuptake inhibitors are used to treat depression. Mania may be treated with carbamazepine, and bipolar disorders can be treated with lithium and antiepileptics.
- Anxiety disorders, such as panic and obsessive-compulsive disorders, can be treated with serotonin reuptake inhibitors.

SECTION OBJECTIVES BOX 47-4

- Correlate CSF glucose, total protein, IgG, IgG index, lactic acid levels and the presence or absence of xanthochromia with CNS disease.
- Explain the significance of xanthochromia in CSF.
- Explain the clinical utility of CSF total protein determinations, increased or decreased IgG index, and performing CSF electrophoresis for oligoclonal bands.
- Explain the clinical utility of CSF glucose determinations.
- Describe the conditions under which a CSF glucose measurement will be useful, as well as when a serum TSH may be useful, and when a urine tox screen may be useful.

CHANGE OF ANALYTE IN DISEASE: NONDRUG ANALYTES (Table 47-7)

Appearance of Cerebrospinal Fluid

CSF is normally crystal clear and free from all pigmentation, that is, "clear and colorless." CSF should be examined in a clear tube together with a tube of water, comparing both tubes in white light against a pure white background. It is best to look down the long axis of the tube. At least 1 mL of fluid should be observed.

An RBC of $500/mm^3$ gives a pink or yellow tinge to the fluid. WBCs of $200/mm^3$ produce a slightly cloudy appearance. Xanthochromia (a yellow tinge) will appear when blood has been mixed with CSF. The xanthochromia does not occur immediately but requires from 2 to 4 hours for the hemoglobin to be degraded. The appearance of xanthochromia after RBCs mix with CSF is directly dependent on the amount of RBC contamination and the length of time that the RBCs are in contact with the CSF. A "traumatic" lumbar puncture occurs when the lumbar puncture needle pierces small blood vessels near the spinal cord coverings, and blood enters the CSF collection tubes. Because blood in the CSF may represent subarachnoid bleeding or simply may result from a traumatic

Table 47-7 Change of Analyte in CNS Disease

	ANALYTE IN CNS					
Disease	Glucose	Total Protein	IgG	IgG Index	Xanthochromia	Lactic Acid
Stroke (cerebral infarction)	N	↑	N	↓	N, ↑	N, ↑
Hemorrhage	N	N, ↑↑	N	N	↑↑	N
Epilepsy	N	N	N	N	N	N
CNS tumor	N, ↓	↑	N, ↑	↓	N, ↑	N, ↑
Infection						
Fungal	↓	↑	↑	↑	N	↑
Viral	N	N	↑	↑	N	N
Coma	↑↑ hyperosmolar ↓ hypoglycemia	↑ (trauma)	N	N	N, ↑ (trauma) N	N
Meningitis, viral	N	N, ↑	N, ↑	↑	N	N

N, Little or no change; ↑, increase; ↑↑, large increase; ↓, decrease.

lumbar puncture (a common occurrence), the CSF sample should be centrifuged immediately. If this is done promptly, bleeding that is caused by a traumatic lumbar puncture should produce no xanthochromia. Xanthochromia indicates that bleeding may have occurred at least 2 to 4 hours before the sample was observed. As many as 10% of patients with subarachnoid hemorrhage actually have clear CSF at 12 hours, but beyond that time, 100% will show xanthochromia if the sample is examined carefully. A more sensitive technique, such as second-derivative spectrophotometry, can enhance the ability to detect low levels of xanthochromia.

Protein concentrations greater than 150 mg/dL also produce a slightly xanthochromic appearance in CSF. When a patient is jaundiced (i.e., when serum bilirubin is elevated, as it may be in liver failure), bilirubin may enter the CSF. However, this requires serum bilirubin levels of at least 10 to 15 mg/dL before CSF xanthochromia is found.

Proteins of Cerebrospinal Fluid

In disease states, local production or modification of proteins within the CNS may lead to diagnostically useful changes in CSF protein patterns. In general, diseases that interrupt the integrity of the capillary endothelial barrier may cause an increase in total CSF protein. Examples include brain tumor, purulent (bacterial) meningitis, cerebral infarction, and trauma.

Immunoelectrophoresis allows further fractionation of CSF protein constituents. The major immunoglobulins in CSF include IgG, IgA, and IgM (with only trace amounts of IgD and IgE). Of all these, IgG is quantitatively the most important. It often is useful for the clinician to know whether an elevated IgG value is caused by local production of that immunoglobulin within the CNS (as may be the case in some demyelinating diseases such as multiple sclerosis) or by the leakage of IgG across a damaged blood-brain barrier (as in some infections). Because normal serum IgG represents 15% to 18% of total serum protein, and because normal CSF IgG consists of only 5% to 12%, the ratio of IgG to total protein sometimes is used to estimate the source of IgG elevation, that is, if the ratio in a sample more nearly approximates the ratio ordinarily found in serum, it is more likely that IgG somehow has been transferred into the CSF from serum. But this is a crude and not especially reliable estimate. A more widely used measure used currently is the IgG-albumin index. The formula for determining it is as follows:

$$\text{IgG index} = \frac{\text{IgG (CSF)} \times \text{Albumin (serum)}}{\text{IgG (serum)} \times \text{Albumin (CSF)}}$$

The upper reference interval for this index must be determined for each laboratory, but generally it ranges between 0.25 and 0.85. The **IgG index** is elevated in diseases in which CNS IgG production is increased and the blood-brain barrier is intact (as in multiple sclerosis). The IgG index is decreased when the blood-brain barrier is compromised, allowing serum proteins to cross into the CSF (as in stroke, tumors, and some forms of meningitis).

An increase in myelin basic protein (MBP) concentration in serum is a potential indicator of demyelination. Myelin is a complex substance that surrounds many CNS axons and is similar to the insulation on a wire cable; it is necessary for normal conduction of nerve impulses down the axon.

Demyelinating diseases comprise a group of disorders in which the primary insult is some form of damage to the myelin coating of CNS axons. MBP, a constituent of normal myelin, has been found to be elevated in a variety of conditions involving myelin damage. Initially, it was believed that MBP was specific for multiple sclerosis, but now it is known to be elevated in many CNS disorders.

γ-Globulin Synthesis

Elevations of CSF γ-globulin may be caused by changes in serum proteins, such as the small-molecular-weight Bence Jones proteins seen in multiple myeloma, which cross the blood-brain barrier and appear in the gamma fraction of CSF proteins. However, evidence indicates that local CNS immunoglobulin production occurs in many diseases. Examples include multiple sclerosis, subacute sclerosing panencephalitis (a rare devastating process of myelin damage that occurs in children and young adults in association with greatly elevated CSF measles titers), many chronic and acute infections (neurosyphilis, tuberculous meningitis, abscess, viral meningoencephalitis, and sarcoidosis), and some brain tumors. As a practical point, in those settings in which CSF total protein rises as a result of increased permeability of the blood-brain barrier, the addition of serum protein (which normally contains 15% to 18% γ-globulin) raises the CSF γ-fraction. It thus becomes difficult to estimate the upper reference interval for γ-globulin as a percentage of total protein when total protein is significantly elevated. In any case, when CSF γ-globulin is elevated, a clinician may order a simultaneous serum protein electrophoresis to help determine the source of the increased CSF γ-fraction.

Oligoclonal Bands

The gamma fraction of CSF is composed of a variety of immunoglobulins. Electrophoresis performed on concentrated CSF combined with immunospecific staining for IgG molecules can demonstrate elevation of a population of proteins within the γ-range. When these proteins all share the same electrophoretic mobility, they are called *oligoclonal bands.* The population of γ-proteins that separates as oligoclonal bands is believed to derive from a few clones of immunocompetent cells. The appearance of oligoclonal bands has been reported in 79% to 90% of patients with multiple sclerosis and in a variety of CNS inflammatory conditions. It is interesting to note that this change in composition of the γ-fraction may occur with no increase in total γ-globulin concentration.

It is important to remember that when blood is present in the CSF as the result of a traumatic lumbar puncture or bleeding within the nervous system, it is expected that the contaminating blood will elevate the CSF protein value. One still can determine the CSF protein level by correcting for the amount of blood present. This can be corrected by subtracting

1 mg/dL of protein for every 1000 RBCs per mm^3. The cell count should be performed as rapidly as possible after lumbar puncture, preferably in the first half hour and certainly not later than 2 hours, because hemolysis will occur after that time.

Glucose in Cerebrospinal Fluid

Determination of CSF glucose helps distinguish bacterial from viral meningitis; the glucose value is often low (less than 40% to 45% of simultaneously analyzed serum glucose) in bacterial meningitis and tuberculous meningitis and generally is normal in viral disease. Carcinomatous meningitis (widespread infiltration of the meninges by tumor cells) also drives CSF glucose values to below the normal range.

Thyroid Function Tests

Diseases of the thyroid gland can result in changes in mood that are difficult to distinguish from psychiatric illness. Therefore, as part of the diagnostic evaluation of patients newly admitted to psychiatric wards, thyroid tests are ordered to rule out thyroid imbalance as a cause (see p. 966 for recommended thyroid testing).

Toxicology Screen

One of the causes of abnormal behavior is the presence of drugs or toxins in the affected patient. A urine drug screen frequently is ordered by emergency unit physicians to establish drugs as a cause of acute psychosis. These tests usually are focused on searching for a limited number of abused stimulant drugs, such as amphetamines, cocaine, and phencyclidine. Less frequent causes of abnormal behavior or neurological symptoms result from heavy metal poisoning. In these cases, analyses of blood lead and urine mercury may be requested.

KEY CONCEPTS BOX 47-4

- Xanthochromia can be detected in stroke, hemorrhage, and brain trauma.
- Increased CSF protein can be associated with stroke, hemorrhage, and brain infection. The IgG index, which measures serum and CSF IgG and albumin levels, can be used to help differentiate among some of these disorders.
- Oligoclonal IgG fractions are associated with multiple sclerosis and CNS inflammatory disease.
- Low CSF glucose is associated with CNS infections and brain tumors.
- A urine tox screen that demonstrates the presence of particular drugs can explain the altered behavior of a patient.

SECTION OBJECTIVES BOX 47-5

- Describe the primary basis for measuring the blood level of a drug used to control a psychiatric disorder.
- List the classes of drugs used to treat psychiatric disorders that require blood monitoring.

CHANGE OF ANALYTE IN DISEASE: THERAPEUTIC DRUG MONITORING

Therapeutic drug monitoring (TDM) is essential for the optimal management of many neurological and psychiatric disorders. The clinician can more readily assess efficacy, toxicity, drug interactions, and the effect of generic substitution when the plasma concentration of the drug is known (see Chapter 14). Measurement of non–protein-bound plasma concentrations of drugs or measurement of active drug metabolites can further refine patient management.

Antiepileptic Drugs

Among neurologists, measurement of plasma concentrations of AEDs is probably the most widely used laboratory test. Table 47-8 presents pharmacokinetic data on the most commonly used AEDs. The "therapeutic range" is an important concept that should be used only as a general guide in patient management. Measurement of AED plasma concentration is indicated to check for compliance if a patient continues to have seizures despite taking the drug, and it is helpful if the patient reports side effects of the medication.

Plasma concentrations of AEDs should always be interpreted within a few weeks of the start of treatment, to ensure that the drug has reached a steady-state concentration, especially with AEDs that have a longer half-life (see Table 47-8). AEDs with a shorter half-life (valproate or carbamazepine) may show substantial variation between peak and trough concentrations. Plasma concentrations of carbamazepine may fall after the first 2 to 3 weeks of use because of the drug's induction of liver enzymes that speed its metabolism.

Measurement of non–protein-bound (free) AED plasma concentrations is useful in patients who receive phenytoin or valproate in combination with other drugs, in patients with renal or hepatic failure, and in those with hypoalbuminemia. In these instances, the free plasma drug concentration may increase and produce toxic symptoms, while the total plasma concentration remains unchanged. Active metabolites of primidone, carbamazepine (especially carbamazepine 10,11-epoxide), and possibly valproate can produce toxicity, and measurement of these metabolites may improve patient management in selected cases.

The most serious side effects associated with ADEs include liver failure, aplastic anemia, bone marrow suppression, and osteoporosis. Monitoring of liver function tests, blood cell counts, and bone densitometry on a regular basis (before drug therapy is started, and then every 6 months, especially during the first year, or when the patient develops related symptoms) is required to detect any subtle changes requiring subsequent adjustment of the medication.

The new generations of AEDs; gabapentin, topiramate, tiagabine, lamotrigine, levetiracetam, oxcarbazepine, pregabalin, and zonisamide; have fewer side effects and drug-drug interactions, making them likely to be well tolerated by the patient.

Table 47-8 Commonly Used Antiepileptic Drugs

Antiepileptic Drug	Trade Name	Recommended Therapeutic Range, mg/mL*	Approximate Time to Steady State, Days	Protein Binding	Other
Phenytoin	Dilantin	10-20	3-21[†]	High	
Carbamazepine	Tegretol Carbatrol	4-12	3-5	Medium	Active metabolite (10-11 epoxide)
Primidone	Mysoline	5-12	1-2	Low	Metabolized to PEMA and phenobarbital
Phenobarbital		10-40	15-25	Low	
Valproate/Divalproex	Depakene Depakote	50-120	2-5	High	Saturable protein binding
Ethosuximide	Zarontin	40-100	7-13	Low	
Felbamate	Felbatol	30-60	4-5	Low	Associated with aplastic anemia and hepatic failure
Gabapentin	Neurontin	2-10	1-2	None	Not liver metabolized
Topiramate	Topamax	5-20	4-5	Low	
Tiagabine	Gabatril	NE	1-2	High	
Lamotrigine	Lamictal	2-20	4-5	Low	Concentrations increased 2-fold when used with valproate
Levetiracetam	Keppra	5-30	1-2	None	Not liver metabolized
Oxcarbazepine	Trileptal	4-12	2-3	Low	Rapidly metabolized to active compound
Pregabalin	Lyrica	NE	1-2	None	No liver metabolism
Zonisamide	Zonegran	10-40	10-15	Low	

NE, Not established; *PEMA,* phenylethylmalonamide.
*See text under "Antiepileptic Drugs."
†Exhibits saturable metabolism, so time to steady state increases as plasma concentration increases.

Antipsychotic Drugs

Antipsychotics, also known as neuroleptics, comprise a heterogeneous group of medications used to treat psychosis associated with schizophrenia, depression, dementia, and nonspecific agitation. They also may be useful in a variety of movement disorders such as Huntington's disease, tic disorders, and Tourette's syndrome. Neuroleptics include the drug class phenothiazines, all of which share the three-ring phenothiazine structure but differ in terms of side-chain varieties.

Clozapine (a dibenzodiazepine), quetiapine (a dibenzothiazepine), olanzapine (a thienobenzodiazepine), risperidone (a benzisoxazole), and ziprasidone (a benzothiazolylpiperazine) are atypical compounds used in the United States. None of these medications require therapeutic blood levels for effective dosing, but patients receiving clozapine are followed through bimonthly CBC and WBC counts because of the risk of aplastic anemia associated with this compound.

Another major group of neuroleptics includes the butyrophenones such as droperidol, haloperidol, and pimozide, which have structures dissimilar to those of the phenothiazines. At present, haloperidol is the most widely prescribed conventional neuroleptic in the United States. Atypical antipsychotics, with their lower risks for extrapyramidal syndrome (EPS) and tardive dyskinesia (TD), soon may replace conventional antipsychotics in the treatment of most patients.

No correlation has been noted between blood concentrations of neuroleptic drugs and clinical response.

It has been suggested that a plasma level of 5 to 20 ng/mL is the optimal therapeutic window for haloperidol treatment of psychotic symptoms and schizophrenia. Haloperidol levels above 20 ng/mL are linked to subjective and objective medication side effects such as dysphoria, hypotension, and parkinsonian effects, which may inhibit a therapeutic response. In clinical practice, blood concentrations of neuroleptics are rarely obtained.

Antidepressant Drugs

The selective serotonin reuptake inhibitors include fluoxetine, sertraline, paroxetine, fluvoxamine, and citalopram. The norepinephrine-serotonin reuptake inhibitors include venlafaxine, mirtazine, and nefazodone. The only dopaminergic antidepressant is bupropion. Typical doses and side effects of these medications are listed in Table 47-9. Therapeutic drug monitoring is not typically useful with these medications. The possibility exists for interactions based on cytochrome P-450 enzyme subtypes used to metabolize each drug. For instance, the competition for SSRI metabolism by CYP 3A4 means that if tricyclics are used concurrently, blood concentrations of the tricyclics will be elevated by as much as 50%. Blood monitoring is not necessary as a rule, but clinicians must be alert to reported side effects and must use caution when giving tricyclics to any patient with compromised myocardium.

Tricyclic Antidepressants

Apart from reuptake blockade of serotonin and norepinephrine, the tricyclic antidepressant medications block

Table 47-9 Antidepressant Medications

Medication	Typical Dose Range, mg	Dosing	Common Side Effects
Fluoxetine	5-80	qd, usually AM	Insomnia, agitation in patients with anxiety, emotional blunting
Paroxetine	5-80	qd, usually HS	Sedation, possible weight gain
Sertraline	12.5-250	qd	± Agitation in anxious patients
Fluvoxamine	25-300	qd, usually HS	Insomnia or sedation
Citalopram	10-80	qd	Sedation
Venlafaxine, extended release	37.5-375	qd, usually AM	Sweating, insomnia, early nausea
Bupropion, sustained release	100-450	bid, 2nd dose before 6 PM	Agitation, insomnia, no antianxiety effect
Nefazodone	50-600	bid, although may be given HS only	Agitation (mCPP metabolite may be anxiogenic) or sedation
Mirtazapine	15-90	qhs	Sedation, weight gain
Tricyclics (imipramine, clomipramine, desipramine, amitriptyline, nortriptyline)	10-150 for nortriptyline, 10-300 for all others	qd, usually HS	Dry mouth, increased heart rate, orthostatic hypotension, dizziness, constipation, increased sweating, blurred vision, weight gain
Monoamine oxidase inhibitors	30-60 for Parnate 60-90 for Nardil	tid	Dry mouth, blurred vision, constipation, weight gain, orthostatic hypotension Hypertensive crisis if combined with tyramine-containing foods or serotonergic/stimulant medications
Trazodone	25-600	qhs	Sedation Often used as hypnotic in subtherapeutic doses

HS, Bedtime dosing.

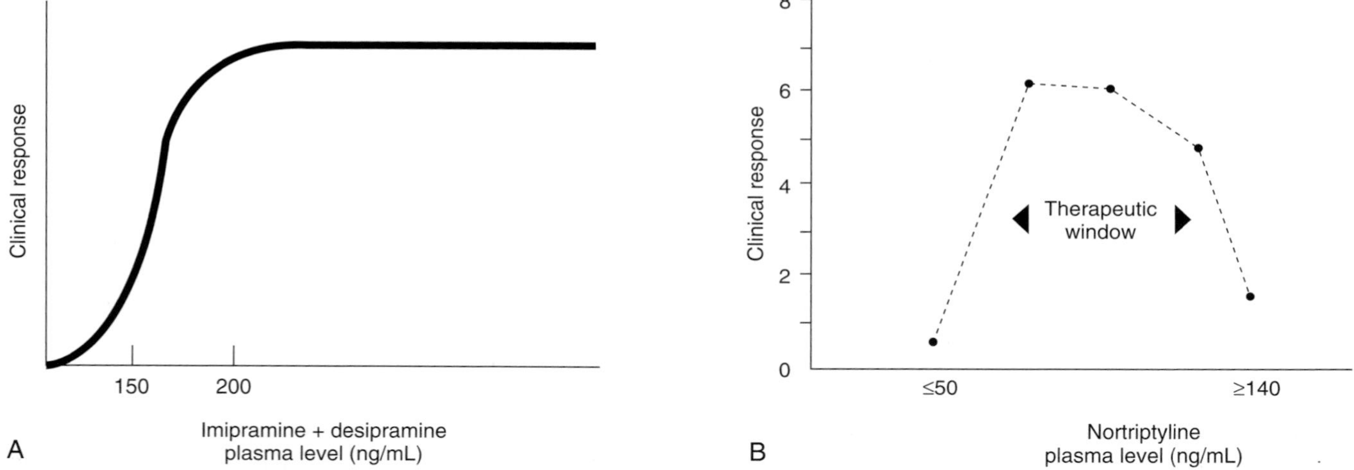

Fig. 47-6 A, Sigmoidal relationships between clinical response and imipramine plus desipramine plasma levels. **B,** Curvilinear relationship between clinical response and nortriptyline plasma levels. (From Schatzberg AF, Cole JO: *Manual of Clinical Psychopharmacology,* Washington, DC, 1986, American Psychiatric Press.)

α-adrenergic, muscarinic, and histaminic receptors to variable degrees, resulting in medication side effects such as orthostatic hypotension, dry mouth, constipation, and sedation (see Table 47-9). Tricyclic antidepressants are absorbed from the gastrointestinal tract to a variable and incomplete degree. Protein binding appears to occur at a rate of 75%, and the medications are highly lipid soluble. In the liver, tertiary amines (amitriptyline and imipramine) are desmethylated to secondary amines (nortriptyline and desipramine) that are active metabolites. Half-lives are between 10 hours and 70 hours and can be even longer, as with nortriptyline and protriptyline. Steady-state plasma levels are achieved within 5 to 7 days, and once-a-day dosage is possible.

The dosage for most tricyclic antidepressants usually ranges between 50 and 300 mg/day, depending on age, body weight, and liver and renal function. Notable exceptions include nortriptyline and protriptyline, both of which have dosage requirements between 50 and 150 mg/day. The linkage between plasma levels of tricyclics and their clinical response appears clearest in patients with major depression. For most tricyclic antidepressants, the relationship between response and plasma level appears sigmoidal (Fig. 47-6, *A*). Yet, for nortriptyline and to a lesser extent protriptyline, the relationship is curvilinear, and when plasma levels are above the therapeutic range, clinical response falls dramatically and side effects are more prominent (Fig. 47-6, *B*).

Monoamine Oxidase Inhibitors

Two classes of monoamine oxidase inhibitors (MAOIs) are known: the hydrazine class, which includes isocarboxazid and phenelzine, and the nonhydrazine class, which includes tranylcypromine. The clinical effects of these and other antidepressant medications take 2 to 3 weeks to develop for reasons that are not understood. MAOIs are completely absorbed in the gastrointestinal tract and are metabolized in the liver by acetylation. The half-life is extremely variable because up to 50% of Caucasians and more than 50% of people of Asian descent are slow acetylators. Dosage ranges from 30 to 60 mg/day for isocarboxazide and tranylcypromine, and from 45 to 90 mg/day for phenelzine.

The side effects and dietary restrictions required for patients receiving the MAOIs have limited use of this class of drug. Tyramine, which usually is broken down in the gastrointestinal tract by monoamine oxidase A, must be eliminated from the diet; otherwise rapid and dangerous elevation of blood pressure can occur. Tyramine is found in large quantities in cured foods such as beer, wine, cheese, and sausage. Another factor that limits the use of MAOIs is the potential for dangerous interactions with other antidepressants. MAOIs cannot be used concurrently with the SSRIs, nefazodone, venlafaxine, mirtazapine, or bupropion. If these drugs are being used, they must be tapered off before MAOI treatment is started. This is not a serious problem for drugs with shorter half-lives, but the long half-life of fluoxetine means that the patient must be off fluoxetine for at least 4 weeks before beginning an MAOI. Tricyclics can be combined with the MAOIs, typically with the tricyclic started first and the MAOI added. No relationship has been established between MAOI plasma level and response rate.

Anxiolytics

As was mentioned above, the SSRI and SNRI medications, as well as the tricyclics and MAOIs, all are effective anxiolytics, and the newer agents now are used as first-line treatment for the anxiety disorders. The benzodiazepines and buspirone sometimes are used as sole treatment for anxiety disorders, but they are used more commonly as adjunctive treatment for anxiety, affective, and psychotic disorders. Benzodiazepines also are given to aid in alcohol withdrawal.

All benzodiazepines share the same three-ring structure but differ mainly in substitutions on the heptagonal ring. Three subgroups have been established: (1) the 2-ketobenzodiazepines, including chlordiazepoxide, diazepam, and prazepam, which are oxidized in the liver to desmethyldiazepam (active metabolite) with a half-life of 60 hours; (2) the 3-hydroxybenzodiazepines (oxazepam, lorazepam, and temazepam), which are metabolized in the liver with a half-life of 9 to 15 hours; and (3) the triazolobenzodiazepines (alprazolam and triazolam), which are metabolized in the liver with a 3- to 8-hour half-life. Oxazepam is the safest benzodiazepine to use in patients with liver disease, because it is excreted by the kidney after glucuronidation.

The most common side effects include sedation at low doses, ataxia at higher doses, and respiratory suppression at toxic doses. Generally, it is believed that these drugs have a wide safety margin, and overdose only rarely leads to lethal outcome. The benzodiazepine antagonist flumazenil can be used acutely in benzodiazepine overdose.

Maximum doses for the individual benzodiazepines differ widely, ranging from 6 mg/day for alprazolam to 200 mg/day for chlordiazepoxide. In contrast to other psychiatric medications discussed in this section, benzodiazepines have potentially strong addictive properties, causing psychological and physical drug dependence and possible withdrawal upon cessation of the drug. Therapeutic plasma concentrations of benzodiazepines have not been established, except for clonazepam, which also is used as an antiepileptic.

Apart from the benzodiazepines, buspirone is the other commonly used class of anxiolytics. It is a nonbenzodiazepine, nonsedating anxiolytic. This drug probably does not act directly through the GABA receptor complex. It is believed that dopaminergic pathways might mediate its anxiolytic effects. Daily dosage ranges from 5 to 40 mg. Side effects upon use include nausea and headaches. Plasma levels are not in use at the present time.

Mood Stabilizers

This group of drugs includes lithium carbonate, carbamazepine, valproate, olanzapine, lamotrigine, gabapentin, and topiramate. Their therapeutic use in psychiatry involves the treatment of bipolar disorder, schizoaffective disorder, intermittent explosive disorder, post-traumatic stress disorder, and unstable behavior related to personality disorder.

Physiologically, lithium ions are indistinguishable from sodium, and they replace sodium along cell membranes. The exact mode of lithium action is unknown. Because lithium replaces sodium throughout the whole body, its side effects may involve most organ systems. Neurological effects such as tremor, ataxia, confusion, sedation at higher and toxic levels, and encephalopathy in conjunction with haloperidol administration have been described. Long-term lithium treatment can result in hyperthyroidism from a nontoxic goiter. Renal effects such as polyuria with secondary polydipsia, renal diabetes insipidus, and interstitial nephritis are seen occasionally.

Dosage ranges from 600 to 2100 mg/day in two or three divided doses. Plasma levels should be measured approximately 12 hours after the previous dose to obtain a trough value. Plasma levels from 0.8 to 1.5 mEq/L have been shown to produce a therapeutic response in the treatment of acute mania. Slightly lower lithium levels have been recommended for maintenance treatment of bipolar disorders and treatment of other conditions. The maintenance plasma level of lithium often is limited by subjective side effects and by the development of thyroid or renal impairment. Lithium is used frequently in conjunction with other mood stabilizers in patients with severe forms of bipolar disorder.

Carbamazepine, valproate, lamotrigine, gabapentin, and topiramate are used as antiepileptics but also are used increasingly in psychiatry for disorders such as rapid cycling bipolar disorder, depressed bipolar disorder, and intermittent explosive disorder. Although these medications may be used in addition to lithium and can be used in combination with one another, only valproate and carbamazepine are recommended for use as first-line medications for mood stabilization; lamotrigine is recommended for first-line treatment of bipolar depression.

Dosage and plasma level ranges, particularly for valproate and carbamazepine, are similar to those that apply when they are used as antiepileptics, although few available data correlate plasma concentrations of antiepileptic drugs with psychiatric efficacy.

KEY CONCEPTS BOX 47-5

- Measurement of blood levels of a drug requires that a known relationship has been established between drug concentration and the clinical effect (therapeutic or toxic) of that drug.
- Commonly measured drugs used to treat psychiatric disorders include the tricyclic antidepressants, antiepileptics (phenytoin, carbamazepine, phenobarbital, valproate, etc.), and lithium.

BIBLIOGRAPHY

Addington J, Cadenhead KS, Cannon TD, et al: North American prodrome longitudinal study: a collaborative multisite approach to prodromal schizophrenia research, Schizophrenia Bulletin 33:665, 2007.

American Psychiatric Association: *Diagnostic and Statistical Manual of Mental Disorders, Fourth Edition, Text Revision (DSM-IV-TR),* Washington, DC, 2004, American Psychiatric Publishing.

Berrettini WH: Are schizophrenic and bipolar disorders related? A review of family and molecular studies, Biol Psychiatry 48:531, 2000.

Bhugra D: The global prevalence of schizophrenia, PLoS Med 2005. Available at http://www.pubmedcentral.nih.gov/articlerender.fcgi?artid=1140960.

Blackwood DHR, Visscher PM, Muir WJ: Genetic studies of bipolar affective disorder in large families, Br J Psychiatry 178(suppl 41): s134, 2001.

Bremner JD, Narayan M, Anderson ER, et al: Hippocampal volume reduction in major depression, Am J Psychiatry 157:115, 2000.

Davis KL, Charney D, Coyle JT, et al, editors: *Neuropsychopharmacology,* Philadelphia, 2002, Lippincott, Williams & Wilkins.

Fishman RA: *Cerebrospinal Fluid in Diseases of the Nervous System,* Philadelphia, 1980, Saunders.

Gabbard GO, editor: *Gabbard's Treatments of Psychiatric Disorders,* ed 4, Washington, DC, 2007, American Psychiatric Publishing.

Garvey M, Rubeis R, Hollon S, et al: Response of depression to very high plasma levels of imipramine plus desipramine, Biol Psychiatry 30:57, 1991.

Graves P and Sidman R. *Xanthochromia is not pathognomonic for subarachnoid hemorrhage. Acad Emerg Med* Feb; 11:131-135, 2004.

Kaplan H, Sadock B: *Synopsis of Psychiatry,* ed 9, Baltimore, MD, 2003, Williams and Wilkins.

Kendler KS, Thornton LM, Gardner CO: Genetic risk, number of previous depressive episodes, and stressful life events in predicting onset of major depression, Am J Psychiatry 158:582, 2001.

Pesce AJ, Kaplan LA: *Methods in Clinical Chemistry,* electronic version 5.2, Cincinnati, 2006, Pesce Kaplan Publishers.

Posner JB, Saper CB, Schiff N, et al: *Plum and Posner's Diagnosis of Stupor and Coma,* ed 4, New York, 2007, Oxford University Press.

Privitera MD, Cavitt J, Ficker DM, et al: *Clinician's Guide to Antiepileptic Drug Use,* Philadelphia, 2006, Lippincott, Williams & Wilkins.

Rowland LP, editor: *Merritt's Textbook of Neurology,* ed 9, Philadelphia, 1994, Williams & Wilkins.

Sanchez-Juan P, Green A, Ladogana A: CSF tests in the differential diagnosis of Creutzfeld-Jakob disease, Neurology 67:637, 2006.

Seeman P, Weinshenker D, Quirion R, et al: Dopamine supersensitivity correlates with D2 high states, implying many paths to psychosis, Proc Natl Acad Sci U S A 102:3513, 2005.

Stahl SM, Stahl SM: *Stahl's Essential Psychopharmacology: Neuroscientific Basis and Practical Applications,* Cambridge, 2005, Cambridge University Press.

Stanley B, Molcho A, Stanley M, et al: Association of aggressive behavior with altered serotonergic function in patients who are not suicidal, Am J Psychiatry 157:609, 2000.

Thapar A, Harold G, Rice F, et al: The contribution of gene-envionment interaction to psychopathology, *Developmental Psychopathology* 19(4):989-1004, 2007.

Tsuang MT, Taylor L, Faraone SV: An overview of the genetics of psychotic mood disorders, J Psychiatry Res 38:3, 2004.

Yoshimura R, Nakamura J, Shinkai K, et al: Clinical response to antidepressant treatment and 3-methoxy-4-hydroxyphenylglycol levels: mini review, Prog Neuropsychopharmacol Biol Psychiatry 28:611, 2004.

INTERNET SITES

http://www.iasp-pain.org/AM/Template.cfm?Section=General_Resource_Links&Template=/CM/HTMLDisplay.cfm&ContentID=3058

http://www.anzca.edu.au/resources/books-and-publications/acutepain_update.pdf

http://faculty.washington.edu/chudler/introb.html#dr

http://emedicine.medscape.com/article/286342-overview—Soreff S, Bipolar affective disorder

General Endocrinology

Gregory A. Clines and Laurence M. Demers

48 Chapter

Chapter Outline

Key Terms

acromegaly A pathological state in adults that is associated with hypersecretion of growth hormone.

adenohypophysis The anterior lobe of the pituitary gland, which secretes trophic hormones.

amenorrhea The absence of a menstrual cycle and menstrual period.

autocrine factor A cellular factor that interacts with receptors found on the same cell that released the factor.

bioavailable hormone A hormone in the circulation, whether free or weakly bound to plasma proteins, that is available for tissue receptor binding and cell uptake.

Cushing's disease A pathological state that is associated with excessive pituitary secretion of adrenocorticotropic hormone (ACTH).

cytokines Peptides synthesized and released by white blood cells and tissue macrophages that stimulate or suppress the functional activity of lymphocytes, monocytes, neutrophils, fibroblast cells, and endothelial cells.

endocrine gland A specialized gland that releases hormones into the circulation, thereby affecting a tissue or an organ at a distal site.

feedback loop A loop that integrates the functions of two endocrine glands by means of a positive or negative hormone signal.

galactorrhea Uncontrolled secretion of fluid from the breast.

G-protein A regulatory protein found in the membrane of all mammalian cells that acts to transmit an extracellular hormone signal to inner membrane factors as part of a cell membrane transduction signaling system.

hormone A chemical substance released by an endocrine gland into the circulation.

hormone transport The mechanism by which hormones are carried in the bloodstream, bound to protein carriers.

intracrine factor A cytosolic factor made by a cell that travels to the nucleus and binds to a specific receptor on DNA to regulate gene activity.

juxtacrine factor A membrane-bound growth factor that interacts with the membrane receptor of a neighboring cell via direct cell-to-cell contact.

neurohypophysis The posterior part of the pituitary gland that is an extension of the central nervous system.

paracrine factor A factor that is released by one cell within a tissue and binds to receptors of a different cell within that same tissue.

peptide hormones Hormones that are made from amino acids by specialized endocrine glands and are released into the circulation to interact with membrane-bound receptors of other tissues and organs.

pituitary adenoma A tumor of the pituitary that produces excessive amounts of a particular pituitary hormone.

pituitary portal circulation The vascular channel that connects the hypothalamus with the anterior pituitary.

pulsatile release The release of hypothalamic and pituitary hormones in short bursts, or pulses, during the course of a 24-hour day. The amplitude and frequency of the pulse are unique to each hormone.

receptors Specific cytosolic and membrane proteins that bind a hormone or growth factor with high specificity and affinity.

releasing factors Peptides synthesized by the hypothalamus and released into the pituitary portal circulation to affect pituitary hormone synthesis and secretion.

steroids Hormones that are made by endocrine glands from cholesterol and that have as a basic structure the cyclopentanophenanthrene nucleus.

Methods on Evolve

Adrenocorticotropic hormone (ACTH)
Aldosterone
Beta-hCG (beta-human chorionic gonadotropin)
Catecholamines
Cortisol
Dehydroepiandrosterone and its sulfate (DHEA and DHEA-S)
Estradiol
Follicle-stimulating hormone (FSH)
Insulin and C-peptide
Luteinizing hormone (LH)
Parathyroid hormone (parathyrin) (PTH)
Progesterone
Prolactin
Renin
Testosterone
Thyroid hormones: T3 uptake, thyroxine (total), thyroxine free and free triiodothyronine
Thyroid-stimulating hormone (TSH)

SECTION OBJECTIVES BOX 48-1

- List the chemical types of hormones and their modes of action.
- Describe the mechanisms of action of steroid and peptide hormones.
- Describe the regulatory control of hormone biosynthesis and release, especially the concept of feed-back control.
- Describe mechanisms for controlling the availability of free hormones.

FUNDAMENTALS OF ENDOCRINOLOGY

The endocrine system comprises part of the extracellular communication system within the body that links the brain to organs and functions that control body metabolism, growth and development, and reproduction. The other two major components of this communication system, the central nervous system and the immune system, also are linked to the endocrine system as part of the brain's overall control of bodily function. The endocrine system itself functions through an elaborate network of chemical messengers called **hormones** that are produced by highly specialized endocrine organs. The location of the endocrine glands is shown in Fig. 48-1. Hormones enter the circulation to exert their action at a site usually distant from the site of production. Hormones interact with specific receptors within or on the target cell, conferring the selectivity of hormone action. The traditional definition of endocrinology, that is, the study of hormone action distal to the site of hormone production, has become obscured in recent years because we now recognize the important local, or autocrine, effects of hormone metabolism and action within a given **endocrine gland** or tissue. In addition, many growth factors produced locally by specific cells elicit a network of cellular communication akin to the hormone receptor interactive event. Many of the biological effects of hormones are produced at the target site through local metabolism of hormone precursor substances. The local biosynthesis of estrogen from steroid precursor substrates such as androstenedione and the formation of triiodothyronine from T_4 are examples of local hormone synthesis at the target cell.

Control of the endocrine system is affected primarily by its linkage to the central nervous system through the hypothalamus and pituitary glands. This aspect of the endocrine system is referred to as the neuroendocrine system and involves an intimate relationship between neurosecretory chemicals formed in the brain and hormonal factors produced by the endocrine organs located within the brain. It now is evident that the immune system also acts at nerve centers of the brain to facilitate the orchestration of hormone signals, both positive and negative, through the elaboration of a network of **cytokine** factors produced by endocrine tissues and immunocompetent cells that reside in the brain.

The Chemical Nature of Hormones

Hormones are divided into basically two broad classes: peptides and steroids. Most hormones are amino acid and peptide in nature, ranging from complex carbohydrate–polypeptide molecules, such as human chorionic gonadotropin, to single amino acid moieties such as the catecholamines. **Steroids** all are derived from cholesterol and are subdivided into two types: those containing an intact cyclopentanophenanthrene

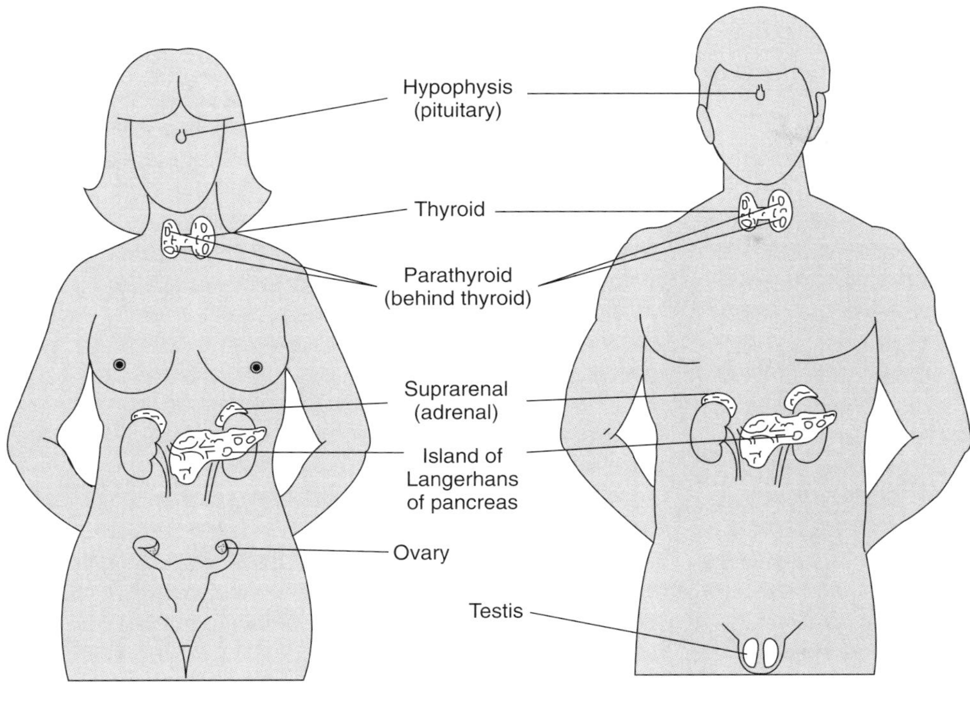

Fig. 48-1 Location of endocrine glands. (From Toporek M: *Basic Chemistry of Life*, St. Louis, 1980, Mosby.)

nucleus, such as adrenal and gonadal steroids, and those such as vitamin D that have an alteration in the B ring of the basic phenanthrene nucleus. It is the chemical makeup of the hormone that is integral to its ability to interact with a specific tissue-based receptor to bring about hormone action. For example, the simple lack of a methyl group between the A and B rings of a steroid molecule, along with a saturated A ring, determines the difference between a female steroid hormone such as estradiol and the male hormone testosterone. It is this subtle chemical difference and the presence of highly specific protein receptors in tissues that allow the hormone to recognize a particular tissue or organ and invoke its biological effect. A list of the major peptide and steroid hormones and their primary sites of action is shown in Table 48-1.

Mechanisms of Hormone Action

All hormones act on their respective target glands and tissues through highly specific binding proteins, called **receptors,** located on the surface of the cell membrane or within the cytosol of the target cell. The binding of a hormone to its specific receptor serves as an initial signal to a cell. An amplification of the signal then ensues, involving many intermediate messenger signals. These signals ultimately influence the nucleus of the target cell to elicit an alteration in gene expression, resulting in the synthesis of a specific mRNA message and new protein synthesis. Figs. 48-2 and 48-3 provide examples of hormone binding and the mechanism of hormone action as they currently are understood.

Steroid Hormones

All steroid hormones interact with their target cells by binding to specific protein receptors located in both the cytoplasmic and nuclear fractions of the cells (see Fig. 48-2). Each steroid-responsive tissue contains a finite concentration of receptor protein with an affinity constant that is greater than that of other steroid binders such as the transport proteins. Transport proteins, which are found in the circulation, carry steroids from the organ of synthesis to the target organ or tissue. The higher affinity of the receptor protein enables the tissue to sequestrate a specific steroid from the hormone's specific carrier protein as the tissue is perfused with blood that contains the circulating steroid.

Steroids enter the cell primarily through diffusion, bind to the receptor molecule, and produce a conformational change in the receptor structure. This conformational change in the receptor activates the receptor complex, forming a transformed receptor-steroid activated complex. This complex has a high affinity for nuclear binding sites on chromatin and binds to both regulatory and nonregulatory DNA sequences in the 5-prime end of the responsive gene element. Binding of the transformed receptor-steroid complex to the regulatory elements of the gene leads to gene activation and subsequent synthesis of specific proteins. The net result is altered cell metabolism, which can lead to cell growth and differentiation and the secretion of specific cell products. All steroid hormones interact with their receptor complexes in a similar fashion. Thus the interaction is much the same for a cortisol-activated event as it is for estrogen that acts to promote uterine cell growth.

Although we speak of cytosol receptors for steroids, it is important to understand that thyroid hormone also exerts its biological effect through a cytosol-receptor complex with translocation of the complex to the nucleus in a fashion similar to that of the steroid hormones. For certain malignacies, tissue steroid receptor levels are measured so the clinician can determine the appropriate course of treatment. In the case of breast

Table 48-1 Steroid and Peptide Hormones

Hormone	Source	Target Organ	Circulating Level	Biological Effect
Steroid Hormones				
Androgens				
Testosterone (dihydrotestosterone)	Testis	Accessory sex glands	3 to 10 ng/mL	Male, secondary sex characteristics, protein anabolism
DHEAS (dehydroepiandrosterone sulfate)	Adrenal	Liver, fat tissue	1500 to 4000 ng/mL	Androgen substrate
Estrogens				
Estradiol	Ovary	Accessory sex glands, liver, brain	50 to 300 pg/mL	Female, secondary sex characteristics
Estriol	Fetal placental unit	Liver, uterus	<1 to 30 μg/mL	Pregnancy hormone
Estrone	Ovary, fat tissue	Accessory sex glands	50 to 200 pg/mL	Estradiol substrate
Progesterone	Ovary	Uterus, breast, brain	5 to 20 ng/mL	Pregnancy hormone
Adrenal Steroids				
Cortisol	Adrenal	Liver, muscle, brain, fat tissue	50 to 250 μg/L	Gluconeogenesis, immune system control
Aldosterone	Adrenal	Kidney	50 to 300 ng/L	Salt homeostasis
Peptide Hormones				
Anterior Pituitary				
TSH (thyroid-stimulating hormone)	Anterior pituitary	Thyroid gland	0.4 to 4.0 μU/mL	Biosynthesis of thyroid hormones
ACTH (adrenocorticotropic hormone)	Anterior pituitary	Adrenal	25 to 80 pg/mL	Biosynthesis of adrenocortical hormones
FSH (follicle-stimulating hormone)	Anterior pituitary	Ovary/testis	5 to 20 mIU/mL	Follicular development, ovary and sperm formation, testis
LH (luteinizing hormone)	Anterior pituitary	Ovary/testis	5 to 25 mIU/mL	Corpus luteum, ovary, Leydig cell, testis
Prolactin	Anterior pituitary	Mammary gland, uterus, ovary, testis	5 to 20 ng/mL	Mammary gland development, ovary and testis steroid production
GH (growth hormone)	Anterior pituitary	All tissues	2 to 5 ng/mL	Tissue growth, fat and carbohydrate metabolism
Posterior Pituitary				
AVP (arginine vasopressin)	Posterior pituitary	Kidney	2 to 8 pg/mL	Water homeostasis
Oxytocin	Posterior pituitary	Breast, uterus	1 to 5 pg/mL	Milk secretion, uterine contractility
Gonadal Hormone				
Inhibin	Granulosa cells, Sertoli cells	Anterior pituitary	Men: 50 to 300 pg/mL Women: 40 to 400 pg/mL	Inhibition of FSH secretion
Calcitropic Hormones				
PTH (parathyroid hormone)	Parathyroid	Bone, kidney, intestine	10 to 55 pg/mL	Calcium homeostasis
Calcitonin	Thyroid	Bone	0 to 50 pg/mL	Calcium regulation
Pancreatic Hormones				
Insulin	Pancreas	Most tissues	6 to 25 μU/mL	Carbohydrate metabolism
Glucagon	Pancreas	Liver	50 to 100 pg/mL	Glycogenolysis
Gastrointestinal Hormones				
Gastrin	Stomach	Stomach	30 to 150 pg/mL	Acid secretion
Secretin	Small intestine	Stomach, pancreas	0 to 50 pg/mL	Stomach and pancreatic fluid secretion
VIP (vasoactive intestinal polypeptide)	GI tract, pancreas, lung	GI tract	0 to 75 pg/mL	GI tract secretion and sphincter relaxation
Adipose Tissue Hormone				
Leptin	Fat cells	Brain, other tissues	0.7 to 18.3 ng/mL	Reduced food intake
Thyroid Hormones				
T_4 (thyroxine)	Thyroid	All tissues	4 to 12 μg/dL	Basal metabolism
T_3 (triiodothyronine)	Thyroid	All tissues	80 to 220 ng/dL	Basal metabolism

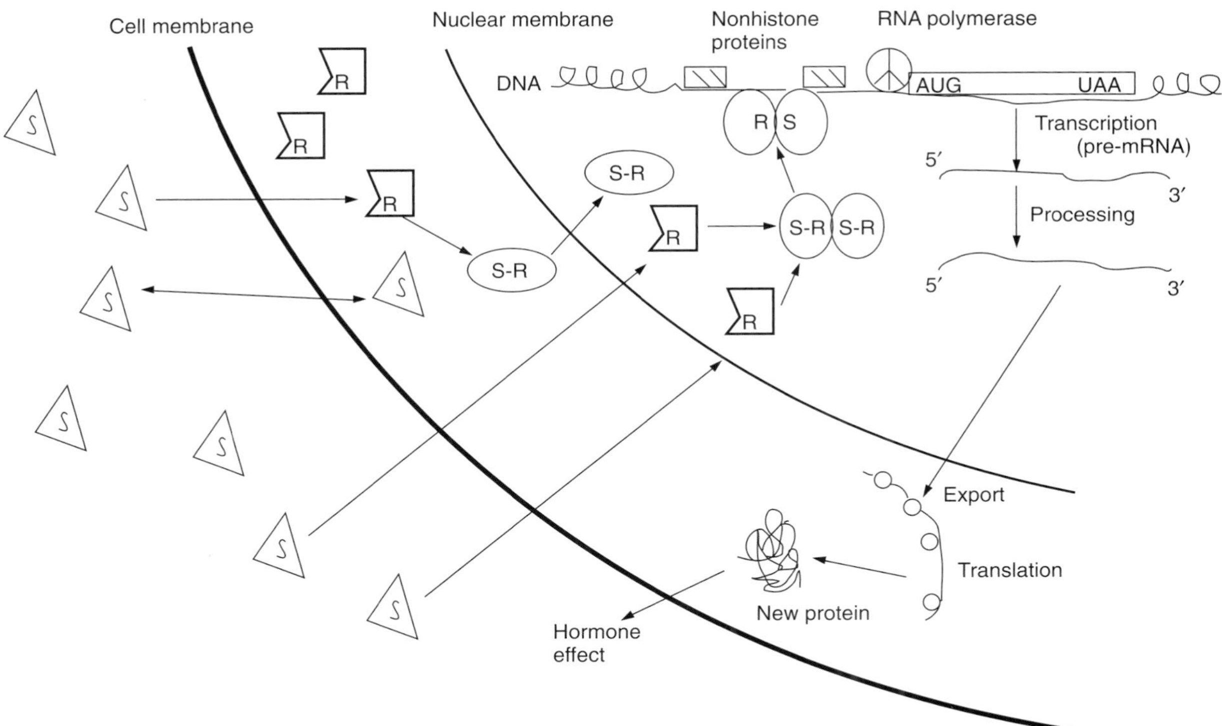

Fig. 48-2 Current proposed mechanism of action of steroid hormones (estrogens, androgens, progesterone, glucocorticoids, aldosterone). Steroids (S) diffuse across the plasma membrane and bind to a cytosolic or nuclear protein receptor (R). Steroid binding activates the receptor complex (S-R), which then translocates to the nucleus of the cell, where it interacts with chromatin at a specific binding site on DNA called the *steroid response element*. This binding activates the transcription of specific genes involved in steroid hormone action. Transcription of messenger RNA then takes place with the eventual synthesis of specific proteins by cells that are linked to steroid hormone action.

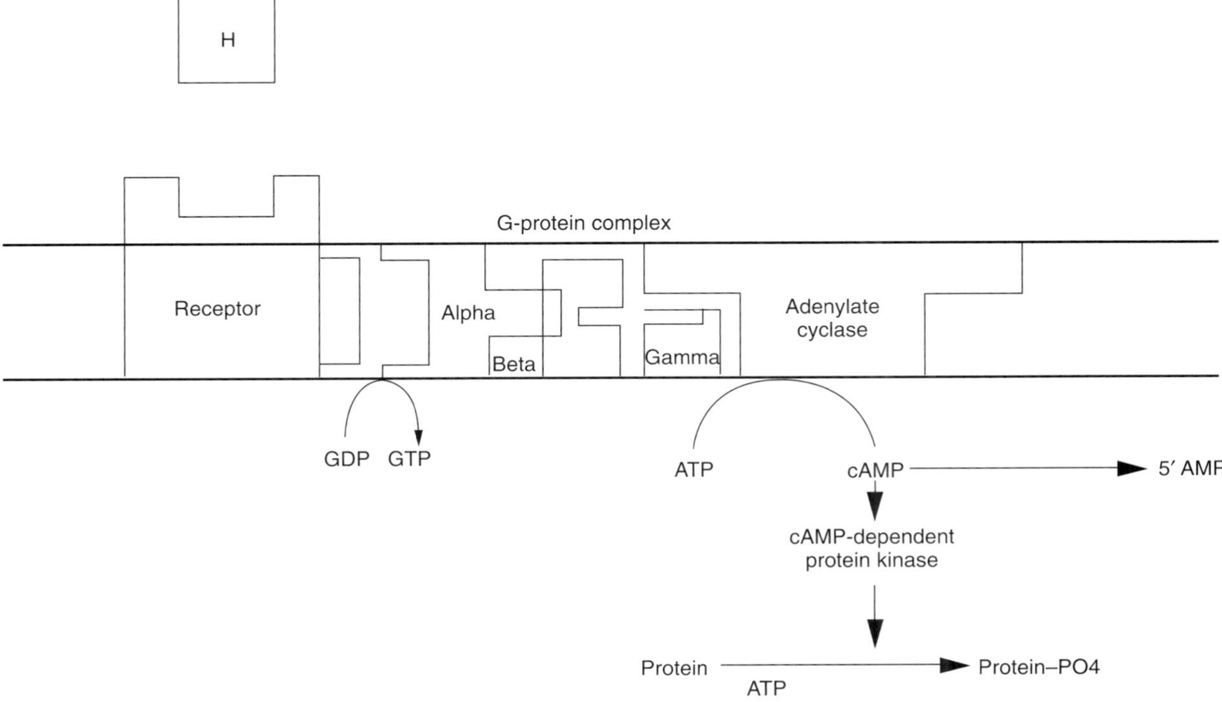

Fig. 48-3 Current proposed mechanism of action of peptide hormones. Peptide hormones bind to a specific receptor on the external domain of the plasma membrane. Hormone binding causes activation of a G-protein complex in the cell membrane that is coupled to and activates the enzyme adenylate cyclase. When the catalytic component of adenylate cyclase is activated, adenosine triphosphate (ATP) is converted into cyclic adenosine monophosphate (cAMP), which in turn activates cAMP-dependent protein kinase, resulting in protein phosphorylation and expression of the peptide hormone effect.

cancer, estrogen and progesterone tissue receptor levels are important prognostically, and they facilitate categorization of the subtype of breast cancer. Normal breast tissue contains very small quantities of estrogen and progesterone-receptor proteins. Certain forms of breast cancer demonstrate an increase in the level of breast tissue steroid-receptor protein. These breast cancers are termed hormone dependent. They require a particular modality of antihormonal therapy for the patient. Hormone ablative therapy (reduction of hormone levels) thus becomes an alternative means of chemotherapy for the patient. This therapy is based on the use of drugs that inhibit the binding of estrogen to its receptor or inhibit the biosynthesis of estrogenic hormones. Thus measurement of breast tissue steroid-receptor protein content has proved to be an important clinical tool in categorizing the subtype of hormone-dependent breast cancer and in facilitating the selection of appropriate antihormonal therapy.

Peptide Hormones

Peptide hormones interact with cellular receptors located on the surface of the cell membrane, in contrast to the intracellular cytoplasmic receptors, which bind steroid and thyroid hormones. The receptor protein for peptide hormones comprises three areas, or domains: an extracellular hormone-binding domain, a transmembrane spanning domain, and the intracellular kinase domain. The receptor mechanism located within the cell membrane appears to be much more complex than the cytosolic-based receptor mechanism. The signaling mechanism involved with peptide hormone-receptor interaction includes intracellular postreceptor cascade events that involve multiple effector systems such as the cyclic nucleotides, arachidonic acid metabolites, G-proteins, and inositol phospholipids. These signaling systems act as secondary messengers that transmit the signal of the initial receptor-hormone interaction to other areas of the cell. In many cases, when the hormone binds to the extracellular domain of the membrane-bound receptor, a membrane-bound intermediate signal is activated that translates the signal to an intracellular event. This membrane-bound signal transducer is often a guanine nucleotide–binding regulatory protein **(G-protein).** The G-protein is coupled to the adenylate cyclase and phospholipase enzyme systems that activate subsequent intracellular protein kinases to transmit the biological response. Some receptor systems contain the effector component as part of the intrinsic structure of the receptor. Most of the growth factors, such as insulin, insulin-like growth factor, and epidermal growth factor, interact with a surface receptor that has inherent protein tyrosine kinase enzyme activity within the intracellular domain of the receptor. An example of the G-protein–membrane receptor complex and the activation sequence by a peptide hormone is shown in Fig. 48-3.

Regulatory Control of Hormone Synthesis and Release

Feedback Control Mechanism

A unique feature of the endocrine system is its ability to regulate itself by providing negative- or positive-feedback stimuli to each gland that produces a secretory hormone. All hormone production comes under some form of feedback control. A "feedback" control system requires two production units, in which the product of one unit directly affects production of the other unit. The products of the two units make up the two halves of a continuous **feedback loop.** The product of one unit usually causes the second unit to increase production of its product. The second unit's product "feeds back" to the original unit to control the output of that unit. Most often, the feedback is negative, that is, the product of the second gland causes a decrease in hormone release from the first gland. This negative-feedback loop, in turn, results in diminished stimulation of the second gland. Under normal physiological conditions, the overall effect of the two parts of the feedback loops within the endocrine system is to maintain relatively constant levels of circulating hormones.

Hormone feedback to the hypothalamic-pituitary axis from endocrine glands is the most well-known feedback loop; however, other feedback loops are known to be involved in endocrinology, for example, calcium feedback to the parathyroid glands to reduce parathyroid hormone (PTH) secretion and glucose feedback control of pancreatic insulin secretion. When endocrine feedback control is studied, however, the paradigm is usually the hypothalamic-pituitary-endocrine gland axis (Fig. 48-4). Hormone output from a target endocrine gland, such as the thyroid gland, the adrenal gland, or the gonads, is controlled primarily by negative feedback to the hypothalamus and the pituitary, which maintain central nervous system (CNS) control over the circulating level of each gland's hormone. When circulating hormone levels decline, the hypothalamus rapidly senses the decline in hormone output and increases its production of hypothalamus-based **releasing factors** that enter the **pituitary portal circulation** in the brain to stimulate pituitary hormone synthesis and secretion and reestablish normal hormone output. This stimulus is termed a positive-feedback loop. Conversely, when hormone output from the endocrine gland becomes excessive, high levels of circulating hormone provide negative feedback to the hypothalamic-pituitary axis, thereby reducing the synthesis of hypothalamic releasing factors and hence pituitary hormone secretion. Reduced pituitary secretion leads to a reduction of the original stimulus of the target glands, to maintain hormone levels.

Negative-feedback control predominates in endocrinology, although positive feedback is also important. An example of positive feedback is the ovarian estradiol-pituitary positive-feedback event, which occurs at the midpoint of the monthly menstrual cycle, during which ovarian estradiol stimulates the ovulatory surge of pituitary gonadotropin release. The surge of pituitary gonadotropins stimulates further estradiol production; this positive-feedback loop continues until the ovary releases an ovum reducing estradiol output.

Each target organ controls its own biosynthetic rate and promotes the synthesis of hormone when needed through attenuation of the negative-feedback loop that decreases hypothalamic-pituitary secretions. Examples of the feedback and stimulus loops that tie the hypothalamic-pituitary axis to

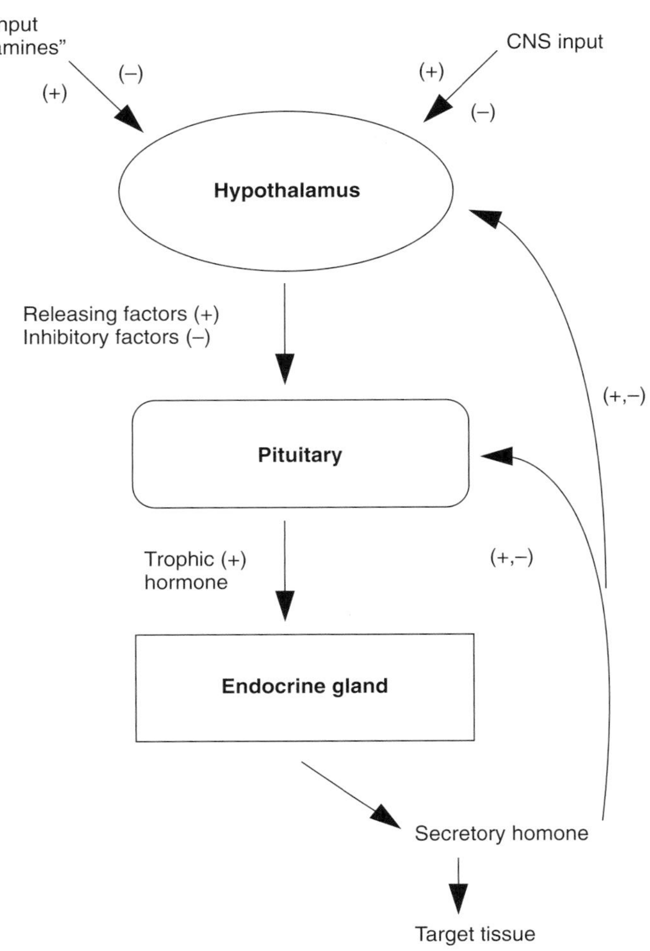

Fig. 48-4 Regulatory feedback loops of the hypothalamic-pituitary–target organ axis. The hypothalamus receives neural and sensory input to produce pituitary hormone–releasing and inhibitory peptides and factors. The pituitary responds by releasing trophic hormones that act on specific endocrine glands or tissues to promote primary gland hormone synthesis and release. The secretory hormone from the endocrine organ negatively feeds back to the higher centers of control to maintain a homeostatic balance of hormone in the circulation.

the primary endocrine organ or tissue are shown in Figs. 48-5 through 48-9.

The hypothalamic and pituitary hormones are secreted in cyclical patterns that vary in duration. Studies in recent years have focused on the pulsatile and circadian release of pituitary hormones. It now is evident that virtually all hypothalamic and pituitary hormones are synthesized and released in a minute-to-minute pulsatile fashion. For example, in both men and women, pituitary release of FSH and LH occurs every 30 to 40 minutes as a consequence of the **pulsatile release** of gonadotropin-releasing hormone (GnRH) from the hypothalamus.

Overlaying this shorter, pulsatile cycle, pituitary hormone secretion also exhibits a cyclical change in secretion rates that occurs over a 24-hour period, termed a *circadian rhythm*. The frequency and magnitude of circadian release are different among the individual pituitary hormones. For example, in the case of pituitary adrenocorticotropic hormone (ACTH) secretion, a characteristic circadian rhythm occurs during the course of the 24-hour day, with much higher output in the early morning hours that reaches a nadir around midnight. Growth hormone output exhibits increased amplitude and frequency during periods of rapid eye movement (REM) sleep, a period from about midnight to 4 AM. In women, there is the added factor of menstrual cyclicity of the pituitary reproductive hormones, luteinizing hormone (LH), and follicle-stimulating hormone (FSH), which occurs over the course of a 30-day menstrual cycle (see Chapter 50). Pulsatility and variable hormone secretory behavior are important considerations for the interpretation of circulating levels of hormones within the context of normal biological rhythms.

Control of Hormone Availability

Hormones are potent, biologically active compounds. The physiological activity of hormones is controlled by changing their rates of synthesis and release. In addition, however, two other mechanisms act by limiting the availability of hormones after they have been released into the circulation. These mechanisms are rapid catabolism (breakdown) and sequestration.

Catabolism-Peptide Hormones

Except for the thyroid hormones, peptide and amino acid–derived hormones are water soluble and are found free in plasma. However, rapid catabolism of these hormones to inactive compounds by tissue and plasma enzymes reduces the availability of the original intact hormone and gives it a relatively short half-life. For example, PTH is released from parathyroid glands as an 84-amino acid, intact peptide. Within a few minutes, it is acted upon by proteolytic enzymes in the circulation, to reduce this hormone to inactive fragments.

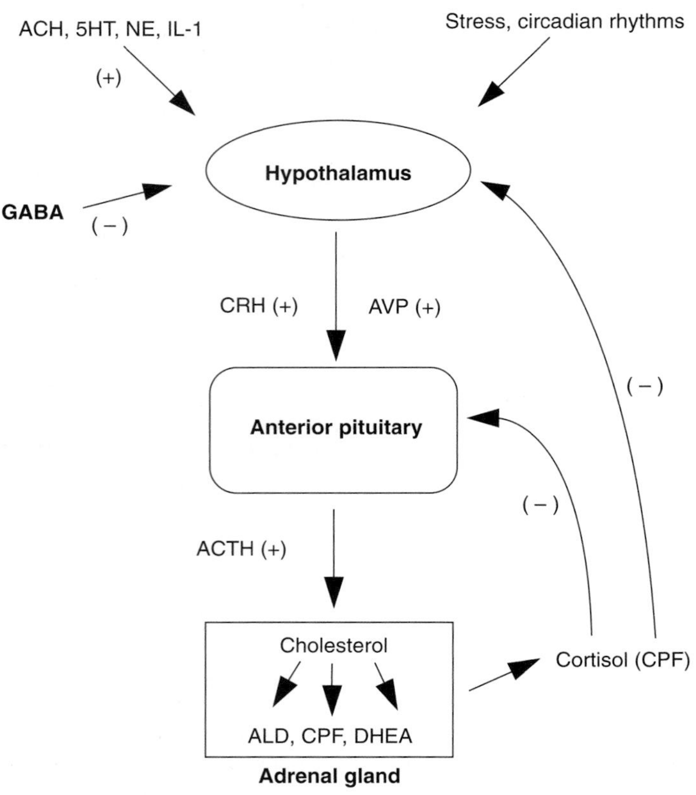

Fig. 48-5 The regulatory feedback loop of the hypothalamic-pituitary-adrenal axis. Several neurotransmitters, including acetylcholinesterase (ACh), 5-hydroxytryptamine (5-HT), norepinephrine (NE), and the cytokine interleukin-1 (IL-1), have a positive effect on the release of corticotropin-releasing hormone (CRH) from the hypothalamus. Gamma-aminobutyric acid (GABA) has a negative influence. Stress and circadian rhythm also influence the release of CRH from the hypothalamus. Both CRH and arginine vasopressin (AVP) stimulate the pituitary to release adrenocorticotropic hormone (ACTH), which in turn stimulates the adrenal gland to synthesize and release three major classes of hormones (aldosterone [ALD], cortisol [CPF], and dehydroepiandrosterone [DHEA]). Cortisol is the only adrenal steroid to feed back negatively to the hypothalamic-pituitary axis to control its own biosynthetic rate.

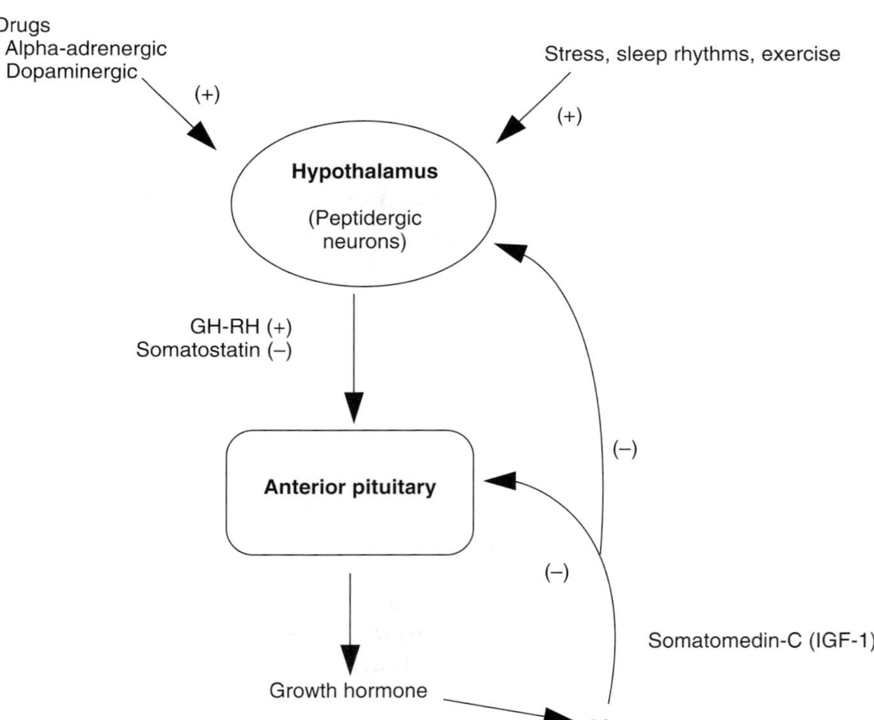

Fig. 48-6 The regulatory feedback loop of the hypothalamic-pituitary–growth hormone axis. Growth hormone release from the pituitary is driven primarily by growth hormone–releasing hormone (GH-RH) from the hypothalamus. GH-RH release from the hypothalamus is influenced positively by alpha-adrenergic and dopaminergic drugs, and by stress, sleep patterns, and exercise. Growth hormone acts on the liver to produce somatomedin-C, or insulin-like growth factor (IGF-I). This factor in turn negatively feeds back to the hypothalamic-pituitary axis to maintain homeostatic control over growth hormone secretion.

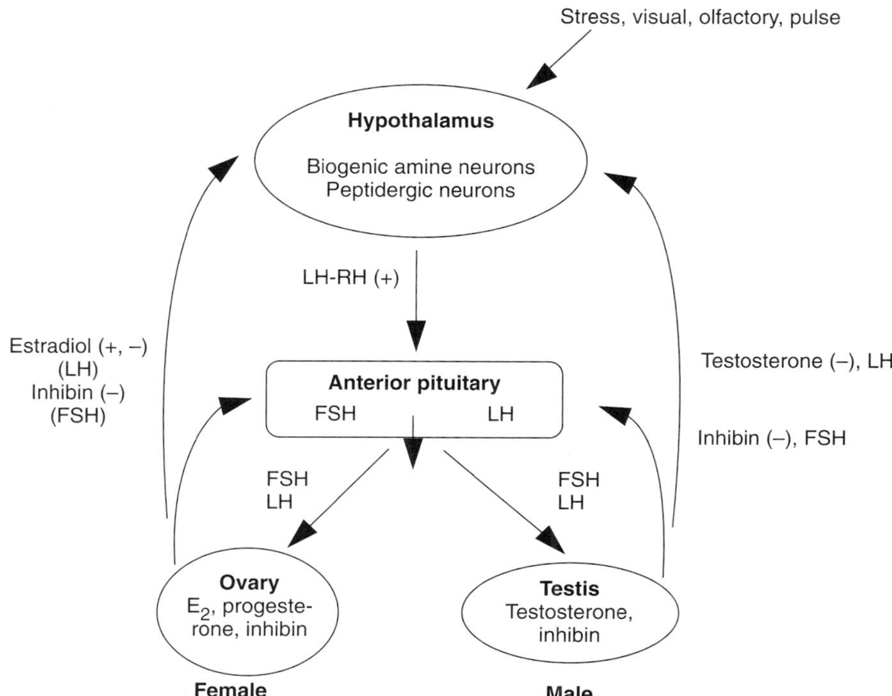

Fig. 48-7 The regulatory feedback loop of the hypothalamic-pituitary-gonadal axis. Biogenic amine and peptidergic neurons in the hypothalamus respond to neural and sensory input from the brain to elicit the release of gonadotropin hormone (luteinizing hormone–releasing hormone [LH-RH]). This input can be visual and olfactory in origin and occurs in a pulsatile fashion. Stress can override these inputs in a negative fashion. LH-RH in turn acts on the pituitary to synthesize and release the gonadotropins follicle-stimulating hormone (FSH) and luteinizing hormone (LH). In the female, FSH causes ovarian follicular development and the production of estradiol (E_2), whereas LH causes corpus luteum development and the secretion of progesterone. Estradiol feeds back both negatively and positively to the hypothalamic-pituitary axis to control the menstrual cycle and LH secretion. FSH release feedback control is orchestrated by an ovarian peptide called *inhibin*. In the male, FSH causes testicular spermatogenesis, whereas LH stimulates testosterone production by the testes. Testosterone negatively feeds back to the hypothalamic-pituitary axis to control LH release, whereas a testicular peptide, inhibin, feeds back to control FSH release.

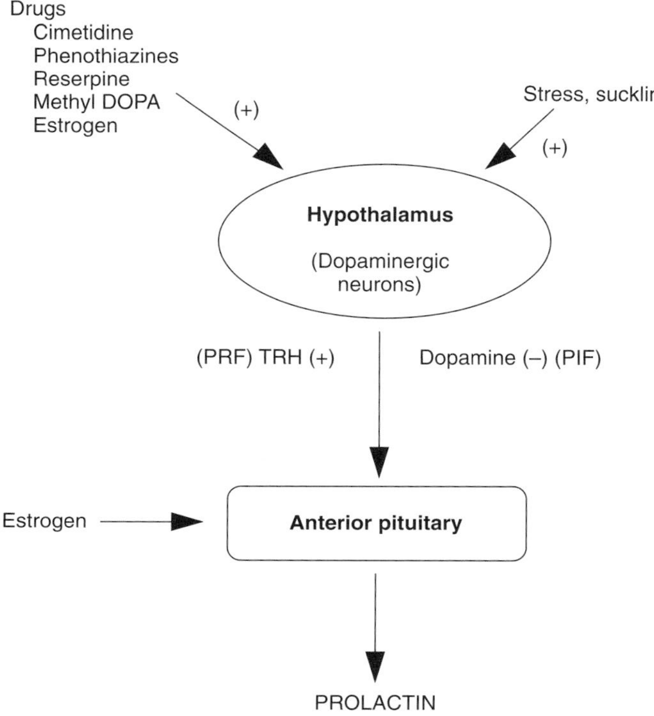

Fig. 48-8 The regulatory feedback loop for prolactin secretion. Prolactin release from the pituitary is under tonic inhibitory control by hypothalamus-derived dopamine, or prolactin inhibitory factor (PIF). Thyrotropin-releasing hormone (TRH) in turn is stimulatory to prolactin release. Prolactin release is affected by many factors that influence dopamine release. Drugs, estrogen, and stress are overriding factors that can produce an augmentation in prolactin release from the pituitary. Estrogen can directly sensitize the pituitary to release prolactin.

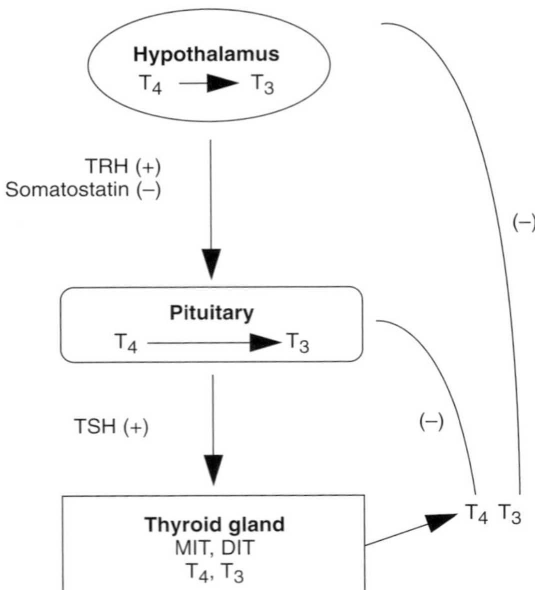

Fig. 48-9 The regulatory feedback loop of the hypothalamic-pituitary-thyroid axis. The hypothalamus secretes thyrotropin-releasing hormone (TRH) to stimulate the synthesis and release of thyroid-stimulating hormone (TSH) from the pituitary. TSH in turn stimulates the thyroid gland to grow, vascularize, and produce the thyroid hormones tetraiodothyronine (T_4) and triiodothyronine (T_3). T_3 is formed primarily from T_4 outside the thyroid gland. T_4 (through hypothalamic and pituitary conversion to T_3) and T_3 (directly) feed back to the hypothalamic-pituitary axis to maintain a homeostatic balance of circulating thyroid hormone.

Thus control of plasma circulatory levels of active hormone requires a balance between new hormone synthesis and release from tissues and the metabolic inactivation of existing hormone.

Sequestration: Free and Bound Transport of Steroid and Thyroid Hormones

Immediate control of the activity of steroid and thyroid hormones in plasma is exercised by sequestration of most of the steroid and thyroid hormones into a protein-bound, inactive form. Because steroid hormones are themselves water insoluble, plasma proteins also serve as the transport medium for these hormones. The transport/binding proteins, which are synthesized in the liver, are listed in Table 48-2. Generally, three circulating pools of hormones are known; they are listed here in order of increasing bioavailability: those bound to specific proteins with high affinity for the hormone; those bound to proteins with low affinity for the hormone; and those totally free in the plasma. An example of the binding of testosterone to its respective carrier proteins is shown in Fig. 48-10. In the case of thyroid hormone, three different proteins, each with different binding affinities, participate in the transport of T_4 and T_3 within the circulation: thyroxine-binding globulin, thyroxine-binding prealbumin, and albumin (see Chapter 49).

Table 48-2 Hormone Transport Proteins

Protein	Hormone
CBG (cortisol-binding globulin)	Cortisol
SHBG (sex hormone–binding globulin)	Estradiol, testosterone
TBG (thyroid-binding globulin)	T_3, T_4
TBPA (thyroxine-binding prealbumin)	T_4
VDBG (vitamin D–binding globulin)	Vitamin D
ALB (albumin)	All hormones

Free and Protein-Bound Hormone Transport

Several proteins serve as carriers of hormones in plasma and as a form of hormone storage within the circulation (see earlier). Albumin and prealbumin serve as general **hormone transport** proteins for steroid hormones and thyroid hormones. Binding of thyroid hormones and steroid hormones to albumin and prealbumin is weak, however, with an affinity constant that is much lower than that of the tissue receptor. Thus hormones bound to albumin and prealbumin are regarded as a weakly bound form of free hormones and are considered to be readily bioavailable to tissues—a phenomenon that contrasts with the previously held belief that only hormones absolutely free of carrier proteins could gain access to tissue receptors. This concept has led to the description of free hormone as inclusive of both free and weakly bound hormone.

In addition to general, low-affinity transport proteins such as albumin, specific transport proteins are known to exist. These specific transport proteins have high affinity for the hormones they carry, which closely parallels the binding and specificity characteristics of intracellular receptors; thus they significantly influence the metabolic clearance rate for hormones. Several important considerations underscore the role of all transport proteins that carry hormones within the circulation. High-affinity binding proteins act as reservoirs for the storage and transport of hormones within the circulation. Once free or weakly bound hormone enters the tissue, rapid circulatory adjustments to the free hormone level are made through exchange and reequilibration between specific transport protein–bound hormone and weakly bound transport protein–bound hormone. The overall decline in circulatory hormone then is eventually compensated for through activation of positive feedback to higher centers of control, as occurs in the hypothalamic-pituitary axis. This keeps available sufficient quantities of life-sustaining hormones such as thyroxine and cortisol continuously with a significant circulating reservoir that is available as soon as it is needed.

Many laboratories now measure **bioavailable hormone** (i.e., free and albumin- or prealbumin-bound hormone), in contrast to previous measurements, which included only the free concentration of hormone. An example of the utility of measuring both free and weakly bound hormone can be seen in the measurement of free and weakly bound testosterone (Fig. 48-10). Testosterone is carried in the circulation bound tightly to its specific carrier protein, sex hormone–binding globulin (SHBG), and bound weakly to albumin. Only a small (<10%) fraction of testosterone in the circulation is actually free. When blood perfuses an organ that contains testosterone

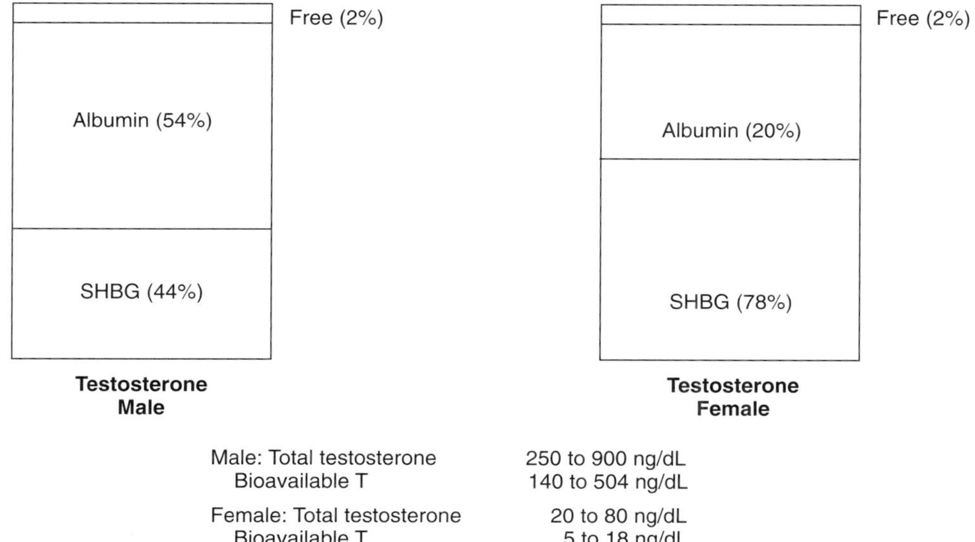

Fig. 48-10 Free and weakly bound testosterone. Testosterone circulates while bound to two proteins: a specific binding protein, sex hormone–binding globulin (SHBG), and albumin. Only a small fraction of testosterone circulates in a free state. Total testosterone levels reflect the combination of SHBG-bound, albumin-bound, and free testosterone. The bioavailable form of circulating testosterone, the form that "sees" the tissue receptor, is composed of the free fraction and that portion that is bound to albumin. Thus bioavailable testosterone is the biologically active form of the hormone that is found in the circulation.

receptors, both free and albumin-bound fractions of testosterone are available for immediate binding to an available receptor. Hence, the term *bioavailable testosterone* is used to describe the free and albumin-bound fractions of total hormone in the circulation.

Some steroid hormones, like dehydroepiandrosterone (DHEA), a major androgenic steroid produced by the adrenal gland, lack a specific transport protein. To compensate for the lack of a specific carrier protein for this steroid, DHEA is sulfated at the 3-hydroxyl position of the basic steroid molecule. This step increases the solubility of this steroid for general transport in the circulation. Thus DHEA circulates within the blood primarily as a sulfated derivative (i.e., DHEA-S).

Local Hormone and Growth Factor Action

The classical understanding of endocrinology and hormones states that a hormone is produced by a specialized gland in one part of the body and travels through the bloodstream to a distant site to elicit a biological effect. A family of peptide growth factors serves as extracellular regulators of cell growth and function but do not act at distant sites. They act locally and rely on cell-to-cell communication within the tissue and cellular environment. Terms such as ***autocrine factor*** and ***paracrine factor*** have been coined to describe the local synthesis and release of growth factors that interact with receptors on neighboring cells within the same tissue (paracrine effect) or with receptors from the same cell that release the growth factor (autocrine effect) (Fig. 48-11 and Color Plate 12).

The gastrointestinal tract is a prime site of local regulatory interactions between hormones, growth factors, and neurotransmitters that influence cell function through cell-to-cell communication (see Chapter 35). An analogy for this system of communication is the cytokine network of communication that exists between the lymphoid cells of the immune system and the cells of a particular tissue, such as tissue macrophages and epithelial cells.

Two additional terms have been used to describe growth factor communication within the local cellular environment. **Intracrine factor** refers to an intracellular cytosolic factor that travels to the nucleus in the same cell to bind to a specific receptor within the DNA-binding region of chromatin (see Color Plate 12).

The term **juxtacrine factor** refers to direct cell-to-cell communication elicited by growth factors that are still anchored to each cell's membrane. When cells come into contact with each other, this membrane-bound growth factor directly influences its neighboring cell. As the family of growth factors continues to expand, a reclassification of the nomenclature will be needed to assign hormones, growth factors, and neural peptides to their proper locations and functions.

KEY CONCEPTS BOX 48-1

- Chemically, hormones are amino acids, peptides, or steroids.
- Steroid and thyroid hormones act by binding first to cytosol or nuclear receptors, and then to chromatin.
- Protein hormones act by binding to cell membrane receptors, which then activate a series of "second messengers" within the cell.
- Feedback (usually negative feedback) loops are the primary mechanism for regulating hormone release.
- Primary mechanisms for controlling the availability of active hormone are rapid catabolism and sequestration.
- Free and weakly bound hormones are the most biologically active form of steroid hormone.
- Autocrine, paracrine, and juxtacrine hormones act locally to regulate cell activity.

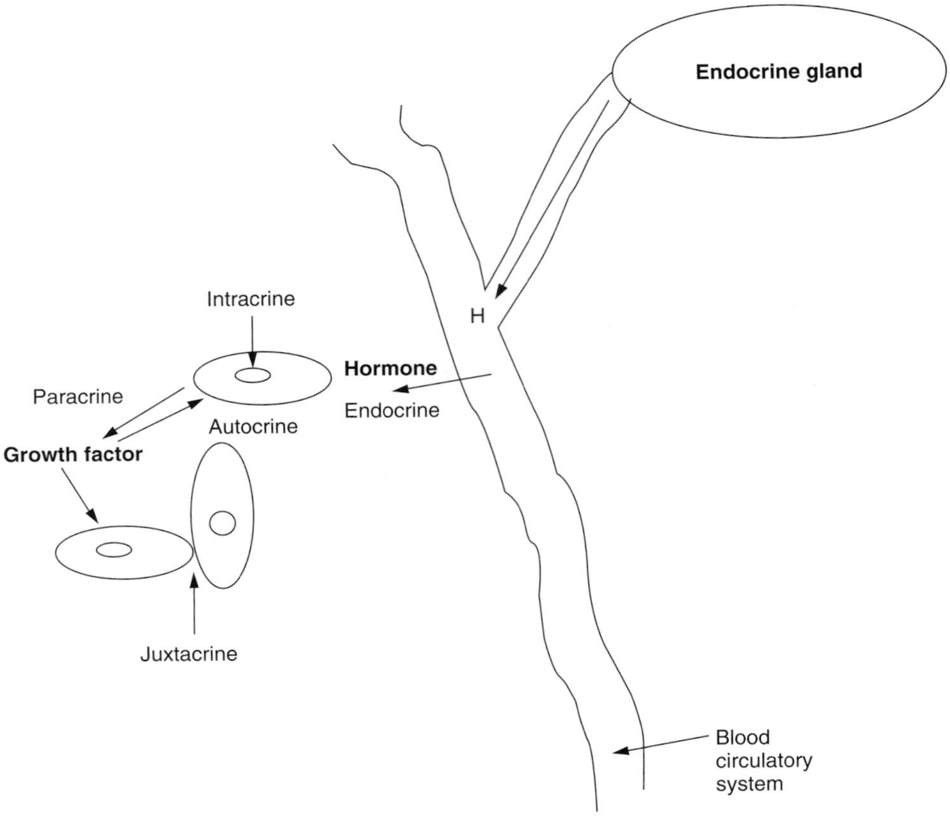

Fig. 48-11 Local and systemic modalities of hormone and growth factor action. Hormones (H) are the chemical messengers that are released into the circulation by endocrine glands to effect a response.

SECTION OBJECTIVE BOX 48-2

- List the hypothalamic factors and the pituitary hormones they control.

THE HYPOTHALAMIC-PITUITARY AXIS

Hypothalamus

The hypothalamus exerts control over pituitary function through direct neurostimulation and neurosecretion events from the hypothalamus. The anatomical positioning of the hypothalamus at the base of the brain with both neural and anatomical connections to the pituitary through the pituitary stalk and the pituitary portal circulation ensures a close interdependence of these two important organs. The pituitary is configured anatomically with a posterior and an anterior lobe (Fig. 48-12). The hypothalamus directly innervates the posterior lobe (**neurohypophysis**), and hypothalamic stimulation causes the posterior pituitary to release stored peptide hormones such as arginine vasopressin (AVP) and oxytocin. These two hormones are synthesized by the neurosecretory cells of the hypothalamus and are stored in the neurohypophysis. In contrast, the anterior lobe (**adenohypophysis**) responds to hypothalamus-derived neuropeptides, which, when released directly into the pituitary portal circulation, cause the release of the corresponding pituitary hormones (see Table 48-1).

In addition to the classical hypothalamic releasing factors, a hypothalamic peptide, somatostatin, exerts a negative influence on thyroid-stimulating hormone (TSH), growth hormone (GH), and several other hormone secretions, including gastrointestinal and pancreatic hormones. Somatostatin is a peptide that is synthesized not only by the hypothalamus but also within the lumen of the gastrointestinal tract and the pancreas. Different isoforms are synthesized in the brain and gastrointestinal tract. This neurohormone exerts a profound inhibitory effect on the synthesis of GH and TSH and the secretion of these hormones from the pituitary. Somatostatin inhibits virtually all endocrine secretions (including gastrin, insulin, glucagon, and secretin) of the gastrointestinal tract, pancreas, and gallbladder. Its primary role is to attenuate hypersecretion of these hormones in pathological states, for example, endocrine-secreting tumors such as insulinomas and carcinomas. Somatostatin analogs have been used as effective therapeutic agents to treat endocrine-secreting pituitary tumors such as acromegaly and pancreatic tumors such as insulinomas.

Neurohypophysis

The neurosecretions of vasopressin and oxytocin have specialized roles in mammalian physiology that involve water-conserving (antidiuretic) and nonvascular smooth muscle contracting properties, respectively. Arginine vasopressin (AVP, also known as antidiuretic hormone [ADH]) is the major homeostatic factor that maintains normal water

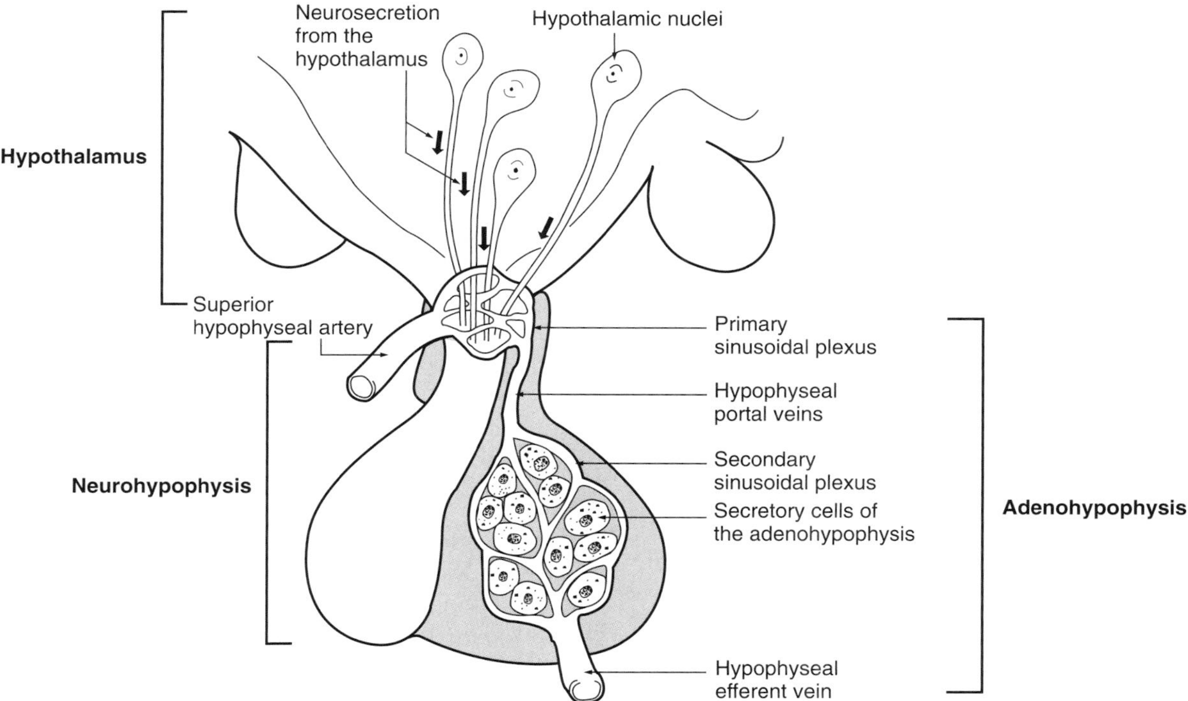

Fig. 48-12 Sinusoidal portal system of the pituitary gland.

concentration in the blood, keeping plasma volume and blood osmolality tightly controlled. Control of blood volume plays an important role in the maintenance of normal blood pressure. (see pp. 533-535). The release of AVP occurs immediately in response to increases in plasma osmolality, and AVP acts in the kidney to increase water reabsorption by the distal kidney tubules and the collecting ducts. AVP also participates in volume regulation. A sudden reduction in blood volume of greater than 10%, as can occur with a massive hemorrhage, can evoke a rapid release of AVP. Volume receptors for AVP are located in the heart and the carotid sinus. Under normal conditions, AVP is released in response to changes in plasma osmolality. Severe volume depletion, however, can override the influence of osmolality on AVP release.

Oxytocin appears to have a role in mammalian physiology that transcends reproductive behavior. Release of oxytocin generally is brought about through a neurogenic reflex transmitted primarily from nerve endings in the nipple of the breast. The stimulus is transmitted through the spinal cord, midbrain, and ultimately, to the hypothalamus. Suckling of the breast induces the release of oxytocin, which causes contraction of epithelial cells that encircle mammary acini. This produces expulsion of milk from the milk ducts of the breast, termed *milk letdown*, which is a key event in breast feeding. Oxytocin also plays a role in the induction of labor in pregnancy by stimulating the nonvascular smooth muscle of the uterus to contract. Although the exact signal precipitating the onset of human labor has not yet been identified, oxytocin receptors in the uterus translate the oxytocin signal to produce rhythmical myometrial contractile changes and the physical events of labor. Secretion of oxytocin from the posterior pituitary occurs independent of AVP secretion; thus it is believed that both fall under independent control mechanisms.

Adenohypophysis

The anterior lobe of the pituitary is responsible for the secretion of trophic hormones that govern virtually the entire endocrine system. As was noted previously, pituitary cell differentiation, proliferation, and hormone synthesis are controlled by neurosecretory factors of hypothalamic origin. All the releasing factors are peptides except dopamine (Table 48-3), a neurotransmitter that also is synthesized and released from the hypothalamus and plays an important regulatory role over pituitary hormone secretion. Dopamine is believed to be the major regulator of prolactin secretion, exerting continuous and sustained inhibition on its release from the pituitary. In addition to its effect on prolactin, dopamine inhibits the secretion of TSH, FSH, LH, and GH.

Although each hypothalamic-releasing factor has a targeted hormone, some integration of hormone release does occur. For example, thyrotropin-releasing hormone (TRH) causes synthesis and release of not only TSH but prolactin as well. Similarly, luteinizing hormone–releasing hormone (LH-RH) stimulates the release of both FSH and LH. Only corticotropin-releasing hormone (CRH) and growth hormone–releasing hormone (GH-RH) act through a single pituitary hormone release mechanism. All releasing factors interact with the pituitary through the same common receptor mechanism used by other peptide hormones. Although they generally are restricted to the pituitary portal circulation, several releasing factors have been measured in blood and urine. Direct target organ effects have been described for LH-RH in the ovary and testis. The exact physiological meaning of this interaction is still unclear.

KEY CONCEPTS BOX 48-2

- The hypothalamus and the pituitary glands are located within the brain. The hypothalamus is composed of both neural and glandular cells, and is responsive to CNS stimulation.
- The hypothalamus and the pituitary endocrine glands are the primary regulators of all other endocrine glands.

Table 48-3 Human Hypothalamic Neurosecretory Factors

Vasopressin	cys-tyr-phe-gln-asn-cys-pro-arg-gly-NH_2 (1084.38 daltons)
Oxytocin	cys-tyr-ile-gln-asn-cys-pro-leu-gly-NH_2 (1007.35 daltons)
CRH	ser-glu-glu-pro-pro-ile-ser-leu-asp-leu-thr-peh-his-leu-leu-arg-glu-val-leu-glu-met-ala-arg-ala-glu-gln-leu-ala-gln-gln-ala-his-ser-asn-arg-lys-leu-met-glu-ile-ile-NH_2 (4758.14 daltons)
GH-RH	try-ala-asp-ala-ile-phe-thr-asn-ser-tyr-arg-lys-val-leu-gly-gln-leu-ser-ala-arg-lys-leu-leu-gln-asp-ile-met-ser-arg-gln-gln-gly-glu-ser-asn-gln-glu-arg-gly-ala-arg-ala-arg-leu-NH_2 (5040.40 daltons)
LH-RH	pglu-his-trp-ser-tyr-gly-leu-arg-pro-gly-NH_2 (1182.39 daltons)
TRH	pglu-his-pro-NH_2 (362.42 daltons)
Somatostatin	ala-gly-cys-lys-asn-phe-phe-trp-lys-thr-phe-thr-ser-cys (1638.12 daltons)
Dopamine	3,4-dihydroxyphenylmethylamine

CRH, Corticotropin-releasing hormone; *GH-RH*, growth hormone–releasing hormone; *LH-RH*, luteinizing hormone–releasing hormone; *p-*, pyrido-; *TRH*, thyrotropin-releasing hormone.

SECTION OBJECTIVES BOX 48-3

- List the primary causes of hypo- and hyper-functioning pituitary and hypothalamus glands.
- Which tests can be they can be used to distinguish between hypo- and hyper-functioning pituitary and hypothalamus glands.
- Describe the procedure used to test for growth hormone deficiency in children.

PATHOLOGICAL CONDITIONS

Diseases and disorders of the hypothalamic-pituitary axis can strike at any age and can produce a myriad of symptoms that often are subtle in presentation. A number of genetic causes for pituitary dysfunction have been described. Table 48-4 lists those genetic abnormalities that are currently known. Many early forms of endocrine disease are detected only with provocative testing. Bacterial infections, tumors, and head trauma are the most usual causes of alterations in central hormone regulation in the young. In older adults, vascular disease, inflammatory disease, and nutritional deficiency are additional causes of neuroendocrine disorders (Box 48-1). Associated with these diseases are deficits in the autoregulatory feedback loop from the target organs. The loss of circadian rhythm, for example, of ACTH secretion with bacterial infection brings about subsequent compromise in pituitary-adrenal function. This effect can be subtle but nevertheless important, in that cortisol production is a key factor in the control of immune cell function. Because we cannot easily determine the local hormone environment of the pituitary portal circulation, we rely on the measurement of pituitary hormones in the systemic circulation to provide a clinical picture of events at the hypothalamic level in health and disease.

Abnormalities of hormone secretion usually are defined in terms of serum levels of the hormone, that is, high or low levels, and the endocrine gland directly demonstrating the abnormality. In addition, the disease is defined by whether the hormone abnormality is the result of the endocrine gland producing the hormone (primary disease), a disease of the

Table 48-4 Genetic Causes of Pituitary Disease

Gene Function	Disease/Associated Conditions	Hormone Abnormalities
Pituitary Hormone Deficiency		
HESX1	Pituitary organogenesis, septo-optic dysplasia	GH, PRL, TSH, LH, FSH
LHX3	Rigid cervical spine	
LHX4		
PROP1	Pituicyte development, common mutation	GH, PRL, TSH, LH, FSH
POU1F1 (PIT1)	Pituicyte development	GH, PRL
TBX19 (TPIT)	Corticotroph development	ACTH
KAL1	GnRH neuron migration, Kallmann's syndrome, anosmia	LH, FSH
Pituitary Hormone Excess		
MEN1	Multiple endocrine neoplasia 1, tumor suppressor	GH, PRL, ACTH (rare)
GNAS	G-protein signaling, McCune-Albright syndrome	GH, PRL
PRKAR1A	Protein kinase, Carney complex	GH

Box 48-1

Disorders of the Hypothalamic-Pituitary Axis

Hypopituitarism
- Congenital
  - Gene deletions
  - Aplasia/hypoplasia
  - Disconnection of pituitary stalk
  - Hypoxia
- Acquired
  - Apoplexy
  - Infection
  - Trauma
  - Radiation
  - Neoplasm
  - Drugs
  - Surgery
- Functional defects
  - Isolated hormone deficiency
  - Severe illness
  - Multiple hormone defects
- Secondary hypothyroidism
- Secondary hypoadrenalism
- Hyposomatotropism
- Hypogonadotropic hypogonadism

Hyperpituitarism
- Hypothalamic
  - Irradiation
  - Infection
  - Tumor
- Primary pituitary
  - Hyperplasia or adenoma
- Hypersomatotropism
  - Acromegaly
  - Starvation
  - Infection
- Adrenocorticotropin
  - Pituitary adenoma
  - Addison's disease*
- Thyrotropin
  - Primary hypothyroidism*
- Hypergonadotropism
  - Primary organ failure*
- Hyperprolactinemia
  - Pituitary stalk section
  - Pregnancy
  - Pituitary adenoma
  - Hypothyroidism

*Hyperpituitarism secondary to primary organ failure.

pituitary gland controlling the primary gland (secondary disease), a disease of the hypothalamus controlling the pituitary (tertiary disease), or an inability of the hormone's target tissue to respond to the hormone (end-organ, or quaternary, disease). For example, increased levels of thyroxine that result from a pituitary gland that produces excessive TSH defines secondary hyperthyroidism.

Pituitary Hormone Deficiency

Deficiencies in a specific pituitary cell type can result in primary pituitary failure. A list of primary causes of hypopituitarism can be found in Box 48-1.

Secondary pituitary failure can occur as a result of a deficiency or excess in one or more hypothalamic-releasing factors brought on by infection, brain tumor, head trauma, brain surgery, or a congenital defect. Hypothalamic tumors, such as a craniopharyngioma, or inflammatory episodes in the brain, such as meningitis, can result in inappropriate synthesis of certain hypothalamic-releasing factors, leading to a decrease in pituitary hormone synthesis and release. Hypothalamic hypothyroidism, for example, is a deficiency syndrome of TRH secretion that is diagnosed initially by observation of a suppressed circulating level of TSH of unknown origin. Provocative testing in the form of an intravenous TRH stimulation test can help the clinician to determine whether the suppressed TSH level is due to hypothalamic disease or is a result of pituitary dysfunction. An isolated deficiency in LH-RH is the most common form of hypothalamic-releasing hormone deficiency and is caused by a congenital defect in the development of LH-RH–containing neurons in embryonic life. A deficiency in GH-RH is yet another example of a hypothalamic disorder that results in idiopathic dwarfism. This disorder typically is diagnosed by observation of inappropriate blood levels of circulating growth hormone before and after provocative testing. Deficiencies in the availability of TRH, LH-RH, GH-RH, and CRH all have been described in patients and usually are categorized as tertiary endocrine disease.

Pituitary Hormone Excess

Primary Hyperpituitarism

Pituitary hypersecretion most commonly is caused by the presence of a **pituitary adenoma** or a benign tumor of pituitary origin. Although nonfunctioning adenomas are the most common type of pituitary lesion, prolactin-secreting pituitary adenoma is by far the most common form of hypersecreting pituitary disease. Prolactin, the secretion of which is usually under continuous negative control by the neurosecretory factor dopamine, is produced and secreted in uncontrollably large amounts by pituitary prolactinomas. Prolactin-secreting tumors are diagnosed more readily in women, because disruption of the normal menstrual cycle and **amenorrhea** usually herald a potential problem early in the manifestation of the disease. Women with prolactinomas also can manifest **galactorrhea,** that is, an abnormal secretion of fluid from the nipple of the breast. Males who develop a prolactinoma, in contrast, are less fortunate and usually do not present at a microadenoma stage as females do. Growth of the prolactin-secreting pituitary tumor usually continues in the male without overt symptoms, and the tumor eventually reaches the size of a macroadenoma before symptoms appear. Headache, impotence, and visual field disturbances that occur as consequences of tumor extension that compresses the optic nerve are the classical symptoms that result from a pituitary macroadenoma. The diagnosis of a prolactinoma usually is confirmed by the appearance of blood levels of prolactin in excess of 200 ng/mL.

Growth hormone– and ACTH–producing pituitary tumors are also relatively common pituitary disorders, although of lower prevalence than prolactin-secreting tumors. Growth hormone excess is characterized by the development of acromegalic features, including soft tissue and cartilaginous growth, which result in the characteristic facial features of gigantism. This growth hormone excess disease entity is called **acromegaly.** The major effect of growth hormone is that it induces the synthesis of an insulin-like growth factor (IGF-1) by the liver. In patients with acromegaly, IGF-1 levels are raised to a greater extent than those of growth hormone itself. The availability of commercial immunoassays for IGF-1 has permitted the routine measurement of this circulating growth factor for the diagnosis and management of patients with acromegaly.

Pituitary adenomas that hypersecrete ACTH are also common and lead to the condition known as **Cushing's disease** (see Chapter 51). This syndrome is associated with bilateral adrenal hyperplasia and clinical manifestations of cortisol overproduction as a consequence of excessive ACTH. TSH-producing pituitary adenomas leading to thyroid gland hyperstimulation have been described but are very rare.

Secondary Hyperpituitarism

Pituitary hypersecretion can be induced by numerous factors, including neurogenic tumors of the hypothalamus. Overproduction of releasing factors will hyperstimulate the pituitary, leading to excessive pituitary hormone release that overrides the usual negative-feedback mechanisms. LH-RH hypersecretion associated with precocious puberty, GH-RH–secreting gangliocytomas causing acromegaly, and CRH-secreting tumors producing Cushing's disease are examples of releasing factor hypersecretion and secondary causes of hyperpituitarism. Hypothalamus-based disorders are relatively rare, however, compared with the hypersecretion that occurs with primary pituitary disease.

Inappropriate release (hypersecretion) of AVP (ADH) from the posterior region of the pituitary gland can bring about excessive water retention and a dangerous expansion of plasma volume. Brain injury resulting from physical trauma, infection, or tumors in the brain can bring about excessive AVP release, leading to the clinical condition known as SIADH (syndrome of inappropriate secretion of antidiuretic hormone). The ectopic production of AVP by certain tumors can also lead to inappropriate water retention. The thirst mechanism in the brain also is linked to AVP secretion from the neurohypophysis. Both drinking behavior and AVP release are believed to be activated by similar hyperosmotic stimuli, resulting in repletion of plasma water in states of dehydration. SIADH is associated with dilutional hyponatremia and the production of urine that is hypertonic relative to plasma, despite normal renal and adrenal function. Clinically, SIADH is associated with symptoms of muscle weakness, malaise, and poor mental status, ultimately progressing to convulsions.

KEY CONCEPTS BOX 48-3

- Diseases of the hypothalamus and of the pituitary glands can present as primary excess or deficiency of releasing factors and hormones, respectively, with secondary effects on the endocrine glands they control.
- Secondary disease of the hypothalamus and pituitary glands, excess or deficiency, usually is caused by disease of the other endocrine glands, deficiency or excess.
- Measurement of these factors and hormones can help in diagnosing the nature of the disorders.

SECTION OBJECTIVES BOX 48-4

- Describe how the measurement of endocrine hormones such as prolactin, ACTH, GH, TSH, FSH, and LH can be used to determine hypothalamus/pituitary function.
- Describe the use of the dexamethasone suppression test and the insulin challenge test.

TESTS OF HYPOTHALAMIC AND PITUITARY FUNCTION

Evaluation of pituitary disease very often is difficult because of subtle disease presentation. The diagnosis usually requires some form of provocative testing of gland function by suppression or stimulation of the pituitary gland through exogenous hormone treatment, or by provocation of symptoms with stress or exercise. These challenge tests then are followed by measurement of specific pituitary hormones. For each suspected type of pituitary adenoma, a specific testing protocol usually is employed to confirm the clinical suspicion. Many factors, however, must be considered when one is interpreting these functional tests. The pulsatile nature of pituitary hormone secretion, the time of day the test is performed, whether stress or infection might be present, and the concentration of circulating hormone all are factors that affect the interpretation of pituitary function test results. In addition, clinical laboratories have access to a wide variety of immunoassays with differing specificities and sensitivities that affect interpretability of provocative hormone testing.

ACTH Excess

Dexamethasone Suppression Tests (see p. 1016)

The presence of a tumor that is secreting ACTH usually is suspected when an abnormal elevation in urine or blood cortisol levels is observed. In these patients, cortisol determinations are made after a low-dose dexamethasone suppression test is performed. Lack of cortisol suppression is suggestive of a pituitary tumor. One then gives a higher dose of dexamethasone, which will elicit modest but still incomplete suppression of cortisol output in the patient with a functional pituitary adenoma. Cortisol output in patients with ACTH from an ectopic (nonpituitary) source will not be suppressed by either low- or high-dose dexamethasone.

Inferior Petrosal Sinus Sampling (http://www.cushings-help.com/petrossal.htm)

The sensitivity of the high-dose dexamethsone suppression test for detecting ACTH-secreting tumors is near 70%, and this test will fail to identify Cushing's disease accurately in some patients. Because endogenous cortisol excess in most patients results from excess ACTH pituitary secretion, some endocrinologists do not advocate use of the high-dose dexamethasone suppression test. The most reliable test for the diagnosis of Cushing's disease is inferior petrosal sinus sampling of the pituitary. This procedure involves catheterization of bilateral femoral or jugular veins into both petrosal sinus veins. A peripheral catheter is also placed. Blood ACTH is measured simultaneously from both petrosal veins and the peripheral site. In Cushing's disease, the central-to-peripheral ACTH ratio is expected to be greater than or equal to 2.0, or greater than or equal to 3.0 after administration of 1 μg/kg body weight of CRH. The sensitivity and specificity of this diagnostic test are greater than 90%.

GH Excess

Oral Glucose Tolerance Test

The most reliable test for the diagnosis of GH excess—acromegaly in adults or gigantism in children—is the oral glucose tolerance test. After administration of 75 g of glucose, GH is expected to fall to less than 1 ng/mL within 2 hours after ingestion. Most patients with GH excess will have GH levels in excess of 2 ng/mL after glucose ingestion.

GH Deficiency

Insulin Challenge Test

The most commonly performed challenge test for a growth hormone deficiency is the insulin challenge test, which is used to determine the presence of a GH deficiency in adults and young children. For adult patients, endocrinologists use the insulin-induced hypoglycemia test exclusively. Insulin is administered at a dose of 0.1 unit per kilogram body weight with a target glucose of less than 50 mg/dL. Individuals with normal GH production will have a prompt increase in serum GH concentration. For pediatric patients, endocrinologists often use a combination of insulin-induced hypoglycemia and the drug levodopa (L-dopa), which acts in the CNS to induce pituitary release of GH. Insulin usually is administered first, and blood is collected at 30-minute intervals for 90 minutes for the assessment of GH. This is followed by the administration of L-dopa over the subsequent 120 minutes, with additional collection of blood for GH measurement every 30 minutes. As a result of the influence of stress, baseline levels can be raised slightly because of the venipuncture, which sometimes can lead to misinterpretation of results. The recent availability of the releasing factor GH-RH for clinical use has allowed a better clinical workup of patients with a subtle manifestation of pituitary growth hormone deficiency. Administration of GH-RH and measurement of GH are useful in discerning growth deficiencies of hypothalamic origin.

Secondary Hypogonadism

LH-RH Challenge

LH-RH usually is given intravenously to stimulate pituitary secretion of FSH and LH; low FSH and LH levels after this challenge are suggestive of hypopituitary function. LH-RH analogs are available for use in provocative testing and in the treatment of a variety of reproductive disorders and malignancies, such as endometriosis and prostate cancer.

KEY CONCEPTS BOX 48-4

- The dexamethasone suppression test is used to test for pituitary or ectopic, tumor-derived ACTH. Questionable results can be followed by inferior petrosal sinus sampling of the pituitary gland to determine excess production.
- The insulin challenge test is used to detect the presence of a GH deficiency in young children.

CHANGE OF ANALYTE IN DISEASE

Prolactin

The pulsatile secretion of prolactin has little effect on its measurement or interpretation for the diagnosis of a prolactinoma because of the high levels of prolactin that usually are achieved in this disease. Prolactin hypersecretion usually is established simply by the observation of an elevated basal level. A prolactin level above 200 ng/mL is virtually diagnostic of a prolactinoma. Mild elevations of prolactin (25 to 50 ng/mL), however, can be achieved easily in response to the stress of venipuncture or simply after physical examination and examination of the breasts. Repeated measurement of mild elevations in prolactin will confirm the presence of a prolactinoma. Levels up to 150 ng/mL, which are elevated approximately 10-fold, can be achieved in normal individuals who are receiving certain medications. The phenothiazines, atypical antipsychotics, metoclopramide, and methyldopa can produce a significant increase in prolactin secretion, thus a careful drug history is important when one is assessing a patient with raised levels of prolactin. A pituitary magnetic resonance imaging (MRI) scan of a patient with raised prolactin levels is required to confirm the presence of a pituitary tumor.

ACTH

Patients with an ACTH-producing pituitary adenoma usually are diagnosed by an elevation in basal blood cortisol levels; ACTH measurements are not routinely needed in these cases. ACTH measurements are used more commonly for patients requiring localization of the tumor within the pituitary before surgical removal of the pituitary adenoma. In these cases, blood samples are collected from the petrosal sinus. Occasionally, patients with a suspected ectopic source of ACTH, from an ACTH-producing tumor, are candidates for blood ACTH measurements. The highest values for ACTH usually are found in patients who are producing this peptide from a tumor source. The dexamethasone suppression test is used for this diagnosis (see earlier). Sustained high levels of ACTH can be helpful in establishing the presence of a nonpituitary source for ACTH. Tumors of the lung, particularly oat cell carcinoma, are commonly associated with nonpituitary sources of ACTH. Blood levels of ACTH in a patient with a pituitary adenoma rarely exceed 1000 pg/mL; however, with an ectopic source, levels are frequently in excess of this concentration. Pancreatic tumors also are commonly associated with ectopic ACTH release.

ACTH measurements are not used routinely. The short half-life of ACTH, stringent collection requirements because of the lability of this peptide (antiproteases are required in the collection vial), and the need for immediate sample storage at −20°C are factors that impede the routine use and the interpretation of an ACTH result.

Growth Hormone

Growth hormone is secreted in healthy individuals in a pulsatile fashion, with the greatest amounts produced during rapid eye movement sleep. During the day, blood levels of GH may range from undetectable to 5 ng/mL. However, GH levels can be influenced greatly by stress and by the recent ingestion of food, with carbohydrates suppressing and proteins stimulating GH secretion. Thus a single determination of GH is not particularly useful in establishing inadequate or excessive release of GH from the pituitary. When a GH deficiency is suspected, provocative testing usually is required to confirm this suspicion (see earlier).

One method used to evaluate the possibility of pituitary hypersecretion of growth hormone in a patient suspected of having acromegaly is to measure the concentration of somatomedin C, or IGF-1. The concentration of this liver factor, which mediates the effects of growth hormone, is raised in the circulation in patients with acromegaly, and its measurement can be useful in confirming the diagnosis in borderline cases. IGF-1 measurements are also helpful in monitoring therapy of patients treated for acromegaly.

TSH

The availability of ultrasensitive TSH assays has greatly enhanced the usefulness of TSH measurements in the diagnosis of hypofunction or hyperfunction of the pituitary-thyroid axis. Before the advent of these highly sensitive tests, TRH stimulation tests were important provocative tests that helped distinguish hypothalamic from pituitary disease as the cause of thyroid dysfunction. This is particularly important when hyperthyroidism and euthyroidism are being distinguished. The newer, highly sensitive TSH assays can reasonably be expected to distinguish between depressed and normal TSH secretion, thus obviating, in most patients, the need to carry out TRH provocative testing. Basal TSH level becomes the important parameter to measure when the adequacy of pituitary TSH release is being assessed. A basal serum TSH level of less than 0.05 μIU/mL, for example, indicates with virtual certainty that primary hyperthyroidism exists for whatever clinical reason. TRH testing has been abandoned for the most part and has been reserved for establishing the differential diagnosis of suspected hypothalamus-based thyroid disease in patients who have a complex disease presentation (see p. 964). Patients who have a TSH level in excess of 10 μIU/mL are strongly suspected of having hypothyroidism, and when the TSH level exceeds 25 μIU/mL, the diagnosis usually is established as primary hypothyroidism.

FSH/LH

Of all the pituitary hormones influenced by pulsatile release, the gonadotropins are the most affected. In males, this pulsatility does not interfere with the clinical utility of gonadotropin measurements, because assessment of primary gonadal disease is the usual reason for determining gonadotropin levels in the male. Testosterone measurements provide the initial biochemical indication for the diagnostic workup of the hypogonadal male. Measurement of the gonadotropins with LH-RH provocative testing can be useful in the diagnosis of males with hypogonadotropic hypogonadism, or secondary hypogonadism (see earlier).

In women, the situation is more complex because the menstrual cycle, menopausal status, and the pulsatility and frequency of hypothalamic LH-RH secretion all affect the interpretation of serum FSH and LH levels. A single gonadotropin measurement is of little practical use in the female unless one simply wants to determine the probability of menopause. In this case, FSH serves as a better test than LH in confirming menopause. In more intricate cases of infertility, amenorrhea, and the many disorders that influence the hypothalamic-pituitary-ovarian axis, multiple blood measurements of the gonadotropins are necessary to pinpoint the disorder (see pp. 980 and 982). An alternative to this is the use of timed urine gonadotropin measurements, which can effectively integrate the pulsatile secretion of gonadotropins and concentrate the gonadotropins for use in the different clinical diagnoses. Pediatric endocrinologists routinely use urinary gonadotropin measurements to diagnose delayed puberty, precocious puberty, and functional disorders of the pituitary-ovarian and pituitary-testicular axis in young girls and boys.

In general, dynamic testing of pituitary function takes on the uniqueness of the specific disorder. With the current clinical availability of the four hypothalamic-releasing factors—GH-RH, CRH, LH-RH, and TRH—direct pituitary responses now can be monitored via measurement of the corresponding pituitary peptide. This allows the clinician to distinguish between hypothalamic and pituitary disease and to determine adequacy of the hypothalamic-pituitary-endocrine axis.

KEY CONCEPTS BOX 48-5

- Elevations in serum prolactin are used to diagnose prolactinemia.
- TSH is the most useful test in screening for pituitary-based thyroid disease.
- FSH and LH are used to determine whether hypothalamic or pituitary dysfunction is the cause of hypogonadal or hypergonadal disease.

BIBLIOGRAPHY

Belchetz P, Hammond P, editors: *Mosby's Color Atlas and Text of Diabetes and Endocrinology*, St. Louis, 2003, Mosby.

Besser GM, Thorner MO: *Clinical Endocrinology* (including CD-ROM), ed 3, St. Louis, 2002, Mosby.

DeGroot LJ, Jameson JL: *Endocrinology*, ed 5, Philadelphia, 2006, Elsevier/Saunders.

Gardner DG, Shoback DM, editors: *Greenspan's Basic & Clinical Endocrinology*, ed 8, New York, 2007, McGraw Hill.

Hall R: *Color Atlas of Endocrinology*, ed 2, St. Louis, 1990, Mosby.

Kronenberg HM, Melmed S, et al, editors: *Williams' Textbook of Endocrinology/Comprehensive Clinical Endocrinology*, ed 11, Philadelphia, 2008, Elsevier.

Strauss J, Barbieri R, editors: *Yen and Jaffe's Reproductive Endocrinology: Physiology, Pathophysiology, and Clinical Management*, ed 6, Philadelphia, 2009, Saunders.

INTERNET SITES

www.endo-society.org—The Endocrine Society Home Page

www.mic.ki.se/Diseases/c19.html—Karolinska Institute (a list of sites providing information on a wide variety of endocrine disorders)

www.aace.com/—American Association of Clinical Endocrinologists

http://www.endocrine.niddk.nih.gov/—National Institute of Diabetes & Digestive & Kidney Diseases

www.euro-endo.org—European Federation of Endocrine Societies

www.ncbi.nlm.nih.gov/sites/entrez?db=OMIM—Online Mendelian Inheritance in Man

http://www.hormoneproblems.com/Gen_Endo.htm

http://www.hormoneproblems.com/Gen_Endo.htm

http://emedicine.medscape.com/article/120767-overview—Growth hormone deficiency

http://emedicine.medscape.com/article/122287-overview—Hypopituitarism (panhypopituitarism)

http://emedicine.medscape.com/article/124634-overview—Prolactinoma

Thyroid

Sally Newsome and Peter E. Hickman

Chapter 49

Chapter Outline

Methods on Evolve

T3 uptake
Thyroglobulin (Tg)
Thyroid autoantibodies
Thyroid-stimulating hormone (TSH)
Thyroxine (total)
Thyroxine, free and free triiodothyronine

Key Terms

colloid The material found within the follicles of the thyroid and containing thyroglobulin, which include precursors of the thyroid hormone.

deiodinases Enzymes that remove iodine from T_4 (to make active T_3) and T_3 (to make inactive diiodotyrosine [DIT]).

diiodotyrosine (DIT) An intermediate in the synthesis and metabolism of thyroid hormones.

follicles Vesicles within the thyroid that comprise thyroid hormone–producing cells.

fT_4 Free T_4; the portion of T_4 that is not protein bound.

goiter Enlargement of the thyroid gland.

Graves' disease Immune disorder caused by the binding of antibodies to thyroid-stimulating hormone (TSH) receptors, resulting in an unregulated increase in thyroid hormone production and release.

Hashimoto's thyroiditis Inflammatory process of the thyroid caused by a derangement of the immune system, which may or may not lead to abnormal thyroid function.

hyperemesis gravidarum Prolonged vomiting in pregnancy.

hyperthyroidism Metabolic and clinical state caused by an increase in circulating active thyroid hormone.

hypothyroidism Metabolic and clinical state caused by decreased levels of circulating active thyroid hormone or increased tissue resistance; primary—decreased thyroid function caused by disease of the thyroid gland; secondary—decreased thyroid function caused by disease of the pituitary gland; tertiary—decreased thyroid function caused by disease of the hypothalamus.

medullary thyroid cancer Cancer of the C-cells of the thyroid gland.

monoiodotyrosine (MIT) An intermediate in the synthesis and metabolism of thyroid hormones.

nodule Localized enlargement of a portion of the thyroid gland.

ophthalmopathy Protrusion of the eye seen in Graves' disease.

organification Incorporation of ionic iodine into the molecular structure of tyrosine.

prealbumin (transthyretin) A protein that binds to and transports thyroid hormones in the blood.

resin-uptake test Measurement of the number of available binding sites on plasma thyroid hormone–transporting proteins.

thyroglobulin A glycoprotein of molecular weight 660,000 D produced by the follicular cells and containing the precursors of T_3 and T_4.

thyroiditis A general term for inflammation of the thyroid gland.

thyrotoxicosis Condition caused by excess thyroid hormone secretion; often used as a synonym for hyperthyroidism.

thyroxine T_4, a thyroid hormone with iodine atoms in positions 3, 5, 3′, and 5′ (tetraiodothyronine).

thyroxine-binding globulin (TBG) A glycoprotein with α-mobility that transports thyroid hormone in the blood.

transthyretin (prealbumin) A protein that binds to and transports thyroid hormones in the blood.

TRH (thyrotropin-releasing hormone) A hypothalamic tripeptide that promotes release of TSH from the pituitary.

triiodothyronine Thyroid hormone with iodine atoms in positions 3, 5, and 3′.

TSH (thyroid-stimulating hormone, thyrotropin) A glycoprotein composed of α- and β-subunits that is released from the pituitary. TSH promotes thyroid hormone production and release.

TSI Thyroid-stimulating immunoglobulin.

Wolff-Chaikoff effect Decreased formation and release of thyroid hormone in the presence of excess iodine.

The function of the thyroid is the production and secretion of thyroid hormones. These hormones have multiple metabolic actions in most cells of the body. Synthesis and release of thyroid hormones are under the control of **thyroid-stimulating hormone (TSH)** produced by the pituitary gland. Thyroid hormones in turn inhibit the secretion of TSH.

Deficiency of thyroid hormone has many adverse effects, particularly in children in whom deficiency is associated with mental retardation and reduced growth, and in adults who have mental and physical slowing, impaired metabolism, and cold intolerance. Excess thyroid hormone leads to a hypermetabolic state, with tachycardia and increased heat production.

SECTION OBJECTIVES BOX 49-1

- Describe the steps that lead up to the synthesis and secretion of thyroid hormones.
- Explain the hypothalamic and pituitary regulation of thyroid hormone concentration, mechanism of action in target cells, and thyroid hormone catabolism.
- List the three thyroid hormone binding proteins and their relative affinities for T_4 and T_3.
- Discuss the general, physiological, metabolic, cardiovascular, central nervous system, and gastrointestinal effects of thyroid hormone, relating the normal effects to symptoms noted in patients with hyper- or hypothyroidism.

ANATOMY

The thyroid gland is located in the front of the neck. It usually comprises two small lobes joined by an isthmus at the midline. In Western countries with adequate iodine intake, the weight of the gland is commonly 10 to 20 g, but in countries where iodine deficiency is common, the gland may be much larger.

The fine structure of the thyroid gland is shown in Fig. 49-1. The thyroid gland is composed of many **follicles.** These are of variable size and resemble a spheroidal sac lined by follicular cells. Within the sac is a gelatinous **colloid,** which contains the stored **thyroglobulin** made by the follicular cells. The follicles are separated by a delicate fibrous tissue stroma, and interspersed among the fibrous tissue are parafollicular or C-cells, which secrete the hormone calcitonin.

PHYSIOLOGY

Synthesis and Secretion of Thyroid Hormones

Three important and interrelated functions involved in the synthesis and secretion of thyroid hormones include synthesis of the tyrosine amino acid–containing protein thyroglobulin, incorporation of iodine into tyrosine residues of this protein, and regulation of thyroglobulin hydrolysis and thyroid hormone secretion. The latter steps are controlled predominantly by the action of thyroid-stimulating hormone (TSH) released from the pituitary gland.

Synthesis and Storage of Thyroglobulin

Thyroglobulin (Tg), a glycoprotein with a molecular weight of about 660,000 daltons, is synthesized by the follicular cells,

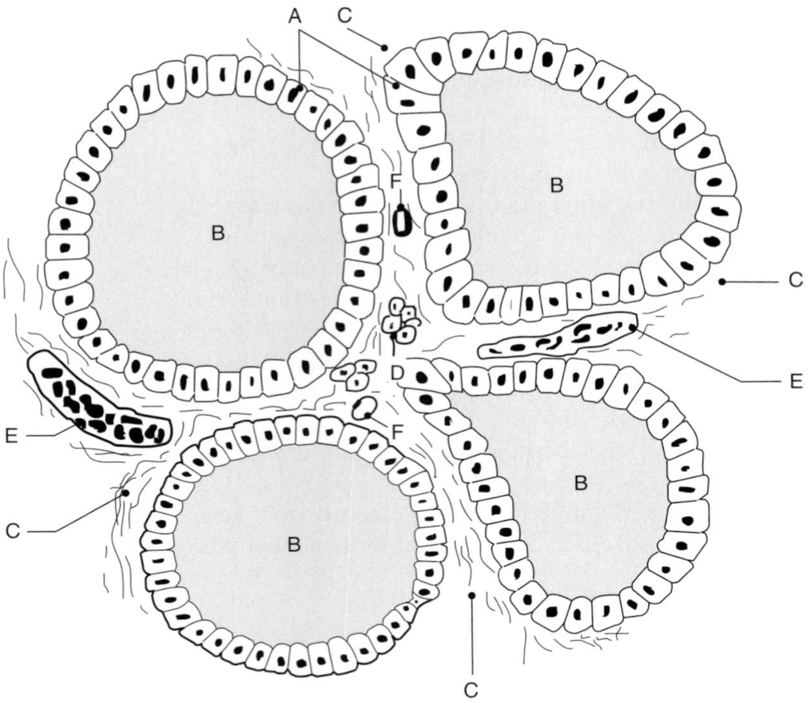

Fig. 49-1 Thyroid gland structure consists of follicular cells *(A)* that enclose colloid *(B)* and parafollicular C-cells *(D)* in the interstitium *(C)*. *E,* Venule; *F,* capillary.

carried within secretory vesicles toward the apical portion of the follicular cells, and discharged into the lumen of the follicle through a process of exocytosis. Intracellular Tg serves as a pre-formed matrix containing 123 tyrosine residues to which reactive iodine is attached to form **monoiodotyrosine (MIT)** and **diiodotyrosine (DIT).** Most iodination occurs when Tg is within the exocytic vesicles of the follicular cells. After their formation, enzymatic coupling of MIT and DIT takes place to form intrathyroglobulin triiodothyronine (T_3) and thyroxine (T_4). Coupling appears to occur between two iodotyrosine residues located in separate thyroglobulin chains or within folds of the same protein strands. Only a small portion (≈10%) of the tyrosine residues within Tg are iodinated. The structures of the thyroid hormones and their precursors are shown in Fig. 49-2. Iodinated Tg serves as a storage pool of thyroid hormone.

Iodine Uptake and Incorporation into Thyroglobulin

Ingested iodide is absorbed by the small intestine and is distributed throughout the extracellular water. Its predominant fate is urinary excretion or uptake into thyroid follicular cells against a concentration gradient that is energy dependent and is stimulated by TSH.

Iodide may be absorbed similarly by several other tissues within the body, notably the placenta and the mammary gland, for the purpose of ensuring adequate iodide delivery to the fetus and newborn. For other tissues that absorb iodide against a concentration gradient, such as the salivary glands and the gastric mucosa, the purpose is less certain.

Within the thyroid follicular cell, iodide is oxidized to iodine while it is bound to tyrosine residues within the thyroglobulin molecule (**organification**) through the action of the enzyme thyroid peroxidase, forming MIT or DIT.

The intrathyroid iodine compartment contains about 90% of total body iodine, which can amount to as much as 6000 to 12,000 μg. Recommended iodine intake is 90 μg/day in infants, 120 μg/day in children between 6 and 12 years, 150 μg/day in adults, and 250 μg/day in pregnant and lactating women. Even minor iodine deficiency can cause thyroid gland enlargement.[1]

Thyroid Hormone Secretion

TSH from the pituitary gland binds to the TSH receptor on the basal membrane of the follicular cell and via a cyclic adenosine monophosphate (cAMP)-dependent mechanism stimulates the uptake of thyroglobulin from stored colloid into cellular lysosomes, where the thyroglobulin is hydrolyzed and T_4, T_3, MIT, and DIT are released. Intracellular MIT and DIT are deiodinated immediately, and their iodine is reused in subsequent thyroid hormone synthesis. T_3 and T_4 are resistant to intrathyroid deiodination and are secreted immediately. The daily secretion of thyroid hormone includes about 80 to 100 μg of T_4 and about 7 μg of T_3 per day. The sequence of events, from iodide uptake into the follicular cell through to release of thyroid hormones into the circulation, is shown in Fig. 49-3.

Although all T_4 production takes place within the thyroid gland, approximately 80% of T_3 is produced by extrathyroidal deiodination of T_4. Although the liver and the kidney are the major organs for production of T_3 from T_4, many other tissues have the capacity for production of some T_3.

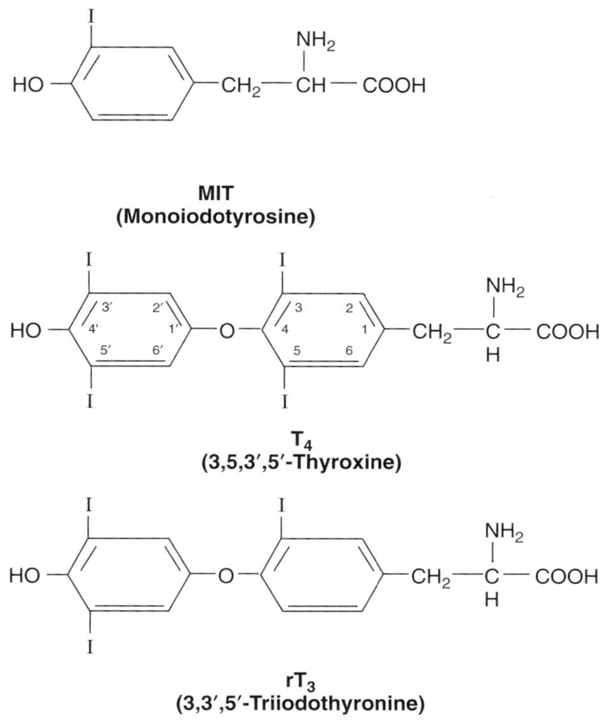

MIT
(Monoiodotyrosine)

DIT
(Diiodotyrosine)

T_4
(3,5,3′,5′-Thyroxine)

T_3
(3,5,3′-Triiodothyronine)

rT_3
(3,3′,5′-Triiodothyronine)

Fig. 49-2 Chemical structure of thyroid hormones and iodinated precursors and metabolites.

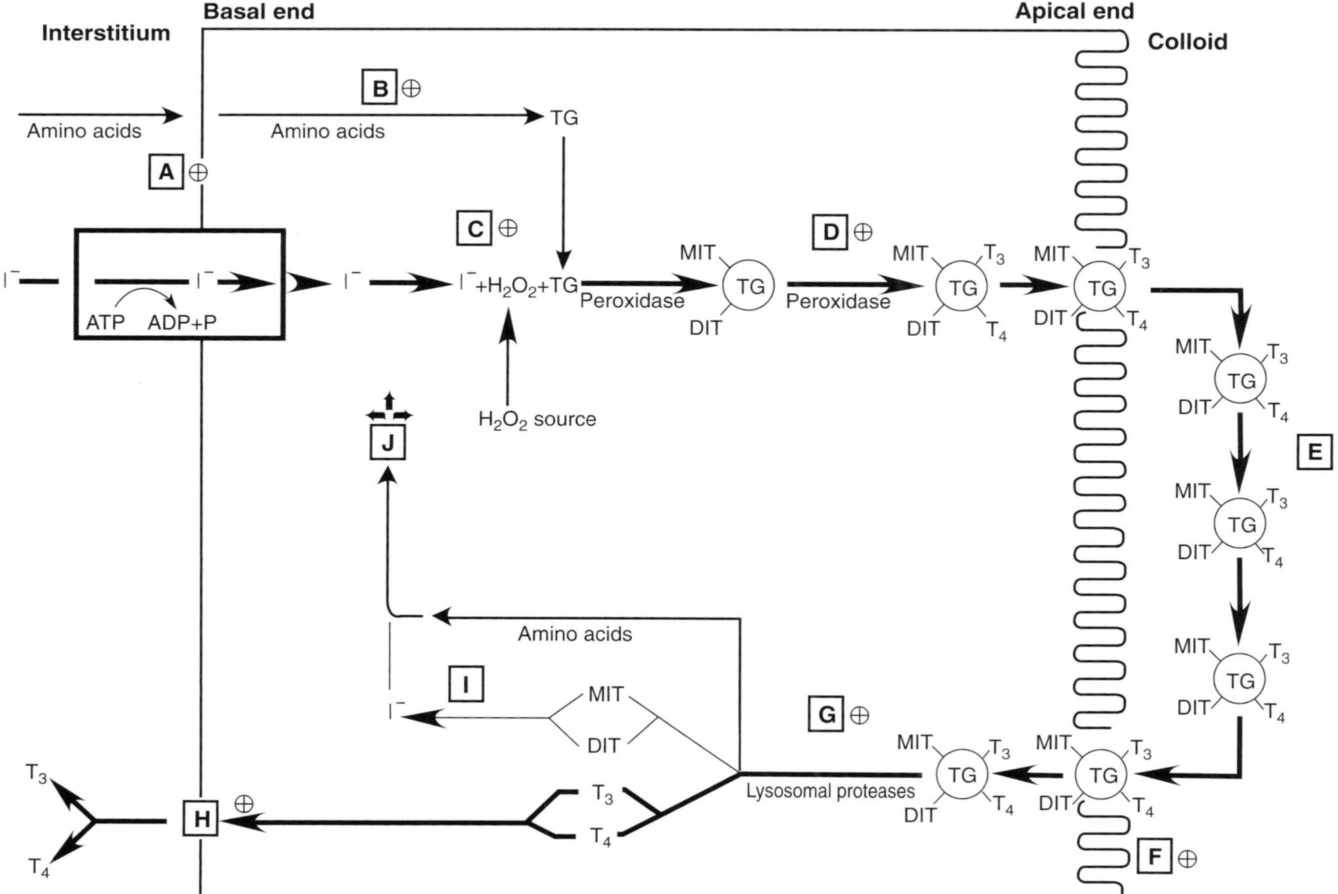

Fig. 49-3 Thyroid cell. Schema depicting stages of thyroid hormonogenesis and intrathyroidal iodine metabolism. *A,* Iodine transport; *B,* thyroglobulin (TG) synthesis; *C,* iodide organification; *D,* intrathyroglobulin oxidative coupling; *E,* storage. *F,* endocytosis; *G,* hydrolysis; *H,* hormone secretion; *I,* intrathyroidal deiodination; *J,* recycling. Steps influenced by the thyroid-stimulating hormone (TSH) are indicated by the symbol ⊕.

Regulation of Thyroid Hormone Secretion

Hypothalamic-Pituitary-Thyroid Axis (HPTA) and Its Regulation

The HPTA consists of a group of physiologically interrelated neuroendocrine and endocrine organs that regulate and control the secretion of thyroid hormone through a highly integrated feedback system, as shown in Fig. 49-4. The central role in this axis is performed by the thyroid gland, which produces, stores, and secretes the hormones T_4 and T_3.

Thyrotropin-releasing hormone (TRH) is a tripeptide produced in the paraventricular nucleus of the hypothalamus and secreted into the portal venous system, which then drains to the pituitary. TRH binds to receptors in the pituitary, causing increased production and secretion of TSH.

TSH is a 28 kd glycopeptide that is structurally composed of two subunits, α and β. The α-subunit is common to several pituitary peptide hormones, namely TSH, luteinizing hormone (LH), follicle-stimulating hormone (FSH), and human chorionic gonadotropin (hCG). It is the β-subunit that confers on TSH the specific physiological properties that differentiate it from other glycopeptides. The primary stimulus for TSH release from the pituitary is TRH binding to pituitary thyrotroph cells. At the thyroid, TSH binds to specific cell membrane receptors, thereby activating adenylate cyclase and increasing intracellular levels of cAMP. The increased levels of cAMP have two main actions. The first trophic action involves the stimulation of cell reproduction and growth (hypertrophy). The second effect is the stimulation of production and secretion of thyroid hormones by thyroid follicular cells. These hormones in turn feed back to the hypothalamus and pituitary to reduce the secretion of TRH and TSH. TSH secretion is exquisitely sensitive to this feedback inhibition by thyroid hormone. A twofold change in free thyroxine (**f**$\mathbf{T_4}$) concentration results in an approximately 100-fold inverse change in the concentration of TSH, as is shown in Fig. 49-5. The net result is that thyroid hormone concentration is regulated within a narrow range.

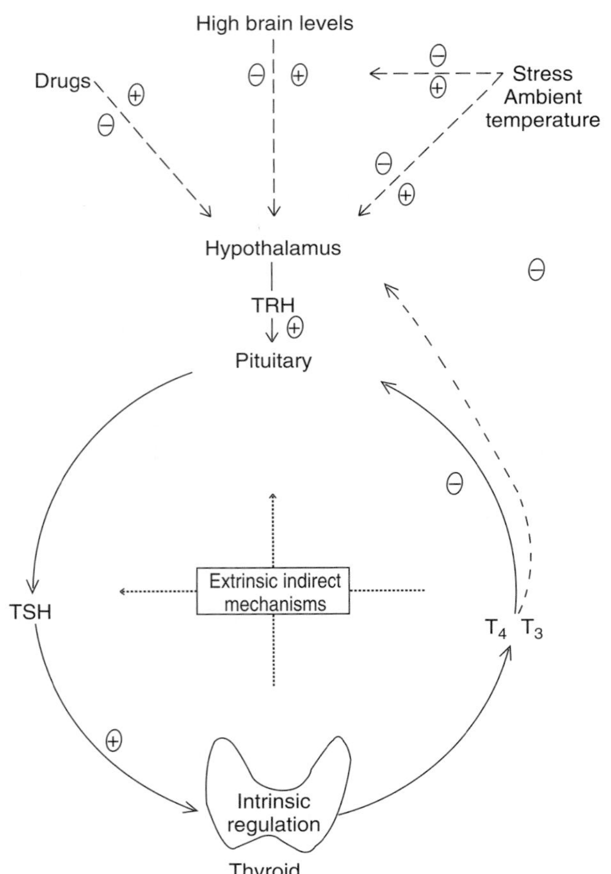

Fig. 49-4 Hypothalamic-pituitary-thyroid axis (HPTA). Stimulatory, ⊕, or inhibitory, effect of agent.

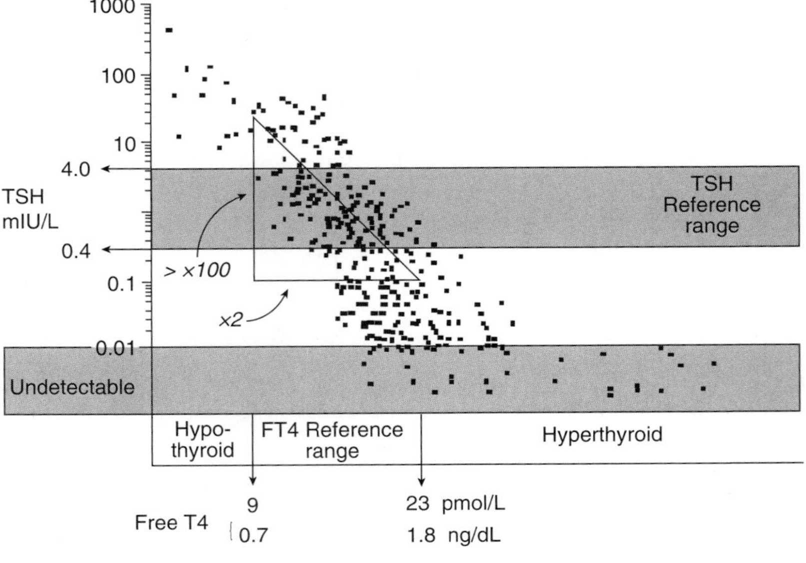

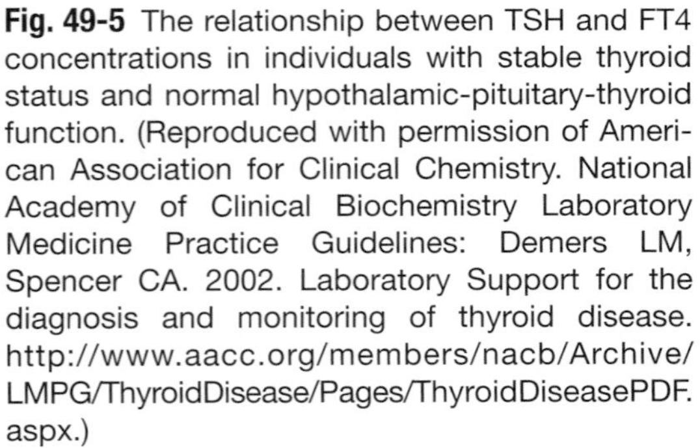

Fig. 49-5 The relationship between TSH and FT4 concentrations in individuals with stable thyroid status and normal hypothalamic-pituitary-thyroid function. (Reproduced with permission of American Association for Clinical Chemistry. National Academy of Clinical Biochemistry Laboratory Medicine Practice Guidelines: Demers LM, Spencer CA. 2002. Laboratory Support for the diagnosis and monitoring of thyroid disease. http://www.aacc.org/members/nacb/Archive/LMPG/ThyroidDisease/Pages/ThyroidDiseasePDF.aspx.)

Some evidence of autocine/paracrine regulation (see p. 941) of TSH release has been found, along with pituitary neuromedin B, a TSH release inhibitor that is upregulated by thyroid hormones and downregulated by TRH.[3]

Transport of Thyroid Hormones

After release from the thyroid, both T_4 and T_3 circulate within the blood, primarily bound to one of three binding proteins, with thyroid hormones distributed in equilibrium among all binding proteins. The most important of the thyroid hormone–binding proteins is the 54 kd **thyroxine-binding globulin (TBG).** This protein has a higher binding affinity for T_4 than for T_3. **Transthyretin (prealbumin,** thyroxine binding prealbumin [TBPA]), a 55 kd protein, has a lower affinity for T_4 than does TBG. Albumin has low affinity but high capacity for the thyroid hormones. Under physiological circumstances, TBG transports 60% to 75% of total T_4. TBPA and albumin transport 15% to 30% and 10% of T_4, respectively. As is true for T_4, most (99.7%) plasma T_3 circulates in the bound form. The affinity of TBG for T_3 is lower than its affinity for T_4, and binding of T_3 to TBPA is negligible. T_3 is bound mostly to TBG and to a lesser extent to albumin.

Approximately 0.02% of total T_4 and approximately 0.3% of total T_3 is unbound. It is these unbound fractions that are readily available for cellular uptake and are physiologically active, particularly T_3.

Mechanism of Action of Thyroid Hormones

T_3 has more biological activity than does T_4; indeed, T_4 can be considered more as a prohormone to T_3. Peripheral tissue deiodination of T_4 to T_3 (see later) leads to increased amounts of biologically active T_3. This peripheral conversion can vary markedly from tissue to tissue.

T_3 and T_4 probably enter cells through a mixture of diffusion and active transport.[4] The classical actions of T_3 are mediated through regulation of gene transcription. Within the nucleus, T_3 binds to thyroid hormone nuclear receptors (TRs), and this complex in turn binds to specific DNA sequences called thyroid hormone response elements (THREs), causing stimulation or inhibition of gene transcription.

Numerous actions of T_3 occur very rapidly and appear to be independent of gene transcription. These include cellular transport of Ca^{2+}, Na^+, and glucose; alterations in activity of kinases and phospholipases[5]; and activation of cytochrome C oxidase in mitochondria. The latter perhaps is an effect of 3,5-diiodo-L-thyronine (T_2).[6]

General Metabolic and Physiological Effects of Thyroid Hormones

Thyroid hormones exhibit widespread actions within the body; these are summarized in Table 49-1. The effects of thyroid hormone can be classified according to their clinical expression into (1) general metabolic effects, (2) growth and maturation effects, and (3) organ-specific effects. Generally speaking, both intermediary metabolic pathways and specific metabolic pathways are stimulated by T_3, resulting in increased oxygen consumption and calorigenesis (generation of body heat). Thyroid hormone has important actions as a promoter of cell differentiation, growth, and maturation. Deficiency of thyroid hormone in early life results in severe impairment of physical growth, maturation, and brain development. The third class of thyroid hormonal effects represents many direct effects exerted on specific organs and systems; these effects are particularly important in heart, bone, and the nervous system.

In the heart, T_3 affects cardiac gene expression, for example, by stimulating myosin α–heavy chain synthesis and depressing myosin β–heavy chain synthesis. T_3 influences the sensitivity of the heart to the sympathetic nervous system, for example, by stimulating synthesis of β_1-adrenergic receptors, and causes peripheral hemodynamic alterations that influence cardiac function.[7]

T_3 stimulates bone to produce cytokines, growth factors, and angiogenic factors that influence bone development and growth. Excess of serum thyroid hormone is associated with osteoporosis and bone fractures. The precise mechanism is not clear, but increased bone turnover and associated bone microarchitectural changes with increased fragility appear to be involved.[8]

The developing fetus requires thyroid hormone for normal brain development.[9] The fetus is dependent upon the mother until midgestation, when it begins to produce thyroid hormones independently. Insufficient first-trimester levels of maternal thyroid hormone have been demonstrated to increase the risks for mental[10] and psychomotor deficits in the newborn.[11] The late second and early third trimesters appear to be critical transition periods in fetal thyroid hormone metabolism, as the fetal thyroid axis develops increasing autonomy.[12]

In the adult brain, most T_3 is produced locally from T_4 through the action of D2 deiodinase (see later).[13] Although the mechanisms are not well understood, cerebral blood flow to regions that mediate attention, memory, and visuospatial processing is decreased in hypothyroid patients.[14] Indeed, brain size physically changes with abnormalities of thyroid homeostasis, increasing in hyperthyroidism and decreasing in hypothyroidism.[15]

Deiodinases and the Metabolism of Thyroid Hormones

Thyroid hormones are metabolized predominantly by deiodination (see later), although small amounts of T_4, T_3, and reverse T_3 (rT_3) are conjugated with glucuronide or sulfate in the liver and excreted in the bile, or are metabolized to the acetic acid analogs tetrac and triac.[16]

Three **deiodinases,** called D1, D2, and D3, are known. D1 is present in high concentrations in liver and kidney and converts T_4 to T_3 and rT_3 in equimolar quantities. This enzyme, which is the main source of T_3 in hyperthyroid patients, is inhibited by the antithyroid drug propylthiouracil (PTU). D2

Table 49-1 Basic Physiological Effects of Thyroid Hormone and Their Relationship With Syndromes of Thyroid Dysfunction

		USUAL SYMPTOMS	
System	**Thyroid Hormone Effects**	**Hyperthyroidism**	**Hypothyroidism**
Metabolic	Increased calorigenesis and O_2 consumption	Heat intolerance	Cold intolerance
		Flushed skin	Dry and pale skin
	Increased heat dissipation	Increased perspiration	Coarse skin
	Increased protein catabolism	Increased appetite and food ingestion	Lethargy
	Increased glucose absorption and production (gluconeogenesis)	Muscle wasting and proximal weakness	Generalized weakness
			Weight gain
	Increased glucose use	Weight loss	Voice coarsening, slow speech
		Onycholysis (nail disease)	Myxedema
		Lid lag	
		Proptosis (exophthalmos)	
	Lipid metabolism	$\downarrow$ Serum HDL	
Cardiovascular	Increased adrenergic activity and sensitivity	Palpitations	Slow heart rate (bradycardia)
		Fast heart rate (tachycardia)	Low blood pressure
	Increased heart rate	Bouncy, hyperdynamic arterial pulses	Heart failure
	Increased myocardial contractility (inotropy)	Shortness of breath	Heart enlargement
			Atrial fibrillation
	Increased cardiac output	Widened pulse pressure ($\uparrow$ systolic BP, $\downarrow$ diastolic BP)	
	Increased blood volume		
	Decreased peripheral vascular resistance		
Central nervous	Increased adrenergic activity and sensitivity	Restlessness, hypermotility	Apathy
		Nervousness	Mental sluggishness
		Emotional lability	Depressed reflexes
		Fatigue	Mental retardation
		Exaggerated reflexes	
		Tremor	
GI	Increased motility	Hyperdefecation	Constipation

BP, Blood pressure; *HDL,* high-density lipoprotein.

is present in high concentration in muscle, brain, skin, and placenta. D3 is present in brain and placenta and inactivates T_4 by converting it to rT_3 and inactivates T_3 by converting it to 3,3′-diiodothyronine (DIT). The activities of D2 and D3 are sensitive to changes in serum T_4 and T_3; they change in a reciprocal manner to hormone concentration to maintain homeostasis.[17] Most circulating T_3 in euthyroid persons is produced by deiodinase activity in liver, kidney, and muscle, although most cells in the body can produce some T_3. Reverse T_3 is an inactive product of thyroid hormone metabolism; it is formed by removal of an iodine residue from the 5 position, making 3,3′,5′-triiodothyronine (see Fig. 49-2). The metabolic pathways for thyroid hormones are shown in Fig. 49-6.

During severe illness, T_3 and T_4 concentrations in plasma typically fall, and TSH concentration remains constant. This is similar to the pattern seen during starvation, where the change is thought to reflect an adaptation to reduce energy expenditure. It is unclear whether a reduction in T_3 is a protective mechanism against hypercatabolism, or an overreaction by the body.[18]

KEY CONCEPTS BOX 49-1

- Thyroid hormones, T_4 (thyroxine), and T_3 are iodinated tyrosine molecules that are connected in tandem within the thyroglobulin (TG), which is stored in thyroid colloid. These hormones are released after proteolysis of TG.
- After stimulation by hypothalamic TRH, the pituitary secretes TSH; this stimulates the thyroid to release T_4 and T_3. Rising levels of T_4 and T_3 feed back on the hypothalamus and pituitary to inhibit TRH and TSH release.
- T_4 and T_3 are transported to target cells bound to the plasma proteins TBG prealbumin, and albumin.
- In target cells, T_4 is converted to active T_3, which binds to receptors that bind to DNA, thereby changing gene activity. T_4 and T_3 are metabolized to inactive, deiodinated form.
- T_3 increases the metabolic rate by increasing glucose metabolism and gluconeogenesis. T_3 increases cardiac output and heart rate and enhances the sensitivity of the CNS.

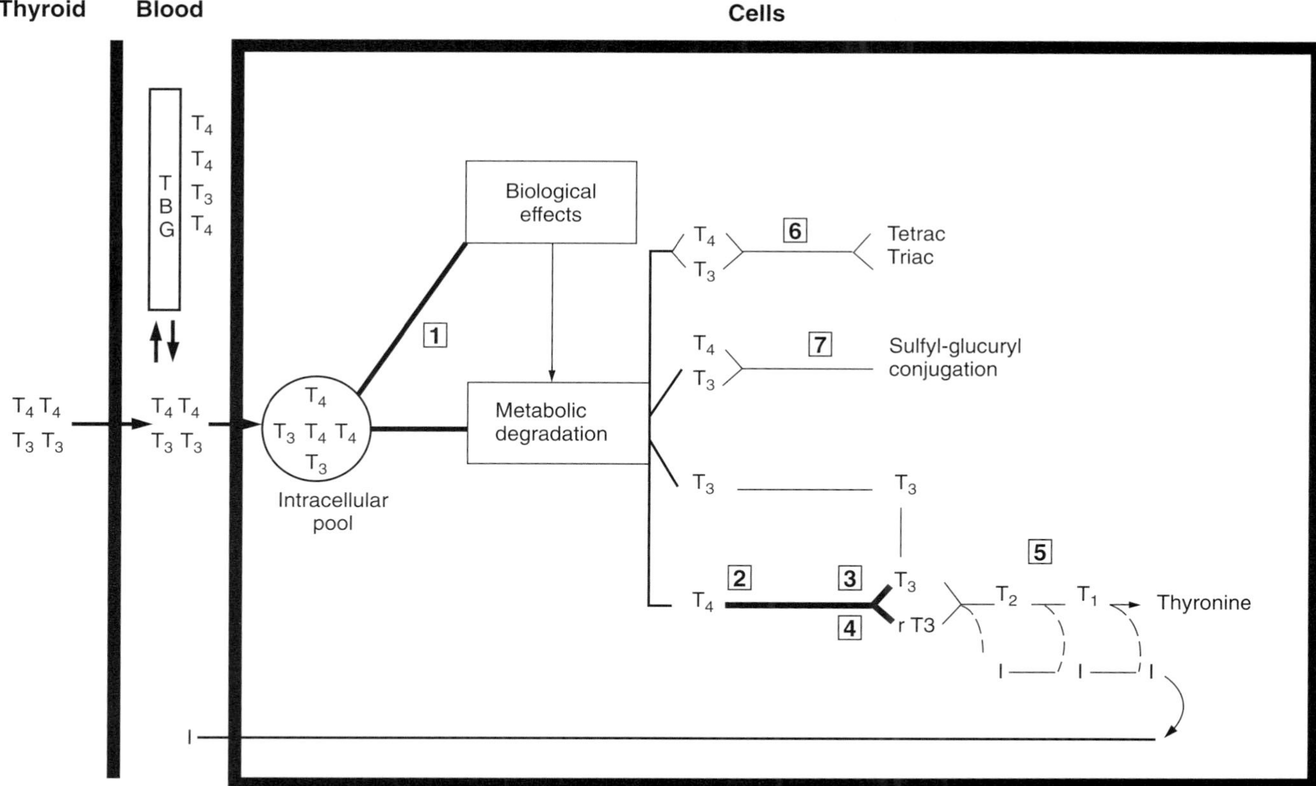

Fig. 49-6 Metabolic pathways of thyroid hormone. *1,* Biological effects through binding to intracellular receptors; *2,* main deiodinative pathway for thyroxine (T_4); *3,* conversion of T_4 into triiodothyronine (T_3); *4,* conversion of T_4 to reverse triiodothyronine (rT_3); *5,* serial deiodinations of T_3 and rT_3; *6,* deamination and decarboxylation pathway; *7,* conjugative pathway.

SECTION OBJECTIVES BOX 49-2

- Discuss the usefulness of population screening for thyroid disease.
- Discuss Graves' disease, nodular thyroid disease, thyroiditis, thyrotoxicosis, and subclinical hyperthyroidism according to prevalence, etiology, symptoms, typical laboratory findings, and treatment.
- Discuss Hashimoto's thyroiditis and other causes of hypothyroidism discussed in this section according to etiology, symptoms, typical laboratory findings, and treatment.
- Discuss the changes in thyroid function that occur during pregnancy, including the effects of this change on TBG, T_3 and T_4, free T_3 and free T_4, and TSH concentrations.
- Discuss thyroid function in the fetus and the newborn and the need to screen for pre- or perinatal hypothyroidism.
- Discuss the euthyroid-sick syndrome according to proposed pathogenesis and typical laboratory results.

PATHOLOGICAL CONDITIONS

Disorders of thyroid function can be divided into two main groups: **hyperthyroidism,** in which there is overproduction of thyroid hormones, and **hypothyroidism,** which is characterized by underproduction. Both hyperthyroidism and hypothyroidism can be further categorized as primary thyroid disease, in which the disease process originates within the thyroid gland, or secondary thyroid disease, in which pituitary dysfunction is the source of thyroid abnormalities. Secondary thyroid disease is very uncommon.

The Third National Health and Nutrition Examination Survey (NHANES III) examined the prevalence of thyroid disease in the United States. Of that study population, 4.7% self-reported that they had thyroid disease or goiter, or were taking thyroid medications. An additional 4.6% of remaining subjects were found to be hypothyroid (0.3% overt and 4.3% subclinical), and 1.3% hyperthyroid (0.5% overt and 0.7% subclinical). This equates to 11.2 million persons with clinical thyroid disease (including the self-reported group) and an additional 7.9 million with subclinical disease.[19]

Iodine is essential for normal thyroid function. Worldwide, the most common cause of thyroid dysfunction is iodine deficiency. In parts of the world where there is iodine sufficiency, the most common pathological mechanism is autoimmunity.

Hyperthyroidism

Hyperthyroidism most accurately refers to an overactive thyroid gland. **Thyrotoxicosis** is a term that often is used

Box 49-1

Causes of Hyperthyroidism

- Autoimmune
  - Graves'
  - Hashitoxicosis
- Thyroiditis (often transient hyperthyroidism)
  - Painless sporadic
  - Postpartum
  - Subacute
  - Suppurative
  - Radiation
  - Drug-induced
- Nodular disease
  - Toxic multinodular goiter
  - Toxic adenoma
- Thyroid-stimulating hormone (TSH)-mediated
  - TSH-producing pituitary adenoma
- Human chorionic gonadotropin (hCG)-mediated
  - Hyperemesis gravidarum
  - Trophoblastic disease
- Exogenous thyroid hormone intake
  - Excessive replacement therapy
  - Intentional suppressive therapy
  - Factitious hyperthyroidism

interchangeably with hyperthyroidism, although it is a broader term that refers to any condition in which excess circulating thyroid hormone is present. Thyrotoxicosis therefore includes excessive **thyroxine** ingestion, whereby the patient will manifest clinical features of hyperthyroidism with no abnormality within the thyroid gland. A vast majority of cases of hyperthyroidism result from primary thyroid disease (Box 49-1). Many of these diseases are autoimmune in nature.

Excess thyroid hormone leads to an increase in the body's metabolism, which can lead to a number of different symptoms. Common symptoms and signs are listed in Table 49-1. In addition, some women experience menstrual irregularity or amenorrhea, and some men notice tender or enlarged breasts, or erectile dysfunction. Other important clinical associations of hyperthyroidism include atrial fibrillation, osteoporosis and lipid changes including lowered HDL concentrations.

Graves' Disease

Graves' disease, the most common cause of hyperthyroidism, accounts for 60% to 80% of all cases of hyperthyroidism. Graves' disease is much more prevalent in women than in men and commonly occurs between the ages of 40 and 60 years. It is strongly heritable, with 80% of total predisposition to Graves' disease resulting from genetic factors.[20] It is an autoimmune disorder in which serum autoantibodies bind to TSH receptors on the thyroid cell and stimulate the production and release of thyroid hormone. These antibodies comprise a heterogeneous group of serum immunoglobulin G (IgG) components that are generically termed *thyroid-stimulating immunoglobulins (TSI).*[21] Graves' disease shares many immunological features with autoimmune hypothyroidism, and patients often have high serum concentrations of antibodies against thyroglobulin and thyroid peroxidase.

Graves' disease is characterized clinically by symptoms and signs of hyperthyroidism (see Table 49-1), the presence of diffuse **goiter, ophthalmopathy,** and, much less commonly, dermopathy (pretibial swelling of the shins). Graves' ophthalmopathy is characterized by a myxedematous infiltration of the tissues (swelling observable by pressing on the tissue) and muscles of the orbit, resulting in protrusion of the eyes (exophthalmos) and ocular muscle dysfunction. The ophthalmopathy may exist without accompanying thyroid hyperfunction, and the severity and clinical course of the ophthalmopathy are unrelated to those of hyperthyroidism. Similar to many autoimmune disorders, Graves' disease often is less severe or even remits during pregnancy, but a postpartum return of the disease may occur. TSH receptor antibodies can cross the placenta and cause transient neonatal Graves' disease. This condition is reported in about 2% of pregnancies in women with a background of Graves' disease.[22] The higher the serum levels of maternal TSH receptor antibodies in the third trimester, the greater is the likelihood of neonatal Graves' hyperthyroidism.[23] Recent clinical guidelines have suggested that women with a history of Graves' should be tested for the presence of TSH receptor antibodies during the second half of pregnancy, so that those at risk of having a baby with neonatal Graves' disease can be identified.[24]

Nodules

Nodular thyroid disease is very common, and the incidence of **nodules** increases with increasing age. Approximately 5% of adults in the United States have a palpable thyroid nodule.[25] An overwhelming majority of these nodules are benign. A multinodular goiter (MNG) may be defined as a structurally and functionally heterogeneous thyroid enlargement. Thyroid function in patients with an MNG often becomes less responsive to normal thyroid homeostatic mechanisms (autonomous) with increasing age; these individuals may develop subclinical (suppressed TSH with normal thyroxine, see later) or overt hyperthyroidism. This is known as a toxic multinodular goiter and is the second most common cause of hyperthyroidism overall and the most common cause in older patients.

Solitary thyroid nodules can be benign colloid nodules, adenomas, cysts, or, less commonly, carcinomas. Many apparently solitary nodules are actually the largest of multiple colloid nodules in small MNGs. Adenomas can become autonomous and may cause hyperthyroidism, although most patients with adenomas will be euthyroid. Thyroid cancer is a very rare cause of hyperthyroidism.

Thyroiditis

Thyroiditis is a general term that is used to describe inflammation of the thyroid gland. All forms of thyroiditis (Box 49-2) can potentially cause hyperthyroidism, because large quantities of hormone can be released from inflamed and

Box 49-2

Types of Thyroiditis

Autoimmune
Hashimoto's (chronic lymphocytic thyroiditis)
Postpartum
Painless sporadic thyroiditis

Infectious/Postviral
Subacute
Suppurative

Other
Radiation thyroiditis
Drug-induced

disrupted follicles. Postpartum, painless sporadic, and subacute thyroiditis may result in triphasic changes in thyroid function with initial thyrotoxicosis, followed by a period of euthyroidism and then hypothyroidism. Some patients subsequently will develop permanent hypothyroidism. **Hashimoto's thyroiditis** (also known as chronic lymphocytic thyroiditis) is associated most commonly with permanent hypothyroidism but occasionally is associated with transient thyrotoxicosis.

Postpartum thyroiditis occurs in 5% to 7% of women after delivery in iodine-sufficient areas[26] and typically occurs 1 to 6 months postpartum. The thyroid gland often becomes enlarged, especially in women from iodine-deficient areas. Postpartum thyroiditis and painless sporadic thyroiditis are indistinguishable except by the relation of the former to pregnancy. Most women with postpartum thyroiditis will not require treatment because this type of thyroiditis is transitory. However, they have a higher than average incidence of permanent hypothyroidism later in life.

Sudden release of hormone may be seen after irradiation of the thyroid gland (radiation thyroiditis). Thyroid hyperfunction caused by radiation thyroiditis usually is mild and self-limited. Some drugs can cause thyroiditis and thyrotoxicosis. See the section on drugs and the thyroid.

Other Causes of Thyrotoxicosis

Tumors that originate from the trophoblast, or the outer cellular layer of the forming embryo, can secrete large amounts of hCG, which exhibits weak TSH-like activity. As a result, trophoblastic tumors may cause increased secretion of thyroid hormones. Both normal pregnancy and **hyperemesis gravidarum** (excessive vomiting of pregnant women) can be associated with mild hyperthyroidism (see thyroid function in pregnancy later). Secondary hyperthyroidism caused by pituitary tumors that secrete high levels of TSH is a rare occurrence.

Some iodine-deficient patients develop hyperthyroidism after iodine has been replaced through diet or after the administration of radiographic iodine-containing contrast material. This condition, known as the Jod-Basedow phenomenon, is believed to occur in patients with occult Graves' disease or multinodular goiter.

Thyrotoxicosis can be caused by administration of excessive thyroid hormone by the physician (iatrogenic), or as the result of surreptitious intake of thyroid hormone by patients (factitious).

Subclinical Hyperthyroidism

The availability of sensitive assays for **thyrotropin** (TSH) has resulted in the identification of patients with low TSH concentration (<0.5 mU/L) but normal thyroid hormone concentration. These patients generally do not have any symptoms of hyperthyroidism and are classified as having subclinical hyperthyroidism. Common causes of subclinical hyperthyroidism are the same as those for overt hyperthyroidism—autonomously functioning thyroid nodules and multinodular goiters. Excessive replacement of thyroxine and Graves' (especially in those over 55 years of age) are much less common causes.[27]

The prevalence varies considerably between different studies. The NHANES III survey identified 0.7% of more than 16,000 subjects, but other studies have reported prevalence of up to 12%. Progression to overt hyperthyroidism occurs at between 1% and 4% per year and is more likely with underlying multinodular goiter or an autonomously functioning nodule.[28,29]

The clinical importance of subclinical hyperthyroidism lies in its effects on the cardiovascular system, particularly increased rates of atrial fibrillation. Overt hyperthyroidism is associated with low bone density and an increase in fractures. Whether subclinical hyperthyroidism is associated with adverse skeletal outcomes has been a topic of debate, although some studies have shown decreased bone density in postmenopausal women on suppressive doses of T_4 for thyroid cancer or goiter.[30,31] Some studies have shown an increase in all-cause mortality as well.[32]

Laboratory Findings (see Table 49-2)

Laboratory findings in hyperthyroidism include elevated thyroid hormones (total [T]T_4, fT_4, TT_3, and fT_3) and low or suppressed TSH. Some patients may have isolated T_3 toxicosis or T_4 toxicosis, in which only T_3 or T_4, respectively, is increased. In the rare case of TSH-induced hyperthyroidism (e.g., pituitary tumor–producing excess TSH), patients will have elevated TSH and high thyroid hormone concentrations. Patients with low or suppressed TSH but normal fT_4 and fT_3 are likely to have subclinical hyperthyroidism.

In patients with thyroid disease of an autoimmune origin, thyroid antibodies like thyroid peroxidase antibody (TPO-Ab) may be positive. Some patients with Graves' disease will have a positive TSI or thyroid receptor antibody. The newer second-generation assay for TSH receptor antibodies has a high sensitivity of up to 99% for the diagnosis of Graves' disease.[33]

After treatment with medication or radioactive iodine has been initiated for hyperthyroidism, disease activity is best

Table 49-2 Changes in Thyroid Function Tests in Different Disease States

Clinical Entity	TSH	T_4 or fT_4	T_3 or fT_3	T_3RU	TSI	TPO-ab	Thyroid Scan Uptake
Graves' disease	↓	↑	↑	↑	Positive	May be positive	Uniformly increased
Toxic multinodular goiter/ toxic thyroid adenoma	↓	↑	↑	↑	Negative		Patchy, increased
Autoimmune thyroiditis (may have triphasic TFT changes)	↓ N ↑	↑ N ↓	↑ N ↓	↑ N ↓	Negative	Likely to be positive	Usually decreased, may be increased in Hashimoto's thyrotoxicosis
Subacute/suppurative thyroiditis	↓	↑	↑	↑	Negative	Unlikely to be positive	Decreased
Pregnancy thyrotoxicosis/ trophoblastic disease	↓			N ↓	Negative		Contra-indicated in pregnancy
Secondary (pituitary) hyperthyroidism	↑ (or normal, not suppressed)	↑	↑	↓	Negative	Unlikely to be positive	Increased
Excess T_4 therapy	↓	↑	↑	↓		Depends on underlying cause	Decreased uptake
Primary hypothyroidism	↑	↓	↓	↓ N	Negative	May be positive	
Secondary (pituitary) hypothyroidism	↓ (or normal)	↓	↓	↓	Negative	Unlikely to be positive	
Nonthyroidal illness*	N	N ↓	N ↓	N	Negative	Negative	

fT_3, Free triiodothyronine; *fT_4*, free thyroxine; *T_3*, triiodothyronine; *T_4*, thyroxine; *TFT*, thyroid function tests; *TPO-ab*, thyroid peroxidase antibody; *T_3RU*, T_3 resin uptake; *TSH*, thyroid-stimulating hormone; *TSI*, thyroid-stimulating immunoglobulin; *N*, normal.
*Nonthyroidal illness—rarely, any pattern may be seen.

monitored initially with fT_4 and fT_3, because TSH will take several weeks or longer to return toward the reference interval.

Treatment

Three main treatment modalities are available for hyperthyroidism. Antithyroid drugs like methimazole or propylthiouracil (PTU) inhibit the production of thyroid hormone in the thyroid. Surgical thyroidectomy and radioactive iodine both aim to eliminate excess functioning thyroid tissue. All these methods are used currently, and selection depends on the cause of hyperthyroidism, specific clinical situations, and the physician's personal preferences. Large regional variation in their use has been noted, for example, radioactive iodine is favored in North America, and antithyroid drugs are preferred in most other parts of the world.[34]

A number of medications are used when patients with high thyroxine levels need to be treated quickly (e.g., before surgery). Saturated solution of potassium iodide (SSKI) and Lugol solution, both of which contain high doses of iodine, decrease the synthesis of new thyroid hormone (Wolff-Chaikoff effect) and reduce the release of pre-formed hormone from the thyroid. Large doses of glucocorticoids like dexamethasone sometimes are used to treat thyrotoxicosis because they reduce T_4 to T_3 conversion peripherally, and possibly decrease T_4 concentrations in Graves' disease.[35] β-Blockers suppress the symptoms of hyperthyroidism and often are used while one is waiting for other treatments to become effective. Propranolol has some impact on peripheral conversion of T_4 to T_3 at high doses, which is not seen with other β-blockers, but the clinical significance of this is probably small.[36]

Hypothyroidism

A clinical state of hypothyroidism develops whenever insufficient amounts of thyroid hormone are available to tissues. The most common group of conditions causing hypothyroidism are those that involve the thyroid gland itself (i.e., primary hypothyroidism), as shown in Box 49-3.

The severity of symptoms and signs (see Table 49-1) will depend on the magnitude of thyroid hormone deficiency and the acuteness with which the deficiency develops. Many of the clinical manifestations reflect a generalized slowing of metabolism (e.g., fatigue, cold intolerance, weight gain, bradycardia) or an accumulation of matrix glycosaminoglycans in the interstitial spaces of many tissues, which can lead to coarse hair and skin and puffy face. Other associated clinical and laboratory findings include carpal tunnel syndrome, menstrual irregularities, anemia, hyponatremia, and hypercholesterolemia.

Hashimoto's Thyroiditis

Hashimoto's thyroiditis (chronic autoimmune thyroiditis) is probably the most common cause of hypothyroidism in iodine-sufficient areas. It is caused by cell- and antibody-mediated destruction of thyroid tissue and can be enlarged (goitrous) or atrophic. More than 90% of patients will have antibodies to thyroglobulin or thyroid peroxidase. These antibodies exhibit little if any functional activity. In an occasional patient with Hashimoto's, thyrotoxicosis will alternate with hypothyroidism, most likely because of the intermittent presence of thyroid-stimulating and thyroid-blocking antibodies.[37]

Box 49-3

Causes of Hypothyroidism

Primary Hypothyroidism
- Hashimoto's thyroiditis/chronic autoimmune thyroiditis
- Iatrogenic/treatment-related
  - Post-thyroidectomy
  - Post–radioactive iodine treatment
  - Previous external neck irradiation
  - Use of antithyroid drugs
- Transient thyroiditis
  - Painless sporadic thyroiditis
  - Postpartum thyroiditis
  - Subacute thyroiditis
- Congenital hypothyroidism
  - Thyroid agenesis/dysgenesis
  - Defects in hormone synthesis
- Infiltrative thyroid disease (Reidel's thyroiditis, hemochromatosis, sarcoidosis, amyloidosis)
- Iodine deficiency or excess
- Drugs (antithyroid drugs, interferon [IFN]-α, amiodarone, lithium, interleukin [IL]-2, sunitinib)

Central (Secondary or Tertiary) Hypothyroidism
- Thyroid-stimulating hormone (TSH) deficiency
- Thyroid-releasing hormone (TRH) deficiency

Thyroid Hormone Resistance

Other Causes of Hypothyroidism

Hypothyroidism can result from treatment for hyperthyroidism. Total thyroidectomy results in hypothyroidism within 2 to 4 weeks of surgery. Subtotal thyroidectomy will result in hypothyroidism in many patients, particularly those with Graves' disease, presumably because of superimposed chronic autoimmune thyroiditis. Destruction of the thyroid gland by radioactive iodine (RAI) treatment and external neck irradiation can result in hypothyroidism. The rate of hypothyroidism depends on the dose given, and hypothyroidism can develop many months or years after administration of the initial dose. Drugs used to treat hyperthyroidism also can cause hypothyroidism (see later).

Iodine deficiency and excess can cause hypothyroidism. Iodine deficiency is the most common cause of hypothyroidism worldwide, affecting approximately 2 billion people. Iodine deficiency is rare in North America because of inclusion of iodized salt in the diet, but it persists in Europe and many other countries because of low utilization of iodized salt. In certain regions (Africa, South America), the effect of low dietary iodine intake is magnified by consumption of cassava roots that contain cyanoglucosides. These substances are metabolized to thiocyanate, which has antithyroid properties.[38] Iodine excess can cause hypothyroidism by inhibiting iodide organification and T_4 and T_3 synthesis (the Wolff-Chaikoff effect). Subjects with normal thyroid glands "escape" from this effect and maintain normal thyroid function. However, those with abnormal thyroid glands (e.g., Hashimoto's or other thyroiditis, previous partial thyroidectomy or RAI) are at risk for iodine-induced hypothyroidism. Excess iodine can be derived from iodine supplements, kelp tablets, iodine-containing medicines like amiodarone or some cough medicines, or radiographic contrast agents.[39] It is interesting to note that iodine fortification of salt in areas of Denmark with previous mild to moderate iodine deficiency has led to an increase in both hyperthyroidism and hypothyroidism. The mechanism behind the increase in hypothyroidism remains unknown.[40,41]

Numerous drugs can cause hypothyroidism. See section on drugs that affect thyroid function, later in the chapter.

Congenital Hypothyroidism

Congenital hypothyroidism occurs in approximately 1 in 4000 newborns and is one of the most common treatable causes of mental retardation.[42] Most newborns with congenital hypothyroidism have few or no clinical manifestations of thyroid deficiency. For this reason, newborn screening programs in which T_4 and/or TSH is measured in heel-prick blood specimens were developed in the mid-1970s to detect this condition as early as possible.[43] The most common causes of congenital hypothyroidism are agenesis and dysgenesis of the thyroid. A few individuals have inherited defects in thyroid hormone biosynthesis or were delivered by mothers who were receiving an antithyroid drug for hyperthyroidism. Among children who become hypothyroid later, the most common cause is Hashimoto's thyroiditis (chronic autoimmune thyroiditis).

Secondary Hypothyroidism

Secondary hypothyroidism is that caused by TSH deficiency (i.e., pituitary disease); tertiary hypothyroidism is caused by TRH deficiency (i.e., hypothalamic disease). These two causes of hypothyroidism are rare and account for less than 1% of all cases of hypothyroidism. They usually occur in conjunction with other deficiencies of pituitary hormones.[44]

Subclinical Hypothyroidism

Subclinical hypothyroidism is defined as a high TSH concentration with normal thyroid hormone levels. Most patients are asymptomatic; however, some may have mild, nonspecific symptoms of hypothyroidism. The causes are the same as for overt hypothyroidism, including chronic autoimmune thyroiditis, previous treatment for hyperthyroidism, and undertreatment of known overt hypothyroidism. Developing evidence suggests that persons with subclinical hypothyroidism have a higher cardiovascular mortality than euthyroid persons.[45]

In contrast to subclinical hyperthyroidism, a substantial number of patients with subclinical hypothyroidism, particularly those with positive thyroid-peroxidase antibodies, will develop overt hypothyroidism. It remains contentious whether patients with normal fT_4 levels should be treated with thyroxine, or simply monitored.

Thyroid Hormone Resistance

Resistance to thyroid hormone is an inherited condition (usually autosomal dominant inheritance) that is characterized by reduced responsiveness of target tissues to thyroid hormone. It is caused by mutations in the gene for one of the T_3 nuclear receptors that lead to a decreased affinity for T_3. More than 100 different mutations have been discovered. Variable severity of hormonal resistance has been noted in different tissues in the same patient and among different patients with the same mutation.

Laboratory Findings (see Table 49-2)

In general, all patients with hypothyroidism will have low thyroid hormone concentrations, and in the commonest form, primary hypothyroidism, TSH will be elevated. Secondary (or tertiary) hypothyroidism will have low or normal levels of TSH with low thyroid hormone concentrations. Most patients with chronic autoimmune thyroiditis will have positive thyroid antibodies, most commonly antibodies against TPO. Approximately 10% of the general population will be positive for TPO antibodies, many of whom will not have thyroid disease. Some of these individuals will develop hypothyroidism later in life. In thyroid hormone resistance, thyroid hormone concentrations are elevated, and TSH is variably normal or high.

Treatment

Treatment for patients with hypothyroidism consists of oral thyroid hormone replacement, which reverses abnormal laboratory findings and clinical symptoms and signs if no abnormalities occur in the transport and peripheral use of thyroid hormones. The agent most commonly used is levothyroxine (T_4), which is converted peripherally to T_3.

Although thyroxine is converted to the metabolically active **triiodothyronine** by widespread peripheral monodeiodination, some physicians advocate treating hypothyroid patients with both T_4 and T_3. Part of the problem with using T_3 is that it is absorbed rapidly and has a short half-life that can lead to unwanted serum peaks, sometimes with accompanying symptoms of palpitations.

Goiter

Goiter is a generic reference to an enlargement of the thyroid gland. It may be associated with a hyperthyroid, hypothyroid, or euthyroid state. Diffuse goiter is characterized by uniform enlargement of the thyroid gland. In multinodular goiter, the thyroid gland is enlarged in a nonuniform fashion, resulting in nodules that are located both superficially and deep within the gland.

Solitary Nodule

A solitary nodule refers to the presence of a solitary localized enlargement of a portion of the thyroid gland. Although most of these nodules represent benign conditions, such as cysts, localized hemorrhage, focal thyroiditis, and adenomas, they also may represent malignant tumors of the thyroid. External radiation therapy, used in the past for acne and enlarged tonsils and other conditions of the head, neck, and chest, has been associated with increased risk for the development of thyroid cancer and benign thyroid neoplasms.[46]

Thyroid adenomas can become autonomous and cause hyperthyroidism (see section on hyperthyroidism).

Thyroid Cancer

Cancer of the thyroid gland is an uncommon tumor, with an annual incidence in the United States of 30,000 cases.[47] The age- and gender-adjusted incidence of thyroid cancer is increasing faster than for any other malignancy in recent years. Increased screening and earlier detection are important contributors to this.

Thyroid epithelial cell–derived cancers are divided into three categories: papillary, follicular (both considered well-differentiated carcinomas), and anaplastic (undifferentiated). Clinical outcome is significantly worse for undifferentiated carcinomas. Other malignancy-associated diseases of the thyroid include **medullary thyroid cancer** (MTC) (originating from the parafollicular C-cells of the thyroid), primary thyroid lymphoma, and metastases from breast, colon, or renal cancer, or melanoma.

Most patients with thyroid cancer present with a thyroid nodule, but a few present with cervical lymphadenopathy or distant metastases. Patients with thyroid cancer usually do not present with significant abnormalities in thyroid function. Thyroid carcinomas can synthesize thyroid hormones and cause hyperthyroidism, but this is rare.

Thyroid epithelial cell–derived carcinomas often release thyroglobulin into the circulation, where it may be followed as a tumor marker. Because benign thyroid diseases can cause increased concentrations of thyroglobulin, the best use of thyroglobulin as a tumor marker is for monitoring disease in patients already diagnosed with thyroid cancer after treatment. Because anti-thyroglobulin antibody invalidates the use of the thyroglobulin assay, the presence of anti-thyroglobulin antibodies must be ascertained each time serum thyroglobulin is measured.

Medullary thyroid carcinomas secrete calcitonin that may be used as a tumor marker for both the diagnosis and therapeutic response of these tumors.

Useful Tests in Thyroid Nodules and Thyroid Cancer

Because thyroid nodules can be hyperfunctioning, it is important to monitor thyroid function tests. In the case of a nodular gland and hyperthyroidism, a thyroid nuclear medicine scan may show a "hot" (hyperfunctioning) nodule with suppression of the rest of the thyroid gland.

Monitoring of patients with thyroid cancer can be complex. After thyroidectomy and destruction of remnant thyroid tissue with radioiodine, progress can be monitored through serum thyroglobulin levels and iodine nuclear medicine scans. Both thyroglobulin levels and iodine scans are more sensitive when the patient's TSH level is elevated. Before these tests are given, patients are requested to stop their thyroxine for 4 to 6 weeks to allow TSH to rise. An alternative to thyroxine withdrawal is to administer recombinant TSH (rTSH) 1 day before the tests are given. rTSH is expensive and currently is not widely available.

Multiple Endocrine Neoplasia Syndromes

Multiple endocrine neoplasia (MEN) syndromes are rare conditions in which several endocrine glands develop benign or malignant tumors. These syndromes are heritable with autosomal dominant inheritance. They are classified into two types (MEN type 1 and MEN type 2), with MEN 2 having three subtypes (MEN 2A, MEN 2B, and familial medullary thyroid carcinoma [FMTC]) (Box 49-4). FMTC is actually a variant of MEN 2A that is characterized by a strong predisposition to medullary thyroid carcinoma, in the absence of the other tumors associated with MEN 2A or 2B. Recognition of MEN is important for treatment and for evaluation of family members, especially in cases of MEN 2, in which MTC can cause considerable morbidity and mortality. Family members found to have an RET protooncogene mutation (which causes MEN 2) may choose to undergo elective thyroidectomy as a preventative strategy before developing MTC.

Drugs That Affect Thyroid Function

Numerous drugs can cause thyroid dysfunction (Table 49-3).

Interferon-Alpha

Approximately 1% to 5% of patients who receive interferon-alpha (IFN-α) develop thyroiditis, with or without thyrotoxicosis. Other thyroid abnormalities, including Graves' disease, permanent hypothyroidism, or increased serum antithyroid antibody concentrations without thyroid dysfunction, can also occur.[48] The risk for any form of thyroid dysfunction is greater in those patients who have increased serum antithyroid antibody concentrations before initiation of IFN-α.

Amiodarone

Amiodarone, a drug that contains 37% iodine, can affect thyroid function in several different ways. It can produce hyperthyroidism by causing thyroiditis or iodine-induced hyperthyroidism (usually in patients with preexisting nodular goiter). It also can cause hypothyroidism via the antithyroid

Box 49-4

Classification of Multiple Endocrine Neoplasia

MEN 1
Primary hyperparathyroidism (>90%)
Pituitary tumors (10% to 20%), including prolactinomas, growth hormone (GH)-secreting, corticotropin-secreting, nonfunctioning adenomas
Enteropancreatic tumors (60% to 70%): gastrinoma, insulinoma, glucagonoma, nonsecreting tumors

MEN 2A
Medullary thyroid cancer (>90%)
Pheochromocytoma (40% to 50%)
Parathyroid hyperplasia (10% to 20%)

MEN 2B
Medullary thyroid cancer
Pheochromocytoma
Other: neuromas, ganglioneuromas, marfanoid habitus

Table 49-3 Drugs That Affect Thyroid Function and Thyroid Function Tests

Drugs That Cause Clinical Thyroid Dysfunction

Drugs	Mechanism
Thionamides (carbimazole, methimazole), propylthiouracil, perchlorate, iodine, iodine-containing drugs including amiodarone, radiographic agents, kelp tablets, saturated potassium iodide solutions (SSKI)	Inhibition of thyroid hormone synthesis
Lithium	Inhibition of thyroid hormone release
Iodine-containing drugs, amiodarone	Stimulation of thyroid hormone synthesis and/or release
Cholestyramine, iron sulfate, aluminium hydroxide, omeprazole and other gastric acid inhibitors	Decreased absorption of thyroxine (i.e., can cause hypothyroidism in those taking oral thyroxine)
Interferon-α, interleukin-2	Immune dysregulation
Sunitinib	Presumed destructive thyroiditis

Drugs That Cause Abnormal Thyroid Function Tests without Clinical Thyroid Dysfunction

Drugs	Mechanism
Salicylates, furosemide, heparin, phenytoin	Decreased T_4 binding to TBG $\rightarrow$ N fT_4, $\downarrow TT_4$
Phenytoin, carbamazepine, rifampicin	Increased T_4 clearance
Dobutamine, glucocorticoids	Suppression of TSH secretion
Amiodarone, glucocorticoids, propylthiouracil, propranolol, iopanoic acid	Impaired conversion of T_4 to T_3 (i.e., decreased type 1 and 2 deiodinases)

fT_4, Free thyroxine; *T*, total; *T_3*, triiodothyronine; *T_4*, thyroxine; *TBG*, thyroxine binding globulin; *TSH*, thyroid-stimulating hormone; *N*, normal.

action of iodine (especially in patients with preexisting thyroid disease). Amiodarone-induced hyperthyroidism seems to occur more frequently in iodine-deficient areas, and hypothyroidism occurs more frequently in iodine-sufficient areas, such as the USA.[49] Amiodarone also can inhibit the peripheral conversion of T_4 to T_3. As a result, serum T_3 concentration in patients with amiodarone-induced hyperthyroidism may not be increased above the reference interval.

Lithium

Lithium inhibits the coupling of iodotyrosine residues to form T_4 and T_3, and it inhibits secretion of T_4 and T_3. Lithium treatment can cause goiter in up to 50% of patients. Approximately 20% to 30% develop hypothyroidism. Most have subclinical hypothyroidism, but a few will develop overt hypothyroidism.[50] Lithium also is associated with chronic autoimmune thyroiditis, thyroid antibody positivity, and possible hyperthyroidism because it induces a painless thyroiditis.

Sunitinib

Sunitinib, an anti-cancer tyrosine kinase inhibitor, has been associated with hypothyroidism in 15% to 42% of patients.[51] Another study found a high prevalence of hypothyroidism (46%) without evidence of thyroid autoimmunity preceding hyperthyroidism or destructive thyroiditis, and suggested that sunitinib impairs iodine uptake.[52]

Antithyroid Drugs (Methimazole, Carbimazole, Propylthiouracil)

Excessive use of these drugs in the treatment of hyperthyroidism can cause hypothyroidism, and patients who are receiving these drugs should have their thyroid function checked regularly. Ethionamide, which is used to treat tuberculosis, is structurally similar to methimazole and is a rare cause of hypothyroidism.

Other Causes

Excessive thyroxine or tertroxin (T_3) ingestion can lead to thyrotoxicosis. Carbamazepine can increase the clearance of T_4, in hypothyroid patients who are taking oral T_4. These patients should have their thyroid function checked after starting these medications. Interleukin-2 has been associated with painless thyroiditis in a few cases.

Pregnancy and Thyroid Function

Striking changes in thyroid function occur during pregnancy. Serum TBG concentration increases almost twofold because estrogen increases hepatic TBG production and TBG sialylation; the latter results in decreased clearance of TBG. As a result, total TT_4 and TT_3 are increased. However, fT_4 and fT_3 remain unaffected.

Human chorionic gonadotropin (hCG) has weak TSH-like activity as the result of similarities in primary structure for the two hormones. Serum hCG concentrations increase soon after fertilization and peak at 10 to 12 weeks. During this period, serum fT_4 and fT_3 concentrations increase slightly, usually within the reference interval, and serum TSH concentrations usually fall compared to pre-pregnancy levels, but usually in the reference interval. In 10% to 20% of pregnant women, serum TSH concentration will be below the reference range in the first trimester, with no clinical consequences.

Hyperemesis gravidarum is a syndrome that is defined as nausea and vomiting associated with weight loss of greater than 5% during early pregnancy. It may be caused by high serum concentrations of hCG and estradiol. Many afflicted women have subclinical or mild overt hyperthyroidism, which resolves as the hCG concentration falls after the first trimester, and rarely requires antithyroid treatment.[53]

Trophoblastic tumors (hydatidiform molar pregnancies, choriocarcinomas) are associated with very high levels of hCG and can cause biochemical and clinical hyperthyroidism. Removal of the molar pregnancy or effective chemotherapy for the choriocarcinoma cures the hyperthyroidism.[54]

Thyroid Function in the Fetus and Newborn (see Chapter 45)

Although TSH is circulating in the fetus from around 10 to 12 weeks of gestation, little thyroid hormone synthesis occurs before 18 to 20 weeks of gestation. Thereafter, fetal thyroid secretion increases gradually. At term, TSH is higher and T_4 and T_3 concentrations are lower in the newborn than in the mother. Within 30 to 60 minutes of delivery, TSH surges and then settles to 6 to 10 U/L by 1 week of age. The TSH surge stimulates thyroidal T_4 secretion, and TT_4, fT_4, and T_3 peak at 24 to 36 hours post delivery and then gradually fall over the first 4 weeks of life.

The extent to which maternal thyroid hormones cross the placenta is controversial. In infants with congenital absence of the thyroid, cord serum concentrations range from 20% to 50% of normal.[55] TSH-receptor antibodies can cross the placenta and cause thyroid dysfunction in the offspring of women with Graves' disease. Little TSH crosses the placenta.

Maternal iodine deficiency during pregnancy can result in cretinism and mental retardation in the offspring. Women are recommended to consume 250 µg iodine/day during pregnancy and lactation.[56]

Inadequately treated hypothyroidism and hyperthyroidism during pregnancy can have adverse effects on both mother and child. Women with a history of thyroid disease should be euthyroid before the time of conception with a TSH <2.5 mU/L. Women given a diagnosis of thyroid disease during pregnancy should be treated expeditiously until they are euthyroid. Screening of pregnant women for thyroid disease remains controversial. Universal screening is not recommended; however, screening of high-risk individuals is suggested. Women need more thyroid hormone during pregnancy, and women who are being treated with thyroxine for hypothyroidism often need a dosage increase, sometimes as early as the fifth week of gestation.[57]

Screening

In screening for thyroid disease in an asymptomatic population such as the elderly, it is widely recommended[58,59] that the initial test be a serum TSH measurement (see later). An abnormal TSH result should be followed up by repeated measurement of TSH and fT_4.

The value of routine screening for hypothyroidism remains controversial. One recent clinical consensus group recommended against population-based screening but suggested aggressive case finding, particularly in women older than 60 years and others at high risk for thyroid dysfunction (e.g., previous radiation treatment to the thyroid, previous thyroid surgery or thyroid dysfunction, personal history of type 1 diabetes or other autoimmune disease, family history of thyroid disease, atrial fibrillation).

Genetics and Thyroid Disease

Genetic predisposition is an important causative factor for autoimmune thyroid disease (AITD) such as Graves' disease and Hashimoto's thyroiditis. In contrast to the monogenic MEN cancer syndromes (see earlier), however, AITD consists of polygenic disorders that result from the combination of genetic predisposition and environment. Genetic susceptibility to AITD is thought to be determined by a series of interacting susceptibility alleles from several different genes. Some of these alleles/genes have been identified, and others remain elusive. AITD is associated with other autoimmune disorders, including type 1 diabetes, Addison's disease, and premature ovarian failure. These disorders are likely to share susceptibility alleles.[60]

Thyroid Function in Nonthyroidal Illness (Euthyroid-Sick Syndrome)

Assessment of thyroid function is difficult in patients with significant nonthyroidal illness. These individuals often have low T_3, T_4, and TSH levels. Debate continues as to whether these patients are clinically euthyroid (hence the term *euthyroid-sick syndrome*) or may have acquired transient central hypothyroidism. In some cases, prescribed medications may be influencing thyroid function test results. Treatment remains controversial and appears to offer little benefit.[61]

The pathogenesis of this phenomenon is unknown but may include decreased peripheral conversion of T_4 to T_3, decreased clearance of rT_3, and decreased binding of thyroid hormones to thyroxine-binding globulin (TBG). Proinflammatory cytokines, including tumor necrosis factor-alpha (TNF-α), IL-1, and IL-6, may be responsible for some of the changes.[62]

KEY CONCEPTS BOX 49-2

- Primary disease of the thyroid gland causes most hypothyroid and hyperthyroid disease. Secondary disease (pituitary disease) or tertiary (hypothalamic) thyroid is rare. Some types of primary thyroid disease may have an autoimmune nature.
- The best single test for detecting thyroid disease is TSH. Tests given to follow up on abnormal TSH assess free thyroid hormone levels.
- Because of severe consequences of maternal hypothyroidism for the fetus, many pregnant women are given tests for thyroid disease early in pregnancy.
- Screening of asymptomatic but high-risk populations for thyroid disease is best accomplished with TSH measurements.

SECTION OBJECTIVES BOX 49-3

- Name the best thyroid function test used to investigate the thyroid axis.
- List static and dynamic tests of thyroid function.
- Predict a diagnosis of hyperthyroidism or hypothyroidism, given TSH, total and free T_4 and T_3, T_3RU, TSI, TPO antibody, and thyroid scan uptake test results.

THYROID FUNCTION TESTING

Because thyroid disease may be subtle, and because signs and symptoms of thyroid disease are often very nonspecific, thyroid function testing is an important element in assessing the patient with possible thyroid disease.

Nuclear medicine imaging of the thyroid, with the use of isotopes of iodine or technetium 99m (^{99m}Tc), is an important part of clinical investigation of thyroid disease. Both isotopes are taken up by active thyroid tissue, and such investigations may be of importance in investigation of thyrotoxicosis, nodular goiters, and malignancy.

Static Tests of Thyroid Function

The major thyroid function tests (TFTs) are listed in Table 49-2, along with characteristic changes seen in different disease states. TSH is still the single most requested and most important test for investigation of the thyroid axis. Moreover, significant changes have taken place over the past few years in the selection of supporting tests to be used. Europe and Australasia moved early to measurement of free thyroid hormones. Within the United States, a steady move has been made to the use of free thyroid hormone assays; these now are used more widely than are measures of total thyroid hormones and calculations of free thyroid hormone indices.

TSH

TSH is regulated tightly by negative feedback by free thyroid hormone concentration. Because thyroid disease is almost always primary, that is, because it usually is caused by a disorder of the thyroid gland itself rather than occurring as a result of disorders of the pituitary, changes in TSH are invariably a reliable indicator of thyroid status.

Total Thyroid Hormones

Changes in total thyroid hormone concentration are far less sensitive indices of thyroid function than is TSH (see Fig. 49-5); for this reason, they should not be measured alone.

Free Thyroid Hormones

Free thyroid hormone, the biologically active moiety,[63] can be estimated by measuring total thyroid hormone concentration plus some measure of binding protein concentration and calculating a free thyroid hormone index, or by directly measuring the free thyroid hormone concentration.

The free T_4 index (FT_4I) indirectly estimates the level of free T_4 in blood and adjusts for most interferences caused by binding-protein abnormalities.[64] The FT_4I is determined from total T_4 and resin-uptake values obtained on the sample.

Calculation of the free T_3 index is similar to that used for FT_4I, except that total serum T_3 is used.[65] It has applications and significance similar to those of the FT_4I.

Thyroid Antibodies

Anti-Thyroid Peroxidase Antibodies (Anti-TPO Antibodies, Previously Called *Antimicrosomal Antibodies*)

In Western societies, the primary cause of hypothyroidism is autoimmune disease. The primary antigen involved is thyroid peroxidase.

Anti-Thyroglobulin Antibodies (Anti-Tg Ab)

Tg is synthesized in the follicular cells of the thyroid and is stored in the follicle as colloid (see section on physiology). Low concentrations of Tg may be found in the circulation of normal individuals. An important use of anti-Tg antibody assays is as an adjunct to Tg assays, because anti-Tg antibodies may interfere with this assay.

Thyroglobulin (Tg)

Thyroglobulin is made uniquely by the thyroid. Measurement of Tg is of particular use in assessing the presence of any remnant thyroid tissue after thyroidectomy is performed for malignancy.

Thyroid Receptor Antibodies (TR Ab)

Autoantibodies may be directed against the TSH receptor, the so-called long-acting thyroid stimulator, or LATS.[66] These autoantibodies may stimulate or inhibit thyroid gland activity. In the latter case, they prevent TSH binding and action. Both blocking and stimulating thyroid receptor antibodies have high affinity for and bind to similar epitopes on the TSH receptor.[67] Only bioassays can differentiate stimulating from blocking antibodies. Such assays are only available through research laboratories.

Dynamic Tests of Thyroid Function

TRH Stimulation Test

TRH is the hypothalamic tripeptide that stimulates TSH release from the pituitary. The TRH stimulation test was important until the early 1980s, when TSH assays did not have the capacity to measure down to the lower end of the euthyroid reference interval. Since the advent of TSH assays that can detect TSH to well below the lower limit of the euthyroid reference interval, the TRH stimulation test is used rarely, and TRH for intravenous use is now virtually unobtainable.

rTSH Stimulation Test for Identifying Residual Malignant Thyroid Cancer Tissue

Thyroid cancer usually is treated by total thyroidectomy coupled with high-dose radioiodine, followed by replacement with thyroxine to suppress TSH secretion, so that any remaining ectopic/metastatic thyroid tissue is not stimulated. Follow-up for the presence of any residual thyroid tissue is accomplished by measurement of Tg, which is produced only by thyroid tissue. This procedure requires cessation of thyroxine therapy for several weeks so that the patient becomes hypothyroid, TSH rises, and any ectopic thyroid tissue is stimulated to produce Tg. This is an unpleasant procedure for patients, and there is a move to use recombinant TSH (rTSH) to stimulate any ectopic tissue and eliminate the need for the patient to become hypothyroid. This procedure is expensive and is used to a very limited extent at present, but use of rTSH is likely to increase.[68]

KEY CONCEPTS BOX 49-3

- TSH is the first test used to detect most types of thyroid disease.
- Total T_4 is not an important test, but it may be used in conjunction with estimates of TBG saturation to estimate free thyroid hormone levels.
- Direct measurement of free T_4 or T_3 is best used as a follow-up to TSH measurements or to monitor treatment for thyroid disease.

SECTION OBJECTIVES BOX 49-4

- Discuss expected changes in serum free T_4, total T_4, TSH, and thyroid antibodies in the following states:
  - Primary hyperthyroidism and hypothyroidism
  - Secondary hyperthyroidism and hypothyroidism
  - Thyroid cancer
  - Euthyroid-sick syndrome
- Discuss the reasons for discordant results between TSH and fT_4.
- Explain the clinical utility of serum TSH measurements in the diagnosis and management of thyroid disease.
- Explain why variations in the concentration of thyroid hormone binding proteins limit the usefulness of total T_4 and total T_3 measurements.
- List conditions that increase or decrease thyroid hormone binding protein levels.
- Discuss the clinical utility of thyroid antibody testing.

CHANGE OF ANALYTE IN DISEASE

See Table 49-2 for a summary of typical changes seen in the major thyroid function tests in different disease states. Nonthyroidal illness with its highly varied results is covered in the section on pathology.

TSH

A principal use of thyroid-stimulating hormone (TSH) determinations in serum is the diagnosis of hyperthyroidism or hypothyroidism. Patients with untreated hypothyroidism stemming from intrinsic thyroid defects (primary hypothyroidism), regardless of the cause, have elevated serum levels of TSH. Hypothyroidism caused by pituitary lesions (secondary) or hypothalamic (tertiary) lesions will occur with normal or low TSH concentrations, but secondary hypothyroidism is extremely rare. Most patients with hyperthyroidism have low or undetectable TSH levels in serum, reflecting the inhibitory effects of high levels of circulating thyroid hormone on the hypothalamic-pituitary axis.

Serum TSH levels are used to monitor treatment of thyroid disease. Treatment for a hypoactive thyroid gland can be monitored by tracking elevated TSH down into the reference range. Although serum TSH measurements are not useful when TSH is severely depressed in hyperthyroidism, once the TSH begins to be detectable, tracking of serum TSH into the reference interval suggests a proper response. A stable serum TSH level within the reference interval is a marker for long-term successful treatment of thyroid disease.

Serum Total T_4

Increases in total serum T_4 can occur because of increased hormone synthesis, increased hormone release from thyroid cells, or increased binding capacity of plasma proteins, especially TBG. Causes of changes in thyroxine-binding globulin concentration are shown in Box 49-5. Increased hormone secretion is seen most frequently in states of hyperthyroidism. Causes of hyperthyroidism are listed in Box 49-1. Decreases in serum total T_4 occur in cases of hypothyroidism (see Table 49-2).

Serum total T_4 and T_3 are clinically meaningful only if the functional levels of thyroid hormone–binding proteins in blood are known. This is achieved by use of the **resin-uptake test** (see later), which does not measure a specific analyte per se but measures the functional state (ability to bind hormone) of the hormone-binding proteins (such as TBG).

Increased T_4 release from the thyroid gland occurs because of cellular damage caused by subacute thyroiditis and Hashimoto's thyroiditis, and after radiation treatment to the gland. Increased concentration of serum TBG results in increased total serum T_4, but the concentration of fT_4 remains constant, and these conditions are not accompanied by hyperthyroidism.

Serum Total T_3

In general, increases in total T_3 are proportionately greater than the increases in T_4 that are seen in most states of hyperthyroidism. Routine measurements of total T_3 are not necessary. In approximately 5% of hyperthyroidism cases with reduced levels of serum TSH, elevation of T_3 occurs while serum T_4 levels remain normal. This condition is termed *T_3 thyrotoxicosis.*[69] Total T_3 measurements are needed for thyroid disease to be diagnosed and treatment monitored in these cases.

Estimates of Free Thyroid Hormone Concentration

Concentrations of total thyroid hormones may vary markedly in the presence of constant concentrations of free hormones because of changes in the concentrations of thyroid hormone–binding proteins unrelated to thyroid disease. Because of the limited utility of total thyroid hormone measurements, the American Thyroid Association recommended in 1990 that free thyroid hormones should be measured directly or estimated indirectly.[58]

Box 49-5
Causes of Abnormalities in Thyroxine-Binding Globulin (TBG)

Quantitative

Increased TBG serum levels
- Pregnancy
- Estrogen therapy
- Clofibrate treatment
- Oral contraceptives
- Perphenazine
- Abuse of heroin or methadone
- Acute hepatitis
- Hypothyroidism
- Neonatal period
- Acute intermittent porphyria
- Genetic TBG excess

Decreased TBG serum levels
- Androgens
- Anabolic agents
- Cirrhosis
- Acute illness
- Surgical stress
- Severe chronic illness
- Severe hypoproteinemia
- Protein malnutrition
- Nephrotic syndrome
- Hyperthyroidism
- Corticosteroid therapy
- L-Asparaginase therapy
- Active acromegaly
- Klinefelter's syndrome
- Cushing's syndrome
- Down syndrome
- Type III hyperlipidemia
- Chronic metabolic acidosis
- Genetic deficiency (usually X-linked)

Qualitative

Genetic
- Genetically determined increase in binding affinity
- Genetically determined decrease in binding affinity

Drugs Competing With T_4 and T_3 for TBG-Binding Sites
- Phenytoin (diphenylhydantoin, Dilantin)
- Dicumarol
- Heparin (causes release of fatty acids, which affect hormone binding to TBG)
- Atromid S
- Aspirin
- Phenylbutazone

T_3 Resin Uptake

Hyperthyroidism is characterized by complete or almost complete saturation of binding sites on TBG; in hypothyroidism, relatively less binding of free hormone to binding proteins is seen.

If TBG in plasma is increased, total T_4 will be increased, but fT_4 will be normal. Added labeled T_3 will bind to TBG, and less will be available for binding to the resin. Conversely, if the TBG that is present in blood is decreased, uptake of labeled hormone by the resin will be increased. Artifactual changes in T_3 resin uptake (T_3RU) can occur when abnormalities in thyroxine-binding proteins are present.[70]

Certain drugs (e.g., salicylates, phenytoin, furosemide, and fenclofenac) compete with thyroid hormone for TBG-binding sites. This phenomenon is reflected by normal free T_4, low total T_4, and high resin-uptake values.

Calculated Free Thyroid Hormone Indices

The FT_4I is elevated in hyperthyroidism and is decreased in hypothyroidism. The FT_3I may be helpful for excluding T_3 toxicosis in some patients who are taking oral contraceptives in whom isolated serum T_3 increases are found without corresponding elevations of T_4. In general, the FT_3I offers no advantages over the FT_4I, and it is used less frequently in clinical practice.

Free Thyroid Hormones

In hyperthyroidism, fT_4 is increased, and in hypothyroidism, it is decreased. Direct estimation of free thyroid hormone concentration appears to provide more reliable estimates of true thyroid status than do calculated indices, although results may be artifactually changed when significant abnormalities in binding proteins occur, or when heterophile and autoantibodies are present.[71] Free T_3 measurements do not yield as clinically useful information as fT_4 in most cases and should be used only for special circumstances, such as when T_3 toxicosis is suspected.

Thyroid hormone binding proteins are frequently present in abnormal concentrations in physiological states such as pregnancy, or in association with drug therapy, and abnormalities in binding proteins that affect hormone binding are also common. For this reason, artifactual changes in total thyroid hormone concentration in euthyroid individuals may be common, while free hormone measurements will better reflect true thyroid status.

Serum levels of free hormones, which are increased in cases of hyperthyroidism and decreased in hypothyroidism (see Table 49-2), are used to corroborate findings of an abnormal serum TSH. In addition, free thyroid measurements can be used to supplement TSH measurements when treatment for thyroid disease is monitored, especially during early recovery of hyperthyroidism when depressed serum TSH levels may be unmeasurable.

Thyroid Antibodies

Anti-TPO Ab

The NHANES III study reported on thyroid disease in the U.S. population. In an apparently disease-free population, 11.3% of persons had anti-TPO antibodies, and 10.4% had Tg antibodies.[19] A correlation was evident between TPO-Ab concentration and TSH concentration, which suggested that developing thyroid disease may be present.

Tg-Ab

A small number of persons have positive Tg-Ab with no evidence of thyroid disease,[19] and Tg-Ab measurement offers little useful information for patients with autoimmune thyroid disease. Patients with thyroid malignancies that are secreting Tg may develop a progressively rising titer of Tg-Ab, and this may be a useful tool for detection of tumor recurrence.[72]

Tg

Measurement of Tg is an important tool in assessment of patients with differentiated thyroid malignancies. After successful thyroidectomy for thyroid malignancy, Tg concentration in blood will fall to undetectable levels. The reappearance of Tg in blood is strongly suggestive of tumor recurrence. For the purpose of stimulating Tg secretion, patients will be taken off replacement thyroxine for several weeks to render them briefly hypothyroid, with the subsequent TSH rise stimulating any ectopic thyroid tissue to produce Tg. This procedure is unpleasant for patients, and stimulation with recombinant TSH is progressively replacing this procedure (see earlier).

Because Tg-Ab interferes with modern assays for Tg, resulting in underestimation of Tg concentration, it is highly desirable to measure Tg-Ab whenever Tg is being measured.[73]

Thyroid Receptor Antibodies (TR-Ab)

TR-Ab assays in most cases do not offer much more useful information over TSH and thyroid hormone measurements. However, TR-Ab can cross the placenta and can render a fetus thyrotoxic, and TR-Ab estimation is useful in this clinical setting.[22]

Discordance Between fT_4 and TSH Concentrations

Because of the strong feedback regulation of thyroid hormones on TSH secretion, an inverse relationship should be established between these moieties. If one moiety is high, then the other should be low. Occasionally, results will be obtained where there is discordance (i.e., both are inappropriately high or inappropriately low). Possible causes that should be considered in such a circumstance are listed in Box 49-6.

Nonthyroidal illness is a frequently encountered cause of discrepant thyroid test results. This has been discussed in the section on pathology.

Recommendations for Thyroid Testing

The American Thyroid Association and the National Academy of Clinical Chemistry have put forth a series of recommendations on thyroid disease, including screening. These can be found at http://www.thyroid.org/professionals/index.html and at http://www.aacc.org/AACC/members/nacb/LMPG/OnlineGuide/PublishedGuidelines/ThyroidDisease/, respectively.

TSH Reference Intervals

Most laboratories provide an upper limit for reference intervals for TSH concentration between 4.0 and 5.0 mU/L. Clinicians have expressed concern that this upper limit is too

Box 49-6

Causes of Discordance Between TSH and fT_4

Increased TSH Without Low fT_4
Subclinical hypothyroidism
Recent change in thyroid hormone dosage
Drugs
Inappropriate secretion of TSH
Laboratory problem (e.g., heterophile antibody interference)

Subnormal TSH Without Increased fT_4
Subclinical hyperthyroidism
Recent decrease in thyroid hormone dose
Recent treatment of thyrotoxicosis
Nonthyroidal illness
Drugs
Central hypothyroidism

fT_4, Free thyroxine; *THS,* thyroid-stimulating hormone.

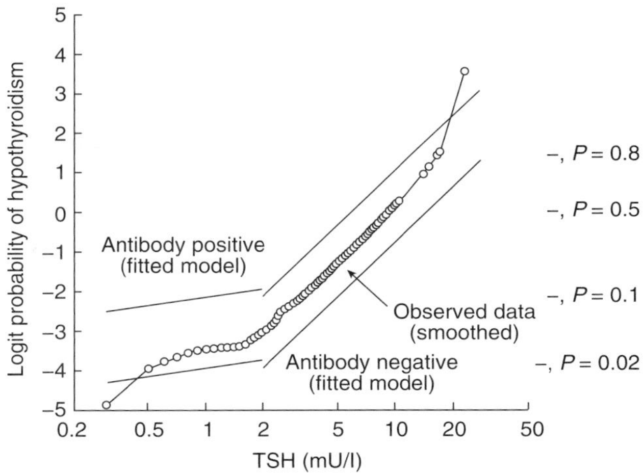

Fig. 49-7 Logit probability (log odds) for development within twenty years of hypothyroidism with increasing values of TSH as measured at first survey in 912 female survivors. (Reproduced with permission of Blackwell Publishing from Vanderpump MPJ, Tunbridge WMG, French JM, Appleton D, Bates D, Clark F et al: The incidence of thyroid disorders in the community: a twenty-year follow-up of the Whickham Survey. Clin Endocrinol 43:55-68, 1995.)

high and includes persons with subtle hypothyroid disease. The Whickham Survey showed that TSH concentrations above 2.0 mU/L were associated with an increased likelihood of subsequent development of hypothyroidism, as shown in Fig. 49-7.[74] NHANES III data[19] show that persons apparently free from thyroid disease but who had increased TPO antibodies had a higher TSH reference interval than did persons who were TPO antibody negative. It has been suggested that the upper reference interval for TSH should be reduced to 3.0 mU/L, or even 2.5 mU/L.[59]

Because several nonpathological reasons for a mild TSH increase, such as natural circadian rhythm, acute stress,[75] and confounders such as heterophile antibodies, have been put forth, it has been disputed whether treatment is warranted in this group of persons with TSH concentration between 2.5 and 4.0 mU/L, although it is suggested that TSH should be followed on a regular basis.[76]

KEY CONCEPTS BOX 49-4

- Primary hyperthyroidism includes elevated thyroid hormones (total and free) and decreased TSH. Primary hypothyroidism consists of decreased thyroid hormones (total and free) and increased TSH.
- Rare secondary and tertiary types of hyperthyroidism are associated with elevated thyroid hormones (total and free) and increased TSH. Secondary and tertiary forms of hypothyroidism include decreased thyroid hormones (total and free) and decreased TSH.
- Anti-TPO Abs are increased in autoimmune disease involving thyroiditis which is common.
- Whilst Graves' disease is common and caused by immunoglobulins binding to, and stimulating the TSH receptor, measurement of antibodies to the TSH receptor is less commonly used.

REFERENCES

1. Knudsen N, Laurberg P, Perrild H, et al: Risk factors for goiter and thyroid nodules, Thyroid 12:879, 2002.
2. Harjai KJ, Licata AA: Effects of amiodarone on thyroid function, Ann Intern Med 126:63, 1997.
3. Pazos-Moura CC, Ortiga-Carvalho TM, de Moura EG: The autocrine/paracrine regulation of TSH secretion, Thyroid 13:167, 2003.
4. Jansen J, Friesma EC, Milici C, et al: Thyroid hormone transporters in health and disease, Thyroid 15:757, 2005.
5. Kavok NS, Krasilnikova OA, Babenko NA: Thyroxine signal transduction in liver cells involves phospholipase C and phospholipase D activation: genomic independent action of thyroid hormone, BMC Cell Biol 2:5, 2001.
6. Bassett JHD, Harvey CB, Williams GR: Mechanisms of thyroid hormone receptor–specific nuclear and extra nuclear actions, Mol Cell Endocrinol 213:1, 2003.
7. Kahaly GJ, Dillmann WH: Thyroid hormone action in the heart, Endocr Rev 26:704, 2005.
8. Murphy E, Williams GR: The thyroid and the skeleton, Clin Endocrinol 61:285, 2004.
9. Boyages SC: The neuromuscular system and brain in hypothyroidism. In Braverman LE, Utiger RD, editors: *Werner & Ingbar's The Thyroid: A Fundamental and Clinical Text,* ed 8, Philadelphia, 2000, Lippincott Williams & Wilkins.
10. Haddow JE, Palomaki GE, Allan WC, et al: Maternal thyroid deficiency during pregnancy and subsequent neuropsychological development of the child, N Engl J Med 341:549, 1999.
11. Pop VJ, Kuijpens JL, van Baar AL, et al: Low maternal free thyroxine concentrations during pregnancy are associated with impaired psychomotor development in infancy, Clin Endocrinol 50:149, 1999.
12. Hume R, Simpson J, Delahunty C, et al: Human fetal and cord serum thyroid hormones: developmental trends and interrelationships, J Clin Endocrinol Metab 89:4097, 2004.
13. Courtin F, Zrouri H, Lamirand A, et al : Thyroid hormone deiodinases in the central and peripheral nervous system, Thyroid 15:931, 2005.

14. Krausz Y, Freedman N, Lester H, et al: Regional cerebral blood flow in patients with mild hypothyroidism, J Nucl Med 45:1712, 2004.
15. Oatridge A, Barnard ML, Puri BK, et al: Changes in brain size in patients with hyper- or hypothyroidism, Am J Neuroradiol 23:1539, 2002.
16. Chopra IJ, Solomon DH, Chopra U, et al: Pathways of metabolism of thyroid hormones, Recent Prog Horm Res 34:521, 1978.
17. Bianco AC, Kim BW: Deiodinases: implications of the local control of thyroid hormone action, J Clin Invest 116:2571, 2006.
18. Peeters RP, Debaveye Y, Fliers E, et al: Changes within the thyroid axis during critical illness, Crit Care Clin 22:41, 2006.
19. Hollowell JG, Staehling NW, Flanders WD, et al: Serum TSH, T4 and thyroid antibodies in the United States Population (1988-1994): National Health and Nutrition Examination Survey (NHANES III), J Clin Endocrinol Metab 87:489, 2002.
20. Brix TH, Kyvik KO, Christensen K, et al: Evidence for a major role of heredity in Graves' disease: a population-based study of two Danish twin cohorts, J Clin Endocrinol Metab 86:930, 2001.
21. McKenzie JM, Zakarija M, Sato A: Humoral immunity in Graves' disease, Clin Endocrinol Metab 7:31, 1978.
22. McKenzie JM, Zakarija M: Fetal and neonatal hyperthyroidism and hypothyroidism due to maternal TSH receptor antibodies, Thyroid 2:155, 1992.
23. Peleg D, Cada S, Pele A, et al: The relationship between maternal serum thyroid-stimulating immunoglobulin and fetal and neonatal thyrotoxicosis, Obstet Gynecol 99:1040, 2002.
24. Abalovich M, Amino N, Barbour LA, et al: Management of thyroid dysfunction during pregnancy and postpartum: an Endocrine Society Clinical Practice Guideline, J Clin Endocrinol Metab 92:s1, 2007.
25. Utiger RD: The multiplicity of thyroid nodules and carcinomas, N Engl J Med 352:2376, 2005.
26. Muller AF, Drexhage HA, Berghout A: Postpartum thyroiditis and autoimmune thyroiditis in women of childbearing age: recent insights and consequences for antenatal and postnatal care, Endocrine Rev 22:605, 2001.
27. Diez JJ: Hyperthyroidism in patients older than 55 years: an analysis of the etiology and management, Gerontology 49:316, 2003.
28. Sawin CT, Geller A, Kaplan MM, et al: Low serum thyrotropin (thyroid stimulating hormone) in older patients without hyperthyroidism, Arch Intern Med 151:165, 1991.
29. Toft AD: Subclinical hyperthyroidism, N Engl J Med 345:512, 2001.
30. Baldini M, Gallazzi M, Orsatti A, et al: Treatment of benign nodular goitre with mildly suppressive doses of L-thyroxine: effects on bone mineral density and on nodule size, J Intern Med 251:407, 2002.
31. Faber J, Galloe AM: Changes in bone mass during prolonged subclinical hyperthyroidism due to L-thyroxine treatment: a meta-analysis, Eur J Endocrinol 130:350, 1994.
32. Parle JV, Maisonneuve P, Sheppard MC, et al: Prediction of all-cause and cardiovascular mortality in elderly people from one low serum thyrotropin result: a 10-year cohort study, Lancet 358:861, 2001.
33. Costaliola S, Morgenthaler NG, Hoermann R, et al: Second generation assay for thyrotropin receptor antibodies and superior diagnostic sensitivity for Graves' disease, J Clin Endocrinol Metab 84:90, 1999.
34. Wartofsky L, Glinoer D, Solomon B, et al: Differences and similarities in the diagnosis and treatment of Graves' disease in Europe, Japan and the United States, Thyroid 1:129, 1991.
35. Panzar C, Beazley R, Braverman L: Rapid preoperative preparation for severe hyperthyroid Graves' disease, J Clin Endocrinol Metab 89:2142, 2004.
36. Langley RW, Burch HB: Perioperative management of the thyrotoxic patient, Endocrinol Metab Clin North Am 32:519, 2003.
37. Pearce EN, Farwell AP, Braverman LE: Thyroiditis, N Engl J Med 348:2646, 2003.
38. Bourdoux P, Delange F, Gerard M, et al: Evidence that cassava ingestion increases thiocyanate formation: a possible etiologic factor in endemic goiter, J Clin Endocrinol Metab 46:613, 1978.
39. Roti E, Minelli R, Gardeini E, et al: Impaired intrathyroidal iodine organification and iodine-induced hypothyroidism in euthyroid women with a previous episode of postpartum thyroiditis, J Clin Endocrinol Metab 73:958, 1991.
40. Pedersen IB, Laurberg P, Knudsen N, et al: Increase in incidence of hyperthyroidism predominantly occurs in young people after iodine fortification of salt in Denmark, J Clin Endocrinol Metab 91:3830, 2006.
41. Pedersen IB, Laurberg P, Knudsen N, et al: An increased incidence of overt hypothyroidism after iodine fortification of salt in Denmark: a prospective population study, J Clin Endocrinol Metab 92:3122, 2007.
42. Delange F: Neonatal screening for congenital hypothyroidism: results and perspectives, Horm Res 48:51, 1997.
43. Fisher D: Editorial: next generation newborn screening for congenital hypothyroidism? J Clin Endocrinol Metab 90:3797, 2005.
44. Samuels MH, Ridgway EC: Central hypothyroidism, Endocrinol Metab Clin North Am 21:903, 1992.
45. Walsh JP, Bremner AP, Bulsara MK, et al: Subclinical thyroid dysfunction as a risk factor for cardiovascular disease, Arch Intern Med 165:2467, 2005.
46. Maxon HR, Saenger EL, Thomas SR, et al: Clinically important radiation associated thyroid disease: a controlled study, JAMA 244:1802, 1980.
47. Jemal A, Siegal R, Ward E, et al: Cancer statistics, 2006, CA Cancer J Clin 56:106, 2006.
48. Preziati D, La Rosa L, Covini G, et al: Autoimmunity and thyroid function in patients with chronic active hepatitis treated with recombinant interferon alpha-2a, Eur J Endocrinol 132:587, 1995.
49. Martino E, Bartalena L, Bogazzi F, et al: The effects of amiodarone on the thyroid, Endocr Rev 22:240, 2001.
50. Perrild H, Hegedus L, Baastrup PC, et al: Thyroid function and ultrasonically determined thyroid size in patients receiving long-term lithium treatment, Am J Psychiatry 147:1518, 1990.
51. Desai J, Yassa L, Marqusee E, et al: Hypothyroidism after sunitinib treatment for patients with gastrointestinal stromal tumors, Ann Intern Med 145:660, 2006.
52. Mannavola D, Coco P, Vannucchi G, et al: A novel tyrosine-kinase selective inhibitor, sunitinib induces transient hypothyroidism by blocking iodine uptake, J Clin Endocrinol Metab 92:3531, 2007.
53. Goodwin TM, Montoro M, Mestman JH: Transient hyperthyroidism and hyperemesis gravidarum: clinical aspects, Am J Obstet Gynecol 167:648, 1992.
54. Hershman JM: Human chorionic gonadotropin and the thyroid: hyperemesis gravidarum and trophoblastic tumors, Thyroid 9:653, 1999.
55. Vulsma T, Gons MH, de Vijlder JJ: Maternal-fetal transfer of thyroxine in congenital hypothyroidism due to a total organification defect or thyroid agenesis, N Engl J Med 321:13, 1989.
56. International Council for Control of Iodine Deficiency Disorders (ICCDD): Iodine requirements in pregnancy and infancy, IDD Newsletter 23:1, 2007.
57. Alexander EK, Marquee E, Lawrence J, et al: Timing and magnitude of increasing levothyroxine requirements during pregnancy in women with hypothyroidism, N Engl J Med 351:241, 2004.

58. Surks MI, Chorpa IJ, Mariash CN, et al: American Thyroid Association guidelines for the use of laboratory tests in thyroid disorders, JAMA 263:1529, 1990.
59. Demers LM, Spencer CA: Laboratory support for the diagnosis and monitoring of thyroid disease, NACB Laboratory Medicine Practice Guidelines, 2002. Available at www.nacb.org/lmpg/thyroid_lmpg_pub.stm.
60. Vaidya B, Kendall-Taylor P, Pearce SHS: Genetics of endocrine disease: the genetics of autoimmune thyroid disease, J Clin Endocrinol Metab 87:5385, 2002.
61. Adler SM, Wartofsky L: The nonthyroidal illness syndrome, Endocr Metab Clin North Am 36:657, 2007.
62. Papanicolaou DA: Euthyroid sick syndrome and the role of cytokines, Rev Endocr Metab Disord 1:43, 2000.
63. Ekins RP: Free hormones in blood: the concept and the measurement, J Clin Immunoassay 7:163, 1984.
64. Stein RB, Price L: Evaluation of adjusted total thyroxine (free thyroxine index) as a measure of thyroid function, J Clin Endocrinol Metab 34:225, 1972.
65. Sawin CT, Chopra D, Albano J, et al: The free triiodothyronine (T3) index, Ann Intern Med 88:474, 1978.
66. McKenzie JM, Zakarija M: Antibodies in autoimmune thyroid disease. In Braverman LE, Utiger RD, editors: *Werner and Ingbar's The Thyroid,* Philadelphia, 1996, JB Lippincott, p 416.
67. Morgenthaler NG, Ho SC, Minich WB: Stimulating and blocking thyroid-stimulating hormone (TSH) receptor autoantibodies from patients with Graves' disease and autoimmune hypothyroidism have very similar concentration, TSH receptor affinity, and binding sites, J Clin Endocrinol Metab 92:1058, 2007.
68. Cooper DS, Doherty GM, Haugen BR, et al: Management guidelines for patients with thyroid nodules and differentiated thyroid cancer, Thyroid 16:109, 2006.
69. Figge J, Leinung M, Goodman AD, et al: The clinical evaluation of patients with subclinical hyperthyroidism and free triiodothyronine (free T3) toxicosis, Am J Med 96:229, 1994.
70. Ray RA, Howanitz PJ, Howanitz JH: Controversies in thyroid function testing, Clin Lab Med 4:671, 1984.
71. Spencer CA: Assay of thyroid hormones and related substances, Thyroid Disease Manager. Available at www.thyroidmanager.org/index.html. Accessed 9-11-07.
72. Pacini F, Mariotti S, Formica N, et al: Thyroid autoantibodies in thyroid cancer: incidence and relationship with tumor outcome, Acta Endocrinol 119:373, 1988.
73. Spencer CA: Editorial: challenges of serum thyroglobulin (Tg) measurement in the presence of Tg autoantibodies, J Clin Endocrinol Metab 89:3702, 2004.
74. Vanderpump MPJ, Tunbridge WMG, French JM, et al: The incidence of thyroid disorders in the community: a twenty-year follow-up of the Whickham Survey, Clin Endocrinol 43:55, 1995.
75. Hickman PE, Yu S, Price L, et al: Thyroid-stimulating hormone secretion is a dynamic process, Ann Clin Biochem 38:147, 2001.
76. Surks MI, Goswami G, Daniels GH: The thyrotropin reference range should remain unchanged, J Clin Endocrinol Metab 90:5489, 2005.

The Gonads

Shenaz Seedat and Elisabeth Nye

Chapter 50

Chapter Outline

Normal Ovary and Ovarian Function
- *Early Development of the Ovary*
- *Ovary of the Reproductive Years*
- *The Menstrual Cycle*
- *The Menopause*

Pathological States
- *Amenorrhea*
- *Dysfunctional Uterine Bleeding*
- *Polycystic Ovary Syndrome*
- *Other Disorders Associated With Androgen Excess*
- *Ovarian Hyperfunction*

Normal Testes and Testicular Function
- *Early Development*
- *The Mature Testes*

Pathological States
- *Hypogonadism*
- *Testicular Hyperfunction*
- *Erectile Dysfunction*

Change of Analyte in Disease: Evaluation of the Infertile Couple
- *Evaluation of Infertility*
- *Female Infertility*
- *Male Infertility*
- *Infertility Treatment*

Methods on Evolve

α-Fetoprotein
Beta-hCG (beta-human chorionic gonadotropin)
Dehydroepiandrosterone and its sulfate (DHEA and DHEA-S)
Estradiol
Estriol
Follicle-stimulating hormone (FSH)
Luteinizing hormone (LH)
Progesterone
Prolactin
Testosterone

Key Terms

amenorrhea Absence or abnormal cessation of menstruation.

androgens Sex steroid hormones responsible for the development of male secondary sex characteristics.

anovulation Failure of the ovary to produce ova.

corpus luteum Transient endocrine organ that arises from the granulosa and theca cells of the ovarian follicle and secretes progesterone during the luteal phase of the menstrual cycle.

cryptorchidism Failure of the testes to descend into the scrotum.

dihydrotestosterone Metabolite of testosterone with potent androgenic activity.

diploid Cell that contains the full complement of 46 chromosomes.

dysfunctional uterine bleeding Unpredictable menstrual bleeding in association with anovulatory cycles.

dysmenorrhea Cramping and pain associated with menstruation.

endometrium Tissue that forms the inner lining of the uterus.

epididymis Elongated, cordlike structure of the testis that contains ducts capable of storing spermatozoa.

estrogens Sex steroid hormones responsible for the development of female secondary sex characteristics. Most bioactive is estradiol.

fallopian tubes Long, slender tubes that extend from the uterus toward the ovaries.

fecundability The probability of achieving pregnancy within one menstrual cycle (20% to 25% per cycle).

gonadotropins Glycoprotein hormones (FSH and LH) that are secreted by anterior pituitary cells (gonadotropes) and stimulate the gonads.

gonadotropin-releasing hormone (GnRH) Decapeptide hormone that is secreted by hypothalamic neurons and stimulates gonadotropin secretion by the pituitary.

gynecomastia Glandular enlargement of the mammary glands in males.

haploid Cell that contains 23 chromosomes, the haploid number.
hirsutism Excess terminal (thick pigmented) body hair that occurs in a male distribution pattern in women.
hypogonadism Abnormally low activity of the gonads.
infertility Involuntary failure to conceive after 1 or more years of unprotected intercourse.
inhibin Glycoprotein hormones secreted by the testes and the ovary whose principal role is probably to exert negative feedback on pituitary FSH secretion.
***in vitro* fertilization (IVF)** Assisted reproductive technique in which oocytes are extracted and fertilized in the laboratory, and embryos are transferred transcervically into the uterus.
Kallmann's syndrome Inherited defect in hypothalamic gonadotropin-releasing hormone (GnRH) secretion that causes hypogonadotropic hypogonadism.
Klinefelter's syndrome Sex chromosome abnormality in males (XXY) that produces primary hypogonadism and infertility.
Leydig cells Interstitial cells of the testes that produce testosterone.
luteal phase deficiency Abnormal corpus luteum function that results in inadequate progesterone production.
meiosis Process of cell division in which specialized cells called gametes are produced (spermatozoa in males and ova in females) that contain half the diploid number of chromosomes, that is, the haploid number.
menarche Onset of menstruation.
menopause Cessation of menstruation.
mosaicism The presence of two populations of cells with different genotypes that have developed from a single fertilized egg in one individual.
polycystic ovary syndrome (PCOS) Condition characterized by hyperandrogenism, menstrual irregularities, and anovulation.
premature ovarian failure Amenorrhea, infertility, estrogen deficiency, and elevated gonadotropins in a woman younger than 40 years of age.
premenstrual syndrome (PMS) Behavioral changes associated with the menstrual cycle.
pronucleus A haploid set of chromosomes from the female or male gametes. The male pronucleus is the sperm nucleus after it has entered the ovum at fertilization but before fusion with the female pronucleus; the latter is the nucleus of the ovum before fusion with the male pronucleus.
pseudohermaphroditism Conditions in which the individual has sex chromosomes and gonads that are characteristic of one sex but has some phenotypical features (such as external genitalia) of the other sex.
sex hormone–binding globulin (SHBG) A protein produced by the liver that binds testosterone and estradiol in blood.
spermatozoa Male reproductive cells produced in the testes.
testicular feminization syndrome Failure of virilization in a genetic and gonadal male caused by an X-linked defect in the androgen receptor.
testosterone Principal male sex hormone.
Turner's syndrome Chromosomal abnormality (45 X) in girls associated with gonadal dysgenesis.
virilization Development of male phenotypical features in a female.

SECTION OBJECTIVE BOX 50-1

- Describe the normal development of the ovary and mature ovum, and the accompanying biochemical changes.
- Describe the changes associated with normal female puberty and the accompanying biochemical changes.

NORMAL OVARY AND OVARIAN FUNCTION

Early Development of the Ovary

Fetal Ovary

Formation of the gonads occurs early in fetal development; primordial germ cells can be identified in the 4.5-day-old human blastocyst. This process is identical in male and female embryos. By 42 days of gestation, sexual dimorphism becomes apparent. In male embryos, the developing gonad switches to the male pattern, and seminiferous cords can be identified in the fetal testes. The gene that controls testicular differentiation is located on the Y chromosome. In its absence, ovarian development will occur; however, it takes longer (about 70 days) for developing ovarian tissue in a female embryo to become histologically identifiable.

The ovary is composed of three principal cell types: (1) coelomic epithelial cells, which differentiate into granulosa cells; (2) mesenchymal cells, which give rise to the ovarian stroma; and (3) primordial germ cells (oogonia). These primordial cells continue to proliferate in the fetal ovary through successive mitotic division and reach the maximum number of 6 to 7 million oogonia by the 20th week of gestation. Thereafter, the number of germ cells decreases (a process known as atresia), so that only about 1 million are present at birth, about 400,000 are present at **menarche,** and only a few remain by the **menopause.** Oogonia continue to undergo mitosis (cell division that produces two genetically identical daughter cells) until they are converted to primary oocytes.

The primary oocytes begin a unique form of cell division called **meiosis,** which occurs only in the germ cells of the gonads. Meiosis involves two cell divisions (meiosis I and II), in which only the first is preceded by duplication of the chromosomes. Gonadal germ cells contain the full complement of 46 chromosomes, the **diploid** number. After the process of meiosis, however, specialized cells called *gametes* are produced that contain only half the diploid number of chromosomes (the **haploid** number). Reproduction involves the fusion of male and female gametes to form a zygote, which once again will contain the diploid number of chromosomes. In the female fetus, meiosis I is initiated by primary oocytes during the second trimester of gestation, but this process is arrested during the resting phase, when each cell contains a duplicate set of chromosomes. Meiosis I does not resume until after menarche, at which time it will proceed in an individual ovum at the time of ovulation.

The daughter cells from meiosis I each contain one of the duplicated sets of chromosomes (i.e., they are diploid), but the cell cytoplasm is distributed unequally, thus producing one normal cell and a DNA-containing structure called the *first polar body*. Meiosis II is initiated at the time of fertilization but is not preceded by duplication of the chromosomes, so the ensuing gamete is haploid, and a second polar body is formed. Fusion of the female pronucleus with the male pronucleus within the fertilized ovum then restores the chromosome number to diploid. In contrast to the process of mitosis, which produces genetically identical daughter cells, during meiosis I, an exchange of alleles (alternate gene forms coding for the same characteristic) occurs between the chromatids of homologous pairs of duplicated chromosomes, resulting in chromosomes with a different genetic constitution from those of the mother cell.

In the fetal ovary, primary oocytes become surrounded by a layer of primitive granulosa cells, and together these make up the primordial follicle. This process continues until 6 months after birth. Oocytes that are not incorporated into follicles undergo degeneration. Most of the enzymes required for steroid hormone synthesis from cholesterol are present in human fetal ovaries; however, significant quantities of steroid hormones are not secreted in utero.

The primordial genital ducts—*Wolffian ducts* (male) and *Müllerian ducts* (female)—temporarily coexist in all embryos during the ambisexual period of development (up to 8 weeks). Critical factors in determining which of the duct structures stabilizes or regresses are two secretions from the testes: antimüllerian hormone and **testosterone.** In the absence of these factors, the wolffian duct system regresses, and müllerian duct development takes place. The **fallopian tubes,** the uterus, and the upper third of the vagina develop from the Müllerian ducts.

Childhood and Premenarchal Ovary

After birth, the ovaries increase in size and weight, from about 250 mg to 4000 mg by menarche. Increases in the amount of ovarian stroma, the size of individual follicles, and the number of follicles all contribute to ovarian growth. Hormonal regulation of both male and female reproductive function is dependent on a complex system that involves the hypothalamus, the pituitary, and the gonads. As will be discussed later in greater detail, the hypothalamus secretes a decapeptide hormone, **gonadotropin-releasing hormone (GnRH),** which stimulates the anterior pituitary to secrete the glycoprotein hormones, luteinizing hormone (LH), and follicle-stimulating hormone (FSH) (the **gonadotropins**). Plasma gonadotropin levels vary markedly in females during different stages of life. During the second trimester of pregnancy, they rise progressively to levels that are similar to those observed during menopause. During the latter part of the second trimester, the fetal hypothalamic-pituitary axis matures, becoming progressively more sensitive to the suppressive effects of high levels of estriol and progesterone secreted by the placenta. Fetal plasma gonadotropin concentrations therefore decrease to virtually undetectable levels by birth. After delivery, with removal of the placenta, plasma gonadotropin levels once again increase markedly because of the abrupt decrease in estriol and progesterone levels. Elevated gonadotropin levels persist for the first few months, decreasing to low levels again within 1 to 3 years. During the childhood years, the hypothalamic-pituitary axis remains highly sensitive to the negative-feedback effects of gonadal steroids, so that gonadotropin levels remain low despite the low levels of circulating gonadal steroids. Although basal gonadotropin secretion is low in prepubertal females, there is still a distinct pulsatile rhythm of secretion, with pulses occurring every 2 to 3 hours—a pattern similar to that observed in adults.

Puberty is characterized by three major events: (1) adrenarche, the onset of adrenal androgen secretion; (2) decreased sensitivity of the hypothalamic-pituitary axis to negative feedback by gonadal steroids, leading to increased activity of the GnRH-secreting hypothalamic neurons and increased pituitary gonadotropin secretion; and (3) gonadarche, increased ovarian estradiol secretion and the onset of ovulatory cycles. The increase in secretion of adrenal **androgens** occurs before maturation of gonadotropin secretion. Plasma levels of androstenedione, dehydroepiandrosterone (DHEA), and dehydroepiandrosterone sulfate (DHEAS) begin to increase in children between the ages of 6 and 8 years. Although a close relation between onset of adrenarche and initiation of gonadarche has been noted, the control mechanisms for these two events are independent. The precise factor that initiates the onset of puberty is unknown; it may involve disinhibition or enhanced stimulation of hypothalamic neuronal activity. Regardless of the mechanism, puberty is characterized by decreased sensitivity of the hypothalamic-pituitary axis to circulating levels of gonadal steroids.

Pulsatile secretion of GnRH is critical in the initiation of puberty. In girls, FSH levels increase earlier than LH levels do. Because of increased FSH concentrations, plasma estradiol levels (more than 90% derived from the ovary) increase progressively throughout puberty. Estradiol accelerates linear growth and stimulates development of female secondary sex characteristics (i.e., breast growth, maturation of the urogenital tract, and development of the female body habitus). Adrenal androgens regulate axillary and pubic hair development. The culmination of puberty is the advent of cyclical, regular (and hence ovulatory) menses; however, the age of menarche is influenced by many factors, including general health, nutrition, body weight, and genetic factors.

Ovary of the Reproductive Years

Structural Organization of the Mature Ovary

Mature human ovaries are paired, oval-shaped organs with a combined weight during the reproductive years of 10 to 20 g (average, 14 g). The ovaries are attached to the posterior surface of the broad ligament by a fold of peritoneum called the *mesovarium* and lie in proximity to the posterior and lateral pelvic wall. Blood vessels, nerves, and lymphatics reach the ovaries via the mesovarium, entering each organ via the hilum.

Histologically, the ovary consists of three distinct regions: (1) an outer cortex that contains the germinal epithelium and the follicles; (2) a central medulla that consists of stroma; and (3) a hilar area around the mesovarium attachment. Ovarian follicles can be divided into two functional types: nongrowing, or primordial, and growing. Most follicles remain nongrowing throughout the reproductive period. Following recruitment of a growing follicle, significant changes in growth, structure, and function occur. The follicle undergoes five histologically distinct stages of development: primary, secondary, tertiary, mature, or graafian and atretic. When mature, an ovarian follicle consists of three layers of cells: (1) the *theca externa*, (2) the *theca interna*, and (3) the granulosa cells (Fig. 50-1). The oocyte is contained within, surrounded by an accumulation of granulosa cells and a cavity that contains antral fluid. As the follicle matures, the oocyte also grows, accumulating nutritional stores and completing the process of meiosis I. The mature graafian follicle then is ready to release the ovum through the process of ovulation. The average time period for development of a primary follicle to the point of ovulation is 10 to 14 days. Recruited primordial follicles either develop into a dominant, mature graafian follicle destined to ovulate, or they degenerate and die via the process of atresia.

After rupture of the follicle and release of the ovum, clotting leads to the formation of the *corpus hemorrhagicum*. The granulosa and theca cells of the follicle then proliferate to form the **corpus luteum.** The *corpus luteum* is a transient endocrine organ that predominantly secretes progesterone for about 14 days. The purpose of the *corpus luteum* is to prepare an estrogen-primed endometrium for acceptance of a newly fertilized ovum and the establishment of early pregnancy. In the absence of pregnancy, the *luteum* begins to degenerate about 4 days before the next menses, and eventually it is transformed into a fibrous scar, the *corpus albicans*.

KEY CONCEPTS BOX 50-1

- The ovaries began development in fetal life.
- Increased secretion of adrenal androgens (DHEA, DHEAS) stimulates increased secretion of pituitary hormones (LH and FSH), development of ovarian estradiol secretion, and ovulatory cycles.
- Female puberty is associated with physical secondary sexual changes, increased production of adrenal androgens, decreased sensitivity of the hypothalamus and pituitary glands to estradiol, and increased ovarian estradiol secretion.
- Rupture of the mature ova lead to the formation of the corpus luteum, which secretes progesterone to prepare the uterus for a fertilized egg.

SECTION OBJECTIVES BOX 50-2

- Describe the hypothalamic-pituitary-gonadal axis and its regulation.
- Outline the pathways of biosynthesis, transport, and metabolism of sex hormones.
- Describe the function of inhibins and activins.

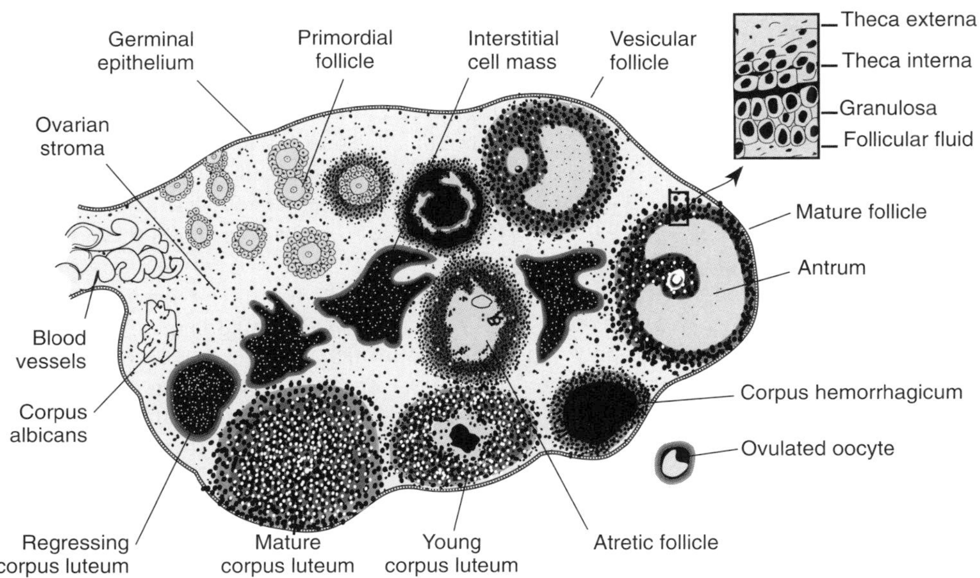

Fig. 50-1 Diagram of ovary, showing sequential development of a follicle and formation of corpus luteum. Section of wall of a mature follicle is enlarged at upper right. (From Gorbman A, Bern HA: *A Textbook of Comparative Endocrinology,* New York, 1962, Wiley & Sons.)

The Hypothalamic-Pituitary-Ovarian Axis: An Overview

Cyclical ovarian function depends on appropriately timed secretion of the anterior pituitary gonadotropins, FSH and LH, in response to hypothalamic GnRH. Coordination of the menstrual cycle also depends on positive- and negative-feedback relationships between the ovarian hormones, estradiol and progesterone, and GnRH, FSH, and LH secretion (Fig. 50-2).

The release of pituitary FSH and LH requires the constant pulsatile secretion of GnRH from the hypothalamus. Gonadotropin-releasing hormone regulates (1) synthesis and storage of gonadotropins, (2) movement of gonadotropins from a reserve pool ready for secretion, and (3) immediate release of FSH and LH. The gonadotropins are glycoproteins that are composed of two polypeptide chains, designated α and β. The α-chain is common to both, whereas the β-subunit is unique, thus endowing specific biological activity for each hormone.

The release of FSH and LH is affected both positively and negatively by estradiol and progesterone. Whether estradiol or progesterone stimulates or inhibits gonadotropin secretion depends on the concentration of the hormone and the duration of exposure of the pituitary. Estradiol exerts its inhibitory effect on both the hypothalamus and the pituitary. Some inhibition of FSH and LH release occurs at low levels of estradiol, but it is more complete at high concentrations. Progesterone in high concentrations inhibits gonadotropin secretion through suppression of hypothalamic GnRH release.

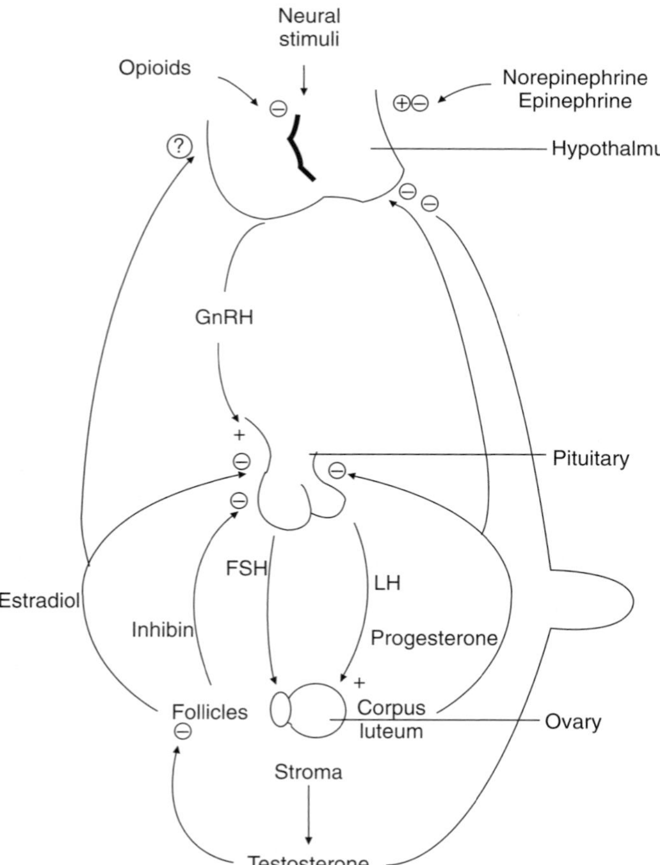

Fig. 50-2 Diagram of hypothalamic-pituitary-ovarian axis. *FSH,* Follicle-stimulating hormone; *GnRH,* gonadotropin-releasing hormone; *LH,* luteinizing hormone; +, positive effect; –, negative effect. (Modified from Greenspan FS: *Basic and Clinical Endocrinology,* East Norwalk, CT, 1991, Appleton & Lange.)

In addition to negative-feedback effects, female gonadal steroids have a positive effect on pituitary gonadotropin secretion. Positive feedback is triggered by a sharply rising plasma level of estradiol and is critical in promoting the LH surge required to initiate ovulation. The two essential attributes are (1) estradiol concentrations greater than 700 pmol/L (200 pg/mL), and (2) maintenance of elevated estradiol levels for at least 48 h. Progesterone at low concentrations also stimulates LH release but only after the pituitary has been exposed to prolonged high levels of estradiol.

Hypothalamic-pituitary regulation of ovarian function is also influenced by neural stimuli from the central nervous system. The hypothalamus receives both neural and hormonal signals, which can affect GnRH secretion and the menstrual cycle. This type of input can disrupt the pattern of GnRH secretion and lead to **anovulation** and **amenorrhea.** These manifestations may be observed in situations of chronic stress or profound weight loss.

Ovarian Steroid Hormones

The ovarian steroid hormones belong to a large family of steroid compounds, whose composition is based on a four-ring structure that contains three cyclohexane rings and one cyclopentane ring (Fig. 50-3). Steroid hormones have diverse biological effects that vary according to the nature of numerous chemical modifications of the basic steroid structure, such as unsaturation of carbon-carbon bonds within the rings, or attachment of hydroxyl or ketone groups to specific carbon atoms. Ovarian hormones are classified on the basis of their structure and principal biological functions into three major types: estrogens, progestagens, and androgens.

Estrogens

The naturally occurring **estrogens** are C_{18}-steroids. They are characterized by an attached hydroxyl group (estradiol) or ketone group (estrone). The principal and most potent estrogen secreted by the ovary is estradiol-17β. In contrast, relatively small amounts of estrone are secreted by the ovary, most of which originates from extraglandular conversion of androstenedione (and estradiol to a lesser extent) in peripheral tissue, mainly adipose tissue. Increased extraglandular estrone formation can occur in simple obesity or in conditions such as polycystic ovary syndrome, in which increased androstenedione secretion occurs. Estrogen formed by this route then can interfere with normal feedback mechanisms and cause disturbances in the menstrual cycle. Estrogens promote the development of female secondary sex characteristics, as well as uterine growth, thickening of the vaginal mucosa, thinning of the cervical mucus, and development of the ductal system of the breast.

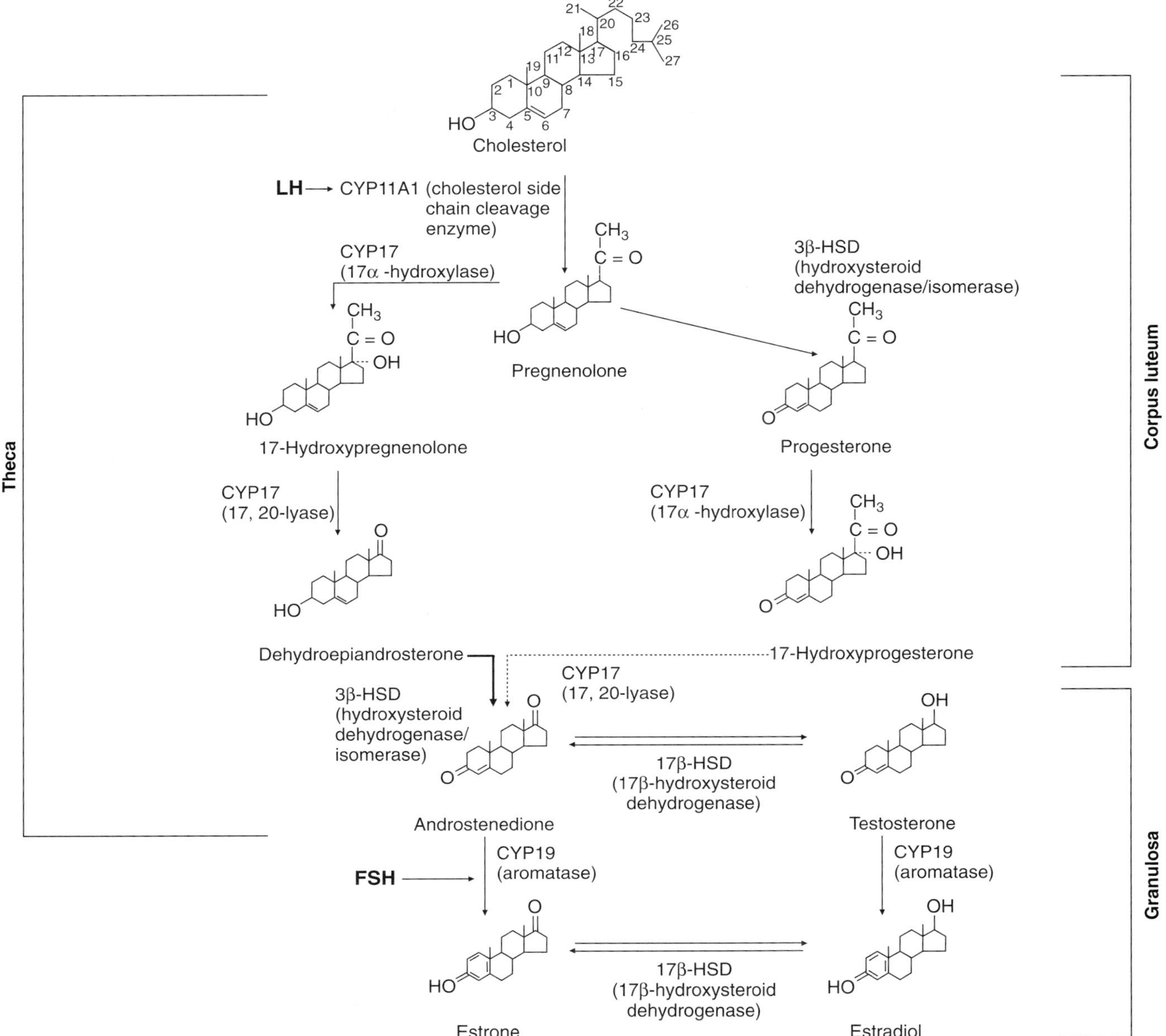

Fig. 50-3 Principal pathways of steroid hormone biosynthesis in the human ovary. Although each cell type of the ovary contains the complete enzyme complement required for the formation of estradiol from cholesterol, the amounts of the various enzymes and consequently the predominant hormones formed differ among cell types. The major enzyme complements for the corpus luteum, theca, and granulosa cells are shown in *brackets;* these cells produce predominantly progesterone and 17-hydroxyprogesterone (corpus luteum), androgen (theca), and estrogen (granulosa). The major sites of action of luteinizing hormone (LH) and follicle-stimulating hormone (FSH) in mediating this pathway are shown by the *horizontal arrows*. The *dotted line* emphasizes that the metabolism of 17-hydroxyprogesterone is limited in the human ovary. (From Wilson JD, et al: *Williams' Textbook of Endocrinology,* ed 9, Philadelphia, 1999, Saunders.)

Progestagens

The progestagens, which are C_{21}-steroids, include pregnenolone, progesterone, and 17-hydroxyprogesterone (17-OHP). Pregnenolone is the precursor of all ovarian steroid hormones (see Fig. 50-3). Progesterone is the primary secretory product of the corpus luteum and is required for the induction of secretory activity in an estrogen-primed uterus, implantation of a fertilized ovum, and maintenance of early pregnancy. The corpus luteum also secretes 17-OHP; however, this steroid has little or no biological activity.

Androgens

The ovarian thecal cells and, to a lesser extent, the stromal cells produce a variety of C_{19}-steroids in small amounts, including dehydroepiandrosterone (DHEA), androstenedione, testosterone, and **dihydrotestosterone.** Only testosterone and dihydrotestosterone are true androgens capable of interacting with the androgen receptor. The major C_{19}-steroid produced is androstenedione, some of which is released into plasma; the remainder is converted into testosterone or estrogen within the ovary. Circulating androstenedione also can be converted to testosterone or estrogen in extraglandular tissue.

Biosynthesis of Ovarian Steroid Hormones

All steroid hormones are derived from cholesterol (see Fig. 50-3). Cholesterol may be synthesized de novo within the ovary, or it may be derived from pre-formed sources (e.g., circulating plasma lipoproteins). The primary source is the uptake of plasma low-density lipoprotein (LDL) cholesterol. Little hormone is stored in the ovary, so secretory activity is closely related to synthetic activity and substrate availability. The main steroid-producing cells of the ovary (i.e., the granulosa, theca, and corpus luteum cells) contain the full complement of enzymes required for the synthesis of any of the ovarian steroid hormones. However, the predominant steroid that is produced differs among cell types. The granulosa cells primarily produce estradiol, the thecal and stromal cells secrete androgens, and the corpus luteum produces progesterone and 17-OHP. Several factors determine which steroid is secreted by each cell type, including the levels of gonadotropin and the relative numbers of cell gonadotropin receptors, the local expression of steroidogenic enzymes, and the availability of LDL cholesterol. Both FSH and LH are required for estrogen synthesis. The rate-limiting step in ovarian steroidogenesis is the initial conversion of cholesterol to pregnenolone. This process is regulated by LH, which stimulates thecal cell uptake of LDL cholesterol and the subsequent synthesis of pregnenolone. FSH controls the conversion of androgens to estrogens. In response to LH, the thecal cells produce androstenedione and small amounts of testosterone. These steroids diffuse into the granulosa cells, in which (in response to FSH) they are aromatized to produce estrone and estradiol-17β.

Transport of Steroid Hormones

After secretion, gonadal steroids circulate in a free (unbound) state, or weakly or strongly bound to plasma proteins. Steroid transport molecules include specific globulins and albumin. **Sex hormone–binding globulin (SHBG)** is a β-globulin that is synthesized by the liver and exhibits high-affinity, low-capacity binding. Albumin has a low affinity but a high capacity. Approximately 60% of plasma estradiol is weakly bound to albumin and 38% to SHBG, and 2% to 3% is free. Progesterone binds strongly to cortisol-binding globulin (CBG) and weakly to albumin. The general consensus is that the biological activity of steroid hormones is proportional to the concentration of free hormone in plasma, not to the concentration of protein-bound hormone. However, the globulin-binding proteins may have specific functional properties related to tissue delivery, in addition to steroid transport. The metabolic clearance rate of gonadal steroids is inversely related to the binding affinity for SHBG; therefore, alterations in the concentration of SHBG can affect gonadal steroid metabolism and target tissue activity. The level of SHBG may be altered by a variety of clinical conditions. SHBG concentrations are increased by estrogens (pregnancy, oral contraceptive pills, hormone replacement therapy) and hyperthyroidism, and are decreased by androgens, hypothyroidism, and obesity.

Mechanisms of Action of Steroid Hormones

Steroid hormones have a low molecular weight and diffuse readily across cell membranes down a concentration gradient because of their high lipid solubility. Steroid receptors are localized within the cytoplasm and the cell nucleus. After steroid binding to its specific receptor, conformational changes occur within the hormone-receptor complex that expose high-affinity DNA-binding sites that then can interact with chromosomal DNA to alter rates of transcription of specific genes. This process is followed by mRNA synthesis, transport of mRNA to ribosomes in the cytoplasm, and synthesis of appropriate proteins that direct cell function. Low levels of steroid hormones produce specific biological effects because of the high affinity, specificity, and concentration of steroid receptors within cells. Specificity is determined partially by the relative numbers of receptors within a cell, for example, in estrogen target tissues such as the uterus, estradiol action is greater and more prolonged, because each target cell contains large numbers of estrogen receptors.

Metabolism of Ovarian Hormones

Plasma estradiol is converted rapidly in the liver to estrone. Some of this estrone reenters the circulation; however, the majority is metabolized further to estriol or 2-hydroxyestrone, conjugated, and then excreted by the kidney. Progesterone is cleared rapidly, having a half-life of about 5 minutes. It is converted in the liver to pregnanediol, conjugated to glucuronic acid, and excreted via the kidneys.

Nonsteroidal Hormones

Steroidogenesis and the development of the dominant ovarian follicle with each menstrual cycle are modulated by many local nonsteroidal factors such as cytokines, growth factors, and neuropeptides. Most important is the inhibin-related family of multifunctional glycoproteins, which act locally to influence the development of the ovarian follicle. They are also present in the circulation and play an important role in the regulation of gonadotropin secretion.

Two forms of **inhibin** have been identified, namely, inhibin A ($\alpha\beta_A$) and inhibin B ($\alpha\beta_B$). These glycoproteins are dimers of two subunits linked by disulfide bonds. The α-subunit is common to both forms of inhibin, whereas the β-subunits are specific for each hormone. In the male, the principal circulating form of inhibin is inhibin B. In the female, serum levels of inhibin A and B fluctuate during the menstrual cycle. Inhibin A levels are low in the early follicular phase and rise in the late follicular phase to reach maximum concentrations during the luteal phase. Changes in inhibin B levels parallel those in FSH, in that they rise rapidly at the onset of the follicular phase, peak just after the midcycle FSH rise, and then progressively fall during the remainder of the luteal phase. These cyclical changes in inhibin concentrations suggest that circulating inhibin B is produced by the granulosa cells during follicular development, whereas inhibin A is secreted mainly by corpus luteum cells. The major local effect of ovarian inhibin is to increase theca cell androgen production. Granulosa cells secrete inhibin into follicular fluid, enabling it to diffuse into thecal cells and positively modulate LH-induced androgen synthesis. Circulating inhibins (A and B) contribute to ovarian-pituitary negative-feedback relationships by decreasing FSH secretion.

The activins are disulfide-linked dimers of the β-subunits of inhibin. Three forms have been identified, namely, activin A ($\beta_A\beta_A$), activin B ($\beta_B\beta_B$), and activin AB ($\beta_A\beta_B$). All the activins have the capacity to stimulate FSH secretion from the pituitary gland; however, their precise roles have yet to be determined. The activins appear to act primarily at a local level. Plasma activin A concentrations do not change significantly during the menstrual cycle, suggesting that circulating activin is not important in the regulation of pituitary FSH secretion. In the ovary, however, locally produced activin A may augment the effects of FSH, as it has been shown to enhance the proliferation of cultured granulosa cells and induce the expression of FSH receptors. Gonadotropes produce activin B in the pituitary, where it may act directly to increase FSH secretion.

KEY CONCEPTS BOX 50-2

- The menstrual cycle requires coordinated secretion from the hypothalamus (GnRH) and pituitary (LH and FSH), and negative- and positive-feedback control by estradiol.
- Estradiol (E_2) is a steroid sex hormone that is produced by the ovaries from cholesterol and is transported in blood mostly bound to the liver proteins SHBG and albumin.
- E_2 acts on cells by binding to cytoplasmic receptors; the E_2-receptor binds to DNA to change gene activation.
- Inhibins are gonadal peptides that help regulate pituitary gonadotropins and also act locally to stimulate androgen production.

SECTION OBJECTIVES BOX 50-3

- List the parts of the menstrual cycle.
- Describe the hormonal changes that regulate the menstrual cycle and discuss the investigation of absent/abnormal menstruation.
- Define *dysmenorrhea* and the premenstrual syndrome.
- Describe the physical and biochemical changes of the menopause.

The Menstrual Cycle

The development of regular, ovulatory menstrual cycles depends on complex interactions between the hypothalamus, pituitary, ovaries, and genital tract. The menstrual cycle is usually divided into two phases: the follicular or proliferative phase, and the luteal or secretory phase (Fig. 50-4). The length

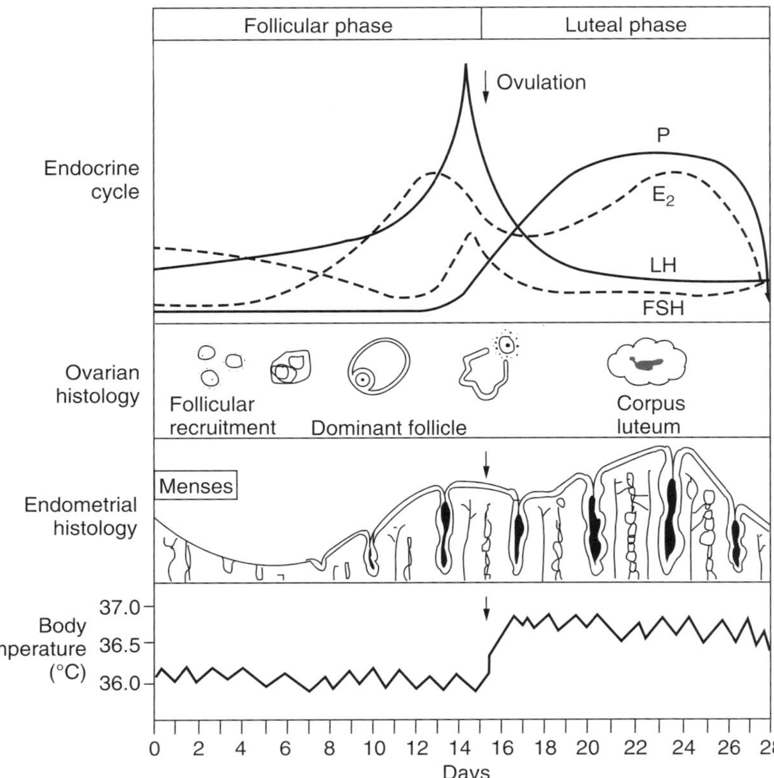

Fig. 50-4 Hormonal, ovarian, endometrial, and basal body temperature changes and relationships throughout the normal menstrual cycle. *E₂,* Estradiol; *FSH,* follicle-stimulating hormone; *LH,* luteinizing hormone; *P,* progesterone. (From Braunwald E, et al: *Harrison's Principles of Internal Medicine,* ed 15, New York, 2001, McGraw-Hill.)

of the menstrual cycle is defined as the period dating from the onset of one menstrual bleed (day 1) until the onset of the next. The average normal cycle length is 28 days. The greatest variability in cycle length occurs after menarche and before the menopause, because of inadequate follicular development that results in anovulatory cycles. Variation in the length of the menstrual cycle between individual women results from variability in the length of the follicular phase, from 10 to 16 days. In contrast, the duration of the luteal phase (approximately 14 days) is remarkably constant.

Follicular Phase

The initiation of follicular growth begins during the last few days of the luteal phase of the preceding menstrual cycle. During this period, the corpus luteum is degenerating, and plasma progesterone and estrasdiol levels are declining. With the reduction in negative feedback, FSH concentrations increase, stimulating the growth of new follicles and estradiol secretion. During menstruation, levels of estradiol, progesterone, and LH are relatively constant and low, whereas FSH concentrations are rising. Several follicles are recruited during days 1 through 4 of the menstrual cycle in response to FSH. Selection of the dominant follicle occurs between cycle days 5 and 7. This follicle then continues to grow and releases factors that suppress the maturation of the other recruited follicles. During the early follicular phase, FSH levels continue to rise. However, estradiol concentrations increase in parallel with follicular growth, thereby exerting a negative-feedback effect on hypothalamic and pituitary hormone secretion, and resulting in a fall in FSH levels by the midfollicular phase. In contrast, LH levels, which are low during the first part of the follicular phase, begin to rise in the midfollicular phase as a result of the positive-feedback effects of rising estradiol concentrations.

Ovulation

Just before ovulation, estradiol secretion by the preovulatory follicle increases dramatically, initiating the LH surge. LH enhances follicular progesterone secretion, which stimulates the midcycle increase in FSH release. Onset of the LH surge occurs 34 to 36 hours before release of the ovum from the follicle. The peak LH level occurs about 10 to 12 hours before ovulation. Ovulation usually occurs at around day 14 in a 28-day cycle. Immediately before the LH peak, estradiol levels fall precipitously, slowly rising again after ovulation. The precise mechanism of follicular rupture is unknown. Just before ovulation, the follicle becomes extensively vascularized, and proteolytic enzymes such as collagenase and plasmin digest collagen in the follicular wall, leading to thinning and distension. Prostaglandin concentrations reach a peak in follicular fluid just before ovulation and are thought to play a role in the rupture of the follicle.

Luteal Phase

After ovulation, the ruptured follicle undergoes changes in structure and function to become the corpus luteum. The corpus luteum is the site of steroid secretion by the ovary during the luteal phase; progesterone and some estradiol are primarily produced. Progesterone produced by the corpus luteum begins to increase 3 days after ovulation, and rising progesterone levels rapidly inhibit LH secretion. Progesterone concentrations reach a maximum about 8 to 9 days after the LH peak. Estradiol levels also increase during the luteal phase and, together with progesterone, cause a progressive decline in LH and FSH concentrations. In the last few days of the luteal phase, as the corpus luteum begins to regress, the levels of estradiol and progesterone decrease. Loss of negative feedback results in rising FSH levels once more, and the recruitment of a new batch of follicles for the next cycle.

The Effect of Ovarian Hormones on the Uterus/Endometrium

Fluctuations in estradiol and progesterone levels during the menstrual cycle produce characteristic changes in the **endometrium** (the tissue that lines the uterus) (see Fig. 50-4). In the initial phase, these changes relate to preparation of the endometrium to receive and implant a fertilized ovum. During the follicular phase of the menstrual cycle, rising levels of estradiol stimulate reconstruction of the endometrium following the preceding menstrual period. This phase of endometrial growth is termed the *proliferative phase,* during which endometrial thickness increases from about 0.5 mm to 3.5 to 5.0 mm. Following ovulation, the endometrium continues to respond to the combined effects of estradiol and progesterone. Overall endometrial thickness remains constant, but individual components continue to grow, so a progressive increase in the tortuosity of the endometrial glands and intensified coiling of the spiral blood vessels occur. This phase corresponds with the luteal phase of the menstrual cycle but is called the secretory phase because of the significant increase that occurs in endometrial gland secretion. The endometrial glands secrete many substances, including numerous peptide growth factors, cytokines, and prostaglandins, the functions of which have yet to be elucidated fully. Implantation of a fertilized ovum (now a blastocyst) occurs about 6 days after ovulation, and by this stage, the endometrium is of sufficient depth, vascularity, and nutritional richness to support the early development of the placenta, that is, invasion of the trophoblastic cells to create the trophoblast–maternal blood interface. The peak endometrial gland secretory activity coincides with the time of blastocyst implantation.

In the event of successful implantation, human chorionic gonadotrophin (hCG) is produced by the trophoblastic cells, and the corpus luteum is maintained. If this does not happen, the corpus luteum begins to regress about 9 days after ovulation, and estradiol and progesterone levels decrease. Withdrawal of these hormones initiates several events within the endometrium. Arteriolar vasomotor changes result in rhythmical vasoconstriction and vasodilatation within the spiral vessels. Each successive vasoconstrictive spasm is more severe, ultimately leading to tissue necrosis and interstitial hemorrhages caused by capillary breakdown. As ischemia and tissue weakness progress, bleeding into the endometrial cavity occurs, and menstruation begins.

Premenstrual Syndrome

Many women experience a variety of cyclical premenstrual symptoms that occur after ovulation and disappear after menstruation. The most frequently encountered symptoms include abdominal bloating, anxiety, breast tenderness, crying spells, depression, fatigue, irritability, headache, thirst, and appetite changes, all of which occur during the last 7 to 10 days of the menstrual cycle. In some women, the combination of symptoms known as the **premenstrual syndrome (PMS)** is more severe for unknown reasons. Although the cause is unknown, prevention of ovulation through the use of oral contraceptives often is helpful. Other treatments that may relieve some symptoms include drug therapy with bromocriptine (a dopamine agonist), prostaglandin synthetase inhibitors (nonsteroidal anti-inflammatory agents), mild diuretics, or antidepressants, if symptoms are severe.

Dysmenorrhea

Dysmenorrhea, or painful menstruation, is very common, affecting at least 50% of women at some time during their reproductive life. Primary dysmenorrhea is associated with ovulatory cycles and is caused by uterine smooth muscle contractions induced by prostaglandins, especially prostaglandin $F_{2\alpha}$, which is formed in the secretory endometrium. Patients with primary dysmenorrhea often have additional symptoms, which may include headache, nausea and vomiting, diarrhea, and emotional disorders. This form of dysmenorrhea can often be treated through prevention of ovulation with oral contraceptives or through the use of prostaglandin synthetase inhibitors. Secondary dysmenorrhea is associated with a variety of conditions such as endometriosis, pelvic inflammatory disease, congenital defects in uterine development, and the presence of intrauterine devices. Secondary dysmenorrhea sometimes requires surgical therapy; however, about 80% of women with either form of dysmenorrhea experience some relief with the use of prostaglandin synthetase inhibitors. A further benefit of these agents is a reduction in the amount of blood lost with menstrual flow.

The Menopause

The menopause is the permanent cessation of menstruation that results from loss of ovarian follicular function. Clinically, the menopause is recognized as having occurred after 12 consecutive months of amenorrhea, so the time of the final menses is determined retrospectively. The perimenopause, or the *climacteric,* includes the period immediately before the menopause, when the endocrinological, biological, and clinical features of approaching menopause commence, through the first year after menopause. The mean age at which menopause occurs is about 51 years. No correlation between age of menarche and age of menopause has been found. Socioeconomic circumstances, race, parity, and weight have no effect on the timing of the menopause, but women who smoke may experience an earlier menopause.

The major underlying pathophysiology of the menopause is the loss of ovarian follicles. Ovarian primordial follicle numbers decrease steadily with increasing age up to about the age of 38, and their number declines much more rapidly during the last decade of reproductive life. At the time of the menopause itself, few if any follicles can be found in the ovaries. The ovary of the postmenopausal women is reduced in size, weighs less than 2.5 g, and is wrinkled in appearance. Microscopically, the cortical area is reduced because of follicular loss, the stroma becomes hyperplastic, and interstitial and hilar cells are more prominent.

The normal menstrual cycle is characterized by changing levels of plasma gonadotropins, ovarian steroids, and inhibins, as described earlier. No endocrine event clearly differentiates the time just before and just after the final menses. FSH levels begin to rise a year or two before the final menses, coinciding with the onset of cycle irregularity, whereas estradiol levels are well maintained until just a few months before the cessation of menses. It is only after a woman has experienced more than 3 months of amenorrhea that the rise in FSH is accompanied by a substantial fall in estradiol levels. Indeed, during the perimenopause, FSH concentrations may be raised to the postmenopausal range during some cycles but may return to premenopausal levels during subsequent cycles. Thus, in menstruating women, laboratory measurement of FSH cannot reliably determine menopausal status. LH levels remain largely unchanged during the perimenopausal period.

A major hormonal event of the menopausal transition is a decline in inhibin B levels during the first half of the cycle. This decrease in inhibin B produces a reduction in negative feedback on the pituitary, thereby allowing a rise in FSH that is sufficient to stimulate follicular development and maintain dominant follicle function and estradiol production for as long as possible. The observed fall in inhibin B levels in older women may reflect a decrease in the size of the recruited cohort of follicles at the onset of each cycle, or a decrease in the ability of granulosa cells to secrete inhibin B. As cycles become irregular, menstrual bleeding may occur at the end of an inadequate luteal phase, or after an estradiol peak, without subsequent ovulation or corpus luteum formation. However, ovulation and the formation of a functional corpus luteum can occur, and the perimenopausal woman is not safe from unexpected pregnancy until elevated levels of both FSH and LH can be demonstrated. In the postmenopausal state, a 10- to 15-fold increase in circulating FSH levels is seen, along with a 4-5-fold increase in LH and a more than 90% decrease in circulating estradiol. Inhibin levels are undetectable postmenopausally. FSH levels are higher than LH levels because LH is cleared from the blood much faster (half-lives are about 30 minutes for LH and 4 hours for FSH). Gonadotropin levels reach a maximum some 1 to 3 years after the final menses, and elevated levels of both FSH and LH provide conclusive evidence of ovarian failure.

Classical symptoms of the menopause such as hot flushes, vaginal dryness, and urinary frequency are thought to result from falling or low estradiol levels. Hot flushes are associated with a sensation of warmth that commonly is accompanied by skin flushing and perspiration. These can be occasional or frequent, can last from seconds to an hour, and may be associated with mild warmth or profound sweating. Hot flushes diminish spontaneously as time from the menopause increases; therefore, the primary indication for treatment is to relieve distressing symptoms. In some women, hot flushes are a major problem, disrupting work, sleep, or daily activities. Other clinical consequences of the postmenopausal state include significantly increased risks of developing coronary heart disease and osteoporosis. Postmenopausal women are estimated to have a twofold higher risk of developing coronary heart disease than premenopausal women, after adjustment is made for age. The adverse change in age-adjusted plasma lipid and lipoprotein profiles that occurs after the menopause is a significant factor in this association. A causal relationship between the menopause and osteoporosis is evident in the higher rates of osteoporotic fractures observed in postmenopausal women and the loss of bone mineral density that has been documented after the menopause. Longitudinal cohort studies suggest that maximum changes in bone mineral density occur during the late perimenopause and the early postmenopause, corresponding to the time of maximum decrease in circulating estradiol levels (Burger, 1999).

Until recently, hormone replacement therapy (HRT) was routinely prescribed for the alleviation of postmenopausal symptoms and for the prevention of postmenopausal coronary heart disease (CHD) and osteoporosis. However, data from the Women's Health Initiative (WHI) and the Heart and Estrogen/Progestin Replacement Study (HERS) trial have dramatically changed these recommendations, although this long-range trial is ongoing.

Estrogen therapy (alone or combined with progestin) still is regarded as the most effective option for the short-term relief of menopausal symptoms in women without a history of breast cancer, CHD, stroke, or thromboembolic disease. Progestin should always be added for women with an intact uterus because increased rates of endometrial hyperplasia and cancer associated with unopposed estrogen therapy is seen within as little as 6 months following commencement. Treatment is not recommended for longer than 2 to 3 years, and routine mammograms and breast examinations must be pursued, given the increased incidence of abnormal mammograms reported in patients on short-term HRT studied in the WHI.

KEY CONCEPTS BOX 50-3

- Menstrual cycle phases include the follicular (proliferative) and luteal.
- In the former, FSH stimulates new follicles; E_2 and LH levels are rising and one of the follicles ruptures, releasing an ova.
- In the luteal phase, progesterone is secreted, decreasing LH production. At the end of this phase, the corpus luteum regresses, causing a decrease in progesterone and E_2.
- High levels of E_2 and progesterone stimulate thickening of the uterus; if no fertilized egg implants, the uterine growth regresses (menstruation). Implantation causes production of hCG, which maintains the uterus during pregnancy.
- Dysmenorrhea, or painful menstruation, may be associated with uterine disorders and pelvic inflammatory disease.
- Menopause, the cessation of the menstrual cycle, is noted by decreased E_2 and elevated FSH and LH. Estrogen replacement therapy will reduce the effects of E_2 withdrawal.

SECTION OBJECTIVES BOX 50-4

- Define *amenorrhea.*
- List genetic causes of ovarian dysfunction.
- Define *premature ovarian failure.*
- List two disorders of the pituitary that affect ovarian function.
- Describe the primary features of the polycystic ovarian syndrome.

PATHOLOGICAL STATES

Amenorrhea

As was described earlier, normal menstrual function depends on the complex hormonal interactions between the hypothalamus, pituitary, and ovaries. An intact outflow tract and the existence and development of the endometrium also are required for normal menstrual flow. Abnormalities in any of these hormonal or anatomical systems may cause amenorrhea (absence of bleeding). The clinical problem of amenorrhea may be defined by the following criteria:

1. No period by age 14 in the absence of growth or development of secondary sex characteristics.
2. No period by age 16, regardless of the presence of normal growth and development with the appearance of secondary sex characteristics.
3. In a woman who has been menstruating, the absence of periods for a length of time equivalent to a total of at least three of the previous cycle intervals, or 6 months of amenorrhea.

Assessment of a patient with amenorrhea requires a careful history and examination. Pregnancy must always be excluded. Further investigation depends to some extent on the history and examination findings, for example, in a young woman with primary amenorrhea and abnormal development, initial investigations should include a karyotype and pelvic ultrasound. The presence of normal secondary sex characteristics implies that estradiol production was adequate in the past. The progestin withdrawal test provides a functional assessment of current estradiol status in women. In the following sections, various disorders that may cause amenorrhea and how the clinical laboratory contributes to the diagnostic process will be described. The causes of amenorrhea are shown in Box 50-1, and a proposed clinical workup is summarized in Fig. 50-5.

Disorders of the Outflow Tract or Uterus

Congenital abnormalities of the organs that develop from the müllerian duct system must always be considered in the evaluation of primary amenorrhea. Many different müllerian anomalies can occur, including imperforate hymen, obliteration of the vaginal orifice, absence of the uterine cavity or endometrial lining, and absence of the uterus itself or the cervix. Some of these anomalies are apparent on physical examination; others can be identified via pelvic ultrasound. Patients with complete müllerian agenesis have an absent vagina and varying uterine abnormalities, ranging from virtual absence of the uterus with the presence of rudimentary uterine

Box 50-1

Causes of Amenorrhea

Disorders of the Outflow Tract or Uterus
Müllerian duct anomalies/complete müllerian agenesis
Complete/partial androgen insensitivity (testicular feminization syndrome)
Endometrial destruction (Asherman's syndrome)

Disorders of the Ovary (Primary Hypogonadism)
Gonadal dysgenesis (Turner's syndrome, mosaics, 45,X/46,XX,47,XXX)
Resistant ovary syndrome
Premature ovarian failure (idiopathic, autoimmune, post irradiation, or chemotherapy)

Disorders of the Anterior Pituitary (Secondary Hypogonadism)
Prolactin-secreting pituitary tumor
Granulomatous infiltration (sarcoidosis, histiocytosis)
Lymphocytic hypophysitis
Primary apoplexy (Sheehan's syndrome)

Central Nervous System Disorders
Kallmann's syndrome
Hypothalamic infiltrative disease (sarcoidosis, histiocytosis, hemochromatosis)
Hypothalamic tumor (craniopharyngioma)
Cranial irradiation

tissue only, to a morphologically normal uterus. Ovarian function is normal in these patients, hence growth and development are also normal. Complete androgen insensitivity (testicular feminization syndrome) produces congenital absence of the uterus and a blind-ending vaginal canal. The patient with testicular feminization has a female phenotype (appearance), including some breast development at puberty, but is a genetic and gonadal male with failure of virilization. Resistance to the action of fetal testicular testosterone means that the male wolffian duct system cannot develop, but antimüllerian hormone produced by the fetal testes acts normally, and hence the female müllerian duct system develops abnormally. The chromosomal karyotype is XY and testicular tissue is present, sometimes intra-abdominally but frequently within an inguinal hernia as antimüllerian hormone mediates testicular descent. The incidence of malignant neoplasia in these gonads is high, and they must be surgically removed. This disorder is transmitted genetically by means of a maternal X-linked recessive gene, which encodes the intracellular androgen receptor. These patients have normal to slightly high male plasma testosterone levels and high LH levels. Incomplete androgen insensitivity occurs more rarely. These individuals also have a female phenotype but show some evidence of androgen effect such as clitoral enlargement.

Secondary amenorrhea can occur after destruction of the endometrium (Asherman's syndrome). This condition usually is the result of an overly aggressive curettage that results in

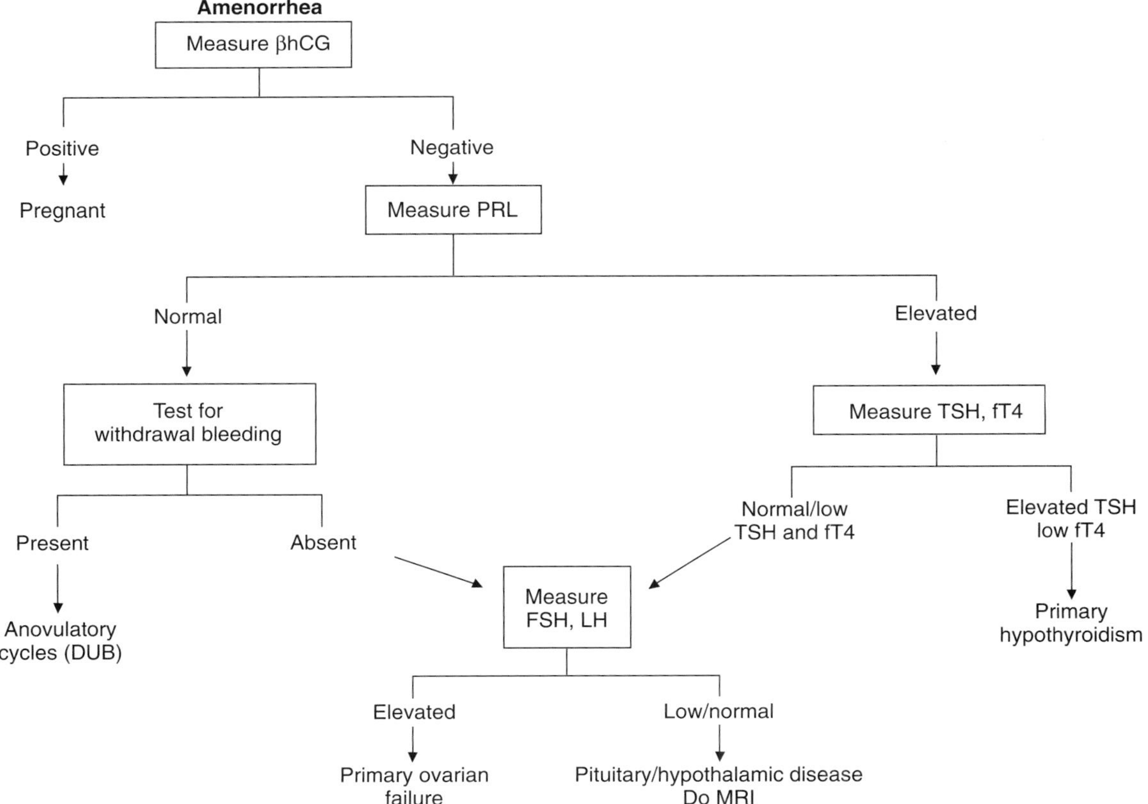

Fig. 50-5 Clinical approach to the investigation of amenorrhea. *DUB,* Dysfunctional uterine bleeding; *FSH,* follicle-stimulating hormone; *fT_4,* free thyroxine; *hCG,* human chorionic gonadotropin; *LH,* luteinizing hormone; *MRI,* magnetic resonance imaging; *PRL,* prolactin; *TSH,* thyroid-stimulating hormone.

intrauterine scarring and adhesions. Rarely, it may occur after intrauterine device (IUD)-related infection or severe generalized pelvic infection.

Disorders of the Ovary

Patients with abnormal gonadal development (gonadal dysgenesis) can present with primary or secondary amenorrhea. Several different chromosomal karyotypes, including 45,X (**Turner's syndrome**), mosaicism (e.g., 45,X/46,XX), deletions of the short or long arms of X, 47,XXX, and, not uncommonly, the normal female karyotype of 46,XX, are associated with gonadal dysgenesis. These individuals have high plasma gonadotropin levels caused by the lack of ovarian estradiol secretion and negative feedback on the pituitary. All patients who present with primary or secondary amenorrhea in conjunction with high gonadotropin levels should have a karyotype determination. Although women with chromosomal defects are more likely to present with primary amenorrhea, individuals with **mosaicism** may have some functional gonadal tissue that gives rise to various degrees of sexual development and transient menstrual cyclicity. Identifying the presence of mosaicism with a Y chromosome is critical. Gonadal tissue in these patients must be surgically removed, because the presence of any testicular component within the gonad carries with it a significant risk of malignant tumor formation. A normal female phenotype does not exclude the presence of a Y chromosome, as about 30% of mosaic patients with a Y chromosome will not develop signs of virilization. Turner's syndrome (an abnormality in or absence of one of the X chromosomes) is relatively common (about 1 in 7000 live female births) and has several well-defined clinical characteristics. The presence of short stature, a webbed neck, a shield chest, and increased carrying angle at the elbow in association with hypergonadotropic hypoestrogenic amenorrhea virtually confirms the diagnosis. A karyotype still must be performed, however, because 30% of patients who present with the classical clinical features of Turner's syndrome are mosaics. In comparison with gonadal dysgenesis, the resistant ovary syndrome is a rare clinical entity. Such patients present with primary amenorrhea in conjunction with high gonadotropin levels and a normal karyotype, but ovarian development occurs and a full-thickness biopsy of the ovary can demonstrate the presence of follicles.

Premature ovarian failure typically is defined as amenorrhea, **infertility,** estradiol deficiency, and elevated gonadotropins in a woman younger than 40 years of age. It affects 1% of women by the age of 40, and 0.1% by age 30 years. Normal menopause is irreversible, whereas premature ovarian failure is associated with intermittent ovarian function in about 50% of cases. Affected women may produce estradiol and ovulate intermittently despite the presence of high gonadotropin levels. Premature ovarian failure therefore may present as primary or secondary amenorrhea. Patients with secondary amenorrhea may experience symptoms of estrogen deficiency such as hot flushes. The underlying cause of premature ovarian failure is unknown in most cases; presumably, the ovarian follicles undergo a process of accelerated atresia. This may be associated with autoimmune endocrine disorders such as primary adrenal failure (Addison's disease), type 1 diabetes mellitus, and hypothyroidism, or it may follow follicle destruction by infections (such as mumps virus) or by physical insults such as irradiation or chemotherapy. Young women with premature ovarian failure, which may occur before peak adult bone mass is achieved, are estrogen deficient for a much longer period than women who undergo a natural menopause. Associated risks of osteoporosis and cardiovascular disease therefore are significantly increased, and appropriate hormone replacement therapy in these patients is critically important. Long-term surveillance is necessary, because hormone replacement should be continued at least until the average age of natural menopause. Young women who desire fertility should be informed that there is a 5% to 10% chance of spontaneous pregnancy, which is not adversely affected by concurrent hormone replacement therapy. The efficacy of hormone ovulation induction regimens in women who fail to conceive naturally is variable in patients with premature ovarian failure.

Disorders of the Anterior Pituitary

Several disorders of the pituitary that can result in estrogen deficiency and amenorrhea are listed in Box 50-2. Despite low concentrations of estradiol in these disorders, plasma gonadotropin levels will be subnormal or within the reference interval (which also provides evidence of abnormal gonadotrope function in view of the coexisting estradiol deficiency), a situation termed *hypogonadotropic* ***hypogonadism.***

Pituitary tumors account for approximately 10% of all intracranial tumors, and prolactin-secreting tumors (prolactinoma) are the most common. Pituitary cells of all types can be transformed into adenomatous lesions, and pituitary tumors may secrete one or more hormones or may be nonfunctioning. Pituitary tumors tend to grow slowly, and when they enlarge, they typically extend superiorly and may impinge on the optic chiasm. Patients therefore may present with the effects of excess hormone secretion, with symptoms of hypogonadism, or with mass effects such as visual field defects.

Women with hyperprolactinemia commonly have amenorrhea and/or galactorrhea; therefore, all patients who present with such symptoms should have a serum prolactin measurement. Not all women with hyperprolactinemia have a prolactinoma, however, and many conditions may be associated with elevations in serum prolactin, including pituitary stalk transection (associated with head injury), hypothalamic granulo-

Box 50-2

Pituitary Disorders Associated With Estrogen Deficiency and Amenorrhea

- Tumors that directly inhibit gonadotropin secretion through the destruction of pituitary gonadotropin-producing cells
- Pituitary apoplexy (spontaneous infarction or necrosis), in the setting of a preexisting pituitary tumor or following severe postpartum hemorrhage and shock (Sheehan's syndrome), causing gonadotrope destruction
- Pituitary tumor secreting prolactin, which then interferes with LH-RH neuron function

matous disease, hypothyroidism, renal failure, and stress. Inhibitory hypothalamic dopaminergic pathways normally regulate prolactin secretion. Many drugs, for example, phenothiazines, metoclopramide, opiates, and the monoamine oxidase inhibitors, exhibit some inhibitory action on the dopamine receptor or deplete central dopamine levels. All these drugs have the potential to produce mild to moderate increases in serum prolactin. The assessment of any patient with hyperprolactinemia therefore requires that a thorough drug history be taken. All patients with elevated prolactin levels in association with amenorrhea and/or galactorrhea require radiological imaging of the pituitary. Magnetic resonance imaging (MRI) is the method of choice, if available, because it is more sensitive than computed tomography (CT) in detecting small pituitary tumors. As with other pituitary tumors, prolactinomas can be divided into microadenomas (<10 mm in diameter) and macroprolactinomas (>10 mm). The serum prolactin level roughly correlates with the size of the tumor; a small elevation in prolactin in association with a large pituitary tumor probably reflects stalk compression rather than tumor prolactin secretion. First-line therapy for prolactinomas is pharmacological. These tumors exhibit a high response rate to treatment with dopamine agonists, bromocriptine, or the longer-acting cabergoline, both biochemically and in terms of tumor shrinkage.

Central Nervous System Disorders

If a pituitary lesion has been excluded, hypothalamic disorders that result in failure of normal pulsatile GnRH secretion must be considered, as these also may produce the clinical syndrome of hypogonadotropic hypogonadism. Deficient GnRH secretion may occur in isolation or as part of a congenital or inherited disorder, or it may result from a variety of structural and functional hypothalamic lesions. A defect in the formation and migration of GnRH neurons is called isolated hypothalamic hypogonadism, or congenital isolated GnRH deficiency. When this condition is associated with anosmia (the inability to smell) and agenesis of the olfactory bulbs, it is called **Kallmann's syndrome.** This genetically heterogenous disorder may be inherited as an autosomal dominant, autosomal recessive, or X-linked trait. The trait is four times more common in males and can be associated with other anomalies such as cleft lip and palate, sensorineural deafness, and renal agenesis. The clinical features of GnRH deficiency typically become apparent at puberty, a time when a marked increase in GnRH secretion normally occurs. Affected women present with primary amenorrhea and failure to develop secondary sex characteristics. Other rare syndromes have a genetic basis in which hypogonadotropic hypogonadism is associated with several other characteristic clinical features; these include the Prader-Willi, Laurence-Moon, and Bardet-Biedl syndromes. These disorders usually are evident in early childhood.

Tumors of the hypothalamus can interfere with the normal pattern of GnRH synthesis, secretion, or stimulation of pituitary gonadotropes. In children, the most common tumor that may result in hypogonadotropic hypogonadism is a craniopharyngioma. In adult patients, gliomas, meningiomas, and germinomas may cause hypothalamic dysfunction. Rarer causes include involvement of the hypothalamus by infiltrative disorders such as hemochromatosis, sarcoidosis, and histiocytosis. Previous cranial irradiation for the treatment of central nervous system tumors or leukemia may result in a gradual deterioration in hypothalamic-pituitary function. Functional forms of hypogonadotropic hypogonadism also exist, in which the disturbance in GnRH secretion is of a transient rather than permanent nature. In susceptible women, amenorrhea may be precipitated by stress, significant weight loss, and participation in regular strenuous exercise. Treatment should be directed at the underlying cause, but cyclical hormone replacement therapy or the oral contraceptive pill can be used to protect against osteoporosis in such women. GnRH suppression due to exogenous anabolic steroids also is reversible, although recovery can take some weeks after steroid withdrawal.

Dysfunctional Uterine Bleeding

Between menarche and the menopause, almost every woman experiences one or more episodes of abnormal uterine bleeding, defined as any bleeding pattern that differs in frequency, duration, or amount from the pattern observed during a normal menstrual cycle. These abnormal bleedings may occur during regular ovulatory cycles. Excessive or prolonged bleeding may be caused by pathological abnormalities of the uterus, such as leiomyomas or endometrial polyps, or by a coagulation disorder. Regular ovulatory cycles characterized by spotting or light bleeding may be due to intrauterine adhesions or cervical scarring. Intermenstrual bleeding or spotting often is caused by endometrial or cervical lesions.

Uterine bleeding during anovulatory cycles is unpredictable with respect to amount, onset, and duration, and is known as **dysfunctional uterine bleeding** (DUB). DUB is usually painless because of the absence of ovulation. This disorder reflects a disruption in the normal maturation and development of the endometrium. In the absence of ovulation, luteal progesterone support of the estrogen-primed endometrium is inadequate; therefore, bleeding occurs at unpredictable and irregular intervals. Exposure of the endometrium to estrogen unopposed by progesterone causes a hyperplastic endometrium, and women with untreated DUB are at increased risk of endometrial cancer. DUB occurs in normal women at the extremes of reproductive life (i.e., post menarche, as anovulatory cycles precede the development of regular ovulatory cycles, and perimenopausally, as follicle depletion leads to anovulatory cycles). In women of reproductive age, the most common cause of chronic anovulation with estrogen present is polycystic ovary syndrome.

Polycystic Ovary Syndrome

The **polycystic ovary syndrome (PCOS)** is a complex disorder that typically is characterized by infertility, **hirsutism,** obesity, and various menstrual disturbances, such as amenorrhea, oligomenorrhea, or DUB. Classic PCOS, as described originally by Stein and Leventhal, is associated with enlarged, sclerotic ovaries with thickened capsules that contain multiple atretic follicles (creating the so-called polycystic appearance), and rare or absent *corpora albicans,* which reflects the lack of ovulation. The presence of this ovarian morphology alone, however, is insufficient to allow the diagnosis of PCOS, as it has been described in 20% to 25% of normal women with regular ovulatory cycles and no evidence of hyperandrogenism (Taylor, 1998). The key features of PCOS therefore include the presence of menstrual irregularity in association with hyperandrogenism, which may be evident clinically (as hirsutism, acne, or male pattern balding) or biochemically (as elevated serum androgen levels). **Hirsutism** is defined as excess terminal (thick pigmented) body hair in a male distribution. It is observed commonly on the upper lip, on the chin, around the nipples, and along the *linea alba* of the lower abdomen. Severe hyperandrogenism may cause increased muscle mass, a deepening voice, and clitoromegaly; however, these signs of **virilization** are associated more commonly with androgen-secreting ovarian or adrenal tumors. Not all women with PCOS are overweight, but at least 50% are obese, and some will resume more regular menstrual cycles after relatively small amounts of weight loss. PCOS also is associated with hyperinsulinemia resulting from relative insulin resistance, which exists independently of body weight but is exacerbated by obesity. About 20% of obese women with PCOS develop impaired glucose tolerance or overt non–insulin-dependent diabetes mellitus by the age of 40 (Taylor, 1998).

Women produce androgens from the adrenal gland and the ovary, as well as from peripheral conversion of less potent androgens to more potent androgens by enzymes such as 5α-reductase located in the skin and fat tissue. The principal source of androgen in PCOS is the ovary. Women with PCOS may have elevated plasma levels of androstenedione, testosterone, and/or DHEA, but considerable individual variation is seen, and androgen levels may be completely normal. Dehydroepiandrosterone sulfate is derived for the most part from the adrenal gland; therefore, it acts as a marker of adrenal androgen hypersecretion. Testosterone is the most potent circulating androgen, but its biological activity is determined by assessing the amount of binding to SHBG, as only the free hormone fraction is biologically active. Androgens and insulin suppress SHBG production by the liver, so women with PCOS tend to have low SHBG levels, and more biologically available testosterone. This can mask the degree of testosterone excess when total testosterone levels are measured. Free testosterone assays are neither widely available nor particularly reliable, therefore the free androgen index (ratio of total testosterone to SHBG) may be used to estimate free testosterone activity. In women with PCOS, total testosterone levels may be normal, but the free androgen index may be elevated. Women with PCOS generally have estradiol levels within the normal range for the early follicular phase but elevated estrone levels. These estrogens are derived in part from numerous small follicles in the polycystic ovary and in part from peripheral aromatization of androgens to estrogens in fat cells. Some women with PCOS have abnormal gonadotropin levels, suggesting a disturbance in the normal pituitary-ovarian relationship. The characteristic pattern is one of relatively high LH levels in conjunction with normal or low FSH levels, resulting in an elevated LH-to-FSH ratio. About 15% to 20% of women with PCOS also have mildly elevated plasma prolactin levels.

Other Disorders Associated With Androgen Excess

The most frequent symptom of hyperandrogenism is hirsutism, a relatively common presenting complaint in women. More than 95% of hirsute women will have the more benign condition of idiopathic hirsutism, which often is familial, or PCOS. However, these conditions should be diagnosed after more serious and potentially life-threatening causes of hirsutism have been excluded. The causes of hirsutism, most of which are associated with hyperandrogenism and menstrual irregularity, are shown in Box 50-3. Less common causes of hirsutism generally can be distinguished from idiopathic hirsutism and PCOS by specific clinical features and biochemical tests. A history of abrupt onset, short duration (less than 1 year), or progressively worsening hirsutism, particularly if associated with signs of virilization, strongly suggests an androgen-secreting ovarian or adrenal tumor. Such patients usually have very high plasma testosterone levels. High levels of DHEAS indicate an adrenal tumor, although a low DHEAS level does not rule out a tumor with 100% sensitivity, as adrenal carcinomas that lack sulfating activity have been reported. In addition, DHEAS secretion decreases after about 30 years of age, so serum levels must be interpreted according to age-specific normal ranges. Transvaginal ultrasound is an effective means of identifying ovarian tumors, but abdominal CT or MRI is required to search for an adrenal mass.

Congenital adrenal hyperplasia (CAH; see p. 1012), specifically, late-onset 21-hydroxylase deficiency, should be considered in women with early onset of hirsutism, hyperkalemia, or a family history of CAH. This diagnosis may be excluded by measuring 17-hydroxyprogesterone (a precursor of cortisol that is converted to 11-deoxycortisol by the 21-hydroxylase enzyme), either randomly or after adrenal stimulation, with exogenous synthetic adrenocorticotropic hormone (ACTH). Testing for Cushing's syndrome should be considered in hirsute women with symptoms and signs suggestive of cortisol excess, such as progressive weight gain with a predominantly central distribution, purple striae, easy bruising, muscle weakness, mood changes, and hypertension. Screening tests include measuring 24-hour urinary excretion of free cortisol and performing an overnight dexamethasone suppression test (see Chapter 51).

Box 50-3
Causes of Hirsutism

Idiopathic (including familial)
Drug-induced (anabolic steroids, minoxidil, phenytoin)
Ovarian
- Polycystic ovary syndrome
- Androgen-secreting ovarian tumors

Adrenal
- Late-onset (nonclassical) 21-hydroxylase deficiency
- Congenital adrenal hyperplasia
- Androgen-secreting adrenal tumors

Cushing's syndrome

Ovarian Hyperfunction

Ovarian neoplasms are organized according to a complex histological classification. Almost any tumor of the ovary may produce an endocrine effect, either through functional activity of the tumor cells themselves or via an effect on reactive nonneoplastic stromal cells. Most clinically functioning tumors are of the sex cord stromal type or are germ cell tumors. Sex cord stromal tumors are thought to be derived from the specialized ovarian stroma; this group includes the granulosa, theca, Sertoli-Leydig, and lipoid cell tumors. The granulosa tumor is the most common malignant functioning tumor of the ovary. Granulosa tumors are almost always estrinizing (increasing secondary female characteristics), although rarely, these tumors produce testosterone and are virilizing. Symptoms differ with the age of the patient; prepubertal girls present with precocious puberty, women in their reproductive years experience disturbances in the menstrual cycle, and postmenopausal women present with irregular vaginal bleeding related to endometrial hyperplasia. Functioning thecomas are almost always estrinizing, whereas Seroli-Leydig and lipoid cell tumors are more often virilizing. In all instances, primary ovarian hyperfunction results in decreased levels of LH and FSH that result from increased negative-feedback effects on the pituitary.

KEY CONCEPTS BOX 50-4

- Amenorrhea, the absence of menstrual bleeding, can be caused by physical, endocrine, and genetic disorders. Lab testing for amenorrhea includes measurement of serum prolactin, LH, FSH, and thyroid hormones.
- Turner's syndrome and genetic mosaicism are common genetic causes of amenorrhea.
- Polycystic ovary syndrome (POCS) is associated with chronic anovulation, hirsutism, and amenorrhea. POCS is usually caused by increased serum androgens.

SECTION OBJECTIVES BOX 50-5

- Describe hypothalamic-pituitary-gonadal axis regulation of testicular function.
- Outline the pathways of biosynthesis, transport, and metabolism of male sex hormones.
- Describe the origin and investigation of male hypogonadism.

NORMAL TESTES AND TESTICULAR FUNCTION

Early Development

Early development of the gonads, up to about 42 days of gestation, is identical in male and female embryos. By this time, in male embryos, the fetal testes become apparent histologically with the development of seminiferous cords in the genital ridge. As in the ovary, three principal cell types are involved in formation of the testes: (1) coelomic epithelial cells that differentiate into Sertoli cells; (2) mesenchymal cells that give rise to interstitial (Leydig) cells; and (3) primordial germ cells. A portion of the Y chromosome is essential for normal male gonadal development. The testes-determining factor has been mapped to a segment on the short arm of the Y chromosome, and the gene isolated from this locus has been called the sex-determining region Y (SRY). Male wolffian duct development is dependent on testicular production of testosterone and antimüllerian hormone. Histological development of the testis is essentially complete by the end of the third month of gestation. Descent of the testes from the abdomen to the scrotum occurs later, and this process is not complete until the seventh month of gestation. Testicular descent depends in part on hormonal factors, such as antimüllerian hormone and androgen, but also on the normal development of abdominal musculature and intra-abdominal pressure. Each testis contains approximately 3×10^5 primordial germ cells, which remain quiescent until puberty, when they divide by mitosis to form spermatogonia. Different from ovarian germ cells, testicular germ cells do not begin the process of meiosis until puberty. As was described previously, the process of meiosis involves two cell divisions; in the male, this ultimately yields cells called *spermatids,* which contain the haploid (23) chromosome number.

Fetal pituitary LH and placental hCG are both important in the regulation of testosterone secretion from the fetal testes, although precise control of testosterone production is not completely understood. In the male embryo, secretion of testosterone by the testes and the level of plasma testosterone begin to rise at the end of the second month of gestation, reaching a maximum level shortly thereafter that is maintained until late in gestation but decreases before birth. At birth, the plasma testosterone level is only slightly higher in males than in females. Shortly after birth, the plasma testosterone level rises in the male infant, remaining elevated for about 3 months but falling to low levels within 1 year. The plasma level then remains low (although higher in males than females) until puberty, when it again increases in boys, reaching adult male levels by about age 17. As in girls, the hypothalamic-pituitary axis in prepubertal boys is highly sensitive to the negative-feedback effects of gonadal steroids; in this instance, testosterone and plasma gonadotropin levels remain low until puberty. However, although basal secretion is low in prepubertal children, the pituitary gonadotropins are secreted in a pulsatile manner, with pulses occurring at 2- to 3-hour intervals. Sleep-associated surges in LH secretion, and to a lesser extent surges in FSH secretion, that occur in response to bursts of GnRH release from the hypothalamus herald the onset of puberty. Later in puberty, pulsatile gonadotropin secretion occurs throughout the day and night, and plasma gonadotropin levels become more sustained, as do resultant increases in plasma testosterone and dihydrotestosterone concentrations. In boys, the anatomical and functional changes of puberty are primarily the result of testicular androgens. Androgens stimulate the development of male secondary sex characteristics and the physical appearance of the male body, accelerate linear growth, and initiate spermatogenesis in the testes.

The Mature Testes

Structural Organization

The adult testes are spheroid organs located within the scrotum. The extra-abdominal location of the testes serves to maintain the testicular temperature about 2 Celsius degrees below core body temperature. The process of spermatogenesis is exquisitely sensitive to alterations in temperature, and temporary increases in systemic or local temperature frequently are followed by brief decreases in sperm production. The macroscopic structure of the testes is shown in Fig. 50-6. The testes contain two functional units: (1) a network of tubules for the production and transport of sperm to the excretory-ejaculatory ducts, and (2) a system of interstitial cells **(Leydig cells)** that constitute the major endocrine component of the testes, as they are responsible for the production of testicular androgens (predominantly testosterone).

Within each testis are about 250 pyramidal lobules that contain coiled seminiferous tubules separated by fibrous septa; this component accounts for 80% to 90% of the testicular mass. The seminiferous tubules are lined with Sertoli cells and germ cells (spermatogonia). The Sertoli cells are large cells, with a basal portion that lies adjacent to the outer basement membrane of the spermatogenic tubule and an inner extensive branching cytoplasm. The process of spermatogenesis takes place within a network of Sertoli cell cytoplasm, and differentiating spermatocytes and spermatids are encompassed by the Sertoli cells (see Fig. 50-6). Thus these cells are thought to provide the necessary environmental conditions for germ cell maturation. Spermatogenesis commences after puberty, when the tubules and interstitial cells become mature. Each spermatogonium that undergoes differentiation gives rise to 16 primary spermatocytes, each of which enters meiosis to give rise to four spermatids. Cell division stops after formation of the spermatids, but a complex series of developmental changes still must occur if these conventional cells are to be transformed into the highly specialized **spermatozoa** capable of flagellum-derived motility. The pituitary gonadotropins play a vital role in the process of spermatogenesis. FSH acts directly on the Sertoli cells in the spermatogenic tubule, whereas LH influences spermatogenesis indirectly by increasing testosterone synthesis in the adjacent Leydig cells. FSH is essential for the initiation of spermatogenesis, but full maturation of spermatozoa also requires adequate local production of testosterone.

The process of spermatogenesis takes approximately 70 days from the beginning of differentiation of the spermatocyte to completion of a motile sperm. The seminiferous tubules empty into a highly convoluted network of ducts called the *rete testis*. Spermatozoa then are transported into a single duct, the **epididymis.** During their 12 to 21 days of passage through the epididymis, the spermatozoa undergo further maturation as required for effective fertilization. The epididymis also serves as a reservoir for sperm, which then enter the vas deferens and are propelled into the ejaculatory duct. In addition to the spermatozoa and secretory products of the testes, the ejaculatory ducts receive fluid from the seminal vesicles. These glands are the source of seminal fructose, which serves as the energy source for spermatozoa, as well as phosphorylcholine, ascorbic acid, and prostaglandins. About 60% of seminal fluid volume derives from the seminal vesicles. The ejaculatory ducts terminate in the prostatic urethra. There, the remaining

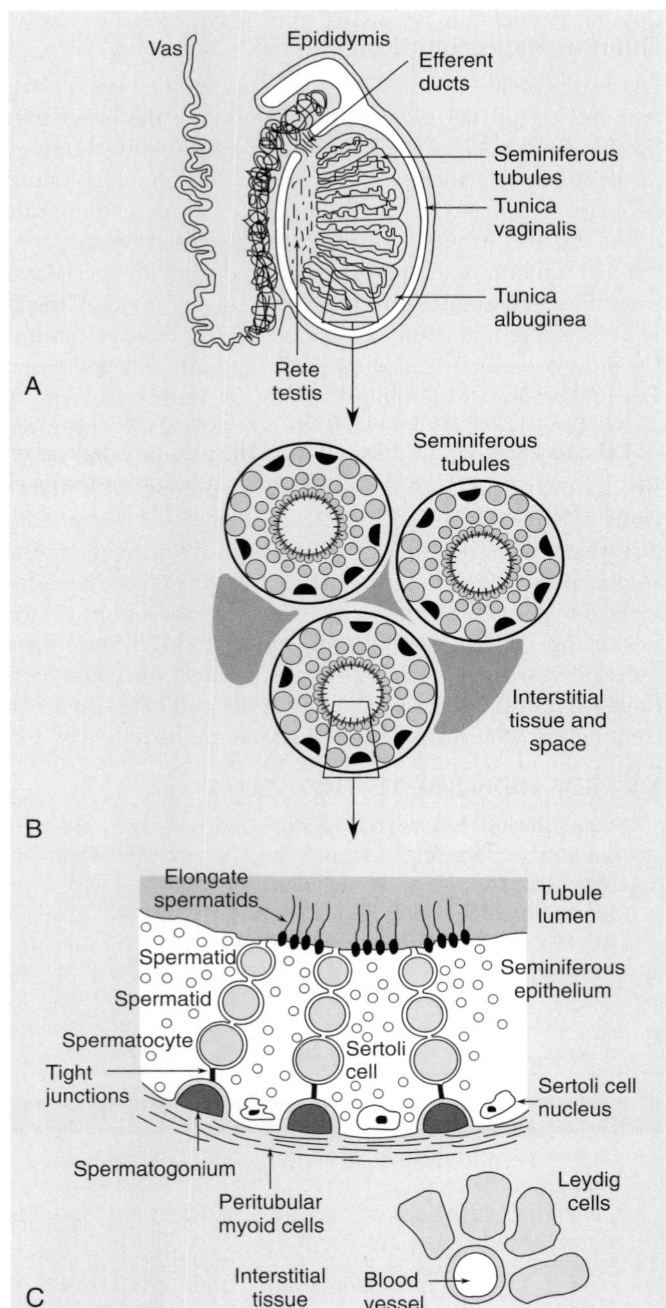

Fig. 50-6 A, Human testis, epididymis, and vas deferens showing efferent ducts leading from the rete testis to the caput epididymis and the cauda epididymis, continuing to become the vas deferens. **B,** Cross section through a seminiferous tubule showing central lumen, seminiferous epithelium, and interstitial space containing Leydig cells. **C,** Anatomical relationships in the seminiferous epithelium between germ cells (spermatogonia, spermatocytes, and spermatids), Sertoli cells, peritubular myoid cells, and Leydig cells. (From Weatherall DJ, et al: *Oxford Textbook of Medicine,* ed 3, Oxford, UK, 1996, Oxford University Press.)

20% of seminal fluid is added by the prostate gland. Constituents of prostatic fluid include spermine, citric acid, fibrinolysin, prostate-specific antigen, and acid phosphatase. Fluid is also added to the seminal plasma by the Cowper glands and by the urethral glands during its transit through the penile urethra.

The Hypothalamic-Pituitary-Testicular Axis: An Overview

As in the female, the control of gonadal function in the male begins with the pulsatile release of GnRH from the hypothalamus. GnRH then is transported via the hypothalamic-pituitary-portal system to the anterior pituitary, where it stimulates the release of LH and FSH. The relative amounts of LH and FSH that are released from the pituitary depend on the frequency of GnRH pulses and on negative-feedback signals from the testes. Optimum amounts of LH and FSH for normal testicular function are released when GnRH pulses occur at a frequency of 3.8 pulses every 6 hours. At a lower pulse rate of GnRH, FSH is released preferentially, whereas a higher pulse frequency of GnRH results in more prominent LH secretion. The major regulator of testosterone production is LH, which specifically binds to high-affinity plasma membrane receptors on the Leydig cells, stimulating testosterone synthesis and secretion. Because of the pulsatile pattern of LH release from the pituitary and its relatively short half-life (30 minutes), plasma LH concentrations normally vary widely in normal men, and a single plasma sample may not provide an accurate estimate of mean LH levels. Plasma FSH levels are more constant because FSH responses to GnRH are more delayed and of a lesser magnitude, and FSH has a significantly longer circulating half-life (4 hours) in comparison with LH. FSH released into the systemic circulation binds specifically to the Sertoli cells, where it has several effects, including increased synthesis of androgen-binding protein and the aromatase enzyme complex, which converts testosterone to estradiol, and increased production of inhibin. During puberty, FSH also stimulates Sertoli cell mitosis and promotes Sertoli cell maturation.

Secretion of LH is controlled by the negative-feedback action of gonadal steroids on the hypothalamus and pituitary. It has been shown in normal males that both testosterone and estradiol may contribute to this inhibition. This may reflect the conversion of testosterone to estradiol within the brain and pituitary, but small amounts of estradiol normally are secreted directly by the testes, and the inhibitory effects of testosterone and estradiol may be independent. Both gonadal peptides and steroid hormones are involved in the negative-feedback inhibition of FSH secretion. Testosterone can inhibit the secretion of both LH and FSH, but the glycoprotein hormone inhibin primarily inhibits the secretion of FSH. In contrast to women, who have fluctuating levels of inhibin A and B during the menstrual cycle, the major circulating form of inhibin in men is inhibin B. Inhibin B is produced by the Sertoli cells, where it may have some local actions within the testes, but its principal role is to provide feedback on the pituitary to inhibit FSH secretion. In the testes, both FSH and testosterone are necessary for normal inhibin production. The activins (dimers of the β-subunit of inhibin) stimulate pituitary FSH secretion in vitro, but their precise role in the physiological regulation of gonadotropin release has yet to be elucidated. The activins may have local actions within the testes; activin β_A- and β_B-subunits have been localized to the Sertoli cells.

Testosterone Synthesis and Secretion

The testis is the primary site of androgen production in the male, and the major circulating androgen is testosterone. As was stated earlier, all steroid hormones are derived from cholesterol (see Fig. 50-3). In the testes (as in the ovary), cholesterol may be synthesized de novo or derived from the systemic circulation by receptor-mediated uptake of LDL. The rate-limiting step in testosterone synthesis is the conversion of cholesterol to pregnenolone. LH regulates the rate of this enzymatic reaction and thus controls the overall rate of testosterone synthesis. The daily production rate of testosterone in normal adult men is approximately 6 mg, but only about 25 μg of testosterone is stored in the testes, indicating that the testes are continuously synthesizing and releasing testosterone into the circulation. A diurnal rhythm in circulating testosterone levels is seen in adult men, with highest levels in the early morning, followed by a progressive fall throughout the day, and reaching the lowest levels at night during the first few hours of sleep. Peak and nadir values may differ by about 30%, and ideally, testosterone concentrations should be measured in the morning. Although testosterone is the major hormone produced, small amounts of dihydrotestosterone, androstenedione, 17-hydroxyprogesterone, progesterone, estradiol, and pregnenolone are secreted by the testes. Testicular estradiol secretion contributes about 20% to 30% of the total circulating estradiol, the remainder being derived from peripheral, extraglandular aromatization of androgenic substrates such as androstenedione. The functions of plasma pregnenolone, progesterone, and 17-hydroxyprogesterone in the male remain unknown.

Testosterone Transport

Of the circulating testosterone in normal men, less than 4% is free (not protein bound), 1% to 2% is bound to cortisol-binding globulin, approximately 50% is loosely bound to albumin, and the remainder (about 45%) is bound with high affinity to SHBG. SHBG levels are increased by estrogens and decreased by androgens; therefore, the normal level of SHBG is about 30% to 50% lower in men than in women, and SHBG levels may be elevated in testosterone-deficient men. In many clinical situations, measurement of the total testosterone concentration (usually by immunoassay) is satisfactory. However, when circulating SHBG levels are altered, this may be reflected by an increase or decrease in the measured total testosterone level. For example, obesity is associated with decreased SHBG levels, and a low total testosterone level in an obese man may be misinterpreted as evidence of androgen deficiency. Because the non–SHBG-bound portion of circulating testosterone is thought to represent the biologically active fraction, methods for estimating the non–SHBG-bound or free testosterone level have been developed (see section on male hypogonadism).

Extraglandular Metabolism of Androgens

Testosterone mediates androgenic effects but also serves as a circulating precursor for the formation of two types of active metabolites. Testosterone can undergo irreversible reduction to generate 5α-reduced steroids, predominantly dihydrotestosterone (DHT), which is a key intracellular mediator of androgen action. The concentration of circulating DHT in adult men is approximately 10% that of testosterone; about 25% of this is secreted directly by the testes, and the remainder arises from the conversion of testosterone in tissues such as the liver, kidney, muscle, prostate, and skin. Two isoenzymes convert testosterone to DHT: 5α-reductase types 1 and 2. The type 1 isoenzyme is found in the liver and skin, and the type 2 enzyme predominates in the male urogenital tract, in which 5α-reduction is a prerequisite for normal androgen-mediated function. Only a small fraction of the DHT generated in target tissues appears in plasma; it is metabolized mainly by 3α-reduction to 5α-androstane 3β-17β-diol, which then enters plasma and is metabolized further by glucuronide conjugation and other pathways.

Most of the estrogens in the circulation of normal adult men are derived through the aromatization of testosterone to 17β-estradiol and androstenedione to estrone. Estrogen formation requires sequential hydroxylation, oxidation, and removal of the carbon at position 19, and aromatization of the A ring of the steroid. Prior 5α-reduction of the steroid A ring prevents completion of aromatization, so DHT and other 5α-reduced steroids are not aromatized. The aromatase enzyme complex is active in many tissues, including muscle, liver, and kidney, but the most significant site is probably adipose tissue. The overall rate of aromatization increases with age and adiposity. In addition to these pathways, testosterone is metabolized to inactive excretory metabolites, including 17-ketosteroids and a series of polar compounds such as diols, triols, and conjugates.

The Androgen Receptor

Cytoplasmic androgen receptors (ARs) are expressed widely in genital and nongenital tissues, and they mediate the cellular effects of testosterone and DHT. The AR binds DHT with a higher affinity than testosterone. Similar to other members of the steroid hormone receptor superfamily, the AR contains a steroid-binding domain, a DNA-binding domain, and a transcription-regulating domain. After androgen binding, the receptor dimerizes and proceeds to the nucleus to bind to DNA target sequences and to initiate or decrease transcription of androgen-responsive genes. AR is encoded by a gene that is located on the X chromosome; therefore, females can be carriers of mutant AR genes, which, when transmitted to male offspring, produce androgen insensitivity syndromes.

Numerous AR mutations in both the steroid-binding and DNA-binding domains have been described that cause complete or partial androgen insensitivity. The AR gene contains a segment of CAG repeats in exon 1 that code for glutamine. Men with spinal and bulbar muscular atrophy (Kennedy disease) have an expansion of this segment to 40 to 60 triplet repeats as compared with an average of 21 in normal men. Such men develop **gynecomastia,** clinical signs of androgen deficiency, and small testes, in association with increased LH and testosterone levels indicative of androgen insensitivity. The mutations are thought to impair activation of androgen-responsive genes.

KEY CONCEPTS BOX 50-5

- Fetal FSH and placental hCG cause production of testosterone, maintaining fetal testes.
- At male puberty, rising testosterone, FSH, and LH levels lead to mature testes and secondary male characteristics.
- A similar hypothalamic-pituitary axis controls testosterone production and secondary male characteristics. GnRH stimulates release of pituitary FSH and LH, which stimulates testosterone production from cholesterol; testosterone in turn exhorts negative-feedback control to diminish hormone production by the pituitary/hypothalamus.
- Testes convert testosterone to the active hormone, dihydrotestosterone (DHT).
- Testosterone is transported in blood to target tissues, mostly (age related, but about 35%) bound to SHBG and albumin.
- Target tissues have cytoplasmic and nuclear androgen receptors.

SECTION OBJECTIVES BOX 50-6

- List the causes of primary and secondary male hypogonadism.
- Describe the genetic cause of Klinefelter's syndrome.
- Describe several other genetic defects that cause hypogonadism.
- List causes of primary and secondary male hypergonadism.
- Define *erectile dysfunction* and discuss its cause.

PATHOLOGICAL STATES

Hypogonadism

Male hypogonadism may be defined as failure of the testes to produce testosterone, spermatozoa, or both. As in women, hypogonadism may be caused by a primary gonadal failure or by an abnormality within the hypothalamic-pituitary axis (Box 50-4; see Fig. 50-7 for clinical workup). The clinical presentation of hypogonadism in males is related directly to the time of development of androgen deficiency. Androgen deficiency during the second to third month of fetal development can cause sexual ambiguity and male **pseudohermaphroditism.** In prepubertal hypogonadism, absence of testosterone production by the testes is associated with persistent infantile genitalia, a barely palpable prostate, poor secondary sexual development, and lack of secondary sex

Box 50-4

Causes of Male Hypogonadism

Primary Hypogonadism

Genetic disorders
- Klinefelter's syndrome
- XX males
- XY/XO gonadal dysgenesis
- Ullrich-Noonan syndrome
- Myotonic dystrophy

Enzymatic defects involving testosterone synthesis
- 5α-reductase deficiency

Androgen receptor defects
- Androgen resistance (testicular feminization syndrome)
- Kennedy syndrome

Testicular damage
- Cryptorchidism
- Infection
- Testicular trauma or torsion
- Chemotherapy

Secondary Hypogonadism

Hypothalamic disorders
- Kallmann's syndrome
- Cranial irradiation
- Systemic illness

Pituitary disorders
- Prolactin-secreting pituitary tumor
- Other pituitary tumor

Hemochromatosis

Lymphocytic hypophysitis

Histiocytosis

characteristics, as well as delayed bone age and eunuchoidal skeletal proportions (crown-to-pubis/pubis-to-floor ratio is decreased, arm span is considerably greater than height). These body proportions result from a failure of epiphyseal fusion and continued growth of long bones. Prepubertal hypogonadism usually is not apparent until the time of puberty, when normal pubertal changes, including genital and secondary sexual development, fail to occur. Postpubertal hypogonadism results in more subtle clinical manifestations. Beard growth may be diminished and body hair thinned, strength and muscle mass may be decreased, libido may be lost, and the testes softened and of decreased volume. Older males may be unaware of any of these changes.

Disorders of the Testes—Primary Hypogonadism

Primary hypogonadism resulting from testicular dysfunction is characterized by low serum testosterone concentrations in conjunction with high gonadotropin levels, which reflect the absence of negative feedback on the hypothalamic-pituitary axis. Abnormal testicular function may be caused by a genetic disorder, defects in testosterone synthesis or metabolism, abnormalities in the androgen receptor, or direct gonadal damage.

The most common genetic disorder that causes primary hypogonadism in men is **Klinefelter's syndrome,** which is associated with the chromosomal pattern of 47,XXY and occurs in about 1 in 400 men. The phenotypical manifestations of Klinefelter's syndrome are characteristic for the classic form of the disorder in which all cell lines carry the XXY karyotype. Many men with this syndrome have a mosaic form, in which some cell lines are XXY and others are XY, so the clinical presentation is variable. This disorder rarely presents before puberty because the only early physical finding is of very small testes (smaller than 1.5 mL after age 6). After puberty, the other characteristic features appear, including gynecomastia, abnormalities in skeletal proportions with exaggerated growth of the lower extremities (decreased crown-to-pubis/pubis-to-floor ratio but no abnormality in arm span/height ratio), reduced androgen-dependent hair growth, central adiposity, poor muscle mass with reduced strength, and infertility. In patients with Klinefelter's syndrome, testosterone concentrations range from low to normal, but postpubertal gonadotropin levels are always elevated, even when testosterone is normal. Other genetic disorders associated with primary hypogonadism include XX males (most due to translocation of the SRY gene to the X chromosome), XY/XO gonadal dysgenesis, Ullrich-Noonan syndrome, and myotonic dystrophy.

Several different enzymes that are involved in testosterone synthesis may be defective, resulting in testosterone deficiency with or without cortisol deficiency. The enzymes that are potentially affected include 20,22-desmolase, 3β-hydroxydehydrogenase, 17α-hydroxylase, 17,20-desmolase, and 17-ketosteroid reductase. Most of these enzyme defects are associated with ambiguous genitalia at birth occurring with a normal male XY karyotype. The 5α-reductase deficiency syndrome is an autosomal recessive disorder that also occurs in males with a normal XY sex chromosome pattern. It arises from absence or instability of the 5α-reductase enzyme, which produces a defect in the conversion of testosterone to DHT. The testes function normally with respect to androgen and antimüllerian hormone production, so the müllerian structure regresses and the normal wolffian system forms, but at birth, these individuals appear to be girls with moderately ambiguous genitalia. At puberty, however, testosterone production by the testes is normal, creating an overall dramatic masculinization with development of a male body habitus and hair distribution, along with penile enlargement. However, those tissues that respond primarily to DHT, such as the scrotum, prostate, and testes, remain prepubertal.

Abnormalities in the androgen receptor have been discussed previously. Complete lack of function results in the testicular feminization syndrome, in which an XY individual has the female phenotype. Variants of this syndrome occur according to the degree of receptor defect. *Kennedy syndrome,* in which primary hypogonadism is associated with a specific muscular dystrophy, is caused by a polynucleotide repeat expansion in the AR gene. The AR sequence is normal, but an expanded polyglutamine region suppresses receptor activity.

Primary hypogonadism that manifests after puberty frequently is the result of testicular damage. Men who are infected with mumps virus during or after puberty have about a 50%

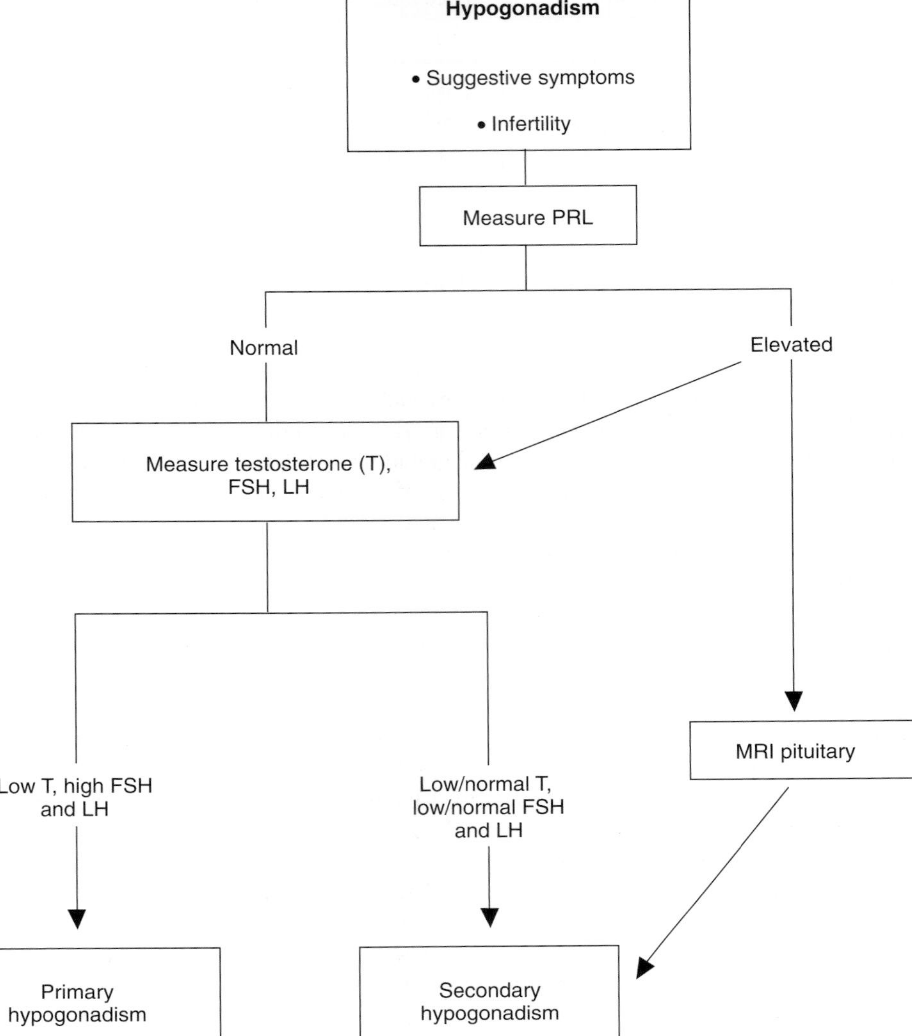

Fig. 50-7 Clinical approach to the investigation of male hypogonadism.

chance of developing orchitis, and as many as 60% of these will be infertile because of extensive seminiferous tubule damage. **Cryptorchidism** (undescended testes) usually results in failure of testicular function on the affected side, and frequently of the nonaffected side also, producing primary hypogonadism. Similarly, unilateral testicular trauma or torsion may cause complete testicular failure, although the mechanism by which the physically undamaged testis is affected is not clear. Therapeutic irradiation and chemotherapy also may damage the testes. Damage to spermatogonia is evident after only 15 rad; at doses greater than 100 rad, extreme oligospermia or azoospermia develops. The likelihood of germ cell recovery is dose dependent, and permanent failure may occur after high-dose therapy, even if the testes are shielded. The main chemotherapeutic drugs that cause infertility are the alkylating agents, such as cyclophosphamide, but other drugs, including chlorambucil, cisplatin, doxorubicin, and vinblastine, can cause germ cell depletion. The toxic effects of chemotherapeutic drugs can be additive, and some combination regimens have particularly profound effects on spermatogenesis.

Secondary Hypogonadism—Hypogonadotropic Hypogonadism

Secondary hypogonadism is characterized by low testosterone concentrations in association with gonadotropin levels that are subnormal or within the reference range, indicating failure of the pituitary to respond normally to lack of negative feedback. Hypogonadotropic hypogonadism may be caused by congenital or acquired defects. As in primary hypogonadism, the clinical presentation of the acquired disorders will depend on whether the individual has gone through puberty, and whether other anterior or posterior pituitary hormone deficiencies are present.

The classic example of congenital hypogonadotropic hypogonadism is Kallmann's syndrome, which is characterized by a defect in hypothalamic GnRH secretion. This syndrome is associated with isolated gonadotropin deficiency and anosmia or hyposmia. Other associated anomalies, such as cleft lip and palate, sensorineural deafness, and cardiac abnormalities, also have been described. *Kallmann's syndrome* is inherited most commonly in an autosomal dominant manner, but autosomal recessive and X-linked modes of inheritance have been reported. The incidence of this syndrome is about 1 in 10,000 male births. These men typically present with failure to go through puberty in association with eunuchoid skeletal proportions. Testicular development remains at prepubertal levels, although, unlike Klinefelter syndrome, the testes are of normal prepubertal size. Basal gonadotropin levels are low normal or undetectable, testosterone levels are low, and serum prolactin levels are normal. If gonadotropin deficiency is the only abnormality and other clinical features such as anosmia are absent, Kallmann's syndrome can be very difficult to distinguish from delayed puberty. Congenital gonadotropin deficiency also is associated with a number of rare genetic syndromes, such as Prader-Willi, Laurence-Moon, and Bardet-Biedl syndromes, which usually are evident in early childhood.

Gonadotropin deficiency may result from numerous acquired disorders that cause pituitary dysfunction (see Box 50-4). Pituitary tumors, granulomatous diseases that affect the pituitary, autoimmune lymphocytic hypophysitis, and hemochromatosis can directly inhibit gonadotropin secretion by damaging the gonadotropin-secreting cells. Prolactin-secreting pituitary tumors can cause hypogonadism without anatomical destruction of gonadotropes; elevated prolactin is thought to interfere with GnRH neuron function. In men, 80% of prolactinomas are macroadenomas, whereas in women, more than 80% are microadenomas. This difference may result from earlier detection in women, in whom hyperprolactinemia is associated with menstrual cycle disturbances and galactorrhea. In contrast, the symptoms of hypogonadism in adult men are often nonspecific. All men with an elevated prolactin level should undergo an MRI of the pituitary. Secondary hypogonadism also occurs in association with any severe systemic illness, in severe uremia, and after therapeutic cranial irradiation.

Testicular Hyperfunction

Testicular tumors account for only about 1% of cancer deaths in American men, but they are the second most common malignancy (after leukemia) in men aged 20 to 35 years. An increased incidence of testicular tumors occurs in men with cryptorchidism, **testicular feminization syndrome** (androgen resistance), and Klinefelter's syndrome. Tumors of the testis may originate from several cell types in the seminiferous tubules or the interstitial tissue, but most testicular neoplasms are germ cell tumors. Germ cell tumors are classified histologically as seminomas or nonseminomas, although approximately 30% of germ cell tumors contain mixed elements. They usually present as a painless scrotal mass. Biochemical markers in serum often are useful in the diagnosis of germ cell tumors and in the detection of residual or recurrent disease following treatment. Overall, about 25% to 30% of germ cell tumors produce hCG, α-fetoprotein (AFP), or both, although the presence of large amounts of hCG or AFP in the serum generally indicates a nonseminomatous tumor. Only a relatively small percentage of seminomas are secretory, whereas about 60% of nonseminomatous germ cell tumors produce significant amounts of hCG, AFP, or both. Non–germ cell tumors are rare. Only 3% of testicular tumors originate from the Leydig cells; 90% of these are benign, and they usually produce steroid hormones (testosterone or estrogen). The production of excessive amounts of androgenic hormones in adult males causes few symptoms, but an estrogen-secreting tumor may cause gynecomastia. In prepubertal boys, excessive testosterone production causes precocious puberty. Primary hypergonadism is characterized by abnormally high testosterone (or estrogen) concentrations in association with suppressed gonadotropin levels.

Secondary hypergonadism also may occur in the setting of altered hypothalamic-pituitary function that results in increased LH/FSH secretion. Premature activation of the hypothalamic-pituitary-gonadal axis produces gonadotropin-dependent precocious puberty in children. In boys, the initial symptom/sign is testicular enlargement; this is followed by further secondary sex development and accelerated linear growth. The most common cause of this disorder is a hypothalamic hamartoma. These non-neoplastic congenital malformations contain ectopic GnRH neurons, which are not subject to the normal central nervous system (CNS) regulation that inhibits activity before puberty; therefore, they may function as autonomous GnRH pulse generators and may initiate puberty. Many other CNS abnormalities can result in gonadotropin-dependent precocious puberty, probably via disruption of tonic inhibitory input to the hypothalamus; these include any space-occupying lesion in the region of the third ventricle and high-dose cranial irradiation administered for childhood tumors.

Erectile Dysfunction

Erectile dysfunction (ED) is defined as difficulty obtaining or maintaining a penile erection sufficient to permit vaginal penetration and satisfactory conclusion of sexual intercourse. Epidemiological data suggest a high prevalence of ED; in the Massachusetts Male Ageing Study, 9.6% of men aged between 40 and 70 years suffered from complete ED, and an additional 25% admitted to moderate dysfunction. Sociological change, the recognition that ED frequently stems from an organic cause, and the availability of better therapies have revolutionized the approach to this disorder. The normal erectile process depends on a complex array of autonomic and somatic nerves that innervate the penis, together with an adequate arterial blood supply. Psychogenic and relationship factors are also important components in normal sexual function. ED can be associated with many systemic diseases, such as diabetes mellitus, aortoilial atherosclerosis, hypertension, previous treatment for benign prostate hyperplasia or prostate cancer, and many neurological disorders. Numerous drugs that act on the central or autonomic nervous system have been associated with ED, including anticholinergic, antidepressant, antipsychotic, and antihypertensive drugs. Differentiating between psychogenic and organic (neurogenic or vascular) causes of ED can be difficult, particularly because the former may frequently arise from the latter. The assessment of a man with ED naturally requires a thorough history and examination. A complete blood count and routine serum chemistries will detect many of the systemic diseases associated with ED. Androgen deficiency and hyperprolactinemia must be excluded by measuring serum testosterone (preferably a morning sample), LH, FSH, and prolactin levels.

Treatment of ED depends to some extent on whether there is an underlying endocrine cause. For example, testosterone replacement therapy should be considered in androgen-deficient men, and those with hyperprolactinemia may require dopamine agonist therapy and/or pituitary surgery. Other therapies for ED are more generic, in that they may be used to treat ED regardless of the underlying cause. Sildenafil (Viagra), a selective inhibitor of cyclical guanosine monophosphate (cGMP)-specific phosphodiesterase type 5 (PDE5), enhances nitric oxide–mediated vasodilatation in the corpus cavernosum by inhibiting cGMP breakdown, thus facilitating smooth muscle relaxation. Nitric oxide release from the noradrenergic noncholinergic nerves that innervate the cavernosal smooth muscle is triggered by sexual stimuli. Therefore, sildenafil potentiates erections induced by physiological mechanisms, and, unlike intracavernosal prostaglandins, it cannot independently invoke an erection. Sildenafil is an effective therapy; clinical trials have shown that about 70% of men with ED of all causes experience significant improvement.

KEY CONCEPTS BOX 50-6

- Male hypogonadism is the failure to produce sperm and/or testosterone.
- Genetic disorders such as Klinefelter's syndrome (47XXY) are a common cause of primary hypogonadism, as are AR defects, and inherited defects of key enzymes needed for testosterone synthesis: 20,22-desmolase, 3β-hydroxydehydrogenase, 17α-hydroxylase, 17,20-desmolase, and 17-ketosteroid reductase.
- Secondary hypogonadism, with low testosterone and low FHS/LH levels, is caused by failure of the pituitary/hypothalamus to respond to low testosterone levels. This failure could be based on inherited defects (Kallmann's syndrome) or tumors.
- Testicular tumors in men 20 to 35 years old are a common cause of primary hypergonadism. These tumors often produce hCG and α-fetoprotein.
- Secondary hypergonadism results from hypothalamic/pituitary activity, usually from a tumor. Testosterone and FHS/LH all are elevated.
- Erectile dysfunction, the inability to maintain an erection, may occur secondarily to vascular problems associated with diabetes, atherosclerosis, etc.

SECTION OBJECTIVES BOX 50-7

- Define *infertility.*
- List the primary male and female causes of infertility.
- List the tests most likely to be used to investigate infertility.

CHANGE OF ANAYLYE IN DISEASE: EVALUATION OF THE INFERTILE COUPLE

Evaluation of Infertility

Infertility is defined as failure to conceive after a year of unprotected intercourse. *Cycle* **fecundability** is the probability that a single cycle will result in pregnancy (20% to 25% in healthy couples), and *fecundity* is the probability that a single cycle will result in a live birth.

The incidence of infertility has increased slightly over the past 30 years, with approximately 10% to 15% of couples in Western nations currently affected. A trend toward increased rates of infertility has been attributed to several factors, including the following:

- Later marriage
- Delayed childbearing
- Greater emphasis on female career
- Improved contraception

Most couples are not truly infertile but rather have decreased fertility. However, a longer duration of infertility and advanced patient age are predictive of a decreased likelihood of subsequently achieving a live birth. Most spontaneous pregnancies occur within 3 years of attempting conception, and success without treatment thereafter is poor. General recommendations are that all couples who seek assistance should be evaluated for infertility after 1 year of unprotected and frequent intercourse.

The causes of infertility (Fig. 50-8) should be considered before any formal evaluation of infertility is commenced, and these should be outlined for the couple.

Evaluation of the infertile couple is heavily dependent on the couple's age and medical history, and whether infertility is primary or secondary. Fig. 50-9 outlines a suggested sequence by which infertility may be evaluated.

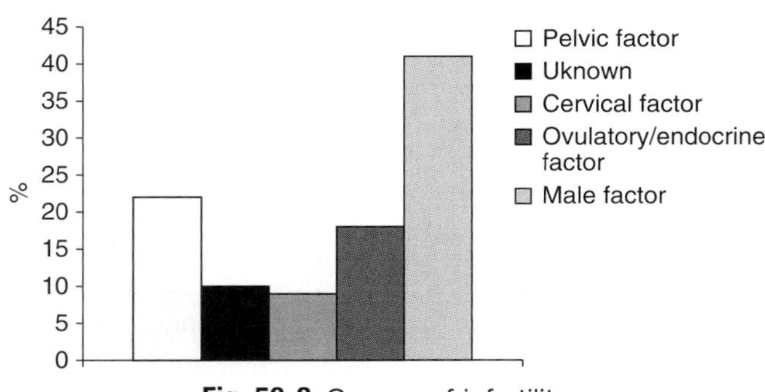

Fig. 50-8 Causes of infertility.

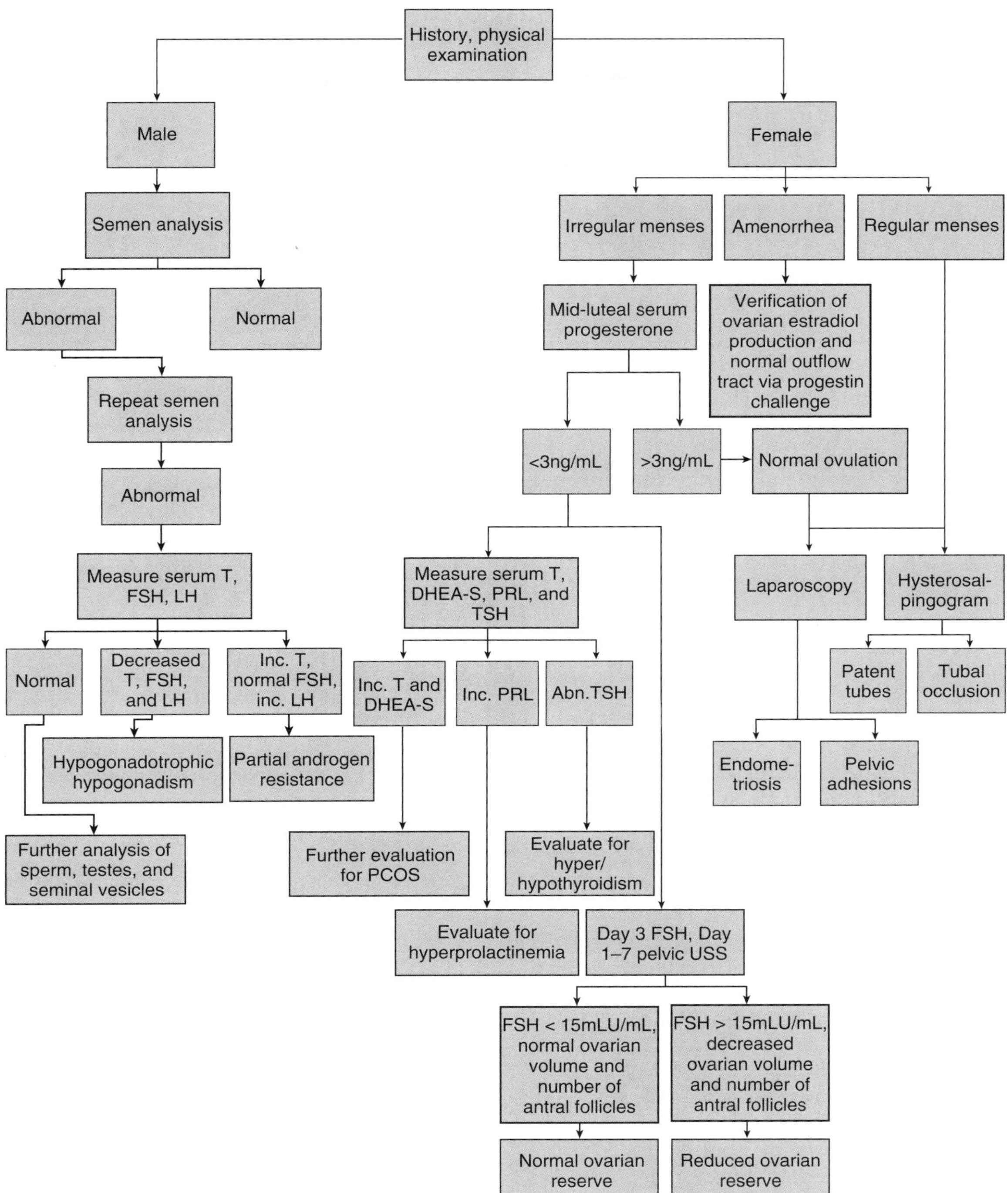

Fig. 50-9 Evaluation of the infertile couple. *DHEA-S,* Dihydroepiandrosterone sulfate; *FSH,* follicle-stimulating hormone; *LH,* luteinizing hormone; *PCOS,* polycystic ovarian syndrome; *PRL,* prolactin; *T,* testosterone; *TSH,* thyroid-stimulating hormone; *USS,* ultrasound scan.

Female Infertility

There are many potential causes of infertility in women (Box 50-5). Several of these, such as congenital abnormalities of the vagina or uterus, gonadal dysgenesis and premature ovarian failure, have already been discussed in preceding sections. The most common causes of infertility in women, however, are tubal pathology and disturbances in ovulation. Normal function of the fallopian tubes is critical to reproduction as the sperm and ovum must unite for fertilization to take place. Tubal disease (Box 50-6) may be evaluated radiologically (hysterosalpingogram) or by laparoscopy.

Disorders of ovulation, ranging from anovulation to **luteal phase deficiency,** account for about 18% of all infertility problems. The investigation and differential diagnosis of

Box 50-5

Causes of Female Infertility

Structural problems
- Tubal pathology
- Uterine abnormalities

Disorders of ovulation
- Anovulation—polycystic ovary syndrome
- Luteal phase deficiency
- Hypogonadism—primary or secondary

Functional problems
- Suboptimal cervical mucus
- Autoimmunity—antisperm antibodies

Box 50-6

Causes of Fallopian Tube Damage

Ectopic pregnancy
Endometriosis
History of pelvic inflammatory disease
Ruptured appendix
Septic abortion
Tubal surgery

amenorrhea and dysfunctional uterine bleeding has been previously discussed. Assessment of ovulation may be done by measurement of daily basal body temperature (BBT). The LH surge (and hence ovulation) typically occurs within 2-3 days of the BBT nadir, although this relationship is not always be reliable. Luteal phase deficiency or a short luteal phase results from insufficient progesterone production from the corpus luteum to support the normal endometrial maturation changes required for implantation of the embryo. Endometrial biopsy is a traditional method of evaluating luteal function but this procedure has some drawbacks in that it is relatively invasive, the biopsy must be appropriately timed within the cycle, and abnormal findings should be confirmed by successive biopsies in two consecutive cycles to make the diagnosis conclusive. Serum progesterone measurements are a more convenient method of assessing luteal function. A midluteal phase progesterone level of greater than 6.5 ng/mL (21 nmol/L), or preferably greater than 10 ng/mL (30 nmol/L), suggests ovulation and normal luteal function. However, progesterone is secreted in a pulsatile fashion, and a single value may not reflect luteal function adequately. Therefore, midluteal phase progesterone measurements may need to be repeated over several cycles.

Uterine abnormalities are rarely a factor in infertility. Intramural and submucosal tumors (myomas) may distort the uterine cavity, or obstruct the tubal lumen or endocervical canal. Infertility and pregnancy loss are thought to result from faulty implantation and compromised placental vascular supply. Uterine scarring (Asherman syndrome) may produce infertility via similar mechanisms. Suboptimal changes in the quality of cervical mucous at midcycle have also been

Box 50-7

Causes of Male Infertility

Structural problems
- Congenital absence of the vas deferens
- Infective epididymitis causing ductal damage
- Cryptorchidism

Hypogonadism
- Primary—testicular damage of any cause
- Secondary—pituitary/hypothalamic disease

Genetic—Y chromosome microdeletions

Functional problems
- Retrograde ejaculation
- Autoimmunity—antisperm antibodies

implicated in infertility. Cervical mucous is normally thick and opaque, except at midcycle when it should become thin, watery and acellular to facilitate sperm penetration. In the post-coital test, sperm motility is assessed in a sample of cervical mucous.

Male Infertility

The medical history of the male partner should focus on identifying factors that are known to impair erectile or testicular function (Box 50-7). Many chronic systemic illnesses are associated with decreased testicular function and reduced sperm production (Handelsman, 1994). Symptoms that suggest primary or secondary hypogonadism must be sought specifically. Key aspects of the physical examination include degree of virilization, any evidence of gynecomastia, and testicular size and consistency.

Any of the causes of primary or secondary hypogonadism previously discussed may present as infertility. Bilateral or unilateral cryptorchidism commonly is associated with infertility (about 70%), even if surgical removal of the undescended testes to the scrotum (orchiopexy) has been performed (Plymate, 1994). Testicular varicoceles are relatively common, with an incidence of around 10%. About 50% of men with varicoceles will have reduced semen quality, some show biochemical evidence of testicular dysfunction, and many have impaired fertility. Ejaculatory dysfunction may cause infertility. Retrograde ejaculation can occur if the sympathetic nerves that mediate closure of the bladder neck sphincter during ejaculation are dysfunctional. A post-ejaculation urine specimen will demonstrate abundant sperm. Diabetic neuropathy, prostatic resection, and extensive pelvic surgery are associated most commonly with retrograde ejaculation.

Sperm transport also can be impaired when abnormalities of the duct system, such as those associated with mutations in the gene responsible for cystic fibrosis (CF), are present. The cystic fibrosis transmembrane conductance regulator gene, located on the short arm of chromosome 7, encodes for a membrane protein that functions as an ion channel and also influences formation of the ejaculatory duct, seminal vesicle, and vas deferens, and the distal two-thirds of the epididymis. More than 400 different mutations in this gene have been described, and these are associated with a spectrum of clinical manifestations. Congenital bilateral absence of the vas deferens is common in men who have CF, but it also can occur in isolation without the other features of CF. Congenital unilateral absence of the vas deferens may be an incomplete form of the bilateral disorder. In polycystic kidney disease, dilated cysts of the seminal vesicles may cause obstruction to semen transport. In addition to mumps virus, which causes a primary orchitis, other infective agents can produce infertility. A variety of organisms, such as *Neisseria gonorrhoea, Chlamydia trachomatis, Mycobacterium tuberculosis, Ureaplasma urealyticum,* and coliform bacteria, can cause chronic epididymitis or prostatitis, which may reduce sperm count or motility directly, or may result in post-infection ductal damage.

Autoimmunity has been postulated to cause infertility. Antibodies to the basement membrane of the seminiferous tubule and, more commonly, to sperm themselves have been described. Whether such antibodies play a directly causative role in infertility remains unclear because upon semen analysis, the presence of anti-sperm antibodies does not correlate with specific abnormalities. Furthermore, not all men who are antibody positive are infertile, and a decrease in antibody titer is not always associated with improved fertility. As was previously discussed, treatment with chemotherapeutic drugs or radiation may lead to infertility.

Not all cases of male infertility can be explained by the above conditions, and up to 40% of cases have been classified previously as idiopathic infertility. However, sequencing of the human genome has led to a new understanding of the genes that regulate spermatogenesis, and many instances of so-called idiopathic infertility may be caused by previously unidentified, subtle genetic defects. Several genes located on the long arm of the Y chromosome that are involved in spermatogenesis have been described. In men with major defects in spermatogenesis and apparently normal chromosome analysis, microdeletions involving genes on the long arm of the Y chromosome have been demonstrated (Hargreaves, 2000). The presence of microdeletions in the Y chromosome has clinical implications if the technique of intracytoplasmic sperm injection (ICSI) is going to be used, because the genetic defect will be transmitted to any male offspring. Testing for Y chromosome microdeletions is undertaken in in vitro fertilization (IVF)/ICSI units, but currently available screening methods that use specific gene probes will not identify all men with microdeletions.

Semen analysis is a critical part of the evaluation of an infertile man. Semen quality is assessed according to sperm count, motility, morphology, and semen volume. Each of these parameters is scored as having good, poor, or equivocal probability of fertility to provide an overall analysis, because no single semen characteristic (except azoospermia) has an absolute correlation with infertility. A total sperm count of <20 million/mL, motility <40%, normal oval morphology <40%, and semen volume <1.0 mL all are associated with impaired fertility. At least three samples collected over a 2- to 4-month period should be analyzed, because semen characteristics can vary considerably in normal men, making interpretation of a single sample difficult. Functional assays, such as the sperm penetration assay, which uses hamster ova to assess the fertilizing capacity of sperm, are laborious and are used only occasionally.

Testicular function also is assessed by measuring serum testosterone, LH, and FSH levels. Four different patterns may be observed in infertile men: (1) frequently, normal values for all three hormones; (2) elevated serum gonadotropins and a low testosterone level, suggesting severe primary testicular failure; (3) elevated FSH, normal LH, and low/normal testosterone, implying a milder form of primary hypogonadism; and (4) low/normal serum gonadotropins and low testosterone levels, indicating secondary hypogonadism. Prolactin levels should be measured in any patient with biochemical evidence of secondary hypogonadism. A biochemical profile consistent with primary hypogonadism in conjunction with any clinical features suggestive of Klinefelter's syndrome should prompt a karyotype assessment. Differentiating between primary and secondary gonadal failure is important because spermatogenesis sometimes can be restored in the secondary syndromes by gonadotropin or GnRH treatment. A testicular biopsy can provide direct information about the degree of spermatogenesis in the region sampled. This procedure is not commonly indicated but may be useful in demonstrating obstructive azoospermia and in enabling sperm retrieval for ICSI.

Testosterone

Measurement of serum testosterone is usually the single most important diagnostic test for investigation of male hypogonadism, because a low value usually is diagnostic. Testosterone within the circulation is bound principally to proteins, the most significant of which is sex hormone–binding globulin (SHBG). Bioavailable testosterone consists of the total of free testosterone (<4%-10% of total testosterone) and that bound weakly to albumin. Only about 35% of total serum testosterone is bioavailable and is able to enter cells and bind to androgen receptors. It is well known that androgen levels decline in men as they age, and as a result of the increase in binding capacity for testosterone in serum, an early and more dramatic decline in free testosterone than in total testosterone concentration is noted. Measurement of free testosterone provides the most accurate reflection of availability or deficiency of physiologically active testosterone; therefore, it now is widely recommended that this be measured in preference or in addition to a total testosterone level (see testosterone method in Evolve).

Infertility Treatment

Ovulation Induction

Clomiphene citrate is the first-line treatment for women with absent or infrequent ovulation and dysfunctional uterine bleeding (oligomenorrhea). Documentation of anovulation via basal body temperature readings is not essential before treatment is provided, but thyroid dysfunction and an elevated serum prolactin level (or pregnancy if there has been no recent menstrual flow) must be excluded; if these are present, specific treatment for an underlying disorder may be indicated. In women with amenorrhea, particularly those who fail to have a withdrawal bleed following the administration of progesterone, estradiol deficiency secondary to hypogonadism (either primary or secondary) must be suspected, and serum estradiol, LH, and FSH levels must be measured. Estradiol-deficient women rarely ovulate in response to clomiphene, and usually, other treatment modalities are pursued at the outset. Ideally, a semen analysis should be performed to exclude azoospermia before any ovulation induction therapy is given.

Clomiphene is an orally active, nonsteroidal agent that has a similar structure to estrogenic compounds but has only a weak biological estrogenic effect. Its structural similarity is sufficient for it to be bound to estrogen receptors, where it remains bound for much longer periods than endogenous estrogens (weeks vs. hours) and acts to inhibit the process of receptor replacement, thereby reducing the number of estrogen receptors on cell membranes. Centrally, this results in lowering of estrogen-related negative feedback on the hypothalamic-pituitary axis, which responds by increasing GnRH, LH, and FSH secretion. Thus, clomiphene does not directly stimulate ovulation but acts to enhance the normal gonadotropin-dependent events that bring it about. Clomiphene treatment therefore is commenced on day 5 of a menstrual cycle, after spontaneous or induced bleeding, and it continues through days 5 to 9, amplifying the normal rise in gonadotropins at a time when the dominant follicle is being selected. If given earlier, multiple follicles may undergo maturation, increasing the risk of multiple pregnancy. Clomiphene may be administered purposely in IVF programs so as to produce more than one oocyte per cycle for collection. In the initial cycle, the dose used is 50 mg/day, but if no ovulation occurs, the dose may be increased to 100 mg or even higher in subsequent cycles, if the woman continues to be anovulatory. The ovulatory surge can occur from 5 to 10 days after the last day of clomiphene administration. The couple is advised to have intercourse every second day for 1 week, beginning 5 days after the last day of medication. About 50% of patients achieve pregnancy with the 50 mg dose and another 20% with the 100 mg dose.

Human menopausal gonadotropin (hMG; a mixture of FSH and LH), used in conjunction with hCG, can stimulate ovulation in anovulatory patients who have potentially functioning ovarian tissue. This treatment usually is used only after maximum doses of clomiphene have failed, because it is expensive, requires careful monitoring, and is associated with the potentially dangerous ovarian hyperstimulation syndrome. Typically, follicular stimulation is achieved within 7 to 14 days of beginning continuous hMG, which is given as a single daily intramuscular injection. Usually, the higher-dose hMG preparation (containing 150 IU of FSH and LH) is used initially, unless the patient has PCOS, in which case the lower hMG dose is used (75 IU of each gonadotropin) because these patients are more responsive than others. Serial estradiol measurements are used to determine the optimum time for administering the ovulatory dose of hCG. Timing of the sample for estradiol measurement in relation to the preceding injection of hMG also must be taken into account. If hMG was administered at between 1700 and 2000 hours on the previous night, and the sample was collected early the following morning, then an estradiol level of 1000 to 1500 pg/mL (3700 to 5500 pmol/L) is optimum. Higher levels indicate a significant risk of ovarian hyperstimulation. Transvaginal ultrasound also may be performed to assess follicular growth and development. Administration of 10,000 IU of hCG (which is structurally and biologically similar to LH) as a single intramuscular injection stimulates ovulation. The couple is instructed to have intercourse on the day of hCG injection and daily for the next 2 days. On occasion, GnRH may be given (0.5 mg subcutaneously for 2 weeks) before a cycle of hMG is administered, so as to suppress endogenous pituitary gonadotropin secretion if disturbed hypothalamic-pituitary-ovarian function is thought to be interfering with successful ovulation induction. In this instance, the aim is to produce a hypogonadal state with estradiol levels <25 pg/mL (90 pmol/L) before hMG is given. Technological advances have resulted in the availability of many different gonadotropin preparations that contain varying proportions of FSH and LH or purified/recombinant FSH alone. The issue of whether hMG or recombinant FSH produces better ovulation/conception rates, or whether timely LH administration (when FSH is used alone) will improve outcome, has yet to be resolved.

Pulsatile GnRH administration is the most physiological means of ovulation induction and is particularly effective in women with hypothalamic amenorrhea, for example, women with Kallmann's syndrome. The advantages of GnRH treatment are that the normal feedback mechanisms that control endogenous gonadotropin secretion are maintained, thus minimizing the amount of biochemical monitoring required and undoubtedly contributing to the low incidence of ovarian hyperstimulation and multiple births caused by this therapy. The major drawback is that it must be given in repeated subcutaneous or intravenous injections via a programmable portable pump for a period of about 3 weeks.

Assisted Reproduction

Assisted reproductive technology (ART) refers to all techniques that involve direct retrieval of oocytes from the ovary. A complete evaluation of both partners is mandatory before any ART therapy is initiated. The most common procedure is **in vitro fertilization (IVF),** but many other techniques are currently available; some are listed below. These procedures can overcome many of the barriers to fertility but at the expense of imposing invasive, costly, and time-consuming protocols. In virtually all cases, ovulation induction protocols as described earlier are used to increase the number of oocytes available for collection within a cycle.

IVF—In vitro fertilization: extraction of oocytes, fertilization in the laboratory, transcervical transfer of embryos into the uterus.

GIFT—Gamete intrafallopian tube transfer: placement of oocytes and sperm into the fallopian tube.

ZIFT—Zygote intrafallopian transfer: placement of fertilized oocytes into the fallopian tube.

ICSI—Intracytoplasmic sperm injection (of a single spermatozoon).

KEY CONCEPTS BOX 50-6

- Infertility is the failure of a couple to produce a conception after 1 year of unrestricted intercourse.
- The cause of infertility can be equally ascribed to male and female factors.
- Common female factors include pelvic disease (blocked tubules), cervical disorders, and ovulatory/endocrine factors.
- Male-based infertility may be caused by physical illness that prevents effective intercourse, reduced or ineffective sperm, and any of the causes of secondary hypogonadism.
- Both males and females require physical examination to rule out physical causes (blocked fallopian tubes, unformed testes), and a complete investigation of the semen and sperm is required.
- For endocrine disorders to be ruled out as the cause of infertility, testosterone, FH, LH, prolactin, and DHEA-S may have to be measured in both males and females.

BIBLIOGRAPHY

Agrawal R, Holmes J, Jacobs HS: Follicle-stimulating hormone or human menopausal gonadotropin for ovarian stimulation in *in vitro* fertilization cycles: a mate-analysis, Fertil Steril 73:338, 2000.

Bhagavath B, Podolsky RH, Ozata M, et al: Clinical and molecular characterization of a large sample of patients with hypogonadotropic hypogonadism, Fertil Steril 85:706, 2006.

Braun M, Wassmer G, Klotz T, et al: Epidemiology of erectile dysfunction: results of the "Cologne Male Survey," Int J Impot Res 12:305, 2000.

Burger H: The endocrinology of the menopause, J Steroid Biochem Mol Biol 69:31, 1999.

Cosman F, Lindsay R: Selective estrogen receptor modulators: clinical spectrum, Endo Rev 20:418, 1999.

De Kretser DM, Meinhardt A, Meehan T, et al: The roles of inhibin and related peptides in gonadal function, Mol Cell Endocrinol 161:43, 2000.

Filicori M, Cognigni GE: Roles and novel regimens of luteinizing hormone and follicle-stimulating hormone in ovulation induction, J Clin Endocrinol Metab 86:1437, 2001.

Greendale GA, Lee NP, Arriola ER: The menopause, Lancet 353:571, 1999.

Grover SA, Lowensteyn I, Kaouache M, et al: The prevalence of erectile dysfunction in the primary care setting: importance of risk factors for diabetes and vascular disease, Arch Intern Med 166:213, 2006.

Handelsman DJ: Testicular dysfunction in systemic disease, Endocrinol Metab Clin North Am 23:839, 1994.

Hargreaves TB: Genetic basis of male infertility, Brit Med Bull 56:650,2000.

Hayes FJH, Seminara SB, Crowley WF: Hypogonadotropic hypogonadism, Endocrinol Metab Clin North Am 27:739, 1998.

Holmes S: Treatment of erectile dysfunction, Brit Med Bull 56:798, 2000.

Kalantaridou SN, Davis SR, Nelson LM: Premature ovarian failure, Endocrinol Metab Clin North Am 27:989, 1998.

Lue TF: Erectile dysfunction, N Engl J Med 342:1802, 2000.

Ory SJ, Barrionuevo MJ: The differential diagnosis of female infertility. In Becker KL, editor: *Principles and Practice of Endocrinology and Metabolism,* ed 3, Philadelphia, 2001, Lippincott Williams & Wilkins.

Pezzani I, Reis FM, Di Leonardo C, et al: Influence of non-gonadotrophic hormones on gonadal function, Mol Cell Endocrinol 161:37, 2000.

Plymate S: Hypogonadism, Endocrinol Metab Clin North Am 23:749, 1994.

Riggs BL, Hartmann LC: Selective estrogen-receptor modulators—mechanisms of action and application to clinical practice, N Engl J Med 348:618, 2003.

Shang Y, Brown M: Molecular determinants for the tissue specificity of SERMs, Science 295:2465, 2002.

Snyder PJ: Clinical features and diagnosis of male hypogonadism, Up to Date, online; Version 15.3.

Speroff L, Fritz MA: *Clinical Gynecologic Endocrinology and Fertility,* ed 7, Baltimore, 2005, Lippincott Williams & Wilkins.

The Royal College of Pathologists: Australia Manual, Version 4.0, 12 March 2004.

INTERNET SITES

http://www.menopause.org/

http://www.nlm.nih.gov/medlineplus/ency/article/000369.htm

http://emedicine.medscape.com/article/1072031-overview—Hirsutism, active 041108

http://video.nationalgeographic.com/video/player/science/health-human-body-sci/human-body/ivf.html

http://www.advancedfertility.com/amenor.htm

http://www.pcosupport.org/—Polycystic Ovarian Syndrome Association

http://www.wdxcyber.com/dxinf001.htm

http://www.inciid.org/

www.fertilityuk.org

http://womenshealth.gov/faq/infertility.htm

http://www.nichd.nih.gov/health/topics/infertility_fertility.cfm

http://kidney.niddk.nih.gov/kudiseases/pubs/impotence/index.htm

http://emedicine.medscape.com/article/444220-overview—Erectile Dysfunction, by Brosman SA

http://www.pms.org.uk/—Premenstrual syndrome

www.ksa-uk.co.uk—Klinefelter's Syndrome Association, UK

http://emedicine.medscape.com/article/922038-overview—Hypogonadism, by Kemp S

Adrenal Hormones and Hypertension

51

Chapter

Morris R. Pudek and Dailin Li

Chapter Outline

Key Terms

ACTH stimulation test An initial screening test used in the assessment of adrenal insufficiency. Also called *short ACTH* or *rapid ACTH* stimulation test.

Addison's disease Primary adrenal insufficiency, most commonly the result of an autoimmune adrenalitis.

adrenal cortex The outer portion of the adrenal gland, which produces various steroid hormones.

adrenal medulla The inner portion of both adrenal glands, which produces catecholamines.

adrenocorticosteroids Term refers to all steroids secreted by the adrenal cortex.

adrenocorticotropic hormone (ACTH) A polypeptide hormone secreted by the anterior pituitary gland, which primarily stimulates the synthesis and release of glucocorticoids from the adrenal cortex.

adrenoleukodystrophy An inherited X-linked disorder in the metabolism of very long chain fatty acids that can lead to severe neurological problems and primary adrenal insufficiency.

autonomous In the context of endocrinology, refers to a gland that does not respond to normal regulatory feedback control mechanisms.

captopril suppression test A test that is useful in the investigation of Conn's syndrome. Captopril is an angiotensin-converting enzyme inhibitor that blocks the formation of angiotensin II, which normally results in a fall in aldosterone.

catecholamines Epinephrine and norepinephrine, which are produced in the adrenal medulla and function to regulate blood glucose levels and to maintain blood pressure.

chromaffin cells Cells found in the adrenal medulla and in other sites throughout the body that produce catecholamines.

clonidine suppression test A function test used in the diagnosis of pheochromocytoma.

congenital adrenal hyperplasia (CAH) Also known as adrenogenital syndrome. A group of hereditary diseases that result from enzyme deficiencies in the steroid hormone production pathways.

Conn's syndrome Another name used to denote primary hyperaldosteronism.

corticosteroid-binding globulin Also known as transcortin. A protein that binds and transports the majority of cortisol in the circulation.

corticotropin-releasing hormone (CRH) A hypothalamic polypeptide that stimulates pituitary ACTH secretion.

Cushing's disease A form of Cushing's syndrome specifically attributable to an ACTH-secreting pituitary adenoma.

Cushing's syndrome A range of specific symptoms that result from the elevation of blood glucocorticoid levels from primary or secondary causes.

dexamethasone suppression test A function test that is used in the diagnosis and differentiation of various causes of Cushing's syndrome.

glucocorticoids A group of steroid hormones secreted by the adrenal cortex that have multiple physiological effects, including regulation of carbohydrate metabolism. Cortisol is the major glucocorticoid in humans.

hyperaldosteronism Increased secretion of aldosterone from the adrenal cortex caused by elevated blood renin levels or autonomous adrenocortical secretion (Conn's syndrome).

hypoadrenalism Adrenal insufficiency resulting in decreased output of steroid hormones from the adrenal cortex.

incidentalomas Tumors found by coincidence *(incidental)* and not associted with overt disease; prevalence increases with age.

mineralocorticoids Steroid hormones secreted by the adrenal cortex that stimulate the resorption of sodium and the excretion of potassium in the distal tubules of the kidneys. Aldosterone is the major mineralocorticoid in humans.

pheochromocytoma A tumor of the chromaffin cells, usually located in the adrenal medulla, that results in hypersecretion of epinephrine and norepinephrine.

primary hypertension, also called **essential hypertension** It is an elevated systemic arterial pressure for which no cause can be found; it often is the only significant clinical finding.

renin-angiotensin system This system is responsible for the regulation of aldosterone secretion from the adrenal cortex.

secondary hypertension Elevated blood pressure associated with several primary diseases, such as renal, endocrine, and vascular diseases.

zona fasciculata The middle portion of the adrenal cortex in which glucocorticoids and various sex hormones are produced.

zona glomerulosa The outer portion of the adrenal cortex in which the mineralocorticoids are produced.

zona reticularis The innermost portion of the adrenal cortex, next to the adrenal medulla, that acts in concert with the zona fasciculata.

Methods on Evolve

Adrenocorticotropic Hormone (ACTH)
Aldosterone
Angiotensin Converting Enzyme (ACE)
Catecholamines (plasma)
Catecholamines (urine)
Cortisol
Dehydroepiandrosterone and its sulfate
Homovanillic acid
Metanephrines
Renin
Sodium and Potassium
Vanillylmandelic acid

PART 1: The Adrenal Hormones

ANATOMY

The adrenal glands are situated at the upper pole of each kidney (Fig. 51-1). In the adult, the adrenal cortex, which constitutes 90% of the gland volume, is made up of three distinct layers. The outer layer is called the **zona glomerulosa.** The wide middle layer and the inner layer are called the **zona fasciculata** and the **zona reticularis,** respectively. These three layers secrete steroid hormones that may have **mineralocorticoid, glucocorticoid,** or androgen functions. The gland is highly vascular with a complex venous circulation that is believed to play a role in regulating steroid hormone synthesis.

The **adrenal medulla** consists of sheets of irregular cells with small nuclei called **chromaffin cells.** These cells synthesize and secrete the **catecholamines.**

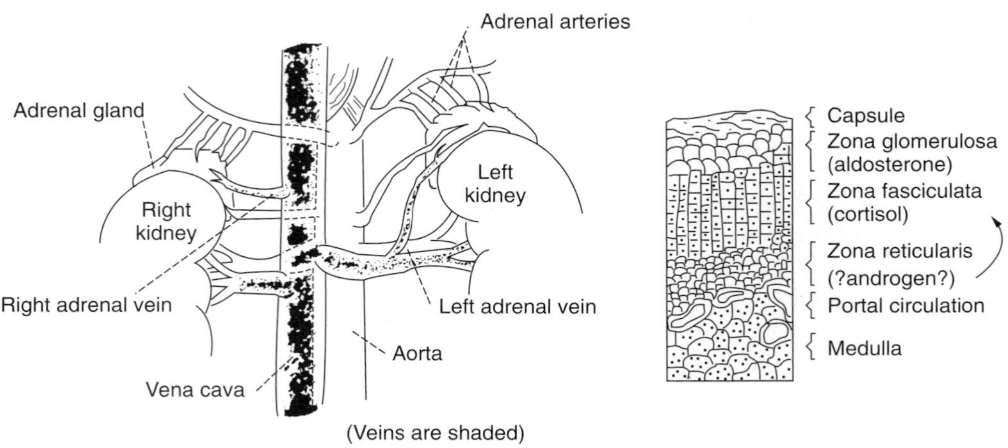

Fig. 51-1 Adrenal gland anatomy and histology. (From Ryan W: *Endocrine Disorders,* St. Louis, 1980, Mosby.)

SECTION OBJECTIVES BOX 51-1

- List the three layers of the adrenal cortex and major hormone classes produced by each layer.
- Explain specific physiological effects of glucocorticoids (especially cortisol) on the intermediary metabolism of glucose and lipids, protein metabolism, blood pressure, the immunological and inflammatory response, red and white cell production and movement, bone metabolism, growth, the gonads, central nervous system, and the thyroid gland.
- Discuss the specific physiological effects of mineralocorticoids (especially aldosterone) on the distal convoluted tubes and collecting ducts of the kidney to regulate sodium and potassium concentrations in the blood and in the regulation of extracellular fluid volume.
- Discuss the specific physiological effects of adrenal androgens (especially DHEA and DHEA-S).
- Discuss the specific physiological effects of norepinephrine and epinephrine from the adrenal medulla.

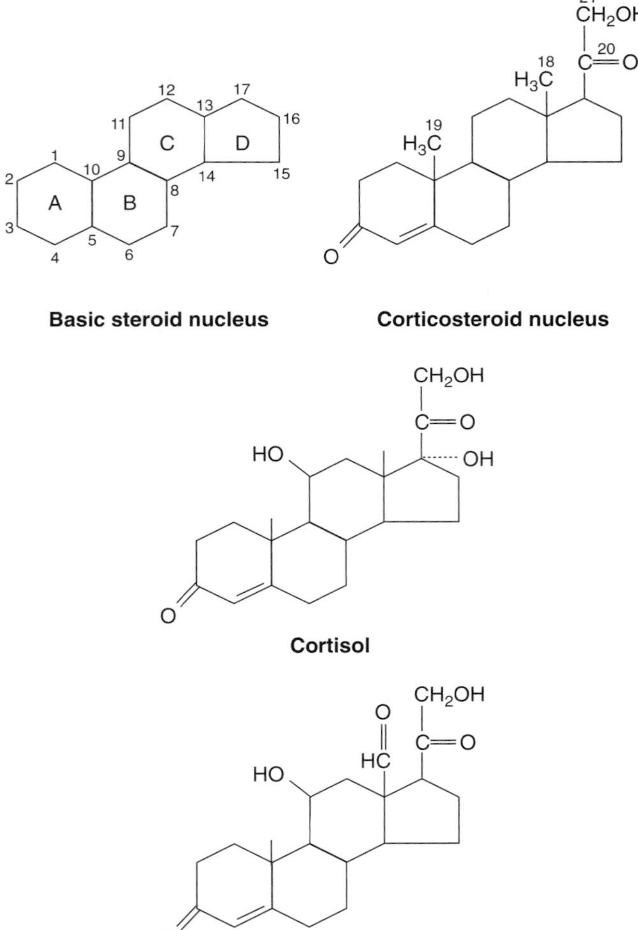

Fig. 51-2 Structures of adrenocortical hormones.

PHYSIOLOGY

All adrenal steroids secreted by the **adrenal cortex (adrenocorticosteroids)** have the same basic cyclopentanoperhydrophenanthrene nucleus consisting of three six-carbon hexane rings and one five-carbon ring. The numbering of the carbon atoms is indicated in Fig. 51-2. The steroid molecules with 21 carbon atoms and a hydroxyl group at the carbon-17 position are termed *17-hydroxysteroids.* The steroid structures with 19 carbon atoms and a ketone group at C-17 are termed *ketosteroids.*

Three major functional groups of steroids are secreted by the adrenal cortex. These consist of the mineralocorticoids secreted by the zona glomerulosa and the glucocorticoids and androgens secreted by the zona reticularis and zona fasciculata. Relatively minor differences in chemical structure result in major differences in the physiological functions of these steroid molecules.

The adrenal medulla secretes the catecholamines. These molecules are not related in structure to the adrenal steroids and have very different physiological functions.

Box 51-1

Physiological Functions of Cortisol

Effects on Intermediary Metabolism
Increases gluconeogenesis
Increases hepatic glycogen synthesis
Increases lipolysis
Increases blood glucose levels
Decreases glucose utilization

Effects on Protein Metabolism
Increases protein catabolism
Decreases protein synthesis

Effects on Blood Pressure
Increases urine flow by increasing glomerular filtration rate (GFR)
At high concentrations acts like aldosterone
Increases synthesis of angiotensinogen
Increases reactivity to vasoconstrictors
Enhances conversion of norepinephrine to epinephrine in adrenal medulla
Modulates effects of kinins and prostaglandins
Promotes movement of sodium out of cells
High concentrations inhibit antidiuretic hormone (ADH) release

Effects on Immunological and Inflammatory Responses
Decreases antibody formation
Decreases circulating lymphocytes, eosinophils, and monocytes
Decreases production and inhibits actions of interleukins and interferons
Stabilizes lysosomes
Inhibits leukocyte migration
Inhibits phagocytosis

Miscellaneous
Bone: Inhibits bone formation, increases resorption, enhances PTH action, and decreases GI calcium absorption
Growth: Decreases growth by inhibiting release of growth hormone and somatomedin C (IGF-I)
Gonads: Inhibits response of pituitary to GnRH, decreasing release of gonadotropins and gonadal steroids
Central nervous system: Chronic high cortisol levels associated with irritability, depression, psychosis, loss of memory and concentration, and decreased libido. Chronic low levels associated with apathy, depression, and decreased appetite.
Thyroid: Increased cortisol inhibits TSH release

GI, Gastrointestinal; *GnRH,* gonadotropin-releasing hormone; *IGF-I,* insulin-like growth factor-I; *PTH,* parathyroid hormone; *TSH,* thyroid-stimulating hormone.

Glucocorticoids

The glucocorticoids (primarily cortisol in humans) are synthesized and secreted by the zona fasciculata and the zona reticularis. These steroid molecules are involved in the regulation of carbohydrate, protein, and lipid metabolism. Cortisol at high concentrations also demonstrates mineralocorticoid activity. Some of the more important physiological effects of the glucocorticoids are summarized in Box 51-1. These hormones are essential for life, especially when the human body is subjected to stress such as surgery, major illness, or severe trauma. Cortisol concentrations increase greatly during these stresses, with the output of cortisol from the adrenal glands increasing from 10 to 30 mg/day in the nonstressed state to as high as 300 mg/day. Stress induces the release of numerous mediator substances such as catecholamines and kinins that can affect cardiovascular function and, if unchecked, can lead to cardiovascular collapse. The glucocorticoids block production and action of such mediator substances and prevent them from becoming life threatening.

Intermediary Metabolism

The overall metabolic action of glucocorticoids is catabolic, promoting protein and lipid breakdown and inhibiting protein synthesis in muscle, connective tissue, adipose tissue, and lymphoid cells. Wound healing is inhibited, and osteoporosis is promoted. Glucocorticoids, however, have an anabolic effect on liver metabolism. The effects of cortisol are antagonistic to those of insulin, increasing the concentration of glucose by stimulating gluconeogenesis. Amino acids and glycerol released through the catabolic action of cortisol on protein and fat are used as gluconeogenic substrates in the liver. Cortisol increases the synthesis and activity of numerous enzymes in the liver that are involved in amino acid and glucose metabolism. Cortisol decreases glucose utilization by muscle and promotes lipolysis in adipose tissue. Paradoxically, central fat stores are increased in states of cortisol excess. The net effects are increased production and conservation of glucose for use by essential tissues such as the brain and red blood cells, at the expense of "less essential" tissues, during times of stress or starvation.

Blood Pressure

Cortisol also contributes to the maintenance of normal blood pressure through several mechanisms. Cortisol increases free water clearance by stimulating the glomerular filtration rate (GFR) and decreasing water reabsorption. At high concentrations, however, cortisol can act like a mineralocorticoid, promoting sodium and water retention and causing hypokalemia. Cortisol interacts avidly with the mineralocorticoid receptor. In fact, free serum cortisol levels are 150-fold higher than free serum aldosterone levels; therefore the mineralocorticoid receptor is saturated by cortisol in most tissues except the kidney. Renal cells rapidly convert cortisol to cortisone, allowing aldosterone to be the predominant regulator of renal sodium reabsorption and potassium excretion. Also, in high concentrations, cortisol may make additional contributions to maintenance of blood pressure homeostasis. These include increasing angiotensinogen (renin substrate) synthesis by the liver; increasing vascular reactivity to vasoconstrictors; maintaining activity of the enzyme responsible for converting norepinephrine to epinephrine in the adrenal medulla, which can affect cardiac output; decreasing the activity of the vasodilatory kinin and prostaglandin systems; and promoting movement of sodium from the cellular compartment to the vascular compartment, leading to extracellular fluid volume expansion.

Immune Function

The hematological effects of cortisol are multiple and include stimulating erythropoiesis and causing leukocytosis by decreasing the movement of polymorphonucleocytes out of the vascular compartment; this results in neutrophilia, lymphocytopenia, monocytopenia, and eosinopenia. Glucocorticoids also suppress the inflammatory and immune responses by stabilizing lysosomes, thereby interfering with leukocyte migration, and inhibiting phagocytosis. Some glucocorticoid action is mediated by its effects on the production and action of mediators such as the interleukins and interferons.

Miscellaneous Functions

Cortisol has a number of miscellaneous physiological effects, many of which are seen at high serum concentrations. These are listed in Box 51-1. The molecular basis for steroid hormone actions is described in Chapter 48.

Mineralocorticoids

Aldosterone is the primary product of the zona glomerulosa, with approximately 200 μg produced per day, roughly 1/100th the amount of cortisol synthesized daily. The major physiological functions of aldosterone include (1) regulation of extracellular fluid volume, and (2) regulation of potassium metabolism. Its actions are mediated through a high-affinity mineralocorticoid receptor found in a variety of tissues. Its most important action is observed in the cells of the renal distal convoluted tubule and the cortical collecting duct, where it promotes sodium reabsorption in exchange for excretion of potassium. Sodium diffuses passively through sodium channels within the apical membranes of the epithelial cells. Aldosterone action increases the number of open sodium channels via methylation of the channels' proteins and promotes synthesis of the channels. Aldosterone also increases potassium conductance through specific channels and enhances the synthesis of sodium-potassium adenosine triphosphatase (ATPase) in the basolateral membranes that generate the electrochemical gradient to drive sodium diffusion across the cell membrane. Water passively follows transported sodium through the membranes (see Chapter 28 and Chapter 30).

The mineralocorticoid receptor is activated by both cortisol and aldosterone. Although the blood concentration of cortisol is 100-fold higher than that of aldosterone, aldosterone is the primary mineralocorticoid because of the presence of 11β-hydroxysteroid dehydrogenase (11β-HSD). 11β-HSD is a microsomal dehydrogenase/reductase that catalyzes the interconversion of biologically active cortisol with its mineralocorticoid inactive form, cortisone. Two tissue specific isoforms of 11β-HDS have been identified: type 1 (11β-HSD1) and type 2 (11β-HSD2), which are coded by different genes. Kidney cells express high concentrations of 11β-HSD2, which rapidly converts cortisol to cortisone, thus inactivating its mineralocorticoid activity. Colon, sweat glands, salivary glands, and placenta also express 11β-HSD2. The mineralocorticoid activity of cortisol and other corticosteroids, such as corticosterone and deoxycorticosterone, can become clinically significant when serum levels of these compounds become elevated, as can be seen in **Cushing's syndrome.** Excess cortisol saturates the inhibiting enzyme 11β-HSD2 in kidney cells, thereby preventing conversion to its inactive form and allowing its mineralocorticoid activity to be expressed. Licorice ingestion or tobacco chewing also inhibits the enzyme and produces clinical manifestations of apparent mineralocorticoid excess. By contrast, in glucocorticoid receptor–expressing tissues, such as liver, adipose tissue, placenta, skin, and eye, 11β-HSD1 converts inactive cortisone to cortisol, thus promoting glucocorticoid receptor hormone action. The liver has the highest concentration of 11β-HSD1. The kidney inactivates cortisol to cortisone, and the liver reactivates cortisone to cortisol, thereby completing the "cortisol-cortisone shunt." Aldosterone has weak glucocorticoid activity, but its concentration is too low to have any physiological effect.

Adrenal Androgens

The predominant androgens secreted by the adrenal cortex include dehydroepiandrosterone sulfate (DHEA-S), dehydroepiandrosterone (DHEA), and androstenedione. Small amounts of testosterone (T) and dihydrotestosterone (DHT) also are secreted. The average daily production rate of DHEA-S is approximately 30 mg in young men and 20 mg in young women. The half-life of DHEA-S is between 8 and 11 hours, whereas it is only 30 to 60 minutes for the unconjugated androgens. Adrenal androgen production reaches a peak at between 20 and 30 years of age and then gradually falls with age to about 20% of peak levels after 70 years. This contrasts with cortisol production, which does not change with age. DHEA-S is also the principal steroid of the fetal adrenal, but serum levels of DHEA-S fall rapidly after birth and then slowly rise in mid-childhood as the zona reticularis matures (adrenarche). At their peak, that is, at ages 20 to 30 years, circulating levels of DHEA-S are 20 times higher than those of cortisol because of increased secretion rates and decreased metabolic clearance. DHEA and DHEA-S levels decrease during illness, depression, and other stresses.

The biological effects of the adrenal androgens may be direct or indirect. These steroids can be converted by peripheral tissues to the primary sex hormones, testosterone, DHT, and estradiol. Adrenal androgens are the major source of testosterone in females. Some direct effects of DHEA have been identified. DHEA can inhibit the enzyme glucose-6-phosphate dehydrogenase, an important factor in controlling the synthesis of nicotinamide adenine dinucleotide phosphate (NADPH), which is required for many important biological reactions, including lipogenesis. DHEA also may be involved in many other broad-based physiological effects, including immune regulation, through possible direct effects on production of cytokines and through its action as a neurosteroid in modulating γ-aminobutyric acid and *N*-methyl-aspartate receptors in the hippocampus area of the brain.

DHEA-S may have an important antiglucocorticoid role and DHEA-S deficiency may result in relative glucocorticoid excess, with impaired memory and negative mood effects. Evidence now suggests that DHEA-S can improve psychological well-being and lean body mass, and may have beneficial effects on bone turnover. Evidence is insufficient to support the general use of DHEA-S in the elderly as an antiaging hormone, but its use in women with **Addison's disease** who traditionally have been treated only with glucocorticoid and mineralocorticoid replacement therapy is supported by clinical studies. Women with primary or secondary adrenal insufficiency have very low DHEA and DHEA-S levels and experience loss of axillary and pubic hair and osteoporosis. Patients not treated with replacement DHEA retain normal longevity but have lower strength and stamina. Studies have shown psychological and sexual function benefits when DHEA was given, resulting in normalization of DHEA-S and androstenedione and low-normal testosterone levels. Also, serum levels of insulin-like growth factor (IGF-1) improved, and serum low-density lipoprotein (LDL) cholesterol levels decreased. Negative effects included acne and hirsutism in a small percentage of women.

Catecholamines

The naturally occurring catecholamines are norepinephrine (NE; noradrenaline), epinephrine (E; adrenaline), and dopamine. The main secretory products of the adrenal medulla are epinephrine and norepinephrine. Production of catecholamines is not restricted to the adrenal medulla, however, and synthesis of these hormones also occurs in the neurons of the sympathetic and central nervous systems (CNS) and in scattered groups of chromaffin cells found in other regions of the abdomen and neck. Norepinephrine is the principal product synthesized in the CNS, and epinephrine is the principal catecholamine produced by the adrenal glands.

The physiological actions of the catecholamines are diverse. Norepinephrine functions primarily as a neurotransmitter. Both norepinephrine and epinephrine influence the vascular system, whereas epinephrine affects metabolic processes such as carbohydrate metabolism. The biological actions of the catecholamines are initiated through their interaction with two different types of specific cell membrane receptors: α-adrenergic and β-adrenergic receptors. These receptors have different affinities for norepinephrine and epinephrine and cause opposing physiological effects. Norepinephrine interacts primarily with α-adrenergic receptors, whereas epinephrine interacts with both α- and β-receptors.

Stimulation of α-adrenergic receptors results in vasoconstriction, decreased insulin secretion, sweating, piloerection (hair standing on end), and stimulation of glycogenolysis in the liver and skeletal muscle, leading to an increase in blood glucose concentration. Stimulation of β-receptors, however, leads to vasodilation; stimulation of insulin release; increased cardiac contraction rate; relaxation of smooth muscle in the intestinal tract; bronchodilation by relaxation of smooth muscles in bronchi; stimulation of renin release, which enhances sodium reabsorption from the kidney; and enhanced lipolysis.

KEY CONCEPTS BOX 51-1

- Glucocorticoids are involved in the regulation of carbohydrate, protein, and lipid metabolism.
- Cortisol at high concentrations also demonstrates mineralocorticoid activity.
- The major physiological functions of aldosterone are (1) regulation of extracellular fluid volume, and (2) regulation of potassium concentration.
- The predominant adrenal androgens are dehydroepiandrosterone sulfate (DHEA-S), dehydroepiandrosterone (DHEA), and androstenedione.
- The adrenal medulla secretes norepinephrine (NE; noradrenaline) and epinephrine (E; adrenaline). Both norepinephrine and epinephrine influence the vascular system, whereas epinephrine affects metabolic processes such as carbohydrate metabolism.

SECTION OBJECTIVES BOX 51-2

- Describe the synthesis of glucocorticoids, mineralocorticoids, adrenal androgens, and medullary hormones.
- List the key or rate limiting enzymes in the biosynthesis of cortisol, aldosterone, and the catecholamines.

BIOSYNTHESIS

Adrenocorticosteroids

All adrenal steroid synthesis begins with cholesterol. Cholesterol in the adrenal tissue may be synthesized in situ from acetate or may come from cholesterol made in the liver and transported to the adrenal glands by LDL.

The biosynthetic pathway that leads to the three major groups of adrenal steroids is outlined in Fig. 51-3. Several of the reactions seen in steroidogenesis involve cytochrome P-450 enzymes, which are heme-containing enzymes that transfer electrons from NADPH to perform hydroxylation reactions with the use of molecular oxygen. The rate-limiting step in the synthesis of all steroids is the conversion of cholesterol to pregnenolone. The enzyme responsible for this side-chain cleavage step (cholesterol desmolase) is a product of the gene CYP11A1. This step is stimulated by **adrenocorticotropic hormone (ACTH)** in the zona fasciculata and zona reticularis and by angiotensin II and III in the zona glomerulosa. The pathway that leads to progesterone is common to both aldosterone and cortisol synthesis. The conversion of pregnenolone to progesterone is catalyzed by 3-β-hydroxysteroid dehydrogenase. In the zona reticularis and zona fasciculata, progesterone is hydroxylated at the 17, 21, and 11 positions to form cortisol. The enzymes responsible are gene products of CYP17, CYP21A2, and CYP11B1, respectively. Under normal circumstances, 10 to 30 mg of cortisol is synthesized per day.

Aldosterone is biosynthesized in the zona glomerulosa from cholesterol by the action of four enzymes: cholesterol desmolase (CYP11A1), 3-β-hydroxysteroid dehydrogenase, 21-hydroxylase (CYP21A2), and aldosterone synthetase (CYP11B2). Cortisol requires a 17-hydroxylation (CYP17), which is expressed only in the zona fasciculata, whereas aldosterone synthetase is expressed only in the zona glomerulosa.

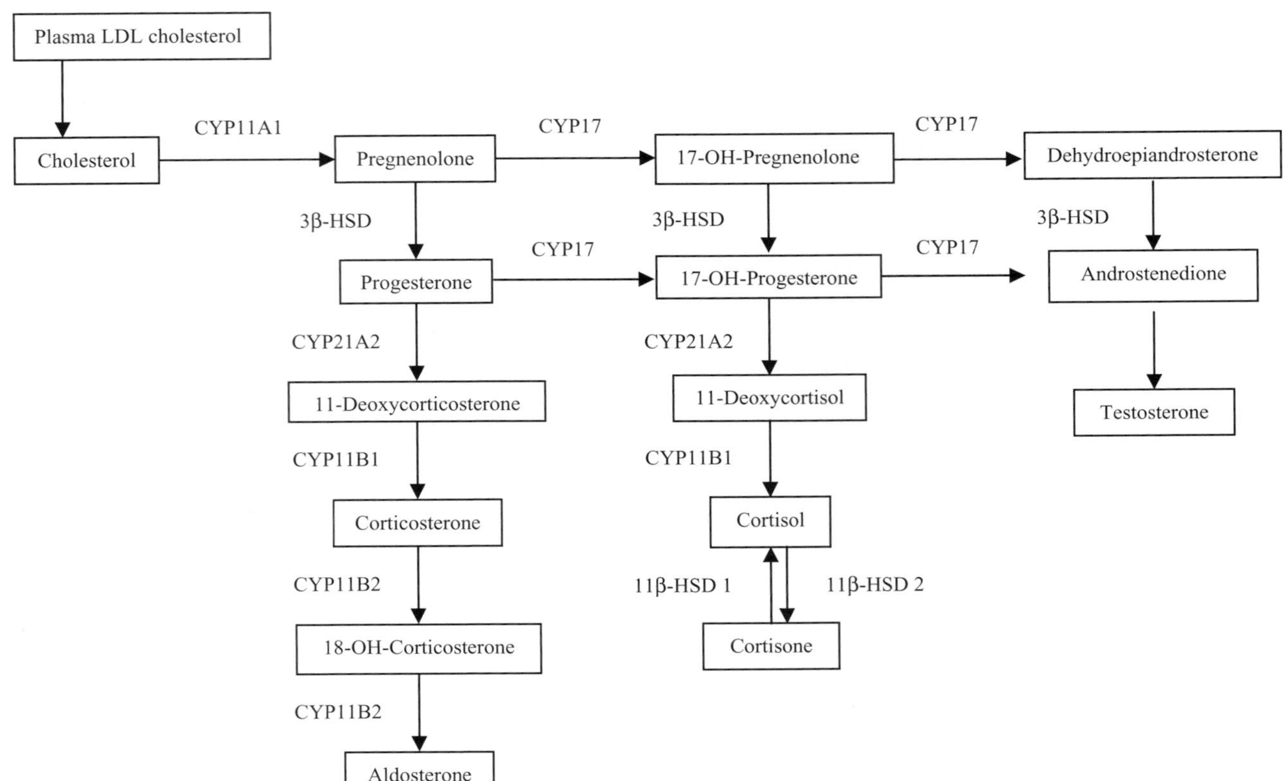

Fig. 51-3 Principal pathways of adrenal steroidogenesis. CYP11A1, mitochondrial cholesterol desmolase, catalyzes the side-chain cleavage of cholesterol. 3β-HSD, 3-β-hydroxysteroid dehydrogenase bound to the endoplasmic reticulum, also catalyzes Δ^5-Δ^4 isomerase activity. CYP17 is responsible for both 17β-hydroxylase activity and 17,20-lyase activity, which cleave off the remaining side chain at the C-17 position. CYP21A2, 21-hydroxylase, catalyzes 21-hydroxylation of progesterone, and 17-hydroxyprogesterone. CYP11B1, 11β-hydroxylase, catalyzes 11 hydroxylation. CYP11B2, aldosterone synthase, catalyzes 18-hydroxylation and 18-methyloxidation. 11β-HSD 2, 11β-hydroxysteroid dehydrogenase type 2, which is mainly expressed in renal distal tubules, catalyzes the conversion of cortisol to cortisone, therefore inactivates the mineralocorticoid activity of cortisol. 11β-HSD 1, 11β-hydroxysteroid dehydrogenase type 1, which is expressed mainly in liver, reactivates cortisone to cortisol.

Androgens are derived from the major pathway of steroid biosynthesis after cleavage of the side chain attached to carbon 17 in ring D (see Chapter 50 for a description of the synthesis of androgens). The adrenal gland production of androgens is significant in that it indirectly generates 60% of circulating testosterone in females, mainly through peripheral tissue conversion of testosterone precursors.

Catecholamines

The biochemical pathway that leads to synthesis of the catecholamines is outlined in Fig. 51-4. The rate-limiting step is the hydroxylation of the amino acid tyrosine, which leads to the formation of dihydroxyphenylalanine (dopa). This step is inhibited by both epinephrine and norepinephrine. Tyrosine is obtained through the diet or through hydroxylation of phenylalanine. Dopa is decarboxylated to form dopamine, which is a major end product in the CNS, where it functions as a neurotransmitter. Dopamine is stored in granules that are present in both neurons and the adrenal medulla. Within the granules, dopamine-β-hydroxylase converts dopamine to norepinephrine. Finally, norepinephrine is released from the storage granules, and phenylethanolamine *N*-methyltransferase (PNMT) methylates the norepinephrine to form epinephrine. PNMT, which is found only in the adrenal medulla, is induced by glucocorticoids (cortisol). High concentrations of cortisol within the adrenal are required for the induction of PNMT in the adrenal medulla. Exogenous steroids suppress endogenous cortisol production, reducing the high concentration of cortisol around the medulla, reducing in turn the production of epinephrine. Adrenocortical insufficiency of whatever cause is associated with reduced epinephrine secretions from the adrenal. The hormones of the adrenal medulla are stored complexed with proteins (chromogranin A, dopamine-β-hydroxylase) and adenosine-5′-triphosphate (ATP) within chromaffin granules. Nerve stimulation results in release of stored catecholamines from these vesicles via the process of exocytosis.

KEY CONCEPTS BOX 51-2

- Cholesterol is the precursor for all adrenal steroid hormones.
- The rate-limiting step in the production of adrenal steroids is the conversion of cholesterol to pregnenolone.
- 17-Hydroxylase activity is expressed in the zona reticularis and zona fasciculata, but not in the zona glomerulosa, resulting in different steroid hormone production in these zones.

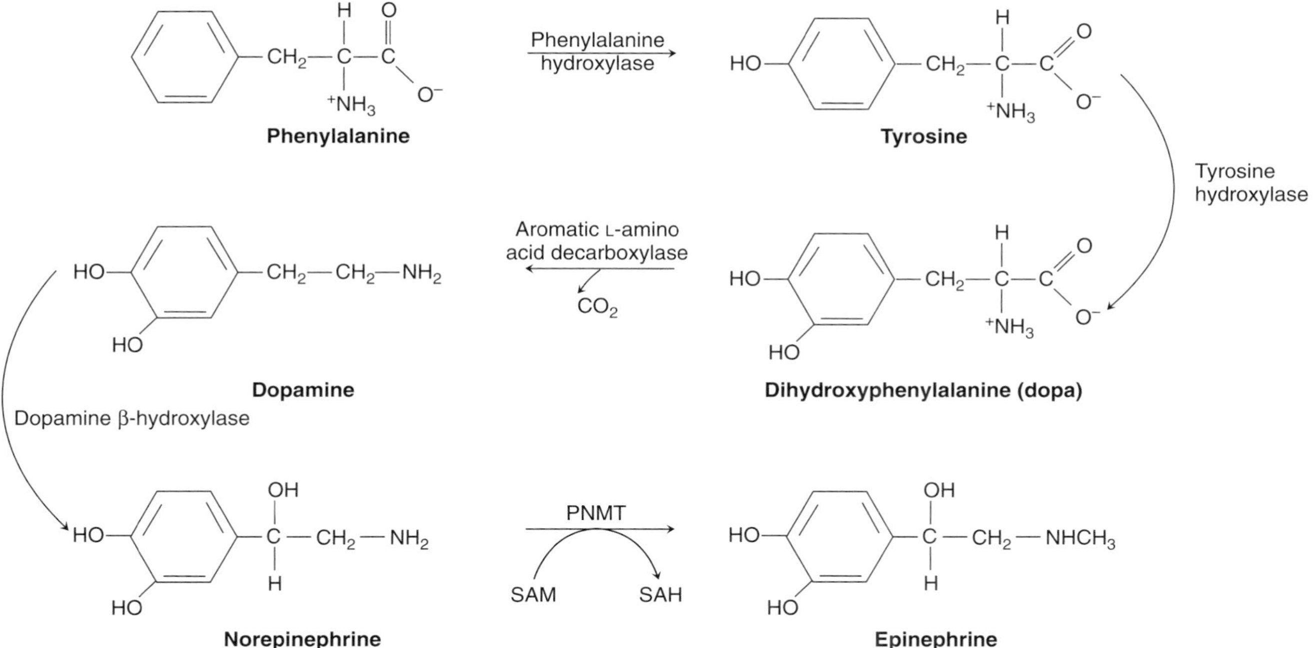

Fig. 51-4 Synthesis of medullary hormones. *PNMT,* Phenylethanolamine *N*-methyl-transferase; *SAH,* S-adenosyl homocysteine; *SAM,* S-adenosylmethionine. (From Orten JM, Neuhaus OW: *Human Biochemistry,* St. Louis, 1982, Mosby.)

SECTION OBJECTIVES BOX 51-3

- List the transport proteins for the glucocorticoids, mineralocorticoids, adrenal androgens, and medullary hormones, and the relative affinities of each protein for the adrenal hormones.
- Describe the catabolism of the glucocorticoids, mineralocorticoids, adrenal androgens, and medullary hormones and their primary excretion products.
- Discuss factors that affect corticosteroid-binding globulin (CBG) levels and binding affinity for cortisol.
- List the two enzymes that degrade catecholamines.

TRANSPORT AND CATABOLISM

Adrenocorticosteroids

In plasma, aldosterone and cortisol are bound to plasma proteins to different degrees. Approximately 40% of plasma aldosterone exists in the free (non-protein bound) state, whereas approximately 4% of cortisol is free in plasma. Albumin and **corticosteroid-binding globulin** (CBG; transcortin, cortisol-binding globulin) account for most of the binding of these two steroids. CBG is a high-affinity, low-capacity steroid binder, which binds 90% of cortisol under normal circumstances, whereas albumin is a low-affinity, high-capacity binding protein. The proportion of cortisol in the free state greatly increases as the concentration of cortisol exceeds the binding capacity of CBG (approximately 550 nmol/L). The binding affinity of CBG for cortisol is reduced in areas of inflammation. This increases the concentration of free cortisol, thereby increasing its effectiveness at that site. CBG levels are increased in hyperestrogenic states such as those found in pregnant women and in women taking estrogen-containing birth control pills. Free cortisol levels remain normal under these circumstances because of a compensatory increase in total cortisol. Aldosterone is much less affected by these hormonally induced changes.

Steroid catabolism is complex, and only a brief discussion of it is necessary to convey an understanding of the pathogenesis and laboratory investigation of adrenal disorders. The liver and the kidneys catabolize most steroids. Examples of the types of reactions that are carried out include further hydroxylation of the steroid nucleus, conjugation with glucuronic acid, and reduction of the double bond in ring A. These transformations increase the water solubility of the steroids, allowing their excretion into the urine. Normally, less than 1% of aldosterone and cortisol is excreted unmetabolized into the urine.

The amount of cortisol that is directly secreted into the urine is related to the proportion of cortisol that circulates in the free form. CBG is saturated at high physiological concentrations of cortisol. Therefore, any increase in cortisol to above this level causes a pronounced increase in the amount of cortisol excreted into the urine; this makes urinary free cortisol a valuable test in the investigation of Cushing's syndrome, as is discussed later.

Catecholamines

Catecholamines are stable within the storage granules of the adrenal medullary cells. However, when they are released, they are degraded rapidly by two enzymes: catechol-O-methyltransferase (COMT) and monoamine oxidase (MAO) (Fig. 51-5). Only a small fraction of catecholamine output

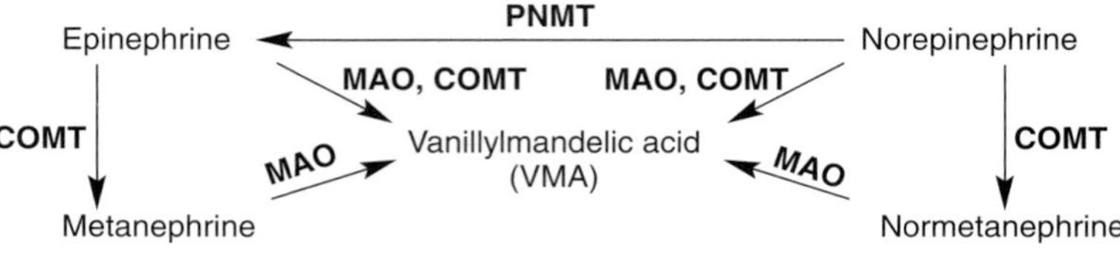

Fig. 51-5 Metabolism of medullary hormones (see text for description of abbreviations).

(2%) is excreted unmetabolized as free catecholamines into the urine. COMT is present in many tissues, especially liver, kidney, and erythrocytes. This enzyme methylates the C-3 hydroxyl group of norepinephrine and epinephrine, producing normetanephrine and metanephrine, respectively. Approximately 20% of catecholamines are excreted into the urine as metanephrines. Most catecholamines, however, are converted further to vanillylmandelic acid (VMA) through the combined action of COMT and MAO; the latter is a ubiquitous enzyme that deaminates these amines. Measurement of free catecholamines, metanephrines, and VMA in the urine may be useful in the diagnosis of adrenal medullary disease. A large proportion of catecholamine metabolites appear in the urine as sulfate conjugates.

KEY CONCEPTS BOX 51-3

- Corticosteroid binding globulin (CBG) is the major tranporter of cortisol and aldosterone. Albumin is a minor transporter of these two hormones. Approximately 40% of aldosterone and 4% of cortisol are in the non-protein bound, free state in serum.
- Variation in CBG levels will affect the level of active free cortisol.
- The catecholamines are metabolized to metanephrines and VMA and are excreted via the kidneys as the free hormones and their metabolites or as sulfate conjugates.

SECTION OBJECTIVES BOX 51-4

- Name the hypothalamic hormones that affect adrenal hormones and describe their functions.
- Decribe the neuronal control over hypothalamic hormones production.
- Describe the effect of aldosterone action on serum sodium and potassium levels.
- Explain the normal hypothalamic-anterior pituitary-adrenal cortex axis for control of glucocorticoid production, including the importance of CRH and ACTH, which glucocorticoid is responsible for negative feedback, normal diurnal variation of cortisol, and the effect of any type of stress on glucocorticoid production.
- Explain the control of mineralocorticoid production, including a detailed discussion of the stimulating factors to activate renin production; biochemical conversions that lead to angiotensin II production; the effect of potassium, ACTH, and natriuretic peptides; and the effect of various drugs on aldosterone and renin levels.
- List six factors that lead to adrenal catecholamine production.

CONTROL AND REGULATION

Glucocorticoids

Cortisol released from the adrenal cortex is regulated by the hypothalamic-pituitary-adrenal axis (Fig. 51-6 and Chapter 48). The hypothalamus synthesizes a 41 amino acid polypeptide, **corticotropin-releasing hormone (CRH)**, which is carried by the circulation to the anterior pituitary gland. There it causes the release of adrenocorticotropic hormone (ACTH), a 39 amino acid polypeptide. The first 18 amino acids of ACTH are essential for its biological activity. The ACTH molecule interacts with membrane receptors of the cells of the adrenal cortex, and through its second messenger, cyclic adenosine monophosphate (cAMP), stimulates the rate-limiting step in steroidogenesis (the conversion of cholesterol to pregnenolone), leading to cortisol secretion. The free circulating cortisol acts in a negative-feedback manner to inhibit the release of ACTH from the pituitary gland. Overriding this system of negative-feedback control are the higher centers of the brain, which establish the normal diurnal variation of cortisol (Fig. 51-7). Serum cortisol levels normally are highest in the morning upon awakening and lowest in the late evening. This pattern is affected mainly by the sleep-wake cycle of the individual. If the sleep-wake cycle is altered, several days are required for the pattern to change. The circadian pattern of ACTH release is controlled by means of CRH secretion from the hypothalamus. Short-term release of cortisol is episodic, following the pattern of ACTH pulses by about 2 to 3 minutes. Stress is another factor that can override the negative feedback of cortisol on ACTH release. Stress stimulates release of neurogenic amines, which, in turn, stimulates the release of CRH. The inflammatory cytokines, tumor necrosis factor-α, interleukin-1, and interleukin-6 also stimulate the release of ACTH. ACTH levels can increase up to 10-fold in times of stress, resulting in high levels of cortisol. Hypoglycemia, which is a form of chemical stress, also can enhance CRH release, ultimately leading to an increase in cortisol. This effect is mediated by glucose receptors within the hypothalamus.

Mineralocorticoids

In healthy individuals, four main factors control the secretion of aldosterone from the zona glomerulosa: (1) the **renin-angiotensin system,** (2) potassium, (3) ACTH, and (4) natriuretic peptides. Under normal circumstances, the renin-angiotensin system predominates. Natriuretic peptides, atrial natriuretic peptide (ANP), and B-type natriuretic peptide (BNP) from the heart may exhibit part of their physiological function through inhibition of aldosterone release (see Chapter 28). Fig. 51-8 outlines the normal regulation of aldosterone secretion. A more detailed description is provided in Chapter 28.

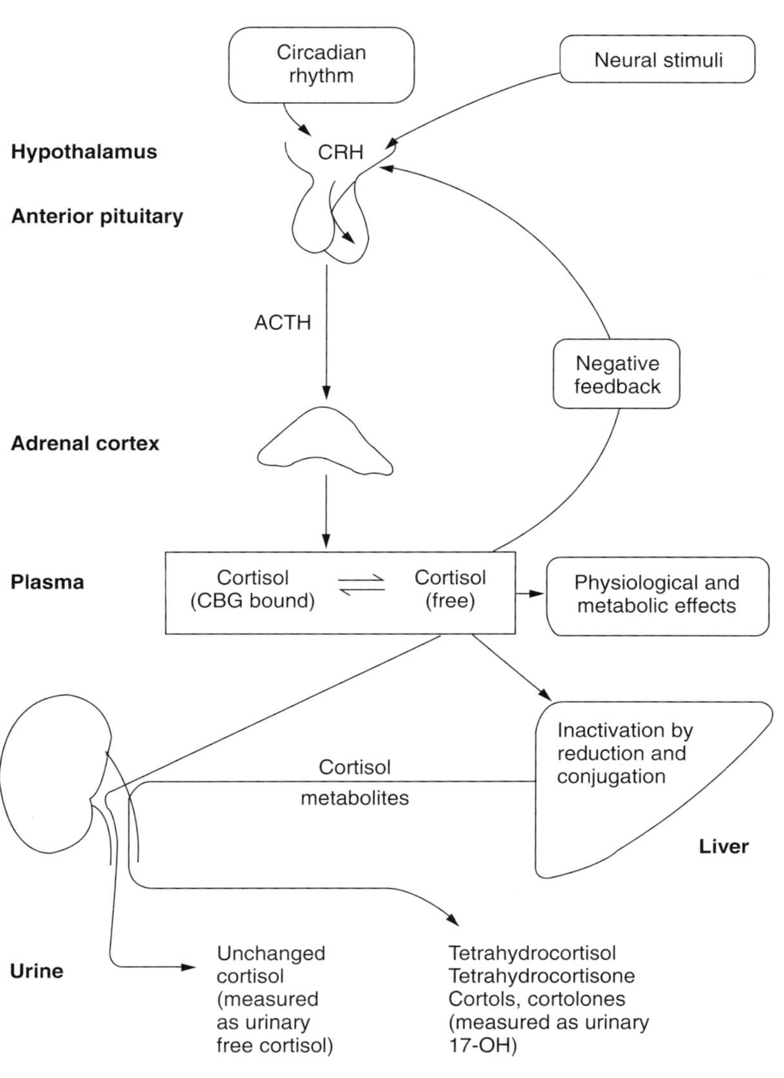

Fig. 51-6 Control and metabolism of glucocorticoids. (From Toft A: *Diagnosis and Management of Endocrine Diseases,* St. Louis, 1981, Blackwell Scientific.)

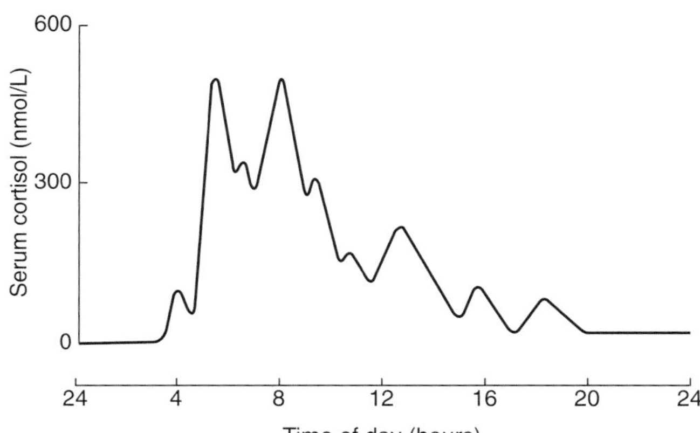

Fig. 51-7 Variation of serum cortisol concentration during 24-hour period in normal individual.

Renin-Angiotensin

Renin is a proteolytic enzyme that is stored by specialized cells in the wall of the afferent arteriole of the glomerulus. These cells are associated with the macula densa, which is part of the juxtaglomerular (JG) apparatus. Two forms of renin are present in the circulation: active renin and its precursor, prorenin. Active renin can be released only from the juxtaglomerular apparatus. Prorenin concentration in the circulation is 10 times higher on average than that of active renin. Extrarenal sources of prorenin also are available.

Three mechanisms regulate renin secretion from JG cells: (1) the JG cell baroreceptor mechanism, which senses blood pressure inside the afferent arteriole; (2) the sympathetic β_1-adrenergic nerve mechanism; and (3) the macula densa mechanism, which senses the amount of sodium chloride inside the renal distal convoluted tubule. A drop in blood pressure or serum sodium concentration results in the release of renin. Renin cleaves a peptide bond in circulating angiotensinogen, a protein secreted by the liver, thus releasing a decapeptide called *angiotensin I.* Angiotensin I in turn is cleaved by angiotensin-converting enzyme (ACE), forming an octapeptide called angiotensin II. Angiotensin II is a potent vasoconstrictor that increases blood pressure directly (pressor) and stimulates aldosterone release through its interaction with a G-protein–coupled receptor on the surfaces of cells in the zona glomerulosa. Aldosterone, which acts through

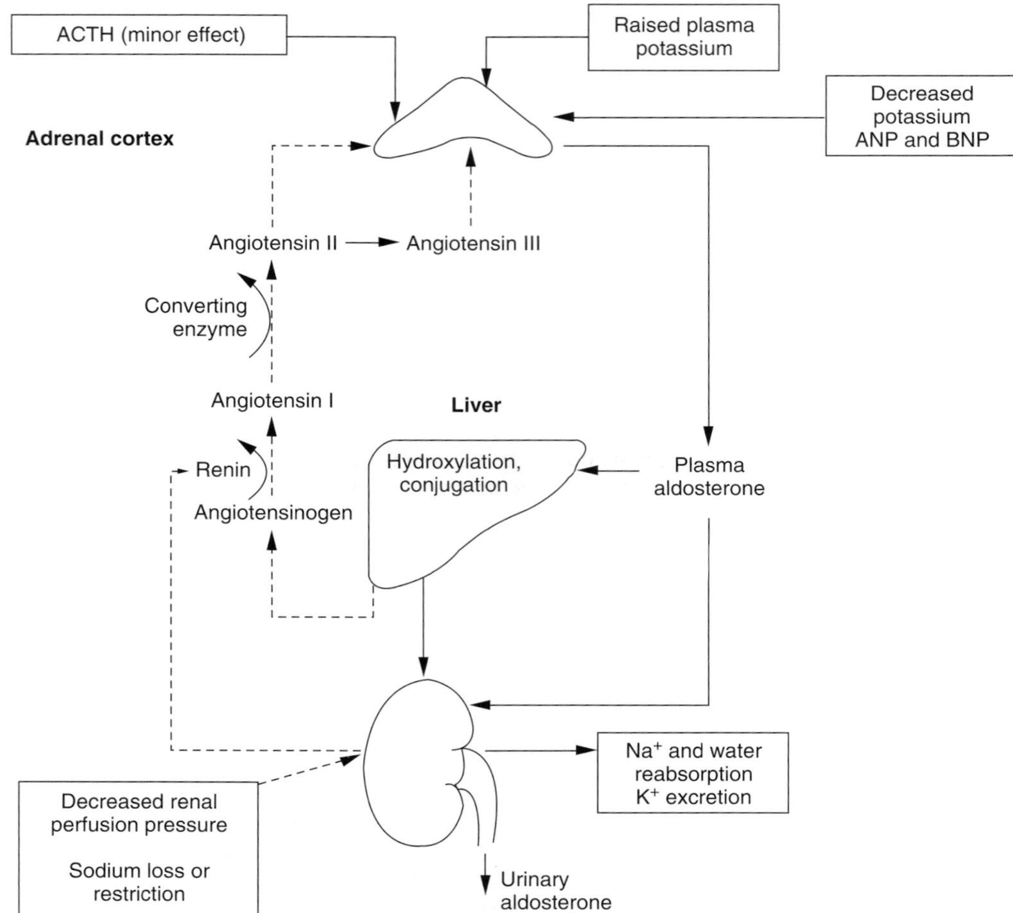

Fig. 51-8 Control and metabolism of aldosterone. (Modified from Toft A: *Diagnosis and Management of Endocrine Diseases,* St. Louis, 1981, Blackwell Scientific.)

the mineralocorticoid receptors within kidney tubular cells, facilitates sodium retention and potassium loss. Finally, angiotensin II is converted to a heptapeptide, angiotensin III, by a carboxypeptidase. Angiotensin III still retains the capacity to stimulate aldosterone release but exhibits little pressor activity.

Potassium and ACTH

Potassium regulates aldosterone secretion directly at the adrenal level. Hyperkalemia stimulates and hypokalemia inhibits aldosterone release. ACTH also can stimulate aldosterone secretion directly; however, this is only an acute phenomenon that is short lived.

Natriuretic Peptides

ANP and BNP inhibit aldosterone secretion, which is responsible for the sodium escape mechanism, to prevent continuous extracellular fluid volume expansion in patients with **hyperaldosteronism.** These peptides also promote natriuresis by the kidneys.

Dopamine, serotonin, γ-melanocyte–stimulating hormone (γ-MSH), β-endorphin, and an unidentified pituitary aldosterone–stimulating factor also participate in aldosterone regulation.

Normally, a circadian rhythm is noted in plasma aldosterone concentration, with highest values occurring in the morning. In addition, alterations in aldosterone levels are associated with postural changes. Plasma levels range from 50 to 150 ng/L (140 to 420 pmol/L) in healthy individuals when recumbent, and from 150 to 300 ng/L (420 to 840 pmol/L) when upright. Approximately 150 to 200 μg of aldosterone is secreted per day under normal circumstances. Several drugs can have physiological effects on the renin-aldosterone system. Nonsteroidal anti-inflammatory agents and β-blockers can decrease aldosterone and renin levels. ACE inhibitors can cause increased renin with decreased aldosterone. Thiazide diuretics and laxatives can increase the concentration of both.

Adrenal Androgens

Androgen secretion is regulated partially by ACTH but not by gonadotropins, which act primarily on the gonads. ACTH stimulation is variable, and dexamethasone (a synthetic corticosteroid) administration decreases adrenal androgen production to a dissimilar degree when compared with administration of cortisol. In other instances, as at adrenarche or during puberty, or with aging or severe illness, cortisol and androgen production diverge; such divergence indicates that other factors are playing a role in the regulation of adrenal androgen secretion. These factors may include arrangement of the blood supply to the adrenal cortex, intrinsic properties of adrenocortical cells, and other unknown factors exogenous to the adrenal, such as factors associated with the pituitary.

Catecholamines

The synthesis of epinephrine and norepinephrine is regulated by the intracellular concentrations of these hormones through negative-feedback inhibition, as was stated previously. The catecholamines are released from the adrenal medulla in response to hypotension, hypoxia, exposure to cold, muscular exertion, pain, and emotional disturbances.

KEY CONCEPTS BOX 51-4

- Cortisol released from the adrenal cortex is regulated by the hypothalamic-pituitary-adrenal axis, involving CRH and ACTH.
- Higher neuronal input can affect the release of CRH from the hypothalamus.
- The free circulating cortisol acts in a negative-feedback manner to control the release of ACTH from the pituitary gland.
- Four main factors control the secretion of aldosterone from the zona glomerulosa: (1) the renin-angiotensin system, (2) potassium, (3) ACTH, and (4) natriuretic peptide.
- One of the functions of aldosterone is to control serum potassium levels by stimulating renal retention of sodium and excretion of potassium.

SECTION OBJECTIVES BOX 51-5

- Relate the clinical findings of hypercortisolism and hyperaldosteronism with the physiological actions of cortisol and aldosterone, respectively.
- Discuss Cushing's syndrome according to iatrogenic and non-iatrogenic causes, a differentiation between ACTH-dependent and ACTH-independent categories, typical clinical symptoms, and features of subclinical Cushing's syndrome with adrenal incidentalomas.
- Discuss hyperaldosteronism according to two principal disorders that cause it, typical clinical symptoms, and secondary causes.
- Discuss congenital adrenal hyperplasia (CAH) or adrenogenital syndrome according to general cause, most common and second most common enzyme deficiency, pathogenesis for the clinical symptoms, and treatment.
- Discuss hypoadrenalism according to three general causes, clinical symptoms of Addison's disease, features of addisonian crisis, pathogenesis of adrenoleukodystrophy, and a differentiation of the symptoms of primary vs. secondary adrenal insufficiency.
- Discuss pheochromocytoma according to pathogenesis and clinical symptoms.
- List the significant laboratory findings for Cushing's syndrome, hyperaldosteronism, congenital adrenal hyperplasia, Addison's disease, and pheochromocytoma.

PATHOLOGICAL CONDITIONS

In this section, the causes and clinical features associated with disorders of the adrenal cortex and the adrenal medulla are discussed. In general, the gland may hyperfunction and produce excessive quantities of bioactive molecules, or the gland may hypofunction and secrete too few molecules that are essential for the normal maintenance of life. The pathological cause of these disorders may be neoplastic, hyperplastic, vascular, inflammatory, autoimmune, infectious, hereditary, or idiopathic.

Disorders of the Adrenal Cortex

Hyperadrenalism

Three basic conditions are associated with hyperadrenalism, each of which may have more than one cause. These include Cushing's syndrome, which results from excess cortisol production; primary hyperaldosteronism, or **Conn's syndrome;** and congenital adrenal hyperplasia, which is caused by an enzymatic block in the steroid synthetic pathway.

Cushing's Syndrome

Cushing's syndrome is the term that is used to describe any condition resulting from an increased concentration of circulating glucocorticoid, usually cortisol. The most common cause of excess cortisol is iatrogenic, resulting from high doses of cortisol or other glucocorticoids used in the management of a wide variety of clinical problems. The most common noniatrogenic causes are, in order, pituitary tumors (60%), ectopic ACTH (20%), and adrenal adenoma and adrenal carcinoma (combined 20%). The estimated prevalence of Cushing's syndrome is approximately 1:10,000 women and 1:30,000 men. The most common cause of Cushing's syndrome in children is adrenal tumor.

Cushing's syndrome may be divided into two broad categories: ACTH dependent and ACTH independent. ACTH-dependent Cushing's syndrome, which is caused by excess ACTH, results in bilateral adrenal hyperplasia. This is caused most commonly by **autonomous** ACTH secretion by a benign pituitary adenoma, which is also called **Cushing's disease.** This condition is much more common in women than in men (female-to-male ratio, 3.5:1.0). Ectopic sources of ACTH include carcinoma of the lung (oat cell or small cell) (50%), thymic cancer (10%), pancreatic carcinoid (10%), neural crest tumors (5%), bronchial carcinoid (2%), medullary carcinoma of the thyroid (5%), and miscellaneous tumors (18%). It is now known that many nonendocrine tissues of the body can synthesize small amounts of proopiomelanocortin (POMC), the precursor to ACTH. Very few tissues can actually metabolize POMC and release bioactive ACTH. Most lung tumors produce POMC, but only 3% of these have the appropriate proteolytic enzymes to release active ACTH, thus causing Cushing's syndrome.

In ACTH-independent Cushing's syndrome, serum ACTH levels are low because of the negative inhibition that results from increased cortisol production of adrenal adenomas and carcinomas. Adrenal carcinoma has a particularly bad prognosis, with most patients dying within 3 years despite surgical intervention. Adrenal neoplasms usually are unilateral. In adults, about half of these are malignant, whereas in children, neoplasms of the adrenal are more often malignant.

Rare causes of Cushing's syndrome include ectopic CRH secretion, primary pigmented nodular adrenal disease (isolated or with Carney complex), and ACTH-independent macronodular adrenal hyperplasia. This last disorder is characterized by ectopic expression of functional cell membrane receptors by the adrenal cells for gastric inhibitory polypeptide (GIP) (food-dependent Cushing's syndrome), vasopressin, catecholamines, interleukin-1, leptin, luteinizing hormone (LH), or serotonin, with normal increases in serum levels of these hormones stimulating cortisol secretion.

Cushing's syndrome in advanced stages may be easy to recognize (Box 51-2). In early stages of the disease, however, patients can have a wide variety of clinical symptoms that may be confused with other common problems such as essential hypertension, glucose intolerance, depression, and obesity. The laboratory plays a major role in the diagnosis. Cushing central obesity is a characteristic redistribution of adipose tissue with increased deposition around the face (moon facies), in the supraclavicular region, in the interscapular region (buffalo hump), and in the mesenteric bed (truncal obesity). The reason for this is not known. Less common findings include neuropsychiatric dysfunction, pigmentation (ACTH-dependent cause only), acne, and hypokalemic alkalosis. Polyuria may be seen because cortisol in high concentrations may suppress antidiuretic hormone (ADH) release. Neuropsychiatric problems include depression, manic behavior, psychoses, and attempts at suicide.

The catabolic effects of glucocorticoids on protein metabolism can account for bruising, striae (stretch marks), osteoporosis, and muscle weakness. Hypertension and hypokalemia may be explained by the mineralocorticoid actions of excess cortisol. Hirsutism, acne, and menstrual dysfunction, which may result from excess adrenal androgen production, may be seen most dramatically in some cases of adrenal carcinoma. Hyperpigmentation sometimes occurs in association with ectopic ACTH, when high levels of ACTH, which exhibits some melanocyte-stimulating hormone (MSH) activity, cause generalized hyperproduction of melanin. Some patients may suffer from impotence, decreased libido, and infertility.

Several key clinical clues might suggest an ectopic source for ACTH. Some patients may not present with some of the physical findings of Cushing's syndrome because of rapid onset of symptoms, which may occur with oat cell carcinoma. Symptoms are more common with slow-growing tumors such as bronchial, thymic, or pancreatic carcinoids. Because of the very high ACTH and cortisol levels seen in some of these patients, they may be hyperpigmented, may have more profound hypokalemia, or may demonstrate glucose intolerance, weakness, and edema. Other signs associated with malignant disease such as anorexia and weight loss also may be obvious. Opportunistic infections may be a key feature of ectopic ACTH because of the immunosuppressive effects of large concentrations of cortisol. Pneumocystic pneumonia is a possible complication.

Box 51-2

Major Causes and Clinical Features of Cushing's Syndrome

Causes

ACTH independent
- Adrenal adenoma
- Adrenal carcinoma

ACTH dependent
- Pituitary adenoma secreting ACTH (Cushing's disease)
- Ectopic ACTH
- Ectopic corticotropin-releasing hormone

Nodular hyperplasia
- ACTH-independent macronodular hyperplasia

Cortisol secretion is mediated by ectopic expression of functional membrane receptors in adrenal glands for:
- Gastric inhibitory polypeptide
- Vasopressin
- Catecholamines
- Interleukin-1
- Leptin
- LH
- Serotonin

Primary pigmented nodular adrenal disease
- Sporadic
- Part of Carney complex

Iatrogenic

Glucocorticoid therapy
ACTH therapy

Clinical Features

Truncal obesity (buffalo hump, superclavicular fat)
Hypertension
Glucose intolerance
Plethoric facies (moon face)
Skin atropy (bruising, purple striae [stretch marks])
Muscle (proximal) weakness
Menstrual and gonadal dysfunction
Acne
Hirsutism
Osteoporosis
Psychiatric problems

ACTH, Adrenocorticotropic hormone; *LH,* luteinizing hormone.

The frequent findings of Cushing's syndrome are seen in Box 51-2. Less common findings at diagnosis include osteoporosis, edema, polyuria and polydipsia, and fungal infection. Some patients have only isolated symptoms, and diagnosis can be missed for a long time. Other laboratory abnormalities associated with Cushing's include neutrophilia, leukocytosis, increased cholesterol, and hypercoagulability. Any child with recent weight gain and stunted linear growth should be investigated for Cushing's syndrome.

Recently, recognition of subclinical Cushing's syndrome associated with adrenal **incidentalomas** has improved. Patients present with apparently clinically nonfunctioning adrenal adenoma, whereas their cortisol secretion becomes autonomous and dysregulated and is not fully restrained by pituitary feedback. The better term for this condition might be *subclinical autonomous glucocorticoid hypersecretion*. The prevalence of adrenal incidentaloma is approximately 4%, and it is estimated that 75% of these patients are nonfunctional; 5% to 20% may hypersecrete cortisol, bringing the prevalence of subclinical Cushing's syndrome to as high as 2 to 8 per 1000, depending on the testing methods and criteria used to define subclinical cortisol excess. By definition, these individuals should be asymptomatic; however, subclinical Cushing's syndrome may have long-term consequences, such as central obesity, hypertension, and diabetes. Women with subclinical Cushing's syndrome are at greater risk of vertebral fracture independent of their gonadal status. Subclinical Cushing's syndrome may contribute to development of insulin resistance and metabolic syndrome, thereby increasing the risk of atherosclerosis and cardiovascular complications.

Hyperaldosteronism

Primary autonomous hypersecretion of aldosterone by the zona glomerulosa is caused mainly by two disorders: (1) aldosterone-producing adrenal adenoma (APA), or Conn's syndrome; and (2) idiopathic hyperaldosteronism (IHA), caused by bilateral adrenal hyperplasia. The use of the serum or plasma aldosterone concentration–to–plasma renin activity (or renin mass) ratio (ARR) as a screening test, followed by salt-loading aldosterone suppression confirmatory testing, has resulted in detection of milder cases of primary aldosteronism, such as IHA. It now is recognized that IHA accounts for approximately 60%, and APA accounts for 35%, of cases of hyperaldosteronism. Primary (unilateral) adrenal hyperplasia, which is indistinguishable biochemically from APA, may account for 2% of patients with hyperaldosteronism, and pure aldosterone-producing adrenocortical carcinomas are even more rare (<1%). A rare form of primary hyperaldosteronism, glucocorticoid-remediable aldosteronism (GRA; <1% of cases), also called dexamethasone-suppressible hyperaldosteronism but now officially renamed *familial hyperaldosteronism type 1 (FH type 1)*, has clinical features of Conn's syndrome but results from ectopic expression of aldosterone synthase (AS), the gene product of CYP11B2. A chimeric gene is formed at meiosis between two homologous genes on chromosome 8: CYP11B1 and CYP11B2; this allows the gene product of CYP11B2 aldosterone synthase, which normally is expressed only in the zona glomerulosa, to be expressed partially in the zona reticularis and to be kept under ACTH control rather than under angiotensin II control. Another genetic cause of increased mineralocorticoid activity includes apparent mineralocorticoid excess (AME). AME is an autosomal recessive disorder caused by deficiency of the 11β-HSD2 enzyme resulting from mutations in the 11β-HSD2 gene located on chromosome 16q22. Defective 11β-HSD2 fails to inactivate cortisol. Cortisol now is free to interact with the mineralocorticoid receptor, causing hypertension and hypokalemia. Both of the above hereditary causes of hypertension are treatable with dexamethasone.

Box 51-3

Major Causes and Clinical Features of Primary Hyperaldosteronism (Conn's Syndrome)

Causes

Adrenal aldosterone-producing adenoma, APA (35% of cases)
Idiopathic hyperaldosteronism, IHA (60% of cases)
Primary (unilarteral) adrenal hyperplasia (2% of cases)
Pure aldosterone–producing adrenocortical carcinoma (<1% of cases)
Familial hyperaldosteronism (FH)
- Glucocorticoid-remediable aldosteronism (FH type 1) (<1% of cases)
- FH type 2 (APA or IHA) (<1% of cases)

Ectopic aldosterone–producing adenoma or carcinoma (<0.1% of cases)

Clinical Features

Hypertension
Symptoms resulting from hypokalemia
- Muscle weakness
- Polyuria and polydipsia
- Electrocardiographic changes

Glucose intolerance

The major clinical feature of hyperaldosteronism is hypertension. Primary hyperaldosteronism now is recognized as the most common form of **secondary hypertension.** Wide use of the ARR as a screening test in hypertensive patients has resulted in much higher prevalence estimates of this disorder (5% to 13% of all patients with hypertension). The hypertension associated with primary hyperaldosteronism can be explained by the actions of aldosterone that result in retention of sodium and water and a decrease in plasma potassium levels. Spontaneous hypokalemia is reported in only 9% to 37% of patients with Conn's syndrome. The prevalence of primary hyperaldosteronism in patients with hypertension and spontaneous hypokalemia is greater than 50%. The degree of hypokalemia is affected partly by sodium intake. Many patients with hypokalemia do not experience symptoms (Box 51-3). Abnormal glucose tolerance can be observed in more than half of patients, as hypokalemia impairs insulin release from β-cells of the pancreas. The hallmark of primary hyperaldosteronism is inappropriately elevated aldosterone in the presence of suppressed plasma renin activity.

Hyperaldosteronism also may result from secondary causes. In these situations, the adrenal gland is not autonomously secreting aldosterone but is responding to enhanced production and release of renin from the kidney, which may be triggered by sodium loss, decreased renal perfusion, renal artery stenosis, or vascular volume depletion. Rarely, the hypersecretion of renin may be inappropriate, as in Bartter's syndrome, a kidney defect in chloride reabsorption, or in patients with renin-secreting tumors. In contrast to primary aldosteronism in which renin is decreased, plasma renin is elevated in secondary aldosteronism.

Congenital Adrenal Hyperplasia

Congenital adrenal hyperplasia (CAH), or adrenogenital syndrome, describes a group of inborn errors of metabolism that are caused by deficiencies of enzymes in the biosynthetic pathways that lead to cortisol and aldosterone production. At least six distinct inheritable defects have been found in this pathway, the most common of which is 21-hydroxylase deficiency, which accounts for 95% of all cases of CAH. These enzyme defects lead to diminished production of cortisol, which results in increased levels of ACTH, which stimulates adrenal hyperplasia and steroid production as the body attempts to overcome the enzyme deficiency. The block is usually partial, and the patient may be capable of maintaining normal levels of cortisol and aldosterone under normal circumstances, at the expense of the accumulation of steroid precursors that are diverted down other metabolic pathways. Hypersecretion of various androgens, including DHEA and androstenedione, occurs commonly; after peripheral conversion to testosterone, this may lead to precocious puberty in males and varying degrees of masculinization and sexual dysfunction in females.

Symptoms in CAH are related to both the decrease in the final product of metabolism and the accumulation of its precursors. In the case of 21-hydroxylase deficiency, there is an accumulation of 17-hydroxyprogesterone and other precursors. These compounds may exhibit antimineralocorticoid activity by binding to the mineralocorticoid receptor, which can exacerbate the salt-wasting tendency of CAH. Plasma renin levels increase in response, triggering greater demand for aldosterone synthesis, which also requires 21-hydroxylase activity. Severely affected individuals come to medical attention within 1 to 4 weeks of birth. Their nonspecific symptoms, such as poor appetite, vomiting, lethargy, and failure to thrive, may be mistaken for formula intolerance, colic, sepsis, pyloric stenosis, etc. On physical examination, the child may appear gray or mottled with an unobtainable blood pressure value. If the deficiency is partial, the salt-losing tendency is compensated; as little as 2% of normal enzyme activity is sufficient to prevent salt wasting. If loss of enzyme activity is more complete, more severe salt wasting will occur, and an addisonian crisis (see p. 1013) is more likely. The non–salt-wasting variant of this condition, seen in two-thirds of patients with this disorder, is characterized primarily by the problems associated with increased androgens. Less severe deficiencies may not become clinically apparent until after puberty. Without treatment, excess androgen results in precocious development in both males and females, with rapid growth, pubic hair, and acne noted at an early age. Premature epiphyseal closure also may occur. Additional problems for females include clitoromegaly, deepening voice, increased muscle mass, failure of breast development, primary amenorrhea, and facial hair.

The 21-hydroxylase deficiency is inherited through an autosomal recessive trait at an estimated heterozygote frequency of approximately 1 in 50 of the population. The approximate frequency of homozygous 21-hydroxylase deficiency causing CAH is 1 in 10,000 births (male-to-female ratio, 1 : 1). Mild, nonclassic 21-hydroxylase deficiency is much more common, with a prevalence of 1 in 1000 in the general population. The prevalence is much higher in some populations, for example, among Ashkenazi Jews, it may be as high as 1 in 30. Because of the high incidence of nonclassic CAH, some have questioned whether it is a true disease or is simply a common genetic variant (polymorphism). Heterozygous carrier estimates for nonclassic CAH may be as high as 10% of the population.

A deficiency of 11-hydroxylase (gene product of CYP11B1) is the second most common cause of CAH, affecting 1 in 100,000 newborns. However, the prevalence is much higher in Jewish immigrants from Morocco (1 in 5000). Again, depending on the severity of the deficiency, cortisol production may or may not be adequate. A unique feature of this enzyme deficiency is the accumulation of 11-deoxycorticosterone, a precursor in the aldosterone pathway. This steroid and its metabolites promote sodium reabsorption and therefore can cause hypertension. Approximately two-thirds of patients with this deficiency have elevated blood pressure in the first few years of life, along with other complications of hypertension. Most also have hypokalemia, muscle wasting, and cramping. Excess androgen production is another problem and leads to masculinization, abnormal genitalia in females, rapid somatic growth, premature closure of epiphyses, short adult stature, acne, premature adrenarche, amenorrhea, and precocious puberty. Nonclassic forms of 11-hydroxylase deficiency also occur but are much less common than nonclassic 21-hydroxylase deficiency. Treatment for both of these forms of CAH is simply glucocorticoid replacement therapy.

High cortisol concentrations within the adrenal gland are required to induce the enzyme responsible for conversion of norepinephrine to epinephrine within the adrenal. Therefore an additional feature associated with CAH is reduced output of epinephrine from the adrenal because of lower concentrations of cortisol within the adrenal gland. Exogenous glucocorticoid therapy may exacerbate this deficiency because endogenous production by the adrenal is suppressed.

Hypoadrenalism

Adrenal hypofunction or insufficiency can be caused by (1) primary adrenal disease involving the entire adrenal cortex; (2) secondary adrenal insufficiency caused by decreased levels of ACTH or CRH, which result from pituitary or hypothalamic disease; or (3) long-term suppression of the hypothalamic-pituitary-adrenal axis by exogenous glucocorticoids, which leads to adrenal atrophy. Secondary adrenal insufficiency resulting from decreased ACTH or CRH is discussed further in Chapter 48.

Addison's Disease

Primary adrenal hypofunction or insufficiency, also known as Addison's disease, is relatively rare (estimated prevalence, 1 in 50,000). A major cause of Addison's disease today that accounts for 70% of all cases is autoimmune adrenalitis with circulating adrenal antibodies. This disorder may be associated with other autoimmune disorders such as Hashimoto's thyroiditis, hypoparathyroidism, diabetes mellitus, pernicious anemia, vitiligo, and primary ovarian failure. Polyglandular autoimmune disease type II (Schmidt's syndrome) is a form of Addison's that occurs most commonly in females aged 20 to 40. A rarer form, type I, occurs in children and is associated with chronic mucocutaneous candidiasis and hypoparathyroidism. In both forms, an adrenal autoantibody frequently is directed against the enzyme 21-hydroxylase. Other causes of primary adrenal failure are listed in Box 51-4. Tuberculosis was the leading cause of adrenal failure in the first half of the 20th century.

Symptoms of Addison's disease begin to appear after about 90% of the adrenal cortex has been destroyed (see Box 51-4). The disease usually develops slowly with progressive loss of cortisol and increasing ACTH levels, resulting in hyperpigmentation of the patient because of the melanocyte-stimulating hormone properties of ACTH. Sodium loss and potassium retention result from coincident aldosterone deficiency. Hypoglycemia may be caused by cortisol deficiency. These symptoms may be vague and nonspecific. However, after stress caused by illness, surgery, or trauma, some patients may present with an acute life-threatening disease that is termed an *addisonian crisis.* An addisonian crisis, which is the result of an acute deficiency of both mineralocorticoids and glucocorticoids, can evolve rapidly into circulatory shock. Signs of addisonian crisis are listed in Box 51-4. Hyperkalemia and hyponatremia are common laboratory findings, along with hemoconcentration and elevated urea levels that result from fluid loss. Hyperkalemia may be severe enough to induce cardiac arrhythmias and cardiac arrest.

Congenital adrenal hyperplasia, which was discussed in the previous section, can lead to primary adrenal insufficiency. Drugs such as metyrapone, used in the treatment of Cushing's syndrome, *o,p′*-DDD (mitotane), used in the treatment of adrenal cancer, and other therapeutic agents such as ketoconazole and etomidate, which interfere with steroid synthetic pathways, have the potential to cause primary adrenal insufficiency.

The X-linked form of **adrenoleukodystrophy** (ALD) also should be considered in the differential diagnosis of primary adrenal insufficiency in the male patient. ALD occurs more frequently than is recognized, with up to 40% of males with Addison's disease having this problem. The defect is caused by deficiency of a peroxisomal enzyme (lignoceroyl CoA ligase), which results in decreased oxidation and therefore accumulation of very long chain fatty acids (VLCFAs). Pathological changes are noted in the adrenal cortex, testes, CNS white matter, and peripheral nervous system. Cells of the adrenal gland in tissues of the zona fasciculata and zona reticularis become swollen with lamellar inclusions consisting of cholesterol esters of VLCFAs, and they eventually atrophy and die. Patients with ALD may present with adrenal insufficiency alone, a combination of neurological and adrenal problems, or neurological problems alone. Neurological problems include emotional lability, failure at school, and hyperactivity that progresses to visual impairment, diffuse cerebral demyelination, seizures, mental deterioration, and death.

The primary adrenal insufficiency in ALD is mainly the result of diminished cortisol reserve. Primary gonadal insufficiency is a problem in 20% of patients with decreased testosterone and increased gonadotropins. Bone marrow transplantation may arrest progression of the disease in those with mild neurological disorder at the time of treatment.

Patients with secondary adrenal insufficiency usually do not experience symptoms related to hypoaldosteronism because aldosterone synthesis and secretion depend on the renin-angiotensin system rather than on ACTH. Hyperpigmentation is not a feature of this disorder. However, patients with secondary adrenal insufficiency may show other signs of hypothalamic or pituitary disease, including concomitant hypogonadism and hypothyroidism. Symptoms common to both primary and secondary disease of the adrenal cortex include weakness, hypoglycemia, weight loss, and gastrointestinal discomfort.

Box 51-4

Major Causes and Clinical Features of Primary Adrenal Insufficiency

Causes

- Autoimmune adrenalitis
- Granulomatous disease
  - Tuberculosis
  - Histoplasmosis
  - Sarcoidosis
- Neoplastic infiltration
- Hemochromatosis
- Amyloidosis
- Bilateral adrenalectomy
- Infarction
- Infectious disease
- Drugs (metyrapone, ketoconazole, mitotane)
- Adrenoleukodystrophy
- Congenital adrenal hyperplasia

Clinical Features

- Muscle weakness
- Fatigue
- Weight loss
- Orthostatic hypotension
- Pigmentation
- Anorexia
- Addisonian crisis
- Fever
- Dehydration
- Nausea
- Hypotension
- Circulatory shock
- Abdominal pain

Patients prescribed glucocorticoid therapy for 3 weeks or less generally experience only transient hypothalamic-pituitary-adrenal axis suppression. In cases of long-term treatment, dosages must be tapered gradually.

Disorders of the Adrenal Medulla: Pheochromocytoma

Pheochromocytoma, a relatively rare, usually benign tumor that arises from chromaffin cells, results in hypersecretion of the catecholamines, epinephrine and norepinephrine. It is estimated that 0.1% to 0.6% of patients with persistent diastolic hypertension may have this tumor. Although it is a rare cause of hypertension, this tumor is important to diagnose because it is surgically curable, and, even more significant, it can cause death from acute hypertensive attacks. Despite its rarity (prevalence in patients with adrenal incidentalomas is estimated at 5%), all patients with an adrenal mass should be screened for this condition. This tumor can occur as an isolated problem at any age, for example, 10% of pheochromocytomas are reported in children. The overall incidence is estimated at 1 to 2 per 100,000. The autopsy incidence is considerably higher at 0.05%. Pheochromocytomas are discovered most commonly from the third to the fifth decade of life.

Approximately 80% to 85% of pheochromocytomas occur in the adrenal glands, with the remainder occurring in extra-adrenal chromafin cells, anywhere from the base of the brain to the lower abdomen. Tumors from extra-adrenal chromaffin tissue are referred to as paragangliomas. Most of the paragangliomas in the head and neck do not produce catecholamines. Approximately 10% of pheochromocytomas are bilateral or multiple, and approximately 10% are malignant.

Pheochromocytomas can also occur as an inheritable disorder. In this case, they may be associated with multiple endocrine neoplasia (MEN) type 2A syndrome; which manifests as pheochromocytoma, hyperparathyroidism, and medullary carcinoma of the thyroid; or MEN type 2B, which manifests as multiple mucosal neuromas, medullary carcinoma of the thyroid, and pheochromocytoma. Approximately 50% of patients with MEN 2A or B will develop a pheochromocytoma. A significant association with neurofibromatosis (von Recklinghausen's disease) has been noted, with up to 5% of patients developing a pheochromocytoma; and with von Hippel-Lindau disease, with 20% of patients possibly affected. Germline mutations in five genes are responsible for familial pheochromocytoma: the *RET* protooncogene, leading to MEN 2A and 2B; the von Hippel-Lindau gene *(VHL),* causing von Hippel-Lindau syndrome; the neurofibromatosis type 1 gene *(NF1),* which is associated with von Recklinghausen's disease; and recently identified genes that encode the B- and D-subunits of mitochondrial succinate dehydrogenase (*SDHB* and *SDHD*), which are associated with familial paragangliomas and pheochromocytomas. Mutations of each of the *SDHB* and *SDHD* genes have been seen in about 3% to 11% of patients with nonsyndromic pheochromocytoma; they mainly occur as paragangliomas in the head, chest, and abdomen. Head and neck paragangliomas are associated more commonly with *SDHD* than with *SDHB* mutations. *SDHB* mutations in 50% of cases are associated with malignant disease. *SDHD* mutations are imprinted maternally, therefore patients with a mutation inherited from the father develop the disease, and those who inherit from the mother are disease free.

Pheochromocytomas may release their hormones in a sustained or episodic fashion. Clinically, the most significant finding is persistent, labile, or paroxysmal hypertension; other common findings are summarized in Box 51-5. Many of the symptoms may be persistent or episodic, although some patients are totally asymptomatic. Episodes can be as infrequent as once every few weeks or as frequent as 20 to 30 times daily, with attacks persisting for less than a minute or for as long as a week. The symptom pattern depends on the specific catecholamine secreted by the tumor. Rarely, hypotension may be the clinical problem. This is the case if the tumor primarily secretes epinephrine, dopa, or dopamine. Some patients may first present to the physician with cardiac hypertrophy or cardiac failure. It must be emphasized that the clinical symptoms are often subtle and are not specific for pheochromocytoma. Nevertheless, if headaches, palpitations, and sweating are all present together, the specificity of this combination is reported to be greater than 90%. A common cause of death in patients with unsuspected pheochromocytoma is hypertensive or hypotensive crisis precipitated by surgery. Paroxysmal attacks may be precipitated by palpation of the tumor, postural changes, emotional trauma, and even rarely micturition (in the case of a rare bladder tumor).

Box 51-5
Major Causes and Clinical Features of Pheochromocytoma

Causes
Benign adrenal chromaffin cell tumor (80%)
Malignant adrenal chromaffin cell tumor (10%)
Extra-adrenal chromaffin cell tumor (10%)

Clinical Features
Episodic or sustained hypertension
Headache
Sweating
Palpitations with or without tachycardia
Nervousness
Weight loss
Nausea
Weakness or fatigue
Less common:
- Flushing
- Dyspnea
- Dizziness

KEY CONCEPTS BOX 51-5

- Cushing's syndrome resulting from excess cortisol production is caused by iatrogenic treatment, pituitary tumor secreting ACTH, ectopic tumor secreting ACTH, and autonomous secreting adrenal adenoma and carcinoma (ACTH independent).
- Primary hyperaldosteronism (Conn's syndrome) is caused by aldosterone-producing adrenal adenoma and idiopathic hyperaldosteronism associated with bilateral adrenal hyperplasia.
- Congenital adrenal hyperplasia (CAH) is caused by an enzymatic block in the steroid synthetic pathway, most commonly 21-hydroxylase deficiency.
- Primary adrenal insufficiency is also known as Addison's disease. The major cause is autoimmune adrenalitis.
- Pheochromocytoma, a benign tumor arising from chromaffin cells in the adrenal glands or extra-adrenal tissues, is a rare cause of hypertension resulting from hypersecretion of the catecholamines.

SECTION OBJECTIVES BOX 51-6

- Explain the principle and interpretation of the following tests used to diagnose or determine the cause of Cushing's syndrome: salivary cortisol, overnight low-dose dexamethasone suppression, 24-hour urinary free cortisol, morning and afternoon serum cortisol, 2-day low-dose dexamethasone suppression test, plasma ACTH, CT scan, CRH stimulation test.
- Explain the principle and interpretation of the following tests used to diagnose primary hyperaldosteronism: serum aldosterone to plasma renin activity ratio (ARR), oral salt loading test, intravenous saline infusion test, fludrocortisone suppression test, and captopril suppression test.
- Explain the clinical usefulness of serum 17-hydroxyprogesterone assays for the diagnosis of congenital adrenal hyperplasia.
- Explain the principle and interpretation of the following tests used to diagnose primary adrenal insufficiency (Addison's disease): serum ACTH, baseline cortisol, ACTH stimulation test, prolonged ACTH stimulation test, and plasma very long chain saturated fatty acids.
- Explain the clinical usefulness of the following tests used to diagnose pheochromocytoma: urinary VMA, metanephrines, total catecholamines, or fractionated catecholamines; plasma epinephrine, norepinephrine, and free metanephrines; and the clonidine suppression test.

CHANGE OF ANALYTE IN DISEASE
(see Table 51-1)

Hyperadrenalism

Cushing's Syndrome

Patients with the conditions listed in Box 51-2 and on p. 1010 should undergo screening for Cushing's syndrome. Especially at-risk groups are those with poorly controlled diabetes (2% to 5% prevalence of Cushing's syndrome), patients with osteoporosis (3% with mild hypercortisolism), women with polycystic ovary syndrome, and individuals with adrenal incidentalomas (>2 cm; 9% with hypercortisolism). In the laboratory investigation of Cushing's syndrome, the first step is to establish that the patient actually has autonomous cortisol production, or Cushing's syndrome. Once this has been established, the next step is to identify the cause of Cushing's syndrome.

Table 51-1 Change of Analyte With Diseases

Disease	24 Hour Urinary Free Cortisol	17-OHCS	Plasma ACTH	Urinary Aldosterone	Serum Aldosterone	Plasma Cortisol	Plasma Renin Activity	Urine or Plasma Catecholamines	Urine Vanillylmandelic Acid Metanephrine
Hypercortical Disease									
Primary Cushing's syndrome	↑	↑	↓			±			
Cushing's disease (secondary)	↑	↑	±			±			
Ectopic ACTH	↑	↑	↑			±			
Primary hyperaldosteronism				↑	↑		↓		
Secondary hyperaldosteronism				↑	↑		↑		
Hypocortical Disease									
Primary	±	↓	↑			↓			
Secondary	±	↓	↓			↓			
Pheochromocytoma								↑	↑

↑, Elevated; ±, variable response; ↓, diminished.
ACTH, Adrenocorticotropic hormone; *17-OHCS,* 17-hydroxycorticosteroids.

The diagnosis of Cushing's syndrome requires biochemical verification of (1) loss of normal circadian rhythm (a hallmark of Cushing's syndrome); (2) loss of the physiological negative feedback of cortisol, which is assessed by means of the low-dose **dexamethasone suppression test;** and (3) cortisol hypersecretion. Therefore, screening and diagnostic tests for Cushing's syndrome may include late-night salivary cortisol, an overnight low-dose dexamethasone suppression test, and 24-hour urinary free cortisol.

Measurement of salivary cortisol has been proposed for the investigation of Cushing's syndrome; the sample is collected at 11 PM, which is the usual nadir of cortisol secretion. Elevated late-night salivary cortisol levels appear to be the earliest and most sensitive screening test for Cushing's syndrome. Silent hypercortisolism or subclinical Cushing's syndrome may be characterized more frequently by a subtle increase in late-night cortisol secretion than by alteration of 24 hour urine cortisol excretion. False-positive late-night salivary cortisol can occur in patients with hypertension, advanced age, and psychiatric problems; however, repeat testing is often normal in these cases. Elevated levels of late-night salivary cortisol may also be viewed as a predictor of insulin resistance in patients who have a clinically unapparent adrenal adenoma.

Another important test that should be performed initially is the overnight low-dose dexamethasone suppression test. Dexamethasone is a synthetic glucocorticoid that is 30 times as potent as cortisol; it does not cross-react in standard immunoassays for cortisol. The patient takes 1 mg of dexamethasone at 11 PM and comes to the laboratory for a plasma cortisol determination at 8:00 the following morning. A morning cortisol level less than 50 nmol/L (18 μg/L) is normal and usually excludes Cushing's syndrome. Levels greater than 280 nmol/L (100 μg/L) indicate hypercortisolism. False-positive results can be seen in patients with some forms of mental depression, stress-induced hypercortisolism, pseudo–Cushing's syndrome resulting from chronic alcoholism, and increased levels of cortisol-binding globulin associated with pregnancy or the use of birth control pills. False-positive results also are seen in patients given drugs such as phenytoin or rifampin that increase the rate of clearance of dexamethasone. However, the dexamethasone suppression test remains an ideal screening test for Cushing's syndrome, because false-negative results in screening procedures are a more serious problem than false-positive results.

Estimation of a 24-hour urinary free cortisol (UFC) level is another useful initial investigative test. This is in essence a direct measure of the amount of cortisol that is not bound to plasma protein and is excreted unmetabolized in the urine over a 24-hour period. A 24-hour urine cortisol determination is required along with a urine creatinine determination to ensure the adequacy of collection. It also has been suggested by some that up to three separate 24-hour collections should be carried out because of the variability of cortisol output. Immunoassays for urinary free cortisol are not specific enough for accurate estimation. Metabolites of cortisol and their conjugated products cross-react with the antibodies employed and therefore consistently overestimate the true urinary free cortisol concentration. Even if an extraction step is included to remove the more water-soluble conjugates, results may be twice or more as high as the true value. The most accurate way to determine urinary free cortisol is by liquid chromatography tandem mass spectrometry (LC-MS/MS) analysis. Morning cortisol levels are not elevated in many patients with Cushing's syndrome, whereas late-night cortisol usually is increased. Therefore, a small increase in cortisol production at the circadian nadir may not be detected as an increase in UFC. The sensitivity of UFC is 45% to 71% at 100% specificity, so its sensitivity and specificity are not optimal as an initial screening test. Pseudo-Cushing's states may have false-positive UFC testing. UFC however is useful in confirming Cushing's syndrome.

A traditional test that is no longer part of the standard workup for Cushing's syndrome is the morning and afternoon serum cortisol determination. Serum cortisol values usually display diurnal variation, with highest levels occurring in the morning and lowest levels in the early evening. Evening values usually are less than 50% of early morning concentrations. Classically, samples are drawn at 8 AM (reference interval, 140 to 660 nmol/L; 50 to 239 μg/L) and at 4 PM (reference interval, 50 to 330 nmol/L; 18 to 119 μg/L). Many patients with Cushing's syndrome will not show this diurnal variation and will have elevated concentrations at both times. However, the release of cortisol is episodic, and considerable overlap has been noted between healthy individuals and patients with Cushing's syndrome. In differentiating patients with Cushing's syndrome from healthy patients, it is best to take the sample at the time when cortisol is usually at its lowest concentration in the circulation. This happens to occur at midnight, but because it is not always practical to draw blood at this time, the more practical time of 4 PM is often chosen. Midnight plasma cortisol levels less than 50 nmol/L (80 μg/dL) effectively excludes Cushing's syndrome. But this level is not specific. To maximize the specificity of this test, a higher cut-off value of 200 nmol/L (7.5 μg/dL) has been suggested (see Pivonello et al). Loss of diurnal variation also can occur with stress, anorexia, obesity, and emotional disturbances, or it may be caused by sedatives, stimulants, or psychotropic or antiepileptic drugs.

Another variation of the overnight low-dose dexamethasone suppression test is the 2-day low-dose dexamethasone suppression test, which can be used to confirm that the patient has Cushing's syndrome. This test is time consuming and is not included in some of the recent protocols for this disorder. Some now suggest that the high-dose dexamethasone suppression test, which is discussed later, should be performed first. With the classic low-dose dexamethasone suppression test, the patient is given a total dose of 2 mg of dexamethasone per day for 2 days in 0.5 mg doses every 6 hours. This dose is equivalent to about four times the usual adrenal output. During the second day, a 24-hour urine specimen is collected for urinary free cortisol. Plasma cortisol measurements also may be performed. Patients with Cushing's syndrome generally will not show significant suppression of cortisol output with this dose of dexamethasone. Healthy patients should show greater than 50% suppression of urine cortisol output measured before the test is given. Urine cortisol excretion usually falls to less than 50 nmol/day (18 μg/day), and morning serum cortisol to less than 140 nmol/L (50 μg/L). For greater sensitivity, a normal result for serum cortisol could be set at <50 nmol/L. Generally, obesity does result in a normal response, but false-positive results may be seen with psychiatric illness, alcoholism, stress, glucocorticoid resistance, decreased absorbance of dexamethasone, and drugs that stimulate liver metabolism of dexamethasone (phenytoin, phenobarbital), and in people who do not follow instructions for performing the test. False-negative results are associated with chronic renal failure and hypothyroidism.

Once Cushing's syndrome has been confirmed, the cause of the disease must be determined. Several possible approaches can be used to determine the cause of Cushing's syndrome. Plasma ACTH levels, which can be measured by two-site immunometric assay, are essential in determining the specific cause of Cushing's syndrome as ACTH-independent or ACTH-dependent Cushing's syndrome. ACTH is a labile polypeptide hormone, and special precautions are required in its handling. Plasma samples should be collected on ice with an ethylenediaminetetraacetic acid (EDTA) phlebotomy tube, and the plasma should be separated in a refrigerated centrifuge and stored frozen. Assays for ACTH do not measure fragments of ACTH and do not react well with "big" ACTH, a precursor to ACTH that is produced by some tumors. Nondetectable levels of ACTH (<2 pmol/L) are suggestive of an adrenal tumor (ACTH-independent Cushing's syndrome). ACTH levels at the upper half of the reference interval (reference interval <11.4 pmol/L) and up to twice the upper limit of normal are consistent with a pituitary cause of Cushing's syndrome. Very high levels of ACTH (>50 pmol/L) are suggestive of an ectopic source, such as a malignant tumor. Overlap is seen in the plasma concentrations of ACTH associated with ectopic and pituitary causes of Cushing's syndrome.

If the morning plasma ACTH is suppressed in a patient with Cushing's syndrome, a computed tomography (CT) scan usually will identify an adrenal lesion. Adrenal adenomas usually are obvious because adjacent normal adrenal tissue and the contralateral adrenal have become atrophic because of the suppressed ACTH. With adrenal carcinoma, the gland is usually very large, with dimensions that may exceed 6 cm. Other features that help distinguish between adrenal adenoma and carcinoma include increased androgen production associated with adrenal carcinoma.

A single plasma ACTH at the lower end of the reference range does not exclude adrenal Cushing's, particularly in cases of mild or occult disease. When plasma ACTH is at the low end of the reference range, a CRH stimulation test should be performed: (1) the ACTH response to CRH should be blunted in adrenal Cushing's syndrome as the result of continued negative feedback from the elevated serum cortisol, (2) the ACTH response to CRH usually is exaggerated in Cushing's disease if the pituitary tumor expresses the CRH receptor.

The most difficult causes of Cushing's to differentiate are ectopic ACTH production and a pituitary adenoma. This differentiation was not necessary until the 1970s because bilateral adrenalectomy was standard treatment for both. Starting in the late 1970s, transsphenoidal surgery became the treatment of choice for pituitary adenoma.

In distinguishing between Cushing's disease and occult ectopic ACTH syndrome, pituitary imaging with magnetic resonance imaging (MRI) is the required initial study. The presence of an unequivocal pituitary lesion >6 mm on MRI in the absence of clinical features of an ectopic ACTH-secreting tumor usually confirms the diagnosis of Cushing's disease and may justify proceeding with pituitary microsurgery. If the pituitary MRI result is normal or equivocal, bilateral inferior petrosal sinus sampling (IPSS) of the pituitary gland for ACTH should be performed. IPSS for ACTH with CRH stimulation is the only study that has the potential for a diagnostic sensitivity and specificity for Cushing's disease that are higher than its pretest probability. This study must be performed in an experienced center dedicated to performing it safely and correctly.

A high-dose dexamethasone suppression test (HDDST) has been performed to differentiate ACTH-secreting pituitary tumor (Cushing's disease) from ectopic ACTH syndrome. However, recent studies show that continued use of HDDST is not justified because little difference may be evident between the results of HDDST in patients with Cushing's disease and in those with the ectopic ACTH syndrome.

The metyrapone stimulation test has been used to delineate the cause of Cushing's syndrome. Metyrapone acts by inhibiting the enzyme 11-hydroxylase and thereby blocking the synthesis of cortisol. However, most laboratories do not perform this protocol because of the lack of ready availability of an 11-deoxycortisol assay.

The test that is now considered definitive in differentiating pituitary causes of Cushing's syndrome from other causes is bilateral IPSS of the pituitary gland after CRH administration. In this test, a radiologist inserts catheters into both inferior petrosal sinuses, which drain from the anterior pituitary. Venous samples are drawn before and 2, 5, and 10 minutes after 100 μg of CRH has been administered intravenously. The ACTH gradient between the inferior petrosal sinus and peripheral venous sites after CRH stimulation is greater than 3 if the patient has a pituitary tumor. The average gradient seen in patients with a pituitary tumor that is secreting ACTH is about 50. A gradient of less than 2 indicates a nonpituitary source of ACTH. Because samples are taken simultaneously from the right and left sinuses, it is possible to localize the tumor to the right or left side of the anterior pituitary in about 80% of cases. This is useful information for subsequent surgical procedures. If no lesion is identifiable, the surgeon may remove only the left or the right side of the pituitary, thereby lessening the risk of panhypopituitarism.

No widespread agreement suggests that this test should be performed routinely in all patients who are suspected of having pituitary tumors. Data from the National Institutes of Health (NIH) indicate that 50% suppression of cortisol output by high-dose dexamethasone may be inadequate to confirm that the patient has a pituitary tumor. NIH recommends that for confirmation of the diagnosis of a pituitary tumor, urinary free cortisol should be decreased by 90% from baseline value. In NIH experience, no patient with ectopic ACTH has experienced cortisol suppression to this degree. The more invasive petrosal sampling protocol described earlier then may be reserved for those patients who show only partial suppression of urine cortisol excretion.

The pretest probability of Cushing's disease is very high: 90% to 95% of patients with ACTH-dependent Cushing's syndrome having a pituitary microadenoma. Pituitary Cushing's syndrome is much more common in women than in men, with a female-to-male ratio of 7 or 8 : 1, whereas with ectopic ACTH, the ratio is approximately equal. Forty percent of men with Cushing's syndrome may have an ectopic source of ACTH. A woman with mild to moderate hypercortisolism, normal or slightly elevated plasma ACTH, and normokalemia has at least a 95% likelihood of having Cushing's disease. A patient with extreme hypercortisolism, hypokalemia, and marked elevations of plasma ACTH may be more likely to have an occult ectopic ACTH-secreting tumor.

Miscellaneous Tests for the Investigation of Cushing's Syndrome

Other new tests have been developed to aid in the distinction of mild Cushing's from pseudo–Cushing's syndrome. A 48-hour low-dose dexamethasone suppression test is followed by an immediate CRH stimulation test (CRH + 2-day low-dose dexamethasone suppression test [LDDST]). In this test, cortisol should remain suppressed in normal individuals and in those with pseudo–Cushing's syndrome, but not in those with Cushing's syndrome.

In summary, the three diagnostic studies (late-night salivary cortisol, LDDST, and UFC) for Cushing's syndrome are complementary screening tests. Late-night salivary cortisol appears to be the most useful screening test (sensitivity and specificity >90% to 95%, and measurements are easy to repeat). Late-night salivary cortisol is as important in diagnosing mild Cushing's syndrome as thyroid-stimulating hormone (TSH) is in diagnosing mild primary hypothyroidism. UFC and LDDST should be performed to further confirm the diagnosis.

When a salivary cortisol assay is not available, and a patient is suspected of having Cushing's syndrome, begin with an overnight dexamethasone suppression test. Confirm a positive result with a 24-hour urinary free cortisol with or without a subsequent low-dose dexamethasone suppression test. If necessary, a CRH + 2-day low-dose dexamethasone suppression test is performed to exclude pseudo–Cushing's syndrome. In determining the cause of Cushing's syndrome, ACTH measurements are useful. For ACTH-dependent hypercortisolism (a detectable ACTH and increased cortisol), pituitary MRI is performed to identify Cushing's disease resulting from a pituitary adenoma. If pituitary MRI is normal or equivocal, bilateral petrosal sinus sampling for ACTH after CRH administration should provide a definitive diagnosis. See Fig. 51-9 for an outline of the diagnostic protocol.

Primary Hyperaldosteronism

Conn's syndrome, or primary hyperaldosteronism, is an important cause of secondary hypertension. Indications for screening hypertensive patients for primary aldosteronism include (1) spontaneous hypokalemia (<3.5 mmol/L), (2) profound diuretic-induced hypokalemia (<3.0 mmol/L), (3) hypertension refractory to treatment with three or more drugs, (4) adrenal incidentaloma, and (5) onset of hypertension at a young age (<20 y).

The previous, classic approach to screening, confirmation, and localization of the tumor in Conn's syndrome began with detection of hypokalemia. Because it is recognized that many of these patients do not have hypokalemia, it has been suggested that all hypertensive patients who are unresponsive to medical treatment should be screened by determining their random serum aldosterone–to–plasma renin activity (or mass) ratio (ARR). An increased ratio should be confirmed with an acute saline suppression test to demonstrate nonsuppressible aldosterone secretion in the settings of extracellular fluid (ECF) volume expansion. In addition to an elevated ARR, the serum aldosterone level must be increased to above the reference interval to complete the diagnosis of Conn's syndrome. This extra precaution is needed because an increased ARR may be seen when plasma renin activity is low and aldosterone concentration is low-normal. Elevated ARR also may be seen in patients with chronic renal disease and hyperkalemia, which stimulates aldosterone secretion directly. The ARR should be used only as a screening procedure.

An advantage of the ARR is that no posture restrictions are required when the sample is drawn; generally, the patient only needs to be seated for the blood draw. The test may be performed while the patient is taking antihypertensive medications. Mineralocorticoid receptor antagonists (e.g., spironolactone, eplerenone) and the high-dose sodium channel blocker amiloride are the only medications that absolutely interfere with interpretation of the ratio and should be discontinued for at least 6 weeks before patients are assessed. Angiotensin-converting enzyme (ACE) inhibitors may falsely increase renin in some patients with primary hyperaldosteronism. Suppressed renin in the presence of an ACE inhibitor, however, is a strong indicator of primary aldosteronism. ACE inhibitors, angiotensin receptor blockers (ARBs), non–potassium-sparing diuretics, β-adrenergic blockers, and central α_2-agonists do not have to be discontinued.

In patients with suspected primary aldosteronism, screening can be accomplished by measuring a morning (preferably at between 0800 and 1000 hours) ambulatory (sitting position after resting at least 15 minutes) paired random aldosterone and renin activity (or renin mass). A positive test result is defined as the combination of a high ARR and an increased aldosterone. The cutoff for a high ARR is laboratory dependent and, more specifically, renin activity assay dependent. All positive results should be followed by a confirmatory aldosterone suppression test to verify autonomous aldosterone production.

Several approaches can be taken to confirm autonomous aldosterone secretion: the oral salt loading test, the intravenous saline infusion test, and the fludrocortisone suppression test. The principle of these tests is that ECF volume expansion will inhibit renin release and subsequent aldosterone secretion

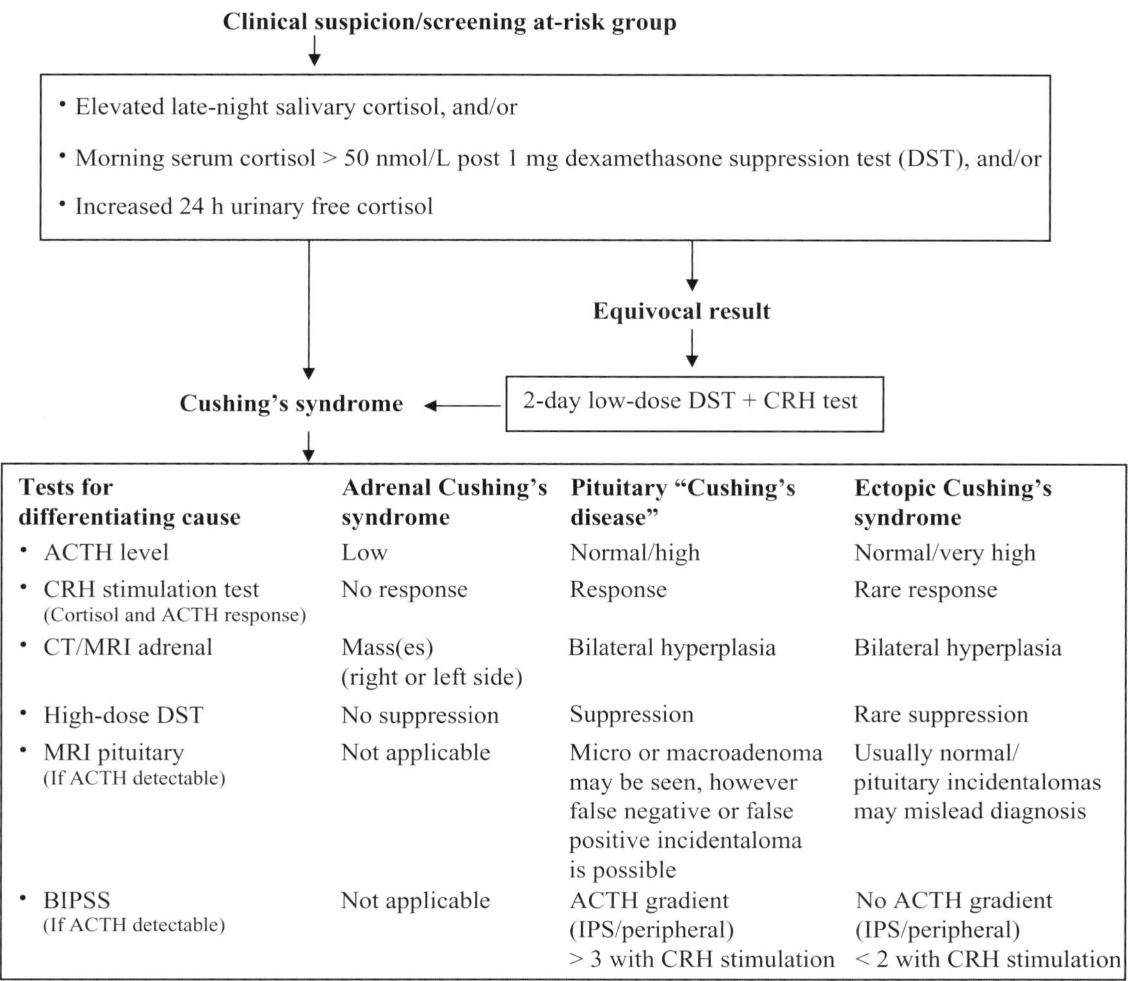

Tests for differentiating cause	Adrenal Cushing's syndrome	Pituitary "Cushing's disease"	Ectopic Cushing's syndrome
• ACTH level	Low	Normal/high	Normal/very high
• CRH stimulation test (Cortisol and ACTH response)	No response	Response	Rare response
• CT/MRI adrenal	Mass(es) (right or left side)	Bilateral hyperplasia	Bilateral hyperplasia
• High-dose DST	No suppression	Suppression	Rare suppression
• MRI pituitary (If ACTH detectable)	Not applicable	Micro or macroadenoma may be seen, however false negative or false positive incidentaloma is possible	Usually normal/ pituitary incidentalomas may mislead diagnosis
• BIPSS (If ACTH detectable)	Not applicable	ACTH gradient (IPS/peripheral) > 3 with CRH stimulation	No ACTH gradient (IPS/peripheral) < 2 with CRH stimulation

Fig. 51-9 Laboratory protocol for the investigation of Cushing's syndrome. See text for details.

in healthy individuals, but not in patients with primary aldosteronism.

Oral Salt Loading Test

The patient is on a high-salt diet with NaCl 12 g/d (200 mmol/d) (supplemented with NaCl tablets if needed) for 3 days. On the third day of the high-salt diet, a 24 hour urine collection for aldosterone excretion, creatinine, and Na^+ is collected. Urinary aldosterone greater than 12 µg/24 hr (33 nmol/24 hr) with concomitant urinary Na^+ excretion >200 mmol/24 hr (to document adequate Na^+ repletion) confirms the diagnosis.

Intravenous Saline Infusion Test

Another approach is to measure supine serum aldosterone before and after infusion of 2 L of normal saline (0.9% NaCl) over a 4-hour time span. Healthy patients and patients with essential hypertension will have serum aldosterone suppressed to <50 ng/L (140 pmol/L). Because hospitalization is required, this is an expensive test to perform.

Fludrocortisone Suppression Test

Fludrocortisone acetate is administered at 0.1 mg every 6 hours for 4 days in combination with NaCl tablets 2 g three times daily with food. On the fourth day, at between 0800 and 1000 hours, while the patient is upright, the serum/plasma aldosterone is measured. Healthy patients will have aldosterone suppressed to <60 ng/L (166 pmol/L).

During aldosterone suppression testing, care must be taken to ensure that K^+ stores are replenished, and blood pressure should be monitored to avoid exacerbation of increased blood pressure. This test is not advised in patients with evidence of heart failure.

The **captopril suppression test** may be used as a confirmatory test. Captopril is a drug that is used to treat some patients with hypertension. Its primary mechanism of action is inhibition of angiotensin-converting enzyme, which converts angiotensin I to angiotensin II. Patients without Conn's syndrome will respond with a drop in serum aldosterone, but patients with Conn's syndrome will not suppress aldosterone levels. Aldosterone usually is measured 2 to 3 hours after a 25-mg oral dose of captopril is given. The expected response is that serum aldosterone should decrease to <100 ng/L (<280 pmol/L).

Once the diagnosis of primary aldosteronism has been established, the cause of the disorder must be determined, so that the proper course of treatment can be chosen.

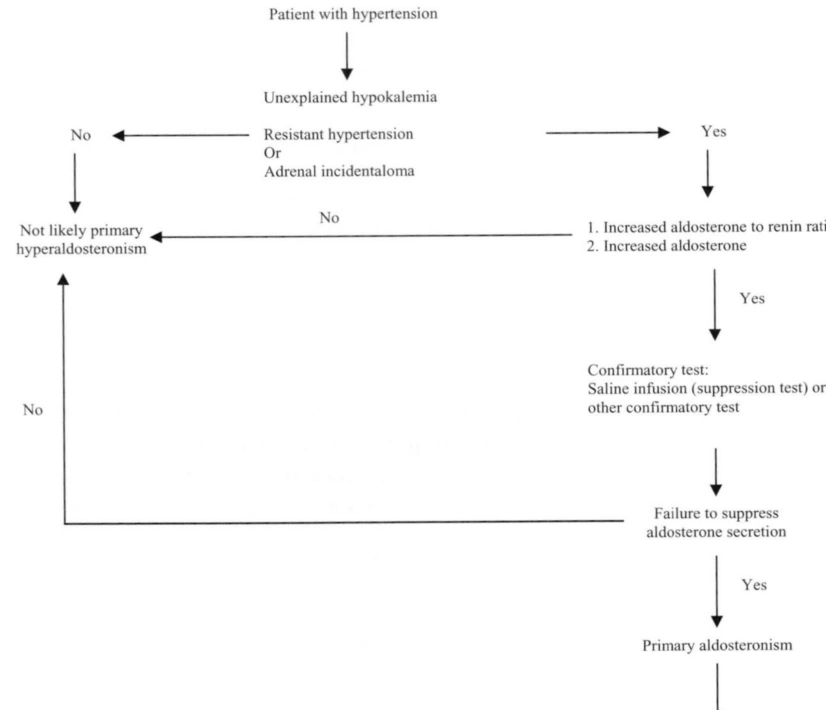

Fig. 51-10 Laboratory protocol for the investigation of a patient with suspected primary hyperaldosteronism (Conn's syndrome).

Radiological imaging is limited because lesions associated with primary aldosteronism may be small (<2 cm). A small adenoma may be labeled incorrectly as IHA on the basis of CT findings of bilateral nodularity or normal-appearing adrenals. Also, apparent adrenal microadenomas actually may represent areas of hyperplasia. In addition, nonfunctioning adrenal masses are common and may produce false-positive results. The overall accuracy of imaging is only 75%.

The best procedure for localizing the lesion is bilateral adrenal venous sampling (AVS). The success of this procedure is dependent on the ability of the radiologist to place the catheter accurately. Results can be improved by simultaneous determination of ACTH-stimulated cortisol from both adrenal veins, which should be symmetrical. The cortisol-corrected ratio of ipsilateral-to-contralateral concentration of serum aldosterone is usually greater than 10:1 in patients with APA, >4:1 in patients with primary (unilateral) adrenal hyperplasia (PAH), and <1.8:1 in patients with IHA. Although this test is considered the standard, it usually is reserved for those cases in which the probability of APA or PAH is high after an adrenal CT scan. After adrenalectomy for APA, 70% of patients are normotensive 1 year later.

A problem with localization and confirmation of Conn's syndrome is the presence of adrenal incidentalomas, which can lead to a false diagnosis of adrenal adenoma when the actual diagnosis is bilateral hyperplasia. Another concern is that in the presence of hypokalemia, aldosterone may be suppressed, giving a false impression of an appropriate level of aldosterone. The test should be repeated after serum potassium has been normalized.

A posture stimulation test has been used in the past to distinguish between APA and IHA. In patients with APA, aldosterone levels may drop after an upright posture is assumed, whereas in those with IHA, aldosterone usually rises. This indicates that plasma renin activity still may be involved in aldosterone regulation in patients with IHA despite low renin levels. However, some patients with APA have a positive response to upright posture (sensitive to renin-angiotensin II). Another biochemical parameter that can be measured is 18-hydroxycorticosterone, the final precursor in the synthesis of aldosterone. The level of this substance is higher in patients with APA than in those with IHA. This test has limited availability, and its accuracy in distinguishing between patients with APA and IHA is less than 80%.

A scheme for the investigation of primary hyperaldosteronism is outlined in Fig. 51-10. The laboratory should play a major part in advising on the collection and handling of specimens required to ensure a successful outcome of these expensive investigations.

Congenital Adrenal Hyperplasia

The reported incidence of congenital adrenal hyperplasia (CAH) ranges from 1:5000 to 1:62,000 births. The most common cause is a 21-hydroxylase deficiency, which accounts for 95% of all cases. A child with this disorder may have evidence of adrenal insufficiency, as was discussed earlier, and may be investigated from this point of view, as is outlined in the next section of this chapter (hypoadrenalism). However, the child also may suffer the biochemical consequences of excess androgen, with females showing signs of virilization and males demonstrating precocious puberty. The definitive test for this condition is the finding in serum of an elevated serum level of 17-hydroxyprogesterone, the immediate precursor to the metabolic block. Measurements of testosterone in serum and pregnanetriol, a metabolite of 17-hydroxyprogesterone, in urine also may be useful. Measurement of serum 17-hydroxyprogesterone is helpful in following the adequacy of glucocorticoid replacement therapy in patients with 21-hydroxylase deficiency. The reference interval for 17-hydroxyprogesterone is 0.5 to 3 nmol/L. Levels may be higher in normal maternal and fetal blood but may drop dramatically after birth and reach adult reference interval levels by 2 to 7 days. Homozygotes for the 21-hydroxylase deficiency have 17-hydroxyprogesterone levels in the 300 to 3000 nmol/L range, whereas heterozygotes have levels between 3 and 30 nmol/L.

An 11-hydroxylase deficiency may also lead to virilization or precocious puberty but is most frequently associated with hypertension and can best be diagnosed by measurement of serum or plasma 11-deoxycortisol. Diagnostic tests for the other forms of congenital adrenal hyperplasia are not discussed because of the rarity of these disorders.

Hypoadrenalism, or Primary Adrenal Insufficiency (Addison's Disease)

When a patient has orthostatic (postural) hypotension, low serum sodium, and increased serum potassium, the possibility of primary adrenal insufficiency, or Addison's disease, should be considered. Samples should be drawn initially for ACTH and baseline cortisol determinations. Aldosterone determinations may be useful but usually are not performed. Patients with **hypoadrenalism** may have cortisol levels within the reference interval even if they have inadequate adrenal reserves. Several tests are now available to assess adrenal reserve capacity. These include the ACTH (synthetic) stimulation test (250 μg and 1 μg), the insulin hypoglycemia stimulation test, the metyrapone stimulation test, and the CRH stimulation test. The insulin hypoglycemia stimulation test and the metyrapone stimulation test are gold standard diagnositic tests. In most cases, an **ACTH stimulation test** is performed.

The ACTH stimulation test uses a synthetic form of ACTH (cosyntropin, Cortrosyn, synacthen) that consists of the first 24 amino acids of ACTH, which is injected intravenously or intramuscularly. The usual dose is 250 μg, which is supraphysiological. The 1 μg dose is apparently more sensitive, but the acceptable response to date is not as well standardized. Blood samples for serum cortisol should be drawn at 30 and 60 minutes after injection. A normal response to this stimulation test manifests as a rise in serum cortisol of at least 280 nmol/L (100 μg/L) to a level greater than 550 nmol/L (200 μg/L), unless the baseline value is already above 550 nmol/L. The fifth percentile for a normal response ranges from 510 to 626 nmol/L, depending on the study and the cortisol assay employed. A low baseline cortisol result with failure to respond to ACTH may be suggestive of primary adrenal failure, or may result from atrophy caused by long-term steroid therapy or pituitary insufficiency. In primary adrenal insufficiency, ACTH levels are greatly elevated (to >50 pmol/L), which in fact may be clinically apparent because of hyperpigmentation of the patient. In secondary adrenal insufficiency or atrophy resulting from exogenous steroids, ACTH levels will be suppressed (to <10 pmol/L). The insulin tolerance test, the metyrapone stimulation test, the CRH stimulation test, and the 4- to 8-hour ACTH infusion test have been advocated to confirm adrenal insufficiency in case of borderline results.

If the response to the cosyntropin stimulation test is abnormal and secondary adrenal insufficiency is suspected, a prolonged (3- to 5-day) ACTH stimulation test or an insulin-induced hypoglycemia stress test may be performed. Intravenous administration of ACTH over several days generally results in a gradual increase in cortisol output if the adrenal insufficiency is a result of long-term deficiency of ACTH from the pituitary. Hypoglycemia ordinarily stimulates release of ACTH from the pituitary. Failure to show increased ACTH or increased cortisol in response to hypoglycemia is suggestive of pituitary or hypothalamic disease. A CRH stimulation test also could be used and would yield results comparable to those of the insulin hypoglycemia test. Although CRH testing generally is not yet available at all diagnostic centers, this test is much safer.

A simplified scheme for the investigation of adrenal insufficiency is shown in Fig. 51-11.

Transient adrenal insufficiency can result from long-term use of glucocorticoids, which inhibit ACTH and CRH release, causing adrenal cortex atrophy. Short-term glucocorticoid therapy is rapidly reversible, but high-dose long-term therapy may result in adrenal insufficiency for as long as 2 years after discontinuation of the steroid medication, and patients are at risk for cardiovascular collapse when severely stressed. It is suggested that any patient who has received more than 20 to 30 mg per day of prednisone or the equivalent for 1 week or longer may be at risk for adrenal insufficiency. It is impossible to predict which patients will have a problem; therefore, a laboratory assessment of adrenal reserve should be routinely performed. If a random cortisol measurement is greater than 400 nmol/L (145 μg/L), the likelihood of a problem is not great. However, the best assessment for reserve capacity is the rapid ACTH stimulation test, which was discussed earlier. One remaining problem is that some patients may respond to acute stimulation but cannot sustain this response in chronic stressed states because of inadequate adrenal reserves. At present, no reliable standard or procedure is available for determining normalcy of the HPA response to sustained severe stress.

Adrenoleukodystrophy, which may be a cause of adrenal insufficiency in males, is diagnosed by measurement of increased levels of very long chain saturated fatty acids ($C_{26:0}$, $C_{25:0}$, $C_{24:0}$) in plasma, red blood cells, white blood cells, or cultured fibroblasts. This assay is available in very few centers. MRI may show characteristic white matter lesions.

Pheochromocytoma

It is important to diagnose pheochromocytoma early because of the potential for a life-threatening hypertensive crisis, which may be triggered by a surgical procedure, a major trauma, or

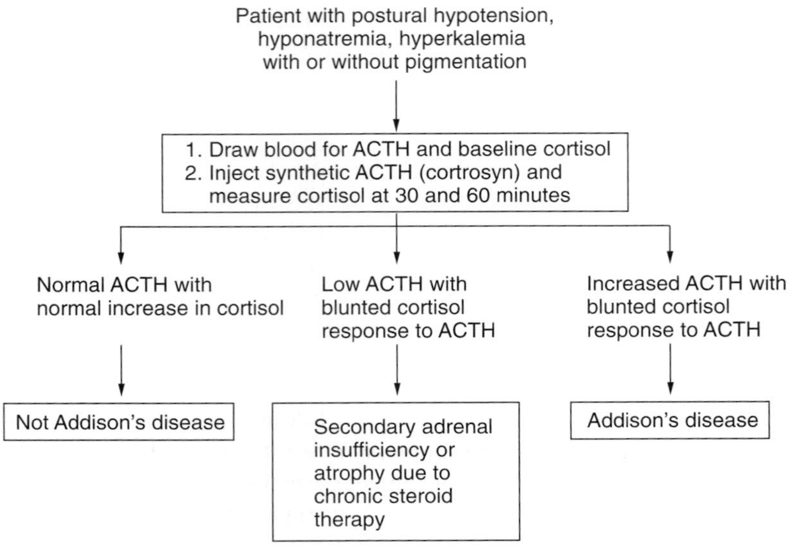

Patient with postural hypotension, hyponatremia, hyperkalemia with or without pigmentation

↓

1. Draw blood for ACTH and baseline cortisol
2. Inject synthetic ACTH (cortrosyn) and measure cortisol at 30 and 60 minutes

Normal ACTH with normal increase in cortisol	Low ACTH with blunted cortisol response to ACTH	Increased ACTH with blunted cortisol response to ACTH
↓	↓	↓
Not Addison's disease	Secondary adrenal insufficiency or atrophy due to chronic steroid therapy	Addison's disease

Fig. 51-11 Laboratory protocol for the investigation of Addison's disease. Please note that secondary adrenal insufficiency is unlikely to occur with hyperkalemia.

certain drugs used in the treatment of depression or hypertension. Indications for testing for pheochromocytoma include (1) paroxysmal, labile, and/or severe sustained hypertension refractory to usual antihypertensive therapy; (2) hypertension and symptoms suggestive of catecholamine excess (two or more of headaches, palpitations, sweating, sudden attacks of anxiety, etc.); (3) paradoxically elevated blood pressure response during anesthesia and surgery; (4) hypertension triggered by β-blockers, monoamine oxidase inhibitors, micturition, or changes in abdominal pressure; (5) adrenal incidentaloma; (6) medullary thyroid carcinoma or a family history of MEN type 2A or type 2B, von Hippel-Lindau syndrome, or von Recklinghausen's neurofibromatosis.

Laboratory tests used to investigate pheochromocytoma include measurement of urinary vanillylmandelic acid (VMA), metanephrines, total catecholamines, or fractionated catecholamines. In addition, measurements can be made of plasma epinephrine and norepinephrine, as well as plasma-free metanephrines (metanephrine and normetanephrine). Dynamic tests include the **clonidine suppression test.** High-performance liquid chromatography (HPLC) methods are considered to be analytically specific, and dietary restrictions are not required. Ideally, a 24-hour urine sample should be collected when the patient is not receiving any drugs, is not under stress, and is medically stable. Many drugs such as monoamine oxidase inhibitors and reserpine can alter catecholamine metabolism and may interfere with interpretation of the results. Increased catecholamine concentrations may be associated with administration of exogenous catecholamines (found in nose drops and appetite suppressants), amphetamines, vasodilators, α-adrenergic receptor antagonists (prazosin and phentolamine), diuretics with hyponatremia, caffeine, cigarette and marijuana smoking, β-blockers, and tricyclic antidepressants. Phenoxybenzamine (α-adrenergic receptor blocker, used to treat patients with suspected pheochromocytoma) and tricyclic antidepressants are major causes of false-positive results. Monoamine oxidase inhibitors will increase metanephrines levels up to fivefold. Other drugs, including clonidine, bromocriptine, and dexamethasone, may decrease catecholamine levels.

Plasma-free metanephrines and urinary-fractionated metanephrines (normetanephrine and metanephrine separately) are the most sensitive tests for diagnosis, and are the most suitable for reliable exclusion of pheochromocytoma. The increased sensitivity of metanephrines compared with catecholamines is because of the continuous production and release of O-methylated metabolites in tumors that contain elevated COMT levels. Although tumors produce and metabolize catecholamines, they do not always release catecholamines. The production and release of O-methylated metabolites is independent of the highly variable release of catecholamines.

One continuing problem is that patients with hypertension from other causes may have borderline deviations of catecholamines and their metabolites. Common findings in patients with essential hypertension include increased norepinephrine, normetanephrine, and VMA. Usually, these values are less than double the upper limit of the normotensive reference interval.

The most common pattern of urine-free catecholamine findings in patients with pheochromocytoma consists of increased levels of norepinephrine with smaller increases or normal levels of epinephrine and dopamine. A less common pattern is a pronounced increase in both norepinephrine and epinephrine with a smaller increase in dopamine, and even less frequent is a pronounced increase in epinephrine with smaller increases or normal levels of norepinephrine and dopamine. This last pattern is seen only in association with adrenal tumors. Some malignant pheochromocytomas may secrete large amounts of dopamine primarily. This is the result of a deficiency of dopamine-β-hydroxylase in malignant cells. An increase in urine norepinephrine is one of the more specific findings associated with pheochromocytoma when a value greater than 900 nmol/day (approximately twice the upper reference level) is used as the decision level. At this concentration, specificity of the assay is greatly improved without loss of sensitivity. Urine norepinephrine measurements are especially useful when the patient has episodic hypertension of short duration. A random urine sample collected shortly after the attack may indicate abnormal catecholamine excretion, whereas metabolite concentrations may be normal.

Considerable interest has been expressed in plasma catecholamine measurements, especially when they are combined with findings of the clonidine suppression test. Many conditions, including volume depletion, anxiety, exercise, anorexia, smoking, renal failure, and obesity, and several drugs such as L-dopa and methyldopa, can cause elevations of plasma catecholamines into the range seen in patients with pheochromocytoma. Sensitivity of plasma catecholamine measurements for the diagnosis of pheochromocytoma may be as high as 95%, but specificity is suboptimal. With plasma catecholamines, despite precautions to minimize stress during the evaluation period, a significant portion of patients with essential hypertension may have plasma norepinephrine concentrations in the equivocal range that could be the result of increased activity of the sympathetic nervous system (SNS).

The measurement of catecholamines in a 24-hour urine sample has several advantages. Urine collections induce minimal stress in the patient, and integration of production of catecholamines over 24 hours minimizes fluctuations in SNS activity.

The clonidine suppression test may be of some use in difficult to diagnose cases. Plasma catecholamines are measured before and 3 hours after administration of 0.3 mg of clonidine. Patients with pheochromocytoma show no suppression, whereas those with essential hypertension suppress their plasma catecholamine levels into the reference interval. Best results are attained with methods that are specific for free catecholamines. If conjugated catecholamines, which have longer half-lives, are included, false-positive results may occur. A recent modification of this protocol involves measurement of plasma normetanephrine instead of plasma norepinephrine after administration of clonidine. The positive and negative predictive values of this test improve from 97% to 100% and from 75% to 96%, respectively. Clonidine may cause severe hypotension, and patients must be observed closely during a clonidine challenge test.

No single test or 24-hour urine sample may be sufficiently sensitive to define the diagnosis of pheochromocytoma. If clinical suspicion is high, it is appropriate to analyze more than one urine sample and to measure free catecholamines and metabolites. Tumors larger than 50 g secrete a preponderance of metabolites because of intratumor metabolism. Tumors smaller than 50 g secrete a larger proportion of free catecholamines directly into the circulation. In our laboratory, we have seen patients with very large adrenal tumors whose free catecholamine output was well within normal limits, but whose catecholamine metabolite values (metanephrine and VMA) were strikingly abnormal. Appropriate patients should be screened with 24-hour urinary fractionated free catecholamines and fractionated urine metanephrines, analyzed by HPLC combined with electrochemical detection. In patients with episodic hypertension, analysis of a random urine sample, associated with the hypertensive episode, for fractionated free catecholamines may be useful. In very difficult cases, a clonidine suppression test combined with plasma catecholamine measurements may be useful. Some literature has suggested that plasma fractionated free metanephrines as the primary test is more sensitive and more specific than determination of urine metanephrines.

In localizing the tumor before surgery, CT scans, MRI, and radioisotope imaging with ^{123}I-metaiodobenzylguanidine (^{123}I-MIBG) are all useful techniques. Anatomical imaging with CT scanning and MRI have similar sensitivity (90% to 100%) and specificity (70% to 80%). Functional imaging with ^{123}I-MIBG has better specificity (95% to 100%) and is valuable for the detection of additional multifocal or metastatic tumors. Therefore, ^{123}I-MIBG scintigraphy is more relevant in patients with extra-adrenal or large (>5 cm) adrenal tumors with increased risk of malignant disease, and in those with a high suspicion of the presence of multifocal disease.

Investigation of the Adrenal Incidentaloma

Adrenal masses are commonly discovered on abdominal CT, at an estimated frequency of 2%. These masses may vary in size and may be functional (20%) or nonfunctional (80%). The mass may occur as an adrenal adenoma, carcinoma, pheochromocytoma, cyst, myelolipoma, or metastatic lesion. Congenital adrenal hyperplasia may cause focal enlargement, or the mass may be the result of an adrenal hemorrhage (usually bilateral). If the lesion is small (<3 cm) and the patient is asymptomatic, CT should be repeated in 6 months. If the lesion is larger and/or the patient is demonstrating symptoms, biochemical testing should be carried out. Signs and symptoms to look for include hypertension (excess cortisol, aldosterone, or catecholamines), hirsutism (excess adrenal androgens), hypokalemia (excess cortisol or aldosterone), and central obesity (excess cortisol leading to insulin resistance).

The patient should be screened for Cushing's syndrome with the use of an overnight dexamethasone suppression test. Urine catecholamines and/or catecholamine metabolites are required to rule out a pheochromocytoma. An aldosterone-to-renin ratio may be useful in ruling out Conn's syndrome. If patient results are positive for any of these, surgical intervention is required.

Approximately 5% to 20% of all adrenal incidentalomas secrete cortisol and may be the cause of subclinical Cushing's; 2% to 3% are found to be pheochromocytomas, and a smaller percentage may secrete aldosterone.

KEY CONCEPTS BOX 51-6

- Cushing's syndrome is screened and confirmed with urinary-free cortisol, late-night salivary cortisol, and the low-dose dexamethasone suppression test.
- The origin of the disease is confirmed by plasma ACTH, pituitary MRI, and bilateral petrosal sinus sampling for ACTH.
- Primary hyperaldosteronism (Conn's syndrome) is screened with the serum aldosterone–to–plasma renin activity (or mass) ratio.
- Conn's syndrome is confirmed by a salt loading suppression test to demonstrate nonsuppressible aldosterone in the settings of extracellular fluid volume expansion. The best procedure for localizing the lesion is bilateral adrenal venous sampling for aldosterone.
- Addison's disease is investigated by ACTH and baseline cortisol tests followed by a rapid ACTH stimulation test.
- Pheochromocytoma is diagnosed by urinary fractionated catecholamines, fractionated metanephrines, and VMA. In patients with renal failure, plasma fractionated catecholamines and plasma metanephrines are the tests of choice.

SECTION OBJECTIVES BOX 51-7

- Describe some of the factors that regulate blood pressure.
- List the major causes and complications of hypertension.
- Describe the minimum laboratory evaluation for the initial workup of a patient with hypertension and the indications for testing for secondary hypertension.
- Explain why renal disease, renal artery or branch stenosis, certain drugs, coarctation of the aorta, and adrenal gland and other endocrine disorders may cause hypertension.
- List common complications of hypertension.

PART 2: Hypertension

DEFINITION AND CRITERIA

Chronic hypertension is a common health problem in industrialized countries, with approximately 25% of the adult population affected. In the United States, African Americans are 1.5 to 2 times more likely to have hypertension than the general population. The higher the individual's blood pressure, the greater is the risk for developing heart disease, stroke, renal failure, and peripheral vascular disease. The risk for development of these complications extends down to blood pressure values below the population mean. Therefore, any definition of hypertension is purely arbitrary. Other factors such as cigarette smoking and hyperlipidemia increase the risk for hypertension-associated complications.

World Health Organization (WHO) and Joint National Committee on Detection, Evaluation, and Treatment of High Blood Pressure (JNC VII) guidelines have defined the criteria

Table 51-2 Classification of Hypertension (JNC VII)*†

Category	Systolic, mm Hg		Diastolic, mm Hg
Normal	<120	and	<80
Prehypertension	120 to 139	or	80 to 89
Stage I	140 to 159	or	90 to 99
Stage II	≥160	or	≥100

*Joint National Committee on Prevention, Detection, Evaluation, and Treatment of High Blood Pressure.
†The stage is defined by the higher of the systolic or diastolic pressure.

for hypertension. These have been subdivided into several categories, defined by the higher of the systolic or diastolic pressure (Table 51-2). Patients with prehypertension are at increased risk for progression to hypertension and require lifestyle modification. It is important not to make the diagnosis of hypertension on the basis of a single measurement, because the stress of visiting a physician may be sufficient to elevate blood pressure in some persons.

It is important to recognize hypertension because it is treatable, and treatment reduces the incidence of complications. Laboratory testing can be used to monitor the course of some complications of hypertension and to screen patients for potentially curable secondary hypertension. This may save the hypertensive patient from lifelong expensive medical therapy; the extent of medical therapy itself may be associated with complications.

FACTORS REGULATING NORMAL BLOOD PRESSURE

To convey a better understanding of the pathophysiology of hypertension, it is necessary to review briefly factors responsible for normal blood pressure regulation. Cardiac output and peripheral vascular resistance are the primary determinants of systemic blood pressure. Cardiac output is determined by plasma volume, cardiac stroke volume (the volume of blood expelled from the heart with each contraction), heart rate, and myocardial contractility. Peripheral vascular resistance is a function of the balance of humoral vasoconstriction (to increase blood pressure) and vasodilation (to decrease blood pressure), adrenergic activity, and arteriolar smooth muscle tone. Ordinarily, blood pressure is adjusted to maintain sufficient organ perfusion without producing organ or vascular damage. Several systems play a role in modulating cardiac output and peripheral vascular resistance. These include the arterial baroreceptor reflex, the body fluid or plasma volume regulatory system, and vascular autoregulation.

Baroreceptors in the aortic arch and carotid arteries sense perfusion pressure and wall tension through the afferent autonomic nervous system. They then signal the brain stem to modulate efferent adrenergic and vagal nerve activity, which, in turn, regulates myocardial contractility, heart rate, and

Table 51-3 Factors That Regulate Blood Pressure

Factor	Site of Synthesis	Mechanism and Sites of Action
Arterial Baroreflex Activators		
Epinephrine	Adrenal medulla	Vasodilation of arterioles of skeletal muscle; vasoconstriction of arterioles of skin, mucous membranes, and viscera; increases in rate and force of cardiac contraction
Norepinephrine	Terminals of sympathetic nervous system	General vasoconstriction
Body Fluid Volume Regulators		
Antidiuretic hormone (ADH)	Neurohypophysis	Enhanced water reabsorption; increased plasma volume
Aldosterone	Adrenal cortex	Renal tubular sodium reabsorption; increased plasma volume
Renin	Juxtaglomerular cells of kidney	Converts angiotensinogen to angiotensin I
Angiotensin-converting enzyme	Lung	Converts angiotensin I to angiotensin II (potent vasoconstrictor, stimulates aldosterone production)
Vascular Autoregulation		
Various	Tissue/organ specific	Local mechanisms to maintain constant tissue perfusion

peripheral vascular resistance. The release of antidiuretic hormone from the hypothalamus is regulated by plasma osmolality and blood pressure. This hormone enhances water reabsorption by the kidney. The renin-angiotensin system stimulates aldosterone release when blood pressure or sodium concentration drops and leads to sodium and water conservation. Angiotensin II generated by this cascade is also a potent vasoconstrictor. This system was described in greater detail earlier in this chapter.

The arterioles have the intrinsic capability to alter muscular tone in response to local perfusion pressures. With this vascular autoregulatory system, when cardiac output rises, the arterioles constrict to protect capillaries and tissues from hyperperfusion. Endothelin, a vasoconstrictor, plays a central role in blood pressure homeostasis. Nitrous oxide (see later discussion) and prostacyclin are locally produced vasodilators. The balance of these factors affects blood pressure.

All these systems work together when a change in blood pressure occurs. Table 51-3 summarizes some of the factors that play a role in regulating blood pressure. Through our improved understanding of the physiology of blood pressure control, newer specific therapeutic agents for treating hypertension have evolved.

Table 51-4 Principal Causes of Hypertension

Cause	Relative Incidence, %
I Primary hypertension	80 to 85
II Renal disease	4 to 5
III Renovascular hypertension	2 to 5
IV Drug- or exogenous agent–induced hypertension	<2
Oral contraceptives	
Sympathetic amines (decongestants)	
Licorice	
High-dose corticosteroids	
V Endocrine	10 to 15
Conn's syndrome	
Cushing's syndrome	
Pheochromocytoma	
Primary hyperparathyroidism	
Hypothyroidism	
Hyperthyroidism	
Acromegaly	
Congenital adrenal hyperplasia (21-hydroxylase and 11-hydroxylase deficiencies)	
VI Coarctation of the aorta	<1

PATHOLOGICAL CONDITIONS

In most patients, the cause of hypertension is unknown. Definable or secondary causes such as renal vascular disease, chronic renal failure, and endocrine abnormalities account for approximately 15% of cases. Unknown genetic and environmental factors may play a role in the approximately 85% of patients with **essential,** or **primary, hypertension.** Evidence indicates that salt intake, alcohol intake, and obesity have important influences. It is beyond the scope of this chapter to review the mechanisms that lead to primary hypertension. It can be stated most simply that the final common pathway is increased peripheral arteriolar resistance. The initiating factor is not known. Because the laboratory is not involved in the diagnosis or management of pimary hypertension, our discussion will focus on the investigation of secondary causes of hypertension.

Secondary Hypertension

Secondary causes of hypertension account for 15% of all cases. They are important to recognize because of the possibility of a more specific medical therapy or surgical cure. Table 51-4 summarizes the major causes of hypertension.

Renal Disease

A leading cause of secondary hypertension is renal disease. Glomerulonephritis, pyelonephritis, polycystic renal disease, renin-secreting tumors, and chronic renal failure all are associated with hypertension.

Renovascular Hypertension

Stenosis, or occlusion of one or both main renal arteries or branches, can cause hypertension by stimulating release of renin from the juxtaglomerular cells of the affected kidney. Greater than 60% occlusion is required to produce a significant hemodynamic effect. In patients who are older than 50 years of age, atherosclerosis is the most important cause of renal artery stenosis; in younger patients, fibromuscular dysplasia (thickening of the arterial wall) is the leading cause. Overall, fibromuscular dysplasia accounts for less than 10% of renal artery stenosis and mainly affects women in the 15 to 50 age bracket. It is an autosomal dominant, progressive disease that can lead to renal atrophy in more than 20% of cases. Renovascular hypertension, or renal artery stenosis, is a frequent cause of curable secondary hypertension, but it is discovered in only about 2% of hypertensive patients. Renovascular hypertension should be suspected when hypertension develops rapidly in those younger than 30 or older than 55 years of age, or when previously stable hypertension suddenly worsens.

Drug-Induced Hypertension

Many drugs may cause hypertension. Oral contraceptives can produce a mild degree of hypertension through an increase in liver production of angiotensinogen (renin substrate). Oral contraceptives also may directly cause some degree of sodium retention. Licorice (glycyrrhizic acid and glycyrrhetinic acid) and carbenoxolone, inhibitors of 11-β-hydroxysteroid dehydrogenase, prevent the inactivation of cortisol to cortisone in renal tubular cells, resulting in increasing levels of cortisol-induced mineralocorticoid activity. Nasal decongestants can cause hypertension through vasoconstriction. Administered glucocorticoids given in excess also increase mineralocorticoid activity. Calcineurin inhibitors (cyclosporine, tacrolimus), tricyclic antidepressants, and illicit drugs such as cocaine and amphetamines are other examples of drug-induced causes of hypertension.

Coarctation of the Aorta

Coarctation of the aorta usually is first identified in childhood. In this condition, an arterial defect with a fibrous aortic stricture reduces blood flow to the lower body and extremities. The result is restricted blood flow to the kidneys and, as a consequence, activation of the renin-angiotensin system.

Endocrine Causes of Hypertension

Several adrenal disorders are associated with hypertension. These include Cushing's syndrome, pheochromocytoma, and Conn's syndrome. The adrenogenital syndrome, resulting from 11-hydroxylase deficiency (a hereditary cause of hypertension), Liddle syndrome, and apparent mineralocorticoid excess are other causes of hypertension that can occur with hypokalemia. The causes, clinical features, and laboratory investigation of these problems are summarized in the first section of this chapter. Other endocrine disorders that may be associated with hypertension include increased pituitary growth hormone (acromegaly), primary hyperparathyroidism, hypothyroidism (rarely hypertensive), renin-secreting tumors, and thyrotoxicosis (high systolic blood pressure).

COMPLICATIONS OF HYPERTENSION

Blood pressure may rise gradually over many years, and the patient may remain asymptomatic for a long time. Hypertension usually is discovered during a routine physical examination. Unfortunately, it is discovered too often after vital organ injury has already occurred. Box 51-6 lists the most frequent complications of hypertensive disease. Headache and lightheadedness, symptoms sometimes associated with hypertension, are seen in less than 25% of patients, and the physical examination is usually unremarkable.

CHANGE OF ANALYTE WITH DISEASE

Once hypertension has been identified in a patient through multiple determinations of blood pressure, a simple minimum evaluation should be initiated. See Box 51-7 for a summary. This evaluation serves three main purposes: (1) to exclude treatable causes of secondary hypertension, (2) to detect evidence of organ damage, and (3) to identify other risk factors that may accelerate cardiovascular disease. This evaluation mainly involves inexpensive, high-volume laboratory tests. The choice of these tests is justified below.

Box 51-6

Complications of Hypertension

Aortic aneurysm
Atherosclerosis acceleration
Cardiac injury: infarction, left ventricular hypertrophy
Kidney disease: glomerulosclerosis with proteinuria, nephrosclerosis, decreased glomerular filtration rate (GFR), and end-stage renal disease
Retinal hemorrhages, exudates, and papilledema
Stroke

Box 51-7

Minimum Evaluation of the Hypertensive Individual

Complete history and physical examination
Serum creatinine, sodium, potassium, glucose, uric acid, cholesterol, and triglyceride concentrations
Hemoglobin
Urinalysis
Electrocardiogram

Urinalysis

Routine urinalysis can detect proteinuria, hematuria, and glycosuria. Proteinuria and hematuria may be attributable to hypertensive nephrosclerosis or to intrinsic renal disease, which in fact may be the cause of the hypertension. A renal biopsy is required to distinguish the cause if an abnormality is observed. The presence of proteinuria in a hypertensive patient may be suggestive of a bad prognosis, and sensitive assays for urinary albumin (microalbuminuria) allow early detection, analogous to diabetic nephropathy. Accumulating evidence suggests that an increased albumin excretion rate is predictive of future cardiovascular disease, as well as renal problems, in hypertensive patients. The use of angiotensin-converting enzyme inhibitors or angiotensin II receptor blockers can reverse the disease process. The presence of glycosuria, which is suggestive of diabetes mellitus, will affect the choice of antihypertensive therapy. For example, thiazide diuretics are contraindicated in diabetes because they can exacerbate glucose intolerance. It is also possible that glucose intolerance may result from other endocrine causes of hypertension such as pheochromocytoma, Cushing's syndrome, or acromegaly.

Sodium

An elevated serum sodium value is not a sensitive or specific test, but it may be elevated in some patients with primary hyperaldosteronism. Another consideration is that serum sodium may be decreased in hypertensive patients receiving thiazide or loop diuretics. This test therefore is also important for monitoring patients who are undergoing diuretic therapy.

Potassium

The finding of a low serum potassium value is a very important clue in a hypertensive patient who is not receiving medication; it is suggestive of the possibility of primary (Conn's syndrome) or secondary (i.e., renal artery stenosis) hyperaldosteronism. Also, serum potassium levels may be raised in patients with acute or chronic renal failure and lowered in patients receiving diuretics. See Table 51-5 for causes and renin/aldosterone findings in patients with hypertension and hypokalemia.

Creatinine

Serum creatinine is a specific screen for renal impairment that may be caused by hypertension or may be the cause of hypertension. Creatinine should be assessed on presentation and annually in all hypertensive patients.

Calcium

The serum calcium level is elevated in primary hyperparathyroidism, which is one of the causes of hypertension. About 50% of patients with this problem will be hypertensive. It is of interest that despite this connection, blood pressure most often does not normalize after surgical cure. Another consideration is that thiazide diuretics can rarely cause hypercalcemia and thus should be excluded before the diagnosis of primary hyperparathyroidism is pursued.

Table 51-5 Causes of Hypertension and Hypokalemia Characterized by Plasma Renin Activity (PRA) and Aldosterone Levels (ALDO)

Finding	Conclusion
Increased PRA, increased ALDO	Secondary hyperaldosteronism from: Renovascular hypertension Diuretic use Renin-secreting tumor Malignant hypertension Coarctation of the aorta
Decreased PRA, increased ALDO	Primary hyperaldosteronism
Decreased PRA, decreased ALDO	Congenital adrenal hyperplasia Exogenous mineralocorticoid DOC-producing tumor Cushing's syndrome 11-β-HSD2 deficiency Liddle syndrome Licorice ingestion

DOC, Deoxycorticosterone; *11-β-HSD2,* 11-β-hydroxysteroid dehydrogenase type 2.

Uric Acid

The uric acid value is elevated in about 40% of patients with essential hypertension. This is more common in patients with renal failure. One explanation for its association with hypertension might be hypertension-induced renal failure. Uric acid levels also may be elevated by thiazide diuretics, in some cases leading to gout. A strong association between the concentration of serum uric acid and the prevalence of the metabolic syndrome has been noted.

Glucose

An elevated fasting plasma glucose value greater than 140 mg/dL (7.0 mmol/L) on two or more occasions is sufficient for the clinician to diagnose diabetes mellitus. About 50% of diabetic patients have hypertension, and up to 10% of hypertensive patients are diabetic. Calcium channel blockers and angiotensin-converting enzyme inhibitors are the preferred antihypertensive drugs for those with diabetes.

Lipid Profile (Total Cholesterol, HDL Cholesterol, LDL Cholesterol, and Triglyceride)

Hyperlipidemia is an important risk factor for atherosclerosis, as is hypertension. The presence of hyperlipidemia is a contraindication for the use of some antihypertensive medications, such as β-blockers and thiazide diuretics, which may exacerbate the lipid problem. Patients with risk factors for cardiovascular disease should be treated very aggressively.

Electrocardiogram

An electrocardiogram should be obtained in all cases to assess cardiac status as a baseline parameter and to determine whether left ventricular hypertrophy is present.

Chest X-Ray Film

A chest x-ray film may identify aortic dilation or elongation and rib notching, which may occur in coarctation of the aorta.

SECONDARY STUDIES

Clues from the history, physical examination, and basic laboratory studies may indicate a possible secondary cause for hypertension. Some of these clues include the following:

1. Abrupt onset of severe hypertension, or onset before 25 years of age or after age 50, may be suggestive of pheochromocytoma or renovascular disease.
2. A history of palpitations, anxiety attacks, sweating, hyperglycemia, and weight loss may be suggestive of pheochromocytoma.
3. An abdominal bruit may be suggestive of renovascular disease.
4. Bilateral upper abdominal masses on physical examination may imply polycystic kidney disease.
5. Abnormal renal function test results may be suggestive of renal insufficiency.
6. Hypokalemia, or easily provoked hypokalemia, in a person with untreated hypertension should be a trigger to investigate primary hyperaldosteronism (Conn's syndrome) or another cause of hypertension and hypokalemia.

The investigation of adrenal disorders with associated hypertension is discussed earlier in this chapter. Other endocrine causes of hypertension are suspected on clinical grounds, and laboratory investigations for these disorders are reviewed in other chapters.

KEY CONCEPTS BOX 51-7

- The major causes of secondary hypertension are renal diseases, drugs, coarctation of the aorta, and endocrine disorders.
- The minimum laboratory evaluation for the initial workup of a patient with hypertension include urinalysis, electrolytes, creatinine, calcium, uric acid, glucose, and lipid profile.
- Clinical features and common laboratory tests may give clues to the presence of secondary causes of hypertension.

BIBLIOGRAPHY

General

Loriaux DL: The adrenal glands. In Becker KL, editor: *Principles and Practice of Endocrinology and Metabolism,* ed 3, Philadelphia, 2001, Lippincott Williams & Wilkins.

Stewart PM: The adrenal cortex. In Kronenberg HM, Melmed S, Polonsky KS, et al: *Williams Textbook of Endocrinology,* ed 11, Philadelphia, 2007, Saunders.

Williams GH, Dluhy RG: Disorders of the adrenal cortex. In Fauci A, Braunwald E, Kasper D, et al, editors: *Harrison's Principles of Internal Medicine,* ed 17, New York, 2008, McGraw-Hill.

Mineralocorticoids

Cartledge S, Lawson N: Aldosterone and renin measurements, Ann Clin Biochem 37:262, 2000.

Kaplan NM: Cautions over the current epidemic of primary aldosteronism, Lancet 357:953, 2001.

Mattsson C, Young WF Jr: Primary aldosteronism: diagnostic and treatment strategies, Nature Clin Practice Nephrol 2:198, 2006.

Mulatero P, Stowasser M, Loh KC, et al: Increased diagnosis of primary aldosteronism, including surgically correctable forms, in centers from five continents, J Clin Endocrinol Metab 89:1045, 2004.

Young WF Jr: Primary aldosteronism: renaissance of a syndrome, Clin Endocrinol 66:607, 2007.

Glucocorticoids

Abdu TAM, Elhadd TA, Neary R, et al: Comparison of low dose short synacthen test (1 μg), conventional dose short synacthen test (250 μg) and insulin tolerance test for the assessment of the hypothalamic-pituitary-adrenal axis in patients with pituitary disease, J Clin Endocrinol Metab 84:838, 1999.

Arlt W, Callies F, van Vlijmen JC, et al: DHEA replacement in women with adrenal insufficiency, N Engl J Med 341:1013, 1999.

Aron DC, Findling JW, Tyrrell JB: Glucocorticoids and adrenal androgens. In Greenspan FS, Gardner DG, editors: *Basic and Clinical Endocrinology,* ed 8, New York, 2007, Lange Medical Books/McGraw-Hill.

Findling JW, Raff H: Screening and diagnosis of Cushing's syndrome, Endocrinol Metab Clin North Am 34:385, 2005.

Findling JW, Raff H: Clinical review: Cushing's syndrome: important issues in diagnosis and management, J Clin Endocrinol Metab 91:3746, 2006.

Henzen C, Suter A, Lerch E, et al: Suppression and recovery of adrenal response after short term high dose glucocorticoid treatment, Lancet 355:542, 2000.

Krasner AS: Glucocorticoid-induced adrenal insufficiency, JAMA 202:671, 1999.

Lindsay JR, Nieman LK: Differential diagnosis and imaging in Cushing's syndrome, Endocrinol Metab Clin North Am 34:403, 2005.

McCann SJ, Gillingwater S, Keevil BG: Measurement of urinary free cortisol using liquid chromatography-tandem mass spectrometry: comparison with the urine adapted ACS:180 serum cortisol chemiluminescent immunoassay and development of a new reference range, Ann Clin Biochem 42:112, 2005.

Newell-Price J, Bertagna X, Grossman AB, et al: Cushing's syndrome, Lancet 367:1605, 2006.

Oelkers W: Adrenal insufficiency, N Engl J Med 335:1206, 1996.

Pivonello R, De Martino MC, Cappabianca P, et al: The medical treatment of Cushing's disease: Effectiveness of chronic treatment with the dopamine agonist cabergoline in patients unsuccessfully treated by surgery, J Clin Endocrinol Metab 94(1):223-30, 2008.

Streeten DHP: What test for hypothalamic-pituitary adrenocortical insufficiency? Lancet 354:179, 1999.

Taylor RL, Machacek D, Singh RJ: Validation of a high-throughput liquid chromatography-tandem mass spectrometry method for urinary cortisol and cortisone, Clin Chem 48:1511, 2002.

Terzolo M, Bovio S, Pia A, et al: Subclinical Cushing's syndrome in adrenal incidentalomas, Endocrinol Metab Clin North Am 34:423, 2005.

Walsh JP, Dayan CM: Role of biochemical assessment in management of corticosteroid withdrawal, Ann Clin Biochem 37:279, 2000.

Werbel SS, Ober KP: Acute adrenal insufficiency, Endocrinol Metab Clin North Am 22:303, 1993.

Adrenal Androgens

Achermann JC, Silverman BL: DHEA replacement for patients with adrenal insufficiency, Lancet 357:1381, 2001.

Arlt W, Callies F, van Vlijmen JC, et al: DHEA replacement in women with adrenal insufficiency, N Engl J Med 341:1013, 1999.

Kroboth PD, Salek FS, Pittenger AL, et al: DHEA and DHEAS: a review, J Clin Pharmacol 39:327, 1999.

Oelkers W: DHEA for adrenal insufficiency, N Engl J Med 341:1073, 1999.

Adrenal Incidentalomas

Bailey RH, Aron DC: The diagnostic dilemma of incidentalomas, Endocrinol Metab Clin North Am 29:91, 2000.

Barzon L, Scaroni C, Sonino N, et al: Risk factors and long term follow-up of adrenal incidentalomas, J Clin Endocrinol Metab 84:520, 1999.

Kievit J, Haak HR: Diagnosis and treatment of adrenal incidentaloma, Endocrinol Metab Clin North Am 29:69, 2000.

Linos DA: Management approaches to adrenal incidentalomas, Endocrinal Metab Clin North Am 29:141, 2000.

Mantero F, Arnaldi G: Management approaches to adrenal incidentalomas, Endocrinol Metab Clin North Am 29:107, 2000.

Young WF Jr: The incidentally discovered adrenal mass, N Engl J Med 356:601, 2007.

Congenital Adrenal Hyperplasia

Speiser PW: Congenital adrenal hyperplasia owing to 21-hydroxylase deficiency, Endocrinol Metab Clin North Am 30:31, 2001.

Therrell BL: Newborn screening for congenital adrenal hyperplasia, Endocrinol Metab Clin North Am 30:15, 2001.

White PC: Steroid ll-β-hydroxylase deficiency and related disorders, Endocrinol Metab Clin North Am 30:61, 2001.

Catecholamines and Pheochromocytoma

Eisenhofer G: Free or total metanephrines for diagnosis of pheochromocytoma: what is the difference? Clin Chem 47:988, 2001.

Eisenhofer G, Goldstein DS, Walther MM, et al: Biochemical diagnosis of pheochromocytoma: how to distinguish true- from false-positive test results, J Clin Endocrinol Metab 88:2656, 2003.

Eisenhofer G, Lenders JW, Linehan WM, et al: Plasma normetanephrine and metanephrine for detecting pheochromocytoma in von Hippel-Lindau disease and multiple endocrine neoplasia type 2, N Engl J Med 340:1872, 1999.

Fitzgerald PA: Adrenal medulla. In Greenspan FS, Gardner DG, editors: *Basic and Clinical Endocrinology,* ed 8, New York, 2007, Lange Medical Books/McGraw-Hill.

Grossman A, Pacak K, Sawka A, et al: Biochemical diagnosis and localization of pheochromocytoma: can we reach a consensus? Ann N Y Acad Sci 1073:332, 2006.

Lenders JW, Eisenhofer G, Mannelli M, et al: Phaeochromocytoma, Lancet 366:665, 2005.

Manger WM: An overview of pheochromocytoma: history, current concepts, vagaries, and diagnostic challenges, Ann N Y Acad Sci 1073:1, 2006.

Neumann HPH: Pheochromocytoma. In Fauci A, Braunwald E, Kasper D, et al, editors: *Harrison's Principles of Internal Medicine,* ed 17, New York, 2008, McGraw-Hill.

Pacak K, Eisenhofer G, Ahlman H, et al: Pheochromocytoma: recommendations for clinical practice from the first international symposium, Nat Clin Pract Endocrinol Metab 3:92, 2007.

Pacak K, Linehan WM, Eisenhofer G, et al: Recent advances in genetics, diagnosis, localization and treatment of pheochromocytoma, Ann Intern Med 134:315, 2001.

Scully RE, Mark EJ, McNeely WE, et al: Case records of the Massachusetts General Hospital, N Engl J Med 344:1314, 2001.

Young WF Jr: Paragangliomas: clinical overview, Ann N Y Acad Sci 1073:21, 2006.

Hypertension

Don BR, Lo JC: Endocrine hypertension. In Greenspan FS, Gardner DG, editors: *Basic and Clinical Endocrinology,* ed 8, New York, 2007, Lange Medical Books/McGraw-Hill.

Harvey JM, Beevers DG: Biochemical investigation of hypertension, Ann Clin Biochem 27:287, 1990.

Hollenberg NK, editor: *Hypertension: Mechanisms and Therapy,* vol 2, *Atlas of Heart Disease,* Philadelphia, 1995, Current Medicine.

Massie BM: Systemic hypertension. In Tierney LM, McPhee SJ, Papadakis MA, editors: *Current Medical Diagnosis and Treatment,* ed 41, New York, 2002, Lange Medical Books/McGraw-Hill.

The Seventh Report of the Joint National Committee on Prevention, Detection, Evaluation and Treatment of High Blood Pressure (JNC-VII), JAMA 289:2560, 2003.

INTERNET SITES

http://www.medhelp.org/nadf/—National Addison's Disease Foundation

http://arbl.cvmbs.colostate.edu/hbooks/pathphys/endocrine/adrenal/index.html—Colorado State Hypertextbook: The Adrenal Gland: Introduction and Index

http://www.nlm.nih.gov/medlineplus/adrenalglanddisorders.html—Medline Plus: Adrenal Gland Disorders

http://www.endotext.com/adrenal/—Physiology and Diseases

http://themedicalbiochemistrypage.org/—Indiana University: Medical Biochemistry

http://cgap.ucdavis.edu—Canine Genetic Analysis: A Research Focus on the Statistics & Molecular Genetics of Diseases in Dogs, Department of Animal Science, University of California—Davis

http://www.cancer.gov/cancer_information/—National Cancer Institute Information

http://www.who.int/en/—World Health Organization

http://www.medhelp.org/—Med Help International: Virtual Medical Center for Patients

http://www.ash-us.org/—American Society of Hypertension

http://hypertension.ca/bpc/resource-center/publications/—The Canadian Hypertension Education Program (CHEP) recommendations

http://www.nice.org.uk/Guidance/CG34/ -NICE Clinical Guidelines: Hypertension: Management of Hypertension in Adults in Primary Care

http://www.hypertensiononline.org/—Baylor College of Medicine

http://emedicine.medscape.com/article/124059-overview—Pheochromocytoma

http://emedicine.medscape.com/article/116716-overview—Adrenal crisis

http://emedicine.medscape.com/article/116467-overview—Addison's disease

Chapter 52

Diseases of Genetic Origin

T. Andrew Burrow, Kejian Zhang, and Gregory A. Grabowski

Chapter Outline

Key Terms

allele Various forms of a gene that occur at a particular locus.

aneuploidy Condition in which one or more chromosomes are missing from or are added to the normal chromosomal constitution of a cell.

anticipation Worsening of phenotype with each successive affected generation.

autosomes The 22 pairs of chromosomes, excluding the sex chromosomes X and Y.

chromosome Microscopically visible physical structure consisting of a large continuous DNA molecule organized into genes and supported by proteins called *chromatin.*

coding region All the exons of a gene that contribute to the protein product(s) of the gene (synonym: open reading frame).

codon A sequence of three consecutive mRNA nucleotides that code for an amino acid or termination signal (stop codon).

digenic inheritance Phenotypical features resulting from the combined effects of mutations in alleles at two separate loci.

diploid Cells that contain two copies (2n) of each chromosome in the genome (i.e., 46 chromosomes in most human cells), as opposed to haploid (n).

dominant A trait that is expressed when an allele is present in the heterozygous or hemizygous (in the case of X-linked inheritance) state.

dominant negative A mutant gene whose product can inhibit the function of the **wild-type** gene product in heterozygotes.

epigenetics Stable, heritable changes in gene expression that do not involve alterations in the DNA sequence.

exon Segments of a gene that code for mature messenger RNA.

expressivity The degree of severity of the disease phenotype.

fluorescence in situ hybridization (FISH) A molecular cytogenetic technique that uses fluorescent-labeled DNA probe hybridization to complement genomic DNA to detect deletions, duplications, translocations, and aneuploid states in interphase and metaphase chromosomes.

frameshift mutation A mutation in which the insertion or deletion of one or more nucleotides, except in multiples of three, disrupts the reading frame of a gene.

gene Segment of DNA that carries the information necessary for the production of specific products (i.e., proteins).

Genetic Association Study Case-controlled analyses that aim to detect associations between one or more genetic polymorphisms and a trait, which might be some quantitative characteristic or a discrete attribute or disease.[1]

genome The sum of the genetic information of an organism.

genotype Refers to the specific nucleotide sequence (allele) present at a particular locus.

haploid Cells that contain a single copy (n) of each chromosome in the genome (i.e., 23 chromosomes in human sperm or egg), as opposed to diploid (2n).

hemizygous A state in which only one copy of a particular gene is present in a diploid organism. Usually refers to X-linked genes in the male, this term also applies to genes on any chromosome segments that are deleted on the homologous chromosome.

heteroplasmy The presence of more than one genotype of mitochondrial DNA in the cellular mitochondria of an individual. The opposite is homoplasmy.

imprinting The phenomenon of different expression of alleles depending on the parent of origin.

intron Non-protein coding segment of DNA that is transcribed into RNA but is removed by splicing before it is translated into proteins.

karyotype An image of a complete set of chromosomes of a single cell, arranged in pairs from largest to smallest.

linkage analysis A technique that uses polymorphic markers that are linked (co-inherited) to a gene in question to map their physical location along a chromosome.

locus The specific location on a chromosome where a gene or nucleotide sequence is located.

lyonization A process of random inactivation of an X chromosome to compensate for the double-gene dosage of two X chromosomes in females.

microarray-based comparative genome hybridization (array CGH) A high-resolution molecular cytogenetics technique that is used to evaluate copy number alterations (deletions and duplications) within the genome.

monosomy Absence of one or a part (partial monosomy) of a chromosome pair from a diploid cell.

multifactorial disorder Condition in which a combination of predisposing multiple genetic factors and environmental conditions contributes to the resulting phenotype; also called *complex disorder.*

mutation A permanent, heritable alteration in the DNA sequence.

nondisjunction Failure of homologous chromosomes (meiosis I) or two chromatids (meiosis II or mitosis) to separate during anaphase, resulting in aneuploidy in the daughter cells.

penetrance The probability that a person who has a particular genotype will express phenotypical characteristics.

phenocopy An environmentally caused phenotype that mimics one produced by a mutant allele.

phenotype Observed trait(s) of the organism under study (physical, behavioral, and biochemical).

pleiotropy The multiple phenotypical effects that a gene has upon an individual.

polymorphism Genetic variation that occurs in at least 1% of the population.

polyploidy A condition in which cells contain more than the diploid (2n) number, or 23 pairs, of chromosomes.

population genetics The study of the distribution of genes in populations and how the frequencies of genes and genotypes are maintained or changed.

recessive A trait that is expressed when an allele is present in the homozygous state.

sex chromosomes The X and Y chromosomes.

single-gene disorder Genetic disease that is caused by mutations in one or both alleles and that usually is inherited in predictable Mendelian patterns.

synonymous (silent) mutation Mutation that does not alter the resulting amino acid sequence.

trisomy The presence of three copies of a particular chromosome in a diploid cell.

wild type The typical form of a gene, phenotype, or organism that occurs in the natural population.

X-linked Traits carried on the X chromosome.

SECTION OBJECTIVES BOX 52-1

- Describe the structure and function of genes and chromosomes.
- Briefly describe the common forms of Mendelian inheritance and the likelihood that a female or male offspring might inherit a trait.
- Distinguish between single gene and mutifactorial genetic disorders.

PRINCIPLES OF GENETICS

In humans, genetic information is stored within the cell nucleus and mitochondria in the form of deoxyribonucleic acid (DNA). Approximately 3.2×10^9 base pairs of DNA in the nuclear haploid **genome** make up the **haploid** number of 23 **chromosomes.** The mitochondrial genome is a single, circular double-stranded molecule of DNA that consists of 16,569 base pairs.

Genes usually refer to segments of DNA that encode the information necessary for the production of specific proteins. About 22,000 genes are present in the nuclear genome, and exactly 37 genes are found in the mitochondrial genome. Genes usually exist in multiple variant forms, or **alleles.** With few exceptions, genes are represented twice in **autosomes** of human **diploid** cells.

Genes consist of intervening, noncoding DNA sequences (**introns** and untranslated regions) and coding sequences or coding regions **(exons),** both of which are transcribed into heteronuclear RNA (hnRNA). hnRNA is processed further into messenger RNA (mRNA) by splicing out the introns and adding a 5′ cap and a 3′ polyadenylate tail. The resultant mRNA strand serves as a template for the translation of a polypeptide product on ribosomes.

Only 1% of the human genome is coding DNA that is used to make mRNA and protein; the remainder is composed of noncoding sequences, that is, introns or structural elements. Highly repeated noncoding human DNA sequences occupy a substantial portion (≈40%) of the human genome. The exact function of the noncoding human DNA sequences is largely unknown. However, in studying 1% (30 megabases) of the genome in the Encyclopedia of DNA Elements (ENCODE), project investigators found essential regulatory functions for non-gene DNA sequences.[2] In comparison, mitochondrial DNA is densely packed with genetic information, of which 93% is coding sequence for 22 tRNA, 2 rRNA, and 13 genes that are mainly in the oxidative phosphorylation/respiratory pathway.

In human diploid cells, 46 chromosomes, or 23 pairs of chromosomes, contain the genes. Twenty-two pairs (numbered 1 to 22) are called *autosomes* (i.e., non–sex determining) and are similar in males and females. They are numbered according to size, from largest (chromosome 1) to smallest (chromosomes 21 and 22). The remaining pair comprises the **sex chromosomes:** XX in females and XY in males. The X chromosome is about 2 times as large as the Y chromosome.

Individual chromosomes may be distinguished on the basis of characteristic banding patterns (see later), or according to the position of the centromere, a constricted region that separates the chromosome into two arms—a short arm (p, for petite) and a long arm (q). Metacentric chromosomes are those in which the centromere is located at or near the center of the chromosome. Submetacentric chromosomes have an off-center centromere, with p and q arms of different lengths. Acrocentric chromosomes have centromeres near one end of the chromosome and satellites on the p arm containing genes that produce ribosomal RNA. The telomeres, which are located at the terminal end of each arm, contain specific repetitive sequences of DNA that "seal" the chromosomes, thus stabilizing and preventing them from joining together.

Chromosomes consist of a complex of DNA and structural proteins (histones and non-histones) called *chromatin,* which exists in two states—euchromatin and heterochromatin. Euchromatin contains the coding DNA and thus is less condensed and more transcriptionally active than heterochromatin.

The average human chromosome is about 140 million bases in size. On average, about 1400 genes are present on each chromosome. Human genes are not distributed evenly on the chromosomes. Functionally similar genes (e.g., cytochrome P-450, *HOX* genes) are clustered occasionally in certain regions of the genome, but more often they are dispersed over different chromosomes (e.g., PAX, NF1). In females, **lyonization** is used as a process to inactivate an X chromosome to compensate for the double-gene dosage of the two X chromosomes.

CATEGORIES OF GENETIC DISORDERS

Single-gene disorders (Table 52-1) result from **mutations** in one or both copies of individual genes. Over 10,000 single-gene disorders have been identified; approximately 2% of the population will be affected by one of these disorders at some point in their lifetime.[3] These disorders usually are inherited in one of four predictable Mendelian patterns (autosomal **dominant,** autosomal **recessive, X-linked** recessive, and X-linked dominant) as determined by whether the allele is dominant or recessive in nature, and whether the gene is located on an autosome or a sex chromosome.

In autosomal dominant inheritance (Fig. 52-1), one allele is abnormal (i.e., mutated) for expression of the disease **phenotype.** The disease frequently involves multiple generations in a family and occurs with equal frequency in males and females. However, such diseases can occur in the absence of family history, suggesting the occurrence of a new mutation or variable **penetrance.** An affected individual has a 1 in 2 chance of transmitting the disease to future offspring. Conditions that demonstrate autosomal dominant inheritance include osteogenesis imperfecta and Marfan, Alagille, and Treacher Collins syndromes.

In autosomal recessive inheritance (Fig. 52-2), for an individual to be affected, he must inherit two copies of a mutant allele at a particular **locus,** one from each parent. If an offspring inherits only one mutant allele, that individual is a carrier and is unaffected. Males and females have an equal likelihood of inheriting the disease. Diseases that are autosomal recessive in inheritance can and do "skip" generations, in contrast to autosomal dominant traits. Because of the need to have two mutant alleles, and because such alleles occur more frequently in relatives, consanguinity is often a factor in this form of inheritance. Each offspring of two carriers for the same autosomal recessive condition has a 25% risk of inheriting both copies of the mutant allele (thus being affected with the disease), a 50% risk of being a carrier, and a 25% risk of inheriting both copies of the normal alleles.

Sickle cell disease is the prototypical autosomal recessive single-gene disorder that occurs at an incidence of approximately 1 in 600 African Americans. It is caused by a missense mutation that encodes a Glu6Val substitution—glutamine changed to valine at **codon** 6—in the hemoglobin beta gene *(HBB).* This substitution results in the production of structurally abnormal hemoglobin S. Clinically, the disorder is characterized by a tendency of red blood cells to assume an abnormal stiff, sickle shape under conditions of low oxygen tension, resulting in hemolysis and acute painful episodes of vascular occlusion, which lead to tissue ischemia and multiorgan dysfunction.[4] The disorder may be diagnosed through biochemical or molecular techniques, including isolation of hemoglobin S through hemoglobin electrophoresis, or identification of the Glu6Val mutation in the *HBB* gene.

In X-linked recessive inheritance (Fig. 52-3), all males who possess a mutant allele demonstrate the disease phenotype and are **hemizygous** (i.e., they have a single X chromosome with the mutant allele). Their Y chromosome does not have such genes. In comparison, females need two copies of a mutant allele to be affected. Exceptions occur in the presence of skewed X inactivation and occasionally in some heterozygous females (e.g., Fabry disease). Thus, phenotypical features occur with greater frequency in males than in females in this form of inheritance. All female offspring of an affected male are carriers of the mutation, whereas male offspring cannot inherit the mutation from their fathers, nor transmit it to their sons. Female offspring of a carrier female have a 50% risk of being carriers, and male offspring have a 50% risk of being affected by the disease. Duchenne muscular dystrophy and

Table **52-1** Common Single Gene Disorders

Disease	OMIM	Gene	Protein	Gene Locus	Inheritance and Incidence	Clinical Features
Cystic Fibrosis	219700	*CFTR*	Cystic fibrosis transmembrane conductance regulator	7q31.2	Autosomal recessive; 1 in 2500	Chronic lung disease, chronic sinusitis, digestion problems, pancreatic insufficiency, meconium ileus, male infertility, poor growth
Sickle Cell Disease	603903	*HBB*	Hemoglobin beta	11p15.5	Autosomal dominant; 1 in 625	Anemia, painful vaso-occlusive crises, cerebrovascular accidents, avascular necrosis of the hip, infection, splenic sequestration crises
Phenylketonuria	261600	*PAH*	Phenylalanine hydroxylase	12q24.1	Autosomal recessive; 1 in 15,000	Mental retardation, microcephaly, seizures, behavioral problems, and eczema
Gaucher Disease	231000	*GBA*	Acid beta glucosidase	1q21	Autosomal recessive; 1 in 100,000 among general population; 1 in 900 among Ashkenazi Jews	Type 1: hepatosplenomegaly, bone lesions, hematological abnormalities, survival into adulthood Type 2: Severe neuronopathic disease, hepatosplenomegaly, death in early childhood Type 3: Subacute neuronopathic disease
Tay-Sachs Disease	272800	*HEXA*	Hexosaminidase A	15q23-24	Autosomal recessive; 1 in 320,000 among general population; 1 in 900 among Ashkenazi Jews	Progressive neurological deterioration, cherry red macules, macrocephaly, death in childhood
Huntington Disease	143100	*HD*	Huntington	4p16.3	Autosomal dominant; 1 in 10,000	Motor disturbances (chorea), behavioral/personality changes, and psychiatric illness
Fragile X Syndrome	300624	*FMR1*	Fragile X mental retardation protein	Xq27.3	X-linked recessive; 1 in 2000 males; 1 in 4000 females	Mental retardation, behavioral problems, characteristic facial appearance, tall stature, macroorchidism, premature ovarian failure, and motor disturbances
Bardet Biedl Syndrome*	209900	*BBS1, BBS2, ARL6/BBS3, BBS4, BBS5, MKKS/BBS6, BBS7, TTC8/ BBS8, B1/BBS9, BBS10, TRIM32/BBS11, and BBS12*	Cilia and intraflagellar transport proteins	20p12, 16q21, 15q22.3-q23, 14q32.1, 12q21.2, 11q13, 9q31-q34.1, 7p14, 4q27, 4q27, 3p12-q13, 2q31	Autosomal recessive; 1 in 100,000	Mental retardation, pigmentary retinopathy, characteristic facial appearance, obesity, postaxial polydactyly, hypogonadism, congenital heart disease, female genitourinary malformations, and renal anomalies and dysfunction
Congenital sensorineural hearing loss*	Several	Several	Several	Several	Variable; 1 in 300 to 1 in 1000	Variable, depending upon gene involved

OMIM, Online Mendelian Inheritance in Man (see p. 1046) disorder number.
*Disease has more than one associated genetic foci.

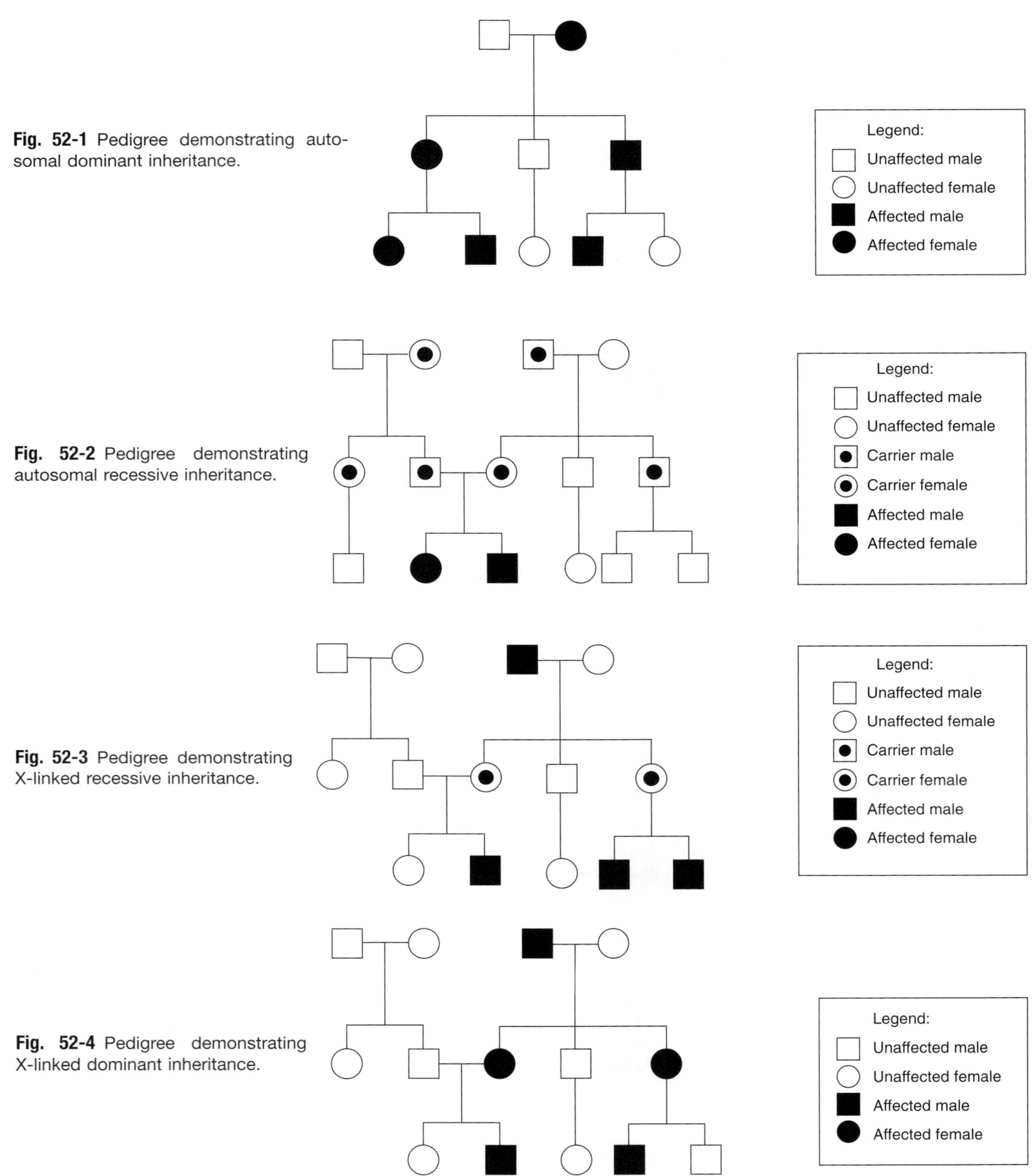

Fig. 52-1 Pedigree demonstrating autosomal dominant inheritance.

Fig. 52-2 Pedigree demonstrating autosomal recessive inheritance.

Fig. 52-3 Pedigree demonstrating X-linked recessive inheritance.

Fig. 52-4 Pedigree demonstrating X-linked dominant inheritance.

hemophilia A and B are additional diseases that demonstrate this pattern of inheritance.

In X-linked dominant inheritance (Fig. 52-4), males and females who possess a single mutant allele on an X chromosome may manifest the disease. Males often are more severely affected than females. Indeed, in some X-linked dominant disorders, affected males do not survive. The male and female offspring of an affected female have a 50% risk of being equally affected. Conversely, all female offspring of an affected male are affected, whereas none of the male offspring are affected.

Incontinentia pigmenti and hypophosphatemic rickets demonstrate X-linked dominant patterns of inheritance.

Genetic disorders may be attributable to mutations at multiple loci. For example, mutations in *GJB2* (Connexin 26) and *GJB6* (Connexin 30) are common autosomal recessive causes of congenital sensorineural hearing loss. *GJB2* and *GJB6* code for two gap junction proteins. Both genes are located in tandem on chromosome 13. Loss of function of these gap junction proteins prevents recycling of toxic ions and metabolites away from hair cells, leading to their death. Treatment includes habilitation with hearing aids or cochlear implants. It is interesting to note that individuals who have mutations in alleles at two separate loci also may exhibit a genetic disorder because of their combined effects (**digenic inheritance**). For example, the *GJB6* mutation D13S1830 is associated with congenital sensorineural hearing loss when present in the homozygous state or in combination with a single *GJB2* mutation.

KEY CONCEPTS BOX 52-1

- Deoxyribonucleic acid (DNA, nuclear or mitochondrial) contains the genetic code, genes, which define the primary structure of proteins by use of a triplet codon for each amino acid. The DNA is packaged into chromosomes along with regulatory and structural proteins. There exist common variants for each gene, called an allel.
- The common Mendialian forms of gene inheritance are autosomal dominant, autosomal recessive, X-linked recessive, and X-linked dominant. All males and homozygous females are usually affected by an X-linked disorder. All female offspring of an affected male become carriers of the disorder.
- Single gene disorders are caused by a mutation in one gene. Disorders that require mutations is multiple genes are multifactorial genetic disorders.

SECTION OBJECTIVES BOX 52-2

- Define the term *aneuploidy,* and describe the types of aneuploidy that can occur.
- Explain the differences among the following factors that promote variable expression among individuals with the same genetic disorders: penetrance, expressivity, pleiotropy, anticipation, and phenocopy.
- Explain the mechanism of inheritance of mitochondrial genes and how it these genes affect male and female offspring.
- Explain the term *epigenetics,* discussing the factors that can affect gene expression. Discuss how gene imprinting can result in genetic disorders.
- Discuss types of DNA mutations and how they can result in polymorphism and disease.

Variations in Mendelian Inheritance

Certain factors alter the predicted patterns of Mendelian inheritance and often promote variable expression among individuals with the same genetic disorders. These factors include penetrance, expressivity, pleiotropy, anticipation, and phenocopy.

Penetrance is the probability that a person who has a particular **genotype** will express phenotypical characteristics. Usually, if a person possesses a mutant allele for a genetic disorder, it is expressed through the phenotype, thus it is completely penetrant. However, this is not always the case. In some genetic disorders (e.g., Treacher Collins syndrome), penetrance is said to be reduced, and a person does not demonstrate an altered phenotype despite possessing the disease genotype. **Expressivity** is the severity of the phenotype. Among individuals with the same genotype, the degree of phenotypical severity can vary (i.e., variable expressivity). **Pleiotropy** describes the multiple phenotypical effects that a gene has upon an individual. For example, mutations in *NF1*, which are associated with neurofibromatosis type 1, may result in multiple phenotypical features, including skin abnormalities, skeletal deformities, and the development of tumors (neurofibromas) on the nerves.

In certain disorders, such as fragile X syndrome and Huntington's disease, anticipation may occur. **Anticipation** implies that the phenotype progressively worsens with passage of the phenotype through each successive generation. Finally, **phenocopy** is an environmentally caused phenotype that mimics one produced by a mutant allele. A classic example of phenocopy is in utero exposure to thalidomide that results in severely shortened/absent upper extremities, similar to those seen in phocomelia, a rare autosomal recessive genetic disorder.

Chromosomal disorders (Tables 52-2 and 52-3) occur in approximately 2% of all live births and in nearly 50% of spontaneous first-trimester miscarriages; they result from numerical and structural abnormalities.[5,6] Imbalances in the levels of multiple gene products encoded on the abnormal chromosome are largely responsible for the phenotypical features observed in individuals with chromosomal aberrations. The clinical features that result from structural or numerical chromosomal abnormalities are variable and depend on the chromosomes involved and the location of the chromosomal abnormality. Clinically, individuals with chromosomal abnormalities may present with some of the following symptoms:

- Multiple congenital anomalies
- Mental retardation
- Multiple unexplained spontaneous abortions
- Ambiguous genitalia
- Primary amenorrhea

Numerical chromosomal abnormalities (e.g., **monosomy, trisomy, polyploidy**) represent the most common type of chromosomal abnormality. Although trisomy 16 is the most common autosomal trisomy identified in miscarriage, trisomies 13, 18, and 21 are identified most commonly in newborns.[5] However, individuals with trisomy 13 and 18 are affected severely, and often, they do not survive.

Down syndrome (trisomy 21) is the most common chromosomal disorder, occurring at an incidence of approximately 1 per 800 live births. As with other trisomies, the risk of having a pregnancy with Down syndrome increases with maternal age. Ninety-five percent of cases are de novo, and 5% are due to translocations involving the acrocentric chromosomes

Table 52-2 Common Chromosomal Disorders

Disease	Chromosome Abnormality	Indicence	Clinical Features
Patau syndrome	Trisomy 13	1 in 5000	Profound mental retardation, holoprosencephaly, cleft lip and palate, polydactyly, seizures, hearing loss, omphalocele, congenital heart defects, and renal anomalies
Edwards syndrome	Trisomy 18	1 in 3000	Profound mental retardation, IUGR, prominent occiput, microphthalmia, micrognathia, congenital heart defects, renal anomalies, clenched hands with overlapping fingers, and rocker bottom feet
Down syndrome	Trisomy 21	1 in 800	Mild-moderate mental retardation, poor muscle tone, growth delay, hearing and vision problems, congenital heart defects, and gastrointestinal defects
Turner syndrome	45,X	1 in 2500 females	Normal intelligence, webbed neck, lymphedema of the hands and feet, short stature, heart and renal anomalies, and infertility
Klinefelter syndrome	47,XXY	1 in 500 males	Learning difficulties, tall stature, gynecomastia, small fibrosed testes, hypogonadism, and azoospermia

IUGR, Intrauterine growth retardation.

Table 52-3 Common Chromosomal Microdeletion Syndromes

Disorder	OMIM	Location	Type	Size	Incidence	Clinical Features
Wolf-Hirschhorn syndrome	194190	4p16.3	Deletion	2.5-30 Mb	1 in 20,000 to 1 in 50,000	Mental retardation, seizures, characteristic facial appearance, congenital heart defects, and genital and renal anomalies
Cri du chat syndrome	123450	5p15.2-p15.3	Deletion	5-40 Mb	1 in 15,000 to 1 in 50,000	Mental retardation, microcephaly, high pitched, "cat-like" cry, and characteristic facial appearance
Williams syndrome	194050	7q11.23	Deletion	2 Mb	1 in 20,000	Mental retardation, loquacious personality, characteristic facial appearance, growth retardation, congenital heart defects, and hypercalcemia
Prader-Willi syndrome	176270	15q11-q13	Deletion (Paternal)	4 Mb	1 in 10,000 to 1 in 15,000	Mental retardation, characteristic facial appearance, hypotonia, poor feeding in infancy with failure to thrive, followed by overeating and obesity, and short stature
Angelman syndrome	105830	15q11-q13	Deletion (Maternal)	4 Mb	1 in 10,000 to 1 in 40,000	Mental retardation, seizures, ataxic gait, absent speech, characteristic facial appearance, hand flapping, happy personality with inappropriate laughter
Smith-Magenis syndrome	182290	17p11.2	Deletion	5 Mb	1 in 25,000	Mental retardation, characteristic facial appearance, self-injurious behaviors, sleep disturbances, congenital heart defects, and renal anomalies
Velo-cardio-facial syndrome	192430	22q11.21	Deletion	3 Mb	1 in 4000	Developmental delays, learning difficulties, characteristic facial appearance, cleft palate, congenital heart disease, absent thymus, hypocalcemia, and renal anomalies

OMIM, Online Mendelian Inheritance in Man (see p. 1046) disorder number.

13, 14, 15, 21, and 22 (Robertsonian translocations), or an isochromosome 21 abnormality (an abnormal metacentric chromosome with two identical arms, e.g., 2 q arms versus a p and a q arm, resulting in a duplication of the q arm and deletion of the p arm). Ninety percent of cases are due to maternal meiosis **nondisjunction** (75% meiosis I error, 25% meiosis II error).

Clinical features include mild to moderate mental retardation, poor muscle tone, growth delay, hearing and vision problems, congenital heart defects, thyroid disease, gastrointestinal defects, early-onset Alzheimer's disease, and an increased risk for certain forms of leukemia. Prenatal abnormalities are detected by ultrasound in 50% of cases. A second-trimester maternal serum screen that demonstrates high beta human chorionic gonadotropin (hCG) and inhibin A and low α-fetoprotein and estriol suggests an increased risk of Down syndrome in the fetus. A **karyotype** that demonstrates trisomy 21 is diagnostic.

Abnormalities in the number of sex chromosomes (e.g., Turner's [45,X], Klinefelter's [47,XXY] syndromes) are commonly identified disorders that may result in significant complications, such as those described earlier. Indeed, 98% of all pregnancies with Turner's syndrome result in miscarriage.[5] Almost all individuals with a sex chromosome abnormality who survive into adulthood are infertile.

Multifactorial (complex) disorders make up the most commonly identified group of genetic disorders (approximately 5% of the pediatric population)[7] and include conditions in which combinations of predisposing genetic factors and environmental conditions contribute to the resulting phenotype. These may include birth defects, such as cleft lip and palate and club foot, as well as adult-onset diseases, such as diabetes mellitus, hypertension, cancer, mental illness, and cardiovascular disease. **Multifactorial disorders** appear to be inherited (i.e., the conditions tend to be observed among multiple individuals within a particular family) but do not follow expected Mendelian patterns of inheritance. Although the risk that a multifactorial disorder will develop in a relative of an affected individual is not as high as would be expected with a single-gene disorder, the more closely related an individual is to an affected person, the more likely that person is to be affected because of more closely shared genes. Additionally, the greater the number of affected relatives, the higher is the recurrence risk.

Multifactorially inherited disorders have been studied classically in monozygotic and dizygotic twins, when both individuals have the condition of interest (concordant) and one is affected and the other is not (discordant). Such studies allow researchers to assess genetic and environmental influences on multifactorial disease. Disease concordance less than 100% in monozygotic twins suggests that environmental factors contribute to disease development. Likewise, greater concordance in monozygotic than dizygotic twins suggests a genetic component to disease development. Additionally, the study of monozygotic and dizygotic twins, who are assumed to share 100% and 50% of their genes, respectively, and are reared together and apart helps to further identify the extent of genetic contributions, that is, heritability, to these diseases.

Mitochondrial DNA disorders (Fig. 52-5) are diseases that arise from mutations in mitochondrial DNA. Males and females may be affected equally, and these disorders may affect multiple generations within a family. However, these diseases are inherited only from the mother. Myoclonic epilepsy with ragged-red fibers (MERRF) and mitochondrial encephalomyopathy, lactic acidosis, and strokelike episodes (MELAS) are examples of disorders that demonstrate mitochondrial inheritance.

Thousands of mitochondrial DNA copies are distributed among the mitochondria in each cell. They are derived solely from the mother's egg at conception (i.e., maternal inheritance). The mitochondria in individuals with mitochondrial DNA diseases usually are composed of mixtures of mutated and normal mitochondrial DNA (i.e., **heteroplasmy**). A critical number (threshold) of mutant mitochondrial DNA strands must be present in a particular cell or organ for the abnormal phenotype to be expressed. Additionally, the number of mutated mitochondrial DNA strands in tissues may change as a result of mitosis (mitotic segregation), which explains why an individual's phenotype may change over time (e.g., an individual whose phenotype transforms from Pearson's syndrome [severe hemopoietic disease] in infancy to Kearns-Sayre syndrome [encephalomyopathy and ophthalmoplegia] at a later age as the proportion of mutated mitochondrial DNA diminishes in hemopoietic cells and increases in brain and muscle cells).[8]

During embryogenesis, the number of mitochondria in the oocytes is reduced before it is subsequently amplified to approximately 100,000 in the mature oocyte. This reduction and amplification of mitochondria (a genetic bottleneck) contributes to mitochondrial DNA variability not only between oocytes, but also between mother and child.[3] Additionally, mothers with higher levels of mutant mitochondrial DNA are more likely to have clinically affected children than mothers with lower levels of mutant mitochondrial DNA.[9] Finally, differences in heteroplasmy among affected family members may help to explain the significant phenotypical variability that can be observed within these families.

Imprinting and Epigenetic Disorders

The term ***epigenetics*** literally means "above the genetics"; it describes stable, heritable changes in gene expression that do not involve alterations in DNA sequence. Genome-wide epigenetic modifications regulate gene expression through such mechanisms as chromatin remodeling, histone modification, and DNA methylation, providing another layer of transcrip-

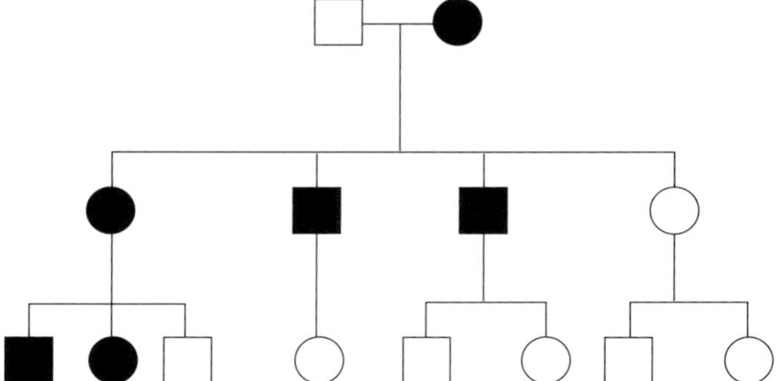

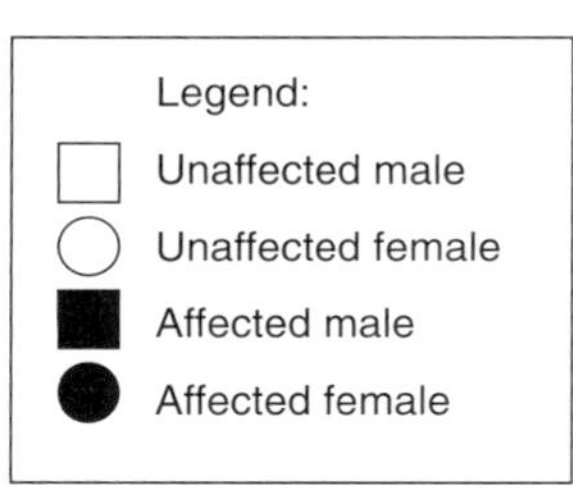

Fig. 52-5 Pedigree demonstrating mitochondrial inheritance.

tional control of gene expression beyond those associated with variation in the sequence of DNA.[10]

Humans inherit two copies of every autosomal gene—one copy from the mother and one from the father, both of which are equally functional for most genes. However, in a small subset, one copy is turned off in a parent-of-origin–dependent manner. The process by which gene expression is altered depending upon whether it was inherited from the mother or the father is called ***imprinting.*** Imprinted genes receive a stable epigenetic mark (e.g., DNA methylation), which provides cells with a memory of the parent of origin of that particular allele. This epigenetic mark determines whether the gene is expressed or not; the allele that receives this imprint, or mark, is silenced. Some imprinted genes are expressed only on the maternally inherited chromosome; others are expressed only on the paternally inherited chromosome.

This epigenetic mechanism is reversible; an imprinted maternally derived allele that is inherited by a male offspring is transformed in his germline so that these alleles are transmitted with a paternal imprint, and vice versa.

Imprinting disorders have been linked to Angelman, Prader-Willi, and Beckwith-Wiedemann syndromes,[11] Alzheimer's disease, autism, bipolar disorder, and diabetes, as well as a number of cancers such as bladder, breast, cervical, colorectal, lung, ovarian, prostate, and testicular, as well as leukemia.

In these disorders, males and females usually are affected equally. However, the disease is manifested only upon inheritance from a parent of one sex. Inheritance from the parent of the opposite sex does not result in the disease because the defective gene is repressed on the chromosome derived from that parent.[12] Both Prader-Willi (PWS) and Angelman (AS) syndromes have been associated with abnormal methylation of imprinted genes at 15q11-q13, including the small nuclear ribonucleoprotein N gene (SNRPN). The promoter region of the SNRPN gene is methylated heavily in the maternally derived allele and is unmethylated in the paternally derived allele, resulting in inactivation and activation of the alleles, respectively. In patients with PWS, the unmethylated allele is absent, whereas in patients with AS, the methylated allele is absent.

Individuals with PWS have small hands and feet, short stature, mental retardation, hypotonia, hypogonadism, and poor feeding at birth, followed by significant overeating and obesity in later childhood. In approximately 70% of individuals with PWS, a deletion of the paternal chromosomal region 15q11-13 occurs. An additional 25% of cases of PWS result from inheriting two maternal copies and no paternal copies of chromosome 15 (maternal uniparental disomy). Less than 1% of cases of PWS result from defects in the regions of DNA that control imprinting (i.e., imprinting center defects).[13]

Conversely, individuals with AS demonstrate severe mental retardation, short stature, characteristic facial appearances, seizures, ataxia, spasticity, and inappropriate laughter. This genetic disorder may result from a deletion in the maternal chromosome at 15q11-13 (70%), a mutation in *UBE3A* (≈11%), paternal uniparental disomy (≈7%), or an imprinting defect (≈3%).[14]

Imprinted genes also are necessary for subsequent normal embryonic development. Reprogramming and resetting of the imprints are tightly controlled by specific genomic regions (imprinting control centers) and methylation enzymes. Several studies have suggested a possible association between imprinting disorders and assisted reproductive techniques.[15] Advances in our understanding of epigenetic mechanisms have been and will be accompanied by new therapeutic options and targets for treatment.[10,16]

GENOMIC VARIATION

Chromosomal Aberrations

Chromosomal aberrations are classified into numerical and structural abnormalities that result in visible alterations of chromosomes by microscopy or change that can be detected by FISH (fluorescence in situ hybridization), CGH (comparative genomic hybridization), or other molecular cytogenetic techniques.

Numerical chromosomal aberrations are usually the result of **aneuploidy,** or abnormal numbers of particular chromosomes. For example, a trisomy has three copies of a particular chromosome or chromosome segment within a cell instead of two. Monosomy has one copy of a chromosome or chromosome segment within a cell instead of the typical two. More rarely, polyploidy may occur, wherein a cell contains more than the diploid (2n) number, or 23 pairs of chromosomes.

Structural chromosomal abnormalities are the result of defects in normal chromosome structure or genomic sequence. These include translocations, deletions, inversions, and duplications, in addition to rarer abnormalities. Structural chromosomal abnormalities may be balanced (a rearrangement occurs, but no genetic material is presumably lost) or unbalanced (genetic material is lost). They usually result from DNA damage caused by exposure to radiation and toxic chemicals, or as an abnormal function of the DNA recombination machinery.

DNA Sequence Variations: Mutations and Polymorphisms

DNA mutations may be classified into several different categories, which are discussed separately in the following sections.

Nucleotide Substitutions, Insertions, and Deletions

Nucleotide substitution involves the replacement of one nucleotide for another. The substitution of a pyrimidine (C or T) for a pyrimidine, or of a purine (A or G) for a purine, is termed a *transition.* If a pyrimidine is substituted for a purine, or vice versa, the term *transversion* applies. Base substitutions are classified further according to the effect that a mutation has upon the DNA coding strand and the ultimate gene product.

Synonymous (silent) mutations generally are single-nucleotide modifications of DNA that change a codon, but the altered codon encodes the same amino acid. This can occur because of redundancy in the genetic code. In comparison, missense mutations alter the DNA sequence and result in a changed codon that encodes a different amino acid. Consequently, the polypeptide sequence is altered; the altered function will depend on the properties of the substituted amino acid and the structure and function of the altered protein. Synonymous and missense mutations can change the RNA splicing consensus (splice site, splicing enhancer, and splicing silencer) sequence, resulting in alternative splicing and creating a nonfunctional protein. Furthermore, both types of mutations may alter mRNA stability or processing. Nonsense mutations alter the DNA sequence, causing the formation of a "stop" codon and prematurely terminating the polypeptide sequence.

Single-nucleotide mutations that occur within conserved sequences at exon/intron boundaries may result in improper splicing by one of several mechanisms: exon skipping, whereby an exon is removed from the RNA sequence; intron retention, whereby an intron is retained within the RNA sequence; and formation of cryptic splice sites, which compete with the normal splice site. RNA splicing mutations may lead to a **frameshift mutation** that disrupts the reading frame, leading to alteration of the amino sequence after that mutation, and possibly resulting in the formation of a "stop" codon. Finally, single-nucleotide mutations also may occur at gene regulatory sites, thereby affecting transcription.

Insertions and deletions of one or more base pairs of DNA alter the DNA sequence and can have a significant impact on the resultant polypeptide product. Inserting or deleting of base pairs that are not multiples of three results in frameshifts and the potential formation of a premature termination codon.

Pathogenic mutations cause disease by producing changes in the quantity or function of the product of an affected gene. Loss-of-function mutations decrease the quantity and/or activity of a protein and usually present as autosomal recessive traits (e.g., phenylketonuria, cystic fibrosis). If 50% of protein quantity or activity is insufficient to maintain normal function (i.e., haploinsufficiency), the resulting trait is autosomal dominantly inherited, for example, Marfan and Alagille syndromes are autosomal dominant genetic diseases that are caused by haploinsufficiency.

Gain-of-function mutations produce products, usually proteins, with new or enhanced activity, increased production, or loss of regulation, and usually occur as autosomal dominant traits (e.g., Huntington's disease, achondroplasia). Abnormal gene products may interfere with the corresponding wild-type products, thereby diminishing the function of the normal gene product (i.e., a **dominant negative** effect). Osteogenesis imperfecta is an example of such a disease.

DNA **polymorphisms** are genetic variations that are defined by **population genetics** as occurring in at least 1% of a population and varying in length from multiple nucleotides to a single nucleotide. Single-nucleotide polymorphisms (SNPs) occur approximately once every 300 bases and constitute the most common class of DNA polymorphism within the human genome. Similar to other DNA polymorphisms, SNPs usually occur in non-coding parts of the genome and therefore usually do not result in disease. They may, however, contribute to enhanced disease susceptibility.

Small copy number variations (e.g., deletions, duplications, insertions, complex multi-site variations) that range in size from kilobases to megabases of DNA represent another significant source of variation in humans. Indeed, a recent study estimated that copy number variations account for 12% of the human genome in European, African, and Asian populations.[17] Similar to SNPs, small copy number variations may contribute to increased disease susceptibility.

KEY CONCEPTS BOX 52-2

- Aneuploidy is the presence or absence of one or more chromosome, resulting in less or more than the normal 23 pairs of chromosomes. For example, trisomy 21 is the result of an extra chromosome #23 (Down syndrome).
- Not all gene mutations will cause disease. The likelihood that a gene mutation results in a disease phenotype is the *penetrance* of the disease, while the degree to which the disease is expressed is the *expressivity*. A single gene can have multiple phenotypic effects in different tissues, called pleiotropy.
- Epignetics describes a number of factors that affect gene expression, independent of the actual DNA sequence. These factors include chromosome structure, alteration in histones, and post-conception DNA modification, such as DNA methylation.
- Epigenetic factors can affect whether genes from the father or mother are expressed, termed *imprinting,* and can sometimes allow the expression of mutant genes.
- A pyrimidine or purine deoxynucleotide can replaced by another pyrimidine or purine (transition mutation) or a pyrimidine can be replaced by a purine (or visa versa, called a transversion mutation). Such base substitutions can have no clinical affect on the final protein product or can result in a protein that is partially or completely defective. The degree of loss of protein function, quantitative or qualitative, will affect the penetrance and expressivity of the mutation.
- Base substitutions or insertions can affect RNA process called frameshift mutation, or produce a code ("stop" codon) that prematurely stops the transcription process.

SECTION OBJECTIVES BOX 52-3

- Briefly discuss the following means to map and identify disease genes: functional cloning, positional cloning, linkage analysis, and genetic association studies.
- Different forms of testing are available for diagnosing genetic diseases.
- Explain the principle, clinical uses, and interpretation of the fluorescence in situ hybridization (FISH) and microarray-based comparative genome hybridization (array CGH) techniques.
- Discuss some of the methods used for molecular genetic testing.
- Recognize genetic disorders that may be identified via newborn screening programs.
- Explain the usefulness of predictive and prenatal genetic testing.
- Outline treatment options currently available for genetic diseases.

MAPPING AND IDENTIFICATION OF DISEASE GENES

The classical approaches to mapping and identifying genes involved in human disease include functional and positional cloning. In functional cloning, physiological function studies precede gene identification and chromosomal mapping. The disease gene usually is isolated only after underlying functional defects have been elucidated. Phenylalanine hydroxylase in phenylketonuria and the β-hemoglobin gene in β-thalassemia are two examples of genes isolated through functional cloning. In positional cloning, gene mapping precedes identification of the disease gene. This approach usually is used when there is little or no understanding about the function of the defective gene. The gene responsible for Duchenne's muscular dystrophy was one of many disease genes isolated via its chromosomal location by positional cloning. Positional cloning requires analysis of samples collected from multiple families in which the genetic disorder segregates.

Linkage disequilibrium and genetic association studies, two important methods for mapping disease-causing genes, require only that the phenotype be well characterized. **Linkage analysis** is a technique used to study the frequency with which two genes remain together (linked) through meiosis as they are passed from one generation to the next. It is used to identify polymorphic markers that are linked (co-inherited) to a gene or trait in question to map its physical location along a chromosome. Genetic association studies are case-controlled analyses that aim to detect an association between one or more genetic polymorphisms and a trait, which might be some quantitative characteristic or a discrete attribute or disease.[1] These studies are particularly useful in the study of complex diseases with sufficient heritability, such as diabetes, arthritis, mental illness, cancer, and heart disease.

The human genome project completed the first working draft of 3 billion base pairs of DNA sequence in the human haploid genome, which provided a vast amount of information for high-resolution genetic mapping. Specifically, millions of polymorphic markers have been identified throughout the entire genome; these data have been and will be used for the discovery of functional biological processes and the isolation of candidate disease-causing genes.

GENETIC TESTING

Genetic testing involves analysis of human DNA, RNA, chromosomes, proteins, and certain metabolites to detect heritable disease–related genotypes, mutations, phenotypes, or karyotypes for clinical purposes.[18] Genetic testing is used in the diagnosis of genetic diseases, prediction of future positive risk of developing manifestations of gene-influenced disease, and assessment of carrier status. However, the results are dependent on reliable laboratory technique and accurate interpretation, which often is complicated.

Diagnostic Genetic Testing

Cytogenetic Testing

Before 1956, it was widely accepted that human cells contained 48 chromosomes. However, in that year, Tjio and Levan, while using a hypotonic solution to process fetal lung tissue, firmly established that human cells contain 46 chromosomes.[19] In the 1960s and the 1970s, staining techniques were developed, allowing for improved visualization of the chromosomes. The first to be developed were whole chromosome stains (i.e., Giemsa, Orcein, and Leishman), which uniformly stain chromosomes.[20,21] However, beginning with the introduction of modern banding techniques in the 1970s (e.g., G-banding, Q-Banding, R-banding), these older staining techniques have been largely replaced.

Cytogenetic analysis is useful for sex determination and identification of abnormalities in chromosome number, such as aneuploidy and polyploidy, as well as chromosomal aberrations, including deletions, duplications, inversions, and translocations. A common method of chromosome analysis involves the culture of peripheral lymphocytes. These mature cells are not actively undergoing mitosis in peripheral blood. Consequently, they are stimulated to divide in vitro by the addition of a mitogen (e.g., phytohemagglutinin) to the culture medium. Toward the end of the culture period, colchicine is added to the culture, which disrupts the mitotic spindle, arresting the cells in the metaphase stage of mitosis. Afterward, the cells may be harvested, prepared on slides, stained by one of multiple techniques (see later), and arranged in a karyotype (Fig. 52-6) for microscopic scrutiny at a magnification of 1000×.[22] This provides a maximum resolution of 3 to 5 megabases for visualization of structural abnormalities.

G-banding is the most common chromosome staining method. This technique involves staining with Giemsa after the slides have been exposed to trypsin, which creates patterns of alternating light and dark bands along the length of the chromosomes, allowing identification of the chromosomes and detection of structural abnormalities.

Approximately 400 bands per haploid set of mid metaphase chromosomes may be identified by conventional staining techniques. However, when high-resolution banding techniques are used on early metaphase and late prophase cells, more than 850 bands per haploid set of chromosomes may be achieved, allowing greater resolution and more precise detection of subtle abnormalities.[21]

Other staining techniques also may be applied in the cytogenetics laboratory. Q-banding stains the chromosomes with dyes, such as quinacrine mustard or quinacrine dihydrochloride, which fluoresces when examined under ultraviolet light, resulting in a banding pattern similar to G-banding. However, the resolution is not as sharp. Q-banding is most useful in identifying Y chromosome heterochromatin, which is highly fluorescent.[21,23] R-banding results in light and dark banding patterns that are the reverse of those observed in G-banding and Q-banding. C-banding techniques stain constitutive heterochromatin in the centromeric regions of all chromosomes and in polymorphic regions of the acrocentric chromosomes,

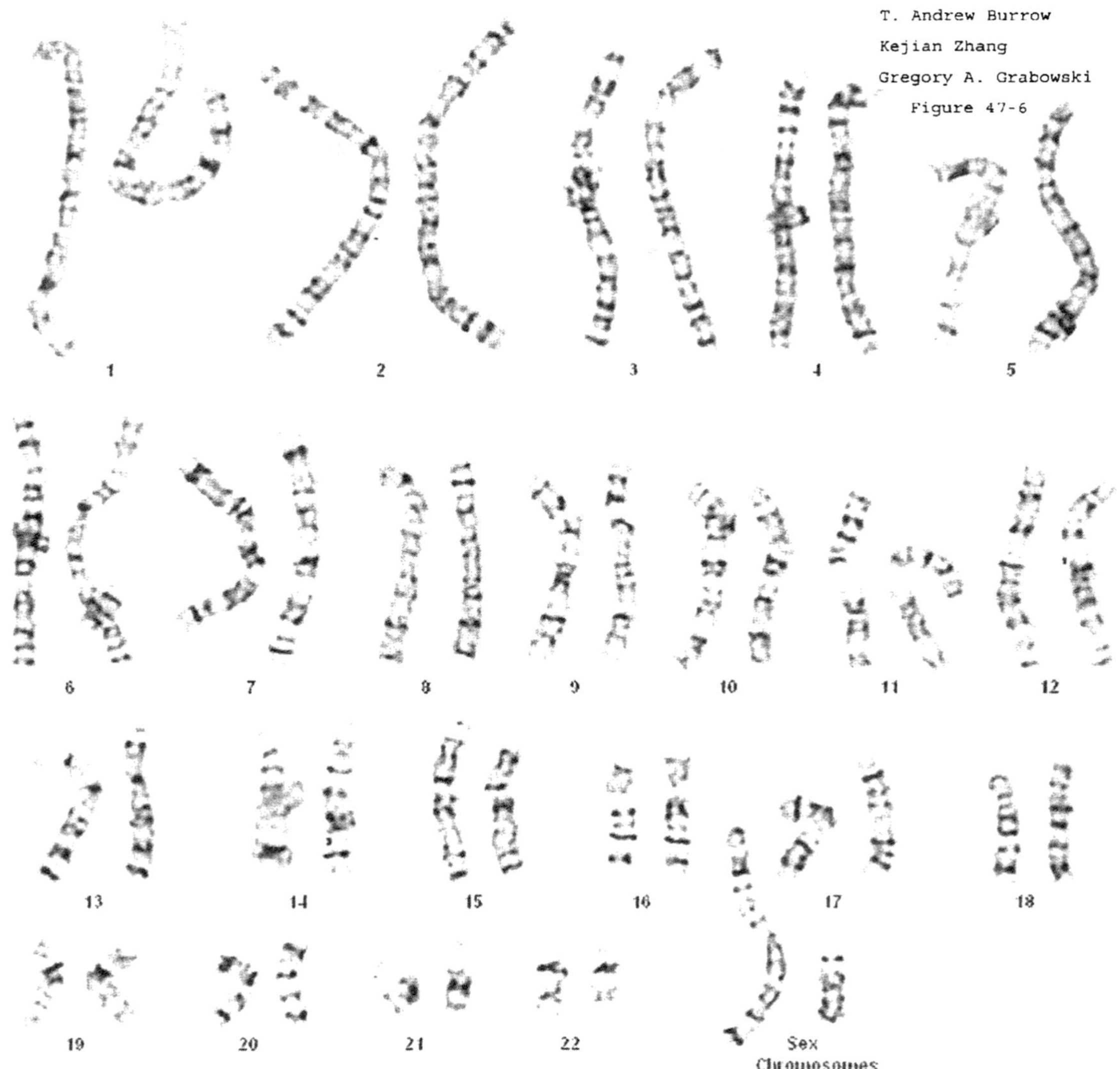

Fig. 52-6 Karyotype of a normal 46,XY male. The G-band technique was performed to stain the chromosomes.

centromeric regions of chromosomes 1, 9, and 16, and the distal portion of the long arm of the Y chromosome.[21]

Fluorescence in situ hybridization (FISH) is a molecular cytogenetic technique that is used to detect deletions, duplications, translocations, and aneuploid states in interphase and metaphase chromosomes. Unlike many other cytogenetic techniques, FISH may be performed on nondividing cells. FISH involves denaturing chromosomal DNA with heat and formamide followed by hybridization to a fluorescently labeled DNA probe, which is synthesized from such sources as complementary DNA (cDNA) and bacterial artificial chromosomes (BACs).[21] The presence or absence of the fluorescent signal, which corresponds to the presence or absence of the complementary chromosomal DNA, is observed with a fluorescent microscope (Fig. 52-7).[21,24] FISH techniques are distinguished by the location on the chromosome at which the probes hybridize, or by the abnormality that they detect; resolution is dependent on the size of the probes.

Locus-specific probes are designed to hybridize to specific areas on chromosomes to detect structural abnormalities (i.e., translocations, deletions, insertions, and duplications) in the chromosomes of interest. For example, failure of locus-specific probes to hybridize at 22q11.2, 7q11.23, and 17p11.2 is diagnostic of velocardiofacial, Williams, and Smith Magenis microdeletion syndromes, respectively. Probes also have been developed for each of the chromosomal subtelomeres, deletions of which may be associated with birth defects and developmental delays.

Centromere-specific probes are designed from unique, repetitive sequences located within the centromere of each chromosome. These probes are used to detect numerical chromosomal abnormalities, to verify the presence of centromeres in structurally abnormal chromosomes, and to serve as controls for other FISH studies.[21]

Dual fusion and break-apart probes are utilized for the detection of reciprocal translocations. Dual fusion FISH probes consist of pairs of two differently labeled probes (i.e., red and green), each binding to a specific region of a different chromosome, and together spanning the breakpoint regions involved in a reciprocal translocation. In

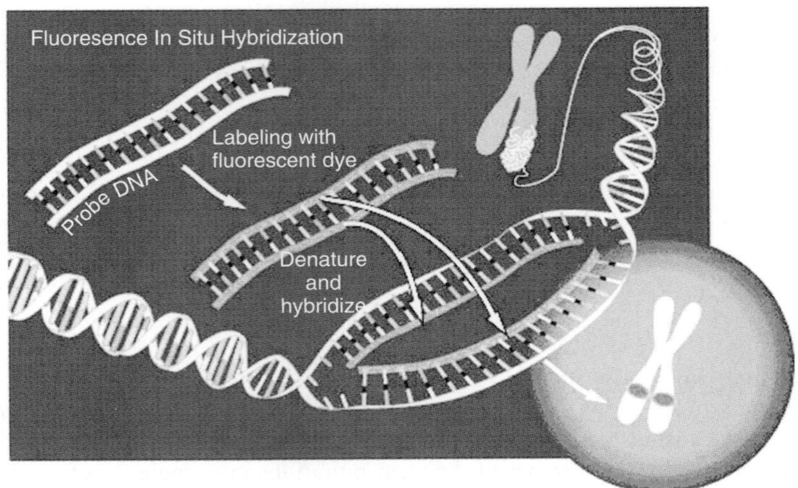

Fig. 52-7 Diagram illustrating the fluorescent in situ hybridization (FISH) technique. (Adapted from the NIH website, http://www.genome.gov/10000206.)

normal cells, two distinct red and green signals are identified. However, in a cell in which a reciprocal translocation is present, a fused red/green signal (which often appears yellow) and a single red and a single green signal are identified.[25] This technique is commonly performed on the bone marrow of individuals with leukemia to evaluate for reciprocal translocations. For example, a reciprocal translocation between chromosomes 22q11.21 and 9q34.1 results in fusion of the *BCR* and *ABL* protooncogenes, respectively, the presence or absence of which has certain diagnostic and prognostic implications.

Conversely, break-away FISH techniques consist of pairs of two differently colored probes (i.e., red and green), each binding to sequences that flank a known breakpoint region. In normal cells, a single, fused red/green signal (which often appears yellow) is observed on each chromosome. Conversely, in abnormal cells in which there is a reciprocal chromosome translocation involving the region flanked by the two probes, a separate red and a separate green signal will be observed, in addition to the normal fused signal.[25]

Whole chromosome painting refers to a form of FISH in which probes hybridize to complementary regions along the entire length of a chromosome. Each probe is labeled with a fluorescent dye the color of which corresponds to a specific chromosome. With the use of combinations of fluorescently labeled probes, each chromosome is "painted" a specific color, creating a spectral karyotype that permits the identification of chromosomes according to color.[22] This technique is useful for the analysis of marker chromosomes and chromosome rearrangements, especially translocations and insertions.

Microarray-based comparative genome hybridization (array CGH) is used in molecular cytogenetics as a high-resolution technique that evaluates for and maps copy number alterations (deletions and duplications) within the genome. Through this technique, whole genomic DNA samples from a patient and a control (normal) individual are labeled differentially with two different fluorophores and are used as probes that competitively co-hybridize onto various nucleic acid targets (i.e., BACs, cDNA, oligonucleotides, and SNPs), which have been applied to a slide. Computer software analyzes the Log2 ratio of fluorescence intensity between reference DNA and test DNA at each target on the array, evaluating for areas of unequal hybridization, which suggests a copy number alteration.[26] In array CGH, resolution is restricted to the size of the clones and the space between the clones.[27]

Two primary array CGH techniques are employed for diagnostic testing: whole genome and targeted arrays. Whole genome arrays include clones selected from throughout the entire genome and provide a high-resolution method of screening for copy number variations throughout the genome. Targeted arrays are designed to evaluate a specific region of the genome (i.e., a specific chromosome or chromosomal region) or to identify and evaluate specific dosage abnormalities in individuals with suspected microdeletion syndromes or subtelomeric abnormalities.[26]

Array CGH has proved particularly important in identifying losses and gains of genetic material ranging in size from kilobases to megabases of DNA that were not identified previously by standard cytogenetic or molecular cytogenetic technologies. Likewise, unlike karyotype analysis, it may be performed in nondividing cells. However, despite its importance as a powerful diagnostic tool, array CGH has some limitations. Balanced chromosome rearrangements, such as true balanced translocations or inversions, will not be detected because these do not result in losses or gains of genetic material. Likewise, this technology will not detect polyploidy (e.g., triploidy), and its ability to detect low levels of mosaicism is limited. Finally, if a clone does not span a chromosomal region in which a copy number variant exists, it will not be detected.

Increasing evidence suggests that DNA copy number variations represent a significant source of variation (i.e., polymorphisms) among individuals. Consequently, it is often difficult to establish whether small copy number alterations are pathogenic or benign polymorphisms. This is particularly the case with results obtained from whole genome microarray CGH. Comparing the patient's and parents' results often helps to clarify whether a particular copy number alteration is likely to be pathogenic. For example, a small copy number variation in a phenotypically abnormal patient that was inherited from a phenotypically normal parent likely represents a polymorphism rather than a pathogenic mutation.

Molecular Genetic Testing (see Chapter 13)

Mutation Screening

Mutation screening is a common strategy for analyzing disease-causing gene variants with a high degree of allelic heterogeneity (the number of different mutations in a single gene). A scanning strategy is also appropriate for analysis of newly identified disease genes for which no or little information is available regarding the number of disease-causing mutations. Techniques used for mutation screen should detect both characterized and uncharacterized mutations. Several previously favored methods (e.g., denaturing high-performance liquid chromatography [DHPLC], single-strand confirmation polymorphism [SSCP]) are used less frequently. DNA sequencing is considered the "gold standard" for screening specific nucleotide alterations associated with genetic disease. Microarray-based resequencing is becoming a very promising new technology for high-throughput mutation screening. However, it has not been used widely in a clinical setting.

Testing for a Specified Sequence Change

Testing for one or a few common mutations offers a cost-efficient way of identifying mutations in diseases that exhibit no or limited allelic heterogeneity (e.g., sickle cell anemia) or in populations in which a limited number of mutations have a high carrier frequency (e.g., cystic fibrosis in Caucasians and Ashkenazi Jews). The methods used for this type of testing are evolving at an unprecedented speed. The most commonly used methods include (1) polymerase chain reaction (PCR) restriction fragment length polymorphism (PCR-RFLP) analysis, (2) DNA sequencing, (3) the amplification refractory mutation system (ARMS), (4) TaqMan Assay by Applied Biosystems Inc. (Foster City, CA), (5) Invader Assay by Third Wave Technologies Inc. (Madison, WI), and (6) the READIT Assay Genotyping System (Promega Corporation, Madison, WI). New technologies for SNP genotyping are evolving rapidly. Ultimately, the technology of genotyping a whole genome for its polymorphic structure through direct resequencing of each individual's genome might be the most comprehensive way to predict and diagnose disease and to provide personalized treatment options.

Testing for DNA Methylation Patterns

Bisulfite modification of genomic DNA, followed by methylation-specific PCR (MSP), has been used to evaluate the methylation status of a segment of DNA (e.g., the SNRPN promoter in Prader-Willi and Angelman syndromes) and to provide accurate and rapid diagnosis of these two syndromes. Sodium bisulfate deaminates cytosine residues in CpG dinucleotides into uracil in genomic DNA, while methylated cytosine residues remain unaffected. After PCR amplification, the uracils are amplified as thymines.[28] Consequently, methylation-dependent changes are introduced into the DNA sequence that can be used to determine the methylation status of a segment of DNA. Similarly, methylation analysis in tumor and normal tissues can help with diagnosis and prognosis in patients with cancer.

Testing for Trinucleotide Repeat Disorders

Trinucleotide repeat expansions are responsible for a number of genetic diseases, such as Huntington's disease, myotonic dystrophy, Friedreich ataxia, and fragile X syndrome (FRAXA). Precise evaluation of the repeat number and methylation status are critical in diagnosing these disorders. For example, fragile X syndrome is the most common form of inherited mental retardation and occurs at an incidence of approximately 1 in 4000 males and 1 in 6000 females. Phenotypical features of fragile X syndrome include mental retardation, large ears, a long and narrow face, increased head circumference, and macroorchidism. The disorder results from CGG repeat expansions in the 5′UTR of the *FMR1* gene, which methylate an adjacent CpG island promoter region, thus decreasing messenger RNA (mRNA) and protein synthesis. CGG repeat expansions greater than 200 repeats in length are considered full mutations and almost always lead to complete expression of the FRAXA syndrome. Individuals with 55 to 200 repeats are called "premutation carriers" and may have minimal or no typical FRAXA abnormalities. However, female premutation carriers can develop premature ovarian failure, and male premutation carriers may develop early-onset ataxia. The premutation is unstable and often leads to further expansion or a full mutation in the subsequent generation, particularly when inherited through the female lineage. PCR, polyacrylamide gel electrophoresis, and Southern blot with methylation-sensitive restrictive enzyme digestion can be used for these types of testing.

Population Screening

Population genetic screening plays an important role in the detection of genetic disease before the onset of symptoms and in the identification of individuals whose offspring are at risk for having a disease.[22] The goal of screening is to identify 100%, or as close as possible to 100%, of individuals at risk for a disease, or whose offspring are at risk for having a disease.[29] However, screening tests have some limitations. A certain number of false-positive and false-negative results will occur, depending on the sensitivity and specificity of the test. Consequently, diagnostic testing must be performed in all individuals who have a positive screen result and in those for whom clinical suspicion of disease is significant despite a negative screen result.[22] One of the largest and most commonly employed population screening tools is the newborn screen. In the United States, newborn screening is mandated in all 50 states, the District of Columbia, Puerto Rico, and other territories. Newborn screening began in the United States in the 1960s with the Guthrie bacterial inhibition assay for phenylketonuria (PKU), a disorder of amino acid metabolism associated with high phenylalanine levels and resulting in mental retardation, if not treated.

Traditionally, newborn screening has relied on the measurement of metabolites (e.g., phenylalanine for phenylketonuria), hormones (e.g., thyroid-stimulating hormone or T_4 for hypothyroidism), and proteins (e.g., galactose-1-phosphate uridyltransferase for galactosemia) for the identification of individuals at risk for having a disease.[29] Recently, new methods such as tandem mass spectrometry (MS/MS) and molecular genetics techniques have revolutionized the field of newborn screening and have greatly expanded the number of identifiable genetic diseases to include more than 25 metabolic, genetic, hematological, and endocrine disorders, as well as hearing impairment (Box 52-1). The actual number of disorders screened varies in each state. However, almost all states screen for PKU, congenital hypothyroidism, and galactosemia. The screening is performed on dried blood specimens obtained on filter paper when newborns are 24 to 48 hours of age.

Other forms of population screening include analysis of the maternal serum biomarkers α-fetoprotein, β-human chorionic gonadotropin (hCG), inhibin A, and estriol during the second trimester of pregnancy (quad screen) to assess the risk for birth defects, such as neural tube defects, and certain chromosomal disorders, such as trisomies 13, 18, and 21, in the current pregnancy, as well as prenatal carrier genetic testing for such diseases as cystic fibrosis in high-risk populations.

Box 52-1

Disorders Commonly Included in Newborn Screening Programs*

Fatty Acid Oxidation Disorders
Carnitine uptake defect
Trifunctional protein deficiency
Medium-chain acyl-CoA dehydrogenase deficiency
Very long chain acyl-CoA dehydrogenase deficiency
Long-chain hydroxyacyl CoA dehydrogenase deficiency

Organic Acid Disorders
Glutaria acidemia type I
Isovaleric acidemia
Propionic acidemia
Methylmalonic acidemia
3-Hydroxy-3-methylglutaryl-CoA lyase deficiency
3-Ketothiolase deficiency
3-Methylcrotonyl-CoA carboxylase deficiency
Multiple CoA carboxylase deficiency

Amino Acid Disorders
Arginonosuccinic acidemia
Citrullinemia
Homocystinuria
Maple syrup urine disease
Phenylketonuria
Tyrosinemia types II and III

Other Metabolic Disorders
Galactosemia
Biotinidase deficiency

Endocrinopathies
Congenital hypothyroidism
Congenital adrenal hyperplasia (21-hydroxylase deficiency)

Other Disorders
Hemoglobinopathies
Cystic fibrosis

CoA, Coenzyme A.
*See National Newborn Screening & Genetics Resource Center http://genes-r-us.uthscsa.edu.

Carrier Genetic Testing

Carrier genetic testing is performed in individuals to determine their carrier status for a particular genetic disorder, usually to determine the individual's risk of having future offspring with that disorder and to assist the person in making informed reproductive decisions. Individuals to whom carrier testing is offered are unaffected by disease; however, their offspring are at risk of inheriting an autosomal recessive or X-linked disorder because of their ethnic background or a family history of a genetic disorder. For example, carrier testing often is offered to individuals of Ashkenazi Jewish descent for several genetic disorders, including Tay-Sachs disease, Gaucher's disease, and cystic fibrosis, because of the significantly increased carrier prevalence within this population. Likewise, carrier testing may be offered to individuals with a family history of a genetic disorder such as Duchenne's muscular dystrophy or fragile X syndrome, to determine a potential carrier's status.

Predictive Genetic Testing

Predictive genetic testing uses genetic testing in an asymptomatic person at risk for a particular disease to predict one's future risk of developing that disease.[30] Predictive genetic testing is subdivided into two categories: presymptomatic and predisposition genetic testing.

Presymptomatic genetic testing is performed in asymptomatic individuals at risk for diseases with delayed onset, such as Huntington's disease, which is a progressive neurodegenerative disease that affects motor and cognitive function with adult onset. An abnormal test result indicates that a person will develop the disease at some point in his or her lifetime, but it does not specify when symptoms will begin to appear. Conversely, a negative result indicates that a person will not develop the disease.[31]

Predisposition genetic testing provides information about an individual's future risk of developing a disease, such as breast or colon cancer. An abnormal result indicates that an individual has an increased (but not certain) risk of developing a disease, and heightened surveillance for the disease is warranted. Conversely, a negative result indicates that an individual's risk of developing the disease is similar to that of the general population.[31]

Predictive genetic testing plays a very important role in risk assessment and treatment of individuals for diseases such as Huntington's disease and cancer; however, it does not provide information regarding age of onset, disease severity, or response to future therapies.

Prenatal Testing

Prenatal testing is used to detect genetic diseases or birth defects in an embryo or fetus before the time of birth. It is indicated any time that a family history, maternal condition, or fetal concern suggests an increased risk that the pregnancy could be affected by a malformation, a chromosomal abnormality, or a genetic disorder.[32]

Prenatal testing may be offered to families known to be carriers of autosomal recessive disorders, such as Tay-Sachs disease, or balanced chromosomal translocations, which increase the risk that the child will be affected with an unbalanced chromosomal translocation. However, in many cases, prenatal testing is offered to couples because of concerns/abnormalities on initial noninvasive routine prenatal screens, such as ultrasonographic examination or maternal serum screening, and to women who become pregnant after 35 years of age (advanced maternal age) because of an increased risk of aneuploidy in the fetus.

Multiple techniques are available for sampling fetal cells and tissues for prenatal genetic testing. These include amniocentesis, chorionic villus sampling (CVS), and percutaneous umbilical blood sampling (PUBS). Using these techniques, one can perform biochemical, molecular, and cytogenetic studies on fetal cells and tissues to establish a diagnosis.

Preimplantation genetic diagnosis (PGD) is a specialized procedure in which genetic diagnosis is performed on an early-stage embryo after in vitro fertilization and before implantation in the uterus. PGD gives at-risk couples the ability to reduce the chance of producing an offspring with the chromosomal or genetic disorder for which it is at risk. Before PGD can be performed, the specific chromosomal abnormality or disease-causing mutation must be known and must have been identified in a previously affected individual or in the carrier parents. Because of the specialized equipment and experience required for this technology, PGD is expensive to perform and is available in only a limited number of centers.

TREATMENT OF GENETIC DISORDERS

Although treatments for many genetic diseases remain primarily symptomatic and preventative, new treatment options for individuals with genetic diseases are emerging rapidly. Examples of currently available clinical treatment options for genetic diseases include transplantation, enzyme replacement therapy, and dietary management.

Bone Marrow and Hematopoietic Stem Cell Transplantation

Bone marrow and hematopoietic stem cell transplantation are performed and indicated for the primary treatment of patients with selected genetic syndromes, including certain lysosomal storage diseases, adrenoleukodystrophies, disorders of bone marrow failure, hemoglobinopathies, and immunodeficiency disorders. Solid organ transplantation is also a treatment option for certain genetic disorders. For example, liver transplantation may be performed in individuals with α_1-antitrypsin deficiency; it not only replaces the damaged organ, but provides a cure for the genetic disease. However, cell and organ transplantation carries a significant risk of complications, the most serious being death, and must be considered carefully for all potential candidates.

Replacement Therapy

Replacement therapy involves the replacement of a gene product, such as an enzyme that is missing or defective as the result of a genetic disease. This usually is done by giving a person an intravenous infusion of purified, recombinant, slightly modified enzyme at regular intervals. Consequently, the recombinant enzyme is taken up by specific cells in the body and is transported to the lysosomes, where it exhibits its biological action. Enzyme replacement therapy is currently available for the following lysosomal storage diseases: Gaucher's disease, Fabry's disease, Pompe's disease, and mucopolysaccharidosis types I, II, and VI. Enzyme replacement therapy is not a cure for these diseases; however, it has been successful in improving or stabilizing the disease course.

The goal of dietary management is to restrict intake in the diet of specific biochemicals that the body is unable to process adequately (e.g., phenylalanine in phenylketonuria), or to replace biochemicals that are deficient as the result of a genetic disease (e.g., biotin in biotinidase deficiency). This is a lifelong treatment modality that does not provide a cure for these diseases but is often capable of preventing many of the severe complications associated with these diseases, including mental retardation and death.

Gene Therapy

Gene therapy involves the introduction of a functioning gene into an individual's DNA to correct the effects of a missing or defective gene. Although gene therapy offers significant potential for the treatment of genetic diseases, the techniques involved are complicated. Significant complications have occurred in patients undergoing gene therapy, and as a result, patient safety is a significant concern. Consequently, this approach to therapy is experimental.

KEY CONCEPTS BOX 52-3

- Determining the chromosomal location after a mutated gene has be disovered is called functional cloning, while in positional cloning the function of the gene product follows the determines of the gene's chromosomal location. Chromosomal location can be deduced by mapping the mutant gene in comparison with nearby known genes ("linkage analysis").
- Genetic association studies in large populations are used to provide linkage between a gene polymorphism and a specific disease.
- Many chemical stains can be used to visualize chromosomes. The FISH DNA hybridization technique employs fluorescent-labeled DNA sequences to visualize specific genes or areas of specific chromosomes. The FISH method can detect chromosomal insertions, deletions, translocations, and duplications.
- The microarray-based comparative genome hybridization (array CGH) technique compares the pattern of DNA hybridization of specific or genome-wide probes for a patient to that of a healthy control to evaluate chromosomal abnormalities.
- A number of molecular techniques are used to screen for mutations, including PCR, ARMS, and TaqMan assays (see Chapter 13 for details of these assays). Modified PCR assays can also detect abnormal DNA methylation patterns. PCR and Southern blot techniques (see Chapter 13) can be used to detect trinuleotide repeat abnormalities.
- Newborns are screened for over 25 treatable, genetic-based metabolic diseases, using filter paper sampling and often GC/MS technology. Population screening of generally healthy populations may also prenatally (Down, hypothyroidism, etc) or for specific high diseases for high-risk populations (e.g., Tay Sachs disease in Ashkenazi Jewish populations). Samples for prenatal testing can be blood, amniotic fluid, or CVS. The healthy population screening identifies individuals at high risk for the genetic disease; follow-up confirmatory testing is then needed.
- Treatment for genetic disease includes diet, to remove a product that can not be metabolized, replacement of the non-functional protein, replacement of a non-functioning organ, or replacement of the defective gene. The latter techniques is still considered an experimental approach.

SECTION OBJECTIVE BOX 52-4

- Be able to access and retrieve information about genes and genetic disorders from Internet resources.

ACCESS TO GENETIC RESOURCES

Since the completion of the Human Genome Project in 2003, a wealth of genetic information has become available. Because of its almost universal availability and limitless capacity, the Internet has become a significant resource for obtaining this information. Despite this, genetic information is often difficult to locate. This section is meant to provide resources to individuals in search of such information.

One of the most important resources for genomic information on the Internet is the National Center for Biotechnology Information (NCBI) website.[33] This site acts as a gateway that provides access to a number of key genetic databases, including the GenBank DNA sequence, Genome, Protein Sequence, SNP, and PubMed databases, all of which are accessible through the Entrez search engine. PubMed contains citations, abstracts, and links to full text of more than 17 million scientific journal articles dating back to the 1950s. Additionally, it contains links to a collection of biomedically related books that can be searched and viewed online.

Online Mendelian Inheritance in Man (OMIM) is a comprehensive searchable catalog of more than 17,000 human genes and genetic disorders that is maintained by Dr. Victor A. McKusick and his colleagues at the Johns Hopkins University and is provided through the National Center for Biotechnology Information (NCBI) website.[34] The database is updated continuously with information obtained from peer-reviewed scientific journals, and it contains links to PubMed abstracts and genomic databases. Each OMIM entry is given a unique 6-digit number, whose first digit indicates the mode of inheritance of the gene involved. A detailed description of the numbering system is available at the OMIM website. For illustrative purposes, Box 52-2 lists some of the information available from the database, and the screen captures in Figs. 52-8 to 52-10 demonstrate some of the search results. Fig. 52-8 is a screen capture from the OMIM website, from which one can search for specific diseases or a class of diseases. In this example, the disease group "lipidoses" is entered. Fig. 52-9 is a screen capture of the partial search result. Fabry's disease is one of the results. Detailed information may be obtained by clicking on the OMIM number associated with Fabry's disease. Fig. 52-10 is a screen capture of detailed information obtained by clicking on the Fabry's disease OMIM number. The information described in Box 52-2 and much more is available through hyperlinks. Thus both members of the public and

Box 52-2

Examples of Information Available on the Online Mendelian Inheritance in Man (OMIM) Website[34]

Website for genetic disease
OMIM number
Common name (e.g., Fabry's disease)
Gene map locus (e.g., Xq22)
Explanation of OMIM number
Clinical feature
Diagnosis
Clinical management
Molecular genetics
Links to references
Links to gene map

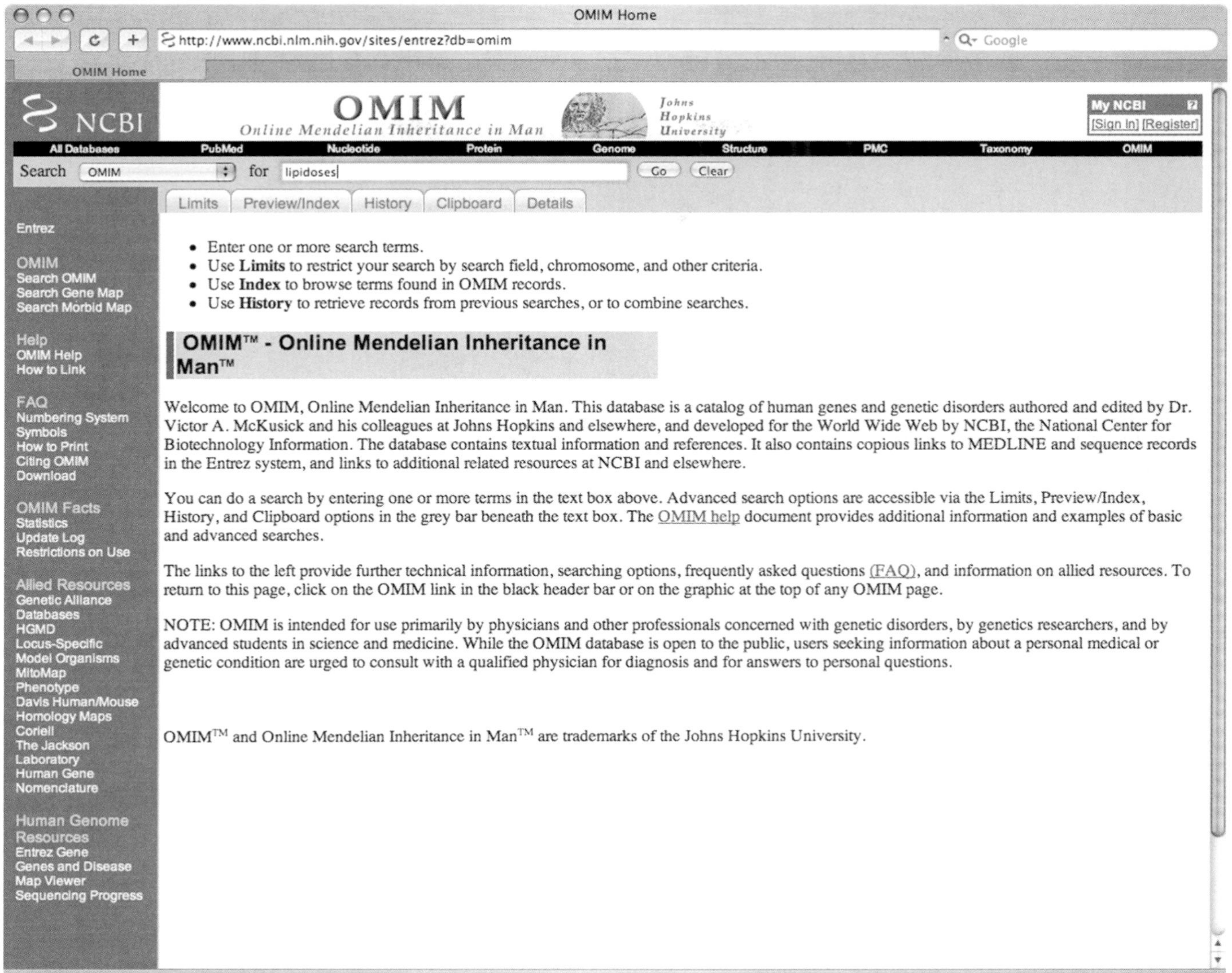

Fig. 52-8 A screen capture from the Online Mendelian Inheritance in Man (OMIM) website, from which one can search for specific diseases or classes of diseases. In this example, the disease group "lipidoses" is entered.

researchers around the world have access to the latest information regarding diagnosis and treatment.

With genome databases and microarray technology, new genetic diseases are being discovered that have no formal name like Fabry's disease; rather, the gene location is used. Work is in progress to predict the likelihood of complex common diseases, such as atherosclerosis, arteriosclerotic heart disease, stroke, cancer, and arthritis. This same information would help the clinician and the patient in selecting appropriate medication. This has given rise to "personalized medicine," in which physicians with knowledge of the patient's genome will prescribe medications known to be effective (http://www.personalizedmedicinecoalition.org/). Attendant to the tremendous advantages that clinical use of genomic science may bring is the specter of misuse of private genetic information. In part, the Health Insurance Portability and Accountability Act (HIPAA) laws were designed to help prevent such misuse (http://www.hhs.gov/ocr/hipaa/). The establishment of standards for privacy and for ethical use of genetic information continues to be an important social goal.

GeneTests[35] is a National Institutes of Health (NIH)-funded website that provides comprehensive expert-authored, peer-reviewed summaries of more than 300 genetic disorders that are updated on a periodic basis. These summaries are structured uniformly and contain sections that describe diagnosis, testing, management, genetic counseling, and resources available for individuals with the specified genetic disorder. Additionally, GeneTests provides a directory of laboratories that offer clinical genetic testing and conduct research studies,

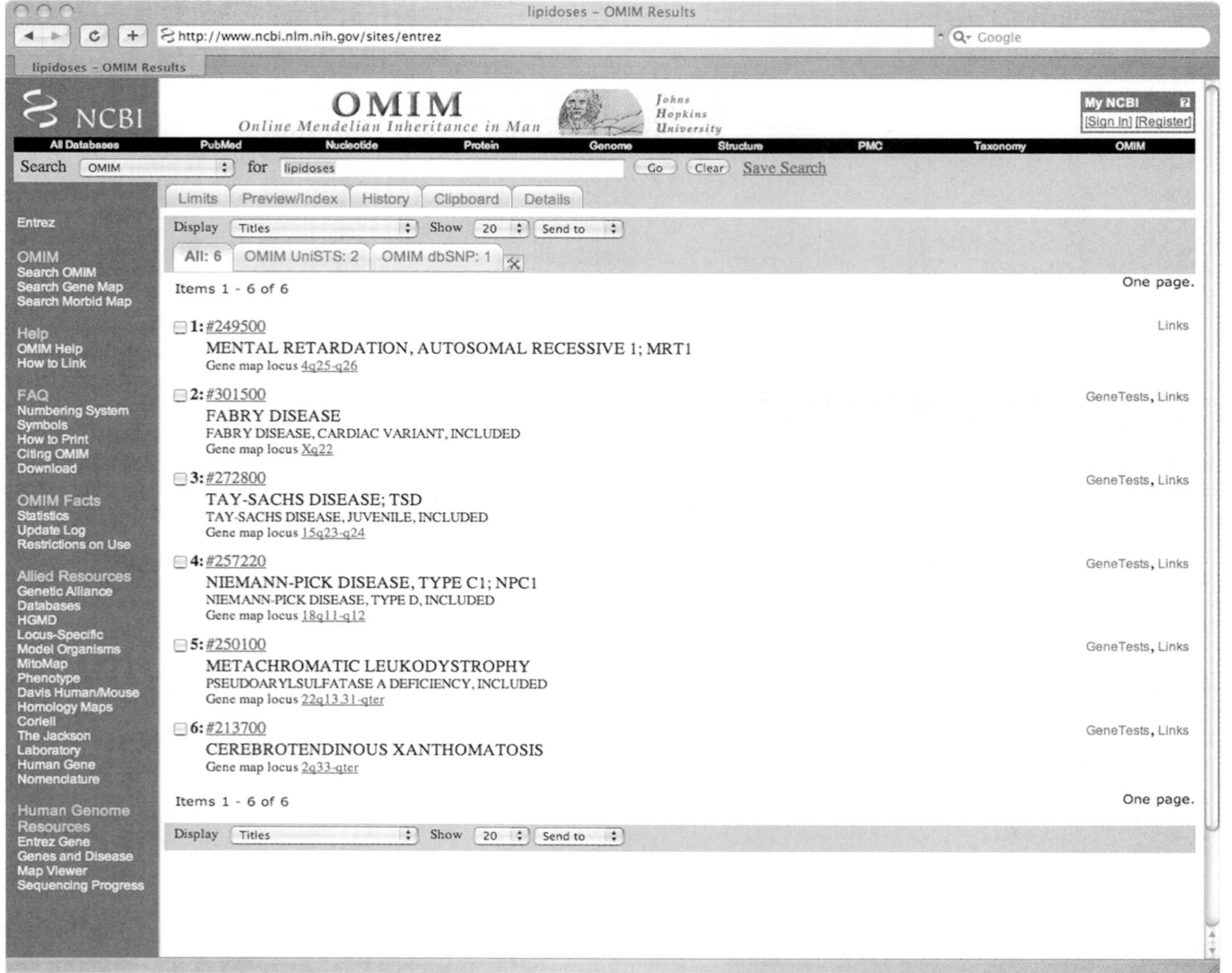

Fig. 52-9 A screen capture of the partial search result. Fabry's disease is one of the results. Detailed information may be obtained by clicking on the Online Mendelian Inheritance in Man (OMIM) number associated with Fabry's disease.

along with a directory of facilities that provide clinical genetics services.

Dozens of other sources, public and private, provide information on medical genetics. The National Organization for Rare Disorders (NORD)[36] is a private organization that maintains a database containing reviews of more than 1150 rare diseases and organizations/support groups dedicated to these diseases. The National Cancer Institute (NCI)[37] provides up-to-date information on genetic cancer disorders, as well as educational materials and updates on current clinical trials related to cancer genetics. Information on current government- and industry-sponsored clinical trials relevant to medical genetics may be found at the website www.clinicaltrials.gov.[38] Furthermore, genetic information can be obtained from professional organizations (e.g., the American College of Medical Genetics) by accessing their websites.[39]

KEY CONCEPTS BOX 52-4

- The Internet is an excellent resource for obtaining information about genetic disorders.
- The Online Mendelian Inheritance in Man (OMIM) Website allows anyone to search for a genetic disease, clinical description of the disease, gene(s) and gene product(s) involved with the disease, and the chromosomal location of the gene.

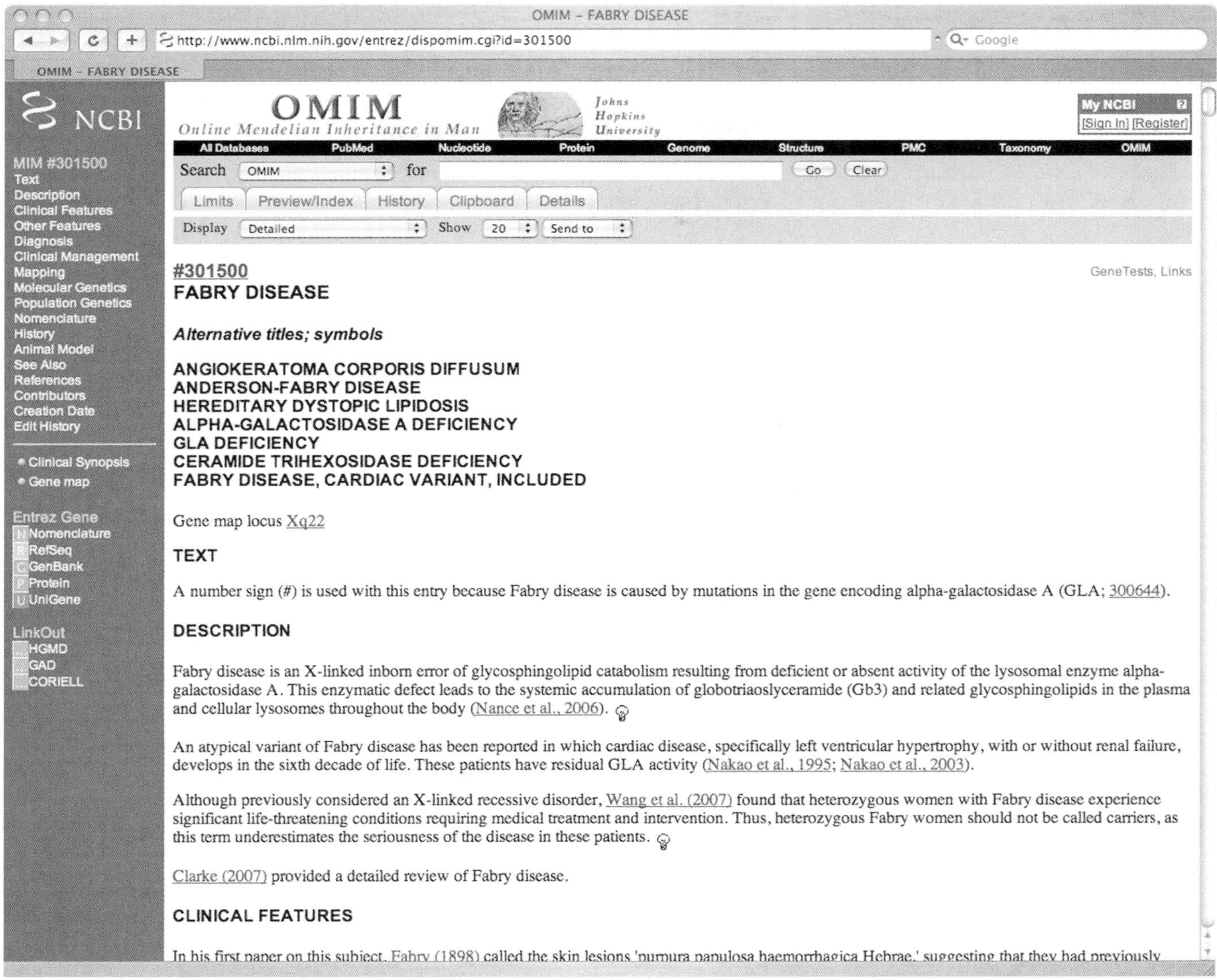

Fig. 52-10 A screen capture of detailed information obtained by clicking on the Fabry's disease Online Mendelian Inheritance in Man (OMIM) number.

REFERENCES

1. Cordell HJ, Clayton DG: Genetic association studies, Lancet 366:1121, 2005.
2. Greally JM: Genomics: encyclopaedia of humble DNA, Nature 447:782, 2007.
3. Nussbaum RL, McInnes RR, Willard HF: *Thompson & Thompson Genetics in Medicine,* ed 6, Philadelphia, PA, 2004, Saunders.
4. Bender MA: Sickle cell disease, March 7, 2006, GeneReviews at GeneTests: Medical Genetics Information Resource (database online), Copyright, University of Washington, Seattle, 1997-2007. Available at http://www.genetests.org. Accessed September 13, 2007.
5. Ensenauer RE, Reinke SS, Ackerman MJ, et al: Primer on medical genomics, Part VIII: Essentials of medical genetics for the practicing physician, Mayo Clin Proc 78:846, 2003.
6. Hamerton JL, Canning N, Ray M, et al: A cytogenetic survey of 14,069 newborn infants, I: Incidence of chromosome abnormalities, Clin Genet 8:223, 1975.
7. Baird PA, Anderson TW, Newcombe HB, et al: Genetic disorders in children and young adults: a population study, Am J Hum Genet 42:677, 1988.
8. DiMauro S, Andreu AL, De Vivo DC: Mitochondrial disorders, J Child Neurol 17(suppl 3):3S35, 2002; discussion 3S46.
9. Chinnery PF, Turnbull DM: Mitochondrial DNA and disease, Lancet 354(suppl 1):SI17, 1999.
10. Waggoner D: Mechanisms of disease: epigenesis, Semin Pediatr Neurol 14:7, 2007.
11. Sparago A, Russo S, Cerrato F, et al: Mechanisms causing imprinting defects in familial Beckwith-Wiedemann syndrome with Wilms' tumour, Hum Mol Genet 16:254, 2007.
12. da Rocha ST, Ferguson-Smith AC: Genomic imprinting, Curr Biol 14:R646, 2004.
13. Cassidy SB, Schwartz S: Prader-Willi syndrome, July 12, 2006, Genereviews at Genetests: Medical Genetics Information Resource (database online), Copyright, University of Washington, Seattle, 1997-2007. Available at http://www.genetests.org. Accessed August 28, 2007.

14. Williams CA, Driscoll DJ: Angelman syndrome, July 30, 2007, GeneReviews at GeneTests: Medical Genetics Information Resource (database online), Copyright, University of Washington, Seattle, 1997-2007. Available at http://www.genetests.org. Accessed August 28, 2007.
15. Paoloni-Giacobino A: Epigenetics in reproductive medicine, Pediatr Res 61(5 Pt 2):51R, 2007.
16. Santos-Reboucas CB, Pimentel MM: Implication of abnormal epigenetic patterns for human diseases, Eur J Hum Genet 15:10, 2007.
17. Redon R, Ishikawa S, Fitch KR, et al: Global variation in copy number in the human genome, Nature 444:444, 2006.
18. Holtzman NA, Watson MS: Promoting safe and effective genetic testing in the United States, September 1997. Available at: http://www.genome.gov/10001733. Accessed July 9, 2007.
19. Tjio JH, Levan A: The chromosome number of man, Hereditas 42:1, 1956.
20. Gardner RJM, Sutherland GR: *Chromosome Abnormalities and Genetic Counseling,* ed 3, New York, NY, 2004, Oxford University Press.
21. Spurbeck JL, Adams SA, Stupca PJ, et al: Primer on medical genomics, Part XI: Visualizing human chromosomes, Mayo Clin Proc 79:58, 2004.
22. Rucknagel DL, Wenstrup R: Diseases of genetic origin. In Kaplan LA, Pesce A, Kazmierczak S, editors: *Clinical Chemistry: Theory, Analysis, Correlation,* ed 4, St. Louis, 2003, Mosby, p. 907.
23. Warburton D: Current techniques in chromosome analysis, Pediatr Clin North Am 27:753, 1980.
24. Price CM: Fluorescence in situ hybridization, Blood Rev 7:127, 1993.
25. Ventura RA, Martin-Subero JI, Jones M, et al: FISH analysis for the detection of lymphoma-associated chromosomal abnormalities in routine paraffin-embedded tissue, J Mol Diagn 8:141, 2006.
26. Bejjani BA, Shaffer LG: Application of array-based comparative genomic hybridization to clinical diagnostics, J Mol Diagn 8:528, 2006.
27. Speicher MR, Carter NP: The new cytogenetics: blurring the boundaries with molecular biology, Nat Rev Genet 6:782, 2005.
28. Ho SM, Tang WY: Techniques used in studies of epigenome dysregulation due to aberrant DNA methylation: an emphasis on fetal-based adult diseases, Reprod Toxicol 23:267, 2007.
29. McCabe LL, McCabe ER: Newborn screening as a model for population screening, Mol Genet Metab 75:299, 2002.
30. Evans JP, Skrzynia C, Burke W: The complexities of predictive genetic testing, BMJ 322:1052, 2001.
31. McPherson E: Genetic diagnosis and testing in clinical practice, Clin Med Res 4:123, 2006.
32. Cunniff C: Prenatal screening and diagnosis for pediatricians, Pediatrics 114:889, 2004.
33. Wheeler DL, Barrett T, Benson DA, et al: Database resources of the National Center for Biotechnology Information, Nucleic Acids Res 35(database issue):D5, 2007.
34. McKusick VA: Mendelian Inheritance in man, and its online version, OMIM, Apr online database by McKusik-Nathans Institute of Genetic Medicine, Johns Hopkins University, Baltimore, MD, and National Center for Biotechnology Information, National Library of Medicine, Bethesda, Maryland. Available at http://www.ncbi.nlm.nih.gov/omim/. Accessed July 24, 2007.
35. GeneTests: Medical genetics information resource, online database by the University of Washington, Seattle, WA. Available at http://www.genetests.org. Accessed July 24, 2007.
36. National Organization for Rare Disorders (NORD), Danbury, CT. Available at http://rarediseases.org. Accessed July 24, 2007.
37. National Cancer Institute, Bethesda, MD. Available at http://www.cancer.gov. Accessed July 24, 2007.
38. ClinicalTrials.gov, National Library of Medicine, Bethesda, MD. Available at http://www.clinicaltrials.gov. Accessed July 24, 2007.
39. American College of Medical Genetics, Bethesda, MD. Available at http://www.acmg.net. Accessed July 24, 2007.

Neoplasia

Barry N. Elkins

53 Chapter

Chapter Outline

Key Terms

angiogenesis A physiological process that involves the generation of new blood vessels from preexisting vessels. It is a normal physiological function of growth and development and also occurs in wound healing. It is an important step when tumors change from a benign state to a malignant state.

apoptosis One of the main types of programmed cell death; it involves a series of biochemical events executed in such a way as to safely dispose of cell debris.

Bence-Jones protein Monoclonal free immunoglobulin light chains found in serum or urine.

carcinoembryonic antigen (CEA) A glycoprotein produced by or associated with cancer cells that also is expressed by fetal cells. Small levels are detected in healthy individuals. Detection occurs by immunochemical analysis.

carcinogen An agent, such as a chemical or a virus, that transforms a cell from a normal to a cancerous state.

clonal selection A widely accepted theory that describes how the immune system responds to infection, and how some B and T lymphocytes are selected for binding to specific antigens that invade the body.

co-carcinogen An agent that by itself does not transform a normal cell into a cancerous state, but in concert with another agent, it can effect the transformation.

confirmation Use of a subsequent test with very high specificity to verify an observation of a less specific test (e.g., a biopsy to verify the presence of a tumor).

dedifferentiation The process by which cells go from a more specific to a more general nature. Usually, such cells lose their morphological architecture and their ability to synthesize specific cell components such as estrogen receptors.

dissemination The phase of cancer in which the cells spread to various parts of the body distant from the site of origin.

estrogen receptor The specific membrane receptor in tissue that binds estrogens. Its presence in breast cancer signifies a differentiated tumor.

heterogeneity Variation in gene expression among cancer cells. Differences between cells exist, and not all cells within a tumor are positive for the same antigen or respond to the same drug.

in situ Confined to the site of origin. Used to describe cancer cells that are localized at their place of origin.

induction phase The period during which a normal cell becomes transformed into a cancerous cell.

invasion The process by which malignant cells move into deeper tissue and through the basement membrane, thereby gaining access to blood vessels and lymphatic channels.

metastases Cancer cells that have spread to other organs and formed colonies that are growing and often invading the organ.

monitoring Measurement of a biochemical marker of cancer after a confirmed diagnosis; used to evaluate the presence or growth of the cancer (e.g., the use of **carcinoembryonic antigen** to monitor colorectal cancer).

neoplasia Literally, new growth; the unrestricted growth of cells that results in cancer.

oncogene A gene whose protein product can cause the development of a cancer when the protein is present (or absent) in abnormal amounts.

Pap (Papanicolaou) smear A common screening test for cancer, in which cells from the cervix are examined for cytological abnormalities consistent with cancer.

staging A process of diagnosis in which the pathologist determines the position of cancer in the progressive cycle of phases: induction, in situ, invasion, and dissemination.

transformation In oncology, the process by which a normal cell becomes malignant, that is, cancerous.

tumor burden The number of tumor cells present in an individual. Tumor markers can estimate tumor burden.

tumor marker A term that implies that certain molecules can be used to screen for or monitor the presence or growth of a cancer. Such markers are usually not specific for cancer and cannot be used for diagnosis.

Methods on Evolve

α-Fetoprotein
Bence Jones proteins
Carcinoembryonic antigens (CEA)
Fecal occult blood
Hormones, various
Immunoelectrophoresis
Immunoglobulins, quantitation, free light chains
Prostate-specific antigen (PSA)
Serum protein electrophoresis
Steroid hormone receptors

CANCER INCIDENCE IN THE UNITED STATES

Increasing longevity, the presence of **carcinogens** in the environment, and other factors have changed the incidence of cancer in the United States; it is the second leading cause of death in the United States. Table 53-1 presents percentages of cancer deaths by organ site and gender, as tabulated in the year 2008 in the United States. The sites associated most strongly with cancer deaths in males of all ages are, in descending order, lung, colorectal, prostate, blood and lymphoid tissues, urinary tract, and pancreas. In females of all ages, the most common cancer sites are lung, breast, colorectal, blood and lymphoid tissues, pancreas, ovary, and uterus. Carcinogens are believed to be responsible for the alterations in cellular genetic material (deoxyribonucleic acid, or DNA) that lead to several cancers, including lung and colorectal cancer. The distribution of deaths by organ site is affected by geographical factors as well. For example, in Japan, unlike in the United States, esophageal and stomach cancers are the most common types of malignancy. In Western countries, cancer is the second leading cause of death. Approximately one in five persons in the United States will die of cancer.

SECTION OBJECTIVES BOX 53-1

- Describe the multi-step process that can lead to cancer.
- Describe the clonal process of cancer.
- Describe oncogenes and the role they play in cancer development.
- Explain the role that genes that control apoptosis can play in cancer development.

CANCER: NATURE OF THE DISEASE

The clonal theory of carcinogenesis states that cancers derive from an original cell that has undergone **transformation.** This transformed cell, or clone, is a normal cell whose genetic material has been altered in such a way that the cell and its progeny lose those regulatory functions that govern cell replication and cell death. Through an evolutionary, multi-step process, cells derived from the initially modified cell begin to multiply, uncontrolled by the usual local inhibitory systems

Table 53-1 Estimated Rates of Cancer Death in 2008 in the United States by Site and Sex

Site	Male, %	Female, %
Breast	*	15
Brain, nervous system	*	2
Colon and rectum	8	9
Non-Hodgkin lymphoma	3	3
Lung and bronchus	31	26
Ovary	NA	6
Pancreas	6	6
Liver	4	2
Prostate	10	NA
Kidney and renal pelvis	3	*
Urinary bladder	3	*
Leukemia	4	3
Esophagus	4	*
All other sites	24	25

Data supplied by the American Cancer Society referenced to the year 2000: http://www.cancer.org/downloads/STT/Cancer_Statistics_2008.
*No data listed.

and often invading other parts of the body. This last phase, called **metastasis,** is usually the cause of death by cancer.

Several points of evidence have led scientists to believe that more than one altered gene must be expressed before a malignant cell is formed. First, the relationship between cancer and age is usually an experiential one, that is, as an individual ages, the likelihood of cancer increases. Time is needed to allow the accumulation of genetic damage, which can lead to the transformed state (see later). Second, cancer cells can be shown to have multiple genetic lesions. Third, cancer is more likely to occur in cells that proliferate. Thus cancer of the heart is very rare, but cancers of the white blood cell are very common. Because white blood cells proliferate, the potential for genetic lesions to be expressed and for the process of cell division to become unregulated is far greater.

Etiology

Cancer as a Multi-Step Process

Cancer has been described as a multi-stage genetic process.[1] The stages of this process include the following:

- Initial DNA damage, and/or
- Chromosome breakdown and rearrangement; gene replication
- Selection of successfully growing mutant cells

Initial changes in cellular DNA can be caused by a variety of carcinogens, including radiation, chemicals, and viruses. This leads to new patterns of gene expression and to faulty control of cell growth. Chromosome breakage and rearrangement occur in several continuous phases after initiation of cell division. This is manifested later in terms of aberrant chromosomal transpositions that lead to genomic rearrangements (see Chapter 52). Changes in the DNA and chromosomes result in a new pattern of gene expression and creates a new phenotype in which previously quiescent genes now are expressed, previously expressed genes now are quiescent, or overexpression of certain key genes occurs. Evidence suggests that the earliest changes in gene expression that can lead to a transformed cell occur in genes that normally regulate cell growth and cell death.[2] These newly expressed or suppressed regulatory genes are known as **oncogenes.**[3] A table that contains a census of more than 363 genes known to be related to cancer occurrence has been published[4] and is being updated constantly. This list is available though the website of the Cancer Genome Project.[5] Assays that detect oncogenes in human tissues are available to help predict the development of oncogene-associated cancers in high-risk groups (see Chapter 13).

Onocogenes[6,7]

An *oncogene* is defined as a gene that, when activated inappropriately, results in the transition from normal, well-regulated cells to the wildly proliferating, uncontrolled cell mass that characterizes cancer. Because only one copy of the gene needs to be mutated for the genotype to affect the phenotype (malignant vs. normal), oncogenes are said to act in a dominant fashion. Most oncogenes are the result of mutations of normal cell regulatory genes (Table 53-2). These normal genes are referred to as *protooncogenes*. The biochemical activities of protooncogenes generally fall into one of three categories: (1) protein kinases and phosphorylases, (2) G-proteins and signal transduction proteins, or (3) transcription factors.[8] When activated, protein kinases and phosphorylases initiate phosphorylation cascades, with the result often being cell growth. Examples include the *erbB* oncogene, which is a mutant form of the epidermal growth factor receptor (EGFR), and the *raf1* gene, a serine kinase that is thought to link signals generated at the cell membrane and nuclear proteins that regulate cell growth.

Table 53-2 Classes of Oncogenes and Their Derived Protein Products

Class of Factor	Factor	Protein Product
Growth factors	*sis*	PDGF B, chain growth factor
Protein tyrosine kinase	*sic*	Membrane-associated, receptor protein tyrosine kinase
Receptors lacking protein kinase activity	*mas*	Angiotensin receptor
Membrane-associated G-proteins	*H-ras*	Membrane-associated GTP-binding/GTPase
Cytoplasmic protein kinases	*rat/mil*	Cytoplasmic protein kinase
Cytoplasmic regulators	*crk*	SH-23 protein
Nuclear transcription co-factors	*myc*	Sequence-specific, DNA-binding protein

GTP, Guanosine triphosphate; *PDGF,* platelet-derived growth factor.

The G-proteins (guanosine triphosphate [GTP]-binding proteins) constitute part of the signal transduction pathways. These pathways connect events at the cell surface, such as the binding of a hormone to its receptor, to events in the nucleus. Activated G-proteins interact with second messenger systems, such as adenyl cyclase and cyclic adenosine monophosphate (cAMP), to stimulate RNA transcription. A well-known example of G-protein oncogenes is the *ras* family of genes. Although normal G-proteins possess a GTPase activity that serves to terminate stimulation, mutant genes are incapable of hydrolyzing GTP and thus are maintained inappropriately in an active state.

The *myc* family of oncogenes, which in the healthy state code for DNA transcription factors, is perhaps the best studied system. *Myc* is overexpressed in several different types of tumors and serves to deregulate the production of cellular growth factors. The presence of activated forms of several oncogenes, for example, the amplification of *N-myc* in neuroblastoma, has been associated with poor prognosis.

The identification of certain mutant or amplified oncogenes will be used increasingly to direct therapy. A current example is the drug Gleevec, which was designed to inhibit the tyrosine kinase activity of the bcr/abl fusion protein in chronic myelogenous leukemia. Detection of amplified copies of the HER2/nue oncogene in breast tumors is used to predict responsiveness to Herceptin therapy (trastuzumab, a humanized anti-HER2/nue monoclonal antibody; Genentech).

Apoptosis

Apoptosis serves two functions in the body: cell termination and homeostasis. Cell termination can be part of normal fetal development and can be used to maintain a relatively constant number of cells throughout the body. Programmed cell death leads to cell shrinkage and fragmentation, which allow cells to be phagocytosed efficiently. In this way, cell components can be reused without the release of potentially damaging intracellular substances.

Apoptosis also can occur when a cell is damaged beyond repair or is infected with a virus; it is used when a cell undergoes stress conditions such as starvation. DNA damage from ionizing radiation or toxic chemicals can induce apoptosis through the action of the tumor suppressor gene *p53*. The signal for apoptosis can come from within the cell, from surrounding tissue, or from a cell that is part of the immune system. Thus apoptosis functions to remove a damaged cell or to prevent the spread of viral infection.

A mutation in the *p53* gene[9] affects a cell's ability to undergo apoptosis; thus a cell with this mutation may continue to divide and develop into a tumor (see later). Germline mutations in *p53* predispose individuals to a wide range of tumor types at an early age; this is known as Li-Fromeni syndrome.[10] Infection with the human papillomavirus interferes with the action of *p53*, potentially leading to the development of cervical cancer.

Expression of the Cancer Phenotype: From Transformation to Cancer

A cell that has been transformed has only the potential to develop into a cancer. Expression of the cancer phenotype requires cell division, which can be induced by additional genetic damage or can result from natural induction of cell division. This can be seen in the inverse relationship between the development of breast cancer and the age at which a woman first carries a pregnancy to near term. This relationship is likely the result of the one-time induction of breast epithelial cell hyperplasia that occurs in a first pregnancy. The later in life that the first pregnancy occurs, the greater is the likelihood that altered genes may accumulate, and a cancer phenotype may be expressed in breast epithelium.

As cancer cells multiply, additional phenotypical changes may occur in the now unstable genetic material. As a result, the process of natural selection allows the most successful cancer cell to proliferate to the greatest extent and to dominate the cancer mass (clonal selection). As the environment surrounding the cancer changes, which may occur as a result of therapy, the selection process continues, often producing a cancer clone that is resistant to therapy.

Diversity of Cancer Cells

Variation of Gene Expression

A broad range of possible combinations of gene expression is seen in the human cell. This range includes normal cells to the most atypical cancer cells. As a result of the genetic changes described earlier, cancer cells exhibit new combinations of gene expression and therefore new phenotypes.

A common phenomenon of cancer is **dedifferentiation,** in which cells go from a more specific cell type (differentiated) to a more general cell type (dedifferentiated) through the process of clonal selection. Thus it is not uncommon for cancer cells to synthesize various compounds that normally are present only in the embryonic or fetal stage. On the other hand, as cells dedifferentiate, they may lose certain specific cellular properties such as receptor activity or enzyme activity. These phenotypical changes can be used as prognostic indicators or as a way to monitor the progress of the disease.

Phenotypical variation is seen not only from cancer cells to normal cells or from cancer type to cancer type, but also within particular cancer types and even within a single tumor. Variable gene expression leads to biological and biochemical diversity of cancer cells; consequently, various tumor-specific markers are not necessarily elaborated by all cancer cells of the same type or even by a single cancer over time. This fact is clinically very important in an investigator's determination of which analyte to follow when **monitoring** patients with known malignancy. For example, in patients with cancer of the breast, **heterogeneity** of genes expressed by various cells occurs, so that not all cells express the **estrogen receptor.**

Cellular diversity within a single tumor also means that a cancer's clinical manifestation, such as the ability of a tumor to metastasize or to respond to therapy, may change with time.

Clinical Manifestations

The clinical manifestations of cancer vary widely, depending on the type of tumor, the tissue affected, and the stage of tumor development. For example, cancer of the gastrointestinal tract is manifested by obstruction, hemoptysis, and bloody stools. Cancer of the lung is manifested by hypoxia, chest pain, and often various neurological symptoms. The clinical manifestations are related to the physiological function of the organ, along with the primary cancer and the effect of the cancer on other organs. For example, cancer of an endocrine gland can result in the production of excess hormone with many systemic hormonal effects. New symptoms are seen with the spread (metastasis) of cancer cells to other organs. Cancer spreads through the lymphatic system and the bloodstream, resulting in liver, bone, and pulmonary metastases.

Time as a Factor: Cancer as a Long-Term Process

Cancer is a long-term process that progresses through four obligatory phases: an **induction phase,** an **in situ** phase, an **invasion** phase, and a **dissemination** phase. During the induction phase, which can last up to 30 years or longer, cells are exposed to one or more gene-altering factors (carcinogens). It has been estimated that approximately three-fourths of all human cancers may be caused by these environmental factors. Not every cell with changed DNA will be transformed, and not everyone who is exposed to the same carcinogen will develop cancer. Additional factors that play a role in the development of cancer include individual (genetic) or tissue susceptibility, the presence of other carcinogens or co-carcinogens,

Box 53-1

Examples of Angiogenic Factors

Angiogenin
Angiopoietin-1
Fibroblast growth factors: acidic (aFGF) and basic (bFGF)
Follistatin
Granulocyte colony-stimulating factor (G-CSF)
Hepatocyte growth factor (HGF)/scatter factor (SF)
Interleukin-8 (IL-8)
Leptin
Placental growth factor
Platelet-derived endothelial cell growth factor (PD-ECGF)
Progranulin
Proliferin
Transforming growth factor-α (TGF-α)
Tumor necrosis factor-α (TNF-α)
Vascular endothelial growth factor (VEGF)/vascular permeability factor (VPF)

From http://www.angio.org/understanding/content_understanding.html.

the site at which the carcinogen may act, the duration of exposure (see earlier), and, of course, the nature, amount, and concentration of the carcinogen under question.

After induction, an in situ phase occurs, during which the transformed cell actually develops into a cancer, but the cancer remains localized within the original site (in situ) and does not invade other tissues. Clonal selection (see earlier) for those cancer cells that grow most successfully occurs during this phase.

The third phase is called the invasion phase. During this phase, as the malignant cells multiply, they invade into deeper tissues through the basement membrane, thereby gaining access to blood vessels and lymphatic channels. One factor that may limit tumor growth during the in situ and invasion phases is the formation of a new blood supply. This process, termed **angiogenesis,** is regulated by the presence of specific angiogenic factors, many of which are normal growth factors (Box 53-1).[11,12]

The fourth stage is the dissemination phase. During this phase, which lasts from 1 to 5 years, the invading cancer spreads to various parts of the body distant from the site of origin, often through the blood and lymphatic systems.

Invasion by Cancer Cells of Surrounding Tissue

Several factors contribute to a cancer's ability to invade surrounding tissue. Such factors include increased motility of the cells, increased pressure within the tumor caused by active multiplication of cells, elaboration by the cancer of lytic substances, lack of intercellular bridges between all normal cells, decreased cohesiveness between cells, and eventual spread of tumor cells to the regional lymph nodes. However, when the metastases are still microscopic (micrometastases), the clinician's ability to detect them is very poor. It has been estimated that approximately half of all patients who appear to be clinically free of metastases do in fact have unrecognized distant micrometastases at the time of initial diagnosis and treatment.

Early detection of cancer, before metastatic spread, is critical to successful treatment of the disease. In fact, it would be ideal to detect cancer during the induction phase; unfortunately, however, this is impossible because before the in situ phase occurs, an investigator cannot be certain whether cancer will actually develop in the individual. The next best approach, then, is to detect cancer during the in situ phase. This has been done with great success in patients with cancer of the cervix, for whom the **Pap (Papanicolaou) smear** technique has been of great benefit. When in situ cancer of the cervix is detected, the prognosis is excellent. Most cancers are detected during the invasion phase. If dissemination has not yet occurred, the prognosis is reasonable. Detection of local spreading with or without involvement of the lymph nodes often leads to a cure. However, if dissemination has already occurred, the prognosis is worse.

Models of Carcinogenesis

Linear Model of Carcinogenesis: Colorectal Cancer Model of Tumorigenesis

A stepwise, or linear, model of colorectal tumorigenesis involving gene mutations for specific molecular pathways and chromosome changes serves as a model for the development of many types of cancers.[13,14] In this model, the following *sequential* steps must occur for colorectal cancer to develop:

1. Mutations in the adenomatous polyposis coli (APC) tumor suppressor gene occur early in the development of polyps.
2. Oncogenic *K-ras* mutations arise during the adenomatous stage.
3. Mutations of tumor suppressor gene *p53* and deletions on chromosome 18q coincide with the transition to malignancy.

The APC/Beta-Catenin Pathway

The *APC* gene encodes a protein, beta-catenin, which, when mutated, results in familial adenomatous polyposis (FAP; Gardner's syndrome); it also plays a critical role in sporadic colon cancer. The *APC* tumor suppressor gene is mutated in more than 70% of all colorectal cancers. The mutated APC protein causes a disruption of the *APC*/beta-catenin complex and increased cytoplasmic levels of free beta-catenin, which translocate to the nucleus, where they activate several oncogenes.

The DNA Mismatch Repair Pathway

Mutations in five different genes have been identified with the hereditary nonpolyposis colorectal cancer (HNPCC) syndrome. Each of the genes encodes a protein involved in DNA mismatch repair, the enzymatic proofreading process that corrects base pair mismatches that arise during DNA replication. These gene defects presumably cause tumor development as a result of widespread mutations that cannot be repaired.

Stochastic Model for Carcinogenesis

For some cancers such as breast and lung cancer, a stochastic or web-of-causation mode seems to best explain the carcinogenic process. In this theory, the order of gene mutation is not important; mutation of any protooncogene or tumor suppressor gene can serve as a first hit. It is not necessary for the first mutational event to be followed by mutation of a specific gene; rather, mutation of some number of genes (a number unknown at the present time) is both necessary and sufficient for the development of a malignant phenotype. Further, the identity of those genes is not fixed; a large number of genes can, in theory, act in concert when mutated to allow the cell to grow in an uncontrollable fashion.

Factors Identified in Promotion of Metastasis

The process of metastasis requires a number of biological and chemical alterations to the cancer cells.[15] These alterations include reduced expression of cellular adhesion molecules (cadherins) and increased degradation of extracellular matrix components by metalloproteases and serine proteases, which allow the cells to detach from one another and move from the primary tumor mass. Finally, interactions among tumor cells and cells of the surrounding environment, mediated by cytokines and growth factors, lead to the establishment of metastases.

KEY CONCEPTS BOX 53-1

- Most cancers develop from a single cell (clone) that expresses one or more mutated genes.
- As the cancer grows, additional genetic changes occur, leading to cancer cells with different combinations of expressed genes that are best able to survive and spread (metastasize). This process can take decades before the cancer is clinically apparent.
- Oncogenes are cellular genes that when mutated or overexpressed or underexpressed can cause the development of a cancer clone.

SECTION OBJECTIVES BOX 53-2

- Describe the four clinical situations in which a laboratory test for a cancer (tumor marker) might be useful.
- List the criteria for a useful tumor marker.
- Describe the natural biologic processes which occur in cancer progression that limit the use of cancer markers

OVERVIEW OF ROLES OF LABORATORY TESTS

Laboratory tests can serve four major functions in the field of **neoplasia:** detection or screening, **confirmation** or diagnosis, classification (**staging**), and monitoring.

Detection (Screening)[16]

A screening test is used to detect a segment of an apparently disease-free population of individuals (asymptomatic) who actually might have the disease for which they are being screened. Common examples of screening tests include blood pressure determination to screen for hypertension and mammography to screen for breast cancer. Because of the limitations of most **tumor markers,** that is, poor sensitivity and specificity, only a few have been approved for use in screening for specific cancers. These include prostate-specific antigen (PSA) for prostate cancer and occult blood for colorectal cancer (see later, pp. 1060 and 1062).

Observations from screening tests can help to classify the individual as diseased (positive) or nondiseased (negative). This rigid classification of test results into positive and negative results sometimes may be too simplistic and error prone. Outcomes of screening tests can be ordered from very negative to very positive, allowing more sophisticated test interpretation in actual screening programs. For example, patients whose results are not negative but are not alarmingly positive enough to justify immediate diagnostic action can be scheduled for repeat screenings or for further diagnostic testing.[17-20]

Sometimes it may be effective to combine two screening tests that are complementary (i.e., directed at different anatomical or biochemical features of the tumor) to enhance the sensitivity of disease detection. Examples of complementary tests include sputum cytological examination and chest x-ray examination for lung cancer.[20]

Confirmation

Individuals who have clinical symptoms or a positive screening test often continue to undergo testing to confirm the presence of cancer. Tests that tend to confirm the presence of cancer include biopsies, radiological procedures such as imaging techniques, and bone marrow examinations. Laboratory tests such as plasma catecholamines for pheochromocytoma and α-fetoprotein for testicular cancer may assist in the diagnosis. For a laboratory test result to be confirmatory, it should possess 100% diagnostic specificity, that is, it should contain no false-positive results.[21] For example, all cases in which the plasma catecholamine level is above a certain value should be associated with pheochromocytoma. Currently, no biochemical tests have been approved for the diagnosis of cancer.

Classification and Staging

Classification of tumors is used to describe the degree of tumor differentiation. Tumors are classified as well differentiated, moderately well differentiated, and poorly differentiated. Poorly differentiated tumors are more aggressive and have a poorer prognosis than others. Tumor staging estimates the extent of disease, based on the size and extent of invasion of surrounding tissues by the tumor, the number of cancer cell–positive lymph nodes, and the presence or absence of metastases. This has been called the TNM (tumor, nodes, metastases) system.[22] The purposes of such staging are to provide reasonable estimates of prognosis (i.e., recurrence of cancer) or of appropriate response to therapy, and to predict the likely course of the disease. Currently, no biochemical tests are used to classify or stage cancers.

Monitoring

Laboratory tests can be used to determine the response of a cancer to treatment. This assessment is based on the concept of tumor burden. The assumption is that if a cancer cell produces a specific biochemical (tumor marker, see later), the level of circulating biochemical may be related to the number of cancer cells. In some cases, such as leukemia, direct laboratory determination of the number of circulating leukemia cells can be used to monitor the disease. Changed levels of a tumor marker or of leukemia cells can be used to detect remission or relapse of the cancer after treatment has been completed.

DEFINITION OF THE IDEAL TUMOR MARKER

An ideal tumor marker should fulfill the following criteria[23]:

1. Ease and affordability of measuring in readily available body fluids
2. Specificity to the tumor studied and frequent association with it
3. Stoichiometric relationship between plasma level of the marker and tumor mass
4. Abnormal level in body fluids in the presence of micrometastases, that is, at a stage at which no clinical or presently available diagnostic methods reveal their presence
5. Body fluid levels that are stable and are not subject to wild fluctuations
6. Much lower concentration than is found in association with all stages of cancer, if present in the body fluid of healthy individuals

It is important to recognize that the evaluation of an ideal tumor marker should relate to the clinical setting. To this end, it has been suggested that all tumor markers also should comply with the following criteria[24]:

1. They should prognosticate a higher or lower risk for eventual development of recurrence.
2. They should change as the current status of the tumor changes over time.
3. They should precede and predict recurrences before they are clinically detectable.

In addition, if a tumor marker is to be used to detect very early stages of cancer, a treatment for that cancer must be available. It might be unethical to detect cancers for which no effective treatment is available (see later).

KEY CONCEPTS BOX 53-2

- Clinical situations that might require a good tumor marker include screening for cancer, diagnosis of a cancer, estimating the aggressiveness of disease (prognosis), and monitoring cancer therapy (estimating tumor burden).
- A good tumor marker should be inexpensive and should reflect the cancer in question and not a healthy state; body fluid levels should reflect the amount of tumor present and the extent of disease.
- In addition, a good tumor marker should indicate the prognosis for curing the disease and should reflect return of disease after treatment.

SECTION OBJECTIVES BOX 53-3

- List three classes of compounds that may be used as tumor markers.
- Define the chemical and biological nature of "oncofetal antigens."
- List the roles in which tumor markers are most likely to be used in screening, diagnosis, prognosis, and monitoring.
- For each of the six biochemical categories of tumor markers, list example tumor markers, current clinical use, and the tumor site they assess.

CHANGE OF ANALYTE IN DISEASE

Classes of Biochemicals Used as Tumor Markers

The types of analytes used as tumor markers are listed in Table 53-3 and are discussed in terms of their clinical applications. The Food and Drug Administration (FDA) regulates which tumor markers can be used. The current FDA-approved list of protein tumor markers includes CEA, AFP, PSA, PAP, CA-125, CA-15-3, and CA-27-29, as well as some others mentioned later in this chapter under specific organ sites. The only tumor marker that is currently approved for screening of the general population is PSA. Reviews that discuss some of these assays in greater depth are recommended for further reading (see, for example, references 24 through 26 and guidelines in reference 27).[24-27]

Oncofetal Antigens

Many of the oncofetal antigens are measured in the laboratory through the use of solid-phase immunometric assays, which employ second antibodies labeled with enzymes and fluorescent or chemiluminescent compounds. These proteins are not recommended for cancer screening.

Antibodies from different reagent vendors will react differently with the antigen. Because these antigens are glycoproteins, and because the carbohydrate portion of the molecule may differ from patient to patient, antibodies from different vendors may react differently from one patient to the next. Therefore, when patients are being monitored, the assay that is used should come from the same manufacturer during the monitoring period. Otherwise, analytically significant changes may occur during serial monitoring as the result of a change in the source of the tumor marker reagent. If it is necessary to change the vendor source, individual patient parallel studies should be performed, in which at least two specimens are analyzed by both methods so the physician can compare individual patient results.

Carcinoembryonic Antigen

Carcinoembryonic antigen (CEA), a glycoprotein that is present in colonic adenocarcinoma and fetal gut, is used to monitor colorectal cancer.[28] The application of CEA is complicated by the presence in these tissues of CEA cross-reacting antigens. In general, CEA plasma levels increase with increasing age and smoking. Neither the sensitivity nor the specificity

Table 53-3 Classes of Biochemicals Used as Tumor Markers

Class of Biochemical	Examples	Use	Tumor Site
Oncofetal protein	CEA	Confirmation, monitoring	Colorectal
	AFP	Confirmation, monitoring	Testicle, liver
	SCC	Confirmation, monitoring	Cervix
Mucin glycoproteins	CA-125	Confirmation, monitoring	Ovary
	CA-19-9	Confirmation, monitoring	Pancreas
	CA-15-3 and CA-27-29	Confirmation, monitoring	Breast
Enzymes	PSA	Screening, confirmation, monitoring	Prostate
	NSE	Confirmation, monitoring	Lung
Hormones	ACTH and others	Confirmation, monitoring	Site specific
	hCG	Confirmation, monitoring	Testicle
Receptors	Estrogen and progesterone receptors	Prognosis, treatment	Breast
	HER-2	Treatment	
DNA markers	*BRCA-1, BRCA-2*	Risk assessment	Breast

ACTH, Adrenocorticotropic hormone; *AFP,* α-fetoprotein; *CEA,* carcinoembryonic antigen; *hCG,* human chorionic gonadotropin; *HER-2,* human epidermal growth factor receptor-2; *NSE,* neuron-specific enolase; *PSA,* prostate-specific antigen; *SCC,* squamous cell carcinoma.

of CEA justifies its use for the definitive diagnosis of cancer, and currently, CEA is approved only for monitoring of colorectal cancer.[29] However, little evidence is available to indicate that monitoring all patients with a diagnosis of colorectal cancer leads to improved patient outcomes or enhanced quality of life.[30]

α-Fetoprotein

α-Fetoprotein (AFP) is an oncofetal glycoprotein. In early embryonic life, it is a predominant component of the serum proteins. It is synthesized first by the yolk sac and later by the fetal liver. Later in life, it is produced mainly in the liver. Serum AFP values should be less than 10 μg/L in healthy subjects. In benign hepatic disorders, moderate elevations (40 μg/L) may be seen. Values above 400 μg/L are almost always associated with hepatocellular carcinoma, germ cell carcinoma (such as testicular carcinoma), chronic aggressive hepatitis, or subacute hepatic necrosis. Currently, AFP is approved only for use with testicular carcinoma and hepatocellular carcinoma.[31]

Carbohydrate Antigen 15-3 and 27-29

Serum carbohydrate antigen (CA) 15-3 (CA-15-3), a glycoprotein antigen, is elevated in the serum of patients with breast cancer. Changes in CA-15-3 concentration in serum after surgery or during chemotherapy mirror the progress of the disease as assessed by clinical and radiological evidence. Just as with the CA-125 antigen, CA-15-3 provides no actual diagnostic assistance, but it does have possible value as a marker for monitoring responsiveness to chemotherapy. It also should be noted that a third of patients with breast cancer who have metastatic disease have CA-15-3 levels within the reference range. The CA-27-29 antigen is detected by an antibody specific for the protein core of the same antigen detected by the antibody to CA-15-3.

Carbohydrate Antigen 19-9

Carbohydrate antigen 19-9 (CA-19-9) occurs in tissue as a monosialoganglioside and in serum as mucin, a high-molecular-weight, carbohydrate-rich glycoprotein. Although CA-19-9 levels may be elevated in pancreatic and colon cancer, its use in these diseases is not recommended.[32,33]

Carbohydrate Antigen 125

Serum carbohydrate antigen 125 (CA-125), a glycoprotein antigen, is elevated in the serum of patients with ovarian cancer. Increased concentrations of CA-125 were found in many patients with epithelial ovarian cancer and with ovarian teratoma. Changes in CA-125 concentration in serum during chemotherapy have mirrored the progress of the disease as assessed by clinical and radiological evidence. It should be noted that CA-125 provides no real assistance for diagnosis; however, it is approved as a marker for monitoring responsiveness to chemotherapy.

TA90

TA90[34] is a glycoprotein that is found in the serum or urine of approximately two-thirds of patients with melanoma. An endogenous humoral (immune globulin [Ig]G) immune response against TA90 has been demonstrated in patients with melanoma.[35] The presence of the TA90-immune complex (IC) has been correlated with recurrence of disease. At a median follow-up of 25 months, TA90-IC status was the only independent prognostic factor in multivariate analysis.[36]

Hormones

Human Chorionic Gonadotropin

Human chorionic gonadotropin (hCG) is a glycoprotein hormone that can be secreted in large amounts by the trophoblastic tissue of tumors of the placenta and the testes. Specific and sensitive assays have revealed that many other cancers can also secrete hCG. hCG determinations are of no value in screening for cancer.

The main clinical use of hCG is related to the diagnosis, therapy, and follow-up study of germ cell tumors.[37]

Table 53-4 presents the World Health Organization (WHO) classification of germ cell tumors and associated markers in

Table 53-4 WHO Classification of Germ Cell Tumors and Associated Tumor Markers

	IMMUNOHISTOCHEMISTRY		*SEROLOGY*		
WHO Classification	**AFP**	**hCG**	**AFP**	**hCG**	**Comments**
Seminoma (S)	–	+	No	± Yes	hCG in giant cells
Embryonal carcinoma (EC)	+	+	± Yes	± Yes	hCG in giant cells
Yolk sac tumor (YST)	+	–	± Yes	No	
Choriocarcinoma	–	+	No	Yes	
Teratoma	–	–	No	No	

From Norgaard-Pedersen B, Hangaard J. In Statland BE, Winkel P, editors: *Laboratory Measurements in Malignant Disease,* Philadelphia, 1982, Saunders; http://www.nature.com/modpathol/journal/v18/n2s/pdf/3800310a.pdf Modern Pathology (2005) 18, S61–S79 & 2005 USCAP, Inc All rights reserved 0893-3952/05.
AFP, α-Fetoprotein; *hCG,* human chorionic gonadotropin.

tissue and serum. In general, AFP and hCG provide the most abundant information about tumor status when they are elevated persistently. The absence of a marker does not preclude the presence of germ cell tumors.

Calcitonin

Calcitonin is secreted by the parafollicular C-cells of the thyroid gland and has as its primary function the lowering of serum calcium levels. It is elevated in medullary thyroid carcinoma (MTC), and its measurement therefore is used to confirm this diagnosis.

Calcitonin levels may be elevated before any clinical evidence of a tumor is noted. In patients with calcitonin levels that are not diagnostic, stimulation testing usually will support a diagnosis of MTC. In addition, MTC can occur as an inherited malignancy; in patients with a family history of MTC, calcitonin stimulation testing can serve as a screening tool. After treatment of MTC by thyroidectomy, calcitonin measurement can serve as an indicator of residual or recurrent disease.

Thyroglobulin

Thyroglobulin levels are elevated in patients with localized or metastatic thyroid carcinoma. After complete thyroidectomy and radioactive iodine ablation therapy, thyroglobulin levels are decreased. Levels less than 1 ng/mL during T_4 therapy, or less than 5 ng/mL without T_4 therapy, are an indication of successful treatment. Elevated levels suggest residual localized disease or recurrence.

A limiting factor in the use of serum thyroglobulin measurement is the potential presence of thyroglobulin autoantibodies, which may cause falsely high or falsely low results in thyroglobulin immunoassays. Thus levels of thyroglobulin autoantibodies should be measured in patients who require serum thyroglobulin levels for monitoring of thyroid carcinoma.[38]

Cellular Markers

Several markers associated with the plasma membrane, cytoplasm, or nuclei of the lymphoid cell have been identified. Various immunological techniques have been used to detect cellular markers; these techniques include cell rosetting, immunofluorescence, and immunoenzymatic testing. The rosetting technique is based on a reaction between an indicator cell (usually an erythrocyte) and the lymphoid cell that causes rosettes to form in cases in which the lymphoid cell carries a particular membrane marker. Through such techniques, the cells may be mixed directly, or the indicator cell may be coated first with antibody or complement to demonstrate receptors for the Fc part of immunoglobulin or complement components. The use of flow cytometry in combination with immunofluorescence has proved to be a powerful technique for detecting cell markers.

It appears that the various antigens demonstrated by these techniques are not tumor-specific antigens but rather are tumor-associated differentiation antigens, which represent the expression of oncofetal antigens that are not normally expressed by differentiated cells.

Lymphocytic leukemias and non-Hodgkin lymphomas have been subdivided into clinical subgroups on the basis of biochemical cell markers. The most striking evidence of the value of typing lymphocytes with a panel of markers has been derived from studies of acute lymphocytic leukemia (ALL). Table 53-5 lists the five prognostically distinct groups of ALL and relevant markers for each. Groups are ordered according to prognosis. Cells of the B-cell type are characterized by the presence of surface membrane immune globulin (SmIg), as are normal mature B cells. Cells of the T-cell type are characterized by the presence of sheep erythrocyte receptors and human thymocyte antigen, as are mature T cells. Cells of the pre–B cell type are characterized by a cytoplasmic IgM heavy chain with no SmIg; this corresponds to the characteristics of an early stage during B-cell differentiation.

The terminal deoxynucleotidyltransferase and the common ALL antigen are of value not only in classifying ALL (see Table 53-5), but also in distinguishing between acute lymphoblastic and myeloblastic leukemia. ALL may be classified into B-cell leukemia (95%), which is characterized by low-density monoclonal surface membrane immune globulins (usually IgM or IgM and IgD with one light chain) and the rarer, but more aggressive, T-ALL (5%). The cells of the last type form E rosettes and have T antigens but lack SmIg.

Table **53-5** Phenotypic Heterogeneity of ALL

ALL	E	HTA	SmIg	Cyμ	CALLA	HLA-DR	TdT
Common ALL	−	−	−	−	+	+	+
Pre-B-ALL	−	−	−	+	+	+	+
Null-ALL	−	−	−	−	−	+	+
T-ALL	+	+	−	−	−	−	+
B-ALL	−	−	+	−	−	+	−

From Plesner T, Wilken M, Avenstrøm S. In Statland BE, Winkel P, editors: *Laboratory Measurements in Malignant Disease,* Philadelphia, 1982, Saunders.
ALL, Acute lymphocytic leukemia; *B-ALL,* B-cell type of acute lymphoblastic leukemia; *CALLA,* common ALL antigen; *Cyμ,* cytoplasmic immune globulin (Ig)M heavy chain; *E,* sheep erythrocyte receptor; *HLA-DR,* human Ia-like antigen; *HTA,* human thymocyte antigen or antigens; *SmIg,* surface membrane immunoglobin; *T-ALL,* T-cell type of acute lymphoblastic leukemia; *TdT,* terminal deoxynucleotidyl transferase.

TUMOR MARKERS FOR SPECIFIC MALIGNANCIES

Prostate Cancer

Prostate cancer (25% of all cancers in males) is the most common malignancy in males in the United States.[39] Prostate-specific antigen (PSA) is an extracellular protease that exists in serum in several molecular forms, including a free or noncomplexed form, and in complexes of PSA with serine protease inhibitors α_1-antichymotrypsin (ACT) and α_2-macroglobulin.[40] Total PSA represents a combination of all immune detectable forms in serum, primarily free PSA and PSA-ACT. The complexed form is the one that is found predominantly in serum. Serum levels of complexed PSA are higher in patients with prostate cancer than in those with benign prostatic hyperplasia (BPH).[41] The percent of free PSA (%fPSA) is lower in patients with cancer and is an accurate means of discriminating between benign and malignant prostate disease.[42]

Although serum PSA levels greater than the reference interval suggest increased risk for prostate cancer, it now is accepted that as many as 25% of men with PSA levels within the reference interval are also at risk.[42,43] Reducing the cutoff from 4 ng/mL to 2.5 ng/mL has been suggested but will lead to a greater number of negative biopsies. %fPSA measurements are used to improve the clinical sensitivity of the total PSA measurement. A total PSA level in the 4.1 to 10.0 ng/mL range is considered to indicate a high likelihood of disease only when the %fPSA is less than 24%. A total PSA in the 3.0 to 4.0 ng/mL range with a %fPSA <19% would suggest that further investigation, such as a biopsy, is needed.

Other calculations, including PSA density (coupled with transrectal ultrasound measurement of prostate volume) and PSA velocity (rate of increase for multiple measurements),[44] as well as age-specific reference ranges, have been suggested as possible approaches to improve PSA specificity.

The American Cancer Society has issued guidelines for the early detection of prostate cancer. The Society recommends that PSA should be used in combination with a digital rectal examination to screen for prostate cancer, beginning at age 50 for men at average risk with a life expectancy of at least 10 years.[45] Screening at an earlier age is warranted for men at high risk. This high-risk group includes all African American men, as well as all men over the age of 40 who have had two relatives diagnosed with prostate cancer. Both high-risk groups may develop prostate cancer several years earlier than the general population. Follow-up testing of high-risk persons initially screened at the age of 40 depends on the PSA result. If the initial PSA is <1 ng/mL, testing would resume at the age of 45. Those with levels from 1 to 2.5 ng/mL would be tested annually. Men with a PSA >2.5 ng/mL would be evaluated further, and a biopsy considered.

The utility of any screening for prostate cancer remains controversial because proper treatment for this disease, when it is detected early, has not been determined. Although some clinicians believe that watchful waiting is sufficient for some prostate cancers, others call for immediate, curative intervention, especially for small, early prostate cancers in men with a life expectancy of longer than 10 years. Because prostate cancer is generally slow growing, and because the PSA test itself has been widely available for only about 15 years, ongoing clinical trials have not been of sufficient duration (15 to 25 years) to provide conclusive data that screening actually improves patient outcome. This ethical question will be resolved through ongoing clinical trials.

PSA is used to monitor response to therapy in treated patients.[45,46] After a prostatectomy has been performed, patients with prostate cancer restricted to the prostate gland should have their serum PSA fall to undetectable limits within 1 to 3 months. In patients treated with internal or external radiation, PSA may take several years to reach a baseline level, which may not approach undetectable limits. A continuous rise in PSA level after treatment indicates local recurrence or distance metastasis; because the cancer is generally so slow growing, the rise may not occur for several years. Clinical trials suggests that the Gleason score (the histopathological grade by which prostate adenocarcinoma is classified) is a better indicator of disease recurrence than are pretreatment levels of PSA.[46] At present, evidence is equivocal regarding the clinical benefit of reporting biochemical recurrence of prostate cancer at PSA levels <0.4 ng/L.[47] However, salvage radiation therapy after prostatectomy has been shown to yield best results when

PSA levels are still very low (<0.5 ng/L).[48] The recurrence limit is less clear after radiation therapy because of the typically slower decline in circulating PSA concentration. The American Society for Therapeutic Radiation and Oncology (ASTRO) has defined biochemical recurrence as three consecutive rises in PSA above the nadir.[49]

Breast Cancer

Breast cancer is the most common malignancy among female individuals (26% of all cases in females) in the United States.[39] Many laboratory tests are available for prognostic and monitoring purposes.

Steroid Receptor Analysis

Both estrogen and progesterone receptor assays are used to assess the prognosis of patients with breast cancer. These tests evaluate the relative concentrations of receptors for estrogen and progesterone in breast tumor tissue excised during surgery, to facilitate selection of patients likely to respond to endocrine therapy. Routine assay of estrogen receptors and progesterone receptors in all newly diagnosed cases of breast cancer has been recommended.[50] Patients who are positive for these receptors respond well to endocrine therapy; receptor-negative patients need alternative therapies.

HER-2 (c-erbB-2)

Human epidermal growth factor receptor (HER)-2 is a cell membrane surface-bound receptor tyrosine kinase that normally is involved in the signal transduction pathways leading to cell growth and differentiation. HER-2 is overexpressed in 25% to 30% of human breast cancers. HER-2 determinations have been recommended in all newly diagnosed breast cancers for selection of patients who may be treated with trastuzumab (Herceptin).[50] However, two types of assays are available for HER-2: immunohistochemistry and fluorescence in situ hybridization (FISH). The possibility of measuring HER-2 in serum has been explored.[51]

Carbohydrate Antigen 15-3 and 27-29

CA-15-3 should not be used alone to monitor therapy in advanced disease.[50] In patients whose disease cannot be evaluated clinically, a confirmed increase in concentration suggests progression of disease. It is recommended that the markers should be assayed before each course of chemotherapy is given and every 3 months thereafter in patients with metastatic disease who are receiving hormone therapy.

Genetic Screening for Breast Cancer

A number of epidemiological studies have documented that a positive family history of breast cancer is a positive predictor of increased risk for this disease. See reference 52 for a detailed complete review of this subject.[52] At least eight genes have been identified that may contribute to an inherited susceptibility to breast and ovarian cancer, the most important of which are *BRCA1* and *BRCA2*. Approximately 5% of breast and ovarian cancers can be attributed to families with mutations in the *BRCA1* gene; this gene has been linked to the 17q21 locus and is thought to be a tumor suppressor gene. It also may be associated with increased risk for ovarian, colon, and prostate cancers. Although numerous mutations in this gene are associated with breast cancer, one specific mutation has a very high frequency among Ashkenazi Jewish women and may account for 16% of breast cancers and 39% of ovarian cancers diagnosed in this population before the age of 50.

Approximately 3% of breast and ovarian cancers have been attributed to families with mutations in the *BRCA2* gene; this gene has been linked to the 13q12-13 locus and is also associated with increased risk for pancreatic cancer and male breast cancer. As with *BRCA1,* one specific mutation of the *BRCA2* gene accounts for a significant number of breast and ovarian cancers in Ashkenazi women, and another specific mutation accounts for a significant number of breast and ovarian cancers in Icelandic women.

DNA testing is available to identify individuals and families who carry these mutations. Although this testing is not recommended for asymptomatic individuals in the general population, it may be used, with appropriate genetic counseling, for members of high-risk families with well-defined syndromes.

The Task Force of the Cancer Genetics Studies Consortium (CGSC) recommends early breast and ovarian cancer screening for individuals with *BRCA1* mutations, and early breast cancer screening for those with *BRCA2* mutations.[53] This group did not make a recommendation for or against prophylactic surgery (e.g., mastectomy, oophorectomy). The guidelines further state that these surgeries are an option for mutation carriers, although evidence of benefit is lacking and case reports have documented the occurrence of cancer after prophylactic surgery has been performed. It is recommended that individuals who are considering genetic testing should be counseled regarding the unknown efficacy of measures taken to reduce risk, and that care for individuals with cancer-predisposing mutations should be provided whenever possible within the context of research protocols designed to evaluate clinical outcomes.[53] These guidelines are based on expert opinion only.

In 2003, an American Society of Clinical Oncology (ASCO) Panel published a detailed policy statement regarding genetic testing for cancer susceptibility.[54] According to the Consensus Panel of the 8th St Gallen Conference, treatment decisions for women with mutations in *BRCA1* or *BRCA2* genes must include consideration of bilateral mastectomy with plastic surgical reconstruction, prophylactic oophorectomy, chemoprevention, and intensified surveillance.[55]

Assessment of Circulating Tumor Cells[56,57]

A recent development is that clinicians now can assess the number of circulating tumor cells (CTC) present in the peripheral blood of patients with metastatic breast cancer. An FDA-approved test enumerates CTC of epithelial origin (CD45-, EpCAM+, and cytokeratin 8, 18+, and/or 19+) in whole blood through the use of flow cytometry. The presence of CTC in peripheral blood is associated with decreased progression-free survival and decreased overall survival in patients with metastatic breast cancer. It is recommended that serial testing for CTC be used in conjunction with other clinical methods for monitoring. The presence of 5 or more CTC in 7.5 mL of whole blood at any time during the course of disease is predictive of shortened progression-free survival and overall survival.

Lung Cancer[58]

Lung cancer is the most frequent cancer in the world, in terms of both incidence (1.2 million new cases, or 12.3% of the world total) and mortality (1.1 million deaths, or 17.8% of the total). Trends in lung cancer incidence and mortality reflect smoking habits and/or exposure to other environmental or occupational carcinogens. Lung cancers can be grouped into two major histological types: non–small cell and small cell lung cancer (NSCLC and SCLC, respectively). NSCLC accounts for 75% to 85% of patients with lung cancer. Small cell lung cancer accounts for 15% to 25% of patients with lung cancer, often has neuroendocrine components, and is treated primarily with chemotherapy and/or radiotherapy.

CEA is elevated in adenocarcinoma and large cell lung cancer, but the increased concentrations found in various benign pathologies and other malignancies preclude its use in screening and limit its diagnostic use. However, CEA may be helpful in the differential diagnosis of NSCLC. CEA may provide prognostic information in NSCLC, particularly in cases of adenocarcinoma of the lung. It also may have a role in monitoring therapy at advanced stages, and in detecting recurrent disease of non–small cell adenocarcinoma. However, it is commonly slightly elevated in tobacco smokers.

Neuron-Specific Enolase

High serum levels of neuron-specific enolase (NSE) (>100 ng/L) in patients with suspicion of malignancy suggest the presence of SCLC, with the differential diagnoses including neuroendocrine tumors, liver cancer, lymphoma, and seminoma. Moderate elevations of NSE also are found in patients with benign lung disease, as well as in some cases of pancreatic, gastric, colorectal, and breast cancer. NSE has been demonstrated to be of use for prognostic purposes in both SCLC and NSCLC. NSE has shown considerable potential for the monitoring of post-treatment SCLC, as well as for the detection of recurrent disease of SCLC after primary therapy.

Colorectal Cancer[59]

Colorectal cancer (CRC) is the third most common cancer worldwide, with an estimated 1 million new cases and half a million deaths each year. In the United States, it is also the third most common malignant disease, with an estimated 153,880 new cases diagnosed in 2008.

Carcinoembryonic Antigen (CEA)

ASCO, the European Group on Tumor Markers (EGTM), and the National Academy of Clinical Biochemistry all recommend against the use of CEA in screening healthy subjects for early CRC. A 2000 College of American Pathologists Expert Panel ranked preoperative serum CEA together with TNM stage, regional lymph node metastasis, blood or lymphatic vessel invasion, and residual tumor after surgery with curative intent as category I prognostic markers for colorectal cancer.[60] According to this group, prognostic factors are those definitely proven to be of prognostic importance on the basis of evidence from multiple statistically robust published trials; they generally are used in patient management.

The 2005 ASCO guidelines state that CEA should be measured every 3 months in patients with Stage II or III CRC for at least 3 years after diagnosis. However, no agreement has been reached as to the magnitude of concentration change that constitutes a clinically significant increase in CEA during serial monitoring. The 2000 ASCO guidelines recommend that CEA should be measured at the start of treatment for metastatic disease and every 2 to 3 months during active treatment, if no other simple test is available to indicate a response. Two values above baseline should be regarded as adequate to document progressive disease even in the absence of corroborating evidence.

Occult Blood Test

The most widely used screening marker for CRC that involves testing for occult blood is the fecal occult blood test (FOBT). The most commonly used FOBT is the guaiac test, which measures the presence of heme in hemoglobin. Because heme is also present in meat and in certain fruits and vegetables, intake of these foods may give rise to false-positive results in the guaiac test. Certain medicines such as non-steroidal anti-inflammatory drugs also can interfere with the test. In contrast, the immunochemical test is not affected by these factors. A number of large randomized trials have shown that screening with the guaiac test reduces mortality from CRC, even with the above mentioned limitations.

Bladder Cancer[61]

Every year in the United States, nearly 56,000 new cases of bladder cancer are diagnosed; approximately 12,000 people die of the disease. Risk factors include tobacco use, exposure to industrial carcinogens, and chronic infection with *Schistosomiasis haematobium.*

Urine cytology may be positive for tumor cells, but the diagnosis usually is established by cystoscopic evaluation, prompted by hematuria or urinary tract symptoms, and by biopsy.

The FDA has cleared six tumor marker tests for use in routine patient care. However, no clinical trial data have demonstrated the usefulness of any of the FDA-cleared markers for increasing survival time, decreasing the cost of treatment, or improving the quality of life of patients with bladder cancer. FDA-approved assays for bladder cancer include the following:

1. The bladder tumor antigen (BTA) STAT and TRAK tests for complement factor H in urine
2. The nuclear matrix protein (NMP22 test) in urine
3. A point-of-care version of the NMP22 test, called Bladder Chek NMP22
4. The ImmunoCyt test, which detects bladder cancer markers present on exfoliated cells

5. Multi-target FISH to detect cancer cells based on the aneuploidy of selected chromosomes. The UroVysion test employs centromere probes specific to chromosomes 3, 7, 17, and 9 to detect aneuploidy associated with bladder cancer.

Monoclonal Gammopathies[62]

The monoclonal gammopathies, also called paraproteinemias or dysproteinemias, consist of a group of disorders characterized by the proliferation of one or more clones of differentiated B lymphocytes, each of which produces an immunologically homogeneous immunoglobulin, commonly referred to as a paraprotein or a monoclonal M-protein. Circulating M-protein may consist of an intact immunoglobulin, the light chain only, (often termed Bence Jones protein) or (rarely) the heavy chain only. The heavy chain is derived from one of the five immunoglobulin classes: G, A, M, D, or E. The light chain is kappa or lambda in type. The monoclonal gammopathies include diseases such as multiple myeloma, Waldenström's macroglobulinemia, plasmacytoma, monoclonal gammopathy of undetermined significance (MGUS), and systemic amyloid light-chain (AL) amyloidosis.

Multiple myeloma has been subclassified into the indolent form (smoldering multiple myeloma, or SMM) and symptomatic systemic disease, often involving end-organ damage to the kidneys, bones, and bone marrow.[63] Indolent disease is characterized by a lack of symptoms, few or no bone lesions, and stable concentrations of M-protein. Waldenström's macroglobulinemia is characterized by elevated levels of monoclonal IgM in the serum, excess lymphoplasmacytoid cells in the bone marrow, and, in contrast to multiple myeloma, involvement of visceral organs, including liver and spleen. Although the number of monoclonal plasma cells found within the bone marrow in AL is usually low, the protein that they produce has an affinity for forming deposits (amyloid) in visceral organs such as heart, kidneys, liver, and spleen, and these protein deposits may cause end-organ dysfunction and early death.

Multiple myeloma arising from plasma cell dyscrasia accounted for approximately 1.4% of new cancer cases and 10% to 15% of all hematological malignancies in the United States in 2008; it was responsible for ≈2.0% of cancer deaths, representing the worst ratio of deaths per new cases for any cancer. Several reviews have estimated the median survival at 3 to 4 years. See Table 53-6 for guidelines in differentiating multiple myeloma from MGUS, Table 53-7 for distribution of diagnoses in patients with monoclonal gammopathies, and Table 53-8 for distribution frequency of monoclonal proteins in patients with multiple myeloma.

Laboratory findings that suggest the possibility of a plasma cell dyscrasia or Waldenström's macroglobulinemia include elevation of the erythrocyte sedimentation rate or serum viscosity, anemia, renal insufficiency with a normal urine sediment, heavy proteinuria in a patient over age 50, Bence-Jones proteinuria (light chains), hypercalcemia, hypergammaglobulinemia, and immunoglobulin deficiency. Clinical symptoms that are suspicious for a plasma cell disorder include back pain, weakness or fatigue, osteopenia, osteolytic lesions, spontaneous fractures, and recurrent infection. However, many patients are asymptomatic and are investigated because of mild anemia or an elevated total protein on routine blood work. M-protein is a tumor marker that is specific for monoclonal gammopathies because it reflects the clonal production of immunoglobulin. The diagnosis of multiple myeloma is made on the basis of several criteria, including the following: a monoclonal M-protein in the plasma or urine, infiltration

Table 53-6 International Guidelines for the Classification of Multiple Myeloma (MM) and Monoclonal Gammopathy of Undetermined Significance (MGUS)

Symptomatic MM
M-protein in serum and/or urine
Bone marrow clonal plasma cells >10% or plasmacytoma
Related organ or tissue impairment (end-organ damage, including bone lesions)

Nonsecretory MM
No M-protein in serum and/or urine with immunofixation
Bone marrow clonal plasma cells >10% or plasmacytoma
Related organ or tissue impairment (end-organ damage, including bone lesions)

Asymptomatic MM (smoldering MM)
M-protein in serum >3.0 g/dL and/or
Bone marrow clonal plasma cells >10%
No symptoms, related organ or tissue impairment

MGUS
M-protein in serum <3.0 g/dL
Bone marrow clonal plasma cells <10%
No evidence of other B-cell proliferative disorders
No related organ or tissue impairment

From Kyle RA, et al: Criteria for the classification of monoclonal gammopathies, multiple myeloma, and related disorders: a report of the International Myeloma Working Group, Br J Haem 121:749, 2003.

Table 53-7 Distribution of Clinical Diagnoses in 1026 Patients With a Monoclonal Protein Detected at the Mayo Clinic in 1992

Condition	Percent
MGUS	56%
Multiple myeloma	18%
Amyloidosis (AL)	10%
Lymphoma	5%
Smoldering myeloma	4%
Solitary or extramedullary plasmacytoma	3%
Chronic lymphocytic leukemia	2%
Waldenström's macroglobulinemia	2%

From Blade J, Kyle RA: Monoclonal gammopathies of unknown significance. In: Malpas JS, Bergsagel DE, Kyle RA, editors: *Myeloma Biology and Management,* New York, 1995, Oxford University Press. *MGUS,* Monoclonal gammopathy of undetermined significance.

Table 53-8 Classification of MM Based on Monoclonal Protein Production from the UK MRC Multiple Myeloma Trials

Classification	Frequency
IgG	59%
IgG1	40%
IgG2	13%
IgG3	4%
IgG4	2%
IgA	21%
Free light chain	15%
IgD	1%
IgE	0.01%
Biclonal	1%
Nonsecretory myeloma	3%

From Bradwell AR: *Serum Free Light Chain Analysis,* ed 4, Birmingham, UK, 2006, The Binding Site Ltd, p. 62.
Ig, Immune globulin; *MM,* multiple myeloma; *MRC,* Medical Research Council; *UK,* United Kingdom.

of plasma cells in the bone marrow, lytic lesions on radiographs of the skeleton, anemia, and hypercalcemia.

Identification of M-Proteins

Protein electrophoresis should be undertaken whenever multiple myeloma, Waldenström's macroglobulinemia, or MGUS is suspected. The monoclonal protein migrates as a single entity in the electric field and is detected by the nonspecific protein stain as a more intensely stained band superimposed on the usual protein pattern. Serum and urine should be tested at the same time; urine electrophoresis is especially valuable in cases of light-chain myeloma, in which most of the intact monoclonal protein is absent from the blood. Protein electrophoresis should always be performed in combination with immunotyping to determine clonality. Immunotyping usually is performed by immunofixation electrophoresis. In addition to aiding in the diagnosis of a monoclonal gammopathy, protein electrophoresis is useful in monitoring the course of disease and the response to therapy among these patients. The concentration of M-protein detected by protein electrophoresis is correlated directly with a patient's tumor burden, except in rare cases of non-secretory myeloma.

Quantitation of Immunoglobulins

Quantitation of IgG, IgA, and IgM (and IgD, if necessary) is clinically useful in determining the tumor burden of an M-protein and in detecting and monitoring the polyclonal hypogammaglobulinemia that may result from functional impairment of normal immunoglobulin-producing cells of the bone marrow through excessive expansion of malignant clone(s).

Free Light Chains

Specific assays for free kappa and free lambda light chains that can generate an accurate free kappa-to-lambda ratio can provide a reliable numerical index of clonality. This assay has changed significantly the way in which patients with so-called non-secretory myeloma and amyloidosis are diagnosed and subsequently monitored during therapy.[64]

Historically, 3% of patients with myeloma have presented with no evidence of monoclonal protein in the serum and urine through traditional immunofixation studies and have been considered to have non-secretory disease. It now is evident that most of these patients have low, but nevertheless abnormal, concentrations of serum free light chains, which are detectable by rate nephelometric techniques.

The advantage of measuring free light chains in serum rather than urine is that the variable reabsorption and subsequent destruction of filtered light chains by tubular cells of the proximal nephron is not a factor. The serum free kappa-to-lambda ratio is also a better indicator of the relative rates of production and is a more dependable indicator of clonality. During chemotherapy, urine free chain levels frequently normalize, whereas serum results may remain abnormal, indicating superior sensitivity for residual disease. Urinary testing is also more difficult to perform in diseases in which large numbers of polyclonal light chains are excreted in the urine (systemic lupus erythematosus, renal insufficiency, tubular dysfunction), potentially obscuring the monoclonal light chains of interest. However urinary light chain assays are more sensitive than urinary immunofixation and provide quantitative results.

KEY CONCEPTS BOX 53-3

- Most tumor markers are proteins such as oncofetal antigens, mucin (CA proteins), receptors, hormones, and enzymes; all are measured antigens. In addition, some endocrine hormones and DNA are used as tumor markers.
- Oncofetal antigens are proteins that most often are active in the fetal stage but often are synthesized in tumors.
- PSA can be used along with other procedures to screen for prostate cancer. The *BRAC* genes are used to determine genetic risk for breast cancer. Most tumor markers are used to monitor disease status.

INVESTIGATION OF NEW CANDIDATE TUMOR MARKERS

Tissue microarray (TMA) techniques are being used currently to isolate and identify potential tumor markers.[65] TMAs consist of up to 1000 tiny cylindrical tissue samples assembled on a routine histology paraffin block of regular size. Sections allow simultaneous analysis of up to 1000 tissue samples in a single experiment. TMAs may be applied over a broad range of cancer research, including prevalence, progression, and prognosis (Table 53-9).[66]

Mass spectrometry[67] is used as a diagnostic or biomarker discovery tool in cancer. The proteins associated with cancer can be analyzed through imaging-based mass spectrometry, and the patterns compared with healthy control tissue to

Table 53-9 Microarray Applications in Cancer Diagnostics

Microarray Technology	Application	Cancer
Comparative genomic hybridization	Classification	Breast
cDNA tissue expression hybridization	Classification	Breast
	Therapeutic response	Lymphoma
Gene expression profiling	Molecular profiling	Prostate
	Prognosis	Breast
		Prostate
		Kidney
	Diagnosis	Rhabdomyosarcoma
		Burkitt lymphoma
		Neuroblastoma
		GI tumor
		Prostate
		Bladder
	Classification	Breast
		Colorectal
		Gastroesophageal
		Kidney
		Ovarian
		Pancreas
		Lung
	Treatment tailoring	Breast
	Molecular profiling	Prostate
	Development stages	B-cell lymphoma
	Mutations	*BRCA1* (breast, ovarian)
Prognostic signature	Prognosis	Breast
		Lung
Genome mining	Biomarker discovery	Ovarian

From Diamandis E, Schmitt M, van der Merwe D: National Academy of Clinical Biochemistry guidelines on the use of microarrays in cancer diagnostics (section 4A). Available at www.aacc.org/AACC/members/nacb/LMPG/OnlineGuide/DraftGuidelines/TumorMarkers/TumorMarkersPDF.htm.

identify cancer-specific changes. Identification of cancer-specific protein patterns in blood by mass spectrometry was demonstrated for ovarian cancer,[68] for breast cancer,[69] and for prostate cancer.[70]

PHARMACOGENOMICS IN CANCER CHEMOTHERAPY

Acute lymphoblastic leukemia (ALL) has provided a model for the use of pharmacogenomics to assist in treating cancer.[71] In some patients with ALL, treatment fails because of drug resistance or adverse drug reactions. It has been demonstrated that in some patients in this subgroup, genetic variants that control the rate of metabolism of chemotherapeutic agents may affect the rate of metabolism of the drug. Germline polymorphisms and gene expression patterns in ALL cells have been linked to the toxicity and efficacy of chemotherapy for ALL and have emerged as useful clinical diagnostic tests. This most likely will be a topic of future laboratory testing.[72-74]

REFERENCES

1. Karakosta A, Golias C, Charalabopoulos A, et al: Genetic models of human cancer as a multistep process: paradigm models of colorectal cancer, breast cancer, and chronic myelogenous and acute lymphoblastic leukaemia, J Exp Clin Cancer Res 24:505, 2005.
2. Aaronson SA: Growth factors and cancer, Science 254:1146, 1991.
3. Cantley LC, Auger KR, Carpenter C, et al: Oncogenes and signal transduction, Cell 64:281, 1991.
4. Futreal PA, Coin L, Marshall M, et al: A census of human cancer genes. Nat Rev Cancer 4:177, 2004.
5. www.sanger.ac.uk/genetics/CGP/Census/Table_1_full_2007-02-13.xls
6. Polosky D, Cordon-Cardo C: Oncogenes in melanoma, Oncogene 22:3087, 2003.
7. Karnoub AE, Weinberg RA: Ras oncogenes: split personalities, Nat Rev Molec Cell Biol 9:517, 2008.
8. Ramsay RG, Gonda TJ: MYB function in normal and cancer cells, *Nat Rev Cancer* 8:523, 2008.
9. Lowe SW, Lin AW: Apoptosis in cancer, Carcinogenesis 21:485, 2000.
10. DeVries A, Flores ER, Miranda B, et al: Targeted point mutations of p53 lead to dominant-negative inhibition of wild-type p53 function, Proc Natl Acad Sci U S A 99:2948, 2002.
11. Liekens S, DeClercq E, Neyts J: Angiogenesis: regulators and clinical applications, Biochem Pharmacol 61:253, 2001.
12. Breier G: Functions of the VEGF/VEGF receptor system in the vascular system, Semin Thromb Hemost 26:553, 2000.
13. Narisawa-Saito M, Yoshimatsu Y, Ohno S, et al: An in vitro multistep carcinogenesis model for human cervical cancer, Cancer Res 68:5699, 2008.
14. www.cancer.gov/cancertopics/pdq/genetics/colorectal.HealthProfessional/page2
15. Yang J, Mani SA, Donaher JL, et al: Twist, a master regulator of morphogenesis, plays an essential role in tumor metastasis, Cell 117:927, 2004.
16. Habbema JDF, van Oortmarssen GJ: Performance characteristics of screening tests. In Statland BE, Winkel P, editors: *Laboratory Measurements in Malignant Disease,* vol 2, Philadelphia, 1982, Saunders.
17. U.K. National Screening Committee: Criteria for appraising the viability, effectiveness and appropriateness of a screening programme. Available at http://www.nsc.nhs.uk/pdfs/criteria.pdf
18. Croyle RT, editor: Psychosocial Effects of Screening for Disease Prevention and Detection, New York, 1995, Oxford University Press.
19. U.S. Preventive Services Task Force: Screening for breast cancer: recommendations and rationale, Ann Intern Med 137:344, 2002.
20. Woolner LB, Fontana RS, Sanderson DR, et al: Mayo Lung Project: evaluation of lung cancer screening through December 1979, Mayo Clin Proc 56:544, 1981.
21. Statland BE: *Clinical Decision Levels for Lab Tests,* Oradell, NJ, 1983, Medical Economics Co.
22. Wittekind C, Sobin LH: *TNM Classification of Malignant Tumours,* New York, 2002, Wiley-Liss.
23. Wu J, Nakamura R: *Human Circulating Tumor Markers, Current Concepts and Clinical Applications,* Chicago, 1997, American Society of Clinical Pathologists Press.
24. Bigbee W, Herberman RB: Tumor markers and immunodiagnosis. In Bast RC Jr, Kufe DW, Pollock RE, et al, editors: *Cancer*

Medicine, ed 6, Hamilton, Ontario, Canada, 2002, BC Decker Inc.

25. Lee P, Pincus MR, McPherson RA: Diagnosis and management of cancer using serologic tumor markers. In McPherson RA, Pincus MR, editors: *Henry's Clinical Diagnosis and Management by Laboratory Methods*, ed 21, Philadelphia, 2007, Saunders Elsevier, p. 1353.
26. Locker GY, Hamilton S, Harris J, et al: ASCO 2006 update of recommendations for the use of tumor markers in gastrointestinal cancer, J Clin Oncol 24:5313, 2006.
27. Sturgeon C: National Academy of Clinical Biochemistry guidelines on quality requirements for the use of tumor markers (section 2). Available at www.aacc.org/AACC/members/nacb/LMPG/OnlineGuide/DraftGuidelines/TumorMarkers/TumorMarkersPDF.htm.
28. Locker GY, Hamilton S, Harris J, et al, American Society of Clinical Oncology: Recommendations for the use of tumor markers in gastrointestinal cancer: CEA (colorectal cancer). Available at http://www.asco.org/ASCO/Downloads/Cancer%20Policy%20and%20Clinical%20Affairs/Clinical%20Affairs%20(derivative%20products)/GI%20TM%20Matrix%20Final.pdf.
29. National Institutes of Health: CEA as a Cancer Marker, vol 3, no 7, Bethesda, MD, 1981, Consensus Development Conference Summary.
30. Duffy MJ: Carcinoembryonic antigen as a marker for colorectal cancer: is it clinically useful? Clin Chem 47:624, 2001.
31. Mizejewski GJ: Biological role of alpha-fetoprotein in cancer: prospects for anticancer therapy, Expert Rev Anticancer Ther 2:709, 2003.
32. Kim JE, Lee KT, Lee JK, et al: Clinical usefulness of carbohydrate antigen 19-9 as a screening test for pancreatic cancer in an asymptomatic population, Gastroenterol Hepatol 19:182, 2004.
33. http://www.asco.org/ASCO/Downloads/Cancer%20Policy%20and%20Clinical%20Affairs/Clinical%20Affairs%20(derivative%20products)/GI%20TM%20Slides%20Final.pdf.
34. Gupta RK: National Academy of Clinical Biochemistry guidelines for the use of tumor markers in malignant melanoma (section 3L). Available at www.aacc.org/AACC/members/nacb/LMPG/OnlineGuide/DraftGuidelines/TumorMarkers/TumorMarkersPDF.htm.
35. Hsueh EC, Gupta RK, Yee R, et al: Does endogenous immune response determine the outcome of surgical therapy for metastatic melanoma? Ann Surg Oncol 7:232, 2000.
36. Chung MH, Gupta RK, Essner RA, et al: Serum TA90 immune complex assay can predict outcome after resection of thick (> or =4 mm) primary melanoma and sentinel lymphadenectomy, Ann Surg Oncol 9:120, 2002.
37. Mazumdar M, Bajorin DF, Bacik J, et al: Predicting outcome to chemotherapy in patients with germ cell tumors: the value of the rate of decline of human chorionic gonadotropin and alpha-fetoprotein during therapy, J Clin Oncol 19:2534, 2001.
38. Thyroglobulin autoantibodies (TgAb) measurements. In *The National Academy of Clinical Biochemistry Laboratory Medicine Practice Guidelines: Laboratory Support for the Diagnosis and Monitoring of Thyroid Disease,* Washington, DC, 2002, NACB, p. 49.
39. http://www.cancer.org/downloads/STT/Cancer_Statistics_2008
40. Stenman UH, Leinonen J, Alfthan H, et al: A complex between prostate-specific antigen and alpha$_1$-antichymotrypsin is the major form of prostate-specific antigen in serum of patients with prostate cancer: assay of the complex improves clinical sensitivity for cancer, Cancer Res 51:222, 1991.
41. Christensson A, Björk T, Nilsson O, et al: Serum prostate-specific antigen complexed to alpha$_1$-antichymotrypsin as an indicator of prostate cancer, J Urol 150:100, 1993.
42. Thompson IM, Pauler DK, Goodman PJ, et al: Prevalence of prostate cancer among men with a prostate-specific antigen level ≤4.0 ng per milliliter, N Engl J Med 350:2239, 2004.
43. Catalona WJ, Smith DS, Ornstein DK: Prostate cancer detection in men with serum PSA concentrations of 2.6 to 4.0 ng/mL and benign prostate examination: enhancement of specificity with free PSA measurements, JAMA 277:1452, 1997.
44. Carter HB, Ferrucci L, Kettermann A, et al: Detection of life-threatening prostate cancer with prostate-specific antigen velocity during a window of curability, J Natl Cancer Inst 98:1521, 2006.
45. Smith RA, Cokkinides V, Eyre HJ: American Cancer Society Guidelines for the early detection of cancer, CA Cancer J Clin 55:31, 2005.
46. Stamey TA: Preoperative serum prostate-specific antigen (PSA) below 10 µg/L predicts neither the presence of prostate cancer nor the rate of postoperative PSA failure, Clin Chem 47:631, 2001.
47. Amling CL, Bergstralh EJ, Blute ML, et al: Defining prostate-specific antigen progression after radical prostatectomy: what is the appropriate cutpoint? J Urol 165:1146, 2001.
48. Stephenson AJ, Scardino PT, Bianco FJ Jr, et al: Salvage therapy for locally recurrent prostate cancer after external beam radiotherapy, Curr Treat Options Oncol 5:357, 2004.
49. Coquard L, Bachaud J: Report of the 38th meeting of the American Society for Therapeutic Radiology and Oncology (ASTRO), Los Angeles, 27-31 October 1996, Cancer Radiother 1:88, 1997.
50. Duffy MJ: National Academy of Clinical Biochemistry guidelines for the use of tumor markers in breast cancer (section 3F). Available at www.aacc.org/AACC/members/nacb/LMPG/OnlineGuide/DraftGuidelines/TumorMarkers/TumorMarkersPDF.htm
51. Asgeirsson KS, Agrawal A, Allen C, et al: Serum epidermal growth factor receptor and HER2 expression in primary and metastatic breast cancer patients, Breast Cancer Res 9:R75, 2007.
52. Greene MH: Genetics of breast cancer, Mayo Clin Proc 72:54, 1997.
53. Burke W, Daly M, Garber J, et al: Recommendations for follow-up care of individuals with an inherited predisposition to cancer, II: BRCA1 and BRCA2 Cancer Genetics Studies Consortium, JAMA 277:997, 1997.
54. American Society of Clinical Oncology: Policy statement update: genetic testing for cancer susceptibility, J Clin Oncol 21:1, 2003.
55. Goldhirsch A, Wood WC, Gelber RD, et al: Meeting highlights: updated international expert consensus panel on the primary therapy of early breast cancer, J Clin Oncol 21:3357, 2003.
56. Budd GT, Cristofanilli M, Ellis MJ, et al: Circulating tumor cells versus imaging—predicting overall survival in metastatic breast cancer, Clin Cancer Res 12:6403, 2006.
57. Cristofanilli M, Budd GT, Ellis MJ, et al: Circulating tumor cells, disease progression, and survival in metastatic breast cancer, N Engl J Med 351:781, 2004.
58. Stieber P: National Academy of Clinical Biochemistry guidelines for the use of tumor markers in lung cancer (section 3P). Available at www.aacc.org/AACC/members/nacb/LMPG/OnlineGuide/DraftGuidelines/TumorMarkers/TumorMarkersPDF.htm.
59. Brunner N: National Academy of Clinical Biochemistry guidelines for the use of tumor markers in colorectal cancer (section 3C). Available at www.aacc.org/AACC/members/nacb/LMPG/OnlineGuide/DraftGuidelines/TumorMarkers/TumorMarkersPDF.htm.
60. Compton CC, Fielding LP, Burgart LJ, et al: Prognostic factors in colorectal cancer, Arch Pathol Lab Med 124:979, 2000.
61. Fritsche HA: National Academy of Clinical Biochemistry guidelines for the use of tumor markers in bladder cancer (section 3H). Available at www.aacc.org/AACC/members/nacb/LMPG/OnlineGuide/DraftGuidelines/TumorMarkers/TumorMarkersPDF.htm.
62. Gupta S, Comenzo RL, Hoffman BR, et al: National Academy of Clinical Biochemistry guidelines for the use of tumor markers in

monoclonal gammopathies (section 3K). Available at www.aacc.org/AACC/members/nacb/LMPG/OnlineGuide/DraftGuidelines/TumorMarkers/TumorMarkersPDF.htm.

63. Criteria for the classification of monoclonal gammopathies, multiple myeloma and related disorders: a report of the International Myeloma Working Group, Br J Hematol 121:749, 2003.
64. Bradwell AR, Carr-Smith HD, Mead GP, et al: Highly sensitive, automated immunoassay for immunoglobulin free light chains in serum and urine, Clin Chem 47:673, 2001.
65. Diamandis E, Schmitt M, van der Merwe D: National Academy of Clinical Biochemistry guidelines on the use of microarrays in cancer diagnostics (section 4A). Available at www.aacc.org/AACC/members/nacb/LMPG/OnlineGuide/DraftGuidelines/TumorMarkers/TumorMarkersPDF.htm.
66. Sawyers CL: The cancer biomarker problem, Nature 452:548, 2008.
67. Chan DW: National Academy of Clinical Biochemistry guidelines on the use of MALDI-TOF mass spectrometry profiling to diagnose cancer (section 4B). Available at www.aacc.org/AACC/members/nacb/LMPG/OnlineGuide/DraftGuidelines/TumorMarkers/TumorMarkersPDF.htm.
68. Petricoin EF, Ardekani AM, Hitt BA, et al: Use of proteomic patterns in serum to identify ovarian cancer, Lancet 359:572, 2002.
69. Li J, Zhang Z, Rosenzweig J, et al: Proteomics and bioinformatics approach for identification of serum biomarkers to detect breast cancer, Clin Chem 48:1296, 2002.
70. Adam BL, Qu Y, Davis JW, et al: Serum protein fingerprinting coupled with a pattern-matching algorithm distinguishes prostate cancer from benign prostate hyperplasia and healthy men, Cancer Res 62:3609, 2002.
71. Cheok MH, Evans WE: Acute lymphoblastic leukaemia: a model for the pharmacogenomics of cancer therapy, Nat Rev Cancer 6:117, 2006.
72. Ansari M, Krajinovic M: Pharmacogenomics in cancer treatment: defining genetic bases for inter-individual differences in responses to chemotherapy, Curr Opin Pediatr 19:15, 2007.
73. Weinshilboum R: Inheritance and drug response, N Engl J Med 348:529, 2003.
74. Gardiner SJ, Begg EJ: Pharmacogenetics, drug-metabolizing enzymes, and clinical practice, Pharmacol Rev 58:521, 2006.

INTERNET SITES

http://www.cancer.org/—American Cancer Society

http://www.cancer.gov/—National Cancer Institute

http://www.cancer.org/docroot/STT/stt_0.asp—American Cancer Society 2008 statistics

http://www.cancer.gov/cancer_information/—CancerNet (current, comprehensive cancer information)

http://www.cancer.gov/clinical_trials/—Cancer trials

http://cis.nci.nih.gov/—Cancer information service

http://medlib.med.utah.edu/WebPath/NEOHTML/NEOPLIDX.html—The Internet Pathology Laboratory for Medical Education, Florida State University College of Medicine

http://www.tmc.tulane.edu/classware/pathology/medical_pathology/New_for_98/Neoplasia_new/5t_Answered/Neoplasia_Cases.html#Case1

http://library.med.utah.edu/WebPath/NEOHTML/NEOPL070.html

http://www.merck.com/pubs/mmanual_home/sec13/149.htm

http://video.google.com/videoplay?docid=-5858291467646146016&q=metastasis&total=64&start=0&num=10&so=0&type=search&plindex=1

http://video.google.com/videoplay?docid=877505047867170592&q=cancer+metastasis&total=36&start=0&num=10&so=0&type=search&plindex=1

http://emedicine.medscape.com/article/204369-overview—Multiple Myeloma, by Grethlein S. Last updated June 16, 2006

http://www.fda.gov/cder/genomics/

http://www.ncbi.nlm.nih.gov/About/primer/pharm.html

Laboratory Evaluation of the Transplant Recipient

Chapter 54

Tiffany Kaiser, Nicole Weimert, Matthew J. Everly, Ruth-Ann Lee, Jason Everly, Adele Rike, and Rita R. Alloway

Chapter Outline

Key Terms

allogeneic Refers to organs or cells from another person, which may or may not have the same histocompatibility antigens as the recipient.

allotransplant An organ or tissue transferred between genetically different individuals of the same species. Also know as **allograft**.

azathiopurine and **6-mercaptopurine** Purine analogs that act on small lymphocytes and dividing cells, thereby blocking development of organ-rejecting T cells.

B cells Lymphocytes that develop in the fetal liver and subsequently in the bone marrow. They respond to antigenic stimuli by dividing and differentiating into plasma cells under the control of cytokines released by T cells.

CD markers This system of nomenclature is used for leukocyte surface molecules as identified by monoclonal antibodies. More than 80 individual molecules are recognized by this series, and some of them are found on cells other than leukocytes.

corticosteroids Agents that have numerous immunosuppressive and anti-inflammatory effects. They interfere with antigen presentation, inhibit the primary antibody response, and reduce the number of circulating T cells.

crossmatch The final pretransplant immunological screening step. With the use of human leukocyte antibody (HLA) antibody screening assays, the potential donor's lymphocytes serve as target cells for the patient's serum. The presence of cytotoxic immune globulin (Ig)G anti-donor HLA antibodies is a strong contraindication to transplantation.

cyclosporine An immunosuppressive drug. Cyclosporine binds to an immunophilin, cyclophilin, and this complex binds to the calcium-dependent calcineurin, which results in inhibition of transcription of cytokines, thereby inhibiting early-stage T-cell activation.

cytokines Substances released by leukocytes and other cells that control the development of the immune response. Often termed the "hormones of the immune system," they modulate the differentiation and division of hematopoietic stem cells and the activation of lymphocytes and phagocytes.

cytotoxicity A general term for the ways in which lymphocytes, mononuclear phagocytes, and granulocytes can kill target cells.

deceased donors Most are brain dead cadavers whose hearts are still beating. However, because of the demand for transplantation, expanded criteria donors now may include deceased donors who were non–heart beating for a short and known period of time.

de novo A descriptor of the first organ transplant that the recipient receives. This term typically denotes a lower immunological risk related to the initial exposure.

donor-specific antibody (DSA) The production of post-transplant antibodies directed to human leukocyte antigens (HLA) of the donor is an indication of an active immune response, with the corresponding risk of graft rejection.

FK506 binding protein (FKBP) A family of proteins (**immunophilins**) that have peptidyl-prolyl isomerase activity and process proline-containing proteins; these proteins are targets for a number of immunosuppressive drugs.

histocompatibility complex Complex of glycoprotein on the surface of cells that is used by the immune system to define self and nonself.

human leukocyte antigen (HLA) The major histocompatibility complex. It is divided into seven main groups: A, B, C, Class III, DR, DQ, and DP.

immunosuppression Measures used to reduce immune responses after transplantation to prevent graft rejection. Most such measures are not specific for the transplant antigens.

interleukin-2 A cytokine that is an essential T-cell growth factor required for division of antigen-activated T cells.

interleukin-2 receptor antibodies Antibodies used to immunosuppress the immune systems of organ recipients. Basiliximab (a chimeric mouse-human interleukin [IL]-2 receptor antibody) and daclizumab (a humanized-mouse IL-2 receptor antibody) bind to the CD25 α-chain subunit of the IL-2 receptor on activated T cells. This renders T cells unable to bind with IL-2 and thus unable to proliferate in response to this cytokine.

laparoscopic donation Refers to the minimally invasive removal of the donated organ via the laparoscopic technique as opposed to the open technique. This method typically improves and shortens postdonation recovery time.

living donor Most live donors are related biologically. Donors and recipients who are human leukocyte antigen (HLA) identical are considered the "perfect match." However, more than 25% of living kidney donors are NOT related biologically. Living donation most frequently involves kidney, but liver and pancreas live donations have been described.

major histocompatibility complex (MHC) A large group of genes, including those encoding class I and II MHC molecules, that are involved in presentation of antigen to T cells.

mTOR A serine/threonine protein kinase that regulates numerous cell functions, including cell growth, cell proliferation, and cell survival. Rapamycin can inhibit this enzyme.

mycophenolic acid Trade name Mycophenolate mofetil (MMF, Cellcept)—An ester prodrug of mycophenolic acid (MPA) that upon absorption is hydrolyzed rapidly to the active form, MPA. MPA reversibly binds and inhibits inosine monophosphate dehydrogenase (IMPDH), an enzyme essential for de novo purine synthesis, thus inhibiting DNA and RNA synthesis and subsequent synthesis of T and B cells.

panel reactive antibody (PRA) A complement-dependent lymphocytotoxicity assay wherein a patient's serum is incubated separately with B cells and T cells from a panel of donors selected to represent the human leukocyte antigens (HLA) commonly found in the local population. The anti-HLA antibodies detected are called panel reactive antibody.

polyclonal anti-lymphocyte agents Immunosuppressive antibodies to human tissue made by injecting human lymphoid material (spleen, thymus, lymph node) into an animal (horse, goat, sheep, rabbit).

rejection A reaction induced by recipient T cells that recognize allogeneic major histocompatibility complex (MHC) molecules. The T cells can activate graft-infiltrating mononuclear cells, damaging the graft. Acute rejection typically is T cell mediated; however, mixed rejections or pure antibody-mediated rejection episodes that are B cell mediated may occur.

sirolimus (Rapamycin, RapamuneR) Sirolimus binds to a specific immunophilin FK506 binding protein (FKBP) similarly to tacrolimus, but it does not exert its immunosuppressive effects by calcineurin inhibition. Sirolimus binds to the enzyme, target of rapamycin (mTOR), and inhibits translation of several cytokines essential for T-cell regulation and proliferation.

sympathetic storm A physiological response to acute brain trauma in which hypothalamic stimulation of the sympathetic nervous system and adrenal glands causes an increase in circulating corticoids and catecholamines. These hormonal changes result in hypertension, pupillary dilation, tachycardia, cardiac arrhythmias, hyperglycemia, and an increased basal metabolic rate.

T cells Lymphocytes that develop in the thymus and whose role is to recognize antigens that originate from within cells of the host as self and foreign antigens as nonself.

tacrolimus (FK506) Tacrolimus binds to an immunophilin FK506 binding protein (FKBP); this complex binds to the calcium-dependent calcineurin, which results in inhibition of transcription of cytokines, thereby inhibiting early-stage T-cell activation.

tissue typing The technique used to determine the major histocompatibility specificities carried on an individual's cells.

tolerance The acquisition of nonresponsiveness to a molecule that normally is recognized by the immune system.

United Network for Organ Sharing (UNOS) A private contractor for the U.S. government that is responsible for data tracking, organ allocation, and recipient tracking.

Methods on Evolve

Cyclosporin (Cyclosporine A)
Cytomegalovirus
Hepatitis B
Hepatitis C virus
Mycophenolic acid
Sirolimus
Tacrolimus

BACKGROUND

Solid-organ transplantation has become the therapy of choice for end-stage diseases of the kidney, liver, and heart. Advances in surgical techniques and diagnostic capabilities, progress in immunology and histocompatibility analysis, development of more specific and potent immunosuppressive agents, improvements in donor management and organ preservation, and new anti-infective agents all have contributed to the success of transplanting solid organs. As a reflection of these improvements, the total number of each type of transplant performed in the United States continues to rise. Although additional types of transplants are being performed, including solid organ (e.g., lung, intestine), cellular (e.g., pancreatic islet cells), and composite tissue (e.g., hand, face, cornea), they are beyond the focus of this chapter. In general, the principles of immunological barriers and **immunosuppression** therapy apply to all types of **allotransplants.**

The term *graft* is used to describe a transplanted organ. *Allograft* refers to tissue that is taken from one individual and used in a second individual. An allograft may come from a live or deceased donor. An allograft from a biological relative is termed a *living related donor graft* (LRD); however, live donors who are not related genetically are acceptable. Individuals from whom allografts are obtained who have been declared legally dead ("brain dead") are termed **deceased donors.**

Transplants are high-risk medical procedures; the major factor that limits transplantation is the shortage of organs. Currently, more than 95,000 patients are awaiting an organ transplant, and just over 8000 donors contributed organs in 2007 (http://www.unos.org/). This represents a continued rise in the demand for transplants in the face of a plateau of deceased donors. In those patients with heart, lung, and liver disease, failure to receive a timely transplant results in death. Brittle diabetic patients, who have difficulty maintaining a euglycemic state, are at high risk for sudden death from hypoglycemia and would benefit from a pancreas transplant. Patients with end-stage kidney disease who are being maintained on dialysis have been shown to have improved survival with a kidney transplant. The percentage of registrants who died while awaiting a transplant increased in 2007 to 6.4%. This has propelled research toward increasing organ availability by liberalizing donor criteria, by using alternative organ sources (e.g., swine, baboon), and by developing new procedures to prolong the primary graft half-life.

As surgical complications and the acute **rejection** rates of transplants have dropped, transplantation programs have focused on improving long-term allograft survival. The role of the clinical laboratory has become increasingly essential to the success of transplant programs. This chapter describes the monitoring of both transplant donors and recipients of solid organs to maximize the success of organ transplantation.

SECTION OBJECTIVES BOX 54-1

- List the types of donors available and the pros and cons of each type.
- Outline the laboratory testing performed before transplantation in potential living and deceased donors, as well as potential transplant recipients.
- List the most important components of laboratory evaluation of the following transplant types: kidney, pancreas, liver, and heart.
- Define the pretransplant immunological assays used to predict the compatibility of a donor with a potential recipient.

PRETRANSPLANT EVALUATION

Before a transplant is performed, potential donors and recipients are thoroughly screened for infection by measurement of viral serologies and are screened for specific immunological markers that will ensure successful transplantation. Each organ has specific criteria that must be reviewed before the transplant is performed.

Deceased Donors

Organ donor management should begin when a donor patient is recognized to have significant neurological damage that is likely to progress to brain death. Organs from deceased donors can potentially be donated to as many as seven individuals. Aggressive medical treatment of these patients is necessary to preserve organ function and facilitate organ transplantation. Before impending death, the brain will produce a **sympathetic storm** in an effort to preserve cerebral blood flow, and patients will become increasingly unstable and will require significant fluid and vasopressor therapy to maintain cerebral perfusion pressure. Once patients progress to brain death, they lose this sympathetic tone and require significant doses of medications, including hormone supplementation, such as **corticosteroid,** thyroid hormone, and vasopressin, to maintain blood pressure and organ perfusion. Frequent monitoring of serum electrolytes and blood gases and pH during this critical time is essential for the successful maintenance of healthy organs.

For donor patients to be declared brain dead, they must have normal laboratory chemistries (Table 54-1) and must have no drug or brain damage that would limit their ability to ventilate spontaneously. Therefore, quick turnaround time of accurate laboratory values is necessary. Aggressive patient management in the intensive care unit and timely use of laboratory data will ensure optimal health of the organs.

Each organ has clinical and laboratory donor criteria (see Table 54-1) that have been associated with improved transplant outcomes. Donors usually are between 2 and 70 years of age. However, kidneys from neonates and donors older than 70 years have been transplanted successfully. In general, donors who are acceptable for renal or liver transplants are also acceptable as pancreas donors. The primary contraindications for the acceptance of a donor for pancreas transplantation include a history of diabetes and acute or chronic pancreatitis.

Table 54-1 Surrogate Laboratory Measures of Healthy Organ Function

Organ	Laboratory Measure	Clinical Rationale
Lung	Arterial Po_2 >300 mm Hg at Fio_2 = 1.0, or Pao_2/Fio_2 >250 to 300 mm Hg	Adequate oxygenation
Heart	Troponin, CKMB	Elevations indicate cardiac injury
Liver	Serum sodium <160 mmol/L; liver function tests (AST, ALT, alk phos, total bilirubin)	Donor serum sodium >160 mmol/L has been linked to early graft loss; elevations of these enzymes, and bilirubin correlate with poor graft function
Pancreas	Serum amylase, lipase, and glucose	Elevation of these enzymes and glucose correlate with poor graft function
Kidney	Serum creatinine, urinalysis	Must be considered in the context of vasopressor requirement, donor age, co-morbid conditions (e.g., hypertension)

ALT, Alanine aminotransferase; *alk phos,* alkaline phosphatase; *AST,* aspartate aminotransferase.

Lung donors must be 65 years of age or younger, with no history of significant lung disease, a clear chest radiograph, and a cumulative cigarette smoking history of less than 30 pack-years. Patients must have sufficiently healthy lung function to maintain adequate organ oxygenation.

Criteria for a useful donor heart include the donor's cardiac assessment, past medical history, physical examination findings, and diagnostic laboratory test results. Donors older than 50 years of age and those who have experienced prominent blunt chest trauma, prolonged hypotension, cardiac arrest, or pre-morbid cardiac symptoms generally are considered unsuitable for heart donation.

Laboratory values, as surrogate markers of healthy organ function (see Table 54-1), often dictate which organs can be procured.

For example, if a potential donor's serum amylase, lipase, and blood glucose are significantly elevated, use of the pancreas is considered carefully. Hyperglycemia is seen frequently in individuals after severe head trauma or as a result of administration of glucose-containing solutions. These factors are not a contraindication for pancreas retrieval if the patient has no history of diabetes. In questionable cases, measurement of glycosylated hemoglobin levels may demonstrate that long-term pancreas function has been normal. An elevated serum amylase is not necessarily indicative of pancreatic trauma. Direct visualization of the pancreas is the best way to assess pancreatic injury in trauma cases. Evidence of pancreatic trauma precludes its retrieval. The age of the potential donor generally is not a factor for pancreatic transplants, although age criteria are slightly more restrictive than for kidney transplants. Moderate elevations in surrogate laboratory measurements are acceptable, especially if these elevations occur in response to decreased blood flow. Each potential donor organ is considered in clinical context to ensure that the recipient will have optimal outcomes. In addition, all potential donors will be checked for transmittable diseases: serum serologies for viral hepatitis (hepatitis B and C), human immunodeficiency virus (HIV), syphilis, and cytomegalovirus, and blood and urine cultures for bacterial infection. History of malignancy, except for nonmelanoma skin cancers, will preclude donation. The donor's blood type and major histocompatibility complex, located on the cell surface of all nucleated cells, will be examined to find suitable recipients who do not have any pre-formed antibodies against the donor tissue. The United Network for Organ Sharing (UNOS) has established mandatory laboratory tests (Table 54-2), although additional tests occasionally may be requested.

Table 54-2 United Network for Organ Sharing: Mandatory Laboratory Testing of the Potential Deceased Donor*

General	Complete blood count
	Electrolytes
	Blood gases
	ABO typing
	Hepatitis screen
	Syphilis screen (VDRL or RPR)
	Screen for antibodies to HIV, HTLV-1, cytomegalovirus
	Blood and urine cultures if hospitalized longer than 72 hours
Renal specific	Serum creatinine and urea, urinalysis
Liver specific	Liver enzymes: transaminases and alkaline phosphatase, total and direct bilirubin, prothrombin time, and partial thromboplastin time
Heart specific	12-Lead electrocardiogram, consultation with cardiologist, chest x-ray film
Pancreas/islet specific	Serum amylase, serum lipase, glucose
Lung specific	Pao_2

HIV, Human immunodeficiency virus; *HTLV,* human T-lymphotropic virus; *RPR,* rapid plasmin reagent; *VDRL,* Venereal Disease Research Laboratory.
*No absolute acceptable ranges are available for these laboratory tests. Aims are to ensure that organs function after transplant, and that no infections or malignancies are passed from donor to recipient.

After procurement, the organs are stored at low temperatures to slow down cellular metabolism and limit injury caused by lack of perfusion.

Live Donors

Because of the significant shortage of organs available for transplantation, other strategies are being used to increase the donor pool. The use of live donors is helping to increase the pool of available donor organs. Although this is not an appropriate strategy for all types of organ transplant, the greatest impact of the use of live donors has occurred in cases of kidney transplantation. Advantages and disadvantages of the procedure are discussed later. As for all types of transplants, live donors must be demonstrated to be free of communicable disease.

Kidney

For several reasons, kidney allograft survival rates are greater when the graft is obtained from a **living donor** versus a deceased donor. These reasons include shortened times when the donor kidney is alternatively warm and cold and ischemic, thereby preventing ischemic reperfusion injury to the kidney after transplant, and enhanced potential for improved immunological match if the recipient is related genetically. A further important advantage of live donor transplants is the elective nature of the procedure, which spares the recipient the long waiting period on dialysis that frequently occurs when one is waiting for a suitable deceased donor transplant. The option of living donation has become more appealing for kidney donors who are undergoing the laparoscopic procedure because this type of surgery is associated with shorter hospitalization, less postoperative pain, and quicker return to work when compared with open nephrectomy donor counterparts. Because most kidneys from living donors are related genetically to the recipient, an immunological advantage and improved long-term graft survival are associated. Regardless of whether the donor is or is not related, living donor allografts are associated with improved long-term graft survival.

All potential donors must be emotionally stable and must fully understand the process and implications of donating a kidney. Kidney donors who have been monitored for up to 20 years after donation exhibit a slight reduction in glomerular filtration rate and a mild increase in urine protein excretion without an increase in hypertension. Potential donors are evaluated to ensure that they are in excellent general health, and that there are no contraindications to the removal of one kidney. The age of the potential living related donor is obviously important. Minors are not eligible for kidney donation, but older donors, up to 70 years of age, may be used if in excellent health.

The potential donor and recipient must be tested to demonstrate ABO blood type compatibility. Although a limited number of transplants are performed across ABO barriers, the risks of organ rejection are greater when this occurs. Another immunocompatibility test, termed a cytotoxic T-cell **crossmatch,** must be performed between the donor and the recipient. This ensures that the recipient has no preformed antibodies against the donor's proteins.

The donor must be free of diseases such as diabetes, hypertension, anemia, renal calculi, or malignancy. Additional studies are performed to assess whether renal function and the structure of the potential renal allograft are completely normal.

Liver

Living donor liver transplantation has been utilized for several years in the pediatric end-stage liver disease population. This procedure involves donation of the lateral segment of the left lobe of the liver from a living donor to a size-matched recipient. More recently, this procedure has been utilized in adults, mainly in the setting of fulminant hepatic failure. Living liver donation involves significant ethical concerns. The surgery involves substantially higher risk in comparison with living kidney donation. The risk of donor mortality is around 1%, and surgical complications range from 5% to 10% based on each individual institution. Donors often are called upon to donate in situations where their child or sibling requires a liver transplant within 24 hours to save their life. Recently, the practice of living donor liver donation has declined as the result of a few highly published cases of donor death during the perioperative process.

Table 54-3 Pretransplantation Evaluation of the Renal Recipient

Complete history and physical examination
Dental evaluation
Gynecological evaluation
Laboratory studies
- Kidney function: serum creatinine and urea
- Liver function: serum AST, ALT, bilirubin, and alkaline phosphatase
- Viral serologies: hepatitis B Ag and Ab; Ab to hepatitis C, CMV, HIV, and EBV
- Urine culture

Immunological testing
X-ray studies
- Chest x-ray film
- Upper gastrointestinal series
- Barium enema (age >40 years)
- Gallbladder ultrasound scan
- Voiding cystourethrogram
- Mammography (female >40 years)

Ab, Antibodies; *Ag,* antigens; *ALT,* alanine aminotransferase; *AST,* aspartate aminotransferase; *CMV,* cytomegalovirus; *EBV,* Epstein-Barr virus; *HIV,* human immunodeficiency virus.

Recipient

A detailed medical and psychological evaluation of all potential transplant recipients is essential. Patients must be sufficiently healthy and motivated to undergo the surgical procedure, to withstand the potential problems of immunosuppressive agents, and to comply with a complex and demanding medical regimen. Oftentimes, they and their families do not realize the burden of frequent laboratory monitoring, clinical appointments, and multiple medications. Noncompliance is a key reason for long-term allograft rejection and failure.

The pretransplantation evaluation example of the recipient of a kidney is listed in Table 54-3. No absolute acceptable ranges are available for the laboratory tests listed in Table 54-3. The aim of such testing is to ensure that the potential recipient is sufficiently healthy to undergo the surgical procedure and to withstand the potential problems associated with immunosuppressive agents.

Not all patients with end-stage renal disease are candidates for transplantation. Patients of advanced age or with prominent systemic illness generally are not acceptable candidates. The American Society of Transplant Physicians has published

Box 54-1

Recipient Contraindications to Renal Transplantation

Active infection
Acute vasculitis or glomerulonephritis
Advanced cardiovascular disease
Advanced pulmonary disease
Age older than 70 years
Drug or alcohol abuse
Malignancy
Morbid obesity
Positive current T-cell crossmatch
Primary oxalosis (oxalate kidney stones)
Severe chronic liver disease
Severe psychosocial problems
Uncorrectable lower urinary tract disease

a list of absolute recipient contraindications to renal transplantation (Box 54-1).

Laboratory tests similar to those listed in Table 54-3 are used to assess potential recipients of liver, heart, pancreas, and lung transplants. Again, the primary goal is to ensure that the patient is healthy enough to survive the surgery and the post-transplantation complications associated with lifelong immunosuppression. Obviously, advanced cardiac disease would not be a contraindication to heart transplantation but would be a contraindication to liver transplantation. Active infection, malignancy, severe psychosocial problems, and any active drug or alcohol abuse are contraindications to all transplants.

Pretransplant Immunological Testing

An individual's unique genetic fingerprint is expressed on the surface of nucleated cells as the **major histocompatibility complex (MHC)** or **human leukocyte antigen (HLA).** The purpose of pretransplant immunological evaluation is to identify an immunologically compatible donor-recipient pair that will enable successful transplantation. Immunological monitoring in the pretransplant period is done to evaluate the sensitivity of the potential recipient's immune system in reacting against potential donor tissue. These laboratory measurements are correlated with clinical and histological findings to determine what type and dose of immunosuppression should be given and to dictate the frequency of monitoring.

Three main immunological areas are evaluated in the pretransplant period: (1) ABO blood group matching, (2) HLA antigen matching, and (3) recipient anti-donor antibodies. ABO blood group matching requires identification of blood group antigens on the surface of erythrocytes. Incompatibility mainly occurs with the major blood group antigens—A, B, AB, and A1—as the result of pre-formed antibodies to blood group proteins not expressed by the recipient's own cells. Transplantation across these blood groups, for example, transplanting an organ from a donor with blood group B into a recipient who is blood group O, would induce hyperacute rejection and traditionally has been a contraindication to transplant.

Today, centers have explored the possibility of transplanting across blood groups by using high doses of immunosuppression and splenectomy before transplantation.

The second pretransplant immunological evaluation is HLA antigen matching. HLA class I antigens are located on the surfaces of all nucleated cells; HLA class II antigens reside on immunological cells. A recipient's pre-formed antibodies against HLA class I or II antigens are responsible for immunological destruction of the allograft once implanted; these antibodies can signal the cellular immune system to induce additional tissue destruction. During the pretransplant period, potential recipients are screened for pre-formed antibodies through a procedure called the **panel reactive antibody (PRA).** This procedure currently is performed by two methods: complement-dependent **cytotoxicity** and flow cytometry.

To assist with organ allocation in liver transplantation, a system was developed to prioritize candidates on the waiting list. This prospective scoring system utilizes patient objective laboratory values to predict survival and to determine who requires a liver transplant most urgently. The **M**odel for **E**nd-stage **L**iver **D**isease (MELD) is used for candidates ages 12 and older, and the **P**ediatric **E**nd-stage **L**iver **D**isease (PELD) for ages 11 and younger. The MELD and PELD scoring systems are used currently by UNOS. Although these systems were designed to help prioritize patients, they do not recognize distinctions in "donor organ quality" such as age, gender, fat content, and heart beating versus non–heart beating status, which ultimately influence outcomes post liver transplantation.

KEY CONCEPTS BOX 54-1

- Two types of organ donors are used: living and cadaver donors. Although grafts from living donors fare better than organs from cadavers, many fewer living donors are available. Living organs are healthier at transplant than are cadaver organs, although the mental status of the living donor is a consideration.
- Laboratory testing must be performed to ensure that donor organs are acceptably functional and free of communicable disease. The recipient must be shown to be healthy enough to accept an organ and survive the transplant process.
- The most common organ-specific tests include the following: kidney, serum creatinine; pancreas, serum amylase and lipase; liver, transaminases and bilirubin; and heart, troponin and CK-MB.
- To ensure tissue antigenic compatibility, both donor and recipient are tested for ABO blood group matching and HLA antigen matching, and the recipient is tested for the absence of anti-donor antibodies.

SECTION OBJECTIVES BOX 54-2

- Discuss immunological testing in the post-transplant recipient and the differences between pre- and post-transplant testing
- Outline recommended laboratory testing of allograft function for the kidney, pancreas, liver, heart, lung, and intestines transplant patient.

POST-TRANSPLANT EVALUATION

Immunological Monitoring

Immunological monitoring is a key laboratory analysis that is undertaken at various time points during the peritransplant and post-transplant periods to optimize graft outcomes. Post-transplant immunological monitoring focuses on gross histological evidence of rejection, correlated with laboratory surrogate and immunological markers. For the purposes of this chapter, only laboratory measures will be evaluated.

Peritransplant and Post-Transplant Immunological Testing

In addition to the methods used for immunological testing in the pretransplant period, novel methods have been used to detect antitransplant immunoreactivity in the peritransplant and post-transplant periods.

Immuknow (Cylex, Inc., Columbia, MD) was the first commercially available assay used to measure the in vivo level of immunosuppression of the transplant recipient. This assay directly measures activated T-cell reactivity through detection of intracellular adenosine-5-triphosphate levels. The AlloMap assay (XDx, South San Francisco, CA) was developed as a noninvasive marker of rejection for heart transplant recipients. AlloMap measures gene expression in peripheral blood mononuclear cells that differentiates between immunoreactive and immunoquiescent states. This assay measures the gene expression profile of 20 genes (11 informative and 9 control) that are involved in T-cell activation and recognition, natural killer cell activation, stem cell mobilization, hematopoiesis, and alloimmune recognition. A gene expression algorithm weighs the contribution of each gene into a score, ranging from 0 to 40, to express the likelihood of a very low to severe acute rejection.

The production of post-transplant antibodies directed to HLA antigens of the donor is an indication of an active immune response, with the corresponding risk of graft rejection. Evidence that anti-HLA antibodies may cause graft loss has led many transplant centers to incorporate routine testing of HLA antibodies after transplantation. Antibodies specific to the donor are detected most commonly at 7 days and 14 days, and at 1, 3, 6, and 12 months after transplant. Early detection of antibodies can reveal those individuals who are at risk for graft loss. One method that is used to detect these anti-HLA antibodies couples individual HLA molecules to microparticles; binding of antibodies to these particles can be detected by flow cytometry.

Post-Transplant Immunological Testing

Many complications associated with transplantation and immunosuppressant medications can be prevented or treated effectively if identified early through vigilant and comprehensive monitoring. During the first 3 to 6 months post transplantation, when the risk for allograft rejection and infection is most intense, frequent monitoring is essential. As time passes and the transplant recipient becomes more stable, concern for rejection and infection lessens while the risk for immunosuppression toxicity and recurrent disease increases. Thus, surveillance over time not only changes focus but usually occurs less frequently. Monitoring involves not only assessment of function of the transplanted allograft, but immunological and pharmacological monitoring as well. Adhering to such strategies will allow continued and superior long-term success in transplantation.

Allograft Function

Extensive laboratory testing is performed to monitor allograft function, infection, recurrent disease, and other related medical conditions. Monitoring strategies for allograft function depend on type of organ and vary in terms of frequency.

Kidney

Reduced kidney allograft function is associated directly with poor graft and patient outcomes. Because clinical signs of dysfunction are unreliable and often nonexistent, laboratory testing is necessary at regular intervals. Both direct and indirect measures of kidney function are used, and any changes within measurements are investigated.

Most kidney allograft dysfunction can be attributed to insufficient glomerular filtration rate (GFR), which describes rate of blood flow through the kidneys. Serial measurements of serum creatinine (SCr) serve as the standard method used to indirectly detect changes in GFR. Within the first few days post transplant, a baseline measure of estimated GFR (eGFR) is determined for each recipient. Multiple donor and recipient factors can affect the recipient baseline GFR. Subsequent surveillance values obtained are compared against the baseline value; elevations in SCr indicate a decrease in GFR and often represent the initial sign of graft complications. Both the degree of SCr elevation and the rate of rise are important in the diagnosis. For calculation of eGFR, the SCr is incorporated into the Modification in Diet in Renal Disease Study Group (MDRD) equation and the Cockcroft Gault (CG) equation, both of which adjust for age, race, gender, and weight (see Chapter 30). Although these measures tend to overestimate GFR to a small degree, they remain helpful for monitoring graft function in kidney transplant recipients.

Urine analyses also are used to monitor kidney function post-transplant. A crucial function of the kidneys is to retain protein by excreting urine that is protein free. Thus, proteinuria (urine containing protein) is another sign of kidney dysfunction. A 24-hour urine collection is the definitive measure; however, this is not always practical, and other less cumbersome measures, such as the urine dipstick test or random urine protein-to-creatinine ratios, are evaluated.

Pancreas

Essential laboratory tests conducted to monitor post-transplant pancreatic function include serum glucose levels and serum and urinary measures of pancreatic enzymes, amylase, and lipase. Control of serum glucose levels is the major goal post transplant; thus serial serum glucose levels are necessary. Based on the levels obtained, hypoglycemic medications can be adjusted appropriately to achieve target glucose serum levels. Pancreatic fluid cytological findings also may be of diagnostic value; an increase in lymphocytes and blast cells is indicative of rejection, whereas a predominance of neutrophils is more characteristic of infection. Functional tests that evaluate insulin response to a glucose load may be useful for assessment of pancreatic reserve.

Although these measures provide information on function of the pancreas, they are unreliable indicators of allograft rejection. Changes in acinar cell exocrine function (see Chapter 34) usually are indicative of rejection; however, these changes are not manifested clinically and cannot be assessed in the laboratory. Typically, when rejection occurs, the graft is inflamed and the patient experiences pain and discomfort, while elevations in serum amylase and lipase may be seen. Because these signs are associated with other pancreas problems as well, additional tests often are required to differentiate among these situations.

Because the pancreas usually is transplanted in combination with the kidney, biochemical markers of kidney function typically are utilized as early indicators of pancreatic function post-transplantation. It is extremely uncommon for an isolated pancreatic rejection to occur in the setting of kidney and pancreas combination transplant. Thus, signs of kidney dysfunction such as elevated SCr are assumed to indicate a likely pancreas rejection.

Liver

Tests routinely used in monitoring liver allograft function are referred to as liver function tests (LFTs; see Tables 54-1 and 54-2). These tests are used to assess the general state of the liver; they do not actually measure function but rather reflect the presence of damage or inflammation. Elevations in aspartate aminotransferase (AST) and alanine aminotransferase (ALT) can be suggestive of hepatocellular necrosis, while elevations in alkaline phosphatase (ALP) and bilirubin suggest cholestasis. These two patterns of abnormality are not mutually exclusive and can occur simultaneously. The observed pattern of abnormality, as well as the timing of occurrence post transplant, may render some causes more suspect than others. Small incremental increases in standard liver tests do not necessarily indicate liver allograft rejection. However, serial increases of >25% over several days are considered a reliable indicator of liver allograft dysfunction. Diagnosis is made by liver biopsy because the clinical signs and symptoms of rejection are extremely variable, nonspecific, and unreliable.

Although elevated liver function tests are indicative of graft dysfunction, these findings do not necessarily reveal graft rejection. Abnormal LFT values may result from other clinical conditions. Usually, further investigation and additional assessments (abdominal ultrasound, liver biopsy, or angiogram) are necessary to determine the exact cause of liver dysfunction. Differential diagnosis of abnormal liver function tests also must include graft dysfunction, technical complications, infection, and recurrence of native disease.

Additional tests may be performed to measure the functional status of the liver, especially early during the post-transplant period. For example, clotting factors and most serum proteins are synthesized in the liver and may be targeted by monitoring strategies used to assess liver function. Factor V is used frequently to assess early liver function post liver transplant because of its short biological half-life and low level in blood replacement products. Serum albumin and international normalized ratio (INR) also are used in the peritransplant period to evaluate the intrinsic functionality of the new liver.

Heart

The use of biochemical markers for the evaluation of cardiac allograft complications is limited by the mechanism of rejection of this organ. In noncardiac allografts, injury to epithelial cells is the cause of observed biochemical alterations. Unlike the kidney, liver, or pancreas, the heart lacks epithelial cells as a primary target for rejection. Thus, in cardiac allograft recipients, changes in the levels of analytes used to measure cardiac function, such as creatine kinase, myoglobin, and troponin, have no clinical correlation with rejection. Electrocardiography, echocardiography, and radionuclide scanning are of value in determining functional status only late in rejection and are not reliable indicators of early allograft rejection. Because of the lack of sensitive and specific markers of rejection, routine serial endomyocardial biopsies serve as the standard for post-transplantation cardiac allograft monitoring.

Lung

Centers vary in their approach to surveillance post lung transplant, but in addition to general laboratory blood tests, blood gases may be monitored. Although this information is useful, it is nonspecific and does not provide precise information on lung function. Therefore, additional non–laboratory-based assessments must be done to evaluate lung function; these include pulmonary function tests (PFTs), which are simple, noninvasive breathing tests used to measure lung function. Radiological examinations such as chest x-rays and computed tomography (CT) scans will be performed. Furthermore, bronchoscopic visualization of the bronchial tubes and lungs may be performed. Compared with other transplanted organs, the lung allograft is more susceptible to rejection, thus serial transbronchial lung biopsies are routine.

Intestines

Post-transplant, no single laboratory test can be performed to monitor intestinal graft function. The D-xylose absorption and fecal fat determination tests may be of diagnostic value. Some transplant center protocols require monitoring of serum electrolytes, fluid status, and stool losses. Additionally, nutritional assessments are required for this patient population, with the goal of eventually discontinuing supplemental feedings.

Clinical manifestations of intestinal graft dysfunction may include fever, abdominal distension, pain, and diarrhea; however, transplant patients with graft dysfunction often present without symptoms. Without a definitive laboratory test and with unreliable clinical symptoms, allograft function and rejection are assessed at regular intervals via ileostomal endoscopy and numerous segmental biopsies.

Infection

Laboratory assessments are conducted to monitor bacterial, viral, and fungal complications post-transplant for recipients of any type of organ. Infectious monitoring protocols generally have involved one of two strategies: prophylaxis or preemptive therapy. *Prophylaxis* refers to administration of therapy to all patients at risk for disease; it is initiated soon after transplant. *Preemptive therapy* involves periodic monitoring for the development of infection in the blood, with therapy initiated once the disease is detected. It is unclear whether one strategy is more advantageous than the other, and transplant centers vary as to which strategy they employ. Regardless of the strategy used, monitoring for infection post-transplant is crucial and is included in most monitoring protocols.

The risk for developing infection varies on the basis of numerous factors, including type of organ transplanted, host and recipient characteristics, length of time post transplant, and type and intensity of immunosuppression. These risks are considered when monitoring protocols are developed, and they account for variability among protocols. Transplant recipients are less likely to exhibit clinical signs of infection because they have decreased immunity; thus hematological blood tests generally are not very useful for diagnosing infection in this patient population. Few transplant recipients demonstrate significant changes in white blood cell (WBC) count that are suggestive of infection. Qualitative tests that directly measure specific proteins produced by invading organisms, along with tissue biopsies, which are the gold standard, provide information necessary for proper diagnosis. When an infectious complication is diagnosed in a transplant recipient, early and aggressive treatment can ensure optimal outcomes. Treatment consists of antimicrobial therapy and, if possible, reduces the overall level of immunosuppression. The balance between over-immunosuppression and under-immunosuppression ultimately is individualized; however, to date, no definitive test has been designed.

Recurrent Disease and Co-Morbid Conditions

The ultimate success of organ transplantation is linked to the overall health of the transplant recipient. Short- and long-term post-transplantation monitoring should include not only the status of the graft, but also screening for recurrent disease or conditions linked directly or indirectly to the patient's pretransplant medical history, immune status, and immunosuppressive therapy. Post-transplant laboratory monitoring may include tests for recurrent disease, hypertension, hyperlipidemia, diabetes mellitus, cardiovascular disease, and cancer. As graft loss rates resulting from acute rejection decrease, monitoring strategies to prevent complications from these chronic diseases should be heightened.

KEY CONCEPTS BOX 54-2

- To ensure that the immunological system is suppressed, testing for T-cell activity and for anti-graft antibodies is performed frequently.
- The same organ-specific laboratory tests used in the pretransplant phase to test organ health are used post-transplant to assess allograft performance and to ensure the absence of recurrent disease.
- Because of the recipient's immunosuppressed state, routine testing is done to ensure the absence of a wide number of communicable diseases.

SECTION OBJECTIVES BOX 54-3

- Explain the immunosuppressive action of the following drugs at the cellular level: corticosteroids, antimetabolites (azathiopurine and mycophenolic acid), calcineurin inhibitors (cyclosporine and tacrolimus), mTOR inhibitors (sirolimus).
- List the types of antibody preparations that are given to assist with immunosuppression, the mode of action, and discuss how this therapy is monitored.

PHARMACOLOGICAL MONITORING

Maintaining a balance between adequate immunosuppression to avert rejection and increased risk of adverse effects associated with treatment is an ongoing challenge for the transplant clinician. Because of the narrow therapeutic window of immunosuppressants, for which toxicity and efficacy levels at times overlap, they are considered "critical dose" drugs. A high degree of interpatient and intrapatient variability in bioavailability and drug metabolism adds to the difficulty involved in achieving a patient-specific therapeutic level.

Therapeutic drug monitoring (TDM; see Chapter 14) is required to individualize the dosage for each patient so as to account for this variability. Factors that affect resulting drug levels are reviewed in Chapter 14. In addition, from a laboratory perspective, a major complication has been the variety of commercial immunoassays and their lack of comparability. See the Evolve website for specific drug assays.

In 2002, the International Association of Therapeutic Drug Monitoring and Clinical Toxicology (IATDMCT) published guidelines on transplant TDM (to be updated after 2009). Pharmacogenetic analysis used with standard pharmacokinetics may allow more effective individualized dosing regimens of immunosuppressive agents. The American Association of Clinical Chemistry (AACC) is actively working to establish laboratory management practice guidelines for the application of pharmacogenetic testing.

Corticosteroids

Corticosteroids were among the first compounds observed to exhibit immunosuppressive activity. Binding of glucocorticoids to their receptors blocks the synthesis or release of lymphokines and **cytokines.** This results in inhibition of T-cell response to stimulation, redistribution of lymphocytes from the vascular to the lymphatic system, and decreased numbers of circulating **T cells** and **B cells.** The cellular immune response is blunted, but almost no immunosuppressive effect is seen in the humoral response (antibody production).

Monitoring in patients receiving corticosteroids is strictly related to detecting an adverse drug reaction. No TDM monitoring for therapeutic efficacy, such as trough level, is done with patients who are receiving corticosteroids.

Antimetabolites

Azathiopurine

Azathiopurine (Imuran, generics), and its sister drug **6-mercaptopurine** are purine metabolism antagonists, exerting immunosuppressive activity through inhibition of DNA, RNA, and protein synthesis. Laboratory monitoring of azathiopurine therapy includes complete WBC and platelet counts weekly for the first post-transplant month, followed by twice monthly counts for 2 months, then monthly counts, to evaluate bone marrow toxicity. Liver function tests (see Tables 54-1 and 54-2) should be evaluated every 2 weeks for the first month, then monthly thereafter, to evaluate hepatic hypersensitivity and, in rare cases, life-threatening hepatic venous occlusive disease.

In addition, patients should be evaluated at baseline for a deficiency in thiopurine methyltransferase (TPMT), which is responsible for S-methylation of azathiopurine to inactive metabolites. Patients who have intermediate to low TPMT activity are predisposed to the hematological toxicities of azathiopurine; lower starting doses are used for patients with low enzyme activity, and avoidance for patients with no activity. TPMT mutations are detected by polymerase chain reaction (PCR).

Mycophenolic Acid

Mycophenolic acid formulations are currently the antimetabolites of choice used in solid organ transplantation. The mechanism of action of mycophenolic acid lies in its ability to reversibly inhibit inosine monophosphate dehydrogenase (IMPDH). This drug has a narrow therapeutic window, and gastrointestinal and bone marrow toxicity has led to limited dose escalation in several patients. Most pharmacokinetic monitoring has been done with mycophenolate mofetil, the formulation that was first released. In heart transplant recipients receiving mycophenolate mofetil, high (>1.5 mg/L) whole blood trough mycophenolic acid (MPA) levels have been correlated with decreased risk of acute rejection. An abbreviated (values measured prior to dose and 0.5 and 2 hours after dose) area under the curve of 30 to 50 mg/L is associated with a 50% to 90% reduction in rejection rates for renal transplant patients. However, MPA exhibits 10-fold interpatient variability in absorption, distribution, and elimination kinetics, making it difficult to establish dosing regimens.

Calcineurin Inhibitors

The calcineurin inhibitors, **cyclosporine** and **tacrolimus,** are widely used immunosuppressive drugs. Most centers use semiautomated immunoassays to measure these drugs, but a trend toward the use of high-performance liquid chromatography (HPLC) with mass-spectroscopy (MS) detection has been noted. With any calcineurin inhibitor level measurement, it is important to remember that it is only a single surrogate marker of overall exposure of the drug. Clinicians usually use the area under the curve (AUC) (see Chapter 14) measure to determine the blood level that best predicts exposure in a specific patient.

Cyclosporine (Sandimmune, Neoral, generics) inhibits the synthesis and release of **interleukin-2** (IL-2) and other lymphokines. It accomplishes this by inhibiting early calcium-dependent events in signal transduction during T-cell activation. Cyclosporine pharmacokinetics is complex, and absorption of cyclosporine after oral dosing is variable. Approximately one-third of the dose is absorbed, but its bioavailability can range from 5% to 90%. Peak blood levels occur 2 to 6 hours after oral dosing. Hydrophobic cyclosporine is distributed widely in tissues and can be detected in tissue as long as 2 weeks after discontinuation of therapy. Approximately 10% of cyclosporine in the blood is carried in leukocytes, whereas 40% to 60% is carried in the red blood cells; the balance is carried in the plasma tightly bound to lipoproteins. Binding to erythrocytes is nonlinear, temperature dependent, and may change with hematocrit. This variability in distribution within blood fractions has necessitated that whole blood anticoagulated with ethylenediaminetetraacetic acid (EDTA) should be the specimen customarily used for clinical analysis.

Cyclosporine undergoes extensive hepatic metabolism. Most identified metabolites have undergone oxidation, or N-demethylation. Elimination of cyclosporine occurs primarily through hepatobiliary excretion with elimination in the feces. Urinary concentrations of cyclosporine and metabolites account for less than 10% of the administered dose.

Serious adverse effects related to cyclosporine treatment include dose-related nephrotoxicity, hypertension, neurotoxicity, gingival hyperplasia, hirsutism, hyperlipidemia, and glucose intolerance. Many of these side effects are similar to the side effects of corticosteroid treatment, adding to their severity with combined therapy. General risks of over-immunosuppression are present as well, with an increased risk of chronic viral infection; although these most often are innocuous in the general population, they can be a threat to the transplant patient. Both acute and chronic nephrotoxicity can occur. In the early post-transplantation period, when the cyclosporine dosage and levels are highest, the probability of occurrence of acute cyclosporine-induced nephrotoxicity is greatest. This toxicity manifests as a reduction in renal blood flow, glomerular filtration rate, and urine output. It may be difficult to distinguish this nephrotoxicity from acute rejection in renal transplants. These short-term effects usually can be reversed when one decreases the cyclosporine dose. Long-term administration of cyclosporine and associated renal vasoconstriction can lead to a nephropathy characterized by interstitial fibrosis. Secondary to the chronic nephropathy are hypertension and hyperuricemia. Decreasing the cyclosporine dose and switching to alternative therapies are the strategies most commonly used to deal with these chronic side effects.

The pharmacokinetic and pharmacodynamic properties of cyclosporine may be affected by many drugs commonly used to treat transplant recipients. Drug interactions with cyclosporine may occur as the result of an alteration of the pharmacokinetic parameters, an alteration of physiological or pharmacological effects, or a combination of these effects. The most common mechanisms for these drug interactions include induction and inhibition of the cytochrome P-450 system, which result in reduced and increased blood cyclosporine levels, respectively. Close monitoring of the patient is suggested when administration of drugs known to interact with cyclosporine is initiated or stopped. This monitoring includes assessment of organ function and the known adverse effects of cyclosporine, as well as the measurement of cyclosporine blood concentrations.

Evolving technology for monitoring cyclosporine and changes in immunosuppressive protocols has made it difficult to establish appropriate therapeutic ranges. Therapeutic ranges are often specific to each institution, with different ranges specific for each organ type, time since transplant, immunosuppressant drug combinations, and recent rejection episodes. It remains very difficult to interpret an individual immunosuppressant concentration without a full understanding of the patient and specifics surrounding dose and level.

Frequent monitoring of cyclosporine levels is particularly valuable when one is following the progress of individual patients. Because of interpatient and intrapatient variability of cyclosporine pharmacokinetic parameters, it is well accepted that monitoring with the AUC calculation more accurately reflects the exposure of a patient to the drug.

When cyclosporine levels are reported, it is recommended that sample type (baseline or 2 hours post dosage), therapeutic range, and assay method also be reported. Changes in cyclosporine assay method or logistics, which may affect the availability of results, should be discussed with the transplant team before implementation.

Tacrolimus (FK506, Prograf), a novel macrolide immunosuppressant, is a powerful and selective anti–T-cell agent that has a similar mode of action to cyclosporine. Tacrolimus binds to an **FK506 binding protein,** and the resultant complex binds to calcium-dependent calcineurin, which results in inhibition of transcription of cytokines. This results in inhibition of early-stage T-cell activation. Tacrolimus is approximately 100 times more potent than cyclosporine and has proved to be more effective than cyclosporine in preventing and treating rejection in various types of organ transplants.

The pharmacokinetics of tacrolimus is similar to that of cyclosporine. It is poorly, erratically, and incompletely absorbed in the gut, although its absorption appears to be less dependent on the availability of bile than is that of cyclosporine. In plasma, the drug binds primarily to α1-acid glycoprotein, whereas in whole blood, it is found mainly in erythrocytes. Tacrolimus is metabolized by the microsomal cytochrome P-450 system of the liver. After hepatic metabolism, more than 95% of the drug is eliminated by the biliary route. Drug interactions between tacrolimus and drugs that inhibit or induce the cytochrome P-450 pathway are very similar to those that occur with cyclosporine. In addition, those drugs that cause nephrotoxicity, such as aminoglycosides and nonsteroidal anti-inflammatory agents, typically are synergistic with tacrolimus.

Nephrotoxicity, neurotoxicity, and hyperglycemia are significant side effects associated with tacrolimus therapy. Nausea, vomiting, and diarrhea are other common side effects that do not occur with cyclosporine. Common neurological side effects associated with tacrolimus include tremor, paresthesia, insomnia, headache, photophobia, and seizures.

Variability in blood concentrations caused by variable pharmacokinetics, drug interactions, and dose-dependent immunosuppressive effects and toxicities justifies careful monitoring of this drug. The correlation between tacrolimus concentrations and efficacy or toxicity is still unclear. However, unlike cyclosporine, tacrolimus trough concentrations accurately reflect tacrolimus AUC concentrations.

mTOR Inhibitors

Sirolimus, Rapamune, Rapamycin

Sirolimus is a macrocyclic triene antibiotic that is produced by fermentation of *Streptomyces hygroscopicus.* Originally developed as an antifungal agent, sirolimus subsequently was noted to have potent immunosuppressive and antiproliferative properties. Everolimus is a structural derivative of sirolimus that currently is undergoing phase 3 trials in the United States. After entry into the cytoplasm, both sirolimus and everolimus bind to the FK506 binding protein 12 (FKBP12), which binds FKBP12-rapamycin–associated protein (modulating the activity of the mammalian target of rapamycin [**mTOR**]), resulting in blockade of T- and B-cell activation by cytokines, thus preventing cell-cycle progression and proliferation.

The principal non-immune toxic effects of sirolimus and everolimus include hyperlipidemia, thrombocytopenia, and impaired wound healing. Other reported effects include delayed recovery from acute tubular necrosis in kidney transplants, reduced testosterone concentrations, aggravation of proteinuria, mouth ulcers, skin lesions, and pneumonitis. Effective strategies to manage these toxicities include dosage reduction; the addition of antihyperlipidemic therapy (i.e HMG-CoA reductase inhibitors) can aid in the treatment of hyperlipidemia.

Routine therapeutic drug monitoring is recommended for most patients who are receiving sirolimus or everolimus; however, because of its different toxicity profile and long half-life, the monitoring frequency is less than that for cyclosporine or tacrolimus. Monitoring is recommended for pediatric patients, patients with hepatic impairment, and patients receiving cytochrome P-450 3A4 inducers or inhibitors, as well as in patients who have had a markedly decreased or discontinued cyclosporine and tacrolimus dose.

Antibody Preparations

Polyclonal Antibodies

Current polyclonal antibody preparations are prepared primarily by injecting human lymphocytes into rabbits and horses. When these polyclonal antibodies are given to transplant recipients, they induce T-cell death and are used for induction therapy with the goals of prolonging graft survival, preventing rejection in patient populations at high immunological risk, and providing rejection rescue.

Polyclonal lymphocyte-depleting antibodies are given intravenously at the time of transplant based on the empirical observation that treatment with these antibodies prevents early acute rejection. The most common side effects of this therapy, which are influenced primarily by rate and dose of antibody administration, include flulike symptoms that can occur during infusion and hematological toxicities. These polyclonal antibody preparations also can produce an antibody response that may limit their efficacy upon repeat administration or may result in rare serum sickness reactions. Detection of the transplant recipient's antibodies to horse, rabbit, or mouse antibodies can prevent such reactions.

Monoclonal Antibodies

Monoclonal antilymphocyte antibodies have better specificity than polyclonal preparations. Instead of targeting all lymphocytes or thymocytes, a specific subset of cells can be chosen for suppression. Although the mouse monoclonal antibody, OKT3, was the first used in transplant patients to prevent and treat acute rejection, its use is limited today. When used, OKT3 is monitored by several means. Measurement of levels of lymphocyte subsets, specifically CD3+ cells, is the primary means of monitoring OKT3 efficacy.

In an effort to circumvent the cytokine release syndrome associated with animal-derived anti-thymocyte preparations, humanized or chimeric antibodies have been developed. Two commercially available chimeric antibodies are directed against the IL-2 receptor. Basiliximab (a chimeric mouse-human IL-2 receptor antibody) and daclizumab (a humanized-mouse IL-2 receptor antibody) bind to the CD25 α-chain subunit of the IL-2 receptor on activated T cells, rendering T cells unable to bind IL-2 and thus unable to proliferate in response to this cytokine. These antibodies have proved to be effective in preventing, but not treating, acute rejection episodes and are used most commonly in the early post transplant period to prevent acute rejection. The subsequent mean time of IL-2 receptor suppression is 36 days for basiliximab and 120 days for daclizumab. Monitoring typically is not performed for these agents.

Alemtuzumab is a humanized murine monoclonal antibody that has been approved by the U.S. Food and Drug Administration (FDA) as a third-line agent for B-cell chronic lymphocytic leukemia. The action of alemtuzumab is directed against the surface protein CD52, which is expressed on the surfaces of many cells, including B and T lymphocytes, natural killer cells, monocytes, and macrophages. It profoundly depletes T cells from peripheral blood for several months, making it an ideal induction agent for use before transplant. Side effects of alemtuzumab include first-dose reactions of neutropenia, anemia, and (rarely) pancytopenia, as well as autoimmunity (e.g., hemolytic anemia, thrombocytopenia, hyperthyroidism). Monitoring is not typically done during alemtuzumab treatment.

Rituximab is a chimeric murine-human monoclonal antibody that is approved in the United States for the treatment of patients with refractory and relapsed B-cell lymphoma or rheumatoid arthritis. The action of rituximab is directed against the surface protein CD20, which is found primarily on the surfaces of naive and immature B cells. Rituximab has emerged as an effective therapy for a variety of antibody-mediated events in kidney transplantation. Rituximab therapy is monitored by measuring the blood levels of surface protein CD19 (which is similar to CD20 but is not inhibited by rituximab). This count provides evidence of depletion of B cells. A single dose of rituximab typically results in 6 to 9 months of B-cell depletion.

KEY CONCEPTS BOX 54-3

- TDM monitoring is performed for mycophenolic acid, cyclosporine and tacrolimus, and sirolimus.
- Laboratory monitoring of azathiopurine therapy is based on WBC and platelet counts.
- Both polyclonal and **monoclonal antilymphocyte** preparations are available. Patients who are receiving polyclonal preparations should be monitored for the development of antibodies to the animal antibodies.

SECTION OBJECTIVES BOX 54-4

- Define the different types of rejection seen in transplant patients with regard to timing and diagnosis.
- List laboratory analytes used to monitor rejection of kidney, liver, and pancreas transplants.
- List the most common infections encountered post transplant.
- Explain how graft organ function and the presence of recurrent and new disease are monitored post transplant.

MONITORING TRANSPLANT OUTCOMES

Transplant Rejection: Types and Mechanisms

Transplant outcomes vary greatly among organ types. For example, unlike kidney allografts, it is reasonable to expect that most liver allografts will serve their recipients throughout the respective life span primarily because of the liver's regenerative ability. In fact, it is speculated that a significant number of patients with a functioning liver allograft die as the result of other co-morbidities (cardiovascular, endocrine, etc.).

Many transplant recipients will have an acute rejection episode within the first year after transplant; many will have additional rejection episodes in subsequent years. Transplant rejection occurs in recipients when the transplanted organ fails to be accepted by the body of the transplant recipient. The immune system then attacks the transplanted organ, in a similar way that it attacks viruses and bacteria. As was discussed earlier, immunosuppressive medications are used to weaken the recipient's immune system to the level at which the recipient is unable to have a strong response to the transplanted organ.

The mechanisms involved in allograft rejection are complex and involve various contributions from the cellular and humoral arms of the immune system. Transplant rejection types can be divided on the basis of time post transplant (Table 54-4). In addition, associated organ-specific classification systems may be used.

The earliest forms of rejection were reportedly hyperacute and acute accelerated rejections. Hyperacute rejection occurs within minutes to hours from the time of transplant because of the presence of preexisting antibodies within the recipient

Table 54-4 Transplant Rejection Types Based on Time of Onset

Rejection Type	Time to Onset of Rejection
Hyperacute	Minutes to hours
Acute accelerated	Few days
Acute	Several days to weeks
Chronic	Months to years

against the transplanted organ tissue. This is called *pre-sensitization.* Pre-sensitization can occur through a previous transplant or blood transfusion, or through pregnancy. Acute accelerated rejection generally occurs in the early days post-transplant. Usually, this type of rejection is associated with graft loss because of the formation of anti-donor antibody. Although these rejections still may occur, they are rare because of advancements in detection techniques for anti-donor antibodies (see previous discussion).

The more common form of rejection is acute rejection. Acute rejection can occur at any time post-transplant but is seen most frequently during the initial months after transplant. Two main forms of acute rejection have been identified: antibody mediated and T cell mediated; these forms are not mutually exclusive in that they can occur simultaneously.

Antibody-mediated rejection (AMR) is similar in pathology to acute accelerated rejection. Across organ groups, a similar incidence of AMR has been reported, as follows: kidneys, 5% to 7%; heart, 7%; and lung, 7%. Manifestations of AMR are driven by B cells of the immune system, which produce antibodies. Antibodies can be donor specific or non–donor specific; the former type is associated with a worse prognosis. In addition to antibodies, glomerular deposition of a complement split product (C4d) serves as a diagnostic marker for antibody-mediated rejection. A common finding in all organs is the presence of acute tissue injury with infiltrates of neutrophils and macrophages. Plasma B cells and organ edema may be found in transplanted tissue, but these findings are nonspecific. Overall, AMR is difficult to treat and has a poor prognosis. Many therapies have little effect on reducing antibody concentrations and therefore only delay rather than eliminate eventual graft rejection.

Similar to AMR, acute T cell–mediated rejection (ACR) generally occurs after the first post-transplant week and most commonly within 3 months after transplantation. In contrast to AMR, in which the antibody is the main immune component, the T cell and its effects are thought to be paramount in ACR. If untreated, ACR can have a poor outcome, as can AMR. However, currently available therapies are very effective in the treatment of acute T cell–mediated rejection; therefore, ACR outcomes generally are not poor.

Chronic rejection usually occurs months or years after transplantation and is defined as progressive deterioration of graft function in the absence of other causes, such as recurrent disease. Similar to acute rejection, chronic rejection can include a cellular and/or humoral component. The form of renal transplant chronic rejection that has been recognized increasingly as problematic is transplant glomerulopathy. This form of rejection is primarily antibody mediated and has a poor prognosis. It is commonly associated with high levels of donor-specific antibodies in the serum and high levels of protein in the urine. To date, chronic rejection as a whole remains one of the major challenges in transplantation.

Acute cellular rejection typically occurs within the first 3 months post-transplant and thereafter becomes less common. Through the use of improved immunosuppressive agents, the incidence of acute rejection has declined; however, the reported incidence remains highly variable (20% to 70%). Chronic rejection has a relatively low incidence (<10%) but a rapid onset with a progressive course.

Monitoring Rejection

Every post-transplant patient is monitored closely for early indicators of rejection. The clinical signs and symptoms of rejection are variable and nonspecific. Observed laboratory abnormalities include elevations in some or all of the following serum analytes: ALT, AST, ALP, and bilirubin. In kidney transplant recipients, serum creatinine serves as a marker. When SCr levels increase by as little as 15%, and other reasons for the rise are excluded, a kidney allograft biopsy may be requested. Pancreas transplant recipients can be monitored through serial measurements of serum amylase and lipase concentrations, as well as by close monitoring of serum blood glucose concentrations. Elevations in these tests indicate that a possible pancreas rejection should be investigated. Lung transplant recipients are not monitored routinely. No single laboratory test can be used to detect rejection of a transplanted intestine; suspicion of rejection is based on clinical evaluation. Typically, instances of intestine rejection are associated with fever, a significant increase in stomal output, and gastrointestinal symptoms. If rejection is suspected, the intestinal graft must be evaluated endoscopically. This evaluation should include as much of the small bowel as possible, along with multiple biopsies from numerous sites, because rejection often can be segmented.

However, these clinical and laboratory parameters cannot distinguish rejection from other causes of organ dysfunction and do not correlate with the severity of rejection. Thus for most transplants, graft biopsy is considered the "gold standard" for assessing possible rejection. Biopsy of the transplanted kidney is the gold standard for diagnosing graft rejection. Most transplant centers adhere to routine biweekly and monthly biopsy for the first year post heart transplant. Liver biopsy remains the gold standard for the diagnosis of liver rejection, although difficulties have been associated with interpretation of biopsy results because many findings are suggestive of more than one cause of liver dysfunction.

The Banff scoring system was developed for use in grading rejection severity. For liver biopsies, once rejection has been diagnosed, three specific biopsy features (portal inflammation, bile duct inflammation, and venular inflammation) are evaluated, scored, and added together to determine a final rejection activity index (RAI). Rejections are defined as mild,

Box 54-2

Infectious Agents Commonly Seen in Transplant Recipients

Bacterial: *Nocardia* species, *Pseudomonas aeruginosa, Serratia marcescens, Proteus rettgeri,* and *Enterobacter cloacae*
Fungal: *Candida albicans* and *Aspergillus fumigatus*
Protozoal: Malaria, leishmania, and nematodes
Viruses: Herpes family (Epstein-Barr virus, CMV, varicella-zoster virus [VZV]), adenovirus, and polyomavirus

moderate, or severe based on the Banff score. Different scoring criteria are used for each organ.

Although no universal treatment protocol is available, most centers do not treat mild rejection episodes (Banff score <2) but may increase the overall level of immunosuppression. Rejections classified as moderate and severe (Banff >2) are treated by increasing the dosage of calcineurin inhibitor or by providing large pulsed doses of methylprednisolone.

COMPLICATIONS OF OVER-IMMUNOSUPPRESSION

The primary problem associated with excessive immunosuppression is an increased risk for infection (Box 54-2) in the transplant recipient. Some of the most common of these are discussed in the following sections.

Infection

Cytomegalovirus (CMV)

Cytomegalovirus (CMV) is a β-herpes virus that infects most humans and is one of the most common viral infections in transplant recipients caused by potent immunosuppressive agents. The direct effects of CMV result from spread of the virus through the blood and its invasion and replication in target organs (e.g., liver, gastrointestinal tract, lung, eye). Risk factors for CMV in the transplant recipient include CMV serostatus of donor and recipient, net state of immunosuppression, concomitant viral infection, and the use of antiviral prophylaxis. CMV infection usually occurs within the first few months post-transplant.

Although most cases are associated with no symptoms, patients with symptoms present with a viral syndrome consisting of fever, low WBC count, pneumonia, and gastrointestinal disease. These indirect viral effects are likely to be seen in transplant recipients and are assumed to be mediated by the ability of CMV to modulate the immune system. Ultimately, if left untreated, CMV results in end-organ damage.

CMV prevention post-transplant generally involves one of two strategies: prophylaxis or preemptive therapy. *Prophylaxis* refers to the administration of antiviral therapy to all patients at risk for CMV disease; this is initiated soon after transplant and is continued for at least 100 days. *Preemptive therapy* on the other hand involves periodic monitoring for the development of CMV infection in the blood and the initiation of therapy once detected. It is unclear whether one strategy is more advantageous than the other, and transplant centers vary as to which strategy they employ.

Multiple antiviral agents are available for the treatment of patients with CMV infection; these include ganciclovir, valganciclovir, foscarnet, and cidofovir. Treatment protocols vary not only in terms of which agent is administered but also in terms of dose and duration.

Table 54-5 World Health Organization Classification of Post-Transplant Lymphoproliferative Disorder

Classification	Subtypes
Early lesions	Reactive plasmacytic hyperplasia
	Infectious mononucleosis-like
Polymorphic post-transplant	Polyclonal
Lymphoproliferative disorder	Monoclonal
Monomorphic post-transplant	B-cell lymphoma
Lymphoproliferative disorder	Diffuse large B-cell lymphoma (immunoblastic, centroblastic, and anaplastic)
	Burkitt/Burkitt-like lymphoma
	Plasma cell myeloma
	T-cell lymphoma
	Peripheral T-cell lymphoma
Other types	Hodgkin's disease–like lesions
	Plasmacytoma-like lesions

Polyomavirus Infection (BKV)

Human polyomaviruses are DNA viruses in the Papovaviridae family that primarily cause disease in hosts with a compromised immune system. BK virus is one of two clinically significant human polyomaviruses and is recognized as a common cause of late kidney graft failure. In organ transplant recipients with a reduced immune system, this virus is able to replicate and cause organ disease.

Clinical features of BK virus–associated kidney disease suggest interstitial nephritis and appear to resemble early graft rejection; disease onset, although variable, typically occurs after the first year post-transplant. As with rejection, SCr levels are elevated, indicating kidney dysfunction and abnormalities. Additionally, the detection of serum antibodies directed against BK virus and urine cytology may aid in the diagnosis. Specific findings on biopsy may be suggestive of BK virus infection.

Post-Transplant Lymphoproliferative Disorder

Post-transplant lymphoproliferative disorder (PTLD) is one of the more devastating complications seen in both **allogeneic** stem cell transplantation and solid organ transplantation. Generally, PTLD refers to B-cell lymphoproliferations that can be subdivided into classifications based on clinical presentation, morphological characteristics, and clonality (Table 54-5). These lymphoproliferations likely occur as the result of interaction with, and regulation of, the immune system by the Epstein-Barr virus (EBV).

EBV, a member of the herpes virus family, is found in the oropharyngeal tissues of nearly all humans. Primary infection with EBV typically is acquired during childhood through infected saliva, as in infectious mononucleosis, or via breast milk. It is estimated that nearly 90% of the global population harbor EBV by the age of 40 years. After infection, the EBV virus commonly remains in the latent state inside B lymphocytes protected by viral proteins that both prevent cell death and cause proliferation. In a non-immunosuppressed patient, EBV generally is not a problematic virus. However, for immunosuppressed transplant recipients, decreased T-lymphocyte activity can lead to EBV-induced dysregulation and uncontrolled B-cell proliferation, ultimately causing PTLD.

PTLD can develop at any time post-transplantation and typically is characterized as early or late. Early PTLD is defined as arising within 1 year following transplantation. PTLD incidence varies widely according to the type of organ transplanted. PTLD is most common among intestinal transplant recipients (19%), followed by lung (8%), heart (3%), and liver (3%) transplant recipients. The lowest PTLD incidence occurs in kidney transplant patients, with less than 1% of recipients affected.

Management of PTLD requires preventative strategies; once the disease is detected, prompt diagnosis and treatment are essential. PTLD is best prevented through risk factor assessment. The two best described PTLD risk factors include EBV serostatus and intensity of immunosuppression.

Although preventative strategies that use less intense immunosuppressive regimens and antiviral prophylaxis are very effective, PTLD still may occur. Diagnosis of PTLD requires close scrutiny of patient clinical complaints. Clinical suspicion for PTLD is increased when post-transplant patients are observed to have a fever over 3 days or longer. A workup consisting of routine laboratory studies, imaging studies, and bone marrow biopsy is required to diagnose PTLD. After diagnosis, tissue biopsy is needed to determine PTLD histology. Additionally, EBV viral loads in the peripheral blood should be measured by EBV polymerase chain reaction (PCR). This level is useful in detecting EBV infection and is helpful in monitoring a patient's response to therapy.

Recurrent Disease or Exacerbation

Acute and chronic rejection and subsequent allograft failure are significant complications post transplant; however, recurrent disease is also a matter of concern. Risk of recurrent disease varies with the type of organ transplanted. Recurrent disease in transplant recipients who receive a kidney is rare; those with a history of systemic lupus or immune globulin (Ig)A nephropathy are at higher risk for recurrence. In general, precautions are taken to ensure that the disease is quiescent before transplantation is begun. In some cases, the addition of immunosuppression to prevent rejection may decrease but not eliminate recurrent disease.

In liver transplant recipients on the other hand, recurrent disease is such a large problem that it is usually the primary cause of morbidity and mortality, rather than allograft dysfunction. The most common diagnosis for end-stage liver failure requiring transplantation is hepatitis C, and the overall recurrence rate of chronic hepatitis C virus (HCV) is greater than 90%, with 5-year patient and graft survival rates of 70% and 57%, respectively.

HCV recurrence is variable and difficult to predict. Patient and graft survival rates tend to vary according to transplant center, yet it is not disputed that liver fibrosis develops at a faster rate in HCV-infected transplant patients, and as many as 20% to 30% of these patients develop cirrhosis within 5 years of transplantation. Rapid progression to cirrhosis and the subsequent decrease in graft survival have led many centers to adjust their post-transplant treatment protocols to include antiviral therapy.

Hepatitis B virus (HBV) recurrence has decreased over the past decade because the number of people who need a liver transplant because of HBV infection has decreased, and because new antiviral agents have been developed for use in combination with hepatitis B immune globulin.

Alcoholic liver disease is a cause of end-stage liver disease and the need for a liver transplant. Alcohol use post liver transplant ranges from 8% to 22% in the first year, with cumulative rates reaching 30% to 40% by 5 years following transplantation. Predictors of resumed alcohol use included pretransplant length of sobriety, a diagnosis of alcohol dependence, a history of other substance use, and previous alcohol rehabilitation. Clinical interviews following transplantation are essential for monitoring alcohol and substance use to detect and prevent relapse.

Aggressive pretransplant therapies for hepatocellular cancer (HCC) have changed the course for these patients, and more patients with HCC are receiving liver transplants. However, liver recipients with HCC continue to remain at risk for recurrence and require vigilant serial imaging and follow-up post-transplantation.

Autoimmune Recurrence

Autoimmune disease recurrence is common post liver transplant, but typically this disease process is manageable. Pharmacological regimens given post transplantation to suppress the immune system not only prevent rejection but also interfere with and inhibit the autoimmune process. Thus, this patient population tends to experience fewer symptoms of recurrent disease.

Post-Transplant Cardiovascular Disease

Although renal transplantation has proved more beneficial than dialysis treatment for end-stage renal disease, overall survival for kidney transplant recipients is significantly influenced by the presence of cardiovascular disease (CVD). CVD is the leading cause of death with a functioning graft in renal transplant recipients and a major reason for graft loss. The risk of death caused by CVD in renal transplant recipients is approximately 3% to 5%, which is 50-fold higher than in the general population. Furthermore, the incidences of stroke, congestive heart failure, and extracranial cerebrovascular atherosclerosis are severalfold higher than in the general population. The metabolic syndrome (see Chapter 38), which now is recognized as a significant risk factor for CVD, is characterized by a constellation of metabolic factors, including central obesity, dyslipidemia, hypertension, and glucose intolerance. The incidence of metabolic syndrome 1 year post-transplant is greater than 50%. Although advances in immunosuppression have drastically improved allograft survival and acute rejection rates, the side effect profile of these agents contributes to cardiovascular risk in such a way that transplant recipients with a functioning graft now are more challenged by the burden of CVD than by complications of acute rejection.

Hypertension is the most prevalent CVD risk factor for individuals undergoing kidney transplantation and for other transplant populations. The pathogenesis of post-transplant hypertension is multifactorial, involving factors such as preexisting hypertension, higher body mass index, calcineurin inhibitor use, corticosteroid use, and primary kidney disease.

Hyperlipidemia is one of the most common cardiovascular complications post-transplantation; it affects more than 50% of kidney transplant recipients. Within the first 3 months post transplantation, increases in serum cholesterol levels are seen, primarily as the result of immunosuppressive medications, particularly the calcineurin inhibitors. Hypertriglyceridemia develops within the first 2 years of transplant, primarily in conjunction with onset of glucose intolerance and increased body weight.

Anemia is a common and significant risk factor for CVD in transplant recipients. Several factors, including female gender, immunosuppressive agents used, age, and infection, contribute to anemia. Therefore, management of anemia through the use of supplementation and pharmacological stimulating agents is essential for the management of post-transplant CVD.

KEY CONCEPTS BOX 54-4

- Graft rejection is defined by the speed at which rejection occurs after transplant: from fastest to slowest, these are; hyperacute, acute accelerated, acute, and chronic.
- Diseases acquired most commonly post-transplant may be bacterial, fungal (*Candida* and *Aspergillus*), protozoal, or viral (herpes family, adenovirus, and polyoma).
- Organ-specific laboratory tests as discussed earlier are used to monitor graft organ failure. To differentiate between organ failure and organ rejection, a biopsy is often required.
- The transplant recipient is at risk for numerous diseases, including cancer, cardiac disease, and hyperlipidemia. Laboratory tests are used to monitor the occurrence of some of these diseases.

BIBLIOGRAPHY

Ansermot N, Fathi M, Veuthey JL, et al: Quantification of cyclosporine and tacrolimus in whole blood: comparison of liquid chromatography–electrospray mass spectrometry with the enzyme multiplied immunoassay technique, Clin Biochem 41:910, 2008.

Arns W, Cibrik DM, Walker RG, et al: Therapeutic drug monitoring of mycophenolic acid in solid organ transplant patients treated with mycophenolate mofetil: review of the literature, Transplantation 82:1004, 2006.

Atwood M: Transplantation chapter summary, *2006 Annual Report*, Chapter 7, p. 148.

Barsoum NR, Bunnapradist S, Mougdil A, et al: Treatment of parvovirus B-19 (PV B-19) infection allows for successful kidney transplantation without disease recurrence, Am J Transplant 2:425, 2002.

Baum C: Weight gain and cardiovascular risk after organ transplantation, JPEN J Parenter Enteral Nutr 25:3, 2001.

Brennan DC, Daller JA, Lake KD, et al: Rabbit antithymocyte globulin versus basiliximab in renal transplantation, N Engl J Med 355:1967, 2006.

Buell JF, Gross TG, Woddle ED, et al: Malignancy after transplantation, Transplantation 80:254S, 2005.

Canadian Multicentre Transplant Study Group: A randomized clinical trial of cyclosporine in cadaveric renal transplantation, N Engl J Med 309:809, 1983.

Ciancio G, Miller J, Gonwa TA, et al: Review of major clinical trials with mycophenolate mofetil in renal transplantation, Transplantation 80:S191, 2005.

Delves PJ, Roitt IM: The immune system, first of two parts, N Engl J Med 343:37, 2000.

Delves PJ, Roitt IM: The immune system, second of two parts, N Engl J Med 343:108, 2000.

Djamali A, Samaniego M, Muth B, et al: Medical care of kidney transplant recipients after the first posttransplant year, Clin J Am Soc Nephrol 1:623, 2006.

Euvrard S, Kanitakis J, Claudy A: Skin cancers after organ transplantation, N Engl J Med 348:1681, 2003.

Figueras J, Busquets J, Grande L, et al: The deleterious effect of donor high plasma sodium and extended preservation in liver transplantation: a multivariate analysis, Transplantation 61:410, 1996.

Fisher AJ, Donnelly SC, Pritchard G, Dark JH, Corris PA: Objective assessment of criteria for selection of donor lungs suitable for transplantation, Thorax 59:434, 2004.

Fishman JA: Infection in solid-organ transplant recipients, N Engl J Med 357:2601, 2007.

Fung JJ: Tacrolimus and transplantation: a decade in review, Transplantation 77:S41, 2004.

Gouarin S, Vabret A, Scieux C, et al: Multicentric evaluation of a new commercial cytomegalovirus real time PCR quantitation assay, J Virol Methods 146:147, 2007.

Halloran PF: Immunosuppressive drugs for kidney transplantation, N Engl J Med 351:2715, 2004.

Han MK, Hyzy R: Advances in critical care management of hepatic failure and insufficiency, Crit Care Med 34:(suppl 9), 2006.

Heeger PS: T-cell allorecognition and transplant rejection: a summary and update, Am J Transplant 3:525, 2003.

Heidelbaugh JJ, Sherbondy MA: Cirrhosis and chronic liver failure, Part II: Complications and treatment, Am Fam Physician 74:767, 2004.

Holt DW, Armstrong L, Griesmacher A, et al: International Federation of Clinical Chemistry/International Association of Therapeutic Drug Monitoring and Clinical Toxicology Working Group on Immunosuppressive Drug Monitoring, Ther Drug Monit 24:59, 2002.

Humar A, Michaels M: American Society of Transplantation recommendations for screening, monitoring and reporting of infectious complications in immunosuppression trials in recipients of organ transplantation, Am J Transplant 6:262, 2006.

Ingi L, Barton TD: Viral respiratory tract infections in transplant patients: epidemiology, recognition and management, Drugs 67:1411, 2007.

Israeli M, Yussim A, Mor, E, et al: Preceding the rejection: in search for a comprehensive post-transplant immune monitoring platform, Transplant Immunol 18:7, 2007.

Iwasaki K: Metabolism of tacrolimus and recent topics in clinical pharmacokinetics, Drug Metab Pharmacokinet 22:328, 2007.

Josephson MA, Gillen D, Javaid B, et al: Treatment of renal allograft polyoma BK virus infection with leflunomide, Transplantation 81:704, 2006.

Kerman RH: Understanding the sensitized patient, Heart Fail Clin 3:1, 2007.

Kirk AD: Induction immunosuppression, Transplantation 82:593, 2006.

Klein J, Sato A: The HLA system, first of two parts, N Engl J Med 343:702, 2000.

Klein J, Sato A: The HLA system, second of two parts, N Engl J Med 343:782, 2000.

Kutsogiannis DJ, Pagliarello G, Doig C, et al: Medical management to optimize donor organ potential: review of the literature, Can J Anesthesiol 53:820, 2006.

Mai ML: The long-term management of pancreas transplantation, Transplantation 82:991, 2006.

McKay DB, Josephson MA: Pregnancy in recipients of solid organs—effects on mother and child, N Engl J Med 354:1281, 2006.

Mehra MR, Uber PA: Genomic biomarkers and heart transplantation, Heart Fail Clin 3:83, 2007.

Miró JM, Laguno M, Moreno A, et al: Management of end stage liver disease (ESLD): what is the current role of orthotopic liver transplantation (OLT)? J Hepatol 44:S140, 2006.

Morris PJ, Russell NK: Alemtuzumab (Campath-1H): a systematic review in organ transplantation, Transplantation 81:1361, 2006.

Morris RG: Immunosuppressant drug monitoring: is the laboratory meeting clinical expectations? Ann Pharmacother 39:119, 2005.

Morris RG, Holt DW, Armstrong VW, et al: Analytic aspects of cyclosporine monitoring on behalf of the IFCC/IATDMCT Joint Working Group, Ther Drug Monit 26:227, 2004.

Mueller AR, Platz KP, Kremer B: Early postoperative complications following liver transplantation, Best Pract Res Clin Gastroenterol 18:881, 2004.

Nashan B: Antibody induction therapy in renal transplant patients receiving calcineurin-inhibitor immunosuppressive regimens, Biodrugs 19:39, 2005.

Ojo A: Cardiovascular complications after renal transplantation and their prevention, Transplantation 82:5, 2006.

Pascual J, Quereda C, Zamora J, et al: Steroid withdrawal in renal transplant patients on triple therapy with a calcineurin inhibitor and mycophenolate mofetil: a meta-analysis of randomized, controlled trials, Transplantation 78:1548, 2004.

Pascual M, Theruvath T, Kawai T, et al: Strategies to improve long-term outcomes after renal transplantation, N Engl J Med 346:580, 2002.

Pei R, Lee J, Chen T, et al: Flow cytometric detection of HLA antibodies using a spectrum of microbeads, Hum Immunol 60:1293, 1999.

Pei R, Lee JH, Shih NJ, Chen M, Terasaki PI: Single human leukocyte antigen flow cytometry beads for accurate identification of human leukocyte antigen antibody specificities, Transplantation 75:43, 2003.

Pescovitz MD: Benefits of cytomegalovirus prophylaxis in solid organ transplantation, Transplantation 82:S4, 2006.

Pham MX, Deng MC, Kfoury AG, et al: Molecular testing for long-term rejection surveillance in heart transplant recipients: design of the Invasive Monitoring Attenuation through Gene Expression (IMAGE) trial, J Heart Lung Transplant 26:808, 2007.

Racusen LC, Solez K, Colvin RB, et al: The Banff 97 working classification of renal allograft pathology, Kidney Int 55:713, 1999.

Randhawa P, Brennan DC: BK virus infection in transplant recipients: an overview and update, Am J Transplant 6:2000, 2006.

Rike AH, Mogilishetty G, Alloway RR, et al: Cardiovascular risk, cardiovascular events, and metabolic syndrome in renal transplantation: comparison of early steroid withdrawal and chronic steroids, Clin Transplant 22:229, 2008.

Staes CJ, Evans RS, Rocha BH, et al: Computerized alerts improve outpatient laboratory monitoring of transplant patients, J Am Med Inform Assoc 15:324, 2008.

Terasaki PI: Humoral theory of transplantation, Am J Transplant 3:665, 2003.

Vanrenterghem YF, Claes K, Montagnino G, et al: Risk factors for cardiovascular events after successful renal transplantation, Transplantation 85:2, 2008.

Vincenti F: A decade of progress in kidney transplantation, Transplantation 77:S52, 2004.

Webster AC, Pankhurst T, Rinaldi F, et al: Monoclonal and polyclonal antibody therapy for treating acute rejection in kidney transplant recipients: a systematic review of randomized trial data, Transplantation 81:(7), 2006.

White DA: *Aspergillus* pulmonary infections in transplant recipients, Clin Chest Med 26:661, 2005.

Wilkinson A, Davidson J, Dotta F, et al: Guidelines for the treatment and management of new-onset diabetes after transplantation, Clin Transplant 19:291, 2005.

Williams R: Global challenges in liver disease, Hepatology 44:521, 2006.

Wood KE, Coursin DB: Intensivists and organ donor management, Curr Opin Anaesthesiol 20:97, 2007.

Yang Z, Wang S: Recent development in application of HPLC-tandem MS in therapeutic drug monitoring of immunosuppressants, J Immunol Methods 336:98, 2003.

Young CJ, Gaston RS: Renal transplantation in black Americans, N Engl J Med 343:1545, 2003.

Zaroff JG, Rosengard BR, Armstrong WF, et al: Consensus conference report: maximizing use of organs recovered from the cadaver donor: cardiac recommendations, March 28-29, 2001, Crystal City, Va, Circulation 106:836, 2002.

INTERNET SITES

http://tpis.upmc.com/TPIShome/—Transplant Pathology Internet Services

http://www.cdc.gov/mmwr/preview/mmwrhtml/rr4910a1.htm—CDC guidelines for immunosuppressed individuals

www.ustransplant.org

www.optn.transplant.hrsa.gov—Location of annual reports prepared by the Scientific Registry of Transplant Recipients (SRTR) in collaboration with the Organ Procurement and Transplantation Network (OPTN) under contract with the Health Resources and Services Administration (HRSA)

An annual publication entitled, *2007 SRTR Report on the State of Transplantation,* is available in the *American Journal of Transplantation,* Issue 4(Part 2):909-1026, 2008.

Toxicology

55 Chapter

Catherine A. Hammett-Stabler

Chapter Outline

Introduction to Toxicology
The Potential for Toxicity
The Dose Makes the Poison
Physical Characteristics of a Toxin
Stereochemistry and Chiral Pharmacology
Mochanisms of Organ Toxicity
Exposure, Kinetics, and Genes
Routes of Exposure
Duration and Frequency of Exposure
Toxicokinetics and Toxicogenetics
Interactions Between Toxins
Toxicology in the Clinical Setting
The Toxicology Laboratory
Choosing Samples and Methods
Medicolegal Challenges
Biological and Chemical Agents of Mass Destruction
The Toxicity of Natural Products
Key Toxins Encountered in the Laboratory
Analgesics
Drugs of Abuse
Amphetamines
Barbiturates
Benzodiazepines
Cannabinoids
Cocaine
Opioids
Phencyclidine
Club Drugs
Gases
Metals
Pesticides
Volatiles

Key Terms

abused drugs Potentially addictive compounds such as alcohol, cocaine, and marijuana that are taken to stimulate or induce pleasure.

acute toxicity The rapid onset (in seconds, minutes, hours) of a harmful effect following exposure to a toxic agent.

analgesics A class of drugs that reduce pain.

antidepressants A class of drugs that alleviate depression.

antidote Any agent that counteracts the effects of a poison.

antipyretic A class of drugs used to reduce fever.

benzodiazepines A group of antianxiety/sedative drugs.

biotransformation The biochemical modification of chemicals as they pass through the body.

chiral drugs Drugs (stereochemical isomers) with four different chemical groups attached to a carbon atom, resulting in nonsuperimposable structures. (The term *chiral* is based on the Greek word for "hand.")

chronic toxicity The appearance of harmful effects weeks, months, or years after exposure or repeated exposure to a toxic material.

club drugs Drugs made popular by their use in the club scene; examples include 3,4-methylenedioxymethamphetamine (MDMA) and gamma hydroxybutyrate.

cutoff concentration The administratively chosen concentration used to determine whether a drug test result is positive or negative. Results equal to or greater than the cutoff concentration are reported as positive. Results less than this concentration are reported as negative.

cytochrome P-450 isoenzymes A superfamily of enzymes responsible for much of drug and toxin biotransformation, usually by oxidation.

dose The amount of a substance given to a patient or received internally into the body.

drug confirmation The process of verifying the identity of a drug or a drug metabolite through the use of a second test method with greater sensitivity and specificity than the first (see **drug screen** and **screening**).

drug interaction The ability of one drug to change the effect of another drug by altering its metabolic fate or by enhancing or opposing its activity at the site of action.

drug screen A test that qualitatively identifies the presence of one or more drugs or classes of drugs.

enantiomers Stereochemical isomers of a compound that are precise mirror images of each other. These isomers demonstrate the ability to rotate polarized light in opposite, but equal, directions.

forensic toxicology Branch of the discipline of toxicology that is concerned with the medical and legal aspects of the harmful effects of chemicals or poisons.

hypnotics A class of drugs often used as sedatives.

LD_{50} The amount of a substance that will cause death in half the animal population tested.

lethal dose The amount of a substance that will cause death after exposure.

opiates or **opioids** A class of drugs with chemical structures similar to those of heroin and morphine. Synthetic opioids include meperidine, oxycodone, and others.

schedule of drug classification Classification scheme used to group drugs according to their potential for abuse. Drugs classified as Schedule I have a very high potential for abuse and no recognized medical use; those classified as Schedule V have a low potential for abuse and are used medically.

screening test A rapid test used to separate samples into those considered presumptively positive for specified drugs and those considered negative.

sympathomimetic amines Drugs that act on the adrenergic nervous system.

therapeutic dose The amount of a substance that will produce a desired pharmacological effect.

toxicant or **poison** A substance that, when taken in sufficient quantity, will cause sickness or death.

toxicogenetics The study of the genetic control of processes involved in the detoxification of poisonous substances (similar to pharmacogenetics).

toxicokinetics The quantitative study of a toxicant's disposition in the body of an affected person over time (similar to pharmacokinetics).

toxicology The study of the adverse effects of chemicals or physical agents on living organisms.

window of detection The period during which a toxin or its metabolites can be detected in a given sample. The term is commonly used to designate the length of time over which a drug of abuse (or the primary metabolite) can be detected in urine.

Methods on Evolve

Acetaminophen
Alcohol
Barbiturates
Benzodiazepines
Drug screen
Ethylene glycol
Lead
Opiates
Salicylates

SECTION OBJECTIVES BOX 55-1

- Define *toxicology.*
- List and explain the specialized branches of toxicology.

INTRODUCTION TO TOXICOLOGY

Toxicology is perhaps the oldest of the modern disciplines of clinical chemistry. The term derives from the Latin *toxicus,* meaning "poisonous," and the Greek *toxikón,* which refers to the **poisons** into which arrows were dipped. Today, toxicology is a broad and diverse science that integrates multiple disciplines, including chemistry, biology, physiology, pathology, pharmacology, and genetics, to study the adverse effects of chemical or physical agents on living organisms.[1-4]

Toxicology has evolved to include a number of specialized, yet overlapping, branches, such as clinical, forensic, environmental, and occupational toxicology. Clinical toxicology focuses on pathological processes that are caused by exposure of a patient to a toxin and includes subsequent medical evaluation and treatment of the patient. Substances encountered range from illicit street drugs to therapeutic drugs to household products to plants and animal-derived substances.[1] At the heart of **forensic toxicology** is its application to the legal system. This area has expanded from investigations of cause of death and criminal investigations to include probation- and parole-related testing, workplace drug testing, and performance (athletic) testing. Since the enactment of state and federal laws to deter drug use in the workplace, many clinical laboratories have expanded their services to include some forensic toxicology by performing workplace drug testing. Workplace drug testing overlaps into occupational toxicology, the discipline concerned with the effects of chemicals encountered in the home and workplace, as safety and accident prevention are major concerns of this branch of toxicology. Environmental toxicologists study chemicals found in the atmosphere, soil, water, or food chain, and the effects of these chemicals on living organisms. Their work includes chemicals that are natural to the environment such as heavy metals or bacteria, as well as those released by man and other species.

As we will see, everything has the potential to be toxic, and this means that other disciplines may cross into toxicology. Consider the patient who is undergoing treatment for an arrhythmia who receives too much of a drug intended to treat his clinical symptoms. Laboratory testing that is begun for the purpose of therapeutic drug monitoring or assessment of electrolyte status may turn into a clinical toxicology investigation. Furthermore, if this investigation determines that the patient was given excessive drug by an individual who intended to inflict harm, a legal investigation could very well ensue, and the case could enter the arena of forensic toxicology.

KEY CONCEPTS BOX 55-1

- Toxicology is the study of the effects of chemicals or physical agents on living organisms.
- The major branches of the science of toxicology include clinical, forensic, environmental, and occupational toxicology.

SECTION OBJECTIVES BOX 55-2

- Define *toxicity* and LD_{50}.
- Describe how physical and chemical factors can influence toxicity.
- List and differentiate the different types of diffusion across cell membranes.
- Discuss the biological and laboratory impact of stereochemistry.
- Explain the mechanisms by which toxins affect body organs.
- Describe the factors that determine the reasons why an organ may be susceptible to a toxin.

THE POTENTIAL FOR TOXICITY

The Dose Makes the Poison

Toxicologists often compare chemicals in terms of their potential to cause harm to a living organism.[5-7] One often used comparison involves documenting the frequency with which an adverse response, such as hepatotoxicity or cardiac arrhythmia, is observed in a population exposed to increasing **doses** of a toxin (Fig. 55-1). Because most chemicals elicit multiple adverse responses, it is important that response(s) that are studied or reported are defined clearly.

For every chemical tested, there should always be a dose below which the toxin does not cause harm. This point, known as the threshold dose, implies that there is a safe level of exposure below this dose for every chemical.[5-7] Above this dose, the defined effect will be observed with increasing frequency of toxicity. This important toxicological concept was stated first by Paracelsus (c. 1493-1541) as "All substances are poisons; there is none which is not a poison. It is the dose that makes a thing not a poison."

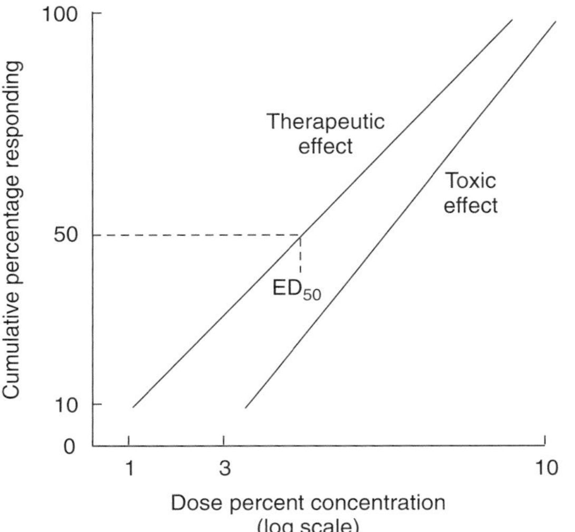

Fig. 55-1 Dose-response curve. Results of therapeutic and toxic effects on a population. ED_{50}, Effective dose for 50% of the population.

The concepts of dose and response can be examined by considering two vastly different chemicals, sarin and water, and their ability to cause death. Sarin, a nerve agent, is recognized as one of the most potent, deadly poisons. But even this highly dangerous poison has been shown to have a concentration or dose below which one can be exposed without significant initial consequences.[7,8] Several terrorist attacks were documented during the 1990s in which gas was released without resulting in numerous deaths. In these cases, wind and other conditions fortunately dispersed and diluted the dose before anyone was harmed.[7,8] Follow-up studies of the victims of these attacks have revealed that some individuals have developed neurological symptoms since the time of exposure. Additional studies are under way to determine whether there is a relationship between low-dose exposure and subsequent symptoms.[9]

Very few would consider water to be a dangerous toxin; in fact, we all would agree that water is necessary to sustain life. Yet numerous cases have been reported in which ingestion of large amounts of water over a short time caused an incapacitating electrolyte imbalance and death.[10] Although exposure to these two diverse chemicals is an extreme example, its purpose is to emphasize that one must define the toxic response, the importance of the dose in acute responses, and the need to consider additional aspects of toxicity such as long-term sequelae.

Death is clearly the most serious harmful effect inflicted by a toxin. For this reason, toxicologists often measure a chemical's potential for toxicity by determining the median **lethal dose,** or $\mathbf{LD_{50}}$ (Table 55-1). This parameter, which represents

Table 55-1 Approximate LD_{50} of Selected Chemicals

LD_{50}, mg/kg	Chemical	Species (Route)
190,000	Water	Mouse (intraperitoneal injection)
29,700	Sucrose	Rat (oral)
14,200	Saccharin	Rat (oral)
11,900	Ascorbic acid	Rat (oral)
7000	Niacin	Rat (oral)
5000	Cimetidine	Rat (oral)
4700	Ethylene glycol	Rat (oral)
3000	Sodium chloride	Rat (oral)
1489	Cyclosporine	Rat (oral)
290	Malathion	Rat (oral)
192	Caffeine	Rat (oral)
51	Nicotine	Rat (oral)
24	Sarin	Human (percutaneous)
20	Arsenic trioxide	Rat (oral)
6.4	Sodium cyanide	Rat (oral)
1.4	Arsenic trioxide	Human (oral)
0.65	Aldicarb	Rat (oral)
0.42	Sarin	Mouse (percutaneous)
0.14	VX (nerve agent)	Human (percutaneous)

LD_{50}, Amount of a substance that will cause death in half the animal population tested.

the dose that causes death to 50% of the population studied, usually is determined in nonhuman models. Data gathered in these studies then are extrapolated to estimate an equivalent dose for humans. In some cases, the human LD_{50} has been verified through documented reports of exposure.

Toxicity studies may be limited in that test species may be more, or less, sensitive to a toxin than humans, or they may exhibit different responses. Perhaps more important, these experiments often are designed to assess acute effects from a single exposure, which may differ considerably from chronic toxicities that result from low-dose, long-term exposure. Despite these limitations, grouping compounds by a clearly defined adverse effect is a useful means of comparing the relative amounts or doses required to cause harm.

Physical Characteristics of a Toxin

A compound's potential for toxicity is highly dependent on the physical state of the compound. Vapors and gases are absorbed quickly via the lungs after inhalation, and liquids must be absorbed through the skin or gastrointestinal tract, or injected. Usually, solids must be ingested and dissolved before they produce an effect. A few compounds, such as mercury, exist in a liquid form but appear in a significant gaseous phase under normal atmospheric conditions. With these, a sufficient amount of the compound may be present in the gaseous phase to induce toxicity through inhalation of the vapor.

Any compound absorbed by the lungs, skin, or GI tract must cross cellular membranes to reach the circulation. An exception to this is those liquids that are injected intravenously. Once in the systemic circulation, a compound may need to enter a cell to exert its effect. Three basic mechanisms are available for crossing body or cell membranes: passive diffusion, active transport, or facilitated transport. Passive diffusion, the primary means by which most drugs and toxins cross membranes, does not require the expenditure of energy; compounds diffuse from an area of high concentration to an area of low concentration. Active transport requires the use of energy because it often moves the toxin across a membrane against a concentration gradient, often with the use of a carrier protein. Facilitated transport also uses a carrier protein that typically is embedded within the membrane lipid bilayer, but it does not require the expenditure of energy. Occasionally, toxins are transported via pinocytosis or phagocytosis, two additional mechanisms that play relatively minor roles in membrane transport.

How readily a molecule moves across the membrane depends on its molecular size, pK_a (degree of ionization), and lipid solubility. Compounds in the ionized form and those that exhibit greater solubility in water do not move very readily across lipid membranes. A toxin that becomes ionized under the conditions of a given body compartment very well may be trapped at that site.

Stereochemistry and Chiral Pharmacology

A number of chemicals and drugs are identical in terms of atomic makeup but differ in the three-dimensional arrangement of their atoms around a *chiral* center (Fig. 55-2). Such compounds are known as stereoisomers. Pairs of stereoisomers that are mirror images of each other are known as **enantiomers.** Although these chemically identical compounds have the same physiochemical properties (melting point, solubility, etc.), they may not be recognized equally in biological systems, because receptors, proteins, and enzymes recognize the specific three-dimensional orientation of each specific chemical group. This means that each stereoisomer may exhibit a different pharmacological action or toxicity (Table 55-2).[11]

Such differences between sterioisomers are illustrated nicely by the properties of methamphetamine. The levo-rotary form of this drug is used as a nasal decongestant, whereas its isomer, D-methamphetamine, is an illegal drug with considerable abuse potential. Both compounds have the same chemical structure, but they clearly exhibit very different pharmacological activities! Many prescribed drugs (see Table 55-2) are found as mixtures (racemic) of both enantiomers. In some cases, each isomer exhibits desired activities; therefore, mixtures may be desirable or advantageous. Stereospecific chromatographic and electrophoretic techniques are used to distinguish between these types of compounds.

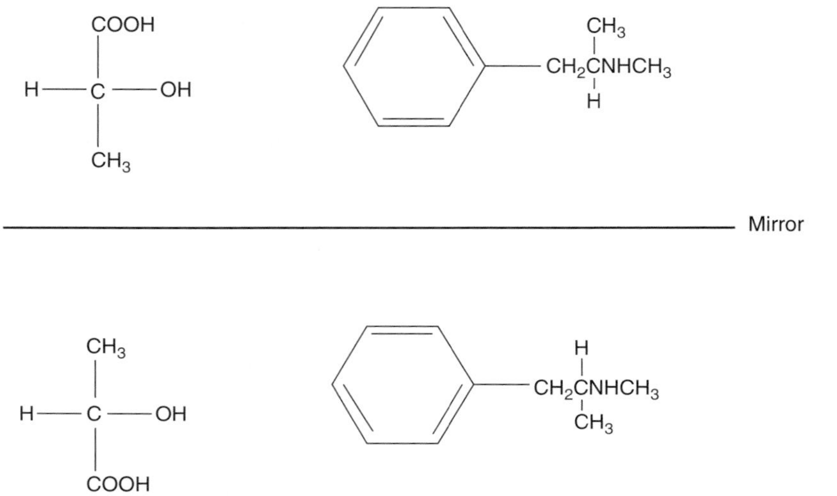

COOH
H—C—OH
CH_3
CH_3 | CH_2CNHCH_3 | H
Mirror
CH_3
H—C—OH
COOH
H | CH_2CNHCH_3 | CH_3

Fig. 55-2 Stereochemistry: enantiomers. The enantiomeric pairs for lactic acid and methamphetamine are shown. When solutions of these are placed in plane polarized light, the *d* or (+) forms rotate the light to the right, whereas the *l* or (–) forms rotate the light to the left.

Table 55-2 Comparison of Pharmacological and Toxicological Differences Between Enantiomeric Pairs

Compound	Properties of *l*-Form	Properties of *d*-Form
Carnitine	—	Produces symptoms of myasthenia gravis
Dopa	Anti-Parkinson's activity	Induces granulocytopenia
Ephedrine (pseudoephedrine)	Decongestant, bronchodilator, pressor activity, naturally occurring as ephedra in plants (ma huang)	Decongestant, bronchodilator (pseudoephedrine)
Fenfluramine	Does not suppress appetite	Appetite suppression (dexfenfluramine)
Methamphetamine	Decongestant	CNS stimulation
Norepinephrine	Increases blood pressure	Less pressor activity
3-Methoxy-*N*-methylmorphinan	Narcotic activity (levomethorphan)	Cough suppression (dextromethorphan)
3-Hydroxy-*N*-methylmorphinan	Narcotic activity (levorphanol)	Minimal narcotic activity (dextromethorphan)
Sotalol	β-Blocker	Class III antiarrhythmic

CNS, Central nervous system.

Mechanisms of Organ Toxicity

The type of organ damage observed is related to the molecular actions of the toxin. Toxins that behave as corrosives or caustics can cause outright tissue injury and destruction, whereas the effects of others are subtle. In numerous cases, the chemical substitutes itself as a substrate for an enzyme that is needed for basic cellular function, as is the case with organophosphate pesticides. Irreversible binding of these chemicals to cholinesterases prevents the enzyme from hydrolyzing acetylcholine released from nerve endings. Acetylcholine then accumulates in nerve cells and overstimulates specific receptors throughout the central and peripheral nervous system. Cyanide exerts its toxic effects by interrupting electron transport in the mitochondrial cytochrome chain. When cyanide binds to the heme group of the final cytochrome in the pathway, the heme molecule is unable to bind oxygen. Electron transfer to molecular oxygen is blocked and cell death occurs. Arsenates and some herbicides act by blocking oxidative phosphorylation. These agents allow electron transport to take place but prevent phosphorylation of adenosine diphosphate (ADP) to adenosine triphosphate (ATP). This action increases oxygen consumption, causing heat production and hyperthermia.

When the action of a toxin involves its reaction with the genetic material within the cell, the DNA or RNA for example, the chemical is classified as a genetic toxin. Depending on the mechanism involved and the outcome, the chemical may be classified further as a carcinogen, mutagen, or teratogen. Chemical carcinogens are those toxins found to promote cancer within a living organism, whereas mutagens and teratogens induce genetic changes that become inheritable (see Chapters 52 and 53). The relationship between the occurrence of specific types of cancer and occupational exposure to a chemical was first observed in the mid-1700s. Shortly after Hill reported an increased incidence of nasal cancer among snuff users, Sir Percival Pott correlated an increased incidence in scrotal cancer among chimney sweeps.[12] Today, we know that in both cases, polycyclic aromatic hydrocarbon products, such as benzo(a)pyrene, are the responsible carcinogens.

The vast blood supply of the liver makes it particularly vulnerable to chemically induced toxic injury.[13] Between 10% and 15% of the total blood supply of the body is estimated to circulate through the liver at any one time. It is simply difficult for the organ to avoid exposure to a circulating toxin. Hepatic injury takes many forms, ranging from cellular degeneration and necrosis to cirrhosis or cholestasis to vascular injury. Also because of the unique morphology of the organ, the location(s) of toxic injury may range from particularly focused areas to sites scattered throughout the organ to the most serious situation, in which the entire organ shows damage. Not all hepatocellular toxicity leads to cell death. In fact, cells may exhibit a variety of significant morphological changes and yet survive. Fortunately, the organ is highly resilient to toxic insult.[13]

Because the kidneys have a rich blood supply, they too are susceptible to injury.[14] Another contributing factor has been identified in the kidney's concentrating properties. Many of the concentrated substances accumulate in the tubular cells, where they cause damage. Although the kidney is by no means as actively involved in drug/toxin metabolism as is the liver, some areas of the kidneys are rich in enzymes involved in detoxification. For example, a significant amount of CYP450 activity is seen in the proximal tubule, one of the sites particularly susceptible to injury.[14]

Pulmonary damage can occur as **toxicants** are inhaled, or as chemicals are circulated through the lung. Types of pulmonary injury include irritation, fibrosis, and destruction of gas-exchanging surfaces (emphysema). As with other organs, some metabolism takes place in the lungs, particularly in the Clara cells of the terminal bronchioles.[15]

Neurotoxicity can be a slow, insidious process or a dramatic one.[8,16,17] At the molecular level, a chemical may interfere with the synthesis of neurotransmitters. The effect of one chemical may lead to an increase in neurotransmitters, while another chemical may inhibit their production or release. Alternatively, a chemical might alter the flow of sodium, potassium, or calcium across ion channels in membranes, thus disrupting transmission of nerve impulses. In other cases, intermediates in signal transduction pathways such as protein kinases and nitric oxide may be affected adversely. With chronic exposure, it may be difficult to determine whether the symptoms are related to toxicity or whether they indicate the presence of a neurodegenerative disease such as Parkinson's or Alzheimer's.[16-18]

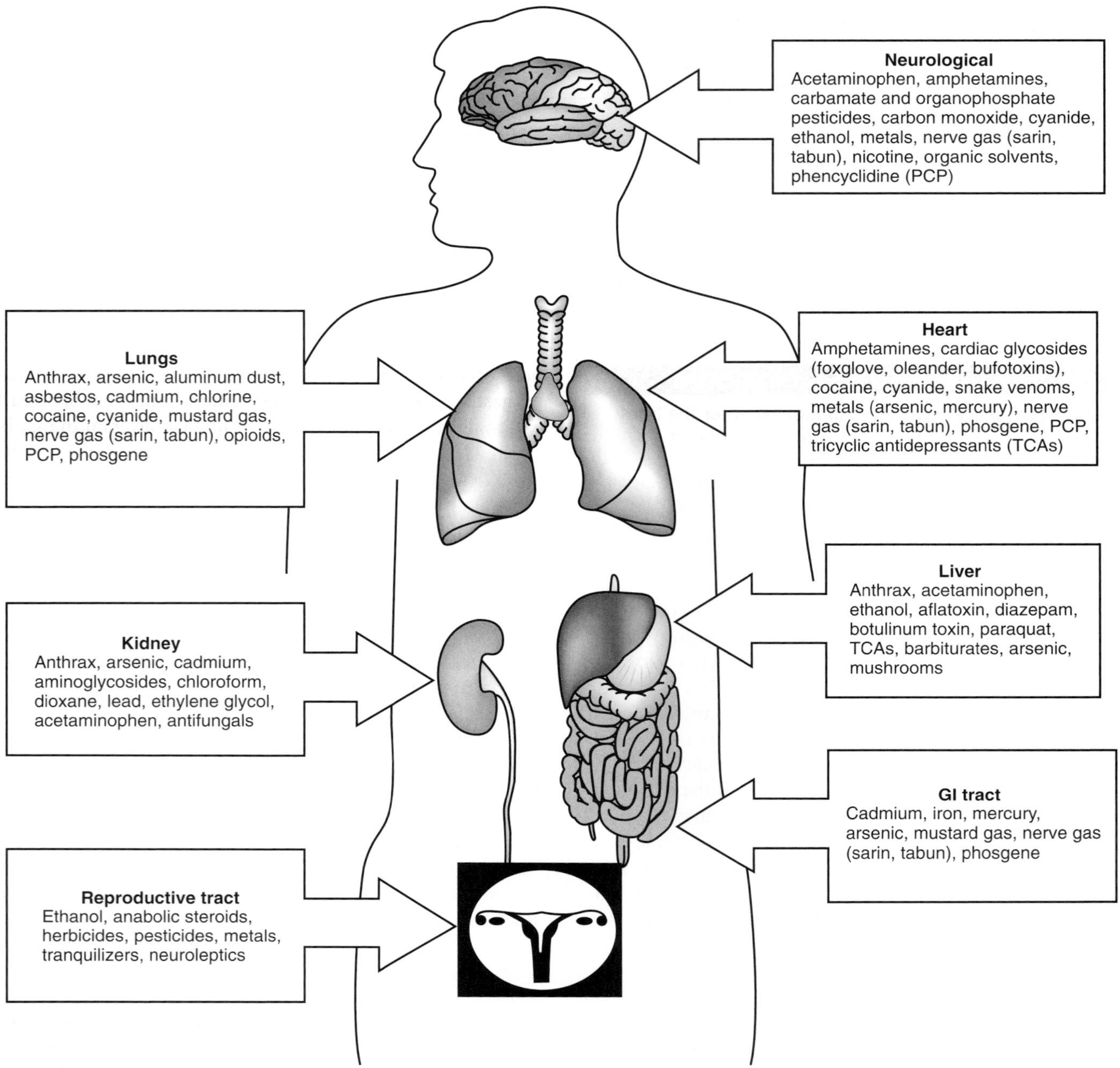

Fig. 55-3 Site of toxicity for various agents.

Because of the complex physiological interactions on which reproduction depends, all steps of reproduction, including ovum and sperm production, fetal organ development and growth, parturition, and lactation, are susceptible to toxins. Exposure of pregnant women to toxins often occurs through the workplace, and so this is an area of focus for many environmental and occupational toxicologists.[17,19,20]

In summary, it is not unusual to find several mechanisms involved in the overall toxicity of a single compound; as a result, several organ systems may be affected adversely (Fig. 55-3). For some toxins, the type of injury is distinctive, that is, microscopic examination of affected tissue obtained by biopsy often will facilitate the identification, or exclusion, of a toxin.

KEY CONCEPTS BOX 55-2

- Degree of toxicity is defined by the frequency of a defined adverse effect in an exposed population.
- LD_{50} is a parameter that describes the dose that causes death to 50% of the population studied.
- Everything is potentially toxic; toxicity depends on the time and dose of exposure.
- The physical state of a toxin—gas, liquid, or solid—and its chemical state—charged, uncharged, lipid soluble—can affect its ease of entry into the body and into cells.
- Ionized toxins cannot move across membranes and may be trapped in the compartment in which they become charged.
- Stereoisomers may differ in terms of pharmacological activity and toxicity.

Table 55-3 Relationship Between Route of Exposure and LD_{50}, mg/kg

	CHEMICAL		
Route of Exposure	Ethanol	Caffeine	Diphenhydramine
Oral	7060	224	114
Subcutaneous	6000	275	99
Intramuscular	—	200	60
Intravenous	1440	58	20
Dermal	20,000	—	60

LD_{50}, Amount of a substance that will cause death in half the animal population tested.

SECTION OBJECTIVES BOX 55-3

- List three routes through which toxins enter the body.
- Describe the relationship between frequency of exposure to a potential toxin and toxicity.
- Describe how pharmacokinetic processes can change with overdose and toxicity.
- Define the terms *pharmacokinetics* and *toxicogenetics.*
- Describe the role of metabolism in toxicity.

EXPOSURES, KINETICS, AND GENES

Routes of Exposure

How a toxin enters the body plays a significant role in the magnitude and speed with which an adverse effect is observed (Table 55-3). The route of exposure also influences how the body metabolizes and eliminates the toxin, in other words, its pharmacokinetics or **toxicokinetics** (see Chapter 14). Most toxins enter the body via the skin, the lungs, and the gastrointestinal tract, but they may be injected or may enter through other routes, such as the eyes, mucous membranes, or rectum. The skin is the most readily accessible organ simply because of its large surface area. Fortunately, it also serves as an efficient barrier, minimizing or even preventing exposure to many toxins. A rapid adverse reaction will be observed when a toxin enters the body through a route that is in direct contact with the toxin's primary target; symptoms may be delayed or even less intense for another toxin that enters through a more remote site.

Cocaine is often used to demonstrate these concepts. When the drug is ingested by insufflation (snorting) or smoking, rapid absorption and distribution produce an intense but brief "high" (euphoria) as the drug reaches receptors in the central nervous system. In contrast, when the drug is applied to the skin of a patient in the medical setting, the patient loses sensation at the administration site but does not experience the "high" sought by those who use the drug illegally. Similarly, individuals who are exposed to low doses of cocaine when drinking coca tea do not experience the euphoria as well.

Duration and Frequency of Exposure

The length of time over which drug exposure occurs and the frequency of exposure (toal dosage) determine the onset and severity of symptoms observed for many toxins.[5,8,18] This relationship between dose and time gives rise to two different types of toxicity: **acute toxicity** and **chronic toxicity.** Acute toxicity refers to the ability of a chemical, above a threshold dose, to cause harm as a result of a one-time exposure; chronic toxicity represents the situation in which the exposure occurs repeatedly over a period of time, frequently at a dose less than that necessary to cause an acute response. Chronic exposure is of greatest concern for those chemicals that are metabolized slowly or are deposited in storage tissues such as bone or fat. In these circumstances, slow accumulation of the toxin occurs over time, and the effects may be apparent only after months or years of exposure. Chronic toxicity cannot be predicted from the responses observed after acute toxicity, and it may in fact affect different organ systems.[18] Acute exposure to a high dose of arsenic ingested accidentally will produce symptoms of gastric distress, respiratory failure, and possibly death within hours to days. On the other hand, a silversmith may be exposed to low doses of arsenic over many years before exhibiting neurological symptoms.[18] The severity of symptoms varies, depending on the agent ingested and the individual's ability to metabolize and excrete the agent. Occasionally, patients experience a delayed hypersensitivity reaction. In these cases, the patient experiences a severe anaphylactic reaction when exposed to a substance, often at a dose normally considered nontoxic. Typically, the patient has been previously exposed to that substance, or something very similar, and has been pre-sensitized.

Toxicokinetics and Toxicogenetics

Pharmacokinetics describes how an individual might process and eliminate a toxic compound (see Chapter 14). For many drugs and chemicals, pharmacokinetic parameters are well defined for the general population. Such data, for example, half-life, volume of distribution, and clearance rates, are useful when the clinician is treating and monitoring patients, provided one remembers two caveats: Pharmacokinetic processes change throughout life, and may change significantly with toxicity. The first caveat explains why newborns and older adults generally are more susceptible to some toxicities.[21] Both of these populations metabolize and clear toxins at a slower rate compared with children and younger adults. Typically, the liver function of the newborn does not reach maturity for several months, after which metabolism and the ability to detoxify may actually exceed those of most healthy adults. In contrast, metabolic and excretion rates begin to decline after the fourth decade of life. Elimination of a drug from a patient in his 80s may be one-half to one-third as rapid as that from a 20-year-old.

Second, in a toxicological situation, the toxic actions of chemicals within a given organ system may cause one or more observed pharmacokinetic processes to be significantly different from those observed in a therapeutic setting. One toxin may delay gastric emptying while another may induce diuresis, such that the known pharmacokinetics of absorption and excretion will not apply. In many cases, the high concentration of a toxin saturates or overwhelms binding proteins, resulting in an increase in the amount of free drug available to act at various target tissues.

Table 55-4 Common Drugs and Toxins Metabolized Via the Cytochrome P-450 Isoenzymes

Cytochrome P450 Enzyme	Drug/Toxin Substrate Metabolized	Inhibitors	Inducers
CYP1A2	Amitriptyline, caffeine, clozapine, haloperidol, imipramine, MDMA, naproxen, phenacetin, phencyclidine, propranolol, theophylline, warfarin	Amiodarone, cimetidine, ciprofloxacin	Tobacco
CYP1B1	Tobacco carcinogens (lung)		
CYP2A6	Nicotine, nitrosamines, aflatoxin		
CYP2C9	Amitriptyline, celecoxib, ibuprofen, naproxen, phenytoin, tolbutamide, warfarin	Amiodarone, fluconazole, fluvastatin, isoniazid phenylbutazone	Rifampin, econazole
CYP2C19	Amitriptyline, diazepam, haloperidol, imipramine, nicotine, omeprazole, phenytoin	Cimetidine, felbamate, indomethacin, ketoconazole	Prednisone
CYP2D6	Amitriptyline, amphetamine, codeine, desipramine, dextromethorphan, haloperidol, heroin, imipramine, methadone, methamphetamine, MDMA, *p*-methoxyamphetamine, nortriptyline, oxycodone, propranolol	Celecoxib, chlorpheniramine, cimetidine, clomiprimine, cocaine, methadone, pentazocine	Amitriptyline, desipramine, imipramine, nortriptyline
CYP2E1	Acetaminophen, caffeine, ethanol, felbamate, fluoxetine, halogenated anesthetics (halothane, isoflurane), halogenated hydrocarbons, isoniazid, methanol, nitrosoamines, propranolol, pyrazole, theophylline	Disulfiram, fluoxetine	Ethanol, isoniazid
CYP3A	Carbamazepine, cocaine, cyclosporine, MDMA, phencyclidine, tacrolimus	Midazolam, erythromycin, methadone	Phenobarbital, dexamethasone

Cytochrome P-450 Drug Interaction Table (http://medicine.iupui.edu/flockhart); Tanaka E, Terada M, Misawa S: Cytochrome P-450 2E1: its clinical and toxicological role, J Clin Pharm Ther 25:165, 2000.
MDMA, 3,4-Methylenedioxymethamphetamine.

Metabolism typically is thought of as the body's primary detoxification mechanism. Although this is true in most cases, several drugs or chemicals are not particularly toxic themselves but are metabolized to compounds (metabolites) that are toxic. In these situations, preventing the formation of toxic metabolite becomes an important part of treatment. This is why patients who ingest ethylene glycol are treated with ethanol or fomepizole. Hepatic alcohol dehydrogenase metabolizes not only ethanol but other alcohol-containing compounds as well. When the ethylene glycol–poisoned patient is given an intravenous dose of ethanol, the two drugs compete for enzymatic metabolism. The enzyme has greater affinity for ethanol and metabolizes it in preference to ethylene glycol. Alternatively, the patient may be treated with fomepizole, a drug that inhibits alcohol dehydrogenase activity. In either case, the patient no longer metabolizes ethylene glycol to its toxic metabolites. The ethylene glycol eventually is excreted by the kidneys.

Similar to the role that genetics plays in an individual's response to a drug used for therapeutic purposes, genetic differences explain some of the different responses observed among individuals exposed to the same toxin at the same dose under the same conditions.[22-24] The toxicologist also must consider situations in which a toxin alters its own metabolism or the metabolism of another compound.[22,23,25] Table 55-4 describes some of the toxins commonly encountered in the clinical laboratory and their relations to various metabolic enzymes; Table 55-5 lists some of the genetic factors that can affect an individual's response to a toxin.

The use of known pharmacokinetic data often is complicated by the fact that the exact chemical, dose, or time of exposure may be unknown, and few poisons are "pure."[26] Household products, cosmetics, pharmaceutical preparations, and street drugs all contain impurities or contaminants. In some cases, the "primary" compound of exposure is not toxic, but the chemicals added as solvents, preservatives, or buffers are toxic. Furthermore, reported toxic exposures typically involve more than one agent.

Interactions Between Toxins

When an individual is exposed to more than one chemical, each chemical may affect the action, metabolism, or clearance of the other. When drugs are involved, this phenomenon is called **drug interaction.** In one case, a drug may inhibit the activity of an enzyme involved in the metabolism of another drug. In another case, two drugs or chemicals may compete for protein binding or for excretion, with one drug or chemical more efficiently metabolized, more tightly bound to the protein, or more rapidly excreted than the other. This may result in different toxicities for both drugs. Drug or chemical interactions may be more intense in patients who are affected by chronic or acute pathological processes that influence metabolism and excretion, such as congestive heart failure, renal disease, and cirrhosis.[19,25]

Table 55-5 Genes and Their Protein Products Responsible for Increased Toxicity

Increased Susceptibility to	Gene	Protein	Gene Locus
Opiate and opioid toxicity	*CYP2D6*	CYP2D6	22q13.1
Barbiturate toxicity	*CYP3A4*	CYP3A4	7q21-q22.1
Mephenytoin toxicity	*CYP2C19*	CYP2C19	10q24.1-q24.3
Polyaromatic hydrocarbons	*CYP1A1*	CYP1A1 (aryl hydrocarbon hydrolase)	15q22-q24
Organophosphates	*PON1*	Paroxonase	7q21.3
Isoniazid Caffeine Sulfonamides Procainamide	*NAT1* *NAT2*	*N*-Acetyltransferases	8p23.1-p21.3
Heavy metals	*SCL4A7*	Bicarbonate transporter	3p22
Heavy metals	*EPB41L1*	Ion transport protein	20q11.2-q12
Heavy metals Acetaminophen Ethanol methamphetamine	*GSTM1, GSTT1, GSTP1*	Glutathionine-S-transferases	1p13.3 22q11.2 11q13
Phenytoin	*EPHX1*	Epoxide hydrolases	1q42.1
Ethanol	*ALADH2*	Acetaldehyde dehydrogenase	12q24.2
Succinylcholine	*CHE1*	Butyrylcholinesterase	3q26.1-q26.2
Ethanol	*ALDH2*	Aldehyde dehydrogenase	12q24.2
Ethanol	*ADH*	Alcohol dehydrogenase	4
Aspirin Fava beans Primaquine	*G6PD*	Glucose-6-phosphate dehydrogenase	Xq28
Acetaminophen Lorazepam	*UGT1A1*	UDP-glucuronosyl-transferase	2q37

KEY CONCEPTS BOX 55-3

- Skin, the lungs, and the gastrointestinal tract are the most frequent routes by which a toxin can enter the body.
- The route of entry can affect the degree of toxicity.
- Severity of toxicity depends on dosage, frequency of dose, and time of exposure.
- Acute and chronic toxicities usually involve single versus chronic exposure.
- Toxins can act over very short times (acute toxicity) or gradually, over long times (chronic toxicity).
- The duration of toxic exposure, as well as the frequency of exposure, can affect the severity of the toxic response.
- Repeated, subtoxic doses of a compound can lead to chronic toxicity.
- An individual's response to a toxin varies with age, gender, and genetic factors.
- Drugs may produce toxic metabolites.
- Toxicokinetic and toxicogenetic parameters can be used to estimate the potency of a toxin.
- Pharmacokinetic parameters identified in a therapeutic setting may not apply in toxicity.
- These parameters may change with the age and health of the individual, and the circumstance of how the toxin was ingested.
- The presence of more than one toxin can enhance or dampen the toxicity of either toxin.

SECTION OBJECTIVES BOX 55-4

- Describe three clinical situations in which toxicology testing is used in patient management.
- List populations at risk for toxic exposure.
- Describe three ways of identifying the presence of toxin; describe their relative accuracy.
- Define *antidote,* and list some examples.

TOXICOLOGY IN THE CLINICAL SETTING

In the clinical setting, the most frequent use of toxicology screens involves the patient who is exhibiting changes in his or her mental status.[1,27-29] When a comatose, confused, or bizarrely acting patient is seen in an emergency setting, drug overdose is one of the possible diagnoses that must be considered by the physician. For the most efficient treatment of this patient, it is important for the physician to try to determine the nature or identity of the drug or drugs used. A history obtained from an alert patient can be helpful, although in general, the patient history is not reliable at least 50% of the time.[30] This means that observing the patient's symptoms is a key requirement for identifying various toxins.

Toxic agents can produce a myriad of symptoms, such as respiratory depression, shock, seizures, arrhythmias, hyperthermia, or hypothermia. The size of pupils, the respiration rate and heart rate, the electrocardiogram, and the condition of organ systems are important signs that can provide infor-

Table 55-6 The Most Common Toxic Syndromes

Anticholinergic Syndromes	
Common signs	Delirium with mumbling speech; tachycardia; dry, flushed skin; dilated pupils; myoclonus; slightly elevated temperature; urinary retention; and decreased bowel sounds. Seizures and dysrhythmias may occur in severe cases.
Common causes	Antihistamines, antiparkinsonian medications, atropine, scopolamine, amantadine, antipsychotic agents, antidepressant agents, antispasmodic agents, mydriatic agents, skeletal muscle relaxants, and many plants (notably Jimson weed and *Amanita muscaria*)
Sympathomimetic Syndromes	
Common signs	Delusions, paranoia, tachycardia (or bradycardia if the drug is a pure α-adrenergic agonist), hypertension, hyperpyrexia, diaphoresis, piloerection, mydriasis, and hyperreflexia. Seizures, hypotension, and dysrhythmias may occur in severe cases.
Common causes	Cocaine, amphetamine, methamphetamine (and its derivatives 3,4-methylenedioxyamphetamine, 3,4-methylenedioxymethamphetamine, 3,4-methylenedioxyethamphetamine, and 2,5-dimethoxy-4-bromoamphetamine), and over-the-counter decongestants (phenylpropanolamine, ephedrine, and pseudoephedrine). In caffeine and theophylline overdoses, similar findings are observed, except for organic psychiatric signs resulting from catecholamine release.
Opiate, Sedative, or Ethanol Intoxication	
Common signs	Coma, respiratory depression, miosis, hypotension, bradycardia, hypothermia, pulmonary edema, decreased bowel sounds, hyporeflexia, and needle marks. Seizures may occur after overdoses of some narcotics, notably propoxyphene.
Common causes	Narcotics, barbiturates, benzodiazepines, ethchlorvynol, glutethimide, methyprylon, methaqualone, meprobamate, ethanol, clonidine, gamma-hydroxybutyrate (GHB)
Cholinergic Syndromes	
Common signs	Confusion, central nervous system (CNS) depression, weakness, salivation, lacrimation, urinary and fecal incontinence, gastrointestinal cramping, emesis, diaphoresis, muscle fasciculations, pulmonary edema, miosis, bradycardia or tachycardia, and seizures
Common causes	Organophosphate and carbamate insecticides, physostigmine, edrophonium, and some mushrooms

mation about the nature of the toxic substance. For this reason, medical toxicologists often group drugs and toxins according to similarities in clinical presentation. These groupings, collectively known as toxidromes, are listed in Table 55-6.[1,27,28,31] As seen, many of the drugs included in each category differ from others within the group in terms of structure or use. Although these classifications are useful, they should be used cautiously because symptoms will vary with dose, ranging from subtle to pronounced, and may be caused by more than one toxin.

Data reported by the American Association of Poison Control Centers (AAPCC) and the Centers for Disease Control and Prevention emphasize that most exposures involve toxins that are readily available in the home.[1,31,32] More than 4.5 million toxic exposures occur annually, resulting in more than a million emergency department visits. Most exposures involving children (defined as younger than age 17 years) are determined to be accidental (Fig. 55-4), and most of those involving adults are determined to be intentional. A review of death statistics reveals that readily available drugs or chemicals contribute to the cause of death in about 11% of suicides, regardless of age.[33]

According to the 2006 National Household Survey on Drug Abuse, more than 20 million individuals admit to using drugs illegally or inappropriately, for example, by using another's prescription.[34] Urine **drug screens** often are performed during the initial evaluation of patients who are seeking substance abuse treatment, because many of these patients also self-medicate with drugs other than the one for which they are seeking treatment. Random screening may be continued to appraise the patient's compliance with the program. Random screening also has become a widely used tool in the management of patients seeking treatment for chronic pain, because this population is recognized as exhibiting a higher incidence of illicit drug use compared with the general population. Pregnant women may be screened for drug use because drug usage surveys indicate that the heaviest use of illicit drugs occurs in persons between 18 and 30 years of age, which for females are the peak childbearing years.[35] It is important to identify and treat pregnant drug abusers to minimize potential drug-induced complications for the mother and the fetus. If it is determined that the woman has not received prenatal care, screening may be done to anticipate potential problems during delivery, because studies have demonstrated that self-reporting leads to underestimation of the true exposure rate.[35] In studies that evaluated cocaine use by pregnant women, the number of positive urine results for the cocaine metabolite was twice the number of patients who admitted to using cocaine.[36]

Treatment of the poisoned patient begins by stabilizing the patient's ABCs—airway, breathing, circulation—and includes assisted ventilation, supplemental oxygen, intravenous access, and maintenance of blood pressure.[1,27,37,38] Supportive therapy is continued until the body is cleared of the drug. Once stabilized, the patient must be decontaminated of any remaining or

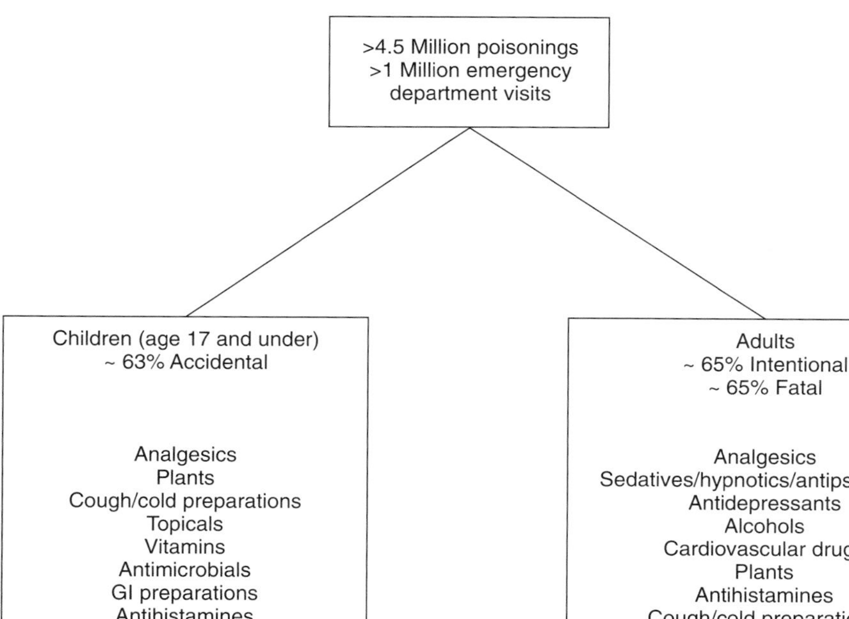

Fig. 55-4 Comparison of poisonings in adults and children. (From www.AAPCC.org.)

unabsorbed toxin. Here, it becomes useful to know the route of entry of the toxin. Skin decontamination may involve washing with soap and water or using vitamin E–laced oils for some pesticides. Treatment options for gastrointestinal decontamination of ingested agents include gastric lavage with large-bore oral or nasal tubes, administration of activated charcoal, and whole bowel irrigation.[1,37,38] The practice of inducing emesis (vomiting) must be used cautiously—the chemical that causes cellular injury while going down causes injury while coming up! Other toxins are eliminated more rapidly by forced diuresis, for example, by increasing urine flow with intravenous administration of a diuretic such as mannitol. This type of therapy would reduce exposure of the kidney to the toxin and thus the potential for nephrotoxicity. Hemodialysis or hemoperfusion also may be effective in removing water-soluble toxins that have a low molecular weight, a low volume of distribution, and low protein binding.

Although it is theoretically possible to trap ionized toxins in the urine by altering the urinary pH, the risks associated with this procedure outweigh the benefits in many cases; therefore, use of this decontamination process tends to be restricted to select situations and is monitored carefully. Chelating agents such as ethylenediaminetetraacetic acid (EDTA), deferoxamine (DFO), and British anti-Lewisite (BAL) are used to bind and remove metals.

The history of poisons is intertwined with that of **antidotes.** Unfortunately, relatively few antidotes are available compared with the number of toxins encountered. Some of the more commonly encountered antidotes are presented in Table 55-7. The use of these antidotes, as with the treatments previously discussed, must be considered carefully because many have their own set of risks, precautions, and contraindications.[1,17,37]

Table 55-7 Examples of Poisons and Antidotes

Poison	Antidote
Acetaminophen	*N*-Acetylcysteine (NAC, Mucomyst)
β-Blockers	Glucagon
Carbon monoxide	Oxygen
Digoxin	Digibind
Ethylene glycol/methanol	4-Methylpyrazole (fomepizole), ethanol
Heavy metals (arsenic, mercury, lead)	Dimercaprol (BAL), EDTA, D-penicillamine, succimer
Iron, aluminum	Deferoxamine
Nitrites, analins, local anesthetics	Methylene blue
Opiates	Naloxone (Narcan)
Organophosphates	Atropine, 2-PAM
Superwarfarins	Phytonadione (vitamin K_1)

BAL, British anti-Lewisite; *EDTA,* ethylenediaminetetraacetic acid; *PAM,* pralidoxime.

KEY CONCEPTS BOX 55-4

- Ways to determine the nature of a toxin in a patient include clinical assessment, laboratory testing, and history of drug use.
- In poisonings and overdoses, patient histories may not be accurate. Classification of symptoms through clinical evaluation often helps point clinicians to specific toxins.
- Drug screens are used most frequently in emergency situations for individuals with changed mental status.
- Antidotes are chemicals that act to counter the toxic effects of another chemical. An example of an antidote is ethanol used in cases of ethylene glycol poisoning.

SECTION OBJECTIVES BOX 55-5

- Discuss the advantages and disadvantages of the various samples available for toxicology.
- Define *meconium,* and describe its role in toxicology testing.
- List the various methods available for toxicology testing.
- Discuss the uses and limitations of immunoassays in toxicology testing.

THE TOXICOLOGY LABORATORY

The extent of services offered by a clinical laboratory depends on available personnel and equipment, as well as the medical services supported. A few patients present to the emergency department with a reliable history of exposure to a toxin, but in many cases, the patient's symptoms could be the result of disease or trauma. Although most clinicians would want firm identification or exclusion of a toxin, it is neither practical nor possible to firmly identify or exclude all suspected toxins in every case.

Fortunately (for the laboratory), most poisonings involve readily available drugs or chemicals and are managed clinically according to the patient's symptoms. Identification is most useful when an antidote is available, a specific treatment is indicated, or the onset of symptoms is delayed. And so, identification represents a small and limited role for most laboratories. If present, identification of an agent may provide reassuring information to the clinician, but other laboratory tests may be even more important for the overall management of the patient's condition.[1,27-30]

Choosing Samples and Methods

The choice of sample depends on a combination of factors and often is dictated by collection limitations and available methods. Serum (or blood) is the sample of choice when a relationship is identified between the concentration of the toxin found in the circulation and toxicity.[39] Examples of drugs for which this relationship exists include acetaminophen, salicylate, ethanol, carbon monoxide, and certain therapeutic drugs. Serum also is preferred when an antidote is available because in these cases, the amount of antidote to be administered is based on the concentration of the toxin that is present in the circulation. Examples of toxins and their corresponding antidotes are provided in Table 55-7.

Unless significant renal toxicity is evident, urine is a readily available, easily collected specimen. For this reason, it is a commonly used sample in the workplace, in pain management and rehabilitation clinics, and in performance testing. However, it should always be remembered that few drugs are found in their original form in urine samples; instead the compounds present in a urine sample typically are metabolic end products, whose presence reflects an exposure that took place in the past.[28,39-41] One of the few situations in which the presence of a toxin in urine can be related to clinical symptoms occurs when it is used to screen for heavy metal exposure.[1,27]

To best interpret the data obtained when urine is used, the toxicologist must have knowledge of the length of time (**window of detection**) that compounds or metabolites are excreted into the urine **after** exposure. If a compound is not found in the urine, this may mean that the person was not exposed, or that the exposure was so recent that metabolism to the detected product has yet to occur. It also could mean that the exposure occurred so far in the past that elimination is complete, or it could mean that the sample is dilute, so that the amount of toxin present is less than the amount that can be detected by the method used.[28,40,41]

Oral fluid (saliva) has gained interest as a sample because it is collected easily and, for a number of drugs, it reflects the concentration of drug in the blood.[32,42] Most drugs of abuse, including ethanol, cocaine, amphetamines, barbiturates, **benzodiazepines,** nicotine, phencyclidine, and cannabinoids, can be measured in this matrix. For some of these drugs, the same methods used for urine testing can be adapted, but for others, the detected metabolites differ. Law enforcement personnel have used breath as a sample for the detection of ethanol ingestion for many years, and point-of-care devices used for this testing have made their way into some emergency and clinical settings.

Meconium accumulates in the fetal intestinal tract from approximately week 12 of gestation until birth and provides a useful sample for assessing a newborn's exposure to drugs in utero during this window of time (see Chapter 45). Drugs and drug metabolites that cross the placenta and enter the amniotic fluid become incorporated into meconium when the fetus swallows the amniotic fluid.[43] In most cases, meconium is not passed until after birth, usually within 5 to 10 days. A urine sample collected from the newborn can reflect exposure during the last trimester, but this sample is often difficult to collect.

Keratinized matrices, such as hair and nails, are other specimen types that are used to detect toxins.[44,45] These matrices complement the more traditional ones of blood, serum, and urine by providing a longer window of detection (weeks to years). In several cases, the analytes are also more stable in these samples because of the way in which they are incorporated into the matrix.[46] However, interpretations of hair and nail results must be performed cautiously because of limited research for some analytes, lack of meaningful reference ranges, and other uncertainties that surround these less used matrices.

Toxicology testing uses all available techniques. The method used should be selected according to the needs and abilities of the laboratory.[2,3,28,39,43] "Spot tests" that use colorimetric or spectrometric methods are described for a few drugs; although rapid, inexpensive, and easy to perform, these methods are very insensitive and notoriously nonspecific. Some of the chemicals required for analysis are hazardous, and interpretation is subjective. For these reasons, spot tests have been replaced by more robust methods.

Chromatography-based techniques such as thin-layer chromatography (TLC), gas chromatography (GC), high-performance liquid chromatography (HPLC), and liquid chromatography-tandem mass spectrometry are used widely (see Chapter 3). These techniques offer the advantage of being adaptable to single- or multiple-analyte testing, as well as being adaptable for multiple matrices (e.g., urine, blood, serum). These techniques are key to the toxicologist's ability to rapidly develop methods to detect and identify new drugs of concern or toxins. Mass spectrometry coupled to GC or HPLC is considered the gold standard for identification. As will be discussed, these methods provide the positive identification so important to forensic testing. Some chromatographic methods require extensive sample preparation and analysis time and therefore may not be suitable for laboratories with few samples, minimal staff, or rapid response needs.

For now, immunoassay techniques are the mainstay of toxicology testing in clinical laboratories, although their use is largely restricted to testing for therapeutic drugs and drugs of abuse. Methods are available in a range of formats from point-of-care devices to reagents used on automated platforms applied for other chemistry testing. Use of these methods allows laboratories to achieve the rapid turnaround times required in the clinical setting or to screen large numbers of samples. Along with these advantages have come limitations that affect the use of these methods within the medical setting, particularly when they are used to test for drugs of abuse in urine (DAU). Confusion can arise if the specificity of the given test is not fully understood and its subsequent limitations in the medical setting are not appreciated. For some immunoassays, specificity is less than that needed for clinical applications, but for others, the opposite is true. It is imperative that this information is available to the staff of the toxicology laboratory, and that staff members understand the limitations of the assays they use for testing.[28,29]

KEY CONCEPTS BOX 55-5

- Drug identification is most useful when an antidote is available, a specific treatment is indicated, or the onset of symptoms is delayed.
- Interpretation of toxicology results requires knowledge of the pharmacological characteristics of the chemicals involved, including their metabolism and excretion.
- Serum and urine are the most frequently used samples for clinical toxicology. Serum is best when the relationship between toxin concentration and toxicity is known. Urine is useful for qualitative detection of a toxin.
- Immunoassays are used most often for drug testing, but they often are limited by their specificity. TLC, HPLC, and GC methods also are used widely.

SECTION OBJECTIVES BOX 55-6

- Describe two key differences between a clinical laboratory and a forensic laboratory.
- Describe the two-step approach for medicolegal testing and the types of methods used for each step.
- Explain confirmatory testing.

MEDICOLEGAL CHALLENGES

Technologists in the clinical toxicology laboratory may become involved in the medicolegal system because results may be subpoenaed for legal proceedings. In these circumstances, the technologist may be required to testify under oath regarding the validity of analytical results. Such testimony usually involves a detailed discussion of the analytical procedures used to conduct the test in question, as well as all other laboratory procedures and policies that might be involved.

Laboratories that perform drug testing for purposes of investigating death, crime, impaired driving, drugs in the workplace, and athletic performance must perform these tests according to good laboratory standards and with impartiality. Forensic laboratories operate under very stringent policies and procedures to make sure this occurs. The methods used by such laboratories, as well as the resulting data, must be legally admissible and defensible.[47] It is common to require forensic laboratories to present additional documents, including personnel training records, instrument maintenance logs, and the specimen's chain-of-custody, during legal testimony.[3,4,47]

Current protocols for medicolegal testing require a two-step approach by which specimens are first tested with the use of rapid, less specific screening procedures, such as immunoassay, to obtain qualitative results. Because most samples are expected to be negative, the initial use of less specific methods is considered a cost-effective means of reducing the number of samples that are subsequently subjected to confirmation testing. Samples that test positive in the screening process are designated as presumptive positive, which must be confirmed by more rigorous confirmatory testing completed by means of a different technique than that used in screening, such as gas chromatography mass spectrometry. In this phase of testing, the amount of drug present is quantified. For workplace and performance testing, the results must be further evaluated and interpreted by a qualified medical review officer (MRO), who makes the final determination of positive or negative.

KEY CONCEPTS BOX 55-6

- Testing for toxins for the purpose of patient care requires less rigorous testing procedures than are used for medicolegal testing, in which legal action might occur as the result of the testing.
- Typically, immunoassays are used for most medical testing.
- Confirmatory testing occurs when the result of an initial assay is confirmed by another, more rigorous procedure. This usually involves HPLC or GC technology, usually with mass spectrometry detection.

SECTION OBJECTIVES BOX 55-7

- Describe the roles played by clinical laboratories in emergency planning and preparedness.
- Describe three herbals that have been found to cause toxicity.
- Describe three pharmaceutical drugs that are derived from plant products.

BIOLOGICAL AND CHEMICAL AGENTS OF MASS DESTRUCTION

The use of chemical and biological agents in warfare is not a modern invention. The first documented use of a chemical agent occurred during the Athenian and Spartan Wars (431 BC), when sulfur was burned beneath the city walls of Plataea and Belium. One of the earliest historical uses of biological warfare dates back to 1348 AD, when Tartar warriors catapulted plague-infected corpses over the city walls of Kaffa in the Crimea.[7,48] Since those times, man has continued to employ poisons and pathogens in domestic and international acts of warfare and terrorism as seen in Fig. 55-5, which lists some successful or potential biological and chemical agents of mass destruction.

Hospitals now include the possibility of a chemical or biological attack when developing emergency preparedness plans.[49] Strategies should include education and increased awareness of personnel, plans for implementation of diagnostic testing for specific agents, performed either onsite or through a designated state or federal facility, and rapid response victim management and treatment. Laboratories should perform organized exercises to test emergency preparedness.

THE TOXICITY OF NATURAL PRODUCTS

The use of alternative medicines continues to rise throughout the world, and in many parts of the world, traditional medicines remain the mainstay of medical care. It is understandable that when people travel or relocate to other countries, they bring such products with them. Many individuals continue to believe that natural products are safe, or at least less toxic, when in fact some include our most potent toxins. Patients use a range of products, including dried materials prepared to brew teas for consumption, tinctures, capsules, and topical creams. Many herbal preparations are purchased over-the-counter, through the Internet, or from international sources, although some are self-grown or are harvested in the wild. As with conventional medications, patients may not understand the proper use of a product and may, for example, ingest a material that was intended to be applied as a salve. Most are not pure products but rather are mixtures of several products, only some of which might be toxic (Table 55-8). For most, little research has been done to determine the active compounds or the mechanism of action.[50-52]

Herbals, like other drugs and toxins, act at multiple sites to produce a myriad of effects. Patients who use comfrey (*Symphytum* spp.), coltsfoot, chaparral *(Larrea tridentata),* mistletoe, and germander have experienced liver dysfunction as the result of alkaloids present in these materials. After using these compounds, patients have experienced effects ranging from mild alterations in liver function tests to more serious conditions such as venoocclusive disease (Budd-Chiari syndrome), hepatitis, and death. Caffeine, kola, and ephedra are commonly found in products purported to promote weight loss or to increase energy. Excessive use of these materials can cause any of the symptoms associated with the sympathomimetic toxidrome, including hypertension and cardiac arrhythmia. Because of its aldosterone-like activity, licorice *(Glycyrrhiza glabra)* and licorice root, often added to teas and other products to sweeten the flavor, can cause hypertension and hypokalemia. Some plants are cultured commercially; however, the practice of harvesting plants in the wild has led to cases of toxicity when another plant has been misidentified as the intended herb.

Toxicity also has resulted from unexpected contaminants such as unreported pharmaceuticals, poisons, and heavy metals. One surprising case of mercury toxicity was found when women in U.S. states bordering Mexico began to demonstrate neurological symptoms. Eventually, heavy metal screening revealed excessive levels of mercury as the toxin. The source was determined to be an herbal beauty cream that originated in Mexico.[52]

The toxicology laboratory should be aware of serious drug–herbal supplement interactions (see Table 55-8). When used with warfarin, products containing feverfew, garlic, gingko, ginger, and ginseng have caused prolonged bleeding times. The interaction of St. John's wort with immunosuppressive drugs and protease inhibitors led the U.S. Food and Drug Administration (FDA) to issue an advisory, warning against the use of this alternative medicine with prescription drugs. Licorice, ginseng, plantain, and hawthorn may interfere with digoxin pharmacodynamically or with drug monitoring.[51] Another complication of herbal toxicity is the shortage of laboratories that can identify these toxins successfully. Most herbals are not detected by routine clinical testing, although methods used for analysis of some of the more toxic metabolites or components are beginning to appear in the literature. Despite these problems, it must be remembered that some of our conventional drugs (e.g., aspirin, taxol, digoxin) originated through herbal practices.

KEY CONCEPTS BOX 55-7

- Laboratories should have plans in place to respond to toxicological disasters.
- A large range of natural products, from heavy metals to herbal products, may have severe toxic effects.
- Laboratories should be aware of these products and should be prepared to assist physicians in measuring them.

SECTION OBJECTIVES BOX 55-8

- Name the common analgesics found in toxicological situations.
- Describe their metabolism, and explain why these analgesics are toxic.

KEY TOXINS ENCOUNTERED IN THE LABORATORY

Analgesics

Acetaminophen is used therapeutically for its **antipyretic** and analgesic activities, but it exhibits very little anti-inflammatory activity. Acetaminophen-containing products became very

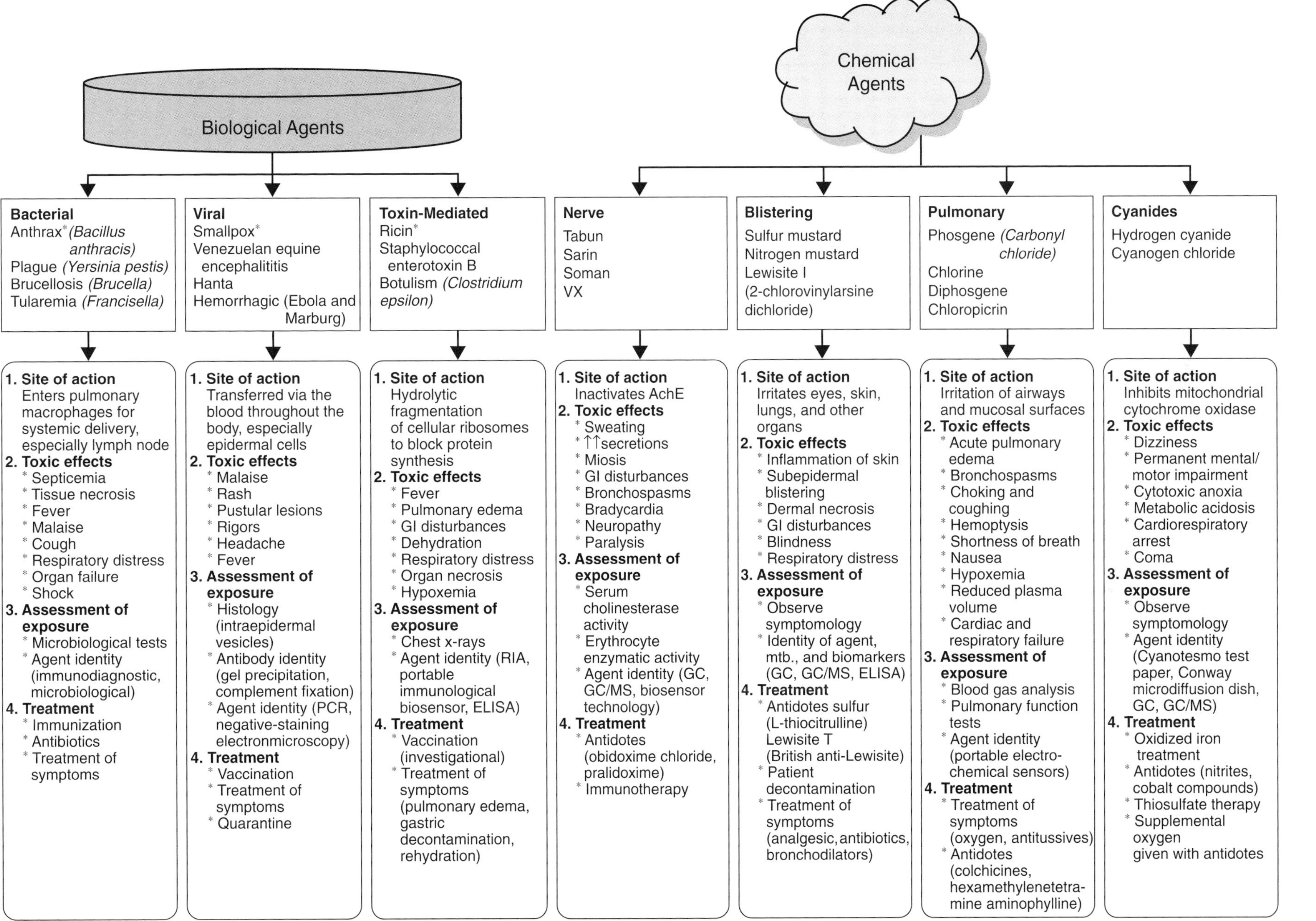

Fig. 55-5 Biological and chemical warfare. *AchE,* Acetylcholinesterase; *GI,* gastrointestinal; ↑↑, increased; *GC,* gas chromatography; *GC/MS,* gas chromatography–mass spectrometry; *ELISA,* enzyme-linked immunosorbent assay; *mtb,* metabolite; *RIA,* radioimmunoassay; *resp.,* respiratory. *For biological agents, the site of action, toxic effects, assessment of exposure, and treatment are discussed for the designated agent. (From Jortani SA, Snyder JW, Valdes RV Jr: The role of the clinical laboratory in managing chemical or biological terrorism, Clin Chem 46:1883, 2000; Budavari S, et al, editors: *The Merck Index: An Encyclopedia of Chemicals, Drugs, and Biologicals,* ed 12, Whitehouse Station, NJ, 1996, Merck Research Laboratories; O'Brien T, et al: The development of immunoassays to four biological threat agents in a bidiffractive grating biosensor, Biosensors and Bioelectronics 14:815, 2000.)

popular following the recognition of a relationship between Reye's syndrome in children and the use of aspirin.

When taken in **therapeutic doses,** acetaminophen is metabolized primarily to nontoxic metabolites that are eliminated readily. Even under these conditions, a very small amount of the drug is metabolized to *N*-acetyl-*p*-benzoquinone imine (NAPQI; Fig. 55-6), a toxic metabolite. Normally, this small amount of toxic metabolite is removed rapidly by reaction with glutathione before significant damage can be done.[53] In an overdose situation, if not enough glutathione is available to remove all of the metabolite, the excess NAPQI becomes available to exert its toxic effects.

The hepatotoxic effects of acetaminophen overdose have received much attention, but other organ systems may be affected, including the kidney and the central nervous system.[53-55] In fact, some patients have had acetaminophen-related renal failure without hepatotoxicity. Symptoms of toxicity often are delayed and initially may be mistaken for influenza, so poisoning may not be suspected. In these cases, toxicity progresses to more serious events, including jaundice, bleeding, neurological changes, hepatic necrosis, and death. A very effective antidote to acetaminophen, *N*-acetylcysteine (Mucomyst), is available for use if the overdose is recognized.[1,27]

Several mitochondrial CYP450 isoenzymes are involved in the formation of NAPQI, and the risk for hepatotoxicity is increased, even under therapeutic conditions, when acetaminophen is co-ingested with any drug that induces these enzymes, especially the CYP2E1 isoenzyme. Ethanol is such a drug, and toxicity has been observed when acetaminophen has been taken after ethanol ingestion. Interpretation of serum levels is more difficult when acetaminophen is combined with other toxic drugs, such as codeine or caffeine, or when it is taken in timed-release or long-acting formulas.

The preferred specimen for analysis is serum. The therapeutic range is 10 to 20 mg/L; toxicity is likely when levels are greater than 150 mg/L at 4 hours or longer after ingestion. If the time of ingestion is known to be longer than 4 hours and ingestion is acute, a single quantitative determination may be adequate. This result can be evaluated by using the Rumack-Matthew nomogram seen in Fig. 55-7. If the time of ingestion

Table 55-8 Herbals of Toxicological Importance

Herbal Preparation	Site of Toxicity
Kava kava, chaparral, coltsfoot, germander, Chinese teas, mistletoe, comfrey, Jin bu huang	Gastrointestinal tract and liver
Ginseng, ephedra, astragalus, salvia, licorice, plantain, oleander, bitter root	Heart
Licorice, dandelion, Aristolochia fangchi, Acorus calamus	Kidney
Red clover, tang-kuel, yarrow, salvia, pau d'arco, feverfew, ginger, gingko	Hematopoiesis
Ephedra, tang-keui, yohimbe, valerian, nutmeg, Jimson weed, mandrake, khat, kava kava, ginseng	CNS

Herbal Preparation	Reported Drug Interactions
St. John's wort	Cyclosporine, tacrolimus, protease inhibitors, digoxin, theophylline, warfarin, oral contraceptives
Ginseng	Warfarin, heparin, aspirin, nonsteroidal anti-inflammatory drugs, corticosteroids
Valerian	Thiopental, pentobarbital, ethanol
Alfalfa	Warfarin
Aloe	Digoxin, diuretics
Feverfew	Aspirin, warfarin
Ma huang	β-Blockers, caffeine, theophylline, decongestants, methyldopa
Kava kava	Alcohol, sedatives

CNS, Central nervous system.

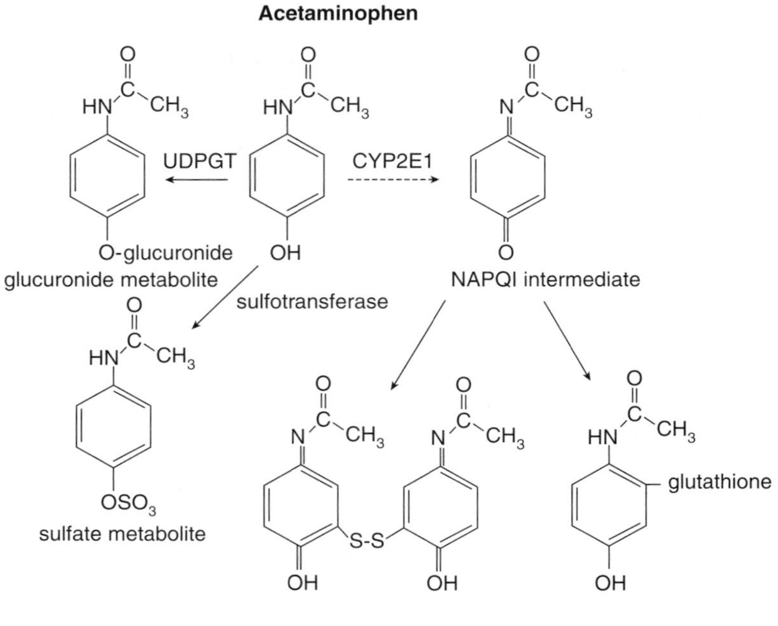

Fig. 55-6 Metabolic pathway for acetaminophen. The metabolic pathways for acetaminophen are shown. Under therapeutic conditions in which CYP2E1 is not induced and glutathione stores are adequate, ≈55% of the drug is metabolized to the glucuronide metabolite, ≈30% to the sulfate metabolite, and ≈6% to the NAPQI metabolite. NAPQI is conjugated rapidly to glutathione and eliminated. *CYP2E1,* Cytochrome P-450 isoenzyme 2E1; *NAPQI, N*-acetyl-*p*-benzoquinone imine; *UDPGT,* uridine diphosphoglucuronosyl transferase. (From Hammett-Stabler CA, et al: Toxicology in the clinical laboratory. In Clarke W, Dufour DR, editors: *Contemporary Practice in Clinical Chemistry,* Washington, DC, 2006, AACC Press.)

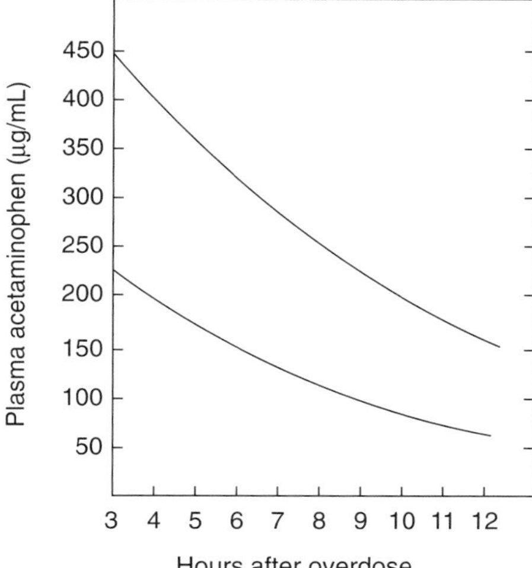

Fig. 55-7 Plasma acetaminophen concentration in relation to time after acute overdose. Liver damage is likely to be severe above the upper line, severe to mild between the lines, and clinically insignificant under the lower line. (From Prescott LF, et al: Cysteamine, methionine, and penicillamine in the treatment of paracetamol poisoning, Lancet 2:109, 1976.)

is unknown, serial measurements are recommended, initially and approximately 2 to 3 hours after decontamination. If the patient is thought to have taken acetaminophen chronically and toxicity is suspected, levels should be determined in two samples collected 3 to 4 hours apart, and the half-life ($t_{1/2}$) should be calculated. The patient's renal and liver function also should be monitored.

Salicylates are ingested most commonly as aspirin (acetylsalicylic acid). This compound is metabolized rapidly to the active drug, salicylic acid. Since the relationship between the drug and the onset of Reye's syndrome has been recognized, the number of aspirin-related poisonings has decreased to about one-third the number of poisonings with acetaminophen. For children, salicylate poisonings usually are acute and involve an overdose, whereas for adults, chronic toxicity may be more common and can go unrecognized for some time.[56]

Even at therapeutic doses, salicylates may cause direct uncoupling of mitochondrial oxidative phosphorylation and direct stimulation of the central nervous system (CNS), resulting in hyperventilation and respiratory alkalosis. Also, because they disrupt the Krebs cycle, these drugs cause a positive anion gap, that is, metabolic acidosis. It is not uncommon to find patients with symptoms of chronic intoxication (e.g., ringing in the ears, nausea, unsteady gait). In cases of overdose, gastric emptying slows, so that half-life increases by about 10-fold. The drug has a low volume of distribution (Vd), so decontamination with charcoal or dialysis is effective. As with acetaminophen, salicylate often is found in combination with other drugs (diphenhydramine [Benadryl], caffeine) and often is formulated as a timed-release preparation.

Serum is the preferred sample, although the compound can be detected in urine. Analytical methods range from spectrophometric to chromatography-based techniques. The therapeutic range depends on use: 20 to 100 mg/L for analgesia and 100 mg/L for anti-inflammatory activity. The reported toxic range is >300 mg/L. Levels should be measured initially or after decontamination and approximately 3 hours later to ensure successful decontamination. Patients also should be monitored by blood gases, pH, electrolytes, and liver function tests.[1,56]

KEY CONCEPTS BOX 55-8

- Overdoses of acetaminophen and aspirin, which are common analgesics, can be life threatening.
- Acetaminophen is metabolized to NAPQI, which is hepatotoxic and renotoxic if protective levels of glutathione are not present.
- The antidote, *N*-acetylcysteine (Mucomyst), is given in cases of overdose.
- Overdose of salicylates (aspirin) and its metabolite, salicylic acid, can cause respiratory and metabolic acidoses, respectively.
- Nomograms are available for the assessment of acetaminophen and salicylate intoxication.

SECTION OBJECTIVES BOX 55-9

- Describe clinical situations in which drugs of abuse testing may occur.
- Describe the sample and testing methods commonly used.
- List the most common classes of abused drugs.
- List the drugs often used as "club drugs."

DRUGS OF ABUSE

Drugs within this group (Table 55-9) range from therapeutic drugs that have a high potential for misuse, such as **opioids,** to those for which no medical or legal uses are known, such as lysergic acid diethylamide (LSD) and phencyclidine (PCP). Because the drugs in this category are often illegal or are used illegally, drugs of abuse testing serves as a good example in which clinical toxicology testing may make a transition to the forensic arena. Testing may be requested when substance abuse is suspected or is being monitored, when compliance with pain management therapies must be confirmed, and when changes in mental status are assessed.

Serum is not used; instead, urine is the sample of choice, hence the term "drugs of abuse in urine," or DAU. When results of these tests are interpreted, it must be recognized that many of these drugs appear in urine as a combination of parent drug and metabolites. Some are detectable in the urine for a few hours, whereas others are excreted for days to weeks. Because most DAU methods are designed to measure specific metabolites, nothing can be concluded about the concentration of active drug in the body, including whether any remains. This sometimes causes confusion when clinicians obtain a report that a drug is present in the urine but the patient does not show clinical symptoms of intoxication.

Table 55-9 Drugs of Abuse in Urine (DAU)

Drug Group	Drugs in Group	Window of Detection	Metabolite Used in Assay	Immunoassay Screen Cut-off*	GC/MS Cut-off*
Amphetamines/ methamphetamines	D-amphetamine, D-methamphetamine, ephedrine, pseudoephedrine, phenylpropanolamine, MDA, MDMA, MDEA, PMA	2 to 4 days (dose/form dependent)	D-amphetamine D-methamphetamine	500/1000	25/50/200/500
Barbiturates	Butalbarbital, talbutal, phenobarbital, pentobarbital, secobarbital, amobarbital	1 to 21 days (dose/form dependent)	Secobarbital	200	100
Benzodiazepines†	Diazepam, flurazepam, oxazepam, nordiazepam	≈72 hours	Nordiazepam	200	50/100
Cannabinoids (THC)	Marijuana	1 to 21 days	THC-acid	20/50	3/15
Cocaine	Cocaine	<72 hours	Benzoylecgonine	150/300	50/150
LSD	LSD	<12 to 24 hours	LSD	0.5	0.5
Methadone	Methadone	3 to 16 days	Methadone	300	100
Opiates†	Heroin, morphine, codeine, oxycodone, hydrocodone, hydromorphone	2 to 5 days	Morphine	300/2000	100
Phencyclidine	PCP	5 to 7 days	PCP	25	25

LSD, Lysergic acid diethylamide; *MDA,* 3,4-methylenedioxyamphetamine; *MDE/MDEA,* 3,4-methylenedioxy-N-ethylamphetamine; *MDMA,* 3,4-methylenedioxymethamphetamine; *PCP,* phencyclidine; *PMA,* paramethoxyamphetamine; *THC,* Δ^9-tetrahydrocannabinol.
*ng/mL; Cut-offs vary according to purpose of testing and regulations.
†Detected benzodiazepines and opiates vary considerably between immunoassays; consult product literature.

Most clinical laboratories use immunoassay-based methods for DAU testing to meet rapid turnaround times demanded in the clinical setting. Because these assays may cross-react with other metabolites, or even with other, unrelated drugs, additional testing may be necessary in some cases. Confirmation testing with more specific and sensitive methods should be available in-house or through a reference laboratory. It also may be necessary to confirm "negative" samples when testing for a drug that is part of a broad class—benzodiazepines or **opiates,** for example—because the antibodies in these assays may not cross-react sufficiently with all drugs or metabolites of the class and may yield a false-negative result. Confirming negative drug screens may be important when these tests are used to monitor compliance, as in pain management clinics or rehabilitation centers.

Amphetamines

Amphetamine, methamphetamine, and their derivatives (methylenedioxyamphetamine, methylenedioxymethamphetamine) are **sympathomimetic amines** that stimulate the CNS, producing excitement, alertness, euphoria, loss of appetite, and reduced sense of fatigue. Both psychological and physiological addiction can occur with amphetamine use. Amphetamines are used therapeutically to treat narcolepsy, obesity, and attention deficit/hyperactivity disorders. Because of the high potential for abuse, the Code of Federal Regulations Controlled Substance Act categorizes most amphetamines as Schedule II substances. Routes of amphetamine administration include oral ingestion, injection, inhalation, and insufflation. Amphetamines are absorbed rapidly from the gastrointestinal tract and are distributed widely throughout the body. In the liver, amphetamines are metabolized to more polar forms to be excreted. Depending on urinary pH, amphetamines are eliminated from the body for the most part within 48 hours.[57] Side effects at low doses include irritability, anxiety, insomnia, blurred vision, hypertension, and cardiac palpitation. Acute toxicity results in agitation, hyperthermia, convulsions, coma, and respiratory and cardiac failure. These drugs are detected by various methods, including immunoassays and gas chromatography (see Method of Analysis on Evolve). Methods are available to distinguish among the racemic forms of amphetamine.

Barbiturates

Barbiturates are CNS depressants that are used medicinally as anxiolytic, anticonvulsant, anesthetic, and muscle-relaxant agents. These drugs bind to the chloride channel molecule of the γ-aminobutyric acid (GABA) receptor, inducing sedation, euphoria, and mood alterations. Barbiturates are taken most commonly through oral and parenteral administration. Depending on their duration of action, barbiturates may be categorized as ultrashort-, short-, intermediate-, or long-acting drugs. Once absorbed, the major pathways of hepatic **biotransformation** include oxidation and glucuronide conjugation. Undesirable effects include drowsiness, mental impairment, dysarthria, and ataxia. At elevated levels, barbiturates can cause coma and cardiovascular and respiratory depression. Immunoassays are used to screen for the presence of this class of agents in urine, but chromatographic methods can be used to identify and quantify specfic barbiturates. Because phenobarbital is used to treat seizures, specific immunoassays are available to quantify this drug in serum.

Benzodiazepines

Benzodiazepines exhibit a pharmacological response similar to that of barbiturates and are used for the same applications. Most benzodiazepines are classified as Schedule IV drugs; flunitrazepam, however, is categorized as a Schedule I drug. Benzodiazepines often are given orally or parenterally. Side effects of these drugs are similar to, but milder than, those of barbiturates. Physical dependence and withdrawal symptoms (including insomnia, agitation, irritability, muscle tension, psychosis, and seizure) may occur with long-term use. Hepatic metabolism reduces benzodiazepines to active and inactive compounds with a half-life equal to or longer than that of the parent drug. Antibodies used in the immunoassays designed to screen for drugs found in the benzodiazepine class often are targeted to nordiazepam. For other benzodiazepines, the degree of cross-reactivity varies considerably. For example, some immunoassays do not detect the presence of flunitrazepam, whereas others may do so if the concentration is sufficient. Chromatographic methods, including GC, gas chromatography/mass spectrometry (GC/MS), HPLC, and liquid chromatography tandem mass spectroscopy (LC/MS/MS) are used to identify and quantify specific benzodiazepines.

Cannabinoids

Δ^9-Tetrahydrocannabinol (THC) is one of at least 61 cannabinoids found in the hemp plant, from which marijuana originates. Binding to the CB1 receptor, THC is the primary psychoactive compound of marijuana that produces the euphoric and relaxant effects for which it is abused.[58] Principal routes of administration include inhalation and ingestion. THC is classified as a Schedule I drug because it has no acceptable medicinal use and high abuse potential. Generally, THC is believed to be nonlethal when used alone, although some patients exhibit adverse effects such as tachycardia, respiratory anomalies, and behavioral and mental impairment. THC is highly lipophilic and is metabolized rapidly to more than 20 metabolites. The primary urinary metabolite, 11-nor-Δ^9-tetrahydrocannabinol-9-carboxylic acid (THC-COOH), is measured to identify THC use. Approximately 70% of a THC dose is excreted in feces and urine within 72 hours; however, in frequent users, half-lives longer than 10 days may occur. THC and its metabolites are detected through immunoassay and chromatographic techniques.

Cocaine

Cocaine is a potent CNS stimulant that is used as a local anesthetic in surgical procedures of the eyes, nose, and throat. Cocaine binds to the dopamine reuptake transporter of the CNS. Because of its high risk for psychological and physical addiction, cocaine is classified as a Schedule II drug. It is available as a hydrochloride salt, which usually is snorted or injected, or as a base that is smoked. The vasoconstrictive action of cocaine can result in myocardial infarct, subdural hemorrhage, cardiac dysrhythmia, and stroke. Other signs of acute toxicity include intense paranoia, bizarre and violent behavior, hyperthermia, pulmonary dysfunction, and sudden collapse.[59,60] Cocaine is metabolized rapidly through enzymatic and nonenzymatic processes to its major metabolites, ecgonine methyl ester (EME) and benzoylecgonine (BE), respectively. When ingested with ethanol, the unique cocaine metabolite cocaethylene is formed. This active metabolite is known to be cardiotoxic. Most of a cocaine dose is excreted in the urine within 24 hours as unchanged parent (1% to 9%), EME (32% to 49%), and BE (35% to 54%). Cocaine and its metabolites are detected through immunoassay and chromatographic techniques.

Opioids

Opioids include the naturally occurring alkaloids of opium (morphine, codeine) and their synthetic derivatives—methadone, heroin, propoxyphene, oxycodone, hydrocodone, hydromorphone, meperidine, and fentanyl. Opioids are prescribed as analgesic, antitussive, and antidiarrheal agents; for relief of acute pulmonary edema; and as suppressants to prevent relapse in heroin addicts (narcotic antagonists such as naltrexone, nalorphine). Opioids such as heroin are classified as Schedule I, and those with medical uses are classified as Schedule II. Because of their CNS effects, which include euphoria, sedation, and relaxation, these drugs are often misused.

Routes of administration include intravenous, intranasal, oral, and parenteral. Patients who use these drugs frequently develop tolerance and physical dependence (see Chapter 56). When unable to obtain the drug, these patients develop symptoms of withdrawal. Adverse effects include hypotension, pulmonary edema, respiratory depression, coma, and death.

Immunoassays are used to screen for drugs found in the opiate class; however, because most immunoassays are designed to target morphine or codeine, these methods may not be adequate for monitoring patients in pain clinics. False negatives often are reported for patients prescribed oxycodone, hydrocodone, and so forth, and these results should be confirmed.[61] Chromatographic methods, including GC, GC/MS, HPLC and LC/MS/MS, are used to identify and quantify specific opiates and metabolites.

Phencyclidine

Phencyclidine (PCP, l-phenylcyclohexylpiperidine) is a potent hallucinogenic agent and dissociative anesthetic that has no medical applications and therefore is classified as a Schedule I substance. It is interesting to note that receptors for PCP in the brain closely resemble or are identical to some of the opioid receptors. In addition, PCP antagonizes the glutamate receptors and may block dopamine uptake. PCP and its analogs—phencyclohexamine (PCE), phenylcyclohexylpyrrolidine (PHP), and thienylcyclohexylpiperidine (TCP)—are snorted, taken orally or intravenously, or smoked in combination with marijuana or tobacco. Tachycardia, psychosis, paranoia, combativeness, mydriasis, and respiratory depression are documented undesirable effects of PCP.[62] Because of its high lipophilicity, PCP can be stored in the brain and adipose tissue for extended periods. Metabolism occurs principally in the liver through oxidative hydroxylation and conjugation followed by renal clearance. Methods of analysis include immunoassay and gas chromatographic techniques.

Club Drugs

This loose category of drugs (listed in Table 55-10), originally named because of its presence and popularity within the dance club scene, includes 3,4-methylenedioxymethamphetamine (MDMA), gamma hydroxybutyrate (GHB), ketamine, and flunitrazepam.[63,64] With the exception of ketamine, these **club drugs** are listed as Schedule I drugs. Diphenhydramine and dextromethorphan, two over-the-counter medications, often are included in this group. Both of these drugs can cause hallucinations when taken in high doses.

MDMA (Ecstasy) is a distant cousin of methamphetamine but does not cause the same physiological and psychotropic effects. Usually taken orally as a tablet or capsule, the drug causes a euphoric sensation about 20 to 40 minutes after ingestion. Most users report no loss of control but find that their memory and mental skills are decreased when challenged. Side effects include hyperthermia, nausea, tooth grinding, and jaw clenching. Users frequently suck on a pacifier or lollipop to lessen soreness in the jaw. Dehydration and heatstroke are common side effects of this drug that result in admission to emergency departments. These conditions are exacerbated further by a combination of increased activity without rest and high room temperature in the typical nightclub environment. Several case reports indicate that hyperthermia and high levels of physical activity can lead to a syndrome of cardiac arrhythmia, rhabdomyolysis, acute renal failure, and disseminated intravascular coagulation, similar to that seen with severe heatstroke. To prevent dehydration, Ecstasy lore dictates drinking large quantities of water while under the influence; this in turn has led to severe water intoxication and hyponatremia.

Another consequence of MDMA use is the sudden onset of fulminant liver failure in some users. Evidence suggests that neurotoxicity may become more evident after long-term use.[63] MDMA may be detected through immunoassay or chromatography-based methods.

GHB, an endogenous chemical, is similar to the neurotransmitter GABA. GHB is a powerful sedative/hypnotic that causes euphoria and loss of inhibitions, similar to the effects of alcohol. Larger doses cause muscle relaxation and hallucinations.[64] Side effects are related to depression of the central nervous system and may include drowsiness, dizziness, nausea, vomiting, loss of muscle control, amnesia, and unconsciousness. The more serious toxic effects associated with higher doses include seizures, bradycardia, and respiratory depression. Chromatographic methods are used to detect the presence of GHB.

Ketamine is used in anesthesia induction before surgery and in veterinary medicine. It is structurally similar to phencyclidine and produces a similar pharmacological effect of dissociation. At higher doses, the drug produces a hallucinogenic state, which users equate to a near-death experience. The use of this drug is associated with hallucinations, nystagmus,

Table 55-10 Pharmacological and Testing Aspects of Club Drugs

Drug	Street Names	Metabolites	Sample	Methods of Detection	Window of Detection	Miscellaneous
Methylene dioxymethamphetamine (MDMA)	Ecstasy, Adam, X, XTC	3,4-methylenedioxyamphetamine (MDA), 4-hydroxy-3-methoxy methamphetamine (HMMA), 4-hydroxy-3-methoxy amphetamine (HMA)	Urine, plasma	Some cross-reactivity of MDA metabolite with amphetamine immunoassays GC; GC/MS	Urine ≈24 hours; plasma ≈5 to 6 hours	Metabolized by CYP2B6 and CYP2D6; other similar drugs include MDEA, PMA
Gamma-hydroxybutyrate (GHB)	Georgia Home Boy, Gamma-OH, Grievous Bodily Harm		Urine, serum	GC-FID; GC/MS	Urine <12 to 24 hours; serum $t_{1/2}$ <1 hour	Detected levels of GHB will increase in citrate-buffered blood
Flunitrazepam (Rohypnol)	Roofie, Roche, La Roche, Rope	7-Aminoflunitrazepam, *N*-Desmethyflunitrazepam, Norflunitrazepam	Urine, plasma	Some cross-reactivity with benzodiazepine immunoassays; GC/MS	Peaks in urine <6 hours; urinary metabolites detectable up to 28 days	
Ketamine (2-[2-chlorophenyl]-2-methylamino-cyclohexanone)	Special K, Cat Valiums, Vitamin K, KitKat	Norketamine, Dehydronorketamine	Urine, plasma	GC/MS		

Adapted from Gulledge C, Phillips J, Hammett-Stabler C: New kids on the block: an update on selected "club drugs," Therapeutic Drug Monitoring and Clinical Toxicology Division newsletter, 15(4):1, 2000.
GC, Gas chromatography; *GC-FIC,* gas chromatography–flame ionization detector; *GC/MS,* gas chromatography–mass spectrometry.

lethargy, tachycardia, and hypertension. It is most dangerous when combined with ethanol, benzodiazepines, or GHB. Ketamine can be detected through chromatographic methods.

KEY CONCEPTS BOX 55-9

- Table 55-9 lists the drugs of abuse in urine (DAU) that are commonly tested for when substance abuse is suspected or is being monitored, when pain management therapy is provided, and when changes in mental status are assessed.
- Immunoassays are the most frequently used screening method for DAU.
- Detection time after dosage for these drugs can vary greatly, from days to months.
- The ingestion of cocaine with ethanol leads to the formation of a unique metabolite, cocaethylene.

SECTION OBJECTIVES BOX 55-10

- Explain the mechanism for the toxicity of CO. Describe its antidote.
- List the heavy metals that commonly cause toxicity.
- Describe the mechanisms by which heavy metals cause toxicity.
- List the samples and methods used for measurement of heavy metals.
- List the three categories of common insecticides; describe their mechanisms of toxicity.
- List the common volatile toxins, and explain how they are measured.

GASES

Carbon monoxide (CO) is one of the leading causes of death in this country through accidental exposure or suicide. CO is a tasteless, odorless gas that is produced when combustion is incomplete. Carbon monoxide binds tightly to iron in hemoglobin and, in doing so, increases the affinity of the hemoglobin for oxygen. As a result, oxygen is not made available to the tissues of the body. Depending on the dose and duration of exposure, symptoms of CO poisoning range from mild headache to seizures and death. The antidote is oxygen. When available, optimal treatment is achieved with hyperbaric oxygen therapy, in which 100% oxygen can be administered under 2 to 3 atmospheres.[65] The level of CO in whole blood is determined by spectrophotometry (cooximetry) or gas chromatography.

METALS

In many cases, poisoning by heavy metals (Table 55-11) is difficult to diagnose unless a clear history of acute exposure is available (see Chapter 42).[14,17,18] Patients often are exposed to these metals at work or in the home, where the exposure may not be realized for some time. With heavy metal poisoning, it is important to identify the source of exposure to prevent reexposure or exposure of other individuals. In the home, possible sources include well water, older pressure-treated lumber, paint, and alternative medicines. In the workplace, occupational exposures are most commonly reported to be the result of inhalation of metallic fumes or dusts.

In many cases, metals exert toxicity by binding to sulfhydryl groups found in various enzymes and proteins, an action that is likely to render the enzyme or protein inactive. An important feature to remember is that the toxic effect may go unnoticed at low doses. Exposure to most metals produces similar symptoms, with neurological changes that include memory loss, mood changes, and loss of coordination, as well as frequent abdominal pain. The optimal specimen type depends on the metal and whether exposure is thought to be recent, chronic, or acute. The use of metal-free sample containers is important, regardless of the specimen type. Methods used to test for heavy metals include atomic absorp-

Table 55-11 Toxicity of Heavy Metals

Metal	Mechanism	Symptoms	Sample
Arsenic	Binds sulfhydryl groups of enzymes and proteins, uncouples oxidative phosphorylation	Acute: garlic odor, gastrointestinal distress, cardiac arrhythmias, uremia Chronic: weakness, malaise, weight loss, hyperpigmentation, Mee's lines, neuropathy, loss of memory	Urine, hair, nails, blood (if exposure within 4 hours)
Cadmium	Binds sulfhydryl groups; binds carboxyl, cysteinyl, histidyl, hydroxyl, and phosphatidyl groups	Gastrointestinal distress, irritability, proteinuria, glycosuria, aminoaciduria, muscle cramps, pulmonary edema, hypertension, loss of memory	Urine, hair
Iron	Corrosive free radical formation, lipid peroxidation	Bleeding, irritability, tachycardia, metabolic acidosis, fever, hepatic necrosis	Serum
Lead	Binds to sulfhydryl groups	Acute: salivation, vomiting Chronic: hematological (basophilic stippling, hypochromic normocytic anemia), ataxia, nausea, constipation, irritability, convulsions, neuropathies, coma, loss of memory	Whole blood, urine (also erythrocyte protoporphyrin)
Mercury	Corrosive; binds to sulfhydryl, carboxyl, amide, and amine functional groups	Chronic: fine muscle tremors, anorexia, weight loss, fatigue, emotional changes, irritability, loss of memory	Urine

tion, inductively coupled plasma emission spectroscopy, and mass spectrometry.

Treatment of the patient includes the use of chemicals that bind directly with metal ions to form stable complexes, as well as such chelators as ethylenediaminetetraacetic acid (EDTA), British anti-Lewisite (dimercaprol), or deferoxamine. These complexes are water soluble and are readily excreted by the kidney.

PESTICIDES

More than 1500 active pesticide ingredients are registered with the U.S. Environmental Protection Agency (EPA).[66] Most studies assessing the toxicity of pesticides focus on the active chemical agent, but in practice, several pesticides may be mixed, or several pesticides may be used sequentially. These practices, coupled with exposure to additives or contaminants, make it difficult to evaluate toxicity possibly related to pesticides. Regional poison control centers and county extension agents are often useful sources of information regarding pesticide products.

Insecticides represent the largest category of toxins found in the home. The three major groups of insecticides, in order of highest to lowest toxicity, are organophosphates, carbamates, and pyrethroids. Most insecticides found in the home contain pyrethrins and growth regulators rather than organophosphates and carbamates. Insecticides of the organophosphate and carbamate categories are neurotoxins that act by phosphorylating pseudocholinesterase (PchE) and acetylcholinesterase (AchE). When this happens, enzymatic activity is inhibited and the cholinergic neurotransmitter, acetylcholine, cannot be hydrolyzed on its release from the nerve ending. Accumulating acetylcholine continues to stimulate muscarinic and nicotinic receptors throughout the central and peripheral nervous system. Most organophosphates are designed so that inhibition of the cholinesterases is irreversible. In contrast, the neurotoxic actions that result from carbamate exposure reverse with time. Clinical signs and symptoms of acute organophosphate poisoning are related directly to the degree of cholinesterase inhibition.[67,68] Pseudocholinesterase activity decreases more rapidly than that of acetylcholinesterase. Clinical symptoms of acute poisoning are experienced when about 40% of the cholinesterase is inhibited; these symptoms include wheezing and increased bronchial secretions. With moderate to larger exposure, muscle weakness, paralysis, tachycardia, headache, ataxia, and confusion may occur. In cases of massive exposure, death occurs when respiration is blocked by a combination of bronchoconstriction, increased bronchial secretion, diaphragmatic contractions, and inhibition of respiratory centers in the brain stem.

Organophosphate exposure is associated with an additional neurotoxic syndrome known as organophosphate-induced delayed neuropathy (OPIDN). This syndrome is not related to cholinesterase inhibition but to inhibition of neurotoxic esterase (NTE).[68] The clinical presentation of OPIDN occurs several days to weeks after exposure, when the cholinergic symptoms have resolved. Symptoms of OPIDN include mild sensory disturbances, ataxia, weakness, fatigue, reduced tendon reflexes, and muscle twitching and tenderness. In severe cases, it may progress to flaccid lower limb paralysis. Frequently, memory and cognitive abilities are impaired. No specific therapy is available; resolution of symptoms may take months or years, or symptoms may persist permanently. Chronic exposure to some organophosphates can cause long-lasting neurological defects involving vision, memory, and learning. These changes have been observed in humans and in other mammals.

For acute exposure, laboratory testing includes monitoring of blood gases and acid-base status, renal and liver function tests, coagulation studies, and measurement of serum pseudocholinesterase activity. Pseudocholinesterase activity has the greatest clinical utility if pre-exposure testing has been done as part of occupational monitoring. When baseline studies are not available, assessing the degree of inhibition is difficult, because activity is related to liver function. Additionally, it should be noted that other chemicals and drugs are known to inhibit cholinesterase.

Rodenticides such as strychnine, arsenic, warfarin, and phosphorus are toxic not only to the targeted pest but also to non-rodents, including humans. Because these products usually are placed in areas accessible to the targeted pest and to livestock, pets, and children, these latter groups are most likely to be involved in cases of accidental poisoning. Intentional poisoning of unsuspecting individuals with rodenticides is rare, but a number of reports on the anticoagulant-based rodenticides, known as superwarfarins, have described their use in simulating bleeding disorders. These particular pesticides, developed to combat the growing resistance of rats and mice to the older formulas, include brodifacoum, bromadiolone, chlorophacinone, and difenacoum. The superwarfarins act by inhibiting the synthesis of coagulation factors II, VII, IX, and X. Symptoms of acute ingestion are consistent with those of other coagulopathies and include transient abdominal pain, vomiting, bruising, hematuria, and heme-positive stools. Although these patients must be watched closely for bleeding, hospitalization may not be necessary. In cases of intentional chronic ingestion, the patient may present with complaints of easy bruising and fatigue and may be found to have heme-positive stools or hematuria.[69]

Few data are available regarding the pharmacokinetic parameters of these agents in humans. Brodifacoum, chlorophacinone, and difenacoum are 100 times more active than regular warfarin. Half-lives are variable but typically extend up to 120 days. The chemicals are metabolized in the liver via the cytochrome P-450 system. Laboratory studies may show a prolonged prothrombin time. The superwarfarins can be measured in serum or plasma with the use of high-performance liquid chromatography.

VOLATILES

By far, ethanol is the drug most commonly encountered in the toxicology laboratory. This drug is readily absorbed from the entire gastrointestinal tract. Because the compound is both water and lipid soluble, it readily crosses most cellular membranes, including the blood-brain barrier and the placenta. The distribution of ethanol follows the water content of the tissue or fluid into which it is moving. As a result, the concentration of ethanol in plasma is ≈1.2 times greater than in whole blood. When ingested with food, the efficiency and rate of absorption are greatly reduced.

Ethanol follows saturation kinetics, so metabolism changes from first order at low concentrations to zero order when the concentration exceeds what the available alcohol dehydrogenase, the primary metabolizing enzyme, can handle. At least two hepatic enzyme systems are involved in the metabolism of ethanol, in addition to alcohol dehydrogenase: the microsomal ethanol oxidizing system and peroxidase-catalase. Other enzymes become involved in ethanol metabolism, depending on the concentration and whether exposure is chronic, as with an alcoholic.[70,71] The acetaldehyde (metabolite) formed is toxic to most tissues. The preferred sample for clinical toxicology is serum or whole blood, but urine, breath, and oral fluid also may be used. Detection occurs through enzymatic methods or gas chromatography. All states have adopted 80 mg/dL (0.08 %) as the legal indication of intoxication. The lethal dose of ethanol varies greatly, depending on whether or not the patient ingests ethanol on a frequent basis. For this reason, the lethal concentration is reported to range between 350 and 500 mg/dL, although death has been reported with much lower concentrations.

Excessive ingestion of ethanol, or alcoholism, is harmful and is considered a serious public health issue. The drug is eliminated rapidly from the circulation in most conditions, and so blood level may not be a good indicator of abstinence. For this reason, other biomarkers of alcoholism have been sought over the years. These have included the use of enzymes such as gamma-glutamyl transferase or the aminotransferases, mean corpuscular volume, and carbohydrate-deficient transferrin. Because each of these has limitations pertaining to sensitivity and specificity, interest has been expressed in using two of the minor metabolites, ethylglucuronide and ethylsulphate, as biomarkers of ingestion. These non-volatile metabolites have longer half-lives than ethanol and are excreted readily into the urine, where each may be detected for several days. However, these markers are not specific to abuse, as evidenced by the recent report that even topical exposure to ethanol leads to their formation.[71] Both may be measured with gas chromatography/mass spectrometry or liquid chromatography/tandem mass spectrometry.

Methanol, isopropyl, and ethylene glycol also are metabolized by alcohol dehydrogenase to form toxic metabolites. As a result, prevention of toxicity is dependent on early identification and treatment with ethanol or fomepazole, an inhibitor of alcohol dehydrogenase. Increases in anion gap and/or osmol gap that are not explainable by other toxins or pathological processes (e.g., diabetic ketoacidosis, renal failure) may help the clinician to recognize ingestion. With ethylene glycol, calcium oxalate crystals, particularly the monohydrate form, often are present and suggestive of poisoning. Serum levels are quantified through gas chromatography. Patients also should be monitored through blood gases and renal and liver function tests.

KEY CONCEPTS BOX 55-10

- CO, created by incomplete combustion, binds to hemoglobin, thus preventing delivery of O_2 to cells. Hyperbaric oxygen is the antidote.
- Hg, Cd, As, and other heavy metals (see Table 55-11) are usually industrial poisons that act by binding to sulfhydryl groups in enzymes, thereby inhibiting enzymatic activity.
- Urine is the best sample for chronic heavy metal exposure; serum is best for acute exposure. Heavy metals usually are measured by atomic absorption spectroscopy.
- Insecticides as a common home poison usually are less toxic pyrethroids.
- Serum cholinesterase activity is a measure of exposure to the neurotoxic organophophates.
- Ethanol, methanol, and isopropanol are volatile alcohols that are metabolized to toxic metabolites by hepatic alcohol dehydrogenase.
- Calcium oxalate crystals are an important laboratory finding, suggesting toxic exposure to ethylene glycol.

REFERENCES

1. Wu AH, McKay C, Broussard LA, et al: National Academy of Clinical Biochemistry Laboratory Medicine Practice Guidelines: recommendations for the use of laboratory tests to support poisoned patients who present to the emergency department, Clin Chem 49:357, 2003.
2. Flanagan RJ: Developing an analytical toxicology service: principles and guidance, Toxicol Rev 23:251, 2004.
3. Drummer OH: Post-mortem toxicology, Forensic Sci Int 165:199, 2007.
4. Levine BA: *Principles of Forensic Toxicology: Revised and Updated,* ed 2, Washington, DC, 2006, AACC Press.
5. Dorato MA, Engelhardt JA: The no-observed-adverse-effect-level in drug safety evaluations: use, issues, and definition(s), Regul Toxicol Pharmacol 42:265, 2005.
6. Aarons L, Graham G: Methodological approaches to the population analysis of toxicity data, Toxicol Lett 12:405, 2001.
7. Sidell F: Chemical agent terrorism, 1996. Available at www.nbc-med.org.
8. Yanagisawa N, Morita H, Nakajima T: Sarin experiences in Japan: acute toxicity and long-term effects, J Neurol Sci 249:76, 2006.
9. van der Schans MJ, Polhuijs M, van Dijk C, et al: Retrospective detection of exposure to nerve agents: analysis of phosphofluoridates originating from fluoride-induced reactivation of phosphorylated BuChE, Arch Toxicol 78:508, 2004.
10. Whitfield AH: Too much of a good thing? The danger of water intoxication in endurance sports, Br J Gen Pract 56:542, 2006.
11. Travis KZ, Pate I, Welsh ZK, Leonard BE: An introduction to enantiomers in psychopharmacology, Hum Psychopharmacol 16:S79, 2001.
12. Geyer SJ: Portrait in history: Percivall Pott, Arch Pathol Lab Med 123:661, 1999.
13. Cullen JM, Miller RT: The role of pathology in the identification of drug-induced hepatic toxicity, Expert Opin Drug Metab Toxicol 2:241, 2006.

14. Sabolić I: Common mechanisms in nephropathy induced by toxic metals, Nephron Physiol 104:107, 2006.
15. Castell JV, Donato MT, Gómez-Lechón MJ: Metabolism and bioactivation of toxicants in the lung: the in vitro cellular approach, Exp Toxicol Pathol 57(suppl 1):189, 2005.
16. Costa LG, Giordano G, Guizzetti M, Vitalone A: Neurotoxicity of pesticides: a brief review, Front Biosci 13:1240, 2008.
17. Kosnett MJ, Wedeen RP, Rothenberg SJ, et al: Recommendations for medical management of adult lead exposure, Environ Health Perspect 115:463, 2007.
18. Vahidnia A, van der Voet GB, de Wolff FA: Arsenic neurotoxicity: a review, Hum Exp Toxicol 26:823, 2007.
19. Bretveld R, Brouwers M, Ebisch I, Roeleveld N: Influence of pesticides on male fertility, Scand J Work Environ Health 33:13, 2007.
20. Winker R, Rudiger HW: Reproductive toxicology in occupational settings: an update, Int Arch Occup Environ Health 79:1, 2006.
21. Benedetti MS, Whomsley R, Canning M: Drug metabolism in the paediatric population and in the elderly, Drug Discov Today 12:599, 2007.
22. Gatzidou ET, Zira AN, Theocharis SE: Toxicogenomics: a pivotal piece in the puzzle of toxicological research, J Appl Toxicol 27:302, 2007.
23. Lynch T, Price A: The effect of cytochrome P450 metabolism on drug response, interactions, and adverse effects, Am Fam Physician 76:391, 2007.
24. Flockhart DA: Cytochrome P450 drug interactions table, 2007. Available at http://medicine.iupui.edu/flockhart.
25. Sweeney BP, Bromilow J: Liver enzyme induction and inhibition: implications for anaesthesia, Anaesthesia 61:159, 2006.
26. Jacobson-Kram D, McGovern T: Toxicological overview of impurities in pharmaceutical products, Adv Drug Deliv Rev 59:38, 2007.
27. Fenton J: *The Laboratory and the Poisoned Patient,* Washington, DC, 1998, AACC Press.
28. Hammett-Stabler CA, Pesce AJ, Cannon D: Urine drug screening in the medical setting, Clin Chim Acta 315:125, 2001.
29. Flanagan RJ, Connally G: Interpretation of analytical toxicology results in life and at postmortem, Toxicol Rev 24:51, 2005.
30. Pohjola-Sintonen S, Kivistö KT, Vuori E, et al: Identification of drugs ingested in acute poisoning: correlation of patient history with drug analyses, Ther Drug Monit 22:749, 2000.
31. Bosse GM, Matyunas NJ: Delayed toxidromes, J Emerg Med 17:679, 1999.
32. Abbruzzi G, Stork CM: Pediatric toxicologic concerns, Emerg Med Clin North Am 20:223, 2002.
33. http://www.nimh.nih.gov/health/publications/suicide-in-the-us-statistics-and-prevention/index.shtml
34. Substance Abuse and Mental Health Services Administration: Results from the 2006 National Survey on Drug Use and Health: National Findings. Available at 0.
35. Miles DR, Lanni S, Jansson L, Svikis D: Smoking and illicit drug use during pregnancy: impact on neonatal outcome, J Reprod Med 51:567, 2006.
36. Das G: Cocaine abuse in North America: a milestone in history, J Clin Pharm 33:296, 1993.
37. Lawrence DT, Bechtel L, Walsh JP, Holstege CD: The evaluation and management of acute poisoning emergencies, Minerva Med 98:543, 2007.
38. Roberts DM, Buckley NA: Pharmacokinetic considerations in clinical toxicology: clinical applications, Clin Pharmacokinet 46:897, 2007.
39. Kraemer T, Paul LD: Bioanalytical procedures for determination of drugs of abuse in blood, Anal Bioanal Chem 388:1415, 2007.
40. Jones AW: Urine as a biological specimen for forensic analysis of alcohol and variability in the urine-to-blood relationship, Toxicol Rev 25:15, 2006.
41. Musshoff F, Madea B: Review of biologic matrices (urine, blood, hair) as indicators of recent or ongoing cannabis use, Ther Drug Monit 28:155, 2006.
42. Samyn N, Laloup M, De Boeck G: Bioanalytical procedures for determination of drugs of abuse in oral fluid, Anal Bioanal Chem 388:1437, 2007.
43. Gray T, Huestis M: Bioanalytical procedures for monitoring in utero drug exposure, Anal Bioanal Chem 388:1455, 2007.
44. Kintz P: Bioanalytical procedures for detection of chemical agents in hair in the case of drug-facilitated crimes, Anal Bioanal Chem 388:1467, 2007.
45. Palmeri A, Pichini S, Pacifici R, et al: Drugs in nails: physiology, pharmacokinetics and forensic toxicology, Clin Pharmacokinet 38:95, 2000.
46. Peters FT: Stability of analytes in biosamples—an important issue in clinical and forensic toxicology? Anal Bioanal Chem 388:1505, 2007.
47. Drummer OH: Requirements for bioanalytical procedures in postmortem toxicology, Anal Bioanal Chem 388:1495, 2007.
48. Jortani SA, Snyder JW, Valdes RV Jr: The role of the clinical laboratory in managing chemical or biological terrorism, Clin Chem 46:1883, 2000.
49. Schwenk M, Kluge S, Jaroni H: Toxicological aspects of preparedness and aftercare for chemical-incidents, Toxicology 214:232, 2005.
50. Cantrell FL: Look what I found! Poison hunting on eBay, Clin Toxicol (Phila) 43:375, 2005.
51. Dasgupta A, Bernard DW: Herbal remedies: effects on clinical laboratory tests, Arch Pathol Lab Med 130:521, 2006.
52. Weldon MM, Smolinski MS, Maroufi A, et al: Mercury poisoning associated with a Mexican beauty cream, West J Med 173:15, 2000.
53. Bessems JG, Vermeulen NP: Paracetamol (acetaminophen)-induced toxicity: molecular and biochemical mechanisms, analogues, and protective approaches, Crit Rev Toxicol 31:55, 2001.
54. Larson AM: Acetaminophen hepatotoxicity, Clin Liver Dis 11:525, 2007.
55. Collins SP, Gesell LB, Zemlan FP: Neurotoxicity in acetaminophen overdose, Acad Emerg Med 8:495, 2001.
56. O'Malley GF: Emergency department management of the salicylate-poisoned patient, Emerg Med Clin North Am 25:333, 2007.
57. Quinton MS, Yamamoto BK: Causes and consequences of methamphetamine and MDMA toxicity, AAPS J 12:E337, 2006.
58. Grotenhermen F: Pharmacology of cannabinoids, Neuro Endocrinol Lett 25:14, 2004.
59. Glauser J, Queen JR: An overview of non-cardiac cocaine toxicity, J Emerg Med 32:181, 2007.
60. Afonso L, Mohammad T, Thatai D: Crack whips the heart: a review of the cardiovascular toxicity of cocaine, Am J Cardiol 100:1040, 2007.
61. Reisfield GM, Salazar E, Bertholf RL: Rational use and interpretation of urine drug testing in chronic opioid therapy, Ann Clin Lab Sci 37:301, 2007.
62. Hoaken PN, Stewart SH: Drugs of abuse and the elicitation of human aggressive behavior, Addict Behav 28:1533, 2003.
63. Gable RS: Acute toxic effects of club drugs, J Psychoactive Drugs 36:303, 2004.
64. Wong CG, Chan KF, Gibson KM, Snead OC: Gamma-hydroxybutyric acid: neurobiology and toxicology of a recreational drug, Toxicol Rev 23:3, 2004.
65. Stoller KP: Hyperbaric oxygen and carbon monoxide poisoning: a critical review, Neurol Res 29:146, 2007.
66. U.S. Environmental Protection Agency (EPA): *Pesticides Industry Sales and Usage,* Washington, DC, 1999, EPA, Publication no. 733-R-99-001.

67. Costa LG: Current issues in organophosphate toxicology, Clin Chim Acta 366:1, 2006.
68. Abou-Donia MB: Organophosphorus ester–induced chronic neurotoxicity, Arch Environ Health 58:484, 2003.
69. Spahr JE, Maul JS, Rodgers GM: Superwarfarin poisoning: a report of two cases and review of the literature, Am J Hematol 82:656, 2007.
70. Zakhari S: Overview: how is alcohol metabolized by the body? Alcohol Res Health 29:245, 2006.
71. Niemelä O: Biomarkers in alcoholism, Clin Chim Acta 377:39, 2007.

INTERNET RESOURCES

http://medicine.iupui.edu/flockhart/—Indiana University's Cytochrome P450 Drug Interaction Table

http://npic.orst.edu/—National Pesticide Information Center

http://ntp-server.niehs.nih.gov/—National Institute of Environmental Health Sciences

http://physchem.ox.ac.uk/MSDS/—The Physical and Theoretical Chemistry Laboratory, Oxford University, Chemical and Other Safety Information

http://toxnet.nlm.nih.gov/—TOXNET, U.S. National Library of Medicine

http://www.aapcc.org/—American Association of Poison Control Centers useful data, educational information, games

http://www.acsmedchem.org/module/acidbase.html—Pharmaceutical Sciences 3320, Principles of Drug Action Functional Groups, Acid Base Chemistry and Physicochemical Properties

http://www.ag.ohio-state.edu/—The Ohio University Pesticide Education Program

http://www.bertholf.net/rlb/Lectures/index.htm—Click on "Clinical and Forensic Toxicology"

http://www.bioterrorism.slu.edu/—Center for the Study of Bioterrorism and Emerging Infections at St. Louis University

http://www.cdc.gov/nchs/deaths.htm—National Center for Health Statistics

http://www.chemhelper.com/tutorials.html—Stereochemistry Tutorial

http://www.epa.gov/—U.S. Environmental Protection Agency

http://www.haz-map.com/—Database of Hazardous Chemicals

http://www.usdoj.gov/dea/concern/concern.htm—U.S. Drug Enforcement Agency

http://www.oas.samhsa.gov/– Substance Abuse and Mental Health Services Administration (SAMHSA), Office of Applied Studies

http://emedicine.medscape.com/article/168139-overview—Toxicity, Salicylate, Azer M (last updated: November 8, 2007)

http://emedicine.medscape.com/article/820200-overview—Toxicity, Acetaminophen, Farrell SE (last updated: October 3, 2007)

Addiction and Substance Abuse

R. Jeffrey Goldsmith

56

Chapter

Chapter Outline

The Addiction Process
Theories to Explain Addiction
Prevalence of Addiction Among Various Groups
Diagnosis of Substance Abuse, Substance Dependence, and Addiction
Recovery and the Treatment Process
The Preemployment or Random Drug Screen
Why Individuals Fail Drug Screens
Change of Analyte in Disease

Key Terms

addiction The compulsive use of a psychoactive chemical, causing problems in the user's life on a physical, psychological, or sociocultural level. Unconscious psychological defenses like denial are a common feature, distorting the addict's self-awareness and confusing the people around him or her. Addiction is a chronic deteriorating process that leads to death or institutionalization if unchecked. Abstinence allows the mind and body to recover sufficiently to work on the social deficits and deteriorated relationships.

contingency contracts Behavioral plans that engage the addict in a carefully delineated treatment program. The consequences of failure to follow through are clearly spelled out in the hope that this will encourage the addict to remain in treatment.

craving An intense urge to use a drug; it may be short lived or tormentingly chronic. Some addicts have environmental triggers for this craving; others have psychological states that evoke the urge, but many have no craving at all.

drug screens Qualitative analyses of the body fluid (urine, blood, saliva, and so forth) of a patient in a search for the possible presence of addictive substances. There usually is a brief list of five to ten drugs for which a sample is screened; however, more comprehensive lists sometimes are requested.

recovery The process of growth and development that occurs after sustained abstinence. Spirituality is an important element in recovery because of the need to transcend the intense self-focus or experience of victimization that many addicts exhibit.

rehabilitation A comprehensive, multicomponent treatment for alcoholics and addicts who are abstinent and are not in withdrawal. It addresses the consequences of alcohol or drug use, the personal problems that are not directly related to use of the chemical, and skills needed for ongoing abstinence and recovery.

substance abuse and **dependence** Two generic terms that pertain to the pathological use of psychoactive substances. Both terms refer to specific diagnoses in the *Diagnostic and Statistical Manual of Mental Disorders, Fourth Edition* (DSM-IV). Dependence includes psychological dependence and physiological dependence; abuse incorporates both psychological and behavioral importance. People use the term *substance abuse* to include alcohol and drug misuse that would not be a DSM-IV diagnosis.

tolerance The behavioral and neurochemical adaptation to the drug effects of a psychoactive substance. It allows the person to experience progressively less toxicity from the substance. Everyone can exhibit some tolerance; however, addicts exhibit a great deal of tolerance.

withdrawal The central nervous system adjustment to the relatively sudden cessation of regular psychoactive substance use. Physical, psychological, and behavioral changes occur in these states. The symptoms of withdrawal are frequently the opposite of the acute effects of the substance.

Methods on Evolve

Alcohol
Drug screen

Addiction and abuse of alcohol and other drugs affect a significant portion of the population of many countries. Alcohol is the most commonly abused substance in Western civilization, and the patterns of behavior seen with alcohol are common to other drugs such as marijuana (marihuana), cocaine, opioids, benzodiazepines, and agents such as glue and petrol (gasoline), which are sniffed. The term *addiction* is defined as "the compulsive use of a psychoactive substance, causing problems in the user's life on a physical, psychological, or sociocultural level." Unconscious psychological defenses against the consequences of addiction, like denial, are common features that distort the addict's self-awareness and confuse the people around him. Addiction is a chronic deteriorating process that leads to death or institutionalization if unchecked. Abstinence from the addictive agent allows the mind and body to recover sufficiently to work on the social deficits and deteriorated relationships that may have pre-dated or resulted from the addiction.

SECTION OBJECTIVE BOX 56-1

- Describe the key steps in the addiction process.

THE ADDICTION PROCESS

It is important to understand that alcohol or other drug use by itself is not addiction. For example, a national survey of eighth to twelfth graders showed that 40.5% of eighth graders, 61.5% of tenth graders, and 72.7% of twelfth graders had tried alcohol.[1] Similarly, 15.7% of eighth graders, 31.8% of tenth graders, and 42.3% of twelfth graders had used marijuana at least once, and 3.4% of eighth graders, 4.8% of tenth graders, and 8.5% of twelfth graders had used cocaine at least once.[1] Drug use within the last month by the same group show considerable decreases in percentage: only 45.3% of twelfth graders had used alcohol recently, 18.3% marijuana, and 2.5% cocaine. Because addiction implies the need to use drugs frequently, it is clear that not all of those who have used these drugs are addicted to them.

For some people, escalating consumption of alcohol, tobacco, or street drugs leads to the development of the clinical syndrome of **substance abuse** or **dependence.**[2] Getting high and calming down when the drug is metabolized in the body is the first experience. If the person continues to use additional drugs within a short time, a number of side effects, usually irritability, tension, depression, and anxiety, may gather unexpectedly. The person must explain to himself how the unwanted feelings happened and often does this by ignoring the drug use and blaming the unwanted feelings on someone else (family, friends, etc.). These negative side effects encourage the person to continue to use the drug to feel "normal." A person who is using excessive alcohol and/or drugs now feels that something is out of control and is not sure what it is. Furthermore, sections of the brain can motivate someone to use the drug at the moment, and learned physiological responses within the brain can influence choices for use in the future. This motivation teams up with the individual's other feelings and can alter self-awareness and desire.

Denial is a psychological defense mechanism that preserves the positive aspects of using alcohol or drugs and splits off the negative side effects to blame on someone else.[3] The chemicals alter behaviors, and the person behaves differently. The discrepancy between the intended behavior and what actually occurs is explained away by excuses and alibis. The person becomes more invested in this denial to understand his or her world in this new fashion. Treatment involves disrupting the denial, so that the person can see his or her actual behavior; this awareness leads to changes in motivation.

Part of the late stage of addiction is the **withdrawal** syndrome, that is, symptoms that occur when no drugs are used. The brain goes through adaptive physiological changes because regular use of drugs alters brain chemistry. A list of withdrawal symptoms that may be observed is presented in Box 56-1. Another aspect of addiction is **craving.** A craving is an intense desire to use a drug.[4] This can occur when the individual is placed in situations that remind him or her of previous drug use, or when a particular mood triggers the urge to get high. Some people do not experience craving.

KEY CONCEPTS BOX 56-1

- A psychological need for drugs may be the initial step in drug addiction.
- Continued drug use may lead to dependence on the drug.
- Denial of addition and the need to shift balm for the addition to another person are also important components of the addition process.
- Addiction and drug craving may lead to withdrawal symptoms late in the process.

SECTION OBJECTIVES BOX 56-2

- Describe the psychological and physiological theories of addiction.
- Describe the recent patterns of drug abuse.

THEORIES TO EXPLAIN ADDICTION

A variety of psychosocial models of addiction have been used to explain the process. All incorporate the addict's high affinity for alcohol and drug use and the large quantities consumed. The models differ in how they explain the individual's movement down the path to addiction and the addicted state once it has been achieved. Each theory has led to different types of treatment interventions. The disease concept proposes that addictions are rooted in a biological vulnerability.[5] Abstinence is the only resolution for the disease, and treatment focuses on understanding loss of control. Treatment provides alternative motivation through problem-solving skills, coping devices, and pharmacotherapy. Attachment theory, self-psychology, and affect regulation theory characterize addiction as an attachment disorder that is induced by a person's attempt to self-repair developmental deficits in psychic structure and early environmental deprivation, leading to ineffec-

Box 56-1

Withdrawal Symptoms

Alcohol and Sedatives
Tremor
Nausea
Vomiting
Tachycardia
Sweating
High blood pressure
Anxiety
Irritability or depressed mood
Orthostatic hypotension

Tobacco
Craving
Irritability
Difficulty in concentrating
Restlessness
Headache

Stimulants and Cocaine
Sleepiness (hypersomnia)
Hyperphagia (abnormally increased appetite)
Depressed mood (±suicidal)

Opiates
Lacrimation (tear production)
Rhinorrhea ("runny nose")
Dilated pupils
Piloerection (involuntary erection of body hair)
Sweating
Diarrhea
Yawning
Mild hypertension
Tachycardia
Fever
Insomnia
Flulike syndrome with myalgia

Caffeine
Headache
Sleepiness
Irritability

Marijuana
Irritability
Loss of appetite
Insomnia

tive attachment styles.[6] Treatment seeks to improve this painful sense of self and shifts the individual's motivation to use alcohol and drugs as a coping mechanism.

PREVALENCE OF ADDICTION AMONG VARIOUS GROUPS

Age groups tell a lot about alcohol and drug use. The use of alcohol and common street drugs usually starts during the teenage years, and national studies recognize 12 to 17 years as the youngest age group involved and 18 to 25 years as the next oldest group.[7] After 25 years of age, most people decrease their drinking and illegal drug use, so that heavy drinking and continued drug use beyond 25 years of age should provide a hint of substance abuse or dependence. Because denial diminishes the consumption history, and because others in the 18- to 25-year-old age group are common drug and alcohol users, it is hard to make a clinical diagnosis in this age group without special training. Table 56-1 describes the various types of alcohol and drug use that are seen among different age groups. The heaviest alcohol use occurs in the 18- to 25-year-old age group, and usage decreases in the older groups.

Studies from 30 years ago provide important evidence of a developmental pattern of drug use.[8] Teenage males use both alcohol and tobacco before using marijuana. Girls vary and use one or the other before trying marijuana. Marijuana use often precedes the use of other illegal drugs. Thus highly addictive and illegal drugs are preceded by less addictive and legal substances. It is probable that these "gateway drugs" sensitize certain parts of the brain.

Misuse of medication is a major cause of morbidity and mortality (see p. 1094, Chapter 55) (Table 56-2).

An increase in pain disorders is seen among older American adults, and inadvertent addiction while taking narcotic medication for valid medical purposes can happen.[9,10] Prescription drug misuse includes drugs diverted for non-medical purposes (both sale and consumption) by the physician or by the patient. Alcoholics and those with medical problems are at high risk for developing substance abuse and dependence. This has led to a new increase in use among teenagers. High school seniors reported increased non-medical use of narcotics between 1991 and 2006 (6.6% up to 13.4%), suggesting that this is a common problem among teens that mimics that seen in older adults who have medical challenges.[1]

Table 56-1 Prevalence of U.S. Alcohol and Drug Use by Age Group in 2006 (percentage of population) in National Survey on Drug Use and Health

U.S. Citizens, Age	Lifetime Alcohol	Past Month Heavy Drinking*	Past Month Tobacco	Past Month Marijuana	Past Month Cocaine
12 to 17	40.4%	2.4%	12.9%	6.7%	0.4%
18 to 25	86.5%	15.6%	43.9%	16.3%	2.2%
26 and over	87.7%	36.0%	29.4%	4.2%	0.8%

*Heavy drinkers had five or more drinks per occasion on 5 or more days over the previous 30 days.

Table 56-2 Examples of Medical Pathophysiology Associated With Chronic Abuse*

Substance	Disease
Alcohol	Liver cirrhosis Cardiomyopathy Fetal alcohol syndrome Trauma of all types Viral infection Gastrointestinal cancer Stroke Insomnia Depression
Cocaine	Nasal septum perforation Viral infection Cardiac arrest Seizure Panic attack Paranoia Premature birth
Opiates	Viral infection Hepatitis Self-poisoning Insomnia Neonatal withdrawal
Tobacco	Pulmonary disorder Cancer of various types Heart attack Osteoporosis Low birth weight

*These occur in addition to withdrawal symptoms.

The substance abuser or dependent person may use more than one drug.[11] About 21% of alcoholics are also dependent on other illegal drugs, and 37% have other psychiatric illness. At least 50% of methadone maintenance patients meet alcohol dependence criteria. The person who is positive for an illegal substance such as cocaine is also likely to be positive for alcohol, opioids, and marijuana on a drug screen.[12]

KEY CONCEPTS BOX 56-2

- There are both psychological and biological theories of addition to explain why some individuals become addicted.
- Prevalence of addiction varies among various age groups; the prevalence of addictions is greater in the 18-25 age range compared to older adults.
- Use of "gateway drugs" by young individuals can lead to use of more addictive drugs.
- Use of legal medications can lead to abuse of those medications and addiction.

SECTION OBJECTIVES BOX 56-3

- Describe the method of diagnosis of addiction.
- Define withdrawal and list some of the key symptoms of withdrawal.
- Describe the role of drug screens in the recovery/treatment process.

Box 56-2

Diagnostic Criteria of Substance Dependence

A maladaptive pattern of substance use that leads to clinical impairment or distress within a 12-month period.
Tolerance: substance is used in larger amounts over a period of time.
Loss of control: A lot of time is spent obtaining, using, or recovering from drugs.
Use despite reasons not to use: Useful activities are given up or reduced because of drug use.
Withdrawal symptoms

DIAGNOSIS OF SUBSTANCE ABUSE, SUBSTANCE DEPENDENCE, AND ADDICTION

The diagnosis of substance abuse or dependence happens quickly at times, if the person identifies loss of control right away, and is difficult at other times, when signs and symptoms are masked by the user. Positive **drug screens** by themselves are not a diagnosis. The use of alcohol and drugs is a very common phenomenon in the United States. Positive drug screens indicate that these substances were used within a certain time period before body fluids were collected. The final diagnosis of abuse or dependence must be made on clinical grounds by a therapist or a physician who takes a history and observes the signs and symptoms of addiction. Long-term use of alcohol or drugs often mimics other psychiatric syndromes. A history of heavy alcohol or drug use is an important diagnostic finding because these are lifetime diagnoses. However, the user's denial is common and often obscures the clinician's awareness of use. Furthermore, other psychiatric disorders are seen frequently, and clinicians focus on these problems rather than on the drug use. Criteria for the diagnosis of substance abuse and dependence are listed in Box 56-2.[2]

Alcoholism is believed to be inherited, and a history of alcoholism in a person's family may place him at high risk for alcohol or drug dependence.[13] Other components of this vulnerability include psychological anxiety, social choices that encourage heavy use, and environmental influences that make drinking or drug use more desirable.

The presence of withdrawal symptoms is important and should raise questions about the user's level of dependence. Long-term regular use of narcotics for pain and sedatives for anxiety or insomnia can produce withdrawal symptoms. Physicians must be careful to examine past history of other illegal drug use and motivation to continue long-term use. Those clinicians who are not well trained in addiction may need expert help to make this clinical decision. The patient, his or her family, and the doctor are all affected by this clarification. Demanding prescriptions early and running out of pills before the proper date may be signs of overuse, not receiving enough, giving pills to others, or selling pills on the street. Long-term daily use of medications like sedatives and narcotics can accidentally lead to physical dependence and withdrawal symptoms. Each scenario is handled differently depending on the patient and the physician involved, and on how collaboratively the patient and family can work with the physician and with each other. A patient can disguise excessive drug use until confronted with positive drug screens or other information. Drug screens can confirm that a patient is using a drug not prescribed by the physician, or is using more than prescribed. A quantitative analysis may be useful when the patient is suspected of escalating the dose or getting prescriptions from other sources. Quantitative analysis over time can monitor how much medication is being taken.

Attempts to employ quantitative laboratory data often meet with mixed success. The combination of tests that includes gamma-glutamyl transferase, mean corpuscular volume, and aspartate aminotransferase can have a diagnostic sensitivity and specificity for alcoholism in the 70% to 95% range.[14] Carbohydrate-deficient transferrin (CDT) has emerged as a new biochemical marker that can be used to measure excessive alcohol consumption. Transferrin is a glycoprotein involved in transporting iron to body tissues. The carbohydrate content of transferrin usually is lower in individuals who are actively drinking alcohol; therefore, the term *carbohydrate-deficient transferrin* was coined. Consumption of four to seven alcoholic drinks per day for at least 1 week can elevate CDT levels significantly in regular drinking individuals. However, it is important to remember that elevated levels are only suggestive of alcoholism, not diagnostic.

RECOVERY AND THE TREATMENT PROCESS

Both inpatient and outpatient programs to stop the addiction cycle have met with considerable success. Almost half (46% inpatient and 30% outpatient) of the alcohol-dependent patients who completed treatment remained abstinent for at least 9 months.[15] The co-occurrence of other psychiatric disorders, other severe physical disorders, chaotic family problems, and serious financial challenges complicates these results. Families can help increase awareness, and external coercion by courts and other agencies can help improve retention of the patient in treatment. When the person appreciates that alcohol or drug use is out of control, and that this is making life unmanageable, he is more likely to commit to abstinence. Along with the commitment to abstinence comes improved cooperation from the patient to reverse the problem; this is the essence of **recovery.** By contract, when the person enjoys the effects of the addictive substances and denies unwanted side effects, even enforced monitoring may result in failed treatment. Treatment attempts to repair the environmental and psychological influences that led to the addiction. Spiritual help may be rallied, and efforts should be made to prevent relapse. Exploring the triggers for drug use allows people to discover alternative, nondrug coping mechanisms for life's problems.

Rehabilitation involves the use of behavioral contracts to overcome ambivalence about stopping drugs. In this particular circumstance, the addict agrees, or contracts, to fulfill a series of rehabilitation steps that may include drug screens, attendance at meetings of group psychotherapy, or Alcoholics Anonymous, and/or individual psychotherapy. The contract also specifies what will happen if the agreement is broken, for example, arranging for an Alcoholics Anonymous sponsor, or a more serious outcome such as reporting prohibited behaviors to the probation officer. Drug screening has many different uses in drug addiction treatment programs. Drug screening is a common component of rehabilitation and may occur on a routine or less regular basis. These screens usually test for a group of the most commonly abused drugs, but less common drugs are added by name if specific concern is expressed. However, if drug misuse is suspected on the basis of positive drug screens, this information is presented to the person for discussion of the use of medications that might show a "false-positive" result, or ongoing drug use. Such a discussion allows the person to stop a relapse early and to resume helpful behaviors and attitudes.

KEY CONCEPTS BOX 56-3

- At least 5 criteria are used by clinicians to diagnosis of substance abuse, substance dependence, and addiction. The diagnosis can only be based on clinical grounds.
- Many people need professional treatment to get into a recovering lifestyle. Drug screens are used to monitor and highlight problems in the recovery process.

SECTION OBJECTIVES BOX 56-4

- Describe the types of drugs screens used in the workplace.
- Describe why people fail drug tests.
- Describe how drug screens are used to detect drug abuse and to monitor rehabilitation.

THE PREEMPLOYMENT OR RANDOM DRUG SCREEN

Many employers use the preemployment drug screen to weed out those potential workers who they believe will introduce risk to their company. The literature has reported costly side effects of employee drug abuse, such as decreased productivity and increased use of health benefits.[16,17]

Various substances are measured in preemployment screens, depending on the situation. By law, those individuals employed by the federal government and those who are under the authority of the Department of Transportation will be screened for those drugs specified by the Substance Abuse Mental Health Service Administration, including opioids, cocaine, barbiturates, marijuana, and phencyclidine. Employers also screen for illegal substances in individuals who are already employed. These screens are performed "for cause," because of actions that introduce the suspicion of drug abuse. Random drug screens are used to increase the likelihood of detecting individuals who are using illegal drugs. In the case of transportation workers, the time and place of the drug screen usually are specified. For other groups, such as the military, screening is often done on a random basis.

WHY INDIVIDUALS FAIL DRUG SCREENS

Even people who know in advance that they will be tested for drugs still fail drug screens. There are several explanations for this. The first is that the person did not understand the physiological aspects of drug testing. The person is not familiar with drug half-lives and does not appreciate how long drugs remain detectable in the blood and urine after the time of last use. Second, an individual who is tested may be in denial about his own addiction and may not comprehend that the drug testing will pick up his drugs of use. The rationale is that drug testing is done "to catch an addict; because I am not an addict, it is not going to catch me." A third reason is that the addicted individual may have no intention of using drugs around the time of the announced drug screen; however, loss of control may cause him or her to use drugs at an inopportune moment. Loss of control may happen in reaction to psychological stress, because of anxiety about the drug test, or in reaction to craving. Withdrawal symptoms can lead people to feel compelled to use drugs to reduce those symptoms. Psychological reasons, such as guilt, may trigger failure of a drug test in order that the guilty person can be caught.

When individuals test positive on a drug screen, someone must be responsible to determine whether the result is caused by a properly prescribed medicine. Therefore, drug screens should be reviewed by a medical review officer (or a knowledgeable physician) who can interpret the drug screen in light of the person's drug and medical history.[16]

CHANGE OF ANALYTE IN DISEASE

A drug screen often is used as part of the diagnostic and treatment process. What is meant by a drug screen is referred to in Chapter 55. In general, drug screens use untimed urine specimens obtained from the patient at random intervals, when certain changes in behavior occur, or at specified intervals. Drug screening has many different uses in drug addiction treatment programs. Identification of drug use is an important function of drug screening, given the unreliability of the alcohol or drug history provided by patients.

Use of drug screens also can be critical in the confrontation of active denial in these patients. Although the purpose is to identify alcohol or drug abuse, the data also may be used to confront the person's denial. Drugs that are screened for, based on earlier discussion, include alcohol, marijuana, cocaine, opioids, and so forth. It must be kept in mind that some agents such as carisoprodol are often not routinely tested.

Drug screening is a very powerful tool in enforcing rehabilitation **contingency contracts** that explicitly require abstinence from certain drugs. Without drug screening, contracts are often unenforceable. Relapse prevention programs use drug screening to monitor ongoing abstinence. The patient in the relapse prevention program has made a commitment to abstinence; however, with certain drugs like nicotine and cocaine, this commitment can be shaken by the experience of craving. Finally, drug screening is a legal requirement of the treatment in methadone maintenance clinics. Patients who are receiving methadone are required by law to get drug screening, and the results frequently are used to determine the future doses of methadone. If the methadone patient is still using opioids, in addition to the prescribed methadone, programs often change the methadone dose to see whether that induces the illegal opioids to be discontinued. Drugs to be screened may consist of only one, such as alcohol, or several, depending on the program. It must be realized that many addicts are multidrug users, and this information is important in the use and interpretation of drug screens.

An important component of drug screens may be the need for confirmation of a positive result (see p. 1096, Chapter 55). Certainly positive results from employment drug screens must be confirmed because livelihoods are at stake; results from certified laboratories also require confirmation.

KEY CONCEPTS BOX 56-4

- The employment screens can occur before and after employment.
- Post-employment drug screen can be random, scheduled, or "for cause."
- Employees for governmental agencies, military personal, and those in the transportation industry usually have routine drug screens.
- Individuals fail drug screens because they do not understand their own illness and do not understand the technical aspects of drug screening.
- Drug screens are important to monitor the comprehensive treatment for addictions.

REFERENCES

1. Johnston LD, O'Malley PM, Bachman JG, Schulenberg JE: *Monitoring the Future: National Results on Adolescent Drug Use: Overview of Key Findings,* Bethesda, MD, 2006, National Institute on Drug Abuse, NIH Publication no. 07-6202.
2. American Psychiatric Association: *Diagnostic and Statistical Manual of Mental Disorders, Fourth Edition,* Washington, DC, 1994, American Psychiatric Association.
3. Shaffer HJ, Simoneau G: Reducing resistance and denial by exercising ambivalence during the treatment of addiction, J Subst Abuse Treat 20:99, 2001.
4. Mezinskis J, Dyrenforth S, Goldsmith RJ, et al: Craving and withdrawal symptoms for various drugs of abuse, Psychiatr Ann 28:577, 1998.
5. Volkow ND: What do we know about drug addiction? Am J Psychiatry 162:1401, 2005.
6. Flores PJ: Addiction as an attachment disorder: implications for group therapy, Int J Group Psychother 51:63, 2001.
7. National Survey on Drug Use & Health. Available at http://www.oas.SAMHSA.gov/NSDUH.
8. Kandel DB, Kessler RC, Margulies RZ: Antecedents of adolescent initiation into stages of drug use: a developmental analysis, J Youth Adolesc 7:13, 1978.
9. Solomon DH, Avorn J, Wang PS, et al: Prescription opioid use among older adults with arthritis or low back pain, Arthritis Rheum 55:35, 2006.
10. Martell BA, O'Connor PG, Kerns RD, et al: Systematic review: opioid treatment for chronic back pain: prevalence, efficacy, and association with addiction, Ann Intern Med 146:116, 2007.
11. Crum RM: The epidemiology of addictive disorders. In Graham AW, Schultz TK, Mayo-Smith MF, et al, editors: *Principles of*

Addiction Medicine, ed 3, Chevy Chase, MD, 2003, American Society of Addiction Medicine, Inc., pp. 17-31.
12. Gorelick DA: Pharmacologic interventions for cocaine, crack, and other stimulant addiction. In Graham AW, Schultz TK, Mayo-Smith MF, et al, editors: *Principles of Addiction Medicine,* ed 3, Chevy Chase, MD, 2003, American Society of Addiction Medicine, Inc., pp. 785-800.
13. Nurnberger JI Jr, Wiegand R, Bucholz K, et al: A family study of alcohol dependence: coaggregation of multiple disorders in relatives of alcohol-dependent probands, Arch Gen Psychiatry 61:1246, 2004.
14. Warner EA: Laboratory diagnosis. In Graham AW, Schultz TK, Mayo-Smith MF, et al, editors: *Principles of Addiction Medicine,* ed 3, Chevy Chase, MD, 2003, American Society of Addiction Medicine, Inc., pp. 337-348.
15. Fuller RK, Hiller-Sturmhofel S: The treatment of alcoholism: a review. In Graham AW, Schultz TK, Mayo-Smith MF, et al, editors: *Principles of Addiction Medicine,* ed 3, Chevy Chase, MD, 2003, American Society of Addiction Medicine, Inc., pp. 409-418.
16. Swotinsky RB, editor: *The Medical Review Officer's Guide to Drug Testing,* New York, 1992, Van Nostrand Reinhold.

INTERNET SITES

http://www.usdoj.gov/dea/—U.S. Drug Enforcement Administration (DEA)

http://www.higheredcenter.org—Higher Education Center for Alcohol and Drug Prevention, a program from the U.S. Department of Education

http://www.oas.samhsa.gov/nsduh.htm—SAMHSA National Survey on Drug Use & Health

http://www.niaaa.nih.gov/—National Institute on Alcohol Abuse and Alcoholism (NIAAA)

http://www.nida.nih.gov/—National Institute on Drug Abuse (NIDA)

http://www.whitehousedrugpolicy.gov/—Office of National Drug Control Policy (ONDCP)

http://www.asam.org/—American Society of Addiction Medicine

http://www.aaap.org/—American Society of Addiction Psychiatry

http://www.casacolumbia.org/—National Center on Addiction and Substance Abuse at Columbia University

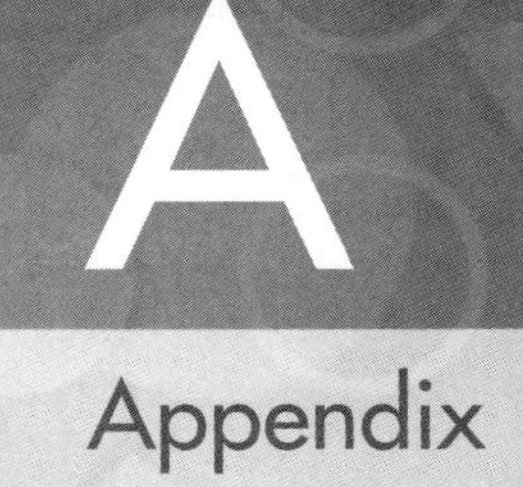

Buffer Solutions*

Appendix A

Buffer solutions (or buffers) are solutions whose pH value to a large degree is insensitive to the addition of other substances. It is important to realize, however, that the pH value of a buffer solution does not change only when acids or bases are added or on dilution, but also when the temperature changes or when neutral salts are added. In accurate work, therefore, it is important to check the pH value electrometrically after all ingredients have been added. The extent to which the pH values of buffer solutions vary when acids or bases are added or the temperature changes is shown in the table that follows. In general, dilution to half the concentration changes the pH value by only some hundredths of a unit (buffer No. 1 in the table opposite is an exception in that the change amounts to approximately pH 0.15); addition of 0.1-molar neutral salt solution may change the pH value to approximately 0.1.

In the table, the solutions are classified into general buffers (most in use for the past 50 years), universal buffers with a low buffering capacity but a wide pH range, and buffers for biological media with a moderate pH range but containing stable ingredients (phosphate and borate, for example, often undergo side reactions with biological media). An important property is often the transparency to ultraviolet light. Occasionally, it is desirable to have a volatile buffer, which can be removed readily[1] (examples are buffers Nos. 20 and 21), but the use of very volatile systems makes close control of the pH essential. Most of the pH data found in the literature relate to the Sørensen scale, and it should be noted that the values given in the table opposite are on the conventional pH scale.

Both stock and buffer solutions should be prepared with distilled water that is free of CO_2. Only standard reagents should be used. If there is any doubt as to the purity or water content of solutions, their molarity must be checked by titration. The amounts x of stock solutions required to make up a buffer solution of the desired pH value are given in the second table in Appendix B, p. 1119.

*This appendix has been compiled by F. Kohler, Department of Physical Chemistry, University of Vienna, and was taken from CIBA-Geigy AG, Basel, Switzerland.

REFERENCES

1. For a list of volatile buffers, see Michl H: In Heftmann E, editor: *Chromatography, Part 1,* New York, 1961, Reinhold, p. 250, also http://www.scrippslabs.com/datatables/reagent_volatile.html, accessed 03/04/09.

No.	Name	pH Range	Temperature	pH Change Per °C
General Buffers				
1	KCl/HCl (Clark and Lubs)[1]	1.0 to 2.2	Room	0
2	Glycine/HCl (Sørensen)[2]	1.2 to 3.4	Room	0
3	Na citrate/HCl (Sørensen)[2]	1.2 to 5.0	Room	0
4	K biphthalate/HCl (Clark and Lubs)[1]	2.4 to 4.0	20°C	+0.001
5	K biphthalate/NaOH (Clark and Lubs)[1]	4.2 to 6.2	20°C	
6	Na citrate/NaOH (Sørensen)[2]	5.2 to 6.6	20°C	+0.004
7	Phosphate (Sørensen)[2]	5.0 to 8.0	20°C	−0.003
8	Barbital-Na/HCl (Michaelis)[3]	7.0 to 9.0	18°C	
9	Na borate/HCl (Sørensen)[2]	7.8 to 9.2	20°C	−0.005
10	Glycine/NaOH (Sørensen)[2]	8.6 to 12.8	20°C	−0.025
11	Na borate/NaOH (Sørensen)[2]	9.4 to 10.6	20°C	−0.01
Universal Buffers				
12	Citric acid/phosphate (McIlvaine)[4]	2.2 to 7.8	21°C	
13	Citrate-phosphate-borate/HCl (Teorell and Stenhagen)[5]	2.0 to 12.0	20°C	
14	Britton and Welford[6]	2.6 to 11.8	25°C	At low pH 0, at high pH −0.02

No.	Name	pH Range	Temperature	pH Change Per °C
Buffers for Biological Media				
15	Acetate (Walpole)[7-9]	3.8 to 5.6	25°C	
16	Dimethylglutaric acid/NaOH[10]	3.2 to 7.6	21°C	
17	Piperazine/HCl[11,12]	4.6 to 6.4	20°C	
		8.8 to 10.6		
18	Tetraethylethylenediamine*[12]	5.0 to 6.8	20°C	
		8.2 to 10.0		
19	Tris-malate[7,13]	5.2 to 8.6	23°C	
20	Dimethylaminoethylamine*[12]	5.6 to 7.4	20°C	
		8.6 to 10.4		
21	Imidazole/HCl[14]	6.2 to 7.8	25°C	
22	Triethanolamine/HCl[15]	7.0 to 8.8	25°C	
23	*N*-Dimethylaminoleucylglycine/NaOH[16]	7.0 to 8.8	23°C	−0.015
24	Tris/HCl[7]	7.2 to 9.0	23°C	−0.02
25	2-Amino-2-methylpropane-1,3-diol/HCl[7,13]	7.8 to 10.0	23°C	
26	Carbonate (Delory and King)[7,17]	9.2 to 10.8	20°C	

From *Geigy Scientific Tables,* ed 8, Basel, Switzerland, 1981, CIBA-Geigy AG.
*Can be combined with tris buffer to give a cationic universal buffer (see reference 12).

TABLE REFERENCES

1. Clark and Lubs: J Bact 2:1, 1917.
2. Sørensen: Biochem Z 21:131, 1909; 22:352, 1909; Ergebn Physiol 12:393, 1912; and Walbum: Biochem Z 107:219, 1920.
3. Michaelis: J Biol Chem 87:33, 1930.
4. McIlvaine: J Biol Chem 49:183, 1921.
5. Teorell and Stenhagen: Biochem Z 299:416, 1938.
6. Britton and Welford: J Chem Soc 1937, 1848.
7. Gomori: In Colowick and Kaplan, editors: *Methods in Enzymology,* vol 1, New York, 1955, Academic Press, p. 138.
8. Walpole: J Chem Soc 105: 2501, 1914.
9. Green: J Am Chem Soc 55:2331, 1933.
10. Stafford et al: Biochim Biophys Acta 18:319, 1955; Krebs, unpublished, 1957.
11. Smith and Smith: Biol Bull 96:233, 1949.
12. Semenza et al: Helv Chim Acta 45:2306, 1962.
13. Gomori: Proc Soc Exp Biol (NY) 68:354, 1948.
14. Mertz and Owen: Proc Soc Exp Biol (NY) 43:204, 1940, quoted by Rauen HM, editor: *Biochemisches Taschenbuch,* ed 2, part 2, Berlin, 1964, Springer, p. 90.
15. Beisenherz et al: Z Naturforsch 8b:555, 1953.
16. Leonis: CR Lab Carlsberg, Sér Chim 26:357, 1948.
17. Delory and King: Biochem J 39:245, 1945.

Preparation of Buffer Solutions

B
Appendix

When not otherwise specified, both stock and buffer solutions should be prepared with water that is free of CO_2. Only standard reagents should be used. If there is any doubt as to the purity or water content of solutions, their molarity must be checked by titration. The amounts of stock solutions required to make up a buffer solution of the desired pH value are given in the table on pp. 1121-1122.

	STOCK SOLUTIONS		
Buffer No.	**A**	**B**	**Composition of the Buffer**
1	KCl 0.2-N (14.91 g/L)	HCl 0.2-N	25 mL A + x mL B made up to 100 mL
2	Glycine 0.1-molar in NaCl 0.1-N (7.507 g glycine + 5.844 g NaCl/L)	HCl 0.1-N	x mL A + (100 − x) mL B
3	Disodium citrate 0.1-molar (21.01 g $C_6H_8O_7 \cdot 1H_2O$ + 200 mL NaOH 1-N per liter)	HCl 0.1-N	x mL A + (100 − x) mL B
4	Potassium biphthalate 0.1-molar (20.42 g $KHC_8H_4O_4$/L)	HCl 0.1-N	50 mL A + x mL B made up to 100 mL
5	Same as No. 4	NaOH 0.1-N	50 mL A + x mL B made up to 100 mL
6	Same as No. 3	NaOH 0.1-N	x mL A + (100 − x) mL B
7	Monopotassium phosphate $^1/_{15}$-molar (9.073 g KH_2PO_4/L)	Disodium phosphate $^1/_{15}$-molar (11.87 g $Na_2HPO_4 \cdot 2H_2O$/L)	x mL A + (100 − x) mL B
8	Barbital sodium 0.1-molar (20.62 g/L)	HCl 0.1-N	x mL A + (100 − x) mL B
9	Boric acid, half-neutralized, 0.2-molar (corr. to 0.05-molar borax: 12.37 g boric acid + 100 mL NaOH 1-N per liter)	HCl 0.1-N	x mL A + (100 − x) mL B
10	Same as No. 2	NaOH 0.1-N	x mL A + (100 − x) mL B
11	Same as No. 9	NaOH 0.1-N	x mL A + (100 − x) mL B
12	Citric acid 0.1-molar (21.01 g $C_6H_8O_7 \cdot 1H_2O$/L)	Disodium phosphate 0.2-molar (35.60 g $Na_2HPO_4 \cdot 2H_2O$/L)	x mL A + (100 − x) mL B
13	To citric acid and phosphoric acid solutions (ca. 100 mL), each equivalent to 100 mL NaOH 1-N, add 3.54 cryst. orthoboric acid and 343 mL NaOH 1-N, and make up the mixture to 1 liter	HCl 0.1-N	20 mL A + x mL B made up to 100 mL
14	Citric acid, monopotassium phosphate, barbital, boric acid, all 0.02857-molar (6.004 g $C_6H_8O_7 \cdot 1H_2O$, 3.888 g KH_2PO_4, 5.263 g barbital, 1.767 g H_3BO_3/L)	NaOH 0.2-N	100 mL A + x mL B
15	Sodium acetate 0.1-N (8.204 g $C_2H_3O_2Na$ or 13.61 g $C_2H_3O_2Na \cdot 3H_2O$/L)	Acetic acid 0.1-N (6.005 g/L)	x mL A + (100 − x) mL B

From *Geigy Scientific Tables,* ed 8, Basel, Switzerland, 1981, CIBA-Geigy AG.

	STOCK SOLUTIONS		
Buffer No.	**A**	**B**	**Composition of the Buffer**
16	ββ-Dimethylglutaric acid 0.1-molar (16.02 g/L)	NaOH 0.2-N	(a) 100 mL A + x mL B made up to 1000 mL (b) 100 mL A + x mL B + 5.844 g NaCl made up to 1000 mL (NaCl = 0.1-molar)
17	Piperazine 1-molar (86.14 g/L)	HCl 0.1-N	5 mL A + x mL B made up to 100 mL
18	Tetraethylethylenediamine 1-molar (172.32 g/L)	HCl 0.1-N	5 mL A + x mL B made up to 100 mL
19	Tris acid maleate 0.2-molar (24.23 g tris[hydroxy-methyl]aminomethane + 23.21 g maleic acid or 19.61 g maleic anhydride/L)	NaOH 0.2-N	25 mL A + x mL B made up to 100 mL
20	Dimethylaminoethylamine 1-molar (88 g/L)	HCl 0.1-N	5 mL A + x mL B made up to 100 mL
21	Imidazole 0.2-molar (13.62 g/L)	HCl 0.1-N	25 mL A + x mL B made up to 100 mL
22	Triethanolamine 0.5-molar (76.11 g/L) containing 20 g/L ethylenediaminetetraacetic acid disodium salt ($C_{10}H_{14}O_8N_2Na_2 \cdot 2H_2O$)	HCl 0.05-N	10 mL A + x mL B made up to 100 mL
23	N-Dimethylaminoleucylglycine 0.1-molar (24.33 g $C_{10}H_{20}O_3N_2 \cdot {}^3/_2H_2O$/L) containing NaCl 0.2-N (11.69 g/L)	NaOH 1-N 100 mL made up to 1 liter with A	x mL A + (100 − x) mL B
24	Tris 0.2-molar (24.23 g tris[hydroxymethyl] aminomethane/L)	HCl 0.1-N	25 mL A + x mL B made up to 100 mL
25	2-Amino-2-methylpropane-1,3-diol 0.1-molar (10.51 g/L)	HCl 0.1-N	50 mL A + x mL B made up to 100 mL
26	Sodium carbonate anhydrous 0.1-molar (10.60 g/L)	Sodium bicarbonate 0.1-molar (8.401 g/L)	x mL A + (100 − x) mL B

The table gives the amounts (x mL) of the stock solutions listed in the first part of Appendix B required to make up a buffer solution of the desired pH value.

pH	1	2	3	4	5	6	7	8	9	10	11	12	13	14	15	16a	16b	17	18	19	20	21	22	23	24	25	26	pH
1.0	54.2	...	...	...	...	...	...	...	...	...	...	...	...	...	...	...	...	...	...	...	...	...	...	...	...	...	...	1.0
1.2	36.0	11.1	9.0	...	...	...	...	...	...	...	...	...	...	...	...	...	...	...	...	...	...	...	...	...	...	...	...	1.2
1.4	23.2	26.4	17.9	...	...	...	...	...	...	...	...	...	...	...	...	...	...	...	...	...	...	...	...	...	...	...	...	1.4
1.6	14.7	36.2	23.6	...	...	...	...	...	...	...	...	...	...	...	...	...	...	...	...	...	...	...	...	...	...	...	...	1.6
1.8	9.3	43.9	27.6	...	...	...	...	...	...	...	...	...	...	...	...	...	...	...	...	...	...	...	...	...	...	...	...	1.8
2.0	5.9	50.7	30.2	...	...	...	...	...	...	...	...	...	74.4	...	...	...	...	...	...	...	...	...	...	...	...	...	...	2.0
2.2	3.8	56.5	32.2	...	...	...	...	...	...	...	...	98.8	68.8	...	...	...	...	...	...	...	...	...	...	...	...	...	...	2.2
2.4	...	62.3	34.1	41.0	...	...	...	...	...	...	...	94.5	64.6	...	...	...	...	...	...	...	...	...	...	...	...	...	...	2.4
2.6	...	68.4	36.0	34.1	...	...	...	...	...	...	...	90.0	61.3	1.6	...	...	...	...	...	...	...	...	...	...	...	...	...	2.6
2.8	...	74.7	37.9	27.8	...	...	...	...	...	...	...	85.1	58.9	3.6	...	...	...	...	...	...	...	...	...	...	...	...	...	2.8
3.0	...	81.0	39.9	21.6	...	...	...	...	...	...	...	80.3	56.9	5.7	...	...	...	...	...	...	...	...	...	...	...	...	...	3.0
3.2	...	86.2	42.1	15.9	...	...	...	...	...	...	...	76.0	55.2	7.8	...	7.0	14.4	...	...	...	...	...	...	...	...	...	...	3.2
3.4	...	90.3	44.8	10.9	...	...	...	...	...	...	...	72.0	53.9	9.9	...	13.3	20.9	...	...	...	...	...	...	...	...	...	...	3.4
3.6	...	...	47.8	6.7	...	...	...	...	...	...	...	68.4	52.9	11.7	...	20.7	26.8	...	...	...	...	...	...	...	...	...	...	3.6
3.8	...	...	51.2	3.3	...	...	...	...	...	...	...	65.1	51.8	13.5	10.9	26.3	32.4	...	...	...	...	...	...	...	...	...	...	3.8
4.0	...	...	55.1	0.0	...	...	...	...	...	...	...	62.0	50.7	15.3	16.6	32.4	36.6	...	...	...	...	...	...	...	...	...	...	4.0
4.2	...	...	60.0	...	3.0	...	...	...	...	...	...	59.1	49.7	17.5	23.9	36.2	40.3	...	...	...	...	...	...	...	...	...	...	4.2
4.4	...	...	66.4	...	6.7	...	...	...	...	...	...	56.4	48.6	19.7	33.5	39.3	43.1	...	...	...	...	...	...	...	...	...	...	4.4
4.6	...	...	74.9	...	11.1	...	...	...	...	...	...	53.7	47.5	21.9	44.9	41.3	45.7	94.3	...	...	...	...	...	...	...	...	...	4.6
4.8	...	...	85.6	...	16.5	...	...	...	...	...	...	51.2	46.4	24.1	56.6	43.5	48.3	91.5	...	...	...	...	...	...	...	...	...	4.8
5.0	...	...	100.0	...	22.6	...	99.2	...	...	...	...	49.0	45.4	26.3	67.8	45.7	51.5	87.8	94.3	...	...	...	...	...	...	...	...	5.0
5.2	...	...	...	...	28.8	87.1	98.4	...	...	...	...	46.9	44.3	28.6	76.8	48.4	53.6	83.6	91.5	3.2	...	...	...	...	...	...	...	5.2
5.4	...	...	...	...	34.4	78.0	97.3	...	...	...	...	44.7	43.2	31.0	84.0	51.3	58.2	77.6	87.8	5.0	...	...	...	...	...	...	...	5.4
5.6	...	...	...	...	39.1	70.3	95.5	...	...	...	...	42.4	42.0	33.4	89.3	55.0	63.6	71.8	83.1	7.3	94.3	...	...	...	...	...	...	5.6
5.8	...	...	...	...	42.4	64.5	92.8	...	...	...	...	40.0	40.8	35.8	...	58.8	68.7	66.5	77.6	9.7	91.7	...	...	...	...	...	...	5.8
6.0	...	...	...	...	45.0	60.3	88.9	...	...	...	...	37.4	39.7	38.3	...	63.9	73.6	61.8	71.7	12.4	88.0	...	...	...	...	...	...	6.0
6.2	...	...	...	...	46.7	57.2	83.0	...	...	...	...	34.5	38.4	40.8	...	69.5	78.5	58.2	66.4	15.2	83.3	43.4	...	...	...	...	...	6.2
6.4	...	...	...	...	...	54.8	75.4	...	...	...	...	31.4	37.0	43.3	...	74.1	83.3	55.5	61.7	17.9	77.9	40.4	...	...	...	...	...	6.4
6.6	...	...	...	...	...	53.2	65.3	...	...	...	...	27.9	35.6	45.8	...	83.5	87.4	...	58.0	20.8	72.0	36.5	...	...	...	...	...	6.6
6.8	...	...	...	...	...	...	53.4	...	...	...	...	23.5	34.2	48.3	...	87.4	91.0	...	55.3	22.2	66.6	31.4	...	...	...	...	...	6.8

The table gives the amounts (x mL) of the stock solutions listed in the first part of Appendix B required to make up a buffer solution of the desired pH value.

pH	1	2	3	4	5	6	7	8	9	10	11	12	13	14	15	16a	16b	17	18	19	20	21	22	23	24	25	26	pH
7.0	...	...	...	...	...	...	41.3	53.3	...	...	...	19.0	32.9	50.9	...	90.0	93.2	...	...	23.7	61.9	25.4	86.2	86.4	...	...	...	7.0
7.2	...	...	...	...	...	...	29.6	55.0	...	...	...	13.8	31.7	53.4	...	91.8	94.9	...	...	25.2	58.1	19.6	79.6	80.6	44.7	...	...	7.2
7.4	...	...	...	...	...	...	19.7	57.6	...	...	...	9.8	30.6	55.8	...	93.0	95.8	...	...	26.7	55.3	14.6	71.3	72.8	42.0	...	...	7.4
7.6	...	...	...	...	...	...	12.8	60.8	...	...	...	6.8	29.6	58.2	...	93.8	96.8	...	...	28.6	...	10.2	62.0	63.2	39.3	...	...	7.6
7.8	...	...	...	...	...	...	7.4	65.2	53.0	...	...	4.6	28.8	60.5	...	...	...	...	...	31.2	...	6.6	52.0	52.1	33.7	43.9	...	7.8
8.0	...	...	...	...	...	...	3.7	70.6	55.4	...	...	...	28.1	62.8	...	...	...	...	...	33.9	...	...	42.0	41.1	27.9	41.6	...	8.0
8.2	...	...	...	...	...	...	...	75.9	58.0	...	...	...	27.6	65.0	...	...	...	...	46.4	36.9	...	...	31.9	31.4	22.9	38.4	...	8.2
8.4	...	...	...	...	...	...	...	81.2	62.1	...	...	...	27.0	67.2	...	...	...	...	43.9	39.9	...	...	22.5	23.0	17.3	34.8	...	8.4
8.6	...	...	...	...	...	...	...	86.2	66.9	94.7	...	...	26.3	69.3	...	...	...	...	40.9	42.7	45.4	...	16.0	15.9	13.0	30.7	...	8.6
8.8	...	...	...	...	...	...	...	90.1	73.6	92.0	...	...	25.2	71.3	...	...	...	45.5	36.8	...	42.8	...	11.7	10.3	8.8	23.3	...	8.8
9.0	...	...	...	...	...	...	...	93.2	83.5	88.4	...	...	24.0	73.2	...	...	...	43.2	31.8	...	39.2	...	...	...	5.3	17.7	...	9.0
9.2	...	...	...	...	...	...	...	...	95.6	84.0	...	...	22.6	75.1	...	...	...	40.0	26.2	...	34.7	...	...	...	...	13.3	10.0	9.2
9.4	...	...	...	...	...	...	...	...	...	78.9	87.0	...	21.4	77.0	...	...	...	35.8	20.4	...	29.3	...	...	...	...	9.2	18.4	9.4
9.6	...	...	...	...	...	...	...	...	...	73.2	75.5	...	20.2	78.8	...	...	...	30.8	15.2	...	23.6	...	...	...	...	5.2	29.3	9.6
9.8	...	...	...	...	...	...	...	...	...	67.2	65.1	...	19.0	80.4	...	...	...	25.0	10.8	...	19.0	...	...	...	...	4.1	42.0	9.8
10.0	...	...	...	...	...	...	...	...	...	62.5	59.6	...	18.1	81.8	...	...	...	19.4	7.4	...	13.1	...	...	...	...	2.3	53.4	10.1
10.2	...	...	...	...	...	...	...	...	...	58.8	56.4	...	17.1	83.1	...	...	...	14.3	...	...	9.2	...	...	...	...	...	63.7	10.2
10.4	...	...	...	...	...	...	...	...	...	55.7	54.1	...	16.5	84.3	...	...	...	10.0	...	...	6.2	...	...	...	...	...	73.1	10.4
10.6	...	...	...	...	...	...	...	...	...	53.6	52.3	...	16.0	85.4	...	...	...	6.9	...	...	...	...	...	...	...	...	81.2	10.6
10.8	...	...	...	...	...	...	...	...	...	52.2	...	...	15.5	86.5	...	...	...	...	...	...	...	...	...	...	...	...	87.9	10.8
11.0	...	...	...	...	...	...	...	...	...	51.2	...	...	14.7	87.8	...	...	...	...	...	...	...	...	...	...	...	...	...	11.0
11.2	...	...	...	...	...	...	...	...	...	50.4	...	...	13.5	89.3	...	...	...	...	...	...	...	...	...	...	...	...	...	11.2
11.4	...	...	...	...	...	...	...	...	...	49.5	...	...	11.7	91.3	...	...	...	...	...	...	...	...	...	...	...	...	...	11.4
11.6	...	...	...	...	...	...	...	...	...	48.7	...	...	9.1	94.5	...	...	...	...	...	...	...	...	...	...	...	...	...	11.6
11.8	...	...	...	...	...	...	...	...	...	47.6	...	...	5.5	99.0	...	...	...	...	...	...	...	...	...	...	...	...	...	11.8
12.0	...	...	...	...	...	...	...	...	...	46.0	...	...	1.3	...	...	...	...	...	...	...	...	...	...	...	...	...	...	12.0
12.2	...	...	...	...	...	...	...	...	...	43.2	...	...	...	...	...	...	...	...	...	...	...	...	...	...	...	...	...	12.2
12.4	...	...	...	...	...	...	...	...	...	39.1	...	...	...	...	...	...	...	...	...	...	...	...	...	...	...	...	...	12.4
12.6	...	...	...	...	...	...	...	...	...	31.8	...	...	...	...	...	...	...	...	...	...	...	...	...	...	...	...	...	12.6
12.8	...	...	...	...	...	...	...	...	...	21.4	...	...	...	...	...	...	...	...	...	...	...	...	...	...	...	...	...	12.8

From *Geigy Scientific Tables,* ed 8, Basel, Switzerland, 1981, CIBA-Geigy AG.

Concentrations of Common Acids and Bases*

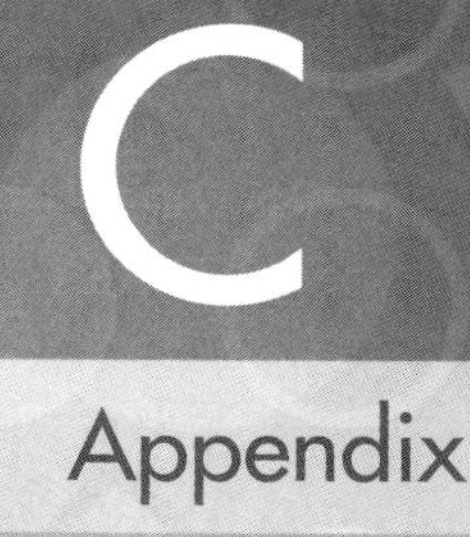

Compound	Molecular Weight	Specific Gravity	Weight, %	Normality	mL/Liter for 1N* Solution
HCl	36.46	1.19	36.0	11.7	85.5
HNO_3	63.02	1.42	69.5	15.6	64.0
H_2SO_4	98.08	1.84	96.0	35.9	28.4
CH_3COOH	60.03	1.06	99.5	17.6	56.9
NH_4OH	35.04	0.90	58.6	15.1	66.5
H_3PO_4	98.00	1.69	85.0	44.1	22.7
Thioglycolic acid	92.12	1.26	80.0	10.9	91.3
HCOOH	46.03	1.21	97.0	25.5	39.2
	46.03	1.19	88.0	22.7	44.1
$HClO_4$	100.50	1.67	70.0	11.65	85.7
Pyridine	79.10	0.98	100.0	12.4	80.6
2-Mercaptoethanol	78.13	1.14	100.0	14.6	68.5

From Brewer JM, Pesce AJ, Ashworth H: *Experimental Techniques in Biochemistry,* Englewood Cliffs, NJ, 1974, Prentice-Hall, Inc.
M, Molecular weight; *s,* specific gravity.
To calculate concentration (c) from the weight percent (w) of a compound, use the following formula: $\frac{10\ ws}{M} = c$

*Remember, the normality (N) is not the same as the molarity (M) for sulfuric and phosphoric acid.

Major Plasma Proteins*

D

Appendix

Protein	Molecular Weight	Concentration, mg/100 mL	Electrophoretic† Mobility	Biological Function
Prealbumins				
Thyroxine-binding (TBPA)	55,000	10 to 40	7.6	Thyroxine transport
Retinol-binding (RBP)	21,000	3 to 6		Vitamin A transport
Albumin	66,300	3500 to 5500	5.92	Maintains osmotic pressure, transport of bilirubin, free fatty acids, anions, and cations, cell nutrition
α_1-Globulins				
α_1-Acid glycoprotein (α_1-S)	42,000	55 to 140	5.7	Acute phase protein
α_1-Antitrypsin (α_1-AT)	54,000	200 to 400	5.42	Antiserine type of protease
α_1-Glycoprotein (9.5S, α_1M)	308,000	3 to 8	α_1	Unknown
α_1-Glycoprotein B (α_1B)	50,000	15 to 30	α_1	Unknown
α_1-Glycoprotein T (α_1T)	60,000	5 to 12	α_1	Unknown, tryptophan-poor
α_1-Antichymotrypsin (α_1X)	68,000	30 to 60	α_1	Chymotrypsin inhibitor
α_1-Lipoproteins, high-density (HDL)	28,000	254 to 387	α_1	Lipid transport
α_2-Globulin				
G_0-Globulin (Gc)	51,000	40 to 70	α_2	Vitamin D transport
Ceruloplasmin (Cp)	134,000	15 to 60	4.6	Copper transport, peroxidase activity
α_2-Glycoprotein, histidine-rich (HRG)	58,000	5 to 15	α_2	Unknown
Zn-α_2-glycoprotein (Znα_2)	41,000	2 to 15	4.2	Unknown, binds Zn^{2+}
α_2-HS-glycoprotein (α_2HS)	49,000	40 to 85	4.2	Unknown, binds Ba^{2+}
α_2-Macroglobulin (α_2M)	725,000	150 to 420	4.2	Inhibitor of thrombin, trypsin, and pepsin
Transcortin (TC)	49,500	<7	α_2	Cortisol transport
Haptoglobins (Hp)				
Type 1-1	100,000	100 to 200	4.1	Binds hemoglobin, prevents loss of iron
Type 2-1	200,000	160 to 300	α_2	
Type 2-2	400,000	120 to 260	α_2	
α_2-Lipoproteins (VLDL)	250,000	150 to 230	Pre-β	Lipid transport
Thyroxine-binding protein (TBG)	58,000	1 to 2	α_2	Thyroxine transport
β-Globulins				
Hemopexin (Hpx)	57,000	50 to 100	3.1	Binds heme
Transferrin (Tf)	76,500	200 to 320	3.1	Iron transport
β-Lipoproteins (LDL)	250,000	280 to 440	3.1	Lipid transport
C4 complement component (C4)	206,000	40 to 80	β_1	Complement system
β_2-Microglobulin ($\beta_2\mu$)	11,818	Trace	β_2	Common portion of the HLA transplantation antigen
β_2-Glycoprotein I (β_2 I)	40,000	15 to 30	1.6	Unknown
β_2-Glycoprotein II (GGG)	63,000	12 to 30	β_2	C3 activator (activates properidin)

*Does not include clotting factors, complement factors, or enzymes except fibrinogen, C3, and C4 of complement, which occur in substantial concentrations.

†Tiselius moving boundary electrophoresis in Tiselius units ($cm^2\ V^{-1}\ sec^{-1} \times 10^5$, at 0°C, ph 8.6, and ionic strength 0.15).

Protein	Molecular Weight	Concentration, mg/100 mL	Electrophoretic[†] Mobility	Biological Function
β_2-Glycoprotein III (β_2 III)	35,000	5 to 15	β_2	Unknown
C-reactive protein (CRP)	118,000	1	β_2	Opsonin, motivates phagocytosis in inflammatory disease
C3 complement component (C3)	180,000	55 to 180	β_2	Complement system
Fibrinogen (ϕ, Fib.)	341,000	200 to 600	2.1	Blood clotting
γ-Globulins				
Immunoglobulin M (IgM)	950,000	60 to 250	2.1	Antibodies, early response
Immunoglobulin E (IgE)	190,000	0.06	2.1	Reagin of the allergy system
Immunoglobulin A (IgA)	160,000	90 to 450	2.1	Tissue antibodies
Immunoglobulin D (IgD)	160,000	15	1.9	Cell surface and plasma antibodies
Immunoglobulin G (IgG)	160,000	800 to 1800	1.2	Antibodies, long range

From Natelson S, Natelson EA: *Principles of Applied Chemistry,* vol 3, New York, 1980, Plenum Publishing Corp.

Conversions Between Conventional and SI Units

Appendix

	Conventional Units	× Factor	= SI Units
Gram	g/mL	$\frac{10^{15}}{mw}$	pmol/L
	g/100 mL	10	g/L
	g/100 mL	$\frac{10}{mw}$	mol/L
	g/100 mL	$\frac{10^4}{mw}$	mmol/L
	g/d	$\frac{1}{mw}$	mol/d
	g/d	$\frac{10^3}{mw}$	mmol/d
	g/d	$\frac{10^9}{mw}$	nmol/d
Microgram	µg/100 mL	$\frac{10}{mw}$	µmol/L
	µg/d	$\frac{1}{mw}$	µmol/d
	µg/d	$\frac{10^3}{mw}$	nmol/d
Picogram	pg	$\frac{10^3}{mw}$	fmol
	pg/mL	$\frac{10^3}{mw}$	pmol/L
Milliequivalent	mEq/L	$\frac{1}{valence}$	mmol/L
	mEq/kg	$\frac{1}{valence}$	mmol/kg
	mEq/d	$\frac{1}{valence}$	mmol/d
Milligram	mg/100 mL	10^{-2}	g/L
	mg/100 mL	$\frac{10^{-2}}{mw}$	mol/L
	mg/100 mL	$\frac{10}{mw}$	mmol/L
	mg/100 mL	$\frac{10^4}{mw}$	µmol/L
	mg/100 g	10	mg/kg
	mg/100 g	$\frac{10}{mw}$	mmol/kg
	mg/d	$\frac{1}{mw}$	mmol/d
	mg/d	$\frac{10^3}{mw}$	µmol/d
Milliliter	mL/100 g	10	mL/kg
	mL/min	1.667×10^{-2}	mL/s
Millimeters of mercury	mm Hg	1.333	mbar
	mm Hg	0.133	kPa
Minute	min	60	s
	min	0.06	ks
Percent	%	10^{-2}	1 (unit)
	% (g/100 g)	10	g/kg
	% (g/100 g)	10^{-2}	kg/kg
	% (g/100 mL)	10	g/L
	% (g/100 mL)	$\frac{10}{mw}$	mol/L
	% (g/100 mL)	$\frac{10^4}{mw}$	mmol/L
	% (mL/100 mL)	10^{-2}	L/L

Modified from Campbell JM, Campbell JB: *Laboratory mathematics,* ed 5, St Louis, 1997, Mosby.
d, Day; *Eq,* equivalent; *g,* gram; *L,* liter; *min,* minute; *mw,* molecular weight; *Pa,* pascal; *s,* second; *f,* Femto (10^{-15}); *p,* pico (10^{-12}); *n,* nano (10^{-9}); *µ,* micro (10^{-6}); *m,* milli (10^{-3}); *k,* kilo (10^3).

Conversions Between Conventional and SI Units for Specific Analytes

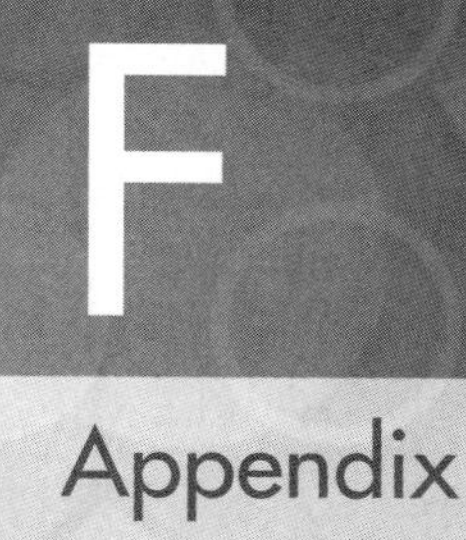

Appendix

Analyte	Conventional Units	MULTIPLY BY Conventional to SI	MULTIPLY BY SI to Conventional	SI Unit
Acetaminophen	µg/mL	6.61	0.151	µmol/L
Albumin	g/100 mL	144.9	0.0069	µmol/L
Ammonia	µg/100 mL	0.59	1.7	µmol/L
Anticonvulsant drugs				
Carbamazepine	µg/mL	4.32	0.23	µmol/L
Ethosuximide	µg/mL	7.08	0.14	µmol/L
Phenobarbital	µg/mL	4.31	0.23	µmol/L
Phenytoin	µg/mL	3.96	0.25	µmol/L
Primidone	µg/mL	4.58	0.22	µmol/L
Valproic acid	µg/mL	6.93	0.14	µmol/L
Bilirubin	mg/100 mL	17.1	0.059	µmol/L
Bromide	µg/mL	0.0125	80	mmol/L
Calcium	mg/100 mL	0.25	4	mmol/L
Chloride	mEq/L	1	1	mmol/L
Cholesterol	mg/100 mL	0.026	38.7	mmol/L
Cortisol	µg/100 mL	0.0276	36.2	µmol/L
Creatinine	mg/100 mL	88.4	0.0113	µmol/L
Digoxin	ng/mL	1.28	0.781	nmol/L
Estriol	µg/L	3.47	0.288	nmol/L
Ferritin	µg/L	2.2	0.445	pmol/L
Folic acid	µg/100 mL	22.7	0.044	nmol/L
Gentamicin	µg/mL	2.22	0.45	µmol/L
Glucose	mg/100 mL	0.055	18	mmol/L
Haptoglobin	mg/100 mL	0.118	8.47	µmol/L
hCG	U/L	—	—	—
HDL cholesterol	mg/100 mL	0.026	38.7	mmol/L
5-HIAA	mg	5.23	0.19	µmol/L
Ig A	mg/100 mL	0.0625	16	µmol/L
D	mg/100 mL	0.054	18.5	µmol/L
E	ng/mL	0.005	200	nmol/L
G	mg/100 mL	0.067	15	µmol/L
M	mg/100 mL	0.011	91	µmol/L
Insulin	pg/mL	0.174	5.74	nmol/L
	µU/mL	7.25	0.138	nmol/L
Iron	µg/100 mL	0.179	5.58	µmol/L
Ketones (acetoacetate)	mg/L	0.111	9.01	mmol/L
LDL cholesterol	mg/100 mL	0.026	38.7	mmol/L
Lead	µg/L	4.83	0.207	nmol/L
Lithium	mEq/L	1	1	mmol/L
Magnesium	mg/100 mL	0.41	2.43	mmol/L
Phenylalanine	mg/L	6.05	0.165	µmol/L
Phosphorus	mg/100 mL	0.323	3.1	mmol/L
Potassium	mEq/L	1	1	µmol/L
Quinidine	µg/mL	3.09	0.324	mmol/L
Salicylate	mg/100 mL	0.0724	13.8	mmol/L
Sodium	mEq/L	1	1	µmol/L
Theophylline	µg/mL	5.55	0.180	mmol/L
Thyroid-stimulating hormone	mU/L	—	—	—
Thyroxine	µg/100 mL	12.9	0.078	nmol/L
TIBC	µg/100 mL	0.179	5.58	µmol/L

Analyte	Conventional Units	MULTIPLY BY		SI Unit
		Conventional to SI	SI to Conventional	
Transferrin	mg/100 mL	0.11	9.09	μmol/L
Triglycerides	mg/100 mL	0.0114	87.5	mmol/L
Urea	mg/100 mL	0.166	6.01	mmol/L
Urea N	mg/100 mL	0.356	2.81	mmol/L
Uric acid	mg/100 mL	59.5	0.0168	μmol/L
Vanillylmandelic acid	mg	5.03	0.20	μmol
Vitamin B_{12}	pg/mL	0.738	1.36	pmol/L
VLDL cholesterol	mg/100 mL	0.026	38.7	mmol/L
Gases	mm Hg	0.133	7.51	kPa
Enzymes	U/L	1.67×10^{-8}	0.6×10^{8}	katal/L

hCG, Human chorionic gonadotropin; *HDL,* high-density lipoprotein; *5-HIAA,* 5-hydroxyindoleacetic acid; *Ig,* immunoglobulin; *LDL,* low-density lipoprotein; *TIBC,* total iron binding capacity; *VLDL,* very low-density lipoprotein.

Index

Note: Page numbers followed by "f" refer to illustrations; page numbers followed by "t" refer to tables; page numbers followed by "b" refer to boxes.

B

D

E

F

G

I

L

O

P

Q

S

U

V